Greenfield's
Neuropathology

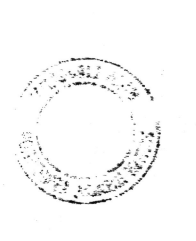

Greenfield's Neuropathology

NINTH EDITION

VOLUME 2

Edited by

Seth Love MBBCh PhD FRCP FRCPath
Professor of Neuropathology
Institute of Clinical Neurosciences
School of Clinical Sciences
University of Bristol
Southmead Hospital
Bristol, UK

Herbert Budka MD
Professor of Neuropathology
Consultant, Institute of Neuropathology
University Hospital Zurich
Zurich, Switzerland

James W Ironside CBE BMSc FRCPath FRCPEdin FMedSci FRSE
Professor of Clinical Neuropathology and Honorary
Consultant in Neuropathology
National Creutzfeldt–Jakob Disease Surveillance Unit
University of Edinburgh
Western General Hospital
Edinburgh, UK

Arie Perry MD
Professor of Pathology and Neurological Surgery
Director of Neuropathology
Director of Neuropathology Fellowship Training Program
University of California, San Francisco
San Francisco, CA, USA

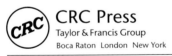
CRC Press
Taylor & Francis Group
Boca Raton London New York

CRC Press is an imprint of the
Taylor & Francis Group, an **informa** business

CRC Press
Taylor & Francis Group
6000 Broken Sound Parkway NW, Suite 300
Boca Raton, FL 33487-2742

© 2015 by Taylor & Francis Group, LLC
CRC Press is an imprint of Taylor & Francis Group, an Informa business

No claim to original U.S. Government works

Printed on acid-free paper
Version Date: 20141203

Printed and bound in India by Replika Press Pvt. Ltd.

International Standard Book Number-13: (Volume 2) 978-1-4987-2111-0 (Hardback)
(Two-volume set) 978-1-4987-2128-8 (Hardback)

Visit the Taylor & Francis Web site at
http://www.taylorandfrancis.com

and the CRC Press Web site at
http://www.crcpress.com

Contents

Preface

Greenfield's Neuropathology holds a special place in the heart of most neuropathologists. It has long been a standard-bearer of our specialty. In 1921, Joseph Godwin Greenfield and Edward Farquhar Buzzard published *Pathology of the Nervous System*, which had a key role in defining neuropathology as a distinct specialty. The authors set out to 'describe clearly the anatomical changes which are associated with disorders of nervous function, to discuss briefly questions of pathogenesis, and to indicate in a few words, where it is possible, the relationship between structural alterations and clinical signs and symptoms.' In 1958, a book entitled simply *Neuropathology*, by Greenfield, William Blackwood, William McMenemy, Alfred Meyer and Ronald Norman, updated and greatly expanded on most of the content of *Pathology of the Nervous System*. Unlike *Pathology of the Nervous System*, however, *Neuropathology* did not cover neoplastic diseases (dealt with instead in a companion book, Russell and Rubinstein's *Pathology of Tumours of the Nervous System*). However, tumours of the nervous system have been included in *Greenfield's Neuropathology* since the seventh edition in 1997.

Readers of a succession of editions over many decades have dipped into this venerable reference book seeking definitive advice and instruction on all matters neuropathological. Producing a new edition of *Greenfield's Neuropathology* has therefore been both a huge privilege and a massive responsibility. It has also been a balancing act, in which we have had to reconcile the tension between the physical constraints of a two-volume book and the ever-expanding amount of information encompassed within our field. Indeed, this may be the last edition of *Greenfield's Neuropathology* that can be produced in hardcover printed format. Accommodating the additional information has largely involved a combination of reorganisation and restraint, together with considerably increased use of photographs and diagrams.

The reorganisation has involved the merging of vascular disease, hypoxia and related conditions into a single chapter; the subdivision of movement disorders into separate chapters on extrapyramidal disorders, ataxias and motor neuron diseases; the inclusion of separate chapters on ageing and dementia, the latter encompassing an expanded section on vascular dementia; and the further subdivision of the tumour section from two chapters in the previous edition to twenty-one in the present one, which we hope will make this part of the book easier to navigate. The total number of chapters in the book has increased from twenty-four to forty-six. Restraint has been applied in relation to the inclusion of references and of some very detailed molecular genetic and phenotypic information that is readily accessible through online resources such as OMIM, the database of Genotypes and Phenotypes (dbGaP), AlzGene and PDGene. We expect readers to look to *Greenfield's Neuropathology* for guidance and perspective rather than as a substitute for bibliographic databases and search engines.

The changes have involved a great deal of work on the part of our authors, who have shown unfailing courtesy and forbearance in responding to requests to condense prose, reorganise chapters and be selective in the inclusion of references. We are in their debt. Throughout, our objectives, much like those of Greenfield and Buzzard, have been to describe clearly the neuropathological changes that underlie neurological diseases, to discuss briefly their pathogenesis, and to try to relate molecular genetic, structural and biochemical alterations to clinical and neuroradiological manifestations.

Once a full account has been taken of the clinical and neuroradiological manifestations of neurological disease in a particular patient, a detailed visual examination of the diseased tissue is the starting point for almost all neuropathological investigations. Much of the excitement of neuropathology comes from discovering visual clues to disease, macroscopic or microscopic, whether in a section stained simply with haematoxylin and eosin, a series of confocal laser scanning images or a transmission electron micrograph. Neuropathology remains a highly visual specialty and most of us neuropathologists obtain immense aesthetic gratification from our work. Not surprisingly, therefore, we have placed a strong emphasis on visual aspects of this reference book, which includes over one thousand completely new photographs and drawings. It also incorporates new design elements such as the alternate colour coding of chapters that is intended to allow their easier navigation. To this same end, both volumes now include full indexes to the whole book. There are also improved search, annotation and bookmarking facilities in the bundled bonus e-book version of this edition. The e-book frees users from most of the physical limitations (not least of which are the size and weight) of the printed version and can be downloaded to a wide range of mobile and electronic devices, so that it is not necessary to be online to have full access to *Greenfield's Neuropathology*.

Publication of this ninth edition of *Greenfield's Neuropathology* would not have been possible without the support of many people, initially at Hodder Arnold and subsequently at Taylor and Francis. At Hodder Arnold, Joanna Koster, Editorial Director; Caroline

Makepeace, Head of Postgraduate and Professional Publishing; Mischa Barrett, Project Editor; and Miriam Trent, Editorial Assistant, were closely involved in the early stages. At Taylor and Francis, Barbara Norwitz, Executive Editor; Amy Blalock, Supervisor, Editorial Project Development; Rachael Russell, Senior Editorial Assistant; and Linda Van Pelt, Senior Project Manager, Medical, all worked on different stages of the title, and one person who merits special thanks is Sue Hodgson for her invaluable help as Executive Editor. Glenys Norquay provided freelance support and Jayne Jones designed the cover and interior pages.

We are pleased to present the ninth edition of *Greenfield's Neuropathology*. We hope you obtain as much satisfaction from reading this book as we have from editing it.

S Love
H Budka
J W Ironside
A Perry

November 2014

Contributors

Knarik Arkun, MD
Director
Neuropathology and Autopsy Service
Assistant Professor
Department of Pathology
Tufts Medical Center
Boston, MA, USA

Sylvia L Asa, MD, PhD
Medical Director
Laboratory Medicine Program
University Health Network
Lakeridge Health & Women's College Hospital
Senior Scientist
Ontario Cancer Institute
Professor
Department of Laboratory Medicine and Pathobiology
University of Toronto
Toronto, ON, Canada

Juan M Bilbao, FRCP (Canada)
Professor Emeritus of Neuropathology
St Michael's and Sunnybrook Hospitals
University of Toronto
Toronto, ON, Canada

Daniel J Brat, MD, PhD
Professor and Vice Chair
Translational Programs
Department of Pathology and Laboratory Medicine
Emory University School of Medicine
Georgia Research Alliance Distinguished Cancer Scientist
Atlanta, GA, USA

Susan C Brown, PhD
Reader in Translational Medicine
Comparative Biomedical Sciences
Royal Veterinary College
London, UK

Herbert Budka, MD
Professor of Neuropathology
Consultant, Institute of Neuropathology
University Hospital Zurich
Zurich, Switzerland

Steven A Chance, DPhil
Associate Professor in Clinical Neurosciences
Department of Neuropathology
University of Oxford
Oxford, UK

Leila Chimelli, MD, PhD
Professor of Pathology
Federal University of Rio de Janeiro
Rio de Janeiro, Brazil

Patrick F Chinnery,
　BMedSci, MBBS, PhD, FRCP, FRCPath, FMedSci
Professor of Neurogenetics
Newcastle University
Newcastle upon Tyne, UK

H Brent Clark, MD, PhD
Director of Neuropathology
Professor of Laboratory Medicine and Pathology,
　Neurology, and Neurosurgery
University of Minnesota Medical School
Minneapolis, MN, USA

Tim J Crow, MBBS, PhD, FRCP, FRCPsych, FMedSci
SANE POWIC
University Department of Psychiatry
Warneford Hospital
Oxford, UK

Matthew D Cykowski, MD
Neuropathology Fellowship Program
Houston Methodist Hospital/MD Anderson Cancer Center
Houston, TX, USA

Jean Debarros, PhD, MBPsS
Research Clinical Psychologist
Counselling Service
University of Oxford
Oxford, UK

Martina Deckert, MD
Professor
Department of Neuropathology
University Hospital of Cologne
Cologne, Germany

Marc R Del Bigio, MD, PhD, FRCPC
Canada Research Chair in Developmental
　Neuropathology
Professor
Department of Pathology (Neuropathology)
University of Manitoba
Winnipeg, MB, Canada

Salvatore DiMauro, MD
Lucy G Moses Professor
Department of Neurology
Columbia University Medical Center
New York, NY, USA

Ann-Christine Duhaime, MD
Director
Pediatric Neurosurgery
Massachusetts General Hospital
Nicholas T Zervas Professor of Neurosurgery
Harvard Medical School
Boston, MA, USA

Charles Eberhart, MD, PhD
Professor of Pathology, Ophthalmology and Oncology
Director of Neuropathology and Ophthalmic Pathology
Johns Hopkins University School of Medicine
Baltimore, MD, USA

Margaret M Esiri, DM, FRCPath
Neuropathology Department
John Radcliffe Hospital
Emeritus Professor of Neuropathology
Nuffield Department of Clinical Neurosciences
University of Oxford
Oxford, UK

Phyllis L Faust, MD, PhD
Associate Professor of Clinical Pathology and Cell Biology
Department of Pathology and Cell Biology
Columbia University
New York, NY, USA

Isidro Ferrer, MD, PhD
Professor
Institute of Neuropathology
Bellvitge University Hospital and University of Barcelona
Hospitalet de Llobregat
Barcelona, Spain

Rebecca D Folkerth, MD
Director of Neuropathology
Department of Pathology
Brigham and Women's Hospital
Consultant in Neuropathology
Boston Children's Hospital
Associate Professor of Pathology
Harvard Medical School
Boston, MA, USA

Christine E Fuller, MD
Professor
Pathology and Neurology
Director
Neuropathology and Autopsy Pathology
Department of Pathology
Virginia Commonwealth University
Richmond, VA, USA

Gregory N Fuller, MD, PhD
Professor and Chief
Section of Neuropathology
The University of Texas
MD Anderson Cancer Center
Department of Pathology
Houston, TX, USA

Bernardino Ghetti, MD, FANA, FAAAS
Distinguished Professor
Indiana University
Chancellor's Professor
Indiana University-Purdue University Indianapolis
Department of Pathology and Laboratory Medicine
Division of Neuropathology
Indiana University School of Medicine
Indianapolis, IN, USA

Jeffrey A Golden, MD
Chair
Department of Pathology
Brigham and Women's Hospital
Ramzi S Cotran Professor of Pathology
Harvard Medical School
Boston, MA, USA

Glenda M Halliday, PhD
Professor of Neuroscience and NHMRC Senior Principal
    Research Fellow
School of Medical Sciences and Neuroscience Research
    Australia
University of New South Wales
Sydney, NSW, Australia

Brian N Harding, MA, DPhil, BM, BCh, FRCPath
Department of Pathology and
    Laboratory Medicine
Children's Hospital of Philadelphia
Perelman School of Medicine
University of Pennsylvania
Philadelphia, PA, USA

John B Harris, PhD, BPharm, FSoCBiol, MRPharmSoc
Emeritus Professor of Experimental
    Neurology
Medical Toxicology Centre
Newcastle University
Newcastle upon Tyne, UK

Jason F Harrison, MD, PhD
Neurosurgery Resident
Department of Neurosurgery
Virginia Commonwealth University
Richmond, VA, USA

Mark W Head, BSc, PhD
Reader
University of Edinburgh
Deputy Director
National CJD Research & Surveillance Unit
Edinburgh, Scotland

J Robin Highley, DPhil, FRCPath
Senior Clinical Lecturer in Neuropathology
Department of Neuroscience
Sheffield Institute of Translational Neuroscience
University of Sheffield
Sheffield, UK

Janice L Holton, BSc, MBChB, PhD, FRCPath
Professor of Neuropathology
Department of Molecular Neuroscience
University College London Institute of Neurology
London, UK

Henry H Houlden, MD, PhD
Professor of Neurology and Neurogenetics
Department of Molecular Neuroscience
University College London Institute of Neurology
London, UK

Paul G Ince, MBBS, MD, FRCPath
Professor of Neuropathology
Head of Department of Neuroscience
University of Sheffield
Sheffield, UK

James W Ironside, CBE, BMSc, FRCPath,
  FRCPEdin, FMedSci, FRSE
Professor of Clinical Neuropathology and Honorary
  Consultant in Neuropathology
National Creutzfeldt–Jakob Disease Surveillance Unit
University of Edinburgh
Western General Hospital
Edinburgh, UK

Thomas S Jacques, PhD, MRCP, FRCPath
Higher Education Funding Council for England
  Clinical Senior Lecturer
Honorary Consultant
Paediatric Neuropathologist
University College London Institute of Child Health and
  Great Ormond Street Hospital
Department of Histopathology
Great Ormond Street Hospital for Children NHS
  Foundation Trust
London, UK

Evelyn Jaros, PhD
Clinical Scientist in Neuropathology
Neuropathology/Cellular Pathology
Newcastle upon Tyne Hospitals NHS Foundation Trust
Honorary Senior Research Associate
Institute of Neuroscience and Institute for Ageing
Newcastle University
Campus for Ageing and Vitality
Newcastle upon Tyne, UK

Martin Jeffrey, BVMS, DVM, Dip ECVP,
  MRCVS, FRCPath
Consultant Pathologist
Pathology Department
Animal Health and Veterinary Laboratories Agency
  (AHVLA-Lasswade)
Penicuik, UK

Anne Jouvet, MD, PhD
Associate Professor of Pathology
Centre de Pathologie et Neuropathologie Est
Centre de Biologie et Pathologie Est
Groupement Hospitalier Est
Hospices Civils de Lyon
Lyon, France

Raj Kalaria, PhD, FRCPath
Professor of Cerebrovascular Pathology
  (Neuropathology)
Institute of Neuroscience
Newcastle University
National Institute for Health Research Biomedical
  Research Building
Campus for Ageing and Vitality
Newcastle upon Tyne, UK

B K Kleinschmidt-DeMasters, MD
Professor of Pathology, Neurology, and
  Neurosurgery
Department of Pathology
University of Colorado School of Medicine
Aurora, CO, USA

Jillian Kril, PhD, FFSc (RCPA)
Professor of Neuropathology
Sydney Medical School
The University of Sydney
Sydney, NSW, Australia

Nichola Z Lax, PhD
Research Associate
Wellcome Trust Centre for Mitochondrial
  Research
Institute of Neuroscience
Newcastle University
Newcastle upon Tyne, UK

David N Louis, MD
Pathologist-in-Chief
Massachusetts General Hospital
Benjamin Castleman Professor of
  Pathology
Harvard Medical School
James Homer Wright Pathology
  Laboratories
Massachusetts General Hospital
Boston, MA, USA

Seth Love, MBBCH, PhD, FRCP, FRCPath
Professor of Neuropathology
Institute of Clinical Neurosciences
School of Clinical Sciences
University of Bristol
Southmead Hospital
Bristol, UK

James Lowe, DM, FRCPath
Professor of Neuropathology
University of Nottingham
Honorary Consultant in Neuropathology to
  the Nottingham University Hospitals
  NHS Trust
School of Medicine
Faculty of Medicine and Health Sciences
University of Nottingham
Nottingham, UK

Sebastian Lucas, FRCP, FRCPath
Emeritus Professor of Histopathology
Department of Histopathology
St Thomas' Hospital
London, UK

Susan S Margulies, PhD
George H Stephenson Professor
Department of Bioengineering
University of Pennsylvania
Philadelphia, PA, USA

Michelle Fevre Montange, PhD
Centre de Recherche en Neuroscience de Lyon
    INSERM U1028
CNRS UMR 5292
Equipe Neuro-oncologie et Neuro-inflammation
Université de Lyon
Lyon, France

G R Wayne Moore, BSC, MD, CM, FRCPC, FRCPath
Clinical Professor
Department of Pathology and Laboratory Medicine
International Collaboration on Repair Discoveries (ICORD)
University of British Columbia
Vancouver General Hospital
Vancouver, BC, Canada

Christopher M Morris, PhD
Senior Lecturer
Medical Toxicology Centre
National Institutes of Health Research
Health Protection Research Unit in Chemical and
    Radiation Threats and Hazards
Institute of Neuroscience
Newcastle University
Newcastle upon Tyne, UK

Francesco Muntoni, FRCPCH, FMedSci
Director
Dubowitz Neuromuscular Centre
MRC Centre for Neuromuscular Diseases
University College London Institute of Child Health and
    Great Ormond Street Hospital for Children (GOSH)
London, UK

Arie Perry, MD
Professor of Pathology and Neurological Surgery
Director of Neuropathology
Director of Neuropathology Fellowship Training Program
University of California, San Francisco
San Francisco, CA, USA

Rahul Phadke, MBBS, MD, FRCPath
Consultant Neuropathologist
University College London Institute of Neurology
National Hospital for Neurology and Neurosurgery and
    Dubowitz Neuromuscular Centre
Great Ormond Street Hospital for Children
London, UK

Pedro Piccardo, MD
Senior Investigator
Chief Transmissible Spongiform Encephalopathy
    Pathogenesis Section
Laboratory of Bacterial and TSE Agents
Office of Blood Research and Review
Center for Biologics Evaluation and Research
U.S. Food and Drug Administration
Silver Spring, MD, USA
Professor
Neurobiology Division
The Roslin Institute
University of Edinburgh
Easter Bush, UK

James M Powers, MD
Professor Emeritus
Department of Pathology
University of Rochester School of Medicine
    and Dentistry
Rochester, NY, USA

Robin Reid, BSc, MBChB, FRCPath
Formerly Consultant Pathologist
Western Infirmary
Glasgow, UK

Guido Reifenberger, MD
Professor
Department of Neuropathology
Heinrich Heine University
Düsseldorf, Germany

Tamas Revesz, MD, FRCPath
Professor Emeritus in Neuropathology
UCL Institute of Neurology
University College London
London, UK

Hope T Richard, MD, PhD
Neuropathology Fellow
Department of Pathology
Virginia Commonwealth University
Richmond, VA, USA

Marc K Rosenblum, MD
Founder's Chair and Chief
Neuropathology and Autopsy Service
Memorial Sloan-Kettering Cancer Center
Professor of Pathology and Laboratory
    Medicine
Weill Medical College of Cornell
    University
New York, NY, USA

Robert E Schmidt, MD, PhD
Professor of Pathology and Immunology
Director
Division of Neuropathology
Medical Director
Electron Microscope Facility
Washington University School of Medicine
St Louis, MO, USA

Caroline A Sewry, PhD, FRCPath
Professor of Muscle Pathology
Dubowitz Neuromuscular Centre
Institute of Child Health and Great Ormond Street
    Hospital
London
Wolfson Centre for Inherited Neuromuscular
    Diseases
Robert Jones and Agnes Hunt Orthopaedic
    Hospital
Oswestry, UK

Sanjay Sisodiya, MA, PhD, FRCP, FRCPEdin
Professor of Neurology
Department of Clinical and Experimental Epilepsy
UCL Institute of Neurology
London
Consultant Neurologist
Epilepsy Society
National Hospital for Neurology and Neurosurgery
Chalfton St Peter, UK

Colin Smith, MD, FRCPath
Reader in Pathology
University of Edinburgh
Edinburgh, UK

Christine Stadelmann-Nessler, MD
Professor
Department of Neuropathology
University Medical Center Göttingen
Göttingen, Germany

Kinuko Suzuki, MD
Emeritus Professor of Pathology and Laboratory Medicine
University of North Carolina at Chapel Hill
Chapel Hill, NC, USA
Neuropathology
Tokyo Metropolitan Institute of Gerontology
Tokyo, Japan

Kunihiko Suzuki, MD
Director Emeritus
Neuroscience Center
University of North Carolina
Chapel Hill, NC, USA

Robert W Taylor, PhD, DSC, FRCPath
Professor of Mitochondrial Pathology
Wellcome Trust Centre for Mitochondrial Research
Institute of Neuroscience
Newcastle University
Newcastle upon Tyne, UK

Maria Thom, BSC, MBBS, MRCPath
Senior Lecturer
Institute of Neurology
University College London
London, UK

Douglas M Turnbull, MD, PhD, FRCP, FMedSc
Professor of Neurology
Director
Wellcome Trust Centre for Mitochondrial Research
Director
LLHW Centre for Ageing and Vitality
Newcastle University
Newcastle upon Tyne, UK

Alexandre Vasiljevic, MD
Associate Professor of Pathology
Centre de Pathologie et Neuropathologie Est
Centre de Biologie et Pathologie Est
Groupement Hospitalier Est
Hospices Civils de Lyon
Lyon, France

Harry V Vinters, MD
Professor of Pathology and Laboratory Medicine,
 Neurology
Chief of Neuropathology
Division of Neuropathology
Member of Brain Research Institute ACCESS
 Program
Department of Cellular and Molecular
 Pathology
University of California, Los Angeles
Los Angeles, CA, USA

Steven U Walkley, DVM, PhD
Director
Rose F Kennedy Intellectual and Developmental
 Disabilities Research Center
Head
Sidney Weisner Laboratory of Genetic
 Neurological Disease
Departments of Neuroscience, Pathology and
 Neurology
Albert Einstein College of Medicine
Bronx, NY, USA

Stephen B Wharton, BSC, MBBS, PhD, FRCPath
Professor and Honorary Consultant in Neuropathology
Department of Neuroscience
Sheffield Institute of Translational Neuroscience
University of Sheffield
Sheffield, UK

Clayton A Wiley, MD, PhD
Professor of Pathology
Director of Neuropathology
PERF Endowed Chair
Univeristy of Pittsburgh Medical Center
 Presbyterian Hospital
Pittsburgh, PA, USA

Robert G Will, MA, MD, FRCP
Professor of Clinical Neurology
National Creutzfeldt–Jakob Disease Surveillance Unit
University of Edinburgh
Western General Hospital
Edinburgh, UK

Abbreviations

AA	anaplastic astrocytoma
AACD	age-associated cognitive decline
AAMI	age-associated memory impairment
ABC	ATP-binding cassette
ABCA1	ATP-binding cassette transporter 1
ABRA	Aβ-related angiitis
ACA	anterior cerebral artery
ACC	adrenocortical carcinoma
ACCIS	Automated Childhood Cancer Information System
ACh	acetylcholine
AChR	acetylcholine receptor
ACTH	adrenocorticotropin
AD	Alzheimer disease
ADAMTS13	a disintegrin and metalloproteinase with a thrombospondin type 1 motif, member 13
ADC	apparent diffusion coefficient
ADCA	autosomal dominant cerebellar ataxia
ADEM	acute disseminated encephalomyelitis
ADK	adenosine kinase
ADNFLE	autosomal dominant nocturnal frontal lobe epilepsy
ADP	adenosine diphosphate
AFP	alpha-fetoprotein
AGA	aspartylglucosaminidase
AGE	advanced glycosylation end product
AGPS	alkylglycerone phosphate synthase
AGS	Aicardi-Goutières syndrome
AGU	aspartylglucosaminuria
AHLE	acute haemorrhagic leukoencephalitis
AHT	abusive head trauma
AIDP	acute inflammatory demyelinating polyneuropathy
AIDS	acquired immunodeficiency syndrome
AIP	aryl hydrocarbon receptor-interacting protein
AIS	axon initial segment
AISS	axonal index sector score
AL	amyloidosis
ALCL	anaplastic large cell lymphoma
ALD	adrenoleukodystrophy
ALK	anaplastic lymphoma kinase
ALL	acute lymphoblastic leukemia
ALS	amyotrophic lateral sclerosis
ALT	alternative lengthening of telomeres
AMAN	acute motor axonal neuropathy
AMN	adrenomyeloneuropathy
AMPA	α-amino-3-hydroxy-5-methyl-4-isoxazolepropionic acid
AMSAN	acute motor sensory axonal neuropathy
ANA	antinuclear antibody
ANCA	antineutrophil cytoplasmic autoantibody
ANCL	adult neuronal ceroid lipofuscinosis
Ang-1	angiopoietin-1
Ang-2	angiopoietin-2
ANI	asymptomatic neurocognitive impairment
AOA1	early-onset ataxia with oculomotor apraxia, type 1
APGBD	adult polyglucosan body disease
APLA	antiphospholipid antibody
ApoE	apolipoprotein E
APP	amyloid precursor protein
APrP	amyloid prion protein
APUD	amine precursor uptake and decarboxylation
AQP4	aquaporin-4
AR	androgen receptor
ARBD	alcohol-related brain damage
ARFGEF2	adenosine diphosphate (ADP)-ribosylation factor guanine exchange factor 2
ASA	arylsulfatase A
ASDH	acute subdural haematoma
ASE	acute schistosomal encephalopathy
ASL	arterial spin labelling
AT	ataxia telangiectasia
ATP	adenosine triphosphate
ATRT	atypical teratoid/rhabdoid tumour
ATTR	amyloid transthyretin
AVM	arteriovenous malformation
BA	Brodmann area
BACE	β-site APP-cleaving enzyme
BAC	bacterial artificial chromosome
BAV	Banna virus
BBB	blood-brain barrier
BDNF	brain-derived neurotrophic factor
BDV	Borna disease virus
BEAN	brain expressed protein associated with NEDD4
bFGF	basic fibroblast growth factor
BGC	basal ganglia calcification
BHC	benign hereditary chorea
BMAA	β-N-methylamino-L-alanine
BMD	Becker muscular dystrophy
BMP	bone morphogenetic protein
BOLD	blood oxygenation dependent
bp	base pair
BPAU	bromophenylacetylurea

BRC	brain reserve capacity	CLL	chronic lymphatic leukaemia
BRRS	Bannayan-Riley-Ruvalcaba syndrome	CM	cerebral malaria
BSE	bovine spongiform encephalopathy	CMD	congenital muscular dystrophy
CAA	cerebral amyloid angiopathy	CMRgl	cerebral metabolic rate for glucose
CADASIL	cerebral autosomal dominant arteriopathy with subcortical infarcts and leukoencephalopathy	$CMRO_2$	cerebral metabolic rate for oxygen
		CMROGl	cerebral metabolic rates of oxygen and glucose
CAE	childhood absence epilepsy	CMT	Charcot–Marie–Tooth
CAHS	chronic acquired hepatocerebral syndrome	CMV	cytomegalovirus
		CN	cystic nephroma
CAMTA1	calmodulin-binding transcription activator 1	CNC	Carney's complex
		CNP	2′,3′-cyclic nucleotide 3′-phosphodiesterase
c-ANCA	cytoplasmic antineutrophil cytoplasmic antibody	CNS	central nervous system
CANOMAD	chronic ataxic neuropathy, ophthalmoplegia, M-protein agglutination, disialosyl antibodies	CNS PNET	central nervous system primitive neuroectodermal tumour
		CNTF	ciliary neurotrophic factor
CAR	coxsackievirus and adenovirus receptor	CO	carbon monoxide
CARASIL	cerebral autosomal recessive arteriopathy with subcortical infarcts and leukoencephalopathy	COL4A1	collagen, type IV, alpha 1
		COX	cytochrome c oxidase
		COX-2	cyclooxygenase-2
cART	combined antiretroviral therapy	CP	choroid plexus
CASK	calcium-dependent serine protein kinase	CPCS	chronic post-concussion syndrome
CBD	corticobasal degeneration	CPM	central pontine myelinolysis
CBF	cerebral blood flow	CPP	cerebral perfusion pressure; central precocious puberty
CBS	corticobasal syndrome	CPT	carnitine palmitoyltransferase
CBTRUS	Central Brain Tumor Registry of the United States	CR	cognitive reserve
		CR3	complement receptor type 3
CCM	cerebral cavernous malformation	CRABP	cellular retinoic acid binding protein
CCSVI	chronic cerebrospinal venous insufficiency	CRBP	cytoplasmic retinol binding protein
		CREB	cyclic adenine dinucleotide phosphate response element binding protein
CD	Cowden disease		
CDE	common data elements		
CDI	conformation dependent immunoassay	CRH	corticotropin-releasing hormone
CDK5	cyclin-dependent kinase 5	CRIMYNE	critical illness myopathy and neuropathy
CDKI	cyclin-dependent kinase inhibitor		
CDKN2C	cyclin-dependent kinase inhibitor 2C	CRMP-5	collapsing response mediator protein 5
CDV	canine distemper virus	CRV	cerebroretinal vasculopathy
CEA	carcinoembryonic antigen	CSDH	chronic subdural haematoma
CESD	cholesteryl ester storage disease	CSF	cerebrospinal fluid
CGH	comparative genomic hybridization	CSPα	cysteine string protein α
cGMP	cyclic guanosine monophosphate	CT	computed tomography
CGRP	calcitonin gene-related peptide	CTD	connective tissue disease
CHD5	chromodomain helicase DNA binding domain 5	CTE	chronic traumatic encephalopathy
		CTF	Colorado tick fever
CHN	congenital hypomyelinating neuropathy	CTL	cytotoxic lymphocyte
CHS	classical hippocampal sclerosis	CUP	cancer of unknown primary
CIM	critical illness myopathy	CUTE	corticotropin upstream transcription-binding element
CIP	critical illness polyneuropathy		
CIPD	chronic inflammatory demyelinating polyneuropathy	CuZnSOD	copper- and zinc-containing superoxide dismutase
CIS	clinically isolated syndrome		
CISP	chronic immune sensory polyradiculopathy	CVD	cardiovascular disease
		CVS	chorionic villus sampling
CK	cytokeratin; creatine kinase	CVST	cerebral venous sinus thrombosis
CLA2	X-linked cerebellar ataxia	CVT	cerebral venous thrombosis

CWD	chronic wasting disease
CX32	connexin 32
DAB	diaminobenzidine
DAG	dystrophin-associated glycoprotein
DAI	diffuse axonal injury
DAPAT	dihydroxyacetonephosphate acyltransferase
DASE	developmentally arrested structural elements
DAWM	diffusely abnormal white matter
DCX	doublecortin
DEHSI	diffuse excessive high-signal intensity
DFFB	DNA fragmentation factor subunit beta
DHA	docosahexaenoic acid
DHAP	dihydroxyacetone phosphate
DHPR	dihydropyridine receptor
Dil	dioctadecyl-tetramethylindocarbacyanine perchlorate
DILS	diffuse infiltrative lymphocytosis syndrome
DIR	double inversion recovery
DLB	dementia with Lewy bodies
DLBCL	diffuse large B cell lymphoma
DLK	dual leucine kinase
DM	dermatomyositis
DMD	Duchenne muscular dystrophy
DMNV	dorsal motor nucleus of the vagus
DMPK	dermatomyositis protein kinase
DNER	delta/notch-like epidermal growth factor-related receptor
DNL	disseminated necrotizing leukoencephalopathy
DNMT	DNA methyltransferase
DNT	dysembryoplastic neuroepithelial tumour
DPR	dipeptide repeat
DPX	di-n-butylphthalate-polystyrene-xylene
DRD	dopa-responsive dystonia
DRPLA	dentatorubropallidoluysian atrophy
DSD	Dejerine-Sottas disease
DSPN	diffuse sensory polyneuropathy
DTI	diffusion tensor imaging
DTICH	delayed traumatic intracerebral haemorrhage
DWI	diffusion weighted imaging
DXC	doublecortin
EA	episodic ataxia
EAAT	excitatory amino acid transporter
EAN	experimental allergic neuritis
EBP	elastin-binding protein
EBV	Epstein-Barr virus
EC	endothelial cell; entorhinal cortex
ECGF1	endothelial cell growth factor 1 (platelet-derived)
ECM	extracellular matrix
ECMO	extracorporeal membrane oxygenation

EDH	extradural haematoma
EEE	eastern equine encephalitis
EEG	electroencephalogram
EET	epoxyeicosatrienoic acid
EF HS	end folium hippocampal sclerosis
EGA	estimated gestational age
EGB	eosinophilic granular body
EGFR	epidermal growth factor receptor
EGL	external granule cell layer
EGR2	early growth response 2 gene
EIEE	early infantile epileptic encephalopathy
EL	encephalitis lethargica
ELBW	extreme low birth weight
ELISA	enzyme-linked immunosorbent assay
EM	electron microscopy
EMA	epithelial membrane antigen
EME	early myoclonic encephalopathy
EMG	electromyography
EMT	epithelial-mesenchymal transition
eNSC	embryonic neural stem cell
ENU	ethylnitrosourea
EPC	endothelial progenitor cell
EPMR	epilepsy with mental retardation
ER	endoplasmic reticulum
ERG	electroretinogram
ERK	extracellular signal-regulated kinase
ERM	ezrin, radixin and moesin
ESAM	endothelial cell-selective adhesion molecule
ESR	erythrocyte sedimentation rate
ETANTR	embryonal tumour with abundant neuropil and true rosettes
ETMR	embryonal tumor with multilayered rosettes
EVOH	ethylene-vinyl alcohol copolymer
FA	Friedreich's ataxia
FACS	fluorescence-activated cell sorting
FAD	familial Alzheimer's disease
FAF	familial amyloidosis of the Finnish type
FAK	focal adhesion kinase
FALS	familial amyotrophic lateral sclerosis
FAP	familial amyloid polyneuropathy; familial polyposis
FBD	familial British dementia
FBXO7	F-box only protein 7
FCD	focal cortical dysplasia; follicular dendritic cell
FCE	fibrocartilaginous embolism
fCJD	familial Creutzfeldt-Jakob disease
FDD	familial Danish dementia
FDF-2	fibroblast growth factor 2
FFI	fatal familial insomnia
FFPE	formalin-fixed paraffin-embedded tissue

FG	fast-twitch glycolytic		GIST	gastrointestinal stromal tumour
FGF	fibroblast growth factor		GLAST	glutamate/aspartate transporter
FHL1	four and a half LIM domains protein 1		GLB1	galactosidase, beta 1
FILIP	filamin-A-interacting protein		GLD	globoid cell leukodystrophy
FIPA	familial isolated pituitary adenoma		GLM	glial limiting membrane
FISH	fluorescence *in situ* hybridization		GM	gliomesodermal tissue
FKRP	fukutin-related protein		GOM	granular osmiophilic material
FLAIR	fluid-associated inversion recovery		GP	globus pallidus
FLNA	filamin A		GPI	glycosylphosphatidylinositol
FMD	fibromuscular dysplasia; Fukuyama muscular dystrophy		GROD	granular osmiophilic deposit
fMRI	functional magnetic resonance imaging		GSC	glioma stem cell
FOG	fast-twitch oxidative glycolytic		GSD	glycogen storage disease
FPS	fasciitis-panniculitis syndrome		GSN	gelsolin
FR	fatigue resistant		Gsp	G-protein oncogene
FS	febrile seizure		GSS	Gerstmann-Sträussler-Scheinker disease
FSH	follicle stimulating hormone		gTSE	genetic transmissible spongiform encephalopathy
FSHD	facioscapulohumeral muscular dystrophy		GU	genitourinary
FTBSI	focal traumatic brain stem injury		GWAS	genome wide association studies
FTD	frontotemporal dementia		HAART	highly active antiretroviral therapy
FTL	ferritin light		HACE	high altitude cerebral oedema
FTLD	frontotemporal lobar degeneration		HAD	HIV-associated dementia
FUPB1	far-upstream element binding protein 1		HAM	HTLV-1-associated myelopathy
FUS	fused-in-sarcoma protein		HAN	hereditary neuralgic amyotrophy
FXTAS	fragile X tremor/ataxia syndrome		HANAC	hereditary angiopathy with nephropathy, aneurysms and muscle cramps
G-CIMP	glioma CpG island methylator phenotype		HAS	high-altitude stupid
GABA	gamma-aminobutyric acid		HAT	human African trypanosomiasis
GAD	gracile axonal dystrophy; glutamic acid decarboxylase		HB-EGF	heparin-binding epidermal growth factor
GAG	glycosaminoglycan		HCG	human chorionic gonadotropin
GALT	gut-associated lymphoid tissue		HCHWA-D	hereditary cerebral haemorrhage with amyloid angiopathy of the Dutch
GAP-43	growth-associated protein 43		HCHWA-F	hereditary cerebral haemorrhage with amyloid angiopathy of the Flemish
GAT1	glutaric aciduria type 1		HCHWA-I	hereditary cerebral haemorrhage with amyloid angiopathy of the Icelandic
Gb Ose3 Cer	globotriaosylceramide		HCMV	human cytomegalovirus
GBE	glycogen branching enzyme		HD	Huntington's disease
GBM	glioblastoma		HDL	high density lipoprotein
GBS	Guillain–Barré syndrome		HDL1	Huntington disease-like type 1
GC	granule cell		HDL2	Huntington disease-like type 2
GCA	giant cell (or temporal) arteritis		HDL3	Huntington disease-like type 3
GCD	granule cell dispersion		HE	hepatic encephalopathy
GCI	global cerebral ischaemia; glial cytoplasmic inclusion		H&E	haematoxylin and eosin
GCL	granule cell layer		HERNS	hereditary endotheliopathy with retinopathy, nephropathy and stroke
GCS	Glasgow Coma Scale		HERV	human endogenous retrovirus
GDAP1	ganglioside-induced differentiation-associated protein 1		HES	hairy/enhancer of split
GDNF	glial cell-derived neurotrophic factor		HES-1	hairy/enhancer of split 1
GEMM	genetically engineered mouse model		hGH	human growth hormone
GFAP	glial fibrillary acidic protein		HH	hypothalamic hamartoma
GFP	green fluorescent protein		HHV-8	human herpesvirus 8
GH	growth hormone		HIF	hypoxia inducible factor
GHR	GH receptor			
GI	gastrointestinal			

HIHRATL	hereditary infantile hemiparesis, retinal arteriolar tortuosity and leukoencephalopathy	IIM	idiopathic inflammatory myopathy
HIMAL	hippocampal malrotation	IL-1β	interleukin-1 beta
HIV	human immunodeficiency virus	ILAE	International League Against Epilepsy
HLA	human leukocyte antigen	ILOCA	idiopathic late-onset cerebellar ataxia
HLH	helix-loop-helix	ILS	isolated lissencephaly sequence
HMEG	hemimegalencephaly	IMAM	inflammatory myopathy with abundant macrophages
HMERF	hereditary myopathy with early respiratory failure	IMD	inherited myoclonus-dystonia
HMG	high mobility group	IML	inner molecular layer
HMGCR	3-hydroxy-3-methylglutaryl-coenzyme A reductase	IMNM	immune-mediated necrotizing myopathy
H-MRS	proton magnetic resonance spectroscopy	IMT	inflammatory myofibroblastic tumour
HMSN	hereditary motor and sensory neuropathy	INAD	infantile neuroaxonal dystrophy
		INCL	infantile neuronal ceroid lipofuscinosis
HNE	hydroxy-2-nonenal	iNOS	inducible nitric oxide synthase
HNPCC	hereditary nonpolyposis colorectal cancer	ION	inferior olivary nucleus
HNPP	hereditary neuropathy with liability to pressure palsy	IPI	initial precipitating injury
		iPSC	induced pluripotent stem cell
H_2O_2	hydrogen peroxide	IPSP	inhibitory postsynaptic potential
HPC	haemangiopericytoma	IRD	infantile Refsum's disease
HPE	holoprosencephaly	IRES	internal ribosomal entry site
HPF	high-power field	IRIS	immune reconstitution inflammatory syndrome
HPS	haematoxylin-phloxine-safranin		
HPV	human papillomavirus	IRS	insulin receptor substrate
HRE	hypoxia response elements	ISF	interstitial fluid
HRP	horseradish peroxidase	ISPD	isoprenoid synthase domain-containing
HS	hippocampal sclerosis	ISSD	infantile sialic acid storage disease
HSA	hereditary systemic angiopathy	ITPR-1	inositol triphosphate receptor type 1
HSAN	hereditary sensory and autonomic neuropathy	IUGR	intrauterine growth restriction
		IVH	intraventricular haemorrhage
HSP	heat-shock protein; hereditary spastic paraplegia	JAK/STAT	Janus kinase and downstream signal transducer and activator of transcription
HSV	herpes simplex virus		
5-HT	5-hydroxytryptamine	JAM	junctional adhesion molecule
hTERT	human telomerase reverse transcriptase	JME	juvenile myoclonic epilepsy
HTLV-I	human T-cell lymphotropic virus I	JNCL	juvenile neuronal ceroid lipofuscinosis
HVR	hereditary vascular retinopathy	JXG	juvenile xanthogranuloma
IBM	inclusion body myositis	kb	kilobase
ICA	internal carotid artery; internal cerebral artery	KO	knockout
		KPS	Karnofsky performance status
ICAM-1	intercellular adhesion molecule-1	KRS	Kufor Rakeb syndrome
ICD	I-cell disease; intracellular domain	KS	Korsakoff's syndrome
ICE	interleukin-converting enzyme	KSS	Kearns-Sayre syndrome
ICH	intracerebral haematoma	LA	lupus anticoagulant
iCJD	iatrogenic Creutzfeldt-Jakob disease	LB	Lewy body
ICP	intracranial pressure	LCH	Langerhans cell histiocytosis
IDH	intradural haemorrhage	LCMV	lymphocytic choriomeningitis virus
IENF	intra-epidermal nerve fibre	LDD	Lhermitte-Duclos disease
IFS	isolated familial somatotropinoma	LDL	low-density lipoprotein
IGF	insulin-related growth factor	LEAT	long-term epilepsy-associated tumour
IgM	immunoglobulin M	LFB	Luxol fast blue
IHC	immunohistochemistry	LFB-CV	Luxol fast blue-cresyl violet
IHI	incomplete hippocampal inversion	LGI1	leucine-rich glioma-inactivated 1
		LGMD	limb-girdle muscular dystrophy
		LGN	lateral geniculate nucleus

LH	luteinizing hormone
LIF	leukaemia inhibitory factor
LINCL	late infantile neuronal ceroid lipofuscinosis
LMNA	lamin A/C
LNMP	last normal menstrual period
LOH	loss of heterozygosity
LPH	lipotropin
LRPN	lumbosacral radioplexus neuropathy
LSA	lenticulostriate artery
L-SS	Lewis-Sumner syndrome
LTD	long-term depression
LTP	long-term potentiation
MAG	myelin-associated glycoprotein
MAGE-A	melanoma-associated cancer-testis antigen
MAP	microtubule-associated protein
MAPK	mitogen-activated protein kinase
MATPase	myofibrillar adenosine triphosphatase
MBD	Marchiafava-Bignami disease
MBEN	medulloblastoma with extensive nodularity
MBP	myelin basic protein
MCA	middle cerebral artery
MCB	membranous cytoplasmic body
MCD	malformation of cortical development
MCI	mild cognitive impairment
MCM2	minichromosome maintenance 2
MCP-1	monocyte chemoattractant protein 1
MDC1A	merosin-deficient CMD
MELAS	mitochondrial encephalomyopathy, lactic acidosis and stroke-like episodes
MEN	multiple endocrine neoplasia
MEN2	multiple endocrine neoplasia type 2
MERRF	myoclonic epilepsy with ragged-red fibres
MFN2	mitofusin 2
MFS	Miller Fisher syndrome; mossy fibre spouting
MGUS	monoclonal gammopathy of unknown significance
MHC	myosin heavy chain
MHC-I	major histocompatibility complex class I
MHV	mouse hepatitis virus
MIBE	measles inclusion body encephalitis
MJD	Machado-Joseph disease
ML	mucolipidosis
MLC	myosin light chain
MLD	metachromatic leukodystrophy
MLI	mucolipidosis I
MM	methionine homozygosity
MMN	multifocal motor neuropathy
MMP	matrix metalloproteinase
MMR	mismatch repair; measles-mumps-rubella
MNCV	motor nerve conduction velocity
MND	motor neuron degeneration; mild neurocognitive disorder; motor neuron disease
MNGC	multinucleated giant cell
MNGIE	mitochondrial neuro-gastrointestinal encephalomyopathy
MnSOD	manganese-containing superoxide dismutase
MNU	methylnitrosourea
MOG	myelin-oligodendrocyte protein
MPNST	malignant peripheral nerve sheath tumour
MPO	myeloperoxidase
MPS	mucopolysaccharidosis
MPT	mitochondrial permeability transition
MPTP	N-methyl-4-phenyl-1,2,3, 6-tetrahydropyridine
mPTS	membrane peroxisomal targeting sequence
MPZ	myelin protein zero
MR	magnetic resonance
MRC	Medical Research Council
MRI	magnetic resonance imaging
mRNA	messenger ribonucleic acid
MRS	magnetic resonance spectroscopy
MRT	malignant rhabdoid tumour
MS	multiple sclerosis
MSA	multiple system atrophy; myositis-specific autoantibody
MSA-C	cerebellar form of multiple system atrophy
MSB	Martius scarlet blue
MSD	multiple sulphatase deficiency
MSH	melanotropin
MSI	microsatellite instability
mtDNA	mitochondrial DNA
MTI	magnetization transfer imaging
MTLE	mesial temporal lobe epilepsy
MTMR2	myotubularin-related protein 2
mTOR	mammalian target of rapamycin
MTR	magnetization transfer ratio
MuSK	muscle-specific kinase
MV	valine heterozygous
MVE	Murray Valley encephalitis
NAA	N-acetylaspartate
NAD+	nicotinamide adenine dinucleotide
NADH-TR	nicotinamide adenine dinucleotide-tetrazolium reductase
NAHI	non-accidental head injury
NALD	neonatal adreno-leukodystrophy
NAM	necrotizing autoimmune myopathy
NARP	neuropathy, ataxia and retinitis pigmentosa
NAT	non-accidental trauma
NAWM	normal-appearing white matter

NBCCS	naevoid basal cell carcinoma syndrome
NBIA	neurodegeneration with brain iron accumulation
NBIA1	neurodegeneration with brain iron accumulation, type 1
NBIA2	neurodegeneration with brain iron accumulation, type 2
NCAM	neural cell adhesion molecule
NCI	neuronal cytoplasmic inclusion
NCIPC	National Center for Injury Prevention and Control
NCL	neuronal ceroid lipofuscinosis
NCM	neurocutaneous melanosis
NECD	notch extracellular domain
NF	neurofilament protein
NF1	neurofibromatosis type 1
NF2	neurofibromatosis type 2
NFL	National Football League
NFP	neurofilament protein
NFT	neurofibrillary tangle
NGF	nerve growth factor
NHNN	National Hospital for Neurology and Neurosurgery
NIFID	neuronal intermediate filament inclusion disease
NIID	neuronal intranuclear inclusion disease
NINDS	National Institute of Neurological Disorders and Stroke
NINDS-PSP	National Institute of Neurological Disorders and Stroke and the Society for Progressive Supranuclear Palsy
NIRS	near-infrared spectroscopy
NK	natural killer
NMDA	N-methyl-D-aspartate
NMDAR	N-methyl-D-aspartate receptor
NMO	neuromyelitis optica
nNOS	neuronal nitric oxide synthase
NO	nitric oxide
NOS	not otherwise specified
NOTCH3	notch homolog 3
NPC	Niemann-Pick disease type C
NPH	normal pressure hydrocephalus
NPY	neuropeptide Y
NSAID	non-steroidal anti-inflammatory drug
NSC	neural stem cell
NSE	neuron specific enolase
NTD	neural tube defect
NTE	neuropathy target esterase
NTS	nucleus of the solitary tract
OCT	optimal cutting temperature; optical coherence tomography
OEF	oxygen extraction fraction
O-FucT-1	O-fucosetransferase 1
OH	hydroxyl radical
OMIM	Online Mendelian Inheritance in Man
OML	outer molecular layer
OPC	oligdendrocyte precursor cell
OPCA	olivopontocerebellar atrophy
OPIDPN	organophosphate-induced delayed polyneuropathy
ORF	open reading frame
PACNS	primary angiitis of the central nervous system
PAFAH	platelet activating factor acetyl hydrolase
PAMP	pathogen-associated molecular pattern
PAN	polyarteritis nodosa; perchloric acid naphthoquinone
p-ANCA	perinuclear ANCA
PARK1	Parkinson's disease and alpha-synuclein
PAS	periodic acid–Schiff
PB	pineoblastoma
PBD	peroxisome biogenesis disorder
PBH	parenchymal brain haemorrhage
PBP	progressive bulbar palsy
PC	pineocytoma
PCD	Purkinje cell degeneration
PCNA	proliferating cell nuclear antigen
PCNSL	primary central nervous system lymphoma
PCP	planar cell polarity
PCR	polymerase chain reaction
PCV	packed cell volume
PD	Parkinson's disease; pars distalis
PDC	parkinsonism/dementia complex
PDCD	programmed cell death
PDD	Parkinson's disease dementia
PDGF	platelet-derived growth factor
PDGFB	platelet-derived growth factor beta
PDH	pyruvate dehydrogenase
PECAM	platelet-endothelial cell adhesion molecule
PEM	protein-energy malnutrition
PEO	progressive external ophthalmoplegia
PEP	postencephalitic parkinsonism
PERM	progressive encephalomyelitis with rigidity and myoclonus
PES	pseudotumoural encephalic schistosomiasis
PET	paraffin-embedded tissue; positron emission tomography
PGNT	papillary glioneuronal tumour
PGP	protein gene product
PHF	paired helical filament
PHP	pseudo-Hurler polydystrophy
PhyH	phytanoyl-CoA hydroxylase
PI	pars intermedia
PiB	Pittsburgh compound B
PICA	postero-inferior cerebellar artery
PKAN	pantothenate kinase-associated neurodegeneration

PKC	protein kinase C
PLA2G6	phospholipase A2, group VI
PLAN	PLA2G6-associated neurodegeneration
PLP	proteolipid protein
PLS	primary lateral sclerosis
PMA	pilomyxoid astrocytoma; progressive muscular atrophy
PMCA	protein misfolding cyclic amplification
PMD	Pelizaeus-Merzbacher disease
PME	progressive myoclonic epilepsy
PML	progressive multifocal leukoencephalopathy
PMNS	post-malaria neurological syndrome
PMP	peroxisomal membrane protein
PMP2	peripheral myelin protein 2
PMS	psammomatous melanotic schwannoma
PN	pars nervosa
PNDC	progressive neuronal degeneration of childhood with liver disease
PNET	primitive neuroectodermal tumour
PNMA	paraneoplastic Ma antigen
PNS	peripheral nervous system
pO_2	partial pressure of oxygen
POEMS	polyneuropathy, organomegaly, endocrinopathy, M-protein, skin changes
POLG	polymerase γ
POMC	proopiomelanocortin
PPA	primary progressive aphasia
PPB	familial pleuropulmonary blastoma
PPCA	protective protein with cathepsin A-like activity
ppm	parts per million
pPNET	peripheral primitive neuroectodermal tumour
PPS	pentosan polysulphate; post-polio syndrome
PPT	pineal parenchymal tumour
PPTID	pineal parenchymal tumour of intermediate differentiation
PR	progesterone receptor
PRBC	parasitized red blood cell
PRES	posterior reversible encephalopathy syndrome
PRL	prolactin
PRNP	PrP gene
PROMM	proximal myotonic myopathy
PROP-1	prophet of Pit-1
ProtCa	activated protein C
ProtS	protein S
PrP	prion protein
PrP-CAA	PrP-cerebral amyloid angiopathy
PRR	pattern recognition receptor
PSAP	prosapson
PSD	post-stroke dementia
PSIR	phase-sensitive inversion recovery
PSP	progressive supranuclear palsy
PSP-CA	progressive supranuclear palsy with cerebellar ataxia
PSP-CST	atypical progressive supranuclear palsy with corticospinal tract degeneration
PSP-P	progressive supranuclear palsy with parkinsonism
PSP-PAGF	pure akinesia with gait freezing with subsequent development of typical signs of progressive supranuclear palsy
pSS	primary Sjögren's syndrome
PTAH	phosphotungstic acid haematoxylin
PTC	periodic triphasic complex
PTD	primary (idiopathic) torsion dystonia
ptd-FGFR4	pituitary tumour-derived FGFR4
PTLD	post-transplant lymphoproliferative disorder
PTPR	papillary tumour of the pineal region
PTRF	polymerase I and transcript release factor
PTS	peroxisomal targeting signal
Ptx2	pituitary homeobox factor 2
PVH/IVH	periventricular/intraventricular haemorrhage
PVL	periventricular leukomalacia
PWI	perfusion weighted imaging
PXA	pleomorphic xanthoastrocytoma
QuIC	quaking induced conversion
RALDH	retinaldehyde dehydrogenase
RANO	response assessment in neuro-oncology
RAR	retinoic acid receptor
RARE	retinoic acid response element
RC2	reaction centre type 2
RCA-1	*Ricinus communis* agglutinin 1
rCBF	regional cerebral blood flow
rCBV	regional cerebral blood volume; relative cerebral blood volume
RCC	renal cell carcinoma
RCDP	rhizomelic chondrodysplasia punctata
RDD	Rosai-Dorfman disease
RDP	rapid onset dystonia-parkinsonism
RE	Rasmussen encephalitis
REM	rapid eye movement
rhNGF	recombinant human nerve growth factor
RIG	radiation-induced glioma
RIM	radiation-induced meningioma
RING	Really Interesting New Gene
RIP1	receptor-interacting protein 1
RIS	radiologically isolated syndrome
RNI	reactive nitrogen intermediate
ROS	reactive oxygen species
RPLS	reversible posterior leukoencephalopathy syndrome
RPS	rhabdoid predisposition syndrome
Rpx	Rathke's pouch homeobox
RRF	ragged-red fibre

RRMS	relapsing-remitting form of multiple sclerosis
RSMD1	rigid spine muscular dystrophy type 1
RSV	Rous sarcoma virus
RTA	road traffic accident
RTK	receptor tyrosine kinase
RVCL	retinal vasculopathy with cerebral leukodystrophy
RXR	retinoid X receptor
SAH	subarachnoid haemorrhage
SANDO	sensory ataxic neuropathy, dysarthria and ophthalmoparesis
SAP	serum amyloid P
Sap-A	sapsosin-A
Sap-B	sapsosin-B
Sap-C	sapsosin-C
SAR	specific absorption rate
SBF2	set binding factor 2
SBMA	spinal and bulbar muscular atrophy
SBP	systemic blood pressure
SBS	shaken baby syndrome
SCA	spinocerebellar ataxia
SCAR1	spinocerebellar ataxia recessive type 1
SCD	subacute combined degeneration
SCI	spinal cord injury
sCJD	sporadic Creutzfeldt-Jakob disease
SCLC	small cell lung cancer
SCMAS	subunit c of mitochondrial ATP synthase
SCO	subcommissural organ
SCS	spinal cord schistosomiasis
SDF-1	stromal cell-derived factor 1
SDH	subdural haematoma; succinate dehydrogenase
SDS	Shy-Drager syndrome
SE	spin echo; status epilepticus
SEER	Surveillance, Epidemiology and End Results
SEGA	subependymal giant cell astrocytoma
SF-1	steroidogenic factor-1
sFI	sporadic fatal insomnia
SFT	solitary fibrous tumour
SFV	Semliki forest virus
Shh	Sonic hedgehog
SIADH	syndrome of inappropriate antidiuretic hormone secretion
SIS	second impact syndrome
SKL	serine-lysine-leucine
SLD	sudanophilic (orthochromatic) leukodystrophy
SLE	systemic lupus erythematosus; St. Louis encephalitis
Sm	Smith
SMA	spinal muscular atrophy
SMARD	spinal muscular atrophy with respiratory distress
SMC	smooth muscle cell
SMN	survival motor neuron
SMNA	sensorimotor neuropathy with ataxia
SMTM	sulcus medianus telecephali medii
SN	substantia nigra
SNAP	sensory nerve action potential
SNARE	soluble N-ethylmaleimide-sensitive factor attachment protein receptor complex
SND	striatonigral degeneration
SNP	single nucleotide polymorphism
SNPC	substantia nigra pars compacta
SNPR	substantia nigra pars reticulata
SO	slow-twitch oxidative
SOD	superoxide dismutase
SPECT	single photon emission computed tomography
SPLTLC1	serine-palmitoyltransferase 1
SPS	stiff-person syndrome
SRP	signal recognition protein
SSPE	subacute sclerosing pan-encephalitis
SUDEP	sudden unexpected death in epilepsy
SVD	small vessel disease
SVZ	subventricular zone
SWI	susceptibility-weighted imaging
SYN	synaptophysin
TACE	TNFα converting enzyme
TAI	traumatic axonal injury
TBI	traumatic brain injury
TBP	TATA box-binding protein
TCGA	The Cancer Genome Atlas
TCI	total contusion index
TCR	T-cell receptor
TEF	thyrotroph embryonic factor
TGA	transposition of the great arteries
TGF	transforming growth factor
TGM6	transglutaminase 6
THCA	trihydroxycholestanoic acid
TIA	transient ischaemic attack
TLE	temporal lobe epilepsy
TLR	Toll-like receptor
TME	transmissible mink encephalopathy
TMEV	Theiler's murine encephalomyelitis virus
TNF	tumour necrosis factor
TOCP	triorthocresylphosphate
Topo II alpha	topoisomerase II alpha
TPNH	triphosphopyridine nucleotide
TPP	thiamine pyrophosphate
TS	Tourette's syndrome; Turcot syndrome
tSAH	traumatic subarachnoid haemorrhage
TSC	tuberous sclerosis complex
TSE	transmissible spongiform encephalopathy
TSH	thyrotrophin

TSP	tropical spastic paraparesis		VLM	visceral larva migrans
TTF-1	thyroid transcription factor 1		VM	vacuolar myelopathy
TTP	thrombotic thrombocytopenic purpura		VMB	vascular malformation of the brain
TTR	transthyretin		VPF	vascular permeability factor
UBO	unidentified bright object		VPSPr	variably protease sensitive prionopathy
UCH-L1	ubiquitin carboxy-terminal hydrolase		VSMC	vascular smooth muscle cell
uPA	urokinase plasminogen activator		VV	valine homozygous
UPDRS	Unified Parkinson's Disease Rating Scale		vWF	von Willebrand factor
UPR	unfolded protein response		VZ	ventricular zone
UPS	ubiquitin-proteasome system		WBC	white blood cell
UV	ultraviolet		WE	Wernicke's encephalopathy
VaD	vascular dementia		WEE	western equine encephalitis
VCAM-1	vascular cell adhesion molecule 1		WHO	World Health Organization
VCI	vascular cognitive impairment		WKS	Wernicke-Korsakoff syndrome
vCJD	variant Creutzfeldt-Jakob disease		Wlds	wallerian degeneration slow
VCP	vasolin-containing protein		WM	white matter
VEE	Venezuelan equine encephalomyelitis		WNV	West Nile virus
VEGF	vascular endothelial growth factor		WSM	widely spaced myelin
VEP	visual evoked potential		XMEA	X-linked myopathy with excessive autophagy
VGKC	voltage-gated potassium channel		YAC	yeast artificial chromosome
VHL	Von Hippel-Lindau		ZASP	Z-line alternatively spliced PDZ protein
VLBW	very low birth weight		ZPT	zinc pyridinethione
VLCFA	very-long-chain fatty acid		ZS	Zellweger syndrome
VLDL	very low density lipoprotein			

Psychiatric Diseases

Margaret M Esiri, Steven A Chance, Jean Debarros and Tim J Crow

INTRODUCTION

This chapter reviews the current evidence on aetiology and the nature of the brain changes in the psychoses, incorporating the spectrum of affective and schizophrenic illness. We include also schizotypal personality disorder and autism, as well as dyslexia and attention deficit–hyperactivity disorder. Emphasis is placed on the dimension of symmetry–asymmetry and its correlate in language as possible defining features of the human brain. We note that in both post-mortem and imaging studies, sex differences are prominent in relation to major psychiatric syndromes.

Categories or Dimensions?

Since Kraepelin introduced the distinction between dementia praecox (which later became called schizophrenia) and manic–depressive insanity, the notion that there are two major and independent categories of psychosis has been deeply embedded in the literature. Textbooks are organized around separate chapters on schizophrenia and manic–depressive illness; but Kraepelin himself had doubts. In 1920 he wrote that 'No experienced psychiatrist will deny there is an alarmingly large number of cases in which it seems impossible, in spite of the most careful observations, to make a firm diagnosis. It is becoming increasingly clear that we cannot distinguish satisfactorily between these two illnesses and this brings home the suspicion that our formulation of the problem may be incorrect'.[268]

Whereas there is little doubt that Kraepelin's prognostic distinction between illnesses that present with a major affective component, which often are associated with a relatively complete recovery between episodes, and those with a worse outcome that present with psychotic symptoms that cannot be understood as secondary to mood changes, is sound, there are considerable doubts whether the distinction can be regarded as categorical. Are we dealing with discrete disease entities or with continua?

Alternative systems of classification have been proposed. For example on the basis of a latent class analysis of a large database of families with psychosis, Kendler et al.[256] argued that as many as six separate categories (Figure 17.1) could be justified. However, no pathognomonic feature or distinctive aetiology for any of these putative entities has been established. Rather, they consist of varying combinations of features (thought disorder, delusions, hallucinations, affective change and negative symptoms) that are present with differing degrees of stability across the spectrum of psychosis.

There are consistencies in epidemiology. The psychoses are conditions that are unusual in that they present from early adult life (which one might expect to be the healthiest phase) onwards. There is a tendency for those conditions that are more 'schizophrenic' in form (i.e. those characterized by mood-incongruent delusions and hallucinations, thought disorder and negative symptoms) to have an earlier onset and generally worse outcome than those that are more 'affective' in form (i.e. with features more readily understood as related to a change in mood) (see Figure 17.1). The general rule is that notwithstanding great individual variation, schizophrenic illnesses with negative symptoms have an earlier onset and worse outcome than those without such features, and that schizoaffective illnesses (i.e. illnesses with an affective component but mood-incongruent psychotic symptoms) have a slightly later onset and less severe outcome followed by bipolar and unipolar affective illnesses. Thus, there is a spectrum of illness from early onset 'schizophrenic' to later onset and better outcome affective psychoses and delusional states. Overlying this is an influence of sex. Whereas earliest onsets of schizophrenic illness are more likely to be in males, the sex difference is minimal for bipolar (manic–depressive) illness and reverses to an excess of females in later-onset depressive

975

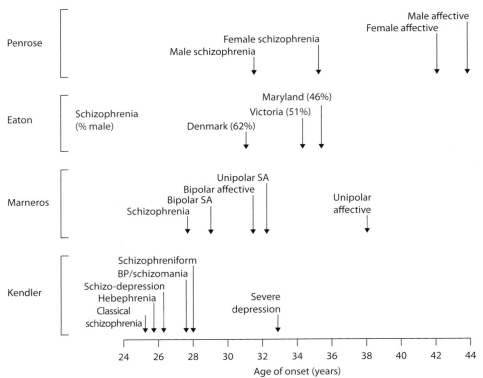

17.1 Age of onset in relation to diagnostic category of psychosis in four different studies. Penrose's data relate to 5456 pairs of relatives with mental illness admitted to the mental hospitals in Ontario, Canada, between 1926 and 1943.[338] Eaton and colleagues included data from three case registers relating to schizophrenia.[157] Marneros and colleagues included 355 cases of psychosis in a long-term follow-up study in Germany.[288] The data of Kendler and colleagues were obtained in an analysis of a family study in Roscommon, Ireland.[256] Although different categories of psychosis have been adopted in the different studies, illnesses with a worse outcome (often labelled 'schizophrenic') generally have an earlier age of onset than those described as 'affective' and, at least for schizophrenic psychoses onset, are earlier in males (as in the studies by Penrose[338] and Eaton et al.[157]). BP, bipolar; SA, schizoaffective.

and paraphrenic (delusional states with minimal negative symptoms) illnesses. These relationships between outcome of symptom pattern and sex are unexplained but consistent with the manifestations of psychosis as boundary phenomena of late and sex-influenced developmental processes.

SCHIZOPHRENIC PSYCHOSES

Notwithstanding the problems of the original Kraepelinian dichotomy, some form of classification is necessary. Medical practice and research require a diagnosis. A system that has acquired increasing influence is the definition of 'first rank' or 'nuclear' symptoms of schizophrenia by Schneider.[370] Although these by no means identify a discrete disease entity, such as is implied by a naïve interpretation of the original Kraepelinian distinction, they do define a boundary of severity or non-understandability that is useful in practice and leads to interesting theoretical conclusions. The symptoms can be reliably assessed, and several have been incorporated in the Vth (current) version of the *Diagnostic and Statistical Manual of Mental Disorders* of the American Psychiatric Association.[8]

Schneider's first-rank symptoms are:

i. Auditory hallucinations: hearing one's thoughts spoken aloud; hearing voices speaking about one in the third person;

ii. Primary experiences concerning one's thoughts: that they are removed from one's head; that thoughts that are not one's own are inserted into one's head; that one's thoughts are broadcast to others;

iii. Similar (passivity) experiences concerning one's actions, sensations and emotions (i.e. that they are controlled or imposed from outside);

iv. Primary delusions: the conviction based on sensory experience that a particular set of events has special meaning.

Epidemiology of Schizophrenia

These symptoms are important for two reasons. First, they cast light on the nature of the underlying disturbance; specifically, they suggest a failure of the mechanism by which self-generated activity (e.g. in speech) is distinguished from that which comes from outside (symptom 1), more generally they constitute anomalies of the transition from thought to speech (symptom 2), of autonomy and control of action and experience (symptom 3), and of the acquisition of meaning (symptom 4). Second, they have played a critical role in defining the epidemiology of psychosis. Psychoses with these characteristics occur in populations as widely separated as the Eskimo Inuit and the Nigerian Yoruba.[311] The World Health Organization (WHO) Ten-Country Study of the Incidence, Manifestations and Outcome of

Schizophrenia[229] concluded that, at least when a restrictive definition (i.e. one based on the presence of nuclear symptoms) was adopted, 'schizophrenic illnesses are ubiquitous, appear with similar incidence in different cultures and have clinical features that are more remarkable by their similarity across cultures than by their difference' (Figure 17.2).

These conclusions suggest that the phenomena of psychosis are intrinsic to human populations and unrelated to environmental variables. Similar conclusions have been drawn on the basis of cross-cultural studies of bipolar (manic–depressive) illness,[428] which arguably represents a contiguous and related segment of the psychotic spectrum. The lifetime risk of schizophrenia is often estimated at 1 per cent[190] and that for bipolar (manic–depressive) disorder is somewhere around 0.8 per cent,[428] whereas that for major depression is greater at between 3 per cent and 5 per cent.

The conclusion that the incidence of psychosis is uniform across populations has been challenged by Hare,[195] on the basis that the rapid expansion of the mental hospitals in the nineteenth century suggests that there was a real increase in the incidence of schizophrenia, and by Torrey[404] on the grounds that, contrary to the WHO study, there are true geographical variations. However, neither claim was based on an operational definition. If the psychoses represent a continuum of disorders rather than discrete categories, it may be that only with a definition based on specific identifiable features such as the first-rank symptoms or the presence of bipolar mood swings can the true population characteristics be ascertained. What is not in doubt is that illnesses with essentially the same characteristics have been identified in all populations in which they have been sought, for example the African Bantu,[356] the Australian Aborigines[310] and the Iban of Central Borneo,[20] populations that have been separated for tens of thousands of years, both from each other and from those included in the WHO studies (e.g. Indian, Japanese and European). The discovery of a population that was free from psychotic illness would have significant implications for theories of aetiology.

Relative uniformity across populations has been challenged also by Saha *et al.*[363] who collected prevalence estimates from 188 studies. They estimated median values for 1000 people (10–90 per cent quantiles) for the distributions of point, period, lifetime and lifetime morbid risk of 4.6 (1.9–10.0), 3.3 (1.38–2.0), 4.0 (1.6–12.1) and 7.2 (3.1–27.1), respectively. McGrath[295] concludes that 'there is prominent variation in the incidence of schizophrenia between sites. The incidence … is significantly higher in males than in females (male:female ratio =1.4)'. A problem with this conclusion is that if, as suggested earlier, we are dealing with continua of variation rather than discrete categories, then where one draws a boundary to define the category of schizophrenia is essentially arbitrary. Endicott *et al.*[162] applied different sets of operational criteria to a consecutive series of patients admitted to the Psychiatric Institute in New York and found variations between sets of criteria differing by a factor of 6. If different criteria are applied in different centres then substantial variations in incidence or prevalence will be expected, even though the underlying phenomena are relatively uniformly distributed across populations. The WHO findings suggest that when the criteria for a diagnosis of schizophrenia are drawn more tightly (focusing on nuclear symptoms), the incidence across centres is more uniform. This is not what would be expected if the variations were independent of diagnostic criteria. Although excesses of admissions in Afro-Caribbean people are frequently reported in the UK, it is not clear that the problem of accurately assessing the base population (i.e. the numbers of individuals of the same age and sex in the general population) as the denominator has been solved. This part of the population, particularly males, tends to be mobile and elusive to census enumeration.

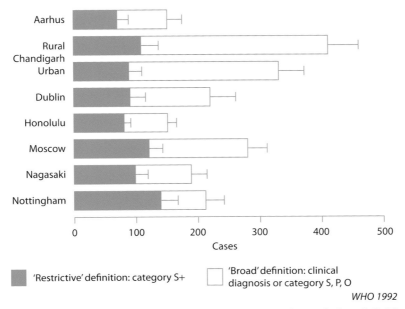

WHO 1992

17.2 Incidence of schizophrenia in seven centres according to broad and restrictive definitions in the World Health Organization Ten-Country Study.[229] By the broad definition (which included diagnoses allocated by the hospital clinicians together with those of researchers adopting liberal criteria), there were significant differences between countries in incidence. When the criteria were defined more narrowly, specifically by the presence of nuclear or first-rank symptom features, the differences between the centres became less and, in this comparison, were not significant. O, ordinary psychosis; P, paranoid psychosis; S, schizophrenia.

Are There Environmental Precipitants?

The view that prevalence is uniform across populations implies an intrinsic (i.e. primarily genetic) origin of psychosis; this is somewhat problematic (see The Nature of the Genetic Core, p. 979) and perhaps for this reason has not been widely entertained. The alternative notion is that psychosis is, at least sometimes, the consequence of an environmental insult. Several such factors have been suggested, including perinatal complications and infections.

Pregnancy and Birth Complications

There have been many investigations of the hypothesis that one or another complication of pregnancy is associated with an increase in the risk of schizophrenic psychosis, but no specific complication can be regarded as an established correlate of later psychosis. A study that reinvestigated a previous positive finding with the use of a more closely matched control group illustrates the nature of the problem. The authors report that they are convinced that the results of their earlier study were seriously misleading, and that the data they now present fail to yield 'any substantial evidence that the incidence of obstetric complications in people who subsequently develop schizophrenia is raised'.[255]

The British Perinatal Mortality Survey recorded systematic data on the antenatal courses and births of 16 980 individuals born in the week 3–9 March 1958. Those who developed schizophrenia by either broad or narrow criteria by the age of 28 years were no more likely than the cohort as a whole to have experienced perinatal complications.[106] Nor were those 945 mothers who were recorded as suffering from influenza in the second trimester in the autumn of 1957 more likely to have children who later developed schizophrenia.[104,106] A subsequent analysis of the many variables recorded for this cohort[362] suggested that those few indices that distinguished patients from controls related more to the characteristics of the mother (e.g. she more often had psychosocial problems, more often weighed less than 51 kg and had fewer antenatal attendances) than to complications of the birth. Low birth weight (<2500 g) was more frequent in the patient group, as it was also in the recent cohort study of Jones et al.[242] who concluded that the differences they found 'appeared to be due largely to the characteristics of the child, not the delivery'. The mothers of individuals who later develop psychosis themselves have an increased incidence of psychiatric problems, and the early development of children who later suffer from psychosis departs from the mean of the population (see later). These facts make it clear that such deviations as are present in fetal and early development in these children are by no means necessarily evidence of an environmental contribution to aetiology.

A meta-analysis of case control studies[58] casts further light on the problem. In a comparison of 1923 individuals with schizophrenia and 527 925 births in the general population, Cannon and colleagues reported that three classes of complication were 'significantly associated with schizophrenia: complications of pregnancy (bleeding, diabetes, rhesus incompatibility, pre-eclampsia); abnormal fetal growth and development (low birth weight, congenital malformations, reduced head circumference); complications of delivery (uterine atony, asphyxia, emergency caesarean section)'. They also write, however, 'The findings from the population-based studies were mostly negative and surprisingly contradictory' and that at 'no stage (had) a causal relationship been established for any one obstetric factor'.

Viral Infection

Both Hare[195] and Torrey[404] considered that the variations in incidence that they discerned were evidence for horizontal transmission (i.e. a contagious agent). An argument against this theory is that when two siblings are affected the onset of illness tends to be at the same age, as would be expected on the basis that it is intrinsic to a developmental programme, rather than simultaneously, as expected if both were exposed to an environmental agent or that such an agent was passed from one to the other sibling.[120] Such considerations suggest an origin consistent with the uniformity of incidence observed in the WHO study. However, another version of the viral hypothesis is that the exposure to the agent occurs *in utero* and that this has an effect that is not expressed as illness until maturity is reached. The particular agent for which such claims have been made is the influenza virus (as noted earlier), originally on the basis that an increase in births of individuals who later developed schizophrenia occurred in Finland after the 1957 epidemic.[296] However, evidence relating to this claim is inconsistent across populations.[100,405] Studies, including the 1957 epidemic, which have examined rates of psychosis in the offspring of 945 mothers who actually suffered from influenza during the putative risk period of the second trimester have yielded no evidence of an effect.[104,121] Where 26.5 cases were predicted by the Mednick-O'Callaghan hypothesis, only three were observed, almost exactly the population expectation; see also Cannon et al.[57] The general absence of evidence that infection early in life predisposes to later schizophrenia was confirmed in the UK National Child Development Study cohort.[274] There was no excess of any of the childhood infections (measles, chickenpox, mumps, German measles, whooping cough, scarlet fever, infectious hepatitis or rheumatic fever) in pre-schizophrenic or pre-affective individuals relative to controls. One possible exception should be mentioned – one case of meningitis was observed in each of the pre-schizophrenic and pre-affective groups when none would have been expected in the sample studied. That this may be a real association is suggested by the observations of Abrahao et al.[1] who followed up 190 individuals affected by meningitis in Sao Paulo and observed 8 cases of schizophrenia versus none in a control sample of 156 siblings. Although it may be rare, this possible association deserves further investigation.

Psychopharmacologic Agents

It has long been recognized that amphetamine-related compounds can provoke acute psychotic disturbances that resemble those seen in schizophrenia (see section on Neurohumoral Theories, p. 981). However these remit on cessation of intake. Long-term effects and the negative symptoms that are so disabling a feature of so many schizophrenic illnesses are not seen.[83] More recently it has been suggested that ingestion of cannabis and cannabinoids contributes significantly as an aetiological factor to long-term illness. A problem in assessing this hypothesis is that the use of such substances is widespread in many populations, difficult to assess accurately and, like other psychotropic agents and tobacco, generally somewhat increased in populations suffering from or at risk of psychotic disorder. However, given that there are substantial cross-national differences in the consumption of these agents it would appear that comparisons across populations linked to census or case register data would cast light on the question.

The Nature of the Genetic Core

That there is a genetic factor in predisposition to schizophrenia is attested by an increase in risk to first-degree relatives of approximately 10 per cent relative to a lifetime expectation of 1 per cent in the general population, and a relative risk of 48 per cent to the monozygotic twin compared with 17 per cent to the dizygotic twin of an affected individual.[190] The case is further supported by studies of the adopted-away offspring of affected individuals[209] and the rates of psychosis in the biological and adoptive families of adoptees who develop schizophrenia.[259] These findings are compatible with a genetic influence, although the mode of transmission has been obscure. Hopes have run high that a systematic linkage approach within families will identify the relevant gene. There have been a number of genome scans, that is searches for linkage between polymorphic markers spaced across the genome and transmission of illness within families with schizophrenia, schizoaffective disorder and bipolar and unipolar affective illness.

There have been a number of claims for linkage. The genes in question, together with their chromosomal locations, are summarized in Table 17.1.

These candidates are viewed optimistically by some reviewers – 'Thus the discovery of susceptibility genes this summer opens the door to improved understanding of the pathogenesis of schizophrenia';[78] 'The evidence of several of the genes is now strong';[201] 'The identification of these and other susceptibility genes will open up new avenues for research aimed at understanding pathogenesis ...;[327] and 'The emerging evidence suggests the possibility of relatively specific relationships between genotype and psychopathology'.[93] However, a more cautious appraisal is suggested by the following considerations:

- Although these genes were originally identified in whole or in part by linkage studies there is considerable doubt concerning the reproducibility of the findings.[118]
- Association studies (investigations of whether specific alleles at polymorphic sites are associated with disease within populations rather than within families) have not supported earlier 'candidate' genes and have yielded new 'positives'[324] that have not themselves been replicated in subsequent association studies.[82]

TABLE 17.1 Putative genes for psychosis

Candidate gene	Chromosomal location	Putative function	Positive reviews	Negative reviews	Consistent linkage in sibling pair genome scans	Consistent finding in genome-wide association studies
Dysbindin	6p22.3	Dystrobrevin-binding protein	78, 92, 93, 200, 201, 327		No	No
Neuregulin	8p	Growth factor	78, 92, 93, 200, 201, 327		No	No
Catechol-O-methyl-transferase (COMT)	22q11	Monoamine degrading enzyme	78, 92, 93, 200, 201, 327		No	No
D-Amino acid oxidase (DAAO)	12q24	Oxidative catalytic enzyme	78, 92, 200, 327	201	No	No
G72 (D-amino acid oxidase activator, DAOA)	13q34	Activator of above	78, 92, 93, 200, 201, 327		No	No
RGS4	1q21–22	Regulator of G-protein signalling	200, 201	78, 92, 93	No	No
GRM3	7q21	Glutamate receptor	201	92, 93, 200	No	No
DISC1	1q	Phosphodiesterase binding factor	92, 201, 327	78, 200	No	No
ZNF804A	2q	Zinc finger protein		82	No	Yes
CACNAIC	15q	L-type voltage-gated calcium channel		82	No	Yes
PCDH11XY gene pair	Xq21.3 and Yp11.2	Cell adhesion molecules	529		No	No

For these reasons considerable caution is advisable before accepting any of the candidates as causative. The failure to establish DNA sequence variation in the presence of strong evidence from twin and adoption studies that genetic predisposition is present and indeed is the major contribution to aetiology, requires some explanation. There are two possibilities:

i. The predisposition to psychosis is dependent upon multiple genes, each of sufficiently small effect to escape detection in the linkage studies conducted so far. On the basis of an analysis of the aggregated findings of genome-wide association studies, it has been argued that a large number of genes, perhaps as many as a thousand across the genome are involved.[345]

ii. The predisposition is not genetic in the strict sense of relating to variations in the DNA sequence, but 'epigenetic' in that it relates to the ill-understood mechanisms that regulate gene expression in different tissues. The relative consistency of the morphological changes (see p. 984) (e.g. in post-mortem studies and the apparent uniformity of incidence across populations are arguments against the multiple genes explanation). With respect to incidence, for example, it can be argued that if many genes were involved the frequency of the variants would vary independently in different populations.

An appraisal[80] of the International Schizophrenia Consortium genome-wide association studies material identified only six relatively weak findings, surprisingly all on chromosome 6. The authors concluded 'These results suggest, but do not prove, that many traditional ideas about the genetic basis of SCZ may be incorrect. Indeed, the singular advantage of genomic surveys is that they are unbiased by prior knowledge and can yield novel and unexpected findings. Given current knowledge of the genetic architecture of schizophrenia (SCZ) and the capacity to assess common and rare variations across the genome, it is possible that the next few years will lead to marked changes in major hypotheses about the genetic basis of SCZ'.

A problem for any genetic theory is discordance in monozygotic twins. Differences in environmental factors between ill and well twins have been sought, but not found.[406] One possibility is that discordance reflects 'epigenetic' (i.e. stochastic processes in central nervous system [CNS] development)[110] (see later).

One twin finding relates to morphology. Since the rediscovery by Geschwind and Levitsky[186] of asymmetry of the planum temporale, there has been interest in the posterior segment of the Sylvian fissure. Falkai and colleagues[164] reported a loss of the normal length asymmetry of the fissure. Although no change in the length was reported in a study of discordant monozygotic twins,[24] reanalysis of the length measurements relating to the posterior segment defined anteriorly by Heschl's sulcus revealed an accentuation of the asymmetry in the well twin relative to controls and a loss of asymmetry in the ill twin.[111] This finding (Figure 17.3) suggests that at least a component of the change associated with schizophrenia relates to those areas of the brain that have evolved most recently (in relation to language) and develop latest in ontogeny and

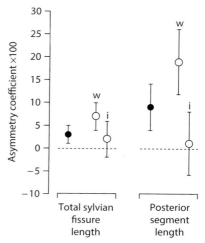

17.3 Deviations in asymmetry in twins discordant for schizophrenia. Data are from the National Institute of Mental Health twin study.[24] Asymmetry coefficients [(L 2 R)/(L 1 R) 3 100] (where L is left and R is right) of total and posterior fissure lengths are presented for twin pairs where both twins are well (•), and for ill (i) and well (w) members of discordant pairs.

are distributed asymmetrically between the hemispheres. However, because the difference is between twins who may be expected to have identical gene sequences – and is seen in the absence of environmental differences between the twins – this suggests that the key difference that relates to psychosis is epigenetic (i.e. related to gene expression rather than to gene sequence).

If, as argued later (see Anomalies of Asymmetry, p. 984), the evidence indicates that schizophrenia is an anomaly in the development of asymmetry, the findings provide a clue to the genetic basis and its significance. Further, if asymmetry is the defining characteristic of the human brain,[114] the phenomena of psychosis and the genetic transition from a prior hominid species to modern *Homo sapiens* are related.

Where is the asymmetry gene? Based on the manifestations of sex chromosome aneuploidy, it has been argued that a determinant of asymmetry is present in a region of homology between the X and Y chromosomes.[101] The evidence is that Turner's syndrome is associated with deficits in spatial ability (i.e. attributable to the right hemisphere), whereas extra X syndromes (e.g. XXY Klinefelter's, XXX and XYY syndromes) are associated with verbal delays, such as are expected with left hemisphere impairment. This supports the hypothesis that the determinant of asymmetry is on both the X and the Y chromosomes because: (i) deficits in Turner's syndrome are generally attributable to genes that are subject to X inactivation (i.e. have a homologue on the Y chromosome) and (ii) the deficits in XYY syndrome appear similar to those seen in XXY and XXX syndromes.[184] The case for an XY homologous asymmetry gene is reinforced by the finding of congruent anomalies of anatomical asymmetry in Turner's and Klinefelter's syndromes.[355]

The earlier argument illustrates an alternative to the 'polygenes of small effect' hypothesis – that there is a major gene in the class that is present on the X chromosome and in homologous form in the non-recombining region of the Y chromosome. Such genes are subject to epigenetic modification by the process of 'meiotic suppression of unpaired chromosomes'.[410] The inactivation is widely assumed to occur in order to achieve dosage compensation between males and females, but it has also been pointed out[119] that the message passed to the fertilized ovum encodes information that relates to the latest evolved species characteristic. In humans, this characteristic is postulated to be cerebral asymmetry.

The findings summarized earlier relating to sex chromosome aneuploidies draw attention to the region of Xq21.3/Yp homology that arose 6 million years ago around the time of origin of the hominid lineage.[343,429] Within this region is located the Protocadherin 11XY gene pair that codes for two cell surface adhesion proteins, one from the X and one from the Y. Relative to the sequences in the other great apes, there have been 16 coding changes in the Y and 5 in the X sequence.[429] The hypothesis proposed is that the pattern of asymmetry that is characteristic of the modern human brain arose in its present form from the interaction of Protocadherin 11X and Y generated by changes in the sequence of both genes that occurred at the time of the speciation event.[107,108,114,117,343] For an alternative view of cerebral asymmetry, see Sun et al.[395] The case for an XY homologous gene for cerebral dominance predisposing to psychosis has recently been reviewed.[119a]

Psychosis Over the Life Span

The natural history of schizophrenia has been much debated. Although Kraepelin's original concept that schizophrenia is a disease that is inevitably associated with a persisting defect is pessimistic for the spectrum as usually conceived, the clinical rule that one-third can be expected to recover, one-third will have a stable deficit and one-third will progress is still a fair generalization, at least in the early years of illness. A small minority progress to a state of temporal disorientation (i.e. of dementia).[122,279] At the other end of the spectrum, however, in long-term follow-up studies, there are patients who do well. There is a relationship between age at onset and outcome, those with earlier onset tending to worse outcome.[157] Those who are male and single do worse, probably reflecting the sex difference in age of onset: onset is 2–3 years earlier in males, who are thus less likely to marry. Across the spectrum of psychosis there is a relationship between form of illness and outcome; for example, a favourable prognosis was found in between 7 per cent and 41 per cent of patients with a schizophrenic illness (the first figure indicating the percentage without any psychological deficit and the latter the percentage with preservation of full autonomy), whereas the figures for schizoaffective illness were 50 per cent and 78 per cent, and 65 per cent and 93 per cent for affective disorders.[287]

Three general classes of theory of pathogenesis – neurohumoral, neurodegenerative and neurodevelopmental – can be distinguished, each with a different origin and some support in the recent literature and each with implications for aetiology.

Neurohumoral Theories

These are generally based on observations of psychotomimetic compounds and attempts to explain the established efficacy of neuroleptic treatments. Neurohumoral theories have the attraction of explaining the lability (e.g. onset and recovery) of what were previously described as 'functional' psychoses in terms of the chemical physiology of the nervous system. Serotonergic,[404] dopaminergic[350] and glutaminergic[99,325] theories have been developed on the basis of psychoses induced by lysergic acid diethylamide (LSD), amphetamines and phencyclidine, respectively. Particularly in the latter two cases, the symptoms resemble some positive schizophrenic symptoms quite closely. The dopamine hypothesis, that schizophrenia is due to overactivity in the dopamine pathways, retains the advantage of providing the only viable explanation (through D2 receptor blockade) of the antipsychotic effects of the range of neuroleptic medication. However, these theories do not predict the presence of structural changes in the brain or intellectual impairment, nor do they account for the negative symptoms (affective flattening and poverty of speech) that contribute substantially to poor long-term outcome. Further weaknesses are a lack of evidence of a primary disturbance in any of the putatively affected neurotransmitter systems and the lack of an aetiological theory. Although there have been many predictions that genetic variation in one or other neurotransmitter receptor or synthetic enzyme might be correlated with susceptibility to psychosis, none has yet been established.

Neurodegeneration or Neurodevelopment?

Documentation of structural change (reviewed later) lent apparent support to the view that psychosis was the outcome of a chronic viral or other exogenous insult to the brain. The neurodegeneration concept is compatible with negative symptoms and intellectual impairment but has difficulty explaining positive symptoms. Ventricular enlargement, and possibly a decrease in brain size, can be accounted for, but loss of asymmetry is more difficult to explain. Gliosis, which was detected in some earlier studies of schizophrenia, was thought to lend support to the neurodegeneration theory, but later, more rigorous studies failed to detect such changes (see Glial Cell Changes, p. 999). Most telling is the absence of evidence for any specific exogenous agent that can be correlated with psychosis – as already noted the case for any complication of birth or pregnancy is not strong, and a specific viral agent has not been incriminated. Moreover it is difficult to account for the epidemiological characteristics. What environmental agent is distributed uniformly across populations without respect for geographical, climatic or sociocultural variation?

Although there are earlier precedents,[79,333,388] neurodevelopmental theories have flourished since Weinberger[426] pointed out how such a theory could account for the timing of onset of illness and also might explain the brain changes. It is at first surprising that a disorder occurring initially in early to middle adult life or even later, has an origin in developmental CNS pathways. Most would suppose that development is programmed early and completed sometime in adolescence at the latest. However, the human brain has a complex topography. Aspects of its growth (e.g. the myelination of the corpus callosum) continue well into adult life. Whereas the original neurodevelopmental hypothesis proposed that 'a fixed lesion early in life interacts with normal brain maturational events that occur much later',[426] one must also consider genetic influences on the lifetime course of development, including adult neuroplasticity and ageing.[119,149,261]

Although neither neurohumoral deviation nor neurodegeneration is able to account for the relative selectivity of the impairment in schizophrenia to higher nervous system function, theories that invoke dysfunction in specific sets of cortical connections are more convincing. Thus, negative symptoms are plausibly accounted for by a disturbance of dorsolateral or orbital prefrontal cortex or of cortical projections to the amygdala, and some positive symptoms (including thought disorder) are reasonably attributed to deviations in language-related areas (e.g. asymmetrically distributed or connected systems). The general notion[304,333,388] that it is the structures that are latest evolved and most specific to *Homo sapiens* that are the most vulnerable explains the selectivity of the disease process to higher functions. Because these phylogenetically recent systems are also those that develop latest in an individual organism, such theories (in a connectionist formulation) provide a possible explanation of age of onset.

Consistent with a developmental perspective are childhood precursors of psychosis. In population cohorts, those children who later develop schizophrenic and affective disorders deviate from the mean of the populations of which they are a part in certain informative respects. As a group, these children are mildly impaired on a number of assessments of educational attainment (in the range of 0.2–0.6 standard deviations), are delayed in some motor milestones (e.g. walking[240] and in learning to read[126]) and are more likely to have speech difficulties at the ages of 7 and 11 years (32 per cent versus 8 per cent of controls and 41 per cent versus 11 per cent, respectively). Some of these impairments, although of lesser degree, have been reported in children who later developed major affective disorders.[415]

Pre-psychotic children also differ from their peers with respect to certain behavioural characteristics. On assessments made by their teachers, male pre-schizophrenic children were more likely to be rated as anxious and hostile toward adults and other children at the age of 7 years, and at the age of 11, in addition, were more likely to be described as withdrawn and depressed as also were pre-schizophrenic females at this age. Pre-affective psychotic patients did not deviate in these respects, although they were more likely to be rated as restless at the age of 7 years. A group of children who were later admitted to psychiatric facilities but who did not receive diagnoses of psychosis deviated from the norms of the population at the age of 11 in a pattern that resembled that seen in psychosis, but in this group the deviation was in females rather than in males.[126]

These patterns suggest that there are significant variations in the trajectories of development (with possible correlates in brain structure) that relate to cognition as well as behaviour, and that those predisposed to psychosis represent a subset that deviates in a systematic way from the population as a whole. The challenge is to determine the origin and functional significance of the variations and the nature of the structural correlates in the brain.

Dyskinesias in Schizophrenia

Orofacial dyskinesias are commonly observed in patients with chronic schizophrenia and are sometimes attributed to neuroleptic medication, being explained as an alteration at the level of the dopamine receptor. However, such movement disorders were observed long before the introduction of chlorpromazine[420] and are present in patients who have never received neuroleptic medication.[170,292,328]

Therefore, considerable doubt exists as to whether such movements are an irreversible consequence of neuroleptic medications, as is implied by the widely held concept of 'tardive dyskinesia'.[123] It seems likely that the movements are a component of the disease process, sometimes being associated with negative symptoms and intellectual impairments (type II syndrome[98]). In a post-mortem study, the movements were not found to be associated with an increase in D2 ligand-binding sites.[123]

Animal Models of Schizophrenia

It may seem futile to attempt to model such a complex human disease as schizophrenia, with the characteristic disruption of thought and social behaviour, in animals. If schizophrenia is a disease of the specific capacity of *Homo sapiens* for language,[103] then it can be argued that such models are irrelevant. However, the early pharmacological evidence that drugs affecting dopaminergic, serotonergic and glutaminergic neurotransmission can mimic the symptoms of schizophrenia in normal humans, encouraged the development of animal models of the disease based on the effects of agonists and antagonists of dopamine, 5-hydroxytryptamine (5-HT) and glutamate.[137,248,305,325,398] Lesion studies in small mammals and primates have possible relevance for schizophrenia.[368] More recently, transgenic animals with altered expression of receptors for some of these neurotransmitters have been investigated for their relevance to schizophrenia.

Brain Structure in Schizophrenia

No specific (and therefore diagnostic) brain alterations have yet been identified in schizophrenia at either the macroscopic or microscopic level: the brains from most cases appear outwardly normal. The changes that have been detected apply to groups of cases and the overlap with the (often wide) normal range for all parameters (with the possible exception of asymmetry, see later) is considerable.

In vivo brain imaging has been important in uncovering disease-associated structural differences. Imaging studies, however, can point only to macroscopic differences in brain structure. Neuropathology is needed to delve into the microscopic and molecular differences that underpin these gross changes. In the following account of brain structure in schizophrenia, the evidence from neuro-imaging and post-mortem macroscopic examination will be reviewed.

Evidence from In Vivo Imaging Studies

The best established finding (although in general neither lateralized nor reliably related to sex) is a degree of ventricular enlargement. This was noted by Southard: 'the coarse atrophy is usually of moderate degree, and often does not appreciably alter the brain weight, at least outside the limits of expected variation. More remarkable is the high proportion of cases of internal hydrocephalus …'.[388] Enlargement of the ventricles was later documented by air encephalography. The limitation of air encephalography studies (i.e. that they included few normal controls), was overcome by the introduction of the less hazardous technique of computed tomography (CT). The first CT scan study[235,236] demonstrated clearly that a group of institutionalized patients with a diagnosis of schizophrenia by restrictive diagnostic criteria had ventricular areas that were enlarged relative to a control group matched for age and premorbid occupation. Ventricular enlargement was unrelated to past or current physical treatments, a conclusion documented in subsequent systematic studies of larger populations. Weinberger and colleagues[427] extended their sample to include a range of ages, and demonstrated that for each decade from the age of 20 years onwards the difference between patients and controls was approximately the same. Consistent with a developmental concept, this suggests that the changes are present early in the disease course.

An important conclusion is that within the group of patients with broadly defined schizophrenia, ventricular enlargement is relatively constant. The variance for ventricular size is not increased relative to that in the control group and there is no evidence of bimodality within the patient group.[135,203,329,417] A subgroup with an 'organic' type of schizophrenia cannot be separated from the rest of the population with psychosis. Ventricular enlargement is not focal[366] and is not clearly linked to volume reduction in surrounding structures.[45,252] But in an analysis of variance of a magnetic resonance imaging (MRI) study, the component parts of ventricular enlargement have been found to depend upon hemisphere (left or right), the anteroposterior dimension and sex of the individual.[316] Such a finding suggests that enlargement of the ventricles in psychosis is a complex function of the variables that influence the origins of the cerebral cortex in the subventricular zone.

Evidence has accumulated for a reduction in brain size. A reduction of the order of 1–2 per cent in brain area has been reported in CT scan studies,[237,335] although these have not defined the anatomical site of the loss. More precise information comes from MRI assessments, findings reviewed by Shenton[379] and Wright.[435] A meta-analysis[435] concluded that whereas there was a mean increase in ventricular size of 26 per cent in patients with schizophrenia, mean cerebral volume was reduced by 2 per cent. A meta-analysis of brain weight[202] in post-mortem studies, including the brains of 540 individuals with schizophrenia and 794 controls, found a mean difference of 24 grams, or about 2 per cent ($p = 0.04$ 95% CI 1–47 controlling for age and sex). The reduction was similar in male and female patients and there was no correlation with duration of illness.

Does structural change progress? In a careful comparison of 72 patients at the time of the first episode with 78 controls, a significant increase in ventricular volume was not found,[319] suggesting that the later presence of such change is evidence of progression of the disease process (i.e. contrary to some earlier conclusions noted earlier).[146] In their first-episode series, Narr et al.[319] found an interaction indicating expansion of the dorsal superior horn of the lateral ventricle in female patients compared with same sex controls that may indicate the first evidence of the disease process. That there is indeed progressive change is also documented in recent longitudinal studies.[138,145,146,434] Van Haren et al.[412] obtained two MRI brain scans over a 5-year interval from 96 patients with schizophrenia and 113 healthy subjects between ages 16 and 56 years. The trajectory of brain volume changes differed between patients and healthy individuals. Before the age of 45 years (the first 20 years of illness), cerebral and grey matter loss and lateral ventricle increase were excessive in patients relative to controls, and greater in patients with a poor outcome. The normally curved trajectory of grey matter volume change with age was absent in patients. Later in life, the degree of volume change in patients was similar to that observed with normal ageing.

A meta-analysis[254] found evidence of progressive ventricular enlargement after illness onset greater than that seen in controls (effect size = 0.45, 95% CI 0.19–0.71, $p = 0.0006$) that was also present in a sub-analysis of chronic patients with a mean duration of illness of 7.6 years at baseline scan ($p = 0.002$). The results were unaffected by variation in the diagnostic inclusion criteria; no significant effect of age of onset, duration of illness, or age at baseline scan, was found in the meta-regression analysis. Progressive change in ventricular volume a number of years after illness onset challenges an exclusively neurodevelopmental model.

Recent meta-analyses of structural MRI studies in psychosis have confirmed a modest reduction in brain size and located it in part in the insula and limbic system. A review of meta-analyses of MRI studies[128] concluded that:

i. The structure most frequently recognized as reflecting a patient-control difference is the *insula* (22 of 24 group by hemisphere comparisons), followed by *thalamus* (13 of 24 comparisons) and the *anterior cingulate gyrus* (12 out of 24).

ii. The *right* insula is involved in each of the schizophrenia categories, first-episode schizophrenia and bipolar disorder; the *left* insula is additionally implicated by each of the analyses relating to schizophrenia with the exception of one meta-analysis of first-episode schizophrenia,[47] and was not identified in the bipolar sample of Yu et al.[439]

iii. In addition to the previously recorded deficits in superior temporal gyrus[221,379] the medial temporal lobe and the parahippocampal gyrus, both on the left, were noted as frequently reduced by Honea et al.,[221] and the uncus/amygdala as showing deficits to the left by Ellison-Wright and Bullmore[160] and by Yu et al.[177] in relation to schizophrenia. Although the uncus was not identified by Glahn et al.,[187] Fornito et al.[177] or Bora et al.,[47] reduction of the parahippocampal gyrus on the left was recorded by Glahn et al.[187] as well as by Ellison-Wright et al.[161] and reductions in the posterior cingulate gyrus on the left were recorded by Fornito et al.,[177] Ellison-Wright and Bullmore[160] and Bora et al.,[47] each in relation to their groups of schizophrenia patients.

iv. No study found such posterior reductions in bipolar disorder. Thus if the 'posterior limbic system' is defined as the medial temporal lobe, uncus, parahippocampal and posterior cingulate gyri (see Table 17.2), each of the analyses including chronic schizophrenic illnesses finds deficits to the left. In first-episode schizophrenia, one study (Ellison-Wright et al.[161]) found reduction on both sides and one (Bora et al.[47]) in neither hemisphere.

TABLE 17.2 Macroscopic post-mortem changes in schizophrenia (not present in all studies)

Modest decrease (2–8 per cent) in brain weight

Modest decrease in brain volume

Modest decrease in brain length

Regional alterations:

    Temporal lobe reduced in volume and length

    Left superior temporal gyrus reduced in volume

    Reduction in parahippocampal gyrus volume and cortical thickness (left > right)

    Reduction in volume of mediodorsal and anteroventral nuclei of thalamus

    Enlargement of striatum

Enlargement of lateral ventricles, especially temporal horns (sometimes left > right)

Cavum septum pellucidum

Schizencephaly

Partial agenesis of corpus callosum

v. The anterior cingulate gyrus is diminished on the right in all analyses of schizophrenia with the exception of Yu et al.[439] Bora et al.[47] and Ellison-Wright and Bullmore[160] identified additional deficits in the left hemisphere but the other analyses of schizophrenia from Honea,[221] Ellison-Wright,[161] Glahn[187] and Fornito[177] did not. In contrast to the predominant right-sidedness of the deficits in schizophrenia, Ellison-Wright and Bullmore[160] located a region in the anterior cingulate gyrus on the left in which the reduction was specific to bipolar disorder.

These findings suggest localization and an element of lateralization (see Anomalies of Asymmetry, this page) of the psychotic disease process. With a focus on the cortical segment of the limbic circuit (Broca's grand lobe limbique) it appears that schizophrenic illnesses have a degree of selectivity to anterior structures on the right side and to posterior structures (e.g. parahippocampal gyrus) on the left. Bipolar illness has a degree of affinity for anterior structures on the left side. On grounds of symmetry one might predict that these are accompanied by selectivity to the right side posteriorly, and a recent study of quadrantic volume[283] supports this.

Evidence from Post-Mortem Studies

Recent post-mortem studies have added to the evidence from *in vivo* imaging for relatively consistent changes in macroscopic brain structure (Table 17.2). Thus, consistent with a modest decrease in brain weight (2% in a recent meta-analysis),[202] some studies have also found brain volume and length to be slightly reduced. Regional alterations have also been reported: temporal lobe reduction in volume or length reduction in the volume of the superior temporal gyrus, and reduction in volume or thickness of the cortex of the parahippocampal gyrus, both of which sometimes selective to the left side and correlated with ventricular enlargement.[65]

Reduction in volume of the mediodorsal and anteroventral nuclei of the thalamus, and enlargement of the striatum are also reported. However, other studies did not find differences from controls in some of these regions.[15,131,198] Although some negative findings may reflect the small number of brains examined, others are the result of respectably large, seemingly well-executed studies. For example, from

the studies of others[206] as well as our own, we conclude that the structure of the hippocampus is not changed with respect to either the volumes of the subfields[421] or the size and cell densities of its constituent pyramidal neurons.[217] On the basis of these studies we find it difficult to believe that there is a gross structural abnormality in the hippocampus itself, by contrast with the parahippocampal gyrus. By contrast with the post-mortem literature, in a review of MRI studies of the hippocampus, Nelson et al.[321] concluded that there was an overall 4 per cent reduction, and in their meta-analysis of regional brain volumes, Wright et al.[435] stated that the volume of the hippocampus was reduced to 93 per cent on the left and 95 per cent on the right. No such trends were apparent in the post-mortem studies of Heckers et al.[205] and Walker et al.[421] as noted earlier.

One possible explanation is that MR image analysis techniques have difficulty in defining the boundary between the hippocampus and the temporal horn of the ventricle that, according to a consensus of MRI and post-mortem studies, is enlarged. A review comparing post-mortem and MRI studies suggests that partial volume effects may be of critical significance.[64] A recent MRI study of 56 subjects with DSM-IIIR schizophrenia, 26 patients with other psychoses and 104 comparison subjects in a well-documented birth cohort from North Finland found that when corrected for total brain volume, the volumes of the hippocampus and amygdala were not significantly reduced.[399]

Anomalies of Asymmetry

Since the observations of Broca and Dax in the 19th century,[51,142] it has been known that in most individuals some aspect of language is located on the left side of the brain. The theoretical implications of this observation have become apparent only slowly.

Although the human brain is in subtle respects an asymmetrical structure (and therefore speech lateralization has a possible anatomical basis), a fact known to Cunningham[133] and Eberstaller[158] in the late 19th century, the knowledge had to a large extent been lost until the asymmetry of the planum temporale was rediscovered by Geschwind and Levitsky[186] (Figure 17.4). That hemispheric lateralization is founded in a genetic mechanism that is specific to humans has been appreciated more recently. Population-based

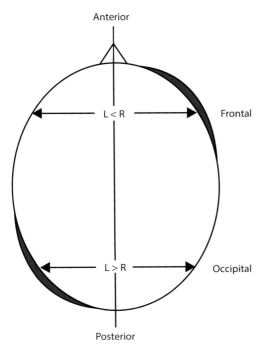

Anterior

L < R — Frontal

L > R — Occipital

Posterior

17.4 Width asymmetries in the human brain from right (R) frontal to left (L) occipital. This is sometimes known as the 'Yakovlevian torque'. These asymmetries are reflected in the asymmetry to the left of the planum temporale, as described by Geschwind and Levitsky.[186]

directional handedness is characteristic of humans, and in spite of claims to the contrary, it has not been clearly established in other primate species. In those ape species that are closest to humans (e.g. the gorilla[12] and chimpanzee[285]), the systematic bias to the right is absent. As Annett[11] has consistently argued, this is the feature that is most characteristic of humans as a species. It can be attributed to a single gene. Its correlate is language, the function that, it has been argued,[40,73] has features that are qualitatively distinct from those of the communicative systems of other primates. Thus, it is conceivable that the capacity for language arose as a result of a discrete genetic event that allowed the brain to lateralize, which occurred at some time after the separation of the chimpanzee and hominid lineages.[112,114]

Awareness of the lateralization of the human brain had an early influence on thinking about the evolutionary origins of mental illness. In 1879, Crichton-Browne conducted some of the first post-mortem studies of psychosis. He prefaced the report of his study with the statement that 'It seemed not improbable that the cortical centres, which are the most highly evolved and voluntary and which are supposed to be located on the left side of the brain, might suffer first in insanity'.[96] Thirty-five years later Southard, in describing his own post-mortem studies, took the line of thought one step further: 'The atrophies and aplasias when focal show a tendency to occur in the left cerebral hemisphere ... Aside from the left-sidedness of the lesions very striking is their preference for the association centres of Flechsig – for this there is probably good *a priori* reason in the structure, late evolutionary development and relatively high lability of these regions'.[388]

Much of the evidence relevant to the nature of the disease process in psychosis comes from gross morphological studies, both radiological and post mortem (Fig 17.5). Some of the evidence (summarized later) is directly relevant to the speculations of Crichton-Browne and Southard that these changes are in some way related to asymmetries of cortical anatomy. However, a puzzling feature is that aspects of the changes differ in the two sexes. It appears that the morphological changes in psychosis are related to interactions between sex and asymmetry.

A number of investigators have reported anomalies of width asymmetry in schizophrenia. In CT scan studies, Crow et al. found lesser asymmetries in the half of patients with earlier onset compared with those with later onset and controls,[125] and in a large series Falkai et al.[166] described a systematic reduction of width asymmetries across all categories of patients with psychosis. In an MRI study of 87 first-episode patients compared with 52 normal controls, DeLisi et al. found width asymmetries to be reduced in the posterior third ($p = 0.02$) and occipital ($p = 0.05$) quarters of the brain.[145] In a similar series of 70 first-episode patients compared with 51 normal controls, Bilder et al. studied regional hemispheric volumes in five consecutive coronal slices and found that the normal asymmetry to the right in premotor, prefrontal and temporal regions, and to the left in sensorimotor and occipitoparietal regions was reduced in patients.[41] In Table 17.3 we summarize the findings in five studies with diverse methodologies, and each draws the conclusion that an anomaly of cerebral asymmetry is central to the disease process.

Subjects in the comparison group had significant lateral asymmetries in each region: their occipitoparietal and sensorimotor regions were larger on the left, and their premotor, prefrontal and temporal regions were larger on the right. Patients lacked lateral asymmetries and showed significantly less asymmetry than healthy subjects in occipitoparietal, premotor and prefrontal regions. Absence of the normal asymmetry was more common among patients initially diagnosed with the undifferentiated than with the paranoid subtype of schizophrenia and was associated with more severe negative symptoms among men. Asymmetries were related to sex and handedness regardless of diagnosis; specifically, dextral men showed more asymmetry than non-dextral men or dextral women. The absence of normal hemispheric asymmetries suggests an anomaly in the development of laterally specialized cerebral systems in schizophrenia, and this may be associated with an initial presentation of non-paranoid psychosis.

Some studies indicate a change in asymmetry of ventricular structure. In a study in which the ventricle was filled with radio-opaque material after the brain had been fixed in formalin, Crow et al.[124] observed that the relative change in the temporal horn area on a radiograph from the lateral aspect was greater than for other components of the ventricle and that it was confined to the left side (side by diagnosis interaction $F1,65 = 11.02$, $p < 0.02$). By contrast, the enlargement in Alzheimer-type dementia is bilateral. In MRI studies of first episodes, De Greef et al.[144] found correlations with clinical indices of severity that clustered around the temporal horn on the left side and Narr et al.[315] also found ventricular enlargement was greater on the left and in the posterior horn, the measure that was most variable

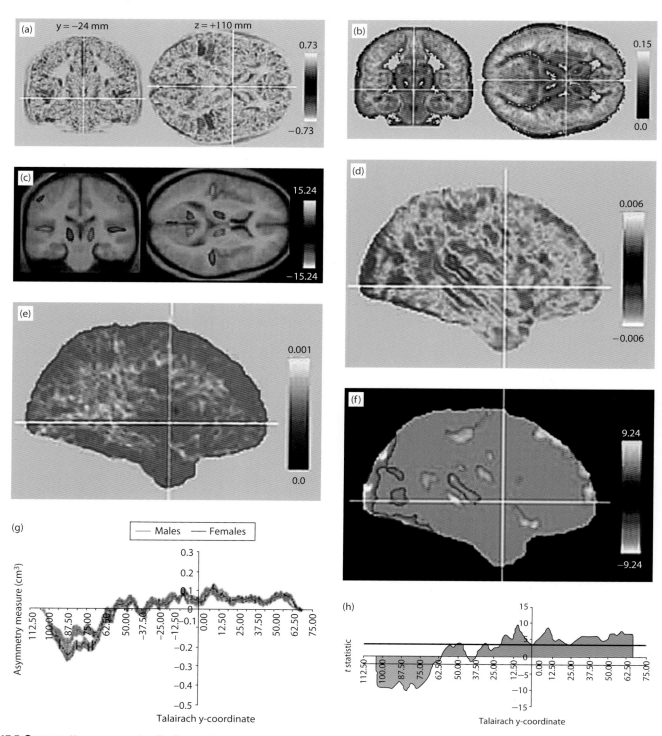

17.5 Grey matter asymmetry findings. Average grey matter asymmetry images **(a,d)** and standard error images **(b,e)** are shown above significance maps of the t statistics **(c,f)** for the reflection and column map analyses of the technique according to Barrick and colleagues.[21] Reflection asymmetry results are illustrated through coronal (Talairach slice $y = -224$ mm) and axial (Talairach slice $z = +110$ mm) slices in standard space with statistically significant results overlain on the mean T1-weighted image computed across 30 subjects. All three-dimensional images are displayed using the neurological convention. Average grey matter slice profiles are illustrated for male (green) and female (orange) subjects, with standard error bars marked **(g)** above a graph of the t statistic across the male and female subjects combined **(h)**. The black horizontal bars above and below the x-axis in graph **(h)** represent the t statistic threshold beyond which sliced profile asymmetries are significant. Hot and cold colours represent larger and smaller regions for the ipsilateral hemisphere in the reflection results and rightward and leftward asymmetries in the column map and slice profile results respectively.

Reprinted from Barrick TR, Mackay CE, Prima S et al.,[21] with permission from Elsevier.

TABLE 17.3 Salient findings in selected studies of asymmetry in psychosis

17

	Patients	Methods	Main findings	Conclusions
Crow et al. 1989[124,125]	27 schizophrenia by Feighner criteria; 26 controls; 30 Alzheimer dementia	Post-mortem radiographic examination of ventricular component volumes	Temporal horn enlargement selective to left hemisphere in schizophrenia, but bilateral in Alzheimer dementia	'The findings are consistent with the view that schizophrenia is a disorder of the genetic mechanisms that control the development of cerebral asymmetry'
Bilder et al. 1994[41,42]	70 patients with first-episode schizophrenia; 51 healthy controls	Structural magnetic resonance imaging of four (25 per cent of total) cerebral coronal sections	In healthy controls: occipitoparietal and sensorimotor regions were larger on the left, and premotor, prefrontal, and temporal regions were larger on the right. Patients lacked lateral asymmetries in occipitoparietal, premotor, and prefrontal regions	Absence of normal hemispheric asymmetries suggests an anomaly in the development of laterally specialized cerebral systems in schizophrenia
Narr et al. 2001[315]	Patients with first-episode schizophrenia (n = 50) compared with demographically matched healthy comparison subjects (n = 50)	High-resolution magnetic resonance images were used to examine differences in gyral complexity, measured three-dimensionally in five separate hemispheric regions covering the entire cortical surface	Significant main effects of hemisphere were found in frontal, parietal and occipital regions in directions complementary to cerebral torques	'... Sexually dimorphic developmental processes and differences in hemispheric connectivity, which ....influence the organization and/or frequency of cortical folding, seem to be disturbed during gyral formation *in utero*'
Csernansky et al. 2008[129]	33 individuals with schizophrenia and 30 healthy individuals group matched for age, gender, race and parental socioeconomic status	T1-weighted magnetic resonance scans, sulcal depth was measured across the entire cerebral cortex by reconstructing surfaces of cortical mid-thickness (layer 4) in each hemisphere and registering them to the human PALS cortical atlas	In the parietal operculum average sulcal depth was shallower in individuals with schizophrenia. In individuals with schizophrenia, sulcal depth in the left hemisphere was correlated with the severity of impaired performance on tests of working memory and executive function	'Group differences in sulcal depth showed significant bilateral symmetry across much of the occipital, parietal, and temporal cortices'
Kawasaki et al. 2008[253]	120 right-handed subjects comprising four groups of 30 subjects (i.e. male and female schizophrenia, male and female control)	Voxel-based morphometry with magnetic resonance images	A skew towards rightward asymmetry in the pars triangularis and a reduction in leftward asymmetry in the planum temporale in patients relative to control subjects	'A disturbance of cerebral asymmetry in schizophrenia .... might reflect a perturbation in the lateralization process underlying left cerebral dominance for language'

between individuals. Superior and posterior horn enlargement was greater in males. Thus these findings suggest that there is a change in some structure within the temporal lobe and that this relates to onset of illness.

Some authors have reported losses or reversals of asymmetry in cortical structures in schizophrenia, whereas others have not. In a study of three different definitions of the planum temporale, Meisenzahl et al.[297] failed to show significant differences between 30 men with and 30 men without schizophrenia in planum temporale volumes. A possible resolution is suggested by Harasty et al.[194] who analysed histological data from 21 post-mortem adult individuals and found that the neocortex of the left planum temporale is thinner but longer than that on the right side. The volumes of the left and right plana were approximately equal, leading these authors to conclude that hemispheric differences arise from a 'ballooning' of cortex on one side relative to the other. Such an explanation of asymmetry had been suggested by Barta et al.[23] This appears to be a potentially important generalization, although there are apparent discrepant findings,[165] wherein a post-mortem study of 24 patients versus 24 age and sex-matched controls found a reduction in anteroposterior diameter of the planum temporale by 20% on the left side (p=0.008), consistent with Harasty's hypothesis, but also found a reduction of the volume asymmetry coefficient. The discrepancies are puzzling, although two meta-analyses concluded that asymmetry is reduced.[377] If the generalization holds it seems that the changes in the planum temporale should be considered in the wider context of the cortex as a whole. As Harasty et al. indicate,[194] a change in the separation of the cortical minicolumns may have physiological significance, as also may a reduction in the ratio of apical to basal dendrites of pyramidal cells (see the section on microscopic changes later).

Change in asymmetry of structures within the parietal lobe is suggested by two MRI studies; in one a reversal of asymmetry in the inferior parietal lobule was localized to the angular gyrus[322] and in the other there was a reduction in volume of the inferior parietal lobule on the left and a reversal of asymmetry in males but not in females.[179] Highley et al.[215] found bilateral reduction of parieto-occipital white matter volume in females whereas in males this volume was greater than in controls. In an MRI study of post-mortem brain, the anteroposterior position of the maximum cross-sectional area was further anterior on the left than on the right side in controls but further posterior in schizophrenic subjects.[66] The findings are consistent with the generalization that the key changes in schizophrenia are in late-developing neocortex and that they interact with sex.

In a further post-mortem study of the brains of 31 patients with schizophrenia and 27 comparison subjects, volume reductions (in the order of 5–10 per cent) were detected in the superior temporal gyrus[213] and parahippocampal and fusiform gyri[293] on the left side (Figure 17.6). The effect of these reductions was that the normal asymmetry to the left was lost or even reversed. A significant difference was observed between the sexes in the relationship of these changes to age of onset. With increasing age of onset in males but decreasing age of onset in females, the

asymmetry became more anomalous (i.e. discrepant to the comparison group). Further evidence that the changes in psychosis are lateralized comes from the meta-analysis of voxel-based morphometry studies. In this analysis the most lateralized findings were in the medial temporal lobe and parahippocampal gyrus to the left, and in the anterior cingulate gyrus on the right (i.e. approximating to the cerebral torque).

In the anterior cingulate region a subdivision into cingulate and paracingulate gyrus is more frequent on the left than on the right side of the brain in normal subjects.[228,334] In a series of 131 MRI scans of patients with first episodes of schizophrenia, this asymmetry was lost in male but not in female patients.[440] In an earlier post-mortem study in seven female patients, a loss of the weight and surface rightward asymmetries of the cingulate gyrus were observed.[5] By contrast, in a stereological study no differences between the sides or between patients and controls were observed in volume assessments of the anterior cingulate gyrus.[214] However, these measures included both cingulate and paracingulate gyri and it is possible that these gyri carry asymmetries that are reciprocally related – to the right in the cingulate and to the left in the paracingulate. Moreover, there are subtle differences in cortical structure between patients and controls in the frontal lobes. That these relate to sex and laterality is suggested by the finding that asymmetries are present in the distances measured over the superior surface from frontal pole to central sulcus, which are to the right in males and to the left in females[210] (reciprocal changes are seen in central sulcus to occipital pole distances), and that in each sex these asymmetries are reversed in patients. Given the absence of volume changes related to illness in the gross gyral structure of the frontal lobes,[214] such changes may reflect asymmetries in shape and fine surface structure. The cingulate and paracingulate cortices thus constitute one region in which interindividual and interhemispheric variation is present. Given their lateralized activation in a verbal fluency task[389] and possible anomalies of this lateralization in psychosis,[113] the precise anatomical differences between these areas in the two hemispheres is a focus of particular interest.

An interesting approach to cortical gyral asymmetries was proposed by Bullmore et al.[56] who measured radius of gyration (an index of the dispersion of points in a radially organized structure about its centre of gravity) in relation to the subcortico–cortical boundary. There were significant differences between the hemispheres that were related to handedness in controls, the radius of gyration being greater in the non-dominant hemisphere. In male, but not female, patients with schizophrenia, this difference was reversed.

Commissural Changes

The commissures (corpus callosum and anterior commissure) are of interest in the context of the previously mentioned work suggesting that hemispheric differences are relevant to the pathophysiology of psychosis. It is possible that the primary change is in interhemispheric fibre connections. Witelson and Nowakowski[430] suggested that cortical areas that are more lateralized have fewer interhemispheric connections. This principle has been used in the interpretation of sex differences in the corpus callosum, and the sex difference in age of onset. For example,

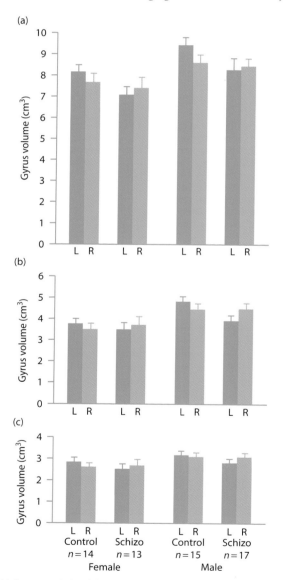

17.6 Volumes of the (a) superior temporal, (b) fusiform and (c) parahippocampal gyri in post-mortem brain from female and male patients with schizophrenia. In each case, there is an asymmetry to the left (L) in controls, and loss of asymmetry or an asymmetry to the right (R) in patients with schizophrenia.

From Highley et al.[213] and McDonald et al.[293]

Pujol et al.[344] and Cowell et al.[91] report that the corpus callosum goes on increasing in size into the third and even fourth decades of life, and that the increase goes on later in females. One can speculate that the sex difference is somehow related to the degree of lateralization according to the Witelson and Nowakowski principle, for example, that the greater anatomical asymmetry in males reflects greater loss of interhemispheric fibres and perhaps thereby an earlier encounter with a critical threshold of myelination.

Many MR investigations, including some with diffusion tensor imaging (DTI), have now been completed on the corpus callosum in schizophrenia. In a meta-analysis, Woodruff et al.[432] found that in 313 patients compared with 281 controls, there was a significant ($p>0.02$) reduction in cross-sectional area, although this difference was not controlled for possible differences between the groups in cortical mass (see Anomalies of Asymmetry, p. 984). Using voxel-based morphometry in 159 patients with schizophrenia or schizophreniform disorder and 158 healthy comparison subjects,[223] significant decreases in white matter density in the genu and truncus of the corpus of the corpus callosum in left and right hemispheres and in the right anterior internal capsule and anterior commissure, with no interactions between diagnosis and age, were reported. These authors considered the findings consistent with aberrant interhemispheric connectivity in the anterior regions of the brain, reflecting decreased hemispheric specialization. A frequent finding has been upward bowing (i.e. increased curvature of the corpus callosum as a whole).[314,317] This correlated with, and has generally been considered to be secondary to, lateral ventricular enlargement and therefore not to reflect directly on pathophysiology. In 50 male and 50 female normal adults Suganthy et al.[393] found that the length of the corpus callosum was greater in males and increased with age in both sexes, whereas the width of the trunk and genu decreased with age in males but not females.

A diffusion tensor imaging study of the corpus callosum found an increase in mean diffusivity and a decrease in fractional anisotropy in the splenium but not in the genu of the corpus callosum.[176] A systematic review of DTI studies found 14 to show a reduction in fractional anisotropy, and 2 to show a loss of normal asymmetry.[245] Using a modification of DTI designed to isolate the precise anatomy of the fibre distribution Savadjiev et al. (unpublished data) identified a single sexually dimorphic and lateralized change in the genu of the corpus callosum in adolescent onset schizophrenia that was correlated with negative symptoms in opposite directions in the two sexes.

Cortical Gyrification

If schizophrenia is a disorder of the cerebral cortex and is developmental in origin, abnormalities of sulcogyral structure may be expected, and according to the asymmetry hypothesis, would be differentially distributed to the two hemispheres. Vogeley et al.[418] reported an increase in gyrification index in male but not female patients selective to the right side. Similar lateralized increases were reported by Harris et al.[196] and Narr et al.,[318] and in the latter study were also confined to male subjects. Sallet et al.,[365] however, observed reductions in cortical volume relative to healthy comparison subjects, and found these reductions bilateral

and related to disorganization in general, but left sided in relation to paranoid subtype of illness. Gyrification index was reported as reduced on the left side in adolescent onset psychosis by Jou et al.[243] However, some investigations have looked for and failed to observe a change in gyrification – for example Highley et al.,[215] using a stereological technique for randomly sampling the cortical surface, found no difference between 60 individuals with psychosis and 42 comparison subjects.

Clinicopathological Correlations

Some clinicopathological correlations have been reported (Table 17.4), although not all can be regarded as established. Some, but not all, studies have suggested that patients with prominent negative symptoms have larger lateral ventricles or progressive ventricular enlargement.[143] Positive symptoms have been related to temporal lobe structure. Clinical correlates include an association between fusiform gyrus volume and Liddle's 'disorganization' factor,[77] correlation between the degree of thought disorder and size of the planum temporale in the superior temporal gyrus,[378] and change in auditory cortex in Heschl's gyrus has been associated with hallucinations.[394] One feature of the disease that is relatively easy to define and has been related to pathology in several studies is the age of onset (see Table 17.4). This tends to be earlier for males than for females and may explain why males have a more severe course of the disease.[143,157,237] The main findings of an ambitious attempt to determine the neural correlates of the three major symptom patterns in schizophrenia are represented in Figure 17.7.

Conclusions on Macroscopic Brain Structure in Schizophrenia

Taken together, the evidence from both *in vivo* imaging and post-mortem studies indicate that the lateral ventricles are enlarged, an enlargement that is most marked in the temporal and occipital horns. The third ventricle is also enlarged, but not the fourth. This change in ventricular size is accompanied by a modest reduction (around 2 per cent) in brain volume and weight, along with comparable reductions in cerebral hemisphere volume, weight and length, whole temporal lobe volume and length, and superior temporal, fusiform and parahippocampal gyrus volumes. All of these reductions are small in size and the gyral changes tend to be more marked on the left side. The changes are present at disease onset and there is evidence for progression,[146,250,254,433] particularly in childhood-onset cases[146,231,312] Basal ganglia enlargement, if present, probably reflects the effects of neuroleptic treatment, although there is a suggestion that the basal ganglia can also be reduced in size in drug-naïve patients.[258] Thalamic volume reduction has been reported (but there are also significant negative findings both in MRI and post-mortem studies) as has loss or reversal of the normal asymmetry to the right of the pulvinar.[216] The cerebellum has rarely been studied and the evidence is conflicting, but there may be some tissue deficits, particularly of the vermis.[10,230,251] The brain stem may be slightly reduced in size but this needs to be studied further. A number of findings have

TABLE 17.4 Some clinicopathological correlations in schizophrenia

Pathology	Clinical correlate	Reference
Ventricles		
Temporal horn volume increase	Negative symptoms	444
Right temporal horn volume increase	Negative symptoms in first-episode patients	143
Third ventricle volume increase	Hallucinations	130
Cerebral weight/length/volume		
Decreased brain length	Poor premorbid brain function, more severe negative symptoms	239
Decreased brain weight	Poor premorbid brain function and academic record	239
Left temporal lobe length	Age of onset	25
Prefrontal white matter volume	Negative symptoms	366
Volume of left frontal lobe white matter	Negative symptoms	429
Medial temporal lobe volume	Positive symptoms	46
Superior temporal gyrus volume	Positive symptoms	23, 173, 290, 299
Left anterior superior temporal gyrus volume	Severity of hallucinations	378
Left posterior superior temporal gyrus volume	Severity of hallucinations	22, 290, 347
Basal ganglia volume	Positive symptoms	383
Caudate volume increase	Impairment on finger tapping and Hebb's recurring digits neuropsychological tests	220
Measures of asymmetry		
Reversal of superior frontal lobe asymmetry	Age of onset	211
Reversal of parahippocampal and fusiform gyrus asymmetry	Age of onset	293
Frontal lobe cortical volume asymmetry	Age of onset	214
Disturbed hippocampal asymmetry	Age of onset	181
Other features		
Increased synaptic protein markers in cingulate cortex	Severity of symptoms	342
Loss of NMDA receptor subunit NRI mRNA in superior temporal gyrus	Intellectual impairment	224

NMDA, N-methyl-D-aspartate.

been reported in relation to the corpus callosum both in structural MRI and DTI studies. A frequently reported finding of upward bowing seems likely to reflect ventricular enlargement, and may have added to the difficulty of defining intrinsic change. Given the problem of age and sex-related change, it appears that no definitive conclusions concerning interhemispheric transmission can yet be drawn. A meta-analysis of corpus callosum size measured with MRI found a small reduction in the size of this structure,[433] possibly reflecting a change in cortical volume, but recent DTI studies raised the possibility of systematic changes in fibre tracts in this structure.

Ventricular enlargement, the most reproducible of the macroscopic brain changes in schizophrenia, is consistent with increased ventricular pressure as well as decreased tissue volume. The evidence of modest brain tissue reduction, however, indicates that the latter is its cause in schizophrenia. The enlargement of sulcal spaces over the surface of the cerebral hemispheres bears out this interpretation.[444] The reduced tissue volume appears to apply more to grey than to white matter. There is a suggestion of altered sulcogyral patterns in the temporal[211] or frontal lobes[418] and of altered cerebral asymmetry,[196,318] but there are also negative findings.[215] As with the findings in the corpus callosum, those concerning sulcogyral patterns give support to the conclusion that the disease process is at the level of cortical folding, and late in development. A number of findings are asymmetrical and therefore consistent with the view that schizophrenia is an anomaly of development of asymmetry, with a primary focus in the cerebral cortex.

The conclusion that emerges from recent meta-analyses of MRI examination is that the most striking change is in the insula (somewhat lateralized to the right) followed by a reduction of volume of the anterior cingulate to the right, and the parahippocampal gyrus to the left.

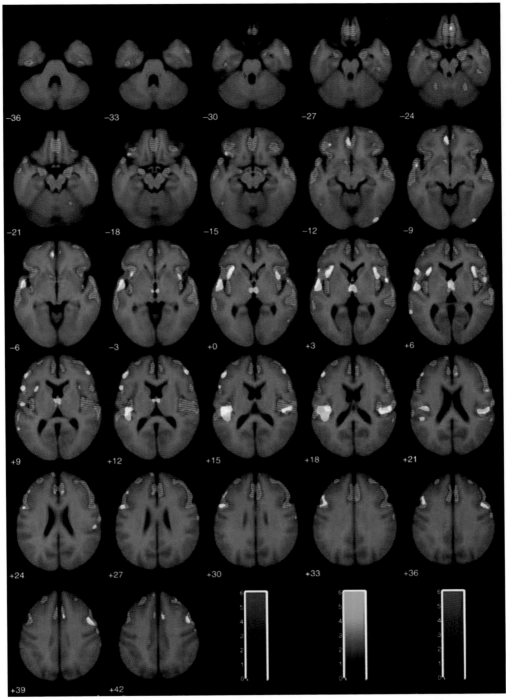

17.7 Neural correlates of syndromes in schizophrenia. Brain areas with significant volume-based reductions in grey matter in relation to dimensional syndromes in schizophrenia. Red signifies negative, green positive and blue disorganization syndromes respectively. Findings of note are (i) all three syndromes are represented within the cortex around the lateral sulcus including the insula; (ii) negative symptoms are associated with grey matter density reductions in dorsolateral prefrontal cortex, perhaps more on the right than the left, and also in cingulate and paracingulate gyri on both sides; (iii) disorganization is seen most clearly associated with the posterior lateral sulcus on the left; and (iv) there is a relatively discrete locus for positive symptoms on either side of the midline close to the fornix.[266]

Thus of those changes that have been discussed (ventricular enlargement, a modest reduction in cortical mass and loss of asymmetry) it seems that the last (i.e. a change along the dimension of symmetry–asymmetry) has the strongest claim as the most characteristic of schizophrenic psychosis. It almost certainly reflects an anomalous course of development, and could plausibly account for the other two changes.

AFFECTIVE PSYCHOSES

Brain Structure: Evidence from *In Vivo* Imaging

With the background of evidence (see Introduction, p. 975) for a continuum of psychotic illness that encompasses both the spectrum of schizophrenic psychoses and those described as affective or manic–depressive, the question arises whether morphological changes are present in the latter conditions and, if so, how they relate to those seen in schizophrenic psychoses. An answer to this question could cast light on the functional meaning of the brain changes in psychosis, and indeed on the general question of the relationship between affect and the associative functions of the cortex.

The literature is smaller than that on the more characteristically schizophrenic illnesses, and post-mortem validation is less substantial. Elkis et al.[159] conducted a series of meta-analyses incorporating 912 patients and 932 controls. In a comparison of patients with mood disorders to normal controls, the former were found to have moderate enlargement of the ventricles (d statistic = 0.44) and increased sulcal prominence (d = 0.42).

By comparison with patients with schizophrenia the degree of ventricular enlargement was of lesser magnitude (p = 0.002) and the effect size of the difference (d = -0.20) was small. The data were insufficient to support a comparison between the groups with respect to sulcal prominence. The authors concluded that 'One interpretation of the findings is that there is a common pathophysiology underlying ventricular enlargement in schizophrenia and mood disorders, but it is more potent in the former.'

The finding of a reduction in cortical volume in bipolar disorder that is similar but of lesser magnitude to that seen in schizophrenia reinforces this conclusion. It is consistent with the concept that in the spectrum of psychosis as a whole the primary pathology reflects population variation in the trajectory of development of the cerebral cortex. An early meta-analysis that included 26 studies comprising volumetric measurements on up to 404 patients with bipolar disorder enlargement of the right lateral ventricle, but no other volumetric deviations reached significance. There was heterogeneity across studies, especially with respect to the third ventricle, the left subgenual prefrontal cortex, the amygdala and the thalamus.[294]

Sulcal widening, although age dependent and difficult to quantify, has often been reported as a correlate of ventricular enlargement in schizophrenia. It is also present in bipolar disorder. For example, Young et al.[438] reported an increase in cortical sulcal widening in 30 patients with geriatric-onset manic disorder in comparison with 18 age-matched controls, and found the change to be related to age at onset of illness. However, similar changes are reported at the other end of the age spectrum. Friedman et al.[180] compared 20 patients with schizophrenia and 15 with bipolar disorder (aged 10–18 years) to 6 age-matched controls, and found that the two patient groups were distinguished from controls by a reduction in intracranial volume and an increase in frontal and temporal sulcal size; they also found that the schizophrenic and bipolar groups could not be distinguished. These findings are consistent with the concept of a continuum of psychosis. However, the possibility of qualitative difference is raised by an application of fractal analysis to the white/grey matter boundary in 39 patients with schizophrenia, 23 with manic–depressive illness and 31 control subjects.[55] The fractal dimension (a measure of complexity) was found to be correlated with subcortical volume and with anterior cerebral volume, and negatively correlated with sulcal fluid volume. Patients with manic–depressive illness were significantly increased relative to controls, whereas patients with schizophrenia showed a decrease.

Third ventricular enlargement in schizophrenic psychosis is generally correlated with the lateral ventricles, and in some series has been reported to be greater in those with a late onset.[238] It might have been predicted that the change would be of a lesser magnitude or of later onset in affective illness. This does not seem to be the case. When assessed in parallel series, the increase in volume is similar in the two diagnoses.[337]

If the affective and schizophrenic psychoses are part of a single spectrum and the key to its origin is in laterality, then variation in the form of psychosis should relate in some way to the hemispheric dimension. This line of thought originated in Flor-Henry's original observation of the relationship between temporal lobe epilepsy and psychosis. When the lesion was on the left side the form of the psychosis was more often schizophrenic and when on the right side it was more often affective in form.[174] The association of schizophrenic features with a focus in the dominant hemisphere is supported by subsequent studies as reviewed earlier, consistent with the view that Schneiderian first-rank symptoms are indicators of pathology in the dominant temporal lobe.[409] The association of affective features with the non-dominant hemisphere is less clear. Studies after traumatic and vascular lesions are relevant. Mania has been observed particularly in association with lesions of the right temporal lobe.[337] After stroke an excess of depressive reactions was observed following lesions of left prefrontal cortical and subcortical structures.[309] These observations suggest that affect is lateralized in the human brain, although the mechanism is obscure.

With respect to the morphological changes associated with the affective disorders themselves, Pearlson et al.[337] observed that whereas there was a shift in asymmetry (loss of left-sided predominance) of the superior temporal gyrus, such as has been previously observed in patients with schizophrenia,[22,213,378] no such change was observed in patients with bipolar affective disorder. Comparable findings (reduced grey matter volume in the posterior superior temporal gyrus on the left side) were reported in 17 patients with first episodes of schizophrenic psychosis relative to 16 patients with affective psychosis and 18 control subjects.[218] This suggests a differentiation of forms of psychosis along an axis of asymmetry. However, Chu et al.[76] reported an increase in temporal horn volume that was selective to the left side in both schizophrenia and bipolar disorder. In a study of cerebral volume asymmetries, Bilder et al.[41] found that a group of 81 patients with affective or schizoaffective disorders were intermediate between 61 healthy volunteers with the most marked anteroposterior torques and 87 patients with schizophrenia or schizophreniform disorders who had the least marked asymmetries. The authors considered their findings compatible with a 'continuum' hypothesis in which reduction of asymmetry constituted a risk factor for major mental illness.

Some studies across diagnostic categories are relevant to the spectrum concept. McDonald et al.[294] obtained MRI scans from 25 people with schizophrenia, 37 with bipolar disorder who had experienced psychotic symptoms, and 52 healthy volunteers. Deficits in grey matter were reported in frontotemporal neocortex, medial temporal lobe, insula, thalamus and cerebellum in schizophrenia, whereas there were no significant regions of grey matter abnormality in bipolar disorder. The findings in schizophrenia are in agreement with the literature (e.g. Honea et al.[221]) with respect to the medial temporal lobe and the insula, and the negative findings in bipolar disorder can be seen in relation to a literature in which change is smaller and sometimes inconsistent. But in an interesting extension of their study McDonald et al.[294] included 36 unaffected first-degree relatives of the schizophrenic probands and 50 unaffected first-degree relatives of the bipolar probands, and calculated an index of genetic risk within families. Genetic risk for schizophrenia was specifically associated with grey matter deficits in fronto-striato-thalamic and left lateral temporal regions (the latter) consistent with the literature as a whole,[221] whereas genetic risk for bipolar disorder was associated with deficits in the right anterior cingulate gyrus (also pinpointed in the meta-analysis in relation to schizophrenia) and ventral striatum. There is a hint here that schizophrenic symptoms were more closely associated with left posterior and affective symptoms with right anterior deficits, consistent with some earlier formulations,[175] but more recent meta-analyses (see Brain Structure in Schizophrenia, p. 982) raise the possibility of right-sided change in the anterior cingulate in schizophrenia and left-sided change in bipolar disorder. Most of the literature at this point is based upon volumetric assessment. The possibility that relative change in surface area and thickness is the critical variable and that sex is also relevant requires more detailed assessment.

Electrophysiological studies cast light on the problem. In a magneto-encephalographic (MEG) study, the 100-ms component of the auditory field potential in the superior temporal gyrus was found to be lateralized with the source in the right hemisphere anterior to that in the left, the asymmetry being greater in males than females.[351] In 20 patients with schizophrenia the asymmetry was altered, being lost in males, but accentuated in females. Similar anomalies of asymmetry have been observed in other MEG studies. Tiihonen et al.[402] observed that the asymmetry present in all normal subjects (left source posterior to right) was reversed in six of 19 patients with schizophrenia, with greater dispersal of the asymmetries in patients compared with controls. In patients with reversed asymmetry the distance between the auditory potential and the temporal pole (assessed on MRI) was reduced on the left side. Thus, a body of MEG evidence is consistent with a loss or reversal of asymmetry in the auditory pathways in schizophrenia that relates to the anatomical structure of the temporal lobe. Salisbury et al. showed that the P300 electrical evoked potential amplitude was reduced over the left temporal lobe in their group of first-episode patients with schizophrenic psychoses relative to those with affective psychoses

and normal controls.[364] That these changes in asymmetry are not confined to schizophrenic psychoses is suggested by a study of the somatosensory evoked potential in which an asymmetry (right anterior to the left) was observed in controls and subjects with bipolar disorder without a history of psychotic symptoms, but was lost in 12 bipolar subjects with a history of psychotic symptoms.[352] A similar reversal of asymmetry of the somatosensory evoked potential had previously been demonstrated in 16 patients with schizoaffective disorder.[353] These MEG findings suggest, therefore, that the differences in pathophysiology between manic–depressive and schizophrenic psychoses are quantitative rather than qualitative, consistent with the hypothesis that the primary determinant lies along the axis of symmetry–asymmetry.

Interest in the cingulate gyrus in affective disorder was raised by Drevets et al.[153] who found decreased blood flow in subgenual cingulate cortex in patients with bipolar and unipolar depression. An MRI investigation revealed a volume reduction in this region of 39 per cent in 21 patients with bipolar disorder and 48 per cent in 17 patients with unipolar disorder, in both cases selective to the left side, relative to a group of 21 controls.[153] The location of the change in affective disorder anterior to and beneath those described in the cingulate gyrus in schizophrenic psychoses is of particular interest, and their relationship to the subtle sulcogyral structure in this region (see earlier section) requires careful comparative studies.

In conclusion, the changes in affective psychosis are similar to, but of lesser degree than those seen in schizophrenic psychoses. They include enlargement of the lateral and third ventricles, with perhaps decreased overall cortical mass. That the affective psychoses are associated with anomalies of asymmetry is supported by MRI and MEG investigations. One possibility is that affective and schizophrenic psychoses reflect deviations in the course of development of the cerebral cortex that are separated by the dimension of asymmetry and that this difference is reflected in differences in psychopathological expression (e.g. in age of onset and outcome).

Interpretation of Macroscopic Changes in Affective Psychoses

There is a broad measure of agreement that the disorder has a neurodevelopmental origin, even if a precise timing for the aberrant process cannot be determined yet. There is agreement that lateral and third cerebral ventricles are enlarged and the cerebral grey matter volume is slightly reduced, probably most significantly in the temporal lobes, and that some of these changes are present at the time of disease onset. The evidence from post-mortem studies is that the changes are distributed widely and primarily at the level of the cerebral cortex. Ventricular enlargement may reflect anomalies in timing of cortical development. Alterations in cerebral asymmetry appear important, and these interact with sex and age in a complex and at present, poorly understood way. One possibility is that targeted areas include the 'hetero-modal association cortex'[336] involved with language that has evolved in the transition from a hominid precursor to modern Homo sapiens.[102,103,105,109,112]

CELLULAR STUDIES IN PSYCHOSIS

To understand the significance of the brain volume reduction in schizophrenia, the evidence for microscopic alterations must be examined. In other diseases associated with reduced volume of a brain structure, this is often due to reductions of neurons and/or white matter myelin and axons. With the expectation that the same may be true of schizophrenia, many of the quantitative studies of the microscopic pathology have concerned possible alterations in neuron number. Some such studies have used stereological methods to arrive at an estimate of cell number that reflects both cell density and the regional volume. This gives the most accurate quantitative account of a cell population.[80,192] However, this is not always achievable because of constraints imposed by tissue deficiencies or processing and the fact that the margins of cortical areas are not readily determined. A compromise position has been taken in some studies[374] and simpler cell density measurements have been made in others. This has the unsatisfactory consequence that it is difficult to make direct comparisons between studies in which, not surprisingly, the findings differ considerably (Figure 17.8).

Quantitative Studies of Neurons in Schizophrenia

Figure 17.8 summarizes data from quantitative studies of neuron density in various brain regions, and Figure 17.9 summarizes the data available on neuronal size. By far the most intensively studied regions are the hippocampus and the frontal lobe. This emphasis reflects the frequently expressed view that limbic and frontal lobe malfunction can best explain the symptoms of schizophrenia. Functional imaging studies have also lent weight to this idea. One global assessment of cortical neuron number found values within normal limits. However, other studies suggest reductions in schizophrenia, with a mean of ~15 per cent fewer neurons. Of these, five out of six record a reduction in mean neuron number of more than 5 per cent, although the effect did not reach statistical significance in the small samples of two studies.[270,401] It must be noted that estimates of total cell number compound data on cell density and region volume and of the two components, reduced region volume is the more replicated.

Studies of cell density are far more numerous than estimates of total number. Figure 17.10 illustrates a meta-analysis of the majority of quantitative studies of neuron density. These report contradictory findings, both positive (indicating both increased and decreased cell density) and negative, with no effect overall shown by meta-analysis.[18] The instances of reduced density in several studies are unlikely to be a result of an increase in reference volume as grey matter volume is generally found to be reduced in schizophrenia in imaging and post-mortem studies. However, a unifying interpretation is indicated by some individual studies[62,69,149] that showed that the contrast between patients and controls depended on when in adulthood the cell organization is measured. Normal neuron density in cortex increased with age in controls, whereas it was unchanged with age in patients. Patients <50 years

therefore had increased density (reduced spacing), whereas patients >60 years had reduced density (increased spacing). The relationship is detected by meta-regression (see Figure 17.10) although the interaction is often not seen in individual studies (32 studies each had a patient sample size of fewer than 15 subjects). The results indicate that, in normal adulthood, ageing is associated with a restructuring of neuropil (the space between cells) such that the neurons are closer together in old age. In schizophrenia, the neurons do not become more closely packed, possibly due to abnormal neuroplasticity in adulthood.

Findings in subregions of the brain are summarized briefly later.

Hippocampal Neurons

This subject has been reviewed by Harrison.[199] The majority of studies of neuronal number/density indicate that there is little or no change in this parameter, although a few studies have reported reductions or increases (see Figure 17.8). There is more consistency in the smaller number of studies of hippocampal neuron size, with two small studies reporting no change and three larger studies reporting a modest decrease in the size of neurons in various hippocampal subfields. Some early studies indicated that hippocampal neurons were misaligned, particularly at the boundaries between subfields, but later studies were unable to confirm this. Slight distortion of the shape of the hippocampus has been suggested as an explanation. Cells containing immunoreactive reelin are reported to be significantly reduced in number[167] as are cells containing parvalbumin.[443] In elderly subjects, there is reported to be increased evidence of oxidative DNA damage in hippocampal neurons in schizophrenia.

Entorhinal Cortex

Much prominence has been given to reports of qualitative differences in the localization and form of layer II pre-α clusters of neurons in the entorhinal cortex. They were described as less tightly clustered, atrophic and more deeply situated than normal in schizophrenia. With greater recognition of the large normal variability in the cytoarchitecture of this region and the fact that negative as well as positive findings continue to be reported, there is some caution about the significance of these observations (reviewed by Harrison).[199] A relatively early study describing significantly reduced neuronal numbers in the entorhinal cortex has not been confirmed, although there may be a change in cluster pattern.

Frontal Cortex

Most studies of neurons in the frontal cortex have been performed in Brodmann areas (BA) 9, 46, 4 and 10, and in the anterior cingulate cortex (BA24). Studies of neuronal density have yielded inconsistent findings of no change in, increased and decreased neuronal densities. These findings variously refer to pyramidal or non-pyramidal neurons or neurons immunoreactive for calcium-binding proteins (see Figure 17.8). A clear picture has yet to emerge. As with the hippocampus, the few studies of cell size have provided more consistency, with normal or slightly reduced neuron size being found (see Figure 17.9).

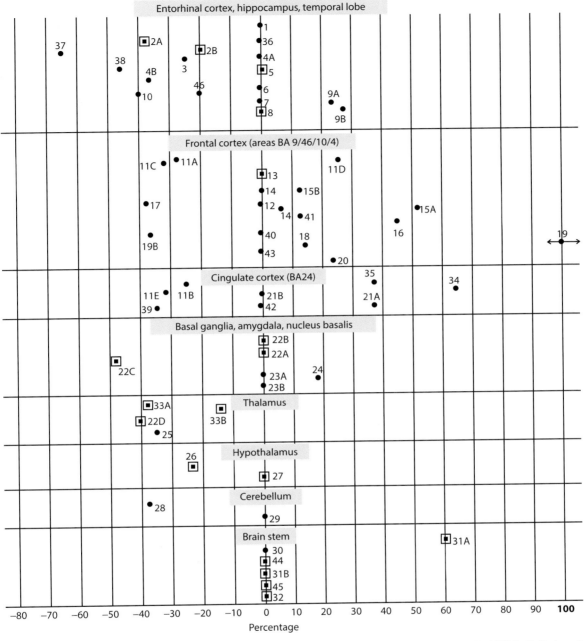

17.8 Studies of neuronal number (□) and density (•) in schizophrenia: 1, Kovelman and Scheibel;[267] 2, Falkai and Bogerts (A, entorhinal cortex; B, hippocampus);[163] 3, Jeste and Lohr;[234] 4, Benes *et al.* (A, CA2–4; B, CA1);[35] 5, Heckers *et al.*;[206] 6, Arnold *et al.*;[16] 7, Cotter *et al.*;[84] 8, Krimer *et al.*;[271] 9, Zaidel (A, CA3; B, CA1);[441] 10, Benes *et al.* (non-pyramidal neurons in CA2);[38] 11, Benes *et al.* (A, layer VI neurons, prefrontal cortex; B, cingulate cortex; C, BA10 small neurons, layer 2; D, pyramidal neurons layer V; E, BA24 interneurons layers 2–6);[33] 12, Woo *et al.* (parvalbumin neurons);[431] 13, Pakkenberg;[133] 14, Akbarian *et al.*;[3] 15, Davis and Lewis (A, calbindin neurons; B, calretinin neurons);[140] 16, Anderson *et al.*;[9] 17, Beasley and Reynolds (parvalbumin neurons, layers III/IV);[28] 18, Selemon *et al.*;[374] 19, Rajkowska *et al.* (A, small neurons; B, very large neurons in layer IIIC);[348] 20, Selemon *et al.*;[375] 21, Kalus *et al.* (A, parvalbumin cells, layer V; B, total neuronal density);[244] 22, Pakkenberg (A, basolateral-amygdala; B, ventral pallidum; C, nucleus accumbens; D, mediodorsal thalamus);[330] 23, Arendt *et al.* (A, globus pallidus; B, nucleus basalis);[14] 24, Beckmann and Lauer (striatum);[31] 25, Danos *et al.* (parvalbumin neurons in anteroventral thalamus);[136] 26, Bernstein *et al.* (nitric oxide synthase neurons in paraventricular nucleus);[39] 27, Briess *et al.* (mammillary bodies);[50] 28, Reyes and Gordon (cerebellar vermis; Purkinje cells expressed per unit length);[354] 29, Tran *et al.* (Purkinje cells);[408] 30, Lohr and Jeste (locus coeruleus)[281] 31, Garcia-Rill *et al.* (A, mesopontine nucleus; B, locus coeruleus);[183] 32, German *et al.*;[185] 33, Young *et al.* (A, mediodorsal thalamus; B, anteroventral/medial thalamus);[437] 34, Chana *et al.* (layer 6);[62] 35, Chana *et al.* (layer 5);[62] 36, Walker *et al.*;[421] 37, Zhang and Reynolds (CA2 parvalbumin neurons);[443] 38, Fatemi *et al.* (dentate cortex, Brodmann area 4 reelin neurons);[167] 39, Cotter *et al.* (layer 2 calbindin neurons);[85] 40, Beasley *et al.* (white matter neurons);[29] 41, Eastwood and Harrison (superficial white matter neurons);[156] 42, Cotter *et al.* (calretinin and parvalbumin neurons);[85] 43, Cotter *et al.*;[86] 44, Craven *et al.*;[94] 45, Craven *et al.*;[95] 46, Chance *et al.*[67]

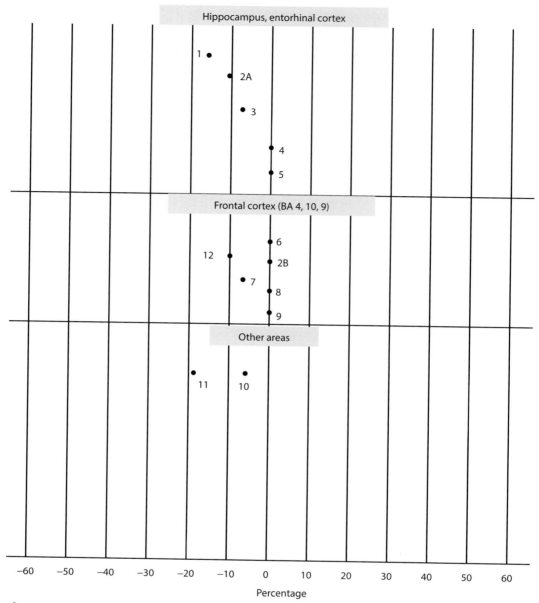

17.9 Studies of neuronal size measurements in schizophrenia. 1, Benes *et al.* (posterior hippocampus CA1–4);[36] 2, Arnold *et al.* (A, hippocampus; B, frontal cortex/BA4);[17] 3, Zaidel *et al.*;[442] 4, Christison *et al.*;[75] 5, Benes *et al.*;[38] 6, Benes *et al.*;[33] 7, Rajkowska *et al.*;[348] 8, Bene *et al.*;[35] 9, Woo *et al.*;[431] 10, Tran *et al.* (Purkinje cells);[408] 11, Chana *et al.* (layer 5, anterior cingulate cortex);[62] 12, Pierri *et al.*[340]

Much interest was generated by studies of the location of nicotinamide adenine dinucleotide phosphate diaphorase histochemically reactive cells, which are believed to represent residual neurons from the developmentally early formed cortical subplate. Most of these cells undergo programmed cell death once the cortical structure is in place, although some persist into adult life in superficial subcortical white matter.[7] Initial studies suggested that these cells were dispersed more deeply in frontal and temporal lobe white matter in schizophrenia than in normal controls,[2] the implication being that cortical development is faulty in schizophrenia. However, later studies showed less dramatic or opposite results, casting doubt on this concept.[4,9] A further cell type of interest is the reelin-containing cell, which is decreased in frontal and temporal cortices (or there is less reelin expressed per cell) and in the hippocampus in schizophrenia.

Some consistency and coherence, and a possible way forward, emerge from a study that investigated the earlier reports of Selemon and colleagues that the density of pyramidal cells in areas 9 and 44 of dorsolateral prefrontal cortex was increased, a result held to be consistent with the 'reduced neuropil' hypothesis.[376] Cullen and colleagues examined cell density in area 9 in both hemispheres and found no evidence of an overall increase in density, but they did find an asymmetry of density with a relative increase in density in the left hemisphere in controls that was reversed (i.e. a greater density on the right compared with the left in

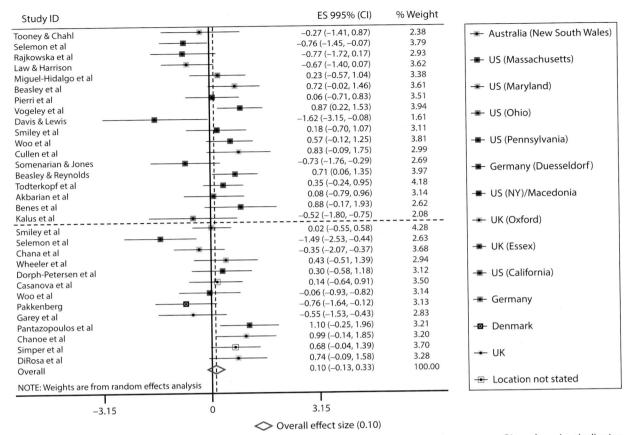

Study ID	ES 995% (CI)	% Weight
Tooney & Chahl	−0.27 (−1.41, 0.87)	2.38
Selemon et al	−0.76 (−1.45, −0.07)	3.79
Rajkowska et al	−0.77 (−1.72, 0.17)	2.93
Law & Harrison	−0.67 (−1.40, 0.07)	3.62
Miguel-Hidalgo et al	0.23 (−0.57, 1.04)	3.38
Beasley et al	0.72 (−0.02, 1.46)	3.61
Pierri et al	0.06 (−0.71, 0.83)	3.51
Vogeley et al	0.87 (0.22, 1.53)	3.94
Davis & Lewis	−1.62 (−3.15, −0.08)	1.61
Smiley et al	0.18 (−0.70, 1.07)	3.11
Woo et al	0.57 (−0.12, 1.25)	3.81
Cullen et al	0.83 (−0.09, 1.75)	2.99
Somenarian & Jones	−0.73 (−1.76, −0.29)	2.69
Beasley & Reynolds	0.71 (0.06, 1.35)	3.97
Todterkopf et al	0.35 (−0.24, 0.95)	4.18
Akbarian et al	0.08 (−0.79, 0.96)	3.14
Benes et al	0.88 (−0.17, 1.93)	2.62
Kalus et al	−0.52 (−1.80, −0.75)	2.08
Smiley et al	0.02 (−0.55, 0.58)	4.28
Selemon et al	−1.49 (−2.53, −0.44)	2.63
Chana et al	−0.35 (−2.07, −0.37)	3.68
Wheeler et al	0.43 (−0.51, 1.39)	2.94
Dorph-Petersen et al	0.30 (−0.58, 1.18)	3.12
Casanova et al	0.14 (−0.64, 0.91)	3.50
Woo et al	−0.06 (−0.93, −0.82)	3.14
Pakkenberg	−0.76 (−1.64, −0.12)	3.13
Garey et al	−0.55 (−1.53, −0.43)	2.83
Pantazopoulos et al	1.10 (−0.25, 1.96)	3.21
Chanoe et al	0.99 (−0.14, 1.85)	3.20
Simper et al	0.68 (−0.04, 1.39)	3.70
DiRosa et al	0.74 (−0.09, 1.58)	3.28
Overall	0.10 (−0.13, 0.33)	100.00

NOTE: Weights are from random effects analysis

−3.15   0   3.15

◇ Overall effect size (0.10)

- Australia (New South Wales)
- US (Massachusetts)
- US (Maryland)
- US (Ohio)
- US (Pennsylvania)
- Germany (Duesseldorf)
- US (NY)/Macedonia
- UK (Oxford)
- UK (Essex)
- US (California)
- Germany
- Denmark
- UK
- Location not stated

17.10 Effect sizes from a meta-analysis of 31 studies.[18] Studies are organized by control mean age. Size of marker indicates relative sample size of each study; colour indicates geographical location of brain samples. Studies that were completed in the frontal lobe are listed above the dotted line, whereas studies that were completed in other brain regions are below the dotted line. This is to show that there is a similar trend in both groups. There were 18 studies in the frontal lobe and 13 studies in other brain areas.

patients), the significance of the patient–control difference being greatest in layer 3.[132] In addition, a difference in cell size (larger on the left) and cell shape (more spherical) was observed in control subjects that was absent in patients. In the prefrontal cortex, a selective reduction of large pyramidal neurons in schizophrenia was found by Rajkowska et al.,[348] indicating particular vulnerability among the magnopyramidal neurons. The findings thus can be seen as consistent with the concept that the torque is a major characteristic of human association cortex that has an influence on interhemispheric connections and that is relevant to the pathophysiology of psychosis.

An observation on the anterior cingulate gyrus that remains to be confirmed independently is that the lamina II neurons are divided into smaller, more widely spaced clusters than normal, separated by larger bundles of vertically running axons detectable with antibodies to 200-kDa neurofilament protein or glutamate.[32,34,37] These observations suggest that this region of cortex may be oversupplied with excitatory afferents from other cortical regions. In view of the evidence from imaging studies and the previously mentioned study on dorsolateral prefrontal cortex, particular interest relates to whether the apparent changes in this region are lateralized.

Temporal Cortex and Other Cortical Regions

Negative correlations between superior temporal gyrus and lateral ventricles, and parahippocampal gyrus and lateral ventricles in schizophrenia support the notion that key changes in the temporal lobe are linked to diffuse enlargement of the lateral ventricles.[65] Most cytoarchitectural studies of the temporal lobe have focused on the superior temporal plane (the planum temporale and Heschl's gyrus) and the medial temporal lobe (the parahippocampal gyrus and entorhinal cortex). The balance of findings (both increased and decreased neuron densities) is consistent with the literature on the frontal lobe and the studies of temporal lobe neocortex contribute to the overall age-dependent contrast between patients and controls suggesting altered neuroplasticity in schizophrenia. Reduced cortical thickness has been found in the planum temporale, although neuron density is reportedly unchanged, so it has been suggested that closer packing of neurons may not always explain reduced cortical volume, and subtly decreased neuron number may be a contributing factor.[386] Altered clustering[30] and reduced volume of layer III pyramidal neurons have been found in this area[396] and a size reduction of the largest pyramidal neurons has been found in the left, but not right planum temporale.[385] It has been suggested that these findings implicate impaired feed-forward connections[396] and altered interhemispheric connections[385] in schizophrenia.

The parietal lobe is relatively underinvestigated in schizophrenia, although one study indicates a slight reduction in the hemispheric asymmetry of cortical depth and neuron density,[387] similar to cortical thickness findings from *in vivo* imaging. Studies of visual cortex (mainly BA17) also find a mix of increased and decreased neuron density, whereas reduced total neuron number appears to be largely dependent on reduced regional volume.[152] Alternative groupings of cortical regions (e.g. 'limbic cortex', including cingulate cortex and entorhinal cortex) also reveal mixed results.

Interneurons

The use of some specific immunohistochemical cell markers has helped to identify effects in subpopulations of neurons. Some consistency has emerged from the use of markers that usually identify inhibitory interneurons in neocortex. Ten studies have reported that the density of this class of cells is reduced by over 10 per cent compared to only three reporting an increase. A few of these studies used the global marker GAD, but most used a mixture of markers for calcium-binding proteins: parvalbumin, calretinin and calbindin, each of which tends to identify a partially separate subpopulation. The densities of interneurons identified by parvalbumin and somatostatin are also reduced in the hippocampus[265] and its neighbouring cortical region, the parahippocampal gyrus,[422] although the density of glutamic acid decarboxylase immunopositive neurons here has been found to be increased.[371] Although parvalbumin neurons appear to show the most consistent changes (hypothesized to be linked to NMDA receptor hypofunction and electrophysiological Gamma-band disruption),[189] the discrepancies between markers relate to the unresolved issue of whether the changes reflect the absence of cells or the absence of protein expression in those cells. The absence of interneurons is likely to result in disinhibition of local pyramidal neurons. The alternative scenario, that the cells are still present but that there is a loss of calcium-binding protein expression, would likely also indicate an altered electrophysiological phenotype resulting in disrupted local inhibition.

Other Regions

Of the other regions of the brain, the thalamus has been studied most. Overall, altered neuron number tends to be secondary to grey matter volumetric change. The alterations of neuron density (both increases and decreases; similar to reports from the cerebral cortex) are relatively small (at least seven studies report less than 5 per cent change), and the larger effects that may be reported for total number are usually due to the reductions in thalamic nuclear volumes. Studies of the basal ganglia are fewer but also show inconsistency of findings with regard to neuron number and density. The hypothalamus, cerebellum and brain stem have been little studied. Cell size has been examined only rarely at subcortical sites; there is a suggestion that cerebellar Purkinje cells may be slightly reduced in size,[408] although this is not borne out by another study.[281]

In summary, there is limited evidence of cortical or subcortical neuronal reduction in number in schizophrenia.

Less studied but with more consistent findings to date is a modest and possibly fairly widespread reduction in neuronal size. This finding is suggestive that neurons may have reduced dendritic and/or axonal arborizations and that a reduction in neuropil surrounding a normal complement of neurons may be the explanation for the reduced brain volume documented at the macroscopic level (the 'reduced neuropil' hypothesis). The alternative view, that subtly decreased neuron number may be a contributing factor, has gained some support through slowly accumulating evidence, although coupled with evidence of longitudinal reductions at the macroscopic level it appears to conflict with the prevailing absence of neurodegenerative markers. A possible resolution is that reduced neuropil is present early, followed by a relatively slow, subtle loss of neurons in later life that is difficult to detect. A brief review of synaptic density, dendrites and axons follows. More details can be found in the reviews by Harrison[199] and Lewis *et al.*[277]

Dendrites

The classic Golgi method has been used to study the neuronal dendritic tree in schizophrenia on a few occasions. Unfortunately, the method rarely gives optimal results when used on post-mortem human material.[49] There are reports of neurons showing reduced numbers of dendrites and dendritic spines in schizophrenia in layer III of the cerebral cortex and in the hippocampus.[359] Ultrastructural examination, another means of assessing dendrites, axon terminals and synapses, is similarly very difficult to apply to human post-mortem material, but again there are a few ultrastructural studies of schizophrenia that claim a reduction in size of dendritic spines in the basal ganglia. Use has been made of immunocytochemical markers of somata and dendrites in the subiculum, hippocampus and entorhinal cortex with antibodies to microtubule-associated protein 2 (MAP-2) and 5 (MAP-5), with findings of modestly reduced or unchanged dendritic staining for these antigens. These proteins are important in determining neuronal size, shape and dendritic stabilization. It has been proposed that smaller somal volume is a key change associated with lower basilar dendritic spine density in the auditory cortex in schizophrenia, particularly in deep layer III pyramidal neurons.[276]

Axons

Axons could be affected through excessive or reduced branching (proximally, distally or both). Only recently have studies been performed that have a bearing on the state of proximal axons in schizophrenia. These point to disturbances in axonal routing, but the findings are complex and their interpretation is far from clear. For example, initial studies of the corpus callosum in small cohorts did not show alterations in axonal density[59,282,320] but more recent studies suggest that the large commissural interhemispheric connections are disturbed in a way that alters normal sex differences in these structures. In the Oxford post-mortem series, Highley and colleagues found no change in cross-sectional area of the subdivisions of the corpus callosum, but for axon density, assessed on Palmgren-stained sections, there was a sex by diagnosis interaction ($p = 0.005$) that applied to all regions except for the posterior midbody and splenium.[212] Among controls, females had a greater fibre density than males, but among patients this difference was reversed. The findings suggest a sex-related subtle alteration in interhemispheric connections between areas of cortex that develop late. A comparable change – a reduction in fibre density in females with psychosis relative to controls – was observed in the anterior commissure. The areas in which the changes were seen are those that probably relate to the association areas of the cortex. A normal correlation between the bihemispheric total density of magnopyramidal neurons in layer III of the planum temporale and the number of axons in the connecting region – the isthmus – of the corpus callosum, is absent in schizophrenia. The normal asymmetry of the minicolumnar organization of cells in the planum temporale also reflects axonal connectivity through the isthmus of the corpus callosum.[68] Greater asymmetry is associated with fewer axons, presumably reflecting more independent hemispheric function. This relationship is disturbed in schizophrenia, implicating abnormal connectivity via a different area of the corpus callosum.[148]

Thus, as discussed earlier, most callosal segments normally displayed greater axonal density in females than males, whereas in schizophrenia the fibre counts were reduced in females and increased in males. Similar findings were reported for the anterior commissure, in that in normal females this structure contained more axons than in normal males, whereas in schizophrenia the fibre density was reduced significantly in females but unchanged in males. Sex-dependent, asymmetrical effects have also been found for the limbic connections through the fornix.[63]

Rather than global or regional reduction in axons in schizophrenia, these findings suggest a disturbance that includes axons of corticocortical neurons, in part in a sex-dependent fashion. Abnormal axodendritic plasticity, which is most acute in those areas of the brain that go on developing longest (asymmetric association cortex) may be related to altered brain ageing effects on microscopic neuroanatomy. It has been suggested that transcallosal misconnection occurs with a timing of illness onset that reflects the sex difference in maturation of the corpus callosum.[69]

Synapses

There has been a wealth of molecular studies of synaptic features in schizophrenia. To some extent, these have been driven by genetic studies thought to implicate genes involved in synaptic molecules as risk factors for the disease. Detailed analysis can be found in the reviews mentioned earlier. In general, the glutamatergic, gamma-aminobutyric acid (GABA)ergic and dopaminergic systems have been the focus, although no unifying hypothesis has emerged.[407] In keeping with the reduced neuropil hypothesis, where changes have been found in schizophrenia they have usually been in the direction of a reduction, particularly in glutamatergic synapses. However, as in almost all neuropathological investigations of schizophrenia, there are some inconsistencies. As indicated by the data on cell density, which is likely related to neuropil volume, consideration of the lifetime trajectory of synapse formation and plasticity suggests that the size of effect may depend on the age of the subjects. Microarray gene expression profiling has also provided evidence

of an abnormality of presynaptic function, although interpreting the significance of the findings from such studies is complex.[300]

Glial Cell Changes

Much attention has been given to the question of whether or not astrocytosis plays a role in schizophrenia. Although some data are conflicting (see Harrison[199] and Roberts *et al*.[358] for reviews), the current consensus is that there is not an excess of gliosis generally, although there may be a subgroup of demented patients with severe pathology in whom astrocytosis is present. Negative glial fibrillary acidic protein immunocytochemical studies are further supported by studies of glial cells in Nissl-stained sections where no excess has been found.

Detailed attention has been given to this question because it was thought to provide crucial evidence about whether schizophrenia is a neurodevelopmental or a neurodegenerative disease. Gliosis would be expected as a result of a neurodegenerative, but not a developmental, process. The evidence as it stands favours the neurodevelopmental model (see Neurodevelopmental Theories, p. 981). Nonetheless, increasing evidence from brain imaging suggests that schizophrenia is not neuropathologically static during its clinical course.

At the same time, modern microscopy indicates alterations in the numbers of glia and accumulating molecular studies find changed gene expression associated with the late maturing process of myelination. Consequently, interest has switched from astrocytes to oligodendrocytes studied at both light- and electron-microscopic levels. By electron microscopy there were suggestions of apoptosis and necrosis in oligodendrocytes in the prefrontal cortex, and damage to myelin sheaths with formation of concentric lamellar bodies. The latter were also evident in the caudate nucleus. A deficit of oligodendrocytes in the superior frontal cortex[219] and white matter is supported by micro-array studies that found alterations to myelin-related gene expression.[403] The oligodendrocyte changes thought to be accompanied by altered gene expression and abnormal myelination[411] are a possible source of the white matter alterations detected by DTI studies that highlight decreased anisotropy and reduced myelin content in schizophrenia.[54,176,280] However, the different glial cell types have a diversity of functions including myelination, the regulation of glutamate, and a contribution to the immunological response. Because oligodendrocytes are known to express excitatory glutamate receptors, the putative deficits in glutamatergic neurotransmission in schizophrenia (see Harrison and Weinberger[201] for a review) may reflect oligodendroglial changes. Disruption of the glutamate-glutamine cycle, changes in perineuronal nets in late development and altered myelination are all likely to have ongoing effects beyond early development.

Conclusions on Microscopic and Molecular Brain Changes in Schizophrenia

It can be argued that microscopic studies begin to indicate the basis of the macroscopic changes. A reduction in the neuropil, reflecting smaller neurons with less abundantly arborized dendrites and fewer synapses, is a possible explanation for the smaller volume of grey matter (see Figure 17.6). One possibility is that this represents excessive pruning of synapses during developmental maturation;[169] another possibility is that the full complement of synapses fails to develop at an earlier stage. Subsequently failed connectivity may lead to a slow loss of neurons. There is evidence to support a misrouting of axons, as shown by sex-dependent alterations in the fibre content of the corpus callosum and anterior commissure. Where it has been examined, there is both microscopic and macroscopic evidence for altered cerebral asymmetry (e.g. in the study by Cullen et al.[132]). The changes in neurons and their constituents are not accompanied by gliosis but may be related to changes in oligodendrocytes. Other types of neuropathological change are probably no more common in schizophrenic patients than in others.

The microscopic studies suggest that the modest volume reduction in the brain relates to a reduction in size of neurons, their axons and/or dendrites although subtle neuronal loss remains a possible contributing factor. Although it is difficult to reconcile structural and molecular changes with the hyperresponsiveness to dopamine that the effects of neuroleptic medication apparently reveal, it seems likely that neurochemical imbalances are a downstream effect of more global alterations in brain connectivity brought about during development (see p. 999, Synapses).

Cellular Studies of Affective Disorder

Microscopic and molecular studies related to depression have generally reinforced the view derived from *in vivo* imaging that changes similar to but milder than those seen in schizophrenia are present. Attention was directed initially towards the prefrontal cortex by structural and functional imaging studies (see earlier, p. 992). The raphe and locus coeruleus are also obvious sites of interest because antidepressive medication largely influences serotonergic and noradrenergic neurotransmission. A few other sites have also been studied.

Neuropathological studies of the prefrontal cortex have shown a reduction in volume of the subgenual part of BA24 in familial bipolar and depressive disorder, with no change in neuron size or number but reductions in glial cell numbers in this region of 24 per cent in major depression and 41 per cent in bipolar disorder. A further study found a reduction in neuronal size and density, as

well as in glial cell density in the upper cortical layers of rostral orbitofrontal cortex.[349] The dorsolateral prefrontal cortex (BA9) also showed a 20–60 per cent reduction in density of large neurons in supragranular and infragranular layers, as well as a small reduction in neuronal size and a reduction of 20–30 per cent in glial cells in layers III and V.[349] Reduction in 5-HT1A receptor density has been reported.[48,154] Neuropathological changes reported in the raphe and locus coeruleus in depression have been inconsistent. In bipolar disorder and major depression a study of the dorsal raphe in suicide victims found an increase in the number of immunostained serotonergic neurons. Another study of late-onset depression found no change in these neurons.[397] In the locus coeruleus, suicide victims were reported as having lower density and total number of pigmented neurons[13] or no change in the number of these cells.[27] In depression, neurons in the locus coeruleus are variously reported as normal[193,262] or reduced.[27]

Neurochemical Changes in Affective Disorder

The hypothesis that affective disorders are associated with deficits in aminergic transmission originated in observations on depressive states associated with administration of amine-depleting agents such as reserpine, used in the treatment of hypertension, and has been widely accepted in interpretations of the mechanism of action of antidepressant medications (e.g. that these work by blocking neuronal reuptake processes for and thereby facilitating transmission by 5-HT, dopamine or noradrenaline). This hypothesis has received scant support from investigations of aminergic mechanisms in the brains of patients who have suffered from depression or who have committed suicide. Thus, in the brains of 15 patients dying in hospital with depression and 10 individuals who had committed suicide, there were minimal changes in monoamine metabolite concentrations or in ligand-binding capacities for the major monoamine receptors relative to controls.[289] More recent studies using a range of different approaches[121,229,249] have not revealed changes in monoamine parameters that are consistent between brain samples. The suggestion that a polymorphism related to the serotonin reuptake process is at the core of affective change has recently been shown to be unrelated to suicide or depression in a post-mortem study.[284]

OTHER DISORDERS

Autism

Autism, more often regarded now as a range of disorders with common elements, autism spectrum disorders, is a persistent neuropsychiatric syndrome that manifests in early childhood (Box 17.1). It was first described by Leo Kanner.[247] Recent estimates in the USA of autism spectrum disorders have found a prevalence of 1–2.6 per cent, with males being four times more commonly affected than females.[260,264] This suggests that there has been a sizeable increase of cases in recent years, some but not all of which, is estimated to be related to better case recognition. Whether there are environmental factors that play a part in this increase in prevalence is the subject of ongoing research.[207]

TABLE 17.5 Genes in which mutations are reported in rare cases of autism spectrum disorders	
RELN	FMR1
PTEN	GABR3
SHANK3	NRXN1
SHANK2	CNTN4
NL3	NLGN4X
NL4	

- Developmental delays or failure to develop:
  - social interactions, including eye contact
  - language and other communication skills (absent or reduced in Asperger syndrome)
  - sharing of experiences
  - imaginative play
- Narrow range of interests
- Behavioural rigidity, with bizarre, stereotyped behaviour
- Motor manifestations, including toe-walking, hypotonia and repetitive purposeless movements
- Hypersensitivity to some sensations (e.g. auditory) but hyposensitivity to others
- Variable cognitive skills; about half have mental retardation, but some have exceptional talents in narrow domains such as music, art and calculation ('splinter skills')
- Presentation is in early childhood. Parents commonly report regression of acquired skills, e.g. in language and play, at 18–24 months of age
- Epilepsy occurs in up to a third of those affected by adolescence
- Prevalence is 1–2.6 per cent (high recent figures are attributed only in part to improved diagnosis)
- High concordance in monozygotic twins (about 90 per cent), but lower in dizygotic twins (about 10 per cent)
- No simple inheritance pattern
- In a minority of cases there is associated disease with autism spectrum disorder. This includes congenital rubella infection, tuberous sclerosis, fragile X syndrome, Rett syndrome, Angelman's syndrome, Timothy syndrome, dup 15q11-13 and hydrocephalus.[301]

Genetics

The genetics of autism have been the subject of intensive recent study. Findings have been reviewed by Schaaf and Zoghbi[369] and by Marshall and Scherer,[291] Miles,[301] and State and Levitt.[390] Concordance in monozygotic twins is over 90 per cent if allowance is made for variation in severity of manifestation, but less than 10 per cent in dizygotic twins.[369] There are some cases of autism in which a specific gene mutation is present but such cases are estimated to only account for 5–7 per cent of cases (see Box 17.1 and Table 17.5). Fragile X syndrome is the most common of these single gene disorders. Many other genetic abnormalities associated with autism are related to copy number variation. Some variants appear to arise *de novo*. Copy number variants are thought to account for 7–20 per cent of cases and to stem from many different genes, which are mostly related to synaptic development, structure and function. A further 5 per cent or so of cases are thought to be associated with metabolic disorders. That leaves nearly 70 per cent of cases unaccounted for. Transgenic animal models based on some of these rare genetic mutations in autism are beginning to cast light on the mechanisms by which symptoms develop. It is of considerable interest that the emerging evidence of genetic risks for autism show some overlap with other phenotypic neuropsychiatric conditions such as schizophrenia and intellectual disability.

Brain Structure: Macroscopic Changes

Evidence from *In Vivo* Imaging Studies

Many different imaging modalities have been applied to patients with autism, the majority being adolescents or adults. These include studies of T1-weighted MR images that inform about anatomical detail, volumes of grey and white matter and cortical surface and shape, and DTI to investigate the organization of white matter. The fact that most studies have been mainly concentrated on older subjects who are easier to scan represents a shortcoming in a disorder that presents in early childhood. Nevertheless, some important information has been gained even about young children with the condition.

Perhaps the best established finding is that although whole brain volume is within normal limits at birth, it increases in size more rapidly in autistic subjects than in normally developing children in the first few years of postnatal life, following which the growth trajectory levels off so that by adolescence or early adulthood the brain volume can be either enlarged or within normal limits when compared with controls (reviewed by Courchesne et al.[89] and Schumann and Nordahl[373]). This finding fits with earlier evidence that head circumference increases abnormally fast from the end of the first year of life so that 15–20 per cent of cases were macrocephalic by 4–5 years of age.[88,141,147,204] It is also in agreement with post-mortem findings (this page). The explanation for this abnormal growth trajectory is unclear but is discussed later under Microscopic Changes (p. 1002). Altered growth rates of the brain mean that imaging studies undertaken at different ages of subjects are bound to show differing findings, a factor that probably accounts for some of the many inconsistencies in the imaging literature. Some of the main findings that have emerged from these studies are summarized in Box 17.2. The majority of studies indicate an increase in grey matter of amygdala and cortex, particularly dorsolateral and medial prefrontal cortex and temporal cortex with some interesting reversals of normal asymmetry, for example, in inferior frontal cortex. White matter has also been found to be increased, particularly in outer radiate compartments thought to represent short and medium range intrahemispheric connections.[208] The corpus callosum is reported to be reduced in size particularly in its rostral portion.[178,391] DTI studies of white matter have shown additional alterations in asymmetry with the temporal stem showing reversed hemisphere asymmetries in tensor skewness and fractional anisotropy.[272]

Evidence from Post-Mortem Studies

Neuropathological studies in autism have been restricted by a paucity of brains to study. Most studies have been carried out on adult brains which, of course, lack the ability to define important changes in early postnatal life. Fewer than 150 brains have been available for study to date, but efforts are being made to increase the awareness of the need to study post-mortem brains in order to characterize structural changes and regional changes in proteomics and gene expression. Another difficulty in making sense of the pathological changes, which is compounded by the shortage of brains to study, is the marked phenotypic and genetic heterogeneity of the condition. An example of how this heterogeneity can impact on pathology is a recent study that, unusually, defined two autism subgroups: those with idiopathic autism and those with defined genetic abnormalities in chromosome 15q11.2-q13 (dup(15)). The latter group had microencephaly whereas the former had brains of normal or increased weight. Heterotopias in the hippocampal region were found in 89 per cent of the cases in the dup(15) group but in only 10 per cent of the idiopathic group, whereas cortical dysplasia was found in 50 per cent of the idiopathic autism group but in none of the dup(15) group.[425] It will be important in the future for more homogeneous groups of cases, such as these, to be studied separately.

Early studies of autism brains were not able to capture the subtle changes that have more recently been described. Thus, the early pathological studies, reviewed by Bauman and Kemper[26] found no significant changes. However, it is now recognized that, in keeping with head circumference measurements and patient imaging, the brain tends to be larger and heavier than normal, albeit with a wide range in brain weights encountered.

Brain Structure: Microscopic and Molecular Changes

There are no microscopic changes so far described that are specific to autism. Instead, there is a range of non-specific abnormalities and abnormalities associated with epilepsy (which occurs in 30 per cent of subjects with autism), suggestive of deranged development described in multiple regions of the brain,[424] (i.e. minor subependymal nodular changes, cerebellar dysplasias, heterotopias and cerebral cortical irregularities). Most studies have searched for evidence of alterations in size or number of neurons. A few have been stereological, but most have relied on cell density measurements.

The most intriguing question that microscopists have tried to answer is: what is the basis for the early postnatal enlargement of the brain? There is now converging evidence that one answer lies in an increase in neuronal numbers, particularly in the frontal lobes. A recent stereological study indicated that in autistic boys aged 2–16 years there is a 67 per cent excess in prefrontal cortical neurons (79 per cent in dorsolateral prefrontal cortex and 29 per cent in medial prefrontal cortex).[90] However, there was no clear correlation in this study between the number of frontal cortical neurons and the brain weight in autistic subjects, even though such a correlation was found for controls. An automatic counting technique that considers the spacing of mini-columns in the cortex likewise reported an increase in density of mini-columns, and by implication, of the neurons composing them, but with a reduction in dendritic processes occupying the periphery of the mini-columns, in prefrontal cortex in autism.[60] Another possible contributory factor in producing an enlarged brain in autism is an increase in glial cells, as suggested by Vargas et al.[416] and Morgan et al.[306,307] On the other hand, a stereological study of inferior frontal cortex (BA44 and BA45) found no difference in estimated number of pyramidal cells or volumes of the cortical layers, but instead found smaller pyramidal cells in autism.[232]

Other microscopists have concentrated their studies on regions of the brain that appear to be dysfunctional in autism. Thus, a stereological study of the fusiform gyrus in the temporal lobe, that is thought to have impaired function in face recognition in autism, showed a reduced number of pyramidal neurons.[414] This was not confirmed in a non-stereological study.[323] The amygdala has also been studied stereologically and showed, in adolescents and adults, a reduction in neuron number that is at odds with the enlarged size detected early on in postnatal life by imaging studies.[372] This calls to mind the early brain enlargement and later tapering off of brain growth in autism. Findings of reduced neuron numbers in later life in regions that show enlargement early on could reflect more than a simple growth reduction and raise the question of whether neurodegeneration takes place later in autism – a question that at present is unanswered. Von Economo neurons, thought to potentially play a role in higher order cognitive and emotional behaviour because they are unique to great apes and humans, were increased in proportion to cortical pyramidal cells in children,[367] but were unchanged in density in adults.[257]

The cerebellum has been the subject of several studies after attention was drawn to this structure in an early MRI study.[87] The findings have variously shown reduced or unchanged densities of Purkinje cells. However, because reduced density of Purkinje cells is reported in epilepsy, which is a confounding condition in some cases of autism, autism-specific changes in the cerebellum are not yet fully defined. There are many other changes, including in neurotransmitter systems in the cerebellum, reviewed by Fatemi and colleagues.[168]

In terms of regional molecular changes in autism, mention should be made of recent studies of RNA expression and gene splicing.[74,419] Voineagu et al.[419] found that differences in gene transcript expression between frontal and temporal cortex that characterized control subjects were absent or attenuated in autism, suggesting that there is a defect in developmental patterning in autism. In the study by Chow et al.,[74] a whole genome analysis from frozen frontal lobes of autism subjects revealed that genes regulating cell number, genetic integrity and neural patterning were dysregulated in young patients and genes important for signalling, repair and response were dysregulated in older patients, with genes important for development dysregulated in both groups. In the cerebellum and cerebrum, reductions have been found in reelin mRNA with associated upregulation of the reelin receptor, a finding of interest because the *RELN* gene has been implicated in genetic studies of autism and the protein has a major role in neurodevelopment.

A widely explored hypothesis concerning the brain in autism is that there is an imbalance that arises between inhibitory and excitatory influences. Reduction in inhibitory influences exerted by interneurons has been hypothesized to account for the development of epilepsy in 30 per cent of people with autism. One recent study found no difference in the density of parvalbumin or calbindin-positive interneurons (or indeed any cortical neurons) in the posterior cingulate cortex, although the cortex displayed irregularities of cytoarchitecture and poor definition of laminar structure.[323] However, enzymes required for GABA synthesis, glutamic acid decarboxylase types 65 and 67, have shown reduced activity in cerebellum and parietal cortex.[168] and there were also reduced levels of the GABA synthesizing enzyme glutamic acid decarboxylase-67 mRNA in Purkinje cells.[436] GABA receptors are reduced in the cerebellum and parts of the cerebral cortex and hippocampus as well (reviewed by Blatt and Fatemi[44]). In animal models of some syndromal forms of autism (Rett syndrome, mutant mice deficient in the gene *SHANK3)*, disturbance of GABAergic neuronal function seems to play a particularly important part in the phenotype. For example, in a mouse model of Rett syndrome in which the transcription repressor MECP2 is defective, knocking out the gene selectively from forebrain GABAergic neurons almost as effectively reproduces the Rett phenotype (including autistic features) as does knocking out the gene from the entire nervous system (reviewed by Marin[286]). There are also alterations in expression of glutamate system genes in autism as well, for example, upregulation of AMPA receptor subunits GluR1-3 (reviewed by Polsek et al.[341]). Much more research is needed in order to clarify the relative contributions of differing neuronal groups to the overall autistic phenotype, but a start has been made.

Dyslexia

Acquisition of the ability to read text is a key index of educational development and presumably depends in part on the course of CNS development. Relative delay in reading is a matter of concern to parents and educators. Much debate has centred on the notion that there is a specific condition with a defined pathophysiology that perhaps requires special treatment.[97] Proponents of the concept define specific reading retardation as poor reading in relation to intelligence.[361] This definition is consistent with the concept that the condition is at one end of a continuum of variation in the population, but it requires that reading ability and intelligence be defined independently and be measurable.

The absence of an understanding of the cerebral basis of 'intelligence' or the mechanism by which the ability to decode and reproduce words is acquired makes progress difficult. However, the concept proposed by Orton,[326] that delays in reading (and in speech) are related to a delay in hemispheric specialization (as demonstrated e.g. by an increased rate of ambidexterity and difficulty in distinguishing left from right), has attracted support and has the potential to cast light on normal mechanisms of acquisition of speech and reading ability. The concept is supported by observations on an index of relative hand skill at the age of 11 years extracted from the data recorded in the UK National Child Development Study.[127] Children who were close to the point of equal hand skill ('hemispheric indecision') were delayed in reading ability relative to those who were more strongly lateralized, and the former were also disadvantaged in verbal and non-verbal ability. The findings are consistent with the concept that the dimension of lateralization is a major determinant of the rate of development of the ability to formulate and interpret words. Of particular interest are sex differences: girls at the age of 11 years are more lateralized than boys and have a striking advantage in verbal ability. For reading, the sex difference is more complex: boys have a slight overall advantage, except those close to the point of hemispheric indecision (i.e. ambidexterity), who are significantly more impaired. This difference is relevant to the male excess of reading difficulties in the general population,[302] but it also indicates that reading has a more complex relationship to hemispheric lateralization than does the acquisition of spoken words. One can speculate that 'grapheme' to 'phoneme' conversion requires a transition from a spatial representation in one hemisphere to a linear representation in the other in a way that the acquisition of phonemes requires only that the engram is established in the dominant hemisphere.

The concept that ambidexterity ('hemispheric indecision') defines a region of vulnerability with respect to cognitive ability is much strengthened by the findings of a large Internet survey.[339] Those who described themselves with mixed handedness were at significantly increased risk of deficits in spatial ability and dyslexia.

Orton's concept implies that there are variations in symmetry–asymmetry in the population and that those who experience reading difficulties are closer to symmetry. There is anatomical support from MRI and post-mortem studies for some change in the relative development of the two hemispheres. The MR findings include right-sided preponderance in the region of the angular gyrus and larger size of the splenium of the corpus callosum in 21 dyslexic subjects compared with 29 control participants[155] and symmetry or rightward asymmetry of the cross-sectional area of grey matter in the temporal lobe in 17 dyslexic subjects relative to leftward asymmetry in 12 control participants and 6 subjects with delayed reading.[134] A reduction in the ratio of the length of the right planum temporale to that of the right planum parietale in 9 subjects with dyslexia compared with 12 controls is also reported,[275] although in another study no consistent deviation in asymmetry of the planum temporale or planum parietale was found in 16 dyslexic men compared with 14 control subjects.[360] In a post-mortem study of five brains from individuals with dyslexia and seven brains from control subjects, Galaburda and colleagues reported a reduction in neuronal size, with fewer large and more smaller neurons in the left medial geniculate nucleus.[182] In a later study on the same set of brains, the same group found larger neurons in the primary visual cortex (area 17) on the left side in non-dyslexic brains, with a loss of this asymmetry in dyslexia.[233] These findings constitute a *prima facie* case that the primary change in dyslexia relates to asymmetries of the primary sensory and association cortex and adds to the evidence that these asymmetries relate to critical aspects of the human brain's capacity to handle the symbolic forms of language.

Attention Deficit Disorder

What has been referred to as 'attention deficit–hyperactivity disorder' (ADHD) is an ill-defined but apparently common condition associated with educational delay and behaviour disorder. Like other conditions considered in this chapter, it seems likely to represent a quantitative deviation in a dimension of neurodevelopment. In an MRI study of 57 boys with ADHD and 55 healthy, matched controls aged 5–18 years, Castellanos and colleagues reported that subjects with ADHD had 4.7 per cent smaller cerebral volume, smaller globus pallidus and anterior frontal region on the right, loss of the normal right-to-left asymmetry of the caudate, and loss of the normal asymmetry of the lateral ventricles.[61] The findings were interpreted as being consistent with dysfunction of right-sided prefrontal–striatal systems. Anomalies of asymmetry of the head of the caudate had been reported earlier by Hynd and colleagues.[227] In 15 male subjects with ADHD compared with matched controls, Filipek and colleagues similarly found a reversal of asymmetry of the caudate, with loss of substance in the right anterior frontal region, together with a loss of white matter in the parieto-occipital region.[171] Although the precise topography and meaning of the changes are unclear, there is a body of evidence that relates the pathology of ADHD to specific developmental components of the cortex and its connections. As with other disorders discussed in this chapter, there are indications that the poorly understood dimension of asymmetry is critical to pathogenesis.

Schizotypal Personality Disorder

Kretschmer formulated the view that the form of psychotic illness (i.e. whether schizophrenic or manic–depressive) was related to variations in personality and somatotype in the normal population.[269] Whereas the somatic correlates are no longer supported empirically, the concept that there are personality deviations which share characteristics with the features associated with psychotic illness in the absence of unequivocal psychotic symptoms has attracted considerable attention. It is clear that some individuals who later suffer from psychosis have differed from their peers in terms of personality characteristics that go back into childhood[126,241,423] and that an excess of 'schizophrenia spectrum disorders' is seen among the first-degree relatives of patients with typical schizophrenia.[381] The most clearly defined of such deviations is referred to as 'schizotypal disorder'. Individuals so described may suffer from 'positive symptoms', such as the feeling, without necessarily the conviction, that others are talking about or watching them, may entertain unusual beliefs outside the norms of their social group, and may be prone to superstitions and 'magical thinking'. They may also have 'negative features', such as restricted affect and social isolation.

There have been a few investigations of cerebral structure in such individuals. In a CT scan study, Siever and colleagues found that the ventricle-to-brain ratio in 36 male individuals defined as schizotypal was intermediate between that of 42 normal control subjects and 133 male patients with schizophrenia.[382] In an MRI study, Buchsbaum and colleagues observed enlargement of the left anterior and temporal horns of the lateral ventricle in 11 patients with schizophrenia compared with 23 age- and sex-matched controls, and intermediate measurements in 12 patients with schizotypal personality disorder.[53] Consistent with this and with the body of findings in schizophrenia, Dickey and colleagues noted a reduction in left superior temporal gyrus grey matter and reduced left/right asymmetry in 16 right-handed male subjects with schizotypal disorder compared with 14 healthy right-handed males matched for parental socioeconomic status and verbal ability.[150] Thus, brain structure in schizotypal personality disorder deviates in the same direction but to a lesser degree than in overt schizophrenic illness (see also Silverman *et al.*[384]). However, in the sample referred to earlier, Dickey and colleagues found that the increase in cerebrospinal fluid volume was not accounted for by an increase in ventricular size but might reflect an increase in sulcal space.[151] If in schizophrenia there is an anomalous course of development of the cerebral cortex, then this may also be the case in schizotypal disorder. The two conditions may thus represent different points on a dimension of cortical development in the general population, but with a subtle difference in the details of the morphology of the cortex.

Obsessive–Compulsive Disorder

An expanding literature on brain pathology in obsessive–compulsive disorder has arisen mainly from neuroimaging studies. It has been noted in the past that focal lesions in the striatum or pallidum can produce obsessive–compulsive disorder–like behaviour.[273] Meta-analyses of functional imaging studies have implicated the orbitofrontal cortex, the anterior cingulate/medial frontal cortex, the insula, the striatum (the caudate, in particular), and the thalamus. Magnetic resonance spectroscopy has indicated reduced N-acetylaspartate levels, which might suggest reduced neuronal density.[172] The effects of medication on structural changes are unclear. One study on non-medicated subjects found that cortical thickness was reduced in the superior temporal gyrus and the insula.[313] Some neuropharmacological success with serotonin reuptake inhibitors appears to reverse the abnormal metabolic activity seen in these corticobasal ganglia circuits, especially in the orbitofrontal cortex. Myo-inositol levels have also been implicated. MRI studies of white matter using diffusion-weighted imaging have identified altered diffusivity in multiple white matter tracts, particularly the anterior thalamic radiations and the anterior cingulum that are key components of the fronto-striato-thalamic circuits.[72] It has been suggested that there may be neuropathological overlap between obsessive–compulsive disorder, Tourette's syndrome and ADHD with each involving a slightly different combination of basal ganglia and thalamocortical pathways.[380]

Anxiety Disorders, Eating Disorders and Antisocial Behaviour

Several other disorders often characterized as having a less 'organic' aetiology have increasingly been subject to brain imaging investigations seeking to identify a neurobiological basis. Neurobiological theories of anxiety disorders have often focused on the septo-hippocampal system.[191] These have been supported by some evidence of neuroanatomical abnormalities in the hippocampus and the amygdala.[303] Antisocial behaviour, and psychopathy in particular, are often associated with an undue absence of anxiety. Psychopathy has been linked to reduced grey matter in the frontal cortex (orbitofrontal and cingulate), the temporal cortex (the superior temporal gyrus, the hippocampus and the amygdala), increased volume of the striatum, and altered white matter of the corpus callosum and the uncinate fasciculus.[263] The identification of neuropathology in eating disorders is potentially confounded by the brain changes seen as a result of malnutrition, for example sulcal widening and ventricular enlargement that improve with re-feeding in anorexia nervosa. A review of structural MRI data found that anorexia nervosa was associated with reduced grey matter and bulimia nervosa was associated with increased grey matter in the frontal and ventral striatal areas.[413] Longitudinal studies suggest that some of these effects are reduced with recovery.

Psychotic Symptoms in Other Diseases

In most cases, no other organic brain disease is detectable at the time of presentation of schizophrenia or during the course of the disease. However, in a small proportion of patients, there is other accompanying brain pathology. The proportion of cases for which this is true is hard to ascertain, as it depends to some extent on how schizophrenia is defined and on how carefully other brain pathology is sought.[139] Epilepsy, leukodystrophies, cerebral trauma, tumour, narcolepsy and Huntington's disease comprise the main associated conditions. Such organic associations are rare in the presentation of psychotic illness in general (for a critical review, see Lewis[278]) and, with the possible exceptions of epilepsy and metachromatic leukodystrophy, have not led to specific concepts of pathophysiology.

Epilepsy

It has long been recognized that some people with epilepsy also have symptoms that are clinically indistinguishable from schizophrenia. This occurs more frequently than would be expected by chance,[346] with a focus in the temporal lobe being most often associated.[225,246,298] Onset of psychosis usually occurs after the onset of seizures. For cases of temporal lobe epilepsy treated surgically, there is a variable response in terms of reversing schizophrenic symptoms. In a series of 249 temporal lobectomies[52,357] schizophrenia-like psychoses were significantly associated with lesions that (i) originated in the fetus or perinatally; (ii) affected neurons in the medial temporal lobe; and (iii) gave an early first age of seizure. Gangliogliomas were associated disproportionately ($p<0.001$) with risk of psychosis. Most patients show little improvement in their psychosis, but in occasional patients, surgery that abolishes seizures also removes the symptoms of schizophrenia. The reason for the greater-than-chance occurrence of schizophrenia with epilepsy in general, and temporal lobe epilepsy in particular, is not known. The hippocampus and amygdala could be important in generating the symptoms of both conditions, but most patients with temporal lobe epilepsy do not have schizophrenia. Attempts have been made to determine whether there is a definable subgroup of people with temporal lobe epilepsy at risk. Several studies have suggested that a left-sided focus of damage increases the risk.[174,392] A clinical study found that patients with a history of prolonged febrile convulsions in early childhood were also at more risk than others.[246] However, pathological studies have found that schizophrenia is more frequent among people with temporal lobe epilepsy and with low-grade tumours or other focal lesions with mild hippocampal pathology than in those with pure mesial temporal sclerosis, which is the pathology commonly found with prolonged febrile convulsions in infancy (see Chapter 11).[400]

Leukodystrophies

Metabolic diseases presenting in early adult life may cause symptoms initially indistinguishable from those of schizophrenia. Later, with progression of the disease process, these are superseded by frank and progressive neurological symptoms and signs. The disease best known for masquerading initially as schizophrenia is metachromatic leukodystrophy, but other types of leukodystrophy and other metabolic diseases can also present as schizophrenia. These include adrenoleukodystrophy, Kufs' disease (adult neuronal lipofuscinosis), Tay–Sachs disease, Gaucher's disease, Wilson's disease and Fabry's disease (see Chapters 6, 8 and 12).[81,226] The key feature that appears to separate patients with these diseases who do and do not have a schizophrenia-like disorder is the age of onset of symptoms rather than specific aspects of the pathology. Thus, in a review of 129 cases of metachromatic leukodystrophy, Hyde and colleagues found that 53 per cent of patients presenting between the ages of 10 and 30 years had psychotic symptoms, whereas none of the older patients did so.[226]

In considering how it comes about that such diffuse metabolic diseases can give rise, at an early stage and at the age when schizophrenia itself tends to present, to a schizophrenia-like syndrome, it is notable that there is likely to be widespread interference with axonal connectivity. The leukodystrophies often present with dysmyelination of long-distance corticocortical connections and often with axonal loss as well. The corpus callosum as well as the cerebral white matter is affected. In contrast, shorter-projecting subcortical U-fibres and intrinsic interneuronal connections are likely to be spared. An imbalance in cortical connectivity may allow the symptoms of schizophrenia to develop. Also of potential significance is oligodendrocyte pathology and the secondary regenerative effort, visible as increased activity of enzymes required for remyelination in oligodendrocytes, particularly those in the cerebral cortex overlying lesional white matter.[308] Regenerative activity associated with growth factor disturbances could influence neuronal plasticity.

Neurodegenerative Disease

Of the neurodegenerative diseases, the condition associated most frequently with a schizophrenia-like psychosis is Huntington's disease (see Chapter 12). In this condition, a schizophrenia-like disorder is described in 5–10 per cent of cases.[139,332] Huntington's disease and idiopathic schizophrenia affect both mental processes and the extrapyramidal motor system. In some cases of Huntington's disease with schizophrenia, the psychotic symptoms precede the chorea, whereas in others, both manifest around the same time. The psychotic symptoms tend to be superseded by dementia later.

Psychotic symptoms occurring in the course of dementing illness pose a diagnostic and theoretical problem. The distinction between paraphrenic (i.e. delusional) syndromes of late onset, which are more frequent in females and generally are regarded as a component of the psychosis spectrum, and the psychotic syndromes, sometimes transient, that commonly accompany an incipient dementing process is difficult and a potential source of confusion in post-mortem studies. In Alzheimer's disease, Pick's disease and dementia with Lewy bodies, there is a high frequency of psychotic symptoms that may include delusions and flattened affect.[19] If hallucinations occur, they are more commonly visual than auditory and are particularly associated with dementia with Lewy bodies (see Chapter 16, Dementia).

The question has been raised of whether brains from schizophrenia patients are more likely to show other forms of neuropathology, such as vascular lesions and Alzheimer's disease-type pathology. Again, there are conflicting reports in the literature,[197] but the slight excess of vascular lesions is likely to be due to bias in brain selection (the controls representing 'super-controls') and therefore Alzheimer's disease or another defined dementia is seen no more frequently in schizophrenia than in suitably age-matched controls. This leaves unexplained the cognitive impairment in schizophrenia that is well documented in both acute states, in which it is generally mild,[188] and patients (e.g. those with 'age disorientation')[279] in whom it may be severe. One possibility is that the brain in schizophrenia has a diminished reserve that renders age-associated changes (e.g. those related to Alzheimer's disease) capable of producing cognitive decline at levels of severity that are normally asymptomatic, but this seems an unlikely explanation of the phenomenon of temporal disorientation. The schizophrenia disease process sometimes terminates in dementia, for reasons that are unclear at present.

Other neuropathological features that have been associated with schizophrenia are cavum septum pellucidum, schizencephaly and partial agenesis of the corpus callosum.[6,144]

Depression in Alzheimer's Disease

Both the dorsal raphe and the locus coeruleus are subject to neurofibrillary tangle formation and neuron loss in Alzheimer's disease, and depression is commonly encountered in this disease. In such patients, a reduced density of 5-HT endings has been reported in the cerebral cortex,[48,70,445,446] although the extent of neurofibrillary tangle formation and loss of 5-HT neurons in the dorsal raphe was unrelated to depression.[71] Earlier claims that depression in Alzheimer's disease is correlated with the extent of neuronal loss in the locus coeruleus were not confirmed by Hoogendijk and colleagues.[222]

In summary, neuropathological studies have been extended from psychosis to depression to reveal gross morphological and cellular changes in some respects comparable to those seen in psychosis, but the replicability and meaning of these changes is as yet unclear.

CONCLUSIONS

The conditions reviewed in this chapter have some anatomical and pathological features in common. They are all perceived as having an origin in brain development. The dimension of asymmetry has played a critical role in the evolution of the human brain and may be the key to its diversity of structure and the range of deviations in development associated with psychiatric and psychological problems. The case of schizophrenia with a median onset in early adult life and severe impairments is a paradigm. Here, there is evidence for ventricular enlargement that may reflect a delay in cortical development associated with a failure or reversal of lateralization that interacts in an as yet ill-understood way with sex. The sex differences are a possible clue to the genetic basis: a gene in a region of X–Y homology has been postulated to play a role in the evolution of cerebral asymmetry.[112,115,116,429] The psychoses are associated with alterations in brain size – generally a reduction, but enlargement in some cases of autism – and with reduced size, variable between studies and/or conditions, of some neurons. There is generally little or no gliosis associated with these changes.

That bipolar disorder and major depressive disorder show similar but generally less pronounced brain changes to those of schizophrenic psychoses supports the hypothesis that these disorders represent a spectrum of altered development reflected in brain structure and asymmetry. Greater understanding of brain growth and maturation in normal subjects, including the influence of sex, are probably needed before full sense can be made of all the findings in this group of disorders. The absence of major nerve cell deficits in terms of numbers engenders optimism that better control or even prevention may be possible one day. The reduced size of neurons provokes speculation about whether a growth factor or factors may be deficient or whether small size is a consequence of an imbalance of neurotransmission. Progress in documenting neuropathology in these psychiatric disorders should encourage further careful, systematic investigation.

REFERENCES

1. Abrahao AL, Focaccia R, Gattaz WF. Childhood meningitis increases the risk for adult schizophrenia. *World J Biol Psychiatry* 2005;6:44–8.
2. Akbarian S, Bunney WE, Potkin SG, *et al.* Altered distribution of nicotinamide-adenine dinucleotide phosphate-diaphorase cells in frontal lobe of schizophrenics implies disturbances of cortical development. *Arch Gen Psychiatry* 1993;50:169–77.
3. Akbarian S, Kim JJ, Potkin SG, *et al.* Gene expression for glutamic acid decarboxylase is reduced without loss of neurons in prefrontal cortex of schizophrenics. *Arch Gen Psychiatry* 1995;52:258–78.
4. Akbarian S, Kim JJ, Potkin SG, Hetrick WP, Bunney WE, Jones EG. Maldistribution of interstitial neurones in prefrontal white matter in the brains of schizophrenic patients. *Arch Gen Psychiatry* 1996;53:425–36.
5. Albanese AM, Merlo AB, Mascitti TA, Gomez EE, Konopka V, Albanese EF. Inversion of hemispheric laterality of the anterior cingulate gyrus in schizophrenics. *Biol Psychiatry* 1995;38:13–21.
6. Alexander RC, Patkar AA, Lapointe JS, Flynn SW, Honer WG. Schizencephaly associated with psychosis. *J Neurol Neurosurg Psychiatry* 1997;63:373–5.
7. Allendoerfer K, Shatz CJ. The subplate, a transient neocortical structure: its role in the development of connections between thalamus and cortex. *Annu Rev Neurosci* 1994;17:185–218.
8. American Psychiatric Association. *Diagnostic and statistical manual of mental disorders* (DSM-IV). Washington DC: American Psychiatric Association; 1994.
9. Anderson SA, Volk DW, Lewis DA. Increased density of microtubule associated protein 2-immunoreative neurons in the prefrontal white matter of schizophrenic subjects. *Schizophr Res* 1996;19:111–9.
10. Andreasen NC, Rajarethinam R, Cizadlo T, *et al.* Automatic atlas-based volume estimation of human brain regions from mr images. *J Comput Assist Tomogr* 1996;20:98–106.
11. Annett M. *Handedness and brain asymmetry: the right shift theory.* Hove, Sussex: Psychology Press; 2002.
12. Annett M, Annett J. Handedness for eating in gorillas. *Cortex* 1991;27:269–75.
13. Arango V, Underwood MD, Mann JJ. Fewer pigmented locus coeruleus neurons in suicide victims: preliminary results. *Biol Psychiatry* 1996;39:112–20.
14. Arendt T, Bigl V, Arendt A, Tennstedt A. Loss of neurons in the nucleus basalis of Meynert in Alzheimer's disease, paralysis agitans and Korsakoff's disease. *Acta Neuropathol* 1983;61:101–8.
15. Arnold SE, Trojanowski J. Recent advances in defining the neuropathology of schizophrenia. *Acta Neuropathol* 1996;92:217–31.
16. Arnold SE, Hyman BT, Van-Hoesen GW, Damaslo AE. Some cytoarchitectural abnormalities of the entorhinal cortex in schizophrenia. *Arch Gen Psychiatry* 1991;48:625–32.
17. Arnold SE, Franz B, Gur RC, Shapiro R, Moberg P, Trojanowski J. Smaller neuron size in schizophrenia in hippocampal subfields that mediate cortical-hippocampal interactions. *Am J Psychiatry* 1995;152:738–48.
18. Bakhshi K, Borne C, Funchal B, Chance S, editors. *Age effects on brain microstructure in schizophrenia: a meta-analysis and meta-regression of neuron density.* 14th International Congress on Schizophrenia Research; Orlando, FL: April 21-25, 2013.
19. Ballard C, Ayre G, Gray A. Psychotic symptoms and behavioural disturbances in dementia. A review. *Rev Neurol* 1999;55(Suppl 4):544–52.
20. Barrett RJ. Kurt Schneider in Borneo: do first rank symptoms of schizophrenia apply to the Iban? American Anthropological Association 1997; 96th Annual Meeting:84–5.
21. Barrick TR, Mackay CE, Prima S, Vandermeulen D, Crow TJ, Roberts N. Automatic analysis of cerebral asymmetry: an exploratory study of the relationship between brain torque and planum temporale asymmetry. *Neuroimage* 2005;24:678–91.
22. Barta PE, Pearlson GD, Powers RE, *et al.* Auditory hallucinations and superior temporal gyrus volume in schizophrenia. *Am J Psychiatry* 1990;147:1457–62.
23. Barta PE, Pearlson GD, Brill LB, *et al.* Planum temporale asymmetry in schizophrenia: replication and relationship to grey matter abnormalities. *Am J Psychiatry* 1997;154:662–7.
24. Bartley AJ, Jones DW, Torrey EF, Zigun JR, Weinberger DR. Sylvian fissure asymmetries in monozygotic twins: a test of laterality in schizophrenia. *Biol Psychiatry* 1993;34:853–63.
25. Bartzokis G, Neuchterlein KH, Marder SR. Age at illness onset and left temporal lobe length in males with schizophrenia. *Psychiatry Res* 1996;67:189–201.
26. Bauman ML, Kemper TL. Neuroanatomic observations of the brain in autism. In: Bauman ML, Kemper TL, editors. *The neurobiology of autism.* Baltimore: John Hopkins University Press; 1994. p. 119–45.
27. Baumann B, Danos P, Diekmann S, *et al.* Tyrosine hydroxylase immunoreactivity in the locus coeruleus is reduced in depressed non-suicidal patients but normal in depressed suicide patients. *Eur Arch Psychiatry Clin Neurosci* 1999;249:212–9.
28. Beasley CL, Reynolds GP. Parvalbumin-immunoreactive neurons are reduced in thre prefrontal cortex of schizophrenics. *Schizophr Res* 1997;24:349–51.
29. Beasley CL, Zhang ZJ, Patten I, Reynolds GP. Selective deficits in prefrontal cortical GABAergic neurons in schizophrenia defined by the presence of calcium-binding proteins. *Biol Psychiatry* 2002;52:708–15.
30. Beasley CL, Chana G, Honavar M, Landau S, Everall IP, Cotter D. Evidence for altered neuronal organisation within the planum temporale in major psychiatric disorders. *Schizophr Res* 2005;73:69–78.
31. Beckmann H, Lauer M. The human striatum in schizophrenia. II. Increased number of striatal neurons in schizophrenics. *Psychiatry Res* 1997;68:99–109.
32. Benes FM, Bird ED. An analysis of the arrangement of neurons in the cingulate cortex of schiziophrenic patients. *Arch Gen Psychiatry* 1987;44:608–16.
33. Benes FM, Davidson J, Bird ED. Quantitive cytoarchitectural studies of the cerebral cortex of schizophrenics. *Arch Gen Psychiatry* 1986;43:31–5.
34. Benes FM, Majocha RE, Bird ED, Marotta CA. Increased vertical axon numbers in cingulate cortex of schizophrenics. *Arch Gen Psychiatry* 1987;44:1017–21.
35. Benes FM, McSparren J, Bird ED, SanGiovanni JP, Vincent SL. Deficits in small linterneurones in prefrontal and cingulate cortices of schizophrenic and schizoaffective patients. *Arch Gen Psychiatry* 1991;48:996–1001.
36. Benes FM, Sorensen I, Bird ED. Reduced neuronal size in posterior hippocampus of schizophrenic patients. *Schizophr Bull* 1991;17:597–608.
37. Benes FM, Sorensen I, Vincent SL, Bird ED, Sathi M. Increased density of glutamate-immunoreactive vertical processes in superficial laminae in cingulate cortex of schizophrenic brain. *Cereb Cortex* 1992;2:503–12.
38. Benes FM, Kwok EW, Vincent SL, Todtenkopf MS. A reduction of nonpyramidal cells in sector CA2 of schizohrenics and manic–depressives. *Biol Psychiatry* 1998;44:88–97.
39. Bernstein HG, Stanarius A, Baumann B, *et al.* Nitric oxide synthase-containing neurons in the human hypothalamus: reduced number of immunoreactive cells in the paraventricular nucleus of depressive patients and schizophrenics. *Neuroscience* 1998;83:867–75.
40. Bickerton D. *Language and human behavior.* Seattle: University of Washington; 1995.
41. Bilder RM, Wu H, Bogerts B, *et al.* Absence of regional hemispheric volume asymmetries in first episode schizophrenia. *Am J Psychiatry* 1994;151:1437–47.
42. Bilder RM, Wu H, Degreef G, *et al.* Yakovlevian torque is absent in first episode schizophrenia. *Am J Psychiatry* 1994;151:1437–47.
43. Bilder RM, Wu H, Bogerts B, *et al.* Cerebral volume asymmetries in schizophrenia and mood disorders: a quantitative magnetic resonance imaging study. *Int J Psychophysiol* 1999;34:197–205.
44. Blatt GJ, Fatemi SH. Alterations in GABAergic biomarkers in the autism brain: research findings and clinical implications. *Anat Rec* (Hoboken) 2011;294:1646–52.
45. Bogerts B, Ashtari M, Degreef G, Alvir JMJ, Bilder RM, Lieberman J. Reduced temporal limbic structure volumes on magnetic resonance images in first episode schizophrenia. *Psychiatry Res* 1990;35:1–13.
46. Bogerts B, Lieberman JA, Ashtari M, *et al.* Hippocampus-amygdala volumes and psychopathology in chronic schizophrenia. *Biol Psychiatry* 1993;33:236–46.
47. Bora E, Fornito A, Radua J, *et al.* Neuroanatomical abnormalities in schizophrenia: a multimodal voxelwise meta-analysis and meta-regression analysis. *Schizophr Res* 2011;127:46–57.
48. Bowen DM, Najlerahim A, Procter AW, Francis PT, Murphy E. Circumscribed

changes in the cerebral cortex in neuropsychiatric disorders of later life. *Proc Natl Acad Sci U S A* 1999;26:9504–8.

49. Braak H, Braak E. Golgi preparations as a tool in neuropathology with particular reference to investigations of the human telencephalic cortex. *Prog Neurobiol* 1985;25:93–139.

50. Briess D, Cotter D, Doshi R, Everall I. Mamillary body abnormalities in schizophrenia (letter). *Lancet* 1998;352:789–90.

51. Broca P. Remarques sur la sisge de la faculte du langue. *Bull Soc Anatom de Paris* (2nd series) 1861;6:330–57.

52. Bruton CJ. *The neuropathology of temporal lobe epilepsy.* The Maudsley Monograph No 31. Oxford: Oxford University Press; 1988.

53. Buchsbaum MS, Yang S, Hazlett E, *et al.* Ventricular volume and asymmetry in schizotypal personality disorder and schizophrenia assessed with magnetic resonance imaging. *Schizophr Res* 1997;27:45–53.

54. Buchsbaum MS, Tang CY, Peled S, *et al.* MRI white matter diffusion anisotrophy and PET metabolic rate in schizophrenia. *Neuroreport* 1998;9:425–30.

55. *Psychol Med* 1994;24:771–81.

56. Bullmore E, Brammer M, Harvey I, Murray R, Ron M. Cerebral hemispheric asymmetry revisited: effects of handedness, gender and schizophrenia measured by radius of gyration in magnetic resonance images. *Psychol Med* 1995;25:349–63.

57. Cannon M, Cotter D, Coffey VP, *et al.* Prenatal exposure to the 1957 influenza epidemic and adult schizophrenia: a follow up study. *Br J Psychiatry* 1996;168:368–71.

58. Cannon M, Jones PB, Murray RM. Obstetric complications and schizophrenia; historical and meta-analytic review. *Am J Psychiatry* 2002;159:1080–92.

59. Casanova MF, Zito M, Bigelow LB, Berthot B, Sanders RD, Kleinman JE. Axonal counts of the corpus callosum of schizophrenic patients. *J Neuropsychiatry Clin Neurosci* 1989;1:391–3.

60. Casanova MF, van Kooten IA, Switala AE, *et al.* Minicolumnar abnormalities in autism. *Acta Neuropathol* 2006; 112: 287–303.

61. Castellanos FX, Giedd JN, Marsh WL, *et al.* Quantitative brain magnetic resonance imaging in attention-deficit hyperactivity disorder. *Arch Gen Psychiatry* 1996;53:607–16.

62. Chana GS, Landau S, Beasley C, Everall IP, Cotter D. Two-dimensional assessment of cytoarchitecture in the anterior cingulate cortex in major depressive disorder, bipolar disorder, and schizophrenia: evidence for decreased neuronal somal size and increased neuronal density. *Biol Psychiatry* 2003;53:1086–98.

63. Chance SA, Highley JR, Esiri MM, Crow TJ. Fibre content of the fornix in schizophrenia: Lack of evidence for a primary limbic encephalopathy. *Am J Psychiatry* 1999;156:1720–4.

64. Chance SA, Esiri MM, Crow TJ. Amygdala volume in schizophrenia: post-mortem study and review of magnetic resonance imaging findings. *Br J Psychiatry* 2002;180:331–8.

65. Chance SA, Esiri MM, Crow TJ. Ventricular enlargement in schizophrenia: a primary change in the temporal lobe? *Schizophr Res* 2003;62:123–31.

66. Chance SA, Esiri MM, Crow TJ. Macroscopic brain asymmetry is changed along the antero-posterior axis in schizophrenia. *Schizophr Res* 2005;74:163–70.

67. Chance SA, Walker MA, Crow TJ. Reduced density of calbindin-immunoreactive interneurons in the planum temporale in schizophrenia. *Brain Res* 2005;1046:32–7.

68. Chance SA, Casanova MF, Switala AE, Crow TJ. Minicolumnar structure in Heschl's gyrus and planum temporale: asymmetries in relation to sex and callosal fiber number. *Neuroscience* 2006 Dec 28;143:1041–50.

69. Chance SA, Casanova MF, Switala AE, Crow TJ. Auditory cortex asymmetry, altered minicolumn spacing and absence of ageing effects in schizophrenia. *Brain* 2008 Dec;131:3178–92.

70. Chen C, Alder JT, Bowen DM, *et al.* Presynaptic serotonergic markers in community-acquired cases of Alzheimer's disease: correlations with depression and neuroleptic medication. *J Neurochem* 1996;66:1592–8.

71. Chen C, Eastwood SL, Hope T, *et al.* Immunocytochemical study of the dorsal and median raphe nuclei in patients with Alzheimer's disease prospectively assessed for behavioural changes. *Neuropathol Appl Neurobiol* 2000;26:347–55.

72. Chiu CH, Lo YC, Tang HS, *et al.* White matter abnormalities of fronto-striato-thalamic circuitry in obsessive–compulsive disorder: A study using diffusion spectrum imaging tractography. *Psychiatry Res* 2011;192:176–82.

73. Chomsky N. *Knowledge of language: Its nature, origin and use.* New York: Praeger; 1985.

74. Chow ML, Pramparo T, Winn ME, *et al.* Age-dependent brain gene expression and copy number anomalies in autism suggest distinct pathological processes at young versus mature ages. *PLoS Genet* 2012;8:e1002592.

75. Christison GW, Casanova MF, Weinberger DR, Rawlings R, Kleinman JE. A quantitative investigation of hippocampal pyramidal cell shape and variability of orientation in schizophrenia. *Arch Gen Psychiatry* 1989;46:1027–32.

76. Chu O, Olsen SC, Nasrallah HA, Marin R, Lynn M. The left temporal horn is enlarged in both schizophrenia and bipolar disorder. *Biol Psychiatry* 1993;33:122A.

77. Chua SE, Wright I, Poline JB, *et al.* Grey matter correlates of syndromes in schizophrenia: a semi-automated analysis of structural magnetic resonance images. *Br J Psychiatry* 1997;170:406–10.

78. Cloninger CR. The discovery of susceptibility genes for mental disorders. *Proc Natl Acad Sci U S A* 2002;99:13365–7.

79. Clouston TS. *The nature of development* (The Morrison Lectures, 1890). Edinburgh, Scotland: Oliver & Boyd; 1890.

80. Coggeshall RE, Lekan HA. Methods for determining numbers of cells and synapses. A case for more uniform standards of review. *J Comp Neurol* 1996;364:6–15.

81. Coker SB. The diagnosis of childhood neurodegenerative disorders presenting as dementia in adults. *Neurology* 1991;41:794–8.

82. Collins AL, Kim Y, Sklar P, *et al.* Hypothesis-driven candidate genes for schizophrenia compared to genome-wide association results. *Psychol Med* 2012;42:607–16.

83. Connell PH. *Amphetaminepsychosis.* Maudsley Monograph No 5. London 1958.

84. Cotter D, Kerwin R, Doshi B, Martin CS, Everall IP. Alterations in hippocampal non-phosphorylated MAP2 protein expression in schizophrenia. *Brain Res* 1997;765:238–46.

85. Cotter D, Landau S, Beasley C, *et al.* The density and spatial distribution of GABAergic neurons, labelled using calcium binding proteins, in the anterior cingulate cortex in major depressive disorder, bipolar disorder, and schizophrenia. *Biol Psychiatry* 2002;51:377–86.

86. Cotter D, Mackay D, Chana G, Beasley C, Laundau S, Everall IP. Reduced neuronal size and glial cell density in area 9 of the dorsolateral prefrontal cortex in subjects with major depressive disorder. *Cereb Cortex* 2002;12:386–94.

87. Courchesne E, Yeung-Courchesne R, Press GA, Hesselink JR, Jernigan TL. Hypoplasia of cerebellar vermal lobules VI and VII in autism. *N Engl J Med* 1988;318:1349–54.

88. Courchesne E, Carper R, Akshoomoff N. Evidence of brain overgrowth in the first year of life in autism. *JAMA* 2003;290:337–44.

89. Courchesne E, Pierce K, Schumann CM, *et al.* Mapping early brain development in autism. *Neuron* 2007;56:399–413.

90. Courchesne E, Mouton PR, Calhoun ME, *et al.* Neuron number and size in prefrontal cortex of children with autism. *JAMA* 2011;306:2001–10.

91. Cowell PE, Allen LS, Zalatimo NS, Denenberg VE. A developmental study of sex and age interactions in the human corpus callosum. Developmental Brain Research 1992;66:187–92.

92. Craddock N, O'Donovan MC, Owen MJ. The genetics of schizophrenia and bipolar disorder: dissecting psychosis. *J Med Genet* 2005;42:193–204.

93. Craddock N, O'Donovan MC, Owen MJ. Genes for schizophrenia and bipolar disorder? Implications for psychiatric nosology. *Schizophr Bull* 2006;32:9–16.

94. Craven RM, Priddle TH, Cooper SJ, Crow TJ, Esiri MM. The dorsal raphe nucleus in schizophrenia: a post mortem study of 5-hydroxytryptamine neurones. *Neuropathol Appl Neurobiol* 2005;31:258–69.

95. Craven RM, Priddle TH, Crow TJ, Esiri MM. The locus coeruleus in schizophrenia: a postmortem study of noradrenergic neurones. *Neuropathol Appl Neurobiol* 2005;31:115–26.

96. Crichton-Browne J. On the weight of the brain and its component parts in the insane. *Brain* 1879;2:42–67.

97. Critchley M. Developmental dyslexia: a constitutional disorder of symbolic perception. *Res Publ Assoc Res Nerv Ment Dis* 1970;48:266–71.

98. Crow TJ. The two-syndrome concept: origins and current status. *Schizophr Bull* 1985;11:471–86.

99. Crow TJ. The Lieber Award acceptance lecture. September 8, 1989. *Schizophr Res* 1990;3:99–102.

100. Crow TJ. Prenatal exposure to influenza as a cause of schizophrenia; there are inconsistencies and contradictions in the evidence. *Br J Psychiatry* 1994;**164**:588–92.

101. Crow TJ. The case for an X-Y homologous determinant of cerebral asymmetry. *Cytogen Cell Genet* 1994;**67**:393–4.

102. Crow TJ. Constraints on concepts of pathogenesis: language and the speciation process as the key to the etiology of schizophrenia. *Arch Gen Psychiatry* 1995;**52**:1011–4.

103. Crow TJ. Is schizophrenia the price that *Homo sapiens* pays for language? *Schizophr Res* 1997;**28**:127–41.

104. Crow TJ. What was the evidence that prenatal exposure to influenza causes schizophrenia? *Br J Psychiatry* 1997;**169**:790–1.

105. Crow TJ. Schizophrenia as failure of hemispheric dominance for language. *Trends Neurosci* 1997;**20**:339–43.

106. Crow TJ. Influenza and schizophrenia. *Br J Psychiatry* 1997;**170**:578–9.

107. Crow TJ. Why cerebral asymmetry is the key to the origin of *Homo sapiens*: how to find the gene or eliminate the theory. *Curr Psychol Cogn* 1998;**17**:1237–77.

108. Crow TJ. Sexual selection, timing and the descent of Man: a genetic theory of the evolution of language. *Curr Psychol Cogn* 1998;**17**:1079–114.

109. Crow TJ. From Kraepelin to Kretschmer leavened by K Schneider: the transition from categories of psychosis to dimensions of variation intrinsic to *Homo sapiens Arch Gen Psychiatry* 1998;**55**:502–4.

110. Crow TJ. Commentary on Klaening: twin studies of psychosis and the genetics of cerebral asymmetry. *Br J Psychiatry* 1999;**175**:399–401.

111. Crow TJ. Twin studies of psychosis and the genetics of cerebral asymmetry. *Br J Psychiatry* 1999;**175**:399–401.

112. Crow TJ. Did *Homo sapiens* speciate on the Y chromosome? *Psycoloquy* 2000;**11**(001).

113. Crow TJ. Invited commentary on: Functional anatomy of verbal fluency in people with schizophrenia and those at genetic risk. *Br J Psychiatry* 2000;**176**:61–3.

114. Crow TJ. Schizophrenia as the price that *Homo sapiens* pays for language: a resolution of the central paradox in the origin of the species. *Brain Res Rev* 2000;**31**:118–29.

115. Crow TJ. ProtocadherinXY: A candidate gene for cerebral asymmetry and language. In: Wray A, editor. *The transition to language.* Oxford: Oxford University Press; 2002, p. 93–112.

116. Crow TJ editor. *The speciation of modern Homo sapiens.* Oxford: Oxford University Press; 2002.

117. Crow TJ. Sexual selection, timing and an X-Y homologous gene: did *Homo sapiens* speciate on the Y chromosome? In: Crow TJ, editor. *The speciation of modern Homo sapiens.* Oxford: Oxford University Press; 2002, p. 195–216.

118. Crow TJ. How and why genetic linkage has not solved the problem of psychosis: review and hypothesis. *Am J Psychiatry* 2007;**164**:13–21.

119. Crow TJ. Schizophrenia as variation in the sapiens-specific epigenetic instruction to the embryo. *Clin Genet* 2012;**81**: 319–24.

119a. Crow TJ. The XY gene hypothesis of psychosis: origins and current status. *Am J Med Genet B Neuropsychiatr Genet* 2013 Dec;**162**:800–24. doi:10.1002/ajmg.b.32202.

120. Crow TJ, Done DJ. Age of onset of schizophrenia in siblings: a test of the contagion hypothesis. *Psychiatry Res* 1986;**18**:107–17.

121. Crow TJ, Done DJ. Prenatal exposure to influenza does not cause schizophrenia. *Br J Psychiatry* 1992;**161**:390–3.

122. Crow TJ, Mitchell WS. Subjective age in chronic schizophrenia: evidence for a sub-group of patients with defective learning capacity? *Br J Psychiatry* 1975;**126**:360–3.

123. Crow TJ, Owens DGC, Johnstone EC, Cross AJ, Owen F. Does tardive dyskinesia exist? *Mod Probl Pharmacopsychiatry* 1983;**21**:206–19.

124. Crow TJ, Ball J, Bloom SR, et al. Schizophrenia as an anomaly of development of cerebral asymmetry. A postmortem study and a proposal concerning the genetic basis of the disease. *Arch Gen Psychiatry* 1989;**46**:1145–50.

125. Crow TJ, Colter N, Frith CD, Johnstone EC, Owens DGC. Developmental arrest of cerebral asymmetries in early onset schizophrenia. *Psychiatry Res* 1989;**29**:247–53.

126. Crow TJ, Done DJ, Sacker A. Childhood precursors of psychosis as clues to its evolutionary origins. *Eur Arch Psychiatry Clin Neurosci* 1995;**245**:61–9.

127. Crow TJ, Crow LR, Done DJ, Leask SJ. Relative hand skill predicts academic ability: global deficits at the point of hemispheric indecision. *Neuropsychologia* 1998;**36**:1275–82.

128. Crow TJ, Chance SA, Priddle TH, Radua J, James AC. Laterality and sex interat cross the schizophrneia/bipolarity continuum: an interpretation of structural MRI meta-analyses. *Psychiatry Res* 2013;**210**:1232–44.

129. Csernansky JG, Gillespie JG, Gillespie SK, et al. Symmetric abnormalities in sulcal patterning in schizophrenia. *Neuroimage* 2008;**43**:440–6.

130. Cullberg J, Nyback H. Persistent auditory hallucinations correlate with the size of the third ventricle in schizophrenia patients. *Acta Psychiatr Scand* 1992;**86**:469–72.

131. Cullen TJ, Walker MA, Roberts H, Crow TJ, Harrison PJ, Esiri MM. The medio-dorsal nucleus of the thalamus in schizophrenia: a post-mortem study. *Schizophr Res* 2000;**41**:5.

132. Cullen TJ, Walker MA, Eastwood SL, Esiri MM, Harrison PJ, Crow TJ. Anomalies of asymmetry of pyramidal cell density and structure in doroslateral prefrontal cortex in schizophrenia. *Brit J Psychiatry* 2006;**188**:26–31.

133. Cunningham DJ. *Contribution to the surface anatomy of the cerebral hemispheres.* Dublin: Academy House; 1892.

134. Dalby MA, Elbro C, Stodkilde-Jorgenson H. Temporal lobe asymmetry and dyslexia: an in vivo study using MRI. *Brain Lang* 1998;**62**:51–69.

135. Daniel DG, Goldberg TE, Gibbons RD, Weinberger DR. Lack of a bimodal distribution of ventricular size in schizophrenia: A Gaussian mixture analysis of 1056 cases and controls. *Biol Psychiatry* 1991;**30**:886–903.

136. Danos P, Baumann B, Bernstein HG, et al. Schizophrenia and anteroventral thalamic nucleus: selective decrease of parvalbumin-immunoreactive thalamo projection neurons. *Psychiatry Res* 1998;**82**:1–10.

137. Davis KL, Kahn RS, Ko G, Davidson M. Dopamine in schizophrenia: a review and reconceptualization. *Am J Psychiatry* 1991;**148**:1474–86.

138. Davis KL, Buchsbaum MS, Shihabuddin L, et al. Ventricular enlargement in poor outcome schizophrenia. *Biol Psychiatry* 1998;**43**:783–93.

139. Davison K, Bagley CR. Schizophrenia-like psychoses associated with organic disorders of the central nervous system: a review of the literature. In: Herrington RN, editor. *Current problems in neuropsychiatry, schizophrenia, epilepsy, the temporal lobe.* Kent: Headley; 1969, p. 113–84.

140. Daviss SR, Lewis DA. Local circuit neurons of the prefrontal cortex in schizophrenia: selective increase in the density of calbindin-immunoreactive neurons. *Psychiatry Res* 1995;**59**:81–96.

141. Dawson G, Munson J, Webb SJ, Nalty T, Abbott R, Toth K. Rate of head growth decelerates and symptoms worsen in the second year of life in autism. *Biol Psychiatry* 2007;**61**:458–64.

142. Dax M. L'sions de la moitie gauche de l'encephale coincident avec l'oubli des signes de la pensee (Read at congres meridional at Montpelier in 1836). *Gaz Hebdom Med Chirurg* 1865;**11**:259–60.

143. Degreef G, Ashtari M, Bogerts B, et al. Volumes of ventricular system subdivisions measured from magnetic resonance images in first episode schizophrenic patients. *Arch Gen Psychiatry* 1992;**49**:531–7.

144. De Greef G, Bogerts B, Falkai P, et al. Increased prevalence of the cavum septum pellucidum in MRI scans and post mortem brains of schizophrenic patients. *Psychiatry Res Neuroimaging* 1992;**45**:1–13.

145. DeLisi LE, Sakuma M, Tew W, Kushner M, Grimson R. Schizophrenia as a chronic active disease process: a study of progressive structural brain change subsequent to the onset of schizophrenia. *Psychiatry Res* 1997;**74**:129–40.

146. DeLisi LE, Sakuma M, Maurizio AM, Relja M, Hoff AL. Cerebral ventricular change over the first 10 years after the onset of schizophrenia. *Psychiatry Res Neuroimaging* 2004;**130**:57–70.

147. Dementieva YA, Vance DD, Donnelly SL, et al. Accelerated head growth in early development of individuals with autism. *Pediatr Neurol* 2005;**32**:102–8.

148. Di Rosa E, Crow TJ, Chance SA. Axon bundle spacing in the anterior cingulate cortex of the human brain. *J Clin Neurosci* 2008;**15**:1389–92.

149. Di Rosa E, Crow TJ, Walker MA, Black G, Chance SA. Reduced neuron density, enlarged minicolumn spacing and altered ageing effects in fusiform cortex in schizophrenia. *Psychiatry Res* 2009;**166**:102–15.

150. Dickey CC, McCarley RW, Voglmaier MM, et al. Schizotypal personality disorder and MRI abnormalities of temporal lobe gray matter. *Biol Psychiatry* 1999;**45**:1393–402.

151. Dickey CC, Shenton ME, Hirayasu Y, et al. Large CSF volume not attributable to ventricular volume in schizotypal personality disorder. *Am J Psychiatry* 2000;**157**:48–54.

152. Dorph-Petersen KA, Pierri JN, Wu Q, Sampson AR, Lewis DA. Primary visual cortex volume and total neuron number are reduced in schizophrenia. *J Comp Neurol* 2007;**501**:290–301.

153. Drevets WC, Price JL, Simpson JR, et al. Subgenual prefrontal cortex abnormalities in mood disorder. *Nature* 1997;**386**:824–7.

154. Drevets WC, Frank E, Price JL, et al. PET imaging of serotonin 1A receptor binding in depression. *Biol Psychiatry* 1999;**46**:1375–87.

155. Duara R, Kushch A, Gross-Glen K, et al. Neuroanatomic differences between dyslexic and normal readers on magnetic resonance imaging scans. *Arch Neurol* 1991;**48**:410–6.

156. Eastwood SL, Harrison PJ. Interstitial white matter neurons express less reelin and are abnormally distributed in schizophrenia: towards an integration of molecular and morphological aspects of the neurodevelopmental hypothesis. *Mol Psychiatry* 2003;**8**:821–31.

157. Eaton WW, Mortenson PB, Herrman H, Freeman H, Bilker W, Burgess P, et al. Long-term course of hospitalisation for schizophrenia: I. Risk for hospitalisation. *Schizophr Bull* 1992;**18**:217–28.

158. Eberstaller O. Zur oberflächenanatomie des grosshirnhemisphären. *Wiener Medizinische Blätter.* 1884;**7**:479–82.

159. Elkis H, Friedman L, Wise A, Meltzer HY. Meta-analyses of studies of ventricular enlargement and cortical sulcal prominence in mood disorders. *Arch Gen Psychiatry* 1995;**52**:735–46.

160. Ellison-Wright I, Bullmore E. Anatomy of bipolar disorder and schizophrenia: A meta-analysis. *Schizophr Res* 2010;**117**: 1–12.

161. Ellison-Wright I, Glahn DC, Laird AR, Thelen SM, Bullmore E. The anatomy of first-episode and chronic schizophrenia: An anatomical likelihood estimation meta-analysis. *Am J Psychiatry* 2008;**165**:1015–23.

162. Endicott J, Nee J, Fleiss J, Cohen J, Williams JBW, Robert S. Diagnostic criteria for schizophrenia: reliabilities and agreement between systems. *Arch Gen Psychiatry* 1982;**39**:884–9.

163. Falkai P, Bogerts B. Cell loss in the hippocampus of schizophrenics. European Archives of Psychiatry and Neurological Science 1986;**236**:154–61.

164. Falkai P, Bogerts B, Greve B, et al. Loss of Sylvian fissure asymmetry in schizophrenia. A quantitative post-mortem study. *Schizophr Res* 1992;**7**: 23–32.

165. Falkai P, Bogerts B, Schneider T, et al. Disturbed planum temporale asymmetry in schizophrenia. A quantitative post-mortem study. *Schizophr Res* 1995;**14**:161–76.

166. Falkai P, Schneider T, Greve B, Klieser E, Bogerts B. Reduced frontal and occipital lobe asymmetry on the CT scans of schizophrenic patients: its specificity and clinical significance. J Neural Transmission - General Section 1995;**99**:63–77.

167. Fatemi SH, Earle JA, McMenomy T. Reduction in reelin immunoreactivity in hippocampus of subjects with schizophrenia, bipolar disorder and major depression. *Mol Psychiatry* 2000; 5:654–63.

168. Fatemi SH, Aldinger KA, Ashwood P, et al. Consensus paper: pathological role of the cerebellum in autism. *Cerebellum* 2012;**11**:777–807.

169. Feinberg I. Schizophrenia: caused by a fault in programmed synaptic elimination during adolescence? *J Psychiatr Res* 1983;**17**:319–34.

170. Fenn DS, Moussaoui D, Hoffman WF, et al. Movements in never-medicated schizophrenics: a preliminary study. *Psychopharmacology* (Berlin) 1996;**123**:206–10.

171. Filipek PA, Semrud-Clikeman M, Steingard RJ, Renshaw PF, Kennedy DN, Biederman J. Volumentric MRI analysis comparing subjects having attention-deficit hyperactivity disorder with normal controls. *Neurology* 1997;**48**:589–601.

172. Fitzgerald KD, Moore GJ, Paulson LA, Stewart CM, Rosenberg DR. Proton spectroscopic imaging of the thalamus in treatment-naive pediatric obsessive-compulsive disorder. *Biol Psychiatry* 2000;**47**:174–82.

173. Flaum M, O'Leary DS, Swayze VW, Miller DD, Arndt S, Andreasen NC. Symptom dimensions and brain morphology in schizophrenia and related psychotic disorders. *J Psychiatr Res* 1995;**29**:261–76.

174. Flor-Henry P. Psychosis and temporal lobe epilepsy, a controlled investigation. *Epilepsia* 1969;**10**:363–95.

175. Flor-Henry P. Hemispheric laterality and disorders of affect. In: Flor-Henry P, editor. *Cerebral basis of psychopathology.* London: John Right PSG Inc.; 1983, p. 39–61.

176. Foong J, Maier M, Barker GJ, Brocklehurst S, Miller DH, Ron MA. In vivo investigation of white matter pathology in schizophrenia with magnetisation transfer imaging. *J Neurol Neurosurg Psychiatry* 2000;**68**:70–4.

177. Fornito A, Yucel M, Patti J, Wood SJ, Pantelis C. Mapping grey matter reductions in schizophrenia: An anatomical likelihood estimation analysis of voxel-based morphometry studies. *Schizophr Res* 2009;**108**:104–13.

178. Frazier TW, Hardan AY. A meta-analysis of the corpus callosum in autism. *Biol Psychiatry* 2009;**66**:935–41.

179. Frederikse M, Lu A, Aylward EH, Barta P, Sharma T, Pearlson GD. Sex differences in inferior parietal volume in schizophrenia. *Am J Psychiatry* 2000;**157**:422–7.

180. Friedman L, Findling RL, Kenny JT, et al. An MRI study of adolescent patients with either schizophrenia or bipolar disorder as compared with healthy control subjects. *Biol Psychiatry* 1999;**46**:78–88.

181. Fukuzako H, Yamada K, Kodama S, et al. Hippocampal volume asymmetry and age at illness onset in males with schizophrenia. European Archives of Psychiatry and Clinical Neuroscience 1997;**247**:248–51.

182. Galaburda AM, Menard MT, Rosen GD. Evidence for aberrant auditory anatomy in developmental dyslexia. *Proc Natl Acad Sci U S A* 1994;**91**:8010–3.

183. Garcia-Rill E, Riedermann JA, Chambers T, et al. Mesopontine neurons in schizophrenia. *Neuroscience* 1995;**66**:321–5.

184. Geerts M, Steyaert J, Fryns JP. The XYY syndrome: a follow-up study on 38 boys. *Genet Counsel* 2003;**14**:267–79.

185. German DC, Manaye KF, Wu D, Hersh LB, Zweig RM. Mesopontine cholinergic and non-cholinergic neurons in schizophrenia. *Neuroscience* 1999; **94**:33–8.

186. Geschwind N, Levitsky W. Human brain: left-right asymmetry in temporal speech region. *Science* 1968;**161**:186–7.

187. Glahn DC, Laird AR, Ellison-Wright I, et al. Meta-analysis of gray matter anomalies in schizophrenia: Application of anatomic likelihood estimation and network analysis. *Biol Psychiatry* 2008;**64**:774–81.

188. Goldman-Rakic PS. Working memory dysfunction in schizophrenia. *J Neuropsychiatry Clin Neurosci* 1994;**6**:348–57.

189. Gonzalez-Burgos G, Lewis DA. NMDA receptor hypofunction, parvalbumin-positive neurons, and cortical gamma oscillations in schizophrenia. *Schizophr Bull* 2012;**38**:950–7.

190. Gottesman II. *Schizophrenia genesis: the origins of madness.* New York: WH Freeman; 1991.

191. Gray J, McNaughton N. *The neuro-psychology of anxiety: An enquiry into the functions of the septo-hippocampal system,* 2nd edition. New York, NY: Oxford University Press; 2000.

192. Gundersen HJG, Bagger P, Bendtsen TF, et al. The new stereological tools: Dissector, fractionator, nucleator, and point sampled intercepts and their use in pathological research and diagnosis. *APMIS* (Copenhagen) 1988;**96**:857–81.

193. Hankoff LD, Peress NS. Neuropathology of the brain stem in psychiatric disorders. *Biol Psychiatry* 1981;**16**:945–52.

194. Harasty J, Seldon HL, Chan P, Halliday G, Harding A. The left human speech-processing cortex is thinner but longer than the right. *Laterality* 2003;**8**:247–60.

195. Hare EH. Was insanity on the increase? *Br J Psychiatry* 1983;**142**:439–55.

196. Harris JM, Whalley H, Yates S, Miller P, Johnstone EC, Lawrie SM. Abnormal cortical folding in high-risk individuals: A predictor of the development of schizophrenia? *Biol Psychiatry* 2004;**56**:182–9.

197. Harrison PJ. Schizophrenia and its dementia. In: Esiri MM, Morris JH, editors. *The neuropathology of dementia.* Cambridge: Cambridge University Press; 1997, p. 385–97.

198. Harrison PJ. The neuropathology of schizophrenia: a critical review of the data and their interpretation. *Brain* 1999;**122**:593–624.

199. Harrison PJ. The hippocampus in schizophrenia: a review of the neuropathological evidence and its pathophysiological implications. *Psychopharmacol* 2004;**174**:151–62.

200. Harrison PJ, Owen MJ. Genes for schizophrenia? Recent findings and their pathophysiological implications. *Lancet* 2003;**361**:417–9.

201. Harrison PJ, Weinberger DR. Schizophrenia genes, gene expression, and neuropathology: on the matter of their convergence. *Mol Psychiatry* 2005;**10**:40–68.

202. Harrison PJ, Freemantle N, Geddes JR. Meta-analysis of brain weight in schizophrenia. *Schizophr Res* 2003;**64**:25–34.

203. Harvey I, McGuffin P, Williams M, Toone BK. The ventricle-brain ratio (VBR) in functional psychoses: an admixture analysis. *Psychiatry Res Neuroimaging* 1990;**35**:61–9.

204. Hazlett HC, Poe M, Gerig G, et al. Magnetic resonance imaging and head circumference study of brain size in autism: birth through age 2 years. *Arch Gen Psychiatry* 2005;**62**:1366–76.

205. Heckers S, Heinsen H, Heinsen YC, Beckmann H. Limbic structures and lateral ventricle in schizophrenia. A quantitative postmortem study. *Arch Gen Psychiatry* 1990;**47**:1016–22.

206. Heckers S, Heinsen H, Geiger B, Beckmann H. Hippocampal neuron number in schizophrenia. A stereological study. *Arch Gen Psychiatry* 1991;**48**:1002–8.

207. Herbert MR. Contributions of the environment and environmentally vulnerable physiology to autism spectrum disorders. *Curr Opin Neurol* 2010;**23**:103–10.

208. Herbert MR, Ziegler DA, Makris N, et al. Localization of white matter volume increase in autism and developmental language disorder. *Ann Neurol* 2004;**55**:530–40.

209. Heston LL. Psychiatric disorders in the foster-home reared children of schizophrenic mothers. *Br J Psychiatry* 1966;**112**:819–25.

210. Highley JR, Esiri MM, Cortina-Borja M, et al. Anomalies of cerebral asymmetry in schizophrenia interact with gender and age of onset: a post mortem study. *Schizophr Res* 1998;**34**:13–25.

211. Highley JR, Esiri MM, McDonald B, Cooper SJ, Crow TJ. Temporal lobe length is reduced, and gyral folding is increased in schizophrenia: a post mortem study. *Schizophr Res* 1998;**34**:1–12.

212. Highley JR, Esiri MM, McDonald B, Cortina-Borja M, Herron BM, Crow TJ. The size and fibre composition of the corpus callosum with respect to gender and schizophrenia: a post-mortem study. *Brain* 1999;**122**:99–110.

213. Highley JR, McDonald B, Walker MA, Esiri MM, Crow TJ. Schizophrenia and temporal lobe asymmetry. A post mortem stereological study of tissue volume. *Brit J Psychiatry* 1999;**175**:127–34.

214. Highley JR, Walker MA, Esiri MM, McDonald B, Harrison PJ, Crow TJ. Schizophrenia and the frontal lobes: A post mortem stereological study of tissue volume. *Brit J Psychiatry* 2001;**178**:337–43.

215. Highley JR, DeLisi LE, Roberts N, et al. Sex-dependent effects of schizophrenia: an MRI study of gyral folding, and cortical and white matter volume. *Psychiatry Res Neuroimaging* 2003;**124**:11–23.

216. Highley JR, Walker MA, Crow TJ, Esiri MM, Harrison PJ. Low medial and lateral right pulvinar volumes in schizophrenia: a post-mortem study. *Am J Psychiatry* 2003;**160**:1177–9.

217. Highley JR, Walker MA, McDonald B, Crow TJ, Esiri MM. Size of hippocampal pyramidal neurons in schizophrenia. *Brit J Psychiatry* 2003;**183**:414–7.

218. Hirayasu Y, Shenton ME, Salisbury DF, et al. Lower left temporal lobe volume with first episode schizophrenia compared with first episode affective disorder and normal subjects. *Am J Psychiatry* 1998;**155**:1384–91.

219. Hof PR, Haroutunian V, Copland C, Davis KL, Buxbaum JD. Molecular and cellular evidence for an oligodendrocyte abnormality in schizophrenia. *Neurochem Res* 2002;**27**:1193–200.

220. Hokama H, Shenton ME, Nestor PG, et al. Caudate, putamen and globus pallidus volumes in schizophrenia: a quantitative MRI study. *Psychiatry Res* 1995;**61**:209–29.

221. Honea R, Crow TJ, Passingham D, Mackay CE. Regional deficits in brain volume in schizophrenia: a meta-analysis of voxel-based morphometry studies. *Am J Psychiatry* 2005;**162**:2233–45.

222. Hoogendijk WJ, Sommer IEC, Pool CW, et al. Lack of association between depression and loss of neurons in the locus coeruleus in Alzheimer's disease. *Arch Gen Psychiatry* 1999;**56**:45–51.

223. Hulshoff-Pol HE, Schnack HG, Mandl RC, et al. Focal white matter density changes in schizophrenia: reduced inter-hemispheric connectivity. *Neuroimage* 2004;**21**:27–35.

224. Humphries C, Mortimer A, Hirsch S, de Bellroche J. NMDA receptor mRNA correlation with ante mortem cognitive impairment in schizophrenia. *Neuroreport* 1996;**7**:2051–5.

225. Hyde TM, Weinberger DR. Seizures and schizophrenia. *Schizophr Bull* 1997;**23**:611–22.

226. Hyde TM, Ziegler JC, Weinberger DR. Psychiatric disturbances in metachromatic leukodystrophy. *Arch Neurol* 1992;**49**:401–6.

227. Hynd GW, Hern KL, Novey ES, et al. Attention deficit-hyperactivity disorder and asymmetry of the caudate nucleus. *J Child Neurol* 1993;**8**:339–47.

228. Ide A, Dolezal C, Fernandez M, et al. Hemispheric differences in variability of fissural patterns in parasylvian and cingulate regions of human brains. *J Comp Neurol* 1999;**410**:235–42.

229. Jablensky A, Sartorius N, Ernberg G, et al. Schizophrenia: manifestations, incidence and course in different cultures. A World Health Organization Ten Country Study. *Psychol Med* 1992;**20**:1–97.

230. Jacobsen LK, Giedd JN, Berquin PC, et al. Quantitative morphology of the cerebellum and fourth ventricle in childhood-onset schizophrenia. *Am J Psychiatry* 1997;**154**:1663–9.

231. Jacobsen LK, Giedd JN, Castellanos FX, et al. Progressive reduction of temporal lobe structures in childhood-onset schizophrenia. *Am J Psychiatry* 1998;**155**:678–85.

232. Jacot-Descombes S, Uppal N, Wicinski B, et al. Decreased pyramidal neuron size in Brodmann areas 44 and 45 in patients with autism. *Acta Neuropathol* 2012;**124**:67–79.

233. Jenner AR, Rosen GD, Galaburda AM. Neuronal asymmetries in primary visual cortex of dyslexic and nondyslexic brains. *Ann Neurol* 1999;**46**:189–96.

234. Jeste DV, Lohr JB. Hippocampal pathologic findings in schizophrenia: a morphometric study. *Arch Gen Psychiatry* 1989;**46**:1019–24.

235. Johnstone EC, Crow TJ, Frith CD, Husband J, Kreel L. Cerebral ventricular size and cognitive impairment in chronic schizophrenia. *Lancet* 1976;**2**(7992): 924–6.

236. Johnstone EC, Crow TJ, Frith CD, Steven M, Kreel L, Husband J. The dementia of dementia praecox. *Acta Psychiatr Scand* 1978;**57**:305–24.

237. Johnstone EC, Owens DG, Bydder GM, Colter N, Crow TJ, Frith CD. The spectrum of structural brain changes in schizophrenia: age of onset as a predictor of cognitive and clinical impairments and their cerebral correlates. *Psychol Med* 1989;**19**:91–103.

238. Johnstone EC, Owens DG, Crow TJ, et al. Temporal lobe structure as determined by nuclear magnetic resonance in schizophrenia and bipolar affective disorder. *J Neurol Neurosurg Psychiatry* 1989;**52**:736–41.

239. Johnstone EC, Bruton CJ, Crow TJ, Frith CD, Owens DGC. Clinical correlates of postmortem brain changes in schizophrenia: decreased brain weight and length correlate with indices of early impairment. *J Neurol Neurosurg Psychiatry* 1994;**57**:474–9.

240. Jones P, Done DJ. From birth to onset: a developmental perspective of schizophrenia in two national birth cohorts. In: Keshavan MS, Murray RM, editors. *Neurodevelopment and adult psychopathology*. Cambridge: Cambridge University Press; 1997, p. 119–36.

241. Jones P, Rodgers B, Murray R, Marmot M. Child development risk factors for adult schizophrenia in the British 1946 birth cohort. *Lancet* 1994;**344**:1398–402.

242. Jones PB, Rantakallio P, Hartikainen A. Schizophrenia as a long term outcome of pregnancy, delivery and perinatal complications: a 28 year follow up of the 1966 North Finland general population birth cohort. *Am J Psychiatry* 1998;**155**:355–64.

243. Jou RJ, Hardan AY, Keshavan MS. Reduced cortical folding in individuals at high risk for schizophrenia: a pilot study. *Schizophr Res* 2005;**75**:309–13.

244. Kalus P, Senitz D, Beckmann H. Altered distribution of parvalbumin-immunoreactive local circuit neurons in the anterior cingulate cortex of schizophrenic patients. *Psychiatry Res Neuroimaging* 1997;**75**:49–59.

245. Kanaan RAA, Kim JS, Kaufmann WE, Pearlson GD, Barker GJ, McGuire PK. Diffusion tensor imaging in schizophrenia. *Biol Psychiatry* 2005;**58**:921–9.

246. Kanemoto K, Takeuchi J, Kawasaki J, Kawai I. Characteristics of temporal lobe epilepsy with mesial temporal sclerosis with special reference to psychotic episodes. *Neurology* 1996;**47**:1199–203.

247. Kanner L. Autistic disturbances of affective contact. *Nerv Child* 1943;**2**: 217–50.

248. Kapur S, Remington G. Serotonin-dopamine interactions and its relevance to schizophrenia. *Am J Psychiatry* 1996;**153**:466–76.

249. Karlsson J. The rate of schizophrenia in foster-reared close relatives of schizophrenic index cases. *Biol Psychiatry* 1970;**2**:285–90.

250. Kasai K, Shenton ME, Salisbury DF, et al. Progressive decrease of left Heschl gyrus and planum temporale gray matter

volume in first-episode schizophrenia. *Arch Gen Psychiatry* 2003;**60**:766–75.

251. Katsetos CD, Hyde TM, Herman MM. Neuropathology of the cerebellum in schizophrenia - an update: 1996 and future directions. *Biol Psychiatry* 1997;**42**:213–24.

252. Kawasaki Y, Maeda Y, Urata K, *et al.* A quantitative magnetic-resonance-imaging study of patients with schizophrenia. *Eur Arch Psychiatry Clin Neurosci* 1993;**242**:268–72.

253. Kawasaki Y, Suzuki M, Takahashi T, *et al.* Anomalous cerebral asymmetry in patients with schizophrenia demonstrated by voxel-based morphometry. *Biol Psychiatry* 2008;**63**:793–800.

254. Kempton MJ, Stahl D, Williams SCR, DeLisi LE. Progressive lateral ventricular enlargement in schizophrenia: A meta-analysis of longitudinal MRI studies. *Schizophr Res* 2010;**120**:54–62.

255. Kendell RE, McInneny K, Juszczak E, Bain M. Obstetric complications and schizophrenia. Two case-control studies based on structured obstetric records. *Brit J Psychiatry* 2000;**176**:516–22.

256. Kendler KS, Karkowski LM, Walsh D. The structure of psychosis: latent class analysis of probands from the Roscommon Family Study. *Arch Gen Psychiatry* 1998;**55**:492–9.

257. Kennedy DP, Semendeferi K, Courchesne E. No reduction of spindle neuron number in frontoinsular cortex in autism. *Brain Cogn* 2007;**64**:124–9.

258. Keshavan MS, Rosenberg D, Sweeney JA, Pettegrew JW. Decreased caudate volume in neuroleptic-naive psychotic patients. *Am J Psychiatry* 1998;**155**:774–8.

259. Kety SS. Schizophrenic illness in the families of schizophrenic adoptees: findings from the Danish national sample. *Schizophr Bull* 1988;**14**:217–22.

260. Kim YS, Leventhal BL, Koh YJ, *et al.* Prevalence of autism spectrum disorders in a total population sample. *Am J Psychiatry* 2011;**168**:904–12.

261. Kirkpatrick B, Messias E, Harvey PD, Fernandez-Egea E, Bowie CR. Is schizophrenia a syndrome of accelerated aging? *Schizophr Bull* 2008;**34**:1024–32.

262. Klimek V, Stockmeier C, Overholser J, *et al.* Reduced levels of norepinephrine transporters in the locus coeruleus in major depression. *J Neurosci* 1997;**17**:8451–8.

263. Koenigs M, Baskin-Sommers A, Zeier J, Newman JP. Investigating the neural correlates of psychopathy: a critical review. *Mol Psychiatry* 2011;**16**:792–9.

264. Kogan MD, Blumberg SJ, Schieve LA, *et al.* Prevalence of parent-reported diagnosis of autism spectrum disorder among children in the US, 2007. *Pediatrics* 2009;**124**:1395–403.

265. Konradi C, Yang CK, Zimmerman EI, *et al.* Hippocampal interneurons are abnormal in schizophrenia. *Schizophr Res* 2011;**131**:165–73.

266. Koutsouleris N, Gaser C, Jager M, *et al.* Structural correlates of psychopathological symptom dimensions in schizophrenia: a voxel-based morphometric study. *Neuroimage* 2008;**39**:1600–12.

267. Kovelman JA, Scheibel AB. A neurohistological correlate of schizophrenia. *Biol Psychiatry* 1984;**19**:1601–21.

268. Kraepelin E. Die Erscheinungsformen des Irreseins (translated by H Marshall as: Patterns of mental disorder. In: Hirsch SR, Shepherd M, editors. *Themes and variations in European psychiatry*. Wright, Bristol, pp 7–30, l974). *Zeitschrift Gesamte Neurologie Psychiatrie* 1920;**62**:1–29.

269. Kretschmer E. *Physique and character*. London: Kegan Paul, Trench, Trubner & Co Ltd.; 1925.

270. Krimer LS, Herman MM, Saunders RC, *et al.* A qualitative and quantitative analysis of the entorhinal cortex in schizophrenia. *Cereb Cortex* 1997;**7**:732–9.

271. Krimer LS, Hyde TM, Herman MM, Saunders RC. The entorinal cortex: an examination of cyto- and myelo-architectonic organisation in humans. *Cereb Cortex* 1997;**7**:722–31.

272. Lange N, Dubray MB, Lee JE, *et al.* Atypical diffusion tensor hemispheric asymmetry in autism. *Autism Res* 2010;**3**:350–8.

273. Laplane D, Levasseur M, Pillon B, *et al.* obsessive–compulsive and other behavioural changes with bilateral basal ganglia lesions. A neuropsychological, magnetic resonance imaging and positron tomography study. *Brain* 1989;**112**:699–725.

274. Leask SJ, Done DJ, Crow TJ. Adult psychosis, common childhood infection and neurobiological soft signs in a national birth cohort. *Br J Psychiatry* 2002;**181**:387–92.

275. Leonard CM, Voeller KK, Lombardino LJ, *et al.* Anomalous cerebral structure in dyslexia revealed with magnetic resonance imaging. *Arch Neurol* 1993;**50**:461–9.

276. Lewis DA, Gonzalez-Burgos G. Neuroplasticity of neocortical circuits in schizophrenia. *Neuropsychopharmacology* 2008;**33**:141–65.

277. Lewis DA, Hashimoto T, Volk DW. Cortical inhibitory neurons and schizophrenia. *Nat Rev Neurosci* 2005;**6**:312–24.

278. Lewis SW. The secondary schizophrenias. In: Hirsch SR, Weinberger DR, editors. *Schizophrenia*. Oxford: Blackwell; 1995.

279. Liddle PF, Crow TJ. Age disorientation in chronic schizophrenia is associated with global intellectual impairment. *Br J Psychiatry* 1984;**144**:193–9.

280. Lim KO, Hedehus M, Moseley M, de Crespigny A, Sullivan EV, Pfefferbaum A. Compromised white matter tract integrity in schizophrenia inferred from diffusion tensor imaging. *Arch Gen Psychiatry* 1999;**56**:367–74.

281. Lohr JB, Jeste DV. Locus ceruleus morphometry in aging and schizophrenia. *Acta Psychiatr Scand* 1988;**77**:689–97.

282. Machiyama Y, Watanabe Y, Machiyama R. Neuroanatomical studies of the corpus callosum in schizophrenia: Evidence of aberrant interhemispheric fibre connection. In: Takahashi R, Flor-Henry P, editors. *Cerebral dynamics, laterality and psychopathology*. Amsterdam: Elsevier; 1987, p. 411–21.

283. Mackay CE, Roddick E, Barrick TR, *et al.* Sex dependence of brain size and shape in bipolar disorder: an exploratory study. *Bipolar Disord* 2010;**12**:306–11.

284. Mann JJ, Huang YY, Underwood MD, *et al.* A serotonin transporter gene promoter polymorphism (5-HTTLPR) and prefrontal cortical binding in major depression and suicide. *Arch Gen Psychiatry* 2000;**57**:729–38.

285. Marchant LF, McGrew WC. Laterality of limb function in wild chimpanzees of Gombe National Park: comprehensive study of spontaneous activities. *J Hum Evol* 1996;**30**:427–43.

286. Marin O. Interneuron dysfunction in psychiatric disorders. *Nat Rev Neurosci* 2012;**13**:107–20.

287. Marneros A, Diester A, Rohde A. *Affektive, schizoaffektive und schizophrene psychose. Ein vergleichende langseitstudie*. Berlin: Springer; 1991.

288. Marneros A, Rohde A, Deister A. Psychotic continuum under longitudinal considerations. In: Marneros A, Andreasen NC, Tsuang MT, editors. *Psychotic continuum*. Berlin: Springer-Verlag; 1995, p. 17–30.

289. Marsden CD. Cerebral atrophy and cognitive impairment in chronic schizophrenia. *Lancet* 1976;**2**(7994):1079.

290. Marsh L, Harris D, Lim KO, *et al.* Structural magnetic resonance imaging abnormalities in men with severe chronic schizophrenia and an early age at clinical onset. *Arch Gen Psychiatry* 1997;**54**:1104–12.

291. Marshall CR, Scherer SW. Detection and characterization of copy number variation in autism spectrum disorder. *Methods Mol Biol* 2012;**838**:115–35.

292. McCreadie RG, Thara R, Kamath S, *et al.* Abnormal movements in never-medicated Indian patients with schizophrenia. *Br J Psychiatry* 1996;**168**:221–6.

293. McDonald B, Highley JR, Walker MA, *et al.* Anomalous asymmetry of fusiform and parahippocampal gyrus grey matter in schizophrenia: a post-mortem study. *Am J Psychiatry* 2000;**157**:40–7.

294. McDonald C, Zanelli J, Rabe-Hesketh S, *et al.* Meta-analysis of magnetic resonance imaging brain morphometry studies in bipolar disorder. *Biol Psychiatry* 2004;**56**:411–7.

295. McGrath J. Variations in the incidence of schizophrenia: Data versus dogma. *Schizophr Bull* 2006;**32**:195–7.

296. Mednick SA, Machon RA, Huttunen MO, Bonett D. Adult schizophrenia following prenatal exposure to an influenza epidemic. *Arch Gen Psychiatry* 1988;**45**:189–92.

297. Meisenzahl EM, Zetzsche T, Preuss U, Frodl T, Leinsinger G, Moller HJ. Does the definition of borders of the planum temporale influence the results in schizophrenia? *Am J Psychiatry* 2002;**159**:1198–200.

298. Mendez MF, Gran R, Doss RC, Taylor JL. Schizophrenia in epilepsy: seizure and psychosis variables. *Neurology* 1993;**43**:1073–7.

299. Menon RR, Barta PE, Aylward EH, *et al.* Posterior superior temporal gyrus in schizophrenia: grey matter changes and clinical correlates. *Schizophr Res* 1995;**16**:127–35.

300. Miklos GL, Maleszka R. Microarray reality checks in the context of a complex disease. *Nat Biotechnol* 2004;**22**:615–21.

301. Miles JH. Autism spectrum disorders--a genetics review. *Genet Med* 2011;**13**:278–94.

302. Miles TR, Haslam MN, Wheeler TJ. Gender ratio in dyslexia. *Ann Dyslexia* 1998;**48**:27–55.

303. Milham MP, Nugent AC, Drevets WC, Dickstein DP, Leibenluft E, Ernst M, *et al.*

Selective reduction in amygdala volume in pediatric anxiety disorders: a voxel-based morphometry investigation. *Biol Psychiatry* 2005;**57**:961–6.

304. Miskolczy D. Uber das anatomische korrelat der schizophrenie. *Z Neurol* 1933;**147**:509–44.

305. Mohn AR, Gainetdinov RR, Caron MG, Koller BH. Mice with reduced NMDA receptor expression display behaviours related to schizophrenia. *Cell* 1999;**98**:427–36.

306. Morgan JT, Chana G, Abramson I, Semendeferi K, Courchesne E, Everall IP. Abnormal microglial-neuronal spatial organization in the dorsolateral prefrontal cortex in autism. *Brain Res* 2012;**1456**:72–81.

307. Morgan JT, Chana G, Pardo CA, *et al.* Microglial activation and increased microglial density observed in the dorsolateral prefrontal cortex in autism. *Biol Psychiatry* 2010;**68**:368–76.

308. Morris CS, Esiri MM, Sprinkle TJ, Gregson N. Oligodendrocyte reactions and cell proliferation markers in human demyelinating diseases. *Neuropathol Appl Neurobiol* 1994;**20**:272–81.

309. Morris PL, Robinson RG, Raphael B, Hopwood MJ. Lesion location and post-stroke depression. *J Neuropsychiatry Clin Neurosci* 1996;**8**:399–403.

310. Mowry BJ, Lennon DP, De Felice CN. Diagnosis of schizophrenia in a matched sample of Australian aborigines. *Acta Psychiatr Scand* 1994;**90**:337–41.

311. Murphy JM. Psychiatric labelling in a cross-cultural perspective. *Science* 1976;**191**:1019–28.

312. Nair TR, Christensen JD, Kingsbury SJ, Kumar NG, Terry WM, Garver DL. Progression of cerebroventricular enlargement and the subtyping of schizophrenia. *Psychiatry Res Neuroimaging* 1997;**74**:141–9.

313. Nakamae T, Narumoto J, Sakai Y, *et al.* Reduced cortical thickness in non-medicated patients with obsessive–compulsive disorder. *Prog Neuropsychopharmacol Biol Psychiatry* 2012;**37**:90–5.

314. Narr KL, Thompson PN, Sharma T, Moussai J, Cannestra AF, Toga AW. Mapping morphology of the corpus callosum in schizophrenia. *Cereb Cortex* 2000;**10**:40–9.

315. Narr K, Thompson P, Sharma T, *et al.* Three-dimensional mapping of gyral shape and cortical surface asymmetries in schizophrenia: gender effects. *Am J Psychiatry* 2001;**158**:244–55.

316. Narr KL, Thompson PM, Sharma T, *et al.* Three-dimensional mapping of temporo-limbic regions and the lateral ventricles in schizophrenia: gender effects. *Biol Psychiatry* 2001;**50**:84–97.

317. Narr KL, Cannon TD, Woods RP, *et al.* Genetic contributions to altered callosal morphology in schizophrenia. *J Neurosci* 2002;**22**:3720–9.

318. Narr KL, Bilder RM, Kim S, *et al.* Abnormal gyral complexity in first-episode schizophrenia. *Biol Psychiatry* 2004;**55**:859–67.

319. Narr K, Bilder RM, Woods RP, *et al.* Regional specificity of cerebrospinal fluid abnormalities in first episode schizophrenia. *Psychiatry Res Neuroimaging* 2006;**146**:21–33.

320. Nasrallah HA, McCalley-Whitters M, Bigelow LB, Rauscher FP. A histological study of the corpus callosum in chronic schizophrenia. *Psychiatry Res* 1983;**8**:251–60.

321. Nelson MD, Saykin AJ, Flashman LA, Riordan HJ. Hippocampal volume reduction in schizophrenia as assessed by magnetic resonance imaging. *Arch Gen Psychiatry* 1998;**55**:433–40.

322. Niznikiewicz MA, Donnino R, McCarley RW, *et al.* Abnormal angular gyrus asymmetry in schizophrenia. *Am J Psychiatry* 2000;**157**:428–37.

323. Oblak AL, Rosene DL, Kemper TL, Bauman ML, Blatt GJ. Altered posterior cingulate cortical cyctoarchitecture, but normal density of neurons and interneurons in the posterior cingulate cortex and fusiform gyrus in autism. *Autism Res* 2011;**4**:200–11.

324. O'Donovan MC, Craddock N, Norton N, *et al.* Identification of novel schizophrenia loci by genome-wide association and follow-up. *Nat Genet* 2008;**40**:1053–5.

325. Olney JW, Farber NB. Glutamate receptor dysfunction and schizophrenia. *Arch Gen Psychiatry* 1995;**52**:998–1007.

326. Orton ST. *Reading, writing and speech problems in children.* New York: Norton; 1937.

327. Owen MJ, Craddock N, O'Donovan MC. Schizophrenia: genes at last? *Trends Genet* 2005;**21**:518–25.

328. Owens DGC, Johnstone EC, Frith CD. Spontaneous involuntary disorders of movement in neuroleptic treated and untreated chronic schizophrenics - prevalence, severity and distribution. *Arch Gen Psychiatry* 1982;**39**:452–61.

329. Owens DGC, Johnstone EC, Crow TJ, Frith CD, Jagoe JR, Kreel L. Cerebral ventricular enlargement in schizophrenia: relationship to the disease process and its clinical correlates. *Psychol Med* 1985;**15**:27–41.

330. Pakkenberg B. Pronounced reduction of total neuron number in mediodorsal thalamic nucleus and nucleus accumbens in schizophrenics. *Arch Gen Psychiatry* 1990;**47**:1023–8.

331. Pakkenberg B. Total nerve cell number in neocortex in chronic schizophrenics and controls estimated using optical dissectors. *Biol Psychiatry* 1993;**34**:768–72.

332. Panse F. *Die Erbchorea: Eine klinische-gentische studie.* Leipzig: Thieme; 1942.

333. Parfitt DN. The neurology of schizophrenia. *J Ment Sci* 1956;**102**:671–718.

334. Paus T, Tomaiuolo F, Otaky N, *et al.* Human cingulate and paracingulate sulci: pattern, variability, asymmetry, and probabilistic map. *Cereb Cortex* 1996;**6**:207–14.

335. Pearlson GD, Kim WS, Kubos KL, *et al.* Ventricle-brain ratio, computed tomographic density, and brain area in 50 schizophrenics. *Arch Gen Psychiatry* 1989;**46**:690–7.

336. Pearlson GD, Petty RG, Ross CA, Tiens AY. Schizophrenia: a disease of heteromodal association cortex? *Neuropsychopharmacology* 1996;**14**: 1–17.

337. Pearlson GD, Barta PE, Powers RE, *et al.* Ziskind-Somerfield Research Award 1996. Medial and superior temporal gyral volumes in schizophrenia versus bipolar disorder. *Biol Psychiatry* 1997;**41**:1–14.

338. Penrose LS. Survey of cases of familial mental illness. *Eur Arch Psychiatry Clin Neurosci* 1991;**240**:314–24.

339. Peters M, Reimers S, Manning JT. Hand preference for writing and associations with selected demographic and behavioral variables in 255,100 subjects: The BBC internet study. *Brain Cogn* 2006; **62**:177–89.

340. Pierri JN, Volk CL, Auh S, Sampson A, Lewis DA. Decreased somal size of deep layer 3 pyramidal neurons in the prefrontal cortex of subjects with schizophrenia. *Arch Gen Psychiatry* 2001;**58**:466–73.

341. Polsek D, Jagatic T, Cepanec M, *et al.* Recent developments in neuropathology of autism spectrum disorders. *Transl Neurosci* 2011;**2**:256–64.

342. Powchick P, Davison M, Haroutian V, *et al.* Post mortem studies in schizophrenia. *Schizophr Bull* 1998;**24**:325–41.

343. Priddle TH, Crow TJ. The protocadherin 11X/Y gene pair as a putative determinant of cerebral dominance in *Homo sapiens. Future Neurol* 2009;**4**:509–18.

344. Pujol J, Vendrell P, Junque C, Marti-Valalta JC, Capdevila A. When does human brain development end? Evidence of corpus callosum growth up to adulthood. *Ann Neurol* 1993;**34**:71–5.

345. Purcell SM, Wray NR, Stone JL, *et al.* Common polygenic variation contributes to risk of schizophrenia and bipolar disorder. *Nature* 2009;**460**:748–52.

346. Qin P, Xu H, Laursen TM, Vestergaard M, Mortensen PB. Risk for schizophrenia and schizophrenia-like psychosis among patients with epilepsy: population based cohort study. *Br Med J* 2005;**331**:23.

347. Rajarethinam RP, DeQuardo JR, Nalepa R, Tandon R. Superior temporal gyrus in schizophrenia: a volumetric magnetic resonance imaging study. *Schizophr Res* 2000;**41**:303–12.

348. Rajkowska G, Selemon LD, Goldman-Rakic PS. Neuronal and glial somal size in the prefrontal cortex: a postmortem morphometric study of schizophrenia and Huntington disease. *Arch Intern Med* 1998;**158**:215–24.

349. Rajkowska G, Miguel-Hidalgo JJ, Wei J, *et al.* Morphometric evidence for neuronal and glial prefrontal cell pathology in major depression. *Biol Psychiatry* 1999;**45**:1085–98.

350. Randrup A, Munkvad I. Stereotyped activities produced by amphetamine in several animal species and man. *Psychopharmacologia* 1967;**11**:300–10.

351. Reite M, Sheeder J, Teale P, *et al.* Magnetic source imaging evidence of sex differences in cerebral lateralization in schizophrenia. *Arch Gen Psychiatry* 1997;**54**:433–40.

352. Reite M, Teale P, Rojas DC, Arciniegas D, Sheeder J. Bipolar disorder: anomalous brain asymmetry associated with psychosis. *Am J Psychiatry* 1999;**158**:1159–63.

353. Reite M, Teale P, Rojas DC, Sheeder J, Arcinegas D. Schizoaffective disorder: evidence for reversed cerebral asymmetry. *Biol Psychiatry* 1999;**46**:133–6.

354. Reyes MG, Gordon A. Cerebellar vermis in schizophrena (letter). *Lancet* 1981;**2**:700–1.

355. Rezaie R, Roberts N, Cutter WJ, *et al.* Anomalous asymmetry in Turner's and Klinefelter's syndromes - further evidence

for X-Y linkage of the cerebral dominance gene. *Am J Med Genet* 2004;**130**(part B):102–3.

356. Riley BP, Rajagopalan S, Mogudi-Carter M, Jenkins T, Williamson R. No evidence for linkage of chromosome 6p markers to schizophrenia in Southern African Bantu-speaking families. *Psychiatr Genet* 1996;**6**:41–9.

357. Roberts GW, Done DJ, Bruton C, Crow TJ. A "mock up" of schizophrenia: temporal lobe epilepsy and schizophrenia-like psychosis. *Biol Psychiatry* 1990;**28**:127–43.

358. Roberts GW, Royston MC, Weinberger DR. Schizophrenia. In: Graham DI, Lantos PL, editors. *Greenfield's neuropathology*, 6th ed. London: Arnold; 1997, p. 897–929.

359. Rosoklija G, Toomayan G, Ellis SP, *et al.* Structural abnormalities of subicular dendrites in subjects with schizophrenia and mood disorders: preliminary findings. *Arch Gen Psychiatry* 2000;**57**:349–56.

360. Rumsey JM, Donohue BC, Brady DR, Nace K, Giedd JN, Andreason PA. A magnetic resonance imaging study of planum temporale asymmetry in men with developmental dyslexia. *Arch Neurol* 1997;**54**:1481–9.

361. Rutter M, Yule W. Specific reading retardation. *J Child Psychol Psychiatr* 1975;**16**:181–97.

362. Sacker A, Done DJ, Crow TJ, Golding J. Antecedents of schizophrenia and affective illness: obstetric complications. *Br J Psychiatry* 1995;**166**:734–41.

363. Saha S, Chant D, Welham J, McGrath J. A systematic review of the prevalance of schizophrenia. *PLOS Med* 2005;**2**:413–33.

364. Salisbury DF, Shenton ME, Sherwood AR, *et al.* First episode psychosis differs from first episode affective psychosis and controls in P300 amplitude over left temporal lobe. *Arch Gen Psychiatry* 1998;**55**:173–80.

365. Sallet PC, Elkis H, Alves TM, *et al.* Reduced cortical folding in schizophrenia: an MRI morphometric study. *Am J Psychiatry* 2003;**160**:1606–13.

366. Sanfilipo M, Larfargue T, Rusinck H, *et al.* Volumetric measure of the frontal and temporal lobe regions in schizophrenia: relationship to negative symptoms. *Arch Gen Psychiatry* 2000;**57**:471–80.

367. Santos M, Uppal N, Butti C, *et al.* Von Economo neurons in autism: a stereologic study of the frontoinsular cortex in children. *Brain Res* 2011;**1380**:206–17.

368. Saunders RC, Kolachance BS, Bachevalier J, Weinberger DR. Neonatal lesions of the medial temporal lobe disrupt prefrontal cortical regulation of striatal dopamine. *Nature* 1998;**393**:169–71.

369. Schaaf CP, Zoghbi HY. Solving the autism puzzle a few pieces at a time. *Neuron* 2011;**70**:806–8.

370. Schneider K. Primare und Sekundare Symptome bei der Schizophrenie (translated by H Marshall as: Primary and secondary symptoms in schizophrenia. In: Hirsch SR, Shepherd M. *Themes and variations in European psychiatry*. Wright, Bristol, pp 40–44, 1974). *Fortsschritte der Neurologie und Psychiatrie* 1957;**25**:487–90.

371. Schreiber S, Bernstein HG, Fendrich R, *et al.* Increased density of GAD65/67 immunoreactive neurons in the posterior subiculum and parahippocampal gyrus in treated patients with chronic schizophrenia. *World J Biol Psychiatry* 2011;**12**:57–65.

372. Schumann CM, Amaral DG. Stereological analysis of amygdala neuron number in autism. *J Neurosci* 2006;**26**:7674–9.

373. Schumann CM, Nordahl CW. Bridging the gap between MRI and postmortem research in autism. *Brain Res* 2011;**1380**:175–86.

374. Selemon LD, Rajkowska G, Goldman-Rakic PS. Abnormally high neuronal density in the schizophrenic cortex: a morphometric analysis of prefrontal area 9 and occipital area 17. *Arch Gen Psychiatry* 1995;**52**:805–18.

375. Selemon LD, Rajkowska G, Goldman-Rakic PS. Elevated neuronal density in prefrontal area 46 in brains from schizophrenic patients: application of a three-dimensional stereological counting method. *J Comp Neurol* 1998;**392**:402–12.

376. Selemon LD, Mrzljak J, Kleinman JE, Herman MM, Goldman-Rakic PS. Regional specificity in the neuropathologic substrates of schizophrenia: a morphometric analysis of Broca's area 44 and area 9. *Arch Gen Psychiatry* 2003;**60**:69–77.

377. Shapleske J, Rossell SL, Woodruff PW, David AS. The planum temporale: a systematic, quantitative review of its structural, functional and clinical significance. *Brain Res Rev* 1999;**29**: 26–49.

378. Shenton ME, Kikinis R, Jolesz F, *et al.* Abnormalities of the left temporal lobe and thought disorder in schizophrenia. *N Engl J Med* 1992;**327**:604–12.

379. Shenton ME, Dickey CC, Frumin M, McCarley RW. A review of MRI findings in schizophrenia. *Schizophr Res* 2001;**49**:1–52.

380. Sheppard DM, Bradshaw JL, Purcell R, Pantelis C. Tourette's and comorbid syndromes: obsessive–compulsive and attention-deficit hyperactivity disorder. A common etiology? *Clin Psychol Rev* 1999;**19**:531–52.

381. Siever LJ, Gunderson HJG. The search for schizotypal personality: historical origins and current status. *Compr Psychiatry* 1983;**24**:199–212.

382. Siever LJ, Rotter M, Losonczy M, *et al.* Lateral ventricular enlargement in schizotypal personality disorder. *Psychiatry Res* 1995;**57**:109–18.

383. Sigmundsson T, Suckling J, Maier M, *et al.* Structural abnormalities in frontal, temporal and limbic regions and interconnecting white matter tracts in schizophrenic patients with prominent negative symptoms. *Am J Psychiatry* 2001;**158**:234–43.

384. Silverman JM, Smith CJ, Guo SL, Mohs RC, Siever LJ, Davis KL. Lateral ventricular enlargement in schizophrenic probands and their siblings with schizophrenia-related disorders. *Biol Psychiatry* 1998;**43**:97–106.

385. Simper R, Walker MA, Black G, Di Rosa E, Crow TJ, Chance SA. The relationship between callosal axons and cortical neurons in the planum temporale: alterations in schizophrenia. *Neurosci Res* 2011;**71**:405–10.

386. Smiley JF, Rosoklija G, Mancevski B, *et al.* Hemispheric comparisons of neuron density in the planum temporale of schizophrenia and nonpsychiatric brains. *Psychiatry Res* 2011;**192**:1–11.

387. Smiley JF, Konnova K, Bleiwas C. Cortical thickness, neuron density and size in the inferior parietal lobe in schizophrenia. *Schizophr Res* 2012;**136**:43–50.

388. Southard EE. On the topographical distribution of cortex lesions and anomalies in dementia praecox, with some account of their functional significance. *Am J Insanity* 1915;**71**:603–71.

389. Spence SA, Liddle PF, Stefan MD, *et al.* Functional anatomy of verbal fluency in people with schizophrenia and those at genetic risk: focal dysfunction and distributed dis-connectivity reappraised. *Br J Psychiatry* 2000;**176**:52–60.

390. State MW, Levitt P. The conundrums of understanding genetic risks for autism spectrum disorders. *Nat Neurosci* 2011;**14**:1499–506.

391. Stigler KA, McDonald BC, Anand A, Saykin AJ, McDougle CJ. Structural and functional magnetic resonance imaging of autism spectrum disorders. *Brain Res* 2011;**1380**:146–61.

392. Suckling J, Roberts H, Walker MA, *et al.* Temporal lobe epilepsy with and without psychosis: exploration of hippocampal pathology including that in subpopulations of neurons defined by their content of immunoreactive calcium binding proteins. *Acta Neuropathol* 2000;**99**:547–54.

393. Suganthy J, Raghuram L, Antonisamy B, Vettivel S, Madhavi C, Koshi R. Gender and age-related differences in the morphology of the corpus callosum. *Clin Anat* 2003;**16**:396–403.

394. Sumich A, Chitnis XA, Fannon DG, *et al.* Unreality symptoms and volumetric measures of Heschl's gyrus and planum temporal in first-episode psychosis. *Biol Psychiatry* 2005;**57**:947–50.

395. Sun T, Patoine C, Abu-Khalil A, *et al.* Early asymmetry of gene transcription in embryonic human left and right cerebral cortex. *Science* 2005;**308**:1794–8.

396. Sweet RA, Pierri JN, Auh S, Sampson AR, Lewis DA. Reduced pyramidal cell somal volume in auditory association cortex of subjects with schizophrenia. *Neuropsychopharmacology* 2003;**28**:599–609.

397. Syed A, Chatfield M, Matthews F, Harrison P, Brayne C, Esiri MM. Depression in the elderly: pathological study of raphe and locus ceruleus. *Neuropathol Appl Neurobiol* 2005;**31**:405–13.

398. Tamminga CA. Schizophrenia and glutamatergic transmission. *Crit Rev Neurobiol* 1998;**12**:21–36.

399. Tanskanen P, Veijola J, Miettunen J, *et al.* Structural brain differences in schizophrenia and other psychoses in the Northern Finland 1966 birth cohort. *Schizophr Res* 2006;**81**:26–7.

400. Taylor DC. Factors influencing the occurrence of schizophrenia-like psychosis in patients with temporal lobe epilepsy. *Psychol Med* 1975;**5**:249–54.

401. Thune JJ, Uylings HB, Pakkenberg B. No deficit in total number of neurons in the prefrontal cortex in schizophrenics. *J Psychiatr Res* 2001;**35**:15–21.

402. Tiihonen J, Katila H, Pekkonen E, *et al.* Reversal of cerebral asymmetry in schizophrenia measured with

magnetoencephalography. *Schizophr Res* 1998;**30**:209–19.

403. Tkachev D, Mimmack ML, Ryan MM, *et al*. Oligodendrocyte dysfunction in schizophrenia and bipolar disorder. *Lancet* 1972;**362**:798–805.

404. Torrey EF. *Schizophrenia and civilization*. New York: Jason Aronson; 1980.

405. Torrey EF, Bowler AE, Rawlings R. An influenza epidemic and the seasonality of schizophrenic births. In: Kurstak E, editor. *Psychiatry and biological factors*. New York: Plenum; 1991. p. 109–16.

406. Torrey EF, Bowler AE, Taylor EH, Gottesman II. *Schizophrenia and manic-depressive disorder*. New York: Basic Books; 1994.

407. Torrey EF, Barci BM, Webster MJ, Bartko JJ, Meador-Woodruff JH, Knable MB. Neurochemical markers for schizophrenia, bipolar disorder, and major depression in postmortem brains. *Biol Psychiatry* 2005;**57**:252–60.

408. Tran KD, Smutzer GS, Doty RL, Arnold SE. Reduced Purkinje cell size in cerebellar vernis of elderly patients with schizophrenia. *Am J Psychiatry* 1998;**155**:1288–90.

409. Trimble MR. First-rank symptoms of Schneider: a new perspective? *Br J Psychiatry* 1990;**156**:195–200.

410. Turner JMA. Meiotic sex chromosome inactivation. *Development* 2007;**134**:1823–31.

411. Uranova NA, Vostrikov VM, Vikhreva OV, Zimina IS, Kolomeets NS, Orlovskaya DD. The role of oligodendrocyte pathology in schizophrenia. *Int J Neuropsychopharmacol* 2007;**10**:537–45.

412. Van Haren NE, Schnack HG, Cahn W, *et al*. Changes in cortical thickness during the course of illness in schizophrenia. *Arch Gen Psychiatr* 2011;**68**:871–80.

413. Van den Eynde F, Suda M, Broadbent H, *et al*. Structural magnetic resonance imaging in eating disorders: a systematic review of voxel-based morphometry studies. *Eur Eat Disord Rev* 2012;**20**:94–105.

414. van Kooten IA, Palmen SJ, von Cappeln P, *et al*. Neurons in the fusiform gyrus are fewer and smaller in autism. *Brain* 2008;**131**:987–99.

415. van-Os J, Jones P, Lewis G, Wadsworth M, Murray R. Developmental precursors of affective illness in a general population birth cohort. *Arch Gen Psychiatry* 1997;**54**:625–31.

416. Vargas DL, Nascimbene C, Krishnan C, Zimmerman AW, Pardo CA. Neuroglial activation and neuroinflammation in the brain of patients with autism. *Ann Neurol* 2005;**57**:67–81.

417. Vita A, Dieci M, Silenzi C, Tenconi F, Giobbio GM, Invernizzi G. Cerebral ventricular enlargement as a generalized feature of schizophrenia: a distribution analysis on 502 subjects. *Schizophr Res* 2000;**44**:25–34.

418. Vogeley K, Schneider-Axman T, Pfeiffer U, *et al*. Disturbed gyrification of the prefrontal region in male schizophrenic patients: a morphometric study. *Am J Psychiatry* 2000;**157**:34–9.

419. Voineagu I, Wang X, Johnston P, *et al*. Transcriptomic analysis of autistic brain reveals convergent molecular pathology. *Nature* 2011;**474**:380–4.

420. Waddington JL, Crow TJ. Abnormal involuntary movements and psychosis in the pre-neuroleptic era and in unmedicated patients. In: Wolf ME, Mosnaim AD, editors. *Tardive dyskinesia: biological mechanisms and clinical aspects*. Washington: American Psychiatric Press; 1986, p. 51–66.

421. Walker MA, Highley JR, Esiri MM, *et al*. Estimated neuronal populations and volumes of the hippocampus and its subfields in schizophrenia. *Am J Psychiatry* 2002;**159**:821–8.

422. Wang AY, Lohmann KM, Yang CK, *et al*. Bipolar disorder type 1 and schizophrenia are accompanied by decreased density of parvalbumin- and somatostatin-positive interneurons in the parahippocampal region. *Acta Neuropathol* 2011;**122**:615–26.

423. Watt NF. Patterns of childhood social development in adult schizophrenics. *Arch Gen Psychiatry* 1978;**35**:160–5.

424. Wegiel J, Kuchna I, Nowicki K, *et al*. The neuropathology of autism: defects of neurogenesis and neuronal migration, and dysplastic changes. *Acta Neuropathol* 2010;**119**:755–70.

425. Wegiel J, Schanen NC, Cook EH, *et al*. Differences between the pattern of developmental abnormalities in autism associated with duplications 15q11.2-q13 and idiopathic autism. *J Neuropathol Exp Neurol* 2012;**71**:382–97.

426. Weinberger DR. Implications of normal brain developments for the pathogenesis of schizophrenia. *Arch Gen Psychiatry* 1987;**44**:660–9.

427. Weinberger DR, Torrey EF, Neophytides AN, Wyatt RJ. Lateral cerebral ventricular enlargement in chronic schizophrenia. *Arch Gen Psychiatry* 1979;**36**:735–9.

428. Weissman MM, Bland RC, Canino GJ, *et al*. Cross-national epidemiology of major depression and bipolar disorder. *JAMA* 1996;**276**:293–9.

429. Williams NA, Close J, Giouzeli M, Crow TJ. Accelerated evolution of Protocadherin11X/Y : A candidate gene-pair for cerebral asymmetry and language. *Am J Med Genet B Neuropsychiatric Genet* 2006;**141**(Part B):623–33.

430. Witelson SF, Nowakowski RS. Left out axons make men right: a hypothesis for the origins of handedness and functional asymmetry. *Neuropsychologia* 1991;**29**:327–33.

431. Woo TU, Miller JL, Lewis DA. Schizophrenia and the parvalbumin-containing class of cortical local circuit neurons. *Am J Psychiatry* 1997;**154**:1013–5.

432. Woodruff PWR, Pearlson GD, Geer MJ, Barta PE, Chilcoat HD. A computerized magnetic resonance imaging study of corpus callosum morphology in schizophrenia. *Psychol Med* 1993;**23**:45–56.

433. Woodruff PW, McManus IC, David AS. Meta-analysis of corpus callosum size in schizophrenia. *J Neurol Neurosurg Psychiatry* 1995;**58**:457–61.

434. Woods BT. Is schizophrenia a progressive neurodevelopmental disorder? Toward a unitary mechanism. *Am J Psychiatry* 1998;**155**:1661–70.

435. Wright IC, Rabe-Hesketh S, Woodruff PWR, David AS, Murray RM, Bullmore ET. Meta-analysis of regional brain volumes in schizophrenia. *Am J Psychiatry* 2000;**157**:16–25.

436. Yip J, Soghomonian JJ, Blatt GJ. Decreased GAD67 mRNA levels in cerebellar Purkinje cells in autism: pathophysiological implications. *Acta Neuropathol* 2007;**113**:559–68.

437. Young KA, Manaye KF, Liang C, Hicks PB, German DC. Reduced number of mediodorsal and anterior thalamic neurons in schizophrenia. *Biol Psychiatry* 2000;**47**:944–53.

438. Young RC, Nambudiri DE, Jain H, de Asis JM, Alexopoulous GS. Brain computed tomography in geriatric manic disorder. *Biol Psychiatry* 1999;**45**:1063–5.

439. Yu K, Cheung C, Leung M, Li Q, Chua S, McAlonan G. Are bipolar disorder and schizophrenia neuranatomically distinct? An anatomical likelihood meta-analysis. *Front Hum Neurosci* 2010;**4**:189.

440. Yucel M, Velakoulis D, Maruff P, *et al*. Reduced left anterior cingulate fissurization in males with first episode psychoses but not females: a MRI morphometric study. *Schizophr Res* 2000;**41**:6–7.

441. Zaidel DW. Size, shape, and orientation of neurons in the left and right hippocampus: investigation of normal asymmetries and alterations in schizophrenia. *Am J Psychiatry* 1997;**154**:812–8.

442. Zaidel DW, Esiri MM, Harrison PJ. The hippocampus in schizophrenia; lateralized increase in neuronal density and altered cytoarchitectural asymmetry. *Psychol Med* 1997;**27**:703–13.

443. Zhang ZJ, Reynolds GP. A selective decrease in the relative density of parvalumin-immunoreactive neurons in the hippocampus in schiozphrenia. *Schizophr Res* 2002;**55**:1–10.

444. Zipursky RB, Lim KO, Sullivan EV, Brown BW, Pfefferbaum A. Widespread cerebral grey matter volume deficits in schizophrenia. *Arch Gen Psychiatry* 1992;**49**:195–205.

445. Zubenko GS, Moossy J. Major depression in primary dementia: clinical and neuropathological correlates. *Arch Neurol* 1992;**45**:1182–6.

446. Zweig RM, Ross CA, Hedreen JC, *et al*. The neuropathology of aminergic nuclei in Alzheimer's disease. *Ann Neurol* 1988;**24**:233–42.

Prion Diseases

Mark W Head, James W Ironside, Bernardino Ghetti,
Martin Jeffrey, Pedro Piccardo and Robert G Will

INTRODUCTION

Background

Prion diseases, also known as the transmissible spongiform encephalopathies (TSEs), are rare fatal neurodegenerative diseases affecting humans and a range of other mammalian species.[304] In humans, prion diseases are unique among neurodegenerative disorders, because they occur in idiopathic, genetically-determined and acquired forms (Table 18.1).[170,309] As a group, human prion diseases are rare, with an annual mortality rate of 1–1.5 cases per 1 million population.[220]

Sporadic Creutzfeldt–Jakob disease (sCJD) accounts for over 85 per cent of cases of human prion disease and has been identified worldwide, with the exception of some developing countries, in which there may be limited facilities for diagnosis, including neuropathology. The widespread geographical distribution of sCJD implies that any putative risk factor for the development of disease must be ubiquitous and case-control and observational studies have failed to identify an environmental source of infection.[376] The cause of sCJD is unknown, and the current favoured hypothesis is that this condition is due to spontaneous generation of disease-associated prion protein (PrP) in the brain that self-replicates, leading to neuronal dysfunction and death, and the onset of clinical disease.[309]

Genetically determined forms of human prion disease are inherited with an autosomal dominant pattern, usually with almost complete penetrance, and represent about 10 per cent of all cases of human prion disease.[220] Historically classification into different forms – familial Creutzfeldt–Jakob disease (fCJD), Gerstmann–Sträussler–Scheinker disease (GSS), fatal familial insomnia (FFI), and PrP-amyloid angiopathy – was based on clinical and pathological features, which are now augmented through the molecular genetic analyses of the PrP gene (*PRNP*). An increasing number of distinct point, insertion and deletion mutations have been found to be associated with disease.[107,281,282]

Iatrogenic Creutzfeldt–Jakob disease (iCJD) is due to the transmission of prion infection from person to person in the course of medical or surgical treatment, including human pituitary hormones, human dura mater grafts, corneal transplants, depth electroencephalogram (EEG) electrodes and neurosurgical instruments.[43] The presumption is that the hormones or grafts were sourced from individuals dying with Creutzfeldt–Jakob disease (CJD) or that instruments contaminated by use on an individual with CJD were decontaminated inadequately and then reused.

Kuru is restricted to the Fore region of Papua New Guinea and is due to transmission of infection in the course of ritual cannibalism, through either ingestion of human tissues or transdermal spread via superficial wounds or skin scarification.[3] Ritual cannibalism was banned in the late 1950s, but the incubation period can exceed 50 years.[68]

Variant Creutzfeldt–Jakob disease (vCJD) was identified in 1996[380] and is caused by human infection with the cattle disease bovine spongiform encephalopathy (BSE). The disease has occurred predominantly in the United Kingdom, consistent with the link with BSE, but to date (October 2014) a limited number of cases have been identified in the United Kingdom (177) and fears of a large epidemic have receded. Smaller numbers of cases have been identified in eleven other countries. The presumed mechanism of transmission of vCJD is through past infection via the food chain by bovine tissues containing high levels of BSE infectivity.[370] Public health concerns about vCJD however remain with

TABLE 18.1 Human prion diseases

Disease	Incidence and epidemiology	Aetiology
Sporadic Creutzfeldt–Jakob disease (sCJD)	1–1.5 cases per 1 million population per annum, worldwide	Idiopathic
Sporadic fatal insomnia	Extremely rare, previously known as the 'thalamic variant' of sCJD	Idiopathic
Variably protease sensitive prionopathy	Rare: first described in 2008, precise incidence uncertain	Idiopathic
Familial Creutzfeldt–Jakob disease Gerstmann–Sträussler–Scheinker disease Fatal familial insomnia PrP-cerebral amyloid angiopathy	5–10% of all human prion diseases, pedigrees in various locations worldwide, autosomal dominant inheritance	Genetic: linked to *PRNP* mutations, insertions and deletions
Kuru	Fore tribe of New Guinea; first reported in mid-twentieth century, now extinct	Acquired (ritualistic endocannibalism)
Iatrogenic Creutzfeldt–Jakob disease	Primarily France, Japan, UK and USA (>450 cases worldwide)	Acquired by human tissue inoculation or grafting
Variant Creutzfeldt–Jakob disease (vCJD)	UK (177 cases), with an additional 52 cases in 11 other countries (October 2014)	Acquired by dietary exposure to bovine spongiform encephalopathy (BSE), or by red cell transfusion from vCJD-infected asymptomatic donors

evidence of transmission from person to person by blood transfusion and blood products.[155,231,285,286,388]

The most common prion diseases occurring in non-human species are scrapie in sheep, mouflon and goats; chronic wasting disease (CWD) in deer, elk and moose; and BSE in cattle. Prion diseases in animals occur mainly as acquired disorders. Scrapie, CWD and BSE have been transmitted to other species in both experimental and non-experimental settings. Scrapie has been identified for over two centuries in Europe and was long thought to be a transmissible disorder.[37] The first convincing experimental transmission of scrapie was in 1936,[79] and since then there has been an extensive body of research into the nature of the transmissible agent.

Nature of the Transmissible Agent

In the past, the scrapie agent was thought to be a 'slow virus' because of the lengthy incubation periods associated with disease transmission (ranging from months to years) and because the agent was filterable.[89] The agent was also found to possess other unusual biological properties, including a remarkable resistance to conventional means of decontamination that were effective against bacteria and viruses.[83] Alternative suggestions for the nature of the agent to account for these properties included a proposal that the agent might be composed entirely of protein,[125] or a virino.[162] In 1982, Stanley Prusiner published the prion hypothesis, which states that the agent is composed of a modified host protein, the prion protein (PrP), with no nucleic acid component (Box 18.1).[308] This hypothesis was initially the subject of much criticism, because the existence of different strains of the scrapie agent had previously been established following experimental transmission in mice (see Bruce[46] for review). These strains possessed distinctive biological properties, namely their relative incubation periods in selected inbred strains of mice and the pattern of vacuolation in the mouse brain, which were

BOX 18.1. Characteristics of prions

- Prions are unique infectious pathogens that cause a group of fatal neurodegenerative diseases by an unconventional mechanism.
- Prions are transmissible particles that are devoid of nucleic acid and seem to be composed entirely of a modified protein (PrP^{Sc}).
- The normal, cellular PrP (PrP^{C}) is converted into PrP^{Sc} through a post-translational process, during which it acquires a high β-sheet content.
- In contrast to pathogens carrying a nucleic acid genome, prions appear to encipher strain-specific properties in the tertiary structure of PrP^{Sc}.

replicated with fidelity upon serial passage and appeared to imply the presence of an informational molecule to account for their existence.[47] However, no nucleic acid component of the transmissible agent has been confirmed, and the prion hypothesis has gained increasingly widespread acceptance.[305]

History of Prion Diseases in Humans

In the 1920s, Creutzfeldt and Jakob independently reported cases that have subsequently been known as CJD.[76,185] Interestingly, review of Creutzfeldt's original case has suggested that it does not fulfil current diagnostic criteria for a human prion disease, and nor do three of the five cases reported by Jakob in 1921 and 1923.[185,186,243] Although Jakob employed the term 'spastic pseudosclerosis' for this group of diseases,[186] the term 'Creutzfeldt–Jakob disease' was introduced in 1922.[344] In subsequent years, a range of potential causes for CJD were suggested, including neurodegenerative, metabolic and vascular disorders. Because there is no pathological evidence of a conventional inflammatory reaction in the brain in CJD and, because there was no evidence of case-to-case transmission of the disease, an infectious aetiology was not considered likely. However, familial forms of 'spastic pseudosclerosis' were identified as early as 1924,[203] and subsequent reports emphasized the range of clinical and pathological phenotypic variability in sCJD by identifying disease subgroups with particular characteristics, such as the Heidenhain variant, in which cortical blindness is characteristic,[219] and the Brownell–Oppenheimer syndrome, in which cerebellar symptoms predominate and cerebellar pathology is marked.[44]

The initial description of GSS in 1936 did not suggest that this was likely to represent a transmissible disorder, but rather an inherited form of spinocerebellar ataxia with a distinctive neuropathological phenotype that did not appear to be related to CJD.[102] Likewise, the first descriptions of kuru in the late 1950s did not indicate that it might be related to CJD.[98] It was not until the observation by Hadlow on the similarities between the neuropathology of kuru in humans and scrapie in sheep[128] that an infectious aetiology for kuru was considered. This led to the subsequent successful transmission of kuru to a chimpanzee in 1966,[99] followed by transmissions of sCJD in 1968[108] and GSS in 1981.[242]

The recognition of the similarity between scrapie and human prion diseases was a major advance in the understanding of the aetiology of these disorders. The subsequent discovery of PrP in its disease-associated isoforms in these disorders helped to strengthen these links. The identification of the PRNP gene in humans and other species (designated Prnp) demonstrated that the entire open reading frame is contained within a single exon in all species, and the gene is highly conserved within mammals, with only relatively minor differences in the amino acid sequence between species.[307] These major advances have allowed the identification of a widening spectrum of human prion diseases (Table 18.1).[169,170] In particular, the identification of a widening range of PRNP mutations in familial prion diseases in humans has resulted in an ever increasing number of these disorders being identified, sometimes in the apparent absence of a family history of neurological disease.[216]

The recognition of BSE and the subsequent epizootic of this new prion disease in cattle in the United Kingdom and other countries,[343] together with the identification of vCJD as a new human prion disease resulting from exposure to the BSE agent,[380] has rekindled an enormous amount of scientific, medical and political interest in this group of rare and hitherto obscure disorders. The accompanying enhanced surveillance has identified new (or newly described) animal and human prion diseases. This chapter focuses on prion diseases as they occur in humans, with emphasis on the clinical phenotype, criteria for diagnosis and neuropathology. Relevant data on prion diseases in animals will be included, along with a description of the biology and characteristics of prions as essential background information.

PRION BIOLOGY

Definitions: Introducing the Prion Hypothesis

The phenotypic characteristics of prion diseases of humans and animals are heterogeneous in terms of their clinical and pathological features, some elements of which are shared with other neurodegenerative diseases. However, prion diseases are distinct from other human dementias in a number of important respects. First, where there is a known infectious aetiology, the incubation period can be extremely long (measured in years), although the clinical phase of the disease is usually very short indeed (measured in months). Second, the agents responsible do not have the biochemical or biophysical properties commonly associated with conventional infectious agents (Box 18.2). In particular, the extreme difficulty encountered in inactivation of prion infectivity remains a strong argument in favour of an unconventional agent. Third, an unconventional pathogen may be inferred from the observation that human prion diseases occur as acquired, familial and idiopathic disorders and that some familial prion diseases are transmissible under certain conditions. A better understanding of the fundamental aspects of prion disease pathogenesis has come about since 1983 by intense investigation of the role of PrP and the PRNP gene in humans. This has led to the formulation of the prion hypothesis in which PrP occupies a central position in disease pathogenesis (Box 18.1). This hypothesis appears to explain the unconventional biophysical properties of the agent and the unique aetiology of these diseases.[309] Although TSE remains a convenient descriptive and neutral term for these diseases, the majority of researchers now accept the prion hypothesis, at least as a working hypothesis, and the term 'prion disease' is often used in preference to acknowledge this fact.

PrP^C and PrP^{Sc}

Prion diseases are associated with a change in conformation of a normal cellular glycoprotein (termed PrP^C or PrP^{sen}) – a protein that is readily soluble in non-denaturing detergent solutions and sensitive to digestion by proteinase K (Figure 18.1a).[307] PrP^C is a copper-binding glycoprotein that is bound to the outer leaflet of the cell membrane by a glycosylphosphatidylinositol anchor in lipid raft microdomains (Figure 18.1b).[138] It is expressed in a wide variety of cell types, but it is highly expressed in neurons, where it is enriched at the synapse.[153] The normal function of PrP^C is not understood fully, although roles in normal cell function such as synaptic activity, lymphocyte activation, stress resistance and cell signalling have all been proposed.[57,250,330]

In tissues infected with prion agents, some of the normal detergent-soluble and protease-sensitive PrP^C converts into pathogenic 'scrapie-type' or proteinase K-resistant isoform

BOX 18.2. Physicochemical properties of the transmissible agent in prion diseases

- Resistant to inactivation by methods such as ultraviolet (UV) and ionizing radiation that act through modification of a nucleic acid genome.
- Relative sensitivity to inactivation by methods such as chaotropic salts and detergents that act as protein denaturants.
- Resistance to protease inactivation in absence of denaturation.
- A polydispersed size that, at its lowest range, falls below the size of the smallest known viruses.
- Co-purification with low-molecular-weight aggregated forms of PrP^{Sc}.

(a) (b) (c) (d)

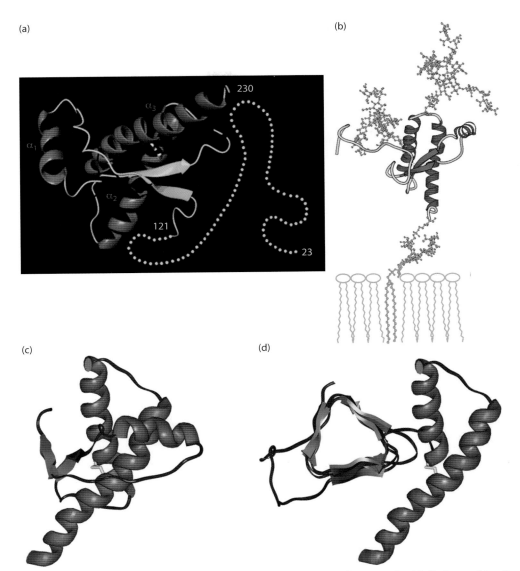

18.1 Structure of the normal (PrP^C) and pathological (PrP^Sc) isoforms of the prion protein. (a) Cartoon of the three-dimensional structure of intact human prion protein, PrP^C (residues 23–230). The α-helices are red, the β-strands are cyan, the segments with non-regular secondary structure within the C-terminal domain are yellow, and the flexibly disordered 'tail' of residues 23–121 is represented by yellow dots.[394] **(b)** Glycosylated PrP^C *in situ*. Schematic representation of the cellular prion protein (residues 93–231) in its glycosylated form, attached to the cell membrane by virtue of its glycosylphosphatidylinositol (GPI) anchor.[322] The three α-helices are shown in red and the short anti-parallel β-sheet region is shown in blue. The two asparagine-linked glycans and the carbohydrate component of the GPI anchor are shown in orange. The lipid component of the GPI anchor and the outer leaflet of the cell membrane are shown in green. **(c)** The structure of PrP^C contains mostly α-helical structures (spiral-shaped red ribbons) and a small portion of β-sheet (blue arrows). The increase in β-sheet upon conversion into the abnormal, prion form is illustrated in **(d)** by a theoretical structure of PrP^Sc. The 90–160 region of amino acid sequence has been remodelled into a α-helical architecture (blue arrows), whereas the C-terminal helices are preserved as in PrP^C (red ribbons) linked by a disulphide bridge (yellow). In addition, it has been proposed that the α-helical PrP forms trimers, which in turn oligomerize to form protofibrils and higher-order structures.[121]

(a) Image courtesy of Professor Kurt Wuthrich, Swiss Federal Institute of Technology, Zurich, Switzerland and the Scripps Research Institute, La Jolla, CA, USA. (b) Image courtesy of Dr Mark Wormald and Professors Pauline Rudd and Raymond Dwek, Oxford Glycobiology Institute, Oxford, UK. (c,d) Images courtesy of Professor Fred Cohen, University of California at San Francisco, San Francisco, CA, USA.

(or isoforms) termed PrP^Sc or PrP^res (Figure 18.1c,d). The prion or 'protein-only' hypothesis proposes that the infectious agent or prion is composed largely or exclusively of PrP^Sc, which when introduced into the organism induces the conversion of further PrP^c into PrP^Sc.[307] The most common form of human prion disease is sCJD. This disease is believed to arise spontaneously, either following the spontaneous conversion of PrP^C into PrP^Sc or from a somatic mutation in PrP that renders it susceptible to conversion to PrP^Sc.[307] It has been proposed that pathogenic mutations favour the spontaneous conversion of PrP^C into PrP^Sc followed by an autocatalytic conversion process.

As described originally, PrP^{Sc} is insoluble in non-denaturing detergents and is partially resistant to protease digestion with proteinase K. This remains largely true; however, proteinase K-sensitive PrP^{Sc} isoforms (senPrP^{Sc}) have been described and implicated in human prion disease pathogenesis.[100,324] Other aberrant isoforms of PrP, such as ^{Ctm}PrP, cyPrP and PrP^{L} have been implicated as those causing prion neurotoxicity.[62,329] The detection of a PrP^{Sc}-like form (PrP*20) in normal human brains have raised the intriguing possibility that PrP^{Sc} is a normal and transitory metabolic products and that prion disease might be thought of as a failure of PrP metabolism.[392] The proliferation of acronyms to identify the increasing number of novel forms of the prion protein is summarized in Table 18.2. Irrespective of the exact nature of the transmissible agent and the mechanism of its neurotoxicity, the prion concept has been highly influential and has been invoked to explain non-mendelian inheritance associated with yeast and filamentous fungal proteins,[360] molecular aspects of long-term potentiation[336] and is currently in the process of being deployed more generally to a wide variety of neurodegenerative diseases.[112]

Advances in Understanding Prion Disease Pathogenesis Using Animal Models

Several prion diseases (scrapie, BSE, CWD, feline spongiform encephalopathy (FSE), sCJD, fCJD, vCJD, kuru, FFI and some but not all forms of GSS) have been transmitted to experimental animals, including primates and rodents. Variable amounts and combinations of the following histopathological lesions have been seen following transmission: (i) vacuolation of neurons, neuropil and, in some instances, the white matter in rodents; (ii) PrP-immunopositivity in a variety of deposits, including amyloid plaques; (iii) neuronal loss; and (iv) activation of astrocytes and microglia (Figure 18.2).[93] The neuropathological diversity, such as the distribution and severity of the vacuolation in mice, together with their relative incubation periods (in selected inbred strains of mice) have been used to identify the strain of the agent.[46] Genetic

TABLE 18.2 Terminology used to denote the increasing number of forms of the prion protein

Prion protein term or acronym	Definition
PrP	Prion protein
PRNP	Gene encoding prion protein in humans
Prnp	Gene encoding prion protein in non-human species
PrP^C	Normal cellular isoform of prion protein
PrP^{Sc}	Abnormal disease-associated form of prion protein (irrespective of its biochemical form, means of detection and the species from which it is derived)
PrP^{sen}	Normal cellular prion protein, as defined by its sensitivity to proteolytic degradation
PrP^{res}	Partially protease-resistant prion protein (often used as an operational definition of PrP^{Sc})
PrP$^{27-30}$	N-terminally truncated form of PrP produced by the action of proteases on tissue samples containing PrP^{Sc} and usually visualized by western blotting
PrP^{Sc} or PrP^{res} isotype (or type)	Classification of disease-associated prion protein according to size of the protease-resistant core fragment, produced by proteinase K treatment under defined conditions and analyzed by western blotting
Glycoforms	Correctly, forms of prion protein differing in the glycans attached; in practice, used to refer to the three forms resulting from variable occupancy of the two N-linked glycosylation sites (non-, mono- and di-glycosylated prion protein)
Glycotype	Classification of disease-associated prion protein according to proportion of the three glycoforms remaining after proteinase K treatment under defined conditions and analyzed by western blotting
senPrP^{Sc}	PrP^{Sc} that is disease-associated, but sensitive to proteolytic degradation under commonly used conditions
PrP*20	A PrP^{Sc}-like form reportedly found at very low levels in normal brain tissue
PrP$^{106-126}$	A cytotoxic synthetic peptide based on conserved residues in PrP at positions 106–126
^{Ctm}PrP	Abnormal protease-sensitive transmembrane form of PrP with its C-terminus in the lumen of the endoplasmic reticulum and proposed to be cytotoxic
cyPrP	Prion protein inappropriately trafficked into the cytoplasm and proposed to be cytotoxic
PrP^L	A form of PrP that accumulates during prion infection and which is neurotoxic (i.e. lethal)
PrP^d or PrP^{TSE}	Disease associated prion protein irrespective of physical form or means of detection. Synonymous with PrP^{Sc} (but lacking the apparent reference to scrapie)

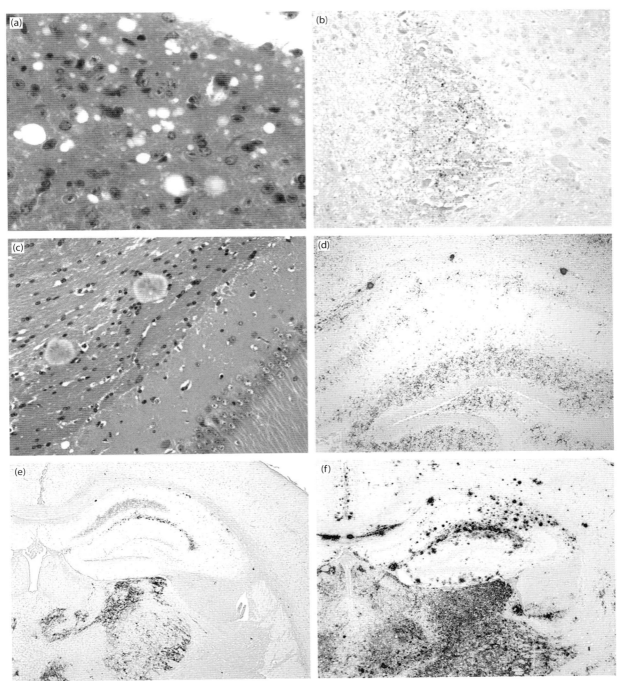

18.2 Creutzfeldt–Jakob disease (CJD) transmission to mice. (a) Vacuolation within the superior colliculus of a wild-type mouse (VM strain) following inoculation with sporadic Creutzfeldt–Jakob disease (sCJD) (MM1 subtype) brain homogenate. **(b)** Prion protein (PrP) deposition within the vestibular nucleus of the medulla in a VM mouse challenged with sCJD (MM1 subtype). **(c)** Plaques within the corpus callosum of a VM mouse challenged with variant Creutzfeldt–Jakob disease (vCJD). **(d)** Widespread PrP accumulation within the hippocampus of a VM mouse challenged with vCJD. **(e)** PrP accumulation following sCJD (MM1 subtype) transmission to transgenic mice expressing human PrP, (homozygous for methionine at codon 129, HuMMTg mouse). **(f)** Intense, widespread PrP accumulation in the corpus callosum and hippocampus, with multiple large florid plaques and smaller cluster plaques in a HuMMTg mouse inoculated with vCJD. 6H4 anti-PrP antibody.

Images (e) and (f) courtesy of Dr Matthew Bishop, University of Edinburgh, Edinburgh, UK.

variation in the murine prion protein gene (*Prnp*) and at other loci is also known to affect incubation period in mice.[1,232]

Rodent models have also been used to define routes of spread of infection from the periphery to the CNS (Figure 18.3), and these studies implicate agent replication in the lymphoreticular system as a key event preceding neuroinvasion.[233] Experimental oral infection with scrapie results in uptake of the agent across the gut wall into lymphoid follicles in the gut, including Peyer's patches. Infectivity appears to replicate in follicular dendritic cells (FDCs) at these sites and then spreads to other lymphoid tissues, including the spleen. Murine scrapie infection results in an abnormal germinal centre reaction in the spleen, which may be associated with increased immune complex trapping by hypertrophic FDCs.[246] However, studies in transgenic mice have revealed that activation of specific complement components is involved in the initial trapping of prions in lymphoreticular organs early after infection.[205]

Follicular dendritic cells play a key role in the peripheral pathogenesis of prion diseases. Functional inactivation of FDCs is associated with a prolonged incubation period following peripheral exposure to prions. From the spleen, infectivity may spread to the spinal cord (and thence to the brain) via retrograde spread along the nerve fibres of the splanchnic plexus.[233] In addition, the agent can spread

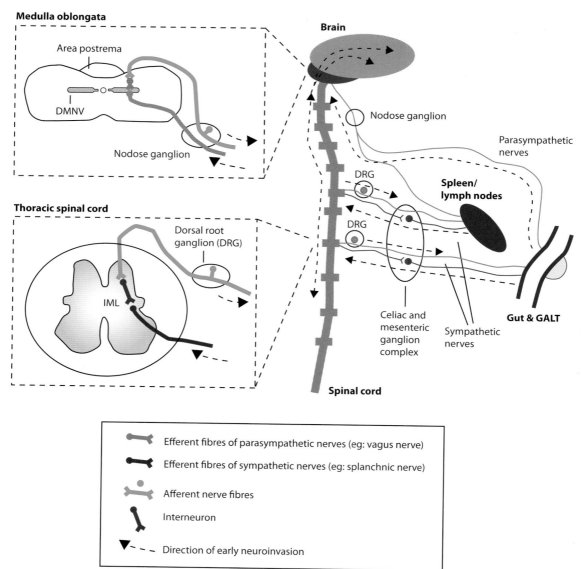

18.3 Following oral inoculation with scrapie, PrP^Sc accumulation indicates the spread of the agent from the gut along two distinct neuroanatomical pathways to the central nervous system (CNS). The agent replicates in the gut-associated lymphoid tissues (GALT) and can then spread to other lymphoid organs, including the spleen. From the spleen, the agent can spread along sympathetic fibres of the splanchnic nerve to the intermediolateral cell column (IML) of the mid-thoracic spinal cord and then to the brain in a caudal-to-cranial direction along the spinal cord. Direct spread from the gut to the CNS can also occur along parasympathetic fibres of the vagus nerve to the dorsal motor nucleus of the vagus (DMNV) within the medulla. DRG, dorsal root ganglion.

Image courtesy of Dr Neil Mabbott, Roslin Institute, University of Edinburgh, Edinburgh, UK.

in a retrograde fashion from the parasympathetic plexi in the gut wall, ascending the vagus nerve and entering the brain stem at the medulla around the dorsal motor vagal nuclei (see Figure 18.3).[233] During the incubation period in experimental scrapie in hamsters and sheep, infectivity can be detected in lymphoid tissues throughout the body, and in whole blood and the buffy coat fraction of blood.[168] Similar events have been demonstrated more recently in sheep experimentally orally infected with BSE.[165] Once infectivity reaches the brain, both infectivity and PrP^{Sc} spread along neuroanatomical pathways, and it seems likely that centrifugal spread can occur from the CNS via peripheral nerves at different stages in the later phases of the disease.

Concept of Prion Agent Strain

The existence of different strains of scrapie agent has been demonstrated and studied for many years in murine models. These strains may be differentiated by their relative incubation periods in selected inbred strains of mice and the precise neuroanatomical pattern of lesions in the brain when an isolate is transmitted and serially passaged in inbred mouse lines (reviewed by Bruce[46]). Once adapted to serial transmission in mice, these phenotypic traits are conserved; however, the primary transmission between species is often inefficient, with only a proportion of the exposed animals succumbing to disease and with variable and sometimes protracted incubation periods. What determines this 'species barrier' is not understood fully, but one component of this may be the degree of structural similarity between the prion proteins of the two species involved (reviewed in Caughey[60]). The identification of the prion protein has led to the concept of molecular strain typing, where different isoforms of PrP^{Sc} are proposed to correspond to individual strains of the transmissible agent (Box 18.3).

Neuropathology

The brain is the organ most affected in prion diseases: despite increasing evidence of PrP^{Sc} accumulation and replication in other tissues and organs, there is scant evidence of either structural or functional disturbances outside the CNS.[80,246] PrP^{Sc} accumulation in the brain in prion diseases is extensive (in most cases) in many grey matter regions, and yet it has been established for many years that not all neurons are equally vulnerable, even within a given brain region, leading to the concept of neuropathological targeting.[94] Histological studies have demonstrated an early loss of parvalbumin

immunoreactivity from a subset of γ-aminobutyric acid (GABA)ergic neurons that precedes spongiform change and reactive astrocytosis in the 263K hamster scrapie model. In this model, the GABAergic neurons appear to be the first population to undergo neurodegeneration and cell death; a similar severe loss of GABAergic neurons has also been observed in CJD,[127] suggesting that this population is selectively vulnerable in prion diseases. A study in the 263K hamster scrapie model found that local accumulation of PrP^{Sc} was followed by dendritic atrophy and a loss of synaptic boutons, with neuronal death occurring after a longer period of time.[27] Sequential analysis of neuropathology suggested that transport of PrP^{Sc} occurred from the thalamus to the cortex along glutaminergic afferent projections. PrP^{Sc} would have then spread trans-synaptically to neurons in layer IV of the cortex and would have undergone orthograde transport to GABAergic presynaptic boutons, where it would have altered synaptic function and resulted in presynaptic bouton degeneration by an unknown mechanism. Spongiform change in the neuropil appears to occur shortly after the accumulation of PrP^{Sc} primarily in the region of synapses, with focal neuritic swelling, loss of internal organelles, splitting of plasma membranes and accumulation of abnormal membranes (Figure 18.4).[221] Altered plasma membrane permeability resulting in spongiform change, at least in its early stages, appears to be a reversible phenomenon that requires the expression of PrP^{C} on neurons.[237]

As PrP^{Sc} accumulates in the brain, there is a loss of antioxidant activity, which may result, at least in part, from a loss of the normal antioxidant activity of PrP^{C} (see Brown[36] for review). Heightened oxidative stress in neurons appears to be associated with increased lipid peroxidation,[35] which increases in time with the accumulation of PrP^{Sc} in the brain. Accumulation of PrP^{Sc} is also reported to result in a dysregulated unfolded protein response, in which sustained translational repression affects neuronal viability.[260] Neuronal

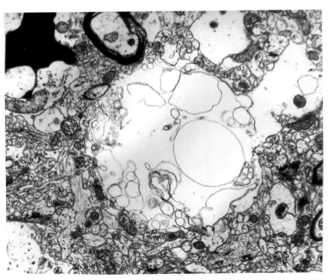

18.4 Electron microscopy of spongiform change in sporadic Creutzfeldt–Jakob disease (sCJD) shows the vacuoles to contain dilated intracellular membrane-bound structures (vacuoles within vacuoles) and amorphous debris.[227]

Image courtesy of Professor Pawel Liberski, Medical University of Lodz, Lodz, Poland.

BOX 18.3. Properties of prion strains

- Prion strains interact with host PrP^{C} to influence characteristics of the disease, such as incubation period and neuropathology.
- Prion strains retain their identity on serial transmission within a species, and after propagation in different host species.
- Prion agents carry their own strain-specific information, which may be encoded in self-perpetuating modifications of PrP^{Sc} or in a separate, unidentified informational molecule that interact with host factors.
- Strain typing in mice can be used to explore links between prion diseases in different species, for example, bovine spongiform encephalopathy (BSE) and variant Creutzfeldt–Jakob disease (vCJD).

damage in prion disease is accompanied by an astrocytic and microglial response early in the disease process.[356] Microglial activation results in the production and release of pro-inflammatory cytokines such as interleukin 1 (IL-1), interleukin 6 (IL-6), interleukin 12 (IL-12) and tumour necrosis factor (TNF), which precede the loss of hippocampal neurones from prion-infected mice. IL-1 and IL-6 may influence the astrocytic response, although interleukin 10 (IL-10) appears to play a particularly prominent role in disease progression: mice deficient in IL-10 are highly susceptible to prion diseases, with a markedly shortened incubation period compared with wild-type mice.[356] The subsequent pathogenic events resulting in cell death in prion diseases are still understood incompletely, but there is an increasing body of evidence to suggest that cell death occurs by apoptosis (see Brandner[31] for review). Several pathways may lead to apoptosis in prion diseases, including oxidative stress, complement activation and cytokine-mediated damage, resulting in increased levels of caspase 3, Fas activation and c-jun upregulation.[95] PrPC appears to have an anti-apoptotic function, the loss of which following conversion to PrPSc may also lead to apoptotic cell death (see Roucou and LeBlanc[320] for review).

Experimental Transmission to Non-Human Primates

Because primates are the closest species to humans, primate transmission has been attempted from a wide range of human prion diseases. According to the National Institutes of Health series, the overall case transmission rate in primates for sCJD, GSS and kuru was over 87 per cent, with higher rates for CJD and kuru and lower rates for familial diseases.[41] In serial passage, incubation times became shorter and stabilized at these shorter times. The route of infection had a significant effect on transmission rate. For example, inocula that reproducibly transmitted disease by the intracerebral route transmitted irregularly after peripheral inoculation. Regarding the distribution of infectivity in human prion diseases, apart from the brain, spinal cord and eye, infectivity was irregularly detectable in other organs (including the spleen, liver and kidney) and in a limited number of experiments was never detected in secretions or excretions.[41] Transmission rates were found to be comparatively low following inoculation of either formalin-fixed specimens or cultured brain tissue. More recently, a macaque model has been established and used to investigate the BSE/vCJD agent strain, its relationship to other human prion diseases, its potential modes of transmission and its unique pathogenesis.[154,223] Squirrel monkeys inoculated with BSE agent develop a spongiform encephalopathy with accumulation of PrPSc and severe tau pathology characterized by the presence of hyperphosphorylated tau in the cerebrum, cerebellum and brain stem.[295] Investigations are underway to determine whether detection of hyperphosphorylated tau in addition to protein 14-3-3 and other molecules in CSF might serve as marker in the ante-mortem diagnosis of vCJD.[123]

Transgenic Models for the Study of Prion Diseases

Over the past few decades, a range of *Prnp* transgenic and knock-out models have been developed to elucidate factors governing the transmissibility of prion diseases between species, to provide efficient bioassays and to study prion pathogenesis (Figure 18.2). Mice in which the *Prnp* has been disrupted (PrP knockout mice or PrP[0/0]) are resistant to prion infection, as shown by the absence of replication of the agent in tissues and the absence of clinical signs of disease or neuropathological lesions.[32] In contrast, mice overexpressing PrP have shorter incubation times than wild-type mice inoculated with the same prion agent, providing useful models for assaying infectivity.[306] Results obtained in mice with high PrP expression levels must be interpreted with caution because in some instances these animals develop a phenotype with necrotizing myopathy and vacuolation of the CNS.[373]

In most cases, transmission of a prion disease from one species to another is less efficient than transmission within the same species, a phenomenon attributed to the 'species barrier'.[45] Transgenic mice expressing PrP genes from a range of species have been used to investigate the molecular mechanisms governing prion disease transmission. Early studies performed in mice carrying hamster transgenes indicated that the efficiency of transmission might depend on the degree of similarity between donor and recipient PrP.[306] However, prion disease has been transmitted in the presence of dissimilar PrP sequences, suggesting that other factors must play a role in susceptibility to infection with prions.[11] Interestingly, study findings indicate that trans-species inoculation of prion-infected material can result in a phenotype characterized by prion-related neuropathological abnormalities, accumulation of PrPSc and propagation of infectivity in the absence of clinical disease.[158,313]

The cell types involved in agent propagation have not been identified completely. It has been assumed that propagation of infectivity and pathology in the brain is neuron-dependent. However, neuron-specific or astrocyte-specific expression of PrP renders PrP knockout mice susceptible to prion infectivity, resulting in astrogliosis and spongiform degeneration, a pattern similar to that seen in wild-type mice. These studies suggest that a common pathway mediated by cytokine overproduction and neuronal dysfunction may be at the base of the neuropathological alterations seen in prion diseases.[311] Another approach to studying prion disease pathobiology has been to graft fetal neural tissue from mice overexpressing PrPC into the brain of PrP knockout mice, followed by inoculation of a prion agent. Infected grafts developed spongiform degeneration and astrogliosis and contained high amounts of PrPSc and infectivity. However, the lifespan of the animal was not reduced and animals remained without neurological symptoms. In addition, no histopathological lesions were observed in PrPC-deficient tissue, even in regions adjoining the graft that contained high amounts of PrPSc, suggesting that PrPC expression is required for neurodegeneration and PrPSc may not be neurotoxic unless newly synthesized from neurons.[32,33]

Transgenic mouse lines have been developed for the study of familial prion diseases. The most extensively studied model expresses a proline (P) to leucine (L) mutation at codon 101 (P101L) of the mouse PrP gene, equivalent to the PrP-P102L mutation present in humans with GSS P102L. Transgenic mice generated by random integration or gene targeting of the mutant gene expressing wild-type or low levels of the mutant PrP do not develop clinical disease or neuropathological lesions.[238] In contrast, overexpression of mutant PrP results in a spontaneous neurological disease with spongiform degeneration and amyloid plaques.[166] It has been suggested that the apparent discrepancy between transgenic P101L models could be explained by transgene copy number and the levels of mutant PrP.[262]

Studies in gene targeted Tg PrP-P101L mice inoculated with brain extracts from two patients with GSS P102L from the same family (one patient with and the other without spongiform degeneration of the brain) showed that efficient transmission of disease was only observed in mice inoculated with brain extracts from the patient with GSS P102L and spongiform degeneration. Serial passage in Tg P101L demonstrated the formation of PrP amyloid in the absence of neurological signs or spongiform degeneration or high levels of infectivity and disease in the apparent absence of PrP^{Sc}.[12,294] A different transgenic model of a familial prion disease was generated by expressing the mouse PrP homologue of a nine-octapeptide insertional mutation (*PG14*) described in humans. Transgenic PG14 mice accumulated a neurotoxic form of PrP that possessed biochemical properties similar to those present in PrP^{Sc}, but which is not associated with infectivity. Models such as these raise an important issue in the pathogenesis of prion diseases: the possible dissociation between toxicity and infectivity.[64]

In contrast, knock-in mice expressing PrP D177N, the mouse equivalent of the *PRNP* mutation associated with human FFI, spontaneously developed a disease reminiscent of FFI in humans that is transmissible to Tg mice expressing both high and wild-type levels of PrP. It was therefore concluded that the D177N mutation in the structured core of PrP was sufficient to generate a specific PrP^{Sc} conformer and infectious prion agent responsible for the pathological hallmarks of FFI.[183]

Membrane attachment of PrP may influence prion disease process. Chesebro *et al.* generated transgenic mice lacking a glycosylphosphatidylinositol moiety (GPI).[63] After scrapie infection the anchorless mice developed high titres of infectivity, extensive PrP^{Sc} amyloid formation without typical clinical signs or spongiform degeneration. This model is reminiscent of the neuropathology seen in certain human familial prion diseases characterized by expression of carboxy-terminal truncated PrP and PrP-cerebral amyloid angiopathy (PrP-CAA).[107]

In Vitro Models of Prion Disease

Recent years have seen remarkable growth in the number and applications of *in vitro* models in which to study particular aspects of the prion disease process. Early attempts at propagating the agent *in vitro* were hampered by the puzzling finding that a very limited number of cell lines could support replication and that this property was agent strain-specific (see Piccardo *et al.* for a recent example involving cell lines commonly employed in vaccine production).[296] Hence, the vast majority of cell culture work has been performed with a single constitutively scrapie-infected mouse neuroblastoma cell line. More recently, cell lines from other species that support prion replication or that can be genetically engineered to do so, have been developed. This area can be anticipated to command a greater importance in the future, with the findings that a) within largely resistant cell populations there can exist a subpopulation of susceptible cells that may be cloned to produce highly susceptible cell lines, b) that such subcloned lines can form the basis of highly sensitive assays for prion infectivity, and c) that the molecular basis of prion diversity and selection can be studies in cell culture.[207,226,235]

Prion replication in cell culture does not appear to result in extensive cell death and is therefore not amenable to investigations of cytotoxic mechanisms. An alternative *in vitro* model in which neuroblastoma cells or neurons are exposed to a synthetic aggregated cytotoxic fragment of the prion protein (PrP$^{106-126}$) has been used extensively to study the cytotoxic mechanism.[91] The cytotoxic effect of PrP$^{106-126}$ depends on cellular PrP expression, which results in activation of various signal transduction pathways, leading to cell damage and apoptosis (see Tagliavini *et al.*[349]). However, the PrP$^{106-126}$ fragment is not known to occur in naturally occurring prion diseases, and therefore it is not certain to what extent this model exactly parallels the events seen *in vivo*.

The past ten years has seen rapid developments cell-free *in vitro* PrP^C to PrP^{Sc} conversion systems.[270] These include an extremely versatile system termed protein misfolding cyclic amplification (PMCA) that uses natural PrP^{Sc} 'seeds' and PrP^C 'substrates' present in tissue homogenates and sequential rounds of sonication and incubation to promote PrP conversion, and a technique termed quaking induced conversion (QuIC), in which shaking replaces sonication and recombinant PrP replaces tissue-derived PrP^C. Interestingly, efficient amplification depends on currently unknown factors present in normal brain extracts, but conversion can also be promoted by polyanions such as short RNA sequences.[81] The PMCA conversion process appears not to have a theoretical limit to the number of cycles of conversion that can be employed, and the protease-resistant PrP thus produced appears to be infectious, albeit with a lower level of associated infectivity than that which accumulates *in vivo*.[58,206] These findings, in combination with the de novo generation of infectivity by chemical refolding of recombinant PrP,[225] and from unseeded PMCA reactions using defined components provide evidence in favour of the prion hypothesis that many consider definitive.[65,368]

Experimental Therapy for Prion Diseases

The development of *in vitro* models has allowed for the screening of candidate therapeutic compounds, often evaluated by their ability to inhibit PrP^{Sc} accumulation in neuroblastoma cells. Compounds with such activities are numerous and chemically heterogeneous and have been the subject of a systematic review.[358] Where the mechanism has been investigated, the compounds appear to directly target PrP^C expression on the cell surface or otherwise interfere with the interaction between PrP^{Sc} and PrP^C. Efforts to evaluate such compounds *in vivo* have shown that some of these compounds, when administered close to the time of experimental challenge, have a measurable effect in prolonging the incubation period in rodents experimentally infected with rodent-adapted scrapie. Once neurological symptoms have appeared, the challenge for any candidate therapy is considerably greater, but perhaps not insurmountable.[266] Despite considerable effort in developing and testing candidate anti-prion agents the evidence from systematic review of therapeutic interventions in human prion disease and from clinical trials is not very encouraging at this point in time.[69,345,359]

Prion Decontamination

The infectious agent causing prion disease shows a remarkable degree of resistance to chemical and physical inactivation procedures that are effective with conventional organisms.[354] For example, it is generally considered that formalin- or glutaraldehyde-fixed tissues are largely free from infectious agents because of the disinfectant properties of aldehydes. However, prion infectivity can survive, in spite of the cross-linking of proteins that occurs during aldehyde fixation. Therefore, in order to reduce the risk of handling infected tissue, small samples (e.g. biopsies) from patients with suspected prion disease are fixed in formalin followed by post-fixation in 96 per cent formic acid for 30 minutes and further fixation in fresh 10 per cent formalin before further processing.[352] Precautions for working with tissues from patients with known or suspected prion diseases are summarized in Box 18.4.

Inactivation procedures that previously have been considered to be completely effective are known to provide a high degree of, but not complete, inactivation. Some examples include exposure to 1M sodium hydroxide for 1 hour at room temperature, gravity-displacement autoclaving at 132°C for 1 hour, and porous-load autoclaving at 134–138°C for 18–60 minutes. In contrast, sodium hypochlorite solutions containing at least 20 000 ppm of available chlorine appear to be an effective method, although this is neither a user-friendly nor a product-friendly method. Numerous studies have indicated that complete inactivation could be achieved by combining these procedures consecutively or simultaneously.[352] Despite the failure of 1M sodium hydroxide at room temperature to completely inactivate the agent, combining 1M sodium hydroxide with heat appears to be a very effective procedure, not only when carried out under steam pressure at 121°C but also when applied as a brief boiling procedure. Novel methods of prion decontamination continue to be investigated, and one such method is the use of radiofrequency gas plasma to sterilize even complex steel surfaces.[13]

A model system has been established that uses prion-contaminated metal wires and rodent bioassay to mimic

---

BOX 18.4. Precautions for working with tissues from patients with known or suspected prion diseases

- Samples should be labelled 'biohazard'.
- Single-use protective clothing is preferred.
- Use disposable equipment wherever possible and dispose by incineration.
- Fixatives and waste fluids should be decontaminated before disposal.
- Effective chemicals and physical agents to reduce prion infectivity include:
  - hypochlorite (20 000 ppm free chlorine)
  - NaOH (1–2N for 1 h)
  - formic acid (100% for 1 h)
  - steam heat (134°C for at least 18 min)

---

potential iatrogenic CJD exposure through contaminated surgical instruments. This model has been of considerable value in determining the relative efficacy of existing and novel decontamination methods for surgical steel instruments, including the combination of denaturing detergents and proteolytic enzymes.[180] The safest method of dealing with instruments and devices used in neurosurgery on patients suspected of having CJD would be to employ, whenever possible, single-use instruments and to dispose of them by incineration. When instruments or equipment cannot be discarded, additional measures should be applied to enhance the level of confidence that the prion agents will be inactivated, or the instruments may be quarantined until a definite diagnosis is available. Recommended measures have been published by the World Health Organization.[387]

Safeguarding the recipients of blood and blood products from accidental exposure to prion infectivity presents particular problems in the area of inactivation,[353] and a more realistic aim might be to develop affinity matrices that could be used to augment the limited ability of leukodepletion filters to reduce infectious titres.[124]

PRION DISEASES IN ANIMALS

Prion diseases have been described in a range of captive and wild animal species (Table 18.3), many of which have been transmitted experimentally to laboratory rodents, ruminants or primates. Until 1998, four prion diseases were recognized in animals: scrapie of sheep and goats, bovine spongiform encephalopathy (BSE) of cattle and related conditions of felids and exotic ruminants in wildlife collections, chronic wasting disease (CWD) of cervids and transmissible mink encephalopathy (TME). This last is extremely rare, with no outbreaks being recorded since the 1980s, and will not be considered further here. Biochemical aspects of TME are referred to later. In 1998 a new sheep disease phenotype, Nor98, was recognized in Norway[17] and in the last decade two further novel prion diseases have been recognized in cattle.[9]

Classic Scrapie

Scrapie occurs as an endemic disorder in Europe, Asia and North America, but certain countries, particularly those of Australasia, are regarded as free from classical scrapie. There is no epidemiological evidence to suggest that scrapie is pathogenic to man.[39]

Scrapie transmission occurs most commonly in the early perinatal period with the efficiency of transmission decreasing with increasing age. Colostrum, milk and placenta are infectious and possibly also other bodily fluids and excreta, but infection of pre-implantation embryos does not occur.[212,312] Direct contact with an infected sheep is not obligatory for transmission as naïve sheep introduced to an infected environment may develop disease and infected placentas probably contribute significantly to environmental contamination.[116] Scrapie has twice occurred in iatrogenic epidemics resulting from contaminated vaccines.

Outbreaks of scrapie have been identified in many different breeds of sheep, goats and mouflon. The clinical features are variable, and include alterations in cardiac

TABLE 18.3 Prion diseases in animals

Disease	Species and epidemiology	Aetiology
Scrapie	Sheep, goats and mouflon, widespread, endemic, identified for 250 years	Acquired, transmission from ewe to lamb
'Nor98' or 'Atypical scrapie'	Sheep; reported in Europe, United States, Asia; mainly single cases on farms	Apparently acquired; mode of transmission unknown
Transmissible mink encephalopathy	Farmed mink; very rare; isolated outbreaks mostly in United States; last reported in 1985	Acquired (source unknown)
Chronic wasting disease	Deer, elk and moose in United States, Canada (captive and wild animals) and Korea (zoological collection); prevalence increasing	Acquired, including horizontal transmission
Bovine spongiform encephalopathy (BSE)	Cattle; large epizootic in United Kingdom since 1980s, now rare; identified worldwide	Acquired (contaminated meat and bone meal animal feed)
Exotic ungulate encephalopathy	Small numbers in wide range of captive species, mostly in United Kingdom since 1980s	Acquired (meat and bone meal animal feed contaminated with BSE agent)
Feline spongiform encephalopathy	Domestic cats and wild felines in zoos, mostly in United Kingdom since 1990s	Acquired (pet food or cattle carcasses contaminated with BSE agent)
L-type BSE or bovine amyloidotic spongiform encephalopathy	Cattle; rare cases in Europe, North America and Japan	Unknown
H-type BSE	Cattle; rare cases in Europe, United States and Japan	Unknown

rhythm and gastrointestinal motility, behavioural changes, incoordination, tremor and pruritus. The duration of the clinical illness can vary from acute death without premonitory signs to around 6 months.[168]

Susceptibility to sheep scrapie and to ovine BSE is heavily influenced by the *Prnp* polymorphisms T112M, A136V, L141F, R154H, P168L and Q171H/R.[115,168] Sheep A136A, R171R appear to be strongly, but not absolutely resistant to classical scrapie, and the risk of disease in sheep of other genotypes is strain dependent. Thus A136A, Q171Q sheep are susceptible, and V136V, Q171Q sheep resistant, to the experimental sheep scrapie strain CH1641 and experimental ovine BSE, whereas the converse situation applies for SSBP/1 scrapie.[168] In goats the polymorphisms I142M, D146S, H154R, R211Q and Q222K influence susceptibility though none provides strong resistance to disease.[115] The use of rams bearing the A136A, R171R allele has been successfully exploited in Europe and the United States to breed resistant alleles into flocks in order to reduce the prevalence of scrapie.

Clinical scrapie is associated with widespread PrP^{Sc} accumulation in brain and viscera. PrP^{Sc} is initially detectable in lymphoid tissues (mainly Peyer's patches) consistent with an oral route of infection.[152,192] With increasing incubation period, there is an incremental involvement in lymphoid tissues and autonomic nerves. Neuroinvasion begins with the parasympathetic dorsal motor nucleus of the trigeminal nerve consistent with an ascending infection from the alimentary tract via the vagal nerves. However, not all sheep genotypes or all scrapie sources show infection in viscera.[192] Infectivity can be demonstrated in blood from early stages of infection[165] and scrapie-affected sheep have an early and consistent involvement of the circumventricular organs, which, lacking a blood-brain barrier, provides for the possibility of an alternative or parallel vascular route of neuroinvasion.[341]

The timing of infectivity or accumulation of PrP^{Sc} in the peripheral tissues is affected by the age at exposure, strain, dose of infection and by *Prnp* polymorphisms, with the most rapid kinetics associated with V136V, Q171Q genotype.[5] In addition to PrP^{Sc} accumulations in nerves and lymphoid tissues, PrP^{Sc} may also be detected in retina, peripheral ganglia, adrenal medulla (Figure 18.5), kidney, muscle spindles and placenta. Kupffer cells of the liver may contain infectivity in ovine BSE[116] and myocytes have been shown to accumulate PrP^{Sc} in goat scrapie.

The neuropathology of scrapie is typical of TSEs comprising vacuolation, neuronal loss and gliosis (Figure 18.6) although clinical scrapie cases can occur where neither vacuolation nor gliosis is histologically apparent. PrP^{Sc} accumulation in scrapie brains occurs in a wider variety of morphological patterns than is encountered in human or rodent TSEs.[192] Electron microscopy has shown that punctate, linear and perineuronal patterns correspond to membrane PrP^{Sc} accumulation by neurons and dendrites whereas stellate, perivascular and sub-pial types relate to glial cells.[192,194] Intra-neuronal, intra-astrocytic and intra-microglial labelling corresponds to lysosomal accumulations in each cell type.[194] Classical or kuru-type amyloid plaques do not occur in scrapie but a distinctive cerebrovascular amyloid is found in a small minority of *Prnp* genotype/source combinations.[192] The distribution and frequency of these PrP^{Sc} types are helpful in characterizing disease phenotypes and discrimination between strains or sources but there is a poor correlation between PrP^{Sc} distribution or accumulation and clinical disease.[117,192]

Immunohistochemical PrP^{Sc} epitope mapping can be used to determine the approximate sites of intra-lysosomal PrP^{Sc} truncation in neurons, glial cells and tingible body macrophages of lymphoid tissues.[192] Ovine, caprine and cervid BSE, and some scrapie strains can be presumptively characterized

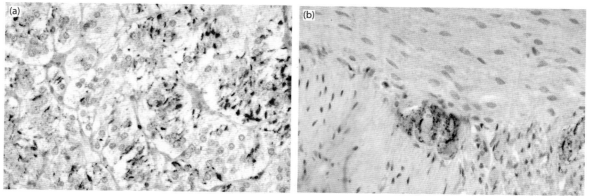

18.5 Natural scrapie in sheep. (a) Prion protein (PrP^{Sc}) accumulation in the adrenal medulla. **(b)** PrP^{Sc} accumulation in ganglion cells within the myenteric plexus of the gut (R145 anti-PrP antibody).

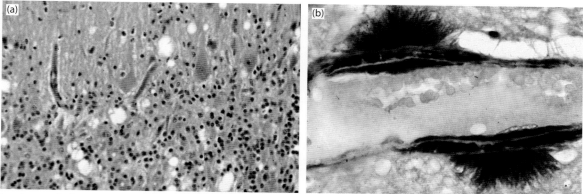

18.6 Natural scrapie in sheep. (a) Spongiform change in the cerebellum, involving both the molecular and granular cell layers with widespread neuronal loss. **(b)** Intense accumulation of prion protein (PrP^{Sc}) around blood vessels in a fibrillary formation and within the blood vessel wall (P2 anti-PrP antibody).

using this approach. Antibodies that recognize epitopes in the 93–99 amino acid sequence of PrP provide specific immunolabelling for intracellular PrP^{Sc} in tissues from several sheep scrapie sources but fail to do so in ovine BSE-infected tissues.[193] Intracellular PrP^{Sc} accumulations in ovine BSE infected sheep can be revealed with antibodies to the C-terminus of PrP. The site of truncation of PrP^{Sc} differs in astrocytes, neurons and macrophages of ovine BSE infected sheep.[193] As differences in truncation presumably correspond with different tertiary or quaternary structures of PrP^{Sc}, this suggests that conformation of PrP^{Sc} may precisely correspond to strain property.

The sub-cellular pathology of scrapie has been extensively studied in rodents and sheep with scrapie. Spongiform changes and process varicosities observed in cell imaging studies correspond to intra-dendritic vacuoles or to parenchymal vacuoles that lack any limiting membrane structure (see Figure 18.4) and contain membranous debris. So-called tubulovesicular bodies (see later, Figure 18.19) are common in rodent TSEs but are less abundant in ruminants.

Immunogold studies suggest that transformation of PrP^{C} to PrP^{Sc} appears to occur on membranes of neurons or glial cells. This initial membrane PrP^{Sc} accumulation does not perturb membrane morphology. However, when PrP^{Sc}, which is attached to the external face of the plasma membrane, is cross-lined to ubiquitin on the cytoplasmic face of the membrane, excess coated vesicles and membrane invaginations, or membrane microfolds are formed (Figure 18.7). PrP^{Sc} may also be released into the extracellular space where it can form amyloid fibrils and plaques. The proportions of these membrane and amyloid changes vary according to strain and/or *Prnp* genotype. Intracellular PrP^{Sc} accumulations are predominantly lysosomal. This membrane pathology is common to different experimental rodent strains, cattle BSE, and probably also to sCJD.[194]

The number of naturally occurring scrapie strains is uncertain. In the absence of any agent-specific nucleic acid or molecular conformational feature of PrP^{Sc}, different prion strains have been identified by their disease phenotypes. Numerous different strains of prion disease originating from animal sources have been defined following multiple passages at limiting dilutions in rodents.[45] These strains are characterized by their relative incubation periods in a panel of inbred mouse strains, the patterns of vacuolation and PrP^{Sc} accumulation, and the mobility and glycoprofile of PrP^{res} on immunoblots. However, it is not clear whether such strains arise by mutation or adaptation on serial passage in rodents.

BSE of cattle, sheep, goats, cats and exotic ruminants as well as vCJD of man all give the same invariable and distinctive disease phenotype when transmitted to rodents.[45,46,48]

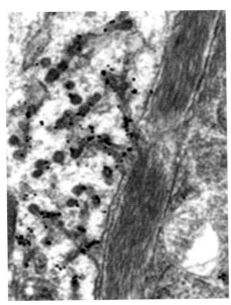

18.7 Natural scrapie in sheep. Dorsal motor nucleus of the vagus showing PrP^{Sc} labelling of dendrite membrane invaginations and sub-plasma membrane coated vesicles (immunogold labelling with 1A8 anti-PrP antibody).

However, this fidelity of rodent phenotype on BSE transmission appears to be exceptional. When naturally occurring sheep scrapie sources are transmitted to sheep, the recipient disease phenotype is influenced by both recipient genotype and donor strain or source. Preservation of the disease phenotype on transmission occurs only where *Prnp* genotypes are homologous.[119] Furthermore, when cloned murine scrapie strains derived from sheep sources were passed back into sheep the disease phenotype in sheep was genotype dependent and the original cloned murine strains were recovered from only one of four strains on further re-isolation and sub-passage in mice.[342] Thus, rodent transmission may reliably be used to provide presumptive BSE strain recognition in a natural host, but cannot be reliably used for other strains and sources. Nevertheless, several distinct disease phenotypes have been identified across Europe within a single *Prnp* sheep genotype supporting evidence for natural as well as experimental strain diversity.[118]

Atypical Sheep and Goat Scrapie

In 1998, a novel clinico-pathological presentation of sheep and goat scrapie was recognized in Norway.[17] Nor98, or atypical scrapie has now been recognized throughout Europe and in North America and Australasia. Clinical cases of atypical scrapie remain rare with most sub-clinical infection detected by active surveillance monitoring. Atypical cases usually occur singly within flocks and target *Prnp* genotypes that are generally considered more resistant to classical scrapie with the F141 allele conferring higher susceptibility than L141.[115]

PrP^{Sc} accumulation patterns are distinct from classical scrapie (Figure 18.8). PrP^{Sc} is usually present as fine punctate deposits[17] and less frequent coarse granular, plaque-like accumulations and linear types of labelling. A distinctive labelling type is found in white matter and consists of PrP^{Sc} in or

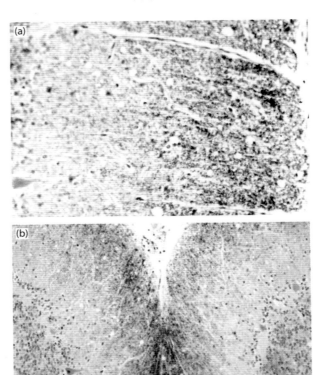

18.8 Nor98 atypical scrapie. (a,b) Cerebellum showing PrP^{Sc} accumulation in diffuse punctuate and granular patterns affecting predominantly the molecular layer with mild spongiform change (F99 anti-PrP antibody).

around axons. PrP^{Sc} accumulation is most consistent in thalamus, cerebellum and cerebral cortex. When present, vacuoles are small and often confluent. In contrast to classical scrapie, vacuolation and PrP^{Sc} are absent from the parasympathetic nucleus of the vagal nerve. Some confirmed atypical cases show no histological or immunohistochemical changes.[18]

Atypical scrapie infections cannot be diagnosed using immunoblotting methods performed using conventional stringent conditions. However, PrP^{res} can be shown by immunoblotting methods that use low concentrations of proteinase digestion and milder conditions of temperature, detergent, chaotropic agents and pH. In such conditions, up to five PrP^{res} bands of between 7 and 31 kDa are obtained.[18] The number and apparent molecular weight of these bands depends on the precise conditions and the antibodies used. A low molecular weight fragment has been mapped at approximately amino-acids 85–90 to 148–155. Further fragments of 85–94 to 233 and 120–233 have also been identified.[18]

Several atypical scrapie cases of varying *Prnp* genotypes have transmitted disease to homologous and heterologous sheep genotypes both by intracerebral and by oral routes of challenge.[339] Despite the apparent absence of lesions, transmissions have also been recorded from lymphoid tissues, nerves and muscles,[6] but evidence from active surveillance programmes suggests that atypical scrapie is probably not horizontally transmitted to other sheep under field conditions.

Bovine Spongiform Encephalopathy

Cattle BSE was first recognized in 1986 and developed into a major epizootic in the United Kingdom with over 180 000 animals developing clinical disease with a further one to three million cattle likely to have been sub-clinically infected and slaughtered for human consumption.[372] Clinical signs of BSE include changes in cardiac rhythm, gastrointestinal motility, apprehension, unsteadiness, incoordination and loss of weight. Epidemiological studies indicated that BSE was transmitted and amplified in the cattle population by the use of meat and bone meal in animal feed.[371] The BSE epizootic was facilitated by changes in rendering practices during the production of meat and bone meal feed that allowed active TSE agents to persist in the final products. It is now unlikely that the original source of the epizootic will ever be proven and both sheep and cattle origins have been suspected. UK meat and bone meal was exported internationally and cases of BSE were reported throughout Europe and in smaller numbers in North America and Asia.[28] It is likely that BSE infections were undetected in other countries that imported meat and bone meal but were unable to mount sensitive surveillance programmes.

BSE is now a rare disease and most remaining infected cattle are detected by active surveillance. The BSE agent was also responsible for novel TSEs in domestic cats and exotic ungulates and felids in zoos (Figure 18.9).[202] The link between cattle BSE and these other novel TSEs was confirmed by strain typing studies in rodents, which demonstrated that a single strain of the TSE agent (the BSE agent) was responsible for all these diseases.[46] BSE is also responsible for vCJD, most likely acquired by the oral route via the consumption of BSE-contaminated meat products.[48,370]

Though varying in magnitude, the nature of cattle BSE lesions is uniform (Figure 18.10). Vacuolation occurs predominantly in the medulla, midbrain and thalamus. PrPSc accumulation follows the same pattern, but is additionally detectable in other brain regions.[371] Within the brainstem, the most intense vacuolation consistently occurs in the nucleus of the spinal tract of the trigeminal nerve and the nucleus of the solitary tract.[372] As in sheep scrapie, initial PrPSc accumulation in brain occurs in the dorsal motor nucleus of the vagal nerve consistent with an ascending infection following oral exposure to infectivity. Unlike scrapie, there is no evidence of PrPSc in viscera of field case BSE, though infectivity can be inconsistently detected in Peyer's patches and enteric nerves plexi of cattle given a massive experimental oral challenge.[355] Immunoblotting reveals a uniform PrPres signature, characterized by a 19-kDa unglycosylated band and predominance of the diglycosylated form of the protein (Figure 18.11).[67] Although these immunoblot features are maintained on transmission of BSE to other species, including man, the neuropathology of felid and exotic ungulate BSE is dissimilar to that of cattle. *Prnp* in cattle, unlike sheep and deer, appears not to contain polymorphic alleles that influence the neuropathology or susceptibility to BSE.

Atypical Bovine Prion Disease

An increased worldwide surveillance for BSE has led to the recognition of at least two other bovine prion-related disorders of cattle in Europe, North America and Japan. Each has distinct histological, biochemical and transmission properties.

Originally detected in older Italian cows,[56] bovine amyloidotic spongiform encephalopathy (BASE or L-type BSE) is mainly characterized by the accumulation of small thioflavin-S fluorescent, kuru-type amyloid deposits accompanied by punctuate and granular PrPSc accumulations affecting thalamus, cerebral cortex and sub-cortical white matter. Mild punctate PrPSc accumulation is also present in several brainstem sites. Limited immunohistochemical studies of H-type BSE are available but show PrPSc in brainstem with predominantly intra-neuronal, intra-glial and perineuronal types of accumulation.

Cattle prion disease can be reliably distinguished by immunoblotting methods. Compared to epidemic BSE, H- and L-type BSE show non-glycosylated PrPres bands that migrate to higher and lower positions, respectively, of the gel in western blots. H- and L-type BSEs are also more sensitive to proteinase digestion when compared to epidemic BSE. Epidemic and L-type BSEs can also be reliably distinguished by glycoform ratio. Epidemic BSE has less unglycosylated and more di-glycosylated PrPres than L-type BSE.[184]

Both L-type and H-type BSE have been transmitted to cattle, sheep, rodents, and in the case of L-type BSE to macaques. In one study serial passage of L-type BSE in mice produced a murine BSE-like phenotype. Although this has led to speculation that BSE may have derived from L-type, as described

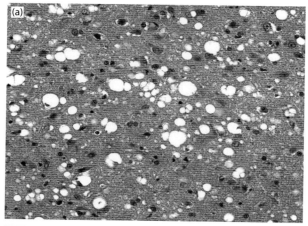

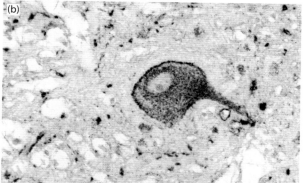

18.9 Feline spongiform encephalopathy in a domestic cat. (a) Spongiform change in the occipital cortex with no amyloid plaque formation. **(b)** Intense prion protein (PrPSc) accumulation within and around a large neurone in the vestibular complex (3F4 anti-PrP antibody).

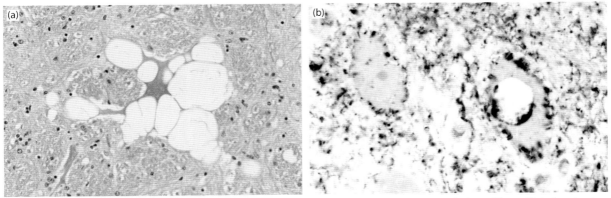

18.10 Brain stem pathology in bovine spongiform encephalopathy (BSE). (a) Intense vacuolation with multiple locules in a neurone within the dorsal motor nucleus of the vagus. **(b)** Punctate, perineuronal and intravacuolar PrP^{Sc} in the dorsal motor nucleus of the vagus (8G8 anti-PrP antibody).

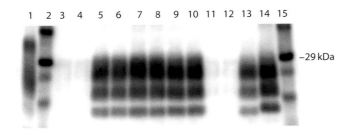

18.11 PrP^{res} profile from natural bovine spongiform encephalopathy (BSE) using a discriminatory western blot. BSE exhibits a lower molecular mass compared with ovine scrapie when the 6H4 anti-PrP antibody is used.
Lanes: 1, control brain – no proteinase K (PK); 2 and 15, biotinylated molecular mass markers (29 kDa marked); 3 and 4, BSE negative controls; 5 and 6, #1 BSE-positive; 7 and 8, #2 BSE-positive; 9 and 10, #3 BSE-positive; 11 and 12, BSE-negative controls; 13, positive BSE control; 14, positive ovine scrapie control.

Image courtesy of Dr Mick Stack and Dr Melanie Chapman, Veterinary Laboratories Agency Weybridge, Addlestone, UK.

earlier, it is premature to assume that there is a one-to-one correlation between rodent disease phenotype and strain, particularly as sheep infected with L-type BSE do not show an epidemic ovine BSE-like phenotype on primary passage.

Chronic Wasting Disease

CWD was first identified as a clinical syndrome in captive North American mule deer in the 1960s, and spongiform encephalopathy was subsequently recognized in affected captive deer and elk in 1978.[384] For the next two decades CWD was apparently restricted to parts of Wyoming but has now been identified in non-contiguous clusters extending to the eastern seaboard of the United States and into Canada. CWD has been diagnosed in four free ranging and captive North American cervid species. Estimates of CWD prevalence vary between 1–30 per cent in free ranging populations with even higher incidences recorded in disease outbreaks in farmed deer.[385]

CWD is the only TSE known to affect free-ranging animals, and appears readily transmissible by horizontal

routes. Although the mechanisms of CWD transmission are uncertain, infectivity has been demonstrated in saliva, faeces, in placenta and in environmental fomites. CWD results in weight loss and behavioural alterations in the early stages of the disease, which are followed by facial hypotonia, excessive salivation, polyuria and polydipsia. Most deer die of aspiration pneumonia 7–8 months after the disease onset.

Prnp polymorphisms affect susceptibility to CWD with different polymorphisms affecting different species. S225F or F225F mule deer and S96S white-tailed deer are at lower risk of developing disease than are S225S mule deer or S96G or G96G white-tailed deer respectively. The *Prnp* polymorphism of elk at codon 132 corresponds to the human 129 codon: M132M and M132L are more susceptible than are L132L elk.[115]

CWD has widespread visceral as well as CNS pathology. The brain shows typical spongiform changes, neuronal loss and gliosis[384] accompanied by PrP^{Sc} accumulation (Figure 18.12). PrP^{Sc} appears in lymphoid tissues within 6 weeks following experimental oral infection, with neuroinvasion of the dorsal motor nucleus of the vagal nerve detected 14 months later. PrP^{Sc} has also been detected in peripheral nerves and ganglia, pancreatic islets, the adrenal medulla, striated muscle, and, uniquely amongst the TSEs, in cardiac muscle.[337]

The increasing prevalence of CWD has given rise to concerns that the disease may transmit to other domestic animals, including cattle and sheep, and that it may also be pathogenic to humans. There is no evidence to date that CWD has transmitted to cattle or sheep living in the vicinity of affected deer. Although TSEs have been reported in deer hunters in the United States (who are likely to have consumed infected deer tissues) these cases appear to represent sporadic CJD rather than a novel human TSE.[16]

PRION DISEASES IN HUMANS
Clinical Diagnosis

Human prion diseases have a wide spectrum of clinical phenotypes and, as with other diseases of this rarity, clinical diagnosis first depends on the recognition of the possibility of this type of disorder. The diagnosis of many cases of sCJD and vCJD can be made with a high degree of accuracy on the

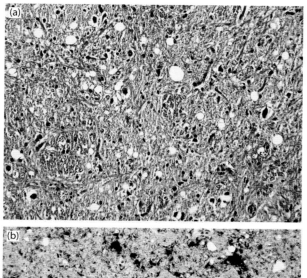

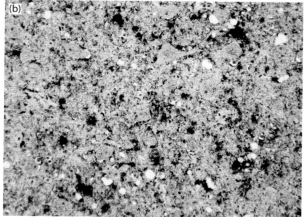

18.12 Brain stem pathology in chronic wasting disease (CWD). (a) Multiple large vacuoles are present within the region of the obex. **(b)** Widespread prion protein (PrP^Sc) in a perineuronal and coarse granular pattern in the obex (Bar 224 anti-PrP antibody).

basis of the characteristic clinical phenotype, and in all prion diseases the typical clinical course is of relentless, often rapid progression in multifocal neurological deficits, usually associated with progressive cognitive impairment. Involuntary movements of the limbs (and sometimes of the trunk and face) and, in particular, myoclonic movements occur in the great majority of cases, and the combination of rapidly progressive dementia and myoclonus is characteristic of sCJD.[379]

Even in sCJD, however, there are atypical clinical presentations, such as cases of long duration[38] and cases with a stroke-like onset,[251] and the clinical phenotypes in genetic forms of human prion disease are markedly varied, with diagnosis in life usually resting on *PRNP* analysis.[216] In many dominantly inherited disorders the identification of a similar disease in other family members is crucial to diagnosis, but in genetic forms of human prion disease a family history is present in only some cases. Iatrogenic CJD is diagnosed on the basis of a progressive neurological disorder in the context of an individual with a recognized risk factor, such as treatment with human pituitary growth hormone or a human dura mater graft. The critical issue in diagnosing iCJD is obtaining, and understanding the implications of, the past medical and surgical history.

The diagnosis of vCJD depends on awareness of the characteristic clinical phenotype, which includes early

psychiatric symptoms[396] followed after an average of 6 months by progressive ataxia and dementia associated with involuntary movements, which may be myoclonic, choreiform or dystonic.[383] The mean age at death in vCJD is only 29 years and, as with recipients of human growth hormone (hGH), a relatively young age at onset of symptoms is often helpful in raising the possibility of this diagnosis. Specialist investigations contribute significantly to the diagnosis of human prion disease and are essential in excluding other conditions. Regardless of the subtype of human prion disease, there is a wide differential diagnosis, which may include some conditions that are potentially treatable, and it is important to exclude other conditions before reaching a diagnosis of human prion disease. Indeed, the possibility of a prion disease may become apparent when routine tests such as computed tomography (CT) brain scan and routine cerebrospinal fluid (CSF) parameters are negative.

The investigations that are most helpful in diagnosis of human prion diseases are the EEG, the CSF 14-3-3 immunoassay and magnetic resonance (MR) imaging brain scan. The EEG shows periodic triphasic complexes (PTCs) at about 1/second in the majority of cases of sCJD, in some genetic CJD cases and in some cases of iatrogenic CJD with a central route of inoculation (e.g. with human dura mater grafts) (Figure 18.13).[377] Although the EEG had not been thought to show these appearances in vCJD, a periodic EEG has been described in two cases late in the course of the illness.[21,389] The 'typical' EEG appearances in CJD are almost diagnostic, as other conditions with a similar abnormality in the EEG (such as lithium toxicity and hepatic encephalopathy) can usually be distinguished on clinical grounds. Although these EEG changes have been described in other neurodegenerative conditions, such as Alzheimer's disease and Lewy body dementia, this is very rare and the EEG findings are a component of the diagnostic criteria for sCJD.

Routine CSF parameters are usually normal, and an elevated white cell count almost excludes the possibility of human prion disease unless this is a second tap or there have been seizures. The CSF protein is elevated in about half the cases of sCJD, but the elevation is usually modest.[379] The most helpful investigation is the 14-3-3 immunoassay, which is positive in over 90 per cent of cases of sCJD, in about 50 per cent of cases of vCJD and in some cases of fCJD and iCJD (Figure 18.14).[381,398] The 14-3-3 test, however, is not specific for the diagnosis of CJD and can be elevated in other conditions, including stroke, Alzheimer's disease and other forms of dementia. The interpretation of a positive test depends upon the clinical context and should be used only to support the diagnosis of CJD in cases in which there is a rapidly progressive illness. The 14-3-3 immunoassay should not be used as a screening test for CJD in populations of individuals with dementing illness. Other CSF proteins, including S100b and tau, are currently the subject of research regarding their potential value in diagnosis, but they have not yet been validated. Amplification of prion protein in the CSF, using the real-time QuIC methodology, promises to have a high sensitivity and specificity for the diagnosis of sCJD and may represent a disease-specific marker.[8,247]

The MR imaging brain scan has become increasingly useful in the diagnosis of vCJD[66] and contributes to the

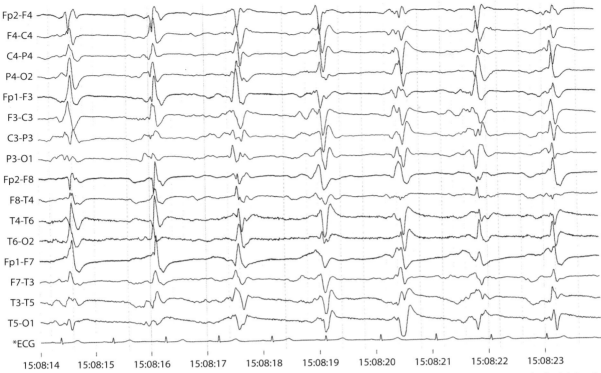

18.13 Electroencephalogram (EEG) in sporadic Creutzfeldt–Jakob disease (sCJD), showing synchronous periodic triphasic complexes in most leads.

18.14 Western blot of cerebrospinal fluid (CSF) 14-3-3 using monoclonal anti-14-3-3 (H-8 Santa Cruz Biotechnology, Santa Cruz, CA, USA), showing the 14-3-3 immunoreactivity seen in three cases of sCJD (A,D,E) and a case of variant Creutzfeldt–Jakob disease (vCJD) (C). A case of Alzheimer's disease (B) is shown, illustrating the lack of CSF 14-3-3 reactivity in this condition. The position of a 30 kilodalton molecular mass marker is shown (30 kDa).

Image courtesy of Dr Alison Green, University of Edinburgh, Edinburgh, UK.

diagnosis of other forms of human prion disease, including sCJD[332] and iCJD. High signal on T2 and fluid-associated inversion recovery (FLAIR) sequences is seen in the posterior thalamus (the pulvinar sign) in over 90 per cent of cases of vCJD (Figure 18.15a), and these changes are, in the appropriate clinical context, highly, but not absolutely, specific for the diagnosis of vCJD.[289] The MR imaging scan can be positive from early in the clinical illness, but serial scans (and serial EEGs in sCJD) may be necessary in order to identify the typical changes. In sCJD, and in some growth hormone-related iCJD cases and genetic CJD cases, the high signal on the MR imaging brain scan is in the caudate and putamen regions of the basal ganglia (Figure 18.15b) and there may also be cortical

hyperintensities (Figure 18.15c), particularly on diffusion-weighted images. These MR imaging changes are present in about 60–70 per cent of sCJD cases and can be present in most subtypes of sCJD, including some clinically atypical cases. MR brain imaging findings are now included in the diagnostic criteria for sCJD.[399]

Invasive diagnostic investigations are not usually carried out in CJD; because clinical diagnosis is relatively accurate, these procedures carry risks and the results rarely alter the management of the patient. However, brain biopsy is carried out in a proportion of patients and, in particular, in those in whom there is real diagnostic doubt or in whom there is the possibility of an alternative treatable condition. As only a small portion of brain is available for examination and because the neuropathological process may be patchy in the early stages of CJD, there is the possibility of negative findings in brain biopsy of patients who do indeed have CJD; this is of importance in relation to public health precautions, as neurosurgical instruments should not be reused until a definitive diagnosis is available.[374] Tonsil biopsy can be useful in supporting the diagnosis of vCJD, as there is a significant accumulation of disease-associated PrP in lymphoreticular tissues in this condition, in contrast to other human prion diseases.[156] Because of the important public health implications of identifying vCJD, tonsil biopsy is often carried out in the initial cases of vCJD in previously unaffected countries, but the procedure has risks, including postoperative haemorrhage,[147] and it is important to consider the welfare of the patient when deciding on invasive diagnostic procedures.

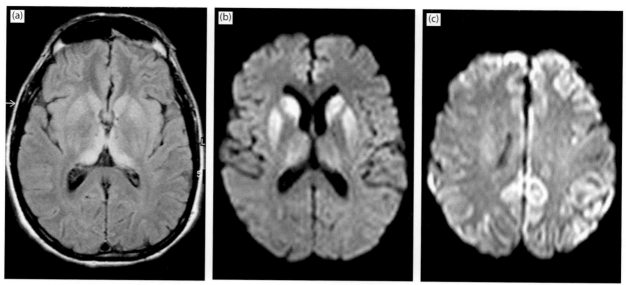

18.15 (a) Axial fluid-associated inversion recovery (FLAIR) magnetic resonance image (MRI) at the level of the basal ganglia demonstrating marked hyperintensity of the dorsomedial and pulvinar nuclei of thalami bilaterally, typical of variant Creutzfeldt–Jakob disease (vCJD). **(b)** Axial diffusion-weighted image showing bilateral caudate head and putamen hyperintensity typical of sporadic Creutzfeldt–Jakob disease (sCJD). **(c)** Axial diffusion-weighted image at the level of corona radiate showing asymmetric, mainly left-sided cortical hyperintensity or 'ribboning', a common finding in sCJD.

Images courtesy of Dr David Summers, Western General Hospital, Edinburgh, UK.

Genetic Techniques for Diagnosis

PRNP gene comprises two exons (in humans) with the entire open reading frame (ORF) contained within exon 2. Numerous single point mutations, as well as deletions and insertions in the octapeptide repeat region of *PRNP*, have been associated with fCJD, GSS and FFI (Figure 18.16). In some instances, the disease phenotype may mimic that present in other, more common neurological disorders (e.g. Alzheimer's disease). Thus, the analysis of the *PRNP* ORF is required to establish the presence of pathogenic mutations and hence to assist in the diagnosis of familial prion diseases,[211] which account for around 10–15 per cent of all human prion diseases. Moreover, certain polymorphisms in the *PRNP* (e.g. at residue 129) appear to influence the disease phenotype.[276] The status of some other very rare polymorphisms (e.g. at residue 171) remains uncertain.[325] Surveillance of prion diseases carried out in Italy has shown that the number of CJD patients carrying *PRNP* mutations is greater than expected.[220] Most of these patients were referred as suspected sCJD cases, without a family history of CJD and with clinical and neuropathological features indistinguishable from sCJD, and so sequencing of the *PRNP* ORF was required to confirm the diagnosis. A large multicentre study in Europe found that a family history of CJD or a similar disorder is absent in 12–88 per cent of genetic CJD cases, depending on the mutation studied.[216] Accordingly, this report suggested the use of the term 'genetic transmissible spongiform encephalopathy' (gTSE). The analysis of the *PRNP* is also important in young patients (younger than age 50 years) for discerning between vCJD and early-presenting familial prion diseases.

Analysis of the *PRNP* is usually performed by extraction of genomic DNA from the patient's blood or from unfixed autopsy tissues, followed by amplification of the *PRNP* ORF using specific primers and PCR techniques. The presence of deletions or insertions can also be determined by the size of the PCR product on gel electrophoresis. In addition, the PCR product can be used for direct sequencing or endonuclease restriction analysis to determine the presence of *PRNP* pathogenic mutations and polymorphisms. A restriction digest will result in a number of DNA fragments, the size of which depend on the exact positions of the recognition sequences for the endonuclease in the original molecule. New methodologies have been described in an attempt to provide rapid and efficient methods for the detection of point mutations by direct sequencing and by the analysis of the coding region of the *PRNP* using denaturing high-performance liquid chromatography.[59] It is also possible to extract DNA for analysis from formalin-fixed paraffin-embedded tissue blocks if no blood or unfixed tissue is available. The extent of the DNA preservation under these circumstances is variable, but the codon 129 polymorphism status can be determined in archival tissues, and some mutations may also be detectable.[42,249] However, this approach requires careful control and is not to be recommended as a routine investigation. The application of genetic screening in clinical practice allows a clear diagnosis in clinically affected patients and may also be used to assess the risk for asymptomatic relatives of developing a prion disease.

Neuropathology and Differential Diagnosis

Neuropathological examination of the brain is essential for a definitive diagnosis of a prion disease. In addition to conventional histology, a range of ancillary techniques, including immunohistochemistry for PrP on paraffin sections and western blotting techniques on homogenates of frozen brain tissue to detect PrP^{Sc}, are used routinely to aid

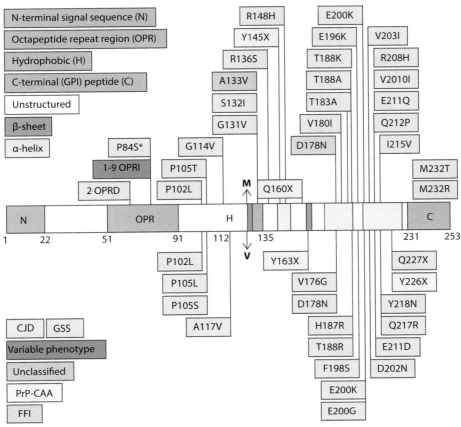

18.16 Diagrammatic representation of the prion protein gene (*PRNP*) open reading frame (codons 1–253) with the structural landmarks of the encoded prion protein marked and the position of pathogenic mutation superimposed using codon number and single letter amino acid codes. X indicates a stop codon. The pathogenic mutations are colour coded with respect to the predominant clinicopathological phenotype and are placed above or below the schematic to indicate the haplotype with respect to codon 129 of the mutated allele. The position of the methionine (M)/valine (V) polymorphism is also shown. An asterisk (*) indicates a currently unknown haplotype. The corresponding figure from the previous edition has been updated for mutations recently found in association with (Creutzfeldt–Jakob disease (CJD)[281] and Gerstmann–Sträussler–Scheinker disease (GSS)[282] and in light of information contained in Beck *et al.*[15]

diagnosis.[51,169] These techniques are usually accompanied by genetic screening for *PRNP* polymorphisms and mutations, which allows the identification of familial prion diseases and the status of the polymorphism at codon 129. The combination of these methods has allowed a widening spectrum of human prion diseases to be identified, many of which are characterized by diverse clinical and pathological phenotypes.[100,175]

Macroscopic examination of the brain in prion disease may reveal no obvious abnormality (Figure 18.17a). However, a degree of cerebral atrophy is not uncommon and may be generalized or localized. The hippocampus is usually spared. Cerebellar atrophy is a particular feature of some cases of sCJD, may also occur in GSS, vCJD and iCJD and was a feature of kuru. The classic histopathological features of human prion diseases comprise spongiform change, neuronal loss, reactive proliferation of microglia and astrocytes, and (in certain subgroups of cases) the formation of amyloid plaques.[50,169] None of these features in itself is absolutely specific for prion diseases, but their occurrence in defined neuroanatomical regions of the brain is both characteristic and of considerable diagnostic importance. In general, the severity of these changes is often related to the duration of the clinical illness, for example in the relatively

rare cases of sCJD with survival of over 1 year. This relationship is not absolute; some cases of sCJD with a short duration of illness can have strikingly severe pathological changes in the brain, including some of the so-called pan-encephalopathic form of sCJD (Figure 18.17b). In contrast, it has been found that several subgroups of human prion diseases, particularly some of the familial disorders (including GSS and FFI), exhibit relatively little or no spongiform change, and so the use of the ancillary investigative techniques mentioned earlier is essential for diagnosis. Brain biopsy is usually reserved for patients in whom a treatable alternative diagnosis, such as cerebral vasculitis, is being considered. However, brain biopsy has been found to be diagnostic in around 95 per cent of CJD in which the diagnosis was subsequently confirmed either at autopsy or on experimental transmission.[50]

Masters and Richardson defined the diagnostic criteria for spongiform change, allowing a clear distinction from other forms of vacuolation in the neuropil, such as status spongiosus, a non-specific coarse vacuolation of grey matter caused by extensive neuronal loss, and gliosis, which can occur in a range of other neurodegenerative disorders, for example frontotemporal lobar degeneration.[240] Spongiform change is characterized by multiple rounded

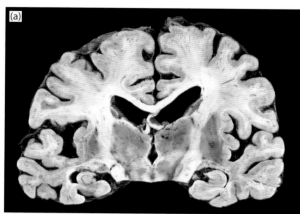

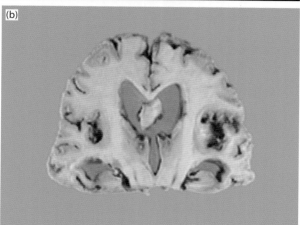

18.17 Macroscopic brain pathology in sporadic Creutzfeldt–Jakob disease (sCJD). (a) Most cases of sCJD show only mild cerebral cortical atrophy, occasionally with cerebellar atrophy and lesser involvement of the basal ganglia and thalamus. **(b)** The pan-encephalopathic form of sCJD shows extensive atrophy of the cerebral cortex, basal ganglia and thalamus, but with relative sparing of the hippocampus.

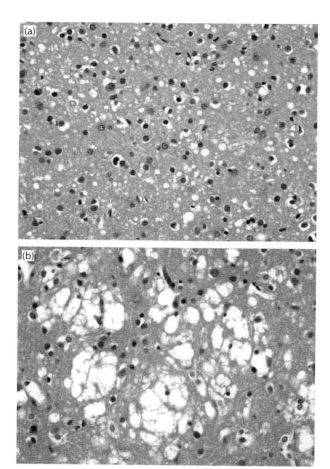

18.18 Spongiform change in sporadic Creutzfeldt–Jakob disease (sCJD). (a) Micro-vacuolar spongiform change with multiple small rounded vacuoles distributed throughout the neuropil. **(b)** Confluent spongiform change occurs as multiple large cyst-like spaces in the neuropil that appear to be formed from coalescing regions of micro-vacuolar spongiform change.

vacuoles within the neuropil, which vary in diameter from 2 to 20 µm, known as micro-vacuolar spongiform change (Figure 18.18a). Vacuolation within neuronal perikarya is extremely uncommon in human prion diseases, in contrast to scrapie and BSE. In some forms of human prion disease, micro-vacuolar spongiform change progresses to the development of larger cystic spaces, usually referred to as confluent spongiform change (Figure 18.18b). On electron microscopy, the spongiform vacuoles consist of distended neuronal process (mainly neurites) containing amorphous and curled membrane fragments (see Figure 18.4).[221] Distended presynaptic terminals also contain tubulovesicular bodies, which measure around 35 nm in diameter and are of higher electron density than synaptic vesicles (Figure 18.19).[227] These structures are a consistent ultrastructural finding in a wide range of human prion diseases, but their precise nature is unknown. Attempts to label tubulovesicular structures with antibodies to PrP have proven negative.[228]

Spongiform change in prion diseases should be readily distinguishable from other forms of neuropil vacuolation, including that seen in cerebral oedema, a range of metabolic disorders and artefacts produced by poor fixation and tissue processing (Table 18.4). However, neuropil

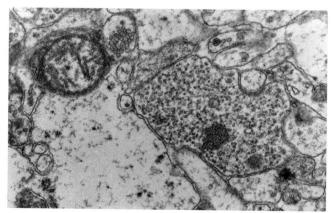

18.19 Tubulovesicular bodies in sporadic Creutzfeldt–Jakob disease (sCJD). Electron microscopy shows tubulovesicular bodies, composed of small oval or tubular structures (approximately 35 nm in diameter) present within the presynaptic terminal, but smaller and more electron-dense than synaptic vesicles and not related to areas of spongiform change.

Image courtesy of Professor Pawel Liberski, Medical University of Lodz, Lodz, Poland.

TABLE 18.4 Other disorders and artefacts associated with spongiform change

Disorder	Distribution
Dementia with Lewy bodies	Temporal cortex (superior and inferior temporal, entorhinal and insular cortex and amygdala)
Pick's disease	Layer 2 in frontal and temporal cortex
Motor neuron disease dementia	Layer 2 in frontal and temporal cortex
Corticobasal degeneration	Layer 2 in frontal and temporal cortex
Other forms of frontotemporal lobar degeneration	Layer 2 in frontal and temporal cortex
Artefact	**Distribution**
Status spongiosus	Transcortical coarse neuropil vacuolation with severe neuronal loss and gliosis; found in a range of disorders (including Creutzfeldt–Jakob disease (CJD), Pick's disease, diffuse hypoxia)
Cerebral oedema	Pericellular and perivascular; grey and white matter
Cerebral hypoxia	Pericellular; grey and white matter
Metabolic encephalopathies	Pericellular and intracellular; grey and white matter
Poor fixation or processing	Pericellular (around retracted cells) and perivascular; grey and white matter
Autolysis	Pericellular, intracellular; most marked in central grey and white matter and the cerebellar granular layer

vacuolation indistinguishable from the micro-vacuolar form of spongiform change has been described in dementia with Lewy bodies, where it may represent degeneration of the terminal axons of large pyramidal neurons.[136,176] In these conditions, the spongiform change is usually confined to the temporal cortex and is not present in the basal ganglia or cerebellum, unlike in most cases of CJD, and the other pathological features of the underlying condition are usually readily apparent on detailed histological assessment. Disorders associated with spongiform change are summarized in Table 18.4.

Spongiform change is usually accompanied by neuronal loss, the degree of which is not necessarily consistent with the degree of vacuolation. Some neuroanatomical regions, for example the medial thalamus in FFI and the pulvinar in vCJD, can exhibit severe neuronal loss and gliosis in the relative absence of spongiform change. The reactive proliferation of astrocytes and microglia in prion diseases usually occurs in association with neuronal loss, but in some cases there seems to be a disproportionately severe gliosis, which has led to the suggestion that astrocytes may be involved in a primary response to PrP^{Sc} accumulation in some forms of prion disease. Reactive astrocytes and microglial cells are also evident within and around amyloid plaques in prion diseases. It is not clear whether this represents a cellular reaction to amyloid deposition or part of the mechanisms of PrP^{Sc} processing that result in plaque formation.

Amyloid plaque formation in human prion diseases is not a consistent neuropathological finding and occurs only in certain well-defined disease subgroups of sCJD and in GSS, iCJD, kuru and vCJD. The plaques contain large fibrillary aggregates of PrP^{Sc} along with other plaque components, such as apolipoprotein J (clusterin)

and amyloid P protein that are not specific for prion diseases. Neuritic dystrophy around PrP plaques has been identified ultrastructurally and by immunohistochemistry for ubiquitin on paraffin sections.[172,228] The first type of amyloid plaque to be identified in a human prion disease was the rounded fibrillary plaques occurring in kuru, particularly in the cerebellum, and the term 'kuru plaque' is used to describe similar structures occurring in other conditions, including certain subtypes of sCJD (Figure 18.20a). A wide range of other plaque morphologies has been described in human prion diseases, including multicentric plaques, which are characteristic of GSS (Figure 18.20b) and the florid plaque in vCJD (Figure 18.20c).[174] Florid plaques have subsequently been identified in small numbers in restricted areas of the brain in other prion diseases, including a subset of iCJD case in recipients of dura mater. The most recently identified form of amyloid plaque in a human prion disease is the microplaque, which is a characteristic and striking feature of the neuropathology of the newly described human prion disease variably protease-sensitive prionopathy (VPSPr) (see later, Figure 18.29b). Some inherited forms of prion disease, particularly the form of GSS occurring in the Indiana kindred (*PRNP* F198S), are associated with neurofibrillary tangle formation in the brain.[107] These tangles are composed of phosphorylated tau aggregates and resemble those occurring in Alzheimer's disease, but their distribution is not confined to the limbic system and neocortex. Amyloid angiopathy composed of PrP^{Sc} is an extremely rare finding in human prion diseases, for example in one uncommon familial form of prion disease, where a stop codon mutation occurs at codon 145 (Figure 18.20d).[106]

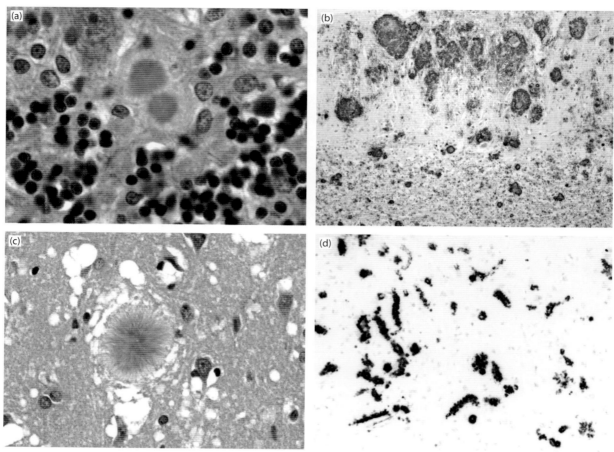

18.20 Plaque formation in human prion diseases. (a) Kuru plaques (centre) are composed of a dense eosinophilic core and a rounded pale fibrillary periphery, most frequently located in the granular layer or the adjacent molecular layer of the cerebellum. **(b)** Multicentric plaques in Gerstmann–Sträussler–Scheinker (GSS) disease can occupy a large volume of the cerebellar cortex, particularly in the molecular layer, where they can merge to form large sheet-like deposits. Smaller multicentric plaques are also present in the granular layer (KG9 anti-PrP antibody). **(c)** A florid plaque in variant Creutzfeldt–Jakob disease (vCJD) (centre) is composed of a fibrillary eosinophilic centre with a pale periphery and surrounded by a rim or halo of spongiform change in an otherwise intact neuropil. **(d)** Amyloid accumulation in PrP-cerebral amyloid angiopathy (PrP-CAA) is best visualized on immunohistochemistry for PrP, showing the characteristic perivascular aggregation both longitudinally and on cross-section (3F4 anti-PrP antibody).

Creutzfeldt–Jakob disease and VPSPr can occur in association with other neurodegenerative conditions, the most common of which is Alzheimer's disease. It is perhaps not surprising that a rare condition can coexist with a far more common condition. Although evidence for functional interactions between the normal form of the prion protein and APP metabolism and Aβ toxicity are starting to emerge (reviewed by Griffiths et al.[126]), there is no direct evidence that indicates any pathogenic relationship between these two conditions. One study on the extent of Alzheimer-type pathology in CJD concluded that in most cases it was likely to represent an age-related change.[134] However, it must be noted that deposition of the amyloid precursor protein (APP) can occur around plaques composed of PrPSc in human prion diseases (often around or within neuritic processes), and an antibody to the Aβ protein labels the periphery of prion amyloid deposits in both the F189S and Q217R variants of GSS.[53] A wide range of other disorders have been reported to occur as chance associations

in patients with human prion diseases, including inflammatory conditions such as meningitis and a range of brain tumours (both primary and metastatic). The differential diagnosis of individual prion diseases is discussed under the relevant headings (later).

Immunohistochemistry for PrP

The identification of PrP has allowed a wide range of antibodies to be produced, most of which do not distinguish between the normal and disease-associated isoforms of the protein in immunohistochemistry. In order to overcome this drawback, a number of pretreatment steps for immunohistochemistry have been devised to improve the sensitivity and specificity of detection methods for PrPSc.[214] This has resulted in a range of protocols that are applicable on formalin-fixed paraffin-embedded brain sections and include the use of a pressure cooker, autoclaving in either water or hydrochloric acid, the use of formic acid to enhance immunostaining and the use of guanidine thiocyanate as a protein denaturant. A number of different patterns of PrP accumulation have been described, ranging from the widespread fine punctate positivity in a synaptic-like, perineuronal (or, more rarely, intraneuronal) pattern of staining (Figure 18.21a,b) to the perivacuolar pattern of accumulation, with more densely aggregated deposits around large coalescent spongiform vacuoles (Figure 18.21c).[175,214] PrP[Sc] plaque positivity is evident in all cases with amyloid plaques, such as kuru plaques in the cerebellum (Figure 18.21d) and the amyloid microplaques in VPSPr, but immunohistochemistry can also reveal small intense plaque-like foci of staining that are not represented by corresponding amyloid plaques (and positivity for Congo red or thioflavin S) in a wider range of cases, particularly in sCJD.

Immunohistochemistry has an advantage over western blot analysis: although the former is less sensitive in the detection of total levels of PrP[Sc] it permits detection of very small quantities of PrP within a tissue, allowing the investigation of the cellular and subcellular localization of PrP[Sc] and its distribution within the brain. However,

problems in the interpretation of an apparently positive result for PrP on immunohistochemistry can arise in disorders associated with oxidative stress in the brain, including ischaemia, and in Alzheimer's disease and other neurodegenerative disorders, where PrP[C] may be upregulated and incompletely denatured by standard pretreatments.[215,250] This can be a particular problem in brain biopsy specimens, especially when protocols optimized for use on autopsy tissues have been employed and no unfixed tissue is available for western blot analysis for PrP[Sc]. To overcome this problem, a recent modification to a previously published protocol for the paraffin-embedded tissue blot has improved the specificity and sensitivity of detection of PrP[Sc] in paraffin sections of prion diseases.[315] This method is particularly suitable for use on brain biopsy specimens, which are generally small and fragmented pieces of tissue. The increasing sensitivity of PrP detection in paraffin sections has allowed the identification of a range of extraneural tissues, particularly lymphoid tissues in vCJD, but also in the peripheral nervous system and intravascular macrophages in a range of human prion diseases (see Budka[50] for review).

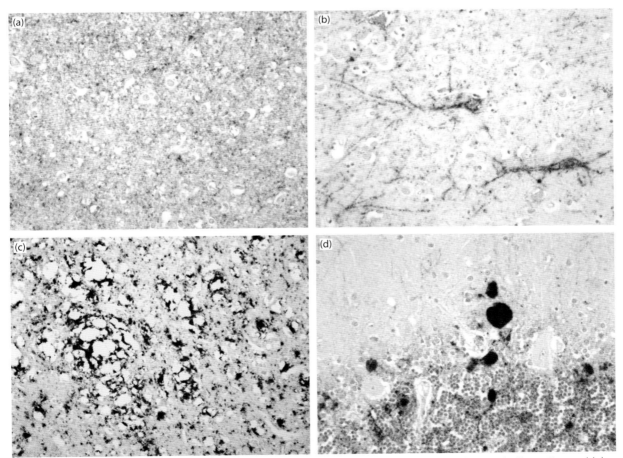

18.21 Patterns of prion protein (PrP) accumulation in human prion diseases. (a) Granular and synaptic-like pattern, which occurs as small aggregates in a relatively regular distribution in the neuropil. **(b)** Perineuronal accumulation can be seen in a variety of sites in the brain, most strikingly around large pyramidal neurons in the cerebral cortex. **(c)** Perivacuolar accumulation of PrP tends to occur around areas of confluent spongiform change. **(d)** Plaque and plaque-like positivity in the cerebellum, with large rounded kuru plaques in the deep molecular layer, which are visible on routinely stained preparations, whereas the plaque-like structures within the granular layer are not evident unless immunohistochemistry for PrP is performed. KG9 anti-PrP antibody.

Western Blot and PrP^res Typing Methods

Western blot analysis of unfixed brain tissue retained at autopsy has become a highly desirable addition to histological and immunohistochemical analysis in the diagnosis of human prion diseases. It may also be performed on peripheral tissues in cases where this is likely to be informative and it is well suited to the analysis of biopsy specimens of brain and tonsil when such tests are required. In variations of this method,[67,143,274] small quantities of frozen tissue (around 100 mg) are homogenized in the presence of non-denaturing detergents, cleared of debris and then digested with proteases, usually proteinase K at 50–100 µg/mL, before being denatured with sodium dodecyl sulphate and separated by polyacrylamide gel electrophoresis. The separated proteins are then transferred on to nitrocellulose or nylon membranes, and protease-resistant PrP (PrP^res) is detected, commonly using mAb 3F4, which binds to an epitope in the protease-resistant core. Under these conditions, the abundant protease-sensitive normal cellular PrP (PrP^C or PrP^sen) is degraded and does not figure on the western blot. Disease-associated PrP (PrP^Sc) survives this treatment, but it is not entirely protease-resistant and proteinase K typically removes 50–80 amino acids from the N-terminus,[277] leaving the protease-resistant core fragment, sometimes referred to as PrP27–39. When applied to samples in which PrP^Sc may be at low levels, such as in the lymphoid tissues, PrP^Sc may be concentrated from a tissue homogenate before analysis by semi-selective precipitation with sodium phosphotungstate[364] or detergent insolubility and centrifugation.[142]

The test can therefore establish in the first instance whether or not abnormal PrP is present, supporting a diagnosis of prion disease or, in its absence, an alternative diagnosis. Although PrP^res is usually detectable in almost all grey matter regions of the brain at end-stage disease, in rare cases, multiple sampling or centrifugal concentration of PrP^res in the sample may be necessary.[142,143] However, western blotting may also be used as a tool to distinguish between different isotypes of PrP^Sc that are characteristic of different forms of human prion disease, in terms of both the sizes of the protease-resistant fragments and the relative abundance of the non-, mono- and di-glycosylated forms.

The paradigm on which PrP typing is based comes from the analysis of two distinct strains of hamster-passaged TME – hyper and drowsy – which were found to differ in the extent of N-terminal truncation, producing diagnostic protease-resistant core fragments differing in 1–2 kDa.[20] This led rapidly to the proposition that different prion strains encipher strain-specific information in the conformation of PrP^Sc,[274] and in the extent of PrP^Sc glycosylation site occupancy.[67]

The majority of researchers recognize two distinct, differently sized non-glycosylated protease-resistant core fragments of the prion protein in CJD termed type 1 and type 2. N-terminal sequencing of these species shows that the 21-kDa type 1 fragment has a major N-terminus at glycine 82, whereas the 19-kDa type 2 fragment has a major N-terminus at serine 97.[277] The N-termini are not uniform but 'ragged' with minor truncation sites

flanking the two major N-termini.[277] The situation is shown diagrammatically in Figure 18.22a. The presence of one or other of these two types in combination with the *PRNP* codon 129 polymorphism was originally proposed to define six phenotypic variants of sCJD.[274,276] In the Parchi and Gambetti nomenclature, the glycosylation site occupancy is considered separately from the fragment size: the suffix A is used to denote PrP^res types in which the mono- or non-glycosylated glycoform predominates such as those found in sCJD, whereas the suffix B is used to denote PrP^res types such as those characteristic of vCJD, where the diglycosylated PrP^res predominates. Typical examples of types 1 (or type 1A), 2A and 2B are shown in Figure 18.22b. Some of the familial or genetic forms of human prion diseases are characterized by type 1 or type 2 PrP^res with a glycoform ratio in which mono- and diglycosylated predominate at the expense of non-glycosylated form.[101] In other familial or genetic forms (most notably) of CAA and some cases of GSS, both N- and C-terminal truncation occurs yielding a low molecular weight protease-resistant core of around 8 kDa.[105] A minority of researchers use an alternative nomenclature in which the glycosylation and fragment size differences are considered together and claim to resolve a greater number of mobility variants than those consistently observed by others.[67] However, the Parchi and Gambetti typing scheme has been shown to be a simple, reliable and transferable method for the PrP^res typing of sporadic CJD and vCJD specimens in an inter-laboratory assessment exercise[278] and will be used throughout this chapter.

The use of alternative methods of distinguishing between PrP^C and PrP^Sc such as conformation dependent immunoassay (CDI) that avoid protease digestion, indicate that up to 90 per cent of the PrP^Sc in CJD brain is protease-sensitive under standard digestion condition (so called senPrP^Sc).[324] CDI is yet to be adopted widely in the diagnosis of human prion disease; however, there is a growing sense of the potential diagnostic significance of senPrP^Sc, particularly in relation to VPSPr – a newly described human prion disease that is characterized by very poorly protease-resistant PrP^Sc that appears on western blots as a faint ladder of PrP^res bands including one at 8 kDa.[100,401]

SPORADIC CREUTZFELDT–JAKOB DISEASE

Definition and Epidemiology

Sporadic Creutzfeldt–Jakob disease is the most frequently occurring human prion disease but, nonetheless, it is a rare idiopathic disorder, with annual mortality rates of 1–1.5 cases per 1 million people and with a worldwide distribution.[220,241] The term 'sporadic' indicates that single cases of sCJD occur in isolation and are not linked causally to other cases. Studies of the geographical distribution of cases within individual countries suggest that the condition is distributed randomly in time and space; clusters of cases have been described only rarely and may reflect the chance aggregation of cases.[71,75] Case-control studies

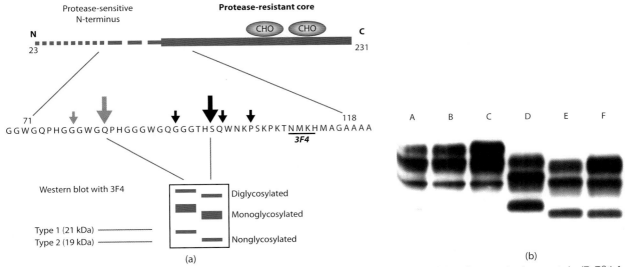

18.22 (a) Schematic representation of the proteinase K-mediated N-terminal truncation of the abnormal prion protein (PrP^{Sc}) found in the Creutzfeldt–Jakob disease (CJD) brain. The full length (23–231) abnormal prion protein consists of a protease-resistant C-terminal core (boxed) and a protease-sensitive N-terminus (dots), between which lies a region of variable protease resistance (dashes). The protease-resistant core contains two consensus N-linked glycosylation sites (CHO) of variable occupancy. The amino acid sequence of the region of variable protease resistance (71–118) is shown in single-letter amino acid code. Arrows denote the N-termini of protease-treated type 1 (grey arrows) and type 2 (black arrows) PrP^{res}, as determined by N-terminal sequencing.[277] The major truncated species is marked with a large arrow and minor species with smaller arrows. The epitope recognized by the monoclonal antibody 3F4 is indicated. The relative mobility of type 1 and type 2 protease-resistant core fragments seen on western blot analysis relates to the difference in the extent of their N-terminal truncation. 3F4 recognizes all three glycoforms (di-, mono- and non-glycosylated PrP^{res}) of both types 1 and 2 PrP^{res}. **(b)** Western blot analysis of prion protein from brain tissue from three different cases of CJD, showing the absence of a diagnostic pattern before protease digestion (A–C) but the appearance of diagnostic differences in fragment mobility and glycoform ratio after digestion with proteinase K (D–F). Lane D shows type 1 PrP^{res} in a case of sCJD (*PRNP* codon 129 MM). Lane E shows type 2A PrP^{res} in a case of sCJD (*PRNP* codon 129 VV). Lane F shows type 2B PrP^{res} in a case of vCJD (*PRNP* codon 129 MM). Western blotting employed the monoclonal antibody 3F4. Approximate molecular mass is shown in kilodaltons.

have failed to identify any consistent risk factor for the development of the disease.[376] Although a higher incidence of prior surgery has been described,[70,369] the possibility of recall bias cannot be excluded as an explanation for these findings. The worldwide distribution, rarity and absence of established risk factors for disease in sCJD led to the hypothesis that it is caused by the formation of disease-associated PrP in the brain as a random event with subsequent self-replication and eventual clinical disease. Although this theory is consistent with the epidemiological data, the age-specific incidence distribution of CJD, with a decline in very elderly people and evidence of geographical clustering of cases in an analysis of past residential history, is not yet explained fully.[229]

Sporadic Creutzfeldt–Jakob disease is predominantly a disease of late middle age and elderly people (Figure 18.23), with a mean age at death of about 65 years. Cases in younger age groups have been described, including four cases in teenagers,[26] and there is an overlap with the age distribution of vCJD. The distribution of cases by sex is equal, with no overall female or male preponderance.

Clinical Features and Diagnostic Criteria

The characteristic clinical course in sCJD is of rapid and relentless progression involving a multifocal neurological disorder and dementia. The most frequent presenting feature is cognitive impairment or ataxia but, typically, there is a rapid decline, with the accumulation of neurological deficits and the development of myoclonic involuntary movements of the limbs and trunk (Table 18.5). The combination of dementia and myoclonus, often with associated cerebellar features, progressing over weeks to a state of total disability is the classic presentation of sCJD and is usually diagnosed readily. Occasional patients may also exhibit a range of other clinical features during the course of the illness, including those of a peripheral neuropathy.[263] Terminally, patients decline to a state of akinetic mutism, in which there is no vocalization, unresponsiveness to external stimuli and rigidity of the limbs, but the eyes may be open and there may be continuing myoclonic movements. Death is usually caused by intercurrent infection such as bronchopneumonia and the mean survival is only about 4 months from symptom onset.

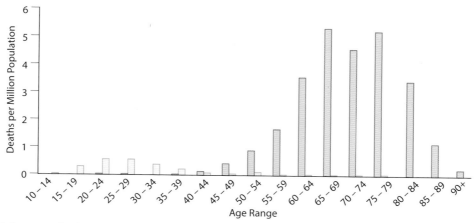

18.23 Age of death in sporadic Creutzfeldt–Jakob disease (sCJD) and variant Creutzfeldt–Jakob disease (vCJD). Most cases of sCJD (lilac) occur in the seventh decade of life, with a declining mortality rate in elderly patients above this age range. sCJD is uncommon under the age of 40 years, but cases in teenagers have been described. By comparison most cases of vCJD (magenta) occur in the third decade of life, with the youngest patient dying at age 14 years and the oldest patient so far identified in the eighth decade of life. UK cases as of December 2013 are shown with mortality rates calculated using UK Office of National Statistics data at mid-2001.

TABLE 18.5 Clinical characteristics of sporadic Creutzfeldt–Jakob disease (sCJD): signs and symptoms at disease onset and during clinical course (percentages)

At onset	%	During clinical course	%
Dementia	35	Dementia	100
Ataxia	35	Involuntary movements (myoclonus)	85
Behavioural disturbance	25		
Dizziness	10	Ataxia	75
Visual	15	Pyramidal	70
Headache	10	Akinetic mutism	60
Involuntary movements (myoclonus)	5	Dysphasia	55
		Visual	40
Dysphasia	5	Cortical blindness	20
Sensory	5	Sensory	10
Cortical blindness	5	Seizures	10

There are, however, a range of atypical presentations, including cases of long duration with an insidious decline in cognitive function reminiscent of Alzheimer's disease, cases with a stroke-like onset,[251] cases presenting with cortical blindness[73] and cases with an early isolated cerebellar syndrome.[44] Variation in the clinical presentation of sCJD is related, at least in part, to the genetic background, the *PRNP* codon 129 genotype and the biochemical properties of PrP deposited in the brain. The combination of three codon 129 genotypes and two types of PrP allows classification of sCJD into six subtypes with differing phenotypic characteristics (Table 18.6).[274,276] The 'typical' forms of

sCJD are represented in the MM1 and MV1 groups and account for over 60 per cent of cases, whereas the other four subtypes are 'atypical' in terms of illness duration, clinical features, investigation results and neuropathology, including two quite distinct phenotypes within the MM2 group.

Diagnostic criteria for sCJD have been formulated and adapted to take account of scientific developments, including the validation of investigations such as the 14-3-3 CSF immunoassay and MR brain scan. A diagnosis of definite sCJD requires neuropathological validation, a classification as probable sCJD (where no neuropathological investigations have been performed) requires a combination of clinical features and positive investigations and a classification as possible sCJD is based on clinical features alone (Box 18.5). A classification of probable sCJD has been estimated to have a specificity of over 95 per cent, but the possible classification is less accurate and most epidemiological studies report only definite and probable cases. The diagnostic criteria are important in allowing comparisons between different studies, but they are not absolute rules for diagnosis, as there are a proportion of cases of sCJD, perhaps 5 per cent, in which the criteria will not be fulfilled in life.[301] It is essential to obtain neuropathological verification of the diagnosis in order to be confident of correct diagnostic attribution, and systematic studies of CJD depend on a high post-mortem rate in suspect cases to achieve adequate case ascertainment.

Clinical Investigations and Genetics

The most useful investigations in sCJD are the EEG, the CSF 14-3-3 immunoassay and MR brain imaging scan. The EEG shows PTC at about 1 per second in the majority of cases (see Figure 18.13),[398] although high rates of about 70 per cent of cases with typical tracings in previous systematic studies have not been maintained in recent years, in which as few as 50 per cent of cases show a typical EEG. This may be because of the development of

TABLE 18.6 Major subtypes of sporadic Creutzfeldt–Jakob disease (sCJD) classified by *PRNP* codon 129 genotype and PrP[res] isotype (data from the UK National Creutzfeldt–Jakob Disease Surveillance Unit)*

Subtype	Frequency (%)	Median age at onset (years)	Median duration of illness (months)	Distribution of vacuolation	PrP deposits
MM1	57	66	3	Cerebral cortex (occipital lobe), cerebellum	Synaptic, perivacuolar
MM2	7	52	17	Cerebral cortex, entorhinal cortex	Perivacuolar
MV1	6	73	5	Cerebral cortex (occipital lobe)	Synaptic, perivacuolar
MV2	14	65	11	Entorhinal cortex, hippocampus striatum, thalamus	Kuru plaques, synaptic
VV1	2	53	10	Cerebral cortex (frontal lobe), entorhinal cortex, striatum	Synaptic
VV2	14	66	6	Cerebellum, striatum, thalamus, hippocampus	Synaptic, perineuronal, plaque-like

*Cases with mixed PrP[res] subtypes are not included.

BOX 18.5. Diagnostic criteria for sporadic Creutzfeldt–Jakob disease (sCJD)*

1 Definite	Neuropathologically/ immunohistochemically confirmed	I	Rapidly progressive dementia
2 Probable	I and 2 of II and III OR I and 2 of II and IV OR Possible and positive 14-3-3	II	A Myoclonus
			B Visual or cerebellar problems
			C Pyramidal or extrapyramidal features
			D Akinetic mutism
3 Possible	I and 2 of II and duration <2 years	III	Typical EEG
		IV	High signal in caudate/putamen on MRI brain scan

*As accepted by the WHO for epidemiological surveillance, updated in 2010.

other diagnostic investigations, which may preclude the need to carry out an EEG or to obtain repeat recordings in order to identify a diagnostic record. The typical EEG features of sCJD are strongly supportive of the diagnosis, as alternative causes of this EEG appearance, such as metabolic disorder and drug toxicity, can be excluded on clinical grounds. There are reports of the characteristic EEG appearances of sCJD in other dementing illnesses such as Alzheimer's disease, but this is unusual and the clinical course often differentiates sCJD. The frequency of a positive EEG in sCJD varies according to age and disease subtype, with higher rates in older people and in the MM1 and MV1 forms of disease. The EEG has a low sensitivity in atypical forms of sCJD.

The CSF 14-3-3 immunoassay is positive in about 90 per cent of cases of sCJD[398] and has a similar level of specificity in the appropriate clinical context – that is, a disease characterized by a rapidly progressive course. The 14-3-3 protein is a marker for neuronal damage and can be elevated in a range of neurological disorders, including stroke and viral encephalitis. The 14-3-3 immunoassay can therefore be used as a diagnostic tool in sCJD only in cases with the appropriate clinical phenotype and will give misleading results if applied indiscriminately. The 14-3-3 immunoassay may be positive in typical cases of sCJD and also in some of the rarer subtypes (see Figure 18.14). The MR brain imaging scan in sCJD shows a high signal in the caudate and putamen on T2 and FLAIR sequences in 60–80 per cent of cases (Figure 18.15b).[332] A recent assessment of the sensitivity and specificity of these changes has led to the inclusion of the MR brain imaging findings into the diagnostic criteria for sCJD. The MR brain imaging changes have been identified in a range of phenotypes of sCJD, including atypical cases in which other investigations are less likely to be positive.

By definition, sCJD is not a familial condition, and sequencing of *PRNP* can exclude any of the mutations associated with genetic disease. This may be important in individual cases, as a family history of CJD is absent in about 50 per cent of cases linked to mutations.[216] Analysis of the codon 129 polymorphism of *PRNP* has demonstrated that methionine homozygosity (MM) is a risk factor for the development of sCJD, with about 70 per cent of cases exhibiting this genotype in white populations.[2] The alternative genotypes, valine homozygous (VV) and heterozygous (MV), both account for about 15 per cent of cases. The valine allele is very rare in the Japanese population, where the great majority of sCJD cases are MM homozygotes and there is evidence of a gradient from west to east across Europe towards Asia and into Africa. Recent studies have indicated that genetic variability in the regulatory region of the *PRNP* gene may have a role in the pathogenesis of sCJD, and genome-wide association studies have suggested several other genetic risk loci, with modest effects, but these require verification.[254,326]

Neuropathology

Macroscopic examination of the brain in sCJD often shows no significant abnormality (see Figure 18.17a). There may be a variable degree of diffuse cerebral cortical atrophy or cerebellar cortical atrophy, the latter particularly involving the vermis. Focal atrophy of the cerebral cortex has also been described in occasional cases; for example, the occipital cortex in the so-called Heidenhain variant of sCJD, and the corpus striatum and thalamus may also appear atrophic. The hippocampus is normally spared in CJD, in contrast to Alzheimer's disease.[50,169] In occasional cases of sCJD, there is widespread severe atrophy of the cerebral cortex and cerebellum, accompanied by secondary degenerative changes in the white matter. Such cases are often referred to as the pan-encephalopathic variant of sCJD, which appears to occur with highest frequency in Japan but are also evident in Europe (see Figure 18.17b).[187,258]

Extensive histological sampling of the brain in sCJD is essential for histological diagnosis and subclassification and should include the frontal, temporal and occipital lobes, the basal ganglia and the cerebellum, as the distribution and severity of the histological features are extremely variable from one area of the brain to another.[51] Brain biopsy is now performed less frequently than in the past and is usually reserved for patients in which an alternative treatable diagnosis, such as cerebral vasculitis, is being considered.

Spongiform change is not entirely specific for sCJD, because similar changes have been described in other neurodegenerative disorders, for example, dementia with Lewy bodies, but the distribution of spongiform change within the brain in these disorders is often restricted to certain anatomical locations, particularly the temporal cortex.[136,176] The spongiform change in sCJD is extremely variable, both from one case to another and between different brain regions within the same case.[175] The diagnostic neuropathological criteria for sCJD have been formulated to take this variability into account and do not include specific details on the precise localization of lesions in the brain (Box 18.6).[51] Studies of the nature and severity of the neuropathological lesions within the brain in sCJD have allowed the identification of distinct disease subtypes. The neuronal loss in sCJD is also variable in its distribution and severity. In some cases the occipital cortex is affected most severely, whereas in other cases the cerebellar cortex bears the brunt of the neuronal loss, with extensive granular cell loss, usually with relative preservation of Purkinje cells. Surviving Purkinje cells do not all appear normal, and both dendritic hypertrophy and axonal torpedoes may be present. Astrocytic and microglial proliferation in sCJD are correspondingly variable in distribution, but in general they reflect the extent of neuronal loss. Severe neuronal loss and gliosis in the cerebral cortex result in status spongiosis, a non-specific finding characterized by collapse of the cortical cytoarchitecture and coarse vacuolation in the surviving neuropil (Box 18.6; Figure 18.24a).

The widespread use of immunohistochemistry and western blot analysis for PrP has allowed the identification of a number of distinct subgroups in sCJD, which appear to be associated with certain combinations of the codon 129 polymorphism and the PrP^res isotype.[276] These different combinations appear to be associated with particular neuropathological and clinical manifestations, but atypical

> **BOX 18.6.** Neuropathological diagnostic criteria for sCJD
>
> • Spongiform encephalopathy in cerebral and/or cerebellar cortex and/or subcortical grey matter; and/or
> • Encephalopathy with PrP immunoreactivity (plaque and/or diffuse synaptic-like and/or patchy/perivacuolar types).

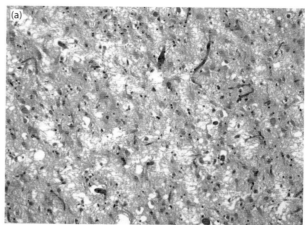

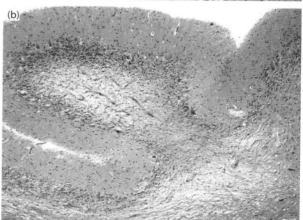

18.24 Severe pathology in sporadic Creutzfeldt–Jakob disease (sCJD). (a) Status spongiosis, with extensive neuronal loss, coarse vacuolation, widespread gliosis and collapse of the cerebral cortical cytoarchitecture after a clinical illness of 41 months. **(b)** Cerebellar pathology in a 64-year-old patient dying from sCJD, showing extreme atrophy and marked neuronal loss in the granular layer with axonal loss and secondary demyelination in the white matter.

sCJD cases occur that do not fit into these subgroups readily (Figure 18.24b).[276] Table 18.6 summarizes the neuropathological features in sCJD according to combinations of codon 129 status and PrP^res type. A fuller description of typical features in each group follows (see Gambetti *et al.*[101] and Budka *et al.*[52] for reviews).

Subtype 1: MM1/MV1
Clinical Features

This is the most common subtype of sCJD, accounting for over 60 per cent of cases, the great majority of which are methionine homozygotes. This subtype corresponds to 'classical' sCJD, with an onset in the seventh decade of life and a short duration of illness of around 4 months. An onset with dementia is followed by rapidly progressive multifocal neurological signs, including myoclonus, ataxia and visual abnormalities. This subtype includes the Heidenhain variant of sCJD, which is characterized by cortical blindness and exhibits severe neuropathological changes in the visual cortex. The EEG exhibits PTC and the 14-3-3 protein is elevated in the CSF.

Neuropathology

Micro-vacuolar spongiform change is present in a widespread distribution in the cerebral cortex, affecting cortical layers 2–6 (Figure 18.25a). The basal ganglia, thalamus and hypothalamus are involved less severely, and the brain stem and hippocampus are relatively spared, although spongiform change is usually severe in the entorhinal cortex. Spongiform change occurs in a patchy distribution in the cerebellar molecular layer, and no amyloid plaques are present. Confluent spongiform change may also occur in the cerebral cortex, particularly in the occipital cortex, with accompanying neuronal loss and gliosis. Immunohistochemistry for PrP shows a predominantly synaptic-like or punctate pattern of PrP accumulation (Figure 18.25b), with varying degrees of severity. Some regions of the cerebral and cerebellar cortex may appear unstained.

Subtype 2: VV2

Clinical Features

This subtype accounts for about 15 per cent of cases, with a mean age of onset around 60–65 years and a duration of illness of about 6 months. The clinical presentation is cerebellar ataxia, with subsequent cognitive impairment and visual abnormalities, but myoclonus is infrequent. The EEG is abnormal but not characteristic for sCJD, and the CSF 14-3-3 levels are increased in around 75 per cent of cases.

Neuropathology

Spongiform change in the cerebral cortex is usually micro-vacuolar in type and occurs in a laminar distribution, usually in layers 4–6, particularly in the frontal and temporal cortex. Spongiform change is usually more severe in the basal ganglia, thalamus and hippocampus, with patchy involvement of the dorsal midbrain regions. The cerebellum is often affected severely (Figure 18.25c), with cortical atrophy and severe spongiform change in the molecular layer

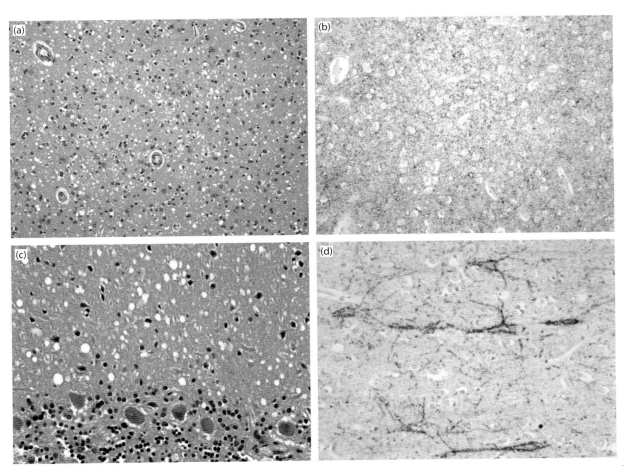

18.25 (a,b) The MM1 subtype of sporadic Creutzfeldt–Jakob disease (sCJD) shows widespread micro-vacuolar change, with a predominantly synaptic pattern of prion protein (PrP) accumulation. **(c,d)** The VV2 subtype of sCJD shows widespread vacuolation and gliosis in the cerebellum and a perineuronal and synaptic pattern of PrP immunoreactivity in the cerebral cortex. KG9 anti-PrP antibody.

and marked loss of granular neurons, with severe gliosis. Immunohistochemistry for PrP shows a characteristic linear pattern of deposition in the cerebral cortex, with intense perineuronal positivity in layers 4 and 5 and decoration of the apical ascending dendrites (Figure 18.25d). Some synaptic positivity is also present in a more widespread distribution in the cortex. In the cerebral cortex, there are numerous plaque-like deposits of PrP, usually in layers 2 and 3. Perineuronal and plaque-like deposits are also evident in the basal ganglia and thalamus, but in the cerebellum the plaque-like deposits can be widespread, involving the molecular and granular layers as well as the white matter and the dentate nucleus. Brain stem involvement can be severe in some cases, with widespread plaque-like deposits and spongiform changes in the pontine nuclei and midbrain.

Subtype 3: MV2

Clinical Features

This subtype occurs at a frequency of around 15 per cent of sCJD cases. The clinical features are similar to those of the VV2 subtype in terms of the age at onset and clinical manifestations at disease onset, with cerebellar ataxia. However, the clinical duration of illness is significantly longer, being around 10–15 months on average. In distinction to the VV2 subtype, myoclonus and pyramidal signs are common, but

visual abnormalities are rare. The EEG is abnormal but not specific for sCJD, and the 14-3-3 assay in the CSF is positive in around 75 per cent of cases.

Neuropathology

The neuropathological hallmark of the MV2 subtype of sCJD is the kuru plaque, a rounded fibrillary amyloid structure with a dense core and pale periphery. These were first described in kuru but are characteristic of this sCJD subtype, occurring most frequently in the cerebellum (molecular and granular layers) (Figure 18.26a). In some cases, these lesions are present in the subcortical grey matter nuclei, but they are relatively uncommon in the cerebral cortex. The other neuropathological features and the patterns of PrP deposition on immunohistochemistry are similar to those in the VV2 sCJD subtype, but perivacuolar accumulation of PrP is more common in the cerebral cortex, and the kuru plaques in the cerebellum stain intensely (Figure 18.26b).

Subtype 4: MM2

Clinical Features

This group occurs at a frequency of around 7 per cent of all sCJD cases and has a younger age at onset than the MM1 subtype (mean age of 52 years in our series), with a

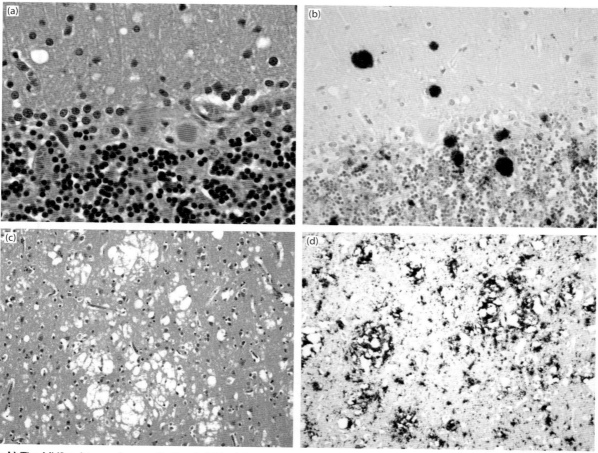

18.26 (a,b) The MV2 subtype of sporadic Creutzfeldt–Jakob disease (sCJD) is characterized by kuru-type plaques in the cerebellum, with both plaque and plaque-like immunoreactivity for prion protein (PrP). **(c,d)** The MM2 subtype of sCJD shows widespread confluent spongiform change in the cerebral cortex, with intense perivacuolar immunoreactivity for PrP. KG9 anti-PrP antibody.

significantly longer duration of illness of 17 months. The onset is usually characterized by cognitive impairment, followed by myoclonus and pyramidal signs, although ataxia is uncommon. The EEG is abnormal, with non-specific slowing, and the 14-3-3 assay in the CSF is less frequently positive than in the MM1 subtype.

Neuropathology

The main histological feature in the MM2 subtype is the presence of widespread confluent spongiform change in the cerebral cortex (Figure 18.26c), which in some cases may be so severe as to result in status spongiosis. Amyloid plaques are not present, but the confluent spongiform change is accompanied by widespread neuronal loss and severe astrocytosis. The spongiform change is less pronounced in the basal ganglia and thalamus, and, although the hippocampus is spared, the entorhinal cortex is usually severely involved. The cerebellum may show only patchy spongiform change, whereas the brain stem shows only minimal pathology. The PrP accumulation on immunohistochemistry is perivacuolar, with intense coarse deposits around and occasionally within the regions of confluent spongiform change (Figure 18.26d).

Subtype 5: VV1

Clinical Features

This is the rarest subtype of sCJD, accounting for only around 1–2 per cent of cases. The age at onset is younger than for the MM1 subtype (53 years in our series, but patients as young as 24 years have been described by Parchi and colleagues[276]), with an average duration of illness of around 10 months. Patients usually have dementia at disease onset, with subsequent myoclonus and pyramidal signs. Cerebellar ataxia and visual abnormalities are less common features. The EEG shows non-specific slowing, and the 14-3-3 assay in the CSF can be positive, but insufficient numbers of cases have been examined to determine the sensitivity and specificity of this investigation in this sCJD subtype.

Neuropathology

Widespread microvacuolar spongiform change occurs in the cerebral cortex, particularly in the frontal and temporal lobes (Figure 18.27a), with less severe involvement of the basal ganglia, thalamus, hippocampus, cerebellum and brain stem. Amyloid plaques are absent, and the pattern of PrP accumulation on immunohistochemistry is synaptic-like or granular (Figure 18.27b).

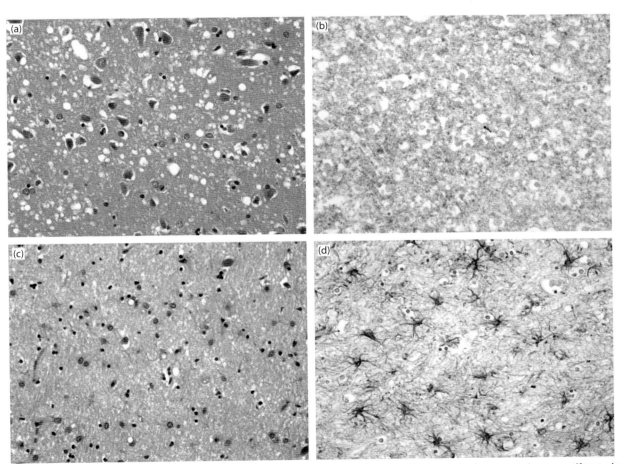

18.27 (a,b) The VV1 subtype of sporadic Creutzfeldt–Jakob disease (sCJD) shows widespread micro-vacuolar spongiform change in the cerebral cortex, and synaptic-like and focal perineuronal positivity for PrP on immunohistochemistry (KG9 anti-PrP antibody). **(c,d)** Sporadic fatal insomnia shows severe neuronal loss and gliosis in the anterior and medial thalamic nuclei, with little spongiform change. The gliosis is best demonstrated by immunohistochemistry for glial fibrillary acidic protein.

Subtype 6: Sporadic Fatal Insomnia (Formerly Known as the MM2 Thalamic Subtype)

Clinical Features

This subtype is rare, accounting for only around 1 per cent of cases, and corresponds to the 'thalamic variant' of sCJD in previous classifications (see Parchi *et al.*[282] for review). The clinical features are similar to those in fatal familial insomnia (hence the current name for this subtype) and *PRNP* sequencing is required to exclude the possibility of this inherited disorder. The mean age at onset is around 50 years, with ataxia, followed by visual signs, dementia and eventually insomnia, with a range of motor abnormalities. The EEG shows non-specific slowing.

Neuropathology

The main neuropathological abnormalities are in the thalamus, with severe neuronal loss and gliosis in the anterior and medial nuclei (particularly the dorsomedial nuclei) and with relative sparing of the posterior nuclei (Figure 18.27c). Spongiform change is usually absent in the thalamus but may be identified in the cerebral cortex, entorhinal cortex and, occasionally, cerebellum. Amyloid plaques are not present, and neuronal loss and gliosis are uncommon outside the thalamus. Immunohistochemistry for PrP appears negative in many regions (including the thalamus), but faint synaptic-like positivity can be identified in the cerebral cortex and entorhinal cortex. The intense gliosis in the thalamus is demonstrated easily by immunohistochemistry for glial fibrillary acidic protein (GFAP) (Figure 18.27d).

The Co-occurrence Phenomenon and a Revised Subclassification System for sCJD

The Parchi and Gambetti system described earlier constitutes the most widely used subclassification system for sCJD and presents a plausible molecular-genetic explanation for the pronounced phenotypic heterogeneity that is found in sCJD.[274,276] It has served well for ten years, but it is perhaps best considered as a working model. The contention that the six subtypes of sCJD correspond to individual definable strains of prion agents has been partially confirmed by the results of limited animal transmission studies.[24,280] These putative human strains comprise sCJD MM1/MV1 (designated strain M1), sCJD VV2/MV2 (designated strain V2), sCJD MM2 (designated strain M2) and sCJD VV1 (designated strain V1) with sporadic fatal insomnia (MM2 thalamic subtype) behaving differently again.[24,259a]

However the contention that the system provides an absolute basis for the sub-classification of sCJD has been brought into doubt by the emerging realization that individual brains contain mixtures of PrP^res types. The original publication of Parchi and colleagues conceded that about 5 per cent of sCJD cases contained both type 1 and type 2 PrP^res.[276] A similar figure was reported by Head and colleagues when a limited sampling protocol was employed.[143] When a more extensive sampling protocol was employed, the number of sCJD cases that can be shown to contain both types rises to about 20–50 per cent, depending on the

codon 129 genotype considerd.[54,143,310,331] An example of this phenomenon is shown in Figure 18.28. Interestingly, type 1 PrP^res was found to predominate in areas with diffuse PrP immunoreactivity, whereas type 2 PrP^res was found to predominate in areas with perivacuolar and plaque-like deposits.[310] The increased sensitivity afforded by antibodies that specifically bind the N-terminal region of protease-digested type 1 PrP^res or type 2 PrP^res on western blots indicates that all samples of PrP^res from cases of sCJD may actually contain both types.[209,299,393]

A revised subclassification system for sCJD recently proposed by Parchi *et al.*[279] identifies six additional mixed subtypes (MM/MV 1+2C, MM/MV 2C+1, VV 2+1, MV 2K+1, MV2 K+C and MM2 T+C) to add to the existing pure types (MM/MV 1, VV2, MV 2K, MM/MV 2C, MM 2T, VV1) making 12 sCJD subtypes in all. It is implicit in this revised classification that cases exist in which a minority type is absent.[54,279] A recent multicentre study of sporadic CJD neuropathology and PrP immunohistochemistry found a high level of concurrence in the recognition of the major sCJD subtypes and some of the mixed subtype, whereas there was less agreement on the classification of atypical cases.[283] A minimal sampling protocol of eight brain regions for neuropathology and four key areas for PrP^res typing has been recommended for correctly classified within this revised subclassification system for CJD,[279] which will add a further incentive for neuropathologists to seek permission to retain the whole brain at autopsy in both fixed and frozen forms.

Distribution of PrP^Sc in Tissues Other than Brain

Consistent with a disease that is thought to arise within the CNS itself, the distribution of PrP^Sc in sCJD appears largely restricted to the brain, cranial nerves and targets that they innervate. Western blot analysis detects PrP^res in the brain, spinal cord, pituitary body, trigeminal ganglion, optic nerve, retina and central olfactory pathway.[142,144,287,395] Immunohistochemistry for PrP has largely confirmed these findings and has also suggested the axonal accumulation of

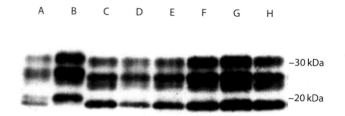

A B C D E F G H

–30 kDa

–20 kDa

18.28 Western blot analysis of PrP^res in cortical regions from a case of sporadic Creutzfeldt–Jakob disease (sCJD) (*PRNP* **codon 129 MM**). The regions of cerebral cortex shown are frontal cortex (A), subfrontal cortex (B), parietal cortex (C), subparietal cortex (D), temporal cortex (E), subtemporal cortex (F), occipital cortex (G) and suboccipital cortex (H). Type 2 PrP^res is seen in all brain regions except subfrontal cortex (B) in which type 1 PrP^res is seen. A mixture of types 1 and 2 is evident in frontal cortex (A). Western blotting employed the monoclonal antibody 3F4. Approximate molecular mass is shown in kilodaltons (kDa).

PrP in peripheral nerves in a small number of sCJD cases. Western blot analysis has, until recently, consistently failed to detect PrP[res] in the lymphoreticular system, dental tissues, non-nervous elements of the eye and peripheral nerve; it was not found in kidney, liver, lung, heart or skeletal muscle in sCJD.[25,140,142,157] However, Brown and colleagues showed that disease transmission by intracerebral inoculation in primates could be achieved from a range of peripheral tissues in sCJD, including lung, liver and kidney, in addition to brain.[41]

The development of more sensitive methods of western blot analysis has shown that low levels of PrP[res] are in fact detectable in spleen and intramuscular nerve fibres in a subset of patients with sCJD.[111,287] The observation that patients with PrP[res]-positive spleen or muscle tend to be those with longer disease duration implies centrifugal spread of PrP[Sc] from the brain, most likely along nerve fibres. However, the demonstration of PrP[res] in paraffin-embedded tissue blot analysis of large arteries in sCJD, with localization to dendritic cells and macrophages in the vessel walls, suggests that other potential routes of spread for PrP[Sc] may exist in sCJD.[213] These findings, allied to the epidemiological evidence for an increased history of surgery in patients with sCJD compared with controls,[70,369] may provide some useful and significant information that could be used for epidemiological modelling and risk assessment.

VARIABLY PROTEASE-SENSITIVE PRIONOPATHY

Definition, Epidemiology and Clinical Features

In 2008 Gambetti and co-workers reported a novel prion disease, which they termed protease-sensitive prionopathy (PSPr), on the basis of eleven cases identified by the National Prion Disease Pathology Surveillance Centre in the United States.[100] The individuals were relatively young compared to typical sCJD, had long disease duration, had no known risk factors for developing CJD, were all of the *PRNP* codon 129 VV genotype and although several had family histories of dementia, none had mutations in the *PRNP* ORF. Subsequent investigation of further individuals exhibiting the PSPr phenotype, including those of MV and MM genotypes, resulted in revision of the name to variably protease-sensitive prionopathy (VPSPr).[401] Prospective identification of individual VPSPr cases in the United Kingdom and elsewhere and retrospective review of atypical sCJD cases indicate that VPSPr is not restricted to America.[145,401] The available evidence suggests that codon 129 VV individuals are disproportionately affected by VPSPr with MV cases rare and MM cases rarer still.[401] The limited numbers of cases in the literature makes defining the common clinical features of VPSPr difficult at this point in time; however, the combination of a long disease duration and the reported atypical neurological signs have been interpreted as evidence that cases of VPSPr may be clinically mistaken for more common neurodegenerative diseases and that VPSPr is under-reported.[100] VPSPr is probably best considered as either a second sporadic human prion disease (after sCJD) or a distinct phenotype within the spectrum of sCJD. Certain aspects of the pathology have led to the suggestion that it represents a sporadic form of GSS.[100,401] Diagnosis of VPSPr rests on neuropathology and critically on PrP biochemistry, but formal diagnostic criteria have yet to be established.

Neuropathology and PrP[res] Detection

Spongiform change is a feature of the neuropathology of VPSPr, particularly in the cerebral cortex and subcortical nuclei, but can also be identified in the cerebellar molecular layer. The vacuoles are generally larger than in the MM1/MV1 form of sCJD, but extensive confluent spongiform change is rare (Figure 18.29a). Neuronal loss and gliosis are variable, but the presence of amyloid microplaques is an important diagnostic feature. These are identifiable on routinely stained sections, but are more easily seen on PrP immunohistochemistry and in PAS-stained sections (Figure 18.29b,c). Microplaques are usually most numerous in the cerebellar cortex, but may also occur in the thalamus, basal ganglia, hippocampus and cerebral cortex (Figure 18.29d). PrP immunohistochemistry shows a different pattern of accumulation than in sCJD, often with a fine granular/synaptic-like background containing rounded target-like aggregates of granules that increase in size towards the periphery of the aggregates. These structures are usually most evident in the cerebellar cortex. The pattern of PrP immunoreactivity in these aggregates may vary according to the antibodies used and the degree of proteolytic predigestion on the tissue sections. The neuropathology of VPSPr varies according to the *PRNP* codon 129 genotype; VV and MV cases tend to have more spongiform change and amyloid microplaques than MM cases, in which there is more of a plaque-like pattern on PrP immunohistochemistry. However, VPSPr can be distinguished from sCJD on histological grounds by the nature and restricted distribution of the spongiform change, and by the characteristic amyloid microplaques and PrP aggregates on immunohistochemistry (Figure 18.29a,b). Coexisting Alzheimer pathology has been described in VPSPr and some cases also have Lewy body pathology, or inclusions that label with antibodies to TDP-43 and FUS.

As its name suggests, one of the defining features of VPSPr is the presence of PrP[Sc] in a form that is markedly less resistant to proteolysis than that which typically characterizes CJD. The typical appearance of VPSPr on western blot analysis is abundant PrP prior to proteinase K digestion, but only a faint 8-kDa PrP[res] band after proteinase K digestion, often accompanied by the presence of an even fainter ladder of higher molecular weight bands (Figure 18.30). Western blot analysis of VPSPr requires electrophoretic separation that includes the low molecular weight range and the enhanced detection sensitivity afforded by PrP[Sc] enrichment methods or particular anti-PrP antibodies.[100,145] The degree of protease sensitivity of PrP[Sc] in VPSPr is reportedly related to codon 129 genotype: greatest in the VV genotype, but less pronounced in the MV and MM genotypes.[401] Moreover, conventionally sized PrP[27-30] PrP[res] fragments may be found in certain brain regions in cases of VPSPr adding to the molecular overlap between VPSPr, GSS and sCJD.[100] Preliminary reports suggest that VPSPr is transmissible to bank voles, segregating as a sCJD-like or a GSS-like strain according to vole *PRNP* genotype.[268]

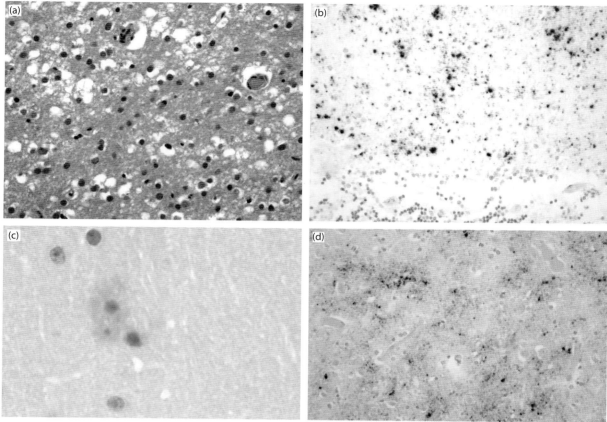

18.29 Pathology in variably protease-sensitive prionopathy (VPSPr). (a) Spongiform change and neuronal loss in the cerebral cortex of an individual homozygous for valine at codon 129 of *PRNP*. **(b)** Intense prion protein (PrP) labelling of microplaques in the cerebellar molecular layer in a codon 129 valine homozygous individual (12F10 anti-PrP antibody). **(c)** Microplaques in the molecular layer of the cerebellum stained with periodic–acid Schiff (PAS). **(d)** Widespread PrP labelling in a granular pattern in the basal ganglia in a methionine/valine heterozygous individual (12F10 anti-PrP antibody).

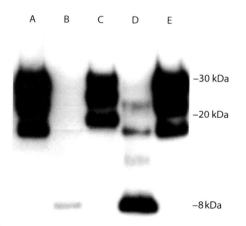

18.30 Western blot analysis of PrPres **from brain tissue of a case of variably protease-sensitive prionopathy (VPSPr) (B and D) with a *PRNP* codon 129 VV genotype.** The VPSPr case is shown flanked by standard samples of variant Creutzfeldt–Jakob disease (vCJD) MM2B (A and E) and sCJD MM1 subtype (c). Lanes A, B, C and E were loaded with a standard amount of brain homogenate, whereas lane D was loaded with a ten-fold excess of VPSPr brain homogenate enriched for PrPres by centrifugation to help clearly visualize the low abundance 8-kDa PrPres band. Western blotting employed the monoclonal antibody 3F4. Approximate molecular mass is shown in kilodaltons (kDa).

FAMILIAL OR GENETIC PRION DISEASES

Definition and Epidemiology

Familial or genetic prion diseases include a group of diseases associated with mutations in the *PRNP* gene that are transmitted in an autosomal dominant manner and include both point mutations and insertion mutations of 24 base pair (bp) repeats located between *PRNP* codons 51 and 91 (see Figure 18.16). Familial prion diseases have four main clinicopathological phenotypes (Box 18.7): (i) fCJD, (ii) GSS, (iii) FFI and (iv) PrP-CAA. Sometimes the clinical and pathological phenotype of the familial prion diseases blends the features of CJD and GSS, but in other cases it lacks the characteristic clinical and histopathological features of prion disease (see Ghetti *et al.*,[107] Kong *et al.*[211] Parchi *et al.*[281,282] for reviews). Current clinical and genetic diagnostic criteria for familial prion diseases are summarized in Box 18.8; these include details of *PRNP* polymorphisms that are known to influence disease phenotype in human prion diseases and others that are of uncertain significance at present.

Familial CJD comprises 10–15 per cent of all human prion diseases, although the percentage varies from one country to another according to the presence of affected kindreds (see Kovacs *et al.*[216] for review). A study of mortality

BOX 18.7. Major clinicopathological phenotypes of familial prion diseases

- Familial Creutzfeldt–Jakob disease (fCJD):
  - Progressive dementia with other neurological signs, including myoclonus, visual abnormalities, ataxia, pyramidal and extrapyramidal signs and akinetic mutism.
  - Spongiform degeneration of the brain with variable neuronal loss and gliosis. Kuru-type amyloid plaques may be present in a minority of cases.
- Gerstmann–Sträussler–Scheinker disease (GSS):
  - Progressive spinocerebellar syndrome, with pyramidal and pseudo-bulbar signs, progressing to dementia and akinetic mutism.
  - Widespread multicentric PrP amyloid plaques in the brain, often in the absence of spongiform change.
- Fatal familial insomnia (FFI):
  - Sleep abnormalities, with dysautonomia, pyramidal signs, myoclonus, dysarthria, dysphagia and ataxia.
  - Severe neuronal loss and gliosis in the anterior and medial thalamus, often with minimal spongiform degeneration in the brain.
- Prion protein cerebral amyloid angiopathy (PrP-CAA):
  - Memory disturbance, disorientation and progressive dementia.
  - PrP amyloid deposition in small and medium-sized vessels, tau-positive neurofibrillary tangle, neuropil threads and dystrophic neurites in the cerebrum.

BOX 18.8. Diagnostic criteria for familial prion diseases

- Definite:
  A. Definite prion disease + definite or probable prion disease in first-degree relative
  B. Definite prion disease with pathogenic Prnp mutation (see later)
- Probable:
  A. Progressive neuropsychiatric disorder + definite or probable prion disease in first-degree relative
  B. Progressive neuropsychiatric disorder + pathogenic PRNP mutation (see later)
- PRNP mutations associated with Gerstmann–Sträussler–Scheinker disease (GSS) neuropathological phenotype: P102L, P105L, P105S, A117V, G131V, S132I, R136S, H187R F198S, D202N, Q212P, Q217R, Y218N, Q227X, M232T
- PRNP mutations associated with Creutzfeldt–Jakob disease (CJD) neuropathological phenotype: P105T, G114V, R148H, D178N-129V, V180I, T183A, T188A, T188K, T118R, E196K, E200K, V203I, R208H, V210I, E211Q, I215V, M232R, 48 bpdel
- PRNP mutations associated with indeterminate neuropathological phenotype: A133V
- PRNP mutations associated with FFI neuropathological phenotype: D178N-129M
- PRNP mutations associated with variable phenotype: 24 bpi, 48 bpi, 72 bpi, 96 bpi, 120 bpi, 144 bpi, 168 bpi, 192 bpi, 216 bpi, 288 bpi
- PRNP mutation associated with vascular PrP amyloid: Y145Stop, Q160Stop, Y163Stop, Y226Stop
- PRNP mutations associated with neuropsychiatric disorder but not proven prion disease: S97N, I138M, G142S, F198V
- PRNP mutations without clinical and neuropathological data: P238S
- PRNP polymorphisms with established influence on phenotype: M129V
- PRNP polymorphisms with suggested influence on phenotype: N171S, E219K, 24 bpdel
- PRNP polymorphisms without established influence on phenotype: P39P, G54S, P68P, A117A, G124G, G127V, Y128Y, Y150Y, V161V, N173N, H177H, T188T, D202D, R208R, Q212Q, R228R, S230S

bpdel, base pair deletion; bpi, base pair insertion.

from CJD and related disorders in Europe, Australia and Canada showed that over 80 per cent of cases were classified as sporadic and up to 15 per cent were familial, of which PRNP codon 200 mutations account for about 50 per cent.[220] Other PRNP mutations are less common, although at least 40 presumably unrelated kindreds who carry the FFI mutation have been published.[282] To date, GSS has been recognized in several countries, including Argentina, Australia, Canada, China, various European countries, Japan, Mexico, the Middle East and the United States. With these countries representing less than 15 per cent of the world's population, an accurate incidence of GSS remains to be determined.[107] Gerstmann–Sträussler–Scheinker disease is probably underdiagnosed, because it may have various presentations, including symptoms of ataxia, spastic paraparesis, parkinsonism, amyotrophy and dementia. Similarly, other familial prion disorders, including FFI and PRNP insertional mutations, have in the past been misdiagnosed as a range of other neurodegenerative disorders, including Alzheimer's disease, Huntington's disease and olivopontocerebellar atrophy.[137] In a significant number of cases (12–88 per cent, depending on the mutation), there is no family history of a neurological disorder, leading to the suggestion that the term 'genetic TSE' is preferable to 'familial prion disease'.[216] Many, but not all, familial prion diseases have been transmitted experimentally; some of those transmitted more recently have used a transgenic mouse with a corresponding mutation to achieve transmission.

In this section, the various familial disorders resulting from mutations and insertions in the PRNP are grouped according to their clinical and pathological phenotypes (see Box 18.7). These are referred to by a designation of both the PRNP mutation or insertion and the codon 129 polymorphism on the mutant allele (such as E200K-129M or

D178N-129V), because both appear to exert an influence on disease phenotype.

Clinical and Neuropathological Features

PRNP E200K-129M

Clinical Features

The most common mutation associated with fCJD is E200K, with methionine at the polymorphic residue 129 (E200K-129M).[216] In families with this haplotype, the mean age at onset is 59–62 years and the mean duration of the disease is 5–7 months. The most common signs at onset include cognitive impairment, psychiatric changes (80–83 per cent), cerebellar signs (43–45 per cent), visual signs (19 per cent) and myoclonus (12 per cent).[101,211] All patients develop dementia and cognitive and psychiatric disturbances. Electroencephalograms showing PTCs typical of sCJD were observed in 75 per cent of cases. The 14-3-3 assay in the CSF is positive in most patients. The only clinical feature that appears to distinguish this group of patients from those with the MM1 subtype of sCJD is the involvement of the peripheral nervous system with motor and sensory neuropathy, which is rare in sCJD.

Neuropathology

The histological features associated with the fCJD E200K-129M haplotype are very similar to those seen in the MM1 subtype of sCJD and include spongiform degeneration, astrogliosis and neuronal loss in the absence of amyloid plaques. The lesions are of variable severity and involve the cerebral cortex, striatum, thalamus and cerebellum (Figure 18.31a). Immunohistochemistry shows PrP deposits with a synaptic-like pattern and sometimes a coarse or perivacuolar pattern of immunoreactivity.[101,211] Coexisting Aβ, tau and α-synuclein pathology has been reported, but TDP-43 and FUS immunoreactive deposits are apparently absent.[217]

PRNP E200K-129V

Clinical Features

Although the number of patients with the E200K-129V haplotype is too small to draw firm conclusions regarding phenotypic characteristics, the patients analyzed showed clinical features that distinguish this group from those with the more common E200K-129M haplotype. These features include early ataxia and late appearance of myoclonus and PTC on EEG.

Neuropathology

The neuropathological features in patients with E200K-129V are characterized by PrP accumulation in the form of plaque-like structures in the cerebellum on immunohistochemistry for PrP (Figure 18.31b).[135] Intracytoplasmic neuronal PrP positivity may also be found particularly in the brain stem (Figure 18.31c).[217]

PRNP D178N-129V

Clinical Features

The clinical presentation and duration of disease in patients with fCJD associated with the D178N-129V haplotype is influenced by the genotype at residue 129 of the normal allele. The mean age at onset of disease is 39 years (range 26–47 years) in 129V homozygous patients and 49 years (range 45–56 years) in heterozygous patients. The duration of disease is shorter – 14 months (range 9–18 months) – for valine homozygotes compared with 27 months (range 7–51 months) for heterozygotes. The typical presentation is with cognitive impairment, depression and abnormal behaviour. The course of the disease is characterized by ataxia, dysarthria, aphasia, tremor and myoclonus, with PTC on EEG examination.

Neuropathology

The neuropathological changes seen in patients with the D178N-129V haplotype include spongiform degeneration, gliosis and neuronal loss. The lesions have a distinctive distribution, with the frontal and temporal cortices generally more affected than the occipital cortex. Within the

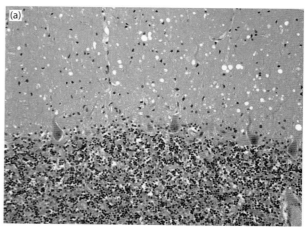

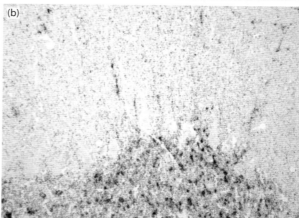

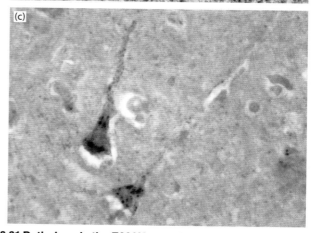

18.31 Pathology in the E200K mutation. (a) Widespread microvacuolar spongiform change is present in the cerebellar molecular layer, but no amyloid plaques are present in the E200K-129M haplotype. **(b)** Immunohistochemistry shows an unusual pattern of PrP accumulation in the cerebellar cortex, with focal intense positivity in the granular layer and irregular linear deposits in the molecular layer in the E200K-129V haplotype (KG9 anti-PrP antibody). **(C)** Focal intracytoplasmic neuronal positivity for PrP in the E200K-129V haplotype (3F4 anti-PrP antibody).

hippocampal region, lesions are prominent in the subiculum and entorhinal cortex. Among the subcortical structures, the putamen and the caudate nucleus show severe spongiosis, whereas the thalamus is affected minimally or moderately. The cerebellum and brain stem are usually spared. PrP immunostaining demonstrates synaptic-like deposits most prominent in areas with severe spongiform lesions, whereas the cerebellum shows minimal immunostaining for PrP. Amyloid plaques have not been reported.[114,211]

PRNP V210I-129M

Clinical Features

The absence of a family history and the existence of asymptomatic carriers at relatively advanced age indicate that the V210I-129M haplotype has low penetrance. The onset of disease among the reported cases is at age 46–80 years, and the duration of disease is 2–24 months. Memory loss and gait disturbance are predominant presenting signs, followed by dementia and myoclonus. Electroencephalographic examination shows PTC.

Neuropathology

Few autopsy cases have been analysed from patients with the V210I-129M haplotype. All show spongiform degeneration and gliosis in the grey matter, which is most prominent in the cerebral cortex and the molecular layer of the cerebellum.[298]

Less Common Mutations Associated with Sporadic Creutzfeldt–Jakob Disease-like Phenotype

PRNP G114V

Clinical Features

A novel *PRNP* mutation, G114V, has been reported in an Uruguayan family and a Chinese family.[230,317] The presentation of the disease included neuropsychiatric disturbances, followed by dementia associated with an extrapyramidal syndrome. All the patients developed the disease at a young age (range 18–40 years), and the duration of the disease was lengthy (range 1–4 years).

Neuropathology

Frontal lobe biopsy in two Uruguayan patients and one Chinese patient showed spongiform degeneration, neuronal loss and gliosis, with synaptic-like PrP immunoreactive deposits similar to those described in sCJD.

PRNP R148H-129M

Clinical Features

The R148H-129M haplotype has been reported in two patients from apparently unrelated families.[218,284] Because in both cases there were no other affected family members, it is probable that this mutation has low penetrance. Detailed analysis in one patient with this mutation showed impaired gait and cognition in the absence of myoclonus or PTC on EEG.

Neuropathology

Neuropathological examination revealed spongiform degeneration, mostly in the cortex and basal ganglia,

whereas PrP immunostaining demonstrated kuru-type plaques associated with synaptic-like immunoreactivity in both patients, similar to the MV2 subtype of sCJD.

PRNP V180I-129M

Clinical Features

The V180I-129M haplotype was described in a few Japanese patients and in one US case (see Kong *et al.*[211] for review). The age at onset for patients with the V180I-129M haplotype varies between 66 and 81 years. Studies on two patients showed cognitive impairment, followed by akinetic mutism, pyramidal and extrapyramidal signs and myoclonus. The EEG failed to show PTC. Pathological laughing and crying has been suggested to be a common sign.[178]

Neuropathology

Neuropathological examination in a few patients showed spongiform degeneration in the cerebrum and weak and diffuse PrP immunoreactivity in the grey matter. Kuru-type plaques were observed in two patients who were heterozygous at codon 129 and in one patient homozygous for methionine at codon 129.[179]

PRNP T183A-129M

Clinical Features

Among the patients reported with T183A-129M haplotype, the mean age at onset was 44 years and the mean duration of disease was 3.7 years.[267] Behavioural disturbances are the predominant presenting signs associated with memory loss, followed by rapid progressive dementia, aggressive behaviour and parkinsonian signs. The EEG examination failed to show characteristic PTC.

Neuropathology

The main histological lesions seen in these patients are spongiform degeneration in the cerebral cortex and basal ganglia. PrP-immunoreactivity was reported to be widespread and punctate, particularly in the cerebral cortex, with a plaque-like pattern in the putamen.

PRNP M232R-129M

Clinical Features

The age of onset of disease for patients with M232R-129M ranges between 54 and 70 years, and the duration of the illness ranges between 4 and 26 months. Presenting signs included memory and gait disturbances, followed by myoclonus and mutism. Electroencephalographic examination showed PTC.

Neuropathology

The few patients with the M232R-129M haplotype who were studied neuropathologically showed spongiform degeneration, astrogliosis and neuronal loss in variable degrees. All three lesions were observed in the cerebral cortex, basal ganglia and brain stem. No spongiform degeneration was reported in the cerebellum. Widespread PrP immunoreactivity was seen in the cerebrum and spinal cord.[163]

Rare Cases

Rare *PRNP* mutations associated with sCJD-like phenotypes are summarized in Table 18.7.

PrPSc Detection in Familial Creutzfeldt–Jakob Disease

The identification of multiple genetic mutations in the *PRNP* gene provides some aetiological basis for phenotypic heterogeneity in inherited prion diseases. However, phenotypic variability is also present within genetic subgroups, even among members of the same family, indicating that epigenetic factors may also play a role. It is likely that the biochemical characteristics of PrPSc modulate the phenotype of familial prion diseases. Two main PrPSc types have been described in patients with fCJD, which correspond to the two major isoforms found in sCJD. Type 1 was detected in patients with the following *PRNP* haplotypes: E200K-129M, D178N-129V, V210I-129M, R208H-129M and T188R-129V. Type 2 was detected in patients with the following *PRNP* haplotypes: E200K-129V, 148H-129M and T183A-129M. The co-occurrence of different PrPSc patterns between brain regions was reported in two patients with the *PRNP* D178N-129V haplotype[131] and two patients with the *PRNP* E200K-129M.[217] In one patient with *PRNP* R208H, a complex pattern of PrPSc isoforms was described, containing three PrPSc isoforms (corresponding to di-, mono- and un-glycosylated species) and an additional 17-kDa PrP fragment.[318]

Fatal Familial Insomnia

PRNP D178N-129M

Clinical Features

Fatal familial insomnia is a disease characterized by alterations in the sleep–wake cycle, dysautonomia and motor signs, associated with thalamic atrophy. Fatal familial insomnia is linked to the D178N-129M haplotype. Patients with FFI who are methionine homozygotes at codon 129 have a disease duration of 12 ± 4 months, whereas the duration is 21 ± 15 months in heterozygous patients.[114] However, the mean age at disease onset does not differ between these two subgroups (mean age 49 years, range 20–72 years). Studies of a large kindred with this mutation have revealed a wide phenotypic spectrum, including variable age of onset.[137] Early symptoms in most patients are insomnia, apathy and enacted dreams. Sleep disturbances are often associated with autonomic alterations, including mild blood pressure elevation, mild pyrexia and increased heart rate.[257] Motor signs, such as diplopia, dysarthria, dysphagia and gait abnormalities and seizures are generally more prominent in heterozygous patients. Spontaneous and evoked myoclonus is often found. Positron emission tomography (PET) with [18F]2-fluoro-2-deoxy-d-glucose shows prominent and selective hypometabolism of the thalamus bilaterally, even in the presymptomatic stage of the disease.[74] The involvement of other areas of the brain is variable. On polysomnography in typical cases, the 24-hour EEG shows a continuous oscillation between the activity of normal wakefulness and sub-wakefulness; as the disease progresses, EEG activities typical of non-rapid eye movement sleep are lost.[257] Laboratory studies to measure the autonomic and endocrine systems show that plasma catecholamines are increased, and cortisol is high in the presence of normal or low plasma corticotrophin levels.

TABLE 18.7 Sporadic Creutzfeldt–Jakob disease (sCJD)-like phenotype in patients with rare *Prnp* mutations (see Kong et al.[178] and Parchi et al.[317] for reviews)

- Three clinically affected members of a family of East India origin were described with dementia, motor decline and ataxia in association with the P105T-129M genotype. The age of the patients was uncharacteristically young, but no autopsy investigation was performed.[319] More recently, a P105T-129V case has been reported with post-mortem examination.[300]
- One 84-year-old man possessed a double *PRNP* mutation, V180I and M232R, on different alleles. The patient developed memory problems followed by dementia in the absence of myoclonus and periodic triphasic complexes (PTCs) on electroencephalography (EEG). No history of dementia was known in the patient's family. Post-mortem examination of the left parietal region showed spongiform degeneration and diffuse PrP immunoreactivity.
- Three mutations have been described at *PRNP* residue 188: T188A was reported in an 82-year-old patient with the clinical diagnosis of Creutzfeldt–Jakob disease (CJD) confirmed at autopsy; T188K in a 59-year-old patient with rapid progressive dementia; and T188R in an individual with an undiagnosed neurological disease. Recently a second patient with the same *PRNP* T188R mutation was reported showing behavioural changes, cognitive and motor impairments. Autopsy findings confirmed the diagnosis of prion disease.[351]
- CJD was diagnosed clinically and confirmed histopathologically in three 69-year-old patients, each with previously unreported *PRNP* haplotypes: E196K-129M, V203I-129M and E211Q-129M. A 71-year-old Chinese patient with rapid progressive dementia without family history and *PRNP* E196K was described.[334] Comprehensive neuropathological analysis shows phenotypic heterogeneity associated with this mutation.[87] An E196A mutation has also been reported associated with a clinical diagnosis of CJD.[400]
- CJD was diagnosed clinically and confirmed histopathologically in a patient with a novel E200G-129V mutation associated with long disease duration and a clinical-pathological phenotype differing from those of the common E200K-129M and the rare E200K-129V mutation cases.[200]
- The R208H-129M haplotype was found in three apparently unrelated individuals. In two patients, the disease phenotype appears to be similar to that described in most patients with sCJD. The third case displayed distinct neuropathological features characterized by tau pathology in the hippocampus and entorhinal cortex and ballooned neurons in the cortex, hippocampus and subcortical grey matter. More recently a fourth case has been described presenting as progressive supranuclear palsy.[244]
- A novel missense mutation (*PRNP* I215V) was recently described in two Spanish families. In two patients CJD was confirmed neuropathologically. Neuropathological studies in the third patient suggested a diagnosis of Alzheimer's disease.[261]
- The P238S mutation was reported in a German patient with possible prion disease. No further information is available.

Neuropathology

The distinctive feature of FFI is severe atrophy of the anterior ventral, dorsomedial and pulvinar thalamic nuclei, with loss of 80–90 per cent of the neurons in the presence of severe gliosis and absence of spongiform change (Figure 18.32). Other thalamic nuclei are affected less severely and more inconsistently (see Kong et al.[211] and Parchi et al.[282] for reviews). Atrophy of the inferior olives is the second most common change. The presence and degree of histopathological changes in the cerebral cortex are a function of the disease duration, which is related in part to the *PRNP* genotype at codon 129. Cases with 7–10 months' duration from the onset of clinical signs usually show focal spongiform degeneration in the entorhinal cortex and minimal gliosis in the deeper layers of the neocortex. In cases with longer disease duration, progressive spongiform degeneration and variable degrees of astrocytosis and neuronal loss are seen in the cerebral cortex. The cerebellar cortex, periaqueductal grey matter, raphe nucleus and reticular formation in the brain stem may also show mild neuronal loss and astrocytosis. Studies on paraffin sections have reported the absence of PrP immunoreactivity in most brain regions analyzed, but PrP accumulation has been reported in the molecular layer of the cerebellum and in the subiculum and entorhinal cortex, particularly in cases with a long clinical duration of illness.[137,282]

PrP^res Detection in Fatal Familial Insomnia

The detection of PrP^res in FFI has in the past been hampered by the relatively low amounts of PrP^res in the brain in some cases. One main isoform has been described in patients with FFI (type 2 PrP^res) but with a characteristic under-representation of the non-glycosylated isoform, compared with sCJD and sporadic fatal insomnia (sFI).[101] A report has shown differences in the PrP^res glycoform ratio between brain regions in one patient, but the clinicopathological significance of this observation remains uncertain.[131]

Gerstmann–Sträussler–Scheinker Disease
PRNP P102L-129M
Clinical Features

The *PRNP* P102L-129M is the most common haplotype among those associated with GSS.[105,107] The clinical phenotype is characterized by a progressive cerebellar syndrome, with ataxia, dysarthria, incoordination of saccadic eye movements and pyramidal and pseudo-bulbar signs. Behavioural and cognitive dysfunctions are seen in most cases, which evolve into dementia or akinetic mutism. Clinical symptoms start in the fourth to sixth decade of life, with a disease duration of a few months to 6 years. In some cases, amyotrophy and an electromyography (EMG) pattern of denervation may be seen early in the course of the disease. Magnetic resonance imaging scans may show brain atrophy (Figure 18.33) and a single photon-emission computed tomography (SPECT) scan might reveal hypoperfusion of the frontal cortex and cerebellum. Myoclonus and PTC in the EEG, characteristics of sCJD, are observed in some individuals, whose disease may have a very rapid clinical course of 5–9 months and with a clinical phenotype indistinguishable from that of sCJD.[211]

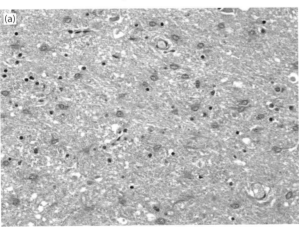

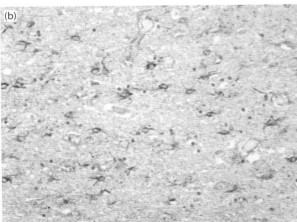

18.32 (a,b) Fatal familial insomnia is characterized by extensive neuronal loss and gliosis in the medial and anterior thalamic nuclei, with relatively little spongiform change and no amyloid plaque formation. The severe gliosis is best demonstrated on immunohistochemistry for the fibrillary acidic protein. The pathological features are very similar to those in sporadic fatal insomnia, shown in Figure 18.27 (c,d).

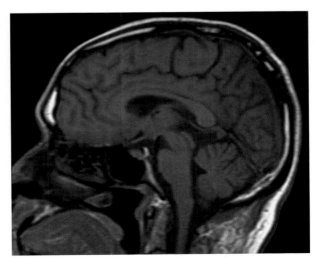

18.33 Sagittal T1-weighted magnetic resonance image of the brain in Gerstmann–Sträussler–Scheinker (GSS) disease shows marked cerebellar atrophy that is particularly obvious in the superior vermis. The cerebral cortex appears relatively spared.

Neuropathology

The *PRNP* P102L-129M haplotype is associated with two neuropathological phenotypes. The first is that of typical GSS; the second is a combination of GSS and CJD features, namely amyloid plaques and spongiform degeneration. The typical GSS features include unicentric and/or multicentric PrP plaques that are most numerous in the molecular layer of the cerebellum; they are also found in the cerebral grey matter (Figure 18.34).[290] Astrocytic proliferation is present in areas with the most severe PrP deposition. Neuronal loss appears to be more severe in cases with spongiform degeneration than in cases with PrP plaques only.[132] It should be noted that the former has been used successfully to induce a spongiform encephalopathy following intracerebral inoculation into transgenic mice with the equivalent mutation (Tg PrP101LL), whereas the latter results in PrP-amyloid deposition in the absence of spongiform degeneration in these same mice.[294]

PRNP P102L-129M-219K

Clinical Features

The clinical presentation is characterized by dementia or cerebellar signs. Magnetic resonance imaging may show severe cerebral atrophy.

Neuropathology

Mild PrP deposition is present in the cerebral and cerebellar cortices and the basal ganglia; however, amyloid and spongiform changes are not observed.[96]

PRNP P102L-129V

Clinical Features

The clinical features are different from those associated with the P102L-129M haplotype and are characterized by the presence of seizures and long tract signs and the absence of dementia. In addition, this mutation is associated with a clinical course that may last up to 12 years, significantly longer than in the P102L-129M haplotype.

Neuropathology

There is moderate to severe loss of fibres in the corticospinal, spinocerebellar and gracilis tracts of the spinal cord (Figure 18.35a). In addition, diffuse PrP deposits are present in the substantia gelatinosa. PrP-amyloid plaques are frequently seen in the cerebellar cortex and, to a lesser extent, in the neocortex (Figure 18.35b,c). No spongiform degeneration is seen.[391]

PRNP P105L-129V

Clinical Features

The age of onset of the clinical signs is in the fourth or fifth decade of life. The duration of the disease ranges from 6 to 12 years. Spastic gait, hyperreflexia and the Babinski sign are prominent in the initial stages. Extrapyramidal signs such as fine finger tremor and rigidity of limbs may be observed. Paraparesis progresses to tetraparesis and is accompanied by emotional incontinence and dementia. Myoclonus, PTC in the EEG and severe cerebellar signs have not been reported. T2-weighted MR imaging scans show hypointensity of the striatum. An EMG may show evidence of denervation, whereas evoked potentials reveal conduction delays in the posterior funiculi and corticospinal tract.[107]

Neuropathology

PrP-amyloid plaques and diffuse deposits are frequently seen in the neocortex, especially the motor area, striatum and thalamus, but rarely in the cerebellum. Neurofibrillary tangles are seen in some cases and may occur in varying amounts. In addition, axonal loss occurs in the pyramidal tracts. No spongiform changes are seen.[390]

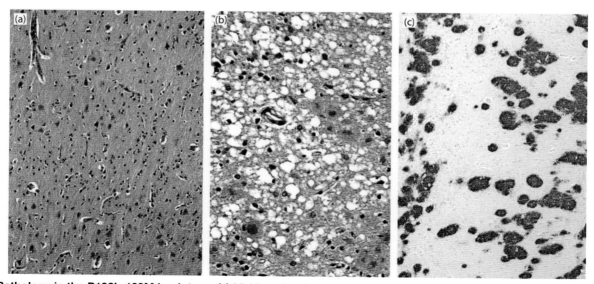

18.34 Pathology in the P102L-129M haplotype. (a) Multicentric plaques in the cerebral cortex, with very little spongiform change. **(b)** Severe confluent spongiform change, with marked neuronal loss and multiple multicentric PrP plaques. **(c)** The multicentric plaques are strikingly demonstrated on immunohistochemistry for PrP. KG9 anti-PrP antibody.

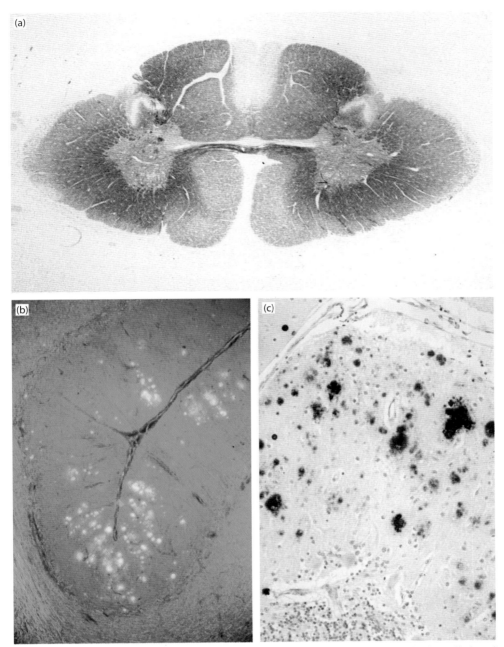

18.35 Pathology in the P102L-129V haplotype. (a) Long tract degeneration, with particularly marked myelin loss in the gracile fasciculus of the spinal cord. Woelcke–Heidenhain stain. **(b,c)** Prion protein (PrP) accumulation in the form of multicentric plaques in the cerebellum demonstrated using thioflavin S (b) and the 3F4 anti-PrP antibody (c).

PRNP A117V-129V

Clinical Features

The *PRNP* A117V-129V haplotype is associated with a variety of clinical phenotypes, ranging from typical GSS disease to classic Alzheimer's disease. The age at onset of clinical signs is in the second to seventh decade of life; the duration ranges from 1 to 11 years. In some individuals, marked extrapyramidal signs with parkinsonian features occur early in the course of the disease, followed by other neurological symptoms.[106,236] Additional signs that may be seen include pyramidal signs, amyotrophy, myoclonus, emotional lability and pseudo-bulbar signs. Behavioural and personality disturbances, such as mood swings, aggressive behaviour and paranoia, frequently present long before neurological signs and symptoms. The phenotypic variability observed among affected individuals even occurs within the same family. The EEG is either normal or non-specifically abnormal, but no PTCs are seen. Results from CT scans vary from normal to moderate cerebral atrophy.

Neuropathology

Cerebral atrophy occurs in some cases. Variable amounts of PrP-amyloid plaques and diffuse deposits are widespread throughout the cerebral cortex (Figure 18.36), hippocampus,

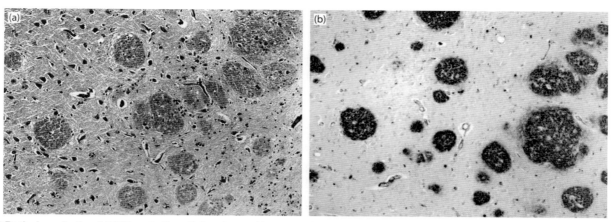

18.36 Pathology in the A117V mutation. Extensive multicentric plaques are present in the cerebral cortex. The larger plaques are evident on routine stains **(a)**, but immunohistochemistry for PrP shows more extensive accumulation with multiple smaller deposits detected **(b)**. 3F4 anti-PrP antibody.

basal ganglia and thalamus; however, in the cerebellum, they may be absent or present in variable amounts. Pyramidal tract degeneration may be present. Spongiform degeneration may also be seen, but, if so, it is focally present in the cerebrum or cerebellum. Neuronal loss, when present, may be severe in the substantia nigra. Neurofibrillary tangles have been seen in individuals with a long disease duration.[107] Recent evidence suggest that GSS A117V is transmissible to transgenic mice expressing human 117V PrP.[7]

PRNP F198S-129V

Clinical Features

A gradual loss of short-term memory, clumsiness in walking evolving into ataxia, bradykinesia, rigidity, mild tremor, dysarthria and cognitive impairment evolving into dementia are the main clinical characteristics. In the early stages of clinical presentation, T2-weighted MR imaging shows cerebellar atrophy and a reduced signal in the substantia nigra and red nucleus. Signs of cognitive impairment and eye-movement abnormalities may be detected before the onset of clinical symptoms. Psychotic depression has been observed in several patients. The symptoms may progress slowly over 5 years or rapidly over as little as 1 year. The age of onset of clinical signs ranges from late in the fourth decade to early in the eighth decade of life. Patients homozygous for valine at codon 129 have clinical signs more than 10 years earlier, on average, than heterozygous patients. The duration of the disease ranges from 2 to 12 years.[103,104,107,211]

Neuropathology

The neuropathological phenotype is characterized by a severe PrP deposition, in the form of PrP-amyloid plaques and diffuse deposits (Figure 18.37), and by the presence of numerous neurofibrillary tangles. This PrP deposition is the most severe seen associated with GSS. Unicentric and multicentric PrP-amyloid plaques and diffuse deposits are distributed in varying degrees throughout most grey matter regions of the brain.[104] The core of the amyloid plaque is immunoreactive to antibodies raised against the mid-region of PrP but is unreactive or weakly reactive to antibodies raised against the amino- and carboxy-terminal regions of PrP. In contrast, there is immunopositivity to antibodies raised against the amino- and carboxy-terminal

regions of PrP in the area adjacent to the amyloid core. Nonfibrillar PrP deposits appear as diffusely immunolabelled areas in the neuropil. By electron microscopy, the amyloid is composed of bundles of fibrils radiating from a central core; each fibril measures 8–10 nm in diameter.[107]

Amyloid deposition is severe in the frontal, insular, temporal and parietal cortices, with the highest concentration of deposits in layers I, IV, V and VI. In the hippocampus, plaques occur predominantly within the stratum lacunosummoleculare of the CA1 sector and subiculum. In the cerebellum, amyloid plaques are most numerous. PrP deposits have also been found in the inner portion of the outer plexiform layer of the neural retina (Figure 18.38). Amyloid deposits are surrounded by astrocytes, astrocytic processes and microglial cells. In the neocortex, many amyloid cores are associated with abnormal neurites, causing them to appear morphologically similar to neuritic plaques of Alzheimer's disease.[103,104] Neurofibrillary tangles and neuropil threads, which are immunoreactive to antibodies raised against the tau protein, are found in cortical and subcortical grey nuclei and in the midbrain and pons (Figure 18.39a,b).[103] They are most numerous in areas of neocortex that have severe PrP-amyloid deposition. Iron deposition in the globus pallidus, striatum, red nucleus and substantia nigra is seen. Spongiform changes are observed rarely. Some of these neuropathological characteristics have also been observed in clinically non-symptomatic individuals with this haplotype (Figure 18.37c,d).

PRNP Q217R-129V

Clinical Features

The phenotype is characterized by gradual memory loss, progressive gait disturbances, parkinsonism and dementia. The neurological signs may be preceded by episodes of mania or depression that respond to antidepressant medications, lithium and neuroleptics. The age at onset of clinical signs varies from the fifth to the seventh decade. The duration of the disease is 2–6 years.[105,107,211]

Neuropathology

The neuropathological phenotype, similar to that associated with the F198S-129V haplotype, is characterized by a severe PrP deposition, in the form of PrP-amyloid plaques

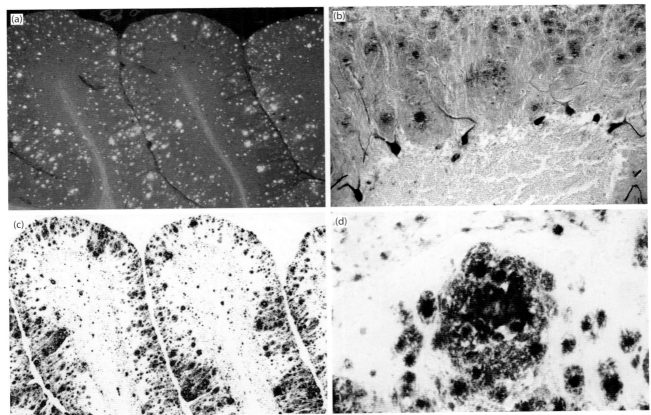

18.37 Pathology in the F198S mutation. Multiple multicentric amyloid plaques are present in the cerebellar cortex: **(a)** thioflavin S; **(c)** immunohistochemistry for PrP. 3F4 anti-PrP antibody. **(b)** The plaques are accompanied by a wide range of abnormalities in the Purkinje cell dendrites. Double immunolabelling with the 3F4 anti-PrP antibody and anti-calbindin. **(d)** The multicentric plaques appear to aggregate to form larger deposits. 3F4 anti-PrP antibody.

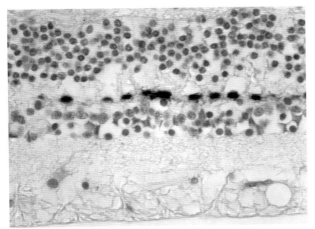

18.38 Prion protein (PrP)-positive deposits in the neural retina in a patient with Gerstmann–Sträussler–Scheinker disease (GSS) associated with the F198S *PRNP* mutation. PrP deposits are found in the inner portion of the outer plexiform layer as shown in the immunohistochemical preparation using an antibody raised against PrP.

and diffuse deposits, and by the presence of numerous neurofibrillary tangles. PrP-amyloid deposits are numerous in the cerebrum and cerebellum. Neurofibrillary tangles are abundant in the cerebral cortex, amygdala, substantia innominata and thalamus. Lewy bodies may be found in the substantia nigra. No spongiform degeneration is seen.[105,211]

Rare Cases

A group of rare *PRNP* gene mutations resulting in a GSS-like phenotype are summarized in Table 18.8. A case with a novel *PRNP* gene mutation (A133V) has been reported with clinical features unlike those of GSS, but with some multicentric plaques confined to the cerebellar cortex.[321] Until the pathological features associated with this mutation can be confirmed in additional cases, it would be prudent to classify this case as having an indeterminate neuropathological phenotype in relation to GSS or fCJD.

PrP^Sc Detection and Characterization in Gerstmann–Sträussler–Scheinker Disease

Several studies using antibodies to the mid-region of the prion protein have shown that the PrP^Sc isoforms in GSS variants are different from those seen in other human prion diseases. In sCJD, vCJD, iCJD and FFI, full-length and N-truncated proteinase K-resistant PrP^res fragments are present on western blot analysis, whereas in GSS full-length as well as N- and C-terminal truncated, non-glycosylated and proteinase K (PK)-resistant PrP^res species are present (Figure 18.40).[275,291–293] In GSS, these fragments can also be detected in non-enzymatically digested brain homogenates, although they are more prominent after proteinase K digestion, suggesting that they are generated *in vivo* by a GSS-specific proteolytic pathway.[291] The

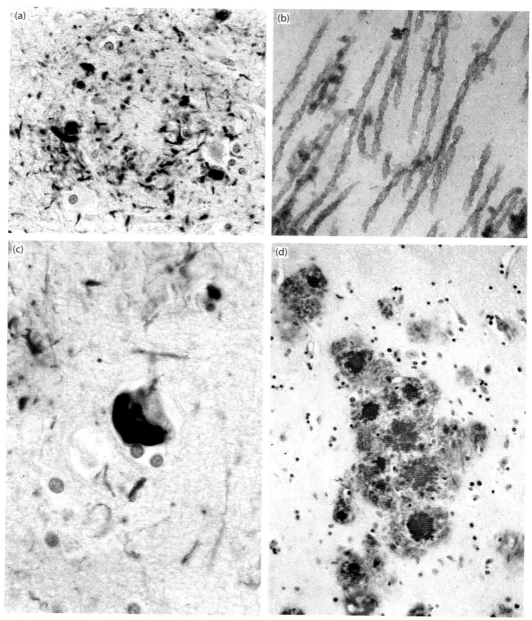

18.39 Pathology in the F198S mutation. (a) Extensive tau accumulation is seen in the form of neurofibrillary tangles and neurites in the cerebral cortex. AT8 anti-tau antibody. **(b)** Electron microscopy of the neurofibrillary tangles shows paired helical filaments with a structure and periodicity similar to those seen in Alzheimer's disease. Presymptomatic pathology in a patient who was assessed as neurologically normal a few months before death following a heart attack. **(c)** Tau accumulation and neurofibrillary tangles in the cerebral cortex. AT8 anti-tau antibody. **(d)** Multicentric PrP plaques in the cerebral cortex. 3F4 anti-PrP antibody.

quantity of fragments present does not correlate with the amyloid burden in the CNS. The molecular mass of the N- and C-truncated PrP^{Sc} fragments may vary according to the specific *PRNP* mutation present (Figure 18.40b).[292,293]

The lowest-molecular-weight N- and C-truncated fragments of PrP^{res} in proteinase K-treated brain extracts are 7 kDa (A117V-129V), 8 kDa (P102L-129M, G131V-129M, F198S-129V, D202N-129V, Q217R-129V) or 10 kDa (Q212P-129M) (Figure 18.40b). The 8-kDa peptides associated with P102L-129M and F198S-129V have the major N-terminus starting at residues 78 and 74, respectively.[275,292,293] The 7-kDa fragment associated with A117V-129V has the major

N-terminus cleavage site at residue 90.[293] These results, coupled with the concept that the pattern of digestion may depend on the tertiary structure of PrP^{Sc}, suggest that the type of conformational isomers present varies according to the *PRNP* mutation present. Another interesting finding is the presence of 21- to 30-kDa PrP^{res} fragments in individuals with P102L-129M and spongiform degeneration.[275,292] This PrP^{res} isoform was originally described in individuals with sCJD, which is characterized by the presence of spongiform degeneration, neuronal loss and gliosis.[308] Studies carried out on GSS A117V have shown the presence of PrP^{res} in some cases but not in others.[151,293] It is important to note that when

TABLE 18.8 Gerstmann–Sträussler–Scheinker disease (GSS)-like and PrP-cerebral amyloid angiopathy (PrP-CAA) phenotypes in patients with rare *PRNP* mutations (see Kong *et al.*[211] and Ghetti *et al.*[107] for reviews)

PRNP mutation	Phenotype
P84S	A patient diagnosed in life with voltage-gated potassium channels (VGKC)-complex-Ab associated encephalitis was found on post-mortem to have Gerstmann–Sträussler–Scheinker disease (GSS) associated with a novel mutation in *PRNP*.[196]
P105S-129V	Slowly progressive behavioural changes with aphasia and cognitive decline without ataxia in a 30-year-old female with an ill-defined family history of neurological disease. Progression with parkinsonism and terminal akinetic mutism. MRI showed high signal intensity in the caudate/putamen 7 years after onset. Electroencephalogram (EEG) did not show periodic triphasic complexes (PTCs). Multicentric prion protein (PrP) amyloid plaques were found in the hippocampus with punctate plaques in the cerebellum and spongiform change in the putamen. A novel PrP^res type was identified.[361]
G131V-129M	Changes in personality, slowly progressive cognitive decline, apraxia, tremor and increased tendon reflexes are the presenting signs. Onset of disease early in fifth decade of life. Magnetic resonance (MR) imaging may show cerebral and cerebellar atrophy. EEG does not show PTCs. In late stages, dementia becomes progressively more severe and ataxia develops. PrP-amyloid plaques and diffuse deposits seen in cortex, subcortical nuclei and cerebellum. Neurofibrillary tangles seen in Ammon's horn and entorhinal cortex, but no spongiform degeneration seen.[107,189]
S132I	In this family, neurological features range from early progressive intellectual impairment to progressive ataxia with terminal dementia for several years prior to death. Cerebellar signs and symptoms present for several years before death. Multicentric PrP plaques present in many brain regions, with little spongiform change.[161]
R136S	Early-onset dementia with psychiatric symptoms followed by ataxia, myoclonus and parkinsonism. Neuroimaging showed no specific abnormalities. EEG abnormal, but with no PTCs. Numerous large multicentric PrP plaques present in the cerebral cortex and cerebellum, with no spongiform change.[273]
Y145Stop	A patient had dementia with a long duration. The *PRNP* Y145Stop mutation was found. Neuropathologically, PrP-amyloid angiopathy is found to be associated with severe neurofibrillary tangle pathology.[106]
Q160Stop-129M	The haplotype was described in patients with dementia of long duration (6–12 years), resulting in reduced brain weight and diffuse cortical atrophy. Neuropathological examination revealed PrP-CAA and numerous tau-positive neurofibrillary tangles and PrP deposition.[191]
Y163Stop-129V	Autonomic failure, peripheral neuropathy and late-onset cognitive decline. Extensive parenchymal and vascular PrP deposition and numerous neurofibrillary tangles were found at post-mortem examination. Extensive and widespread PrP deposition was also found in peripheral tissues.[255]
V176G-129V	Rapidly progressive dementia, cerebellar ataxia and very short disease duration in this 61-year-old patient. Neuropathology showed neuronal loss, scant spongiform change and PrP positive multicentre plaques in the cerebral and cerebellar cortices in conjunction with neurofibrillary tangles and neuritic threads.[340]
H187R-129V	Clinical phenotype characterized by early progressive cognitive impairment, cerebellar ataxia and dysarthria, followed by myoclonus, seizures and occasionally pyramidal and extrapyramidal signs. Neuroimaging shows severe, widespread atrophy of cerebrum and cerebellum. Onset in fourth to six decades of life. Duration 7–18 years. PrP deposition seen in neocortex, hippocampus and cerebellum, with the latter two also having PrP-amyloid plaques. Cortical deposits have a round or elongated, 'curly' appearance. Neurofibrillary tangles also seen in hippocampus. Atrophy and astrogliosis of subcortical white matter present. No spongiform change present in grey matter.
D202N-129V	Cognitive impairment leading to dementia and cerebellar signs is the main clinical feature. Onset early in eighth decade. Duration of clinical illness is about 6 years. Abundant PrP-amyloid deposits present in cerebrum and cerebellum. Neurofibrillary tangles seen in cerebral cortex. No spongiform degeneration observed.
E211D-129V	A kindred with an ataxic phenotype was identified and a patient with typical pathological and molecular features of GSS was described. Comparison with a further two unrelated patients with a E211Q-129M haplotype and a Creutzfeldt–Jakob disease (CJD) clinicopathological phenotype has been used to advance the hypothesis that the alternative substitutions impact differently on PrP stability and control a switch between the CJD and GSS phenotypes.[288]
Q212P-129M	Gradual development of incoordination and slurring of speech are presenting signs, followed by dysarthria and ataxia. Onset late in sixth decade. Duration 8 years. Dementia not reported. PrP-amyloid deposition is mild throughout central nervous system, including cerebellum, which is significantly less affected than that of individuals with any other GSS-associated haplotype. Degeneration of myelinated fibres in anterior and lateral corticospinal tracts in spinal cord. No spongiform degeneration seen.
Y218N	Reported in three Spanish patients, one of which was confirmed neuropathologically. Histopathological studies showed PrP deposits with widespread hyperphosphorylated tau pathology.[4,107]

Continued

TABLE 18.8 Gerstmann–Sträussler–Scheinker disease (GSS)-like and PrP-cerebral amyloid angiopathy (PrP-CAA) pheno-types in patients with rare *PRNP* mutations (see Kong *et al.*[211] and Ghetti *et al.*[107] for reviews) *(Continued)*

PRNP mutation	Phenotype
Y226Stop-129M/V	A 55-year-old man with a 2.5 year duration characterized by cognitive impairment and aphasia with myoclo-nus at later stages. A diffuse amyloid angiopathy, without neurofibrillary tangles was reported at post-mortem examination.[107,188]
Q227Stop-129-129V	An atypical GSS-like phenotype starting with cognitive decline in a patient in the fourth decade of life and lasting 6 years with no evidence of ataxia or pyramidal signs. Numerous multicentric and unicentric plaques and neurofibrillary tangles were found at post-mortem examination.[107,188]
M232T-129M/V	Cerebellar signs and spastic paraparesis are the initial symptoms, followed by dementia. Onset in fifth de-cade. Duration 6 years. PrP-amyloid plaques and diffuse deposits seen in neocortex, subcortical nuclei and cerebellum. Unclear whether spongiform changes are present.

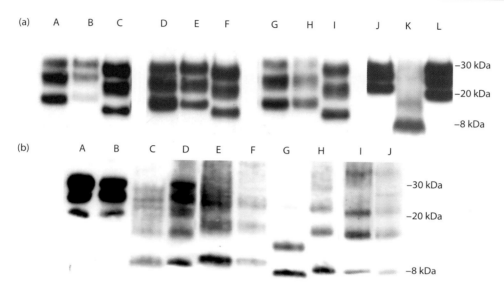

18.40 **(a)** Western blot analysis of PrP[res] in samples of cerebral cortex from cases of familial prion disease. The cases of familial Creutzfeldt–Jakob disease (fCJD) E200K-129MM (B), Gerstmann–Sträussler–Scheinker (GSS) disease P102L-129MM (E) and a two-repeat octapeptide repeat insertion 129MM (H) all show type 1 PrP[res], with typically different glycoform ratios. The case of GSS P102L-129MM shown in (K) lacks type 1 PrP[res], but when an abbreviated electrophoretic separation is performed, abundant low-molecular-weight protease-resistant PrP fragments are detectable. The cases are shown flanked by standard samples of sCJD MM1 subtype (A,D,G,J) and vCJD MM2B (C,F,I,L). Western blotting employed the monoclonal antibody 3F4. Approximate molecular mass is shown in kilodaltons. **(b)** Western blot analysis of PrP[res] in cases of Creutzfeldt–Jakob disease E200K, neocortex (A), GSS P102L, neocortex (B), GSS P102L, cerebellum (C), GSS P102L, neocortex (D), GSS Q212P, neocortex (E), GSS Q212P, cerebellum (F), GSS A117V, neocortex (G), GSS F198S, cerebellum (H), GSS Q217R, neocortex (I) and GSS D202N, neocortex (J). PrP[res] with an electrophoretic mobility of ~21–30 kDa was most abundant in association with spongiform change (A,B), whereas in cases where inconspicuous or no spongiform degeneration was present, distinct 21- to 30-kDa isoforms were not prominent and the PrP[res] pat-tern consisted primarily of distinct ~7- to 15-kDa peptides and variable amounts of poorly defined higher-molecular-weight isoforms (C–J). Western blotting employed the monoclonal antibody 3F4. Approximate molecular mass is shown in kilodaltons.

(b) Reproduced from Piccardo et al.[292] with permission from Lippincott Williams & Wilkins/Wolters Kluwer Health.

PrP[res] is present in GSS A117V, the amount is significantly lower than that found in other GSS variants. It has been pro-posed that a transmembrane PrP isoform plays a central role in the pathogenesis of GSS A117V.[151]

An additional complication in understanding the role of PrP in genetic human prion disease involves the potential role of the wild-type protein (in addition to the gene prod-uct of the mutant allele) in PrP[Sc] formation. For technical reason this aspect of PrP[Sc] formation is rarely performed, but adds a further dimension to understanding PrP[Sc] hetero-geneity in genetic forms and may be directly relevant to the clinico-pathological heterogeneity of GSS.[365]

Amyloid Characterization in Gerstmann–Sträussler–Scheinker Disease

The PrP[Sc]-amyloid filaments in GSS are composed of 7-kDa peptides that extend from about residue 85 to residue 153 in A117V-129V, residue 81 to residue 150 in F198S-129V and residue 81 to residue 146 in Q217R-129V.[283,285] Cases of the GSS F198S-129V haplotype were also found to have an 11-kDa PrP fibrillogenic peptide spanning residues 58–150.[347] Additional studies have shown that the N- and C-truncated peptides present in patients with mutations P102L, A117V, F198S and Q217R originate only from the mutant allele, suggesting that these mutations are a dominant factor for amyloidogenesis.[348,350] The allelic origin of PrP^{Sc} accumulating in the brain of patients with other inherited prion diseases has been investigated. These studies showed that only mutant PrP^{Sc} is detected in FFI and CJD D178N, whereas both wild-type and mutant PrP^{Sc} are present in CJD V210I.[338] Therefore, the recruitment of wild-type isoforms by mutant PrP^{Sc} may depend on mutation-specific PrP configurations that allow interaction between the mutant and normal PrP species.

Data obtained from the study of purified amyloid fractions indicate that in GSS A117V, GSS F198S and GSS Q217R, the minimal PrP^{Sc} segment essential for amyloidogenesis is an N- and a C-truncated fragment spanning residues 88–146.[347,350] The major part of this peptide corresponds to the flexible N-terminal domain of PrP^C, which is thought to undergo conformational changes in the transition of PrP^C into PrP^{Sc}.[314]

PrP-Cerebral Amyloid Angiopathy

PRNP Y145STOP-129M

Clinical Features

The age at onset is in the fourth decade and the duration of illness is 21 years. The clinical phenotype is characterized by memory disturbance, disorientation and a progressive dementia. Electroencephalographic investigations do not show PTC.

Neuropathology

Diffuse atrophy of the cerebrum, enlargement of the lateral ventricles, neuronal loss and gliosis are severe. PrP-amyloid deposits are present in the walls of small and medium-sized parenchymal and leptomeningeal blood vessels and in the perivascular neuropil. PrP-amyloid fibrils are seen adjacent to and within the vessel wall (Figure 18.41a–c). Neurofibrillary tangles, neuropil threads and dystrophic neurites are numerous in the cerebral grey matter.[106] These neurofibrillary lesions are immunoreactive to phosphorylation-dependent and phosphorylation-independent anti-tau antibodies (Figure 18.41d). No spongiform change is present in any area of the grey matter.

Additional Stop Mutations Associated with PrP-CAA

Recently, PrP-CAA associated with tau pathology has been described in patients with the following *PRNP* mutations: Q160X, Y163X and Y226X-129V/M.[107,191] The Y163X mutation is of particular interest following a recent report on a large British kindred with a novel phenotype including diarrhea, autonomic failure and neuropathy associated with widespread PrP deposition in peripheral tissues.[255]

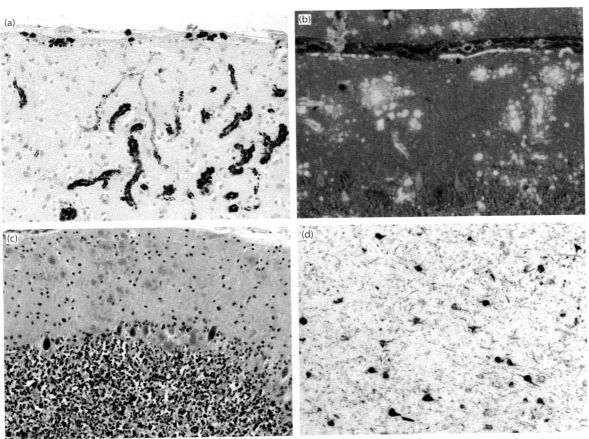

18.41 Pathology in the Y145STOP mutation. Extensive perivascular amyloid deposits are present in the cerebellar cortex, as demonstrated by **(a)** immunohistochemistry for PrP (3F4 anti-PrP antibody) and **(b)** a thioflavin S. **(c)** The amyloid accumulation on a haematoxylin and eosin stain appears faintly basophilic. **(d)** Immunohistochemistry for tau protein reveals multiple neurofibrillary tangles and neurites in the cerebral cortex. AT8 anti-tau antibody.

Amyloid Characterization in PrP-Cerebral Amyloid Angiopathy

It is of interest that in PrP-CAA, the C-terminus of the genetically truncated PrP is similar to the C-terminus of the amyloid peptides found in GSS.[106] Western blot analysis of proteins extracted from purified amyloid fractions shows that the smallest amyloid subunit migrates as a band of about 7.5-kDa. This band is strongly immunoreactive with antibodies to epitopes located within residues 90–147 of PrP and is unreactive with antisera to N- and C-termini.[106] In addition, the amyloid fractions contain higher-molecular-weight PrP peptides migrating as poorly resolved bands of 12–16 and 22–30 kDa. These bands are immunoreactive using the same antibodies that recognize the 7.5-kDa band, suggesting that they probably represent polymers of amyloid protein.[106]

Inherited Prion Disease with Variable Phenotype: the Insertional Mutations

Epidemiology and Genetics

Owen and colleagues were first to report the insertion of extra 24-bp repeats in the PRNP gene in a family with autosomal dominant atypical dementia, in which six 24-bp repeats were inserted.[272] Several additional families with one to nine 24-bp extra repeat insertions have subsequently been identified in the USA, several European countries and Japan. Altogether, at least 31 families are known to have a hereditary prion disease associated with extra 24-bp extra repeats in the PRNP gene. In 26 families, the repeat expansion is coupled with methionine at codon 129, whereas in five other families the inserts were found on the valine allele. In one Japanese case, a novel insertion of three 24-bp extra repeats in the PRNP gene was accompanied by methionine homozygosity at codon 129 and lysine homozygosity at codon 219 (see Table 18.9 for a summary, Kong et al.[211] for review and Croes et al.[78] for an analysis of the effect of the number of repeat insertions on age at onset).

Clinical Features

Clinical data are available on at least 27 families including over 100 affected subjects (see Kong et al.[211] for review). The disease phenotype is highly variable, with age of disease onset ranging between 21 and 82 years and disease duration ranging between 2 months and over 19 years. The clinical and pathological features include either a typical CJD phenotype or a phenotype more consistent with GSS. This phenotypic heterogeneity appears to be related at least in part to the PRNP genotype, because the clinical and neuropathological features become more consistent when cases are grouped according to the number of repeats. Thus, in patients with four or fewer inserted repeats, the mean age at onset is 62 years (range 52–82) and the mean duration is 6 months (range 2–14 months, excluding two cases with an exceptional 7-year duration). The majority of affected subjects have a clinical phenotype with rapidly progressive dementia, ataxia and visual disturbances, myoclonus and PTC on EEG investigation. The disease penetrance appears low in some of these families, in whom the inheritance pattern is unpredictable and recent evidence points towards a susceptibility factor lying upstream from of PRNP.[199] Genetic anticipation does not seem to occur in this group of inherited diseases.

In contrast, the mean age at disease onset in patients with five or more extra repeats is 32 years (range 21–61 years),

TABLE 18.9 Wild-type and disease-associated PRNP alleles with increased and decreased numbers of 24-bp repeats (see Kong et al.[211] for a review)

Repeats[a] (no.)/PRNP codon 129	Sequence of repeat area
Non-pathogenic alleles	
5/Met or Val	R12234
4/Met or Val	R1234
Pathogenic alleles: deletions	
3/Met	R124
3/Met	R134
Pathogenic alleles: insertions	
6/Met	R122234
6/Met[b]	R1223g34
7/Met	R12232a2a4
7/Val	R122a22a2a4
9/Met	R122222234
9/Val	R122322234
9/Met	R122322234
9/Met	R1223g23g234
9/Met	R122232234
10/Met	R122323g2234
10/Met	R1222a22a22234
10/Met	R1223222234
10/Met	R1223g3g3g2234
10/Met	R1223222a234
10/Val	R1223222a234
11/Met	R1222323g2234
11/Met	R122222223g34
11/Met	R1223g223g2234
11/Met	R122323g23g234
11/Met	R12222222234
11/Met	R1222c2222234
12/Met	R122c3232323g34
12/Met	R12232223g2234
12/Met	R122323222234

TABLE 18.9 Wild-type and disease-associated *PRNP* alleles with increased and decreased numbers of 24-bp repeats (see Kong *et al.*[211] for a review) *(Continued)*

Repeats[a] (no.)/*PRNP* codon 129	Sequence of repeat area
13/Val	R1223**22222222**a4
13/Val	R1223**g32222222**34
13/Met	R1223**2222a2222**34
14/Met	R1223**23g2a2223g2**34
14/Met	R1223**233g22a232**34
17/?	R1223**22323g23g223g2**34

[a]Each repeat (R) is a variant 24-bp sequence (R1 is 27bp). For codes, see Goldfarb *et al.* (1991).[113] The insertion is shown in bold.
[b]Two independent families with the same mutation.
Further examples of novel octapeptide repeat insertions continue to accumulate, including: 9/Val (R1223**2234**), 11/Val (R123**3g322**34), 12/Met (R122**2223g-23g2a**34, and 12/Val (R122**22223g2**34).[190,328,363,367]

and the mean disease duration is 6 years (range 3 months to 19 years). The vast majority of patients present with a slowly progressive syndrome characterized by mental deterioration, cerebellar and extrapyramidal signs, often lacking PTC on EEG examination.[114] As in other inherited prion diseases, the amino acid at codon 129 may influence the phenotypic effects of the repeat expansion mutations. In the large British family with six extra repeats, the age at death in patients who were homozygous for methionine at codon 129 was significantly lower than in heterozygous subjects, suggesting a protective role of valine at position 129.[201]

Neuropathology

The pathological phenotype is also different in affected subjects with low and high numbers of octapeptide repeats, although in a slightly different way (see Kong *et al.*[211] for review). All five cases with one, two or four insertions examined at autopsy have a histopathology indistinguishable from classic CJD. The neuropathological features in 20 cases with 5–7 insertions are heterogeneous. Thirteen cases exhibited CJD-like changes, with widespread spongiform degeneration, astrogliosis and variable degrees of neuronal loss; the other seven cases displayed changes that either are consistent with GSS or cannot be easily classified as GSS or CJD. Some rare cases lack the characteristic features of prion diseases, and in one case there were almost no histopathological abnormalities.[201] A histopathological phenotype fully consistent with GSS was observed in all seven cases with eight and nine extra repeats. In addition to various degrees of spongiosis, gliosis and neuronal loss, PrP uni- and multicentric amyloid plaques are present in the molecular layer of the cerebellum (Figure 18.42) and often in the cerebral grey matter. In conclusion, the CJD-like histopathological phenotype seems to be the rule in the presence of up to four extra insertions. In cases with five to seven extra insertions, the histopathology is heterogeneous and includes CJD, GSS-like and indefinable phenotypes. Eight and nine extra-insertions are associated with a GSS-like phenotype. Western blot analysis has found PrP[res] isotypes corresponding to type 1 or type 2 in patients with one and four to seven 24-bp insertional mutations.[211]

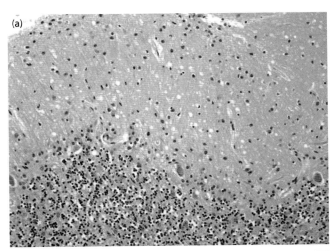

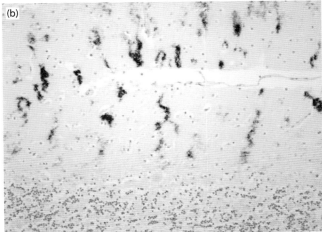

18.42 Pathology in the 144 base pair (bp) insertion mutation. (a) The cerebellum shows extensive micro-vacuolar spongiform change in the molecular layer, with a moderate loss of granular neurons and Purkinje cells. **(b)** Immunohistochemistry for prion protein (PrP) shows branching linear accumulations in the molecular layer that are not evident on routinely stained preparations. KG9 anti-PrP antibody.

Creutzfeldt–Jakob Disease Associated with Deletions in the *PRNP* Octapeptide Repeat Region: Deletions of Two 24-Base Pair Repeats

Until 2001, two types of mutations had been recognized in the *PRNP* gene: point mutations, which result from single amino acid substitutions in PrP (or production of a stop codon resulting in the expression of a truncated PrP isoform), and insertion of 24-bp repeats into the N-terminal region of PrP. Single 24-bp repeat deletions are common polymorphisms and do not appear to predispose individuals to prion disease. However, deletions of two 24-bp repeats have been described in an 86-year-old patient with a clinical diagnosis of possible CJD and in a 62-year-old man with a family history of dementia and histopathological confirmation of CJD, with widespread spongiform change. Western blot analysis showed a PrP[res] type 1 isoform in one of these cases.[14,55]

KURU

Definition and Epidemiology

Kuru is a human prion disease restricted to the Eastern Highlands of Papua New Guinea, mostly in the Fore linguistic group.[3] According to the oral history of the tribe, the epidemic began in the early 1900s. The condition was first investigated by Western medicine in the 1950s,[97] when kuru was the most common cause of death among affected tribes. The disease was spread among families by ritual cannibalism,[3] during which the bodies of deceased relatives were consumed. Infection is likely to have occurred through consumption of infected tissues or through contamination of superficial skin abrasions or lacerations. In the 1950s, most cases of kuru occurred in women and in children and adolescents of both sexes, with only 3 per cent of cases occurring in adult males.[3]

The familial aggregation of disease initially raised the possibility of a complex pattern of inheritance, but the increased risk in women and children is explained by the increased likelihood of exposure of these groups during cannibalistic rituals.[3] With the cessation of cannibalism in 1960, the route of exposure was eliminated and there was subsequently a decline in the number of new cases. The mean age at death in patients with kuru was 49 years in the 1950s, but there has been a gradual increase in this age with time. The last patient under 30 years of age died in 1987, and the last patient under 40 years of age died in 1991.[3] No children born after cannibalism ceased have developed kuru and there is no evidence of vertical transmission of infection. Kuru is now considered extinct; the mean incubation period has been estimated to be around 12 years.[167]

Clinical Features and Diagnostic Criteria

Kuru presented with a cerebellar syndrome, with little evidence of cognitive impairment, perhaps reflecting a peripheral route of infection. There was titubation and truncal instability, followed by progressive ataxia of gait and limbs, often associated with involuntary tremors of the limbs, but not myoclonus.[97] The course was relentlessly progressive, with dysarthria, dysphagia and increasing disability due to ataxia. Pyramidal and extrapyramidal motor dysfunction appeared later in the illness, but no sensory abnormalities were detected.[3] In the terminal stage of the illness, the patient became recumbent but remained conscious and made eye contact and attempted to respond to their environment. In children, there was often a strabismus in association with the cerebellar features. The average duration of the illness is around 12 months.[248] Diagnostic criteria for kuru have not been formulated, but good a working definition is 'a fatal disease with a progressive ataxic course lasting a period of some months diagnosed as kuru by the local people'.[3]

Clinical Investigations and Genetics

Retrospective investigations of the *PRNP* codon 129 polymorphism in kuru found that all codon 129 genotypes have been affected by this disease[61,133] and suggested that methionine homozygosity was a risk factor for the development

of disease, with homozygotes (particularly methionine homozygotes) having a shorter incubation period than heterozygotes.[224,249] Recent cases of kuru with prolonged incubation periods have all belonged to the heterozygous subgroup at codon 129 in the *PRNP* gene, providing additional information on the influence of this polymorphism on disease incubation periods.[253]

Neuropathology

Macroscopic examination of the brain in kuru usually reveals cerebellar atrophy, with no abnormalities detected in the cerebral cortex, basal ganglia or thalamus.[204] Microscopic examination reveals spongiform change present in a relatively uniform distribution in layers 3–5 in the cerebral cortex (Figure 18.43a), with relative sparing of the occipital lobe.[248] The hippocampus is generally spared, but severe spongiform change is present in the subiculum. Marked spongiform change is also present in the caudate nucleus and putamen, with patchy vacuolation occurring in the thalamus and hypothalamus. In the brain stem, spongiform change, neuronal loss and gliosis are present in the periaqueductal grey matter and in the colliculi, with less severe changes in the pontine nuclei, the tegmentum and the olivary nuclei. The spinal cord shows only minimal spongiform change in the substantia gelatinosa, with no obvious neuronal loss; myelin loss has been described in the spinocerebellar and pyramidal tracts.[204]

The molecular layer in the cerebellum shows prominent spongiform change, with degeneration and loss of Purkinje cells and granular neurons and accompanying gliosis (Figure 18.43b). The cerebellum in many cases also shows small rounded fibrillary amyloid plaques up to 30 µm in diameter in the granular layer and, less frequently, the molecular layer (Figure 18.43c).[249] These have become known as 'kuru-type plaques'. Similar plaques are identified in cases of sCJD of the MV2 subgroup[276] and have also been reported in some cases of iCJD occurring in recipients of growth hormone.

Immunohistochemistry for PrP shows intense staining of the amyloid plaques in kuru, with synaptic-like and perineuronal staining also present in the spinal cord, brain stem, basal ganglia and thalamus.[133,249] In the cerebellum, PrP-positive plaques occur most frequently in the granular layer (Figure 18.43d), with synaptic-like positivity also present and perineuronal positivity identified in the dentate nucleus. In the cerebral cortex, synaptic-like positivity is present in layers 3–5, with decoration of occasional apical ascending dendrites. A more widespread pattern of synaptic-like positivity is present in the basal ganglia and thalamus, but the hippocampus shows little positivity. Synaptic-like PrP positivity is also present in the brain stem and spinal cord, with linear PrP accumulation in some white matter tracts. Plaque-like PrP deposits (which do not correspond to fibrillary amyloid plaques in routinely stained sections) are present in the basal ganglia, thalamus, cerebellum and brain stem.[248]

PrPʳᵉˢ Detection in Kuru

PrPʳᵉˢ typing has been reported in only a very limited number of cases, presumably from late in the disease epidemic. The general finding was heterozygosity or homozygosity

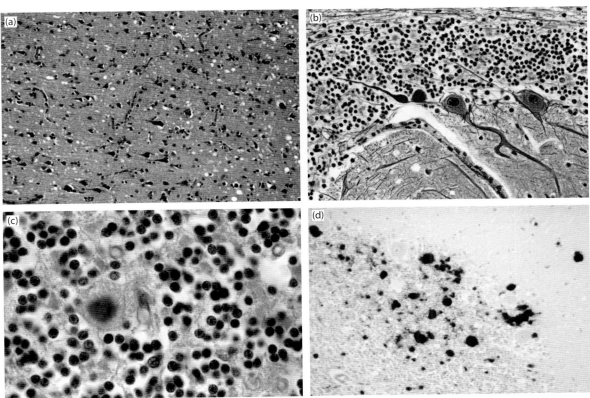

18.43 Pathology in kuru. (a) Micro-vacuolar spongiform change in the cerebral cortex. **(b)** Purkinje cell axonal swellings in the cerebellum. Bodian stain. **(c)** A rounded kuru plaque in the granular layer of the cerebellum. Periodic acid–Schiff stain. **(d)** Intense labelling of kuru plaques and multiple smaller plaque-like deposits in the cerebellar granular and molecular layers. KG9 anti-PrP antibody.

for valine at codon 129 of *PRNP* in conjunction with a type 2A PrP[res].[277,280,366] This is consistent with neuropathological features that are overall not greatly dissimilar from those occurring in the sCJD VV2 subtypes.[276] The tissue distribution in the single case of kuru examined resembles sCJD in that it is largely restricted to the CNS.[34] Transmission to non-human primates and to humanized transgenic mice show strong similarities between the agents involved in kuru and sCJD, suggesting that the kuru epidemic resulted from serial oral exposure to infectivity originating from a case of sCJD, perhaps of the V2 strain.[280,366]

IATROGENIC CREUTZFELDT–JAKOB DISEASE

Definition and Epidemiology

Iatrogenic Creutzfeldt–Jakob disease is caused by the transmission of infection from person to person in the course of medical or surgical treatment. A range of treatments has been implicated in this form of transmission of human prion disease, mainly on the basis of circumstantial evidence (Table 18.10).[43]

Masters and colleagues[241] noted the high frequency of previous neurosurgery in the cases described by Nevin and colleagues[195,264] and subsequent detailed investigation suggested transmission through contaminated neurosurgical instruments.[378] A similar case was subsequently identified in France,[90] but since then no further cases of neurosurgical

transmission have been reported. In 1974, a case of iCJD was reported in a recipient of a corneal graft; the donor was shown to have died from sCJD.[85] One additional probable case of CJD transmission by corneal graft has been reported, with an extended incubation period of 320 months.[150] Other reported cases of CJD in recipients of corneal graft do not have sufficient information to prove a causal link to CJD in the donor. Intracerebral depth electrodes have also transmitted CJD to two individuals in whom the instruments were subsequently used after the index case.[19] The number of cases of iCJD linked to corneal grafts, depth electrodes and neurosurgical instruments is limited, and, despite the resistance of prions to conventional decontamination, there have been no new cases linked to these types of transmission for many years. Although both infectivity and PrP[Sc] are distributed more widely outside the CNS in vCJD than in sCJD, no cases of iatrogenic vCJD transmission by any form of surgery have been identified. However, four instances of probable transmission of vCJD infectivity have been recorded in recipients of non-leukodepleted red blood cells from asymptomatic donors who subsequently died from vCJD. These cases are summarized in Table 18.10 and discussed in more detail later.

The occurrence of CJD in patients of an unusually young age who had been treated hormonally for short stature was the first indication of transmission *via* prior hGH therapy in 1985.[210,302] It is probable that pituitary glands for the production of hGH were obtained from individuals who had died from CJD, and implicated batches of hGH have been transmitted experimentally, confirming the presence of CJD

TABLE 18.10 Cases of iatrogenic Creutzfeldt–Jakob disease (iCJD) transmission worldwide

Mode of transmission	Number of cases	Incubation period (months)
Neurosurgery	4	12–28
Intracerebral electrodes	2	16–20
Corneal transplantation	2	16–320
Dura mater graft	228	15–360
hGH treatment	226	18–504
Human gonadotrophin treatment	4	144–192
Non-leukodepleted packed red blood cell transfusion (variant Creutzfeldt–Jakob disease (vCJD))	4 (only 3 cases manifested clinical features of vCJD)	80–94

Modified from Brown et al.[43]

infectivity.[109] Recombinant hGH was introduced in 1985 in most countries in order to avoid further transmission by this route, but cases are still occurring in the previously treated population with incubation periods exceeding 30 years, including one somewhat controversial case of iCJD reported in an individual who received a low dose of hGH as part of a diagnostic procedure 38 years previously.[77] The risk of developing iCJD varies between countries, with about 6 per cent of treated individuals developing iCJD in France, about 3.5 per cent in the United Kingdom and less than 1 per cent in the USA.[43] These differences may relate to differences in methods of hGH extraction from pituitary glands, the doses used and the duration of treatment in each country.[29,43,92,346] Iatrogenic Creutzfeldt–Jakob disease has also been reported in four recipients of human pituitary gonadotrophin, but no additional cases have been reported for several years.[208]

Transmission of CJD through human dura mater grafts is related mainly to the product Lyodura™. The presumption is that dura from one or more sCJD cases was included in the production process, with cross-contamination through pooling during manufacture.[43] The incubation period varies, with a mean of about 12 years, and the risk appears mainly to relate to grafts produced before 1987, when changes in the manufacturing may have reduced the risk significantly. The majority of cases have occurred in Japan, perhaps reflecting a high level of use of human dura mater grafts. A case of CJD in a porcine graft recipient in the United Kingdom has been reported, but it is uncertain as to whether this represents a chance coincidence or a causal relationship.[148]

Clinical Features and Diagnostic Criteria

The clinical features of iCJD are related to the mechanism of transmission. In cases related to central infection in the CNS, for example neurosurgical instruments, the clinical course is similar to that of sCJD.[40] Human pituitary hormones were given by injection, and with peripheral infection, the clinical illness is characterized by a progressive cerebellar syndrome; cognitive impairment occurs late in the illness, if at all.[239] The clinical features in cases linked to human dura mater grafts are variable, with the majority of cases presenting in a similar way to sCJD and some presenting with a more predominant cerebellar onset.[164] The mean survival in hGH-related CJD is around 1 year.[346]

BOX 18.9. Diagnostic criteria for iatrogenic Creutzfeldt–Jakob disease (iCJD)

1 Definite: Definite CJD with a recognized iatrogenic risk factor

2 Probable:
   A. Progressive predominant cerebellar syndrome in human pituitary hormone recipients
   B. Probable CJD with recognized iatrogenic risk factor

Relevant exposure risks for classification as iatrogenic CJD (relevance of any exposure to disease causation must take into account the timing of the exposure in relation to disease onset):
   – Treatment with human pituitary growth hormone, human pituitary gonadotrophin or human dura mater graft.
   – Corneal graft in which the corneal donor has been classified as having definite or probable human prion disease.
   – Exposure to neurosurgical instruments previously used in a case of definite or probable human prion disease.

This list is provisional, as previously unrecognized mechanisms of human prion disease may occur.

Diagnostic criteria for iCJD have been formulated (Box 18.9), but the most important consideration in making this diagnosis is the awareness of the relevance of specific aspects of past medical or surgical history. Iatrogenic cases of CJD are not associated with *PRNP* mutations, but there is an increased risk of developing this type of human prion disease in association with homozygosity at codon 129 of *PRNP*. Evidence from the French cohort of hGH recipients also suggests that the incubation period in homozygotes is shorter than in heterozygotes.[29]

Neuropathology

The neuropathological findings in iCJD are generally similar to those in sCJD (Figure 18.44a,b), but there are particular differences in dura mater graft and hGH recipients. In dura mater graft recipients, some cases show focally severe pathology in the region of the brain over which the dura mater graft was applied, including cases with selective cerebellar atrophy or parietal and occipital lobe atrophy.[148] A subset of iCJD cases occurring following dura mater graft procedures shows an unusual neuropathology, with florid plaques identified in the cerebral cortex and occasionally the basal ganglia.[335] The florid plaques in these cases are less numerous and not as widespread as the florid plaques in vCJD. One case of dura mater-associated iCJD in a 28-year-old patient also exhibited neuropathological features of Alzheimer's disease, with Aβ plaques, amyloid angiopathy and tau-positive neurofibrillary tangles in the limbic system and cerebral cortex, which were interpreted as possibly related to head trauma in childhood.[303] In hGH recipients with iCJD, the cerebellum is often severely involved, with cortical atrophy, extensive neuronal loss and gliosis in addition to spongiform change and, in some cases, the presence of kuru-type amyloid plaques (Figure 18.44c,d).[346] Spongiform change can also be seen in a widespread distribution and varying severity in the cerebrum (usually most severe in the basal ganglia), and immunohistochemistry for PrP stains the kuru-type plaques as well as smaller plaque-like structures and more diffuse synaptic-like and perineuronal deposits. In the UK series, the neuropathological findings are somewhat similar to those seen in the VV2 and MV2 subtypes of sCJD,[276] but with more severe cerebellar pathology.

PrP^res Detection

Compared with the molecular phenotype of sCJD and vCJD, little has been published concerning iCJD. However, what is known points to close similarities between iCJD and sCJD in a number of important respects: hGH-associated iCJD in the United Kingdom preferentially affects patients who are heterozygous or homozygous for valine at codon 129 of the *PRNP* gene.[29] Our own (Figure 18.45a) unpublished PrP^res typing by western blot of brain tissue from this same cohort shows that the majority of these cases are of the type 2A or have both type 1 and type 2 present (codon 129 VV and MV) and only a small minority have type 1 PrP^res (in codon 129 MV or MM). In contrast to growth hormone-associated iCJD, the very limited numbers of dura mater graft-associated and stereotactic intracerebral EEG needles cases of iCJD have been in patients homozygous for methionine at *PRNP* codon 129 and who have type 1 PrP^res (Figure 18.45b).[148,280,366] Transmission studies conducted in non-human primates using iCJD MM1 (resulting from contaminated stereotactic intracerebral EEG needles) indicate biological characteristics similarly to sCJD MM1 and fCJD E200K implying that the agent is of the M1 type.[24,52,280]

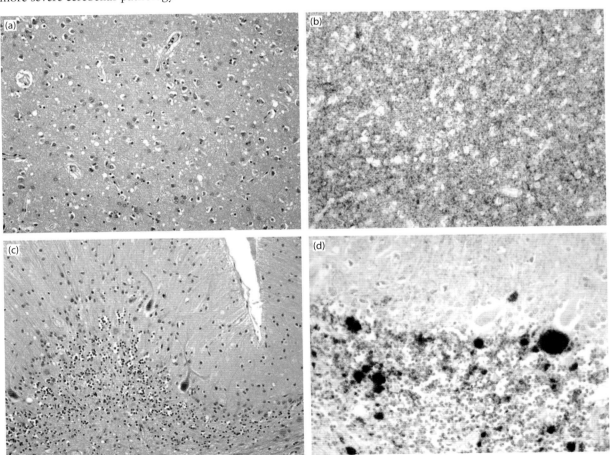

18.44 Pathology in iatrogenic Creutzfeldt–Jakob disease (iCJD). (a) A dura mater graft recipient shows widespread microvacuolar spongiform change in the cerebral cortex with extensive neuronal loss and gliosis. **(b)** A perineuronal and granular pattern of prion protein (PrP) accumulation is present in the cerebral cortex from this case. **(c)** The cerebellum in a case of iCJD following growth hormone therapy shows severe cerebellar pathology, with extensive loss of the granular layer, gliosis, molecular layer vacuolation, cortical atrophy and multiple kuru-like plaques. **(d)** Immunohistochemistry for PrP shows intense labelling of the kuru-type plaques and also demonstrates multiple smaller focal deposits in the granular layer of the cerebellum from this case. (KG9 anti-PrP antibody).

Even though the infection in hGH-associated iCJD is acquired peripherally, the distribution of PrPres in the body resembles that of sCJD. Readily detectable levels of PrPres are restricted to the brain, spinal cord and trigeminal ganglion, with levels below the limits of detection in the lymphoreticular system and most other peripheral tissues.[142,177] However, a study using a highly sensitive western blotting technique has reported the detection of PrPres in skeletal muscle in one of five

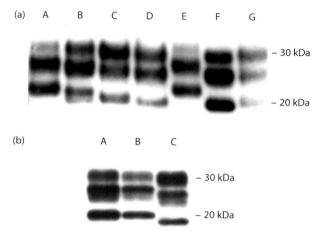

18.45 Western blot analysis of PrPres in samples of cerebral cortex from cases of iCJD associated with growth hormone therapy **(a)** and dura mater grafting **(b)**. The growth hormone-associated cases show type 1 and 2 PrPres together in association with codon 129 valine heterozygosity (B), and type 2 PrPres in association with valine homozygosity (D,F). The dura mater-associated iatrogenic Creutzfeldt–Jakob disease (iCJD) case is a codon 129 methionine homozygous individual showing type 1 PrPres (B). The cases are shown flanked by standard samples of sporadic Creutzfeldt–Jakob disease (sCJD) MM1 subtype (A,E) and vCJD MM2B (C,G). Western blotting employed the monoclonal antibody 3F4. Approximate molecular mass is shown in kilodaltons.

cases of iCJD occurring in recipients of hGH in the United Kingdom.[287] This was not detected in muscles that were likely to be the site of administration of hGH, raising the possibility of centrifugal spread of infectivity in such cases.

VARIANT CREUTZFELDT–JAKOB DISEASE

Definition and Epidemiology

Variant Creutzfeldt–Jakob disease (vCJD) was identified in 1996.[380] vCJD occurs predominantly in the United Kingdom, the country with the largest BSE epidemic in cattle. The neuropathological changes in vCJD resemble those of BSE infection in macaque monkeys, the biochemical properties of PrPres in vCJD are similar to those of PrPres in cattle and other animals infected with BSE, and laboratory transmission studies in wild-type and transgenic mice indicate that the infectious agent in vCJD is almost indistinguishable from the BSE agent.[48,67,222,333] The balance of evidence is consistent with the hypothesis that vCJD represents BSE infection in the human population. The presumed mechanism of human infection is through past exposure to high-titre infectivity in the food chain, a hypothesis supported, but not confirmed, by a case-control study that demonstrated an increased consumption of products containing mechanically recovered meat in cases of vCJD but that was subject to recall bias.[370]

To date (October 2014), 177 cases of vCJD have been identified in the United Kingdom, but the number of annual deaths has declined since 2000, and fears of a large epidemic have receded. Variant Creutzfeldt–Jakob disease has also been identified in a number of other countries (Table 18.11); cases are attributed by country according to the country of normal residence at the time of disease onset and this may not reflect the area in which exposure to BSE occurred. Such exposure may be related to residence in or travel to the United Kingdom, to exported bovines or bovine products from the

TABLE 18.11 Variant Creutzfeldt–Jakob disease (vCJD) cases worldwide (as of October 2014)

Country	Total number of primary cases (number alive)	Total number of secondary cases: blood transfusion (number alive)	Cumulative residence in United Kingdom (>6 months during 1980–1996)
United Kingdom	174 (0)	3 (0)	177
France	27 (0)	–	1
Republic of Ireland	4 (0)	–	2
Italy	2 (0)	–	0
United States	4 (0)	–	2
Canada	2 (0)	–	1
Saudi Arabia	1 (0)	–	0
Japan	1 (0)	–	0
Netherlands	3 (0)	–	0
Portugal	2 (0)	–	0
Spain	5 (0)	–	0
Taiwan	1 (0)	–	0

United Kingdom, or to exposure to indigenous BSE. In some cases of vCJD, there is a history of extended residence in the United Kingdom during the period in which there may have been significant human exposure to BSE (1980–96). This includes the first two patients with vCJD in the United States and the case in Canada, who are likely to have been infected with BSE while in the United Kingdom, although the clinical illness developed many years later while the patients were living in another country. In some cases, however, the source of BSE infection is uncertain, as there was no history of travel to the United Kingdom. This includes the cases in France, Italy, the Netherlands, Spain and Portugal.

Clinical Features and Diagnostic Criteria

Variant Creutzfeldt–Jakob disease is a disease that affects individuals in younger age groups, with a mean age at death of 29 years (range 14–74 years) (Figure 18.23).[383] There is an overlap with the age-specific distribution of sCJD, and young age alone cannot be regarded as indicative of the diagnosis of vCJD.[26] The reason for the young age of patients with vCJD is not known, but it may be due to an increased age-related exposure to BSE and/or age-related susceptibility.[72,362] The disease survival is also distinct from sCJD, with a mean duration of illness of 14 months in vCJD compared with only 4 months in sCJD.

The initial symptoms in vCJD are psychiatric in the great majority of cases, and almost all patients develop psychiatric symptoms as the illness evolves (Table 18.12).[382] Common early complaints include depression, anxiety and withdrawal. Distinction from common psychiatric disorders may

be impossible until frank neurological deficits develop, on average 6 months from disease onset. A minority of patients develop persistent painful sensory symptoms affecting the limbs, face or trunk, and the combination of these symptoms with a psychiatric disorder may be a clue to early diagnosis.[234] All patients develop ataxia, usually affecting gait, which progresses together with increasing evidence of cognitive impairment. All tested patients with vCJD have evidence of neuropsychological deficits, but there may be relative preservation of autobiographical memory.[197] Involuntary movements of the limbs are almost universal, but, in contrast to sCJD, chorea and dystonia occur with a similar frequency to myoclonus. As the disease progresses, there is an accumulation of multifocal neurological impairments, culminating in severe disability and often akinetic mutism. Death is usually due to intercurrent illness such as lung infection.

Diagnostic criteria for vCJD have been formulated (Box 18.10) and validated.[149,382] These criteria include a number of preconditions, a series of clinical features, and the results of diagnostic tests and neuropathological findings. A diagnosis of definite vCJD requires neuropathological validation, and a classification of probable vCJD (where no neuropathological investigations have been performed) is based on a combination of clinical features and either a positive MR imaging brain scan or tonsil biopsy (Box 18.10). Classification as probable vCJD has a high sensitivity and specificity for the diagnosis of vCJD, but the classification of possible vCJD is less precise and, as with sCJD, formal reporting of cases includes definite and probable cases, but not possible cases. The listed criteria have been amended in the light of the report of two cases of vCJD with an EEG recording typical of sCJD in the late stages of the illness.[21,389]

Clinical Investigations and Genetics

The most helpful non-invasive investigation in vCJD is the MR imaging brain scan, which shows high signal in the posterior thalamus on T2 or FLAIR sequences in over 90 per cent of cases (see Figure 18.15a).[66] In some cases with a negative MR imaging brain scan, the images were of poor quality and it may be worthwhile obtaining serial scans if an initial scan is negative. In the clinical context, MR imaging findings are highly, but not absolutely, specific for vCJD, as there is a case report of sCJD with the 'typical' scan appearances.[289] High signal on MR imaging may also be seen in the periaqueductal grey matter and in the caudate and putamen, but for a scan to be judged diagnostic of vCJD the signal intensity should be greatest in the pulvinar region.

Other investigations are less helpful in the diagnosis of vCJD. The EEG may show non-specific slow-wave activity, but many recordings have been normal, including those obtained in individuals with clear evidence of cognitive and neurological impairment. The characteristic changes of sCJD have not been identified in the early stages of the illness, but there is now evidence that such appearances may be identified preterminally. The CSF 14-3-3 immunoassay is positive in only about half the cases of vCJD (in contrast to sCJD) (see Figure 18.14),[122] and there may be an elevated CSF protein in a similar proportion of cases. Levels of tau are increased in the CSF in vCJD, and this finding may be of potential diagnostic value.[120] Tonsil biopsy is discussed later.

TABLE 18.12 Clinical characteristics of variant Creutzfeldt–Jakob disease (vCJD): signs and symptoms at disease onset and during clinical course (percentages)

At onset	%	During clinical course	%
Low mood	60	Dementia	100
Social withdrawal	30	Ataxia	100
Depression	30	Psychiatric symptoms	95
Anxiety	30	Involuntary movements	95
Painful sensory symptoms	30	Myoclonus	70
		Chorea	45
Other sensory symptoms	20	Dystonia	40
		Dysarthria/dysphasia	90
Aggression	15	Sensory symptoms	80
Forgetful	15	Pyramidal	70
Gait abnormality	10	Visual	30
Speech abnormality	5	Headache	20
Visual	5	Seizures	8
Headache	5		

BOX 18.10. Diagnostic criteria for variant Creutzfeldt–Jakob disease (vCJD)

1 Definite: neuropsychiatric 1A and neuropathological confirmation of vCJD[a]	I	A Progressive disorder
		B Duration of illness >6 months
		C Routine investigations do not suggest alternative diagnosis
		D No history of potential iatrogenic exposure
		E No evidence of familial form of transmissible spongiform encephalopathy (TSE)
2 Probable: I and 4/5 of II and IIIA and IIIB I and IVAd	II	A Early psychiatric symptoms[b]
		B Persistent painful sensory symptoms[c]
		C Ataxia
		D Myoclonus or chorea or dystonia
		E Dementia
3 Possible: I and 4/5 of II and IIIA	III	A Electroencephalogram (EEG) does not show typical appearance of sporadic Creutzfeldt–Jakob disease (sCJD)[e] in early stages of illness
		B Bilateral pulvinar high signal on magnetic resonance (MR) imaging
	IV	A positive tonsil biopsy[d]

[a]Spongiform change and extensive PrP deposition with florid plaques throughout the cerebrum and cerebellum.
[b]Depression, anxiety, apathy, withdrawal, delusions.
[c]This includes both frank pain and dysaesthesia.
[d]Tonsil biopsy is not recommended routinely or in cases with EEG appearances typical of sCJD, but it may be useful in suspect cases in which the clinical features are compatible with vCJD and MR imaging does not show bilateral pulvinar high signal.
[e]The typical appearance of the EEG in sCJD consists of generalized triphasic periodic complexes at approximately one per second. Occasionally these are seen in the late stages of vCJD.

Mutations of *PRNP* have not been identified in vCJD, but methionine homozygosity at codon 129 is clearly a risk factor for development of disease, as all tested definite and probable cases to date have this genotype.[397] A possible heterozygous case has been reported but the diagnosis in this case was not confirmed.[198] Whether human BSE infection may yet occur, with longer incubation periods, in the other codon 129 genotypes is unknown. However, one asymptomatic case of apparent transfusion-associated vCJD infection occurred in an individual who was a *PRNP* codon 129 heterozygote,[286] and analysis of DNA extracted from two of the appendix cases that were positive on immunohistochemistry for PrP in a retrospective prevalence study of vCJD infection in the United Kingdom were found to be valine homozygotes.[171] Genome-wide association studies have confirmed that the codon 129 polymorphism in the *PRNP* gene is the main genetic risk factor for vCJD. However, several other loci have been identified, e.g. the *MTMR7* gene, which may be of some significance; further studies are required to assess the full significance of these findings and their relevance to biological pathways involved in vCJD.[252,327]

Neuropathology

The neuropathological features of vCJD allowed it to be identified as a distinct disease,[380] and these findings have remained relatively uniform since then (Box 18.11). The brain in vCJD in most cases is macroscopically normal (Figure 18.46), but in cases with a prolonged disease duration (over 2 years) there is evidence of both cerebellar and cerebral cortical atrophy. No other focal macroscopic lesions are identified.[173,174] Histologically, vCJD shows all the hallmarks of a prion disease, but florid plaques dominate the neuropathological features: large fibrillary amyloid plaques surrounded by a corona or halo of spongiform change (Figure 18.47a,b). These occur in a widespread distribution throughout the cerebral cortex but are most numerous in the occipital cortex and are also identified in the cerebellar cortex (Figure 18.47c,d). Smaller fibrillary plaques without the surrounding spongiform change can be found in other grey matter regions in the brain, including the basal ganglia and thalamus. Florid plaques are particularly characteristic of vCJD but are not entirely specific, as similar lesions have been identified in some cases of iCJD associated with dura mater grafts.[335] However, their large numbers and widespread distribution in vCJD are helpful in establishing a diagnosis. Electron microscopy of florid plaques shows a dense fibrillary core, with amyloid fibrils spaced more loosely at the periphery, and some surrounding dystrophic neurites (Figure 18.48).

Other neuropathological features of vCJD include spongiform change, which is most severe in the basal ganglia (Figure 18.49a,b), particularly the putamen and caudate nucleus, and severe neuronal loss in the posterior thalamic nuclei, particularly the pulvinar (Figure 18.49c).[173] This is accompanied by severe astrocytosis (Figure 18.49d), the neuroanatomical distribution of which appears to correlate with the areas of hyperintensity seen on MR imaging scans (particularly in T2-weighted or FLAIR sequences) within the pulvinar in patients during the clinical stage of the illness.[66]

Immunohistochemistry for PrP shows widespread positivity in vCJD, with a unique pattern of accumulation. In addition to the intense positivity within the florid plaques, there are large numbers of smaller plaque-like lesions frequently occurring in clusters, which are not evident on routine stains (see Figure 18.47b,d). This is accompanied by a widespread pericellular accumulation of PrP in an amorphous or feathery distribution, which appears to be around small neurons and astrocytes.

BOX 18.11. Neuropathological diagnostic criteria for variant CJD

1. Cerebral and cerebellar cortex	Multiple florid plaques in routine stained sections Numerous small cluster plaques in PrP stained sections Amorphous and pericapillary PrP accumulation
2. Caudate nucleus and putamen	Severe spongiform change Perineuronal and periaxonal PrP accumulation
3. Posterior thalamic nuclei	Marked neuronal loss and gliosis Patchy spongiform change
4. Brain stem and spinal cord	Perineuronal and reticular PrP accumulation
5. Biochemistry	Type 2B PrPres on western blot analysis

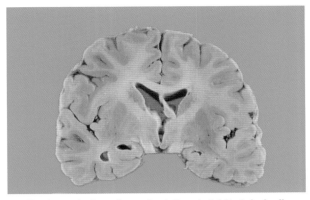

18.46 Brain pathology in variant Creutzfeldt–Jakob disease (vCJD). Macroscopic examination of the brain with vCJD often shows no macroscopic abnormalities, although focal cortical atrophy is evident in patients with a prolonged survival.

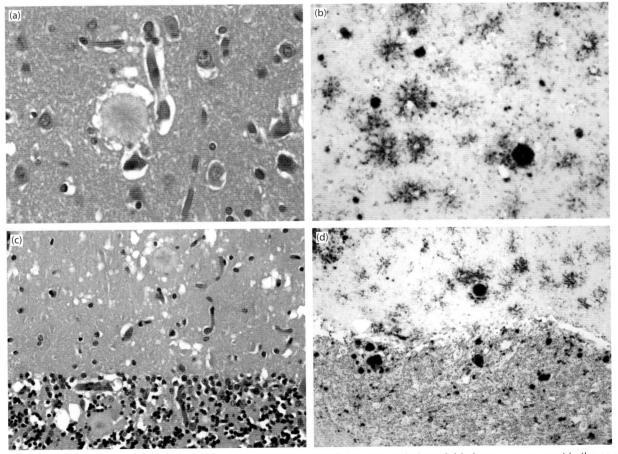

18.47 Plaque pathology in variant Creutzfeldt–Jakob disease (vCJD). Large rounded amyloid plaques are present in the cerebral cortex in the form of florid plaques **(a)**, and in the cerebellum as florid plaques in the molecular layer, but vacuolation occurs around the granular layer plaques **(c)**. Immunohistochemistry for prion protein (PrP) shows intense labelling of these large plaques and also demonstrates multiple smaller cluster plaques in addition to amorphous and pericellular PrP deposits in the cerebral cortex **(b)** and in the cerebellar cortex **(d)**. KG9 anti-PrP antibody.

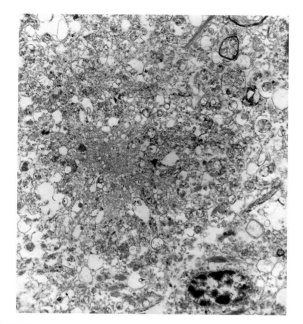

18.48 Electron microscopy of a variant Creutzfeldt–Jakob disease (vCJD) plaque. The plaque has a complex structure with a dense fibrillary centre that is non-homogeneous. This is surrounded by an irregular region of spongiform change, and dystrophic neurites are identified at the plaque periphery.

Occasional perivascular accumulation of PrP is also noted in the cerebral and cerebellar cortex, which may represent accumulation in astrocytic foot processes, but there is no evidence of an amyloid angiopathy. In other brain regions, there is plaque-like positivity and a predominant synaptic-like pattern of PrP accumulation. However, in the basal ganglia, there is an intense perineuronal and periaxonal pattern of positivity, often in a characteristic linear distribution (see Figure 18.49b).[174] Brain biopsy was performed as an investigative procedure in some of the early cases of vCJD, but it is no longer a routine diagnostic tool. The neuropathological features in the brain biopsy are similar to those in the cerebral cortex in autopsy cases, but the extent and severity of the lesions are less pronounced. The characteristic neuropathology of vCJD is clearly recognizable in cases of secondary vCJD attributed to acquisition by blood transfusion.[146,388]

Peripheral Pathology

Variant Creutzfeldt–Jakob disease is also unique among other prion diseases in that PrP^{Sc} accumulation and infectivity can be readily detected outside the CNS.[49] Immunohistochemistry for PrP has shown positivity in a variety of peripheral neural tissues, including sensory and

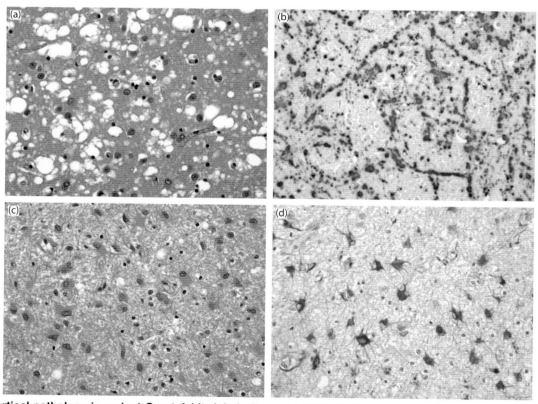

18.49 Subcortical pathology in variant Creutzfeldt–Jakob disease (vCJD). **(a)** The caudate nucleus shows intense spongiform change, but usually there is little evidence of amyloid plaque formation. **(b)** Prion protein (PrP) accumulation in the caudate nucleus and other regions of the basal ganglia shows a distinctive pattern, with multiple small punctate deposits around neurons and also apparently around axons in a linear pattern (KG9 anti-PrP antibody). **(c)** The pulvinar in vCJD shows extensive neuronal loss and gliosis, with patchy spongiform change and little evidence of amyloid plaque formation. **(d)** The intense gliosis is best demonstrated on immunohistochemistry for glial fibrillary acidic protein.

Image courtesy of Professor Pawel Liberski, Medical University of Lodz, Lodz, Poland.

autonomic ganglia (Figure 18.50a).[142] In lymphoid tissues, there is intense positivity for PrP within germinal centres that co-localizes to follicular dendritic cells (Figure 18.50b).[142,157] The accumulation of PrP positivity in lymphoid follicles before the onset of clinical disease has also allowed the use of tonsil biopsy as an aid to pre-mortem diagnosis of vCJD, although some cases may exhibit only very limited lymphoreticular deposition.[256] Studies using highly sensitive detection methods have identified PrP in skeletal muscle in a subset of vCJD patients. Paraffin-embedded tissue blot analysis of the tissues suggested that the PrP was present in peripheral motor nerve fibres, rather than in the skeletal muscle fibres or muscle spindles (Figure 18.50c).[287]

Retrospective review of tissues removed before the onset of clinical disease in vCJD found that PrP positivity could be detected in lymphoid follicles before the onset of clinical disease.[159] This has been exploited in retrospective prevalence studies of anonymized tonsil and appendix tissues, in which the number of positive cases appears to indicate that the number of clinical cases of vCJD to date may not reflect accurately the true number of infections of BSE in the UK population.[160] Two of the three positive appendix cases from an initial study of 12 674 cases had sufficient tissue available for DNA extraction and *PRNP* codon 129 analysis.

Both were shown to be valine homozygotes at codon 129, raising the possibility of prolonged asymptomatic infection in this genetic subgroup.[171] A further study of PrP immunoreactivity in appendix tissues in the United Kingdom has found 16 additional positives out of 32 441 specimens studied, giving an estimated prevalence of around 1 in 2000 of the UK population.[110]

The widespread tissue distribution of PrP and infectivity in vCJD has given rise to concerns that the disease might be transmitted accidentally by medical or surgical procedures.[49,142] There have been four incidences of apparent transmission of vCJD infectivity by blood transfusion, three of which were accompanied by the typical clinical manifestations of vCJD. In the first of these, the recipient developed the clinical features of vCJD 6.5 years after transfusion; in the second and third cases, the patients developed vCJD around 8 years after transfusion.[155,388] The remaining recipient died about 5 years after transfusion, but without clinical features of this illness. However, PrP accumulation was detected biochemically and by immunohistochemistry in lymphoid tissues (spleen and lymph node, but not in tonsil or gut-associated lymphoid tissues), but not in the CNS, indicating an asymptomatic or preclinical infection (Figure 18.50d).[286] Analysis of *PRNP* showed that this patient was a heterozygote, indicating that this genotype

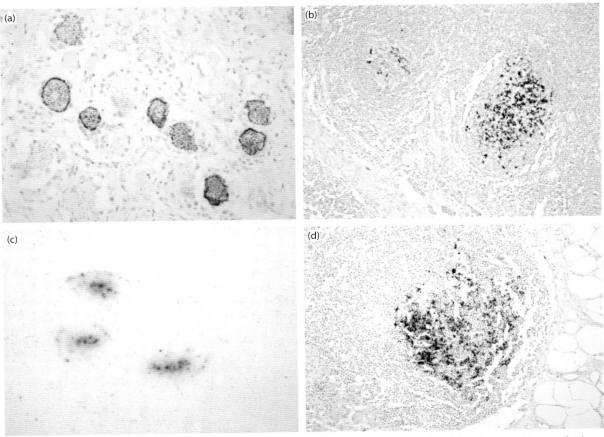

18.50 Peripheral pathology in variant Creutzfeldt–Jakob disease (vCJD). Immunohistochemistry shows evidence of prion protein (PrP) accumulation in **(a)** dorsal root ganglia and **(b)** germinal centres within the tonsil (KG9 anti-PrP antibody). **(c)** Paraffin-embedded tissue (PET) blot preparations for protease-resistant PrP (black) show accumulation in germinal centres within the spleen (6H4 anti-PrP antibody). **(d)** Immunoreactivity for PrP in a cervical lymph node in an asymptomatic patient who had received a blood transfusion from a donor who subsequently died from vCJD, showing evidence of asymptomatic infection at the time of death (12F10 anti-PrP antibody).

is susceptible to vCJD infection. The absence of PrP detection in oral and gut-associated lymphoid tissues suggests that the route of exposure to infectivity (intravenous rather than oral) may have an influence on peripheral disease pathogenesis, but it is possible that the *PRNP* gene codon 129 genotype may also have had an effect. More recently, evidence of vCJD infection was found on high-sensitivity western blot analysis in one region of the spleen of an elderly UK patient with haemophilia, who had received very large quantities of UK-sourced plasma products during his life. This patient was also a *PRNP* codon 129 heterozygote (MV). Although he was a UK resident and had also undergone surgery, endoscopy and received blood transfusions (from donors who did not die with vCJD), a risk assessment indicated that the plasma products were the most likely source of this infection.[285]

PrP^res Detection and Typing

Collinge and co-workers first identified a characteristic PrP^res type common to ten cases of vCJD.[67] The predominance of the diglycosylated band was shown to be characteristic of BSE, and of BSE and vCJD transmitted to other species,[67] leading to the proposition that it represented a BSE/vCJD agent 'glycoform signature'. Classification of the vCJD PrP^res type according to the Parchi and Gambetti system shows mobility identical to type 2 and the predominance of the diglycosylated band resulting in the designation of type 2B. The exact N-termini of type 2B PrP^res from vCJD brain have been mapped by Edman degradation, are found to centre on serine 97 and are not qualitatively different in this respect from other type 2A cases of sCJD, iCJD, kuru and FFI determined by this method.[277]

Type 2B PrP^Sc is a remarkably consistent feature of vCJD, present in all cases of vCJD so far tested, irrespective of national origin, and of the brain region (or lymphoreticular) tissue sampled.[30,143,269] Although type 2B PrP^Sc generally sufficient to distinguish vCJD from sCJD (Figure 18.51a), it is not absolutely specific for vCJD. A protein isotype resembling type 2B can be found in certain forms of genetic human prion disease and in rare atypical cases of sCJD.[135,139] The precise migration and glycoform ratio of type 2B PrP^Sc is subject to tissue specific influence.[140,142,144,157] Type 1-specific antibodies detect a minor type 1B component in vCJD tissue samples.[30,299,393]

Lymphoreticular involvement in general is a consistent feature of vCJD, and one that distinguishes it from other human prion diseases. PrP^Sc is detectable in lymphoid tissues by immunohistochemistry and/or western blotting in tissues obtained at autopsy,[315] in tonsil biopsies taken during the clinical phase of the illness,[157] and even in routine appendicectomy specimens removed before disease onset.[159] PrP^res is readily and consistently detectable in vCJD tonsil, spleen, lymph node, appendix and gut-associated lymphoid tissue (Figure 18.51b).[142,364] Under these same conditions, PrP^res appears undetectable in the lymphoreticular system in other forms of human prion disease, notably sCJD.[142,157]

The use of higher-sensitivity methods shows that this difference between vCJD and sCJD may be quantitative rather than absolute, with the detection of low levels of PrP^res in spleen samples from a subset of Swiss sCJD cases.[111] PrP^res can be found at particularly high levels in the vCJD retina, optic nerve and trigeminal ganglion, but these are features

that vCJD shares with sCJD.[140,142,144] Surprisingly, given the positivity of the trigeminal ganglion, dental tissue specimens appear negative,[141] as do non-nervous tissues in the eye.[140,144,364] Although peripheral nerves have been reported to be negative for PrP^res,[142,364] both the celiac and the stellate ganglia have been shown to be positive in vCJD but negative in sCJD.[129] It seems likely that with the development of ever more sensitive detection methods, further tissues will be found to be positive for PrP^Sc, and this is exemplified by the recent detection of PrP^res in vCJD skeletal muscle tissue.[287] and in the dura mater, liver, pancreas, kidney, ovary, uterus and skin of one thoroughly investigated case.[269] Whether or not all peripheral PrP^res positivity is associated with demonstrable levels of infectivity will require experimental verification, but it seems possible that it will prove to be so, given the report of transmission from vCJD spleen and tonsil.[49]

Close similarity in the transmission properties of BSE and vCJD to mice (and non-human primates) were early indications that the same agent was responsible for both diseases and that the agent was distinct from that involved in scrapie and sCJD.[48,222] The biological properties of the vCJD agent in humans appear consistent between different primary cases (irrespective of national origin), different brain regions and peripheral tissues and between primary

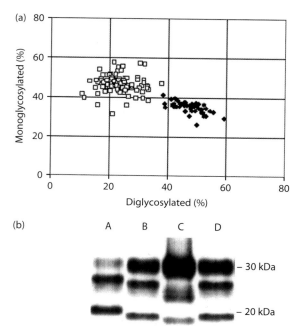

18.51 (a) Scattergram representation of the mean percentage diglycosylated (x-axis) and monoglycosylated (y-axis) PrP^res, as determined by western blot analysis of brain tissue from 108 cases of sporadic Creutzfeldt–Jakob disease (sCJD) (white squares) of all *PRNP* codon 129 genotypes and 46 cases of variant Creutzfeldt–Jakob disease (vCJD) (black circles), all of which were MM at *Prnp* codon 129. Western blotting employed the monoclonal antibody 3F4. **(b)** Western blot analysis of PrP^res in a concentrated tonsil biopsy extract from a case of vCJD (C), standard type 1 PrP^res from autopsy sCJD brain (A) and standard type 2B PrP^res from autopsy vCJD brain (B,D) are shown for comparison. Western blotting employed the monoclonal antibody 3F4. Approximate molecular mass is shown in kilodaltons.

(BSE acquired) and secondary (blood-transfusion-acquired) cases of vCJD.[23,82,316]

FUTURE DEVELOPMENTS

The substantial advances in our understanding of prion diseases have been accompanied by the emergence of this group of hitherto obscure disorders into the wider fields of science, public health, politics and international economics. Despite this, much remains to be answered in terms of the molecular basis, genetic control and pathogenesis of these diseases, including a complete understanding of the nature of the infectious agent and its means of replication and transmission. The decline of BSE and vCJD has, in some minds, indicated that the wider problems for animal and human health associated with prion diseases are no longer as important as in the past 10 years. However, closer study of both of these fields reveals major problems that remain unanswered and, in some cases, poorly controlled.

Prion Diseases in Animals

The spread of CWD in cervids in North America and the emergence of novel prion diseases in sheep and cattle elsewhere continues to present challenges for diagnosis, epidemiology and for the introduction of appropriate control measures. Atypical scrapie has a relatively uniform disease phenotype, but biologically it is very different from classical scrapie. It is not clear whether the novel ruminant prion diseases are variants of the classical form of disease or are different, perhaps sporadic animal prion diseases. Atypical scrapie and the novel prion diseases of cattle are probably not new diseases, but ones that had been overlooked in the past and have only come to light because of the increased awareness and by statutory slaughterhouses testing for PrP[res.] The risks to humans posed by these novel prion diseases are only now beginning to be quantified,[10,386] but the interpretation of such studies is complex: for example, humanized transgenic mice are resistant to infection with BSE,[22] which is a known human pathogen; however, these mice become susceptible to infection with the BSE agent after it has been passaged in sheep.[297] All of these considerations emphasize the need for continued surveillance to identify, monitor and characterize emerging prion agents in ruminants and the assessment of the potential risk posed to other species.

Prion Diseases in Humans

The Uncertain Future of Variant Creutzfeldt–Jakob Disease

Although it is clear that very large numbers of BSE-infected cattle were likely to have entered the human food chain between 1980 and 1996, it is not certain how many humans were infected with BSE over this period. The retrospective prevalence studies of vCJD infection using immunohistochemistry to detect PrP accumulation in lymphoid follicles in appendix tissues have found more positive cases than would have been predicted from the numbers of clinical cases of vCJD so far.[110,160] The finding that positive cases have occurred in individuals who are valine homozygotes at codon 129 in the *PRNP* gene raises the possibility that other *PRNP* codon 129 genotypes are susceptible to vCJD infection, but with longer incubation periods than methionine homozygotes. This possibility is also suggested by the identification of asymptomatic vCJD infections by blood transfusion and factor VIII in a *PRNP* codon 129 heterozygotes.[285,286]

The probability that vCJD infectivity has been transmitted by red blood cell transfusion on four occasions so far[155,231,286,388] has led to further concerns that additional cases of vCJD may occur following secondary transmission through blood and blood products and via contaminated surgical instruments. A study in transgenic mice indicated that such transmissions were influenced substantially by the *PRNP* codon 129 genotype in relation to the incubation period.[22] Continuing surveillance of vCJD is required in order to address these possibilities and to monitor the future occurrence of BSE-related infections (perhaps with a different clinicopathological phenotype to vCJD) in individuals who are valine homozygotes or heterozygotes at *PRNP* codon 129.

Prospects for Treatment of Human Prion Diseases

There is no proven therapy for human prion diseases that influences the underlying disease process, but treatment is available for some of the symptoms of disease. An extensive range of potential treatments for the disease itself have been tried over the years, but drugs such as steroids, antiviral therapy and immune-modulating treatment have proven ineffective. Following the publication of a study indicating the potential efficacy of quinacrine in a cell culture system,[245] it was used on an *ad hoc* basis in cases of human prion disease; however, studies in France and a clinical trial in the United Kingdom failed to demonstrate a significant benefit of quinacrine.[69,130] Similarly, pentosan polysulphate (PPS) influences incubation period and sometimes survival in animal models of prion disease with efficacy related to the timing of treatment relative to exposure.[88] PPS does not cross the blood–brain barrier and following the publication of an article demonstrating efficacy in experimental animals treated by intraventricular infusion,[84] PPS has been given by this route to a small number of patients with human prion disease, including vCJD. Although there is only limited information on outcomes and no formal clinical trials of the efficacy of PPS have been undertaken, there is evidence to suggest that treatment with PPS may have some effect in increasing survival time.[265,357,359,375]

Diagnostic Developments

Given the increasing costs and ethical concerns associated with the use of animals in biomedical research, it seems inevitable that there will be a continuing move away from animal transmission studies and a move towards the development of informative *in vitro* model systems in which to investigate prion disease. Both cellular and cell-free systems are likely to play an increasing role in laboratory research in prion diseases. The development of diagnostic tests and screening assays applicable to readily available biological fluids such as blood is currently the subject of intense investigation, in large measure driven by the perceived needs of the transfusion services in the United Kingdom and elsewhere. Several assays have been shown to be able to detect brain PrP^{Sc} at extremely high dilution factors or to correctly identify clinical, or in some instances preclinical, cases of animal prion disease.[86,271,323] Sensitive and specific detection of PrP^{Sc} in sCJD patient CSF[247] and nasal brushings[269a] and in vCJD patient urine[259] and blood[181,182] have each been reported recently, offering the promise of improved clinical diagnosis for CJD and of a population prevalence or blood donor screening test for vCJD.

CONCLUSION

It is clear that prion diseases continue to represent a formidable challenge to science and medicine. Although many of these challenges lie outside the immediate realms of neuropathology, the fact that prion diseases target the CNS will ensure that neuropathologists in both the veterinary and the medical fields will continue to play a leading role in the identification, study and understanding of these disorders.

ACKNOWLEDGEMENTS

We are grateful to our many colleagues for their provision of expert comments and fine illustrations. We wish to thank Linda McCardle, Suzanne Lowrie, Mags LeGrice and Helen Yull for expert technical assistance, and Dr Diane Ritchie for invaluable help with imaging. The National Creutzfeldt–Jakob Disease Research and Surveillance Unit is funded by the Department of Health and the Scottish Government. The contribution of MWH, JWI and RGW to this chapter constitutes independent research commissioned and funded by the Policy Research Programme in the Department of Health Policy Research Programme (DH121/5061). The views expressed in this chapter are those of the authors and not necessarily those of the Department of Health. PP acknowledges support from NIH-NIAID agreement Y1-A1-4893-02 and FDA agreement 224-05-1307. The findings and conclusion in this article have not been formally disseminated by the Food and Drug Administration and should not be construed to represent any agency determination or policy.

REFERENCES

1. Aguzzi A. Prion diseases of humans and farm animals: epidemiology, genetics and pathogenesis. *J Neurochem* 2006;**97**: 1726–39.
2. Alperovitch A, Zerr I, Pocchiari M, *et al.* Codon 129 prion protein genotype and sporadic Creutzfeldt–Jakob disease. *Lancet* 1999;**353**:1673–4.
3. Alpers MP. The epidemiology of kuru in the period 1987 to 1995. *Commun Dis Intell* 2005;**29**:391–9.
4. Alzualde A, Indakoetxea B, Ferrer I, *et al.* A novel *PRNP* Y218N mutation in Gerstmann–Sträussler–Scheinker disease with neurofibrillary degeneration. *J Neuropathol Exp Neurol* 2010;**69**:789–800.
5. Andreoletti O, Berthon P, Marc D, *et al.* Early accumulation of PrP^{Sc} in gut-associated lymphoid and nervous tissues of susceptible sheep from a Romanov flock with natural scrapie. *J Gen Virol* 2000;**81**:3115–26.
6. Andreoletti O, Orge L, Benestad SL, *et al.* Atypical/Nor98 scrapie infectivity in sheep peripheral tissues. *PLoS Pathog* 2011;**7**:e1001285.
7. Asante EA, Linehan JM, Smidak M, *et al.* Inherited prion disease A117V is not simply a proteinopathy but produces prions transmissible to transgenic mice expressing homologous prion protein. *PLoS Pathog* 2013;**9**:e1003643.
8. Atarashi R, Satoh K, Sano K, *et al.* Ultrasensitive human prion detection in cerebrospinal fluid by real-time quaking-induced conversion. *Nature Med* 2011;**73**:175–8.
9. Balkema–Buschmann A, Ziegler U, McIntyre L, *et al.* Experimental challenge of cattle with German atypical bovine spongiform encephalopathy (BSE) isolates. *J Toxicol Environ Health A* 2011;**74**:103–9.
10. Barria MA, Balachandran A, Morita M, *et al.* Molecular barriers to zoonotic transmission of prions. *Emerg Infect Dis* 2014;**20**:88–97.

11. Barron RM, Thomson V, Jamieson E, *et al.* Changing a single amino acid in the N-terminus of murine PrP alters TSE incubation time across three species barriers. *EMBO J* 2001;**20**:5070–78.
12. Barron RM, Campbell SL, King D, *et al.* High titers of transmissible spongiform encephalopathy infectivity associated with extremely low levels of PrP^{Sc} in vivo. *J Biol Chem* 2007;**282**:35878–86.
13. Baxter HC, Campbell GA, Whittaker AG, *et al.* Elimination of transmissible spongiform encephalopathy infectivity and decontamination of surgical instruments by using radio-frequency gas-plasma treatment. *J Gen Virol* 2005;**86**:2393–9.
14. Beck JA, Mead S, Campbell TA, *et al.* Two-octapeptide repeat deletion of prion protein associated with rapidly progressive dementia. *Neurology* 2001;**57**:354–6.
15. Beck JA, Poulter M, Campbell TA, *et al.* PRNP alleleic sequencing from 19 years of prion protein gene sequencing at the MRC Prion Unit. *Hum Mutat* 2010;**31**:E1551–E1563.
16. Belay ED, Gambetti P, Schonberger LB, *et al.* Creutzfeldt–Jakob disease in unusually young patients who consumed venison. *Arch Neurol* 2001;**58**:1673–8.
17. Benestad SL, Sarradin P, Thu B, *et al.* Cases of scrapie with unusual features in Norway and designation of a new type, Nor98. *Vet Rec* 2003;**153**:202–8.
18. Benestad SL, Arsac JN, Goldmann W, *et al.* Atypical/Nor98 scrapie: properties of the agent, genetics and epidemiology. *Vet Res* 2008;**39**:19–21.
19. Bernoulli C, Siegfried J, Baumgartner G, *et al.* Danger of accidental person to person transmission of Creutzfeldt–Jakob disease by surgery. *Lancet* 1977;**1**:478–9.
20. Bessen RA, Marsh RF. Distinct PrP properties suggest the molecular basis of strain variation in transmissible mink encephalopathy. *J Virol* 1994;**68**: 7859–68.

21. Binelli S, Agazzi P, Giaccone G, *et al.* Periodic electroencephalogram complexes in a patient with variant Creutzfeldt–Jakob disease. *Ann Neurol* 2006;**59**:423–7.
22. Bishop MT, Hart P, Aitchison L, *et al.* Predicting susceptibility and incubation time of human-to-human transmission of vCJD. *Lancet Neurol* 2006;**5**:393–8.
23. Bishop MT, Ritchie DL, Will RG, *et al.* No major change in vCJD agent strain after secondary transmission via blood transfusion. *PLoS One* 2008;**3**:e2878.
24. Bishop MT, Will RG, Manson JC. Defining sporadic Creutzfeldt–Jakob disease strains and their transmission properties. Proc Natl Acad Sci U S A 2010;**107**: 12005–10.
25. Blanquet–Grossard F, Sazdovitch V, Jean A, *et al.* Prion protein is not detectable in dental pulp from patients with Creutzfeldt–Jakob disease. *J Dent Res* 2000;**79**:700.
26. Boesenberger C, Schulz-Schaeffer W, Meissner B, *et al.* Clinical course in young patients with sporadic Creutzfeldt–Jakob disease. *Ann Neurol* 2005;**58**:533–43.
27. Bouzamondo–Bernstein E, Hopkins SD, Spilman P, *et al.* The neurodegeneration sequence in prion diseases: evidence from functional, morphological and ultrastructural studies of the GABAergic system. *J Neuropathol Exp Neurol* 2004;**63**:882–99.
28. Bradley R, Liberski PP. Bovine spongiform encephalopathy (BSE): the end of the beginning or the beginning of the end? *Folia Neuropathol* 2004;**42**:55–68.
29. Brandel JP, Preece M, Brown P, *et al.* Distribution of codon 129 genotype in human growth hormone-treated CJD patients in France and the UK. *Lancet* 2003;**362**:128–30.
30. Brandel JP, Heath CA, Head MW, *et al.* Variant Creutzfeldt–Jakob disease in France and the United Kingdom: evidence of the same agent strain. *Ann Neurol* 2009;**65**:249–56.

31. Brandner S. CNS Pathogenesis of prion diseases. *Br Med Bull* 2003;**66**:131–9.

32. Brandner S, Isenmann S, Raeber A, et al. Normal host prion protein necessary for scrapie-induced neurotoxicity. *Nature* 1996;**379**:339–43.

33. Brandner S, Raeber A, Sailer A, et al. Normal host prion protein (PrPC) is required for scrapie spread within the central nervous system. *Proc Natl Acad Sci U S A* 1996;**93**:13148–51.

34. Brandner S Whitfield J, Boone K, et al. Central and peripheral pathology of kuru: pathological analysis of a recent case and comparison with other forms of human prion disease. *Philos Trans R Soc Lond B Biol Sci* 2008;**363**: 3755–63.

35. Brazier MW, Lewis V, Ciccotosto GD, et al. Correlative studies support lipid peroxidation is linked to PrP(Res) propagation as an early primary pathogenic event in prion disease. *Brain Res Bull* 2006;**68**:346–54.

36. Brown DR. Neurodegeneration and oxidative stress:prion disease results from loss of antioxidant defence. *Folia Neuropathol* 2005;**43**:229–43.

37. Brown P, Bradley R. 1755 and all that: a historical primer of transmissible spongiform encephalopathy. *Br Med J* 1998;**317**:1688–92.

38. Brown P, Rodgers–Johnson P, Cathala F, et al. Creutzfeldt–Jakob disease of long duration: clinicopathological characteristics, transmissibility and differential diagnosis. *Ann Neurol* 1984;**16**:295–304.

39. Brown P, Cathala F, Raubertas RF, et al. The epidemiology of Creutzfeldt–Jakob disease:conclusion of a 15-year investigation in France and review of the world literature. *Neurology* 1987; **37**:895–904.

40. Brown P, Preece MA, Will RG. 'Friendly fire' in medicine: hormones, homografts and Creutzfeldt–Jakob disease. *Lancet* 1992;**340**:24–7.

41. Brown P, Gibbs CJ, Jr, Rodgers–Johnson P, et al. Human spongiform encephalopathy: the National Institutes of Health series of 300 cases of experimentally transmitted disease. *Ann Neurol* 1994;**35**:513–29.

42. Brown P, Cervenakova L, Boellaard JW, et al. Identification of a *PRNP* gene mutation in Jakob's original Creutzfeldt–Jakob disease family. *Lancet* 1994;**344**:130–31.

43. Brown P, Brandel JP, Sato K, Nakamura Y, et al. Iatrogenic Creutzfeldt–Jakob disease: a final assessment. *Emerg Infect Dis* 2012;**18**:901–7.

44. Brownell B, Oppenheimer DR. An ataxic form of subacute presenile polioencephalopathy (Creutzfeldt–Jakob disease). *J Neurol Neurosurg Psychiatry* 1965;**28**:350–61.

45. Bruce ME. Scrapie strain variation and mutation. *Br Med Bull* 1993;**49**:822–38.

46. Bruce ME. TSE strain variation. *Br Med Bull* 2003;**66**:99–108.

47. Bruce ME, McConnell I, Fraser H, et al. The disease characteristics of different strains of scrapie in sinc congenic mouse lines: implications for the nature of the agent and control of pathogenesis. *J Gen Virol* 1991;**72**:595–603.

48. Bruce ME, Will RG, Ironside JW, et al. Transmissions to mice indicate that 'new variant' CJD is caused by the BSE agent. *Nature* 1997;**389**:498–501.

49. Bruce ME, McConnell I, Will RG, et al. Detection of variant Creutzfeldt–Jakob disease infectivity in extraneural tissues. *Lancet* 2001;**358**:208–9.

50. Budka H. Neuropathology of prion diseases. *Br Med Bull* 2003;**66**:121–30.

51. Budka H, Aguzzi A, Brown P, et al. Neuropathological diagnostic criteria for Creutzfeldt–Jakob disease (CJD) and other human spongiform encephalopathies. *Brain Pathol* 1995;**4**:459–66.

52. Budka H, Head MW, Ironside JW, et al. Sporadic Creutzfeldt–Jakob disease. In: Dickson DW, Weller RO (eds). *Neurodegeneration: The molecular pathology of dementia and movement disorders.* Oxford: Wiley–Blackwell, 2011:322–35.

53. Bugiani O, Giaccone G, Verga L, et al. Beta APP participates in PrP-amyloid plaques of Gerstmann–Sträussler–Scheinker disease, Indiana kindred. *J Neuropathol Exp Neurol* 1993;**52**:64–70.

54. Cali I, Castellani R, Alshekhlee A, et al. Co-existence of scrapie prion protein types 1 and 2 in sporadic Creutzfeldt–Jakob disease: its effect on the phenotype and prion-type characteristics. *Brain* 2009;**132**:2642–58.

55. Capellari S, Parchi P, Wolff BD, et al. Creutzfeldt–Jakob disease associated with a deletion of two repeats in the prion protein gene. *Neurology* 2002;**59**:628–30.

56. Casalone C, Zanusso G, Acutis P, et al. Identification of a second bovine amyloidotic spongiform encephalopathy: molecular similarities with sporadic Creutzfeldt–Jakob disease. *Proc Natl Acad Sci U S A* 2004;**101**:3065–70.

57. Cashman NR, Loertscher R, Nalbantoglu J, et al. Cellular isoform of the scrapie agent protein participates in lymphocytes activation. *Cell* 1990;**61**:185–92.

58. Castilla J, Saa P, Hetz C, et al. *In vitro* generation of infectious scrapie prions. *Cell* 2005;**121**:195–206.

59. Castro RM, Landemberger MC, Walz R, et al. High capacity and low cost detection of prion protein gene variant alleles by denaturing HPLC. *J Neurosci Methods* 2004;**139**:263–71.

60. Caughey B. Prion protein conversions: insight into mechanisms, TSE transmission barriers and strains. *Br Med Bull* 2003;**66**:109–20.

61. Cervenakova L, Goldfarb LG, Garruto R, et al. Phenotype–genotype studies in kuru: implications for new variant Creutzfeldt–Jakob disease. *Proc Natl Acad Sci U S A* 1998;**95**:13239–41.

62. Chakrabarti O, Ashok A, Hegde RS. Prion protein biosynthesis and its emerging role in neurodegeneration. *Trends Biochem Sci* 2009;**34**:287–95.

63. Chesebro B, Trifilo M, Race R, et al. Anchorless prion protein results in infectious amyloid disease without clinical scrapie. *Science* 2005;**308**:1435–9.

64. Chiesa R, Piccardo P, Quaglio E, et al. Molecular distinction between pathogenic and infectious properties of the prion protein. *J Virol* 2003;**77**:7611–22.

65. Colby DW, Prusiner SB. *De novo* generation of prions strains. *Nat Rev Microbiol* 2011;**9**:771–7.

66. Collie DA, Summers DM, Sellar RJ, et al. Diagnosing variant Creutzfeldt–Jakob disease with the pulvinar sign: MR imaging findings in 86 neuropathologically confirmed cases. *Am J Neuroradiol* 2003;**24**:1560–69.

67. Collinge J, Sidle KCL, Meads J, et al. Molecular analysis of prion strain variation and the aetiology of 'new variant' CJD. *Nature* 1996;**383**:685–90.

68. Collinge J, Whitfield J, McKintosh E, et al. A clinical study of kuru patients with long incubation periods at the end of the epidemic in Papua New Guinea. *Phil Trans R Soc B* 2008;**363**:3725–39.

69. Collinge J, Gorham M, Hudson F, et al. Safety and efficacy of quinacrine in human prion disease (PRION-1 study): a patient-preference trial. *Lancet Neurol* 2009;**8**:334–44.

70. Collins S, Law MG, Fletcher A, et al. Surgical treatment and risk of sporadic Creutzfeldt–Jakob disease: a case–control study. *Lancet* 1999;**353**:693–7.

71. Collins S, Boyd A, Fletcher A, et al. Creutzfeldt–Jakob disease cluster in an Australian rural city. *Ann Neurol* 2002;**52**:115–18.

72. Cooper JD, Bird SM. Predicting incidence of variant Creutzfeldt–Jakob disease from UK dietary exposure to bovine spongiform encephalopathy for the 1940 to 1969 and post-1969 birth cohorts. *Int J Epidemiol* 2003;**32**:784–91.

73. Cooper SA, Murray KL, Heath CA, et al. Isolated visual symptoms at onset in sporadic Creutzfeldt–Jakob disease: the clinical phenotype of the 'Heidenhain variant'. *Br J Ophthalmol* 2005;**89**: 1341–2.

74. Cortelli P, Perani D, Montagna P, et al. Pre-symptomatic diagnosis in fatal familial insomnia: serial neurophysiological and 18FDG-PET studies. *Brain* 2006;**129**: 668–75.

75. Cousens SN, Harries–Jones R, Knight R, et al. Geographical distribution of cases of Creutzfeldt–Jakob disease in England and Wales 1970–84. *J Neurol Neurosurg Psychiatry* 1990;**53**:459–65.

76. Creutzfeldt HG. Uber eine eigenartige herdformige erkrankung des zentralnervensystems. *Z Gesamte Neurol Psychiatr* 1920;**57**:1–18.

77. Croes EA, Roks G, Jansen GH, et al. Creutzfeldt–Jakob disease 38 years after diagnostic use of human growth hormone. *J Neurol Neurosurg Psychiatry* 2002;**72**:792–93.

78. Croes EA, Thuens J, Houwing–Duistermaat JJ, et al. Octapeptide repeat insertions in the prion protein gene and early onset dementia. *J Neurol Neurosurg Psychiatry* 2004;**75**:1166–70.

79. Cuille J, Chelle PL. Pathologie animale: la maladie dite de la tremblante du mouton est-elle inoculable? *C R Acad Sci (Paris)* 1936;**203**:1552–4.

80. Cunningham C, Wilcockson DC, Boche D, et al. Comparison of inflammatory and acute-phase responses in the brain and peripheral organs of the ME7 model of prion disease. *J Virol* 2005;**79**:5174–84.

81. Deleault NR, Lucassen RW, Supattapone S. RNA molecules stimulate prion protein conversion. *Nature* 2003;**425**:717–20.

82. Diack AB, Ritchie D, Bishop M, et al. Constant transmission proterties of variant Creutzfeldt–Jakob disease in five countries. *Emerg Infect Dis* 2012;**18**:1574–9.

83. Dickinson AG, Taylor DM. Resistance of the scrapie agent to decontamination. *N Engl J Med* 1978;**299**:1413–14.

84. Doh–Ura K, Ishikawa K, Murakami–Kubo I, et al. Treatment of transmissible spongiform encephalopathy by intraventricular drug infusion in animal models. *J Virol* 2004;78:4999–5006.

85. Duffy P, Wolf J, Collins G, et al. Possible person-to-person transmission of Creutzfeldt–Jakob disease. *N Engl J Med* 1974;290:692–3.

86. Edgeworth JA, Farmer M, Sicilia A, et al. Detection of prion infection in variant Creutzfeldt–Jakob disease: a blood based assay. *Lancet* 2011;377:487–93.

87. Eigenbrod S, Frick P, Giese A, et al. Comprehensive neuropathological analysis of genetic prion disease associated with the E196K mutation in *PRNP* reveals phenotypic heterogeneity. *J Neuropathol Exp Neurol* 2011;70:192–200.

88. Farquhar C, Dickinson A, Bruce M. Prophylactic potential of pentosan polysulphate in transmissible spongiform encephalopathies. *Lancet* 1999;353:117.

89. Field EJ. Slow virus infections of the nervous system. *Int Rev Exp Pathol* 1969;8:129–39.

90. Foncin J–F, Gaches J, Cathala F, et al. Transmission iatrogene interhumaine possible de maladie de Creutzfeldt–Jakob avec atteinte des grains de cervelet. *Rev Neurol* 1980;136:280.

91. Forloni G, Angaretti N, Chiesa R, et al. Neurotoxicity of a prion protein fragment. *Nature* 1993;362:543–6.

92. Fradkin JE, Schonberger LB, Mills JL, et al. Creutzfeldt–Jakob disease in pituitary growth hormone recipients in the United States. *J Am Med Ass* 1991;265:880–84.

93. Fraser H. Diversity in the neuropathology of scrapie-like diseases in animals. *Br Med Bull* 1993;49:792–809.

94. Fraser H, Bruce ME, McBride PA, et al. The molecular pathology of scrapie and the biological basis of lesion targeting. *Prog Clin Biol Res* 1989;317:637–44.

95. Fraser JR. What is the basis of transmissible spongiform encephalopathy induced neurodegeneration and can it be repaired? *Neuropathol Appl Neurobiol* 2002;28:1.

96. Furukawa H, Kitamoto T, Tanaka Y, et al. New variant prion protein in a Japanese family with Gerstmann–Sträussler–syndrome. *Mol Brain Res* 1995;30:385–8.

97. Gajdusek DC, Zigas V. Degenerative disease of the central nervous system in New Guinea: the endemic occurrence of 'kuru' in the native population. *N Engl J Med* 1957;257:974–8.

98. Gajdusek DC, Zigas V. Kuru;Clinical, pathological and epidemiological study of an acute progressive degenerative disease of the central nervous system among natives of the Eastern Highlands of New Guinea. *Am J Med* 1959;26:442–69.

99. Gajdusek DC, Gibbs CJ, Alpers DM. Experimental transmission of a Kuru-like syndrome to chimpanzees. *Nature* 1966;209:7946.

100. Gambetti P, Dong Z, Yuan J, et al. A novel human disease with abnormal prion protein sensitive to protease. *Ann Neurol* 2008;63:697–708.

101. Gambetti P, Kong Q, Zou W, Chen SG. Sporadic and familial CJD: classification and characterization. *Brit Med Bull* 2003;66:213–39.

102. Gerstmann J, Sträussler E, Scheinker I. Uber eine eigenartige hereditar-familiare erkrankung des zentralnervensystems.

Zugleich ein beitrag zur frage des vorzeitigen localen alterns. *Z Neurol Psychiat* 1936;154:736–62.

103. Ghetti B, Tagliavini F, Giaccone G, et al. Familial Gerstmann–Sträussler–Scheinker disease with neurofibrillary tangles. *Mol Neurobiol* 1994;8:41–8.

104. Ghetti B, Dlouhy SR, Giaccone G, et al. Gerstmann–Sträussler–Scheinker disease and the Indiana kindred. *Brain Pathol* 1995;5:61–75.

105. Ghetti B, Piccardo P, Frangione B, et al. Prion protein amyloidosis. *Brain Pathol* 1996;6:127–45.

106. Ghetti B, Piccardo P, Spillantini MG, et al. Vascular variant of prion protein cerebral amyloidosis with tau-positive neurofibrillary tangles: the phenotype of the stop codon 145 mutation in *PRNP*. *Proc Natl Acad Sci U S A* 1996;93:744–8.

107. Ghetti B, Tagliavini F, Kovacs G, Piccardo P. Gerstmann–Sträussler–Scheinker disease. In: Dickson DW, Weller RO (eds). *Neurodegeneration: The molecular pathology of dementia and movement disorders*. Oxford: Wiley–Blackwell, 2011:364–77.

108. Gibbs CJ, Jr, Gajdusek DC, Asher DM, Alpers M, et al. Creutzfeldt–Jakob Disease (spongiform encephalopathy): transmission to the chimpanzee. *Science* 1968;161:388–9.

109. Gibbs CJ, Asher DM, Brown PW, et al. Creutzfeldt–Jakob disease infectivity of growth hormone derived from human pituitary glands. *N Engl J Med* 1993;328:358–9.

110. Gill ON, Spencer Y, Richard–Loendt A, et al. Prevalent abnormal prion protein in human appendixes after bovine spongiform encephalopathy epizootic: A large scale study. *BMJ* 2013;347:f5675.

111. Glatzel M, Abela E, Maissen M, et al. Extraneural pathologic prion protein in sporadic Creutzfeldt–Jakob disease. *N Engl J Med* 2003;349:1812–20.

112. Goedert M, Clavaguera F, Tolnay M. The propagation of prion-like inclusions in neurodegenerative diseases. Trends Neurosci 2010;33:317–25.

113. Goldfarb LG, Brown P, McCombie WR, et al. Transmissible familial Creutzfeldt–Jakob disease associated with five, seven, and eight extra octapeptide coding repeats in the *PRNP* gene. *Proc Natl Acad Sci U S A* 1991;88:10926–30.

114. Goldfarb LG, Petersen RB, Tabaton M, et al. Fatal familial insomnia and familial Creutzfeldt–Jakob disease: disease phenotype determined by a DNA polymorphism. *Science* 1992;258:806–8.

115. Goldmann W. PrP genetics in ruminant transmissible spongiform encephalopathies. *Vet Res* 2008;39:30.

116. Gonzalez L, Dagleish MP, Martin S, et al. Factors influencing temporal variation of scrapie incidence within a closed Suffolk sheep flock. *J Gen Virol* 2012;93:203–11.

117. Gonzalez L, Martin S, Begara–McGorum I, et al. Effects of agent strain and host genotype on PrP accumulation in the brain of sheep naturally and experimentally affected with scrapie. *J Comp Path* 2002;126:17–29.

118. Gonzalez L, Siso S, Monleon E, et al. Variability in disease phenotypes within a single *PRNP* genotype suggests the existence of multiple natural sheep scrapie strains within Europe. *J Gen Virol* 2010;91:2630–41.

119. Gonzalez L, Jeffrey M, Dagleish MP, et al. Susceptibility to scrapie and disease phenotype in sheep: cross-*PRNP* genotype experimental transmissions with natural sources. *Vet Res* 2012;43:55.

120. Goodall CA, Head MW, Everington D, et al. Raised CSF phospho-tau concentrations in variant Creutzfeldt–Jakob disease: diagnostic and pathological implications. *J Neurol Neurosurg Psychiatry* 2006;77:89–91.

121. Govaerts C, Wille H, Prusiner SB, Cohen FE. Evidence for assembly of prions with left-handed beta-helices into trimers. *Proc Natl Acad Sci U S A* 2004;101:8342–7.

122. Green AJE, Thompson EJ, Stewart GE, et al. Use of 14-3-3 and other brain-specific proteins in CSF in the diagnosis of variant Creutzfeldt–Jakob disease. *J Neurol Neuosurg Psychiatry* 2001;70:744–48.

123. Green AJE, Andrews MM, Bishop MT, et al. Elevated phosphorylated tau pT-181 in a possible *PRNP* codon 129 MV vCJD case. *J Neurol Neurosurg Psychiatry* 2010;81:1408–9.

124. Gregori L, Lambert BC, Gurgel PV, et al. Reduction of transmissible spongiform encephalopathy infectivity from human red blood cells with prion protein affinity ligands. *Transfusion* 2006;46:1152–61.

125. Griffith JS. Self replication and scrapie. *Nature* 1967;215:1043–4.

126. Griffiths HH, Whitehouse IJ, Hooper NM. Regulation of amyloid-β production by prion protein. *Prion* 2012;6:217–22.

127. Guentchev M, Hainfellner JA, Trabattoni GR, et al. Distribution of parvalbumin-immunoreactive neurons in brain correlates with hippocampal and temporal cortical pathology in Creutzfeldt–Jakob disease. *J Neuropathol Exp Neurol* 1997;56:1119–24.

128. Hadlow WJ. Scrapie and Kuru. *Lancet* 1959;2:289–90.

129. Haik S, Faucheux BA, Sazdovitch V, et al. The sympathetic nervous system is involved in variant Creutzfeldt–Jakob disease. *Nat Med* 2003;9:1121–3.

130. Haik S, Brandel JP, Salomon D, et al. Compassionate use of quinacrine in Creutzfeldt–Jakob disease fails to show significant effects. *Neurology* 2004;63:2413–15.

131. Haik S, Peoc'h K, Brandel JP, et al. Striking PrP^{Sc} heterogeneity in inherited prion diseases with the D178N mutation. *Ann Neurol* 2004;56:909–11.

132. Hainfellner JA, Brantner–Inthaler S, Cervenakova L, et al. The original Gerstmann–Sträussler–Scheinker family of Austria: divergent clinicopathological phenotypes but constant PrP genotype. *Brain Pathol* 1995;5:201–11.

133. Hainfellner JA, Liberski PP, Guiroy DC, et al. Pathology and immunocytochemistry of a kuru brain. *Brain Pathol* 1997;7:547–53.

134. Hainfellner JA, Wanschitz J, Jellinger K, et al. Coexistence of Alzheimer-type neuropathology in Creutzfeldt–Jakob disease. *Acta Neuropathol* 1998;96:116–22.

135. Hainfellner JA, Parchi P, Kitamoto T, et al. A novel phenotype in familial Creutzfeldt–Jakob disease: prion protein gene E200K mutation coupled with valine at codon 129 and type 2 protease-resistant prion protein. *Ann Neurol* 1999;45:812–16.

136. Hansen LA, Masliah E, Terry RD, et al. A neuropathological subset of Alzheimer's disease with concomitant Lewy body disease and spongiform change. *Acta Neuropathol* 1989;78:194–201.

137. Harder A, Jendroska K, Kreuz F, et al. Novel twelve-generation kindred of fatal familial insomnia from Germany representing the entire spectrum of disease expression. *Am J Med Genet* 1999;87:11–16.

138. Harris DA, Peters PJ, Taraboulos V, et al. Cell Biology of Prions. In: Prusiner SB ed. *Prion biology and diseases*, 2nd edn. New York: Cold Spring Harbor Laboratory Press, 2004:483–544.

139. Head MW, Tissingh G, Uitdehaag BM, et al. Sporadic Creutzfeldt–Jakob disease in a young Dutch valine homozygote: atypical molecular phenotype. *Ann Neurol* 2001;50:258–61.

140. Head MW, Northcott V, Rennison K, et al. Prion protein accumulation in eyes of patients with sporadic and variant Creutzfeldt–Jakob disease. *Invest Ophthalmol Vis Sci* 2003;44:342–6.

141. Head MW, Ritchie D, McLoughlin V, et al. Investigation of PrPres in dental tissues in variant CJD. *Br Dent J* 2003;195:339–43.

142. Head MW, Ritchie D, Smith N, et al. Peripheral tissue involvement in sporadic, iatrogenic and variant Creutzfeldt–Jakob disease: an immunohistochemical, quantitative and biochemical study. *Am J Pathol* 2004;164:143–53.

143. Head MW, Bunn TJR, Bishop MT, et al. Prion protein heterogeneity in sporadic but not variant Creutzfeldt–Jakob disease: UK cases 1991–2002. *Ann Neurol* 2004;55:851–9.

144. Head MW, Peden AH, Yull HM, et al. Abnormal prion protein in the retina of the most commonly occurring subtype of sporadic Creutzfeldt–Jakob disease. *Br J Ophthalmol* 2005;89:1131–3.

145. Head MW, Knight R, Zeidler M, et al. A case of protease sensitive prionopathy in a patient in the United Kingdom. *Neuropathol Applied Neurobiol* 2009;35:628–32.

146. Head MW, Yull HM, Ritchie DL, et al. Pathological investigation of the first blood donor and recipient pair linked by transfusion-associated variant Creutzfeldt–Jakob disease transmission. *Neuropathol Applied Neurobiol* 2009;35:433–6.

147. Heath C, Cooper SA, Murray K, et al. Reply to comment by Lukic et al on validation of diagnostic criteria for variant Creutzfeldt–Jakob disease. *Ann Neurol* 2011;69:212.

148. Heath CA, Barker RA, Esmonde TFG, et al. Dura mater-associated Creutzfeldt–Jakob disease: experience from surveillance in the UK. *J Neurol Neurosurg Psychiatry* 2006;77:880–82.

149. Heath CA, Cooper SA, Murray K, et al. Validation of diagnostic criteria for variant Creutzfeldt–Jakob disease. *Ann Neurol* 2010;67:761–70.

150. Heckmann JG, Lang CJG, Petruch P, et al. Transmission of Creutzfeldt–Jakob disease via a corneal transplant. *J Neurol Neurosurg Psychiatry* 1997;63:388–90.

151. Hegde RS, Mastrianni JA, Scott MR, et al. A transmembrane form of the prion protein in neurodegenerative disease. *Science* 1998;279:827–34.

152. Heggebo R, Gonzalez L, Press C M, et al. Disease-associated PrP in the enteric nervous system of scrapie-affected Suffolk sheep. *J Gen Virol* 2003;84:1327–38.

153. Herms J, Tings T, Gall S, et al. Evidence of presynaptic location and function of the prion protein. *J Neurosci* 1999;19:8866–75.

154. Herzog C, Riviere J, Lescoutra–Etchegaray N, et al. PrPTSE distribution in a primate model of variant, sporadic, and iatrogenic Creutzfeldt–Jakob disease. *J Virol* 2005;79:14339–45.

155. Hewitt PE, LLewelyn CA, Mackenzie J, Will RG. Creutzfeldt–Jakob disease and blood transfusion: results of the UK Transfusion Medicine Epidemiological Review study. *Vox Sang* 2006;91:221–30.

156. Hill AF, Zeidler M, Ironside J, et al. Diagnosis of new variant Creutzfeldt–Jakob disease by tonsil biopsy. *Lancet* 1997;349:99–100.

157. Hill AF, Butterworth RJ, Joiner S, et al. Investigation of variant Creutzfeldt–Jakob disease and other human prion diseases with tonsil biopsy samples. *Lancet* 1999;353:183–9.

158. Hill AF, Joiner S, Linehan J, et al. Species-barrier-independent prion replication in apparently resistant species. *Proc Natl Acad Sci U S A* 2000;97:10248–53.

159. Hilton DA, Fathers E, Edwards P, et al. Prion immunoreactivity in appendix before clinical onset of variant Creutzfeldt–Jakob disease. *Lancet* 1998;352:703–4.

160. Hilton DA, Ghani AC, Conyers L, et al. Prevalence of lymphoreticular prion protein accumulation in UK tissue samples. *J Pathol* 2004;203:733–9.

161. Hilton DA, Head MW, Singh V, et al. Gerstmann–Sträussler–Scheinker disease: a new mutation. *Neuropathol Appl Neurobiol* 2007;33:265.

162. Hope J. The nature of the scrapie agent: the evolution of the virino. *Ann N Y Acad Sci* 1994;724:282–9.

163. Hoque MZ, Kitamoto T, Furukawa H, et al. Mutation in the prion protein gene at codon 232 in Japanese patients with Creutzfeldt–Jakob disease: clinicopathological, immunohistochemical and transmission study. *Acta Neuropathol* 1996;92:441–6.

164. Hoshi K, Yoshino H, Urata J, et al. Creutzfeldt–Jakob disease associated with cadaveric dura mater grafts in Japan. *Neurology* 2000;55:718–21.

165. Houston F, McCutcheon S, Goldmann W, et al. Prion diseases are efficiently transmitted by blood transfusion in sheep. *Blood* 2008;112:4739–45.

166. Hsiao KK, Scott M, Foster D, et al. Spontaneous neurodegeneration in transgenic mice with mutant prion protein. *Science* 1990;250:1587–90.

167. Huillard D'Aignaux JN, Cousens SN, Maccario J, et al. The incubation period of kuru. *Epidemiology* 2002;13:402–8.

168. Hunter N. Scrapie and experimental BSE in sheep. *Br Med Bull* 2003;66:171–83.

169. Ironside JW. Review: Creutzfeldt–Jakob disease. *Brain Pathol* 1996;6:379–88.

170. Ironside JW. Prion diseases in man. *J Pathol* 1998;186:227–34.

171. Ironside JW, Bishop MT, Connolly K, et al. Variant Creutzfeldt–Jakob disease: prion protein genotype analysis of positive appendix tissue samples from a retrospective prevalence study. *Br Med J* 2006;332:1186–8.

172. Ironside JW, McCardle L, Hayward PA, et al. Ubiquitin immunocytochemistry in human spongiform encephalopathies. *Neuropathol Appl Neurobiol* 1993;19:134–40.

173. Ironside JW, Head MW, Bell JE, et al. Laboratory diagnosis of variant Creutzfeldt–Jakob disease. *Histopathology* 2000;37:1–9.

174. Ironside JW, McCardle L, Horsburgh A, et al. Pathological diagnosis of variant Creutzfeldt–Jakob disease. *APMIS* 2002;11:79–87.

175. Ironside JW, Ritchie DL, Head MW. Phenotypic variability in human prion diseases. *J Neuropathol Appl Neurobiol* 2005;21:565–79.

176. Iseki E, Li F, Kosaka K. Close relationship between spongiform change and ubiquitin-positive granular structures in diffuse Lewy body disease. *J Neurol Sci* 1997;146:53–7.

177. Ishida C, Okino S, Kitamoto T, et al. Involvement of the peripheral nervous system in human prion diseases including dural graft associated Creutzfeldt–Jakob disease. *J Neurol Neurosurg Psychiatry* 2005;76:325–9.

178. Iwasaki Y. Three cases of Creutzfeldt–Jakob disease with prion protein gene codon 180 mutation presenting with pathological laughing and crying. *J Neurolog Sci* 2012;319:47–50.

179. Iwasaki Y, Mori K, Ito, et al. An autopsied case of V180I Creutzfeldt–Jakob disease presenting with panencephalopathic-type pathology and a characteristic prion protein type. *Neuropathol* 2011;31:540–8.

180. Jackson GS, McKintosh E, Flechsig E, et al. An enzyme-detergent method for effective prion decontamination of surgical steel. *J Gen Virol* 2005;86:869–78.

181. Jackson GS, Burk–Rafel J, Edgeworth JA, et al. Population screening for variant Creutzfeldt–Jakob disease using a novel blood test: Diagnostic accuracy and feasibility study. *JAMA Neurol* 2014;71(4):421–8.

182. Jackson GS, Burk–Rafel J, Edgeworth JA, et al. A highly specific blood test for vCJD. *Blood* 2014;123:452–3.

183. Jackson WS, Borkowski AW, Faas H, et al. Spontaneous generation of prion infectivity in fatal familial insomnia knockinmice. *Neuron* 2009;63:438–50.

184. Jacobs JG, Langeveld JP, Biacabe AG, et al. Molecular discrimination of atypical bovine spongiform encephalopathy strains from a geographical region spanning a wide area in Europe. *J Clin Microbiol* 2007;45:1821–9.

185. Jakob A. Uber eigenartige erkrankungen des zentralnervensystems mit bemerkenswertem anatomischen befunde (spastische pseudosklerose-encephalomyelopathie mit disseminierten degenerationsherden). *Z Gesamte Neurol Psychiatr* 1921;64:147–228.

186. Jakob A. Spastische pseudosklerose. *Die Extrapyramidalen Erkrankungen* 1923;215:45.

187. Jansen C, Head MW, Rozemuller AJ, Ironside JW. Panencephalopathic Creutzfeldt–Jakob disease in the Netherlands and the UK: clinical and pathological characteristics of nine patients. *Neuropathol Applied Neurobiol* 2009;35:272–82.

188. Jansen C, Parchi P, Capellari S, *et al.* Prion protein amyloidosis with divergent phenotype associated with two novel nonsense mutations in *PRNP. Acta Neuropathol* 2010;**119**:189–97.

189. Jansen C, Parchi P, Capellari S, *et al.* A second case of Gerstmann– Sträussler– Scheinker disease linked to the G131V mutation in the prion protein gene in a Dutch patient. *J Neuropathol Exp Neurol* 2011a;**70**:698–702.

190. Jansen C, Voet W, Head MW, *et al.* A novel seven-octapeptide repeat insertion in the prion protein gene (*PRNP*) in a Dutch pedigree with Gerstmann– Sträussler– Scheinker disease phenotype: comparison with similar cases from the literature. *Acta Neuropathol* 2011b;**121**:59–68.

191. Jayadev S, Nochlin D, Poorkaj P, *et al.* Familial prion disease with Alzheimer disease-like tau pathology and clinical phenotype. *Ann Neurol* 2011;**69**:712–20.

192. Jeffrey M, Gonzalez L. Classical sheep transmissible spongiform encephalopathies: pathogenesis, pathological phenotypes and clinical disease. *Neuropathol Appl Neurobiol* 2007;**33**:373–94.

193. Jeffrey M, Martin S, Gonzalez L. Cell-associated variants of disease-specific prion protein immunolabelling are found in different sources of sheep transmissible spongiform encephalopathy. *J Gen Virol* 2003;**84**:1033–46.

194. Jeffrey M, McGovern G, Siso S, Gonzalez L. Cellular and sub-cellular pathology of animal prion diseases: relationship between morphological changes, accumulation of abnormal prion protein and clinical disease. *Acta Neuropathol* 2011;**121**:113–4.

195. Jones DP, Nevin S. Rapidly progressive cerebral degeneration (subacute vascular encephalopathy) with mental disorder, focal disturbance and myoclonic epilepsy. *J Neurol Neurosurg Psychiatry* 1954;**17**:148–59.

196. Jones M, Odunsi S, du Plessis D, *et al.* Gerstmann– Sträussler –Scheinker disease: A novel *PRNP* mutation and VGKC-complex antibodies. *Neurology* 2014;**82**:2107-11.

197. Kapur N, Abbott P, Lowman A, *et al.* The neuropsychological profile associated with variant Creutzfeldt–Jakob disease. *Brain* 2003;**126**:2693–702.

198. Kaski D, Mead S, Hyare H, *et al.* Variant CJD in an individual heterozygous for *PRNP* codon 129. *Lancet* 2009;**374**:2128.

199. Kaski DN, Pennington C, Beck J, *et al.* Inherited prion disease with 4-octapeptide repeat insertion: disease requires the interactionof multiple genetic factors. *Brain* 2011;**134**:1829–38.

200. Kim MO, Cali I, Oehler A, *et al.* Genetic CJD with a novel E200G mutation in the prion protein gene and comparison with E200K mutation cases. *Acta Neuropathol Commun* 2013;**1**:80.

201. King A, Doey L, Rossor M, *et al.* Phenotypic variability in the brains of a family with a prion disease characterized by a 144-base pair insertion in the prion protein gene. *Neuropathol Appl Neurobiol* 2003;**29**:98–105.

202. Kirkwood JK, Cunningham AA. Epidemiological observations on spongiform encephalopathies in captive wild animals in the British Isles. *Vet Rec* 1994;**135**:296–303.

203. Kirschbaum WR. Zwei eigenartige erkrankugen des zentralnervensystems nach art der spastischen pseudosklerose (Jakob). *Z Ges Neurol Psychiatrie* 1924;**92**:175–220.

204. Klatzo I, Gajdusek DC, Zigas V. Pathology of Kuru. *Lab Invest* 1959;**8**:799–847.

205. Klein MA, Kaeser PS, Schwarz P, *et al.* Complement facilitates early prion pathogenesis. *Nat Med* 2001;**7**:488–92.

206. Klingeborn M, Race B, Meade–White KD, Chesebro B. Lower specific infectivity of protease-resistant prion protein generated in cell-free reactions. *Proc Natl Acad Sci U S A* 2011;**108**:1244–1253.

207. Klohn PC, Stoltze L, Flechsig E, *et al.* A quantitative, highly sensitive cell-based infectivity assay for mouse scrapie prions. *Proc Natl Acad Sci U S A* 2003;**100**:11666–73.

208. Klug GM, Lewis V, Boyd A, *et al.* Creutzfeldt–Jakob disease surveillance in Australia, January 1970 to December 2003. *Commun Dis Intell* 2004;**28**:356–8.

209. Kobayashi A, Mizukoshi K, Iwasaki Y, *et al.* Co-occurrence of types 1 and 2 PrP(res) in sporadic Creutzfeldt–Jakob disease. *Am J Pathol* 2011;**178**:1309–15.

210. Koch TK, Berg BO, DeArmond SJ, *et al.* Creutzfeldt–Jakob disease in a young adult with idiopathic hypopituitarism. *N Engl J Med* 1985;**313**:731–3.

211. Kong Q, Surewicz WK, Petersen RB, W, *et al.* Inherited prion diseases. In: Prusiner SB ed. *Prion biology and diseases*, 2nd edn. New York: Cold Spring Harbor Laboratory Press, 2004:673–776.

212. Konold T, Moore SJ, Bellworthy SJ, Simmons HA. Evidence of scrapie transmission via milk. *BMC Vet Res* 2008;**4**:14.

213. Koperek O, Kovacs GG, Ritchie D, *et al.* Disease-associated prion protein in vessel walls. *Am J Pathol* 2002;**161**:1979–84.

214. Kovacs GG, Head MW, Hegyi I, *et al.* Immunohistochemistry for the prion protein: comparison of different monoclonal antibodies in human prion disease subtypes. *Brain Pathol* 2002;**12**:1–11.

215. Kovacs GG, Zerbi P, Voigtlander T, *et al.* The prion protein in human neurodegenerative disorders. *Neuroscience Letters* 2002;**329**:269–72.

216. Kovacs GG, Puopolo M, Ladogana A, *et al.* Genetic prion disease: the EUROCJD experience. *Hum Genet* 2005;**118**:166–74.

217. Kovacs GG, Sequin J, Quadrio, *et al.* Genetic Creutzfeldt–Jakob disease associated with the E200K mutation: Characterisation of a complex prionopathy. *Acta Neuropathol* 2011;**121**:39–57.

218. Krebs B, Lederer RM, Windl O, *et al.* Creutzfeldt–Jakob disease associated with an R148H mutation of the prion protein gene. *Neurogenetics* 2005;**6**:97–100.

219. Kropp S, Schulz–Schaeffer WJ, Finkenstaedt M, *et al.* The Heidenhain variant of Creutzfeldt–Jakob disease. *Arch Neurol* 1999;**56**:55–61.

220. Ladogana A, Puopolo M, Croes EA, *et al.* Mortality from Creutzfeldt–Jakob disease and related disorders in Europe, Australia and Canada. *Neurology* 2005;**64**:1586–91.

221. Lampert PW, Gajdusek DC, Gibbs CJ. Pathology of dendrites in subacute spongiform virus encephalopathies. *Adv Neurol* 1975;**12**:465–70.

222. Lasmezas CI, Deslys JP, Demaimay R, *et al.* BSE transmission to macaques. *Nature* 1996;**381**:743–4.

223. Lasmezas CI, Comoy E, Hawkins S, *et al.* Risk of oral infection with bovine spongiform encephalopathy agent in primates. *Lancet* 2005;**365**:781–3.

224. Lee HS, Brown P, Cervenakova L, *et al.* Increased susceptibility to Kuru of carriers of the *PRNP* 129 methionine/ methionine genotype. *J Infect Dis* 2001;**183**:192–6.

225. Legname G, Baskakov IV, Nguyen HO, *et al.* Synthetic mammalian prions. *Science* 2004;**305**:673–6.

226. Li J, Browning S, Mahal SP, *et al.* Darwinian evolution of prions in cell culture. *Science* 2010;**327**:869–72.

227. Liberski PP, Budka H, Sluga E, *et al.* Tubulovesicular structures in Creutzfeldt-Jakob disease. *Acta Neuropathol* 1992;**84**:238–43.

228. Liberski PP, Streichenberger N, Giraud P, *et al.* Ultrastructural pathology of prion diseases revisited: brain biopsy studies. *Neuropathol Appl Neurobiol* 2005;**31**:88–96.

229. Linsell L, Cousens SN, Smith PG, *et al.* A case-control study of sporadic Creutzfeldt–Jakob disease in the United Kingdom: analysis of clustering. *Neurology* 2004;**63**:2077–83.

230. Liu Z, Jia L, Piao Y, *et al.* Creutzfeldt–Jakob disease with *PRNP* G114V mutation in a Chinese family. *Acta Neurol Scand* 2010;**121**:377–83.

231. Llewelyn CA, Hewitt PE, Knight RS, *et al.* Possible transmission of variant Creutzfeldt–Jakob disease by blood transfusion. *Lancet* 2004;**363**:417–21.

232. Lloyd S, Mead S, Collinge J. Genetics of prion disease. *Top Curr Chem* 2011;**305**:1–22.

233. Mabbott NA, MacPherson GG. Prions and their lethal journey to the brain. *Nat Rev Microbiol* 2006;**4**:201–11.

234. Macleod MA, Stewart G, Zeidler M, *et al.* Sensory features of variant Creutzfeldt– Jakob disease. *J Neurol* 2002;**249**:706–11.

235. Mahal SP, Demczyk CA, Smith EW, *et al.* Assaying prions in cell culture: the standard scrapie cell assay (SSCA) and the scrapie cell end point format (SCEPA). *Methods Mol Biol* 2008;**459**:49–68.

236. Mallucci G, Campbell TA, Dickinson A, *et al.* Inherited prion disease with an alanine to valine mutation at codon 117 in the prion protein gene. *Brain* 1999;**122**:1823 –37.

237. Mallucci G, Dickinson A, Linehan J, *et al.* Depleting neuronal PrP in prion infection prevents disease and reverses spongiosis. *Science* 2003;**302**:871–4.

238. Manson JC, Jamieson E, Baybutt H, *et al.* A single amino acid alteration (101L) introduced into murine PrP dramatically alters incubation time of transmissible spongiform encephalopathy. *EMBO J* 1999;**18**:6855–64.

239. Markus HS, Duchen LW, Parkin EM, *et al.* Creutzfeldt–Jakob disease in recipients of human growth hormone in the United Kingdom: a clinical and radiographic study. *Q J Med* 1992;**82**:43–51.

240. Masters CL, Richardson EP. Subacute spongiform encephalopathy (Creutzfeldt– Jakob disease): the nature and progression of spongiform change. *Brain* 1978;**101**:333–44.

241. Masters CL, Harris JO, Gajdusek DC, *et al.* Creutzfeldt–Jakob disease: patterns of worldwide occurrence and the significance

of familial and sporadic clustering. *Ann Neurol* 1979;**5**:177–88.

242. Masters CL, Gajdusek DC, Gibbs CJ, Jr. Creutzfeldt–Jakob disease virus isolation from the Gerstann–Sträussler–syndrome with an analysis of the various forms of amyloid plaque deposition in the virus induced spongiform encephalopathies. *Brain* 1981;**104**:559–88.

243. Masters CL, Gajdusek DC. The spectrum of Creutzfeldt–Jakob disease and the virus-induced subacute spongiform encephalopathies. *Recent Adv Neuropathol* 1982;**2**:139–63.

244. Matej R, Kovacs GG, Johanedisova S, *et al.* Genetic Creutzfeldt–Jakob disease with R208H mutation presenting as progressive supranuclear palsy. *Mov Disord* 2012;**27**:476–9.

245. May BC, Fafarman AT, Hong SB, *et al.* Potent inhibition of scrapie prion replication in cultured cells by bis-acridines. *Proc Natl Acad Sci U S A* 2003;**100**:3416–21.

246. McGovern G, Brown KL, Bruce ME, *et al.* Murine scrapie infection causes an abnormal germinal centre reaction in the spleen. *J Comp Pathol* 2004;**130**:181–94.

247. McGuire L, Peden AH, Orru CD, *et al.* RT-QuIC analysis of cerebrospinal fluid in sporadic Creutzfeldt–Jakob disease. *Ann Neurol* 2012;**72**:278–85.

248. McLean CA. Kuru. In: Dickson DW, Weller RO eds. *Neurodegeneration: the molecular pathology of dementia and movement disorders.* Oxford: Wiley–Blackwell, 2011:378–80.

249. McLean CA, Ironside JW, Alpers MP, *et al.* Comparative neuropathology of kuru with the new variant of Creutzfeldt–Jakob disease: evidence for strain of agent predominating over genotype of host. *Brain Pathol* 1998;**8**:429–37.

250. McLennan NF, Brennan PM, McNeill A, *et al.* Prion protein accumulation and neuroprotection in hypoxic brain damage. *Am J Pathol* 2004;**165**:227–35.

251. McNaughton HK, Will RG. Creutzfeldt–Jakob disease presenting acutely as stroke: an analysis of 30 cases. *Neurol Infect Epidemiol* 1997;**2**:19–24.

252. Mead S, Poulter M, Uphill J, *et al.* Genetic risk factors for variant Creutzfeldt–Jakob disease: a genome-wide association study. *Lancet Neurol* 2009;**8**:57–66.

253. Mead S, Whitfield, Poulter M, *et al.* A novel prion protein variant that colocalizes with kuru exposure. *New Eng J Med* 2009;**361**:2056–65.

254. Mead S, Uphill J, Beck J, *et al.* Genome-wide association study in multiple human prion diseases suggests genetic risk factors additional to *PRNP. Hum Mol Genet* 2012;**21**:1897–906.

255. Mead S, Gandhi S, Beck J, *et al.* A novel prion disease associated with diarrhea and autonomic neuropathy. *N Engl J Med* 2013;**369**:1904–14.

256. Mead S, Wadsworth JDF, Porter M–C, *et al.* Variant Creutzfeldt–Jakob disease with extremely low lymphoreticular deposition of prion protein. *JAMA Neurol* 2014;**71**:340–3.

257. Medori R, Tritschler HJ, LeBlanc A, *et al.* Fatal familial insomnia, a prion disease with a mutation at codon 178 of the prion protein gene. *N Engl J Med* 1992;**326**:444–9.

258. Mizutani T. Neuropathology of Creutzfeldt–Jakob disease in Japan: with special reference to the panencephalopathic type. *Acta Pathol Jpn* 1981;**31**:903–22.

259. Moda F, Gambetti P, Notari S, *et al.* Prion in urine of patients with variant Creutzfeldt-Jakob disease. *N Engl J Med* 2014;**376**:530–539.

259a. Moda F, Suardi S, Di Frede G, *et al.* MM2-thalamic Creutzfeldt–Jakob disease: neuropathological, biochemical and transmission studies identify a distinctive prion strain. *Brain Pathol* 2012;**22**:662–9.

260. Moreno JA, Radford H, Peretti D, *et al.* Sustained translational repression by eIF2a-P mediates prion neurodegeneration. *Nature* 2012;**485**:507–11.

261. Munoz–Nieto M, Ramonet N, Lopez–Gaston, *et al.* A novel mutation I215V in the *PRNP* gene associated with Creutzfeldt–Jakob and Alzheimer's diseases in three patients with divergent clinical phenotypes. *J Neurol* 2013;**260**:77–84.

262. Nazor KE, Kuhn F, Seward T, *et al.* Immunodetection of disease-associated mutant PrP which accelerates disease in GSS transgenic mice. *EMBO J* 2005;**24**:2472–80.

263. Neufeld MY, Josiphov J, Korczyn AD. Demyelinating peripheral neuropathy in Creutzfeldt–Jakob disease. *Muscle Nerve* 1992;**15**:1234–9.

264. Nevin S, McMenemey WH, Behrman S, Jones DP. Subacute spongiform encephalopathy: a subacute form of encephalopathy attributable to vascular dysfunction (spongiform cerebral atrophy). *Brain* 1960;**83**:519–63.

265. Newman PK, Todd NV, Scoones D, *et al.* Postmortem findings in a case of variant Creutzfeldt–Jakob disease treated with intraventricular pentosan polysulfate. *J Neurol Neurosurg Psychiatry* 2014;**85**:9214.

266. Nicoll AJ, Collinge J. Preventing prion pathogenicity by targeting the cellular prion protein. *Infect Disord Drug Targets* 2009;**9**:48–57.

267. Nitrini R, Rosemberg S, Passos–Bueno MR, *et al.* Familial spongiform encephalopathy associated with a novel prion protein gene mutation. *Ann Neurol* 1997;**42**:161–4.

268. Nonno R, Di Bari M, Pirisinu L, *et al.* Variably protease-sensitive prionopathy is transmissible in bank voles. *Prion* 2012;**6S**:6.

269. Notari S, Moleres FJ, Hunter SB, *et al.* Multiorgan detection and characterisation of protease-resistant prion protein in a case of variant CJD examined in the United States. *PLoS One* 2010;**5**:e8765.

269a. Orru CD, Bongianni M, Tonoli G, *et al.* A test for Creutzfeldt-Jakob disease using nasal brushings. *N Engl J Med* 2014;**376**:619–629.

270. Orru CD, Caughey B. Prion seeded conversion and amplification assays. *Top Curr Chem* 2011;**305**:121–33.

271. Orru CD, Wilham JM, Raymond LD, *et al.* Prion disease blood test using immunoprecipitation and improved quaking-induced conversion. *MBio* 2011;**2**:e00078–11.

272. Owen F, Poulter M, Lofthouse R, *et al.* Insertion in prion protein gene in familial Creutzfeldt–Jakob disease. *Lancet* 1989;**1**:51–2.

273. Pacheco P, Orge L, Head M, *et al.* Novel prion disease mutation R136S has an incomplete penetrance dependent upon codon 129 trans allele. In: *Prion 2006: strategies, advances and trends towards protection of society.* Fontenay–aux Roses: NeuroPrion;2006:147.

274. Parchi P, Castellani R, Capellari S, *et al.* Molecular basis of phenotypic variability in sporadic Creutzfeldt–Jakob disease. *Ann Neurol* 1996;**39**:767–78.

275. Parchi P, Chen SG, Brown P, *et al.* Different patterns of truncated prion protein fragments correlate with distinct phenotypes in P102L Gerstmann–Sträussler–Scheinker disease. *Proc Natl Acad Sci U S A* 1998;**95**:8322–7.

276. Parchi P, Giese A, Capellari S, *et al.* Classification of sporadic Creutzfeldt–Jakob disease based on molecular and phenotypic analysis of 300 subjects. *Ann Neurol* 1999;**46**:224–33.

277. Parchi P, Zou W, Wang W, *et al.* Genetic influence on the structural variations of the abnormal prion protein. *Proc Natl Acad Sci U S A* 2000;**97**:10168–72.

278. Parchi P, Notari S, Weber P, *et al.* Inter-laboratory assessment of PrP^{Sc} typing in Creutzfeldt–Jakob disease: a western blot study within the NeuroPrion Consortium. *Brain Pathol* 2009;**19**:384–91.

279. Parchi P, Strammiello R, Notari S, *et al.* Incidence and spectrum of sporadic Creutzfeldt–Jakob disease variants with mixed phenotypes and co-occurrence of PrP^{Sc} types: an updated classification. *Acta Neuropathol* 2009;**118**:659–71.

280. Parchi P, Cescatti M, Notari S, *et al.* Agent strain variation in human prion diseases: insights from a molecular and pathological review of the National Institutes of Health series of experimentally transmitted disease. *Brain* 2010;**133**:3030–42.

281. Parchi P, Gambetti P, Capellari S. Genetic Creutzfeldt–Jakob disease. In: Dickson DW, Weller RO (eds). *Neurodegeneration: the molecular pathology of dementia and movement disorders.* Oxford: Wiley–Blackwell, 2011a:336–43.

282. Parchi P, Capellari S. Gambetti P. Fatal and familial sporadic insomnia. In: Dickson DW, Weller RO eds. *Neurodegeneration: The Molecular Pathology of Dementia and Movement Disorders.* Oxford: Wiley–Blackwell, 2011b:346–49.

283. Parchi P, de Boni L, Saveroni D *et al.* Human prion disease histotype classification allows reliable identification of molecular subtypes: An inter-rate study among surveillance centres in Europe and USA. *Acta Neuropathol* 2012;**124**:517–29.

284. Pastore M, Chin SS, Bell KL, *et al.* Creutzfeldt–Jakob disease (CJD) with a mutation at codon 148 of prion protein gene: relationship with sporadic CJD. *Am J Pathol* 2005;**167**:1729–38.

285. Peden A, McCardle L, Head MW, *et al.* Variant CJD infection in the spleen of a neurologically asymptomatic UK adult patient with haemophilia. *Haemophilia* 2010;**16**:296–304.

286. Peden AH, Head MW, Ritchie DL, *et al.* Preclinical vCJD after blood transfusion in a *PRNP* codon 129 heterozygous patient. *Lancet* 2004;**364**:477–9.

287. Peden AH, Ritchie DL, Head MW, *et al.* Detection and localization of PrP^{Sc} in the skeletal muscle of patients with variant, iatrogenic and sporadic forms of Creutzfeldt–Jakob disease. *Am J Pathol* 2006;**168**:927–35.

288. Peoc'h K, Levavasseur E, Delmont E, *et al.* Substitution at residue 211 in the prion protein drive a switch between CJD and GSS syndrome, a new mechanism governing inherited neurodegenerative disorders. *Hum Mol Genet* 2012;**21**: 5417–28.

289. Petzold GC, Westner I, Bohner G, *et al.* False-positive pulvinar sign on MRI in sporadic Creutzfeldt–Jakob disease. *Neurology* 2004;**62**:1235–6.

290. Piccardo P, Ghetti B, Dickson DW, *et al.* Gerstmann–Sträussler–Scheinker disease (*PRNP* P102L): amyloid deposits are best recognized by antibodies directed to epitopes in PrP region 90–165. *J Neuropathol Exp Neurol* 1995;**54**: 790–801.

291. Piccardo P, Seiler C, Dlouhy SR, *et al.* Proteinase-K-resistant prion protein isoforms in Gerstmann–Sträussler–Scheinker disease (Indiana kindred). *J Neuropathol Exp Neurol* 1996;**55**: 1157–63.

292. Piccardo P, Dlouhy SR, Lievens PMJ, *et al.* Phenotypic variability of Gerstmann–Sträussler–Scheinker disease is associated with prion protein heterogeneity. *J Neuropathol Exp Neurol* 1998;**57**: 979–88.

293. Piccardo P, Liepniedks JJ, William A, *et al.* Prion proteins with different conformations accumulate in Gerstmann–Sträussler–Scheinker disease caused by A117V and F198S mutations. *Am J Pathol* 2001;**158**:2201–7.

294. Piccardo P, Manson JC, King D, *et al.* Accumulation of PrP in the brain that is not associated with transmissible disease. *Proc Natl Acad Sci U S A* 2007;**104**: 4712–7.

295. Piccardo P, Cervenak J, Cervenakova L, *et al.* Squirrel monkeys infected with BSE develop tau pathology. *J Comp Pathol* 2011;**147**:84–93.

296. Piccardo P, Cervenakova L, Vasilyeva I, *et al.* Candidate cell substrates, vaccine production, and transmissible spongiform encephalopathies. *Emerg Infect Dis* 2011;**17**:2262–2269.

297. Plinston C, Hart P, Chong A, *et al.* Increased susceptibility of human-PrP transgenic mice to bovine spongiform encephalopathy following passage in sheep. *J Virol* 2011;**85**:1174–81.

298. Pocchiari M, Salvatore M, Cutruzzola F, *et al.* A new point mutation of the prion protein gene in Creutzfeldt–Jakob disease. *Ann Neurol* 1993;**34**:802–7.

299. Polymenidou M, Stoeck K, Glatzel M, *et al.* Coexistence of multiple PrP^{Sc} types in individuals with Creutzfeldt–Jakob disease. *Lancet Neurol* 2005;**4**:805–14.

300. Polymenidou M, Prokop S, Jung HH, *et al.* Atypical prion protein conformation in familial prion disease with *PRNP* P105T mutation. *Brain Pathol* 2011;**21**:209–214.

301. Poser S, Mollenhauer B, Kraub A, *et al.* How to improve the clinical diagnosis of Creutzfeldt–Jakob disease. *Brain* 1999;**122**:2345–51.

302. Powell–Jackson J, Well RO, Kennedy P, *et al.* Creutzfeldt–Jakob disease after administration of human growth hormone. *Lancet* 1985;**2**:244–6.

303. Preusser M, Strobel T, Gelpi E, *et al.* Alzheimer-type neuropathology in a 28 year old patient with iatrogenic Creutzfeldt–Jakob disease after dural grafting. *J Neurol Neurosurg Psychiatry* 2006;**77**:413–16.

304. Prusiner SB. An introduction to prion biology and diseases. In: Prusiner SB ed. *Prion biology and diseases*, 2nd edn. New York: Cold Spring Harbor Laboratory Press, 2004:1–87.

305. Prusiner SB. Development of the prion concept. In: Prusiner SB ed. *Prion biology and diseases*, 2nd edn. New York: Cold Spring Harbor Laboratory Press, 2004: 89–141.

306. Prusiner SB, Scott M, Foster D, *et al.* Transgenetic studies implicate interactions between homologous PrP isoforms in scrapie prion replication. *Cell* 1990;**63**:673–86.

307. Prusiner SB, Scott MR, DeArmond SJ, *et al.* Prion protein biology. *Cell* 1998;**93**:337–48.

308. Prusiner SB. Novel proteinaceous particles cause scrapie. *Science* 1982;**216**:136–44

309. Prusiner SB. Prions. *Proc Natl Acad Sci U S A* 1998;**95**:13363–83.

310. Puoti G, Giaccone G, Rossi G, *et al.* Sporadic Creutzfeldt–Jakob disease: co-occurrence of different types of PrP(Sc) in the same brain. *Neurology* 1999;**53**: 2173–6.

311. Race R, Priola SA, Bessen RA, *et al.* Neuron-specific expression of a hamster prion protein minigene in transgenic mice induces susceptibility to hamster scrapie agent. *Neuron* 1995;**15**:1183–91.

312. Race R, Jenny A, Sutton D. Scrapie infectivity and proteinase K-resistant prion protein in sheep placenta, brain, spleen and lymph node: implications for transmission and antemortem diagnosis. *J Infect Dis* 1998;**178**:949–53.

313. Race R, Meade–White K, Raines A, *et al.* Subclinical scrapie infection in a resistant species: persistence, replication and adaptation of infectivity during four passages. *J Infect Dis* 2002;**186**(Suppl 2):S166–170.

314. Riek R, Hornemann S, Wider G, *et al.* NMR characterization of the full-length recombinant murine prion protein, mPrP(23–231). *FEBS Lett* 1997;**413**: 282–88.

315. Ritchie DL, Head MW, Ironside JW. Advances in the detection of prion protein in peripheral tissues of variant Creutzfeldt–Jakob disease patients using paraffin-embedded tissue blotting. *Neuropathol Appl Neurobiol* 2004;**30**:360–68.

316. Ritchie DL, Boyle A, McConnell I, *et al.* Transmission of variant Creutzfeldt–Jakob disease from brain and lymphoreticular tissues shows uniform and conserved bovine spongiform encephalopathy-related phenotypic properties on primary and secondary passage in wild-type mice. *J Gen Virol* 2009;**90**:3075–82.

317. Rodriguez MM, Peoc'h K, Haik S, *et al.* A novel mutation (G114V) in the prion protein gene in a family with inherited prion disease. *Neurology* 2005;**64**:1455–7.

318. Roeber S, Krebs B, Neumann M, *et al.* Creutzfeldt–Jakob disease in a patient with an R208H mutation of the *prion protein* gene (*PRNP*) and a 17-kDa prion protein fragment. *Acta Neuropathol* 2005;**109**:443–8.

319. Rogaeva E, Zadikoff C, Ponesse J *et al.* Childhood onset in familial prion disease with a novel mutation in the *PRNP* gene. *Arch Neurol* 2006;**63**:1016–1021.

320. Roucou X, LeBlanc AC. Cellular prion protein neuroprotective function: implications in prion diseases. *J Mol Med* 2005;**83**:3–11.

321. Rowe DB, Lewis V, Needham M, *et al.* Novel prion gene mutation presenting with subacute PSP-like syndrome. *Neurology* 2007;**68**:868–70.

322. Rudd PM, *et al.* Prion glycobiology: structure, dynamics and role for the sugars. *Biochemistry* 2001;**40**:3759–66.

323. Saa P, Castillo J, Soto C. Presymptomatic detection of prions in blood. *Science* 2006;**313**:92–4.

324. Safar J, Geschwind MD, Deering C, *et al.* Diagnosis of human prion disease. *Proc Natl Acad Sci U S A* 2005;**102**:3501–6.

325. Samaia HB, Mari JJ, Vallada HP. A prion-linked psychiatric disorder. *Nature* 1997;**390**:241.

326. Sanchez–Juan P, Bishop MT, Croes E *et al.* A polymorphism in the regulatory region of *PRNP* is associated with increased risk of sporadic Creutzfeldt–Jakob disease. *BMC Med Genet* 2011;**12**:73.

327. Sanchez–Juan P, Bishop MT, Aulchenko YS *et al.* Genome-wide study links MTMR7 gene to variant Creutzfeldt–Jakob disease risk. *Neurobiol Aging* 2012;**33**(7):1487.

328. Sanchez–Valle R, Yague J, Turon A, *et al.* Inherited prion disease with 4-octapeptide repeat insertion linked to valine at codon 129. *Brain* 2012;**135**:1–4.

329. Sandeberg MK, Al-Doujaily H, Sharps B, *et al.* Prion propagation and toxicity *in vivo* occur in two distinct mechanistic phases. *Nature* 2011;**470**:540–2.

330. Santuccione A, Sytnyk V, Leshchyns'ka I, *et al.* Prion protein recruits its neuronal receptor NCAM to lipid rafts to activate p59fyn and to enhance neurite outgrowth. *J Cell Biol* 2005;**169**:341–54.

331. Schoch G, Seeger H, Bogousslavsky J, *et al.* Analysis of prion strains by PrP^{Sc} profiling in sporadic Creutzfeldt–Jakob disease. *PLoS Med* 2006;**3**:e14.

332. Schroter A, Zerr I, Henkel K, *et al.* Magnetic resonance imaging in the clinical diagnosis of Creutzfeldt–Jakob disease. *Arch Neurol* 2000;**57**:1751–7.

333. Scott MR, Will R, Ironside J, *et al.* Compelling transgenetic evidence for transmission of bovine spongiform encephalopathy prions to humans. *Proc Natl Acad Sci U S A* 1999;**96**:15137–42.

334. Shi Q, Chen C, Song XN, *et al.* A Chinese Creutzfeldt–Jakob disease patient with E196K mutation in *PRNP*. *Prion* 2011;**5**:117–20.

335. Shimizu S, Hoshi KI, Muramoto T, *et al.* Creutzfeldt–Jakob disease with florid-type plaques after cadaveric dura mater grafting. *Arch Neurol* 1999;**56**:357–62.

336. Si K, Lindquist S, Kandel ER. A neuronal isoform of the aplysia CPEB has prion like properties. *Cell* 2003;**115**:879–91.

337. Sigurdson CJ. A prion disease of cervids: chronic wasting disease. *Vet Res* 2008;**39**:41.

338. Silvestrini MC, Cardone F, Maras B, *et al.* Identification of the prion protein allotypes which accumulate in the brain of sporadic and familial Creutzfeldt–Jakob disease patients. *Nat Med* 1997;**3**:521–5.

339. Simmons MM, Konold T, Simmons HA, *et al.* Experimental transmission of atypical scrapie to sheep. *BMC Vet Res* 2007;**3**:20.

340. Simpson M, Johanssen V, Boyd A, *et al.* Unusual clinical and molecular-pathogenic

profile of Gerstmann–Sträussler–Scheinker disease associated with a novel *PRNP* mutation (V176G). *JAMA Neurol* 2013;**70**:1180–1185.

341. Siso S, Jeffrey M, Gonzalez L. Neuroinvasion in sheep transmissible spongiform encephalopathies: the role of the haematogenous route. *Neuropath Appl Neurobiol* 2009;**35**:232–46.

342. Siso S, Chianini F, Eaton S, *et al.* Disease phenotype in sheep after infection with cloned murine scrapie strains. *Prion* 2012;**6**:176–85.

343. Smith PG, Bradley R. Bovine spongiform encephalopathy (BSE) and its epidemiology. *Br Med Bull* 2003;**66**:185–98.

344. Spielmeyer W. *Histopathologie des nervensystems.* Berlin: Springer, 1922.

345. Stewart LA, Rydzewska LH, Keogh GF, Knight RS. Systematic review of therapeutic interventions in human prion diseases. *Neurology* 2008;**70**:1272–81.

346. Swerdlow AJ, Higgins CD, Adlard P, *et al.* Creutzfeldt–Jakob disease in United Kingdom patients treated with human pituitary growth hormone. *Neurology* 2003;**61**:783–91.

347. Tagliavini F, Prelli F, Ghiso J, Bugiani O, *et al.* Amyloid protein of Gerstmann–Sträussler–Scheinker disease (Indiana kindred) is an 11 kd fragment of prion protein with an N-terminal glycine at codon 58. *EMBO J* 1991;**10**:513–19.

348. Tagliavini F, Prelli F, Porro M, *et al.* Amyloid fibrils in Gerstmann–Sträussler–Scheinker disease (Indiana and Swedish kindreds) express only PrP peptides encoded by the mutant allele. *Cell* 1994;**7**:695–703.

349. Tagliavini F, Forloni G, D'Ursi P, *et al.* Studies on peptide fragments of prion proteins. *Adv Protein Chem* 2001;**57**:171–201.

350. Tagliavini F, Lievens PM, Tranchant C, *et al.* A 7-kDa prion protein (PrP) fragment, an integral component of the PrP region required for infectivity, is the major amyloid protein in Gerstmann–Sträussler–Scheinker disease A117V. *J Biol Chem* 2001;**276**:6009–15.

351. Tartaglia MC, Thai JN, See T, *et al.* Pathologic evidence that the T188R mutation in *PRNP* is associated with prion disease. *J Neuropathol Exp Neurol* 2010;**69**:1220–7.

352. Taylor DM. Inactivation of transmissible degenerative encephalopathy agents. A review. *Vet J* 2000;**159**:10–17.

353. Taylor DM. Inactivation of TSE agents: safety of blood and blood-derived products. *Transfus Clin Biol* 2003;**10**:23–5.

354. Taylor DM. Preventing accidental transmission of human transmissible spongiform encephalopathies. *Br Med Bull* 2003;**66**:293–303.

355. Terry LA, Marsh S, Ryder SJ, *et al.* Detection of disease-specific PrP in the distal ileum of cattle exposed orally to the agent of bovine spongiform encephalopathy. *Vet Rec* 2003;**152**:387–92.

356. Thackray AM, McKenzie AN, Klein MA, *et al.* Accelerated prion disease in the absence of interleukin-10. *J Virol* 2004;**78**:13697–707.

357. Todd NV, Morrow J, Doh-Ura K, *et al.* Cerebroventricular infusion of pentosan polysulphate in human variant Creutzfeldt–Jakob disease. *J Infect* 2005;**50**:394–6.

358. Trevitt CR, Collinge J. A systematic review of prion therapeutics in experimental models. *Brain* 2006;**129**:2241–65.

359. Tsuboi Y, Doh-Ura K, Yamada T. Continuous intraventricular infusion of pentosan polysulfate: clinical trial against prion disease. *Neuropathology* 2009;**29**:632–6.

360. Tuite MF, Serio TR. The prion hypothesis: from biological anomaly to basic regulatory mechanism. *Nat Rev Mol Cell Biol* 2010;**11**:823–33.

361. Tunnell E, Wollman R, Mallik S, *et al.* A novel *PRNP*–P105S mutation associated with atypical prion disease and a rare PrPSc conformation. *Neurology* 2008;**71**:1431–8.

362. Valleron A–J, Boelle P–Y, Will R, Cesbron J–Y. Estimation of epidemic size and incubation time based on age characteristics of vCJD in the United Kingdom. *Science* 2001;**294**:1726–8.

363. Vital A, Laplanche JL, Bastard JR, *et al.* A case of Gerstmann–Sträussler–Scheinker disease with a novel six octapeptide repeat insertion. *Neuropathol Applied Neurobiol* 2011;**37**:554–9.

364. Wadsworth JD, Joiner S, Hill AF, *et al.* Tissue distribution of protease resistant prion protein in variant Creutzfeldt–Jakob disease using a highly sensitive immunoblotting assay. *Lancet* 2001;**358**:171–80.

365. Wadsworth JD, Joiner S, Linehan JM, *et al.* Phenotypic heterogeneity in inherited prion disease (P102L) is associated with differential propagation protease-resistant wild-type and mutant prion. *Brain* 2006;**129**:1557–69.

366. Wadsworth JD, Joiner S, Linehan JM, *et al.* Kuru prions and sporadic Creutzfeldt–Jakob disease prions have equivalent transmission properties in transgenic and wild-type mice. *Proc Natl Acad Sci U S A* 2008;**105**:3885–90.

367. Wang XF, Guo YJ, Zhang BY, *et al.* Creutzfeldt–Jakob disease in a patient with a novel seven-repeat insertion in *PRNP. J Neurol Neurosurg Psychiatry* 2007;**78**:201–3.

368. Wang F, Wang X, Yuan CG, Ma J. Generating a prion with bacterially expressed recombinant prion protein. *Science* 2010;**327**:1132–5.

369. Ward HJT, Everington D, Croes EA, *et al.* Sporadic Creutzfeldt–Jakob disease and surgery: a case–control study using community controls. *Neurology* 2002;**59**:543–8.

370. Ward HJT, Everington D, Cousens SN, *et al.* Risk factors for variant Creutzfeldt–Jakob disease:a case–control study. *Ann Neurol* 2006;**59**:111–20.

371. Wells GA, Wilesmith JW. The neuropathology and epidemiology of bovine spongiform encephalopathy. *Brain Pathol* 1995;**5**:91–103.

372. Wells GA, Scott AC, Johnson CT, *et al.* A novel progressive spongiform encephalopathy in cattle. *Vet Rec* 1987;**121**:419–20.

373. Westaway D, DeArmond SJ, Cayetano-Canlas J, *et al.* Degeneration of skeletal muscle, peripheral nerves and the central nervous system in transgenic mice overexpressing wild-type prion proteins. *Cell* 1994;**76**:117–29.

374. Whittle IR, Will RG, Ironside JW. Brain biopsy and patients with atypical

presentations of sporadic Creutzfeldt–Jakob disease. *J Neurol Neurosurg Psychiatry* 1997;**63**:547–8.

375. Whittle IR, Knight RS, Will RG. Unsuccessful intraventricular pentosan polysulphate treatement of variant Creutzfeldt–Jakob disease. *Acta Neurochir (Wien)* 2006;**148**:677–9.

376. Wientjens DPWM, Davanipour Z, Hofman A, *et al.* Risk factors for Creutzfeldt–Jakob disease: a reanalysis of case–control studies. *Neurology* 1996;**46**:1287–91.

377. Wieser HG, Schindler K, Zumsteg D. EEG in Creutzfeldt–Jakob disease. *Clin Neurophysiol* 2006;**117**:935–51.

378. Will RG, Matthews WB. Evidence for case-to-case transmission of Creutzfeldt–Jakob disease. *J Neurol Neurosurg Psychiatry* 1982;**45**:235–238.

379. Will RG, Matthews WB. A retrospective study of Creutzfeldt–Jakob disease in England and Wales 1970–79. I: clinical features. *J Neurol Neurosurg Psychiatry* 1984;**47**:134–40.

380. Will RG, Ironside JW, Zeidler M, *et al.* A new variant Creutzfeldt–Jakob disease in the UK. *Lancet* 1996;**347**:921–5.

381. Will RG, Zeidler M, Brown P, *et al.* Cerebrospinal fluid test for new variant Creutzfeldt–Jakob disease. *Lancet* 1996;**348**:955–6.

382. Will RG, Stewart G, Zeidler M, *et al.* Psychiatric features of new variant Creutzfeldt–Jakob disease. *Psychiatric Bull* 1999;**23**:264–67.

383. Will RG, Zeidler M, Stewart GE, *et al.* Diagnosis of new variant Creutzfeldt–Jakob disease. *Ann Neurol* 2000;**47**:575–82.

384. Williams ES. Chronic wasting disease. *Vet Pathol* 2005;**42**:530–49.

385. Williams ES, Young S. Chronic wasting disease of captive mule deer: a spongiform encephalopathy. *J Wildlife Dis* 1980;**16**:89–8.

386. Wilson R, Plinston C, Hunter N, *et al.* Chronic wasting disease and atypical forms of BSE and scrapie are not transmissible to mice expressing wild-type levels of human PrP. *J Gen Virol* 2012;**93**;1624–9.

387. World Health Organization. *WHO infection control guidelines for transmissible spongiform encephalopathies.* http://who.int/csr/resources/publications/bse/whocdscsraph2003.pdf.

388. Wroe SJ, Pal S, Siddique D, *et al.* Clinical presentation and pre-mortem diagnosis of variant Creutzfeldt–Jakob disease associated with blood transfusion: a case report. *Lancet* 2006;**368**:2061–7.

389. Yamada M. The first Japanese case of variant Creutzfeldt–Jakob disease showing periodic electroencephalogram. *Lancet* 2006;**367**:874.

390. Yamada M, Itoh Y, Inaba A, *et al.* An inherited prion disease with a PrP P105L mutation: clinicopathologic and PrP heterogeneity. *Neurology* 1999;**53**:181–8.

391. Young K, Clark HB, Piccardo P, *et al.* Gerstmann–Sträussler–Scheinker disease with the *PRNP* P102L mutation and valine at codon 129. *Mol Brain Res* 1997;**44**:147–50.

392. Yuan J, Xiao X, McGeehan J, *et al.* Insoluble aggregates and protease-resistant conformers of prion protein in uninfected human brains. *J Biol Chem* 2006;**281**:34848–58.

393. Yull HM, Ritchie DL, Langeveld JP, *et al.* Detection of type 1 prion protein in variant Creutzfeldt–Jakob disease. *Am J Pathol* 2006;**168**:151–7.

394. Zahn R, Liu A, Luhrs T, *et al.* NMR solution structure of the human prion protein. *Proc Natl Acad Sci U S A* 2000;**97**:145–50.

395. Zanusso G, Ferrari S, Cardone F, *et al.* Detection of pathologic prion protein in the olfactory epithelium in sporadic Creutzfeldt–Jakob disease. *N Engl J Med* 2003;**348**:711–19.

396. Zeidler M, Johnstone EC, Bamber RWK, *et al.* New variant Creutzfeldt–Jakob disease: psychiatric features. *Lancet* 1997;**350**:908–10.

397. Zeidler M, Stewart G, Cousens SN, *et al.* Codon 129 genotype and new variant CJD. *Lancet* 1997;**350**:668.

398. Zerr I, Pocchiari M, Collins S, *et al.* Analysis of EEG and CSF 14-3-3 proteins as aids to the diagnosis of Creutzfeldt–Jakob disease. *Neurology* 2000;**55**: 811–15.

399. Zerr I, Kallenberg K, Summers DM, *et al.* Updated clinical diagnostic criteria for sporadic Creutzfeldt–Jakob disease. *Brain* 2009;**132**:2659–68.

400. Zhang H, Wang M, Wu L, *et al.* Novel prion protein gene mutation at codon 196 (E196A) in a septuagenarian with Creutzfeldt–Jakob disease. *J Clin Neurosci* 2014;**21**:175–178.

401. Zou WQ, Puoti G, Xiao X, *et al.* Variably protease-sensitive prionopathy: a new sporadic disease of the prion protein. *Ann Neurol* 2010;**68**: 162–72.

Viral Infections

Seth Love, Clayton A Wiley and Sebastian Lucas

INTRODUCTION

This chapter consists of three sections. The first is an introductory section entitled 'General Principles', which includes a general overview of neurovirology and a brief review of some of the stereotyped pathological processes and main patterns of viral infection of the central nervous system (CNS). The next two sections cover first the acute and then the subacute and chronic viral infections. Viral taxonomy provides an organizational framework for these two sections, which contain descriptions of the diseases caused by individual viruses. The descriptions mostly follow a standard format: some background or historical information, followed by an account of the structure of the virus, the epidemiology and pathogenesis of the infection, the clinical features, and the gross and microscopic neuropathological findings. Although logical, this organization has limitations for use in diagnosis; an individual virus may mediate several different types of neurological disease, and, conversely, some of the neurological diseases that are described in this chapter can be caused by more than one virus (or can have both viral and non-viral aetiologies). To address these limitations, the first section of this chapter includes a summary of the principal patterns of viral disease of the CNS and their causes; in subsequent sections, boxes and tables are used to provide information about clinical syndromes that can be caused by several different viruses.

GENERAL PRINCIPLES

Viral Taxonomy

The first system of classifying viruses was based on the species of the infected host and on the associated disease (e.g. hepatitis). With the advent of electron microscopy, this system gave way to a scheme based on the morphological features of the nucleocapsid. The current system of classification is based principally upon the composition and organization of the genetic material.

The International Committee on Taxonomy of Viruses has classified viruses in the following nested categories: families, subfamilies, genera and species.[140] The type of nucleic acid (RNA or DNA) and the presence or absence of an envelope determine the main viral families (Table 19.1). Of the 79 known viral families, 26 infect vertebrates but only a dozen or so contain members that cause CNS disease through direct infection.

Viruses can be subclassified further into serogroups on the basis of the host immune humoral response to the principal viral structural proteins. Although still in use, serological typing is increasingly giving way to molecular definition of viral strains. With the capacity to synthesize recombinant viruses has come the problem of subclassifying the rapidly increasing number of resulting viral strains. There is no universally accepted terminological scheme for these new laboratory constructs.

Biochemical and Biophysical Properties

Viral nucleic acids are contained exclusively within a genome composed of either RNA or DNA. This definition excludes eukaryotic organisms and most microbes, which contain both RNA and DNA, and excludes prions, the replication of which probably does not involve nucleic acids (see Chapter 18).

Viral nucleic acids exist in a variety of forms: linear, circular, segmented, and double- and single-stranded. To a large degree, the physical structure of the genetic material determines the agent's replicative strategy. After entry into the cell cytoplasm, viruses with positive-stranded RNA can immediately use the cellular machinery to synthesize viral proteins. Viruses with genomes composed of DNA

TABLE 19.1 Viral infections of the central nervous system (CNS): classification of viruses

Viral genome	Family name of virus	Family member infecting the CNS	Scale diagram of virus
Double-stranded DNA	Herpesviridae	HSV-1 (HHV-1)	
		HSV-2 (HHV-2)	
		Varicella-zoster virus (HHV-3)	
		Cytomegalovirus (HHV-5)	
		Epstein–Barr virus (HHV-4)	
		Human herpesvirus 6 (HHV-6)	
		Human herpesvirus 7 (HHV-7)	
		Human herpesvirus 8 (HHV-8)	
		Herpes simiae (B-virus)	
	Adenoviridae	Adenovirus	
	Papovaviridae	Simian virus 40	
		JC virus	
Single-stranded DNA	Parvoviridae	Parvovirus B19	
Double-stranded RNA	Reoviridae	Coltivirus (Colorado tick fever)	
		Seadornavirus (Banna)	
Single-stranded sense non-segmented RNA	Retroviridaea	Deltaretrovirus (HTLV-1, HTLV-2)	
		Lentivirus (HIV-1, HIV-2)	
	Coronaviridae	Coronavirus (JC virus)	
	Togaviridae	Alphavirus (EEE, WEE, VEE, Chikungunya, Semliki Forest)	
		Rubivirus (rubella)	
Viral genome	Family name of virus	Family member infecting the CNS	
	Flaviviridaea	Flavivirus (JE, SLE, MVE, Kunjin, Rocio, TBE, West Nile, Louping ill, Dengue, Omsk, Kayasnur Fores , Wesselbron, Ilheus, Usutu, Rio Bravo, yellow fever)	
	Picornaviridae	Enterovirus (polioviruses, group A coxsackie, group B coxsackie, echovirus, enterovirus) Human parechovirus	

TABLE 19.1 Viral infections of the central nervous system (CNS): classification of viruses *(Continued)*

Viral genome	Family name of virus	Family member infecting the CNS	Scale diagram of virus
Single-stranded antisense segmented RNA	Bunyaviridae	Orthobunyavirus (La Crosse)	
		Phlebovirus (Rift Valley fever)	
	Arenaviridae	Arenavirus (LCMV)	
Single-stranded antisense non-segmented RNA	Orthomyxovirusa	Influenza viruses	
	Paramyxoviridae	Henipavirus (Hendra, Nipah)	
		Morbillivirus (measles)	
		Rubulavirus (mumps)	
	Rhabdoviridae	Rabies	
		Borna	
	Filoviridae	Ebola	

EEE, eastern equine encephalitis; HHV, human herpes virus; HIV, human immunodeficiency virus; HSV, herpes simplex virus; HTLV, human T-cell leukaemia/lymphoma virus; JE, Japanese encephalitis; LCMV, lymphocytic choriomeningitis virus; MVE, Murray Valley encephalitis; SLE, St Louis encephalitis; TBE, tick-borne encephalitis; VEE, Venezuelan equine encephalomyelitis; WEE, western equine encephalitis.
Adapted from Johnson R. *Viral infections of the nervous system*. Philadelphia: Lippincott-Raven, 1998.

must be transported into the nucleus in order to initiate transcription.

Most viral genomes are complexed with a protein nucleocapsid, in an economical modular structure. Electron microscopy reveals a myriad of nucleocapsid forms and sizes (see Table 19.1). All are composed of self-assembling subunits that encapsulate the viral genome. The nucleocapsid not only acts as a protective shell, shielding the nucleic acids from the environment, but, for many viruses, also directs the entry, unpacking and intracellular transport of viral nucleic acids.

Although the nucleocapsid is essential for non-enveloped viruses to bind to cell surface receptors, other viruses have delegated these surface interactions to protein ligands incorporated within a lipid bilayer envelope. The lipids of the envelope are derived from host cell membranes, whereas the virus encodes the ligands. Apart from their role in viral attachment to the cell surface, some viral envelope proteins promote fusion of the viral envelope and cytoplasmic membrane and are crucial to the entry of viral nucleic acids from the virion into the cell.

Once within the cell cytoplasm, different viruses have evolved a diverse range of strategies to complete their replication. Sense-stranded RNA viruses can complex with cellular ribosomes to synthesize viral proteins and, subsequently, nucleic acids. The replication of other forms of virus may require the introduction into the host cell of accessory viral proteins in addition to the nucleic acids. Because no host cell protein can reverse-transcribe RNA into DNA, retroviruses must bring this enzyme into the cell to support infection.

General Strategies of Viral Replication

The strategies of viral replication can be conveniently divided into two parts: (1) infection of, and replication within, individual cells and (2) spread to new cells and new hosts. Investigations in cell biology and biochemistry have substantially elucidated the mechanisms of viral infection of host cells. Although the process varies somewhat for different viruses, in broad outline the replication cycle of all viruses follows a stereotypical sequence of adsorption, penetration, uncoating, transcription, translation, replication, assembly and budding. However, elucidating the mechanisms of viral spread to new cells (and hosts) presents a continuing challenge and involves almost the entire gamut of biological sciences.

Infection and Replication

The first barrier to infection of the host cell is the cell surface—a complex array of lipids, proteins and carbohydrates whose electrical charge repels the approach of similarly charged surfaces. For the virus to infect a cell, it must first attach itself to the cell surface. It achieves this by exploiting the fact that cells, particularly those of multicellular organisms, communicate with and attach to neighbouring cells by means of specific surface molecules. These are used as viral receptors, the viruses having nucleocapsid or envelope ligands that are complementary to the particular host cell surface molecules. The presence of these complementary molecules on the surface of the virus and its target host cell greatly increases the probability that a chance encounter between virus and cell will lead to adsorption of the virus to the cell surface and subsequent infection of the cell. Once attached to the cell surface, the virus inserts its genetic material into the cell by co-opting normal cellular processes (e.g. endocytosis), by the action of unique fusogenic viral proteins or by a combination of these processes (e.g. by the action of fusogenic viral proteins that are activated upon entry into the low-pH environment of lysosomal vesicles).

One of the most enigmatic phases in the lifecycle of some viruses begins after entry of the genome and before replication commences. Rather than starting replication immediately, some viruses (e.g. herpesviruses) may enter variable periods of latency. Precisely what occurs during viral latency is not understood well and differs between viruses.

After entry into the cell, the viral genes must be transported to the appropriate intracellular locations for transcription and replication. Depending on the nature of the viral genetic material, this may require direct transport to the nucleus (for DNA viruses), transport to the nucleus only after a cytoplasmic interregnum during which the viral RNA genome is reverse-transcribed into DNA (in the case of retroviruses), or transport to the rough endoplasmic reticulum. For single-stranded RNA viruses, the orientation of the viral genome relative to coding mRNA has significant implications for subsequent replication steps. RNA viruses with genomes in an antisense orientation must contain an RNA-dependent RNA polymerase to synthesize the sense strand required for translation of RNA into viral proteins.

Most viruses do not simply share the cellular machinery for transcription and translation but actively inhibit the cell's use of this machinery, the better to direct it to viral replication. Viral replication can occur at the expense of the cell (as in lytic infection) or can progress in a more controlled fashion, compatible with prolonged survival of the host cell. For non-enveloped viruses, release from the cell usually requires cytolysis, whereas enveloped viruses acquire their envelope by actively budding from cell membranes. Budding is not a random process, but rather a carefully orchestrated part of the replication cycle. The precise site of budding determines not only the coat envelope proteins but also the route of subsequent viral dispersion. It is likely that by co-opting specific intracellular transport mechanisms, viruses can target their release to regions advantageous for their subsequent spread (e.g. from the apical surface of epithelial cells for entry into a gland lumen or release into the external environment, or from the basal surface for entry into the bloodstream).

Spread within the Host or Spread to New Hosts

Lacking any form of motility, viruses depend upon host and environmental factors for spreading both within and between hosts. Most viral infections begin with inoculation of only a minute quantity of infectious particles. To secure infection of the new host, this inoculum is usually expanded by an initial round of viral replication at the site of entry. Several routes are then available for dissemination within the host. The most common of these is haematogenous. Viraemia is established by passive leakage of locally accumulated virions or by active transfer of virus into the bloodstream (e.g. by polarized budding of the virus). The lymphatics offer a second avenue of dissemination, usually through the movement of infected leukocytes. The virus that causes acquired immunodeficiency syndrome (AIDS), human immunodeficiency virus (HIV), not only uses the latter mode of transport for systemic dissemination, but also, through the trafficking of infected monocytes, may achieve a 'Trojan horse' entry into the CNS (see Human Immunodeficiency Viruses).

A third route of viral transport into the CNS uses the inherent connectivity of the nervous system: small amounts of virus enter peripheral nerve processes and exploit axonal retrograde and anterograde transport to achieve entry into the brain. Intracellular transport has several advantages over extracellular transport. Within the cell, viruses are protected from the environment and from many host defences, the immune system in particular. Because transport within the axon is accurate and efficient, small amounts of virus are able to achieve rapid, targeted dissemination. Once within the CNS, the virus may continue to be transported within neurites and across synapses (trans-synaptic spread) or, after further replication, may enter and be disseminated by the cerebrospinal fluid (CSF).

In spreading between hosts, viruses use a variety of strategies to circumvent a harsh environment that would otherwise rapidly cause their inactivation: drying can destroy viral ligands and enzymic proteins, whereas low pH and ultraviolet (UV) light damage viral nucleic acids. The structure of some non-enveloped virions provides resilience against specific environmental hazards (e.g. by conferring acid stability to viruses that pass through the stomach). Adsorption of the virus to a variety of materials and surfaces (fomites), and exploitation of their biophysical properties, may protect it from damaging environmental effects such as drying. The indiscriminate release in respiratory secretions or faeces of massive amounts of virus increases the chances of one infectious virion finding a portal into a new host. More discriminant transfer may be mediated by the release of virus into bodily fluids such as saliva and semen, which are exchanged between hosts with minimal external environmental contact and dilution. Arboviruses occupy a unique ecological niche, employing an insect vector to effect their transfer in viraemic blood, without exposure to the external environment. Changes in host behaviour have led to 'unnatural' means of viral spread in which environmental hurdles are bypassed through novel means of exchange of infectious materials (e.g. blood transfusions, organ transplantation and the sharing of needles for intravenous drug abuse). In addition to achieving horizontal spread within a host community, some viruses have developed the means to spread vertically from parent to offspring. In mammals, the relationship between mother and child provides potential avenues of transmission across the placenta, within the birth canal and through breast milk.

Maintenance of Infection within the Population

As relevant to viral infections as the factors sustaining the virus within a host are the factors that sustain the virus within the host population. Each virus occupies a unique ecological niche. Viruses can be endemic (i.e. present continuously within a population) with or without mediating significant disease. Epidemics arise when a large proportion of a population that has not been infected previously is suddenly exposed to a pathogenic virus (or strain of virus) for the first time. Many viruses sustain endemic infections by continuous horizontal spread to naive hosts. Viruses can also maintain endemic infection by vertical spread, through materno-fetal routes. A further means of vertical spread, germline transmission, has been well documented in murine systems, but to date has not been observed in humans. In temperate climates, arboviruses have evolved several novel means of maintaining endemic infection and surviving the winter (overwintering), by transovarial (virus passed to eggs) or trans-stadial (virus passed from larvae to nymphs) infection of the insect vector.

The Immune Response and Viral Infections of the Central Nervous System

Viral infection initiates a contest between the replicating virus and an immune response aimed at abrogating the infection. In some cases, a curious symbiosis develops between the two contestants, but most infections proceed to the demise of either virus or host. The virus uses a range of molecular strategies for usurping the host cell machinery and energy and achieving rapid replication. The host counters with an intricate system of defences that can be divided broadly into innate and adaptive immune responses. The following is but a brief account of the interaction between viruses that infect the CNS and key elements of the immune response. A detailed description of the immune response in the CNS is beyond the scope of this chapter. Where relevant, aspects of the immune response that are peculiar to individual viruses are noted in the section on that virus.

The Innate Immune Response

Its immediacy and relatively 'uneducated' nature distinguish innate from adaptive immunity (Box 19.1). Physical barriers are important first-line defences against viral infections. The intact epidermis is impervious to most infectious agents and its continually shedding, acellular, keratinized outer layer is a particularly hostile environment for intracellular pathogens. The gastrointestinal and respiratory secretions contain chemicals that trap and inactivate pathogens. The nervous system has evolved a blood–brain barrier that prevents the ingress of many blood-borne infectious and toxic agents. Unfortunately, the blood–brain barrier also limits the access of some of the host defences against infection; for example under normal circumstances, immunoglobulin and complement levels are much lower in the CSF than in the blood. The degree to which the blood–brain barrier limits cellular immunity is still open to question. The brain lacks lymphatics but it does not necessarily follow that this limits cellular immune surveillance. Although transplantation experiments have suggested that the brain is, to some extent, an immunologically restricted or privileged environment, the blood–brain barrier does not seem to curtail the immune response to most infections of the CNS.

Other contributors to the innate immune response are neutrophils, haematogenous and tissue macrophages, and natural killer cells. These cells are rapidly mobilized to sites of infection and release many chemicals, including proteases and nucleases, that create an inhospitable microenvironment for viral replication and spread. This non-specific response has the advantage that it can be mustered within hours. Of course, it also has the disadvantage of being non-specific in nature and, were it not locally contained, would be highly detrimental to the host. Further non-specific defence is provided by interferons. These are synthesized by most cells in response to viral infection and interfere with the synthesis of viral genes. The objective of all of these elements of the innate response is to slow down viral

---

BOX 19.1. Innate immunity

Within the past decade, there has been an explosion of knowledge regarding the responses of individual cells to threats in general and viral infection in particular. Cellular innate immunity involves first the sensing of the threat (the recognition of non-self or altered-self structures) and then the metabolic response. The former process is mediated by cellular receptors that recognize pathogen-associated molecular patterns (PAMPs) and damage-associated molecular patterns (DAMPs) (for review see Ross,[968] Takeuchi et al.[1108] and Gordon[391]).

The sensing of threats at cell membranes depends largely on Toll-like receptors (TLRs), which have an extracellular or intraluminal ligand-binding domain consisting of leucine-rich repeat regions (LRRs) capable of detecting specific PAMPs/DAMPs, such as those of viruses or virus-infected cells. The types and distributions of different TLRs vary according to their function. Those on the surface of the cell detect surface pathogens whereas TLRs on internal membranes (e.g. lysosomes) are adapted to detecting endosomal pathogens. Intracellular signalling is mediated by the Toll/IL-1 receptor cytoplasmic domain through the recruitment of adaptor proteins, leading to activation of protein kinases, transcription factors and eventual gene transcription (for example, of IL-1β and IL-18).

TLRs are not the only sensing component of the innate immune response. Cytoplasmic receptors such as retinoic acid-inducible gene (RIG)-I-like receptors (RLRs) and nuclear oligomerization domain (NOD)-like receptors (NLRs) are also key components of the innate immune response. Unlike TLRs, they are exclusively cytoplasmic and recognize cytosolic viruses and bacterial products. Like TLRs, however, they contain LRRs capable of binding many different ligands. After binding specific ligands, NLRs recruit additional cytoplasmic proteins to form a multiprotein complex known as an inflammasome, that is capable of activating caspase-1. Caspase-1 then cleaves cellular proteins such as those transcribed by TLR activation (e.g. IL-1β and IL-18) to their active forms that, upon secretion, contribute to the inflammatory cascade.

replication and thereby give the adaptive immune response enough time to remove the virus selectively, before infection has progressed too far. Patients with specific deficiencies in innate immunity (e.g. deficient TLR-3) are particularly prone to HSV-1 infection.[994,1270]

The Adaptive Immune Response

The adaptive immune response comes into effect only after the immune system has been primed or 'educated' to react to the invading pathogen (or to antigenic determinants of that pathogen) and is directed specifically against it. Once educated, the adaptive response exhibits memory and is mounted more rapidly if confronted for a second time with the same pathogen; hence, the utility of vaccinations. Historically, the adaptive response has been divided into humoral and cellular components, although it is now recognized that these are closely interrelated. The initial priming of the immune response takes days to weeks. During this time, antigen-presenting cells (APCs), such as macrophages and dendritic cells, migrate to lymph nodes and present viral antigens, in conjunction with specific co-stimulatory signals, to particular subpopulations of lymphocytes. Lymphocytes with the capacity to recognize the specific antigenic determinants of the virus, when presented together with the co-stimulatory signal from the APCs, are induced to proliferate and influence the properties of other lymphocytes and also of nearby cells other than lymphocytes (such as endothelial cells and macrophages) and can thereby augment or limit the immune response. After they have proliferated, and under the influence of cytokines released by helper T-lymphocytes, activated B-lymphocytes differentiate into plasma cells and synthesize antibodies that target and in some cases neutralize the virus. Specific populations of cytotoxic T-lymphocytes, which recognize and destroy infected cells before the virus can replicate and spread, are also expanded.

The outcome of infection is, to a large extent, determined by the speed and effectiveness of the immune response. Although much has been elucidated about the factors that initiate and regulate the response, much remains to be determined, especially about the mechanisms for halting the response after the virus has been eliminated and before substantial host damage occurs. Once educated, the immune system is usually highly effective in preventing reinfection. Unfortunately, some viruses adapt by mutating, so that critical antigenic determinants are no longer recognized by antibodies or lymphocytes primed to react to the virus in its initial guise and therefore infection by the new mutants is possible. This phenomenon is illustrated well by the influenza virus, which mutates to cause epidemics with disturbing frequency. Other viruses, such as HIV, mutate so rapidly that new strains evolve repeatedly during the course of a single infection.

Innate and Adaptive Immunity within the Central Nervous System

As noted already, the bulk of the CNS is protected by the blood–brain barrier. Immediately adjacent to the blood–brain barrier, and also in the brain parenchyma away from the blood vessels, are numerous APCs (microglia)

capable of identifying infectious agents and initiating an immune response. Elegant experiments in rodents have demonstrated that activated lymphocytes enter and exit the nervous system with a high frequency.[572,829] Once these activated cells encounter their target antigen in the appropriate context, an intense immune cascade is initiated. Locally elaborated cytokines induce the expression of adhesion molecules on the surface of endothelial cells and the further recruitment of innate and adaptive immune-response cells. Inflammatory mediators soon disrupt the blood–brain barrier, allowing the immune response to proceed unimpeded.

Timely termination of the immune response is of particular importance in the CNS, where oedema and other bystander effects of inflammation can be more damaging than the infection itself. The most common forms of therapeutic intervention in neurovirology are concerned with limiting both the acute immune response and viral replication. A further hazard of some viral infections is their potential to initiate a cascade of autoimmune responses that may continue to damage the host nervous system even after the virus has been eliminated. During the primary immune reaction, lymphocytes may be activated by viral antigens that resemble normal constituents of the CNS (so-called molecular mimicry). This may provoke an autoimmune response to those same constituents. Alternatively, the inflammatory response may expose host antigens that were previously hidden from the immune system and are capable of eliciting an autoimmune response. Such mechanisms have been invoked to explain post-viral acute disseminated encephalomyelitis (Box 19.2, Table 19.2) and multiple sclerosis (see Chapter 23).

BOX 19.2. Acute disseminated encephalomyelitis and viral infections

Acute disseminated encephalomyelitis (ADEM) is a multifocal inflammatory disorder of the central nervous system (CNS), characterized histologically by acute perivenular inflammation and demyelination. It is usually preceded by a systemic viral, mycoplasma or bacterial infection or, more rarely, by vaccination, and it is believed to be due to a T-cell-mediated hypersensitivity reaction. The pathogenesis, clinical features and pathological findings are discussed in detail in Chapter 23.

Infections by many different viruses have been reported to precede ADEM, but a small number stand out as being implicated most commonly (Table 19.2). In general, the frequency is very much less after vaccination than after infection with wild-type virus.

Acute disseminated encephalomyelitis has been associated rarely with Epstein–Barr virus (EBV)[751,1040] and parainfluenza virus type 3 infection,[743] with influenza vaccination[267,931,992,1197] and with vaccination with inactivated Japanese encephalitis (JE) virus prepared from infected mouse brain.[347a] Acute disseminated encephalomyelitis occurs in approximately 1 in 200–20,00 patients given inactivated rabies vaccines made from the brain tissue of adult animals and 1 in 8000 patients given suckling mouse brain vaccine, but this complication can be prevented by the use of cell culture-derived rabies vaccines.[982, 460a] Acute disseminated encephalomyelitis probably occurred in some patients with smallpox and affected a significant proportion of patients immunized with vaccinia.

TABLE 19.2 Acute disseminated encephalomyelitis and viral infections

Virus	Approximate relative frequency of acute disseminated encephalomyelitis (ADEM)	Reference
Measles	1:1000	
Measles vaccine	1:2 000 000	167
Mumps	1:1000	621,667
Mumps vaccine	0.4:1 000 000	171
Rubella	1:5000–10.000	68
Rubella vaccine	Probably not associated with ADEM	
Varicella	Approximately 1:10 000	539a, 1035a

Diagnosis of Viral Infections of the Central Nervous System

The signs and symptoms of most viral infections of the CNS are relatively non-specific and are attributable largely to the inflammatory reaction rather than the virus itself: severe headache, stiff neck and fever usually signify meningitis; nausea and vomiting are indicators of elevated intracranial pressure; alterations in the level of consciousness tend to occur with progression to frank encephalitis. With some exceptions, such as poliomyelitis and herpes simplex encephalitis, localizing neurological signs are unusual and their relationship to particular viruses inconsistent. The development of a rash, myositis or arthritis may suggest viral infection, but most systemic manifestations are non-specific (e.g. fever, elevated peripheral blood leukocyte count). Serology is of value for retrospective diagnosis, but it is rarely helpful in the acute stage; assays for virus-specific immunoglobulin M (IgM) antibodies may support a diagnosis of recent infection, but a positive serological diagnosis usually requires comparison of antiviral titres during the acute infection with those during convalescence, typically 2–3 weeks later.

During infection, examination of CSF obtained by lumbar puncture is often informative. In viral meningitis, CSF protein is usually elevated and there is a modest pleocytosis, characteristically lymphocytic, although neutrophils may be present in the early stages. Cerebrospinal fluid glucose is usually normal, and this, together with the modest degree of pleocytosis and paucity of neutrophils, tends to distinguish viral meningitides from other microbial infections of the CNS, although there are many exceptions to this general rule. For many years, viral culture of CSF was a mainstay of diagnosis. However, for routine diagnosis of viral infections, culture has largely been supplanted by polymerase chain reaction (PCR) amplification of viral nucleic acids. Neuroimaging studies are useful to exclude abscesses, neoplasms and other non-viral processes, and the demonstration of focal abnormalities in the temporal and frontal lobes may help in diagnosing herpes simplex encephalitis. Imaging can also help to determine the most

promising sites for brain biopsy. In the past, brain biopsy was regularly used to diagnose viral infections, particularly herpes encephalitis. Nowadays most viral encephalitides can be diagnosed by PCR of CSF. Multiplex PCR assays on CSF specimens are capable of establishing a viral aetiology in up to two thirds of patients with aseptic meningitis.[306,636] Enteroviruses are most frequently detected, followed by herpesviruses Epstein–Barr virus, herpes simplex virus and varicella-zoster virus.[306,352,636] Brain biopsy is still used occasionally in the diagnostic work-up of atypical encephalitides and for exclusion of non-infective processes.

Polymerase chain reaction has greatly facilitated the diagnosis of CNS infections in general, but particularly those caused by viruses. In acute infections, traditional antibody assays have an inherent lag time, dependent upon the stimulation of adaptive immunity. Specific IgM is detectable within the serum by about 1 week, and rising immunoglobulin G (IgG) titres soon thereafter. An increase in the level of antibodies in the CSF may be delayed by up to a week compared with the response in the serum. In contrast, PCR of viral nucleic acids in CSF allows early detection of most viral infections of the CNS,[218,494] although the PCR may become negative as antibody titres rise. Multiplex nucleic acid micro-arrays allow rapid simultaneous screening of CSF for large numbers of viruses.[619] Chronic and subacute viral diseases, and those that result from reactivation rather than primary infection, offer particular diagnostic challenges: antibody titres are often difficult to interpret, and quantitative PCR may be needed to assess the significance of viral nucleic acids in the CSF.[813]

General Pathological Features of Viral Infections of the Central Nervous System

The neuropathological manifestations of most viral infections fall into a limited number of stereotyped patterns (Table 19.3). These depend primarily on the specific virus and on the age and immune status of the patient. However, other factors such as the route and site of entry of virus into the body and the presence of other neurological disease, including other infections, can influence the pattern of disease. The following are brief descriptions of the principal patterns of viral disease of the CNS, and the viruses most often responsible. More detailed accounts are included in the sections relating to the individual viruses.

Inflammation Restricted to the Meninges

Most viral infections of the CNS cause meningeal inflammation, and in many cases of viral meningitis this is the only histological abnormality apart from scanty perivascular lymphocytic infiltrates in the superficial cortex and choroid plexus. The presentation is usually of a short-lived meningitic illness that is not due to any of the common bacterial causes of meningitis: so-called 'aseptic meningitis' (see Aseptic Meningitis). The most common viral causes of this pattern of disease (in approximately descending order of frequency, although this varies in different parts of the world) are echoviruses, coxsackieviruses, other enteroviruses, herpes simplex virus type 2 (HSV-2), mumps virus,

TABLE 19.3 General pathological features of some of the more common viral infections of the central nervous system (CNS)

Pattern of disease	Pathological features	Viruses usually responsible	Main differential diagnoses
Inflammation restricted to the meninges	Lymphocytic meningeal infiltrate Perivascular inflammation in superficial cortex	Echoviruses Coxsackie viruses, other enteroviruses HSV-2 Mumps HIV LCM Other viral causes of aseptic meningitis (see Table 19.4)	Acute bacterial meningitis, especially if partially treated Other bacterial and infective meningitis, especially due to tuberculosis or Lyme disease Neoplastic meningitis Reaction to intrathecal drug administration Other non-viral causes of aseptic meningitis (see Table 19.5)
Disease restricted to the grey matter (polioencephalitis/poliomyelitis)	Predominantly mononuclear inflammation of grey matter, with perivascular cuffing of blood vessels, but these may be absent in rabies Neuronophagia Usually some meningeal inflammation, but may be absent in rabies	Polioviruses Coxsackieviruses – mainly A4, A7, A9 and B1–5, but also A6, A7, A9, A11, A14, A21 and B6 Echoviruses – mainly 2, 4, 6, 9 and 11, but also 1, 3, 7, 14–16., 18, 19, 22, 30 and 33 Enteroviruses 70 and 71 Rabies Arboviruses (especially West Nile virus, JE and TBE)	Paraneoplastic (autoimmune) encephalitis, Rasmussen's encephalitis
Disease restricted to white matter (leukoencephalitis, leukoencephalopathy)	Multiple well-demarcated foci of demyelination, pleomorphic astrocytes, enlarged oligodendroglial nuclei containing amphophilic inclusions, and scant lymphocytic inflammation Diffuse leukoencephalopathy, usually associated with low-grade chronic inflammation and multinucleated giant cells Vacuolar myelopathy	Papovavirus (JC virus) HIV	Multiple sclerosis Pontine and extrapontine myelinolysis Acute disseminated encephalomyelitis Multifocal necrotizing leukoencephalopathy Drug toxicity (amphotericin B, BCNU, cisplatin, cytosine arabinoside, methotrexate) X-irradiation Previous CO, cyanide or methanol poisoning, global cerebral hypoxia, white matter ischaemia Mitochondrial disorders Subacute combined degeneration

TABLE19.3 General pathological features of some of the more common viral infections of the central nervous system (*Continued*)

Pattern of disease	Pathological features	Viruses usually responsible	Main differential diagnoses
Disease of both grey and white matter (pan-encephalitis/pan-myelitis) U.C. *Inflammation*	Necrotizing destructive disease Usually associated with mononuclear Inflammation and sheets of foamy macrophages Non-necrotizing disease Microglial nodules in grey and white matter, and variable perivascular lymphocytic inflammation	HSV-1, HSV-2 VZV CMV Arboviruses (rarely) HIV CMV Measles Arboviruses Early HSV infection Atypical herpes simplex encephalitis	Bacterial and other non-viral infections Ischaemic and hypoxic lesions Toxic and metabolic disorders Hypoxic, ischaemic or toxic brain damage Paraneoplastic encephalitis/myelitis Rasmussen's encephalitis (although predominantly involves cortex) Rickettsial infections Syphilis Lyme disease

HIV and lymphochoriomeningitis virus (LCMV). Other viruses that can cause aseptic meningitis are listed in Table 19.4, whereas non-viral causes of this syndrome are listed in Table 19.5.

Disease Restricted to the Grey Matter (Polioencephalitis/Poliomyelitis)

The principal viruses in this category are the enteroviruses (poliovirus; coxsackieviruses A4, A7 and B3; echoviruses 2 and 9; enteroviruses 70 and 71), some arboviruses (West Nile fever, Japanese encephalitis (JE), tick-borne encephalitis (TBE) and rabies. The enteroviruses produce disease that is largely restricted to the spinal cord, brain stem and primary motor cortex. Inflammation is marked, initially polymorphonuclear but later mononuclear, with prominent cuffing of blood vessels and parenchymal infiltration by lymphocytes and macrophages. Neuronophagia occurs and is characterized by the accumulation of microglia and macrophages around dying neurons. Also present within the perineuronal infiltrate may be T-cells that target specific neuronal antigens. The sites of destroyed neurons are marked for days to weeks afterwards by residual clusters of microglia, forming microglial nodules. In viral pan-encephalitis (see Disease of Both Grey and White Matter [Pan-encephalitis/Pan-myelitis]), similar or, in some cases, larger, less discrete, microglial nodules also occur in the white matter.

Rabies predominantly affects the hippocampus, medial temporal neocortex and cerebellum, but it can involve the spinal cord, brain stem and cerebral cortex. Infected neurons may contain distinctive cytoplasmic inclusion bodies (Negri bodies). There is usually evidence of neuronophagia, but inflammation may be very scanty or absent. Arboviral infections such as TBE, West Nile fever and JE often cause inflammation that is predominantly of the grey matter.

The main pathological differential diagnosis of viral polioencephalitis is paraneoplastic (autoimmune) encephalitis, which can involve the limbic system (particularly medial temporal lobe structures and the cingulate gyrus), the brain stem, the cerebellum or, less frequently, the spinal cord (see Chapter 24). Another, rare, differential diagnosis is Rasmussen's encephalitis, in which the abnormalities are confined to one cerebral hemisphere and consist of chronic inflammation, perivascular lymphocytic cuffing of blood vessels, formation of microglial nodules, rarefaction and, in some cases, cavitation of the affected cortex. The inflammation in Rasmussen's encephalitis often extends into the superficial white matter (see also Chapter 11).

Disease Restricted to the White Matter (Leukoencephalitis or Leukoencephalopathy)

JC virus, a papovavirus, is the cause of progressive multifocal leukoencephalopathy (PML), a disease that usually occurs in patients with depressed cell-mediated immunity. The pathological characteristics of this disease include multifocal demyelination, pleomorphic, often bizarre, astrocytes, enlarged oligodendrocyte nuclei containing amphophilic inclusions, and usually little or no lymphocytic inflammation. Occasionally, and particularly in patients with HIV receiving highly active antiretroviral therapy (HAART), PML may be associated with infiltration by large numbers of lymphocytes, as well as numerous macrophages.

Infection with HIV may be associated with several patterns of white matter disease. These include cerebral leukoencephalopathy characterized by diffuse gliosis and pallor of myelin staining; vacuolar myelopathy, with vacuolation and breakdown of myelin in the posterior and lateral spinal funiculi; and multifocal necrotizing leukoencephalopathy, with foci of necrosis, reactive gliosis and dystrophic calcification. In addition, patients with AIDS receiving HAART rarely develop severe inflammatory demyelination that is unrelated to PML.

The differential diagnosis of demyelinating viral disease includes multiple sclerosis and extrapontine myelinolysis. Acute disseminated encephalomyelitis also causes multifocal demyelination, associated with perivenous inflammation. Multifocal necrotizing leukoencephalopathy often involves the pons, but can also affect cerebral white matter and is characterized by foci of white matter vacuolation, dystrophic axonal swelling and mineralization, and loss of myelin staining; inflammation is usually restricted to small numbers of macrophages. The causes of diffuse leukoencephalopathy are numerous and include ischaemia, hypoxia, previous carbon monoxide, cyanide or methanol poisoning, drug toxicity and X-irradiation; most of these can also cause or simulate necrotizing leukoencephalopathy. Several mitochondrial disorders cause white matter lesions. These are characterized by intramyelinic vacuolation or by gliosis and cavitation. Calcification may occur, but this is usually related to blood vessels rather than dystrophic axons.

Disease of Both Grey and White Matter (Pan-encephalitis/Pan-myelitis)

This can be subdivided into necrotizing and non-necrotizing disease, according to whether or not there is destruction of all tissue elements in affected regions of CNS. Necrotizing viral infections of the CNS are most often due to herpesviruses: HSV-1, HSV-2, cytomegalovirus (CMV) or varicella-zoster virus (VZV). HSV-1 is the most common cause of necrotizing viral pan-encephalitis in immunocompetent individuals. HSV-2 can cause necrotizing pan-myelitis. Various patterns of necrotizing CMV and VZV infection can occur in the brain and spinal cord of patients with depressed cell-mediated immunity, particularly in AIDS. All of these viruses cause lytic infection of neurons, glia and endothelial cells, and the formation of eosinophilic nuclear and cytoplasmic inclusions. Cytomegalovirus causes the formation of enlarged, 'cytomegalic' cells, with large intranuclear eosinophilic inclusions surrounded by a clear halo. The necrotizing infections are associated with a prominent mononuclear inflammatory cell reaction that includes many foamy macrophages. Occasionally, arboviruses, such as JE virus and the equine encephalitis viruses, cause necrotizing CNS infection.

The differential diagnosis of necrotizing disease affecting both grey and white matter is wide and includes bacterial and other non-viral infections, ischaemic and hypoxic lesions, vasculitides, several drugs, toxins and metabolic disorders. Necrotizing myelopathy is also a rare non-infective paraneoplastic manifestation of systemic carcinoma (see Chapter 11).

Many viruses cause non-necrotizing pan-encephalitis or pan-myelitis. The appearance and distribution of the lesions may give an indication of the specific aetiology. The presence of scattered microglial nodules in white or grey matter is suggestive of HIV or CMV encephalitis, but these may also be a feature of arbovirus infection. Multinucleated giant cells suggest a diagnosis of HIV encephalitis, and cytomegalic inclusion cells indicate CMV. Human T-cell lymphotropic virus type I (HTLV-I) causes a chronic, largely non-necrotizing pan-myelitis, most severe in the thoracic region. In addition to a post-infectious acute disseminated encephalomyelitis, measles can cause two distinct patterns of infective encephalitis: subacute sclerosing pan-encephalitis (SSPE) and, in immunosuppressed patients, measles inclusion body encephalitis. The former is characterized by widespread chronic inflammation, rarefaction and gliosis, with only sparse intranuclear inclusion bodies, whereas the latter is characterized by multiple, relatively circumscribed foci of hypercellularity containing reactive astrocytes and microglia but very few lymphocytes, and numerous intranuclear and cytoplasmic inclusions in neurons, glia and microglia. Tissue necrosis may not be evident in early herpes simplex encephalitis, and inflammation may be sparse and limited to the meninges and small perivascular infiltrates. Immunosuppressed patients occasionally develop atypical, non-necrotizing herpes simplex encephalitis.

Reactive inflammation in relation to hypoxic, ischaemic or toxic brain damage can mimic non-necrotizing pan-encephalitis or pan-myelitis. The differential diagnosis also includes paraneoplastic encephalitis/myelitis, which predominantly affects the grey matter but can also involve the white matter, and Rasmussen's encephalitis, described earlier (see also Chapter 11). Rickettsial infections may cause perivascular lymphocytic cuffing and microglial nodules in the grey and white matter, with or without vascular thrombosis and haemorrhages. Syphilis and Lyme disease also come into the differential diagnosis of non-necrotizing pan-encephalitis.

ACUTE VIRAL INFECTIONS
Aseptic Meningitis
Aetiology

The term 'aseptic meningitis' is used to describe a benign, short-lived illness characterized by meningitic symptoms and signs (headache, photophobia, neck stiffness) and a CSF pleocytosis (mild, moderate or marked), the cause of which is not evident on routine microscopy and culture. The pleocytosis consists predominantly of lymphocytes, but samples of CSF taken very early in the course of the illness may contain moderate numbers of neutrophils. Non-poliovirus infections of the genus Enterovirus account for over 80 per cent of cases of aseptic meningitis, but a wide range of other viruses can cause this syndrome, as, much less commonly, may some bacteria, other microorganisms and some non-infective disorders (Table 19.5).[225,445,971] There is considerable geographical and seasonal variation in the causes of aseptic meningitis. In the United States, viral meningitis is responsible for an estimated 26 000–42 000 hospitalizations each year.[582] In parts of the world where poliovirus infection remains endemic (see later under Poliomyelitis and Polioencephalitis), this virus remains a significant cause of aseptic meningitis, as well as of acute flaccid poliomyelitis and polioencephalitis. Enteroviral infections occur throughout the year but are most common during summer and early autumn. Children are more susceptible than adults, those under 1 year of age being at greatest risk. PCR-based techniques are generally used to confirm enteroviral meningitis.

Several other viruses are common causes of aseptic meningitis (see Table 19.4). Aseptic meningitis is a frequent

TABLE 19.4 Viral causes of aseptic meningitis

Common causes	Less common causes
Non-polio enteroviruses (responsible for 80% of cases of aseptic meningitis)	Varicella-zoster virus
	Epstein–Barr virus
	Cytomegalovirus
Herpes simplex virus type 2	Herpes simplex virus type 1
Mumps	Human herpesvirus 6
Human immunodeficiency virus	Poliomyelitis virus (in regions without effectively implemented immunization programmes)
Lymphocytic choriomeningitis virus	
Arboviruses	
Measles	
Parainfluenza	Influenza
Adenovirus	Rubella
	Rotavirus

TABLE 19.5 Non-viral causes of aseptic meningitis

Infective causes	Partially treated bacterial meningitis
	Borrelia burgdorferi
	Leptospira sp.
	Mycobacterium tuberculosis
	Cryptococcus neoformans
	Treponema pallidum
Rare infective causes	*Mycoplasma pneumoniae*
	Rickettsia sp., *Coxiella burnetti*, *Ehrlichia* sp.
	Chlamydia psittaci, trachomatis
	Listeria monocytogenes, *Brucella* sp., *Bartonella henselae* (cat-scratch bacillus)
	Nocardia sp., *Actinomyces* sp.
	Coccidioides immitis, *Histoplasma capsulatum*, rarely other fungi
	Parasites: *Angiostrongylus cantonensis*, *Toxoplasma gondii*, *Taenia solium*, *Echinococcus granulosus*, *Strongyloides stercoralis*, *Schistosoma* sp., *Trypanosoma* sp. and others
	Parameningeal infections: epidural abscess, osteomyelitis
Adverse reactions to medications	Antibiotics: trimethoprim–sulfamethoxazole, trimethoprim, penicillin, isoniazid
	Non-steroidal anti-inflammatory drugs, especially ibuprofen
	Intravenous immunoglobulins, OKT3 (murine monoclonal antibody to CD3)
	Various cytotoxic drugs, carbamazepine, long-term antibiotics
Miscellaneous	Intracranial tumours, especially epidermoid and dermoid cysts, but also glial and metastatic tumours
	Post-neurosurgery, intrathecal injections, spinal anaesthesia, chymopapain injection
	Systemic illness, especially autoimmune/connective tissue diseases
	Heavy metal poisoning, especially lead intoxication

Adapted Hammer and Connolly.[445]

complication of primary genital HSV-2 infection.[231] HSV-2 is also the chief cause of recurrent aseptic meningitis (Mollaret's meningitis), with HSV-1 accounting for a small proportion of cases of this disorder.[635,899,1252] Over 50 per cent of patients with mumps virus infection have a CSF lymphocytosis, although only 1–10 per cent develop clinical features of meningitis. This complication affects a higher proportion of males than females with mumps. It usually manifests days to weeks after the onset of parotitis, but it can precede the parotitis or occur in the absence of other systemic manifestations.[545,667] The Urabe vaccine-associated strain of mumps virus caused meningitis in a small proportion of those vaccinated, but this complication is not associated with the Jeryl Lynn strain that has been used since 1992.[765] Since the 1980s, HIV has become an increasingly common cause of aseptic meningitis. The meningitis is usually part of an infectious mononucleosis-like illness that occurs at the time of HIV seroconversion, within a few weeks of exposure to the virus,[229,884] and may be associated with acute facial paralysis–'Bell's palsy' (Box 19.3). Lymphocytic choriomeningitis virus is an occasional cause of aseptic meningitis after human contact with infected guinea pigs or their excreta.[978] Other viral causes of aseptic meningitis include arboviruses (in endemic areas), measles, parainfluenza virus (mostly type 3) and adenovirus.[36,37,427,1059]

Pathological Findings

Because the course of aseptic meningitis is benign, there are few reports of the neuropathological features. Occasionally, patients with aseptic meningitis die as a result of concurrent systemic illness (e.g. viral myocarditis), and histological examination of the CNS reveals a scanty infiltrate of lymphocytes in the meninges (Figure 19.1), in the perivascular space surrounding some of the superficial cortical blood vessels and in the choroid plexus.[911] Autopsy examination of the brain of a patient who died 15 days after contracting HIV by intravenous infusion of infected blood revealed only mild perivascular cuffing and leptomeningeal infiltration by lymphocytes.[256]

Human Parechovirus

Human parechovirus (HPeV) was first isolated during a summer epidemic of diarrhea in 1956.[1229a] Initially classified as echovirus 22, the isolate was reclassified as HPeV1 in 1999[1076a] on the basis of distinguishing molecular characteristics. The prevalence of serological evidence of infection suggests that neonates are highly susceptible to infection, with antibody-positive sera appearing in the first months of life.[1a,1106a] By 1 year of age more than 90 per cent of sera contain neutralizing antibody.[545a] Primary infection of neonates is predominantly associated with diarrhea; however, respiratory disease is also seen.[1076b] HPeV has been associated with myocarditis[985a] and isolated from cardiac muscle of an agammaglobulinaemic individual who died of myocarditis.[719a] Two large PCR-based studies of CSF from children under 5 years of age who presented with sepsis detected HPeV in 2.3 to 4.2 per cent of the specimens.[901a,1239a] In additional studies, subtyping of CSF HPeV isolates consistently demonstrated HPeV3.[90a,452a] Given the protean clinical manifestations and high prevalence of HPeV infection, diagnosis is a laboratory challenge. HPeV is difficult

---

BOX 19.3. Bell's palsy

The term 'Bell's palsy' refers to acute, non-traumatic facial paralysis, usually maximal within 2 days of onset and largely reversible, although recovery may be incomplete and may take several months. In some patients, weakness is preceded by ipsilateral sensory disturbances in the distribution of the facial nerve.[373a] These disturbances include retro-auricular pain and loss of taste on the anterior two-thirds of the tongue. Occasionally, the sensory and motor dysfunction also involves cranial nerves V, VIII, IX and X and the second cervical nerve.[373a] The paralysis is associated with swelling of the nerve within the facial canal.[1258] In a few cases, the facial nerve has been subjected to pathological examination, which has shown lymphocytic infiltration, oedema and variable nerve fibre degeneration.[678,734,762]

There is strong circumstantial evidence that many cases of Bell's palsy are caused by reactivation of latent herpes simplex virus type 1 (HSV-1) or varicella-zoster virus (VZV) in the geniculate ganglion of the facial nerve. Furuta and colleagues demonstrated HSV-1 DNA by in situ hybridization in a relatively high proportion of neurons (5.3 per cent) in 11 of 15 geniculate ganglia obtained at autopsy.[350] Subsequently, Murukami and colleagues detected HSV-1 DNA in samples of facial nerve endoneurial fluid and posterior auricular muscle in 11 of 14 patients with Bell's palsy, but not in patients with Ramsay Hunt syndrome (see later) or in other controls.[807] Furuta and colleagues analysed the saliva of patients with Bell's palsy, Ramsay Hunt syndrome and HSV-seropositive and -seronegative controls, and found that 40 per cent of patients tested within 7 days of onset of Bell's palsy shed HSV-1 in their saliva (compared with figures of 19 per cent for HSV-seropositive controls and 7 per cent for patients with Ramsay Hunt syndrome), and that most of these had ceased to shed HSV-1 by the second week.[349b] These data are in keeping with a large number of anecdotal reports and serological surveys linking Bell's palsy to HSV-1 infection.[551,820,1056] To date, however, conclusive evidence is lacking that antiviral drugs are of any benefit in patients with Bell's palsy and questions remain as to the pathogenic relevance of virus in the geniculate ganglia or the specificity of the serological findings.[577]

Although latent HSV-1 infection most often involves the trigeminal and geniculate ganglia, over 50 per cent of vestibular and spiral ganglia in the inner ear have also been reported to contain HSV-1 DNA and may represent reservoirs of latent virus that, on reactivation, may cause vestibular neuritis or sudden hearing loss.[34,348,351,1015]

Acute facial paralysis is a component of Ramsay Hunt syndrome[500a] in which reactivation of VZV from the geniculate ganglion also causes pain in the ear, followed by the eruption of herpetic vesicles within the external auditory meatus and, in some cases, the anterior pillar of the fauces. Other manifestations can include tinnitus, hyperacusis, vertigo, decreased hearing and involvement of cranial nerves V, XI and X.[6] The presence of a mucocutaneous vesicular eruption was previously used to distinguish the zoster-related facial paralysis of Ramsay Hunt syndrome from 'idiopathic' Bell's palsy. However, it is now recognized that vesicles may not be present in facial paralysis due to zoster and that VZV is a major cause of Bell's palsy. Evidence for reactivation of VZV in such cases comes from serological surveys[788,950] and the detection of VZV DNA in saliva.[349c,349d] It should be noted that J Ramsay Hunt also described a separate syndrome, of progressive myoclonic ataxia, described in Chapter 13.

Other viruses that have been reported to be associated with acute facial paralysis include human immunodeficiency virus (HIV), either during seroconversion or in later stages of the disease,[84,1154] human T-cell lymphotropic virus I (HTLV-I),[76]

rubella,[528a] mumps virus,[79] Epstein–Barr virus (EBV),[422a] human herpesvirus 6 (HHV-6) and 7 (HHV-7),[1107] and hepatitis C virus infection in conjunction with interferon-α therapy.[477a]

Apart from viruses, the most common infective cause of acute non-traumatic facial paralysis is Lyme disease.[113,228,550] Facial nerve palsy has also been reported in association with *Mycoplasma pneumoniae* infection[596] and cat-scratch disease[191] (caused by infection with *Bartonella henselae*). Non-infective differential diagnoses include sarcoidosis (see Chapter 20), diabetes mellitus, chronic alcoholism, connective tissue diseases, tumours, pregnancy and Melkersson–Rosenthal syndrome. The last of these is an autosomal dominant disorder, possibly linked to chromosome 9p11[1054] and comprising recurrent unilateral or bilateral facial palsy, facial oedema and lingua plicata ('scrotal tongue'), with onset in childhood or young adulthood.[1273] Orofacial biopsies reveal granulomatous cheilitis.

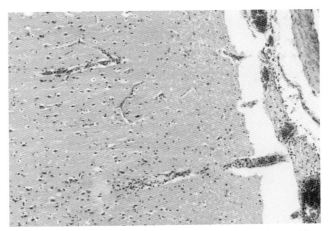

19.1 Coxsackievirus meningitis. Scanty perivascular and leptomeningeal infiltration by lymphocytes in a patient with aseptic meningitis due to coxsackievirus infection. The patient died from coxsackievirus-associated myocarditis.

Reproduced from Ellison and Love.[308a] © Elsevier, 1998.

to isolate *in vitro* and laborious to characterize by serotyping, so most laboratories rely on RT-PCR for identification. The recent design of degenerate primers to the 5'NTR has allowed detection of all currently known HPeVs.[839a,839b] In the most extensive clinical study to date,[1177a] HPeV infection accounted for approximately two thirds of neonates admitted to intensive care units for encephalitis. In the clinical setting of possible meningoencephalitis, evaluation of CSF was considered 'aseptic' (no pleocytosis and unremarkable protein and glucose concentrations). To date there have been no autopsy reports of HPeV3 infection, but evaluation of cases by a variety of neuroimaging modalities[667a,1177a] showed extensive periventricular lesions.

Poliomyelitis and Polioencephalitis

The terms 'poliomyelitis' and 'polioencephalitis' are used to describe inflammatory disease of grey matter in the spinal cord and brain, respectively.

Aetiology

Poliomyelitis and polioencephalomyelitis are most often caused by viruses of the genus Enterovirus.[539,800,970] These icosahedral, non-enveloped viruses measure 28–30 nm in diameter and contain single-stranded positive-sense RNA. Spread of virus is predominantly faeco-oral and is facilitated by crowding and poor sanitation. Infections are most common during summer and early autumn. The genus comprises the polioviruses (of which there are three serotypes), group A coxsackieviruses (23 serotypes), group B coxsackieviruses (6 serotypes), echoviruses (31 serotypes) and several further enteroviruses, including serotypes 68–71. More recent identification of additional serotypes of Enterovirus has been by analysis of genome sequence, and the classification of viruses within this genus is increasingly based on sequencing of the nucleotide sequence encoding the VP2 protein. This has identified four major phylogenetic groups of Enterovirus: cluster A, composed of coxsackie A16-like viruses and including several newly identified enteroviruses; cluster B, containing most coxsackie B and echoviruses as well as coxsackie A9 and enterovirus 69; cluster C, comprising the polioviruses and some coxsackie A viruses; and cluster D, composed of enteroviruses 68 and 70.[803,847,848]

Until the development and widespread use of poliovirus vaccines, these viruses were responsible for almost all cases of poliomyelitis and polioencephalomyelitis, including the epidemics of paralytic poliomyelitis in Europe and North America in the latter half of the nineteenth century. Paradoxically, these epidemics were probably related partly to improvements in hygiene and sanitation, which delayed exposure of children and adults to the virus; exposure at an early age carries a lower risk of paralytic disease and confers protective immunity in later life.[824,1215] The introduction in the 1950s of the Salk vaccine, containing inactivated virus, and in the early 1960s of the Sabin vaccine, comprising live attenuated poliovirus, caused a sharp decline in poliomyelitis.[824,989,993,1089] Paralytic infection by wild-type (i.e. non-vaccine) poliovirus still occurs in a few parts of South Asia and Africa, where poliovirus infection remains endemic.[38] The Global Polio Eradication Initiative began in 1998. Nevertheless, in 2008 a total of 1652 cases of paralytic polio were reported worldwide. Wild-type polio remains endemic in parts of Africa and Asia. In vaccinated populations, poliomyelitis is usually caused either by the rare reversion to neurovirulence of attenuated vaccine-related strains of poliovirus, or by other non-polio enteroviruses. The risk of paralytic disease after use of the oral poliovirus vaccine is approximately 1 in 2.5 million and is largely associated with the first or second dose of the vaccine.[840,1089] To eliminate the risk of vaccine-associated poliomyelitis, vaccination in the United States has, since 2000, been based on the exclusive use of inactivated poliovirus vaccine.[15] In the United Kingdom, this change was made in 2004.[271]

Non-polio enteroviruses do, very occasionally, cause encephalitis, paralytic poliomyelitis or transverse myelitis (Box 19.4). Of particular note in this regard are enteroviruses 70 and 71. Enterovirus 70 has been responsible for several epidemics of acute haemorrhagic conjunctivitis. Approximately 1 in 10 000 of the patients developed paralytic poliomyelitis, and about half of these also developed

BOX 19.4. Acute transverse myelitis and viral infections

The term 'transverse myelitis' (TM) refers to inflammation that extends horizontally across most of the spinal cord but is restricted vertically to only a few segments. Developmental, compressive, neoplastic, traumatic, metabolic, degenerative and non-inflammatory vascular causes of transverse myelopathy are usually excluded. Some definitions of TM also exclude disease that is attributable directly to infection of the cord (i.e. infective myelitis) and confine the diagnosis to the following categories of inflammatory myelopathy:[902,988,1018,274,1142]

- myelopathy due to multiple sclerosis (individual lesions usually spare the grey matter and extend over no more than two segments);
- myelopathy as part of the spectrum of neuromyelitis optica/anti-aquaporin-4 disease (see Chapter 23) (usually extending over more than three segments and involving spinal grey as well as white matter);
- myelopathy due to systemic vasculitis and connective tissue diseases, such as systemic lupus erythematosus, Sjögren's disease, Behçet's disease, scleroderma, mixed connective tissue disease, primary biliary sclerosis and anti-phospholipid syndrome;[649,1035]
- para-infectious and vaccine-associated inflammatory myelopathies (TM has, rarely, been reported to occur after hepatitis B, measles–mumps–rubella, diphtheria–tetanus–pertussis rabies, poliovirus, typhoid or Japanese B encephalitis vaccination);[103]
- paraneoplastic myelitis, particularly in association with anti-collapsin response-mediator protein-5 (CRMP)-5 IgG in small cell carcinoma of the lung, or anti-amphiphysin IgG in patients with carcinoma of the breast;[902]
- idiopathic TM.

Idiopathic TM accounts for a minority of cases of TM (10 to 45 per cent according to one review[103] and just 15.6 per cent in a large retrospective series).[275] Consensus criteria for diagnosis of idiopathic TM are:[1142]

- the development of bilateral (but not necessarily symmetrical) spinal cord dysfunction that has a clearly defined sensory level and worsens to maximum between 4 hours and 21 days after onset;
- an absence of neurological symptoms or signs attributable to brain disease, or of MRI abnormalities of the brain;
- exclusion of cord compression by MRI and exclusion of any other cause of transverse myelopathy;
- spinal inflammation demonstrated either by CSF pleocytosis or elevated immunoglobulin G index, or by MRI with gadolinium enhancement, at onset or within 7 days.

Patients usually present with increasing flaccid weakness, segmental sensory abnormalities that often include pain or paraesthesiae, and disturbances of bladder and bowel function.[627] Spinal MRI and lumbar puncture show evidence of acute inflammation. The neurological manifestations worsen over 1–3 weeks, during which time the lower limb weakness tends to become spastic and many patients lose all leg movement. Recovery can take many months: one-third to two-thirds of patients are left with few neurological sequelae, and the remainder have moderate to severe disability.[13,627]

Several viruses can cause infective myelitis. These include many of the enteroviruses, and the herpesviruses herpes simplex virus 1 (HSV-1) and 2 (HSV-2), varicella-zoster virus (VZV) and cytomegalovirus (CMV). In addition, myelitis that is probably not due directly to infection of the cord (i.e. para-infectious TM) occasionally complicates infection by echovirus, coxsackievirus or hepatitis A virus, varicella, Epstein–Barr virus (EBV), measles, mumps and rubella. Reports of the pathological findings are sparse, but most suggest that para-infective and idiopathic TM represent a localized form of post-infective acute disseminated encephalomyelitis (see Box 19.2, Acute disseminated encephalomyelitis and viral infections, and Chapter 23).[13,627]

cranial nerve palsies.[877,1189] Enterovirus 71, a cause of hand, foot and mouth disease and herpangina, has also been responsible for outbreaks of neurological disease, manifesting variably as meningoencephalitis, paralytic poliomyelitis, bulbar polioencephalitis, cranial neuritis and ascending radiculitis, in several parts of the world, including Australia, Brazil, Bulgaria, Hungary, Japan, Malaysia, Taiwan and the United States.[14,371,477,495,1037] A significant number of children with enterovirus 71 infection have developed fulminant fatal brain stem encephalitis.[492,495,690,841] Sporadic cases of encephalitis, poliomyelitis and transverse myelitis have been associated with a range of echoviruses (especially echovirus 30) and coxsackieviruses. Most patients have been children, infants or neonates. Neonates are susceptible to severe enteroviral infections involving the lungs, liver, heart, pancreas and adrenal glands, as well as the CNS.[778]

Because the clearance of enteroviruses from the CNS is antibody-dependent, enteroviral infection of patients with impaired B-cell function, usually due to X-linked agammaglobulinaemia or combined variable immunodeficiency, can cause a chronic meningoencephalitis or myelitis (see later under Subacute and Chronic Viral Infections).[441,753,983]

Flaccid paralysis resembling that caused by the enteroviruses is, rarely, a manifestation of arbovirus infection (see later under Arboviruses), particularly West Nile fever,[344,861,1022] TBE[364] and JE.[1062] Brain stem encephalitis and transverse myelitis have been described in patients infected with hepatitis A virus,[132,1151] which, like the enteroviruses, is a member of the Picornavirus family but in a separate genus, Hepatovirus. Species B adenoviruses have also been associated occasionally with a poliomyelitis-like illness.[262,862]

Pathogenesis

Infection of the CNS by poliovirus and non-polio enteroviruses is probably haematogenous in most cases. After initial intestinal infection and replication of virus in Peyer's patches and other gastrointestinal tract-associated lymphoid tissue, there is a primary (minor) viraemia, with spread to the lymphoreticular system and other systemic tissues. After further replication, a secondary (major) viraemia ensues, during which virus enters the CNS, if it has not already done so during the primary viraemia. The neurotropism of the neuropathogenic enteroviruses depends on their attachment to specific neuronal receptors. The attachment initiates steric alterations in the conformation of the capsid and release of the viral RNA into the cytoplasm.[421,921,969] In the case of polioviruses, the receptor is CD155. Decay-accelerating factor (DAF) is a cell-surface receptor for several echoviruses.[93] Echoviruses 1 and 8 bind to the $_2$-subunit of very late activation antigen 2 (VLA-2/2β1 integrin).[92] Coxsackievirus A21 binds to intercellular adhesion molecule 1 (ICAM-1)[1250] and group B coxsackieviruses to coxsackievirus–adenovirus receptor (CAR) and DAF.[1026] CD155, ICAM-1 and CAR are all members of the immunoglobulin superfamily.

Although in most cases enterovirus infection of the CNS is thought to be haematogenous, retrograde axonal transport of poliovirus has been demonstrated in transgenic mice carrying the human poliovirus receptor gene.[854,934] Poliovirus receptor protein has been demonstrated on denervated and regenerating fibres in human muscle and at motor end plates, and intra-axonal transport from injured muscle has been suggested as the explanation for the clinical observation that skeletal muscle injury and injection increase the risk of neurological disease in patients with concurrent poliovirus infection.[410,420,660]

Although poliomyelitis has been recognized for centuries, much remains unknown regarding its pathogenesis, e.g. which cells are infected in gastrointestinal tract, why the virus preferentially infects lower motor neurons, and what role cellular immunity plays in recovery or protection from infection.[823]

Clinical Features

These are predominantly diseases of young children. The initial intestinal infection and primary viraemia that occur during the first few days after exposure to the virus may be asymptomatic but are often accompanied by mild, non-specific symptoms that can include sore throat, gastrointestinal upset, mild pyrexia, headache and general malaise. In patients with enterovirus 70 infection, the initial presentation usually includes conjunctivitis and subconjunctival haemorrhages. Patients with enterovirus 71 infection may present with hand, foot and mouth disease, characterized by a vesicular rash on the palms of the hands and soles of the feet, and mouth ulcers. In children, the onset of encephalitis or paralytic disease is usually heralded by increasing pyrexia, headache, vomiting, neck stiffness and irritability, often several days after resolution of the initial non-specific illness. In adults, the prodromal symptoms tend to be less pronounced than in children.

Patients may experience muscle pain or stiffness before the development of paralysis. The distribution of paralysis depends on the distribution of the lesions within the CNS. The spinal cord is usually involved. The paralysis is typically asymmetrical, and the lower limbs are involved more often than the upper limbs and trunk.[539] Bulbar disease occurs in 10–15 per cent of patients. Cranial nerve palsies most frequently involve the glossopharyngeal and vagus nerves. Involvement of the reticular formation can cause cardiac arrhythmias, sleep apnoea and abnormal patterns of breathing.[539] In recent epidemics of enterovirus 71 infection, many children presented with myoclonus, tremor, ataxia, cranial nerve palsies, or pulmonary oedema and sudden cardiorespiratory collapse.[495,690]

Particularly during the first 10 days of life, neonates infected with enteroviruses are at risk of developing severe, multiorgan disease.[4,778] Group B coxsackievirus serotypes 2–5 cause an acute myocarditis with or without meningoencephalitis, pneumonia, hepatitis, pancreatitis or adrenalitis. Several echoviruses (echovirus 11, in particular) can cause necrotizing neonatal hepatitis with or without pneumonia and meningoencephalitis.

Pathological Findings
Acute Phase: Macroscopic Features

The brain and spinal cord are usually macroscopically normal. In severe cases, vascular congestion, petechial haemorrhages and focal necrosis may be evident in the spinal grey matter or brain stem.

Acute Phase: Microscopic Features

The extent of histological involvement almost always exceeds that predicted by the clinical manifestations. The distribution of lesions is variable. In classic poliomyelitis/polioencephalitis, the spinal grey matter, particularly the anterior horns, is usually involved most severely (Figure 19.2a–c). Other parts of the CNS for which the disease shows a predilection include motor nuclei in the pons and medulla, the inferior olivary complex (Figure 19.2d), the reticular formation and the deep cerebellar nuclei. Apart from the precentral gyrus, the cerebral cortex is usually spared. Bulbar encephalitis in children with poliovirus or enterovirus 71 infection occasionally may be associated with necrotizing lesions in the dorsomedial pons and medulla (Figure 19.3); this pattern of lesions has been noted in patients with neurogenic pulmonary oedema and acute cardiovascular collapse, probably related to the damage to vasomotor centres in the brain stem.[62,690]

There is intense inflammation in the leptomeninges and affected grey matter (Figure 19.2), particularly during the first few days. Neutrophils are present initially, but lymphocytes and macrophages soon predominate in perivascular cuffs and parenchymal infiltrates. Small blood vessels in areas of inflammation are congested and, very occasionally, give rise to small haemorrhages. Neuronophagia is prominent from a very early stage, as lymphocytes and microglia, accompanied initially by neutrophils, aggregate around infected, dying neurons. Clusters of microglia remain at sites of neuronal destruction for several weeks after the rest of the inflammation has subsided.

Chronic Phase: Macroscopic Features

In patients who die and are autopsied months or years after the acute illness, there is wasting of affected muscles, and thinning and grey discolouration of the corresponding anterior nerve roots.

Chronic Phase: Microscopic Features

Examination of affected regions shows obvious loss of motor neurons (Figure 19.4), atrophy and fibrosis of anterior nerve roots, and neurogenic atrophy of the corresponding muscles (see Chapter 25). There may be scanty perivascular lymphocytic cuffing, and an increase in microglia and anterior horn gliosis, but the parenchyma of the affected spinal cord or brain stem is usually remarkably well preserved.

Pathological Findings in Neonatal Enteroviral Infection
Macroscopic Features

Autopsy examination in fatal infections reveals evidence of multiple organ involvement, although the macroscopic abnormalities are often minor and non-specific. In some cases, however, the liver is extensively necrotic and haemorrhagic, and foci of softening and haemorrhage may be macroscopically visible in the myocardium, adrenal glands, pancreas and other tissues, including the brain and spinal cord.

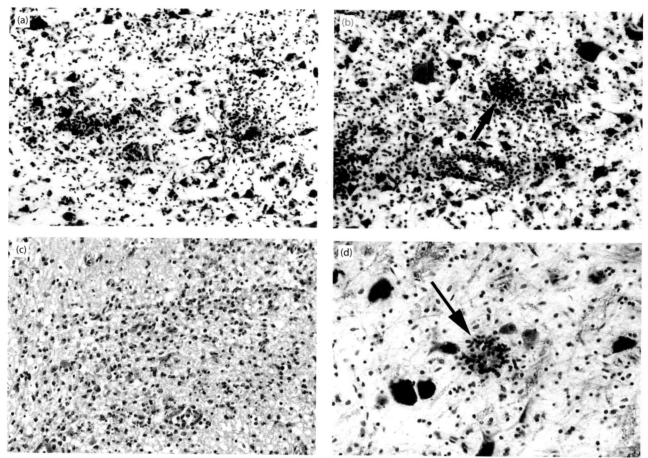

19.2 Poliomyelitis and polioencephalitis. (a) Patchy infiltrate of lymphocytes, neutrophils and microglia in the precentral gyrus in an adult with acute poliovirus encephalitis. Luxol fast blue/cresyl violet. **(b)** Neuronophagia: a dense cluster of inflammatory cells (arrow) marks the site of degeneration of an infected neuron. Luxol fast blue/cresyl violet. **(c)** Mixed infiltrate of macrophages, lymphocytes and neutrophils in the spinal grey matter of a child with acute poliomyelitis due to coxsackievirus B3. **(d)** Neuronophagia (arrow) of a neuron in the inferior olive of a patient with brain stem encephalitis caused by coxsackievirus. Luxol fast blue/cresyl violet.

(c) Courtesy of Dr D Hilton, Derriford Hospital, Plymouth, UK.

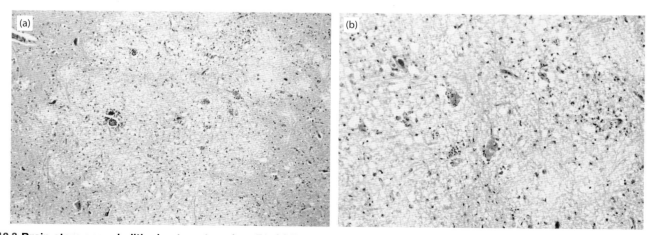

19.3 Brain stem encephalitis due to enterovirus 71. (a) Rarefaction of the dorsal medulla in a child with enterovirus 71 polioencephalomyelitis. **(b)** Necrosis of neurons and other parenchymal elements.

Section courtesy of Dr KT Wong, University of Malaya, Kuala Lumpur, Malaysia.

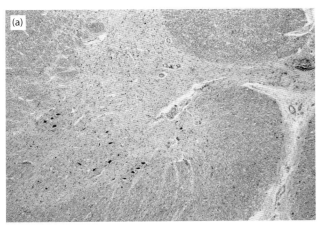

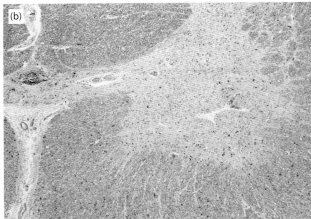

19.4 Old poliomyelitis. Preserved **(a)** and affected **(b)** anterior horns at the same level of spinal cord from a patient with longstanding unilateral weakness after poliomyelitis. Note the absence of anterior horn cells in (b).

Microscopic Features

Affected organs contain foci of necrosis and haemorrhage (Figure 19.5). The extent of inflammation varies. Fulminant hepatic necrosis may be associated with a relatively scanty infiltrate of macrophages and lymphocytes. Cardiac involvement consists of multiple foci of myofibre necrosis and inflammation, confluent in areas, and in some cases haemorrhagic. Viral inclusions are rarely discernible, although the systemic lesions usually contain abundant viral antigen and RNA (Figure 19.5c).

The distribution of lesions in the CNS is variable (Figure 19.6). A mononuclear cell inflammatory infiltrate is usually present in the meninges, and there are clusters of lymphocytes and microglia in the parenchyma of the brain and spinal cord. Unlike in immunocompetent older children and adults, the lesions can involve the white as well as the grey matter and may be necrotizing or haemorrhagic. The brain stem (Figure 19.6a,d) and spinal cord are often involved severely, but lesions may be scattered throughout the cerebellum (Figure 19.6b) and cerebrum (Figure 19.6c). Viral antigen and RNA are generally much scantier in lesions in the CNS (Figure 19.6d,e) than in other infected organs.

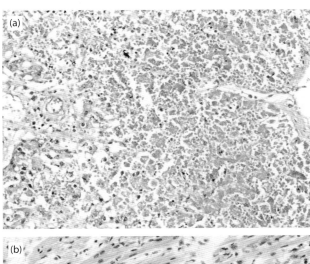

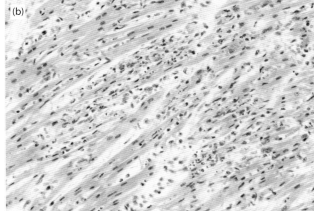

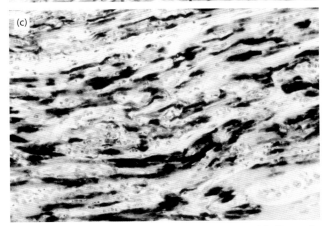

19.5 Neonatal coxsackievirus B3 infection. (a) Extensive hepatic necrosis. **(b)** Cardiac myofibre necrosis and infiltration by inflammatory cells. **(c)** *In situ* hybridization reveals abundant coxsackievirus RNA within the muscle fibres.

Original material courtesy of Dr A Charles, Bristol Children's Hospital, Bristol, UK.

Post-Polio Syndrome

Clinical Features

This is a syndrome of newly manifesting weakness, dyspnoea and musculoskeletal pain in survivors of acute poliomyelitis who do not have any other neuromuscular disease. Sleep hypoventilation and apnoea are frequent[493,1171] and

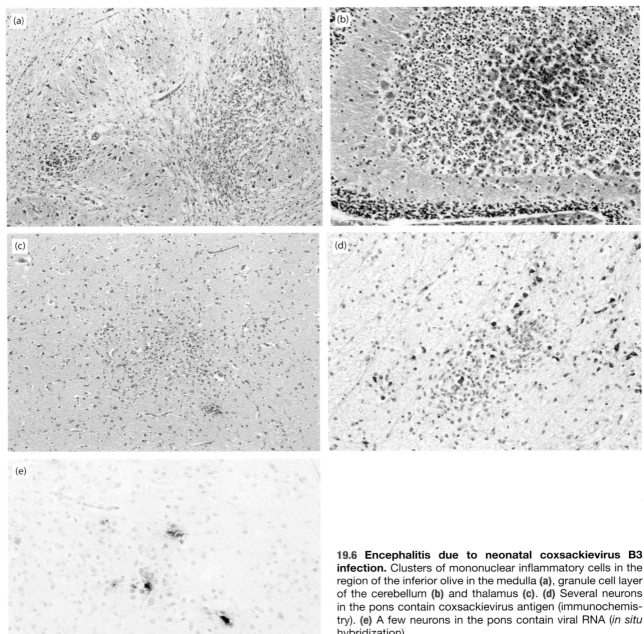

19.6 Encephalitis due to neonatal coxsackievirus B3 infection. Clusters of mononuclear inflammatory cells in the region of the inferior olive in the medulla **(a)**, granule cell layer of the cerebellum **(b)** and thalamus **(c)**. **(d)** Several neurons in the pons contain coxsackievirus antigen (immunochemistry). **(e)** A few neurons in the pons contain viral RNA (*in situ* hybridization).

Original material courtesy of Dr A Charles, Bristol Children's Hospital, Bristol, UK.

progressive bulbar disease can occur.[488,1064] The proportion of survivors developing this syndrome has varied considerably in different studies, ranging from under one-third[493,1131] to over two-thirds.[584] The figure depends on the precise criteria that are used and the duration of survival: the interval between the acute disease and the onset of post-polio syndrome ranges from about 5 to 65 years, with a mean of 35–40. years.[584,1131]

Pathogenesis

Electrophysiological and enzyme histochemical studies in survivors of acute poliomyelitis have revealed much more extensive initial denervation, axonal sprouting and reinnervation of muscle fibres than is suspected clinically.[243,689] The development of the post-polio syndrome has been attributed to an inability of motor neurons to support an extensive arbour of axonal sprouts over a long period.[243] Other contributing factors are the long-term stresses on joints and tendons, caused by modifications in posture and gait, and the overactivity of those muscles that are used to compensate for weakness in others.[892] The presence of lymphocytic infiltrates in the spinal cord of some long-term survivors of acute poliomyelitis[561,898] has led to the suggestion that post-polio syndrome is an autoimmune disorder, although the inflammation is certainly not restricted to patients with progressive disease. There is evidence that enteroviruses can cause persistent neuronal infection in patients with impaired B-cell function (see later under Subacute and Chronic Viral Infections), and persistent infection has been suggested as another possible explanation for this syndrome.[243,659,801] Polymerase chain reaction-based attempts to detect enteroviral RNA in the cerebrospinal fluid of patients have yielded contradictory results, including, in some cases, the demonstration of enteroviral RNA sequences in neurologically normal controls.[243,801,802] A variety of therapies have been tried for post-polio syndrome, including intravenous immunoglobulin; however, none has shown consistent benefit.[616]

Herpesviruses

The herpesviruses are large, enveloped, spherical viruses, ranging from 120 to over 200 nm in diameter. The virions have a toroidal (i.e. doughnut-shaped) core comprising linear double-stranded DNA wound around a fibrillar proteinaceous spool. The core is surrounded by an icosahedral capsid, an amorphous protein tegument that coats the outer aspect of the capsid, and a loose outer lipid envelope. The envelope includes a number of glycoproteins that interact with cell-surface receptors and other host proteins.

The family Herpesviridae is divided into three subfamilies, which include several viruses that are pathogenic to humans:

- α-herpesviridae:
  - HSV-1/human herpesvirus 1;
  - HSV-2/human herpesvirus 2;
  - VZV/human herpesvirus 3;
  - B virus/cercopithecine herpesvirus 1/herpesvirus simiae.
- β-herpesviridae:
  - CMV/human herpesvirus 5;
  - human herpesvirus 6 (HHV-6);
  - human herpesvirus 7 (HHV-7).
- γ-herpesviridae:
  - Epstein–Barr virus (EBV)/human herpesvirus 4;
  - human herpesvirus 8 (HHV-8).

Herpes Simplex Virus
Aseptic Meningitis and Mollaret's Meningitis

Seroprevalence studies have suggested that 45 million people in the United States have been infected with HSV-2, with an annual incidence of 1 million new infections per year.[96] As noted (see earlier under Aseptic Meningitis), aseptic meningitis is a relatively frequent complication of primary genital infection by HSV-2 and an occasional complication of recurrences of genital disease.[231] In addition, HSV-2 DNA can be identified in the CSF of most patients who experience recurrent aseptic meningitis (Mollaret's meningitis), with HSV-1 accounting for a small proportion of cases of this disorder.[635,899,1252]

Classic Herpes Simplex Encephalitis

Herpes simplex virus is the most common cause of acute necrotizing encephalitis in immunocompetent individuals. The estimated annual incidence is 2–4 cases/million per year.[980] Records indicate about 150 cases per year in England[259] and 2100 cases per year in the United States.[581]

Aetiology and Pathogenesis   Classic herpes simplex encephalitis is usually caused by HSV-1, but HSV-2 is responsible for a small proportion of cases (see later for aetiology of herpes simplex encephalitis in neonates).[269,980,1052] Spread of HSV-1 is by contact with infected saliva or respiratory secretions. In most patients, initial infection by HSV-1 involves the oropharyngeal mucosa. Less common sites include the skin of the fingers (e.g. in medical and dental personnel, as a result of contact with oral secretions of an infected patient)[332] and the shoulders of wrestlers (herpes gladiatorum, caused by the contact of abraded skin with infected saliva).[967] The primary infection can be asymptomatic but may be associated with a painful vesicular eruption. Serological studies indicate that at least half of the population has been infected by the age of 15 years and 90 per cent by adulthood.[539] Rarely, primary infection is complicated by widespread cutaneous or systemic dissemination, in association with malnutrition, immunodeficiency, dermatitis or pregnancy.[172,465,539]

Replication of HSV involves a complicated series of molecular and cellular events. The interaction of glycoproteins in the viral envelope with cell-surface receptors leads to fusion of the envelope with the outer cell membrane and release of the nucleocapsid into the cytoplasm. The nucleocapsid is transported to the nucleus, where linear DNA is released, circularized and transcribed. The transcription proceeds in a series of cascades, starting before protein synthesis with (1) the immediate–early genes, which encode non-structural proteins that regulate the transcription of viral DNA and activate (2) the early genes. These encode further regulatory proteins and enzymes involved in viral transcription and replication and also initiate the transcription of (3) the late genes. These last genes encode the major structural proteins of the virus. The capsid proteins are synthesized in the cell cytoplasm, transported into the nucleus and packaged with viral DNA to form nucleocapsids. The envelope is formed by translocation of the virus through a modified region of nuclear membrane.

After local replication, the virus is conveyed by retrograde axonal transport along sensory fibres to the primary sensory ganglia, where, after further replication, latent infection is established. In the case of HSV-1, latency is established most often in the trigeminal ganglia. In adults, virus can be isolated from over 50 per cent of trigeminal ganglia and viral DNA demonstrated by PCR in about two-thirds of unselected trigeminal ganglia and in a higher proportion in seropositive patients.[71,72,1084] The virus has also been rescued from explants of superior cervical and nodose (vagal) ganglia,[1203] and HSV-1 DNA has been demonstrated in geniculate,[350,1015] spinal,[846] ciliary,[147] coeliac,[375] vestibular and spiral ganglia.[348,351,1015,1123]

Of possible relevance to the pathogenesis of herpes encephalitis are the observation of latency-associated viral transcripts (see later) in the olfactory bulbs of mice several weeks after corneal or intranasal inoculation of HSV-1[301,1090] and the detection by Liedtke and colleagues of HSV-1 DNA in 15.5 per cent[672] and by Baringer and Pisani in 17.5 per cent of olfactory bulbs in humans.[71] In several experimental models of HSV infection, viral DNA and latency-associated transcripts (LATs) can also be detected within the brain itself, well after resolution of the acute illness.[311,697,952] In humans, HSV-1 DNA is readily demonstrable in the brain after herpes encephalitis.[822,832,835] Perhaps more surprisingly, by use of nested PCR on unfixed, frozen tissue, small amounts of HSV-1 DNA have been detected in brain tissue from about one-third to one-half of individuals without a history of encephalitis.[71,518] The biological significance of low levels of HSV DNA in the brain of adults without a history of encephalitis is unclear. Although explant co-cultivation allows the recovery of HSV from latently infected sensory ganglia in the peripheral nervous system (PNS), this has not been achieved from CNS tissue. Itzhaki and colleagues reported a significant association between the possession of an apolipoprotein E ε4 allele, the presence of HSV-1 DNA within the CNS and the development of Alzheimer's disease (as well as an association between 4 and recurrent cold sores).[518] For further discussion of the pathogenesis of Alzheimer's disease, see Chapters 15 and 16.

During latency, only a small proportion of neurons in infected peripheral sensory ganglia harbour viral genomes, which take the form of circularized or concatameric episomes (i.e. not integrated into the host cell DNA).[217,757,953] The factors involved in establishing and maintaining latency are still unclear. Viral transcription is restricted to a small part of the genome that encodes the LATs, comprising a large (8.3 kb), unstable transcript[1241] that is cleaved to form an abundant, 2.0-kb, stable, poorly polyadenylated transcript, from which smaller, less abundant transcripts are spliced.[217,1072,1190] The LATs are encoded by the strand of the viral genome that is antisense to the gene for the immediate–early protein, ICP0, and that partly overlaps the 39-end of that gene. Although the LATs contain several putative open reading frames (ORFs), most evidence indicates that these are not translated.[300,1190] The precise role of LATs in the establishment, maintenance and reactivation of latent infection is unclear. When the LATs were discovered to be antisense to the ICP0 transcript, the assumption was made that they functioned as an antisense control mechanism[1083] but this has not been substantiated. Subsequent studies suggested that LATs are needed for the maintenance and reactivation of latent infection.[470,654] Detailed analysis has shown this to be an oversimplified view, and it seems that only the first 1.5 kb of the primary (8.3 kb) LAT, a region that does not overlap any other known HSV-1 gene, is needed for efficient reactivation.[329] Several investigators have reported that LATs protect HSV-infected neurons from apoptosis.[128,510,891]

Reactivation of the virus within the trigeminal or other peripheral sensory ganglia results in local multiplication of virus, and its anterograde axonal transport to the skin or mucosa, where lytic epithelial infection ensues. This usually manifests with the development of cold sores. The mechanisms of reactivation are unclear and involve several viral genes. The probability of reactivation in experimental infections increases with the number of latently infected neurons.[1003] Reactivation may seem to be spontaneous, may be precipitated by local stimuli involving skin or mucosa innervated by latently infected neurons, or may result from a range of systemic factors. Effective local stimuli include trauma and UV irradiation; systemic precipitants include pyrexia, emotional stress, physiological fluctuations in hormone levels during the menstrual cycle, and immunosuppression.

The route of entry of HSV-1 into the CNS to cause herpes encephalitis has been much debated. Serological studies suggest that in approximately one-third of non-neonatal cases of herpes encephalitis, the encephalitis is a complication of the patient's first exposure to HSV-1.[816,1226] In the remaining two-thirds of patients, who have serological evidence of previous HSV-1 infection, the encephalitis is thought to result either from reactivation of the latent virus or from primary infection by a different strain of HSV-1.[1226] Whitley and colleagues used restriction enzyme analysis of viral isolates to show that the strain of HSV-1 in the trigeminal ganglia differed from that in the brain in approximately half of the cases of fatal herpes encephalitis that they examined.[1223] As described later, with few exceptions, the distribution of disease within the brain is relatively stereotyped, suggesting a consistent route of entry and mechanism of spread.

Proposals to explain the route of entry into the brain and consequent pattern of disease are as follows:

- *Spread of virus along olfactory nerve fibres and tracts.* In theory, this could occur during primary nasopharyngeal infection or as a complication of recrudescent nasopharyngeal infection resulting from reactivation of latent virus in the trigeminal ganglion. As noted earlier, there is latent HSV-1 infection in the trigeminal ganglia in most people. Evidence of olfactory spread of virus into the CNS after nasopharyngeal infection comes from animal experiments[301,1090] and the occasional observation of HSV-related histological changes in the olfactory mucosa[1150] or of virus in the olfactory nerves[856] in cases of fatal herpes encephalitis. Viral antigen is present in the olfactory bulbs and tracts in a high proportion of patients with herpes encephalitis,[282,283,321] and has been demonstrated to spread posteriorly from the olfactory bulbs along the olfactory tracts after intranasal inoculation of virus in mice.[1132]

- *Reactivation of latent virus in the trigeminal ganglia,* and its spread along either the centrally projecting nerve roots into the brain stem or the peripherally projecting sensory fibres that innervate the meninges of the anterior and middle cranial fossae. The distribution of lesions in classic herpes encephalitis argues against direct spread from the trigeminal ganglia into the brain stem, but this pathway may account for the infrequent cases of herpes encephalitis that present with brain stem involvement.[444,966,1152] Although spread of virus along peripherally projecting trigeminal fibres to the meninges over the frontal and temporal lobes has been suggested,[255] no direct evidence has been produced in support of this route of entry into the brain.

- *Reactivation of virus that has previously established latent infection within the brain.* Several studies have demonstrated HSV-1 DNA within the brain of patients dying from diseases other than herpes encephalitis.[71,518] Some support for the hypothesis that this may represent a source of virus in herpes encephalitis comes from the observation of Baringer and Pisani that the HSV-1 DNA could be detected in the frontal and temporal lobes but not the occipital lobe or cerebellum (i.e. in a distribution corresponding to that of herpes encephalitis).[71] However, in many of their cases, viral DNA was also present in the medulla, a region largely spared in herpes encephalitis. It remains to be demonstrated that the viral DNA within the CNS represents virus that is susceptible to reactivation.

Clinical Features and Laboratory Findings Patients present with a combination of non-specific features of encephalitis, and focal neurological signs due to involvement of the temporal and frontal lobes. Most patients develop fever, headache and confusion,[539,578,1227] and relatively frequent focal neurological signs include dysphasia, hemiparesis, ataxia and focal seizures. Although the onset may be fulminant, many patients have an influenza-like prodromal illness,[578] and some patients present with the insidious development of personality changes and behavioural abnormalities over several days.

Examination of the CSF usually reveals a moderate leukocytosis, variable numbers of red blood cells and an elevation of protein, usually to 80–100 mg/dL, although in the early stages the CSF may be normal. Computed tomography (CT) scans, magnetic resonance imaging (MRI) and electroencephalography (EEG) show focal abnormalities that usually involve one or both temporal lobes, but the changes are not specific and may not be present until relatively late. Because of the high prevalence of HSV seropositivity in the population at large, serological diagnosis depends on the demonstration of a significant (usually taken to be four-fold or greater) rise in the titre of HSV antibodies in the CSF, but the sensitivity is relatively poor and serological confirmation may not be possible for some weeks.[1226] Culture of CSF is usually negative for HSV, although viral antigen can be demonstrated in the CSF in a high proportion of cases.[643] For many years, brain biopsy was regarded as the most sensitive and only specific means of diagnosing herpes encephalitis, but PCR-based detection of HSV DNA in the CSF has now supplanted biopsy and serology as the diagnostic method of choice. Polymerase chain reaction allows the detection of HSV-1 or HSV-2 DNA in the CSF in over 95 per cent of patients at presentation, with a specificity approaching 100 per cent, and remains positive for several days after the commencement of treatment with aciclovir.[50,587,1226] Aurelius and colleagues detected HSV DNA in the CSF for up to 27 days after the onset of neurological disease.[50]

Without treatment, classic herpes encephalitis is usually fatal (a review by Longson and Bailey of previous surveys of the literature yielded overall mortality figures of 51–76 per cent)[683] and most survivors have behavioural abnormalities, memory disturbances and other neurological deficits of varying severity.[468,642,683] Since the introduction of vidarabine and later aciclovir, the mortality and morbidity rates have fallen substantially, although approximately 20 per cent of patients die despite aciclovir treatment. The mortality and morbidity are greatest in patients under 3 years, the elderly and patients whose level of consciousness is severely depressed when treatment is started.[517,578,642,1228] Despite a lack of randomized trials, steroids are often given

together with antiviral therapy.[336] Many survivors have persistent neurological dysfunction, especially dysnomia and impairment of memory, although these may be evident only on formal neuropsychological testing. A small proportion of patients experience a clinical deterioration or relapse weeks, months or, very rarely, years after cessation of antiviral therapy.[268,592,605,901] The relapse rate is higher in children: a figure of 25% has been reported.[630] Rarely, relapse may be precipitated by surgery for epilepsy.[126,685] Some patients respond to further treatment with aciclovir. Viral DNA or antigen may be detectable in the CSF and brain during relapses.[592] In other patients, a post-infectious immune mechanism has been proposed to explain the clinical deterioration.[75,901] Of possible relevance in this regard is the demonstration by Aurelius and colleagues of a persistent inflammatory response in the CSF for many years after acute herpes encephalitis.[51]

Pathological Findings

Acute Phase: Macroscopic Features The macroscopic appearances are stereotyped and distinctive. There is bilateral, usually asymmetrical, haemorrhagic necrosis involving the temporal lobes, especially anteriorly and inferiorly, and, to a greater or lesser extent, the insulae, cingulate gyri, posterior orbital frontal cortex and underlying white matter (Figure 19.7). The brain is usually swollen, the haemorrhagic regions particularly so, and transtentorial herniation of the medial part of the affected temporal lobe or lobes is relatively common. In most cases, examination of serial coronal slices through the cerebrum shows the lesions in the temporal lobe, the posterior orbital frontal cortex and the insula to be contiguous. In the early phase, the disease is often quite limited in macroscopic extent—so much so that the petechiae and softening may appear to be confined to the inferomedial part of one temporal lobe only. The brain may even appear grossly normal (Figure 19.7a).

Acute Phase: Microscopic Features The lesions of herpes encephalitis extend from the pial surface through the cerebral cortex and well into the white matter (Figure 19.8a–e). The earliest lesions contain little or no parenchymal inflammation (Figure 19.8a,b). Small numbers of neutrophils and lymphocytes may be present in the perivascular spaces, and moderate numbers of lymphocytes and macrophages in the overlying leptomeninges. The affected neurons, glia and endothelial cells tend to have slightly hypereosinophilic cytoplasm. In some cells, the nuclear chromatin appears to be finely dispersed or disintegrating, with loss of basophilia. Other nuclei contain more clearly defined homogeneous eosinophilic inclusions, some surrounded by an irregular rim of condensed, marginated chromatin (Figure 19.8d). The eosinophilic material may be separated from the marginated chromatin by a clear zone, forming classic Cowdry type A inclusions. Clumps of eosinophilic inclusion material may also be visible in the cytoplasm. Inclusions are usually most abundant in cells towards the edge of the lesions. The affected neurons bear a superficial resemblance to the hypereosinophilic neurons of ischaemia, and the lesions may be mistaken for acute infarcts. However, this impression is dispelled by immunohistochemistry, which in early herpes encephalitis reveals

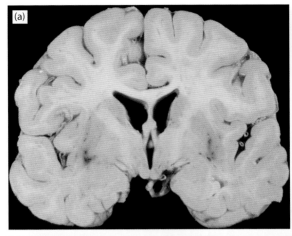

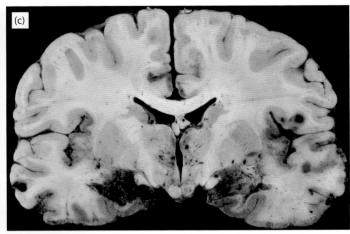

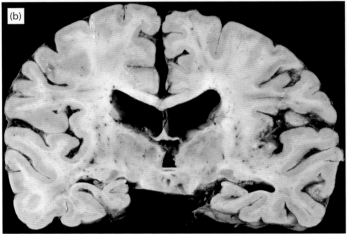

19.7 Herpes encephalitis. Coronal slices through the cerebrum in cases of herpes encephalitis. **(a)** Slice from a patient with very early disease and no lesions visible on macroscopic examination (see also Figure 19.8b,c). **(b)** In another case, lesions are limited to the parahippocampal gyri and right insula. **(c)** Extensive haemorrhagic necrosis involving the temporal lobes, insulae, cingulate gyri, anteromedial part of the thalamus and adjacent part of the hypothalamus. This patient had jaundice (for reasons not related directly to the encephalitis), which has caused green discolouration of the brain in regions of inflammation and disruption of the blood–brain barrier.

(a) Courtesy of Dr D Hilton, Derriford Hospital, Plymouth, UK.

abundant viral antigen within the nucleus and throughout the cytoplasm of many neurons, glia and endothelial cells (Figure 19.8b,c). Immunolabelled cells may extend well into the subcortical white matter and can involve the corpus callosum and internal capsule. Although virus is not usually demonstrable in the trigeminal nuclei or tracts in the brain stem, it may be present in the locus coeruleus and raphe nuclei, possibly reflecting retrograde axonal transport along brain stem neurons with cortical projections. Rarely, herpes encephalitis is confined to the brain stem. This is usually caused by HSV-1 and carries a high mortality: 41 per cent in a review by Livorsi *et al*.[680]

In most autopsied cases, the disease is at a more advanced stage. Affected regions of brain contain sheets of necrotic cells, foci of haemorrhage, and an intense perivascular and interstitial infiltrate of lymphocytes and foamy macrophages (Figure 19.8e). The blood vessels are often themselves infiltrated by inflammatory cells or completely necrotic. Neuronophagia and, later, microglial nodules may be present. Nuclear inclusions are sparse at this stage.

HSV antigen is demonstrable for up to about 3 weeks after the onset of encephalitis,[321] but the number of immunopositive cells declines considerably after 2 weeks; immunolabelling may be confined to ghost-like remnants of neurons and foamy macrophages in regions of necrosis. Immunohistochemistry is much less likely to demonstrate viral antigen after treatment with

aciclovir. Especially during the first 2 weeks, electron microscopy is often successful in revealing herpesvirus nucleocapsid particles within the nuclei of infected cells (Figure 19.8f). Viral DNA can be detected in frozen or paraffin sections by *in situ* hybridization or PCR amplification.[578,832,833]

Chronic Phase: Macroscopic Features In patients dying some weeks after the onset of untreated or unsuccessfully treated disease, the haemorrhagic necrosis will have progressed to cavitation and atrophy, with indentation or collapse of the affected temporal lobes and yellow or brown discolouration of the surrounding brain tissue and overlying meninges (Figure 19.9a). In longer-term survivors, the affected parts of the brain appear shrivelled and brown.[832,833]

Chronic Phase: Microscopic Features The normal grey and white matter in the affected parts of the temporal and frontal lobes and insula are replaced by cavitated glial scar tissue, containing an occasional microglial nodule (Figure 19.9b,c). Clusters of lymphocytes are usually present in the meninges and brain parenchyma.[45,832,833,835] Similar changes have been observed in brain tissue obtained from a few patients with clinical relapse of encephalitis weeks or longer after treatment with aciclovir.[75,126] Although at autopsy inflammation is most pronounced in the temporal lobes, sparse perivascular and parenchymal aggregates of mononuclear inflammatory cells

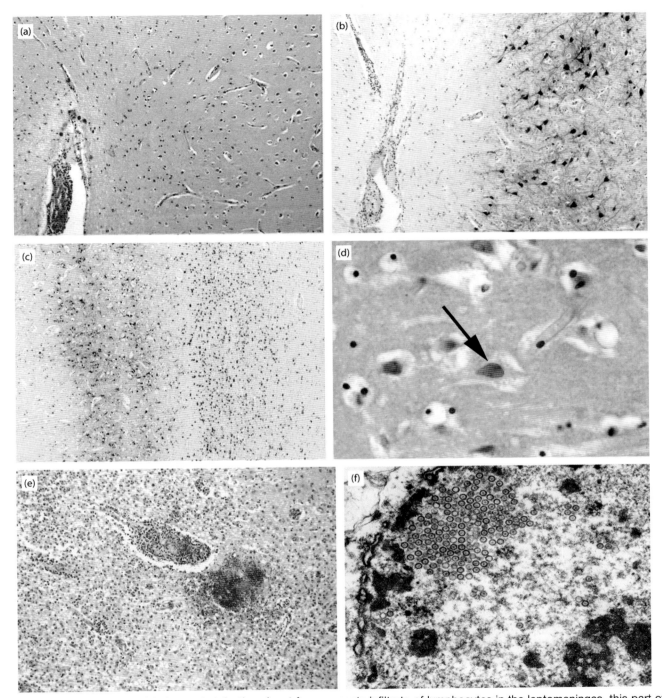

19.8 Herpes encephalitis. (a) Very early infection. Apart from a scanty infiltrate of lymphocytes in the leptomeninges, this part of the parahippocampal gyrus appears normal. **(b)** In an adjacent section, immunohistochemistry reveals abundant herpes simplex virus type 1 (HSV-1) antigen within most neurons. These sections are from the brain illustrated in Figure 19.7a. **(c)** At lower magnification, viral antigen is seen to be present not only in neurons but also in many cells within the underlying white matter. **(d)** A neuron containing an intranuclear viral inclusion (arrow). **(e)** Extensive necrosis and acute haemorrhage in a section of temporal lobe from a patient with established herpes encephalitis. Some of the blood vessels are cuffed by inflammatory cells, and the intervening parenchyma contains numerous foamy macrophages. **(f)** Electron micrograph of herpesvirus particles within the nucleus of an infected neuron.

may be present in all parts of the cerebral hemispheres, and foci of inflammation are commonly found in the brain stem, including the loci coerulei.[835]

Virus is no longer demonstrable by culture, electron microscopy or immunohistochemistry, but in most cases viral DNA is readily detectable, even in paraffin-embedded material, by PCR.[45,533,834,835] The distribution of viral DNA in the cases studied by Nicoll and colleagues[835] corresponded more closely to that of the inflammatory infiltrates (i.e. predominantly in the temporal lobes and

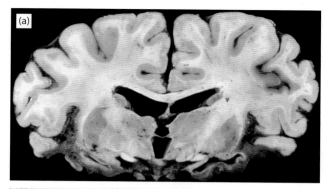

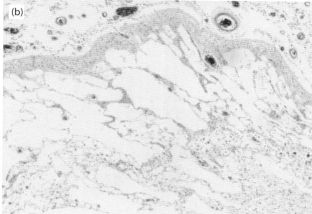

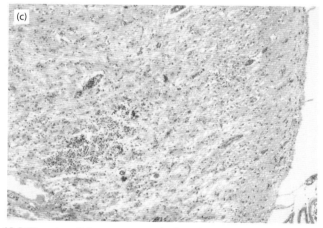

19.9 'Burnt-out' herpes encephalitis. (a) There is marked atrophy and brown discolouration of the temporal lobes and insulae in a long-term survivor of herpes encephalitis. **(b,c)** Temporal lobe from patients with burnt-out herpes encephalitis shows severe astrocytosis with extensive cavitation in **(b)** and clusters of mononuclear inflammatory cells in **(c)**.

Reproduced from Ellison and Love.[308a] © Elsevier, 1998.

brain stem, and absent from the cerebellum) than to the destructive lesions. The distribution of HSV-1 DNA was similar to that in the normal brains studied by Baringer and Pisani,[71] although in the latter cases the DNA was demonstrated in frozen rather than paraffin-embedded tissue, and by nested rather than one-stage PCR, so that much smaller quantities could be detected. The rare late relapses that occur many years after the initial encephalitis are thought to result from local reactivation of latent HSV.[1070]

Atypical Herpes Simplex Encephalitis

Occasional patients develop non-necrotizing, atypical forms of herpes simplex encephalitis due to HSV-1 or HSV-2.[198,601,818,96] This may involve a site other than the temporal or frontal lobes, usually the brain stem, and is often more slowly progressive than classic herpes encephalitis, with persistence of viral antigen as well as DNA. Although the likelihood of developing herpes encephalitis is probably not increased by immunosuppression, this does seem to predispose to atypical forms of the disease, most cases of which have been reported in patients with AIDS.[198,339,444,834] In addition, the increasing use of PCR to detect HSV-1 DNA in the CSF has led to the identification of immunocompetent patients in whom the disease is relatively mild and recovery complete without administration of antiviral drugs.[292,339,731]

Granulomatous Herpes Simplex Encephalitis

This very rare form of herpes encephalitis has been recorded only in children.[533,685] In most cases, an initial episode of 'typical' acute herpes encephalitis has been complicated by the development of intractable seizures, progressive neurological deficits and enlarging regions of abnormality on neuroimaging, in some cases after an interval of several years. Neuropathological examination reveals chronic granulomatous inflammation with foci of necrosis and mineralization (Figure 19.10).

Spinal Cord Disease Associated with Herpes Simplex Virus

Both HSV-1 and HSV-2 can cause myelitis and radiculitis, although HSV-2 is more often responsible. Initial infection with HSV-2 usually involves the genital skin or mucosa and occurs as a result of venereal contact with infected genital or cutaneous lesions. Latent infection is established within the second, third and fourth sacral ganglia, from which virus can be recovered by explant co-cultivation.[70] Although latent HSV-2 is probably most abundant within the sacral ganglia, HSV-2 DNA can also be detected in other posterior root ganglia.[846] Reactivation of latent HSV-2 leads to recurrent genital lesions, and, in conjunction with these mucocutaneous recurrences, patients may experience radiculitis and meningitis.[101] As noted earlier, HSV-2 is also the chief cause of recurrent aseptic meningitis (Mollaret's meningitis), most episodes of which occur in the absence of genital lesions.

Herpes myelitis is a relatively rare complication of HSV infection. In some cases, the spinal cord disease is limited to a few segments and is followed by complete clinical recovery, suggesting a non-necrotizing inflammatory process,[819,894,1041] although, not surprisingly, there are scant pathological data from such cases. HSV-2 occasionally causes an ascending necrotizing myelopathy, usually in patients who are immunosuppressed.[135,519,819,1232] Histology reveals extensive coagulative necrosis of the cord parenchyma and mononuclear inflammation in the spinal leptomeninges and roots (Figure 19.11). Herpes simplex antigen is usually abundant within the cord, and viral particles may be visible on electron microscopy.

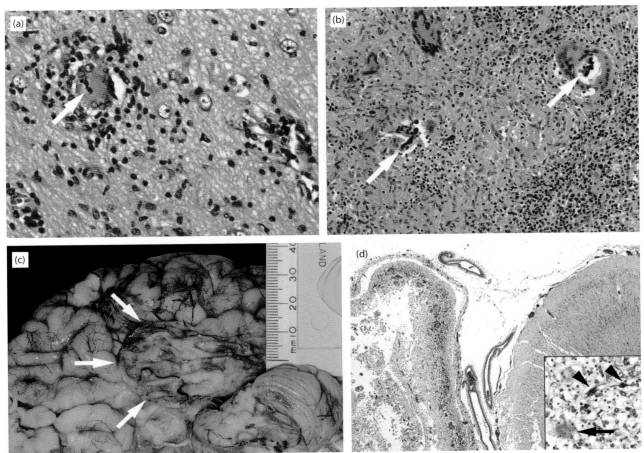

19.10 Granulomatous herpes encephalitis. (a) Temporal lobe biopsy from a 6-year-old who had herpes encephalitis at 18 months of age. He was treated with aciclovir and made a good initial recovery, but his psychomotor development was delayed and at 2 years he developed complex partial seizures that did not respond to antiepileptic medications. The biopsy contained clusters of lymphocytes and small, discrete, non-necrotizing granulomas within the gliotic cerebral cortex and superficial white matter in the region of neuroradiological abnormality at the time of his initial herpes encephalitis. Some of the giant cells contained mineralized material (arrow). He was given aciclovir postoperatively and made a good recovery. **(b)** This biopsy was from an 11-year-old who had herpes encephalitis at the age of 5 months. His subsequent psychomotor development was delayed, and at 2 years he developed simple and complex partial seizures that did not respond to medical treatment. After a previous biopsy that showed granulomatous encephalitis, herpes simplex virus type 1 (HSV-1) DNA and elevated titres of HSV immunoglobulin M (IgM) antibodies were detected in the cerebrospinal fluid. He responded well to a short course of aciclovir, but some months later he developed a hemiparesis, and this further biopsy was taken. It shows extensive granulomatous inflammation that includes scattered multinucleated giant cells, some with mineralized cytoplasmic inclusions (arrows). He was given a prolonged course of aciclovir, as well as rifampicin and iso-niazid (although no mycobacteria were cultured or detected by polymerase chain reaction), and he was much improved clinically at 1 year's follow-up. **(c)** View from below of the brain from an 11-week-old child who died of an encephalitic illness. Cutaneous herpes simplex virus type 2 (HSV-2) infection 9 weeks previously had seemed to respond to topical aciclovir. The left temporal lobe (arrows) has a collapsed appearance. **(d)** A low-magnification photomicrograph shows a severely abnormal gyrus (left) adjacent to a relatively preserved gyrus (right). The abnormal gyrus is cavitated and the cortex reduced to a layer of gliotic inflammatory tissue containing numerous foci of mineralization. An adjacent section immunostained for HSV-2 and viewed at higher magnification (inset) reveals viral antigen (arrowheads) and granulomatous inflammation, with multinucleated giant cells (arrow).

Reproduced from Love et al.,[676] with permission from Lippincott Williams & Wilkins/Wolters Kluwer Health..

Neonatal Herpes Simplex Encephalitis

Neonatal herpes encephalitis is acquired *in utero*, during delivery or the first 4 weeks of life, and differs in its pathogenesis and clinical and pathological manifestations from the adult disease. The incidence is approximately 1 in 3200–5000 live births.[138,1226]

Aetiology and Pathogenesis Between one-half and three-quarters of neonatal HSV infections are due to HSV-2.[138,869,1134,1226] About 5 per cent of cases are acquired *in utero*, 85 per cent during delivery by contact of the fetus with infected maternal genital lesions, and the remaining 10 per cent by contact with infected secretions from the mother or another source during the early postnatal period. Primary maternal HSV-2 infection during late pregnancy, and prolonged rupture of membranes or the use of inva-sive fetal monitors in a woman with active genital infection, are risk factors for neonatal infection.[138,589] However, most infected neonates have a young primiparous mother whose

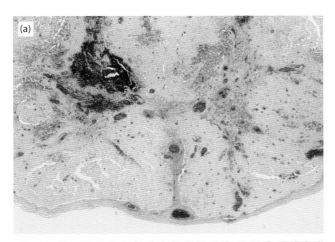

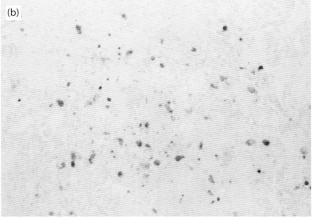

19.11 Herpes myelitis. (a) Haemorrhagic necrosis of the spinal cord in a patient with acquired immunodeficiency syndrome (AIDS) with herpes myelitis. **(b)** Immunohistochemistry reveals abundant herpes simplex viral antigen (red reaction product) within the necrotic cord parenchyma.

herpesvirus genital disease is, although active, subclinical; in about 70 per cent of cases, neither the mother nor her partner has a history of recurrent genital lesions.[137,869,1225] Almost half of neonatal herpesvirus infections occur in infants of low birth weight, usually premature.[137,138,1225] This is probably because active, genital, HSV-2 infection tends to induce premature labour but it is also possible that premature infants are more susceptible to infection.

As noted later, encephalitis may be one component of a disseminated infection or an isolated manifestation of neonatal infection with HSV. The pathogenesis of the encephalitis probably differs in these two circumstances. During disseminated infection, HSV is thought to enter the CNS haematogenously and is thus distributed widely throughout the CNS and other organs.[415,588,836,1224,1226] In isolated encephalitis, the initial pattern of cerebral disease is often similar to that in adults, with localized involvement of the temporal lobes, suggesting a similar, intra-axonal mechanism of entry into the brain.

Clinical Features and Laboratory Findings Three main patterns of neonatal herpesvirus infection have been delineated.[588] In approximately 45 per cent of cases, the disease is clinically confined to the skin, eyes and mouth and the CNS appears not to be affected, although a small proportion of these children have long-term neurological sequelae.[1225] Of the remaining 55 per cent or so, 20 per cent develop encephalitis as one component of a disseminated disease (which also involves the liver, lungs, adrenal glands and, less consistently, other organs) and in 35 per cent encephalitis is the only manifestation of HSV infection. Those with disseminated disease tend to present at about 1 week of age and have a worse prognosis than those with isolated encephalitis, who usually present at about 2 weeks of age. Vesicular skin lesions and keratoconjunctivitis are present in approximately two-thirds of neonates with disseminated disease.[589] Involvement of the CNS usually manifests non-specifically, with poor feeding, irritability, lethargy and seizures. HSV DNA can be demonstrated in the CSF,[588,591] and, unlike in children and adults with herpes encephalitis, viral DNA can usually be detected in the serum, even in neonates with isolated encephalitis.[591]

The introduction of aciclovir has improved the outcome of neonatal herpes simplex encephalitis, but the disease still carries significant morbidity and mortality.[589] Although the mortality of isolated neonatal herpes simplex encephalitis has been reduced to under 15 per cent, over 50 per cent of survivors have persistent neurological disability, usually greater in those surviving HSV-2 than HSV-1 infection. The mortality of disseminated infection is much higher—approximately 50 per cent—but neurological development in most of the survivors is normal.[589,1134] Long-term neurological complications of neonatal herpes simplex encephalitis include microcephaly, seizure disorders, ophthalmological defects, cerebral palsy and mental retardation. The efficacy of antiviral therapy in neonatal HSV infection is controversial.[547]

Pathological Findings
Macroscopic Features The brain is usually swollen, congested and extensively softened, sometimes with parenchymal or ventricular haemorrhage. Long-term survivors, especially of HSV-2 infection, may show cystic encephalomalacia.[177,302,1173]

Microscopic Features At least by the time of autopsy, the lesions of neonatal herpes encephalitis tend not to be restricted to any particular part of the brain and can involve grey and white matter in the cerebrum, cerebellum, brain stem or any combination of these. The features are of a necrotizing encephalitis, associated with meningeal and parenchymal infiltration by lymphocytes and macrophages (Figure 19.12). Some lesions may be haemorrhagic. Particularly during the first few days of infection, nuclear inclusions, viral antigen and DNA are abundant.[415,836] Using *in situ* PCR, Gressens and colleagues were able to demonstrate viral DNA within the brain of an infant who had survived 7 weeks with neonatal herpes encephalitis, at which time there were already changes of cystic encephalomalacia.[416]

Varicella-Zoster Virus

Varicella-zoster virus mediates two distinct clinical diseases—chickenpox and shingles. Chickenpox is a common

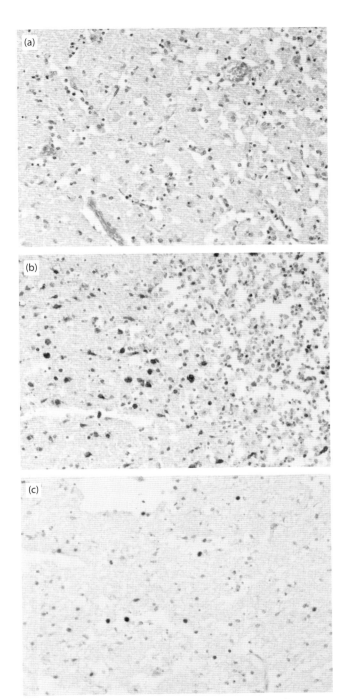

19.12 Neonatal herpes encephalitis. (a) Infiltration by macrophages in a region of cerebral cortex that is starting to cavitate. **(b)** Immunohistochemistry shows many cells containing herpes simplex virus type 2 (HSV-2) antigen. **(c)** Demonstration of HSV-2 DNA in the adjacent white matter by *in situ* hybridization.

childhood exanthematous disease of widespread cutaneous distribution, whereas shingles is less common, is limited largely to elderly people and causes an exanthem that is usually of restricted distribution. Because the distribution of the chickenpox rash is, like that of smallpox (variola), generalized, but its course usually benign (unlike that of smallpox), the disease was termed 'varicella', the diminutive of variola. Zoster derives its name from the Greek for 'girdle', because of the dermatomal distribution of the rash.

Aetiology

Varicella-zoster virus (VZV) is difficult to purify and study. It is highly cell-associated and, until quite recently, good small animal models of VZV infection did not exist.[184,443,814] *In vitro* preparations contain only scanty cell-free virus that is very poorly infective. Experimental infection has usually required the inoculation of virus-infected cells. Morphologically, VZV is indistinguishable from HSV, and at the molecular level there is considerable homology between the unique short segments of these herpesviruses, suggesting derivation from a common ancestor.[258] Of the two viruses, the biology of VZV is the less well understood. Most of the genes and proteins have similar functions to those of HSV. Entry of cell-free VZV into the cell is mediated by the binding of envelope protein-associated mannose 6-phosphate groups to the mannose 6-phosphate receptor on the cell surface.[185] Infection also occurs by direct contact with infected cells; this is not dependent on the expression of mannose 6-phosphate receptor. Dendritic cells[2a] and T-cells[629] may be responsible for the spread of cell-associated virus from infected respiratory mucosa to local lymphoid tissue, and T- and B-cells and monocytes for its subsequent haematogenous dissemination.[717]

Varicella

Pathogenesis   Primary VZV infection (varicella or chickenpox) is usually acquired by inhalation or mucosal contact with infected secretions. Primary viraemia occurs after replication of virus at the site of entry and is followed by a more robust secondary viraemia after further amplification in the lymphoreticular system. The prodromal symptoms accompany the secondary viraemia, which also leads to infection of endothelial cells. The successive crops of cutaneous and mucosal lesions result from spread of virus from infected endothelial cells to the overlying epithelium. Although multiple classes of immunoglobulins can be detected within a week of infection, cell-mediated immunity is essential for control of the viral infection.

Clinical and Pathological Features   Varicella is a highly contagious generalized exanthematous disease with marked seasonality, the incidence peaking in winter and spring. Before the 1995 introduction of a live-attenuated vaccine, the annual incidence in the United States was 1500 per 100 000 population per year.[362] Infection of children is generally benign, and complications are more likely in adults.[425] Vaccine development was spearheaded in Japan, for the treatment of children with leukaemia.[1105] The live attenuated vaccine, now administered routinely in many countries, is 70–90 per cent effective in preventing primary infection, and those who develop varicella despite vaccination usually experience milder disease.

In healthy children, varicella manifests about 2 weeks after exposure, with mild fever, malaise and rapid appearance of the typical rash, first on the scalp and then on the trunk and limbs. Successive crops of vesicles appear every 2–4 days. It has been estimated that less than 4 per cent of infections are subclinical.

The CNS is involved in approximately 1 in 1000 cases of varicella. In most of these cases, otherwise healthy children develop transient acute cerebellar ataxia beginning 5–12 days after the rash.[223,502] MRI shows cerebellar oedema and, in some cases, changes that may reflect demyelination, but because fatal cases of acute cerebellar ataxia have not been reported, the pathological substrate of the cerebellar ataxia remains unclear. Whereas VZV can be detected by PCR of CSF, assessment of specific IgG in CSF is more sensitive (30 versus 93 per cent).[815] Rare complications of varicella include aseptic meningitis, transverse or ascending myelitis,[742,1159,1272] Guillain–Barré syndrome,[811] CNS vasculitis[454,489] and post-infectious acute disseminated encephalomyelitis (see Box 19.2).[29] Most of these complications are more common in adults, in whom approximately 20 per cent of varicella-related deaths are due to CNS involvement.

A further potential complication of exanthematous illnesses in children, and of varicella in particular, is Reye's syndrome.[603] This encephalopathic condition manifests several days after the appearance of the rash, with severe headache, vomiting, seizures and coma. Fatty degeneration of the liver (pan-lobular micro-vesicular steatosis) and cerebral oedema are the pathological hallmarks of the syndrome. Even with aggressive treatment, the mortality approaches 20 per cent.[1093] In most cases, the development of Reye's syndrome in children with exanthematous illnesses has been precipitated by the ingestion of salicylates; since this association was first reported, the incidence of Reye's syndrome has fallen markedly.[83]

In immunocompromised patients, varicella is more severe and more likely to result in complications.[141,334,1204] In patients with HIV infection or other illnesses that compromise the immune system, such as leukaemia, Hodgkin's disease, and cancers and conditions requiring chronic steroid use, the incubation period of the disease is shorter and the rash may be chronic or recurrent.[365,1074] Complications of primary varicella that are more likely in this population include meningitis,[1195] myelitis and meningoencephalitis.[1106] In children with leukaemia, the mortality of primary varicella infection ranges from 7 to 28 per cent.[334] Fatal systemic dissemination can occur without skin lesions – varicella *sine herpete*.[397,1080]

Neonatal Varicella

The consequences of varicella infection *in utero* depend on the stage of gestation. If maternal varicella is acquired during the first two trimesters of gestation, the fetus is at risk of developing varicella embryopathy (fetal varicella syndrome), a syndrome of limb hypoplasia, eye damage, gastrointestinal and genitourinary anomalies and cicatricial scarring.[16,1112] Combined data from several cohort studies indicated a rate of varicella embryopathy after maternal infection of 0.55 per cent for the first trimester, 1.4 per cent for the second trimester and zero for the third trimester.[1112] There are, however, reports of varicella embryopathy complicating maternal infection up to 28 weeks of gestation.[1112] Maternal administration of pooled varicella-zoster immunoglobulin reduces but does not eliminate the risk of transplacental infection and embryopathy.[882]

The pathogenesis of the embryopathy is not entirely clear. It has been suggested that most of the fetal damage is due not to the initial fetal varicella but to zoster myelitis or encephalomyelitis complicating reactivation of virus *in utero*.[469] This would account for the segmental distribution of anomalies of the skin, peripheral nervous system, autonomic nervous system and musculoskeletal system, all of which receive innervation from the same levels of the spinal cord; the short latent period between primary fetal varicella and the development of fetal zoster is thought to reflect the lack or immaturity of cell-mediated immunity during the first and second trimesters.

The few reports of the neuropathological findings in congenital varicella syndrome describe destructive lesions involving the cerebral grey and white matter in the cerebrum, basal ganglia, brain stem and spinal cord, occasionally with accompanying inflammation but without viral inclusions or antigen.[451,638,711]

Intrauterine varicella infection during the third trimester is usually subclinical but may lead to infantile zoster, which usually involves the thoracic dermatomes and follows a benign course with good recovery. Neonatal varicella generally results from primary maternal infection during the last 3 weeks of pregnancy;[1001] that occurring within 4 days of birth tends to be mild, but neonatal varicella developing between about 5 and 12 days postnatally often results in disseminated neonatal infection, with mortality of 20–30 per cent.[910,1001]

Zoster

Pathogenesis After the primary infection, VZV establishes latent infection in the dorsal root, cranial nerve and autonomic ganglia.[375,377,712,776] Infection of the ganglia is probably by a combination of axonal transport of virus along sensory nerves innervating affected skin and haematogenous spread within infected mononuclear cells. Within the ganglia, latent VZV DNA is predominantly in neurons.[776] The molecular basis of VZV latency is still being elucidated. Several immediate–early and early genes are transcribed during latency. A protein encoded by *IE63* (immediate–early gene 63) is expressed in both acute and latent infection and has been shown to elicit humoral and cellular immunity.[713,990] Sadzot-Delvaux and colleagues suggested that the response of T-cells to IE63 and other proteins of VZV may regulate its reactivation from latency.[990] Other viral genes transcribed during latency include ORFs 21, 29 and 62 and possibly 4 and 18.[776] Proteins corresponding to ORFs 21, 29, 62, 63 and 4 were detected immunohistochemically within dorsal root ganglia from patients with latent VZV; these proteins localized to the nucleus during lytic infection but were predominantly cytoplasmic in latently infected neurons.[693]

Zoster is a relatively frequent complication of many conditions associated with depressed cellular immunity, including Hodgkin's disease, leukaemias, AIDS and particularly bone marrow and organ transplantation, but not of depressed humoral immunity, such as hypogammaglobulinaemia.[2,42] The reactivation of VZV, unlike HSV, is not triggered by cutaneous stimuli such as trauma or UV radiation. The observation that herpes zoster is predominantly a disease of elderly people has been ascribed to an age-related decline in cellular immune function, although why this should apply to VZV and not to other herpesviruses is unclear.[144]

Clinical Features The overall annual incidence of zoster ranges from 1.2 to 4.8 per 1000.[1125] Herpes zoster most often affects elderly people, in whom the annual incidence exceeds 10 per 1000.[1125] However, approximately 5 per cent of patients with zoster are children or neonates.[293] By 60 years, about half of people destined to develop zoster will have experienced at least one attack. Unfortunately, this does not confer protection from further attacks. Most patients do not have an identifiable cause for reactivation. Patients with depressed cell-mediated immunity have an increased incidence of zoster and are more likely to develop complications.[447,499] On the basis of CSF PCR positivity for VZV, CNS infection is estimated at 1.8/100 000.[893] Vaccination against VZV reduces the incidence and morbidity of zoster (including post-herpetic neuralgia) in older adults.[870]

Blocking viral thymidine kinase activity with aciclovir is the most efficacious therapy for active CNS disease.[1082] Brink et al.[134] detected a mutation in VZV thymidine kinase in three stem cell transplant patients who were resistant to aciclovir. Despite its potential immunosuppressive potential, oral corticosteroids are often given along with antiviral drugs.[855]

Before the eruption of the characteristic rash, there is often pain, tingling or pruritus in the affected dermatome. This may precede the rash by up to 100 days. The rash appears over several days and is usually unilateral, involving a single dermatome. Thoracic and sacral dermatomes are most often involved, but 10–15 per cent of cases involve the ophthalmic division of the trigeminal nerve. The rash may last up to 4 weeks or even longer and is accompanied by pain and discomfort, which usually resolve over months but can persist for years. A herpes zoster eruption can transmit the virus to susceptible individuals, who then develop varicella, but the likelihood of transmission of virus is much lower than from patients with varicella. Reactivation of VZV with the development of severe systemic or CNS complications can occur in the absence of a rash – zoster *sine herpete* (Figure 19.13).[374,622,739]

Diagnosis is aided by analysis of CSF; timing of sampling relative to disease onset influences the diagnostic sensitivity.[412] Fewer than half of patients with CNS disease and CSF positivity for VZV by PCR have a skin rash.[876]

In addition to the neuralgia, reactivation of VZV can cause a range of rarer neurological complications. These include ophthalmic zoster, Ramsay Hunt syndrome (acute facial neuropathy associated with an ipsilateral painful, erythematous vesicular rash in and around the external auditory meatus and sometimes the palate and tongue),[593,1187] meningoencephalitis and myelitis, which can present before, or several months after, the shingles. The onset of zoster encephalitis or myelitis is usually acute and accompanied by fever and meningeal signs and impairment of consciousness.

Rarely, ophthalmic zoster is complicated by development of contralateral hemiplegiaas a result of vasculitis with resultant thrombosis and brain infarction.[299] The vasculitis probably results from spread of virus along branches of the trigeminal nerve that supply the ipsilateral basal blood vessels. Support for this comes from the demonstration of viral particles and antigen within the vascular smooth muscle rather than the endothelium of affected vessels,[299,312] and

from the detection of VZV DNA in CSF and in the affected arteries but not in those from the contralateral cerebral hemisphere.[755]

Since the early 1990s, it has become evident that the clinical spectrum of zoster-related CNS vasculopathy and infarction is wider than previously recognized, particularly (but not only) in patients with AIDS. The zoster rash may involve dermatomes of the trigeminal nerve other than the ophthalmic division or may not occur at all, and zoster-related granulomatous vasculitis or necrotizing vasculopathy can involve any part of the CNS.[115,199,376,403] Often, the pattern of disease within the CNS seems to be determined by the pathogenesis and distribution of vascular infection. Bilateral or diffuse involvement of meningeal blood vessels[984] is likely to be haematogenous or secondary to seeding of the CSF, rather than to spread along trigeminal nerve fibres. Patients may develop a vasculopathy associated with infection of intracranial vessels.[569] Infection of small parenchymal vessels may also be caused by contiguous spread of virus from infected brain tissue.

Pathological Findings Disease of the CNS associated with the recrudescence of VZV can take several forms, depending on the immune status of the patient and, probably, the mechanism of spread of the virus to the CNS. The principal types of VZV-related CNS lesion that occur, albeit rarely, in immunocompetent patients are (1) bulbar encephalitis or transverse myelitis, as a result of spread of virus from the trigeminal or corresponding dorsal root ganglion, respectively, and usually associated with a dermatomal zoster rash and ganglioradiculitis (a) and (2) vasculitis, usually granulomatous, with infarcts (Figure 19.14b,c). The lesions of bulbar encephalitis and transverse myelitis show infiltration by lymphocytes, macrophages and microglia, tend to undergo necrosis and may be haemorrhagic. However, some patients develop a non-necrotizing brain stem encephalitis characterized by the presence of scattered microglial nodules.[1010] The granulomatous vasculitis involves large basal and parenchymal arteries. The blood vessels show mural and perivascular infiltration by macrophages and occasional multinucleated giant cells,[199,279,403,603] segmental necrosis and thrombosis. The histological appearances may be indistinguishable from those associated with primary angiitis of the CNS. In other cases, there is vascular necrosis and thrombosis, with little or no inflammation.

Most reports of the CNS complications of zoster concern patients with AIDS, in whom the patterns of CNS disease can be divided as follows:[199,403]

- bulbar encephalitis or transverse myelitis due, as in immunocompetent patients, to spread of virus from the corresponding trigeminal or dorsal root ganglion. The lesions are usually necrotizing and occasionally haemorrhagic;
- ventriculitis (Figure 19.15), often associated with, and possibly secondary to, periventricular vasculitis;
- multifocal lesions in the deep or subcortical cerebral white matter (Figure 19.16), often associated with vasculitis and thought to be due to haematogenous spread of infection. In some cases, the lesions are partly

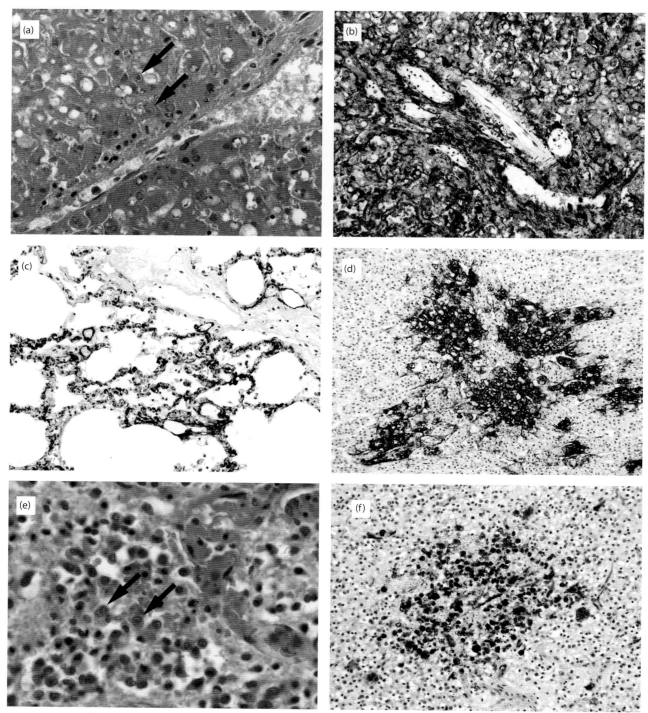

19.13 Disseminated zoster in a 12-year-old. This child, who had serological evidence of previous varicella and had been treated for acute lymphoblastic leukaemia, developed an oligodendroglioma. After making a good initial response to subtotal resection of the tumour, he developed fatal disseminated zoster without a rash (zoster *sine herpete*). **(a)** The liver was extensively necrotic, but in better preserved areas intranuclear viral inclusions could be identified (arrows). **(b)** The liver contained abundant varicella-zoster virus (VZV) antigen. Immunohistochemistry also revealed zoster infection of the lung **(c)**, adrenal gland **(d)** and many other tissues. **(e)** Intranuclear viral inclusions (arrows) in degenerate-looking brain tissue in the region of previous surgery. **(f)** Varicella-zoster virus antigen in a focus of necrosis within residual oligodendroglioma.

demyelinating, and viral inclusions and antigen can be found in oligodendrocytes;

- leptomeningeal vasculitis or vasculopathy, often associated with haemorrhagic infarcts in the brain or spinal cord (Figure 19.17). Spinal cord involvement may take the form of an extensive haemorrhagic meningomyeloradiculitis and vasculitis; in some patients, this has occurred in conjunction with necrotizing ventriculitis

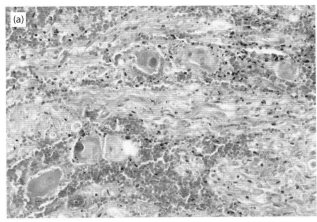

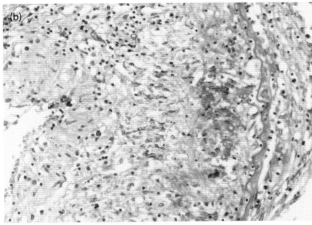

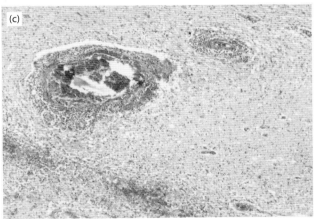

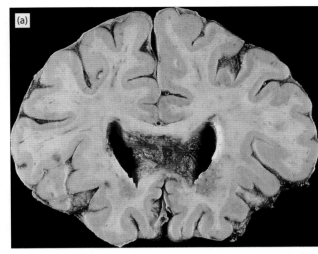

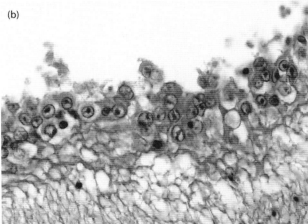

19.15 Varicella-zoster virus (VZV) ventriculitis in a patient with acquired immunodeficiency syndrome (AIDS). (a) Coronal slice at the level of the genu of the corpus callosum. The lining of the lateral ventricles is replaced by an irregular layer of soft brown tissue. The softening extends several millimetres into the adjacent brain parenchyma. **(b)** In places where the ependyma is still intact, histology shows VZV inclusion bodies in almost all of the ependymal cells.

Courtesy of Professor F Gray, Hôpital Lariboisière, Paris, France.

19.14 Varicella-zoster virus (VZV) infection in immunocompetent patients. (a) Necrotizing ganglionitis due to VZV. **(b)** Focal fibrinoid necrosis and mononuclear cell infiltration in the wall of the posterior cerebral artery of a patient who developed vasculitis and contralateral hemiplegia a few days after ophthalmic zoster. **(c)** Necrotizing vasculitis associated with an infarct in the basal ganglia of the same patient.

Reproduced from Ellison and Love.[308a] © Elsevier, 1998.

and may have been due to seeding of CSF by infected ependymal cells.

There is often overlap between the patterns of disease in an individual patient.

In patients with AIDS, the combination of aciclovir and recovery of immune function due to HAART, may modify the findings in zoster-related neurological disease, resulting in 'burnt-out' lesions (Figure 19.18).[264,407] These are centrally necrotic or cavitated and contain foamy macrophages but lack the acute astrocytic reaction and the viral inclusions and antigen that are present in active disease.

Epstein–Barr Virus

Epstein–Barr virus (EBV) is a γ-herpesvirus first identified in cultures of lymphoblasts from Burkitt's lymphoma.[317] Primary infection may be associated with the development of infectious mononucleosis, and a combination of latent and low-level productive infection probably causes or contributes to the development of Burkitt's lymphoma in Africa, B-cell lymphoproliferative diseases in patients

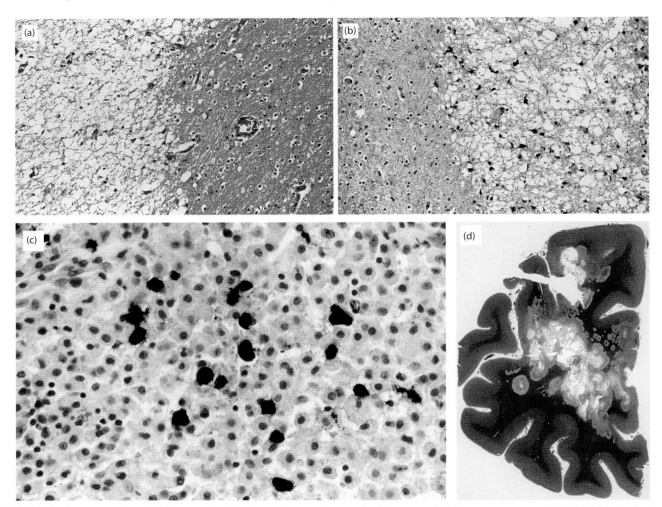

19.16 Varicella-zoster virus (VZV) encephalitis in a patient with acquired immunodeficiency syndrome (AIDS). (a) Lesion in the deep cerebral white matter, sharply demarcated from adjacent, uninvolved white matter. The paucity of inflammation reflects the patient's immunosuppression. **(b)** Immunohistochemistry for VZV reveals several infected oligodendrocytes at the edge of the lesion. **(c)** An acutely involved region of white matter shows extensive infiltration by macrophages. Most of the residual oligodendrocytes are infected with VZV. **(d)** The white matter of the frontal lobe of a patient with VZV encephalitis contains multiple sharply demarcated lesions. These are predominantly demyelinating, but several of the lesions have become confluent and undergone central cavitation. The lesions extend into the deep part of the cortical ribbon. Loyez.

Courtesy of Professor F Gray, Hôpital Lariboisière, Paris, France.

with congenital or acquired immunodeficiencies (including AIDS), some types of Hodgkin's disease (particularly of mixed cellularity type) and nasopharyngeal carcinoma.[707,726] In a proportion of cases, EBV DNA can be detected in several other types of lymphocytic, epithelial and soft tissue tumours, T-cell/natural killer (NK) cell lymphoma, primary effusion lymphoma, lymphoepithelial-like carcinoma, gastric carcinoma and leiomyosarcoma, but the possible role of the virus in the genesis of these neoplasms is still uncertain.[237,707] Infection with EBV is a cause of lymphocytic interstitial pneumonitis and hairy leukoplakia in patients with AIDS.[411,1014] The role of EBV in the development of primary cerebral lymphomas and soft tissue tumours affecting the nervous system is considered in Chapter 40. Epstein–Barr virus has also been associated with diverse non-neoplastic neurological diseases (see later), but pathological data are limited.

Pathogenesis

Spread occurs through oropharyngeal contact with infected saliva. The virus can be detected, at least intermittently, in the saliva of most seropositive people.[1261] Virus has also been detected in urethral discharges and exfoliated cervical cells, raising the possibility of venereal transmission in some cases.[515,1050,1242] Primary infection is usually asymptomatic, although some patients develop the clinical syndrome of infectious mononucleosis (glandular fever). The virus is usually acquired during childhood or adolescence, the average age of infection being earlier in lower socioeconomic groups and in crowded living conditions.[457,562,837,1094] Approximately 90 per cent of all adults are seropositive for EBV.

Cell entry results from the binding of gp350/220 glycoprotein in the viral envelope to the complement 3d

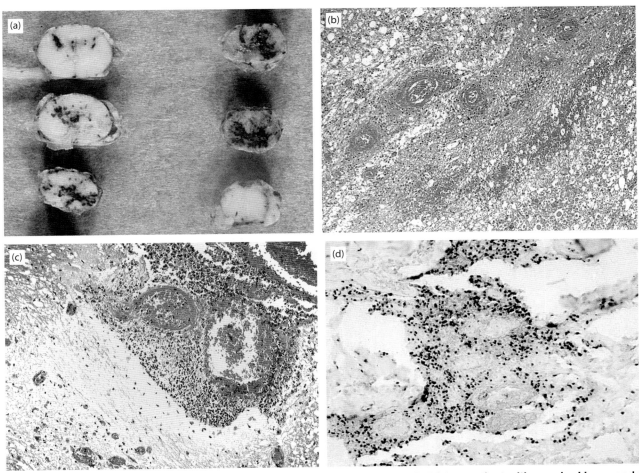

19.17 Haemorrhagic meningomyeloradiculitis caused by varicella-zoster virus (VZV) in a patient with acquired immunodeficiency syndrome (AIDS). (a) Transverse slices through the affected spinal cord reveal foci of haemorrhage and extensive necrosis. **(b)** Vascular and parenchymal necrosis and patchy parenchymal haemorrhage. **(c)** Necrotic spinal leptomeningeal blood vessels surrounded by a chronic inflammatory infiltrate. **(d)** Demonstration of VZV by *in situ* hybridization in large numbers of cells surrounding necrotic vessels in the spinal parenchyma.

Courtesy of Professor F Gray, Hôpital Lariboisière, Paris, France.

receptor (CD21 antigen) in the cytoplasmic membrane, and cross-linking of adjacent complement 3d receptor proteins.[1051,1115] Endocytosis of the virus also requires membrane fusion, mediated by interaction between virion gp42 and cellular human leukocyte antigen (HLA) class II molecule HLA-DR, -DP or -DQ.[429] EBV proliferates in oropharyngeal epithelium and salivary glands, where it establishes a persistent low-level productive infection.[656,766] The virus spreads to B-cells and establishes latent infection in resting memory B-cells, within which the viral genome is maintained episomally.[599] During latency, the virus exploits the normal regulation of transcription by the B-cell, so that the pattern of viral gene expression varies according to the stage of differentiation of the cell.[55,337] The latency-associated viral genes expressed at one or more stages of B-cell differentiation are *EBNA1*, *EBNA2*, *EBNA3A*, *EBNA3B*, *EBNA3C*, *EBNA LP*, *LMP1* and *LMP2*. The expression of five of these, *EBNA1*, *EBNA2*, *EBNA3A*, *EBNA3C* and *LMP1*, is capable of immortalizing infected B-cells.[599,707]

Clinical Features

The features of infectious mononucleosis develop 4–7 weeks after exposure and usually resolve gradually over subsequent weeks, although the duration is variable and the disease may last for days or months (see Box 19.5 for a discussion of the relationship to chronic fatigue syndrome).[707] Patients develop headache, lassitude, anorexia and, typically, a triad of fever, sore throat and tender lymphadenopathy. The pharynx is severely inflamed and may show petechial haemorrhages. About half of patients develop splenomegaly. Splenic rupture is a rare complication. Mild hepatitis is common. Jaundice sometimes occurs but hepatomegaly is unusual. Laboratory investigations reveal a lymphocytosis and, later, enlarged, atypical lymphocytes. Occasional systemic complications include autoimmune haemolytic disease, thrombocytopenia, myocarditis and nephritis.[580] EBV infection of patients with X-linked lymphoproliferative syndrome (caused by mutations in the *SH2D1A* gene at Xq25) results in fatal infectious mononucleosis,

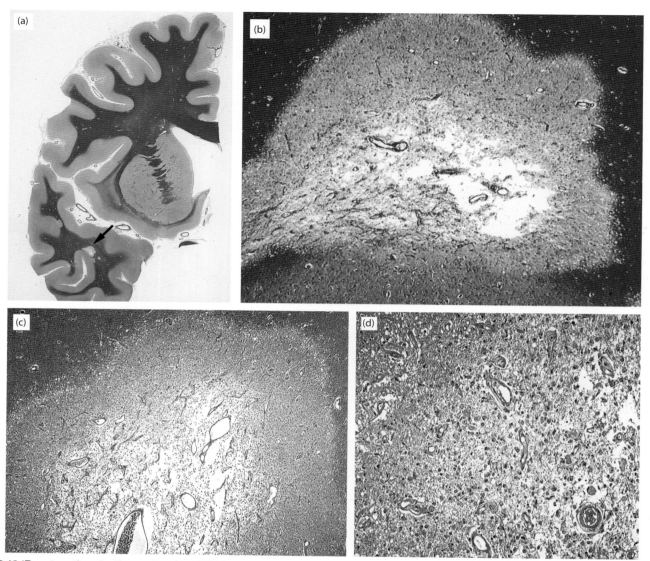

19.18 'Burnt-out' varicella-zoster virus (VZV) encephalitis. These illustrations are from a patient with acquired immunodeficiency syndrome (AIDS) who developed an encephalitis with multiple cerebral lesions visible on magnetic resonance imaging, and VZV in the cerebrospinal fluid. He was treated with high doses of aciclovir and highly active antiretroviral therapy (HAART), which resulted in an increased CD4 count, decreased human immunodeficiency virus (HIV) load and disappearance of VZV from the cerebrospinal fluid. His neurological status did not improve, however, and he died from aspiration pneumonia. **(a)** Necrotic subcortical lesion (arrow) in the temporal lobe. Luxol fast blue/cresyl violet. **(b)** The lesion has a targetoid appearance, typical of VZV infection. Luxol fast blue/cresyl violet. **(c)** The central region consists of loosely arranged blood vessels and scattered macrophages. **(d)** Higher magnification shows some of the blood vessels to have thickened walls, possibly reflecting previous vasculitis. Note the paucity of lymphocytes. Varicella-zoster virus was not detectable, either immunohistochemically or by *in situ* hybridization.

Reproduced from De la Grandmaison et al.,[260] with permission from the Royal College of Radiologists.

agammaglobulinaemia or B-cell lymphoma, complicating uncontrolled polyclonal expansion of T- and B-cells.[214,917] EBV also causes or contributes to the development of post-transplantation lymphoproliferative and other neoplastic disorders.[599,707,918]

Headache is a very frequent in infectious mononucleosis and often associated with a CSF pleocytosis and neck stiffness.[54,233,289] Epstein–Barr virus DNA and specific antibodies are present in the CSF during the acute illness but disappear during convalescence.[509,1007] Much rarer complications include painful lumbosacral radiculopathy, polyradiculopathy, transverse myelitis, optic neuritis and encephalitis.[233,422,1029] Most patients make a good recovery but some have persistent neurological deficits.[289,546] In some cases, the encephalitis is probably a post-infectious hypersensitivity reaction (see Box 19.2).[20] Criteria for the diagnosis of neurological disease associated with primary EBV infection were reviewed by Bathoorn *et al.*[78] A variety of neurological complications, from meningitis to haemorrhagic encephalitis,[82,1108] have been associated with EBV reactivation and the presence of the virus in the CSF.

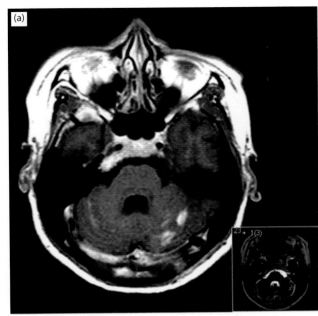

BOX 19.5. Chronic fatigue syndrome

Chronic fatigue syndrome (CFS, also sometimes referred to in the United Kingdom as myalgic encephalomyelitis, ME) came to prominence and was given this specific label in the mid-1980s, with reports of clusters of patients, mostly women, who had chronic relapsing fatigue, recurrent low-grade fever, sore throat, lymphadenopathy, myalgia, arthralgia, headaches, sleep disturbances and an impaired ability to concentrate.[737] Although the designation of this disorder as CFS is relatively recent, the symptoms correspond to descriptions of 'neurasthenia' and 'nervous exhaustion' that go back at least as far as the mid-nineteenth century. The currently accepted clinical definition of CFS is:[681]

- clinically evaluated, unexplained, persistent or relapsing, self-reported fatigue, lasting for at least 6 consecutive months and that is of new or definite onset; is not the result of ongoing exertion; is not substantially alleviated by rest; and results in substantial reduction in previous levels of occupational, educational, social or personal activities; and
- four or more of the following concurrent and persistent symptoms:
  - impaired short-term memory or concentration;
  - sore throat;
  - tender cervical or axillary lymph nodes;
  - muscle pain;
  - multi-joint pain without arthritis;
  - headaches of a new type, pattern or severity;
  - unrefreshing sleep;
  - post-exertional malaise lasting for more than 24 hours.

A syndrome of fatigue lasting for longer than 6 months has been reported in a small proportion of patients after various viral or presumed viral infections, particularly infectious mononucleosis.[681,1221,1222] However, most studies have not found evidence of an association between CFS and viral infection.[668,681,738] Subtle alterations in immune and endocrine function have been noted in some studies of patients with CFS.[610,736] It has been suggested that these alterations may lead to persistent viral infection or 'incomplete' expression of latent virus, but the evidence is inconclusive.

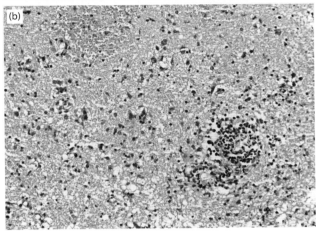

Sparse neuropathological data are available. Sworn and Urich illustrated florid, non-necrotizing mononuclear cell inflammation in the cerebral cortex of an 8-year-old who developed a fatal encephalitis during the second week of infectious mononucleosis.[1102] Francisci and colleagues reported fatal necrotizing haemorrhagic encephalitis in an immunocompetent young adult; EBV-DNA was present in his CSF and post-mortem brain tissue.[342] We have seen EBV encephalitis and vasculitis in a patient with HIV infection (Figure 19.19); MRI showed multiple enhancing lesions in the cerebellum and overlying meninges, thought to be tuberculous but biopsy revealed T-cell infiltration of blood vessels and cerebellar parenchyma and abundant EBV-encoded small RNA (EBER). The findings in most cases that have been examined neuropathologically have been mild and non-specific, including cerebral or cerebellar oedema, sparse petechial haemorrhages in the spinal cord or cerebrum, and mild inflammation of the meninges or nerve roots.[100,288,944,975] EBV infection has occasionally been associated with the development of Guillain–Barré syndrome (see Chapter 24).

Several epidemiological and serological studies have suggested a role for EBV infection in the development of multiple sclerosis (see Chapter 23).

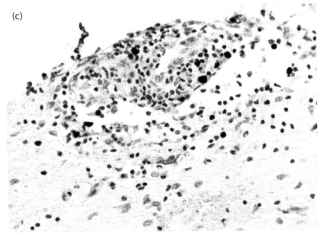

19.19 EBV encephalitis and vasculitis in HIV disease. **(a)** MRI scan of brain showing cerebellar meningeal and parenchymal lesions, thought to be tuberculous meningitis. **(b)** Abundant lymphocytes in the vessel wall and adjacent parenchyma. Immunohistochemistry showed almost all of these to be T-cells. **(c)** *In situ* hybridization with a probe for EBV-encoded small RNA (EBER), shows strong labelling of lymphocytes.

Cytomegalovirus

Many mammals are infected by species-specific β-herpesviruses. Most adult humans have been infected by CMV. However, it is only the immunosuppressed host that develops significant CNS pathology. CMV has a worldwide distribution. Its presence even in isolated populations, such as indigenous people of the Brazilian rainforest,[1086] indicates that the virus–host relationship predates early human migrations.

Aetiology

This is the largest of the herpesviruses, measuring approximately 200 nm in diameter. The name 'cytomegalovirus' is derived from the morphological changes it induces in infected cells, which enlarge markedly and develop characteristic nuclear and cytoplasmic inclusions. The genomic organization and replication of CMV share many similarities with those of the other herpesviruses. Multiple strains of CMV have been identified, initially on the basis of antigenic variation and subsequently by identification of differences in nucleotide sequence. Sequencing of part of the envelope glycoprotein B (gB) gene in a range of different strains has revealed four main groups, each with a characteristic nucleotide and peptide sequence.[195] More recently, polymorphisms in short tandem repeats within the viral genome have been used for rapid characterization of different strains of CMV.

Heparan sulphate (sulfate) proteoglycans serve as initial tethering sites for CMV on the cell surface.[221] On many permissive cells, subsequent docking of the virus is mediated by its binding to epidermal growth factor receptor (EGFR).[1199] Integrin v3 functions as a co-receptor for CMV.[1200] Activated EGFR and v3-integrins co-localize in lipid rafts, where they interact to form multimeric complexes, a process that seems to initiate viral endocytosis. Binding and endocytosis of the virus are accompanied by the activation of toll-like receptors (TLR), TLR2 in particular, and induction of innate immunity, but this is probably not involved directly in the entry of the virus into the cell.[221]

Pathogenesis

The virus spreads both horizontally and vertically. Horizontal spread is facilitated by close contact and crowded living conditions. The virus is excreted for long periods in most bodily fluids and is usually acquired by oral or respiratory routes. However, CMV can also be transmitted venereally, through blood transfusion and by organ transplantation. Multiple infections by different strains can occur in a single host,[760,1069] particularly if immunocompromised.[64]

The virus readily crosses the human placenta. The incidence of congenitally acquired CMV ranges from 0.5 to 2.2 per cent of live births in developed countries.[1143] Transmission can also occur in the postnatal period, especially if the infant is breastfed by the infected mother.[1076] Subsequent waves of infection occur at the time of entry into school[1032] and at puberty. Over half of the population is seropositive by 25 years and over 80 per cent by 35 years. The figures are higher in lower socioeconomic groups. In some high-risk groups (e.g. homosexual people) seropositivity approaches 100 per cent.

From its site of primary infection, CMV is disseminated haematogenously throughout the body, including the brain. Latent CMV infection is established in myeloid progenitor cells in the bone marrow and transmitted to the progeny myelomonocytic cells in the blood and other tissues.[607,613,699] Myeloid dendritic cell progenitors are reservoirs of latent infection.[927] *Ex vivo* differentiation of these cells to a mature dendritic cell phenotype causes chromatin remodelling of the viral major immediate-early promoter/enhancer and reactivation of infectious virus. Unlike VZV and HSV, CMV is not transported axonally and does not establish latent neuronal infection. The effects of CMV on the CNS are due to entry into the CNS of haematogenous cells harbouring replicating virus, and subsequent infection and destruction of resident cells.

Clinical Features

Primary infection of young children with CMV can cause pneumonia or anicteric hepatitis. In older children and adults, primary CMV infection can cause an infectious mononucleosis-like syndrome of fever, lymphocytosis with atypical lymphocytes, lymphadenopathy and hepatitis, which is usually subclinical but very occasionally becomes severe.[552] In immunocompetent patients, CNS complications are rare but can include meningitis, encephalitis,[56] transverse myelitis,[379,763] radiculomyelitis[553] and retinitis.[1085] A more common complication is Guillain–Barré syndrome,[1011,1185] which may be related to the development of antibodies that cross-react with GM2 ganglioside (see Chapter 24).[512]

Cytomegalovirus is a significant source of morbidity after kidney, heart, heart–lung, liver and bone marrow transplantation;[981] a mononucleosis syndrome and pneumonia are the most common problems related to CMV infection or reactivation in this population. Up to 30 per cent of bone marrow and 60 per cent of solid organ transplant patients develop CMV infection.[338,531] The risk of CMV-related disease is reduced by prophylactic aciclovir or ganciclovir before transplantation.[235] Symptomatic CNS disease is unusual in transplant patients, even when infection of the brain can be shown at autopsy,[295,937] but CMV retinitis is a significant problem and can lead to blindness.

Much of the literature on the neuropathological manifestations of CMV infection relates to patients with AIDS. Cytomegalovirus is the most common opportunistic viral infection in patients with AIDS and affects numerous organ systems. Cytomegalovirus colitis, adrenalitis, hepatitis and pneumonitis are important causes of morbidity in these patients. Some 10–40 per cent of patients with AIDS have CNS involvement by the time of autopsy,[597,896,976] although symptomatic CMV-related neurological disease is infrequent.[353] Before the introduction of effective antiviral agents, CMV chorioretinitis affected one-fifth of patients with AIDS[793] and often led to unilateral or complete blindness. The use of better antiviral drugs has substantially improved the outcome of CMV retinitis in AIDS.[698,961]

The CNS manifestations of CMV infection in AIDS are difficult to distinguish from those of HIV itself and from those of other opportunistic infections. The two main clinical syndromes relate to (1) CMV encephalitis with widespread microglial nodules, which can cause subacute dementia, delirium, confusion, apathy and focal neurological deficits[478,721] and (2) CMV ventriculoencephalitis, which may present insidiously or rapidly with progressive encephalopathy, cranial nerve palsies and nystagmus, and is associated with high CSF protein and increasing ventriculomegaly.[398,558,721] Some patients develop the ophthalmoplegia, ataxia, memory impairment and confabulation of Wernicke–Korsakoff syndrome.[1136] Involvement of the spinal cord and nerve roots is uncommon but can lead to ascending motor weakness, areflexia, loss of sphincter control, paraesthesiae and sensory impairment.[85,349,396] Some patients develop peripheral neuropathy, usually patchy and multifocal, and manifesting with numbness and painful paraesthesiae;[349,977] the mechanisms may include direct infection of anterior horn cells and dorsal root ganglia, and ischaemic nerve damage resulting from infection of endothelial cells.[232,991] The virus can usually be detected by PCR of CSF,[1036] although interpretation is complicated by the ubiquity of CMV infection in patients with AIDS. CMV infection is usually treated with ganciclovir but, as in other human herpesvirus infections, treatment may be complicated by the emergence of thymidine kinase mutants, necessitating the use of alternative drugs, such as foscarnet.[40]

Pathological Findings

The neuropathological appearances are varied (Figure 19.20).[1184] Some patients develop a low-grade encephalitis in which there is widespread formation of microglial nodules (Figure 19.20a). Scattered cytomegalic cells can usually be identified, most of which are associated with microglial nodules, but detection of CMV-infected cells is facilitated by immunostaining for viral antigens. CMV infection in patients with AIDS is often accompanied by HIV encephalitis and can also occur in association with concurrent HSV infection.[1163] CMV-related lesions may involve any part of the nervous system and are almost always found in other organs as well.

In advanced AIDS, CMV can also cause necrotizing ventriculoencephalitis, in which numerous cytomegalic cells line the ventricles and largely replace the normal ependyma (Figure 19.20b–d). The subependymal tissue may be extensively necrotic and usually contains large numbers of cytomegalic inclusion cells. Apart from an infiltrate of macrophages, there may be little inflammation. Other unusual patterns of CMV-related disease include widespread microvascular endothelial infection in the spinal cord and nerve roots, necrotizing myeloradiculopathy,[197] and large necrotizing cerebral lesions that present with mass effect and later cavitate to resemble infarcts. CMV-related peripheral neuropathy is associated with foci of endoneurial necrosis, infiltrates of polymorphonuclear and mononuclear inflammatory cells, and cytomegalic inclusions in macrophages, fibroblasts and endothelial cells.[232,991] Axonal degeneration usually predominates, but segmental demyelination is seen in some cases.

Neonatal Cytomegalovirus Infection

Pathogenesis Symptomatic disease of the CNS in neonates is usually due to infection *in utero*. The risk of transmitting CMV to the fetus during primary maternal infection is 30–60 per cent, which is much greater than during latent or reactivated disease, when the risk is under 2 per cent.[8,242,1076,1143] Because horizontal transmission of CMV is facilitated by crowded living conditions, most women in lower socioeconomic groups will have acquired CMV in childhood. The risk of primary maternal infection during pregnancy and of consequent fetal infection is therefore greater in higher socioeconomic groups, within which up to 50 per cent of pregnant women may still be susceptible.

Infants can acquire CMV postnatally, through infected genital secretions, saliva and breast milk, but this does not usually lead to neurological disease.

Clinical Features Most CMV infections *in utero* are asymptomatic, but 5–15 per cent of infected fetuses develop congenital disease of variable severity.[94] The risk of fetal complications is highest if infection is acquired during the first trimester. The most severe form of congenital infection is disseminated cytomegalic inclusion disease,[826] which manifests shortly after birth with petechiae (in 80 per cent of cases), hepatosplenomegaly (75 per cent), jaundice (65 per cent), microcephaly (50 per cent) and chorioretinitis (12 per cent) and often runs a fatal course within days or weeks. Surviving infants may have microcephaly, severe metal retardation, seizures, spasticity, severe hearing loss, chorioretinitis and optic atrophy.[745,880] Hydrocephalus is uncommon. Infants with less severe perinatal disease may present in later infancy with ophthalmic and auditory impairment, and microcephaly. In milder cases, deafness, or minimal brain dysfunction with intellectual and behavioural problems, may become apparent only later in life.[449,756] Infants infected *in utero* continue to shed virus in saliva and urine for several years, in amounts much higher than after infection in childhood or adulthood.[1075]

Infection of full-term infants in the postnatal period is usually subclinical or associated with only minor morbidity.[805] However, postnatal infection of premature infants may cause severe disease, with chronic respiratory difficulties, anaemia, hepatosplenomegaly and an atypical lymphocytosis.[67]

Pathological Findings Infants coming to autopsy after neonatal cytomegalic inclusion disease usually have evidence of widespread infection commencing *in utero* and involving many organs. The brain is usually small and may show porencephaly or polymicrogyria; less frequent findings include hydrocephalus, lissencephaly and cerebellar hypoplasia.[73,890] On sectioning, the brain may feel gritty, owing to foci of calcification, which are most prominent in the periventricular region (Figure 19.21). The larger foci of calcification are macroscopically visible as granules of hard white material. Cystic spaces may be present in the brain parenchyma. The degree of residual inflammation on microscopic examination depends on the timing of examination in relation to the acute neonatal disease. Most cases show obvious meningoencephalitis, and cytomegalic inclusions can be found in all cellular elements of the brain, including

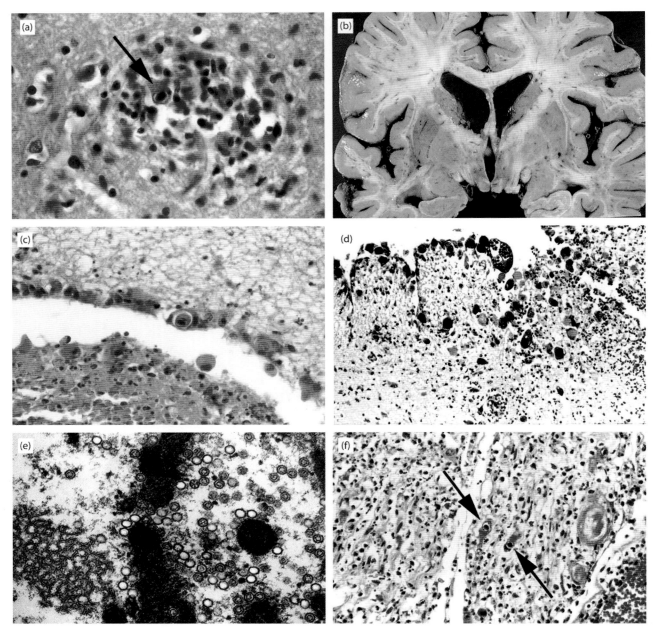

19.20 Cytomegalovirus (CMV) infection in patients with acquired immunodeficiency syndrome (AIDS). (a) The microglial nodule in this section includes a cytomegalic cell (arrow). (b) Coronal slice through the brain of a patient with AIDS with CMV ventriculitis. There is mild ventricular dilation, and discolouration and sloughing of the ependymal surface. (c) Histology shows the ventricle to be partly denuded of ependyma and covered by necrotic debris. The residual ependymal lining contains several cells with CMV inclusions. The subependymal tissue is markedly oedematous. (d) CMV ventriculitis immunostained for CMV. The partially ulcerated ependymal surface and oedematous subependymal tissue contain numerous immunolabelled cytomegalic cells (red). The inflammatory response consists predominantly of macrophages. (e) Electron micrograph of the nucleus of an infected cell reveals abundant non-enveloped CMV nucleocapsids. (f) CMV radiculitis: two cytomegalic cells (arrows) are seen within the necrotic nerve root.

neurons. Cytomegalic cells are most numerous in periventricular regions, particularly around the lateral ventricles. Foci of mineralization are present in the grey and white matter, most with little associated inflammation. There may be astrocytosis, especially in the subependymal region.

Central nervous system disease complicating postnatal infection is characterized histologically by the presence of numerous microglial nodules scattered throughout the brain. These are not usually associated with mineralization and contain only occasional cytomegalic cells with inclusions. A similar pattern of CMV encephalitis, occurring several months after birth, has also been reported as a complication of congenital co-infection with HIV and CMV.[86]

Human Herpesvirus 6

Human herpesvirus 6 is a ubiquitous β-herpesvirus that closely resembles HHV-7 and, to a lesser extent, CMV, in its genomic organization and biological properties.

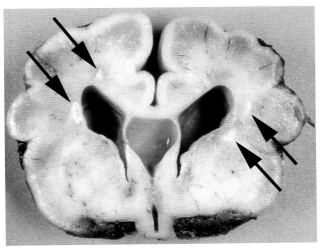

19.21 Congenital cytomegalovirus (CMV) encephalitis. The ventricles are moderately dilated, and several foci of calcification are visible in the periventricular region (arrows).

Courtesy of Dr Helen Porter, Bristol Children's Hospital, Bristol, UK. Reproduced from Ellison and Love.[308a] © Elsevier, 1998.

Aetiology

Two antigenically distinct variants, HHV-6A and HHV-6B, are recognized.[286] Most HHV-6-related clinical infections in immunocompetent hosts are caused by HHV-6B, but most neurological disease and infections in immunocompromised hosts are caused by HHV-6A. The cellular receptor for HHV-6 is CD46 (membrane cofactor protein),[996] a regulator of complement activation.

Pathogenesis

Spread of HHV-6 is usually from close contacts within the family.[286,1091,1269] The virus is probably transmitted through infected saliva or respiratory secretions. The incidence of HHV-6 infection peaks between the ages of 6 and 21 months, and by 2 years of age most children are seropositive.[157,1269] Rarely, infection is acquired *in utero*, as evidenced by the demonstration of HHV-6 DNA in umbilical cord blood in a small percentage of neonates,[5] and possibly intrapartum, as the virus is present in the cervix in about 20 per cent of pregnant women.[859] The virus is tropic for T-lymphocytes, within which it replicates.[286] It also infects monocytes[611] and bone marrow progenitor cells, from which it may be transmitted to myeloid progeny.[694] Latent infection is probably established in monocytes and possibly other cells, including cells in the CNS (see review see Yao *et al.*)[1260] In one study, brain tissue from 34 of 40 consecutive autopsies on patients 20–95 years in age contained HHV-6 DNA: only variant A in 4 cases, only variant B in 23 cases, and both variants in 7 cases.[175] HHV-6 latency-associated transcripts have been identified that are oriented in the same direction as the immediate–early 1 and 2 genes and share their protein-coding regions, but that have distinct transcription start sites and exons.[614] Reactivation of the virus occurs under conditions of impaired cell-mediated immunity.[222,286,1049]

Clinical and Pathological Features

Primary infection by HHV-6 is the principal cause of roseola infantum (exanthem subitum),[286,1253] a disease of infants and children that is characterized by a fever and, as the fever subsides, a faint maculopapular rash. The other cause of this disease is HHV-7 (see later under Human Herpesvirus 7). Only a minority of infected children develops roseola infantum. Infection with HHV-6 frequently occurs in the absence of a rash and is an important cause of febrile seizures in young children.[437] Rarely, primary infection is complicated by meningitis or encephalitis,[10,43,496,513,1257] and viral DNA is detectable in the CSF during most primary infections.[155,612] An acute disseminated encephalomyelitis-like illness has been reported.[560] In older children, HHV-6 infection may cause an infectious mononucleosis-like illness, although whether this is a manifestation of primary infection or reactivation is unclear.[1079]

Reactivated infection with HHV-6 occurs in about half of recipients of bone marrow transplant and one-third of recipients of solid organ transplant.[286] The manifestations include fever, rashes, bone marrow suppression and meningitis or limbic encephalitis. Symptomatic HHV-6-related disease is rare in HIV-infected patients, but pneumonitis and encephalitis have been reported.[157]

There is scant information on the pathological findings in HHV-6 encephalitis. Reports describe multifocal lymphohistiocytic inflammation of grey and white matter and, in some cases, haemorrhage or necrosis.[10,908,1191] Viral DNA can usually be detected in the CSF, and both viral DNA and antigen have been demonstrated in neurons, oligodendrocytes and astrocytes.[9,340,341,1124]

The contribution of HHV-6 to other neurological diseases is still unclear. There has been considerable interest in the potential role of HHV-6 in multiple sclerosis (see Chapter 23),[1260] but the interpretation of most of the relevant studies is complicated by the fact that the virus often persists asymptomatically in the CSF and even the brain after primary infection, which may itself be asymptomatic.[155,209,1146] In a few studies of brain tissue from patients with multiple sclerosis, immediate–early and late HHV-6 gene transcripts and protein were detected in oligodendrocytes in demyelinating lesions and, in some cases, in normal-appearing white matter.[174,389,842,863] Viral DNA and antigen have also been detected in astrocytes in temporal lobectomy specimens from some patients with temporal lobe epilepsy.[294]

Human Herpesvirus 7

Human herpesvirus 7 is a β-herpesvirus that shares several biological features with HHV-6.[280] Most children will have been infected with HHV-7 by 3 years, usually through contact with infected saliva or breast milk,[156,347,1251] or possibly by contact with infected cervical secretions during parturition in a small proportion of cases.[859] The virus is tropic for CD4 lymphocytes and, like HIV but unlike HHV-6, binds to the actual CD4 receptor protein.[696] Primary infection with HHV-7 can cause roseola infantum (exanthem subitum), febrile infection in the absence of a rash, febrile seizures, an infectious mononucleosis-like syndrome and, rarely, an encephalitis or myelitis.[1167,1201] The series reported by Torigoe and colleagues included two children in whom HHV-7 infection was complicated by seizures, hemiplegia and brain atrophy.[1137] Both encephalitis and myelitis have been reported as complications of HHV-7 reactivation in haematopoietic cell transplant patients.[176,1002,1202]

Human Herpesvirus 8

Human herpesvirus 8 was initially identified in association with Kaposi's sarcoma,[21] and later with primary effusion/body cavity lymphoma and Castleman's disease. The virus was eventually classified as a γ-herpesvirus.[270] Seroprevalence studies indicate that HHV-8 has a more limited geographical distribution than the other herpesviruses.[536,575] The overall prevalence of infection has been estimated at under 5 per cent, but certain populations have a seroprevalence as high as 50 per cent. The virus is transmitted both non-sexually, probably through saliva, and sexually, particularly among homosexual men.[270,536] Several HHV-8 genes are capable of disrupting the normal cellular control of proliferation and apoptosis. Symptomatic infection is confined to immunosuppressed people (especially patients with AIDS) and manifests with benign or malignant proliferative disorders. HHV8 is not known to infect the CNS.[378]

B Virus

B virus (cercopithecine herpesvirus 1/herpesvirus simiae) is endemic in certain Old World primates, particularly those of the genus *Macaca* (macaques). This genus includes several species of macaque that are used in biomedical research and some that have been kept as domestic pets.[867]

Aetiology

The amino acid sequence, mode of replication and lifecycle of B virus are similar to those of HSV-1 and HSV-2 (see earlier).[498] The virus infects mucosal or cutaneous epithelium, where its replication involves the sequential transcription of α, β and γ genes. The virus is conveyed by retrograde axonal transport along sensory fibres to the primary sensory ganglia, where, after further replication, latent infection is established. Reactivation from latency involves the replication and anterograde spread of virus to skin or mucosa, and subsequent lytic epithelial infection. Between 70 and 100 per cent of adult macaques in captivity are seropositive for B virus.[498,1212] Like HSV-1 infection in humans, primary infection with B virus in macaques may result in gingivostomatitis but often occurs without such signs, and is followed by the establishment of a latent infection with intermittent reactivation and shedding of the virus in saliva or genital secretions, particularly under conditions of stress or immunosuppression.

Pathogenesis of Human Infection

Most human infections result from monkey bites or scratches, but laboratory workers have also been infected by laceration with glass from a culture tube containing contaminated monkey kidney cells,[250] by needlestick injury[41] and by splashing

of contaminated biological material (possibly faeces) into the eye.[166] Human-to-human transmission has occurred when the wife of an infected patient applied hydrocortisone cream first to her husband's skin lesions and then to her own skin in an area of contact dermatitis.[165] To date, B virus encephalomyelitis has been reported in over 30 patients.

Clinical and Pathological Features

The incubation period for human disease usually ranges from 2 to 5 weeks but may be shorter. Patients present with pain, dysaesthesiae or numbness at the site of exposure, after which they rapidly develop encephalomyelitis, with headache and pyrexia, sensory disturbances and weakness, confusion, coma and death.[481,498] The distribution of sensory and motor disturbances is partly dependent on the site of initial infection and may predominantly affect one side of the body, at least initially. In the absence of antiviral treatment, B virus infection in humans is usually fatal, and the few survivors have had severe neurological deficits. The pathological findings in fatal cases have been of widespread necrotizing pan-encephalomyelitis with foci of haemorrhage, and perivascular and parenchymal infiltration by mononuclear inflammatory cells. Eosinophilic intranuclear inclusions are sparse. Both aciclovir and ganciclovir have been successful in ameliorating or reversing the neurological manifestations in some patients, and valaciclovir has been recommended for prophylaxis after moderate- to high-risk exposure to B virus (e.g. after mucosal exposure or a bite with puncturing of the skin).[216]

Adenovirus

Aetiology

The virions of adenovirus are non-enveloped, icosahedral particles that are 60–90 nm in diameter and contain double-stranded DNA. The genus is subdivided into several subgenera (A–F), in which there are currently 51 known serotypes.[608,652] Many of these are common causes of human diseases, especially in children. Infection may be transmitted by respiratory, faeco–oral and, possibly, venereal[1101] routes. Protruding from pentons (pentagonal capsid subunits/capsomeres) at the 12 vertices of the icosahedral capsid are fibre proteins, the binding of which to specific cell surface receptors initiates endocytosis. The CAR protein serves as a receptor for most of the adenoviruses,[956] but group B viruses bind to CD46[1020] and group D serotype 37 uses sialic acid as a cellular receptor.[39] Endocytosis of bound virus is initiated by interaction of viral pentons with v1, v3 or v5 integrins on the cell surface.[670,827] Mild lowering of pH within endosomes containing the virus particles causes partial disassembly of the capsids and disruption of the endosomal membrane, and allows entry of the virus into the cell cytoplasm. The virus is then translocated along microtubules to the nuclear pore complex, where the genome is released and viral transcription and replication occur.

Clinical and Pathological Features

Most adenovirus infections are asymptomatic or cause only minor illness. Some serotypes can, however, cause pharyngitis, bronchitis, otitis media, pneumonia, gastroenteritis, hepatitis, keratoconjunctivitis, mesenteric adenitis, acute haemorrhagic cystitis and coagulopathy.[206,873,986,1172] Adenovirus infection with resulting hyperplasia of mucosal and submucosal lymphoid tissue in the distal part of the small intestine is a well-documented cause of intussusception in infants and young children.[831,1233] The virus can establish low-grade persistent or possibly latent infection in tonsillar and other lymphoid tissue.[357,830] Symptomatic, in some cases severe, adenovirus infections are relatively frequent in recipients of organ transplant and other immunosuppressed patients, with children being particularly susceptible.[608,652]

Encephalitis is a rare complication of adenovirus infection, occurring predominantly (although not exclusively) in immunosuppressed patients, and there are few descriptions of the neuropathological findings in this condition. In one patient, necrosis, perivascular and parenchymal haemorrhage, focal lymphocytic inflammation and microglial nodule lesions were found in the occipital lobe.[194] Bilateral haemorrhagic inflammatory lesions were present in the temporal lobes in a bone marrow transplant patient with adenovirus encephalitis; the lesions also involved the infundibular region of the hypothalamus, the supraoptic nuclei, the superior colliculi and periaqueductal grey matter, and the sensory nuclei of the trigeminal nerve, lateral vestibular nuclei and nuclei ambiguus.[253] Necrotizing adenovirus ependymitis was documented in a child with AIDS,[23] and perivascular mononuclear cell infiltrates were noted in the periventricular white matter in neonatal disseminated adenovirus infection.[866] A basal forebrain mass in an HIV-infected female patient was found at autopsy to contain adenovirus.[1182] In most of these cases, the sections of inflamed brain tissue have included intranuclear viral inclusions in neurons and glia (Figure 19.22). The inclusions appear homogeneously basophilic, with ill-defined edges, and cause enlargement of the affected nuclei. Electron microscopy reveals large paracrystalline arrays of icosahedral virus particles within neuronal and, less frequently, glial nuclei. Virus particles may also be present in the cytoplasm.

Orthomyxoviruses

The orthomyxoviruses are enveloped viruses with a single-stranded negative-sense segmented RNA genome. Known for endemic and pandemic human pulmonary infections around the world, of the five genera only influenza A is thought to have the potential to cause neurological disease. Influenza A is further classified into subtypes based upon the antigenicity of two of its envelope proteins: hemagglutinin (HA) and neuraminidase (NA). With 16 subtypes of HA and 9 of NA, there is a broad spectrum of possible recombinant serotypes. In recent years, H1N1 and H3N2 serotypes have been responsible for seasonal influenza. Antigenic drift and shift result in periodic pandemics. The 1918/1919 pandemic of 'Spanish' influenza was notable for its impressive virulence (it caused 25–50 million deaths) and temporal association with the neurological disease: encephalitis lethargica (von Economo's disease).[741] There has been much speculation regarding the capacity of influenza to infect the human brain. During pandemics, many people have been hospitalized with encephalopathy or encephalitis.[1135] However, H1N1 has not been recovered from the CSF or brain of human patients, raising the possibility that the neurological disease is secondary to the immune response to the virus.[11]

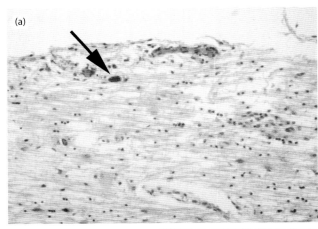

(a)

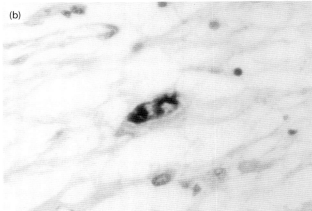

(b)

19.22 Adenovirus encephalitis in a child with acquired immunodeficiency syndrome (AIDS). (a) The periventricular white matter is inflamed and reactive. Several glial cells have enlarged nuclei containing basophilic viral inclusion bodies (arrow). **(b)** Higher magnification of an enlarged glial nucleus immunostained for adenovirus.

Courtesy of Professor H Vinters, University of California, Los Angeles, CA, USA.

Avian influenza (H5NX) expresses a hemagglutinin molecule known to bind to glycosylation sites in the CNS. This virus has been detected in bird, vertebrate animal and human brain tissue, where it mediates an acute encephalitis. In 8 years since the outbreak of H5N1 in 2003, there have been approximately 600 reported cases of human encephalitis, over half of them lethal. This relatively small number of cases reflects the fact that the avian influenza virus has not developed the capacity to spread from human to human. However, unlike other serotypes, H5N1 has the capacity to spread systemically and to infect numerous organs in addition to the brain. In human autopsies, the virus was detected in multiple organs and tissues, including lung, bowel, lymph node, neurons and placenta.[355,423] Experimental infection of laboratory animals (mice and ferrets) confirmed the neurotropism of this virus (Figure 19.23).[110]

Paramyxoviruses

The paramyxoviruses are large, enveloped, pleomorphic viruses, ranging from 100 to 300 nm in diameter and

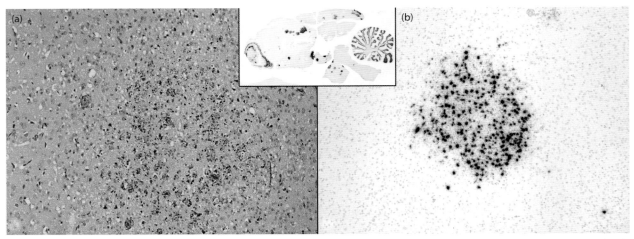

19.23 H5N1 influenza virus encephalitis in a ferret. (a) Focus of viral infection in the deep cerebral grey matter, 6 days after intra-nasal infection with H5N1 (VN04). There is abundant neuronal karyorrhexis and early infiltration by mononuclear inflammatory cells. **(b)** *In situ* hybridization with 35S-labeled probe for viral M protein RNA reveals strong signal (black grains) localized to neurons. The inset is a whole-mount scan of a sagittal brain slice, showing severe infection of olfactory cortex and multiple foci of viral infection in other parts of the brain.

containing a core of single-stranded, non-segmented, neg-ative-sense RNA. The family Paramyxoviridae is currently subdivided into two subfamilies, Paramyxovirinae and Pneumovirinae.[914] The Paramyxovirinae include four gen-era: Respirovirus (formerly Paramyxovirus), Rubulavirus, Morbillivirus and Henipavirus.[1198] The Pneumovirinae com-prise two genera: Pneumovirus and Metapneumovirus. The paramyxoviruses that are known to cause human neuro-logical disease are mumps virus (in the genus Rubulavirus), measles virus (in the genus Morbillivirus), and Hendra and Nipah viruses (in the genus Henipavirus).

Mumps

Humans are the only known natural host of this virus, of which 10 genotypes (A–J) have been identified.[799] The genotyping is based on the sequence of the *SH* (small hydrophobic protein) gene, the most variable part of the viral genome. Genotypes C–E, G and H have tended to pre-dominate in the western hemisphere, and genotypes B, F and I in Asian countries, but the dominant genotype var-ies at different times in different regions. Spread occurs by contact with infected respiratory secretions and saliva. The virus replicates in the upper respiratory tract and then in regional lymphoid tissue before a viraemia occurs, with sys-temic dissemination. During the viraemia, the virus spreads to the choroid plexus and ependyma and can be detected in the CSF.[466] Enhanced neurovirulence has been associated with some genotypes (C, D, H, J) and some vaccine strains (Urabe Am9, Leningrad–Zagreb and Hoshino).[248,298,583] The molecular basis of this is not known.[799]

Clinical and Pathological Features

The usual incubation period is 2–3 weeks. Clinical pre-sentation usually consists of headache, low-grade fever and malaise. Over 50 per cent of patients develop ten-der enlargement of the parotid glands, and in a minor-ity of cases other salivary glands are similarly affected. Orchitis occurs in 20–30 per cent of post-pubertal males with mumps, but rarely results in testicular atrophy. Mild

mastitis is common in post-pubertal females. Less frequent complications include pancreatitis, oophoritis and thyroid-itis. Sensorineural deafness occurs in 1 in 15 000–20 000 cases, probably due to cochlear infection.[1219]

As noted (see earlier under Aseptic Meningitis), most patients with mumps virus infection have a CSF lympho-cytosis, and up to 10 per cent develop aseptic meningitis. Males are more susceptible than females. Meningitis usu-ally manifests days to weeks after the onset of parotitis but can precede the parotitis or occur in its absence.[545,667] Some vaccine strains can cause aseptic meningitis, but the frequency is much lower (about 1 in 5000–20 000 vac-cine recipients) than that in association with wild-type viral infection.[248,298,583] Approximately 1 in 1000 patients develops acute disseminated or brain stem encephalomy-elitis (see Chapter 23 and Box 19.2), from which as many as a quarter of patients suffer permanent neurological sequelae.[621] Some of these patients show evidence of con-tinued synthesis of anti-mumps virus antibodies in the CSF for several years after the acute infection. There is both clinical and immunological overlap between such patients and the very few cases in which mumps has been associated with the development of a chronic, progressive encepha-litis.[432,505,516] Other, rare complications include transverse myelitis,[844,1177] lower motor neuron paralytic disease (which is usually transient, although permanent sequelae have been reported),[657] facial palsy and Guillain–Barré syn-drome.[369,905] For the most part, mumps is preventable by vaccination, although compliance has not been sufficient to achieve herd immunity. Moderate salivary gland and CNS involvement (largely subclinical) is a known complication of live-attenuated vaccination.[1] In countries without vac-cination, the incidence of mumps is over 100/100 000 per annum with a peak at 5–9 years of age. The relationship between measles–mumps–rubella (MMR) vaccination and autism is discussed later (see under Measles).

The induction of aqueduct stenosis and hydrocephalus in suckling hamsters infected with mumps virus was first demonstrated by Johnson and co-workers[542] and has since been confirmed by others.[1106] Subsequently, hydrocephalus has been reported as a rare complication of mumps in children.[851,1068,1126]

Measles

This highly contagious virus is transmitted by inhalation of droplets of infected respiratory secretions and usually causes a short-lived febrile disease with a typical maculopapular rash. Involvement of the CNS, when it occurs, usually takes the form of aseptic meningitis or acute disseminated encephalomyelitis.[541] The latter complicates about 1 in 1000 cases of measles and 1 in 2 000 000 patients receiving measles vaccination (see Box 19.2 and Chapter 23).[167] Much less commonly, measles causes a subacute infective encephalitis, of which there are two types: measles inclusion body encephalitis and subacute sclerosing pan-encephalitis; these disorders, and the pathogenesis of measles virus infection of the CNS, are described in detail later in this chapter (see later under Subacute and Chronic Viral Infections).

In 1998, Wakefield and colleagues reported a series of 12 children with lymphoid nodular hyperplasia of the terminal ileum and non-specific, non-granulomatous colitis.[1193] Ten of the children had also been diagnosed as having autism or autistic spectrum disorder, of onset 1 day to 18 months after combined MMR vaccination. This report caused widespread public concern about the safety of the MMR vaccine. However, the possibility of an aetiological link to the combined vaccine, or indeed to measles virus, was refuted conclusively in several subsequent epidemiological studies.[244,277,486,573,709]

Henipaviruses

The genus Henipavirus comprises two members of the subfamily Paramyxovirinae: Hendra virus and Nipah virus.[1198] These have longer genomes than other members of the subfamily and differ also in showing broad species tropism, with the ability to cause fatal disease in both animals and humans. The zoonotic paramyxoviruses have a natural reservoir in pteropids: fox-bats (Megachiroptera).[205,701,1180] Emergence of Henipavirus epidemics in livestock and humans has been linked to climate change and disruption of natural ecosystems. Deforestation and El Nino cycles led to fruit tree failures and the migration of forest fox-bats to commercial orchards and pig farms.[684] Most human infections have been caused by close contact with infected animals (horses in the case of Hendra virus and pigs in the case of Nipah virus), probably through inhalation of infected droplets of either respiratory secretions or urine, but other routes of infection have been documented and there is increasing evidence of human-to-human transmission of Nipah virus. Ephrin-B2 and -B3 were shown to be cellular receptors for both viruses.[121,650,718]

Hendra

This paramyxovirus was first identified in Australia in 1994 after an outbreak of severe respiratory disease affecting racehorses in the Brisbane suburb of Hendra.[700] The trainer and stablehand were also infected; the trainer died. A separate, smaller outbreak in Queensland was associated with the death of two horses and a 35-year-old man who had cared for them.[868] The patient made an initial recovery from aseptic meningitis but 13 months later presented with irritability, low back pain and seizures. Over the next few days he developed low-grade pyrexia, dense hemiplegia, brain stem dysfunction and depressed consciousness. He remained obtunded and pyrexial until his death 25 days after admission. Post-mortem examination revealed necrotizing meningoencephalitis, with foci of necrosis in the neocortex, basal ganglia, brain stem and cerebellum, and occasional multinucleated endothelial cells in the brain and other organs. Hendra virus was demonstrated within the brain by immunohistochemistry, PCR and electron microscopy. A further case of human disease occurred in Queensland in November 2004, when a veterinarian suffered a 'mild Hendra infection' after performing an autopsy on a horse that had had clinical symptoms consistent with Hendra infection.[220]

Nipah Virus

A paramyxovirus related to, but distinct from, Hendra virus was shown to be the cause of outbreaks of encephalitis in several parts of peninsular Malaysia and Singapore between 1998 and 1999.[204,883,1111] As the virus was first isolated from patients who came from the Nipah River Village, it was named Nipah virus. Subsequent serological and epidemiological studies indicated that the virus was predominantly transmitted to humans from infected pigs.[1111] Dogs, cats, horses and goats were also infected, probably from pigs, and instances of human-to-human and dog-to-human infection were documented.[1111]

Several further outbreaks have occurred in Bangladesh, with mortality rates up to 70 per cent.[220,682] Outbreaks in 2001 and 2003 were not related to obvious zoonotic sources of infection; clustering of cases in several households and the increased incidence in those handling, or exposed to secretions of, sick patients suggested person-to-person transmission. A subsequent outbreak in the Tangail district, in 2005, is thought to have resulted from the ingestion of fruit that had been partially eaten and contaminated by fruit bats.

Clinical Features

Most patients present with symptoms and signs of an acute encephalitis, including fever, severe headache, vomiting, an altered level of consciousness, myoclonus and, in some cases, prominent brain stem dysfunction.[203,204,383,883] MRI reveals multiple discrete hyperintense lesions in the subcortical and deep cerebral white matter, best demonstrated using fluid-attenuated inversion recovery (FLAIR) sequences.[883,1111] Some patients also develop atypical pneumonia. Overall mortality is of the order of 30–40 per cent,[383,1111] but the prognosis varies according to the pattern of clinical disease: in patients with brain stem involvement the mortality is very high, whereas most patients who retain a normal level of consciousness during the acute illness survive.[383] About 15–20 per cent of patients have persistent neurological deficits, seizures or personality changes.

Late-onset or recurrent encephalitis was reported in a minority of patients who had previously recovered from acute encephalitis (7.5 per cent) or who initially had asymptomatic or non-encephalitic infection (3.4 per cent).[1111] The interval between initial and recurrent infection was several months. Recurrence manifested with rapid onset of fever, headache, seizures and focal neurological signs, and was fatal in 4 of 22 patients.[1111]

Pathological Features

Post-mortem examination of a few cases revealed widespread necrotizing vasculitis involving arterioles, capillaries and venules, with associated thrombosis and ischaemic damage or small foci of frank infarction. The vasculitis was most extensive in the brain but the lungs, heart, kidneys and other organs were also affected.[204,1111,1240] Other features included endothelial syncytia, eosinophilic inclusion bodies within the nucleus and cytoplasm of neurons adjacent to vasculitic blood vessels, and occasional neuronophagia and microglial nodules (Figure 19.24). Immunohistochemistry with anti-Hendra antibodies (which cross-react with Nipah virus) confirmed endothelial as well as parenchymal infection in the brain and other organs. Viral antigen was also detected in the brain after recurrent encephalitis; perivenous demyelination was not a feature.[1111] Neuropathological examination of a case of fatal relapse of Nipah encephalitis revealed large, confluent destructive parenchymal lesions, some haemorrhagic. Viral inclusions were larger and more abundant than in patients with acute disease, filling most of the cytoplasm of many macrophages, neurons and glia, including ependymal cells.

Rubella

Rubella virus is a small, enveloped RNA virus, the only member of the genus Rubivirus (in the family Togavirus). The virus is spherical, with an outer diameter of approximately 70 nm and an electron-dense core, 30–35 nm in diameter, which contains single-stranded, positive-sense RNA. The envelope includes protruding, spike-like heterodimers of two glycoproteins, E1 and E2. E1 is responsible for haemagglutination and probably for the binding of the envelope to cell-surface receptors, leading to entry of the virus into the cytoplasm within endosomes.[897] Sequencing of E1 has revealed two major phylogenetic groups of rubella virus (clades 1 and 2), which have been subdivided further into genotypes 1B, 1C, 1D, 1E, 1F, 2A and 2B and three provisional genotypes (1a, 1g and 2c).[1246] These have distinct geographical distributions:[1246,1271] 1B has been found in Europe and along the eastern coast of South America, 1C in Central America and along the western coast of South America, 1D in Asian countries, 1F in China and 1C in a single outbreak in Japan. Genotype 1a, the most frequently isolated form of rubella before 1984, has now almost disappeared, except in Mongolia and Myanmar. Genotype 1D was previously found in Canada and the United States, but was last detected in Canada in 1987 and in the United States in 1988. Genotype 1E, first identified in 1997, now has a global distribution. Genotype 2B is distributed widely in Africa, Asia and Europe. Genotype 2A was isolated in China in 1979 and 1980 but has not reappeared since. Genotype 2c has been found in the Russian Federation only.

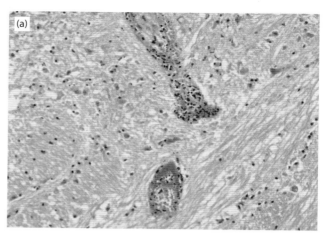

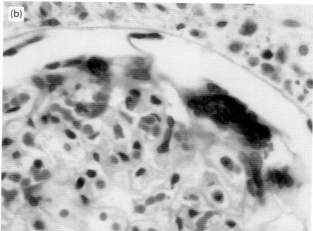

19.24 Nipah virus infection. (a) Necrotizing vasculitis, with ischaemic damage to the surrounding brain tissue. **(b)** Endothelial syncytia in a renal glomerulus.

Courtesy of Professor KT Wong, University of Malaya, Kuala Lumpur, Malaysia.

Postnatal Rubella

Pathogenesis

Humans are the only known host of rubella virus. Postnatal infection occurs by inhalation of infected respiratory secretions.[68] After initial replication of the virus in the upper respiratory tract and spread to regional lymphoid tissue, a minor viraemia occurs, with spread to systemic lymphoreticular tissues. After further replication, a secondary (major) viraemia ensues, which disappears soon after the onset of the rash, coincident with the appearance of neutralizing antibodies. During the viraemia, virus spreads to many tissues, including the placenta in pregnant women, and the CNS.[1074]

Clinical and Pathological Features

In children and adults, rubella virus usually causes German measles, but 25–50 per cent of infections are subclinical.[459] The incubation period is 12–23 days. This benign exanthematous disease presents with headache, low-grade fever, conjunctivitis and catarrh. Many patients develop posterior cervical and post-auricular lymphadenopathy, and a maculopapular rash that spreads downwards from the face and neck to the trunk and limbs. Rubella is often complicated by arthralgias or arthritis, particularly in women, and rarely by thrombocytopenia.

Approximately 1 in 5000–10 000 patients develops a post-infectious encephalomyelitis,[68] in some cases with optic neuritis;[224,459] the risk is greater in adults than children. Other unusual neurological complications of postnatal infection include myelitis[224] and Guillan–Barré syndrome. Central nervous system disease due to documented direct infection occurring postnatally is very rare. Connolly and colleagues reported a patient in whom rubella was complicated by the development of internal carotid artery thrombosis and cerebral infarction, as well as liver necrosis; at autopsy, rubella virus antigen and virus particles were found in the brain.[224] A few patients with intrauterine or childhood rubella infection have developed a progressive encephalitis some years later. This disorder, progressive rubella panencephalitis, is described in more detail later (see under Subacute and Chronic Viral Infections). For comment on the relationship of MMR vaccination and autism, see earlier under Measles.

Congenital Rubella

Epidemiology

Since the introduction of a live rubella vaccine in 1969, congenital rubella has declined dramatically in incidence; in several countries, indigenously acquired congenital infection has almost been eliminated.[1133] The incidence of congenital rubella remains high in some parts of Europe (particularly in central and eastern areas),[878,935,1245] Asia,[570] South America (especially Brazil)[648,947] and Africa, reflecting the varying effectiveness with which vaccination has been implemented.[68]

Pathogenesis

Congenital infection results from transplacental spread of the virus during the viraemia associated with maternal infection. In the vast majority of cases, this occurs in women who have not been vaccinated or previously infected by rubella virus. In very few cases, congenital rubella has resulted from maternal reinfection during pregnancy.[3,1210] The pathogenesis of the teratogenic effects is not entirely clear. The virus infects endothelial cells and causes damage to blood vessels, and this may produce ischaemia in the CNS and other tissues during critical stages of development.[487,965] Direct infection by virus can also cause cell-cycle arrest and apoptosis.[47,290,915] In congenital rubella infections, virus may persist within the CNS for months and, in some cases, can still be isolated from the CSF when the child is over 1 year of age.[276,346]

Clinical Features

The risk of teratogenic fetal damage declines from approximately 80 per cent during the first 8–12 weeks of gestation to 50 per cent towards the end of the first trimester.[764,886] The risk falls to about 25 per cent by the end of the second trimester, and fetal damage is rarely evident if infection occurs after the 20th week. The classical rubella syndrome is almost exclusively a complication of first-trimester infections and comprises a variety of neurological, ophthalmological and cardiovascular manifestations.[68,276,886,1024] In early second-trimester infections, fetal damage, when it occurs, is usually limited to sensorineural deafness. As noted earlier, very rarely congenital or postnatal rubella infection manifests up to a decade or more later as a slowly progressive pan-encephalitis (see Subacute and Chronic Viral Infections).

The most common neurological abnormalities are sensorineural deafness (present in two-thirds to three-quarters of patients) and encephalitis. With increasing age, patients may show psychomotor retardation. The head circumference is often smaller than expected for the age but usually proportionate to the child's reduced stature. Ophthalmological abnormalities are present in up to 90 per cent of patients and include various combinations of cataracts, pigmentary chorioretinitis and microphthalmia. Later manifestations can include glaucoma. The most common cardiovascular malformations in congenital rubella are patent ductus arteriosus, peripheral pulmonary artery stenosis, and atrial or ventricular septal defects.

Affected neonates may manifest an expanded rubella syndrome of continuing infection, which includes pneumonitis, hepatosplenomegaly, thrombocytopenia and a purpuric rash. There may also be anaemia and leukopenia. This syndrome may persist for several months after birth. Occasionally, it develops after an initial period of apparent quiescence. Many patients have abnormalities of T-cell function, which are probably related to the increased incidence of autoimmune diseases, particularly insulin-dependent diabetes mellitus and hypothyroidism. Birth weight is usually low and postnatal growth retarded. Radiography may reveal skeletal lucencies and other bony abnormalities.

Pathological Features

The brain is usually small (Figure 19.25a). Other macroscopic abnormalities, such as aqueduct stenosis and hydrocephalus, polymicrogyria, agenesis of the corpus callosum and neural tube defects, have been described but are so infrequent as probably to be coincidental. Histology reveals collagenous thickening and mineralization of scattered blood vessels in the deep white matter, basal ganglia and thalamus.[965] Foci of parenchymal necrosis, with accumulation of lymphocytes and macrophages, may be present in the vicinity of the affected blood vessels (Figure 19.25b).

Rabies

Aetiology

Rabies viruses are enveloped RNA viruses of the genus Lyssavirus in the family Rhabdovirus. The Lyssavirus genus includes seven established genotypes: classic rabies virus (RABV, genotype 1), Lagos bat virus (genotype 2), Mokola virus (genotype 3), Duvenhage virus (genotype 4), European bat lyssavirus 1 (EBLV-1, genotype 5), European bat lyssavirus 2 (EBLV-2, genotype 6) and Australian bat lyssavirus (ABLV, genotype 7).[60] These fall into two phylogroups: group I, which includes genotypes 1, 4, 5, 6 and 7, and

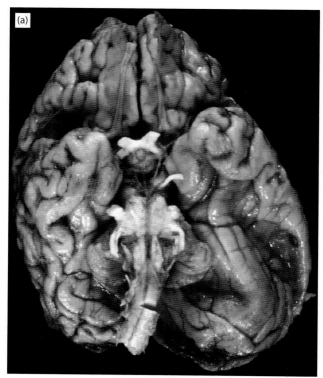

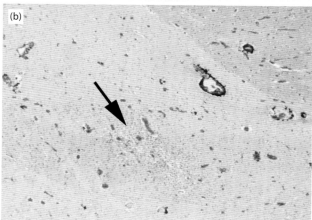

19.25 Congenital rubella. (a) The inferior aspect of the brain shows atrophy, involving the cerebrum and cerebellum. The distortion of the cerebrum is due to aqueduct stenosis and hydrocephalus. **(b)** The caudate nucleus and internal capsule include a focus of parenchymal necrosis (arrow), with accumulation of mononuclear inflammatory cells. Foci of mineralization are present in the walls of several of the blood vessels and adjacent parenchyma.

group II, which includes the divergent African genotypes 2 and 3. Other distinct genotypes–Aravan virus (ARAV), Khujand virus (KHUV), Irkut virus (IRKV) and West Caucasian bat virus (WCBV)–have yet to be classified. The precise reservoir/vector of genotype 3, MOKV, remains to be determined. Of the other classified lyssaviruses, bats are reservoirs and exclusive vectors for five. Genotype 1 (classic rabies; RABV) also has terrestrial vectors, mainly dogs and other carnivores, and is spread in domestic and wild animals worldwide. Genotypes 2–7 are mostly confined to the Old World and Australia. The viruses are bullet-shaped

(Greek *rhabdos*, rod), 70–85 nm in diameter and 180 nm in length. The genome comprises non-segmented, single-stranded, negative-sense RNA. Included within the envelope are externally protruding spikes of viral glycoprotein (G-protein). The binding of these to cell-surface receptors initiates fusion of the envelope with the cytoplasmic membrane and endocytosis of the virus. Nicotinic acetylcholine receptor (nAChR) has been shown to be a receptor for viral entry at the neuromuscular junction.[639,658] Other viral receptors include neural cell adhesion molecule (NCAM) and p75 neurotrophin receptor (p75NTR).[639,1128,1145] Replication occurs in the cytoplasm, within a circumscribed region that corresponds to the Negri body.[628] First, a series of five monocistronic mRNAs is transcribed from sequential ORFs along the genome; a positive-sense RNA genomic intermediate is then synthesized, and this acts as a template for the synthesis of new genomes. Virus particles are assembled within the cytoplasm and acquire an envelope as they bud through the modified cytoplasmic membrane or endoplasmic reticulum of the host cell, to form mature rabies virions.

Epidemiology

Most cases of rabies result from the introduction of infected saliva through a bite wound inflicted by a rabid animal. Human mortality from endemic canine rabies in Asia and Africa, where the great majority of cases occurs, has been estimated to be approximately 55 000 deaths per year[606]: approximately 56 per cent of these are in Asia and 44 per cent in Africa. The disease is endemic in animals in the Americas, large parts of Europe, Africa and Asia. Several island countries and states, including Ireland, Japan, Australia, New Zealand, Iceland and Hawaii, have long been free of indigenous rabies. Other countries listed as rabies-free in the World Health Organization (WHO) RABNET databank in 1999 included Norway, Sweden, Portugal, Greece and Uruguay.[1244] No deaths from indigenously acquired human rabies had occurred in Britain for a century before 2002, when an unvaccinated bat conservationist in Dundee died after infection by EBLV-2; he had not received post-exposure prophylaxis.[825] Four other EBLV-2-infected bats were identified in Britain between 1986 and 2005.

Dog bites account for most cases of human rabies. However, in parts of Europe and North America, where government programmes have largely eliminated stray dogs and vaccination has limited or eradicated rabies in domestic pets, wild animals are usually responsible for transmitting the disease. The principal wild-animal reservoirs of infection are foxes (particularly in Europe, but also in parts of North America, Africa and the Middle East); raccoons, skunks and coyotes (mainly in North America); wolves (in Asia and parts of Europe); jackals (in Africa); mongeese (in Africa and parts of Asia); and bats. Rabies may also be spread by ferrets and domestic cats.

Insectivorous bats are increasingly implicated as a source of human disease. They accounted for 21 of the 36 cases (58 per cent) diagnosed in the United States between 1980 and 1999.[168] Insectivorous bats have also caused human rabies in Canada, South America and Europe. The bites inflicted by bats are small and may go unnoticed. Although the risk of infection usually depends on the severity of the wound and the amount of virus in the saliva, even superficial bat-inflicted wounds carry a high risk because of the unique ability of bat rabies variants to infect and multiply within fibroblasts and epithelial cells.[461,792] Haematophagous (vampire) bats are an important source of human rabies in parts of Central America and South America, including Trinidad, Guyana, Mexico, Brazil, Bolivia, Argentina, Surinam, Belize and Peru.[59,386] In Australia, fruit bats have been the source of ABLV that has caused two fatal infections in humans;[705] in one case the incubation period was 27 months, but viral RNA was detected in the patient's saliva, post-mortem examination revealed necrotizing encephalitis with cytoplasmic inclusion bodies in the hypothalamus, viral antigen and RNA were demonstrated in brain tissue, and virus was recovered by culture.[448]

Rarely, human rabies is transmitted by means other than a bite wound. There are rare reports of aerosol transmission: two probable instances in laboratories and two in humid bat-infested caves.[226,227,1235] Transmission has also occurred by corneal[61,380,490,532,1243] and organ transplantation.[146,963]

Pathogenesis

In most cases, rabies virus replicates within skeletal muscle at the site of inoculation before being taken up by axons at the neuromuscular junction and transported centripetally to the CNS.[527,628,798] This usually occurs within days (see Incubation Period) but may be delayed for several months, probably because of prolonged sequestration of virus within muscle.[180] Once within the CNS, the virus replicates and spreads rapidly between neurons and along axons through the spinal cord and brain stem to the cerebrum and cerebellum.

The early behavioural changes that occur in furious rabies, such as agitation, aggressiveness and abnormal sexual behaviour, are thought to reflect early infection of limbic structures, with relative sparing of the neocortex.[540] However, whether the clinical presentation is of furious or paralytic rabies seems to be related largely to the immune response of the patient to the virus. Hemachudha and colleagues found that patients with furious rabies had mounted a T-cell response to rabies virus, whereas patients with paralytic rabies showed no such response.[463] In addition, the latter patients were less likely to have raised serum levels of soluble interleukin 2 (IL-2) receptor and interleukin 6 (IL-6).[462] In contrast, in experimental rabies, the development of paralytic disease was found to depend on an intact T-cell response.[1092,1214] Electrophysiological studies have demonstrated severe peripheral nerve dysfunction in paralytic but not furious rabies.[463]

Once infection has spread through the CNS, virus is also transported centrifugally along axons to a wide range of peripheral tissues, including the salivary and lacrimal glands (from which virus is shed in saliva and tears), cornea and nuchal skin (of use in diagnosis; see Pathological Findings), heart, lungs, gastrointestinal tract, adrenal glands, kidneys and urinary bladder.

Clinical Features and Laboratory Findings

Incubation Period

The incubation period is very variable.[461,644] In about 50 per cent of cases, it is between 30 and 90 days, but the range extends from under 10 days to over 1 year. The incubation period is shorter in children than adults and also varies according to the proximity of the site of inoculation to the CNS, the onset of symptoms being most rapid after bites on the head. Very short incubation periods (under 1 week) may result from direct inoculation of virus into peripheral nerve.[461] In the majority of cases, the incubation period is sufficiently long to allow the development of a protective immune response to rabies vaccine administered soon after exposure. Immediate immunity can be provided during the interim period by local and systemic administration of rabies immune globulin. Most deaths from rabies involve patients who do not receive post-exposure vaccination.[241,461]

Prodrome

The onset of CNS disease is usually heralded by non-specific 'flu-like, symptoms which can include headache, fever, malaise, nausea and vomiting, and in many cases pain or paraesthesiae at the site of the bite. This prodromal period lasts up to 2 weeks (usually 2–10 days).

Acute Neurological Disease

Approximately 70–80 per cent of patients develop furious (also termed encephalitic) rabies, characterized by insomnia, episodes of agitation and aggressive behaviour (which can include biting), autonomic dysfunction (hypersalivation, pupillary dilatation, piloerection and, later, cardio-respiratory disturbances), hallucinations, hydrophobia, dysphagia, dysarthria and nystagmus. The clinical presentation differs somewhat in patients with bat rabies variant infection, some of whom develop focal neurological signs (focal limb weakness, hemiparesis, hemi-anaesthesia), myoclonus and cranial nerve palsies.[461] About 20–30 per cent of patients develop paralytic (also termed dumb) rabies, which can include paralysis of one or more limbs, or ascending paralysis simulating Guillain–Barré syndrome (see Chapter 24). Sensory loss and incontinence may be present. The two forms of rabies may overlap.

Terminal Stage

The acute neurological disease progresses to stupor, coma and death over a period of 1–2 weeks. The average survival is 5 days in encephalitic rabies and 13 days in paralytic rabies.[461] Complications that may occur during the terminal stage include inappropriate antidiuretic hormone (ADH) secretion, diabetes insipidus, haematemesis, and cardiac and respiratory failure. Occasionally, the course is more protracted, but survival has been reported in only six patients: one had been vaccinated against rabies[163] and four had received post-exposure prophylactic vaccination,[19,453,708,906] but only one, a 15-year-old female, has survived without any anti-rabies prophylaxis.[170]

Pathological Findings

The brain and spinal cord may appear swollen, but are usually macroscopically normal. The microscopic appearances are of a widespread polioencephalomyelitis (Figure 19.26). The classic histological feature is the Negri body: a sharply delineated, round or oval, eosinophilic inclusion in the neuronal cytoplasm.[628,798] Some neurons contain more pleomorphic, less clearly circumscribed (although ultrastructurally similar) eosinophilic cytoplasmic inclusions, termed lyssa bodies. The inclusions may be seen in most parts of the CNS but tend to be easiest to find in Purkinje cells (Figure 19.26a,b), hippocampal pyramidal cells and brain stem nuclei. Electron microscopy shows the Negri and lyssa bodies to contain a matrix of granular or filamentous nucleocapsid material, within which bullet-shaped virus particles may be visible. These are often concentrated at the periphery, budding into surrounding cisternae of the endoplasmic reticulum.

Leptomeningeal and perivascular lymphocytic infiltrates and neuronophagia are usually present (Figure 19.26c), but there is often a striking disparity between the abundance of virus and the limited degree of inflammation. The clusters of microglia that remain after destruction of neurons are known as Babes' nodules. Immunostaining of virus usually shows them to be much more abundant than is evident on conventional microscopy, particularly in the spinal cord, brain stem, thalamus and basal ganglia.[461,1130] Although by conventional light microscopy inclusion bodies are rarely evident in astrocytes and almost never seen in oligodendrocytes, Tirawatnpong and colleagues demonstrated viral antigen in oligodendrocytes in three patients with paralytic rabies and one of four patients with encephalitic rabies, and in occasional astrocytes in all seven cases.[1130]

There is no consistent relationship between the clinical presentation and the distribution of virus or extent of inflammation within the CNS. However, in paralytic rabies, peripheral nerves show either segmental demyelination and remyelination, or axonal degeneration,[192] and an infiltrate of T-cells can be demonstrated in dorsal and spinal nerve roots.[463] The nerve root inflammation tends to be most pronounced at the level of the bitten dermatome. In both paralytic and furious rabies, inflammation may be present in the spinal grey matter and dorsal root ganglia.[463]

Once the virus has spread centrifugally to peripheral tissues, it can be identified ante-mortem in corneal cells and cutaneous nerve fibres. This allows the diagnosis to be confirmed by immunofluorescent staining of corneal impressions or nuchal skin biopsies (in which viral antigen can be demonstrated in small nerve fibres surrounding hair follicles).[108,1265]

Arboviruses

The arboviruses evolved from a common ancestor approximately 20 000 years ago.[1060] The first human disease shown to be caused by a filterable agent that was transmitted through the bite of an insect was yellow fever, in 1901. This mode of transmission was subsequently demonstrated for many viruses, which were grouped together under the designation arboviruses (short for 'arthropod-borne viruses'). From a taxonomic perspective, this grouping together of

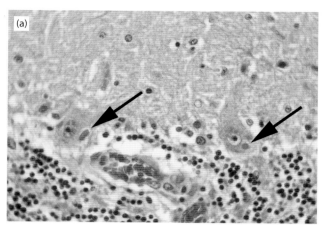
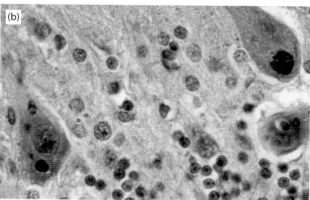
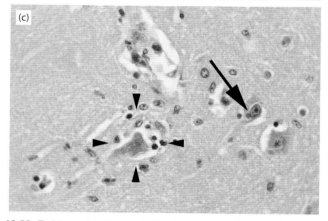

19.26 Rabies. (a) Both of the Purkinje cells contain Negri bodies–sharply demarcated eosinophilic cytoplasmic inclusions surrounded by clear 'haloes' (arrows). Note the paucity of inflammation. **(b)** Immunohistochemical demonstration of rabies viral antigen within infected Purkinje cells. **(c)** Scanty inflammation and early neuronophagia (arrowheads) in the subiculum. Note the presence of a Negri body in an adjacent neuron (arrow).

(a) Courtesy of Dr L Chimelli, Universidade Federal do Rio de Janeiro, Rio de Janeiro, Brazil. (b) Courtesy of Professor F Gray, Hôpital Lariboisière, Paris, France. (c) Courtesy of Professor F Gray, Hôpital Lariboisière, Paris, France.

Reproduced from Ellison and Love,[308a] © Elsevier, 1998.

heterogeneous viruses from several families is irregular, but the term 'arbovirus' is nonetheless a convenient label for a group of infectious agents that share several epidemiological and clinical features.

Rather than adapting to a single host, the arboviruses have evolved lifecycles that take advantage of the long lifespan of the mammalian or bird host (particularly its capacity to live through winter) and the wide distribution and feeding habits of the insect vector. Transmission is linked tightly to host viraemia.[716,1148] Most host–vector combinations are unperturbed by viral infection; however, when a new host (e.g. horse, human) enters the cycle, the virus itself or the host immune response often leads to disease.[284,686] In most cases, viral replication in the new host is without utility to the virus, which is prevented from completing its lifecycle. The viruses have adapted to a specific environmental niche in which the insect vector and host are tightly linked. It is particularly when the environment is perturbed that arboviruses are likely to be diverted into replicating in significant numbers in dead-end mammalian hosts ('spillover').[1205] The annual incidence of arboviral encephalitis varies widely, presumably because variations in the environmental conditions alter the quantity and distribution of the insect vectors.[261,1027] Changes to the environment over the past few decades have been accompanied by a dramatic expansion in the geographical distribution of arboviral infections.[190,679,924] A single arthropod vector can carry multiple infectious agents (e.g. *Ixodes ricinus* can transmit both tick-borne encephalitis virus (TBEV) and *Borrelia burgdorferi*), infection by one of these occasionally masking infection by another.[500] Mosquito saliva contains proteins that suppress local immunity and probably thereby facilitate transmission of arboviruses.[1012]

Arboviruses are derived from four families of virus: Togaviridae, Flaviviridae, Bunyaviridae and Reoviridae. Arboviruses constitute only a small fraction of the viruses in these families. Other viruses in these families infect only insects or only birds and mammals. An example of the last of these categories of virus is rubella, a member of the genus Rubivirus in the family Togaviridae. From a molecular genetic perspective, the four families that contain arboviruses have little in common, apart from the fact that all are RNA viruses. Only those arboviruses that cause human neurological disease are considered later.

Currently, human vaccines are available for JE and TBEV only.[821] There are no approved antiviral drugs for treating arboviral infections.[257,307,881,1081] Arboviruses have been intensively studied in the hospital and laboratory. It is not therefore surprising that accidental infections have occurred in these settings.[887] In the hospital setting, accidental transmission of arboviruses has usually occurred percutaneously. In the laboratory, most have occurred through the aerosol route. Such unconventional modes of transmission are often associated with atypical and severe clinical manifestations.

Togaviridae

In this family, only the genus Alphavirus harbours arboviruses. All were initially isolated in the 1930s, from horses that had died during epidemics of equine encephalitis.

Western equine encephalitis (WEE) was discovered and named in a 1930 epidemic in the San Joaquin Valley of California.[759] Three years later, eastern equine encephalitis (EEE) was isolated on the US Atlantic seaboard. Serological studies showed that these viral isolates and that from a Venezuelan epidemic (Venezuelan equine encephalomyelitis, VEE) were related. Normally, these three equine encephalitis viruses cycle between mosquitoes and birds. Encephalitis occurs only in the dead-end hosts (humans or horses).

Alphaviruses are enveloped viruses with an icosahedral nucleocapsid 60–65 nm in diameter. Laminin-binding protein has been identified as a possible receptor for VEE virus.[122,123] The cell receptor for WEE and EEE viruses is not known. Entry into the cell is by endocytosis. Each virion contains a single strand of polyadenylated positive-sense RNA that has a methylated cap at the 5′ end and can be transcribed on cellular ribosomes. The solitary polypeptide transcribed from the 5′ end is cleaved by host proteases into four non-structural proteins that together form the viral RNA-dependent RNA polymerase responsible for transcribing full-length antisense RNA. Full-length genomic RNA as well as shorter fragments of mRNA encoding the structural nucleocapsid and envelope proteins are synthesized from this strand. The nucleocapsid assembles around the genomic RNA. The envelope proteins are glycosylated and transported to the cell surface, where they bind to the nucleocapsid and direct the budding of mature virus from the cell surface.[1046]

Eastern Equine Encephalitis Virus

Epidemiology and Pathogenesis This disease is endemic along the Atlantic seaboard of the Americas.[783,1206] The virus is normally transmitted by mosquitoes that feed exclusively on birds. Most infected bird species do not develop disease, but others suffer a high mortality.[263,595] Mosquitoes with a more diverse feeding behaviour occasionally transmit the virus to horses and humans. EEE is uncommon in humans, and fewer than 5 per cent of human infections are clinically symptomatic.[384] However, in those who develop symptomatic disease, the mortality and morbidity are high: of 36 cases reported in the United States between 1988 and 1994, 13 died and 8 of the survivors had moderate to severe neurological disability.[272] Aerosol infection (of experimental animals or, accidentally, of humans as a result of a laboratory accident) is associated with increased neurovirulence.[1077]

Clinical Features In symptomatic cases, symptoms of meningoencephalitis appear 1–2 weeks after infection and progress rapidly, with the development of focal signs, seizures and, in many cases, coma and death within days. Neuroradiology typically shows focal lesions in the basal ganglia and thalamus.[272]

Pathological Findings On neuropathological examination, little distinguishes EEE from other acute viral meningoencephalitides (Figure 19.27). The brain is usually swollen. Histology reveals a pan-encephalitis with a predilection for the basal ganglia and brain stem.[77,328] Widespread oedema and perivascular inflammation may be accompanied by vascular thrombosis and focal parenchymal necrosis. Neuronophagia and microglial nodules are often prominent. In longer-surviving cases, the white matter may contain foci of demyelination and gliosis. Virus can be demonstrated within the acutely infected brain by electron microscopy, immunofluorescence and *in situ* hybridization and is particularly prominent in oligodendrocytes.[356,413,585]

Western Equine Encephalitis Virus

Epidemiology and Pathogenesis Although largely confined to the western United States and Canada, WEE has also been reported in South America, the Caribbean and the eastern United States.[148,1206] Like EEE, WEE infects feral avian populations and is transmitted by mosquitoes. WEE virus is more prevalent than its eastern counterpart, epidemics occurring in the summer and early autumn. Epidemics of WEE have higher attack and fatality rates in humans (50 in 100 000 and 8–15 per cent, respectively) compared with those of EEE.[930] The likelihood of human infection causing symptomatic disease varies with age, from almost 100 per cent in infected infants to under 0.1 per cent in adults.

Clinical Features In adults, neurological disease associated with WEE virus infection is usually limited to aseptic meningitis. A minority of patients develop encephalitis, manifesting with nausea and vomiting, confusion progressing to stupor, and flaccid or spastic paralysis. *In utero* infection has been described.[230,1038] Long-term neurological sequelae are common in infants, but fatalities rare. The encephalitis is most likely to be fatal in elderly patients.[746]

Pathological Findings The pathological features of WEE are similar to those of EEE.[455,920,979] Damage may be disproportionately severe in the white matter.

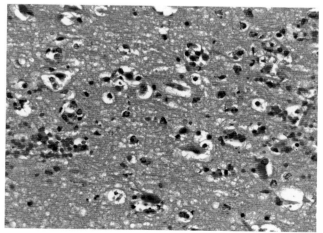

19.27 Eastern equine encephalitis. In this case, the cerebral cortex contains an inflammatory infiltrate that consists predominantly of neutrophils, some of which are clustered around neurons. At later stages of disease, lymphocytes and macrophages predominate and neuronophagia is often prominent.

Courtesy of Dr David Louis, Massachusetts General Hospital, Boston, MA, USA.

Venezuelan Equine Encephalitis Virus

A group of related togaviruses in the Caribbean basin and South America causes encephalitis that has been termed VEE. The viruses can be subdivided on the basis of their epidemiological patterns as enzootic (present in feral species at all times but in low numbers)[1207] and epizootic (occurring in epidemics). The usual mammalian hosts of enzootic strains of VEE viruses are rodents, with mosquitoes being the insect vectors. Infection of horses and humans by enzootic strains is common (the prevalence of antibodies is 100 per cent in some areas) but usually subclinical. Neuropathological findings in human infection range from congestion and mild leptomeningeal inflammation to necrotizing pan-encephalitis. In a series of 21 patients with fatal VEE, histology revealed inflammatory cell infiltrates in the leptomeninges and perivascular spaces in 14 patients, cerebritis in 5 patients and meningoencephalitis associated with necrotizing vasculitis in 2 patients.[265]

Epizootic strains of VEE viruses cause outbreaks of disease in horses and are spread by a variety of insect vectors.[485] Humans are highly susceptible to infection. The symptoms are usually limited to fever, chills and myalgias, but fatal lymphoreticular disease has been described in children. Rarely, children develop encephalitis, but neurological sequelae and fatalities are exceptional and little is known of the neuropathology. *In utero* infection with massive CNS necrosis has been reported.[1217] There is no licensed human vaccine or antiviral drug of proven effectiveness.[1208]

Other Togaviruses Reported to Cause Human Neurological Disease

Chikungunya virus-associated disease was originally described in tropical Africa in the 1960s. Transmitted by *Aedes* mosquitoes, the virus causes an acute disease with high fever, skin rash, arthralgia and occasionally meningoencephalitis.[247,703,839] In 2004, Chikungunya fever re-emerged in Africa and quickly spread through countries around the Indian Ocean, infecting more than 6 million people. Because of the high viraemia in vertebrate hosts including humans (10^9–10^{12} virus/mL blood), the spread of virus reflects the movement of tourists. Despite the severe acute disease, only 1 in 100 infections is fatal. Neurological infection is most often severe in infants and the elderly. Chikungunya derives its name from its Mozambican origin: in Makonde the word means 'to walk bent over', the result of neurological infection. For the first week of infection, virus is readily detected by PCR and afterwards by persistent viral IgG. Experimental inoculation of mice reveals glial tropism with a lesser degree of neuronal involvement. The cell receptor for the virus is unknown.

In sub-Saharan Africa, Semliki Forest virus is a known human pathogen. Willems and colleagues described a case of fatal Semliki Forest virus encephalitis in a laboratory worker.[1234]

Flaviviridae

Although the Flaviviridae family of viruses was formally classified as such only in 1984,[1218] these viruses are a major cause of human disease (more than 170 million people, 3 per cent of the world population, are chronically infected with hepatitis C virus[669]), and have played an important role in human history. Several attempts to build the Panama Canal were abandoned because of outbreaks of yellow fever. The family Flaviviridae includes many clinically important arboviruses with the capacity to cause encephalitis or lethal haemorrhagic disease. Nine serologically defined groups of flavivirus are recognized, and these include over 50 species and many more subspecies and strains.[139] These viruses use a range of insect vectors that vary in different parts of the world.

Flaviviridae are enveloped viruses with smaller (37–50 nm) nucleocapsids than those of Togaviridae. The cellular receptors vary according to the species and strain of flavivirus, as well as the type of host cell, and many are still unidentified. v3 integrin can serve as a receptor for both JE and West Nile fever viruses.[202] After binding to receptors, entry into the cell occurs by clathrin-mediated endocytosis followed by fusion of endosomes with cellular lysosomes and release of the viral genome.[201] Because the viral RNA is in a sense orientation, it can be translated immediately by cellular ribosomes. The genome codes for 12 non-structural proteins. A matrix (M) protein surrounds the nucleocapsid. The viral envelope, complete with envelope (E) protein, is acquired by budding through modified Golgi and endoplasmic membranes, and includes determinants of neurovirulence.[179]

During natural infection, IgM peaks at 2 weeks[480]; survivors develop higher antibody titres than non-survivors.[1061,1236] Multiplex PCR assays can be used to detect clinically important flaviviruses.[1181] Currently available commercial vaccines[916] to JE and yellow fever offer some protection against other flaviviruses (e.g. West Nile virus, WNV); this protection declines to undetectable levels by 4 years but recovers well after booster immunization.[1254] Production of endogenous -interferon seems to influence the outcome of flaviviral infections, but no benefit has been demonstrated from interferon treatment.[1061,1063]

Japanese Encephalitis Virus

Epidemiology and Pathogenesis   In terms of global incidence, morbidity and mortality, JE is the most important of the arboviral encephalitides.[1060,1158] It is the principal cause of viral encephalitis in Asia, with an estimated incidence of 30 000–50 000 and mortality of 10 000 per annum.[576] The extent of endemic infection is probably underestimated, given the low ratio of symptomatic to asymptomatic disease (1:25 to 1:1000),[775] particularly in vaccinated populations.[615,706] Japanese encephalitis is spread by several genera of mosquito. The implementation of measures to eradicate mosquitoes and a mass immunization programme have reduced the incidence of JE in Japan to under 20 cases per year. Other Asian nations have been less successful in preventing JE.

The feral reservoir of JE virus is not known, but the virus can survive through winter in female mosquitoes. The domestic pig is an important amplifying host during epidemics. In tropical regions, JE occurs throughout the year, but in temperate regions infections occur in late summer and early autumn. In endemic areas, the vast majority of the population has been infected and is immune; thus, new cases occur predominantly in children. In naive populations, all age groups are susceptible.[828] As for other arboviruses,

disruption of the ecosystem by cultivation of rice and domestic husbandry provides new breeding grounds for the vector and amplification of the virus.[1205] The mortality associated with clinical infections can be high (70 per cent), but is substantially lower with adequate medical support (e.g. 10 per cent in US military personnel). Fortunately, most infections are subclinical.[88] The use of vaccines based on inactivated virus has greatly decreased the incidence of JE.[310,1266]

Newer live-attenuated vaccines and viral-vector-based vaccines have been developed that may eventually replace the inactivated vaccines.[442,958,1263]

Clinical Features   Clinical disease is heralded by a prodrome of headache, fever, chills and nausea 1–2 weeks after infection. Most patients with JE are infants or children, in whom gastrointestinal complaints may predominate. Neurological disease begins with symptoms of meningeal irritation but progresses rapidly to encephalomyelitis, the manifestations of which can include prominent extrapyramidal movement disorders, cranial nerve palsies, and weakness or flaccid paralysis of the upper and lower limbs. The disease may simulate Guillain–Barrè syndrome or poliomyelitis.[773,774,1062] As in other arboviral encephalitides, children frequently develop seizures. Because viral recovery from the CSF is difficult and PCR has a yield of only about 50 per cent in JE, confirmation of the diagnosis is usually based on serological studies.[145,503] Approximately 30 per cent of survivors of symptomatic infection have neurological sequelae, which can include epilepsy, motor disturbances, and intellectual and behavioural abnormalities.[359,501,632]

Pathological findings   The brain usually appears swollen and congested. Microscopy reveals a chronic inflammatory infiltrate throughout the brain. The inflammation tends to be particularly severe in the grey matter of the thalamus, substantia nigra, pons, medulla and spinal cord (Figure 19.28) and occasionally is necrotizing. Immunohistochemistry has shown viral antigen within neurons in the cerebral cortex, thalamus and brain stem.[520,543,590] Foci of rarefaction and glial scarring have been noted in the substantia nigra and thalamus and, to a lesser extent, cerebral cortex of long-term survivors.[514]

St Louis Encephalitis Virus

Epidemiology and Pathogenesis   St Louis encephalitis (SLE) virus is a member of the same antigenic group of flaviviruses as JE virus. Discovered in its city namesake in 1933, the virus occurs throughout the United States.[260] It shares many epidemiological features with other flaviviruses, humans representing a dead-end host, the incidence of infections peaking in late summer and early autumn, and overwintering occurring in hibernating mosquitoes. The virus is endemic in bird populations throughout much of North America and tropical Central America and South America. In the eastern United States, SLE is predominantly an urban disease spread by the *Culex pipiens* mosquito, whereas in the western United States it is a rural disease spread by *Culex tarsalis*. In some parts of the eastern United States, the seroprevalence approaches 4 per cent.[418]

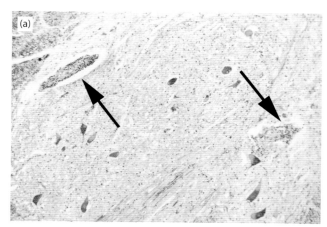

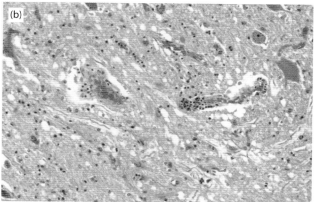

19.28 Japanese encephalitis. (a) Perivascular inflammation (arrows) in the spinal grey matter of a patient with Japanese encephalitis who had predominantly spinal disease. Luxol fast blue/cresyl violet. **(b)** Higher magnification of the spinal grey matter reveals reactive astrocytes and parenchymal infiltration by mononuclear inflammatory cells.

Courtesy of Professor F Scaravilli, Institute of Neurology, London, UK.

Clinical Features Most SLE virus infections are subclinical. Symptomatic encephalitis is more common in people over 60 years. Convulsions occur in about 10 per cent of clinical cases and are a poor prognostic sign. In symptomatic patients, the case-fatality rate can be as high as 10 per cent. Early administration of interferon-2b was reported to decrease the severity of CNS disease.[923] Severe neurological sequelae, which can include gait and speech impairment, tremors, depression and memory loss, affect about 25 per cent of survivors. Viral isolation is unusual, and diagnosis is usually serological.[784]

Pathological Findings The neuropathological features are of a non-necrotizing pan-encephalitis. Inflammation may be particularly marked in the thalamus and midbrain. Chu and colleagues reported two cases of flavivirus infection, one of which was confirmed to be due to SLE, developed meningoencephalitis with relatively discrete regions of abnormality on MRI, involving cerebral cortex and subjacent white matter.[200] Inflammation was prominent in the meninges and around small penetrating blood vessels, some of which had undergone fibrinoid necrosis; the authors also noted neuronophagia and microglial nodules in the cerebral cortex (Figures 19.29 and 19.30a,b). Viral antigen can be demonstrated by immunofluorescent staining of brain sections[936] and viral particles by electron microscopy (Figure 19.30c,d).[200]

Murray Valley Encephalitis Virus

Murray Valley encephalitis (MVE) occurs mostly in southeastern Australia, but cases have been reported as far away as New Guinea. Most infections are subclinical. In affected areas, up to one-third of the population may be seropositive.[287] The mosquito vector spreads the virus from large water birds to humans. Epidemics occur every 5–10 years, depending on the rainfall.[704,729] The peak incidence is from late spring to early autumn. Central nervous system disease ranges from mild meningoencephalitis to severe encephalitis with paralysis, respiratory failure and coma. Patients who recover from severe disease are usually left with neurological deficits.[90] Recovery of virus from serum and CSF is difficult, and the diagnosis is usually confirmed serologically.[1229] Neuropathological examination reveals non-specific features of a pan-encephalitis.[949] Animal studies have suggested that subneutralizing antibody titres predispose to severe CNS disease.[1194]

Kunjin

Kunjin has a distribution overlapping that of MVE and extending into South East Asia.[438] Wild birds and small mammals serve as viral reservoirs, from which mosquitoes transmit the virus to humans. Encephalitis has been reported.[438,702,804,1168]

Rocio Virus

Rocio virus is endemic in wild birds in the São Paulo State of Brazil. Mosquito vector transmission results in approximately 50 human cases of encephalitis each year.[540] The case-fatality rate is about 4 per cent, with neurological impairment in approximately 20 per cent of survivors. The neuropathological findings in fatal cases are similar to those of other flavivirus encephalitides.

Tick-Borne Encephalitis Virus

Epidemiology and Pathogenesis The term 'tick-borne encephalitis virus' refers to a complex of closely related flaviviruses. The best characterized of these are European (Central European encephalitis virus) TBE, endemic in many parts of Central Europe and transmitted by *Ixodes ricinus* ticks; Far Eastern (Russian spring–summer encephalitis) TBE, endemic in southern Russia and the Far East and transmitted by *Ixodes persulcatus* ticks; and Siberian TBE, endemic in the western Siberian region of Russia.[414,419,609] Powassan encephalitis virus, endemic in Canada, northern United States and parts of Russia, is probably closely related. Feral insectivores (such as shrews, voles and hedgehogs) are the principal reservoirs, but TBE viruses are unique among arboviruses in achieving adequate titres in cows and goats to allow transmission through infected milk and milk products. Several thousand cases occur annually – at least 11 000 in Russia and about 3000 in the rest

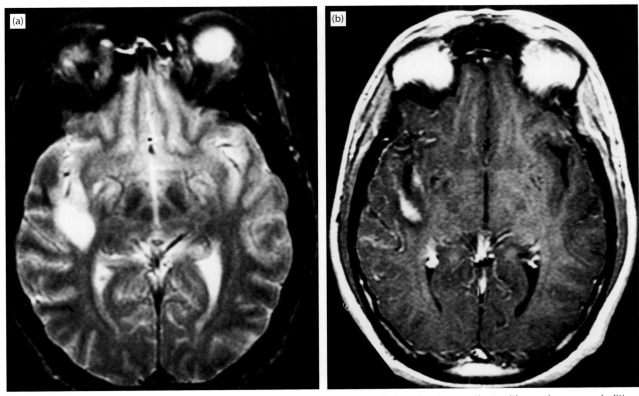

19.29 St Louis encephalitis (SLE) virus infection: MRI. (a) T2-weighted MR imaging in a patient with meningoencephalitis due to SLE virus. Note the strong signal in the right temporal lobe. **(b)** T1-weighted MRI after administration of gadolinium. There is enhancement in the leptomeninges and underlying temporal lobe in the same region that was abnormal in the T2-weighted images.

Courtesy of Dr C Chu, University of Pittsburgh, Pittsburgh, PA, USA, and Dr S Miller, Duke University, Durham, NC, USA. Reproduced from Chu et al.,[197] with permission from Lippincott Williams & Wilkins/Wolters Kluwer Health.

of Europe.[285,419] Most patients are adults who have been working outdoors in endemic areas in late spring and early autumn. Diagnosis is usually made by serological testing.[957] PCR on serum permits diagnosis before seroconversion, but the diagnostic yield of this technique then falls off rapidly.[484]

Clinical Features Febrile, meningeal, meningoencephalitic, poliomyelitic, polioradiculoneuritic and chronic forms of TBE are recognized. Patients typically present 1–2 weeks after infection with headache and fever and may develop a meningoencephalitis of variable severity, ranging from mild meningitis to a rapidly progressive, in some cases fatal, encephalitis.[427,555] Common manifestations include ataxia, impairment of consciousness, and cranial and peripheral nerve palsies.[427,556] Tick-borne encephalitis virus-induced poliomyelitis often involves the neck, shoulders and upper limbs, causing drooping of the head ('hanged-head syndrome').[419] Powassan encephalitis has been reported to cause cerebellar and vestibular abnormalities,[309,661] but has also been confused clinically with herpes simplex encephalitis.[315]

The different subtypes of TBE tend to be associated with different patterns of disease.[419] Far Eastern TBE virus causes meningoencephalitis, with case-fatality rates of 20–60 per cent and particularly severe disease in children. Siberian TBE virus characteristically causes a non-paralytic febrile form of encephalitis, with relatively low mortality (less than

8 per cent), but a tendency for patients to develop chronic encephalitis. European TBE virus tends to cause a biphasic illness, with initial fever and subsequent neurological disease of variable severity; mortality and residual morbidity are low (1–2 per cent), and the disease is generally milder in children than adults.

Neurological sequelae of TBE can include intellectual and behavioural abnormalities, dysphasia, ataxia and weakness.[427,434,435,556] A low-grade chronic progressive encephalitis with seizures (Kozhevnikov's epilepsy) may, rarely, complicate acute Russian spring–summer encephalitis.[852]

An effective inactivated-virus vaccine has been available in Europe for 30 years.[310,460,634] In Austria, where previously more than 50 per cent of all viral meningoencephalitides were due to TBE virus, vaccination programmes have covered close to 90 per cent of the population. Although 'breakthrough' disease has occurred in older age groups, because the introduction of vaccination only a single case of TBE has been seen in a patient under 20 years of age.[634]

Pathological Findings The neuropathological features are of a polioencephalomyelitis that can involve the grey matter of the cerebral cortex, basal ganglia, cerebellum, brain stem and spinal cord (often with accentuation in the anterior horns) (Figures 19.31 and 19.32).[364,620,1021] Affected parts of the brain show infiltration by lymphocytes and macrophages, neuronophagia, and marked microglial activation. Foci of haemorrhage and necrosis may be present. Electron

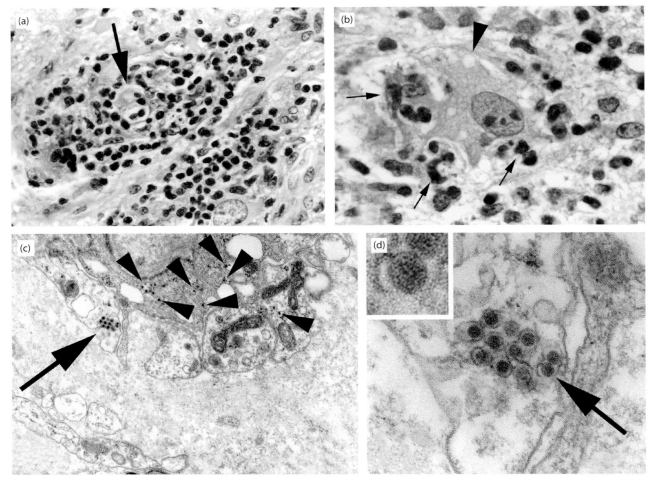

19.30 Flavivirus encephalitis. (a) Brain biopsy reveals intense perivascular inflammation (arrow) and **(b)** neuronophagia within the brain parenchyma (the arrowhead indicates a neuron and the arrows indicate inflammatory cells). **(c)** Low-power electron micrograph, showing scattered cytoplasmic virions (arrowheads). A cluster of virions (arrow) is shown at higher magnification in **(d)**. A single virion is shown in the inset.

Reproduced from Chu et al.,[197] with permission from Lippincott Williams & Wilkins/Wolters Kluwer Health.

microscopy has shown viral particles in neurons and glia.[740] Gelpi and colleagues demonstrated viral antigens immuno-histochemically in autopsy brain tissue from patients with disease of up to 35 days' duration.[364] Large neurons were preferentially immunolabelled. The regions of grey matter with most marked neuronal damage contained the densest inflammatory infiltrates, composed mostly of cytotoxic T-cells, macrophages and microglia, but only sparse immunolabelled structures–mostly clusters of granular material marking the remains of infected neurons that were undergoing neuronophagia. Viral persistence for over a year within the CNS has been reported.[633]

West Nile Virus

Epidemiology and Pathogenesis West Nile virus is antigenically related to JE, SLE and MVE viruses. More than 150 species of birds and 30 species of mammals are susceptible.[1169] Studies of antigenic variations among strains of WNV in Europe, Africa and Asia indicate that there is frequent intercontinental exchange of West Nile viral strains by migrating birds.[913,925] The potential effects of environmental changes on the dissemination of mosquito-borne diseases were highlighted by the outbreak of West Nile fever in the boroughs surrounding the city of New York in 1999,[537] resulting in 60 confirmed human infections and 7 deaths.[382] Initial projections that WNV might not become established in the USA[925] soon proved overoptimistic, as evidenced by the frequent isolation of WNV nucleic acids from dead crows and trapped *Culex* mosquitoes in the New York city area.[1078] It is presumed that migrating birds carried the virus to the United States and that subsequent feeding by local mosquitoes gave the strain a beachhead on the eastern coast. Annually in the US there are up to 1000 reported cases of WNV infection, two thirds of which are neuroinvasive and approximately 0.5 per cent fatal. During the past decade, screening of blood donations for WNV in the United States revealed viraemia in over 100 donations annually.

In endemic regions, in parts of Africa, Central Europe and Asia, up to 60 per cent of adults are seropositive.[246,333] Epidemics occur when avian vectors spread

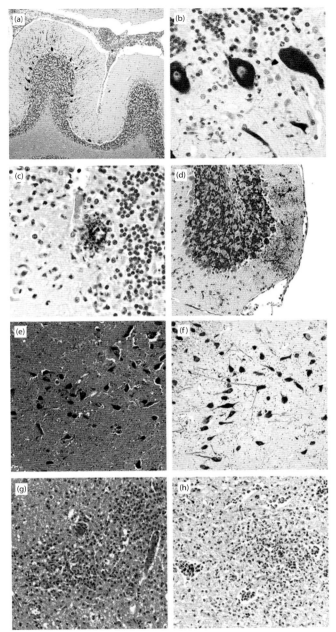

19.31 Tick-borne encephalitis (TBE): involvement of cerebellum and midbrain. (a) Immunohistochemistry for TBE viral antigen shows patchy distribution of the infected Purkinje cells, with labelling of the neuronal somata and apical dendrites. **(b)** Strong labelling of Purkinje cells for TBE virus, with little associated inflammation. **(c)** Granular immunopositivity for TBE virus marks the remains of an infected Purkinje cell that is undergoing neuronophagia. **(d)** Patchy distribution of Purkinje cell immunopositivity for TBE virus in an experimentally infected mouse. **(e)** The substantia nigra in this patient is inflamed only mildly, but it contains abundant TBE viral antigen **(f)**. **(g)** Dense inflammatory infiltrate in another part of the substantia nigra, with only scanty residual vital antigen at sites of neuronophagia **(h)**.

Courtesy of Professor H Budka, Medical University of Vienna, Vienna, Austria.

Reproduced from Gelpi et al.,[358] with permission from Lippincott Williams & Wilkins/Wolters Kluwer Health.

the virus to naive populations. In general, under 15 per cent of human infections cause aseptic meningitis or encephalitis.[497] A 1996–97 outbreak of West Nile fever in Romania was unusual in that, of 393 serologically confirmed cases, 352 developed encephalitis,[162] although these serological data may have underestimated the total number of patients infected with WNV during that epidemic. The proportion of reported patients with WNV infection in whom encephalitis occurred has also been relatively high in epidemics in the United States (2946 of 4156 reported to the Centers for Disease Control and Prevention in 2002, and 2600 of 9100 reported in 2003). Molecular epidemiological studies suggested that envelope protein glycosylation sites were important determinants of neuroinvasiveness that differed between US and African outbreaks.[81,361] Although most human infections are acquired through mosquito bites, patients develop high circulating levels of virus, and consequently infection has been transmitted through breast milk, organ transplantation and blood transfusion (Box 19.6) and transplacentally.[169,631] Early systemic humoral immunity is critical in preventing neurological disease,[845,955] but an intact cellular immune response is required to clear the virus from the host.[316] Serology and PCR are used for diagnosis.[181,333,962]

An effective WNV vaccine is available for horses but not, at present, for humans, although JE and yellow fever vaccines may offer some protection.[80,1254] Treatment is largely supportive. Three of seven patients treated with interferon-2b showed neurological improvement.[1006] Infection in two patients following renal transplant was treated successfully by a combination of supportive measures and a reduction of immunosuppression.[452]

Clinical and Pathological Features Most WNV infections are asymptomatic or cause a self-limited acute febrile illness. The incubation period is 1–6 days. A rash occurs in approximately half of clinically recognized cases. Other clinical features can include lymphadenopathy, pharyngitis, nausea and vomiting. A range of ocular manifestations has been described.[63,554] The disease usually lasts 3–6 days, and recovery is complete. In the minority of patients who develop encephalitis, the clinical features tend to be relatively non-specific – mainly headache and altered mentation.[133] A minority of patients develop polioencephalomyelitis or parkinsonism.[395,535,1023]

Before 2003, little information was available on the neuropathological findings in patients with WNV encephalitis. A therapeutic trial in patients with cancer and infected with passaged WNV[1065] produced histological changes of acute, non-necrotizing encephalitis. Since the introduction of WNV into the Americas, several detailed neuropathological reports have appeared.[604,861] Many, but not all, of the patients have had some impairment of immune function, as a result of age, HIV infection or organ transplantation.[102,604,810,926] The principal histological changes are of non-necrotizing polioencephalomyelitis. The virus has a predilection for certain groups of neurons, such as anterior horn cells in the spinal cord, nigral neurons in the midbrain, and Purkinje cells in the cerebellum.[125,344,861] Viral inclusions are not detectable by light microscopy, but the virus can be demonstrated immunohistochemically in infected neurons.[333,861]

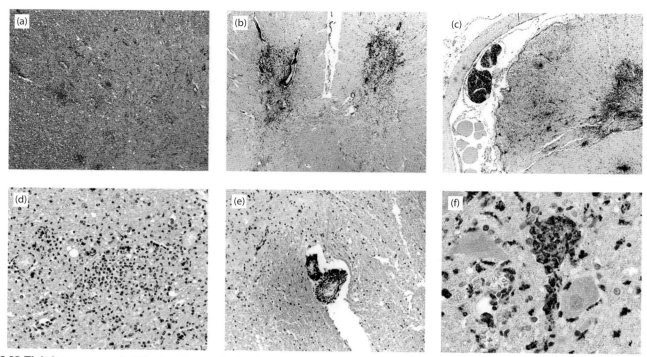

19.32 Tick-borne encephalitis: involvement of spinal cord. (a) Prominent inflammatory infiltrate in anterior horn of spinal cord. **(b)** Labelling of macrophages and microglia for HLA-DR confirms that inflammation is largely restricted to the spinal grey matter, with particularly severe involvement of the anterior horns. **(c)** The anterior roots are also infiltrated by macrophages and microglia, whereas the posterior roots are spared. Antibody to HLA-DR. **(d)** Most of the lymphocytes in the affected spinal grey matter are CD8-positive cytotoxic T-cells. **(e)** B-cells are mostly confined to perivascular cuffs. **(f)** Neuronophagia of an anterior horn cell. The macrophages and microglia have been labelled with anti-CD68.

Reproduced from Gelpi et al.,[358] with permission from Lippincott Williams & Wilkins/Wolters Kluwer Health.

Other Flaviviruses That Can Cause Human Neurological Disease

Louping III Virus Endemic in northern parts of the United Kingdom, louping is a tick-borne disease of sheep (hence its other name, ovine encephalomyelitis).[285] Birds can become infected by eating the insect vector,[373] but there is no evidence of significant small-mammal infection.[372] Humans are occasionally infected and develop a mild meningoencephalitis. Fewer than 100 human cases have been reported.[251,1055] A small animal model of the disease shows widespread neuronal degeneration distinct from the more localized lesions seen in lambs.[1031]

Haemorrhagic Fever Many other flaviviruses cause haemorrhagic, febrile disorders that are rarely complicated by non-fatal meningoencephalitis. These include dengue, Omsk haemorrhagic fever,[987] Kayasnur Forest disease,[1209] Wesselbron,[748] Ilheus,[240] Usutu,[1175] Rio Bravo and yellow fever. Their names indicate the sites of original isolation or the regions of their predominance.

Bunyaviruses

The Bunyaviridae comprise five genera, of which two, Orthobunyavirus and Phlebovirus, contain species of virus that mediate significant neurological disease in humans: California encephalitis virus (in the genus Orthobunyavirus) and Rift Valley fever virus (in the genus Phlebovirus). Bunyaviruses are negative-stranded RNA viruses. Their genome is subdivided into three strands (large, medium and small) that are packaged into a 80- to 120-nm enveloped spherical nucleocapsid. The largest strand codes for the viral RNA polymerase, the intermediate-length strand for the two envelope glycoproteins, and the smallest strand for the nucleocapsid proteins.[114] Viral particles are synthesized in the cytoplasm but, rather than budding from the plasma membrane, they bud into intracytoplasmic vesicles associated with the Golgi apparatus. A non-structural protein with homology to the pro-apoptotic Reaper protein of Drosophila[219] promotes cytolysis and viral release.[124] Viral glycoproteins bind to an uncharacterized cell-surface protein and initiate acid-dependent membrane fusion to infect new cells.

Like the other arboviruses, Bunyaviruses divide their lifecycle between haematophagous insects and warm-blooded hosts. Small mammals constitute the wild reservoir. Transovarial transmission permits overwintering.[66] Humans are dead-end hosts. The California serogroup is so named because of its initial isolation in Kern County, California.[446] Since then, the virus has been rarely associated with encephalitis in various western states of the United States.

La Crosse Encephalitis Virus

This virus, in the California encephalitis virus serogroup, is the bunyavirus that is most pathogenic for humans. It was isolated in La Crosse, Wisconsin, in 1960.[1129] The distribution of

BOX 19.6. Transmission of viral infection by blood transfusion or tissue transplantation

Infection by several viruses with the potential to cause neurological disease can be acquired from an infected donor by transfusion of blood or blood products or by tissue or organ transplantation.

Because latent infection by herpesviruses is so common, it is difficult to distinguish transmission of infection by transfusion or transplantation from reactivation of latent virus. This applies particularly after transplantation, as patients are almost inevitably receiving immunosuppressive treatment that is conducive to viral reactivation. However, there is good evidence that both herpes simplex 1 (HSV-1) and 2 (HSV-2) can be transmitted by means of corneal grafts,[111,932,948] and there are rare reports of HSV-2 infection acquired by organ transplantation.[389a] Acquisition of varicella-zoster has been reported as a complication of cardiac transplantation,[327b] and cytomegalovirus can be transmitted by blood or blood products and through transplants of organs or tissues.[196, 327a, 574,761] Human herpesvirus 8 (HHV-8) transmitted by organ transplantation is a risk factor for Kaposi's sarcoma or HHV-8-associated lymphoma in the recipient.[695,728,928]

Rabies has been transmitted through both corneal[61,380,490,532,1243] and organ transplantation.[146,963] Transmission of infection by transfusion of blood or blood products has been documented for tick-borne encephalitis[1192] and West Nile fever.[106,885,1033] West Nile virus has also been transmitted from an organ donor to four transplant recipients.[519a] Lastly, the retroviruses human T-cell lymphotropic virus I (HTLV-I) and II (HTLV-II) and human immunodeficiency virus (HIV) are readily transmitted by transfusion of blood and blood components[25,600,758,946] and have also been transmitted through transplants of tissues or organs from infected donors.[796,933,1045,1267]

La Crosse virus is defined by the distribution of its insect vectors *Aedes triseriatus* and *Aedes albopictur* (treehole-breeding woodland mosquitoes).[320] La Crosse encephalitis is predominantly a disease of children,[24] and in endemic regions (US mid-Atlantic and mid-western states) has an annual incidence of 20–30 per 100 000 children under 15 years.[750] Approximately 70 cases of La Crosse encephalitis are reported in the United States each year.[66] The peak incidence of human disease is from June to September, coincident with the period of maximum human outdoor activity. It is estimated that there are more than 1000 subclinical infections for every reported case and that by middle age approximately a quarter of the population in endemic regions is seropositive.[66,1196]

Clinical and Pathological Features An incubation period of about 1 week is followed by a 1- to 2-week illness characterized by symptoms of aseptic meningitis that can progress to encephalitis. The neurological disease tends to be more severe than that due to enteroviruses, the main clinical differential diagnosis in young children. In one series of 127 patients,[750] 20 per cent developed hyponatraemia and 13 per cent had cerebral oedema and evidence of raised intracranial pressure (in some cases to the extent of causing internal herniation). In the same cohort, 12 per cent had persistent neurological deficits at the time of discharge. These included sixth nerve palsy, hemiparesis, poor balance, and problems with speech, short-term memory and behaviour. Long-term sequelae vary depending upon the severity of illness during the acute stage.[65] Seizures are relatively common, particularly in children who experience seizures during the acute stage. Fewer than 1 per cent of symptomatic infections are fatal. Reported autopsy findings include leptomeningitis, perivascular cuffs of mononuclear inflammatory cells, scattered microglial nodules and, occasionally, foci of necrosis, predominantly in the cerebral cortex and brain stem.[559]

Rift Valley Fever Virus

Bunyaviruses in the Rift Valley fever virus group, such as Toscana virus (a serotype of sandfly fever Naples virus)[1164] and Rift Valley fever virus itself,[507] have a wide geographical distribution that includes southern Europe, Africa, the Arabian peninsula, Central Asia and the Americas.[18,182] Gould and Higgs[394] point to the increasing frequency of Rift Valley fever epidemics in the Arabian peninsula as a probable effect of global climate change. Human infections are usually asymptomatic or mild. However, these viruses can cause haemorrhagic fever, retinitis and meningoencephalitis. In a fatal case,[749] neurohistology revealed perivascular cuffing and parenchymal infiltration by mononuclear inflammatory cells. Considerable effort has been made to produce effective vaccines.[508]

Reoviridae

The term 'Reoviridae' is derived from an acronym of respiratory, enteric, orphan viruses. Of the nine genera in this family, only five include viruses that infect animals, few are associated with diseases in humans, and little is known about the neuropathology. The principal causes of human disease are Colorado tick fever (CTF) virus, in the genus Coltivirus, and Banna virus (BAV), in the genus Seadornavirus (South Eastern Asia dodecaRNA viruses).[49] The viral genome comprises double-stranded RNA divided into 10–12 segments. The virion consists of a non-enveloped double protein capsid. The inner core is a symmetrical icosahedral nucleocapsid. The structure and composition of the outer capsid vary among the different genera. Colorado tick fever virus and BAV are icosahedral, with a diameter of 60–70 nm. All enzymes necessary for viral transcription are carried within the virion.

Colorado Tick Fever Virus

Colorado tick fever was first recognized as a distinct entity in the 1930s, when its clinical manifestations were distinguished from those of the rickettsial disease Rocky Mountain spotted fever. The distribution of CTF throughout the Rocky Mountain forest of the United States and Canada reflects the distribution of its principal vector, the wood tick *Dermacentor andersoni*. Human infection results from the bite of adult wood ticks. Because CTF virus is not spread vertically in the tick, only ticks that have passed into the nymph stage and have dined on blood from an infected mammal can transmit the virus. Small mammals have prolonged viraemia, possibly extending through hibernation. Human infection peaks in late spring and early summer, when emerging adult ticks seek out new hosts. The estimated annual incidence is approximately 100 cases, with only rare fatalities. However, epidemiological data are limited because CTF is not a notifiable disease, the clinical symptoms may be confused with other entities, and confirmation of the diagnosis depends on serological analysis.[48,960]

Clinical Features After an incubation period of 4 days, patients have abrupt onset of fever, chills, headache, retro-orbital pain, photophobia, myalgia, abdominal pain, and generalized malaise.[49] Viral replication within erythroblasts leads to sequestration and circulation of virus within mature erythrocytes. Perturbation of other bone marrow elements presumably accounts for the leukocytopenia and thrombocytopenia that accompany acute infection. Severe forms of CTF occur mainly in children and can include pericarditis, myocarditis, orchitis, haemorrhagic fever and, in fewer than 10 per cent of cases, meningitis or meningoencephalitis.[49,390,1073] Most patients recover fully after 5–10 days.

Banna Virus

Banna virus was first isolated in 1987 from the CSF and serum of patients with encephalitis in Yunnan province of southern China.[49,1116] Numerous isolates were subsequently obtained from other patients with encephalitis. Underdiagnosis is likely, because of misattribution to Japanese encephalitis, which is also prevalent in these regions.[49] Vectors for the genus include *Anopheles*, *Culex* and *Aedes* mosquitoes.

Clinical Features Patients were reported to develop a 'flu-like illness, with myalgia, arthralgia, fever, and clinical features of encephalitis.[49,1116]

SUBACUTE AND CHRONIC VIRAL INFECTIONS

Some viral infections of the CNS progress over months or years rather than days or weeks. The incubation period is usually considerably longer than that of acute viral infections. In the past, the so-called 'slow virus infections', Creutzfeldt–Jakob disease and other transmissible spongiform encephalopathies, previously included in this category, are now known to be caused by the accumulation of abnormal prion protein and not by viral infection and are considered separately in Chapter 18.

Chronic Enteroviral Encephalomyelitis
Aetiology

The clearance of enteroviruses from the CNS depends on intact humoral immunity. Patients with X-linked agammaglobulinaemia or combined variable immunodeficiency are at risk of developing a chronic meningoencephalitis or myelitis due to enteroviral infection.[753,771,871,983,1233] Chronic enteroviral meningoencephalitis has also been reported as a complication of immunosupressive treatment for neoplasia, bone marrow transplantation, and AIDS.[35,99,335,343,]

[874,919,1008] The virus most frequently recovered is echovirus 11. On review of the literature, Archimbaud and colleagues list, in decreasing order of frequency, echovirus 30, 3, 5, 9, 25, 2, 7, 17, 19, 24, 29, 30 and 33, and coxsackievirus B3, B4 and A15 as also occasionally responsible, and recovered echovirus 13 from the CSF of their patient with lymphoma.[35] As in this last case, the enterovirus may be detected by culture of CSF, but this is often unrewarding and the diagnosis is more often based on the demonstration of enteroviral RNA by PCR.

Clinical and Pathological Features

The age at presentation is very variable. In the series of Rudge and colleagues, the mean age of onset in patients with X-linked agammaglobulinaemia was 16 years and in patients with combined variable immunodeficiency 39 years.[983] Patients may develop (1) a myelopathy with paraparesis, ascending sensory loss and bladder dysfunction, (2) an encephalopathy with insidious development of headache, lethargy, intellectual decline, seizures, optic atrophy, and pyramidal and extrapyramidal motor disturbances, or (3) a combination of myelopathic and encephalopathic features. A persistent CSF pleocytosis is usually present. Many patients have dermatomyositis or other systemic manifestations of chronic enteroviral infection. The neurological disease usually progresses over several years, but periods of clinical improvement may occur. Beneficial responses to intravenous or intraventricular immunoglobulins have been reported in some cases,[318,871] but not others.[771,983] The anti-enterovirus drug pleconaril has been of some success in treating this disease.[35,972]

The histological appearances are of a patchy, non-necrotizing, chronic meningoencephalitis of variable severity and distribution (Figure 19.33). Lymphocytes and macrophages are present in the subarachnoid space. Examination of affected regions of the CNS reveals perivascular cuffs of lymphocytes, microglial nodules and, in some cases, marked neuronal loss and gliosis.[430,983,1004,1233] The inflammation affects both grey and white matter. Immunohistochemical demonstration of echovirus 11 within astrocytes and neurons was reported.[430]

Subacute Measles Encephalitides

Measles virus is responsible for two subacute encephalitides: measles inclusion body encephalitis (MIBE) and subacute sclerosing pan-encephalitis (SSPE).

Aetiology

Measles virus is a pleomorphic enveloped virus of the genus Morbillivirus in the Paramyxovirus family. The virus particles may be spherical or filamentous, 100–300 nm in diameter and up to 1000 nm in length. The nucleocapsid contains single-stranded, negative-sense RNA that is complexed with the nucleocapsid protein (N) and two other proteins, large protein (L) and phosphoprotein (P), which together confer RNA-dependent RNA polymerase activity. On the inner aspect of the surrounding envelope is the matrix (M) protein and on the outer aspect the haemagglutinin (H) and fusion (F) proteins.

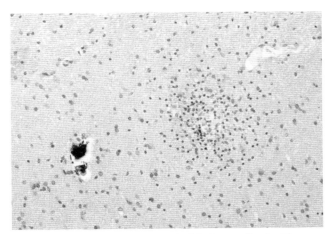

19.33 Chronic enteroviral encephalitis in a patient with combined variable immunodeficiency. A large microglial nodule and focal mineralization are present at the junction of cerebral cortex and white matter. There is moderate gliosis of the surrounding parenchyma.

Courtesy of Dr D Ellison, Southampton General Hospital, Southampton, UK.

CD46 (membrane cofactor protein) was the first identified measles virus receptor,[296,822] but serves this function for laboratory-adapted strains only[1256] and probably not *in vivo*.[943] Signalling lymphocyte-activation molecule (SLAM), expressed by T and B cells, macrophages, dendritic cells and thymocytes, is an established receptor for measles virus *in vivo*,[943,1117,1118,1255,1256] but is not expressed by respiratory tract epithelial cells, endothelial cells or neurons, which are nonetheless also infected by this virus. Poliovirus receptor-related 4 protein (PVRL4, nectin 4), may serve as the measles virus receptor for epithelial cells,[843] and the substance P receptor, neurokinin-1 (NK-1), as the viral receptor for neurons.[719] Upon binding of the virus, F protein initiates fusion of the envelope with the cell membrane, leading to release of the nucleocapsid into the cytoplasm. There the RNA is transcribed to produce multiple copies of the viral proteins, before a positive-sense RNA genomic intermediate is synthesized, which acts as a template for the synthesis of new genomes. The nucleocapsids are assembled in large numbers in the cytoplasm and also accumulate within the nucleus. The H and F envelope proteins are transported to and incorporated in the cell membrane. The M protein is needed for association of the nucleocapsid with the envelope proteins at the cell surface and the subsequent budding of the virus through the modified cytoplasmic membrane to form a mature virion.[473] M protein is also an inhibitory regulator of measles virus ribonucleoprotein transcriptional activity.[1098] In addition to their role in the budding of the virus, the H and F proteins are involved in mediating local fusion of adjacent cells.[107,943,1104]

Measles Inclusion Body Encephalitis

Pathogenesis

Measles inclusion body encephalitis (MIBE) develops in patients with depressed cell-mediated immunity, usually associated with leukaemia or lymphoma or its treatment but occasionally due to other causes of immunosuppression.[7,12,143,345] Very rarely, MIBE has been reported to occur in patients with apparently intact immune function;[112,173] in one such case a vaccine strain of measles virus was responsible.[112] The relatively few detailed serological and molecular genetic studies that have been conducted in MIBE suggest that, as in SSPE (see Subacute Sclerosing Pan-encephalitis), the clones of virus that are present in the CNS have undergone mutation of the genomic sequences encoding the M, H and F proteins, with the result that the expression of these proteins is restricted or abnormal.[57,964,1098] The mechanisms of persistence and spread of the virus within the brain are probably the same in the two diseases, with the more rapid course, much greater abundance of viral inclusions and relative paucity of lymphocytic inflammation in MIBE being due to the depression of cell-mediated immunity. The relationship between these viral genomic mutations and the persistence and spread of virus within the CNS is discussed later (see Subacute Sclerosing Pan-encephalitis).

Clinical Features

MIBE usually develops within a few months of acute measles. Most patients make a good clinical recovery from the acute illness and then present weeks or months later with seizures or confusion. Patients may develop myoclonus and a variety of focal neurological deficits. The disease progresses to coma and, in most cases, death within a few weeks of onset. A few patients have survived, but with severe neurological dysfunction. The nucleoside analogue ribavirin was used successfully to treat subacute measles encephalitis in a 4-year-old girl with leukaemia.[812] Turner *et al.*[1149] reported two children who had received a single dose of measles, mumps and rubella vaccine in the first year of life, developed probable MIBE after kidney transplantation for nephrotic syndrome but made partial neurological recoveries, which the authors attributed to a combination of prior vaccination, reduction of immunosuppressive therapy and the use of intravenous immunoglobulin and ribavirin.

Pathological Findings

The brain usually appears macroscopically normal, although foci of softening and discolouration may be noted. Histology reveals scattered foci of hypercellularity, within which many neurons and occasional astrocytes and oligodendrocytes contain eosinophilic inclusion bodies (Figure 19.34). Outside these lesions, which can involve any part of the brain, the parenchyma appears normal. Within the lesions, both nuclear and cytoplasmic inclusion bodies are present. The intranuclear inclusions largely fill the nucleus, apart from a few pyknotic clumps of marginated chromatin (Figure 19.34a,b). The cytoplasmic inclusions are also eosinophilic but are less well defined and more difficult to discern in haematoxylin and eosin preparations. The nucleocapsids are demonstrated readily by electron microscopy (Figure 19.34e) and the abundant viral antigen by immunohistochemistry (Figure 19.34c). The lesions contain reactive astrocytes and microglia and may include scanty perivascular lymphocytes and macrophages

(Figure 19.34d). Also present, in some lesions, are sparsely scattered multinucleated cells that contain viral inclusion bodies (Figure 19.34b).

Subacute Sclerosing Pan-encephalitis

Pathogenesis

Subacute sclerosing pan-encephalitis is a disease of patients who usually do not have immunological impairment and occurs years or even decades after an initial infection by measles virus. Estimates of the risk vary from 4 to 11 per 100 000 patients with measles.[149] The male to female ratio is approximately 2:1.[308,780] The risk is several-fold greater in patients who contract measles in the first year of life and is reduced 10- to 20-fold by measles vaccination.[330,780] The annual incidence of SSPE has declined steadily in countries with measles vaccination programmes, typically to below 0.05 per million population, but remains high in countries with poor measles control, such as India and Papua New Guinea, at over 20 per million.[149,428,727,772] Key factors in the pathogenesis of SSPE are thought to be the inadequate nature of the cellular immune reponse, allowing the virus to persist within infected cells, and the hypermutation of certain particularly susceptible regions of the viral genome that encode the M, H and F proteins, and subsequent clonal expansion of the mutated virus within the brain.[58,158,159,942,1009,1042] In SSPE, the M protein is not produced at all, the cytoplasmic domain of the F protein is altered, and the H protein is poorly transported to the cell membrane, so that the virus is incapable of budding to the exterior, but the cell-fusion function of the F and H proteins is maintained, allowing the virus to spread within the brain by local cell fusion.[107,439,1009] By this manner of spread, the virus evades the immune system, which in SSPE produces high titres of antibodies to viral proteins other than the M protein.[440,1211] This strong humoral immune response provides a continuing selective pressure that favours clonal expansion of the mutated virus. The immaturity of the cellular immune system in early life combined with the presence of circulating maternal antibodies to measles virus during the first few months of life may similarly promote the emergence of mutant clones and contribute to the increased risk of SSPE that follows infection at a very early age.

Clinical Features

Patients usually present between 5 and 15 years, but the range extends from 1 to 35 years. Most patients have a history of measles, usually at an early age (before 2 years in about 50 per cent of patients).[779] Rarely, SSPE occurs during infancy as a complication of maternal infection shortly before delivery.[249] The average interval from measles to SSPE is 7 years,[779] but in cases complicating maternal infection the latent period is reduced to a few months[249] and in older-onset cases the interval may be as long as 22 years.[1048] For reasons that are not understood, most adult-onset SSPE is in males.[1048]

The scheme of Jabbour and colleagues is often used to subdivide the disease into four stages.[526] The first stage comprises the insidious development of intellectual impairment and behavioural abnormalities. At least 50 per cent of patients develop visual disturbances as a result of a macular chorioretinitis, which may be the earliest manifestation of the disease.[213,409] In adult-onset SSPE visual symptoms may predate motor manifestations by up to 5 years.[909,1048] However, after about 1–2 months, a majority of patients enters the second stage, lasting 2–3 months, during which intellectual decline accelerates and episodic motor disturbances become prominent. Patients often show repetitive, symmetrical myoclonic jerks every 5–10 seconds and associated with characteristic EEG changes. During the third stage, which usually lasts 1–4 months, patients become uncommunicative and develop various combinations of ataxia, spasticity, choreoathetosis and dystonias, with gradual disappearance of the myoclonus. The fourth, final stage may last for months to years, during which patients develop stupor, autonomic disturbances and coma, leading eventually to death.

The progression of disease is very variable. In some patients death occurs within months, whereas in others the disease seems to progress only intermittently. Survival in excess of 10 years is well documented, and some patients experience periods of clinical improvement or stabilization that can last several years.[212,997] There are rare reports of multiple cases of SSPE within families, suggesting genetic susceptibility;[1030,1179] such patients have been reported to have more rapidly progressive disease.

Pathological Findings

In many cases, the brain is macroscopically normal. In cases of longer duration, there is usually moderate to marked generalized brain atrophy, and the white matter may have an abnormally firm texture and a mottled grey appearance (Figure 19.35a).

The histological features are of chronic encephalitis, with leptomeningeal, perivascular and parenchymal infiltration by lymphocytes and macrophages (Figure 19.35b,c). The distribution and severity of lesions are variable. The affected grey matter shows patchy inflammation and striking microglial hyperplasia, astrocytosis, loss of neurons, occasional neuronophagia and, in most cases, sparse intranuclear inclusions. Inflammation tends to be less marked in longstanding disease, although the destructive changes are more pronounced. The inclusions are sharply defined intranuclear eosinophilic bodies, which may have a surrounding clear space ('halo'). The inclusions are readily demonstrated immunohistochemically, but neither inclusions nor antigen may be detectable at all in very longstanding disease, although viral RNA can still be demonstrated by *in situ* hybridization.[17] The cerebral cortex, white matter, basal ganglia, thalamus and brain stem are usually involved and, particularly in longstanding disease, the neuronal loss, microglial activation and gliosis may be widespread and severe, and the disease process may involve the cerebellum and spinal cord. The affected white matter is severely gliotic, with predominantly perivascular inflammation, and patchy loss of myelinated fibres that is most marked in disease of several years' duration.

Another finding that is largely restricted to cases of several years' duration is the presence of neurofibrillary tangles (Figure 19.35d,e).[722,723] As in Alzheimer's disease, the tangles tend to involve the hippocampus and cerebral cortex, the nucleus basalis of Meynert, the hypothalamus

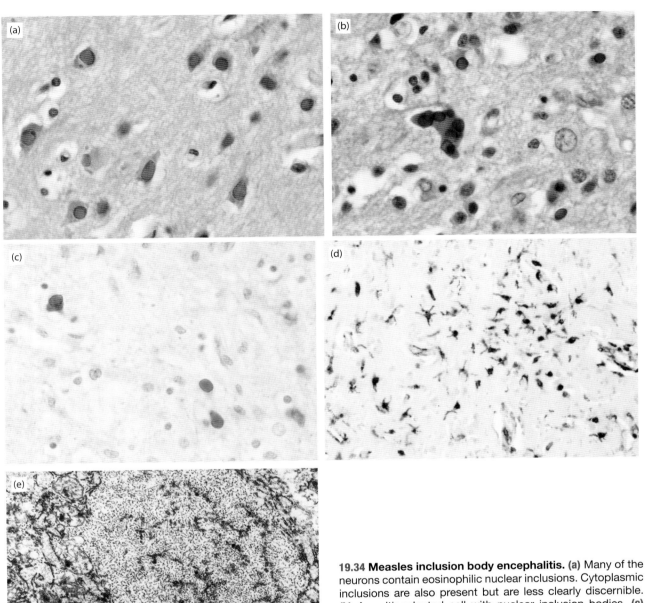

19.34 Measles inclusion body encephalitis. (a) Many of the neurons contain eosinophilic nuclear inclusions. Cytoplasmic inclusions are also present but are less clearly discernible. **(b)** A multinucleated cell with nuclear inclusion bodies. **(c)** Immunohistochemistry reveals abundant measles viral antigen. **(d)** Reactive microglia immunolabelled for CD68. **(e)** On electron microscopy, the nuclear inclusions are seen to contain numerous filamentous virus particles.

(b) Reproduced from Ellison and Love.[308a] © Elsevier, 1998.

and the brain stem raphe nuclei. Electron microscopy shows the tangles in SSPE to consist of paired helical filaments. They have a similar antigenic profile to the tangles of Alzheimer's disease[1071] and may be accompanied by scattered tau-immunopositive neurites in the adjacent grey matter. The distribution of tangles bears no obvious relationship to that of viral antigen,[69] but McQuaid and colleagues observed frequent co-localization of measles virus genome and neurofibrillary tangles.[754] Ikeda and colleagues reported the occurrence of numerous argyrophilic, tau-immunopositive tangles in oligodendroglia in two autopsy cases of SSPE.[506]

Progressive Rubella Pan-encephalitis

This very rare encephalitis presents several years after the initial, usually congenital, rubella infection (the pathogenesis and manifestations of which are described under Rubella).

Pathogenesis

This is still a poorly understood disorder. Rubella virus has been isolated from brain tissue in only one case[238] and from peripheral lymphocytes in one other.[1238] Patients have normal cell-mediated and humoral immunity, with

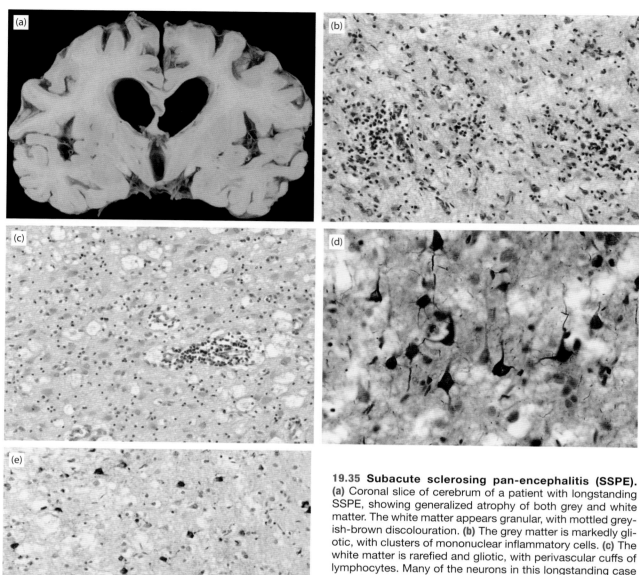

19.35 Subacute sclerosing pan-encephalitis (SSPE). **(a)** Coronal slice of cerebrum of a patient with longstanding SSPE, showing generalized atrophy of both grey and white matter. The white matter appears granular, with mottled greyish-brown discolouration. **(b)** The grey matter is markedly gliotic, with clusters of mononuclear inflammatory cells. **(c)** The white matter is rarefied and gliotic, with perivascular cuffs of lymphocytes. Many of the neurons in this longstanding case contain neurofibrillary tangles, as demonstrated by modified Bielschowsky impregnation **(d)** and immunohistochemistry for tau **(e)**.

(a) and original sections courtesy of Dr D Hilton, Derriford Hospital, Plymouth, UK.

high levels of antibodies against rubella virus in the serum and CSF and evidence of antibody synthesis within the CNS.[1170,1239] Coyle and Wolinsky found the serum in two patients and CSF in one patient to contain high levels of immune complexes, which included antibody directed against rubella virus.[236] These may contribute to the vascular abnormalities in the CNS. Many T-cells in the CSF of another patient with progressive rubella pan-encephalitis were found to react against autologous antigens, such as myelin basic protein, proteolipid protein and galactocerebrosides.[730] Some of the cells that reacted to myelin basic protein also responded to rubella antigen, raising the possibility that autoimmune brain damage may be triggered by molecular mimicry between viral and host epitopes.

Clinical Features

In most cases, the initial infection is congenital, but progressive rubella pan-encephalitis has occurred after childhood rubella.[1141,1237] Patients usually present between 8 and 20 years with insidious dementia and ataxia.[1139,1213,1237] Other manifestations can include seizures, spasticity, choreoathetosis and myoclonus. A perimacular pigmentary retinopathy may develop.[1213] The disease progresses slowly and intermittently, in most cases over several years, until the patient becomes decerebrate and, eventually, dies.

Pathological Findings

Very few cases have been studied neuropathologically.[1139–1141,1213] On macroscopic examination, the white matter appears gelatinous and reduced in volume, and the ventricles are correspondingly dilated (Figure 19.36a,b). The cerebellum may be disproportionately shrunken with atrophy of all layers.[1140] Microscopy reveals widespread neuronal loss and gliosis in the grey matter, with perivascular lymphocytic aggregates and microglial nodules (Figure 19.36c). The white matter is severely gliotic and rarefied. A consistent feature in reported cases has been the presence of amorphous, periodic acid–Schiff (PAS)-positive, mineralized material within blood vessel walls (Figure 19.36d) and forming globules in the white matter of the cerebrum and cerebellum. No viral inclusions are seen.

Progressive Multifocal Leukoencephalopathy

First described in 1958,[46] PML was suggested by Richardson to be the result of an opportunistic viral infection.[938] Virus particles were later identified by electron microscopy in the brain of patients with PML.[1043,1275] In 1971, the polyomavirus responsible for PML, JC virus, was cultured from brain tissue.[875]

JC virus is a species that was previously in the genus Polyomavirus in the family Polyomaviridae. The human Polyomaviridae include simian virus 40 (SV40), BK polyomavirus (BKV) and JC polyomavirus (JCV). Apart from very rare instances of low-grade meningoencephalitis caused by BK virus in patients with AIDS,[129,662,1166] only JCV is associated with CNS disease. Early reports of PML due to SV40 infection probably reflected confusion of SV40 with JC virus.[313,1088] The recent identification of seven additional human polyomaviruses less closely related to JCV, BKV and SV40 prompted the subdivision of the family Polyomaviridae into three genera: Orthopolyomavirus (including JCV, BKV and SV40), Wukipolyomavirus (which includes the newly identified human viruses), and Avipolyomavirus (these infect birds, not humans).[1121]

The incidence of PML rose dramatically with the onset of the AIDS epidemic,[95] prior to which PML was a rare disease that occasionally complicated leukaemia, lymphoma or organ transplantation. Between 1979 and 1994, 3894 deaths due to PML were reported in the United States.[479] Of these, 89 per cent were associated with HIV infection, and 2.1 per cent of patients who died from AIDS had PML. Between 1984 and 1994, the proportion of deaths due to PML increased 20-fold, from 0.2 to 3.3 per 1 million. Although the great majority of these deaths have been in adults, children with inherited or acquired immunodeficiency are also at risk of PML.[26,795] PML has been reported in up to 10 per cent of AIDS patients, and HIV infection in 55–85 per cent of patients with PML.[98,1220]

PML has, very rarely, been reported in patients without identifiable underlying disease,[954,1044] but is largely restricted to immunocompromised hosts. Although initially described as a complication of lymphoproliferative malignancies, PML can complicate any form of immunodeficiency, including that due to genetic disorders and chronic inflammatory and infectious diseases, such as tuberculosis, sarcoidosis and rheumatoid arthritis. Progressive multifocal leukoencephalopathy may result from iatrogenic immunosuppression (e.g. for the treatment of autoimmune disorders or for organ transplantation). Progressive multifocal leukoencephalopathy has been reported in patients being treated for multiple sclerosis or Crohn's disease with natalizumab;[211,602,646,1109,1167] this humanized monoclonal antibody binds to the 4 subunit of very late antigen-4 integrin and thereby blocks the trafficking of lymphocytes, including those responsible for immune surveillance within the CNS. PML has also complicated the treatment of plaque psoriasis with efalizumab (since withdrawn, a humanized antibody directed at the subunit of CD11), and has occurred in patients receiving rituximab (a chimeric IgG1 monoclonal antibody that targets CD20+ B lymphocytes), mostly for treatment of lymphoma.[602,1109] Surprisingly, PML is relatively unusual in patients receiving a bone marrow transplant.

Progressive Multifocal Leukoencephalopathy and Brain Tumours

JCV can induce neoplasms in several non-mammalian species, including rodents and monkeys.[710] This, the presence of bizarre malignant-looking astrocytes in PML and the observation that *in vitro* infection can transform cultured human glia as well as the detection of JCV DNA or T antigen in a range of tumours, have led to the speculation that JCV may be tumourigenic in humans. However, the causality of this association has not been established.[710] CNS glial tumours, medulloblastomas and lymphomas have occurred only rarely in conjunction with PML.[1039,370,476,1044] See Chapter 26 for further discussion of the aetiology of neuroepithelial tumours.

Aetiology

Polyomaviridae are non-enveloped icosahedral viruses measuring approximately 45 nm in diameter. The viral genome comprises double-stranded circular DNA, complexed with cellular histones and wound in a super-helix. The viral proteins are encoded by overlapping genes on both strands of DNA. The super-helix is surrounded by a nucleocapsid composed of 72 capsomeres, each composed of three proteins (VP1, VP2, VP3). These are needed for initial attachment of the virus to sialic acid (SA) residues on the cell surface.[154,467] The serotonin 2A receptor was shown to serve as a receptor for JCV entry.[314] However, it is probably not the receptor for all types of cell; the serotonin 2A receptor blocker risperidone did not reduce infection of primary human fetal glial cells by JCV(Mad-1),[178] the prototypical type of JCV associated with PML (see later). Subsequent viral endocytosis is dependent on the presence of 4 integrin, which probably serves as a post-attachment receptor.[163] Once within the cell, the virus is transported rapidly to the nucleus, where uncoating occurs. Cellular transcription factors bind to viral promoters and initiate the transcription of early proteins. JCV early mRNA is alternatively spliced to yield five transcripts, encoding small tumour antigen (t), large tumour antigen (T) and three further proteins: T'_{135}, T'_{136}, and T'_{165}. The early proteins are needed for viral multiplication and for transcription of the late coding region, which encodes the viral capsid proteins VP1, VP2 and VP3, and the viroporin, agnoprotein.

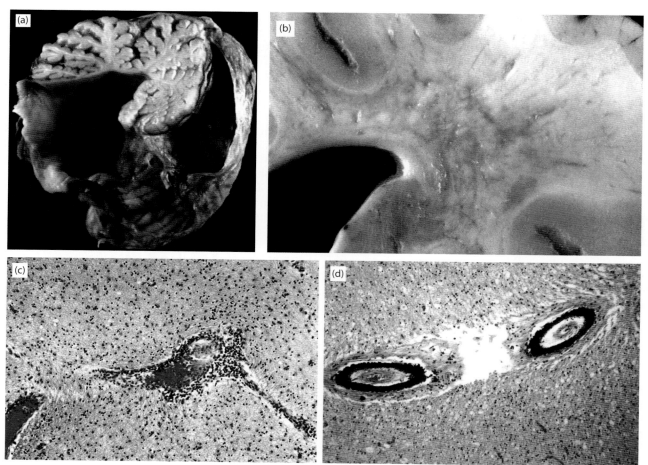

19.36 Progressive rubella pan-encephalitis. (a) The cerebellum is severely atrophic and the fourth ventricle is dilated. **(b)** The cerebral white matter appears grey and gelatinous, with a pitted surface. **(c)** Perivascular and parenchymal infiltrate of mononuclear inflammatory cells. **(d)** There is extensive mineralization of blood vessels in the striatum.

Courtesy of Dr JJ Townsend, University of Utah, Salt Lake City, UT, USA.

The transcription of early and late viral proteins is regulated by the non-coding control region (NCCR), which requires cell type-specific transcription factors present in glial cells, as well as transcription factors that are expressed in all cell types.[1121] Oligodendrocytes support productive JC virus infection, which leads to cell lysis and consequent demyelination. Productive infection can also occur in cerebellar granule cells.[304] Astrocytes do not support productive infection by JC virus, but non-permissive infection of these cells leads to their morphological transformation and resulting bizarre appearance (see Pathological Findings).

There are two main genetic forms of JCV: the archetypal form, found in kidney, urine and sewage, and the PML-associated or prototypical forms, which are associated with PML and typified by the Mad-1 strain.[602,1109,1120,1221] Prototypical forms of JCV differ from the archetypal form in having duplications, tandem repeats, insertions and deletions in the NCCR.

Pathogenesis

Over 50 per cent of adolescents and 66–90 per cent of adults have serological evidence of polyomavirus infection. JC virus is highly stable in the environment.[117] Spread of infection probably occurs by oral and respiratory routes.[297,1220] JCV DNA can be detected in tonsillar tissue from over one-third of children and adults.[569,782] The virus infects B-lymphocytes, CD34+ haematopoietic progenitor cells and kidney epithelium, probably establishing latent or low-grade persistent infection in bone marrow, spleen, lymph nodes, kidney, gastrointestinal epithelium and possibly the CNS.[303,491,602,640, 1109,1110,1162,1220] The infection is usually entirely benign. It remains unclear whether the development of PML involves entry into the brain of bone marrow-derived CD34+ cells or B-lymphocytes, or the reactivation of JCV already present within the brain. There is evidence that immunosuppression promotes the rearrangement of the NCCR and the emergence of PML-associated strains of JCV.[602,1109,1110] Other than the NCCR, the only polymorphic part of the JCV genome is in the VP1 genotyping region.[1121] VP1 loop mutations and substitutions probably influence the rate of disease progression.[1121] HIV-1 transactivator protein (tat) may have a role in the development of PML in AIDS patients, through stimulation of JCV transcription[245] and replication.[1103]

Clinical Features

The onset of PML is usually insidious. Patients present with diverse neurological deficits that vary according to the site of disease within the CNS but often include neuropsychological deficits, apraxia, retrochiasmal visual deficits and motor problems.[1216] Seizures were reported in 18 per cent and were association with lesions abutting the cerebral cortex.[673] Conventional examination of the CSF is usually normal. Before the introduction of cART, PCR analysis for JCV nucleic acids had a sensitivity of 72 to 92 per cent and specificity approaching 100 per cent,[27,118,119,785] but in HIV patients treated with cART the sensitivity was reported to be only 57.5 per cent,[732a] probably because of improved clearance of virus by immune cells. The clinical and radiological findings at presentation may simulate those of a primary brain tumour,[141] but mass effect is uncommon. MRI is more sensitive than CT scanning for demonstrating the multiple small lesions in the white matter.[319,1188] Patients typically have asymmetrical, multifocal, bihemispheric lesions in the subcortical white matter in early disease, later involving deep white matter and sometimes contiguous deep grey matter structures.[1121] Lesions appear hypointense on T1 sequences and hyperintense on T2 and FLAIR sequences and do not show contrast enhancement.[1121,1220]

Until the late 1990s, PML was usually fatal within 6 months, although occasional remissions had been reported, usually after effective treatment of the cause of the underlying immunosuppression.[239,458,912] Indeed, the restoration of immune function is the central plank of treatment of PML. In PML associated with HIV infection, the prognosis has been greatly improved by the introduction of cART, which is often effective in slowing or even halting the progression of PML.[210,358,602,674,770,1109,1116,1121] In patients receiving natalizumab, restoration of immune function is achieved by withdrawal of natalizumab; because the immunosuppressive effects of this drug last for several weeks, patients are usually also treated by plasma exchange or immunoabsorption.[211] Reversal of immunosuppression in other clinical contexts may have to be balanced against the risk of tumour recurrence or organ transplant rejection.

Restoration of immunity in patients with PML is often complicated by immune reconstitution inflammatory syndrome (IRIS—in the context of PML sometimes designated PML-IRIS), in which there is worsening of the clinical disease, at least temporarily, because of the development of an inflammatory reaction to JCV. Neuroimaging often shows contrast enhancement and oedema of lesions, reflecting their infiltration by inflammatory cells. Although in general the inflammatory response heralds a favourable outcome,[97,305,786] PML-IRIS may cause significant morbidity and sometimes mortality,[208,211] particularly when lesions affect the brain stem or cerebellum.[674] Patients on natalizumab who develop PML usually require aggressive treatment with corticosteroids, sometimes over several months.[211] Although most often seen in the context of HAART, an inflammatory variant of PML was occasionally noted in patients with AIDS before the introduction of effective treatment,[436] and in patients with immunosuppression due to diseases other than AIDS,[939] and was associated with prolonged survival. Recovery from PML seems to depend on the development of a JC virus-specific CD8+ cytotoxic T-cell response.[617]

JCV Neuronopathy and Meningitis

Productive infection of cerebellar granule cells by JCV (JCV granule cell neuronopathy) can cause subacute or chronic cerebellar dysfunction, including gait ataxia, dysarthria, and incoordination.[602,1109] MRI shows cerebellar atrophy. JCV infection (and consequent loss) of granule cells is relatively common in PML and is often found in association with typical demyelinating lesions in the immediately adjacent cerebellar white matter. However, JCV granule cell neuronopathy can occur in the absence of white matter disease.[618] Wuthrich et al.[1248] detected JCV-infected cells in the granule cell layer in post-mortem or biopsy tissue from 28 of 43 patients with PML. In three cases, no lesions were found in the cerebellar white matter. In addition, JCV infection of cerebellar granule cells was demonstrated in tissue from a further, HIV-positive patient who did not have PML anywhere in the CNS.

JCV has occasionally been detected in the CSF of both immunocompromised and immunocompetent patients who present with symptoms of meningitis and have no parenchymal lesions detected on neuroimaging.[602,1109] Wuthrich et al.[1249] also reported a lung cancer patient who developed an encephalopathy associated with productive infection of pyramidal neurons in the cerebral cortex and necrosis at the junction with underlying white matter.

Pathological Findings

Macroscopic Features

The brain is externally unremarkable, but sectioning reveals multiple small or larger confluent foci of grey discolouration (Figure 19.37a). These are usually best seen in the white matter or at the junction of white matter and cerebral cortex, but they can sometimes be discerned within the grey matter as well. The lesions may cause pitting or gelatinous softening of the cut surface of the brain. Confluent lesions may cavitate (Figure 19.37a).

Microscopic Features

Many more lesions can usually be discerned histologically than macroscopically. The lesions most often involve the cerebral white matter and myelinated fibres within the cerebral cortex, but the cerebellum, deep grey nuclei, brain stem and, occasionally, the spinal cord can be affected. The lesions typically show loss of myelin, with axonal sparing. In larger lesions, however, loss of axons may be considerable. There are numerous foamy macrophages, particularly in active lesions. In classic PML, the inflammatory infiltrate consists almost exclusively of macrophages, with only scanty lymphocytes. However, as noted earlier, the lesions in patients with AIDS can show intense inflammation and necrosis, particularly after initiation of combined antiretroviral treatment (cART; also termed high active antiretroviral treatment or HAART) (Figure 19.38). This finding correlates with the presence of lesions that show contrast-enhancement on neuroimaging.[97,319,1241] Oligodendrocytes at the margins of the lesions have enlarged nuclei filled with homogeneous, amphophilic or basophilic material (Figure 19.37c). The lesions and immediately adjacent brain tissue may contain astrocytes with enlarged, hyperchromatic, bizarrely shaped nuclei and abundant eosinophilic cytoplasm (Figure 19.37b). These resemble malignant astrocytes and can cause confusion in biopsies, particularly during intraoperative cytological or histological assessment. Rarely, PML and glioma coexist.[426,1044]

Cerebellar granule cell infection by JCV is evidenced by the presence of cells with large vesicular nuclei and central nucleoli in the granule cell layer (Figure 19.39). In some cases, there is focal loss of granule cells. JCV infection of granule cells is usually but not always associated with PML in the adjacent white matter.

The presence of JC virus can be confirmed by several techniques, including electron microscopy, immunohistochemistry (Figure 19.37d) and in situ hybridization. These methods usually reveal the virus to be distributed more widely within the brain than is suggested by conventional histological examination. Ultrastructural examination shows the enlarged oligodendroglia to contain numerous intranuclear viral particles. Virus particles are rarely, if ever, detected in astrocytes. Viral nucleic acids can be demonstrated by in situ hybridization in oligodendrocytes and astrocytes[1188] and are usually distributed more widely within the brain than is suggested by conventional histological examination.

In patients who have been successfully treated with cART, the resolution of PML may leave foci of gliosis and inflammation without any detectable viral inclusions. A neuropathological diagnosis of 'burnt-out' PML is usually based on a combination of previous clinical and radiological findings, the prior detection of JCV in the CSF, and the presence of well-demarcated foci of chronic demyelination, astrocytic gliosis and varied amounts of lymphocytic inflammation (Figure 19.40).

Retroviruses

Retroviruses were first identified in association with sarcomas, lymphomas and leukaemias in animals.[215] An intensive

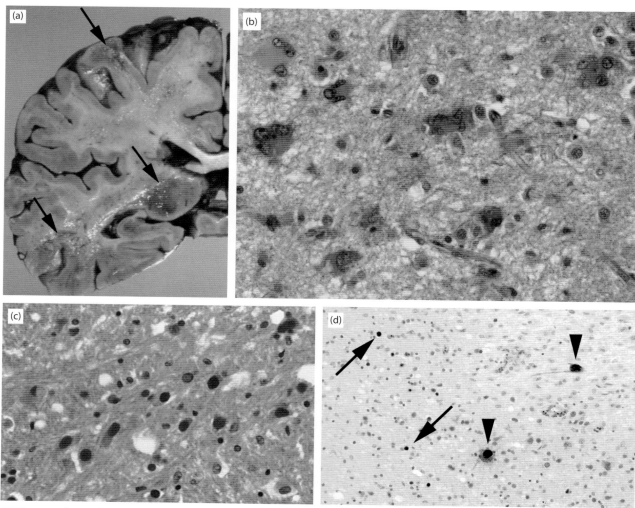

19.37 Progressive multifocal leukoencephalopathy (PML). **(a)** In this florid example of PML, the affected white matter has a pitted appearance and includes multiple foci of grey-brown discolouration. Confluent, partly cavitated lesions are present in the superficial white matter and overlying cortex and in the thalamus (arrows). **(b)** Bizarre-looking multinucleated astrocytes in PML. These should not be mistaken for neoplastic cells. In a small biopsy, the distinction can be difficult to make. **(c)** The white matter at the edge of a focus of active demyelination includes many oligodendrocytes with enlarged nuclei, filled with homogeneous, amphophilic material. **(d)** Immunohistochemistry reveals viral antigen (brown reaction product) in several oligodendroglial nuclei (arrows) around the edge of a focus of demyelination, and in some of the bizarre-looking astrocytes (arrowheads).

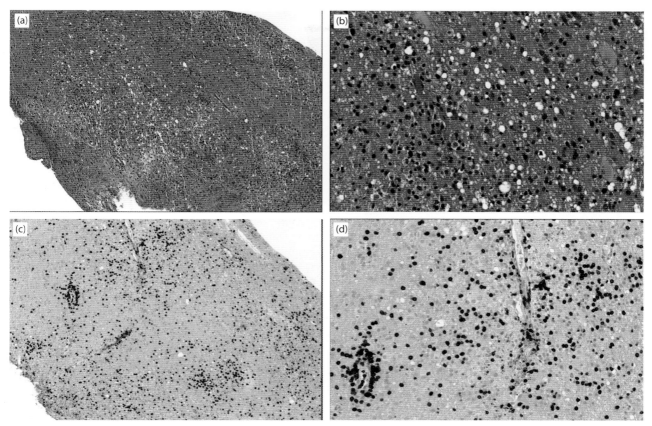

19.38 Florid inflammatory reaction to JCV in an AIDS patient after administration of combined antiretroviral treatment (PML-IRIS). (a) Multiple foci of increased cellularity are visible in this biopsy of cerebral white matter. **(b)** At higher magnification, the infiltrate is seen to comprise a mixture of astrocytes (some with abundant eosinophilic cytoplasm), macrophages and lymphocytes. **(c)** Many of the lymphocytes are CD3-positive T-cells. **(d)** High-magnification view of the CD3-positive cells. Some are cuffing small blood vessels, others are scattered within the abnormal parenchyma. There are also small fragments of immunopositive apoptotic debris.

search for possible retroviruses associated with human cancer led to the discovery of human T-cell leukaemia/lymphoma viruses HTLV-1 and HTLV-2, both associated with rare forms of adult T-cell leukaemia. Decades later, HTLV was found to be the aetiological agent of a slowly progressive neurological disorder (HTLV-1-associated myelopathy). Human T-cell lymphotropic virus-related disease is still relatively rare. Another human retrovirus, HIV, was identified only in the 1980s, but has already infected more than 40 million people worldwide.

Retroviridae were initially divided into the genera Oncovirus, Spumavirus and Lentivirus on the basis of their biological effects.[215] Subsequent genomic sequencing and the identification of further retroviruses led to their subdivision into two subfamilies: Orthoretrovirinae (containing the genera Alpharetrovirus, Betaretrovirus, Gammaretrovirus, Deltaretrovirus, Epsilonretrovirus and Lentivirus) and Spumaretrovirinae (containing the genus Spumavirus). Of these, the known causes of human disease are two of the deltaretroviruses (HTLV-1 and HTLV-2) and two of the lentiviruses (HIV-1 and HIV-2). On the basis of genomic sequence variation, HIV-1 and HIV-2 have both been subdivided into multiple clades.

All retroviral virions are composed of two identical copies of a single-stranded RNA genome surrounded by a nucleocapsid and envelope. A minimum protein complement of reverse transcriptase, protease and integrase is incorporated within the nucleocapsid. Lentiviruses contain, in addition, several other accessory proteins, some of which are crucial to infectivity. The nucleocapsid consists of multiple proteins, including the group-associated antigens (gag proteins) that were of historical importance in classifying the retroviruses. Surrounding the nucleocapsid is a lipid bilayer studded with envelope (env) viral glycoprotein. The env protein is encoded by a single gene, but during viral maturation the protein backbone is cleaved so that the mature protein comprises a small transmembrane protein and a non-covalently associated surface protein. The surface portion of the env protein contains the binding sites for the cell receptor, whereas the transmembrane portion of the protein is involved in membrane fusion.

After binding of envelope proteins to the cell receptor, retroviruses enter the cytoplasm either through direct fusion with the plasma membrane[1080] or by receptor-mediated endocytosis and fusion with lysosomes.[907] Cells already infected with a particular retrovirus are highly resistant to super-infection by the same species of retrovirus or other retroviruses that use the same receptor (this phenomenon, termed 'interference', was helpful in classifying some groups of retroviruses, such as

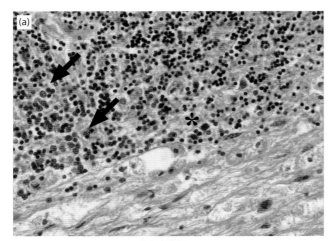

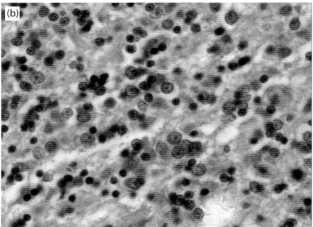

19.39 Cerebellar granule cell infection by JCV. (a) Demyelination of the cerebellar white matter is associated here with infection of granule cells in the adjacent cortex. The infected cells are most numerous towards the left of the figure, where many have enlarged vesicular nuclei and a prominent central nucleolus (arrows). Note the contrasting appearance of the nuclei of infected oligodendrocytes (asterisk). **(b)** The altered appearance of the nuclei of infected granule cells is more obvious at higher magnification.

the murine leukaemia viruses[929]). Once within the cytoplasm, the viral reverse transcriptase initiates DNA synthesis from the genomic RNA template.[127] Viral DNA and parts of the nucleocapsid[127] are then transported to the host nucleus, where a second viral protein randomly integrates viral DNA into the host genome. This stably integrated complex (provirus) directs all subsequent viral synthesis.

Strong promoters and viral transcription factors enhance the transcription of viral genes. If integration places a cellular proto-oncogene under the control of retroviral promoters, then cellular transformation may occur.[456] Early viral transcripts appear to be limited to potent transcription factors that regulate transcription from the provirus and control RNA splicing. The transcription factors are synthesized from double-spliced subgenomic mRNA.[150] Subsequently, full-length viral RNA is transcribed, producing gag, polymerase (pol) and env proteins. The transcripts coding for env proteins are translated on membrane-bound ribosomes, facilitating the incorporation of these proteins into the cell membrane. The remaining genes are translated on free polyribosomes. Retroviral assembly occurs at the cell membrane, the packaging of genomic RNA occurring simultaneously with the budding of virus.

The complex virus entry, replication and release pathways of the retroviruses have enabled the development of five classes of antiretroviral drugs active against HIV: nucleoside/nucleotide reverse transcriptase inhibitors, non-nucleoside/nucleotide reverse transcriptase inhibitors, protease inhibitors, entry inhibitors and integrase inhibitors.

Human Immunodeficiency Viruses

Human immunodeficiency viruses (HIV), of which the most important and common type is HIV-1, have been established as the cause of the acquired immunodeficiency syndrome (AIDS) since the mid-1980s. The syndrome was officially first recognized in 1981.[164]

Recent molecular archaeology studies enable the tracing back in time to when mankind was first infected with these viruses, through matching dated HIV samples with the known virus mutation rates to arrive at common ancestor virus. HIV-1 first crossed into man in central Africa, about 1920, by accident, from a chimpanzee infected with simian immunodeficiency virus (SIVcpz). This became the HIV-1 group M virus, the most successful of the HIVs, and the cause of 99 per cent of HIV infections. The other HIV-1 groups (O, N, P viruses) arose from other, later transmissions of SIVcpz but have remained localized, with few patients. Group M viruses have since mutated in man further into numerous subtypes, with subtype B dominating infections transmitted within Europe and North America, and subtype C dominating in southern Africa.[888]

The West African HIV-2 has only 40 per cent sequence homology with HIV-1, and crossed from sooty mangabey monkeys into man some time in the early twentieth century. Again, there have been several transmissions to man, and the evolution of several virus subtypes within HIV-2. A comprehensive account of the origins of the HIVs, their clinical disease recognition from the 1970s, and how they became disseminated around the globe is given by Pepin.[888]

Epidemiology

Up-to-date epidemiological and transmission data on the HIV pandemic are available from UNAIDS (www.unaids.org). Currently there are, globally, about 33 million people living with HIV infection, with about 1.8 million deaths and 2.6 million new infections per year. Sub-Saharan Africa is the region the most affected; Eastern Europe and Asia have the fastest growing epidemics. Because each part of the world suffers from its own HIV epidemic, with different risk factors, co-infections and medical responses, the following account is necessarily generalized.

While discussing the pathogenesis of HIV-related brain disease, mainly as seen at autopsy, this section is also intended to assist pathologists who receive brain biopsies from patients with clinical and radiological abnormalities where the diagnosis is unclear (Box 19.7).

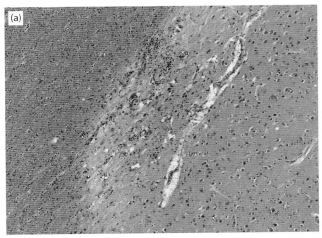

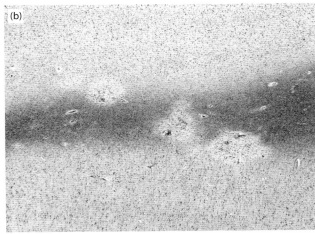

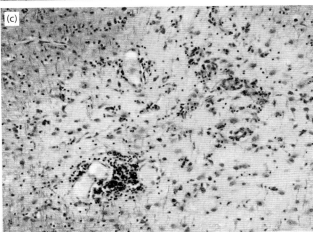

19.40 'Burnt-out' PML. This AIDS patient had presented with clinical and neuroradiological features of PML a year earlier, and JCV DNA had been detected in his CSF. After successful treatment of his HIV infection with cART, his PML resolved clinically. He died of unrelated disease. **(a)** Post-mortem examination revealed multiple circumscribed foci of myelin pallor, gliosis and lymphocytic inflammation at the junction of cerebral cortex and white matter. Note the paucity of oligodendrocyte nuclei. **(b)** The lack of myelin in these foci gave them a punched-out appearance in sections stained with Luxol fast blue and cresyl violet. **(c)** Higher magnification revealed clusters of lymphocytes and many reactive astrocytes.

Pathogenesis

Ultrastructurally, HIV can be distinguished from other retroviruses. However, as HIV spend little of their life-cycle as extracellular particles, electron microscopy is of minimal diagnostic utility. The genomic structure of HIV is similar to that of other retroviruses, except for the inclusion of genes encoding accessory proteins such as *tat, nef, rev, vif, vpr* and *vpu*. Whether these contribute to specific features of HIV-related neurological disease is unclear.

HIV enters host cells via receptors on the surface membrane. The CD4 protein, present on helper T-lymphocytes and monocytes, is crucial, along with one of the chemokine co-receptors, of which CCR5 appears most important for monocytes/macrophages. Infection of both CD4+ T-cells and microglial cells in the brain and spinal cord are key aspects of HIV disease.

HIV infection of T-cells causes their destruction (particularly in the gut) via complex immunological cell-mediated processes.[781] The result is defective T-cell mediated cell mediated immunity (CMI) and the flourishing of opportunistic infections of all types (viruses, bacteria, mycobacteria, fungi, protozoa and a few worms). HIV infection of monocyte-derived cells damages their general immune functions.

The various HIV-2s are less virulent than HIV-1, and are restricted to those who live on the west coastal areas of Africa,

BOX 19.7. Guidance on the interpretation of brain biopsies from HIV-infected patients with focal or diffuse lesions

- Obtain the clinical and radiological information on the case. Ascertain whether the patient is a new HIV presentation or is on cART, and his or her recent blood CD4 count and HIV viral load.
- Consider and look for lymphoma, tuberculosis, viral inclusion bodies, *Toxoplasma* trophozoites and cysts, and fungi (*Cryptococcus, Aspergillus*).
- Stain for acid-fast bacilli and fungi routinely.
- Routinely immunolabel for JC virus, CMV, HSV, *Toxoplasma* and HIVp24
- Perform differential immunohistochemistry for B-cells (CD20), T-cells (CD3 and possibly CD4 and CD8) and macrophages (CD68).
- Consider IRIS if the patient is on cART and CD8+ T-cells are abundant—if granulomatous inflammation, it could be IRIS to an infection; if no infection, then CNS-HIV-IRIS.
- Obtain the microbiology and molecular diagnostic data on contemporary blood and CSF.
- Discuss the case with clinical colleagues—and seek expert pathological advice if the diagnosis is still not evident.

now or in the past. The pathology of HIV-2 is broadly similar to that of HIV-1, which is the main focus of this section.

The generation of effective anti-HIV drugs since the mid-1990s has been the most important advance in managing the disease. Zidovudine monotherapy had transient beneficial effects and now the drugs are used in combination, to reduce the development of resistance; hence 'combination antiretroviral therapy' (cART – this term is used in preference to the earlier 'highly active antiretroviral therapy' (HAART)). As a result, most people diagnosed before a life-terminating complication can be treated and restored to reasonable or better health; and expect to live a life-expectancy that approaches normal. This is important when considering the chronic neurocognitive diseases encountered in HIV disease. Because the clinicopathological complications that characterize AIDS can now be reversed, the old term 'AIDS' is being supplanted by the more appropriate term 'HIV disease'.

Brain Entry and Location of HIV

Central and peripheral nervous system diseases are important aspects of clinical HIV disease from infection unto death. This is because HIV enters the central neuraxis early during infection (at seroconversion)[475] and remains there in microglial cells and macrophages – even in very low non-replicating and barely detectable quantities – as a latent infection forever despite cART.[1127] From here, it can re-emerge systemically, if anti-HIV treatment is stopped or drug resistance develops.[109]

Two important points – precisely where in the brain HIV remains and replicates, and in how many cells types – are still controversial.[1013] High-tech investigations indicate that HIV is in astrocytes, parenchymal microglia, and perivascular macrophages; and that trafficking of latent virus via the latter cells increases with immunosuppression.[1127] Second, the various cART drugs differ in their penetration into the CSF and (presumably) the brain parenchyma – they have different CNS penetration effectiveness (CPE) scores.[663] This may impact on the chronic neurocognitive disorders in treated patients.

General Clinical Features of HIV Infection

Primary infection is often accompanied by constitutional symptoms similar to those of infectious mononucleosis or influenza, including an aseptic meningitis syndrome. This so-called HIV seroconversion illness occurs within a few weeks of infection by the virus, and coincides with the very high initial blood HIV viral load (often millions of copies per mL of blood), a drop in blood CD4+ T-cells, and development of the antibodies that are the basis for standard HIV blood tests.[781] HIV virus is found in the CSF from this point on in HIV disease, disappearing only if the patient is effectively treated with cART.

After the acute infection, usually the viral load drops and the CD4 count rises. Patients then enter a long asymptomatic phase; this may last a few years to two decades or more, depending on the individual's host response to HIV. However, in the absence of drug intervention, all those infected eventually develop HIV disease. HIV viral replication and consequent depletion of T-cells through apoptosis continue, and the host cell-mediated immune system collapses. When blood CD4+ T-cell counts drop below 200/mm³, systemic symptoms may develop, and opportunistic infections and tumours progress – this is advanced HIV disease. In the 30 years since recognition of the diseases caused by HIVs, there has been an

ever-broadening range of HIV-associated conditions: infections and pathological processes that either are directly caused by HIV or occur where HIV infection alters the cadence of 'normal' pathologies. In these later phases, various HIV-associated brain syndromes, both acute and chronic, present.

From the mid-1990s, everything changed with the introduction of cART. The aim is reduction of blood (and tissue – including brain – HIV load) to undetectable, and restoration of the blood CD4+ T-cell counts to more normal levels. As well as profoundly altering the prognosis of HIV infection, cART has introduced its own complications. The neuromuscular system is a significant target of these unintended events. However, it must be emphasized that in large HIV patient cohorts, cART has greatly reduced the incidence of the classic HIV-associated brain infections and of HIV encephalopathy/dementia;[1122] and it has reduced the overall prevalence of the mild non-specific pathologies seen in autopsy brains.[326] The major milestones in our understanding of HIV CNS neuropathology are summarized in Box 19.8.

Patterns of HIV-Related Neuromuscular Disease

Broadly, these HIV-related diseases are categorized into three groups:

1. Central nervous system (brain and spinal cord):
   a. Directly or indirectly related to HIV infection, with or without modification by cART:
      i. Early brain involvement (around or soon after seroconversion illness).[402,404]
      ii. Later brain disease.
   b. HIV-related opportunistic infections and tumours (described elsewhere in this chapter and book).
   c. Co-morbidities, such as age-related neurodegenerative disease, vascular disorders (stroke), metastatic non-AIDS-associated cancers, chronic liver disease, HCV infection.
2. Peripheral neuropathy.
3. Myopathy.

This section focuses on the CNS processes directly related to HIV. Adult HIV disease is far more investigated than paediatric (which is considered at the end of this section). The pathology is not straightforward, because of:

1. A now-historical classification.[142]
2. The emphasis on autopsy brain pathology rather than *in vivo* brain biopsies for systematic explication.
3. Numerous case reports of HIV-infected patients with complicated, highly variable and often unexplained brain pathology. There is a lack of correlative consensus of the clinical, imaging and microbiological investigations with the underlying pathology. Neuroimaging cannot always indicate specific pathologies.[768]
4. The effects, mainly indirect, of cART on brain pathology, including the immune reconstitution inflammatory response syndrome (IRIS).
5. Common mild non-specific neuropathological features found in brains of most patients dying with or from HIV disease: such as aseptic lymphocytic meningitis,

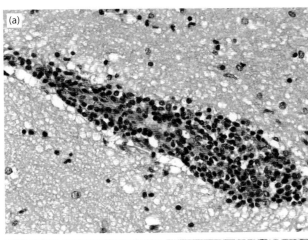

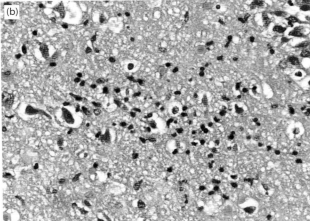

19.41 HIV-seroconversion illness and encephalitis (autopsy case from suicide). (a) Vascular infiltration–these were all T-cells. (b) Hippocampus with an encephalitis reaction, including microglial activation.

perivascular inflammation,[404,1005] microglial and astrocyte activation,[326] accumulation of amyloid precursor protein to indicate axonal breakdown.[22]

6. Confounding effects of cerebrovascular disease, HCV infection, chronic liver disease, and history of intravenous drug use, all of which influence assessment of pathology attributable to HIV infection.

Clinical Pathology of HIV CNS Disease

Seroconversion Illness

Clinically acutely infected, many patients have headache and an aseptic meningitis syndrome: HIV testing is now a standard diagnostic work-up for this syndrome, but opportunities to study the pathology are rare. A personally observed case showed CD8+ T-cell infiltration of meninges, vessels and the parenchyma, but without microglial nodules or giant cells, nor demonstrable HIV on immunohistochemistry (Figure 19.41). We presume that such mild, non-destructive meningo-encephalitis is common and resolves as the seroconversion phase passes (it is not fatal *per se*). However, it may explain the dystrophic deposition of calcium in cerebral vessels and in the parenchyma, frequently found at autopsy many years later.[404]

Rare cases of an acute inflammatory demyelinating leukoencephalopathy (like ADEM) are reported at seroconversion, with HIV found in the CSF.[549] Autoimmune encephalitis (limbic encephalitis) has also been described during seroconversion illness, with typical temporal lobe features.[1019] Treatment with intravenous immunoglobulin and cART resulted in significant improvement. It is likely that in such uncommon patients, acute HIV infection combines with an inherited predisposition to produce florid inflammatory disease.

CNS Disease Presenting after Seroconversion

The various syndromes are divided into those presenting before any anti-HIV therapy has been given, and those that follow effective cART. Necessarily, many of the syndromes overlap.

Pre-antiretroviral Treatment – Chronic Neurocognitive Disorders

Historically, up to 30 per cent of patients with late HIV disease developed motor and cognitive deficits that were not attributable to opportunistic infection or tumour. Originally termed the 'AIDS dementia complex' (ADC), this has been reclassified into the 'HIV-associated neurocognitive disorders' (HAND)[28,529] with clinical case definitions for stages of increasing severity:

1. HIV-associated asymptomatic neurocognitive impairment (ANI).
2. HIV-associated mild neurocognitive disorder (MND).
3. HIV-associated dementia (HAD).

HAD, at its extreme spectral end, results in a vegetative state. Cognitive impairment, poor concentration, forgetfulness, apathy, confusion, and other functions are tested with standardized neuropsychometric tests. Part of the problem in understanding the underlying neuropathology is the overlap–particularly for ANI and MND–with similar clinical impairments in 'the normal population' as HIV-infected cohorts on cART are ageing, because these deficits increase naturally with age.

The major pathological entity is HIV encephalitis, which was delineated in the 1980s and correlated, to an extent, with HIV-associated dementia, and certainly with brain atrophy.[142] Its definition is histopathological (Table 19.6, Figure 19.42). The multinucleated giant cells (MNGC) resemble Langhans' giant cells, although the nuclei are more hyperchromatic. Immunostaining shows they contain HIV antigen. These cells, with associated microglial proliferation and activation, are most abundant in subcortical cerebral structures–cerebral and cerebellar white matter and the basal ganglia.

Epidemiologically, the prevalence of HIV encephalitis in autopsy brain is highly variable. Earlier studies of demented HIV patients could find it in virtually all cases; in contrast, a large autopsy study in Africa found it in only 1 per cent of adult patients.[687] An international retrospective study found an overall prevalence of one quarter.[252] Much depends on case selection. There is no doubt that with widespread availability of cART, the frequency has diminished.[87]

The second lesion formally defined,[142] HIV leukoencephalopathy, has been less studied and compared (Table 19.6). It seems often to represent myelin pallor rather than demyelination, and the important differential diagnosis is JC virus encephalitis. Where there is myelin damage, oligodendrocytes under reactive proliferation.[322]

What Is the Neuropathological Substrate of the HAND Syndromes?
This is a controversial subject. There are increasing clinical and neuroimaging investigations as increasing numbers of HIV-infected patients are managed on cART and present with neurocognitive defects, and yet correlative neuropathology is hardly involved. Certain things are clear:

- HIV encephalitis and HIV leukoencephalopathy do not consistently correlate with HIV-associated dementia.[188,326,1122]

- With cART, HAD rates are lower, but rates of the milder syndromes of ANI and MND have not changed much.[663]

Other histomorphological explanations–linked to HIV infection–have been sought to explain HAND:

- neuron loss with or without HIV encephalitis: detailed neuron counts in the frontal cortex have shown losses of nearly 40 per cent compared with HIV-uninfected controls;[324]
- microglial cell activation associated with neuronal apoptosis and axonal damage;[406] the activated microglia effect damage via oxidative stress;
- dendritic and synaptic damage, without frank neuronal loss[325] and neuron spatial cluster pattern abnormalities–both correlating with clinical dementia.[44]

In summary, no classic HIV neuropathology features correlate well with HAND syndromes (in contrast to what was believed 10 years ago).[326] The subtle neuronal loss, network and architectural abnormalities indicated earlier may be important. It may be that the background neuroactivation–mild microglial cell activation and astrogliosis[207]–commonly seen in those living long with HIV as the critical aetiology is most significant. There is much emphasis on 'chronic systemic inflammation' in HIV disease, with microbial translocation from the gut as a driving force, linked to CNS inflammation. It remains to be seen whether improving cART strategies can suppress this inflammation and reduce neurocognitive defects in HIV-infected patients.[354]

Pre-antiretroviral Treatment–Acute Neuropathological Presentations
There are a large number of case reports of unusual acute presentations in HIV-infected people with inflammatory and degenerative brain lesions, which are difficult to fit into a coherent pathogenetic framework, although many probably represent similar conditions (e.g. ADEM-like),

TABLE 19.6 HIV: The main neuropathological entities in the 1991 systematic classification[142,399]

Pathological lesion	Location	Histopathology	Clinical correlation
HIV encephalitis	Brain	Multiple disseminated foci of microglia, macrophages and multinucleated giant cells (MNGCs)	HIV-associated dementia and HAND syndromes?
		If MNGCs are not found, the presence of HIV antigen or nucleic acids is required, as determined by *in situ* hybridization or immuno-histochemistry	
HIV leukoencephalopathy	Brain	Diffuse white matter damage including myelin loss, reactive astrogliosis, macrophages and MNGCs, but little or no inflammatory infiltrates	HIV-associated dementia and HAND syndromes?
		If MNGCs are not found, HIV demonstration is required	
Vacuolar myelopathy	Spinal cord	Multiple areas of the cord, predominantly in the dorsolateral tracts, exhibit vacuolar myelin swellings and macrophages; some macrophages typically reside within vacuoles	Clinical or subclinical myelopathy
Microglial nodules	Neuraxis	Small nodules of microglial cells, without MNGCs	Some may be due to HIV; CMV and *Toxoplasma* infections are also common aetiologies.[838]

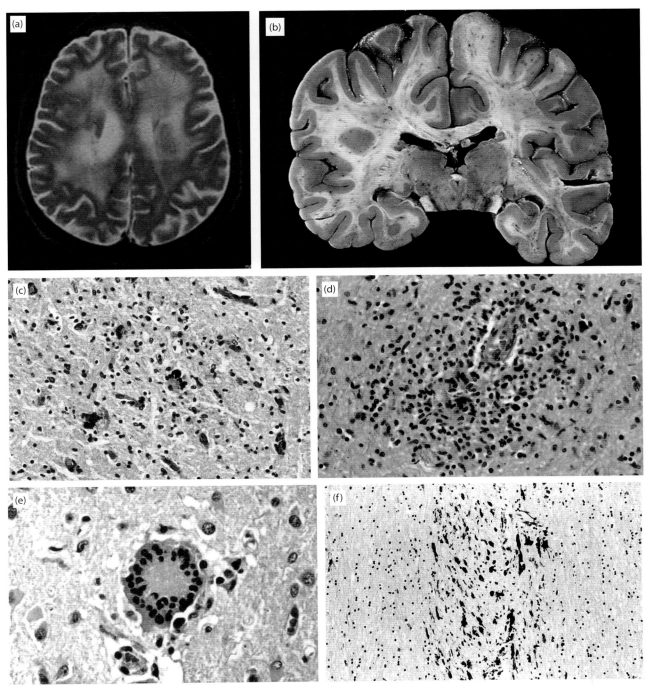

19.42 HIV encephalitis (a) MRI brain scan of a patient with HIV-associated dementia. There is diffuse white matter signal intensity. **(b)** Coronal slice of cerebrum from a patient with acquired immunodeficiency syndrome (AIDS) with dementia. There is ill-defined grey discolouration of the deep white matter. **(c)** Severe HIV encephalitis: diffuse infiltration by macrophages, some of which have fused to form multinucleated giant cells. **(d)** The basal ganglia show mononuclear inflammatory cells around blood vessels and within the brain parenchyma. Most of these cells are of monocyte/macrophage lineage, and some have fused to form multinucleated giant cells. **(e)** Solitary multinucleated giant cell of 'foreign body' type. **(f)** The white matter contains numerous HIV-infected macrophages, immunostained for the envelope protein gp41. This severe degree of infection is unusual.

Continued

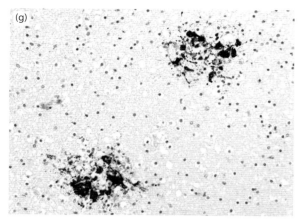 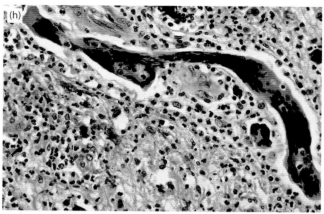

19.42 (*Continued*) (g) Paediatric HIV encephalitis: large deposits of HIV virus in microglial nodules in the parietal lobe white matter. HIV-p24 immunohistochemistry. **(h)** HIV-2 bizarre HIV encephalitis. An enormous microglial giant cell among acute inflammation, from a 2 cm nodule in the cerebellum. *In situ* hybridization showed HIV-2 within the cell.

described differently. Some of them are indicated here; some of the patients recovered on cART:

- *Acute fulminating fatal leukoencephalopathy.* Pathologically: cerebral myelin pallor, focal haemorrhages, preserved axons, no multinucleate giant cells or lymphocytic infiltration;[549]
- *Acute relapsing brain oedema with diffuse blood–brain barrier alteration.* Pathologically: cerebral swelling, white matter oedema, axonal damage, no HIV encephalitis;[405]
- *Fulminant multiple sclerosis-like leukoencephalopathy.* Pathologically: demyelination and perivenous lymphocytosis;[400]
- *Tumefactive demyelination with focal cerebral damage.* Pathologically: clearly defined demyelination, axonal preservation, perivenous lymphocyte (CD8+) infiltration.[1160] Also termed acute transient inflammatory leukoencephalopathy,[1120] and perhaps representing an intermediate entity between classic multiple sclerosis and acute demyelinating encephalomyelitis (ADEM);
- *Occipital posterior reversible leukoencephalopathy syndrome (PRES)*[1114] (no pathology, only imaging);
- *Focal pontine leukoencephalopathy, with typical pons histopathology;*[1183]
- *Rapidly progressive degeneration of auditory, visual and corticospinal tract.* Pathologically: vacuolar degeneration of the pyramidal tracts in the medulla, myelin destruction, astrogliosis, no lymphocytic infiltration.[598]

Perhaps some of these are variants of the originally depicted HIV leukoencephalopathy,[142,399,401] except that the definition excluded inflammatory infiltration, and included multinucleate giant cells and demonstrable HIV on immunohistochemistry. As with the severe atypical seroconversion syndromes, individual host response genes may be critical.

Brain Disease in Those Treated with Anti-HIV Therapy

Antiretroviral therapy, by reversing in part the immunosuppressive consequences of HIV infection, has significantly reduced the frequency of brain opportunistic infections and severe neurocognitive disorders.[1122] Conversely, it has

introduced a new set of aberrant immunopathological disorders, which are still being described.

HIV Encephalitis and Leukoencephalopathy Progressing Despite cART

Antiretroviral therapy is not always effective. A series of patients on cART was described, with HIV-associated dementia, whose autopsy brain pathology showed a continuation of HIV encephalitis with MNGC and demonstrable HIV antigens, plus myelin loss and axonal injury (HIV leukoencephalopathy).[647] Notably, nearly all the patients had high blood and CSF HIV viral loads and low blood CD4 counts. Although there was discussion of possible direct toxicity in the brain from the cART drugs, it seems more likely that ineffective anti-HIV treatment was more important.

CNS-IRIS

The other syndrome is the immune reconstitution inflammatory syndrome (IRIS) phenomenon, whereby there is clinical deterioration despite successful virological and immunological recovery in HIV-infected patients following treatment with antiretroviral therapy. Usually, IRIS develops within 2–3 months of commencing cART, some cases occur as late as 2 years after. Up to a quarter of patients may be affected, depending on geographical location.[544]

CNS-IRIS is defined as unexpected worsening of the neurological condition, consistent with inflammation, and opportunistic infection and drug toxicity are excluded; the blood HIV viral load has decreased from baseline and the blood CD4 count has increased.[744] It is mediated by activated CD8+ T-cells trafficking into the CNS[544] and represents a hyperinflammatory and oedematous flare due to improved host immune responses to the infection antigens.

The infections that prompt IRIS include the usual HIV-associated infections (JC virus, tuberculosis, cryptococcosis, etc.). IRIS is further subdivided into 'paradoxical' IRIS, where the underlying infection was known and being treated prior to commencing cART; and 'unmasking IRIS' where the causative infection was not known before. Importantly, HIV itself in the brain can precipitate IRIS, and this is the subject of this subsection.

The case reports of CNS-IRIS, due to HIV, are clinically and pathologically heterogeneous.[234,408,482,676,744,769,849,922,945,985,1176] They include autopsy and biopsy pathology. Broadly, the patients, within weeks or months of commencing cART, develop headache, focal neurological signs or dementia (slow presentation), or an acute presentation with seizures. Neuroimaging usually shows diffuse white matter damage, sometimes multiple ring enhancement, with or without cerebral swelling. A few cases have more focal cerebral lesions.

Pathologically, the consistent feature is severe perivascular and parenchymal infiltration by CD8+ T-cells (Figure 19.43). The acutely presenting cases also show demyelination with axonal preservation, and sometimes necrosis[676,744,922] resembling HIV leukoencephalopathy. Only a few patients also have residual HIV encephalitis histology with MNGC and scanty detectable HIV antigen.

Thus, in CNS-IRIS due to HIV *per se*, there is an augmented immune response, to HIV or perhaps myelin, with a variable breakdown of the blood–brain barrier, affecting all parts of the brain, with massive influx of CD8+ T-cells. Drug toxicity seems most unlikely, given the heterogeneity of the treatment regimes the patients are taking. Some of the biopsied patients were treated with steroids and recovered.

When brain biopsies of such patients are examined, clinical correlation and exclusion of other pathogeneses is critical. In one case, where in addition to the T-cells there was also influx of B-cells, a provisional diagnosis of B-cell lymphoma was made (Figure 19.43).[482]

Finally, there is a recently recognized syndrome of acute and fatal cerebral swelling developing in adults on successful long-term cART, i.e. more than 4 years–which is beyond the usual case definition of IRIS–with undetectable blood viral loads and good CD4 counts. All patients so far described are African. Clinically, the patients deteriorate neurologically over days to 2 weeks; pre-mortem brain scans show diffuse swelling without focal lesions. At autopsy, there is a florid white matter diffuse and perivascular infiltrate of CD8+ T-cells, no demyelination or neuron damage, no MNGCs and no demonstrable HIV infection or any community-acquired encephalitis virus infection (Figure 19.44).[688] The aetiopathogenesis is obscure, but it may be a very slow form of IRIS and/or a sudden leakage

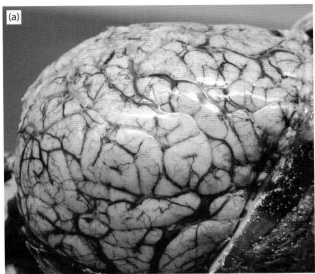

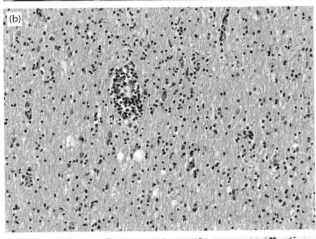

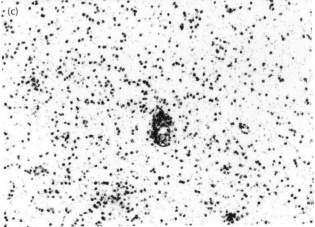

19.44 Fatal late onset acute CD8+ T-cell encephalitis in a patient treated successfully with cART. (a) Autopsy brain showing cerebral swelling. The pre-mortem neuroimaging indicated diffuse oedema without focal lesions. **(b)** White matter encephalitis without demyelination. **(c)** Nearly all the inflammatory cells are CD8+ T-cells. Immunohistochemistry for CD8.

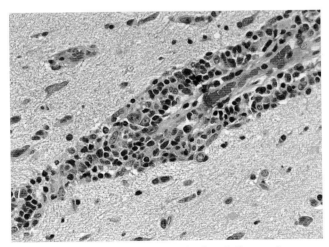

19.43 HIV-IRIS (immune reconstitution inflammatory syndrome) causing transient neurological deficits following anti-retroviral treatment. Brain biopsy showing vascular and perivascular infiltration by cells shown on immunohistochemistry to comprise a mixture of CD20+ B-cells and CD8+ T-cells. This was initially misinterpreted as lymphoma.

of the blood–brain barrier. The uniform African ethnicity suggests that host genetic factors also play a role. Some cases have been clinically diagnosed in time to be treated with massive steroid doses and have recovered, although with subsequent functional brain damage (personal observation). The syndromes discussed in this CNS-IRIS section are referred to as 'CD8 encephalitis'.

Vacuolar Myelopathy

At autopsy, up to 30 per cent of autopsied patients with advanced HIV disease have vacuolar myelopathy (VM), but usually the process is subclinical. Clinically, there is leg weakness, spastic paraparesis, sensory ataxia and incontinence. VM does not occur early in HIV disease.

The histopathology of VM is vacuolation of of the spinal cord white matter in the posterior and lateral columns (Figure 19.45).[1113] It is very like subacute combined degeneration of the cord associated with vitamin B12 deficiency (see Chapter 9).[895] However, in HIV disease, vitamin deficiency is not the cause. The vacuolation is associated with scattered lipid-containing macrophages (well visualized with CD68 immunostaining), but little gliosis and no lymphocytic infiltration. As the disease progresses, the vacuolation leads to breakdown of myelin and degeneration of axons.[974] Macrophage activation is probably the key pathogenetic event.[1153]

There is no productive HIV infection in VM, and there are no multinucleate giant cells and usually no HIVp24 immunopositivity. If microglial nodules with some detectable HIV are seen, this is better termed 'HIV myelitis' not VM; and the severity of VM does not correlate with local HIV antigen.[1113] Occasionally, the cerebral white matter shows a similar pathology, but note that brain removal and fixation artefact can produce a pseudo-VM picture.

Peripheral Neuropathies and Myopathies

Peripheral Neuropathy Several types of peripheral neuropathy and myopathy have been observed in HIV disease, and can affect up to 40 per cent of patients.[951] The most common

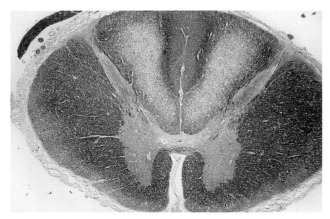

19.45 Vacuolar myelopathy due to human immunodeficiency virus (HIV). The posterior columns show extensive symmetrical vacuolation, whereas the involvement of the lateral columns is minimal. Luxol fast blue and periodic acid–Schiff.

neuropathy is a chronic progressive symmetrical distal polyneuropathy with bilateral tingling, numbness or neuropathic pain. Nerve conduction studies indicate mixed axonal degeneration and demyelination.[879] However, there are probably several processes going on, including HIV itself and its cART treatment.

Early in the disease, some patients experience an inflammatory demyelinating polyneuropathy with acute motor weakness and areflexia. Cerebrospinal fluid pleocytosis distinguishes this syndrome from Guillain–Barré syndrome.

The distal polyneuropathy can be caused by HIV *per se*, and also by its treatment, particularly the neurotoxic d-NRTIs such as ddI and d4T (see www.i-Base.info). Overall, up to one third of HIV patients suffer from it, and ageing is a risk factor.[323] The pathogenesis, like that of HAND and vacuolar myelopathy, may involve macrophage activation.[1153]

Patients with more advanced disease may also develop progressive polyradiculopathy, transient myeloradiculopathy and cranial neuropathies due to infection by CMV, HSV and VZV. Among the differential diagnosis is vasculitis of the nerves or roots, which can be caused by HIV.[367]

Myopathy Several types of myopathies are reported in advanced HIV disease, classified into four groups:[52,951]

1. HIV-associated myopathy including polymyositis, inclusion body myopathy, nemaline myopathy, HIV-wasting syndrome.
2. Muscle complications of cART (NRTI drugs), HIV-associated lipodystrophy syndrome.
3. Opportunistic infections and tumour infiltrations.
4. Rhabdomyolysis.

Antiretroviral therapy has modified some of these, but the NRTI drugs are mitochondrial toxic; they produce a histologically similar degenerative myopathy to that seen in HIV disease alone.[1047] The clinical and pathological features of these disorders are considered further in Chapters 7 and 25.

Paediatric HIV CNS Disease

Children infected with HIV have nearly all acquired the infection from their mothers perinatally: *in utero* transmission, during birth and from breast milk. Without cART, more than half such infected children are dead by the age of 2 years. Prevention of mother-to-child transmission, through antenatal HIV testing and targeted antiretroviral therapy, has been very successful and could almost eliminate paediatric HIV disease. Without antiretroviral prophylaxis, the maternal-child transmission rate is about 25 per cent. In the United Kingdom, the majority of such infected children were born in Africa (data from the Health Protection Agency, www.hpa.org.uk).

HIV-infected children not on cART can develop all the standard opportunistic infections and lymphoma as do adults.[360,623] The incidence of specific lesions, such as HIV encephalitis, is variable: up to 44 per cent in US series,[624] but only 6 per cent in West African children.[87] Case selection is crucial, and presence of severe encephalopathy has declined since the introduction of antiretroviral treatment.[777] Like adults, children can present with an acute demyelinating encephalomyelitis as the first indication of HIV disease.[1147]

However, children differ significantly from adults because of their neurodevelopment. The classic triad of paediatric HIV encephalopathy is: developmental delay, secondary microcephaly and pyramidal tract neuromotor deficits.[777] The pathology has been reviewed in the pre-cART era.[1096] Opportunities to study the brains of such children are unfortunately scarce, and we know little of the chronic, lifetime pathology of HIV in adolescents infected perinatally.

Other HIV-Associated Disease of the CNS

This section has focussed on pathology directly attributable to the HIV virus and its complex interactions with the immune system in the brain and spinal cord. The numerous HIV-associated opportunistic infections and tumours (lymphomas) are discussed elsewhere in this chapter and in Chapter 40. There are other major co-morbidities that also contribute to CNS disease in HIV-infected people, which need to be borne in mind when assessing individual cases: ageing, stroke and vasculopathy, and hepatitis C virus (HCV) co-infection.

With cART, HIV-infected cohorts are ageing and the ageing processes in the brain undoubtedly interact with those of chronic HIV infection, and complicate the assessment of HAND syndromes. In addition, HCV has an ill-understood impact on brain function in all people, and there is a growing HCV epidemic among the HIV-infected.

Stroke

Assessment of the relationship between stroke and HIV disease is complicated by coexistence of other risk factors, particularly intravenous drug use, but epidemiological data indicate that in HIV-infected people, stroke is more common than in HIV-negative controls.[327] Ischaemic stroke is more common than haemorrhagic. A major contributory factor is thought to be endothelial cell dysfunction, caused directly by HIV and perhaps also by cART drugs. In addition, some of the cART regimes induce a metabolic hyperlipidaemia, and there are prothrombotic coagulopathies associated with HIV. Cerebral HIV-vasculopathy is an evolving concept (Table 19.7), also including cerebral HIV vasculitis,[189] which overlaps with the better-known VZV vasculitis syndrome.[900]

For a comprehensive review of HIV-related cerebrovascular disease, the reader is referred to Benjamin et al.[89]

Conclusion

Inflammatory HIV brain disease is confusing and heterogeneous–clinically, radiologically and neuropathologically–and much influenced by antiretroviral treatment.[87,1119] There are some agreed specific pathologies, such as HIV encephalitis and vacuolar myelopathy. However, there is a need for more consensus on the other pathologies–acute and chronic (e.g. neurocognitive disorder), spontaneous and cART-related (e.g. CD8 encephalitis)–and thus to integrate

TABLE 19.7 Cerebrovascular causes of stroke in HIV infection

Ischaemic stroke	Large artery atherosclerosis
	Cardio-embolism
	Bacterial endocarditis
	Marantic endocarditis
	Ischaemic heart disease
	HIV-vasculopathy
	Small vessel occlusive disease
	HIV-inflammatory vasculitis
	Infective vasculitis
	Tuberculosis, VZV vasculitis
	Coagulopathy
	Protein S deficiency
	Thrombotic thrombocytopenic purpura
Haemorrhagic stroke	HIV-associated thrombocytopenia
	HIV-vasculitis
	With aneurysm rupture
	Disseminated aspergillosis

Modified from Benjamin et al.[89]

pathogenesis with improving management of HIV-infected patients.

HTLV-1-Associated Myelopathy/Tropical Spastic Paraparesis

Human T-cell leukaemia/lymphoma virus type 1 was the first retrovirus to be identified as a cause of human disease, adult T-cell leukaemia and lymphoma. The virus was later shown to cause tropical spastic paraparesis (TSP), a chronic myelopathy that was subsequently termed HTLV-1-associated myelopathy (HAM). In some patients, HTLV-1 infection is associated with a range of other, mostly inflammatory diseases, such as sialadenitis with keratoconjunctivitis sicca (Sjögren's syndrome), uveitis, vitritis, chronic arthropathy, bronchiolitis and pneumonitis, polymyositis, dermatomyositis and peripheral neuropathy.[385,655,817,1053,1178] It is also associated with an increased frequency and severity of several other infections, including strongyloidiasis, tuberculosis, crusted scabies and chronic infective dermatitis (a complication particularly prevalent in Jamaican children).[641] HTLV-1 co-infection also increases the rate of progression of HIV-1 disease.[424] What determines the manifestations and complications of HTLV-1 infection in individual patients is poorly understood. A closely related human retrovirus, HTLV-2, was first isolated from a patient with hairy cell leukaemia, although the virus is probably not a cause of that disease. HTLV-2 has, rarely, been associated with a chronic myelopathy clinically similar to that caused by HTLV-1.[528,809] Two further human T-cell lymphotropic viruses, HTLV-3 and -4 were recently identified;[714] their possible pathogenicity has yet to be determined.

Aetiology

Human T-cell leukaemia/lymphoma viruses were previously classified as retroviruses in the genus bovine leukaemia virus–human T-cell leukaemia/lymphoma virus (BLV-HTLV), but in 1998 the name of the genus was changed to Deltaretrovirus.[139]

Like HIV, HTLV-1 and HTLV-2 are enveloped viruses measuring 80–100 nm in diameter, each containing two identical copies of single-stranded positive-sense RNA. The ubiquitous vertebrate glucose transporter 1 (GLUT-1) is a receptor for both HTLV-1 and HTLV-2.[724] Receptor binding probably involves other molecules as well, including heparan sulfate proteoglycans[548] and neuropilin-1.[368] The precise mechanism of entry of virus into the cytoplasm is still unclear. Once in the cytoplasm, as in other retrovirus infections, copies of double-stranded DNA provirus are synthesized, transported to the nucleus and integrated into the host DNA. The integration is probably largely random, but there is some evidence of biases in the base composition of the adjacent region of the host genome,[193,1274] and integration seems to occur preferentially within transcriptional units.[872] As noted earlier, transcription of retroviruses is mediated by the machinery of the host cell. The viral particles are assembled in the cytoplasm and acquire their envelope as they bud to the exterior through a modified region of the cell membrane.

Despite the ubiquitous expression of the viral receptor protein GLUT-1, CD4 T-cells constitute the main reservoir of HTLV-1 infection during the lifespan of an infected individual, possibly as a result of the elimination or nonproductive infection of other types of cell into which the virus gains entry.[725] Initial spread of virus within the body is probably mediated largely by direct transfer between immune cells: HTLV-1 usurps the function of the interferon-inducible viral restriction factor tetherin (which normally prevents viral shedding from the cell surface) to form tetherin-containing viral assemblies on the cell surface that are transmitted by cell contact.[860] Later spread is thought to result from clonal expansion of infected cells.

Epidemiology

HTLV-1 infection is endemic in south-western Japan,[571,864] the Caribbean basin,[625,720] Colombia,[959] Brazil,[30,291] Chile,[151] possibly Argentina,[387] Melanesia,[1259] the Seychelles,[715] parts of Africa (including clusters in Zaire and among Zulus in South Africa)[393,1138,1230] and probably parts of India.[787] In some of these regions, the prevalence exceeds 10 per cent. The prevalence is high among Jews originating from Masshad in Iran[767] and may be increased in some Canadian aboriginal groups.[853] In the United States and Europe, the prevalence is highest among immigrants from parts of the world where infection is endemic, but there has been spread of infection to indigenous inhabitants through sexual contact, blood transfusion and drug abuse.[366,530,651,752,797,1034]

HTLV-2 is endemic in many indigenous tribes in North and South America.[105,464] The virus may have entered the New World from Asia with the earliest migration of ancestral Amerindians over 15 000 years ago.[105] Human T-cell lymphotropic virus type II is also prevalent at high levels among intravenous drug abusers in parts of the United States and Europe.[579,651,808] A large serological survey of blood from volunteer donors in the United States followed by interviews with seropositive donors revealed that the major risk factor for HTLV-1 seropositivity was migration from HTLV-1-endemic regions; for HTLV-2 the major risk factor was intravenous drug abuse.[651]

Pathogenesis

The principal modes of transmission of HTLV-1 and HTLV-2 are through breast milk, sexual intercourse, blood transfusion and the sharing of contaminated needles by drug abusers.[291,565,566,579,625,645,1186] Although HTLV can be detected in the cord blood of neonates with infected mothers,[567,999] this rarely leads to established infection; mother-to-child transmission usually results from breastfeeding over several months.[566,1231] Transmission during breastfeeding is probably mediated by infected lymphocytes within the breast milk, although there is evidence that glandular epithelial cells are also susceptible to HTLV infection.[1066] Maternal antibodies to the viral tax protein (see later) are a marker of increased risk of mother-to-child transmission.[1157] Similarly, the presence of anti-tax antibodies in men is associated with a higher risk of venereal transmission of infection to women.[187] HTLV-1 is transmitted venereally more efficiently from males to females than vice versa,[557,1025] leading to higher rates of infection among women than men. HTLV is transmitted particularly efficiently by blood transfusion, the infectivity being associated with the cellular components of the blood. HTLV-2 has also probably been transmitted through a human bite.[120]

A key protein in the pathogenesis of diseases due to HTLV-1 is tax, a transactivating regulatory protein encoded by a gene in the X-region (close to the 3\pm;-end of the viral genome). This protein is a transcriptional transactivator of a 21-base-pair enhancer in the long terminal repeat region of the virus[1099] and also of multiple cellular genes, including tumour necrosis factor, interleukins 1, 2, 6, 8, 10 and 15, and vascular cell adhesion molecule (VCAM).[53,281,472,747,789–791,973,1144] Tax also interacts with, and modifies the activity of, several cell-cycle regulatory genes, causing suppression of p53 and p16INK4A activities[806,1100] and thereby probably promoting the immortalization and malignant transformation of infected T-cells. The actions of tax are mediated by interactions with host proteins in the cyclic adenosine monophosphate (cAMP) response element-binding protein/activating transcription factor (CREB/ATF) and nuclear factor B (NF-B)/c-Rel families, serum response factor and other cellular transcription factors.[534,538] The transactivating actions of tax have been studied most extensively in T-cells but may also involve microglia and possibly other cells in the CNS.

The pathogenesis of the spinal lesions in HAM/TSP has not been resolved, although several observations are probably of relevance. Most, if not all, patients with HAM/TSP show clonal expansion of infected CD4 cells in the peripheral blood.[161,349a] HTLV-1 tax protein induces expression of VCAM-1 by infected T-cells[1165] and may, by activation of this and other genes involved in vascular adhesion and migration, promote entry of the infected CD4 cells into the CNS. The virus is sparse but present within the spinal cord of patients with HAM/TSP.[104,450,735] Double-labelling techniques combining *in situ* hybridization and immunohistochemistry have been used to determine the types of cell that are infected within the spinal cord. In most studies, proviral DNA or viral tax RNA has been localized to perivascular lymphocytes,[450,524] most if not all of which are CD4 cells.[735,794] However, conflicting data were obtained in a study of cases in which tax RNA was found within astrocytes, in spinal parenchyma away from blood vessels.[653]

Although the amount of virus within the cord is small, it seems to be most abundant in the thoracic region, the part of the cord most affected in HAM/TSP. The reasons for this topographical selectivity are not known. Sluggish blood flow in this arterial watershed region of the cord, local production of cytokines, and the expression of cell adhesion molecules may all contribute to the distribution of lesions.[504,865] Increased expression of vascular adhesion molecules and monocyte chemoattractant protein 1 (MCP-1) was demonstrated within the lesions of HAM/TSP.[1156]

A consistent finding in HAM/TSP is the presence of CD8 cytotoxic T-lymphocytes that react specifically with epitopes of HTLV-1, including tax.[74,365a] Tax-specific T-lymphocytes constitute a large proportion of CD8 cells within the CSF and, at least in some cases, greatly outnumber tax-specific T-cells in the blood.[417] Most patients also have markedly elevated, in some cases oligoclonal, anti-HTLV-1 IgG within the serum and CSF.[365a,666,733] There is therefore a vigorous cellular and humoral response directed at HTLV-I-infected CD4 lymphocytes (and possibly astrocytes) in the CNS. Further evidence that infected CD4 lymphocytes are probably targets of the immune response comes from the identification of apoptotic CD4 lymphocytes within the inflamed spinal parenchyma[523,525,1155] and the observation of an increase in the ratio of CD8 to CD4 cells in the spinal cord during progression of the disease.[523,525,1154] The damage to axons and myelin may be due to the release of cytokines and other inflammatory mediators from infected and reactive lymphocytes, macrophages and, possibly, astrocytes. Alternatively, the cytotoxic and humoral response to the infected lymphocytes may cause local autoimmune damage to the spinal parenchyma; support for this hypothesis comes from the finding that serum IgG antibody to HTLV-1 tax in HAM/TSP patients also reacted with heterogeneous ribonuclear protein-A1 (hnRNPA1) in uninfected neurons in CNS tissue.[666]

Clinical Features

The age of onset of HAM/TSP ranges from under 5 to over 75 years, the mean ranging from about 35 to 50 years in different endemic populations.[32,392,571,817] The incubation period is similarly variable, from a few years to several decades. The incubation period depends to some extent on the route of infection: blood transfusion is a much more efficient means of transmitting infection than breastfeeding or sexual

intercourse and tends to be associated with a shorter incubation time before the development of disease—under 1 year in some cases.[186,864,1268] The risk of developing HAM/TSP after infection is relatively small: about one-tenth of that of developing T-cell leukaemia, although both have a similar incubation period. The estimated annual incidence of HAM among HTLV-1-infected people is 3.1 in 100 000; over a lifetime of 75 years, the cumulative incidence is approximately 0.25 per cent.[564] The female:male ratio is approximately 1:4.

The disease manifests as a progressive spastic paraparesis, associated in most cases with sphincter disturbances. In many endemic regions, a high proportion of patients have a history or serological evidence of other sexually transmitted diseases. The onset of paraparesis is usually between 25 and 60 years but can occur in childhood. In a series of 213 Japanese patients, the 21 patients with onset of paraparesis before age 15 years and without a history of blood transfusion tended to be of short stature and to have a relatively slow progression of the disease.[817] Some patients experience backache and mild sensory dysfunction involving the lower limbs, such as paraesthesiae, symmetrical loss of vibration sense in the feet and absent ankle jerks. The CSF may show mild lymphocytic pleocytosis, and the protein level is usually elevated, with an increase in IgG. Depending on the stage of disease, MRI may reveal cord swelling and contrast enhancement or simply atrophy. Small high-signal lesions in T2-weighted images have been noted in the subcortical or deep cerebral white matter in some patients.[381,594] The progression of disability is most rapid during the first year of disease.[33] Progression tends to be faster in premenopausal women, and patients with a high proviral load.[31] The disability may subsequently stabilize for a period, and occasionally function improves slightly.[637] Short-term clinical improvement has been reported after a range of immunomodulatory and other treatments, including the administration of corticosteroids and interferon.[522,829] However, most patients are wheelchair-bound within 10 years.

As noted earlier, the full spectrum of HTLV-1-associated neurological diseases includes not only HAM/TSP but also polymyositis, dermatomyositis and possibly inclusion body myositis (see Chapter 25) peripheral neuropathy (see Chapter 24) and ocular disease, any of which may be present in various combinations in infected patients.

Pathological Findings

The spinal meninges may appear thickened and the cord atrophic, particularly in the lower thoracic region. Lateral funicular degeneration may be grossly discernible. An infiltrate of lymphocytes and macrophages is present in the spinal grey and white matter, most marked in the lower thoracic region (Figure 19.46). The lateral and anterior columns tend to be affected more severely than the posterior columns (Figure 19.46a,b). Small blood vessels usually have thickened hyaline walls, but there may be evidence of capillary proliferation. Intramyelinic vacuolation and demyelination may be evident early in the course of disease,[1262] but these progress to symmetrical degeneration and gliosis involving the long tracts in the spinal cord,

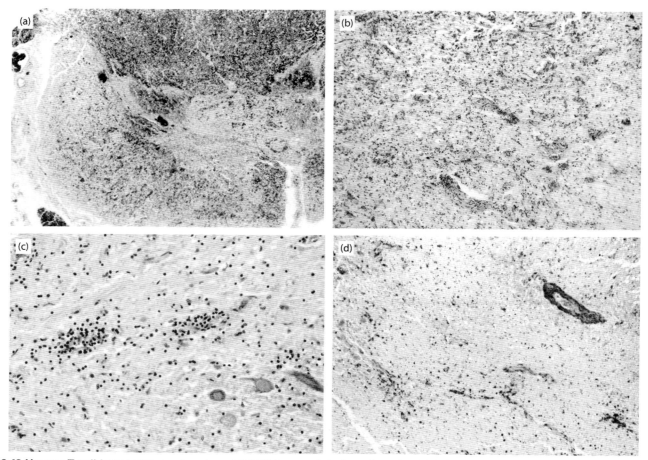

19.46 Human T-cell lymphotropic virus type I (HTLV-I)-associated myelopathy. (a) Solochrome cyanin-stained section through the upper thoracic cord, showing marked loss of myelinated fibres from the lateral and anterior columns, with relative preservation of the posterior column. **(b)** The lateral column showing a patchy infiltrate of lymphocytes as well as the loss of myelinated fibres. Luxol fast blue/cresyl violet. **(c)** Infiltrates of lymphocytes in the grey matter. Note the relative preservation of neurons. **(d)** Low-magnification photomicrograph of a section immunostained for CD45RO, showing large numbers of T-lymphocytes within the cord parenchyma.

especially the lateral columns, although the anterior and posterior columns may also be involved. Dystrophic axonal swellings may be present in the affected spinal white matter.[1247] Proliferation of satellite cells in the spinal root ganglia has been noted in patients with posterior column degeneration.[152] Although the inflammation involves the spinal grey matter as well as the white matter, neurons usually remain relatively well preserved (Figure 19.46c).

Immunohistochemistry shows most of the lymphocytes to be T-cells (Figure 19.46d).[1156,1262] The relative numbers of CD4 and CD8 cells in the spinal cord depend on the duration of illness, both usually being present in approximately equal numbers during the early stages of disease but CD8 cells predominating at later stages.[524,525,1156] There may be scant spinal inflammation in longstanding disease.[998]

Sparse viral nucleic acids may be detectable within the spinal cord by *in situ* hybridization or by PCR. As noted earlier, in most studies proviral DNA or viral tax RNA has been localized to perivascular lymphocytes,[450] most if not all of which are probably CD4 cells.[735,794]

Although the brain is not usually affected in HAM/TSP, in some cases adventitial fibrosis, perivascular gliosis and, rarely, perivascular inflammation and demyelination have been observed in the cerebral white matter, cerebellum and brain stem.[152,850,998]

Borna Virus

Borna virus is the only virus in the family Bornaviridae. It is an enveloped RNA virus with a single-stranded, non-segmented, antisense genome. The first descriptions of Borna as a fatal neurological disease of horses (*Kopfkrankheit de Pferde*) appeared in veterinary handbooks of the late eighteenth century.[388,1087] The name 'Borna' derives from that of a small town in Saxony, Germany, where the equine disease is endemic. Natural Borna occurs in a wide range of other species, including sheep, cattle, cats, ostriches, rabbits, deer, llamas and alpacas. The possible role of Borna virus in human disease is still unclear. Most animal infections are thought to be subclinical, with a relatively high seroprevalence in horses, sheep and cats.[91,563,691]

Pathogenesis

The mechanisms of transmission *in vivo* are unknown. Persistently infected rodents shed virus in the urine, and it has been suggested that susceptible hosts may acquire infection by inhalation. Vertical spread has been documented in mice[858] and horses,[433] and virus can be detected in the colostrum of infected animals. The natural reservoir is not known.

Much of the information on pathogenesis has been derived from experimental studies. The virus has been transmitted experimentally to several species of animal,[626,691,692,857] but most transmission studies have been performed on rats, in which resistance to Borna virus is a dominant trait.[273]

Human Disease

Whether Borna virus infects humans and, if so, causes clinical disease is controversial.[116,671,677,941] Borna virus-specific serum and CSF antibodies of low avidity were found in 1–5 per cent of psychiatric inpatients, a prevalence four times that found in healthy controls.[183,1000,1016] Borna disease virus (BDV) antigen or RNA was detected in human peripheral blood cells in some studies,[521,903,904] but not others.[586,940] The detection of Borna virus antigen and RNA was reported in brain tissue from four of five patients who had presented with memory loss and depression and were to have hippocampal sclerosis.[266] In a subsequent study, Borna virus RNA was demonstrable by nested reverse transcriptase PCR in 2 of 30 normal autopsy brains.[431] Borna virus antigens were detected in the CSF of 3 of 32 patients with recurrent major depression and 2 of 19 patients with multiple sclerosis, but not in a further 179 patients with other psychiatric and neurological diseases.[278] The sequences of Borna virus RNA detected in human blood and brain have been almost identical to those of laboratory strains of Borna virus, raising the possibility that at least some of the isolates may have been contaminants.[1017]

REFERENCES

1. Abdelbaky AM, Channappa DB, Islam S. Unilateral epididymo-orchitis: a rare complication of MMR vaccine. *Ann R Coll Surg Engl* 2008;4:336–7.
1a. Abed Y, Boivin G. Human parechovirus types 1, 2 and 3 infections in Canada. *Emerg Infect Dis* 2006;12(6):969–75.
2. Abendroth A, Arvin A. Varicella-zoster virus immune evasion. *Immunol Rev* 1999;168:143–56.
2a. Abendroth A, Morrow G, Cunningham AL, Slobedman B. Varicella-zoster virus infection of human dendritic cells and transmission to T cells: implications for virus dissemination in the host. *J Virol* 2001;75:6183–92.
3. Aboudy Y, Fogel A, Barnea B, et al. Subclinical rubella reinfection during pregnancy followed by transmission of virus to the fetus. *J Infect* 1997;34:273–6.
4. Abzug MJ, Keyserling HL, Lee ML, et al. Neonatal enterovirus infection: virology, serology, and effects of intravenous immune globulin. *Clin Infect Dis* 1995;20:1201–6.
5. Adams O, Krempe C, Kogler G, et al. Congenital infections with human herpesvirus 6. *J Infect Dis* 1998;178:544–6.
6. Adour KK. Otological complications of herpes zoster. *Ann Neurol* 1994;35:S62–4.
7. Agamanolis DP, Tan JS, Parker DL. Immunosuppressive measles encephalitis in a patient with a renal transplant. *Arch Neurol* 1979;36:686–90.
8. Ahlfors K, Forsgren M, Ivarsson SA, et al. Congenital cytomegalovirus infection: on the relation between type and time of maternal infection and infant's symptoms. *Scand J Infect Dis* 1983;15:129–38.
9. Ahlqvist J, Fotheringham J, Akhyani N, et al. Differential tropism of human herpesvirus 6 (HHV-6) variants and induction of latency by HHV-6A in oligodendrocytes. *J Neurovirol* 2005;4:384–94.
10. Ahtiluoto S, Mannonen L, Paetau A, et al. In situ hybridization detection of human herpesvirus 6 in brain tissue from fatal encephalitis. *Pediatrics* 2000;105:431–3.
11. Akins PT, Belko J, Uyeki TM, et al. H1N1 encephalitis with malignant edema and review of neurologic complications from influenza. *Neurocrit Care* 2010;3:396–406.
12. Alcardi J, Goutieres F, Arsenio-Nunes ML, Lebon P. Acute measles encephalitis in children with immunosuppression. *Pediatrics* 1977;59:232–9.
13. Al Deeb SM, Yaqub BA, Bruyn GW, Biary NM. Acute transverse myelitis. A localized form of postinfectious encephalomyelitis. *Brain* 1997;120:1115–22.
14. Alexander JP Jr, Baden L, Pallansch MA, Anderson LJ. Enterovirus 71 infections and neurologic disease: United States, 1977–1991. *J Infect Dis* 1994;169:905–8.
15. Alexander LN, Seward JF, Santibanez TA, et al. Vaccine policy changes and epidemiology of poliomyelitis in the United States. *J Am Med Assoc* 2004;292:1696–701.
16. Alkalay AL, Pomerance JJ, Rimoin DL. Fetal varicella syndrome. *J Pediatr* 1987;111:320–23.
17. Allen IV, McQuaid S, McMahon J, et al. The significance of measles virus antigen and genome distribution in the CNS in SSPE for mechanisms of viral spread and demyelination. *J Neuropathol Exp Neurol* 1996;55:471–80.
18. Alrajhi AA, Al-Semari A, Al-Watban J. Rift Valley fever encephalitis. *Emerg Infect Dis* 2004;10:554–5.
19. Alvarez L, Fajardo R, Lopez E, et al. Partial recovery from rabies in a nine-year-old boy. *Pediatr Infect Dis J* 1994;13:1154–5.
20. Ambler M, Stoll J, Tzamaloukas A, Albala MM. Focal encephalomyelitis in infectious mononucleosis: a report with pathological description. *Ann Intern Med* 1971;75:579–83.
21. Ambroziak JA, Blackbourn DJ, Herndier BG, et al. Herpes-like sequences in HIV-infected and uninfected Kaposi's sarcoma patients. *Science* 1995;268:582–3.
22. An SF, Giometto B, Groves M, et al. Axonal damage revealed by accumulation of beta-APP in HIV-positive individuals without AIDS. *J Neuropathol Exp Neurol* 1997;56:1262–8.
23. Anders KH, Park CS, Cornford ME, Vinters HV. Adenovirus encephalitis and widespread ependymitis in a child with AIDS. *Pediatr Neurosurg* 1990;16:316–20.
24. Anderson JR, Schneider JR, Grimstad PR, Severson DW. Quantitative genetics of vector competence for La Crosse virus and body size in *Ochlerotatus hendersoni* and *Ochlerotatus triseriatus* interspecific hybrids. *Genetics* 2005;169:1529–39.
25. Anderson KC, Gorgone BC, Marlink RG, et al. Transfusion-acquired human immunodeficiency virus infection among immunocompromised persons. *Ann Intern Med* 1986;105:519–27.
26. Angelini L, Pietrogrande MC, Delle Piane MR, et al. Progressive multifocal leukoencephalopathy in a child with hyperimmunoglobulin E recurrent infection syndrome and review of the literature. *Neuropediatrics* 2001;32:250–55.
27. Antinori A, Ammassari A, De Luca A, et al. Diagnosis of AIDS-related focal brain lesions: a decision-making analysis based on clinical and neuroradiologic characteristics combined with polymerase chain reaction assays in CSF. *Neurology* 1997;48:687–94.
28. Antinori A, Arendt G, Becker J, et al. Updated research nosology for HIV-associated neurocognitive disorders (HAND). *Neurology* 2007;69:1789–99.
29. Appelbaum E, Rachelson M, Dolgopol V. Varicella encephalitis. *Am J Med* 1953;15:223–30.
30. Araujo Ad Q, de Andrada-Serpa MJ. Tropical spastic paraparesis/HTLV-I-associated myelopathy in Brazil. *J Acquir Immune Defic Syndr* 1996;13:S33–7.
31. Araujo AQ, Silva MT. The HTLV-1 neurological complex. *Lancet Neurol* 2006;12:1068–76.
32. Araujo Ad Q, Alfonso CR, Schor D, et al. Clinical and demographic features of HTLV-1 associated myelopathy/tropical

spastic paraparesis (HAM/TSP) in Rio de Janeiro, Brazil. *Acta Neurol Scand* 1993;**88**:59–62.

33. Araujo AQ, Leite AC, Dultra SV, Andrada-Serpa MJ. Progression of neurological disability in HTLV-I-associated myelopathy/tropical spastic paraparesis (HAM/TSP). *J Neurol Sci* 1995;**129**: 147–51.

34. Arbusow V, Schulz P, Strupp M, et al. Distribution of herpes simplex virus type 1 in human geniculate and vestibular ganglia: implications for vestibular neuritis. *Ann Neurol* 1999;**46**:416–19.

35. Archimbaud C, Bailly JL, Chambon M, et al. Molecular evidence of persistent echovirus 13 meningoencephalitis in a patient with relapsed lymphoma after an outbreak of meningitis in 2000. *J Clin Microbiol* 2003;**41**:4605–10.

36. Arguedas A, Stutman HR, Blanding JG. Parainfluenza type 3 meningitis: report of two cases and review of the literature. *Clin Pediatr* 1990;**29**:175–8.

37. Arisoy ES, Demmler GJ, Thakar S, Doerr C. Meningitis due to parainfluenza virus type 3: report of two cases and review. *Clin Infect Dis* 1993;**17**:995–7.

38. Arita I, Nakane M. Road map for polio eradication: establishing the link with Millennium Development Goal no. 4 for child survival. *Jpn J Infect Dis* 2008;**3**:169–74.

39. Arnberg N, Edlund K, Kidd AH, Wadell G. Adenovirus type 37 uses sialic acid as a cellular receptor. *J Virol* 2000;**74**:42–8.

40. Arslan F, Tabak F, Avsar E, et al. Ganciclovir-resistant cytomegalovirus encephalitis in a hematopoietic stem cell transplant recipient. *J Neurovirol* 2010;**2**:174–8.

41. Artenstein AW, Hicks CB, Goodwin BS Jr, Hilliard JK. Human infection with B virus following a needlestick injury. *Rev Infect Dis* 1991;**13**:288–91.

42. Arvin AM, Moffat JF, Redman R. Varicella-zoster virus: aspects of pathogenesis and host response to natural infection and varicella vaccine. *Adv Virus Res* 1996;**46**:263–309.

43. Asano Y, Yoshikawa T, Kajita Y, et al. Fatal encephalitis/encephalopathy in primary human herpesvirus-6 infection. *Arch Dis Child* 1992;**67**:1484–5.

44. Asare E, Dunn G, Glass J, et al. Neuronal pattern correlates with the severity of HIV-associated dementia complex. *Am J Pathol* 1996;**148**:31–8.

45. Asenbauer B, McEntagart M, King MD, et al. Chronic active destructive herpes simplex encephalitis with recovery of viral DNA 12 years after disease onset. *Neuropediatrics* 1998;**29**:120–23.

46. Astrom K, Mancall E, Richardson EJ. Progressive multifocal leukoencephalopathy: a hitherto unrecognized complication of chronic lymphatic leukaemia and Hodgkin's disease. *Brain* 1958;**81**:93–111.

47. Atreya CD, Mohan KV, Kulkarni S. Rubella virus and birth defects: molecular insights into the viral teratogenesis at the cellular level. *Birth Defects Res A Clin Mol Teratol* 2004;**70**:431–7.

48. Attoui H, Billoir F, Bruey JM, et al. Serologic and molecular diagnosis of Colorado tick fever viral infections. *Am J Trop Med Hyg* 1998;**59**:763–8.

49. Attoui H, Mohd Jaafar F, de Micco P, de Lamballerie X. Coltiviruses and seadornaviruses in North America, Europe, and Asia. *Emerg Infect Dis* 2005;**11**:1673–9.

50. Aurelius E, Johansson B, Skoldenberg B, et al. Rapid diagnosis of herpes simplex encephalitis by nested polymerase chain reaction assay of cerebrospinal fluid. *Lancet* 1991;**337**:189–92.

51. Aurelius E, Forsgren M, Skoldenberg B, Strannegard O. Persistent intrathecal immune activation in patients with herpes simplex encephalitis. *J Infect Dis* 1993;**168**:1248–52.

52. Authier FJ, Chariot P, Gherardi RK. Skeletal muscle involvement in HIV-infected patients in the era of HAART. *Muscle Nerve* 2005;**32**:247–60.

53. Azimi N, Brown K, Bamford RN, et al. Human T cell lymphotropic virus type I Tax protein trans-activates interleukin 15 gene transcription through an NF-kappaB site. *Proc Natl Acad Sci U S A* 1998;**95**:2452–7.

54. Baba M, Nakamura Y, Aoki Y, et al. Six cases of aseptic meningitis probably due to Epstein–Barr virus: clinical estimation of anti-EBV titers in serum and spinal fluid. *Rinsho Byori* 1988;**36**:351–6.

55. Babcock GJ, Hochberg D, Thorley-Lawson AD. The expression pattern of Epstein–Barr virus latent genes in vivo is dependent upon the differentiation stage of the infected B cell. *Immunity* 2000;**13**:497–506.

56. Back E, Hoglund C, Malmlund HO. Cytomegalovirus infection associated with severe encephalitis. *Scand J Infect Dis* 1977;**9**:141–3.

57. Baczko K, Liebert UG, Cattaneo R, et al. Restriction of measles virus gene expression in measles inclusion body encephalitis. *J Infect Dis* 1988;**158**:144–50.

58. Baczko K, Lampe J, Liebert UG, et al. Clonal expansion of hypermutated measles virus in a SSPE brain. *Virology* 1993;**197**:188–95.

59. Badilla X, Perez-Herra V, Quiros L, et al. Human rabies: a reemerging disease in Costa Rica? *Emerg Infect Dis* 2003;**9**: 721–3.

60. Badrane H, Bahloul C, Perrin P, Tordo N. Evidence of two Lyssavirus phylogroups with distinct pathogenicity and immunogenicity. *J Virol* 2001;**75**:3268–76.

61. Baer GM, Shaddock JH, Houff SA, et al. Human rabies transmitted by corneal transplant. *Arch Neurol* 1982;**39**:103–7.

62. Baker AB. Poliomyelitis: a study of pulmonary edema. *Neurology* 1957;**7**:743–51.

63. Bakri SJ, Kaiser PK. Ocular manifestations of West Nile virus. *Curr Opin Ophthalmol* 2004;**15**:537–40.

64. Baldanti F, Sarasini A, Furione M, et al. Coinfection of the immunocompromised but not the immunocompetent host by multiple human cytomegalovirus strains. *Arch Virol* 1998;**143**:1701–9.

65. Balfour HH, Seifert GL, Seifert MH, Jr, et al. Meningoencephalitis and laboratory evidence of triple infection with California encephalitis virus, Echovirus II, and mumps. *Pediatrics* 1973;**51**: 680–83.

66. Balkhy HH, Schreiber JR. Severe La Crosse encephalitis with significant neurologic sequelae. *Pediatr Infect Dis J* 2000;**19**:77–80.

67. Ballard RA, Drew WL, Hufnagle KG, Riedel PA. Acquired cytomegalovirus infection in preterm infants. *Am J Dis Child* 1979;**133**:482–5.

68. Banatvala JE, Brown DW. Rubella. *Lancet* 2004;**363**:1127–37.

69. Bancher C, Leitner H, Jellinger K, et al. On the relationship between measles virus and Alzheimer neurofibrillary tangles in subacute sclerosing panencephalitis. *Neurobiol Aging* 1996;**17**:527–33.

70. Baringer JR. Recovery of herpes simplex virus from human sacral ganglions. *N Engl J Med* 1974;**291**:828–30.

71. Baringer JR, Pisani P. Herpes simplex virus genomes in human nervous system tissue analyzed by polymerase chain reaction. *Ann Neurol* 1994;**36**:823–9.

72. Baringer JR, Swoveland P. Recovery of herpes-simplex virus from human trigeminal ganglions. *N Engl J Med* 1973;**288**:648–50.

73. Barkovich AJ, Lindan CE. Congenital cytomegalovirus infection of the brain: imaging analysis and embryologic considerations. *AJNR Am J Neuroradiol* 1994;**15**:703–15.

74. Barmak K, Harhaj EW, Wigdahl B. Mediators of central nervous system damage during the progression of human T-cell leukemia type-associated myelopathy/tropical spastic paraparesis. *J Neurovirol* 2003;**9**:522–9.

75. Barthez-Carpentier MA, Rozenberg F, Dussaix E, et al. Relapse of herpes simplex encephalitis. *J Child Neurol* 1995;**10**:363–8.

76. Bartholomew C, Cleghorn F, Jack N, et al. Human T-cell lymphotropic virus type I-associated facial nerve palsy in Trinidad and Tobago. *Ann Neurol* 1997;**41**:806–9.

77. Bastian FO, Wende RD, Singer DB, Zeller RS. Eastern equine encephalomyelitis: histopathologic and ultrastructural changes with isolation of the virus in a human case. *Am J Clin Pathol* 1975;**64**:10–13.

78. Bathoorn E, Vlaminckx BJ, Schoondermark-Stolk S, et al. Primary Epstein–Barr virus infection with neurological complications. *Scand J Infect Dis* 2011;**2**:136–44.

79. Beardwell A. Facial palsy due to the mumps virus. *Br J Clin Pract* 1969;**23**:37–8.

80. Beasley DW. Vaccines and immunotherapeutics for the prevention and treatment of infections with West Nile virus. *Immunotherapy* 2011;**2**:269–85.

81. Beasley DW, Davis CT, Whiteman M, et al. Molecular determinants of virulence of West Nile virus in North America. *Arch Virol Suppl* 2004;**18**:35–41.

82. Befort P, Gaillard N, Roubille C, Quellec AL. Hemorrhagic leukoencephalitis linked to Epstein–Barr virus in an adult patient. *Clin Neurol Neurosurg* 2010;**9**:829–31.

83. Belay ED, Bresee JS, Holman RC, et al. Reye's syndrome in the United States from 1981 through 1997. *N Engl J Med* 1999;**340**:1377–82.

84. Belec L, Gherardi R, Georges AJ, et al. Peripheral facial paralysis and HIV infection: report of four African cases and review of the literature. *J Neurol* 1989;**236**:411–14.

85. Belec L, Gray F, Mikol J, et al. Cytomegalovirus (CMV) encephalomyeloradiculitis and human immunodeficiency virus (HIV) encephalitis: presence of HIV and CMV co-infected multinucleated giant cells. *Acta Neuropathol* 1990;**81**:99–104.

86. Belec L, Tayot J, Tron P, et al. Cytomegalovirus encephalopathy in an infant with congenital acquired immuno-deficiency syndrome. *Neuropediatrics* 1990;**21**:124–9.

87. Bell JE, Lowrie S, Koffi K, *et al*. The neuropathology of HIV-infected African children in Abidjan, Côte d'Ivoire. *J Neuropathol Exp Neurol* 1997;**56**:686–92.

88. Benenson MW, Top FJ, Gresso W, *et al*. The virulence to man of Japanese encephalitis virus in Thailand. *Am J Trop Med Hyg* 1975;**24**:974–80.

89. Benjamin LA, Bryer A, Emsley H, *et al*. HIV infection and stroke: current perpectives and future directions. *Lancet Neurol* 2012;**11**:878–90.

90. Bennett NM. Murray Valley encephalitis, 1974: clinical features. *Med J Aust* 1976;**2**:446–50.

90a. Benschop KS, Schinkel J, Minnaar RP, *et al*. Human parechovirus infections in Dutch children and the association between serotype and disease severity. *Clin Infect Dis* 2006;**42**(2):204–10.

91. Berg AL, Dorries R, Berg M. Borna disease virus infection in racing horses with behavioral and movement disorders. *Arch Virol* 1999;**144**:547–59.

92. Bergelson JM, St John N, Kawaguchi S, *et al*. Infection by echoviruses 1 and 8 depends on the alpha 2 subunit of human VLA-2. *J Virol* 1993;**67**:6847–52.

93. Bergelson JM, Chan M, Solomon KR, *et al*. Decay-accelerating factor (CD55), a glycosylphosphatidylinositol-anchored complement regulatory protein, is a receptor for several echoviruses. *Proc Natl Acad Sci U S A* 1994;**91**:6245–9.

94. Berger A, Reitter A, Harter PN, *et al*. Problems and challenges in the diagnosis of vertical infection with human cytomegalovirus (CMV): lessons from two accidental cases. *J Clin Virol* 2011;**4**:285–8.

95. Berger JR. Progressive multifocal leukoencephalopathy in acquired immunodeficiency syndrome: explaining the high incidence and disproportionate frequency of the illness relative to other immunosuppressive conditions. *J Neurovirol* 2003;**9**(Suppl 1):38–41.

96. Berger JR, Houff S. Neurological complications of herpes simplex virus type 2 infection. *Arch Neurol* 2008;**5**:596–600.

97. Berger JR, Levy RM, Flomenhoft D, Dobbs M. Predictive factors for prolonged survival in acquired immunodeficiency syndrome-associated progressive multifocal leukoencephalopathy. *Ann Neurol* 1998;**44**:341–9.

98. Berger JR, Pall L, Lanska D, Whiteman M. Progressive multifocal leukoencephalopathy in patients with HIV infection. *J Neurovirol* 1998;**1**:59–68.

99. Berger JR, Fee DB, Nelson P, Nuovo G. Coxsackie B meningoencephalitis in a patient with acquired immunodeficiency syndrome and a multiple sclerosis-like illness. *J Neurovirol* 2009;**3**:282–7.

100. Bergin JD. Fatal encephalopathy in glandular fever. *J Neurol Neurosurg Psychiatry* 1960;**23**:69–73.

101. Bergstrom T, Vahlne A, Alestig K, *et al*. Primary and recurrent herpes simplex virus type 2-induced meningitis. *J Infect Dis* 1990;**162**:322–30.

102. Bhangoo S, Chua R, Hammond C, *et al*. Focal neurological injury caused by West Nile virus infection may occur independent of patient age and premorbid health. *J Neurol Sci* 2005;**234**:93–8.

103. Bhat A, Naguwa S, Cheema G, Gershwin ME. The epidemiology of transverse myelitis. *Autoimmun Rev* 2010;**5**:A395–9.

104. Bhigjee AI, Wiley CA, Wachsman W, *et al*. HTLV-I-associated myelopathy: clinicopathologic correlation with localization of provirus to spinal cord. *Neurology* 1991;**41**:1990–92.

105. Biggar RJ, Taylor ME, Neel JV, *et al*. Genetic variants of human T-lymphotrophic virus type II in American Indian groups. *Virology* 1996;**216**:165–73.

106. Biggerstaff BJ, Petersen LR. Estimated risk of transmission of the West Nile virus through blood transfusion in the US, 2002. *Transfusion* 2003;**43**:1007–17.

107. Billeter MA, Cattaneo R, Spielhofer P, *et al*. Generation and properties of measles virus mutations typically associated with subacute sclerosing panencephalitis. *Ann N Y Acad Sci* 1994;**724**:367–77.

108. Bingham J, Mlambo P. Ante-mortem diagnosis of human rabies by the skin biopsy technique: three case reports from Zimbabwe. *Centr Afr J Med* 1995;**41**:258–60.

109. Bingham R, Ahmed N, Rangi P, *et al*. HIV encephalitis despite suppressed viraemia: a case of compartmentalized viral escape. *Int J STD AIDS* 2011;**22**:608–9.

110. Bissel SJ, Giles BM, Wang G, *et al*. Acute murine H5N1 influenza A encephalitis. *Brain Pathol* 2012;**22**:150–58.

111. Biswas S, Suresh P, Bonshek RE, *et al*. Graft failure in human donor corneas due to transmission of herpes simplex virus. *Br J Ophthalmol* 2000;**84**:701–5.

112. Bitnun A, Shannon P, Durward A, *et al*. Measles inclusion-body encephalitis caused by the vaccine strain of measles virus. *Clin Infect Dis* 1999;**29**:855–61.

113. Bjerkhoel A, Carlsson M, Ohlsson J. Peripheral facial palsy caused by the Borrelia spirochete. *Acta Otolaryngol* 1989;**108**:424–30.

114. Blakqori G, Weber F. Efficient cDNA-based rescue of La Crosse bunyaviruses expressing or lacking the nonstructural protein NSs. *J Virol* 2005;**79**:10420–28.

115. Blue M, Rosenblum W. Granulomatous angiitis of the brain with herpes zoster and varicella encephalitis. *Arch Pathol Lab Med* 1983;**107**:126–8.

116. Bode L, Ferszt R, Czech G. Borna disease virus infection and affective disorders in man. *Arch Virol* 1993;**7**(Suppl):159–67.

117. Bofill-Mas S, Girones R. Role of the environment in the transmission of JC virus. *J Neurovirol* 2003;**9**(Suppl 1):54–8.

118. Bogdan FL, Radu I, Mogoanta L, Frasie M. Meningocerebral lesions in children with iatrogenic AIDS. *Rom J Morphol Embryol* 1996;**42**:53–62.

119. Bogdanovic G, Priftakis P, Hammarin AL, *et al*. Detection of JC virus in cerebrospinal fluid (CSF) samples from patients with progressive multifocal leukoencephalopathy but not in CSF samples from patients with herpes simplex encephalitis, enteroviral meningitis, or multiple sclerosis. *J Clin Microbiol* 1998;**36**:1137–8.

120. Bolton WV, Davis AR, Ge YC, *et al*. Molecular evidence for transmission of human T-lymphotropic virus type II infection by a human bite. *J Clin Microbiol* 1999;**37**:238–40.

121. Bonaparte MI, Dimitrov AS, Bossart KN, *et al*. Ephrin-B2 ligand is a functional receptor for Hendra virus and Nipah virus. *Proc Natl Acad Sci U S A* 2005;**102**:10652–7.

122. Bondarenko EI, Protopopova EV, Konovalova SN, *et al*. [Laminin-binding protein (LBP) as a cellular receptor for the virus of Venezuelan equine encephalomyelitis (VEE): part 1. A study of the interaction between VEE virus virions and the human recombinant LBP.] *Mol Gen Mikrobiol Virusol* 2003;**4**:36–9.

123. Bondarenko EI, Protopopova EV, Konovalova SN, *et al*. [Laminin-binding protein as a cellular receptor for the equine Venezuelan encephalomyelitis virus: report 2. Inhibition of replication of equine Venezuelan encephalomyelitis virus by blocking laminin-binding protein on the surface of Vero cells.] *Mol Gen Mikrobiol Virusol* 2004;**1**:36–40.

124. Borucki MK, Kempf BJ, Blitvich BJ, *et al*. La Crosse virus: replication in vertebrate and invertebrate hosts. *Microbes Infect* 2002;**4**:341–50.

125. Bosanko CM, Gilroy J, Wang AM, *et al*. West Nile virus encephalitis involving the substantia nigra: neuroimaging and pathologic findings with literature review. *Arch Neurol* 2003;**60**:1448–52.

126. Bourgeois M, Vinikoff L, Lellouch-Tubiana A, Sainte-Rose C. Reactivation of herpes virus after surgery for epilepsy in a pediatric patient with mesial temporal sclerosis: case report. *Neurosurgery* 1999;**44**:633–6.

127. Bowerman B, Brown PO, Bishop JM, Varmus HE. A nucleoprotein complex mediates the integration of retroviral DNA. *Genes Dev* 1989;**3**:469–78.

128. Branco FJ, Fraser NW. Herpes simplex virus type 1 latency-associated transcript expression protects trigeminal ganglion neurons from apoptosis. *J Virol* 2005;**79**:9019–25.

129. Bratt G, Hammarin AL, Grandien M, *et al*. BK virus as the cause of meningoencephalitis, retinitis and nephritis in a patient with AIDS. *AIDS* 1999;**13**:1071–5.

130. Deleted in proof.

131. Deleted in proof.

132. Breningstall GN, Belani KK. Acute transverse myelitis and brainstem encephalitis associated with hepatitis A infection. *Pediatr Neurol* 1995;**12**:169–71.

133. Brilla R, Block M, Geremia G, Wichter M. Clinical and neuroradiologic features of 39 consecutive cases of West Nile Virus meningoencephalitis. *J Neurol Sci* 2004;**220**:37–40.

134. Brink AA, van Gelder M, Wolffs PF, *et al*. Compartmentalization of acyclovir-resistant varicella zoster virus: implications for sampling in molecular diagnostics. *Clin Infect Dis* 2011;**8**:982–7.

135. Britton CB, Mesa-Tejada R, Fenoglio CM, *et al*. A new complication of AIDS: thoracic myelitis caused by herpes simplex virus. *Neurology* 1985;**35**:1071–4.

136. Brooks BR, Walker DL. Progressive multifocal leukoencephalopathy. *Neurol Clin* 1984;**2**:299–313.

137. Brown ZA, Benedetti J, Selke S, *et al*. Asymptomatic maternal shedding of herpes simplex virus at the onset of labor: relationship to preterm labor. *Obstet Gynecol* 1996;**87**:483–8.

138. Brown ZA, Wald A, Morrow RA, *et al*. Effect of serologic status and cesarean delivery on transmission rates of herpes simplex virus from mother to infant. *J Am Med Assoc* 2003;**289**:203–9.

139. Blumchen-Osmond C. Deltaretrovirus. In: Blumchen-Osmond C, ed. *ICTVdB: the Universal Virus Database*, version 3. New York: International Committee on

Taxonomy of Viruses, Columbia University, 2004.

140. Blumchen-Osmond C. *The Universal Virus Database of the International Committee on Taxonomy of Viruses.* New York: International Committee on Taxonomy of Viruses, 2005.

141. Buda K, Tubergen DG, Levin MJ. The frequency and consequences of varicella exposure and varicella infection in children receiving maintenance therapy for acute lymphoblastic leukemia. *J Pediatr Hematol Oncol* 1996;**18**:106–12.

142. Budka H, Wiley CA, Kleihues P, *et al.* HIV-associated disease of the nervous system: review of nomenclature and proposal for neuropathology-based terminology. *Brain Pathol* 1991;**1**:143–52.

143. Budka H, Urbanits S, Liberski PP, *et al.* Subacute measles virus encephalitis: a new and fatal opportunistic infection in a patient with AIDS. *Neurology* 1996;**46**:586–7.

144. Burke B, Steele R, Beard O, *et al.* Immune responses to varicella-zoster in the aged. *Arch Intern Med* 1982;**142**:291–3.

145. Burke DS, Nisalak A, Ussery MA, *et al.* Kinetics of IgM and IgG responses to Japanese encephalitis virus in human serum and cerebrospinal fluid. *J Infect Dis* 1985;**151**:1093–9.

146. Burton EC, Burns DK, Opatowsky MJ, *et al.* Rabies encephalomyelitis: clinical, neuroradiological, and pathological findings in 4 transplant recipients. *Arch Neurol* 2005;**62**:873–82.

147. Bustos DE, Atherton SS. Detection of herpes simplex virus type 1 in human ciliary ganglia. *Invest Ophthalmol Vis Sci* 2002;**43**:2244–9.

148. Calisher CH, Shope RE, Brandt W, *et al.* Proposed antigenic classification of registered arboviruses I: Togaviridae, Alphavirus. *Intervirology* 1980;**14**:5–6.

149. Campbell H, Andrews N, Brown KE, Miller E. Review of the effect of measles vaccination on the epidemiology of SSPE. *Int J Epidemiol* 2007;**6**:1334–48.

150. Cann A, Chen I. Human T cell leukemia virus types I and II. In: Fields B, Knipe D, Chanock R, Al E eds. *Fields' virology.* New York: Raven Press, 1990:1501–27.

151. Cartier L, Araya F, Castillo JL, *et al.* Progressive spastic paraparesis associated with human T-cell leukemia virus type I (HTLV-I). *Int Med* 1992;**31**:1257–61.

152. Cartier LM, Cea JG, Vergara C, *et al.* Clinical and neuropathological study of six patients with spastic paraparesis associated with HTLV-I: an axomyelinic degeneration of the central nervous system. *J Neuropathol Exp Neurol* 1997;**56**:403–13.

153. Deleted in proof.

154. Caruso M, Cavaldesi M, Gentile M, *et al.* Role of sialic acid-containing molecules and the alpha4beta1 integrin receptor in the early steps of polyomavirus infection. *J Gen Virol* 2003;**84**:2927–36.

155. Caserta MT, Hall CB, Schnabel K, *et al.* Neuroinvasion and persistence of human herpesvirus 6 in children. *J Infect Dis* 1994;**170**:1586–9.

156. Caserta MT, Hall CB, Schnabel K, *et al.* Primary human herpesvirus 7 infection: a comparison of human herpesvirus 7 and human herpesvirus 6 infections in children. *J Pediatr* 1998;**133**:386–9.

157. Caserta MT, Mock DJ, Dewhurst S. Human herpesvirus 6. *Clin Infect Dis* 2001;**33**:829–33.

158. Cattaneo R, Schmid A, Rebmann G, *et al.* Accumulated measles virus mutations in a case of subacute sclerosing panencephalitis: interrupted matrix protein reading frame and transcription alteration. *Virology* 1986;**154**:97–107.

159. Cattaneo R, Schmid A, Billeter MA, *et al.* Multiple viral mutations rather than host factors cause defective measles virus gene expression in a subacute sclerosing panencephalitis cell line. *J Virol* 1988;**62**:1388–97.

160. Deleted in proof.

161. Cavrois M, Gessain A, Wain-Hobson S, Wattel E. Proliferation of HTLV-infected circulating cells in vivo in all asymptomatic carriers and patients with TSP/HAM. *Oncogene* 1996;**12**:2419–23.

162. Ceausu E, Erscoiu S, Calistru P, *et al.* Clinical manifestations in the West Nile virus outbreak. *Rom J Virol* 1997;**48**:3–11.

163. Centers for Disease Control and Prevention. Rabies in a laboratory worker: New York. *MMWR Morb Mortal Wkly Rep* 1977;**26**:183–4.

164. Centers for Disease Control and Prevention. *Pneumocystis carinii* pneumonia – Los Angeles. *MMWR Morb Mortal Wkly Rep* 1981;**30**: 250–52.

165. Centers for Disease Control and Prevention. B-virus infections in humans: Pensacola, Florida. *MMWR Morb Mortal Wkly Rep* 1987;**36**:289–90, 295–6.

166. Centers for Disease Control and Prevention. Fatal Cercopithecine herpesvirus 1 (B virus) infection following a mucocutaneous exposure and interim recommendations for worker protection. *MMWR Morb Mortal Wkly Rep* 1998;**47**:1073–6.

167. Centers for Disease Control and Prevention. Measles, mumps, and rubella: vaccine use and strategies for elimination of measles, rubella, and congenital rubella syndrome and control of mumps. Recommendations of the Advisory Committee on Immunization Practices (ACIP). *MMWR Morb Mortal Wkly Rep* 1998;**47**:1–57.

168. Centers for Disease Control and Prevention. Human rabies prevention: United States, 1999. Recommendations of the Advisory Committee on Immunization Practices (ACIP). *MMWR Morb Mortal Wkly Rep* 1999;**48**:1–21.

169. Centers for Disease Control and Prevention. Interim guidelines for the evaluation of infants born to mothers infected with West Nile virus during pregnancy. *MMWR Morb Mortal Wkly Rep* 2004;**53**:154–7.

170. Centers for Disease Control and Prevention. Recovery of a patient from clinical rabies: Wisconsin, 2004. *MMWR Morb Mortal Wkly Rep* 2004;**53**:1171–3.

171. Centers for Disease Control and Prevention. Update: vaccine side effects, adverse reactions, contraindications, and precautions: recommendations of the Advisory Committee on Immunization Practices (ACIP). *MMWR Morb Mortal Wkly Rep* 1996;**45**:1–35.

172. Cesario T, Fife LT, Rayhan S, Emmons R. Cutaneous dissemination of herpes simplex virus in individuals fifteen years of age and older. *Am J Med Sci* 1977;**273**:143–6.

173. Chadwick DW, Martin S, Buxton PH, Tomlinson AH. Measles virus and subacute neurological disease: an unusual presentation of measles inclusion body encephalitis.

J Neurol Neurosurg Psychiatry 1982;**45**:680–84.

174. Challoner PB, Smith KT, Parker JD, *et al.* Plaque-associated expression of human herpesvirus 6 in multiple sclerosis. *Proc Natl Acad Sci U S A* 1995;**92**:7440–44.

175. Chan PK, Ng HK, Hui M, Cheng AF. Prevalence and distribution of human herpesvirus 6 variants A and B in adult human brain. *J Med Virol* 2001;**64**:42–6.

176. Chan PK, Li CK, Chik KW, *et al.* Risk factors and clinical consequences of human herpesvirus 7 infection in paediatric haematopoietic stem cell transplant recipients. *J Med Virol* 2004;**72**:668–74.

177. Chang Y, Soffer D, Horoupian DS, Weiss LM. Evolution of post-natal herpes simplex virus encephalitis to multicystic encephalopathy. *Acta Neuropathol* 1990;**80**:666–70.

178. Chapagain ML, Sumitbcay L, Gurjav U, *et al.* Serotonin receptor 2A blocker (risperidone) has no effect on human polyomavirus JC infection of primary human fetal glial cells. *J Neurovirol* 2008;**5**:448–54.

179. Charlier N, Molenkamp R, Leyssen P, *et al.* Exchanging the yellow fever virus envelope proteins with Modoc virus prM and E proteins results in a chimeric virus that is neuroinvasive in SCID mice. *J Virol* 2004;**78**:7418–26.

180. Charlton KM, Nadin-Davis S, Casey GA, Wandeler AI. The long incubation period in rabies: delayed progression of infection in muscle at the site of exposure. *Acta Neuropathol* 1997;**94**:73–7.

181. Charrel RN, de Lamballerie X. [West Nile virus, an emerging arbovirus.] *Presse Med* 2004;**33**:1521–6.

182. Charrel RN, Gallian P, Navarro-Mari J-M, *et al.* Emergence of Toscana Virus in Europe. *Emerg Infect Dis* 2005;**11**: 1657–63.

183. Chen CH, Chiu YL, Wei FC, *et al.* High seroprevalence of Borna virus infection in schizophrenic patients, family members and mental health workers in Taiwan. *Molec Psychiatry* 1999;**4**:33–8.

184. Chen JJ, Gershon AA, Li ZS, *et al.* Latent and lytic infection of isolated guinea pig enteric ganglia by varicella zoster virus. *J Med Virol* 2003;**70**(Suppl 1):S71–8.

185. Chen JJ, Zhu Z, Gershon AA, Gershon MD. Mannose 6-phosphate receptor dependence of varicella zoster virus infection in vitro and in the epidermis during varicella and zoster. *Cell* 2004;**119**:915–26.

186. Chen YC, Wang CH, Su IJ, *et al.* Infection of human T-cell leukemia virus type I and development of human T-cell leukemia lymphoma in patients with hematologic neoplasms: a possible linkage to blood transfusion. *Blood* 1989;**74**:388–94.

187. Chen YM, Okayama A, Lee TH, *et al.* Sexual transmission of human T-cell leukemia virus type I associated with the presence of anti-Tax antibody. *Proc Natl Acad Sci U S A* 1991;**88**:1182–6.

188. Cherner M, Masliah E, Ellis RJ, *et al.* Neurocognitive dysfunction predicts postmortem findings of HIV encephalitis. *Neurology* 2002;**59**:1563–7.

189. Chetty R. Vasculitides associated with HIV infection. *J Clin Pathol* 2001;**54**:275–8.

190. Chevalier V, de la Rocque S, Baldet T, *et al.* Epidemiological processes involved in the emergence of vector-borne diseases: West Nile fever, Rift Valley fever, Japanese encephalitis and Crimean-Congo haemorrhagic fever. *Rev Sci Tech* 2004;**23**:535–55.

191. Chiu AG, Hecht DA, Prendiville SA, et al. Atypical presentations of cat scratch disease in the head and neck. *Otolaryngol Head Neck Surg* 2001;**125**:414–16.

192. Chopra JS, Banerjee AK, Murthy JM, Pal SR. Paralytic rabies: a clinico-pathological study. *Brain* 1980;**103**:789–802.

193. Chou KS, Okayama A, Su IJ, et al. Preferred nucleotide sequence at the integration target site of human T-cell leukemia virus type I from patients with adult T-cell leukemia. *Int J Cancer* 1996;**65**:20–24.

194. Chou SM, Roos R, Burrell R, et al. Subacute focal adenovirus encephalitis. *J Neuropathol Exp Neurol* 1973;**32**:34–50.

195. Chou SW, Dennison KM. Analysis of interstrain variation in cytomegalovirus glycoprotein B sequences encoding neutralization-related epitopes. *J Infect Dis* 1991;**163**:1229–34.

196. Chou SW, Norman DJ. The influence of donor factors other than serologic status on transmission of cytomegalovirus to transplant recipients. *Transplantation* 1988;**46**:89–93.

197. Chretien F, Gray F, Lescs MC, et al. Acute varicella-zoster virus ventriculitis and meningo-myelo-radiculitis in acquired immunodeficiency syndrome. *Acta Neuropathol (Berl)* 1993;**86**:659–65.

198. Chretien F, Belec L, Hilton DA, et al. Herpes simplex virus type 1 encephalitis in acquired immunodeficiency syndrome. *Neuropathol Appl Neurobiol* 1996;**22**:394–404.

199. Chretien F, Belec L, Lescs MC, et al. Central nervous system infection due to varicella and zoster virus in AIDS. *Arch Anat Cytol Pathol* 1997;**45**:142–52.

200. Chu CT, Howell DN, Morgenlander JC, et al. Electron microsocpic diagnosis of human flavivirus encephalitis: use of confocal microscopy as an aid. *Am J Surg Pathol* 1999;**23**:1217–26.

201. Chu JJ, Ng ML. Infectious entry of West Nile virus occurs through a clathrin-mediated endocytic pathway. *J Virol* 2004;**78**:10543–55.

202. Chu JJ, Ng ML. Interaction of West Nile virus with alpha v beta 3 integrin mediates virus entry into cells. *J Biol Chem* 2004;**279**:54533–41.

203. Chua KB. Nipah virus outbreak in Malaysia. *J Clin Virol* 2003;**26**:265–75.

204. Chua KB, Goh KJ, Wong KT, et al. Fatal encephalitis due to Nipah virus among pig-farmers in Malaysia. *Lancet* 1999;**354**:1257–9.

205. Chua KB, Koh CL, Hooi PS, et al. Isolation of Nipah virus from Malaysian Island flying-foxes. *Microbes Infect* 2002;**4**:145–51.

206. Chuang YY, Chiu CH, Wong KS, et al. Severe adenovirus infection in children. *J Microbiol Immunol Infect* 2003;**36**:37–40.

207. Ciardi A, Sinclair E, Scaravilli F, Harcourt-Webster JN, Lucas SB. The involvement of the cerebral cortex in human immunodeficiency virus encephalopathy: a morphological and immunohistochemical study. *Acta Neuropathol* 1990;**81**:51–9.

208. Cinque P, Bossolasco S, Brambilla AM, et al. The effect of highly active antiretroviral therapy-induced immune reconstitution on development and outcome of progressive multifocal leukoencephalopathy: study of 43 cases with review of the literature. *J Neurovirol* 2003;**9**(Suppl 1):73–80.

209. Clark D. Human herpesvirus type 6 and multiple sclerosis. *Herpes* 2004;**11**(Suppl 2):112–19.A.

210. Clifford DB, Yiannoutsos C, Glicksman M, et al. HAART improves prognosis in HIV-associated progressive multifocal leukoencephalopathy. *Neurology* 1999;**52**:623–5.

211. Clifford DB, De Luca A, Simpson DM, et al. Natalizumab-associated progressive multifocal leukoencephalopathy in patients with multiple sclerosis: lessons from 28 cases. *Lancet Neurol* 2010;**4**:438–46.

212. Cobb WA, Marshall J, Scaravilli F. Long survival in subacute sclerosing panencephalitis. *J Neurol Neurosurg Psychiatry* 1984;**47**:176–83.

213. Cochereau-Massin I, Gaudric A, Reinert P, et al. Changes in the fundus in subacute sclerosing panencephalitis: apropos of 23 cases. *J Fr Ophtalmol* 1992;**15**:255–61.

214. Coffey AJ, Brooksbank RA, Brandau O, et al. Host response to EBV infection in X-linked lymphoproliferative disease results from mutations in an SH2-domain encoding gene. *Nat Genet* 1998;**20**:129–35.

215. Coffin J, Hughes S, Varmus H. *Retroviruses*. Cold Spring Harbor, NY: Cold Spring Harbor Laboratory Press, 1997.

216. Cohen JI, Davenport DS, Stewart JA, et al. Recommendations for prevention of and therapy for exposure to B virus (cercopithecine herpesvirus 1). *Clin Infect Dis* 2002;**35**:1191–203.

217. Cohrs RJ, Gilden DH. Human herpesvirus latency. *Brain Pathol* 2001;**11**:465–74.

218. Collazos J. Opportunistic infections of the CNS in patients with AIDS: diagnosis and management. *CNS Drugs* 2003;**17**:869–87.

219. Colon-Ramos DA, Irusta PM, Gan EC, et al. Inhibition of translation and induction of apoptosis by Bunyaviral nonstructural proteins bearing sequence similarity to reaper. *Mol Biol Cell* 2003;**14**:4162–72.

220. Communicable Disease Surveillance Centre. Emerging Infections update: November 2004 to January 2005. *Commun Dis Rep CDR Rev* 2005b;**15**:6–7.

221. Compton T. Receptors and immune sensors: the complex entry path of human cytomegalovirus. *Trends Cell Biol* 2004;**14**:5–8.

222. Cone RW, Huang ML, Corey L, et al. Human herpesvirus 6 infections after bone marrow transplantation: clinical and virologic manifestations. *J Infect Dis* 1999;**179**:311–18.

223. Connolly A, Dodson W, Prensky A, Rust R. Course and outcome of acute cerebellar ataxia. *Ann Neurol* 1994;**35**:673–9.

224. Connolly JH, Hutchinson WM, Allen IV, et al. Carotid artery thrombosis, encephalitis, myelitis and optic neuritis associated with rubella virus infections. *Brain* 1975;**98**:583–94.

225. Connolly KJ, Hammer SM. The acute aseptic meningitis syndrome. *Infect Dis Clin North Am* 1990;**4**:599–622.

226. Conomy JP, Leibovitz A, McCombs W, Stinson J. Airborne rabies encephalitis: demonstration of rabies virus in the human central nervous system. *Neurology* 1977;**27**:67–9.

227. Constantine DG. Rabies transmission by nonbite route. *Publ Health Rep* 1962;**77**:287–9.

228. Cook SP, Macartney KK, Rose CD, et al. Lyme disease and seventh nerve paralysis in children. *Am J Otolaryngol* 1997;**18**:320–23.

229. Cooper DA, Gold J, Maclean P, et al. Acute AIDS retrovirus infection: definition of a clinical illness associated with seroconversion. *Lancet* 1985;i:537–40.

230. Copps S, Giddings L. Transplacental transmission of western equine encephalitis. *Pediatrics* 1959;**24**:31–3.

231. Corey L, Adams HG, Brown ZA, Holmes K. Genital herpes simplex virus infections: clinical manifestations, course and complications. *Ann Intern Med* 1983;**98**:958–72.

232. Cornford ME, Ho HW, Vinters HV. Correlation of neuromuscular pathology in acquired immune deficiency. *Acta Neuropathol* 1992;**84**:516–29.

233. Corssmit EP, Leverstein-van Hall MA, Portegies P, Bakker P. Severe neurological complications in association with Epstein–Barr virus infection. *J Neurovirol* 1997;**3**:460–64.

234. Costello DJ, Gonzalez RG, Frosch MP. A 35-year old HIV-positive woman with headache and altered mental status. *N Eng J Med* 2011;**364**:2343–52.

235. Couchoud C. Cytomegalovirus prophylaxis with antiviral agents for solid organ transplantation. *Cochrane Database Syst Rev* 2000;**2**:CD001320.

236. Coyle PK, Wolinsky JS. Characterization of immune complexes in progressive rubella panencephalitis. *Ann Neurol* 1981;**9**:557–62.

237. Crawford DH. Biology and disease associations of Epstein–Barr virus. *Philos Trans R Soc Lond B Biol Sci* 2001;**356**:461–73.

238. Cremer NE, Oshiro LS, Weil ML, et al. Isolation of rubella virus from brain in chronic progressive panencephalitis. *J Gen Virol* 1975;**29**:143–53.

239. Crowder CD, Gyure KA, Drachenberg CB, et al. Successful outcome of progressive multifocal leukoencephalopathy in a renal transplant patient. *Am J Transplant* 2005;**5**:1151–8.

240. Cruz AC, da Rosa AP, Ferreira I, et al. Ilheus virus (Flaviviridae, Flavivirus) is closely related to Japanese encephalitis virus complex. *Intervirology* 1997;**40**:220–25.

241. Dacheux L, Delmas O, Bourhy H. Human rabies encephalitis prevention and treatment: progress since Pasteur's discovery. *Infect Disord Drug Targets* 2011;**3**:251–99.

242. Daiminger A, Bader U, Enders G. Pre- and periconceptional primary cytomegalovirus infection: risk of vertical transmission and congenital disease. *BJOG* 2005;**112**:166–72.

243. Dalakas MC. Pathogenetic mechanisms of post-polio syndrome: morphological, electrophysiological, virological, and immunological correlations. *Ann N Y Acad Sci* 1995;**753**:167–85.

244. Dales L, Hammer SJ, Smith NJ. Time trends in autism and in MMR immunization coverage in California. *J Am Med Assoc* 2001;**285**:1183–5.

245. Daniel DC, Kinoshita Y, Khan MA, et al. Internalization of exogenous human immunodeficiency virus-1 protein, Tat, by KG-1 oligodendroglioma cells followed by stimulation of DNA replication initiated at the JC virus origin. *DNA Cell Biol* 2004;**12**:858–67.

246. Darwish MA, Ibrahim AH. Prevalence of antibodies to arboviruses in Egypt: results of a serologic survey among 1,113 university students. *Am J Trop Med Hyg* 1975;**24**:981–5.

247. Das T, Jaffar-Bandjee MC, Hoarau JJ, *et al.* Chikungunya fever: CNS infection and pathologies of a re-emerging arbovirus. *Prog Neurobiol* 2010;**2**:121–9.

248. Da Silveira CM, Kmetzsch CI, Mohrdieck R, *et al.* The risk of aseptic meningitis associated with the Leningrad–Zagreb mumps vaccine strain following mass vaccination with measles–mumps–rubella vaccine, Rio Grande do Sul, Brazil, 1997. *Int J Epidemiol* 2002;**31**:978–82.

249. Dasopoulou M, Covanis A. Subacute sclerosing panencephalitis after intrauterine infection. *Acta Paediatr* 2004;**93**:1251–3.

250. Davidson MM, Hummeler K. B virus infection in man. *Ann N Y Acad Sci* 1960;**85**:970–79.

251. Davidson MM, Williams H, Macleod JA. Louping ill in man: a forgotten disease. *J Infect* 1991;**23**:241–9.

252. Davies J, Everall IP, Weich S, *et al.* HIV-associated brain pathology in the UK: an epidemiological study. *AIDS* 1997;**11**:1145–50.

253. Davis D, Henslee PJ, Markesbery WR. Fatal adenovirus meningoencephalitis in a bone marrow transplant patient. *Ann Neurol* 1988;**23**:385–9.

254. Deleted in proof.

255. Davis LE, Johnson RT. An explanation for the localization of herpes simplex encephalitis? *Ann Neurol* 1979;**5**:2–5.

256. Davis LE, Hjelle BL, Miller VE, *et al.* Early viral brain invasion in iatrogenic human immunodeficiency virus infection. *Neurology* 1992;**42**:1736–9.

257. Davis LE, Beckham JD, Tyler KL. North American encephalitic arboviruses. *Neurol Clin* 2008;**3**:727–57.

258. Davison AJ, McGeoch DJ. Evolutionary comparisons of the S segments in the genomes of herpes simplex virus type 1 and varicella-zoster virus. *J Gen Virol* 1986;**67**:597–611.

259. Davison KL, Crowcroft NS, Ramsay ME, *et al.* Viral encephalitis in England, 1989–1998: what did we miss? *Emerg Infect Dis* 2003;**9**:234–40.

260. Day JF. Predicting St Louis encephalitis virus epidemics: lessons from recent, and not so recent, outbreaks. *Annu Rev Entomol* 2001;**46**:111–38.

261. Day JF, Stark LM. Transmission patterns of St Louis encephalitis and eastern equine encephalitis viruses in Florida: 1978–1993. *J Med Entomol* 1996;**33**:132–9.

262. De Azevedo JP, Nascimento LR, Cortinovis MC, *et al.* Characterization of species B adenoviruses isolated from fecal specimens taken from poliomyelitis-suspected cases. *J Clin Virol* 2004;**31**:248–52.

263. Dein FJ, Carpenter JW, Clark GG, *et al.* Mortality of captive whooping cranes caused by eastern equine encephalitis virus. *J Am Vet Med Assoc* 1986;**189**:1006–10.

264. De la Grandmaison GL, Carlier R, Chretien F, *et al.* 'Burnt out' varicella-zoster-virus encephalitis in an AIDS patient following treatment by highly active antiretroviral therapy. *Clin Radiol* 2005;**60**:613–17.

265. De la Monte S, Castro F, Bonilla NJ, *et al.* The systemic pathology of Venezuelan equine encephalitis virus infection in humans. *Am J Trop Med Hyg* 1985;**34**:194–202.

266. De la Torre JC, Gonzalez-Dunia D, Cubitt B, *et al.* Detection of borna disease virus antigen and RNA in human autopsy brain samples from neuropsychiatric patients. *Virology* 1996;**223**:272–82.

267. Denholm JT, Neal A, Yan B, *et al.* Acute encephalomyelitis syndromes associated with H1N1 09 influenza vaccination. *Neurology* 2010;**24**:2246–8.

268. Dennett C, Klapper PE, Cleator GM. Polymerase chain reaction in the investigation of 'relapse' following herpes simplex encephalitis. *J Med Virol* 1996;**48**:129–32.

269. Dennett C, Cleator GM, Klapper PE. HSV-1 and HSV-2 in herpes simplex encephalitis: a study of sixty-four cases in the United Kingdom. *J Med Virol* 1997;**53**:1–3.

270. De Paoli P. Human herpesvirus 8: an update. *Microbes Infect* 2004;**6**:328–35.

271. Department of Health. Improvements to childhood immunisation programme. www.dh.gov.uk/en/Publicationsandstatistics/Pressreleases/DH_4087239. London: Department of Health, 2004.

272. Deresiewicz RL, Thaler SJ, Hsu L, Zamani AA. Clinical and neuroradiographic manifestations of eastern equine encephalitis. *N Engl J Med* 1997;**336**:1867–74.

273. Deschl U, Stitz L, Herzog S, *et al.* Determination of immune cells and expression of major histocompatibility complex class II antigen in encephalitic lesions of experimental Borna disease. *Acta Neuropathol* 1990;**81**:41–50.

274. De Seze J, Stojkovic T, Breteau G, *et al.* Acute myelopathies: clinical, laboratory and outcome profiles in 79 cases. *Brain* 2001;**124**:1509–21.

275. de Seze J, Lanctin C, Lebrun C, *et al.* Idiopathic acute transverse myelitis: application of the recent diagnostic criteria. *Neurology* 2005;**12**:1950–53.

276. Desmond MM, Wilson GS, Melnick JL, *et al.* Congenital rubella encephalitis. Course and early sequelae. *J Pediatr* 1967;**71**:311–31.

277. DeStefano F, Bhasin TK, Thompson WW, *et al.* Age at first measles–mumps–rubella vaccination in children with autism and school-matched control subjects: a population-based study in metropolitan Atlanta. *Pediatrics* 2004;**113**:259–66.

278. Deuschle M, Bode L, Heuser I, *et al.* Borna disease virus proteins in cerebrospinal fluid of patients with recurrent depression and multiple sclerosis. *Lancet* 1998;**352**:1828–9.

279. Devinsky O, Cho ES, Petito CK, Price RW. Herpes zoster myelitis. *Brain* 1991;**114**:1181–96.

280. Dewhurst S, Skrincosky D, van Loon N. Human herpesvirus 7. *Expert Rev Mol Med* 1997;**1**:1–10.

281. Dhib-Jalbut S, Hoffman PM, Yamabe T, *et al.* Extracellular human T-cell lymphotropic virus type I Tax protein induces cytokine production in adult human microglial cells. *Ann Neurol* 1994;**36**:787–90.

282. Dinn JJ. Distribution of herpes simplex virus in acute necrotizing encephalitis. *J Pathol* 1979;**129**:135–8.

283. Dinn JJ. Transolfactory spread of virus in herpes simplex encephalitis. *Br Med J* 1980;**281**:1392.

284. Dobler G. Arboviruses causing neurological disorders in the central nervous system. *Arch Virol* 1996;**11**(Suppl):33–40.

285. Dobler G. Zoonotic tick-borne flaviviruses. *Vet Microbiol* 2010;**3–4**:221–8.

286. Dockrell DH. Human herpesvirus 6: molecular biology and clinical features. *J Med Microbiol* 2003;**52**:5–18.

287. Doherty RL, Carley JG, Filippich C, *et al.* Murray Valley encephalitis in Australia, 1974: antibody response in cases and community. *Aust N Z J Med* 1976;**6**:446–53.

288. Dolgopol VB, Husson GS. Infectious mononucleosis with neurologic complications: report of a fatal case. *Arch Intern Med* 1949;**83**:179–96.

289. Domachowske JB, Cunningham CK, Cummings DL, *et al.* Acute manifestations and neurologic sequelae of Epstein–Barr virus encephalitis in children. *Pediatr Infect Dis J* 1996;**15**:871–5.

290. Domegan LM, Atkins GJ. Apoptosis induction by the Therien and vaccine RA27/3 strains of rubella virus causes depletion of oligodendrocytes from rat neural cell cultures. *J Gen Virol* 2002;**83**:2135–43.

291. Domingues RB, Muniz MR, Jorge ML, *et al.* Human T cell lymphotropic virus type-1-associated myelopathy/tropical spastic paraparesis in Sao Paulo, Brazil: association with blood transfusion. *Am J Trop Med Hyg* 1997;**57**:56–9.

292. Domingues RB, Tsanaclis AM, Pannuti CS, *et al.* Evaluation of the range of clinical presentations of herpes simplex encephalitis by using polymerase chain reaction assay of cerebrospinal fluid samples. *Clin Infect Dis* 1997;**25**:86–91.

293. Donahue JG, Choo PW, Manson JE, Platt R. The incidence of herpes zoster. *Arch Intern Med* 1995;**155**:1605–9.

294. Donati D, Akhyani N, Fogdell-Hahn A, *et al.* Detection of human herpesvirus-6 in mesial temporal lobe epilepsy surgical brain resections. *Neurology* 2003;**61**:1405–11.

295. Dorfman LJ. Cytomegalovirus encephalitis in adults. *Neurology* 1973;**23**:136–44.

296. Dorig RE, Marcil A, Chopra A, Richardson CD. The human CD46 molecule is a receptor for measles virus (Edmonston strain). *Cell* 1993;**75**:295–305.

297. Dorries K. Molecular biology and pathogenesis of human polyomavirus infections. *Dev Biol Stand* 1998;**94**:71–9.

298. Dourado I, Cunha S, Teixeira MG, *et al.* Outbreak of aseptic meningitis associated with mass vaccination with a urabe-containing measles–mumps–rubella vaccine: implications for immunization programs. *Am J Epidemiol* 2000;**151**:524–30.

299. Doyle PW, Gibson G, Dolman CL. Herpes zoster ophthalmicus with contralateral hemiplegia: identification of cause. *Ann Neurol* 1983;**14**:84–5.

300. Drolet BS, Perng GC, Cohen J, *et al.* The region of the herpes simplex virus type 1 LAT gene involved in spontaneous reactivation does not encode a functional protein. *Virology* 1998;**242**:221–32.

301. Drummond CW, Eglin RP, Esiri MM. Herpes simplex virus encephalitis in a mouse model: PCR evidence for CNS latency following acute infection. *J Neurol Sci* 1994;**127**:159–63.

302. Dubois PJ, Heinz ER, Wessel HB, Zaias BW. Multiple cystic encephalomalacia of infancy: computed tomographic findings

in two cases with associated intracerebral calcification. *J Comput Assist Tomogr* 1979;3:97–102.

303. Dubois V, Dutronc H, Lafon ME, *et al.* Latency and reactivation of JC virus in peripheral blood of human immunodeficiency virus type 1-infected patients. *J Clin Microbiol* 1997;35:2288–92.

304. Du Pasquier RA, Corey S, Margolin DH, *et al.* Productive infection of cerebellar granule cell neurons by JC virus in an HIV+ individual. *Neurology* 2003; 6:775–82.

305. Du Pasquier RA, Koralnik IJ. Inflammatory reaction in progressive multifocal leukoencephalopathy: harmful or beneficial? *J Neurovirol* 2003;9(Suppl 1):25–31.

306. Dupuis M, Hull R, Wang H, *et al.* Molecular detection of viral causes of encephalitis and meningitis in New York State. *J Med Virol* 2011;12:2172–81.

307. Dutta K, Nazmi A, Basu A. Chemotherapy in Japanese encephalitis: are we there yet? *Infect Disord Drug Targets* 2011;3: 300–14.

308. Dyken PR, Cunningham SC, Ward LC. Changing character of subacute sclerosing panencephalitis in the United States. *Pediatr Neurol* 1989;5:339–41.

309. Ebel GD. Update on Powassan virus: emergence of a North American tick-borne flavivirus. *Annual Rev Entomol* 2010;95:110.

310. Eckels KH, Putnak R. Formalin-inactivated whole virus and recombinant subunit flavivirus vaccines. *Adv Virus Res* 2003;61:395–418.

311. Efstathiou S, Minson AC, Field HJ, *et al.* Detection of herpes simplex virus-specific DNA sequences in latently infected mice and in humans. *J Virol* 1986;57:446–55.

312. Eidelberg D, Sotrel A, Horoupian D, *et al.* Thrombotic cerebral vasculopathy associated with herpes zoster. *Ann Neurol* 1986;19:7–14.

313. Eizuru Y, Sakihama K, Minamishima Y, *et al.* Reevaluation of a case of progressive multifocal leukoencephalopathy previously diagnosed as simian-virus 40 (sv40) etiology. *Acta Pathol Jpn* 1993;43:327–32.

313a. Ellison D, Love S eds. *Neuropathology*. London: Mosby, 1998.

314. Elphick GF, Querbes W, Jordan JA, *et al.* The human polyomavirus, JCV, uses serotonin receptors to infect cells. *Science* 2004;5700:1380–83.

315. Embil JA, Camfield P, Artsob H, Chase DP. Powassan virus encephalitis resembling herpes simplex encephalitis. *Arch Intern Med* 1983;143:341–3.

316. Engle MJ, Diamond MS. Antibody prophylaxis and therapy against West Nile virus infection in wild-type and immunodeficient mice. *J Virol* 2003;77:12941–9.

317. Epstein MA, Achong BG, Barr YM. Virus particles in cultured lymphoblasts from Burkitt's lymphoma. *Lancet* 1964;i:702–3.

318. Erlendsson K, Swart T, Dwyer JM. Successful reversal of echovirus encephalitis in X-linked hypogammaglobulinemia by intraventricular administration of immunoglobulin. *N Engl J Med* 1985;312:351–3.

319. Ernst T, Chang L, Witt M, *et al.* Progressive multifocal leukoencephalopathy and human immunodeficiency virus-associated white matter lesions in AIDS: magnetization transfer MR imaging. *Radiology* 1999;210:539–43.

320. Erwin PC, Jones TF, Gerhardt RR, *et al.* La Crosse encephalitis in Eastern Tennessee: clinical, environmental, and entomological characteristics from a blinded cohort study. *Am J Epidemiol* 2002;155:1060–65.

321. Esiri MM. Herpes simplex encephalitis: an immunohistological study of the distribution of viral antigen within the brain. *J Neurol Sci* 1982;54:209–26.

322. Esiri MM, Morris CS, Millard PR. Fate of oligodendrocytes in HIV-1 infection. *AIDS* 1991;5:1081–8.

323. Evans SR, Ellis RJ, Chen H, *et al.* Peripheral neuropathy in HIV: prevalence and risk factors. *AIDS* 2011;25:919–28.

324. Everall IP, Luthert PJ, Lantos PL. Neuronal loss in the frontal cortex in HIV infection. *Lancet* 1991;337:1119–21.

325. Everall IP, Heaton RK, Marcotte TD, *et al.* Cortical synaptic density is reduced in mild to moderate HIV neurocognitive disorder. *Brain Pathol* 1999;9:209–17.

326. Everall IP, Vaida F, Khanlou N, *et al.* Cliniconeuropathologic correlates of HIV in the era of antiretroviral therapy. *J Neurovirol* 2009;15:360–70.

327. Evers S, Nabavi D, Rahman A, *et al.* Ischaemic cerebrovascular events in HIV infection: a cohort study. *Cerebrovasc Dis* 2003;15:199–205.

327a. Falagas ME, Snydman DR, Ruthazer R, *et al.* Primary cytomegalovirus infection in liver transplant recipients: comparison of infections transmitted via donor organs and via transfusions. Boston Center for Liver Transplantation CMVIG Study Group. *Clin Infect Dis* 1996;23:292–7.

327b. Fall AJ, Aitchison JD, Krause A, *et al.* Donor organ transmission of varicella zoster due to cardiac transplantation. *Transplantation* 2000;70:211–13.

328. Farber S, Hill A, Connerly M, Dingle J. Encephalitis in infants and children caused by the virus of the eastern variety of equine encephalitis. *J Am Med Assoc* 1940;114:1725–31.

329. Fareed MU, Spivack JG. Two open reading frames (ORF1 and ORF2) within the 2.0-kilobase latency-associated transcript of herpes simplex virus type 1 are not essential for reactivation from latency. *J Virol* 1994;68:8071–81.

330. Farrington CP. Subacute sclerosing panencephalitis in England and Wales: transient effects and risk estimates. *Statist Med* 1991;10:1733–44.

331. Deleted in proof.

332. Feder HM, Jr, Long SS. Herpetic whitlow: epidemiology, clinical characteristics, diagnosis, and treatment. *Am J Dis Child* 1983;137:861–3.

333. Feki I, Marrakchi C, Ben Hmida M, *et al.* Epidemic West Nile virus encephalitis in Tunisia. *Neuroepidemiology* 2005;24:1–7.

334. Feldman S, Lott L. Varicella in children with cancer: impact of antiviral therapy and prophylaxis. *Pediatrics* 1987;80:465–72.

335. Fischmeister G, Wiesbauer P, Holzmann HM, *et al.* Enteroviral meningoencephalitis in immunocompromised children after matched unrelated donor-bone marrow transplantation. *Pediatr Hematol Oncol* 2000;5:393–9.

336. Fitch MT, van de Beek D. Drug insight: steroids in CNS infectious diseases: new indications for an old therapy. *Nat Clin Pract Neurol* 2008;2:97–104.

337. Flano E, Jia Q, Moore J, *et al.* Early establishment of gamma-herpesvirus latency: implications for immune control. *J Immunol* 2005;174:4972–8.

338. Florescu DF, Kalil AC. Cytomegalovirus infections in non-immunocompromised and immunocompromised patients in the intensive care unit. *Infect Dis Drug Targets* 2011;11:354–64.

339. Fodor PA, Levin MJ, Weinberg A, *et al.* Atypical herpes simplex virus encephalitis diagnosed by PCR amplification of viral DNA from CSF. *Neurology* 1998;51:554–9.

340. Fotheringham J, Akhyani N, Vortmeyer A, *et al.* Detection of active human herpesvirus-6 infection in the brain: correlation with polymerase chain reaction detection in cerebrospinal fluid. *J Infect Dis* 2007;3:450–54.

341. Fotheringham J, Donati D, Akhyani N, *et al.* Association of human herpesvirus-6B with mesial temporal lobe epilepsy. *PLoS Med* 2007;5:e180.

342. Francisci D, Sensini A, Fratini D, *et al.* Acute fatal necrotizing hemorrhagic encephalitis caused by Epstein–Barr virus in a young adult immunocompetent man. *J Neurovirol* 2004;10:414–17.

343. Frange P, Michon J, Fromantin I, *et al.* Enterovirus 71 meningoencephalitis during chemotherapy in a child with metastatic osteosarcoma. *J Pediatr Hematol Oncol* 2007;8:566–8.

344. Fratkin JD, Leis AA, Stokic DS, *et al.* Spinal cord neuropathology in human West Nile virus infection. *Arch Pathol Lab Med* 2004;128:533–7.

345. Freeman AF, Jacobsohn DA, Shulman ST, *et al.* A new complication of stem cell transplantation: measles inclusion body encephalitis. *Pediatrics* 2004;114:e657–60.

346. Frey TK. Neurological aspects of rubella virus infection. *Intervirology* 1997;40:167–75.

347. Fujisaki H, Tanaka-Taya K, Tanabe H, *et al.* Detection of human herpesvirus 7 (HHV-7) DNA in breast milk by polymerase chain reaction and prevalence of HHV-7 antibody in breast-fed and bottle-fed children. *J Med Virol* 1998;56:275–9.

347a. Fukuda H, Umehara F, Kawahigashi N, *et al.* Acute disseminated myelitis after Japanese B encephalitis vaccination. *J Neurol Sci* 1997;148:113–15.

348. Fukuda S, Furuta Y, Takasu T, *et al.* The significance of herpes viral latency in the spiral ganglia. *Acta Otolaryngol* 1994;514(Suppl):108–10.

349. Fuller GN, Jacobs JM, Guiloff RJ. Nature and incidence of peripheral nerve syndromes in HIV infection. *J Neurol Neurosurg Psychiatry* 1993;56:372–81.

349a. Furukawa Y, Fujisawa J, Osame M, *et al.* Frequent clonal proliferation of human T-cell leukemia virus type 1 (HTLV-1)-infected T cells in HTLV-1-associated myelopathy (HAM-TSP). *Blood* 1992;80:1012–16.

349b. Furuta Y, Fukuda S, Chida E, *et al.* Reactivation of herpes simplex virus type 1 in patients with Bell's palsy. *J Med Virol* 1998;54:162–6.

349c. Furuta Y, Fukuda S, Suzuki S, *et al.* Detection of varicella-zoster virus DNA in patients with acute peripheral facial palsy by the polymerase chain reaction, and its use for early diagnosis of zoster sine herpete. *J Med Virol* 1997;52:316–9.

349d. Furuta Y, Ohtani F, Aizawa H, *et al.* Varicella-zoster virus reactivation is an important cause of acute peripheral facial paralysis in children. *Pediatr Infect Dis J* 2005;24:97–101.

350. Furuta Y, Takasu T, Sato KC, *et al.* Latent herpes simplex virus type 1 in human geniculate ganglia. *Acta Neuropathol* 1992;84:39–44.

351. Furuta Y, Takasu T, Fukuda S, *et al.* Latent herpes simplex virus type 1 in human vestibular ganglia. *Acta Otolaryngol* 1993;503(Suppl):85–9.

352. Gaeta A. Verzaro S, Cristina LM, *et al.* Diagnosis of neurological herpesvirus infections: real time PCR in cerebral spinal fluid analysis. *New Microbiol* 2009;4: 333–40.

353. Gallant JE, Moore RD, Richman DD, *et al.* Incidence and natural history of cytomegalovirus disease in patients with advanced human immunodeficiency virus disease treated with zidovudine. The Zidovudine Epidemiology Study Group. *J Infect Dis* 1992;166:1223–7.

354. Gannon P, Khan MZ, Kolson DL. Current understanding of HIV-associated neuro-cognitive disorders (HAND) pathogenesis. *Curr Opin Neurol* 2011;24:275–83.

355. Gao R, Dong L, Dong J, *et al.* A systematic molecular pathology study of a laboratory confirmed H5N1 human case. *PLoS One* 2010;10:e13315.

356. Garen PD, Tsai TF, Powers JM. Human eastern equine encephalitis: immunohisto-chemistry and ultrastructure. *Mod Pathol* 1999;12:646–52.

357. Garnett CT, Erdman D, Xu W, Gooding LR. Prevalence and quantitation of species C adenovirus DNA in human mucosal lymphocytes. *J Virol* 2002;76:10608–16.

358. Gasnault J, Taoufik Y, Goujard C, *et al.* Prolonged survival without neurological improvement in patients with AIDS-related progressive multifocal leuko-encephalopathy on potent combined antiretroviral therapy. *J Neurovirol* 1999;5:421–9.

359. Gatus BJ, Rose MR. Japanese B encephalitis: epidemiological, clinical and pathological aspects. *J Infect* 1983;6:213–18.

360. Gavin P, Yogev R. Central nervous system abnormalities in pediatric HIV infection. *Pediatr Neurosurg* 1999;31:115–23.

361. Gea-Banacloche J, Johnson RT, Bagic A, *et al.* West Nile virus: pathogenesis and therapeutic options. *Ann Intern Med* 2004;140:545–53.

362. Gelb L. Varicella zoster virus. In: Fields B, Knipe D, Chanock R, Al E eds. *Fields' virology.* New York: Raven Press, 1990:2011–54.

363. Deleted in proof.

364. Gelpi E, Preusser M, Garzuly F, *et al.* Visualization of Central European tick-borne encephalitis infection in fatal human cases. *J Neuropathol Exp Neurol* 2005;64:506–12.

365. Gershon AA, Mervish N, LaRussa P, *et al.* Varicella-zoster virus infection in children with underlying human immu-nodeficiency virus infection. *J Infect Dis* 1997;176:1496–500.

365a. Gessain A. Virological aspects of tropical spastic paraparesis/HTLV-I associated myelopathy and HTLV-I infection. *J Neu-rovirol* 1996;2:299–306.

366. Gessain A, Gout O, Saal F, *et al.* Epidemiology and immunovirology of human T-cell leukemia/lymphoma virus type I-associated adult T-cell leukemia and chronic myelopathies as seen in France. *Cancer Res* 1990;50:5692s–6s.

367. Gherardi RK, Lebargy F, Gaulard P, *et al.* Necrotizing vasculitis and HIV replication in peripheral nerves. *N Engl J Med* 1989;321:685–6.

368. Ghez D, Lepelletier Y, Lambert S, *et al.* Neuropilin-1 is involved in human T-cell lymphotropic virus type 1 entry. *J Virol* 2006;14:6844–54.

369. Ghosh S. Guillain-Barre syndrome complicating mumps. *Lancet* 1967;i:895–6.

370. GiaRusso MH, Koeppen AH. Atypical progressive multifocal leukoencepha-lopathy and primary cerebral malignant lymphoma. *J Neurol Sci* 1978;35:2–3.

371. Gilbert GL, Dickson KE, Waters MJ, *et al.* Outbreak of enterovirus 71 infection in Victoria, Australia, with a high incidence of neurologic involvement. *Pediatr Infect Dis J* 1988;7:484–8.

372. Gilbert L, Jones LD, Hudson PJ, *et al.* Role of small mammals in the persistence of Louping-ill virus: field survey and tick co-feeding studies. *Med Vet Entomol* 2000;14:277–82.

373. Gilbert L, Jones LD, Laurenson MK, *et al.* Ticks need not bite their red grouse hosts to infect them with louping ill virus. *Proc Biol Sci* 2004;271(Suppl 4):S202–5.

373a. Gilbert SC. Bell's palsy and herpesvi-ruses. *Herpes* 2002;9:70–3.

374. Gilden DH, Dueland AN, Devlin ME, *et al.* Varicella-zoster virus reactivation without rash. *J Infect Dis* 1992;166(Suppl 1):S30–34.

375. Gilden DH, Gesser R, Smith J, *et al.* Presence of VZV and HSV-1 DNA in human nodose and celiac ganglia. *Virus Genes* 2001;23:145–7.

376. Gilden DH, Mahalingam R, Cohrs RJ, *et al.* The protean manifestations of varicella-zoster virus vasculopathy. *J Neurovirol* 2002;8(Suppl 2):75–9.

377. Gilden DH, Cohrs RJ, Mahalingam R. Clinical and molecular pathogenesis of varicella virus infection. *Viral Immunol* 2003;16:243–58.

378. Gilden DH, Mahalingam R, Cohrs RJ, Tyler KL. Herpesvirus infections of the nervous system. *Nat Clin Pract Neurol* 2007;2:82–94.

379. Giobbia M, Carniato A, Scotton PG, *et al.* Cytomegalovirus-associated transverse myelitis in a non-immunocompromised patient. *Infection* 1999;27:228–30.

380. Gode GR, Bhide NK. Two rabies deaths after corneal grafts from one donor. *Lancet* 1988;ii:791.

381. Godoy AJ, Kira J, Hasuo K, Goto I. Characterization of cerebral white matter lesions of HTLV-I-associated myelopathy/tropical spastic paraparesis in comparison with multiple sclerosis and collagen vasculitis: a semiquantitative MRI study. *J Neurol Sci* 1995;133:102–11.

382. Goetz AM, Goldrick BA. West Nile virus: a primer for infection control professionals. *Am J Infect Control* 2004;32:101–5.

383. Goh KJ, Tan CT, Chew NK, *et al.* Clinical features of Nipah virus encephalitis among pig farmers in Malaysia. *N Engl J Med* 2000;342:1229–35.

384. Goldfield M, Welsh JN, Taylor BF. The 1959 outbreak of Eastern encephali-tis in New Jersey. 5. The inapparent infection:disease ratio. *Am J Epidemiol* 1968;87:32–3.

385. Goncalves DU, Proietti FA, Ribas JG, *et al.* Epidemiology, treatment, and prevention of human T-cell leukemia virus type 1-associated diseases. *Clin Microbiol Rev* 2010;3:577–89.

386. Goncalves MA, Sa-Neto RJ, Brazil TK. Outbreak of aggressions and transmission of rabies in human beings by vampire bats in northeastern Brazil. *Rev Soc Bras Med Trop* 2002;35:461–4.

387. Gonzalez LA, Villa AM, Kohler G, *et al.* Further studies on HTLV-I associated myelopathy in Argentina. *Medicina* 1998;58:411–14.

388. Gonzalez-Dunia D, Sauder C, de la Torre JC. Borna disease virus and the brain. *Brain Res Bull* 1997;44:647–64.

389. Goodman AD, Mock DJ, Powers JM, *et al.* Human herpesvirus 6 genome and antigen in acute multiple sclerosis lesions. *J Infect Dis* 2003;187:1365–76.

389a. Goodman JL. Possible transmission of herpes simplex virus by organ transplantation. *Transplantation* 1989;47:609–13.

390. Goodpasture HC, Poland JD, Francy DB, *et al.* Colorado tick fever: clinical, epidemiologic, and laboratory aspects of 228 cases in Colorado in 1973-1974. *Ann Intern Med* 1978;88:303–10.

391. Gordon S. The macrophage: past, present and future. *Eur J Immunol* 2007;37 Suppl 1:S9–17.

392. Gotuzzo E, De Las Casas C, Deza L, *et al.* Tropical spastic paraparesis and HTLV-I infection: clinical and epidemiological study in Lima, Peru. *J Neurol Sci* 1996;143:114–17.

393. Goubau P, Carton H, Kazadi K, *et al.* HTLV seroepidemiology in a central African population with high incidence of tropical spastic paraparesis. *Trans R Soc Trop Med Hyg* 1990;84:577–9.

394. Gould EA, Higgs S. Impact of climate change and other factors on emerging arbovirus diseases. *Trans R Soc Trop Med Hyg* 2009;2:109–21.

395. Gradoth N, Weitzman S, Lehmann EE. Acute anterior myelitis complicating West Nile fever. *Arch Neurol* 1979;36:172–3.

396. Grafe MR, Wiley CA. Spinal cord and peripheral nerve pathology in AIDS: the roles of cytomegalovirus and human immunodeficiency virus. *Ann Neurol* 1989;25:561–6.

397. Grant RM, Weitzman SS, Sherman CG, *et al.* Fulminant disseminated Varicella Zoster virus infection without skin involvement. *J Clin Virol* 2002; 24:7–12.

398. Grassi MP, Clerici F, Perin C, *et al.* Microglial nodular encephalitis and ventriculoencephalitis due to cytomegalo-virus infection in patients with AIDS: two distinct clinical patterns. *Clin Infect Dis* 1998;27:504–8.

399. Gray F. *Atlas of the neuropathology of HIV infection.* Oxford: Oxford University Press, 1993.

400. Gray F, Chimelli L, Mohr M, *et al.* Fulminating multiple sclerosis-like leukoen-cephalopathy revealing HIV infection. *Neurology* 1991;41:105–9.

401. Gray F, Geny C, Lionnet F, *et al.* Etude neuropathologique de 135 cas adultes de syndrome d'immuno-deficience acquise (SIDA). *Ann Pathol* 1991b;11:236–47.

402. Gray F, Hurtrel M, Hurtel B. Early central nervous system changes in HIV infection. *Neuropathol Appl Neurobiol* 1993;19:3–9.

403. Gray F, Belec L, Lescs MC, *et al*. Varicella-zoster virus infection of the central nervous system in the acquired immune deficiency syndrome. *Brain* 1994;117: 987–99.

404. Gray F, Scaravilli F, Everall I, *et al*. Neuropathology of early HIV-1 infection. *Brain Pathol* 1996;6:1–15.

405. Gray F, Belec L, Chretien F, *et al*. Acute, relapsing brain oedema with diffuse blood–brain barrier alteration and axonal damage in AIDS. *Neuropathol Appl Neurobiol* 1998;24:209–16.

406. Gray F, Adle-Biassette H, Brion F, *et al*. Neuronal apoptosis in HIV infection. *J Neurovirol* 2000;6:S38–43.

407. Gray F, Chretien F, Vallat-Decouvelaere AV, Scaravilli F. The changing pattern of HIV neuropathology in the HAART era. *J Neuropathol Exp Neurol* 2003;62: 429–40.

408. Gray F, Bazille C, Adle-Biassette H, *et al*. Central nervous system immune reconstitution disease in AIDS patients receiving highly active antiretroviral treatment. *J Neurovirol* 2005;11:16–22.

408a. Gray F, Lescure FX, Adle-Biassette H, *et al*. Encephalitis with infiltration by CD8+ lymphocytes in HIV patients receiving combination antiretroviral treatment. *Brain Pathol* 2013 Sept; 23(5):525–33.

409. Green SH, Wirtschafter JD. Ophthalmoscopic findings in subacute sclerosing panencephalitis. *Br J Ophthalmol* 1973;57:780–87.

410. Greenberg M, Abramson H, Cooper HM. The relation between recent injections and paralytic poliomyelitis in children. *Am J Publ Health* 1952;42:142.

411. Greenspan JS, Greenspan D, Lennette ET, *et al*. Replication of Epstein–Barr virus within the epithelial cells of oral 'hairy' leukoplakia, an AIDS-associated lesion. *N Engl J Med* 1985;313:1564–71.

412. Gregoire SM, van Pesch V, Goffette S, *et al*. Polymerase chain reaction analysis and oligoclonal antibody in the cerebrospinal fluid from 34 patients with varicella-zoster virus infection of the nervous system. *J Neurol Neurosurg Psychiatry* 2006;8:938–42.

413. Gregory CR, Latimer KS, Niagro FD, *et al*. Detection of eastern equine encephalomyelitis virus RNA in formalin-fixed, paraffin-embedded tissues using DNA in situ hybridization. *J Vet Diag Invest* 1996;8:151–5.

414. Gresikova M, Kaluzova M. Biology of tick-borne encephalitis virus. *Acta Virol* 1997;41:115–24.

415. Gressens P, Langston C, Mitchell WJ, Martin JR. Detection of viral DNA in neonatal herpes encephalitis autopsy tissues by solution-phase PCR: comparison with pathology and immunohistochemistry. *Brain Pathol* 1993;3:237–50.

416. Gressens P, Langston C, Martin JR. In situ PCR localization of herpes simplex virus DNA sequences in disseminated neonatal herpes encephalitis. *J Neuropathol Exp Neurol* 1994;53:469–82.

417. Greten TF, Slansky JE, Kubota R, *et al*. Direct visualization of antigen-specific T cells: HTLV-1 Tax11–19.-specific CD8(1) T cells are activated in peripheral blood and accumulate in cerebrospinal fluid from HAM/TSP patients. *Proc Natl Acad Sci U S A* 1998;95:7568–73.

418. Grimstad PR, Barrett CL, Humphrey RL, *et al*. Serologic evidence for widespread infection with LaCrosse and St Louis encephalitis viruses in the Indiana human population. *Am J Epidemiol* 1987;119:913–30.

419. Gritsun TS, Lashkevich VA, Gould EA. Tick-borne encephalitis. *Antiviral Res* 2003;57:129–46.

420. Gromeier M, Wimmer E. Mechanism of injury-provoked poliomyelitis. *J Virol* 1998;72:5056–60.

421. Gromeier M, Lu HH, Bernhardt G, *et al*. The human poliovirus receptor: receptor–virus interaction and parameters of disease specificity. *Ann N Y Acad Sci* 1995;753:19–36.

422. Grose C, Feorino PM. Epstein–Barr virus and transverse myelitis. *Lancet* 1973;i:892.

422a. Grose C, Henle W, Henle G, Feorino PM. Primary Epstein–Barr virus infections in acute neurologic diseases. *N Engl J Med* 1975;292:392–5.

423. Gu J, Xie Z, Gao Z, *et al*. H5N1 infection of the respiratory tract and beyond: a molecular pathology study. *Lancet* 2007;9593:1137–45.

424. Gudo ES, Bhatt NB, Bila DR, *et al*. Co-infection by human immunodeficiency virus type 1 (HIV-1) and human T cell leukemia virus type 1 (HTLV-1): does immune activation lead to a faster progression to AIDS? *BMC Infect Dis* 2009;9:211.

425. Guess H. Population-based studies of varicella complications. *Pediatrics* 1986;78:723–7.

426. Gullotta F, Masini T, Scarlato G, Kuchelmeister K. Progressive multifocal leukoencephalopathy and gliomas in a HIV-negative patient. *Pathol Res Pract* 1992;188:964–72.

427. Gunther G, Haglund M, Lindquist L, *et al*. Tick-bone encephalitis in Sweden in relation to aseptic meningo-encephalitis of other etiology: a prospective study of clinical course and outcome. *J Neurol* 1997;244:230–38.

428. Gutierrez J, Issacson RS, Koppel BS. Subacute sclerosing panencephalitis: an update. *Dev Med Child Neurol* 2010;10:901–7.

429. Haan KM, Longnecker R. Coreceptor restriction within the HLA-DQ locus for Epstein–Barr virus infection. *Proc Natl Acad Sci U S A* 2000;97:9252–7.

430. Hadfield MG, Seidlin M, Houff SA, *et al*. Echovirus meningomyeloencephalitis with administration of intrathecal immunoglobulin. *J Neuropathol Exp Neurol* 1985;44:520–29.

431. Haga S, Yoshimura M, Motoi Y, *et al*. Detection of Borna disease virus genome in normal human brain tissue. *Brain Res* 1997;770:307–9.

432. Haginoya K, Ike K, Iinuma K, *et al*. Chronic progressive mumps virus encephalitis in a child. *Lancet* 1995;346:50.

433. Hagiwara K, Kamitani W, Takamura S, *et al*. Detection of Borna disease virus in a pregnant woman and her fetus. *Vet Microbiol* 2000;72:207–16.

434. Haglund M, Gunther G. Tick-borne encephalitis: pathogenesis, clinical course and long-term follow-up. *Vaccine* 2003;21:S11–18.

435. Haglund M, Forsgren M, Lindh G, Lindquist L. A 10-year follow-up study of tick-borne encephalitis in the Stockholm area and a review of the literature: need for a vaccination strategy. *Scand J Infect Dis* 1996;28:217–24.

436. Hair LS, Nuovo G, Powers JM, *et al*. Progressive multifocal leukoencephalopathy in patients with human immunodeficiency virus. *Hum Pathol* 1992;23:663–7.

437. Hall CB, Long CE, Schnabel KC, *et al*. Human herpesvirus-6 infection in children. A prospective study of complications and reactivation. *N Engl J Med* 1994;7:432–8.

438. Hall RA, Scherret JH, Mackenzie JS. Kunjin virus: an Australian variant of West Nile? *Ann N Y Acad Sci* 2001;951:153–60.

439. Hall WW, Choppin PW. Measle-virus proteins in the brain tissue of patients with subacute sclerosing panencephalitis. *N Engl J Med* 1981;304:1152–5.

440. Hall WW, Lamb RA, Choppin PW. Measles and subacute sclerosing panencephalitis virus proteins: lack of antibodies to the M protein in patients with subacute sclerosing panencephalitis. *Proc Natl Acad Sci U S A* 1979;76:2047–51.

441. Halliday E, Winkelstein J, Webster AD. Enteroviral infections in primary immunodeficiency (PID): a survey of morbidity and mortality. *J Infect* 2003;46:1–8.

442. Halstead SB, Thomas SJ. New Japanese encephalitis vaccines: alternatives to production in mouse brain. *Expert Rev Vaccines* 2011;3:355–64.

443. Hambleton S. Chickenpox. *Curr Opin Infect Dis* 2005;18:235–40.

444. Hamilton RL, Achim C, Grafe MR, *et al*. Herpes simplex virus brainstem encephalitis in an AIDS patient. *Clin Neuropathol* 1995;14:45–50.

445. Hammer SM, Connolly KJ. Viral aseptic meningitis in the United States: clinical features, viral etiologies, and differential diagnosis. *Curr Clin Top Infect Dis* 1992;12:1–25.

446. Hammon WM, Reeves WC. California encephalitis virus: a newly described agent. I: evidence of natural infection in man and other animals. *Calif Med* 1952;77:303–9.

447. Han CS, Miller W, Haake R, Weisdorf D. Varicella tester infection after bone-marrow transplantation: incidence, risk-factors and complications. *Bone Marrow Transplant* 1994;13:277–83.

448. Hanna JN, Carney IK, Smith GA, *et al*. Australian bat lyssavirus infection: a second human case, with a long incubation period. *Med J Aust* 2000;172:597–9.

449. Hanshaw JB, Scheiner AP, Moxley AW, *et al*. School failure and deafness after 'silent' congenital cytomegalovirus. *N Engl J Med* 1976;295:468–70.

450. Hara H, Morita M, Iwaki T, *et al*. Detection of human T lymphotrophic virus type I (HTLV-I) proviral DNA and analysis of T cell receptor V beta CDR3 sequences in spinal cord lesions of HTLV-I-associated myelopathy/tropical spastic paraparesis. *J Exp Med* 1994;180:831–9.

451. Harding B, Baumer J. Congenital varicella-zoster: a serologically proven case with necrotizing encephalitis and malformation. *Acta Neuropathol* 1988;76:311–15.

452. Hardinger KL, Miller B, Storch GA, *et al*. West Nile virus-associated meningoencephalitis in two chronically immunosuppressed renal transplant recipients. *Am J Transplant* 2003;3:1312–15.

452a. Harvala H, Simmonds P. Human parecho-viruses: biology, epidemiology and clinical significance. *J Clin Virol* 2009;45(1):1–9.

453. Hattwick MA, Weis TT, Stechschulte CJ, et al. Recovery from rabies: a case report. *Ann Intern Med* 1972;76:931–42.

454. Hausler MG, Ramaekers VT, Reul J, et al. Early and late onset manifestations of cerebral vasculitis related to varicella zoster. *Neuropediatrics* 1998;29:202–7.

455. Haymaker WI. Western equine encephalitis: pathology. *Neurology* 1958;8:881.

456. Hayward WS, Neel BG, Astrin SM. Activation of a cellular onc gene by promoter insertion in ALV-induced lymphoid leukosis. *Nature* 1981;290:475–80.

457. Heath CW, Jr, Brodsky AL, Potolsky AI. Infectious mononucleosis in a general population. *Am J Epidemiol* 1972; 95:46–52.

458. Hedley-Whyte E, Smith B, Tyler H, Peterson W. Multifocal leukoencephalopathy with remission and five year survival. *J Neuropathol Exp Neurol* 1966;25:107–16.

459. Heggie AD, Robbins FC. Natural rubella acquired after birth: clinical features and complications. *Am J Dis Child* 1969;118:12–17.

460. Heinz FX. Molecular aspects of TBE virus research. *Vaccine* 2003;21(Suppl 1):S3–10.

460a. Held JR, Lopez Adaros H. Neurological disease in man following administration of suckling mouse brain antirabies vaccine. *Bull World Health Org* 1972;46:321–7.

461. Hemachudha T, Phuapradit P. Rabies. *Curr Opin Neurol* 1997;10:260–67.

462. Hemachudha T, Panpanich T, Phanuphak P, et al. Immune activation in human rabies. *Trans R Soc Trop Med Hyg* 1993;87:106–8.

463. Hemachudha T, Wacharapluesadee S, Mitrabhakdi E, et al. Pathophysiology of human paralytic rabies. *J Neurovirol* 2005;11:93–100.

464. Heneine W, Kaplan JE, Gracia F, et al. HTLV-II endemicity among Guaymi Indians in Panama. *N Engl J Med* 1991;324:565.

465. Hensleigh PA, Glover DB, Cannon M. Systemic Herpesvirus hominis in pregnancy. *J Reprod Med* 1979;22:171–6.

466. Herndon RM, Johnson RT, Davis LE, Descalzi LR. Ependymitis in mumps virus meningitis: electron microscopical studies of cerebrospinal fluid. *Arch Neurol* 1974;30:475–9.

467. Herrmann M, von der Lieth CW, Stehling P, et al. Consequences of a subtle sialic acid modification on the murine polyomavirus receptor. *J Virol* 1997;71:5922–31.

468. Hierons R, Janota I, Corsellis JA. The late effects of necrotizing encephalitis of the temporal lobes and limbic areas: a clinico-pathological study of 10 cases. *Psychol Med* 1978;8:21–42.

469. Higa K, Dan K, Manabe M. Varicella-zoster virus infections during pregnancy: hypothesis concerning the mechanisms of congenital malformations. *Obstet Gynecol* 1987;69:214–22.

470. Hill JM, Sederati F, Javier RT, et al. Herpes simplex virus latent phase transcription facilitates in vivo reactivation. *Virology* 1990;174:117–25.

471. Hilton DA, Love S, Fletcher A, Pringle JH. Absence of Epstein–Barr virus RNA in multiple sclerosis as assessed by in situ hybridisation. *J Neurol Neurosurg Psychiatry* 1994;57:975–6.

472. Hirai H, Suzuki T, Fujisawa J, et al. Tax protein of human T-cell leukemia virus type I binds to the ankyrin motifs of inhibitory factor kappa B and induces nuclear translocation of transcription factor NF-kappa B proteins for transcriptional activation. *Proc Natl Acad Sci U S A* 1994;91:3584–8.

473. Hirano A, Ayata M, Wang AH, Wong TC. Functional analysis of matrix proteins expressed from cloned genes of measles virus variants that cause subacute sclerosing panencephalitis reveals a common defect in nucleocapsid binding. *J Virol* 1993;67:1848–53.

474. Ho DD, Rota TR, Schooley RT, et al. Isolation of HTLV-III from cerebrospinal fluid and neural tissues of. *N Engl J Med* 1985a;313:1493–7.

475. Ho DD, Sarngadharan MG, Resnick L, et al. Primary human T-lymphotropic virus type III infection. *Ann Intern Med* 1985;103:880–83.

476. Ho K, Garancis JC, Paegle RD, et al. Progressive multifocal leukoencephalopathy and malignant lymphoma of the brain in a patient with immunosuppressive therapy. *Acta Neuropathol* 1980;52:81–3.

477. Ho M, Chen ER, Hsu KH, et al. An epidemic of enterovirus 71 infection in Taiwan. *N Engl J Med* 1999;341:929–35.

477a. Hoare M, Woodall T, Alexander GJ. Bell's palsy associated with IFN-α and ribavirin therapy for hepatitis C virus infection. *J Interferon Cytokine Res* 2005;25:174–6.

478. Holland NR, Power C, Mathews VP, et al. Cytomegalovirus encephalitis in acquired immunodeficiency syndrome. *Neurology* 1994;44:507–14.

479. Holman RC, Torok TJ, Belay ED, et al. Progressive multifocal leukoencephalopathy in the United States, 1979–1994: increased mortality associated with HIV infection. *Neuroepidemiology* 1998;17:303–9.

480. Holmes DA, Purdy DE, Chao DY, et al. Comparative analysis of immunoglobulin M (IgM) capture enzyme-linked immunosorbent assay using virus-like particles or virus-infected mouse brain antigens to detect IgM antibody in sera from patients with evident flaviviral infections. *J Clin Microbiol* 2005;43:3227–36.

481. Holmes GP, Hilliard JK, Klontz KC, et al. B virus (Herpesvirus simiae) infection in humans: epidemiologic investigation of a cluster. *Ann Intern Med* 1990;112:833–9.

482. Holmes MV, Desai M, Dosekun O, et al. Is the diagnosis at hand? *Lancet* 2010;375:1134.

483. Holmoy T, Kvale EO, Vartdal F. Cerebrospinal fluid CD41 T cells from a multiple sclerosis patient cross-recognize Epstein–Barr virus and myelin basic protein. *J Neurovirol* 2004;10:278–83.

484. Holzmann H. Diagnosis of tick-borne encephalitis. *Vaccine* 2003;21(Suppl 1):S36–40.

485. Homan EJ, Zuluaga FN, Yuill TM, Lorbacher H. Studies on the transmission of Venezuelan equine encephalitis virus by Colombian simuliidae (Diptera). *Am J Trop Med Hyg* 1985;34:799–804.

486. Honda H, Shimizu Y, Rutter M. No effect of MMR withdrawal on the incidence of autism: a total population study. *J Child Psychol Psychiatry* 2005;46:572–9.

487. Deleted in proof.

488. Hoshino S, Hayashi A, Ohkoshi N, et al. A case of post-poliomyelitis muscular atrophy with cranial nerve signs and widespread muscular atrophy of the extremities. *Rinsho Shinkeigaku* 1997;37:407–9.

489. Hosseinipour MC, Smith NH, Simpson EP, et al. Middle cerebral artery vasculitis and stroke after varicella in a young adult. *South Med J* 1998;91:1070–72.

490. Houff SA, Burton RC, Wilson RW, et al. Human-to-human transmission of rabies virus by corneal transplant. *N Engl J Med* 1979;300:603–4.

491. Houff SA, Major EO, Katz DA, et al. Involvement of JC virus-infected mononuclear cells from the bone marrow and spleen in the pathogenesis of progressive multifocal leukoencephalopathy. *N Engl J Med* 1988;318:301–5.

492. Hsia SH, Wu CT, Chang JJ, et al. Predictors of unfavorable outcomes in enterovirus 71-related cardiopulmonary failure in children. *Pediatr Infect Dis J* 2005;24:331–4.

493. Hsu AA, Staats BA. 'Postpolio' sequelae and sleep-related disordered breathing. *Mayo Clin Proc* 1998;73:216–24.

494. Huang C, Morse D, Slater B, et al. Multiple-year experience in the diagnosis of viral central nervous system infections with a panel of polymerase chain reaction assays for detection of 11 viruses. *Clin Infect Dis* 2004;39:630–35.

495. Huang CC, Liu CC, Chang YC, et al. Neurologic complications in children with enterovirus 71 infection. *N Engl J Med* 1999;341:936–42.

496. Huang LM, Lee CY, Lee PI, et al. Meningitis caused by human herpesvirus-6. *Arch Dis Child* 1991;66:1443–4.

497. Hubalek Z, Halouzka J. West Nile fever: a reemerging mosquito-borne viral disease in Europe. *Emerg Infec Dis* 1999;5:643–50.

498. Huff JL, Barry PA. B-virus (Cercopithecine herpesvirus 1) infection in humans and macaques: potential for zoonotic disease. *Emerg Infect Dis* 2003;9:246–50.

499. Hughes BA, Kimmel DW, Aksamit AJ. Herpes zoster-associated meningoencephalitis in patients with systemic cancer. *Mayo Clin Proc* 1993;68:652–5.

500. Hunfeld KP, Brade V. Zoonotic Babesia: possibly emerging pathogens to be considered for tick-infested humans in Central Europe. *Int J Med Microbiol* 2004;293(Suppl 37):93–103.

500a. Hunt JR. On herpetic inflammations of the geniculate ganglion: a new syndrome. *J Nerv Ment Dis* 1907;34:73–96.

501. Huy BV, Tu HC, Luan TV, Lindqvist R. Early mental and neurological sequelae after Japanese B encephalitis. *Southeast Asian J Trop Med Public Health* 1994;25:549–53.

502. Idrissova Zh R, Boldyreva MN, Dekonenko EP, et al. Acute disseminated encephalomyelitis in children: clinical features and HLA-DR linkage. *Eur J Neurol* 2003;10:537–46.

503. Igarashi A, Tanaka M, Morita K, et al. Detection of west Nile and Japanese encephalitis viral genome sequences in cerebrospinal fluid from acute encephalitis cases in Karachi, Pakistan. *Microbiol Immunol* 1994;38:827–30.

504. Ijichi S, Osame M. Human T lymphotropic virus type I (HTLV-I)-associated myelopathy/tropical spastic paraparesis

(HAM/TSP): recent perspectives. *Int Med* 1995;**34**:713–21.

505. Ike K, Haginoya K, Suzuki Y, *et al.* A case of chronic mumps virus encephalitis manifesting intractable epileptic seizures. *Jpn J Psychiatr Neurol* 1990;**44**:356–7.

506. Ikeda K, Akiyama H, Kondo H, *et al.* Numerous glial fibrillary tangles in oligodendroglia in cases of subacute sclerosing panencephalitis with neurofibrillary tangles. *Neurosci Lett* 1995;**194**:133–5.

507. Ikegami T, Makino S. [Rift Valley fever virus.] *Uirusu* 2004;**54**:229–35.

508. Ikegami T, Makino S. Rift valley fever vaccines. *Vaccine* 2009;**27**(Suppl 4):D69–72.

509. Imai S, Usui N, Sugiura M, *et al.* Epstein–Barr virus genomic sequences and specific antibodies in cerebrospinal fluid in children with neurologic complications of acute and reactivated EBV infections. *J Med Virol* 1993;**40**:278–84.

510. Inman M, Perng GC, Henderson G, *et al.* Region of herpes simplex virus type 1 latency-associated transcript sufficient for wild-type spontaneous reactivation promotes cell survival in tissue culture. *J Virol* 2001;**75**:3636–46.

511. Deleted in proof.

512. Irie S, Saito T, Nakamura K, *et al.* Association of anti-GM2 antibodies in Guillain–Barre syndrome with acute cytomegalovirus infection. *J Neuroimmunol* 1996;**68**:19–26.

513. Ishiguro N, Yamada S, Takahashi T, *et al.* Meningo-encephalitis associated with HHV-6 related exanthem subitum. *Acta Paediatr Scand* 1990;**79**:987–9.

514. Ishii T, Matsushita M, Hamada S. Characteristic residual neuropathological features of Japanese B encephalitis. *Acta Neuropathol* 1977;**38**:181–6.

515. Israele V, Shirley P, Sixbey JW. Excretion of the Epstein–Barr virus from the genital tract of men. *J Infect Dis* 1991;**163**:1341–3.

516. Ito M, Go T, Okuno T, Mikawa H. Chronic mumps virus encephalitis. *Pediatr Neurol* 1991;**7**:467–70.

517. Ito Y, Ando Y, Kimura H, *et al.* Polymerase chain reaction-proved herpes simplex encephalitis in children. *Pediatr Infect Dis J* 1998;**17**:29–32.

518. Itzhaki RF, Lin WR, Shang D, *et al.* Herpes simplex virus type 1 in brain and risk of Alzheimer's disease. *Lancet* 1997;**349**:241–4.

519. Iwamasa T, Yoshitake H, Sakuda H, *et al.* Acute ascending necrotizing myelitis in Okinawa caused by herpes simplex virus type 2. *Virch Archiv A Pathol Anat Histopathol* 1991;**418**:71–5.

519a. Iwamoto M, Jernigan DB, Guasch A, *et al.* Transmission of West Nile virus from an organ donor to four transplant recipients. *N Engl J Med* 2003;**348**:2196–203.

520. Iwasaki Y, Zhao JX, Yamamoto T, Konno H. Immunohistochemical demonstration of viral antigens in Japanese encephalitis. *Acta Neuropathol* 1986;**70**:79–81.

521. Iwata Y, Takahashi K, Peng X, *et al.* Detection and sequence analysis of borna disease virus p24 RNA from peripheral blood mononuclear cells of patients with mood disorders or schizophrenia and of blood donors. *J Virol* 1998;**72**:10044–9.

522. Izumo S, Goto I, Itoyama Y, *et al.* Interferon-alpha is effective in HTLV-

I-associated myelopathy: a multicenter, randomized, double-blind, controlled trial. *Neurology* 1996;**46**:1016–21.

523. Izumo S, Umehara F, Kashio N, *et al.* Neuropathology of HTLV-1-associated myelopathy (HAM/TSP). *Leukemia* 1997;**11**:82–4.

524. Izumo S, Umehara F, Osame M. HTLV-I-associated myelopathy. *Neuropathology* 2000;**20**(Suppl):S65–8.

525. Izumo S. Neuropathology of HTLV-1-associated myelopathy (HAM/TSP). *Neuropathology* 2010;**18**:100–12.

526. Jabbour JT, Garcia JH, Lemmi H, *et al.* Subacute sclerosing panencephalitis: a multidisciplinary study of eight cases. *J Am Med Assoc* 1969;**207**:2248–54.

527. Jackson AC. Rabies virus infection: an update. *J Neurovirol* 2003;**9**:253–8.

528. Jacobson S, Lehky T, Nishimura M, *et al.* Isolation of HTLV-II from a patient with chronic, progressive neurological disease clinically indistinguishable from HTLV-I-associated myelopathy/tropical spastic paraparesis. *Ann Neurol* 1993;**33**:392–6.

528a. Jamal GA, Al-Husaini A. Bell's palsy and infection with rubella virus. *J Neurol Neurosurg Psychiatry* 1983;**46**:678–80.

529. Janssen RS, Cornblath DR, Epstein LG, *et al.* Nomenclature and research case definitions for neurological manifestations of HIV-1 infection. *Neurology* 1991;**41**:778–85.

530. Janssen RS, Kaplan JE, Khabbaz RF, *et al.* HTLV-I-associated myelopathy/tropical spastic paraparesis in the United States. *Neurology* 1991;**41**:1355–7.

531. Jaskula E, Dlubek D, Sedzimirska M, *et al.* Reactivations of cytomegalovirus, human herpes virus 6, and Epstein–Barr virus differ with respect to risk factors and clinical outcome after hematopoietic stem cell transplantation. *Transplant Proc* 2010;**8**:3273–6.

532. Javadi MA, Fayaz A, Mirdehghan SA, Ainollahi B. Transmission of rabies by corneal graft. *Cornea* 1996;**15**:431–3.

533. Jay V, Hwang P, Hoffman HJ, *et al.* Intractable seizure disorder associated with chronic herpes infection: HSV1 detection in tissue by the polymerase chain reaction. *Childs Nerv Syst* 1998;**14**:15–20.

534. Jeang KT, Giam CZ, Majone F, Aboud M. Life, death, and tax: role of HTLV-I oncoprotein in genetic instability and cellular transformation. *J Biol Chem* 2004;**279**:31991–4.

535. Jeha LE, Sila CA, Lederman RJ, *et al.* West Nile virus infection: a new acute paralytic illness. *Neurology* 2003;**61**:55–9.

536. Jenson HB. Human herpesvirus 8 infection. *Curr Opin Pediatr* 2003;**15**:85–91.

537. Jia XY, Briese T, Jordan I, *et al.* Genetic analysis of West Nile New York 1999 encephalitis virus. *Lancet* 1999;**354**:1971–2.

538. Johnson JM, Harrod R, Franchini G. Molecular biology and pathogenesis of the human T-cell leukaemia/lymphotropic virus type-1 (HTLV-1). *Int J Exp Pathol* 2001;**82**:135–47.

539. Johnson R. *Viral infections of the nervous system.* Philadelphia, PA: Lippincott Raven, 1998.

539a. Johnson R, Milbourn PE. Central nervous system manifestations of chicken pox. *Can Med Assoc J* 1970;**102**:831–4.

540. Johnson RT. Experimental rabies: studies of cellular vulnerability and pathogenesis

using fluorescent antibody staining. *J Neuropathol Exp Neurol* 1965;**24**:662–74.

541. Johnson RT. The pathogenesis of acute viral encephalitis and postinfectious encephalomyelitis. *J Infect Dis* 1987;**155**:359–64.

542. Johnson RT, Johnson KP, Edmonds CJ. Virus-induced hydrocephalus: development of aqueductal stenosis in hamsters after mumps infection. *Science* 1967;**157**:1066–7.

543. Johnson RT, Burke DS, Elwell M, *et al.* Japanese encephalitis: immunocytochemical studies of viral antigen and inflammatory cells in fatal cases. *Ann Neurol* 1985;**18**:567–73.

544. Johnson T, Nath A. Immune reconstitution inflammatory syndrome and the central nervous system. *Curr Opin Neurol* 2011;**24**:284–90.

545. Johnstone JA, Ross CA, Dunn M. Meningitis and encephalitis associated with mumps infection: a 10-year survey. *Arch Dis Child* 1972;**47**:647–51.

545a. Joki-Korpela P, Hyypia T. Diagnosis and epidemiology of echovirus 22 infections. *Clin Infect Dis* 1998;**27**(1):129–36.

546. Joncas JH. Epstein–Barr virus encephalitis and neurologic sequelae. *Pediatr Infect Dis J* 1997;**16**:336–7.

547. Jones CA, Walker KS, Badawi N. Antiviral agents for treatment of herpes simplex virus infection in neonates. *Cochrane Database Syst Rev* 2009;**3**:CD004206.

548. Jones KS, Petrow-Sadowski C, Bertolette DC, *et al.* Heparan sulfate proteoglycans mediate attachment and entry of human T-cell leukemia virus type 1 virions into CD4+ T cells. *J Virol* 2005;**20**:12692–702.

549. Jones RH, Ho DD, Forgacs P, *et al.* Acute fulminant fatal leukoencephalopathy as the only manifestation of HIV infection. *Ann Neurol* 1988;**23**:518–22.

550. Jonsson L, Stiernstedt G, Thomander L. Tick-borne Borrelia infection in patients with Bell's palsy. *Arch Otolaryngol Head Neck Surg* 1987;**113**:303–6.

551. Jonsson L, Sundqvist VA, Thomander L. Anti-herpes IgG and IgG subclass antibodies in Bell's palsy. *Acta Otolaryngol* 1988;**106**:1–9.

552. Jordan MC, Rousseau W, Stewart JA, *et al.* Spontaneous cytomegalovirus mononucleosis: clinical and laboratory observations in nine cases. *Ann Intern Med* 1973;**79**:153–60.

553. Kabins S, Keller R, Naragi S, Peitchel R. Viral ascending radiculomyelitis with severe hypoglycorrachia. *Arch Intern Med* 1976;**136**:933–5.

554. Kaiser PK, Lee MS, Martin DA. Occlusive vasculitis in a patient with concomitant West Nile virus infection. *Am J Ophthalmol* 2003;**136**:928–30.

555. Kaiser R. Tick-borne encephalitis in southwestern Germany. *Infection* 1996;**24**:398–9.

556. Kaiser R. The clinical and epidemiological profile of tick-borne encephalitis in southern Germany 1994–98.: a prospective study of 656 patients. *Brain* 1999;**122**:2067–78.

557. Kajiyama W, Kashiwagi S, Ikematsu H, *et al.* Intrafamilial transmission of adult T-cell leukemia virus. *J Infect Dis* 1986;**154**:851–7.

558. Kalayjian RC, Cohen ML, Bonomo RA, Flanigan TP. Cytomegalovirus ventriculoencephalitis in AIDS: a syndrome with

distinct clinical and pathologic features. *Medicine (Baltimore)* 1993;**72**:67–77.

559. Kalfayan B. Pathology of La Crosse virus infection in humans. *Prog Clin Biol Res* 1983;**123**:179–86.

560. Kamei A, Ichinohe S, Onuma R, *et al.* Acute disseminated demyelination due to primary human herpesvirus-6 infection. *Eur J Pediatr* 1997;**156**:709–12.

561. Kaminski HJ, Tresser N, Hogan RE, Martin E. Pathological analysis of spinal cords from survivors of poliomyelitis. *Ann N Y Acad Sci* 1995;**753**:390–93.

562. Kangro HO, Osman HK, Lan YL, *et al.* Seroprevalence of antibodies to human herpesviruses in England and Hong-Kong. *J Med Virol* 1994;**43**:91–6.

563. Kao M, Hamir AN, Rupprecht CE, *et al.* Detection of antibodies against Borna disease virus in sera and cerebrospinal fluid of horses in the USA. *Vet Rec* 1993;**132**:241–4.

564. Kaplan JE, Osame M, Kubota H, *et al.* The risk of development of HTLV-I-associated myelopathy/tropical spastic paraparesis among persons infected with HTLV-I. *J Acquir Immune Defic Syndr* 1990;**3**:1096–101.

565. Kaplan JE, Litchfield B, Rouault C, *et al.* HTLV-I-associated myelopathy associated with blood transfusion in the United States: epidemiologic and molecular evidence linking donor and recipient. *Neurology* 1991;**41**:192–7.

566. Kaplan JE, Abrams E, Shaffer N, *et al.* Low risk of mother-to-child transmission of human T lymphotropic virus type II in non-breast-fed infants. The NYC Perinatal HIV Transmission Collaborative Study. *J Infect Dis* 1992;**166**:892–5.

567. Katamine S, Moriuchi R, Yamamoto T, *et al.* HTLV-I proviral DNA in umbilical cord blood of babies born to carrier mothers. *Lancet* 1994;**343**:1326–7.

568. Katchanov J, Siebert E, Klingebiel R, Endres M. Infectious vasculopathy of intracranial large- and medium-sized vessels in neurological intensive care unit: a clinico-radiological study. *Neurocrit Care* 2010;**3**:369–74.

569. Kato A, Kitamura T, Takasaka T, *et al.* Detection of the archetypal regulatory region of JC virus from the tonsil tissue of patients with tonsillitis and tonsillar hypertrophy. *J Neurovirol* 2004;**4**:244–9.

570. Katow S. Molecular epidemiology of rubella virus in Asia: utility for reduction in the burden of diseases due to congenital rubella syndrome. *Pediatr Int* 2004;**46**:207–13.

571. Kawai H, Nishida Y, Sano Y, *et al.* HTLV-I-associated myelopathy (HAM) in Tokushima Prefecture: geographical and clinical studies in an area between endemic and non-endemic areas of HTLV-I infection. *Jpn J Med* 1991;**30**:534–41.

572. Kawakami N, Lassmann S, Li Z, *et al.* The activation status of neuroantigen-specific T cells in the target organ determines the clinical outcome of autoimmune encephalomyelitis. *J Exp Med* 2004;**199**:185–97.

573. Kaye JA, del Mar Melero-Montes M, Jick H. Mumps, measles, and rubella vaccine and the incidence of autism recorded by general practitioners: time trend analysis. *Br Med J* 2001;**322**:460–63.

574. Kealey GP, Aguiar J, Lewis RW, 2nd, *et al.* Cadaver skin allografts and transmission of

human cytomegalovirus to burn patients. *J Am Coll Surg* 1996;**182**:201–5.

575. Kedes DH, Operskalski E, Busch M, *et al.* The seroepidemiology of human herpesvirus 8. *Nat Med* 1996;**2**:918–24.

576. Keiser J, Maltese MF, Erlanger TE, *et al.* Effect of irrigated rice agriculture on Japanese encephalitis, including challenges and opportunities for integrated vector management. *Acta Trop* 2005;**95**:40–57.

577. Kennedy PG. Herpes simplex virus type 1 and Bell's palsy–a current assessment of the controversy. *J Neurovirol* 2010;**1**:1–5.

578. Kennedy PG, Adams JH, Graham DI, Clements GB. A clinico-pathological study of herpes simplex encephalitis. *Neuropathol Appl Neurobiol* 1988;**14**:395–415.

579. Khabbaz RF, Onorato IM, Cannon RO, *et al.* Seroprevalence of HTLV-1 and HTLV-2 among intravenous drug users and persons in clinics for sexually transmitted diseases. *N Engl J Med* 1992;**326**:375–80.

580. Khanna R, Burrows SR, Moss DJ. Immune regulation in Epstein–Barr virus-associated diseases. *Microbiol Rev* 1995;**59**:387–405.

581. Khetsuriani N, Holman RC, Anderson LJ. Burden of encephalitis-associated hospitalizations in the United States, 1988–1997. *Clin Infect Dis* 2002;**35**:175–82.

582. Khetsuriani N, Quiroz ES, Holman RC, Anderson LJ. Viral meningitis-associated hospitalizations in the United States, 1988–1999. *Neuroepidemiology* 2003;**22**:345–52.

583. Ki M, Park T, Yi SG, *et al.* Risk analysis of aseptic meningitis after measles–mumps–rubella vaccination in Korean children by using a case-crossover design. *Am J Epidemiol* 2003;**157**:158–65.

584. Kidd D, Howard RS, Williams AJ, *et al.* Late functional deterioration following paralytic poliomyelitis. *Q J Med* 1997;**90**:189–96.

585. Kim J, Booss J, Manuelidis E, Duncan C. Human eastern equine encephalitis: electron microscopic study of a brain biopsy. *Am J Clin Pathol* 1985;**84**:223–7.

586. Kim YK, Kim SH, Choi SH, *et al.* Failure to demonstrate Borna disease virus genome in peripheral blood mononuclear cells from psychiatric patients in Korea. *J Neurovirol* 1999;**5**:196–9.

587. Kimberlin DW. Herpes simplex virus infections of the central nervous system. *Semin Pediatr Infect Dis* 2003;**14**:83–9.

588. Kimberlin DW, Whitley RJ. Neonatal herpes: what have we learned. *Semin Pediatr Infect Dis* 2005;**16**:7–16.

589. Kimberlin DW, Lin CY, Jacobs RF, *et al.* Natural history of neonatal herpes simplex virus infections in the acyclovir era. *Pediatrics* 2001;**108**:223–9.

590. Kimoto T, Yamada T, Ueba N, *et al.* Laboratory diagnosis of Japanese encephalitis: comparison of the fluorescent antibody technique with virus isolation and serologic tests. *Biken J* 1968;**11**:157–68.

591. Kimura H, Futamura M, Kito H, *et al.* Detection of viral DNA in neonatal herpes simplex virus infections: frequent and prolonged presence in serum and cerebrospinal fluid. *J Infect Dis* 1991;**164**:289–93.

592. Kimura H, Aso K, Kuzushima K, *et al.* Relapse of herpes simplex encephalitis in children. *Pediatrics* 1992;**89**:891–4.

593. Kin T, Hirano M, Tonomura Y, Ueno S. Coexistence of Ramsay Hunt syndrome and varicella-zoster virus encephalitis. *Infection* 2006;**6**:352–4.

594. Kira J, Fujihara K, Itoyama Y, *et al.* Leukoencephalopathy in HTLV-I-associated myelopathy/tropical spastic paraparesis: MRI analysis and a two year follow-up study after corticosteroid therapy. *J Neurol Sci* 1991;**106**:41–9.

595. Kissling R. Eastern equine encephalitis in pheasants. *J Am Vet Med Assoc* 1958;**132**:466–8.

596. Klar A, Gross-Kieselstein E, Hurvitz H, Branski D. Bilateral Bell's palsy due to Mycoplasma pneumoniae infection. *Isr J Med Sci* 1985;**21**:692–4.

597. Klatt EC, Shibata D. Cytomegalovirus infection in the acquired immunodeficiency syndrome. *Arch Pathol Lab Med* 1988;**112**:540–44.

598. Kleffner I, Wersching H, Schwindt W, *et al.* Triad of visual, auditory and corticospinal tract lesions: a new syndrome in a patient with HIV infection. *AIDS* 2011;**25**:659–63.

599. Klein E. The complexity of the Epstein–Barr virus infection in humans. *Pathol Oncol Res* 1998;**4**:3–7.

600. Kleinman S, Swanson P, Allain JP, Lee H. Transfusion transmission of human T-lymphotropic virus types I and II: serologic and polymerase chain reaction results in recipients identified through look-back investigations. *Transfusion* 1993;**33**:14–18.

601. Kleinschmidt-DeMasters BK, Gilden DH. The expanding spectrum of herpesvirus infections of the nervous system. *Brain Pathol* 2001;**11**:440–51.

602. Kleinschmidt-DeMasters BK, Tyler KL. Progressive multifocal leukoencephalopathy complicating treatment with natalizumab and interferon beta-1a for multiple sclerosis. *N Engl J Med* 2005;**353**:369–74.

603. Kleinschmidt-DeMasters BK, Amlie-Lefond C, Gilden DH. The patterns of varicella zoster virus encephalitis. *Hum Pathol* 1996;**27**:927–38.

604. Kleinschmidt-DeMasters BK, Marder BA, Levi ME, *et al.* Naturally acquired West Nile virus encephalomyelitis in transplant recipients: clinical, laboratory, diagnostic, and neuropathological features. *Arch Neurol* 2004;**61**:1210–20.

605. Knezevic W, Carroll WM. Relapse of herpes simplex encephalitis after acyclovir therapy. *Aust N Z J Med* 1983;**13**:625–6.

606. Knobel DL, Cleaveland S, Coleman PG, *et al.* Re-evaluating the burden of rabies in Africa and Asia. *Bull World Health Organ* 2005;**83**:360–68.

607. Koffron AJ, Hummel M, Patterson BK, *et al.* Cellular localization of latent murine cytomegalovirus. *J Virol* 1998;**72**:95–103.

608. Kojaoghlanian T, Flomenberg P, Horwitz MS. The impact of adenovirus infection on the immunocompromised host. *Rev Med Virol* 2003;**13**:155–71.

609. Kollaritsch H, Chmelik V, Dontsenko I, *et al.* The current perspective on tick-borne encephalitis awareness and prevention in six Central and Eastern European countries: report from a meeting of experts convened to discuss TBE in their region. *Vaccine* 2011;**28**:4556–64.

610. Komaroff AL, Buchwald DS. Chronic fatigue syndrome: an update. *Annu Rev Med* 1998;**49**:1–13.

611. Kondo K, Kondo T, Okuno T, *et al.* Latent human herpesvirus 6 infection of human monocytes/macrophages. *J Gen Virol* 1991;**72**:1401–8.

612. Kondo K, Nagafuji H, Hata A, *et al.* Association of human herpesvirus 6 infection of the central nervous system with

recurrence of febrile convulsions. *J Infect Dis* 1993;**167**:1197–200.

613. Kondo K, Kaneshima H, Mocarski ES. Human cytomegalovirus latent infection of granulocyte-macrophage progenitors. *Proc Natl Acad Sci U S A* 1994;**91**:11879–83.

614. Kondo K, Shimada K, Sashihara J, *et al.* Identification of human herpesvirus 6 latency-associated transcripts. *J Virol* 2002;**76**:4145–51.

615. Konishi E, Suzuki T. Ratios of subclinical to clinical Japanese encephalitis (JE) virus infections in vaccinated populations: evaluation of an inactivated JE vaccine by comparing the ratios with those in unvaccinated populations. *Vaccine* 2002;**21**:98–107.

616. Koopman FS, Uegaki K, Gilhus NE, *et al.* Treatment for postpolio syndrome. *Cochrane Database Syst Rev* 2011;**2**:CD007818.

617. Koralnik IJ. Overview of the cellular immunity against JC virus in progressive multifocal leukoencephalopathy. *J Neurovirol* 2002;**8**(Suppl 2):59–65.

618. Koralnik IJ, Wuthrich C, Dang X, *et al.* JC virus granule cell neuronopathy: a novel clinical syndrome distinct from progressive multifocal leukoencephalopathy. *Ann Neurol* 2005;**4**:576–80.

619. Korimbocus J, Scaramozzino N, Lacroix B, *et al.* DNA probe array for the simultaneous identification of herpesviruses, enteroviruses, and flaviviruses. *J Clin Microbiol* 2005;**43**:3779–87.

620. Kornyey S. Contribution to the histology of tick-borne encephalitis. *Acta Neuropathol* 1978;**43**:179–83.

621. Koskiniemi M, Donner M, Pettay O. Clinical appearance and outcome in mumps encephalitis in children. *Acta Paediatr Scand* 1983;**72**:603–9.

622. Koskiniemi M, Piiparinen H, Rantalaiho T, *et al.* Acute central nervous system complications in varicella zoster virus infections. *J Clin Virol* 2002;**25**:293–301.

623. Kozlowski PB. Pediatric human immunodeficiency virus infection. In: Duckett S ed. *Pediatric neuropathology.* Baltimore, MD: Williams & Wilkins, 1995:435–47.

624. Kozlowski PB, Sher J, Dickson D, *et al.* Central nervous system in pediatric HIV infection: a multicenter study. In: Kozlowski PB, Snider DA, Vietze PM, Wisniewski HM eds. *Brain in pediatric AIDS.* Basel: Karger, 1990:132–46.

625. Kramer A, Maloney EM, Morgan OS, *et al.* Risk factors and cofactors for human T-cell lymphotropic virus type I (HTLV-I)-associated myelopathy/tropical spastic paraparesis (HAM/TSP) in Jamaica. *Am J Epidemiol* 1995;**142**:1212–20.

626. Krey HF, Stitz L, Ludwig H. Virus-induced pigment epithelitis in rhesus monkeys: clinical and histological finds. *Ophthalmologica* 1982;**185**:205–13.

627. Krishnan C, Kaplin AI, Deshpande DM, *et al.* Transverse myelitis: pathogenesis, diagnosis and treatment. *Front Biosci* 2004;**9**:1483–99.

628. Kristensson K, Dastur DK, Manghani DK, *et al.* Rabies: interactions between neurons and viruses: a review of the history of Negri inclusion bodies. *Neuropathol Appl Neurobiol* 1996;**22**:179–87.

629. Ku CC, Padilla JA, Grose C, *et al.* Tropism of varicella-zoster virus for human tonsillar CD4(1) T lymphocytes that express activation, memory, and skin homing markers. *J Virol* 2002;**76**:11425–33.

630. Kullnat MW, Morse RP. Choreoathetosis after herpes simplex encephalitis with basal ganglia involvement on MRI. *Pediatrics* 2008;**4**:e1003–7.

631. Kumar D, Prasad GV, Zaltzman J, *et al.* Community-acquired West Nile virus infection in solid-organ transplant recipients. *Transplantation* 2004;**77**:399–402.

632. Kumar R, Mathur A, Singh KB, *et al.* Clinical sequelae of Japanese encephalitis in children. *Indian J Med Res* 1993;**97**:9–13.

633. Kuno G. Persistence of arboviruses and antiviral antibodies in vertebrate hosts: its occurrence and impacts. *Rev Med Virol* 2001;**3**:165–90.

634. Kunz C. TBE vaccination and the Austrian experience. *Vaccine* 2003;**21**(Suppl 1):S50–55.

635. Kupila L, Vainionpaa R, Vuorinen T, *et al.* Recurrent lymphocytic meningitis: the role of herpesviruses. *Arch Neurol* 2004;**61**:1553–7.

636. Kupila L, Vuorinen T, Vainionpaa R, *et al.* Etiology of aseptic meningitis and encephalitis in an adult population. *Neurology* 2006;**1**:75–80.

637. Kuroda Y, Yukitake M, Kurohara K, *et al.* A follow-up study on spastic paraparesis in Japanese HAM/TSP. *J Neurol Sci* 1995;**132**:174–6.

638. Kustermann A, Zoppini C, Tassis B, *et al.* Prenatal diagnosis of congenital varicella infection. *Prenatal Diag* 1996;**16**:71–4.

639. Lafon M. Rabies virus receptors. *J Neurovirol* 2005;**11**:82–7.

640. Laghi L, Randolph AE, Chauhan DP, *et al.* JC virus DNA is present in the mucosa of the human colon and in colorectal cancers. *Proc Natl Acad Sci U S A* 1999;**13**:7484–9.

641. LaGrenade L, Hanchard B, Fletcher V, *et al.* Infective dermatitis of Jamaican children: a marker for HTLV-I infection. *Lancet* 1990;**336**:1345–7.

642. Lahat E, Barr J, Barkai G, *et al.* Long term neurological outcome of herpes encephalitis. *Arch Dis Child* 1999;**80**:69–71.

643. Lakeman FD, Koga J, Whitley RJ. Detection of antigen to herpes simplex virus in cerebrospinal fluid from patients with herpes simplex encephalitis. *J Infect Dis* 1987;**155**:1172–8.

644. Lakhanpal U, Sharma RC. An epidemiological study of 177 cases of human rabies. *Int J Epidemiol* 1985;**14**:614–17.

645. Lal RB, Gongora-Biachi RA, Pardi D, *et al.* Evidence for mother-to-child transmission of human T lymphotropic virus type II. *J Infect Dis* 1993;**168**:586–91.

646. Langer-Gould A, Atlas SW, Green AJ, *et al.* Progressive multifocal leukoencephalopathy in a patient treated with natalizumab. *N Engl J Med* 2005;**353**:375–81.

647. Langford TD, Letendre SL, Marcotte TD, *et al.* Severe, demyelinating leukoencephalopathy in AIDS patients on antiretroviral therapy. *AIDS* 2002;**16**:1019–29.

648. Lanzieri TM, Parise MS, Siqueira MM, *et al.* Incidence, clinical features and estimated costs of congenital rubella syndrome after a large rubella outbreak in Recife, Brazil, 1999–2000. *Pediatr Infect Dis J* 2004;**23**:1116–22.

649. Lavalle C, Pizarro S, Drenkard C, *et al.* Transverse myelitis: a manifestation of systemic lupus erythematosus strongly associated with antiphospholipid antibodies. *J Rheumatol* 1990;**17**:34–7.

650. Lee B. Envelope–receptor interactions in Nipah virus pathobiology. *Ann N Y Acad Sci* 2007;**51**:65.

651. Lee HH, Swanson P, Rosenblatt JD, *et al.* Relative prevalence and risk factors of HTLV-I and HTLV-II infection in US blood donors. *Lancet* 1991;**337**:1435–9.

652. Leen AM, Rooney CM. Adenovirus as an emerging pathogen in immunocompromised patients. *Br J Haematol* 2005;**128**:135–44.

653. Lehky TJ, Fox CH, Koenig S, *et al.* Detection of human T-lymphotropic virus type I (HTLV-I) tax RNA in the central nervous system of HTLV-I-associated myelopathy/tropical spastic paraparesis patients by in situ hybridization. *Ann Neurol* 1995;**37**:167–75.

654. Leib DA, Bogard CL, Kosz-Vnenchak M, *et al.* A deletion mutant of the latency-associated transcript of herpes simplex virus type 1 reactivates from the latent state with reduced frequency. *J Virol* 1989;**63**:2893–900.

655. Leite AC, Silva MT, Alamy AH, *et al.* Peripheral neuropathy in HTLV-I infected individuals without tropical spastic paraparesis/HTLV-I-associated myelopathy. *J Neurol* 2004;**251**: 877–81.

656. Lemon SM, Hutt LM, Shaw JE, *et al.* Replication of EBV in epithelial cells during infectious mononucleosis. *Nature* 1977;**268**:268–70.

657. Lennette EH, Caplan GE, Magoffin RL. Mumps virus infections simulating paralytic poliomyelitis. *Pediatrics* 1960;**25**:788–97.

658. Lentz TL. Rabies virus binding to an acetylcholine receptor alpha-subunit peptide. *J Mol Recognit* 1990;**3**:82–8.

659. Leon-Monzon ME, Dalakas MC. Detection of poliovirus antibodies and poliovirus genome in patients with the post-polio syndrome. *Ann N Y Acad Sci* 1995;**753**:208–18.

660. Leon-Monzon ME, Illa I, Dalakas MC. Expression of poliovirus receptor in human spinal cord and muscle. *Ann N Y Acad Sci* 1995;**753**:48–57.

661. Leonova GN, Sorokina MN, Krugliak SP. The clinico-epidemiological characteristics of Powassan encephalitis in the southern Soviet Far East. *Zh Mikrobiol Epidemiol Immunobiol* 1991;**3**:35–9.

662. Lesprit P, Chaline-Lehmann D, Authier FJ, *et al.* BK virus encephalitis in a patient with AIDS and lymphoma. *AIDS* 2001;**15**:1196–9.

663. Letendre SL. Central nervous system complications in HIV disease: HIV-associated neurocognitive disorder (HAND). *Top Antivir Med* 2011;**19**:137–42.

664. Deleted in proof.

665. Deleted in proof.

666. Levin MC, Krichavsky M, Berk J, *et al.* Neuronal molecular mimicry in immune-mediated neurologic disease. *Ann Neurol* 1998;**44**:87–98.

667. Levitt LP, Rich TA, Kinde SW, *et al.* Central nervous system mumps. A review of 64 cases. *Neurology* 1970;**20**:829–34.

667a. Levorson RE, Jantausch BA, Wiedermann BL, *et al.* Human parechovirus-3 infection: emerging pathogen in neonatal sepsis. *Pediatr Infect Dis J* 2009;**28**(6):545–7.

668. Levy JA. Viral studies of chronic fatigue syndrome. *Clin Infect Dis* 1994;**18**:S117–20.

669. Leyssen P, De Clercq E, Neyts J. Perspectives for the treatment of infections with Flaviviridae. *Clin Microbiol Rev* 2000;**13**:67–82.

670. Li E, Brown SL, Stupack DG, *et al.* Integrin alpha(v)beta1 is an adenovirus coreceptor. *J Virol* 2001;**75**:5405–9.

671. Lieb K, Staeheli P. Borna disease virus: does it infect humans and cause psychiatric disorders? *J Clin Virol* 2001;**21**:119–27.

672. Liedtke W, Opalka B, Zimmermann CW, Lignitz E. Age distribution of latent herpes simplex virus 1 and varicella-zoster virus genome in human nervous tissue. *J Neurol Sci* 1993;**116**:6–11.

673. Lima MA, Drislane FW, Koralnik IJ. Seizures and their outcome in progressive multifocal leukoencephalopathy. *Neurology* 2006;**2**:262–4.

674. Lima MA, Bernal-Cano F, Clifford DB, *et al.* Clinical outcome of long-term survivors of progressive multifocal leukoencephalopathy. *J Neurol Neurosurg Psychiatry* 2010;**11**:1288–91.

675. Lindberg C, Anderson O, Vahlne A, *et al.* Epidemiological investigation of the association between infectious mononucleosis and multiple sclerosis. *Neuroepidemiology* 1991;**10**:62–5.

676. Lindzen E, Jewells V, Bouldin TW, *et al.* Progressive tumefactive inflammatory central nervous system demyelinating disease in an AIDS patient treated with HAART. *J Neurovirol* 2008;**14**:569–73.

677. Lipkin WI, Schneemann A, Solbrig MV. Borna disease virus: implications for human neuropsychiatric illness. *Trends Microbiol* 1995;**3**:64–9.

678. Liston SL, Kleid MS. Histopathology of Bell's palsy. *Laryngoscope* 1989;**99**:23–6.

679. Liu H, Gao X, Liang G. Newly recognized mosquito-associated viruses in mainland China, in the last two decades. *Virol J* 2011;**1**:68.

680. Livorsi D, Anderson E, Qureshi S, *et al.* Brainstem encephalitis: an unusual presentation of herpes simplex virus infection. *J Neurol* 2010;**9**:1432–7.

681. Lloyd AR, Hickie I, Peterson PK. Chronic fatigue syndrome: current concepts of pathogenesis and treatment. *Curr Clin Top Infect Dis* 1999;**19**:135–59.

682. Lo MK, Rota PA. The emergence of Nipah virus, a highly pathogenic paramyxovirus. *J Clin Virol* 2008;**4**:396–400.

683. Longson M, Bailey A. Herpes encephalitis. In: Waterson A ed. *Recent advances in clinical virology*. Edinburgh: Churchill Livingstone, 1977:1–19.

684. Looi LM, Chua KB. Lessons from the Nipah virus outbreak in Malaysia. *The Malays J Pathol* 2007;**2**:63–7.

685. Love S, Koch P, Urbach H, Dawson TP. Chronic granulomatous herpes simplex encephalitis in children. *J Neuropathol Exp Neurol* 2004;**63**:1173–81.

686. Lowry PW. Arbovirus encephalitis in the United States and Asia. *J Lab Clin Med* 1997;**129**:405–11.

687. Lucas SB, Hounnou A, Peacock CS, *et al.* The mortality and pathology of HIV disease in a West African city. *AIDS* 1993;**7**:1569–79.

688. Lucas SB, Wong KT, Mahadeva, U. Fatal CD8+ T cell encephalitis: an observational study of an emerging complication in HIV-1 infected African patients on effective long term ART. Conference on Retroviruses and Opportunistic Infections (CROI). 2011;Abstract 398.

689. Luciano CA, Sivakumar K, Spector SA, Dalakas MC. Electrophysiologic and histologic studies in clinically unaffected muscles of patients with prior paralytic poliomyelitis. *Muscle Nerve* 1996;**19**:1413–20.

690. Lum LCS, Wong KT, Lam SK, *et al.* Fatal enterovirus 71 encephalomyelitis. *J Pediatr* 1998;**133**:795–8.

691. Lundgren AL, Czech G, Bode L, Ludwig H. Natural Borna disease in domestic animals others than horses and sheep. *Zentralbl Veterinarmed Reihe B* 1993;**40**:298–303.

692. Lundgren AL, Zimmermann W, Bode L, *et al.* Staggering disease in cats: isolation and characterization of the feline Borna disease virus. *J Gen Virol* 1995;**76**:2215–22.

693. Lungu O, Panagiotidis CA, Annunziato PW, *et al.* Aberrant intracellular localization of varicella-zoster virus regulatory proteins during latency. *Proc Natl Acad Sci U S A* 1998;**95**:7080–85.

694. Luppi M, Barozzi P, Morris C, *et al.* Human herpesvirus 6 latently infects early bone marrow progenitors in vivo. *J Virol* 1999;**73**:754–9.

695. Luppi M, Barozzi P, Santagostino G, *et al.* Molecular evidence of organ-related transmission of Kaposi sarcoma-associated herpesvirus or human herpesvirus-8 in transplant patients. *Blood* 2000;**96**:3279–81.

696. Lusso P, Secchiero P, Crowley RW, *et al.* CD4 is a critical component of the receptor for human herpesvirus 7: interference with human immunodeficiency virus. *Proc Natl Acad Sci U S A* 1994;**91**:3872–6.

697. Lynas C, Hill TJ, Maitland NJ, Love S. Latent infection with the MS strain of herpes simplex virus type 2 in the mouse following intracerebral inoculation. *J Neurol Sci* 1993;**120**:107–14.

698. Macdonald JC, Karavellas MP, Torriani FJ, *et al.* Highly active antiretroviral therapy-related immune recovery in AIDS patients with cytomegalovirus retinitis. *Ophthalmology* 2000;**107**:877–81.

699. Maciejewski JP, Bruening EE, Donahue RE, *et al.* Infection of hematopoietic progenitor cells by human cytomegalovirus. *Blood* 1992;**80**:170–78.

700. Mackenzie JS. Emerging viral diseases: an Australian perspective. *Emerg Infect Dis* 1999;**5**:1–8.

701. MacKenzie JS, Field HE. Emerging encephalitogenic viruses: lyssaviruses and henipaviruses transmitted by frugivorous bats. *Arch Virol Suppl* 2004;**18**:97–111.

702. Mackenzie JS, Williams DT. The zoonotic flaviviruses of southern, south-eastern and eastern Asia, and Australasia: the potential for emergent viruses. *Zoonoses Public Health* 2009;**6-7**:338–56.

703. Mackenzie JS, Chua KB, Daniels PW, *et al.* Emerging viral diseases of Southeast Asia and the Western Pacific. *Emerg Infect Dis* 2001;**7**(Suppl):497–504.

704. Mackenzie JS, Barrett AD, Deubel V. The Japanese encephalitis serological group of flaviviruses: a brief introduction to the group. *Curr Top Microbiol Immunol* 2002;**267**:1–10.

705. Mackenzie JS, Field HE, Guyatt KJ. Managing emerging diseases borne by fruit bats (flying foxes), with particular reference to henipaviruses and Australian bat lyssavirus. *J Appl Microbiol* 2003;**94**(Suppl):59–69.S.

706. Mackenzie JS, Gubler DJ, Petersen LR. Emerging flaviviruses: the spread and resurgence of Japanese encephalitis, West Nile and dengue viruses. *Nat Med* 2004;**10**(Suppl):S98–109.

707. Macsween KF, Crawford DH. Epstein–Barr virus: recent advances. *Lancet Infect Dis* 2003;**3**:131–40.

708. Madhusudana SN, Nagaraj D, Uday M, *et al.* Partial recovery from rabies in a six-year-old girl. *Int J Infect Dis* 2002;**6**:85–6.

709. Madsen KM, Hviid A, Vestergaard M, *et al.* MMR vaccination and autism: a population-based follow-up study. *Ugeskr Laeger* 2002;**164**:5741–4.

710. Maginnis MS, Atwood WJ. JC virus: an oncogenic virus in animals and humans? *Semin Cancer Biol* 2009;**4**:261–9.

711. Magliocco A, Demetrick D, Sarnat H, Hwang W. Varicella embryopathy. *Arch Pathol Lab Med* 1992;**116**:181–6.

712. Mahalingam R, Wellish MC, Dueland AN, *et al.* Localization of herpes simplex virus and varicella zoster virus DNA in human ganglia. *Ann Neurol* 1992;**31**:444–8.

713. Mahalingam R, Wellish M, Cohrs R, *et al.* Expression of protein encoded by varicella-zoster virus open reading frame 63 in latently infected human ganglionic neurons. *Proc Natl Acad Sci U S A* 1996;**93**:2122–4.

714. Mahieux R, Gessain A. The human HTLV-3 and HTLV-4 retroviruses: new members of the HTLV family. *Pathol Biol (Paris)* 2009;**2**:161–6.

715. Mahieux R, Gessain A, Truffert A, *et al.* Seroepidemiology, viral isolation, and molecular characterization of human T cell leukemia/lymphoma virus type I from La Reunion Island, Indian Ocean. *AIDS Res Hum Retrovir* 1994;**10**:745–52.

716. Mahmood F, Chiles RE, Fang Y, *et al.* Role of nestling mourning doves and house finches as amplifying hosts of St Louis encephalitis virus. *J Med Entomol* 2004;**41**:965–72.

717. Mainka C, Fuss B, Geiger H, *et al.* Characterization of viremia at different stages of varicella-zoster virus infection. *J Med Virol* 1998;**56**:91–8.

718. Maisner A, Neufeld J, Weingartl H. Organ- and endotheliotropism of Nipah virus infections in vivo and in vitro. *Thromb Haemost* 2009;**6**:1014–23.

719. Makhortova NR, Askovich P, Patterson CE, *et al.* Neurokinin-1 enables measles virus trans-synaptic spread in neurons. *Virology* 2007;**1**:235–44.

719a. Maller HM, Powars DF, Horowitz RE, Portnoy B. Fatal myocarditis associated with ECHO virus, type 22, infection in a child with apparent immunological deficiency. *J Pediatr* 1967;**71**(2):204–10.

720. Maloney EM, Cleghorn FR, Morgan OS, *et al.* Incidence of HTLV-I-associated myelopathy/tropical spastic paraparesis (HAM/TSP) in Jamaica and Trinidad. *J Acquir Immune Defic Syndr* 1998;**17**:167–70.

721. Mamidi A, DeSimone JA, Pomerantz RJ. Central nervous system infections in individuals with HIV-1 infection. *J Neurovirol* 2002;**8**:158–67.

722. Mandybur TI. The distribution of Alzheimer's neurofibrillary tangles and gliosis in chronic subacute sclerosing panencephalitis. *Acta Neuropathol* 1990;**80**:307–10.

723. Mandybur TI, Nagpaul AS, Pappas Z, Niklowitz WJ. Alzheimer neurofibrillary change in subacute sclerosing panencephalitis. *Ann Neurol* 1977;**1**:103–7.

724. Manel N, Kim FJ, Kinet S, *et al.* The ubiquitous glucose transporter GLUT-1 is a receptor for HTLV. *Cell* 2003;**115**: 449–59.

725. Manel N, Battini JL, Taylor N, Sitbon M. HTLV-1 tropism and envelope receptor. *Oncogene* 2005;**24**:6016–25.

726. Manet E, Bourillot PY, Waltzer L, Sergeant A. EBV genes and B cell proliferation. *Crit Rev Oncol Hematol* 1998;**28**:129–37.

727. Manning L, Laman M, Edoni H, *et al.* Subacute sclerosing panencephalitis in Papua New Guinean children: the cost of continuing inadequate measles vaccine coverage. *PLoS Negl Trop Dis* 2011;**1**:e932.

728. Marcelin AG, Roque-Afonso AM, Hurtova M, *et al.* Fatal disseminated Kaposi's sarcoma following human herpesvirus 8 primary infections in liver-transplant recipients. *Liver Transpl* 2004;**10**:295–300.

729. Marshall I. Murray Valley and Kunjin encephalitis. In: Monath T ed. *The arboviruses: ecology and epidemiology.* Boca Raton, FL: CRC Press, 1988:151–90.

730. Martin R, Marquardt P, O'Shea S, *et al.* Virus-specific and autoreactive T cell lines isolated from cerebrospinal fluid of a patient with chronic rubella panencephalitis. *J Neuroimmunol* 1989;**23**:1–10.

731. Marton R, Gotlieb-Stematsky T, Klein C, *et al.* Mild form of acute herpes simplex encephalitis in childhood. *Brain Dev* 1995;**17**:360–61.

732. Martyn CN, Cruddas M, Compston DA. Symptomatic Epstein–Barr virus infection and multiple sclerosis. *J Neurol Neurosurg Psychiatry* 1993;**56**:167–8.

732a. Marzocchetti A, Di Giambenedetto S, Cingolani A, *et al.* Reduced rate of diagnostic positive detection of JC virus DNA in cerebrospinal fluid in cases of suspected progressive multifocal leukoencephalopathy in the era of potent antiretroviral therapy. *J Clin Microbiol* 2005;**43**:4175–4177.

733. Matsui M, Kuroda Y. Aberrant immunity in the central nervous system in relation to disease progression in HAM/TSP. *Clin Immunol Immunopathol* 1997;**82**:203–6.

734. Matsumoto Y, Pyykkö JL, Patterson MJ, Yanagihara N. Facial nerve biopsy for etiologic clarification of Bell's palsy. *Ann Otol Rhinol Laryngol* 1988;**137**(Suppl):22–7.

735. Matsuoka E, Takenouchi N, Hashimoto K, *et al.* Perivascular T cells are infected with HTLV-I in the spinal cord lesions with HTLV-I-associated myelopathy/tropical spastic paraparesis: double staining of immunohistochemistry and polymerase chain reaction in situ hybridization. *Acta Neuropathol* 1998;**96**:340–46.

736. Mawle AC. Chronic fatigue syndrome. *Immunol Invest* 1997;**26**:269–73.

737. Mawle AC, Reyes M, Schmid DS. Is chronic fatigue syndrome an infectious disease? *Infect Agents Dis* 1994;**2**:387–9.

738. Mawle AC, Nisenbaum R, Dobbins JG, *et al.* The seroepidemiology of chronic fatigue syndrome: a case–control study. *Clin Infect Dis* 1995;**21**:1386–9.

739. Mayo DR, Booss J. Varicella zoster-associated neurologic disease without skin lesions. *Arch Neurol* 1989; **46**:313–15.

740. Mázló M, Szántó J. Morphological demonstration of the virus of tick-borne encephalitis in the human brain. *Acta Neuropathol* 1978;**43**:251–3.

741. McCall S, Vilensky JA, Gilman S, Taubenberger JK. The relationship between encephalitis lethargica and influenza: a critical analysis. *J Neurovirol* 2008;**3**:177–85.

742. McCarthy J, Amer J. Postvaricella acute transverse myelitis: a case presentation and review of the literature. *Pediatrics* 1978;**62**:202–4.

743. McCarthy VP, Zimmerman AW, Miller CA. Central nervous system manifestations of parainfluenza virus type 3 infections in childhood. *Pediatr Neurol* 1990;**6**:197–201.

744. McCombe JA, Auer RN, Maingat FG, *et al.* Neurologic immune reconstitution inflammatory syndrome in HIV/AIDS. *Neurology* 2009;**72**:835–41.

745. McCracken GJ, Jr, Shinefield HR, Cobb K, *et al.* Congenital cytomegalic inclusion disease: a longitudinal study of 20 patients. *Am J Dis Child* 1969;**117**:522–39.

746. McGowan JJ, Bryan JA, Gregg MB. Surveillance of arboviral encephalitis in the United States, 1955–1971. *Am J Epidemiol* 1973;**97**:199–207.

747. McGuire KL, Curtiss VE, Larson EL, Haseltine WA. Influence of human T-cell leukemia virus type I tax and rex on interleukin-2 gene expression. *J Virol* 1993;**67**:1590–99.

748. McIntosh B, Gear J. Wesselsbron fever. In: Beran G ed. *CRC handbook series in zoonoses. Section B: viral zoonoses.* Boca Raton, FL: CRC Press, 1981:224–6.

749. McIntosh BM, Russell D, dos Santos I, Gear JH. Rift Valley fever in humans in South Africa. *S Afr Med J* 1980;**58**:803–6.

750. McJunkin JE, de los Reyes EC, Irazuzta JE, *et al.* La Crosse encephalitis in children. *N Engl J Med* 2001;**344**:801–7.

751. McKendall RR, Sadiq SA, Calverley JR. Unusual manifestations of Epstein–Barr virus encephalomyelitis. *Infection* 1990;**18**:33–5.

752. McKendall RR, Oas J, Lairmore MD. HTLV-I-associated myelopathy endemic in Texas-born residents and isolation of virus from CSF cells. *Neurology* 1991;**41**:831–6.

753. McKinney RE, Katz SL, Wilfert CM. Chronic enteroviral meningoencephalitis in agammaglobulinemic patients. *Rev Infect Dis* 1987;**9**:334–56.

754. McQuaid S, Allen IV, McMahon J, Kirk J. Association of measles virus with neurofibrillary tangles in subacute sclerosing panencephalitis: a combined in situ hybridization and immunocytochemical investigation. *Neuropathol Appl Neurobiol* 1994;**20**:103–10.

755. Melanson M, Chalk C, Georgevich L, *et al.* Varicella-zoster virus DNA in CSF and arteries in delayed contralateral hemiplegia: evidence for viral invasion of cerebral arteries. *Neurology* 1996;**47**:569–70.

756. Melish ME, Hanshaw JB. Congenital cytomegalovirus infection. Developmental progress of infants detected by routine screening. *Am J Dis Child* 1973;**126**:190–94.

757. Mellerick DM, Fraser NW. Physical state of the latent herpes simplex virus genome in a mouse model system: evidence suggesting an episomal state. *Virology* 1987;**158**:265–75.

758. Menitove JE. Current risk of transfusion-associated human immunodeficiency virus infection. *Arch Pathol Lab Med* 1990;**114**:330–34.

759. Meyer K, Haring C, Howitt B. The etiology of epizootic encephalomyelitis of horses in the San Joaquin Valley. *Science* 1931;**74**:227–8.

760. Meyer-König U, Ebert K, Schrage B, *et al.* Simultaneous infection of healthy people with multiple human cytomegalovirus strains. *Lancet* 1998;**352**:1280–81.

761. Meyer-König U, Hufert FT, Duffner U, *et al.* G-CSF-mobilised granulocyte transfusion to an ALL patient complicated by cytomegalovirus transmission. *Bone Marrow Transplant* 2004;**34**:1095–6.

762. Michaels L. Histopathological changes in the temporal bone in Bell's palsy. *Acta Otolaryngol* 1990;**470**(Suppl): 114–17, 118.

763. Miles C, Hoffman W, Lai CW, Freeman JW. Cytomegalovirus-associated transverse myelitis. *Neurology* 1993;**43**:2143–5.

764. Miller E, Cradock WJ, Pollock TM. Consequences of confirmed maternal rubella at successive stages of pregnancy. *Lancet* 1982;**ii**:781–4.

765. Miller E, Goldacre M, Pugh S, *et al.* Risk of aseptic meningitis after measles, mumps, and rubella vaccine in UK children. *Lancet* 1993;**341**:979–82.

766. Miller G, Niederman JC, Andrews LL. Prolonged oropharyngeal excretion of EB virus following infectious mononucleosis. *N Engl J Med* 1973;**288**:229–31.

767. Miller M, Achiron A, Shaklai M, *et al.* Ethnic cluster of HTLV-I infection in Israel among the Mashhadi Jewish population. *J Med Virol* 1998;**56**:269–74.

768. Miller RF, Lucas SB, Hall-Craggs MA, *et al.* Comparison of MR imaging with neuropathological findings in the diagnosis of HIV- and CMV-associated central nervous system disease in AIDS. *J Neurol Neurosurg Psychiatry* 1997;**62**:346–51.

769. Miller RF, Isaacson PG, Hall-Craggs MA, *et al.* Cerebral CD8+ lymphocytosis in HIV-1 infected patients with immune restoration induced by HAART. *Acta Neuropathol* 2004;**108**:17–23.

770. Miralles P, Berenguer J, Garcia de Viedma D, *et al.* Treatment of AIDS-associated progressive multifocal leukoencephalopathy with highly active antiretroviral therapy. *AIDS* 1998;**12**:2467–72.

771. Misbah SA, Spickett GP, Ryba PC, *et al.* Chronic enteroviral meningoencephalitis in agammaglobulinemia: case report and literature review. *J Clin Immunol* 1992;**12**:266–70.

772. Mishra B, Kakkar N, Ratho RK, *et al.* Changing trend of SSPE over a period of ten years. *Indian J Public Health* 2005;**4**:235–7.

773. Misra UK, Kalita J. Anterior horn cells are also involved in Japanese encephalitis. *Acta Neurol Scand* 1997;**96**:114–17.

774. Misra UK, Kalita J. Movement disorders in Japanese encephalitis. *J Neurol* 1997;**244**:299–303.

775. Misra UK, Kalita J. Overview: Japanese encephalitis. *Prog Neurobiol* 2010;**2**:108–20.

776. Mitchell BM, Bloom DC, Cohrs RJ, *et al.* Herpes simplex virus-1 and varicella-zoster virus latency in ganglia. *J Neurovirol* 2003;**9**:194–204.

777. Mitchell CD. HIV-1 encephalopathy among perinatally infected children: neuropathogenesis and response to HAART. *Ment Retard Dev Disabil Res Rev* 2006;**12**:216–22.

778. Modlin JF. Update on enterovirus infections in infants and children. *Adv Pediatr Infect Dis* 1997;12:155–81.

779. Modlin JF, Jabbour JT, Witte JJ, Halsey NA. Epidemiologic studies of measles, measles vaccine, and subacute sclerosing panencephalitis. *Pediatrics* 1977;59:505–12.

780. Modlin JF, Halsey NA, Eddins DL, et al. Epidemiology of subacute sclerosing panencephalitis. *J Pediatr* 1979;94:231–6.

781. Moir S, Chun TW, Fauci AS. Pathogenetic mechanisms of HIV disease. *Annu Rev Pathol* 2011;6:223–48.

782. Monaco MC, Jensen PN, Hou J, et al. Detection of JC virus DNA in human tonsil tissue: evidence for site of initial viral infection. *J Virol* 1998;72:9918–23.

783. Monath TP. Arthropod-borne encephalitides in the Americas. *Bull World Health Organ* 1979;57:513–33.

784. Monath TP, Nystrom RR, Bailey RE, et al. Immunoglobulin M antibody capture enzyme-linked immunosorbent assay for diagnosis of St Louis encephalitis. *J Clin Microbiol* 1984;20:784–90.

785. Monno L, Di Stefano M, Zimatore GB, et al. Measurement of viral sequences in cerebrospinal fluid of AIDS patients with cerebral white-matter lesions using polymerase chain reaction. *AIDS* 1998;12:581–90.

786. Montes Santiago J, Perez Fernandez E, Gonzalez Vazquez L, et al. [Progressive multifocal leukoencephalopathy in patients with AIDS: is there a change in patients treated with highly active antiretroviral therapies?] *An Med Interna* 2002;19:230–33.

787. Montgomery RD. HTLV-1 and tropical spastic paraparesis: 1. Clinical features, pathology and epidemiology. *Trans R Soc Trop Med Hyg* 1989;83:724–8.

788. Morgan M, Moffat M, Ritchie L, et al. Is Bell's palsy a reactivation of varicella zoster virus? *J Infect* 1995;30:29–36.

789. Mori N, Prager D. Transactivation of the interleukin-1alpha promoter by human T-cell leukemia virus type I and type II Tax proteins. *Blood* 1996;87:3410–17.

790. Mori N, Gill PS, Mougdil T, et al. Interleukin-10 gene expression in adult T-cell leukemia. *Blood* 1996;88:1035–45.

791. Mori N, Mukaida N, Ballard DW, et al. Human T-cell leukemia virus type I Tax transactivates human interleukin 8 gene through acting concurrently on AP-1 and nuclear factor-kappaB-like sites. *Cancer Res* 1998;58:3993–4000.

792. Morimoto K, Patel M, Corisdeo S, et al. Characterization of a unique variant of bat rabies virus responsible for newly emerging human cases in North America. *Proc Natl Acad Sci U S A* 1996;93:5653–8.

793. Morinelli EN, Dugel PU, Lee M, et al. Opportunistic intraocular infections in AIDS. *Trans Am Ophthalmol Soc* 1992;90:97–108.

794. Moritoyo T, Reinhart TA, Moritoyo H, et al. Human T-lymphotropic virus type I-associated myelopathy and tax gene expression in CD41 T lymphocytes. *Ann Neurol* 1996;40:84–90.

795. Morriss MC, Rutstein RM, Rudy B, et al. Progressive multifocal leukoencephalopathy in an HIV-infected child. *Neuroradiology* 1997;39:142–4.

796. Mortimer JY, Spooner RJ. HIV infection transmitted through blood product treatment, blood transfusion, and tissue transplantation. *Commun Dis Rep CDR Rev* 1997;7:R130–32.

797. Mozzi F, Rebulla P, Lillo F, et al. HIV and HTLV infections in 1305 transfusion-dependent thalassemics in Italy. The COOLEYCARE Cooperative Group. *AIDS* 1992;6:505–8.

798. Mrak RE, Young L. Rabies encephalitis in humans: pathology, pathogenesis and pathophysiology. *J Neuropathol Exp Neurol* 1994;53:1–10.

799. Muhlemann K. The molecular epidemiology of mumps virus. *Infect Genet Evol* 2004;4:215–19.

800. Muir P, van Loon AM. Enterovirus infections of the central nervous system. *Intervirology* 1997;40:153–66.

801. Muir P, Nicholson F, Sharief MK, et al. Evidence for persistent enterovirus infection of the central nervous system in patients with previous paralytic poliomyelitis. *Ann N Y Acad Sci* 1995;753:219–32.

802. Muir P, Nicholson F, Spencer GT, et al. Enterovirus infection of the central nervous system of humans: lack of association with chronic neurological disease. *J Gen Virol* 1996;77:1469–76.

803. Muir P, Kammerer U, Korn K, et al. Molecular typing of enteroviruses: current status and future requirements. The European Union Concerted Action on Virus Meningitis and Encephalitis. *Clin Microbiol Rev* 1998;11:202–27.

804. Muller D, McDonald M, Stallman N, King J. Kunjin virus encephalomyelitis. *Med J Aust* 1986;144:41–2.

805. Muller WJ, Jones CA, Koelle DM. Immunobiology of herpes simplex virus and cytomegalovirus infections of the fetus and newborn. *Curr Immunol Rev* 2010;1:38–55.

806. Mulloy JC, Kislyakova T, Cereseto A, et al. Human T-cell lymphotropic/leukemia virus type 1 Tax abrogates p53-induced cell cycle arrest and apoptosis through its CREB/ATF functional domain. *J Virol* 1998;72:8852–60.

807. Murakami S, Mizobuchi M, Nakashiro Y, et al. Bell palsy and herpes simplex virus: identification of viral DNA in endoneurial fluid and muscle. *Ann Intern Med* 1996;124:27–30.

808. Murphy EL. The clinical epidemiology of human T-lymphotropic virus type II (HTLV-II). *J Acquir Immune Defic Syndr* 1996;13:S215–19.

809. Murphy EL, Fridey J, Smith JW, et al. HTLV-associated myelopathy in a cohort of HTLV-I and HTLV-II-infected blood donors. The REDS investigators. *Neurology* 1997;48:315–20.

810. Murtagh B, Wadia Y, Messner G, et al. West Nile virus infection after cardiac transplantation. *J Heart Lung Transplant* 2005;24:774–6.

811. Murthy JM. Guillain–Barre syndrome following specific viral infections: an appraisal. *J Assoc Physicians India* 1994;42:27–9.

812. Mustafa MM, Weitman SD, Winick NJ, et al. Subacute measles encephalitis in the young immunocompromised host: report of two cases diagnosed by polymerase chain reaction and treated with ribavirin and review of the literature. *Clin Infect Dis* 1993;16:654–60.

813. Mutton K, Guiver M. Laboratory techniques for human viral encephalitis diagnosis. *Infect Disord Drug Targets* 2011;3:206–34.

814. Myers MG, Connelly BL. Animal models of varicella. *J Infect Dis* 1992;166(Suppl 1):S48–50.

815. Nagel MA, Cohrs RJ, Mahalingam R, et al. The varicella zoster virus vasculopathies: clinical, CSF, imaging, and virologic features. *Neurology* 2008;11:853–60.

816. Nahmias AJ, Whitley RJ, Visintine AN, et al. Herpes simplex virus encephalitis: laboratory evaluations and their diagnostic significance. *J Infect Dis* 1982;145:829–36.

817. Nakagawa M, Izumo S, Ijichi S, et al. HTLV-I-associated myelopathy: analysis of 213 patients based on clinical features and laboratory findings. *J Neurovirol* 1995;1:50–61.

818. Nakajima H, Furutama D, Kimura F, et al. Herpes simplex virus type 2 infections presenting as brainstem encephalitis and recurrent myelitis. *Int Med* 1995;34:839–42.

819. Nakajima H, Furutama D, Kimura F, et al. Herpes simplex virus myelitis: clinical manifestations and diagnosis by the polymerase chain reaction method. *Eur Neurol* 1998;39:163–7.

820. Nakamura K, Yanagihara N. Neutralization antibody to herpes simplex virus type 1 in Bell's palsy. *Ann Otol Rhinol Laryngol* 1988;137(Suppl):18–21.

821. Nalca A, Fellows PF, Whitehouse CA. Vaccines and animal models for arboviral encephalitides. *Antiviral Res* 2003;60:153–74.

822. Naniche D, Varior-Krishnan G, Cervoni F, et al. Human membrane cofactor protein (CD46) acts as a cellular receptor for measles virus. *J Virol* 1993;67:6025–32.

823. Nathanson N. The pathogenesis of poliomyelitis: what we don't know. *Adv Virus Res* 2008;71:1–50.

824. Nathanson N, Martin JR. The epidemiology of poliomyelitis: enigmas surrounding its appearance, epidemicity, and disappearance. *Am J Epidemiol* 1979;110:672–92.

825. Nathwani D, McIntyre PG, White K, et al. Fatal human rabies caused by European bat Lyssavirus type 2a infection in Scotland. *Clin Infect Dis* 2003;37:598–601.

826. Nelson CT, Demmler GJ. Cytomegalovirus infection in the pregnant mother, fetus, and newborn infant. *Clin Perinatol* 1997;24:151–60.

827. Nemerow GR. Cell receptors involved in adenovirus entry. *Virology* 2000;274:1–4.

828. Nett RJ, Campbell GL, Reisen WK. Potential for the emergence of Japanese encephalitis virus in California. *Vector Borne Zoonotic Dis* 2009;5:511–17.

829. Neumann H, Wekerle H. Neuronal control of the immune response in the central nervous system: linking brain immunity to neurodegeneration. *J Neuropathol Exp Neurol* 1998;57:1–9.

830. Neumann R, Genersch E, Eggers HJ. Detection of adenovirus nucleic acid sequences in human tonsils in the absence of infectious virus. *Virus Res* 1987;7:93–7.

831. Nicolas JC, Ingrand D, Fortier B, Bricout F. A one-year virological survey of acute intussusception in childhood. *J Med Virol* 1982;9:267–71.

832. Nicoll JA, Maitland NJ, Love S. Autopsy neuropathological findings in 'burnt out' herpes simplex encephalitis and use of the polymerase chain reaction to detect

viral DNA. *Neuropathol Appl Neurobiol* 1991;17:375–82.

833. Nicoll JA, Maitland NJ, Love S. Use of the polymerase chain reaction to detect herpes simplex virus DNA in paraffin sections of human brain at necropsy. *J Neurol Neurosurg Psychiatry* 1991;54:167–8.

834. Nicoll JA, Kinrade E, Love S. PCR-mediated search for herpes simplex virus DNA in sections of brain from patients with multiple sclerosis and other neurological disorders. *J Neurol Sci* 1992;113:144–51.

835. Nicoll JA, Love S, Kinrade E. Distribution of herpes simplex virus DNA in the brains of human long-term survivors of encephalitis. *Neurosci Lett* 1993;157:215–18.

836. Nicoll JA, Love S, Burton PA, Berry PJ. Autopsy findings in two cases of neonatal herpes simplex virus infection: detection of virus by immunohistochemistry, in situ hybridization and the polymerase chain reaction. *Histopathology* 1994;24:257–64.

837. Niederman JC, Evans AS, Subrahmanyan L, McCollum RW. Prevalence, incidence and persistence of EB virus antibody in young adults. *N Engl J Med* 1970;282:361–5.

838. Nielsen S, Petito CK, Urmacher CD, Posner JB. Subacute encephalitis in AIDS: a postmortem study. *Am J Clin Pathol* 1984;82:678–82.

839. Nimmannitya S, Halstead SB, Cohen SN, Margiotta MR. Dengue and chikungunya virus infection in man in Thailand, 1962–1964: I. Observations on hospitalized patients with hemorrhagic fever. *Am J Trop Med Hyg* 1969;18:954–71.

839a. Nix WA, Maher K, Johansson ES, et al. Detection of all known parechoviruses by real-time PCR. *J Clin Microbiol* 2008;46(8):2519–24.

839b. Nix WA, Maher K, Pallansch MA, Oberste MS. Parechovirus typing in clinical specimens by nested or semi-nested PCR coupled with sequencing. *J Clin Virol* 2010;48(3):202–7.

840. Nkowane BM, Wassilak SG, Orenstein WA, et al. Vaccine-paralytic poliomyelitis: United States – 1973 through 1984. *J Am Med Assoc* 1987;257:1335–40.

841. Nolan MA, Craig ME, Lahra MM, et al. Survival after pulmonary edema due to enterovirus 71 encephalitis. *Neurology* 2003;60:1651–6.

842. Novoa LJ, Nagra RM, Nakawatase T, et al. Fulminant demyelinating encephalomyelitis associated with productive HHV-6 infection in an immunocompetent adult. *J Med Virol* 1997;52:301–8.

843. Noyce RS, Bondre DG, Ha MN, et al. Tumor cell marker PVRL4 (nectin 4) is an epithelial cell receptor for measles virus. *PLoS Pathog* 2011;8:e1002240.

844. Nussinovitch M, Brand N, Frydman M, Varsano I. Transverse myelitis following mumps in children. *Acta Paediatr* 1992;81:183–4.

845. Nybakken GE, Oliphant T, Johnson S, et al. Structural basis of West Nile virus neutralization by a therapeutic antibody. *Nature* 2005;437:764–9.

846. Obara Y, Furuta Y, Takasu T, et al. Distribution of herpes simplex virus types 1 and 2 genomes in human spinal ganglia studied by PCR and in situ hybridization. *J Med Virol* 1997;52:136–42.

847. Oberste MS, Maher K, Kilpatrick DR, Pallansch MA. Molecular evolution of the human enteroviruses: correlation of serotype with VP1 sequence and application to picornavirus classification. *J Virol* 1999;73:1941–8.

848. Oberste MS, Maher K, Michele SM, et al. Enteroviruses 76, 89, 90 and 91 represent a novel group within the species Human enterovirus A. *J Gen Virol* 2005;86(Part 2):445–51.

849. Oelschlaeger C, Dziewas R, Reichelt D, et al. Severe leukoencephalopathy with fulminant cerebral oedema reflecting immune reconstitution inflammatory syndrome during HIV infection: a case report. *J Med Case Rep* 2010;4:214.

850. Ogata H, Oka K, Mitsudome A. Hydrocephalus due to acute aqueductal stenosis following mumps infection: report of a case and review of the literature. *Brain Dev* 1992;14:417–19.

851. Ogata A, Nagashima K, Tashiro K, et al. MRI-pathological correlate of brain lesions in a necropsy case of HTLV-I associated myelopathy. *J Neurol Neurosurg Psychiatry* 1993;56:194–6.

852. Ogawa M, Okubo H, Tsuji Y, et al. Chronic progressive encephalitis occurring 13 years after Russian spring-summer encephalitis. *J Neurol Sci* 1973;19:363–73.

853. Oger JJ, Werker DH, Foti DJ, Dekaban GA. HTLV-I associated myelopathy: an endemic disease of Canadian aboriginals of the Northwest Pacific coast? *Can J Neurol Sci* 1993;20:302–6.

854. Ohka S, Yang WX, Terada E, et al. Retrograde transport of intact poliovirus through the axon via the fast transport system. *Virology* 1998;250:67–75.

855. Ohta M, Taga T, Nomura A, et al. Epstein–Barr virus-related lymphoproliferative disorder, cytomegalovirus reactivation, and varicella zoster virus encephalitis during treatment of medulloblastoma. *J Med Virol* 2011;9:1582–4.

856. Ojeda VJ, Archer M, Robertson TA, Bucens MR. Necropsy study of the olfactory portal of entry in herpes simplex encephalitis. *Med J Aust* 1983;1:79–81.

857. Okamoto M, Kagawa Y, Kamitani W, et al. Borna disease in a dog in Japan. *J Comp Pathol* 2002;126:312–7.

858. Okamoto M, Hagiwara K, Kamitani W, et al. Experimental vertical transmission of Borna disease virus in the mouse. *Arch Virol* 2003;148:1557–68.

859. Okuno T, Oishi H, Hayashi K, et al. Human herpesviruses 6 and 7 in cervixes of pregnant women. *J Clin Microbiol* 1995;33:1968–70.

860. Oliere S, Douville R, Sze A, et al. Modulation of innate immune responses during human T-cell leukemia virus (HTLV-1) pathogenesis. *Cytokine Growth Factor Rev* 2011;4:197–210.

861. Omalu BI, Shakir AA, Wang G, et al. Fatal fulminant pan-meningo-polioencephalitis due to West Nile virus. *Brain Pathol* 2003;13:465–72.

862. Ooi MH, Wong SC, Clear D, et al. Adenovirus type 21-associated acute flaccid paralysis during an outbreak of hand-foot-and-mouth disease in Sarawak, Malaysia. *Clin Infect Dis* 2003;36:550–9.

863. Opsahl ML, Kennedy PG. Early and late HHV-6 gene transcripts in multiple sclerosis lesions and normal appearing white matter. *Brain* 2005;128 (Part 3):516–27.

864. Osame M, Janssen R, Kubota H, et al. Nationwide survey of HTLV-I-associated myelopathy in Japan: association with blood transfusion. *Ann Neurol* 1990;28:50–56.

865. Osame M, Nakagawa M, Umehara F, et al. Recent studies on the epidemiology, clinical features and pathogenic mechanisms of HTLV-I associated myelopathy (HAM/TSP) and other diseases associated to HTLV. *J Neurovirol* 1997;3:S50–1.

866. Osamura T, Mizuta R, Yoshioka H, Fushiki S. Isolation of adenovirus type 11 from the brain of a neonate with pneumonia and encephalitis. *Eur J Pediatr* 1993;152:496–9.

867. Ostrowski SR, Leslie MJ, Parrott T, et al. B-virus from pet macaque monkeys: an emerging threat in the United States? *Emerg Infect Dis* 1998;4:117–21.

868. O'Sullivan JD, Allworth AM, Paterson DL, et al. Fatal encephalitis due to novel paramyxovirus transmitted from horses. *Lancet* 1997;349:93–5.

869. Overall JC, Jr. Herpes simplex virus infection of the fetus and newborn. *Pediatr Ann* 1994;23:131–6.

870. Oxman MN, Levin MJ, Johnson GR, et al. A vaccine to prevent herpes zoster and postherpetic neuralgia in older adults. *N Engl J Med* 2005;352:2271–84.

871. Ozawa T, Onodera O, Iizuka O, et al. A case of chronic enteroviral meningitis and hydrocephalus associated with Bruton type agammaglobulinemia. *No to Shinkei* 1998;50:191–6.

872. Ozawa T, Itoyama T, Sadamori N, et al. Rapid isolation of viral integration site reveals frequent integration of HTLV-1 into expressed loci. *J Hum Genet* 2004;49:154–65.

873. Pacini DL, Collier AM, Henderson FW. Adenovirus infections and respiratory illnesses in children in group day care. *J Infect Dis* 1987;156:920–7.

874. Padate BP, Keidan J. Enteroviral meningoencephalitis in a patient with non-Hodgkin's lymphoma treated previously with rituximab. *Clin Lab Haematol* 2006;1:69–71.

875. Padgett BL, Walker DL, ZuRhein GM, et al. Cultivation of papova-like virus from human brain with progressive multifocal leucoencephalopathy. *Lancet* 1971;1:1257–60.

876. Pahud BA, Glaser CA, Dekker CL, et al. Varicella zoster disease of the central nervous system: epidemiological, clinical, and laboratory features 10 years after the introduction of the varicella vaccine. *J Infect Dis* 2011;3:316–23.

877. Pal SR, Dastur DK, Kaiwar R, Prasad SR. Enterovirus-70 antigen in spinal cord cells of patients with poliomyelitis-like illness. *Indian J Med Res* 1986;83:108–10.

878. Panagiotopoulos T, Georgakopoulou T. Epidemiology of rubella and congenital rubella syndrome in Greece, 1994–2003. *Euro Surveill* 2004;9:17–19.

879. Pardo CA, McArthur JC, Griffin JW. HIV neuropathy: insights into the pathology of HIV peripheral nerve disease. *J Periph Nerv Syst* 2001;6:21–7.

880. Pass RF, Stagno S, Myers GJ, Alford CA. Outcome of symptomatic congenital cytomegalovirus infection: results of long-term longitudinal follow-up. *Pediatrics* 1980;66:758–62.

881. Pastorino B, Nougairede A, Wurtz N, et al. Role of host cell factors in flavivirus infection: implications for pathogenesis

and development of antiviral drugs. *Antiviral Res* 2010;3:281–94.

882. Pastuszak AL, Levy M, Schick B, *et al.* Outcome after maternal varicella infection in the first 20 weeks of pregnancy. *N Engl J Med* 1994;330:901–5.

883. Paton NI, Leo YS, Zaki SR, *et al.* Outbreak of Nipah-virus infection among abattoir workers in Singapore. *Lancet* 1999;354:1253–6.

884. Paton P, Poly H, Gonnaud PM, *et al.* Acute meningoradiculitis concomitant with seroconversion to human immunodeficiency virus type 1. *Res Virol* 1990;141:427–33.

885. Pealer LN, Marfin AA, Petersen LR, *et al.* Transmission of West Nile virus through blood transfusion in the United States in 2002. *N Engl J Med* 2003;349:1236–45.

886. Peckham CS. Clinical and laboratory study of children exposed in utero to maternal rubella. *Arch Dis Child* 1972;47:571–7.

887. Pedrosa PB, Cardoso TA. Viral infections in workers in hospital and research laboratory settings: a comparative review of infection modes and respective biosafety aspects. *Int J Infect Dis* 2011;6:e366–76.

888. Pepin J. *The Origin of AIDS.* Cambridge: Cambridge University Press, 2011.

889. Deleted in proof.

890. Perlman JM, Argyle C. Lethal cytomegalovirus infection in preterm infants: clinical, radiological, and neuropathological findings. *Ann Neurol* 1992;31:64–8.

891. Perng GC, Jones C, Ciacci-Zanella J, *et al.* Virus-induced neuronal apoptosis blocked by the herpes simplex virus latency-associated transcript. *Science* 2000;287:1500–503.

892. Perry J, Fontaine JD, Mulroy S. Findings in post-poliomyelitis syndrome. Weakness of muscles of the calf as a source of late pain and fatigue of muscles of the thigh after poliomyelitis. *J Bone Joint Surg Am* 1995;77:1148–53.

893. Persson A, Bergstrom T, Lindh M, *et al.* Varicella-zoster virus CNS disease: viral load, clinical manifestations and sequels. *J Clin Virol* 2009;3:249–53.

894. Petereit HF, Bamborschke S, Lanfermann H. Acute transverse myelitis caused by herpes simplex virus. *Eur Neurol* 1996;36:52–3.

895. Petito CK, Navia BA, Cho E-S, *et al.* Vacuolar myelopathy pathologically resembling subacute combined degeneration in patients with acquired immunodeficiency syndrome. *N Engl J Med* 1985;312:874–9.

896. Petito CK, Cho ES, Lemann W, *et al.* Neuropathology of acquired immunodeficiency syndrome (AIDS): an autopsy review. *J Neuropathol Exp Neurol* 1986;45:635–46.

897. Petruzziello R, Orsi N, Macchia S, *et al.* Pathway of rubella virus infectious entry into Vero cells. *J Gen Virol* 1996;77:303–8.

898. Pexeshkpour GH, Dalakas MC. Long-term changes in the spinal cords of patients with old poliomyelitis: signs of continuous disease activity. *Arch Neurol* 1988;45:505–8.

899. Picard FJ, Dekaban GA, Silva J, Rice GP. Mollaret's meningitis associated with herpes simplex type 2 infection. *Neurology* 1993;43:1722–7.

900. Picard O, Brunereau L, Pelosse B, *et al.* Cerebral infarction associated with vasculitis due to varicella zoster virus in patients infected with HIV. *Biomed Pharmacother* 1997;51:449–54.

901. Pike MG, Kennedy CR, Neville BG, Levin M. Herpes simplex encephalitis with relapse. *Arch Dis Child* 1991;66:1242–4.

901a. Pineiro L, Vicente D, Montes M, *et al.* Human parechoviruses in infants with systemic infection. *J Med Virol* 2010;82(10):1790–6.

902. Pittock SJ, Lucchinetti CF. Inflammatory transverse myelitis: evolving concepts. *Curr Opin Neurol* 2006;4:362–8.

903. Planz O, Rentzsch C, Batra A, *et al.* Persistence of Borna disease virus-specific nucleic acid in blood of psychiatric patient. *Lancet* 1998;352:623.

904. Planz O, Rentzsch C, Batra A, *et al.* Pathogenesis of borna disease virus: granulocyte fractions of psychiatric patients harbor infectious virus in the absence of antiviral antibodies. *J Virol* 1999;73:6251–6.

905. Pollack S, Bar-On E, Enat R. Guillain-Barre syndrome: association with mumps. *N Y State J Med* 1981;81:795–7.

906. Porras C, Barboza JJ, Fuenzalida E, *et al.* Recovery from rabies in man. *Ann Intern Med* 1976;85:44–8.

907. Portis JL, McAtee FJ, Evans LH. Infectious entry of murine retroviruses into mouse cells: evidence of a postadsorption step inhibited by acidic pH. *J Virol* 1985;55:806–12.

908. Portolani M, Tamassia MG, Gennari W, *et al.* Post-mortem diagnosis of encephalitis in a 75-year-old infant associated with human herpesvirus-6 variant A. *J Med Virol* 2005;77:244–8.

909. Prashanth LK, Taly AB, Ravi V, *et al.* Adult onset subacute sclerosing panencephalitis: clinical profile of 39 patients from a tertiary care centre. *J Neurol Neurosurg Psychiatry* 2006;5:630–33.

910. Preblud S, Bergman D. Deaths from varicella in infants. *Pediatr Infect Dis* 1985;4:503–7.

911. Price RA, Garcia JH, Rightsel WA. Choriomeningitis and myocarditis in an adolescent with isolation of Coxsackie B5 virus. *Am J Clin Pathol* 1970;53:825–31.

912. Price RW, Nielsen S, Horten B, *et al.* Progressive multifocal leukoencephalopathy: a burnt-out case. *Ann Neurol* 1983;13:485–90.

913. Price WH, O'Leary W. Geographical variation in the antigenic character of West Nile virus. *Am J Epidemiol* 1967;85:84–7.

914. Pringle CR. Virus taxonomy: San Diego 1998. *Arch Virol* 1998;143:1449–59.

915. Pugachev KV, Frey TK. Rubella virus induces apoptosis in culture cells. *Virology* 1998;250:359–70.

916. Pugachev KV, Guirakhoo F, Monath TP. New developments in flavivirus vaccines with special attention to yellow fever. *Curr Opin Infect Dis* 2005;18:387–94.

917. Purtilo DT, Yang JP, Allegra S, *et al.* Hematopathology and pathogenesis of the X-linked recessive lymphoproliferative syndrome. *Am J Med* 1977;62:225–33.

918. Purtilo DT, Strobach RS, Okano M, Davis JR. Epstein–Barr virus-associated lymphoproliferative disorders. *Lab Invest* 1992;67:5–23.

919. Quartier P, Tournilhac O, Archimbaud C, *et al.* Enteroviral meningoencephalitis after anti-CD20 (rituximab) treatment. *Clin infect Dis* 2003;3:e47–9.

920. Quong T. The pathology of western equine encephalitis. *Can Publ Health J* 1942;33:300–306.

921. Racaniello VR. Early events in poliovirus infection: virus-receptor interactions. *Proc Natl Acad Sci U S A* 1996;93:11378–81.

922. Rackstraw S, Meadway J, Bingham J, Al-Sarraj S, Everall IP. An emerging severe leukoencephalopathy: is it due to HIV disease or highly active antiretroviral therapy? *Int J STD AIDS* 2006;17:205–7.

923. Rahal JJ, Anderson J, Rosenberg C, *et al.* Effect of interferon-alpha2b therapy on St Louis viral meningoencephalitis: clinical and laboratory results of a pilot study. *J Infect Dis* 2004;190:1084–7.

924. Randolph SE. Evidence that climate change has caused 'emergence' of tick-borne diseases in Europe? *Int J Med Microbiol* 2004;293(Suppl 37):5–15.

925. Rappole JH, Derrickson SR, Hubalek Z. Migratory birds and spread of West Nile virus in the Western Hemisphere. *Emerg Infect Dis* 2000;6:319–28.

926. Ravindra KV, Freifeld AG, Kalil AC, *et al.* West Nile virus-associated encephalitis in recipients of renal and pancreas transplants: case series and literature review. *Clin Infect Dis* 2004;38:1257–60.

927. Reeves MB, MacAry PA, Lehner PJ, *et al.* Latency, chromatin remodeling, and reactivation of human cytomegalovirus in the dendritic cells of healthy carriers. *Proc Natl Acad Sci U S A* 2005;102:4140–45.

928. Regamey N, Tamm M, Wernli M, *et al.* Transmission of human herpesvirus 8 infection from renal-transplant donors to recipients. *N Engl J Med* 1998;339:1358–63.

929. Rein A. Interference grouping of murine leukemia viruses: a distinct receptor for the MCF-recombinant viruses in mouse cells. *Virology* 1982;120:251–7.

930. Reisen WK, Chiles RE. Prevalence of antibodies to western equine encephalomyelitis and St Louis encephalitis viruses in residents of California exposed to sporadic and consistent enzootic transmission. *Am J Trop Med Hyg* 1997;57:526–9.

931. Rellosa N, Bloch KC, Shane AL, Debiasi RL. Neurologic manifestations of pediatric novel h1n1 influenza infection. *Pediatr Infect Dis J* 2011;2:165–7.

932. Remeijer L, Maertzdorf J, Doornenbal P, *et al.* Herpes simplex virus 1 transmission through corneal transplantation. *Lancet* 2001;357:442.

933. Remesar MC, del Pozo AE, Pittis MG, *et al.* Transmission of HTLV-I by kidney transplant. *Transfusion* 2000;40:1421–2.

934. Ren R, Racaniello VR. Poliovirus spreads from muscle to the central nervous system by neural pathways. *J Infect Dis* 1992;166:747–52.

935. Revello MG, Gorini G, Zavattoni M, *et al.* Congenital rubella infection following rubella outbreak in northern Italy, 2002: need for an effective vaccination programme. *Eur J Clin Microbiol Infect Dis* 2004;23:780–83.

936. Reyes MG, Gardner JJ, Poland JD, Monath TP. St Louis encephalitis: quantitative histologic and immunofluorescent studies. *Arch Neurol* 1981;38:329–34.

937. Ribalta T, Martinez AJ, Jares P, *et al.* Presence of occult cytomegalovirus infection in the brain after orthotopic liver transplantation: an autopsy study of 83 cases. *Virchows Arch* 2002;440:166–71.

938. Richardson EP, Jr. Progressive multifocal leukoencephalopathy. *N Engl J Med* 1961;265:815–23.

939. Richardson EP, Jr, Johnson PC. Atypical progressive multifocal leukoencephalopathy with plasma-cell infiltrates. *Acta Neuropathol Suppl (Berl)* 1975;(Suppl 6):247–50.

940. Richt JA, Alexander RC, Herzog S, et al. Failure to detect Borna disease virus infection in peripheral blood leukocytes from humans with psychiatric disorders. *J Neurovirol* 1997;3:174–8.

941. Richt JA, Pfeuffer I, Christ M, et al. Borna disease virus infection in animals and humans. *Emerg Infect Dis* 1997;3:343–52.

942. Rima BK, Duprex WP. Molecular mechanisms of measles virus persistence. *Virus Res* 2005;111:132–47.

943. Rima BK, Duprex WP. New concepts in measles virus replication: getting in and out in vivo and modulating the host cell environment. *Virus Res* 2011;1–2:47–62.

944. Ringelstein EB, Sobczak H, Pfeifer B, Hacke W. Polyradiculomeningoencephalitis caused by Epstein–Barr virus infection: description of a case with fatal outcome. *Fortschr Neurol Psychiatr* 1984;52:73–82.

945. Ringelstein A, Oelschlaeger C, Saleh A, et al. Severe aseptic leucoencephalopathy as immune reconstitution inflammatory syndrome in Caucasian and African patients. *AIDS* 2012;23:1435–7.

946. Rios M, Khabbaz RF, Kaplan JE, et al. Transmission of human T cell lymphotropic virus (HTLV) type II by transfusion of HTLV-I-screened blood products. *J Infect Dis* 1994;170:206–10.

947. Rittler M, Lopez-Camelo J, Castilla EE. Monitoring congenital rubella embryopathy. *Birth Defects Res A Clin Mol Teratol* 2004;70:939–43.

948. Robert PY, Adenis JP, Denis F, et al. Herpes simplex virus DNA in corneal transplants: prospective study of 38 recipients. *J Med Virol* 2003;71:69–74.

949. Robertson EG. Murray Valley encephalitis: pathological aspects. *Med J Aust* 1952;i:107–10.

950. Robillard RB, Hilsinger RL, Jr, Adour KK. Ramsay Hunt facial paralysis: clinical analyses of 185 patients. *Otolaryngol Head Neck Surg* 1986;95(Part 1):292–7.

951. Robinson-Papp J, Simpson DM. Neuromuscular diseases associated with HIV-1 infection. *Muscle Nerve* 2009;40:1043–53.

952. Rock DL, Fraser NW. Detection of HSV-1 genome in central nervous system of latently infected mice. *Nature* 1983;302:523–5.

953. Rock DL, Fraser NW. Latent herpes simplex virus type 1 DNA contains two copies of the virion DNA joint region. *J Virol* 1985;55:849–52.

954. Rockwell D, Ruben FL, Winkelstein A, Mendelow H. Absence of imune deficiencies in a case of progressive multifocal leukoencephalopathy. *Am J Med* 1976;61:433–6.

955. Roehrig JT, Staudinger LA, Hunt AR, et al. Antibody prophylaxis and therapy for flavivirus encephalitis infections. *Ann N Y Acad Sci* 2001;951:286–97.

956. Roelvink PW, Lizonova A, Lee JG, et al. The coxsackievirus-adenovirus receptor protein can function as a cellular attachment protein for adenovirus serotypes from subgroups A, C, D, E, and F. *J Virol* 1998;72:7909–15.

957. Roggendorf M, Heinz F, Deinhardt F, Kunz C. Serological diagnosis of acute tick-borne encephalitis by demonstration of antibodies of the IgM class. *J Med Virol* 1981;7:41–50.

958. Rollier CS, Reyes-Sandoval A, Cottingham MG, et al. Viral vectors as vaccine platforms: deployment in sight. *Curr Opin Immunol* 2011;3:377–82.

959. Roman GC, Roman LN. Tropical spastic paraparesis: a clinical study of 50 patients from Tumaco (Colombia) and review of the worldwide features of the syndrome. *J Neurol Sci* 1988;87:121–38.

960. Romero JR, Simonsen KA. Powassan encephalitis and Colorado tick fever. *Infect Dis Clin North Am* 2008;3:545–59.

961. Romeu J, Sirera G, Andreu D, et al. Long-lasting remission of cytomegalovirus retinitis without maintenance therapy in human immunodeficiency virus-infected patients. *J Infect Dis* 1998;177:1080–83.

962. Roos KL. West Nile encephalitis and myelitis. *Curr Opin Neurol* 2004;17:343–6.

963. Roos KL. Fatal encephalitis due to rabies virus transmitted by organ transplantation. *Arch Neurol* 2005;62:855–6.

964. Roos RP, Graves MC, Wollmann RL, et al. Immunologic and virologic studies of measles inclusion body encephalitis in an immunosuppressed host: the relationship to subacute sclerosing panencephalitis. *Neurology* 1981;31:1263–70.

965. Rorke LB, Spiro AJ. Cerebral lesions in congenital rubella syndrome. *J Pediatr* 1967;70:243–55.

966. Rose JW, Stroop WG, Matsuo F, Henkel J. Atypical herpes simplex encephalitis: clinical, virologic, and neuropathologic evaluation. *Neurology* 1992;42:1809–12.

967. Rosenbaum GS, Strampfer MJ, Cunha BA. Herpes gladiatorum in a male wrestler. *Int J Dermatol* 1990;29:141–2.

968. Ross I. A bird's-eye view of macrophage biology. In: Desport M ed. *Lentiviruses and macrophages*. Wymondham, UK: Caister Academic Press, 2010:25–80.

969. Rossmann MG, He Y, Kuhn RJ. Picornavirus-receptor interactions. *Trends Microbiol* 2002;10:324–31.

970. Rotbart HA. Enteroviral infections of the central nervous system. *Clin Infect Dis* 1995;20:971–81.

971. Rotbart HA. Viral meningitis. *Semin Neurol* 2000;20:277–92.

972. Rotbart HA, Webster AD. Treatment of potentially life-threatening enterovirus infections with pleconaril. *Clin Infect Dis* 2001;32:228–35.

973. Rott O, Tontsch U, Fleischer B, Cash E. Interleukin-6 production in 'normal' and HTLV-1 tax-expressing brain-specific endothelial cells. *Eur J Immunol* 1993;23:1987–91.

974. Rottnek M, Di Rocco A, Laudier D, Morgello S. Axonal damage is a late component of vacuolar myelopathy. *Neurology* 2002;58:479–81.

975. Roulet Perez E, Maeder P, Cotting J, et al. Acute fatal parainfectious cerebellar swelling in two children: a rare or an overlooked situation? *Neuropediatrics* 1993;24:346–51.

976. Roullet E. Opportunistic infections of the central nervous system during HIV-1 infection (emphasis on cytomegalovirus disease). *J Neurol* 1999;246:237–43.

977. Roullet E, Assuerus V, Gozlan J, et al. Cytomegalovirus multifocal neuropathy in AIDS: analysis of 15 consecutive cases. *Neurology* 1994;44:2174–82.

978. Rousseau MC, Saron MF, Brouqui P, Bourgeade A. Lymphocytic choriomeningitis virus in southern France: four case reports and a review of the literature. *Eur J Epidemiol* 1997;13:817–23.

979. Rozdilsky B, Robertson HE, Chorney J. Western encephalitis: report of eight fatal cases – Saskatchewan epidemic, 1965. *Can Med Assoc J* 1968;98:79–86.

980. Rozenberg F, Deback C, Agut H. Herpes simplex encephalitis: from virus to therapy. *Infect Dis Drug Targets* 2011;3:235–50.

981. Rubin RH. Cytomegalovirus in solid organ transplantation. *Transpl Infect Dis* 2001;3(Suppl 2):1–5.

982. Rubin RH, Hattwick MAW, Jones S, et al. Adverse reactions to duck embryo rabies vaccine: range and incidence. *Ann Intern Med* 1973;78:643–9.

983. Rudge P, Webster AD, Revesz T, et al. Encephalomyelitis in primary hypogammaglobulinaemia. *Brain* 1996;119:1–15.

984. Ruppenthal M. Changes of the central nervous system in herpes zoster. *Acta Neuropathol* 1980;52:59–68.

985. Rushing E, Liappis A, Smirniotopoulos JD, et al. Immune reconstitution inflammatory syndrome of the brain: case illustrations of a challenging entity. *J Neuropathol Exp Neurol* 2008;67:819–27.

985a. Russell SJ, Bell EJ. Echoviruses and carditis. *Lancet* 1970;1(7650):784–5.

986. Ruuskanen O, Meurman O, Sarkkinen H. Adenoviral diseases in children: a study of 105 hospital cases. *Pediatrics* 1985;76:79–83.

987. Ruzek D, Yakimenko VV, Karan LS, Tkachev SE. Omsk haemorrhagic fever. *Lancet* 2010;9758:2104–13.

988. Sa MJ. Acute transverse myelitis: a practical reappraisal. *Autoimmun Rev* 2009;2:128–31.

989. Sabin AB, Ramos-Alvarez M, Alvarez-Amezquita J, et al. Live, orally given poliovirus vaccine: effects of rapid mass immunization on population under conditions of massive enteric infection with other viruses. *J Am Med Assoc* 1960;173:1521–6.

990. Sadzot-Delvaux C, Arvin AM, Rentier B. Varicella-zoster virus IE63, a virion component expressed during latency and acute infection, elicits humoral and cellular immunity. *J Infect Dis* 1998;178:S43–7.

991. Said G, Lacroix C, Chemouilli P, et al. Cytomegalovirus neuropathy in acquired immunodeficiency syndrome: a clinical and pathological study. *Ann Neurol* 1991;29:139–46.

992. Saito H, Endo M, Takase S, Iie K. Acute disseminated encephalomyelitis after influenza vaccination. *Arch Neurol* 1980;37:564–6.

993. Salk JE. Considerations in the preparation and use of poliomyelitis virus vaccine. *J Am Med Assoc* 1955;158:1239–48.

994. Sancho-Shimizu V, Zhang SY, Abel L, et al. Genetic susceptibility to herpes simplex virus 1 encephalitis in mice and humans. *Curr Opin Allergy Clinl Immunol* 2007;6:495–505.

995. Deleted in proof.

996. Santoro F, Kennedy PE, Locatelli G, et al. CD46 is a cellular receptor for human herpesvirus 6. *Cell* 1999;99:817–27.

997. Santoshkumar B, Radhakrishnan K. Substantial spontaneous long-term remission

in subacute sclerosing panencephalitis (SSPE). *J Neurol Sci* 1998;**154**:83–8.

998. Sasaki S, Komori T, Maruyama S, et al. An autopsy case of human T lymphotropic virus type I-associated myelopathy (HAM) with a duration of 28 years. *Acta Neuropathol* 1990;**81**:219–22.

999. Satow Y, Hashido M, Ishikawa K, et al. Detection of HTLV-I antigen in peripheral and cord blood lymphocytes from carrier mothers. *Lancet* 1991;**338**:915–16.

1000. Sauder C, Muller A, Cubitt B, et al. Detection of Borna disease virus (BDV) antibodies and BDV RNA in psychiatric patients: evidence for high sequence conservation of human blood-derived BDV RNA. *J Virol* 1996;**70**:7713–24.

1001. Sauerbrei A, Wutzler P. Neonatal varicella. *J Perinatol* 2001;**21**:545–9.

1002. Savolainen H, Lautenschlager I, Piiparinen H, et al. Human herpesvirus-6 and -7 in pediatric stem cell transplantation. *Pediatr Blood Cancer* 2005;**45**:820–25.

1003. Sawtell NM. The probability of in vivo reactivation of herpes simplex virus type 1 increases with the number of latently infected neurons in the ganglia. *J Virol* 1998;**72**:6888–92.

1004. Scaravilli F, Coutinho P. Encephalite lymphocytaire dans un cas d'agammaglobulinemie. *Acta Neuropathol* 1973;**25**:787–91.

1005. Scaravilli F, Daniel SE, Harcourt-Webster JN, Guiloff RJ Chronic basal meningitis and vasculitis in acquired immunodeficiency syndrome. *Arch Pathol Lab Med* 1989;**113**:192–5.

1006. Scherret JH, Mackenzie JS, Hall RA, et al. Phylogeny and molecular epidemiology of West Nile and Kunjin viruses. *Curr Top Microbiol Immunol* 2002;**267**:373–90.

1007. Schiff JA, Schaefer JA, Robinson JE. Epstein–Barr virus in cerebrospinal fluid during infectious mononucleosis encephalitis. *Yale J Biol Med* 1982;**55**:59–63.

1008. Schilthuizen C, Berenschot HW, Levin MD. Enteroviral encephalitis in a patient with a marginal zone lymphoma treated with rituximab. *Neth J Med* 2010;**5**:221–3.

1009. Schmid A, Spielhofer P, Cattaneo R, et al. Subacute sclerosing panencephalitis is typically characterized by alterations in the fusion protein cytoplasmic domain of the persisting measles virus. *Virology* 1992;**188**:910–15.

1010. Schmidbauer M, Budka H, Pilz P, et al. Presence, distribution and spread of productive varicella zoster virus infection in nervous tissues. *Brain* 1992;**115**:383–98.

1011. Schmitz H, Enders G. Cytomegalovirus as a frequent cause of Guillain–Barre syndrome. *J Med Virol* 1977;**1**:21–7.

1012. Schneider BS, Higgs S. The enhancement of arbovirus transmission and disease by mosquito saliva is associated with modulation of the host immune response. *Trans R Soc Trop Med Hyg* 2008;**5**:400–408.

1013. Schnell G, Joseph S, Spudich S, Price RW, Swansrom R. HIV-1 replication in the CNS occurs in two cell types. *PLoS Pathog* 2011;**7**:e1002286.

1014. Schooley RT, Carey RW, Miller G, et al. Chronic Epstein–Barr virus infection associated with fever and interstitial pneumonitis: clinical and serologic features and response to antiviral chemotherapy. *Ann Intern Med* 1986;**104**:636–43.

1015. Schulz P, Arbusow V, Strupp M, et al. Highly variable distribution of HSV-1-specific DNA in human geniculate, vestibular and spiral ganglia. *Neurosci Lett* 1998;**252**:139–42.

1016. Schwemmle M. Borna disease virus infection in psychiatric patients: are we on the right track? *Lancet Infect Dis* 2001;**1**:46–52.

1017. Schwemmle M, Jehle C, Formella S, Staeheli P. Sequence similarities between human bornavirus isolates and laboratory strains question human origin. *Lancet* 1999;**354**:1973–4.

1018. Scott TF. Nosology of idiopathic transverse myelitis syndromes. *Acta Neurol Scand* 2007;**6**:371–6.

1019. Scriven J, Davies S, Bannerjee AK, Jenkins N, Watson J. Limbic encephalitis secondary to HIV seroconversion. *Int J STD AIDS* 2011;**22**:236–7.

1020. Segerman A, Atkinson JP, Marttila M, et al. Adenovirus type 11 uses CD46 as a cellular receptor. *J Virol* 2003;**77**:9183–91.

1021. Seitelberger F, Jellinger K. Fruighar-Sommer-Encephalomyelitis in Mitteleuropa: bericht uber verifizierte Beobachtungen aus den Epidemien in Osterreich. *Nervenarzt* 1960;**31**:49–60.

1022. Sejvar JJ. West Nile virus and 'poliomyelitis'. *Neurology* 2004;**63**:206–7.

1023. Sejvar JJ, Haddad MB, Tierney BC, et al. Neurologic manifestations and outcome of West Nile virus infection. *J Am Med Assoc* 2003;**290**:511–15.

1024. Sever JL, Hardy JB, Nelson KB, Gilkeson MR. Rubella in the collaborative perinatal research study: II. Clinical and laboratory findings in children through 3 years of age. *Am J Dis Child* 1969;**118**:123–32.

1025. Seydel J, Kramer A. Transmission and population dynamics of HTLV-I infection. *Int J Cancer* 1996;**66**:197–200.

1026. Shafren DR, Williams DT, Barry RD. A decay-accelerating factor-binding strain of coxsackievirus B3 requires the coxsackievirus-adenovirus receptor protein to mediate lytic infection of rhabdomyosarcoma cells. *J Virol* 1997;**71**:9844–8.

1027. Shaman J, Day JF, Stieglitz M. Drought-induced amplification of Saint Louis encephalitis virus, Florida. *Emerg Infect Dis* 2002;**8**:575–80.

1028. Sharer LR, Cho E-S, Epstein, LG. Multinucleated giant cells and HTLV-III in AIDS encephalopathy. *Hum Pathol* 1985;**16**:760.

1029. Sharma KR, Sriram S, Fries T, et al. Lumbosacral radiculoplexopathy as a manifestation of Epstein–Barr virus infection. *Neurology* 1993;**43**:2550–54.

1030. Sharma V, Gupta VB, Eisenhut M. Familial subacute sclerosing panencephalitis associated with short latency. *Pediatr Neurol* 2008;**3**:215–17.

1031. Sheahan BJ, Moore M, Atkins GJ. The pathogenicity of louping ill virus for mice and lambs. *J Comp Pathol* 2002;**126**:137–46.

1032. Shen CY, Chang BL, Chang SF, et al. Molecular epidemiology of cytomegalovirus infection in kindergarten children. *J Med Virol* 1996;**48**:33–7.

1033. Shepherd JC, Subramanian A, Montgomery RA, et al. West Nile virus encephalitis in a kidney transplant recipient. *Am J Transplant* 2004;**4**:830–33.

1034. Sheremata WA, Berger JR, Harrington WJ, Jr, et al. Human T lymphotropic virus type I-associated myelopathy: a report of 10 patients born in the United States. *Arch Neurol* 1992;**49**:1113–18.

1035. Sherer Y, Hassin S, Shoenfeld Y, et al. Transverse myelitis in patients with antiphospholipid antibodies: the importance of early diagnosis and treatment. *Clin Rheumatol* 2002;**21**:207–10.

1035a. Sherman FE, Michaels RH, Kenny FM. Acute encephalopathy (encephalitis) complicating rubella. *J Am Med Assoc* 1965;**192**:675–81.

1036. Shi J, Wu Y, Cai M, Shang S. Rapid diagnosis of herpetic encephalitis in children by PCR-microarray technology for simultaneous detection of seven human herpes viruses. *Eur J Pediatr* 2010;**4**:421–5.

1037. Shindarov LM, Chumakov MP, Voroshilova MK, et al. Epidemiological, clinical, and pathomorphological characteristics of epidemic poliomyelitis-like disease caused by enterovirus 71. *J Hyg Epidemiol Microbiol Immunol* 1979;**23**:284–95.

1038. Shinefield H, Townsend T. Transplacental transmission of western equine encephalomyelitis. *J Pediatr* 1953;**43**:21–5.

1039. Shiramizu B, Hu N, Frisque RJ, Nerurkar VR. High prevalence of human polyomavirus JC VP1 gene sequences in pediatric malignancies. *Cell Mol Biol* 2007;**3**:4–12.

1040. Shoji H, Kusuhara T, Honda Y, et al. Relapsing acute disseminated encephalomyelitis associated with chronic Epstein–Barr virus infection: MRI findings. *Neuroradiology* 1992;**34**:340–42.

1041. Shyu WC, Lin JC, Chang BC, et al. Recurrent ascending myelitis: an unusual presentation of herpes simplex virus type 1 infection. *Ann Neurol* 1993;**34**:625–7.

1042. Sidhu MS, Crowley J, Lowenthal A, et al. Defective measles virus in human subacute sclerosing panencephalitis brain. *Virology* 1994;**202**:631–41.

1043. Silverman L, Rubinstein LJ. Electron microscopic observations on a case of progressive multifocal leukoencephalopathy. *Acta Neuropathol* 1965;**5**:215–24.

1044. Sima AA, Finkelstein SD, McLachlan DR. Multiple malignant astrocytomas in a patient with spontaneous progressive multifocal leukoencephalopathy. *Ann Neurol* 1983;**14**:183–8.

1045. Simonds RJ. HIV transmission by organ and tissue transplantation. *AIDS* 1993;**7**(Suppl 2):S35–8.

1046. Simons K, Garoff H. The budding mechanisms of enveloped animal viruses. *J Gen Virol* 1980;**50**:1–21.

1047. Simpson DM, Citak KA, Godfrey E, Godbold J, Wolfe DE Myopathies associated with HIV virus and zidovudine: can their effects be distinguished? *Neurology* 1993;**43**:971–6.

1048. Singer C, Lang AE, Suchowersky O. Adult-onset subacute sclerosing panencephalitis: case reports and review of the literature. *Mov Disord* 1997;**12**:342–53.

1049. Singh N, Carrigan DR. Human herpesvirus-6 in transplantation: an emerging pathogen. *Ann Intern Med* 1996;**124**:1065–71.

1050. Sixbey JW, Lemon SM, Pagano JS. A second site for Epstein–Barr virus shedding: the uterine cervix. *Lancet* 1986;**ii**:1122–4.

1051. Sixbey JW, Davis DS, Young LS, et al. Human epithelial cell expression of an Epstein–Barr virus receptor. *J Gen Virol* 1987;**68**:805–11.

1052. Skoldenberg B. Herpes simplex encephalitis. *Scand J Infect Dis* 1996;**100**(Suppl):8–13.

1053. Smadja D, Bellance R, Cabre P, *et al.* Involvements of the peripheral nervous system and skeletal muscles in HTLV1-related paraplegia: study of 70 cases seen in Martinique. *Rev Neurol* 1995;**151**:190–95.

1054. Smeets E, Fryns JP, Van den Berghe H. Melkersson–Rosenthal syndrome and de novo autosomal t(9;21) (p11;p11) translocation. *Clin Genet* 1994;**45**:323–4.

1055. Smith C, Varma M. Louping ill. In: Beran G ed. *CRC handbook series in zoonoses. Section B: viral zoonoses.* Boca Raton, FL: CRC Press, 1981:191–200.

1056. Smith MD, Scott GM, Rom S, Patou G. Herpes simplex virus and facial palsy. *J Infect* 1987;**15**:259–61.

1057. Snider WD, Simpson DM, Nielsen S, *et al.* Neurologic complications of acquired immune deficiency sydnrome: analysis of 50 patients. *Ann Neurol* 1983;**14**:403–18.

1058. Deleted in proof.

1059. Soeur M, Wouters A, de Saint-Georges A, *et al.* Meningoencephalitis and meningitis due to an adenovirus type 5 in two immunocompetent adults. *Acta Neurol Belg* 1991;**91**:141–50.

1060. Solomon T, Mallewa M. Dengue and other emerging flaviviruses. *J Infect* 2001;**42**:104–15.

1061. Solomon T, Winter PM. Neurovirulence and host factors in flavivirus encephalitis: evidence from clinical epidemiology. *Arch Virol Suppl* 2004;**18**:161–70.

1062. Solomon T, Kneen R, Dung NM, *et al.* Poliomyelitis-like illness due to Japanese encephalitis virus. *Lancet* 1998;**351**:1094–7.

1063. Solomon T, Dung NM, Wills B, *et al.* Interferon alfa-2a in Japanese encephalitis: a randomised double-blind placebo-controlled trial. *Lancet* 2003;**361**:821–6.

1064. Sonies BC. Dysphagia and post-polio syndrome: past, present, and future. *Semin Neurol* 1996;**16**:365–70.

1065. Southam CM, Moore AE. Induced virus infections in man by the Egypt isolates of West Nile virus. *Am J Trop Med Hyg* 1954;**3**:19–50.

1066. Southern SO, Southern PJ. Persistent HTLV-I infection of breast luminal epithelial cells: a role in HTLV transmission? *Virology* 1998;**241**:200–14.

1067. Deleted in proof.

1068. Spataro RF, Lin SR, Horner FA, *et al.* Aqueductal stenosis and hydrocephalus: rare sequelae of mumps virus infection. *Neuroradiology* 1976;**12**:11–13.

1069. Spector SA, Hirata KK, Newman TR. Identification of multiple cytomegalovirus strains in homosexual men with acquired immunodeficiency syndrome. *J Infect Dis* 1984;**150**:953–6.

1070. Spiegel R, Miron D, Yodko H, *et al.* Late relapse of herpes simplex virus encephalitis in a child due to reactivation of latent virus: clinico-pathological report and review. *J Child Neurol* 2008;**3**:344–8.

1071. Spillantini MG, Tolnay M, Love S, Goedert M. Microtubule-associated protein tau, heparan sulphate and alpha-synuclein in several neurodegenerative diseases with dementia. *Acta Neuropathol* 1999;**97**:585–94.

1072. Spivack JG, Woods GM, Fraser NW. Identification of a novel latency-specific splice donor signal within the herpes simplex virus type 1 2.0-kilobase latency-associated transcript (LAT): translation inhibition of LAT open reading frame by the intron within the 2.0-kilobase LAT. *J Virol* 1991;**65**:6800–810.

1073. Spruance SL, Bailey A. Colorado tick fever: a review of 115 laboratory confirmed cases. *Arch Intern Med* 1973;**131**:288–93.

1074. Squadrini F, Taparelli F, De RB, *et al.* Rubella virus isolation from cerebrospinal fluid in postnatal rubella encephalitis. *Br Med J* 1977;**ii**:1329–30.

1075. Stagno S, Reynolds DW, Tsiantos A, *et al.* Comparative serial virologic and serologic studies of symptomatic and subclinical congenitally and natally acquired cytomegalovirus infections. *J Infect Dis* 1975;**132**:568–77.

1076. Stagno S, Pass RF, Cloud G, *et al.* Primary cytomegalovirus infection in pregnancy. Incidence, transmission. *J Am Med Assoc* 1986;**256**:1904–8.

1076a. Stanway G, Hyypia T. Parechoviruses. *J Virol* 1999;**73**(7):5249–54.

1076b. Stanway G, Joki-Korpela P, Hyypia T. Human parechoviruses: biology and clinical significance. *Rev Med Virol* 2000;**10**(1):57–69.

1077. Steele KE, Twenhafel NA. Pathology of animal models of alphavirus encephalitis. *Vet Pathol* 2010;**5**:790–805.

1078. Steele KE, Linn MJ, Schoepp RJ, *et al.* Pathology of fatal West Nile virus infections in native and exotic birds during the 1999 outbreak in New York City, New York. *Vet Pathol* 2000;**37**:208–24.

1079. Steeper TA, Horwitz CA, Ablashi DV, *et al.* The spectrum of clinical and laboratory findings resulting from human herpesvirus-6 (HHV-6) in patients with mononucleosis-like illnesses not resulting from Epstein–Barr virus or cytomegalovirus. *Am J Clin Pathol* 1990;**93**:776–83.

1080. Stein BS, Gowda SD, Lifson JD, *et al.* pH-independent HIV entry into CD4-positive T cells via virus envelope fusion to the plasma membrane. *Cell* 1987;**49**:659–68.

1081. Stein DA. Inhibition of RNA virus infections with peptide-conjugated morpholino oligomers. *Curr Pharm Des* 2008;**25**:2619–34.

1082. Steiner I, Budka H, Chaudhuri A, *et al.* Viral meningoencephalitis: a review of diagnostic methods and guidelines for management. *Eur J Neurol* 2010;**8**:999–e57.

1083. Stevens JG, Wagner EK, Devi-Rao GB, *et al.* RNA complementary to a herpesvirus gene mRNA is prominent in latently infected neurons. *Science* 1987;**235**:1056–9.

1084. Stevens JG, Haarr L, Porter DD, *et al.* Prominence of the herpes simplex virus latency-associated transcript in trigeminal ganglia from seropositive humans. *J Infect Dis* 1988;**158**:117–23.

1085. Stewart MW, Bolling JP, Mendez JC. Cytomegalovirus retinitis in an immunocompetent patient. *Arch Ophthalmol* 2005;**123**:572–4.

1086. Stinski M. *Cytomegalovirus and its replication.* New York: Raven Press, 1990.

1087. Stitz L, Bilzer T, Richt JA, Rott R. Pathogenesis of Borna disease. *Arch Virol* 1993;**7**(Suppl):135–51.

1088. Stoner GL, Ryschkewitsch CF. Reappraisal of progressive multifocal leukoencephalopathy due to simian virus 40. *Acta Neuropathol* 1998;**96**:271–8.

1089. Strebel PM, Sutter RW, Cochi SL, *et al.* Epidemiology of poliomyelitis in the United States one decade after the last reported case of indigenous wild virus-associated disease. *Clin Infect Dis* 1992;**14**:568–79.

1090. Stroop WG, Rock DL, Fraser NW. Localization of herpes simplex virus in the trigeminal and olfactory systems of the mouse central nervous system during acute and latent infections by in situ hybridization. *Lab Invest* 1984;**51**:27–38.

1091. Suga S, Yoshikawa T, Kajita Y, *et al.* Prospective study of persistence and excretion of human herpesvirus-6 in patients with exanthem subitum and their parents. *Pediatrics* 1998;**102** (Part 1):900–904.

1092. Sugamata M, Miyazawa M, Mori S, *et al.* Paralysis of street rabies virus-infected mice is dependent on T lymphocytes. *J Virol* 1992;**66**:1252–60.

1093. Sullivan-Bolyai J, Corey L. Epidemiology of Reye's syndrome. *Epidemiol Rev* 1981;**3**:1–26.

1094. Sumaya CV, Henle W, Henle G, *et al.* Seroepidemiologic study of Epstein–Barr virus infections in a rural community. *J Infect Dis* 1975;**131**:403–8.

1095. Deleted in proof.

1096. Sun T, Schwartz NS, Sewel, C, Lieberman P, Gross S. Enterobius egg granuloma of the vulva and peritoneum; review of the literature. *Am J Trop Med Hyg* 1991;**45**:249–53.

1097. Sundstrom P, Juto P, Wadell G, *et al.* An altered immune response to Epstein–Barr virus in multiple sclerosis: a prospective study. *Neurology* 2004;**62**:2277–82.

1098. Suryanarayana K, Baczko K, ter Meulen V, Wagner RR. Transcription inhibition and other properties of matrix proteins expressed by M genes cloned from measles viruses and diseased human brain tissue. *J Virol* 1994;**68**:1532–43.

1099. Suzuki T, Fujisawa JI, Toita M, Yoshida M. The trans-activator tax of human T-cell leukemia virus type 1 (HTLV-1) interacts with cAMP-responsive element (CRE) binding and CRE modulator proteins that bind to the 21-base-pair enhancer of HTLV-1. *Proc Natl Acad Sci U S A* 1993;**90**:610–14.

1100. Suzuki T, Kitao S, Matsushime H, Yoshida M. HTLV-1 Tax protein interacts with cyclin-dependent kinase inhibitor p16INK4A and counteracts its inhibitory activity towards CDK4. *EMBO J* 1996;**15**:1607–14.

1101. Swenson PD, Lowens MS, Celum CL, Hierholzer JC. Adenovirus types 2, 8, and 35 associated with genital infections in patients attending a sexually transmitted disease clinic. *J Clin Microbiol* 1995;**33**:2728–31.

1102. Sworn M, Urich H. Acute encephalitis in infectious mononucleosis. *J Pathol* 1970;**100**:201–5.

1103. Tada H, Rappaport J, Lashgari M, *et al.* Trans-activation of the JC virus late promoter by the tat protein of type 1 human immunodeficiency virus in glial cells. *Proc Natl Acad Sci U S A* 1990;**9**:3479–83.

1104. Tahara M, Takeda M, Shirogane Y, et al. Measles virus infects both polarized epithelial and immune cells by using distinctive receptor-binding sites on its hemagglutinin. *J Virol* 2008;9:4630–7.

1105. Takahashi M. The varicella vaccine. Vaccine development. *Infect Dis Clin North Am* 1996;10:469–88.

1106. Takano T, Mekata Y, Yamano T, Shimada M. Early ependymal changes in experimental hydrocephalus after mumps virus inoculation in hamsters. *Acta Neuropathol* 1993;85:521–5.

1106a. Takao S, Shimazu Y, Fukuda S, et al. Seroepidemiological study of human Parechovirus 1. *Jpn J Infect Dis* 2001;54(2):85–7.

1107. Takasaki T, Higashikawa M, Motoyama S, et al. Serum antibodies to human herpesvirus 7, human herpesvirus 6 and cytomegalovirus in patients with idiopathic facial nerve palsy or sudden deafness. *J Laryngol Otol* 1998;112:617–21.

1108. Takeuchi S, Takasato Y, Masaoka H, et al. Hemorrhagic encephalitis associated with Epstein–Barr virus infection. *J Clin Neurosci* 2010;1:153–4.

1109. Tan CS, Koralnik IJ. Progressive multifocal leukoencephalopathy and other disorders caused by JC virus: clinical features and pathogenesis. *Lancet Neurol* 2010;4:425–37.

1110. Tan CS, Ellis LC, Wuthrich C, et al. JC virus latency in the brain and extraneural organs of patients with and without progressive multifocal leukoencephalopathy. *J. Virol* 2010;18:9200–9.

1111. Tan CT, Wong KT. Nipah encephalitis outbreak in Malaysia. *Ann Acad Med Singapore* 2003;32:112–17.

1112. Tan MP, Koren G. Chickenpox in pregnancy: revisited. *Reprod Toxicol* 2006;21:410–20.

1113. Tan SV, Guiloff RJ, Scaravilli F. AIDS-associated vacuolar myelopathy. A morphometric study. *Brain* 1995;118:1247–61.

1114. Tanioka R, Yamamoto Y, Sakai M, et al. Convalescence of atypical reversible posterior leukoencephalopathy syndrome (PRES) in HIV infection. *J Med Invest* 2007;54:191–4.

1115. Tanner J, Weis J, Fearon D, et al. Epstein–Barr virus gp350/220 binding to the B lymphocyte C3d receptor mediates adsorption, capping, and endocytosis. *Cell* 1987;50:203–13.

1116. Tao SJ, Chen BQ. Studies of coltivirus in China. *Chin Med J (Engl)* 2005;118:581–6.

1117. Tatsuo H, Ono N, Tanaka K, Yanagi Y. SLAM (CDw150) is a cellular receptor for measles virus. *Nature* 2000;406:893–7.

1118. Tatsuo H, Ono N, Yanagi Y. Morbilliviruses use signaling lymphocyte activation molecules (CD150) as cellular receptors. *J Virol* 2001;13:5842–50.

1119. Tavazzi E, Bargiggia V, Pichiecchio A, et al. HIV-related inflammatory leukoencephalopathy of undetermined origin: review of the literature. *Int J Immmunopathol Pharmacol* 2010;23:696–700.

1120. Tavazzi E, Magrassi L, Maccabruni A, et al. Acute transient inflammatory leukoencephalopathy in HIV. *Neurol Sci* 2011;32:899–902.

1121. Tavazzi E, White MK, Khalili K. Progressive multifocal leukoencephalopathy: clinical and molecular aspects. *Rev Med Virol* 2012;22:18–32.

1122. The UK Collaborative HIV Cohort (CHIC) Study Steering Committee. HIV-associated central nervous system diseases in the recent combination antiretroviral therapy era. *Eur J Neurol* 2011;18:527–34.

1123. Theil D, Arbusow V, Derfuss T, et al. Prevalence of HSV-1 LAT in human trigeminal, geniculate, and vestibular ganglia and its implication for cranial nerve syndromes. *Brain Pathol* 2001;11:408–13.

1124. Theodore WH, Epstein L, Gaillard WD, et al. Human herpes virus 6B: a possible role in epilepsy? *Epilepsia* 2008;11:1828–37.

1125. Thomas SL, Hall AJ. What does epidemiology tell us about risk factors for herpes zoster? *Lancet Infect Dis* 2004;4:26–33.

1126. Thompson JA. Mumps: a cause of acquired aqueductal stenosis. *J Pediatr* 1979;94:923–4.

1127. Thompson KA, Cherry CL, Bell JE, McLean CA. Brain reservoirs of latent virus in presymptomatic HIV-infected individuals. *Am J Pathol* 2011;179:1623–9.

1128. Thoulouze MI, Lafage M, Schachner M, et al. The neural cell adhesion molecule is a receptor for rabies virus. *J Virol* 1998;72:7181–90.

1129. Thurnher MM, Thurnher SA, Schindler E. CNS involvement in AIDS: spectrum of CT and MR findings. *Eur Radiol* 1997;7:1091–7.

1130. Tirawatnpong S, Hemachudha T, Manutsathit S, et al. Regional distribution of rabies viral antigen in central nervous system of human encephalitic and paralytic rabies. *J Neurol Sci* 1989;92:91–9.

1131. Tjensvoll AB, Gilhus NE. The post-poliomyelitis syndrome: a real complication. A poliomyelitis material from the Haukeland hospital. *Tidsskr Nor Laegeforen* 1997;117:510–13.

1132. Tomlinson AH, Esiri MM. Herpes simplex encephalitis: immunohistological demonstration of spread of virus via olfactory pathways in mice. *J Neurol Sci* 1983;60:473–84.

1133. Tookey P. Rubella in England, Scotland and Wales. *Euro Surveill* 2004;9:21–3.

1134. Tookey P, Peckham CS. Neonatal herpes simplex virus infection in the British Isles. *Paediatr Perinat Epidemiol* 1996;10:432–42.

1135. Toovey S. Influenza-associated central nervous system dysfunction: a literature review. *Travel Med Infect Dis* 2008;3:114–24.

1136. Torgovnick J, Arsura EL, Lala D. Cytomegalovirus ventriculoencephalitis presenting as a Wernicke's encephalopathy-like syndrome. *Neurology* 2000;55:1910–13.

1137. Torigoe S, Kumamoto T, Koide W, et al. Clinical manifestations associated with human herpesvirus 7 infection. *Arch Dis Child* 1995;72:518–19.

1138. Touze E, Gessain A, Lyon-Caen O, Gout O. Tropical spastic paraparesis/HTLV-I-associated myelopathy in Europe and in Africa: clinical and epidemiologic aspects. *J Acquir Immune Defic Syndr* 1996;13:S38–45.

1139. Townsend JJ, Baringer JR, Wolinsky JS, et al. Progressive rubella panencephalitis: late onset after congenital rubella. *N Engl J Med* 1975;292:990–93.

1140. Townsend JJ, Wolinsky JS, Baringer JR. The neuropathology of progressive rubella panencephalitis of late onset. *Brain* 1976;99:81–90.

1141. Townsend JJ, Stroop WG, Baringer JR, et al. Neuropathology of progressive rubella panencephalitis after childhood rubella. *Neurology* 1982;32:185–90.

1142. Transverse Myelitis Consortium Working Group. Proposed diagnostic criteria and nosology of acute transverse myelitis. *Neurology* 2002;59:499–505.

1143. Trincado DE, Rawlinson WD. Congenital and perinatal infections with cytomegalovirus. *J Paediatr Child Health* 2001;37:187–92.

1144. Tsukada J, Misago M, Serino Y, et al. Human T-cell leukemia virus type I Tax transactivates the promoter of human prointerleukin-1beta gene through association with two transcription factors, nuclear factor-interleukin-6 and Spi-1. *Blood* 1997;90:3142–53.

1145. Tuffereau C, Benejean J, Blondel D, et al. Low-affinity nerve-growth factor receptor (P75NTR) can serve as a receptor for rabies virus. *EMBO J* 1998;17:7250–59.

1146. Tuke PW, Hawke S, Griffiths PD, Clark DA. Distribution and quantification of human herpesvirus 6 in multiple sclerosis and control brains. *Mult Scler* 2004;10:355–9.

1147. Tullu MS, Patil DP, Muranjan MN, Kher AS, Lahiri KR. HIV infection in a child presenting as acute disseminated encephalomyelitis. *J Child Neurol* 2011;26:99–102.

1148. Turell MJ, O'Guinn ML, Dohm DJ, et al. Vector competence of *Culex tarsalis* from Orange County, California, for West Nile virus. *Vector Borne Zoonotic Dis* 2002;2:193–6.

1149. Turner A, Jeyaratnam D, Haworth F, et al. Measles-associated encephalopathy in children with renal transplants. *Am J Transplant* 2006;6:1459–65.

1150. Twomey JA, Barker CM, Robinson G, Howell DA. Olfactory mucosa in herpes simplex encephalitis. *J Neurol Neurosurg Psychiatry* 1979;42:983–7.

1151. Tyler KL, Gross RA, Cascino GD. Unusual viral causes of transverse myelitis: hepatitis A virus and cytomegalovirus. *Neurology* 1986;36:855–8.

1152. Tyler KL, Tedder DG, Yamamoto LJ, et al. Recurrent brainstem encephalitis associated with herpes simplex virus type 1 DNA in cerebrospinal fluid. *Neurology* 1995;45:2246–50.

1153. Tyor WR, Wesselingh SL, Griffin JW, McArthur JC, Griffin DE. Unifying hypothesis for the pathogenesis of HIV-associated dementia complex, vacuolar myelopathy, and sensory neuropathy. *J Acquir Immune Defic Syndr* 1995;9:379–88.

1154. Umehara F, Izumo S, Nakagawa M, et al. Immunocytochemical analysis of the cellular infiltrate in the spinal cord lesions in HTLV-I-associated myelopathy. *J Neuropathol Exp Neurol* 1993;52:424–30.

1155. Umehara F, Nakamura A, Izumo S, et al. Apoptosis of T lymphocytes in the spinal cord lesions in HTLV-I-associated myelopathy: a possible mechanism to control viral infection in the central nervous system. *J Neuropathol Exp Neurol* 1994;**53**:617–24.

1156. Umehara F, Izumo S, Takeya M, *et al.* Expression of adhesion molecules and monocyte chemoattractant protein-1 (MCP-1) in the spinal cord lesions in HTLV-I-associated myelopathy. *Acta Neuropathol* 1996;**91**:343–50.

1157. Umemoto M, Take H, Sawada T. Impact of serum antibodies to p40tax gene product in the intrafamilial transmission of human T cell leukemia virus type I. *Acta Paediatr Jpn* 1994;**36**:62–4.

1158. Umenai T, Krzysko R, Bektimirov TA, Assaad FA. Japanese encephalitis: current worldwide status. *Bull World Health Organ* 1985;**63**:625–31.

1159. Underwood E. The neurological complications of varicella: a clinical epidemiological study. *Br J Child Dis* 1935;**32**:77–96.; 83–107; 241–63.

1160. Uriel A, Stow R, Johnson L, *et al.* Tumefactive demyelination – an unusual neurological presentation of HIV. *Clin Infect Dis* 2010;**51**:1217–20.

1161. Vago L, Castagna A, Lazzarin A, *et al.* Reduced frequency of HIV-induced lesions in AIDS patients treated with zidovudine. *J Acquir Immune Defic Syndr* 1993;**642**–5.

1162. Vago L, Cinque P, Sala E, *et al.* JCV-DNA and BKV-DNA in the CNS tissue and CSF of AIDS patients and normal subjects: study of 41 cases and review of the literature. *J Acquir Immune Defic Syndr* 1996;**12**:139–46.

1163. Vago L, Nebuloni M, Sala E, *et al.* Coinfection of the central nervous system by cytomegalovirus and herpes simplex virus type 1 or 2 in AIDS patients: autopsy study on 82 cases by immunohistochemistry and polymerase chain reaction. *Acta Neuropathol* 1996;**92**:404–8.

1164. Valassina M, Cusi MG, Valensin PE. A Mediterranean arbovirus: the Toscana virus. *J Neurovirol* 2003;**9**:577–83.

1165. Valentin H, Lemasson I, Hamaia S, *et al.* Transcriptional activation of the vascular cell adhesion molecule-1 gene in T lymphocytes expressing human T-cell leukemia virus type 1 Tax protein. *J Virol* 1997;**71**:8522–30.

1166. Vallbracht A, Lohler J, Gossmann J, *et al.* Disseminated BK type polyomavirus infection in an AIDS patient associated with central nervous system disease. *Am J Pathol* 1993;**143**:29–39.

1167. Van den Berg JSP, van Zeihl JH, Rotteveel JJ, *et al.* Neuroinvasion by human herpesvirus type 7 in a case of exanthem subitum with severe neurologic manifestations. *Neurology* 1999;**52**:1077–9.

1168. van den Hurk AF, Craig SB, Tulsiani SM, Jansen CC. Emerging tropical diseases in Australia. Part 4. Mosquito-borne diseases. *Ann Trop Med Parasitol* 2010;**8**:623–40.

1169. Van der Meulen KM, Pensaert MB, Nauwynck HJ. West Nile virus in the vertebrate world. *Arch Virol* 2005;**150**:637–57.

1170. Vandvik B, Weil ML, Grandien M, Norrby E. Progressive rubella virus panencephalitis: synthesis of oligoclonal virus specific, IgG antibodies and homo-geneous free light chains in the central nervous system. *Acta Neurol Scand* 1978;**57**:53–64.

1171. Van Kralingen KW, Ivanyi B, van Keimpema AR, *et al.* Sleep complaints in postpolio syndrome. *Arch Phys Med Rehab* 1996;**77**:609–11.

1172. Van Lierde S, Corbeel L, Eggermont E. Clinical and laboratory findings in children with adenovirus infections. *Eur J Pediatr* 1989;**148**:423–5.

1173. Vasileiadis GT, Roukema HW, Romano W, *et al.* Intrauterine herpes simplex infection. *Am J Perinatol* 2003;**20**:55–8.

1174. Deleted in proof.

1175. Vazquez A, Jimenez-Clavero M, Franco L, *et al.* Usutu virus: potential risk of human disease in Europe. *Euro Surveill* 2011;**16**:ii.

1176. Venkatarama A, Pardo CA, McArthur J, *et al.* Immune reconstitution inflammatory syndrome in the CNS of HIV-infected patients. *Neurology* 2006;**67**:383–8.

1177. Venketasubramanian N. Transverse myelitis following mumps in an adult – a case report with MRI correlation. *Acta Neurol Scand* 1997;**96**:328–31.

1177a. Verboon-Maciolek MA, Groenendaal F, Hahn CD, *et al.* Human parechovirus causes encephalitis with white matter injury in neonates. *Ann Neurol* 2008;**64**(3):266–73.

1178. Verdonck K, Gonzalez E, Van Dooren S, *et al.* Human T-lymphotropic virus 1: recent knowledge about an ancient infection. *Lancet Infect Dis* 2007;**4**:266–81.

1179. Vieker S, Schmitt JJ, Behrens C, *et al.* Subacute sclerosing panencephalitis in two brothers. *Neuropediatrics* 2003;**6**:326–9.

1180. Vigant F, Lee B. Hendra and nipah infection: pathology, models and potential therapies. *Infect Disord Drug Targets* 2011;**3**:315–36.

1181. Vinayagamoorthy T, Mulatz K, Drebot M, Hodkinson R. Molecular typing of West Nile Virus, Dengue, and St Louis encephalitis using multiplex sequencing. *J Mol Diagn* 2005;**7**:152–9.

1182. Vincentelli C, Schniederjan MJ, Brat DJ. 35-year-old HIV-positive woman with basal forebrain mass. *Brain Pathol* 2010;**1**:265–8.

1183. Vinters HV, Anders KH, Barach P. Focal pontine leukoencephalopathy in immunosuppressed patients. *Arch Pathol Lab Med* 1987;**111**:192–6.

1184. Vinters HV, Kwok MK, Ho HW, *et al.* Cytomegalovirus in the nervous system of patients with the acquired immune deficiency syndrome. *Brain* 1989;**112**(Part 1):245–68.

1185. Visser LH, van der Meche FG, Meulstee J, *et al.* Cytomegalovirus infection and Guillain–Barre syndrome: the clinical, electrophysiologic, and prognostic features. Dutch Guillain–Barre Study Group. *Neurology* 1996;**47**:668–73.

1186. Vitek CR, Gracia FI, Giusti R, *et al.* Evidence for sexual and mother-to-child transmission of human T lymphotropic virus type II among Guaymi Indians, Panama. *J Infect Dis* 1995;**171**:1022–6.

1187. Volpi A. Severe complications of herpes zoster. *Herpes* 2007;**14**(Suppl 2):35–9.

1188. Von Einsiedel RW, Fife TD, Aksamit AJ, *et al.* Progressive multifocal leukoenceph-alopathy in AIDS: a clinicopathological study and review of the literature. *J Neurol* 1993;**240**:391–406.

1189. Wadia NH, Wadia PN, Katrak SM, Misra VP. A study of the neurological disorder associated with acute haemorrhagic conjunctivitis due to enterovirus 70. *J Neurol Neurosurg Psychiatr* 1983;**46**:599–610.

1190. Wagner EK, Flanagan WM, Devi-Rao G, *et al.* The herpes simplex virus latency-associated transcript is spliced during the latent phase of infection. *J Virol* 1988;**62**:4577–85.

1191. Wagner M, Muller-Berghaus J, Schroeder R, *et al.* Human herpesvirus-6 (HHV-6)-associated necrotizing encephalitis in Griscelli's syndrome. *J Med Virol* 1997;**53**:306–12.

1192. Wahlberg P, Saikku P, Brummer-Korvenkontio M. Tick-borne viral encephalitis in Finland: the clinical features of Kumlinge disease during 1959–1987. *J Intern Med* 1989;**225**:173–7.

1193. Wakefield AJ, Murch SH, Anthony A, *et al.* Ileal-lymphoid-nodular hyperplasia, non-specific colitis, and pervasive developmental disorder in children. *Lancet* 1998;**351**:637–41.

1194. Wallace MJ, Smith DW, Broom AK, *et al.* Antibody-dependent enhancement of Murray Valley encephalitis virus virulence in mice. *J Gen Virol* 2003;**84**(Part 7):1723–8.

1195. Wallace MR, Hooper DG, Pyne JM, *et al.* Varicella immunity and clinical disease in HIV-infected adults. *South Med J* 1994;**87**:74–6.

1196. Walters LL, Tirrell SJ, Shope RE. Seroepidemiology of California and Bunyamwera serogroup (Bunyaviridae) virus infections in native populations of Alaska. *Am J Trop Med Hyg* 1999;**60**:806–21.

1197. Wang J, Duan S, Zhao J, Zhang L. Acute disseminated encephalomyelitis associated with Influenza A H1N1 infection. *Neurol Sci* 2011;**5**:907–9.

1198. Wang L, Harcourt BH, Yu M, *et al.* Molecular biology of Hendra and Nipah viruses. *Microbes Infect* 2001;**3**:279–87.

1199. Wang X, Huong SM, Chiu ML, *et al.* Epidermal growth factor receptor is a cellular receptor for human cytomegalovirus. *Nature* 2003;**424**:456–61.

1200. Wang X, Huang DY, Huong SM, Huang ES. Integrin alphavbeta3 is a coreceptor for human cytomegalovirus. *Nat Med* 2005;**11**:515–21.

1201. Ward KN, Kalima P, MacLeod KM, Riordan T. Neuroinvasion during delayed primary HHV-7 infection in an immunocompetent adult with encephalitis and flaccid paralysis. *J Med Virol* 2002;**67**:538–41.

1202. Ward KN, White RP, Mackinnon S, Hanna M. Human herpesvirus-7 infection of the CNS with acute myelitis in an adult bone marrow recipient. *Bone Marrow Transpl* 2002;**30**:983–5.

1203. Warren KG, Brown SM, Wroblewska Z, *et al.* Isolation of latent herpes simplex virus from the superior cervical and vagus ganglions of human beings. *N Engl J Med* 1978;**298**:1068–9.

1204. Weaver S, Rosenblum MK, DeAngelis LM. Herpes varicella zoster encephalitis in immunocompromised patients. *Neurology* 1999;52:193–5.

1205. Weaver SC, Reisen WK. Present and future arboviral threats. *Antiviral Res* 2010;2:328–45.

1206. Weaver SC, Powers AM, Brault AC, Barrett AD. Molecular epidemiological studies of veterinary arboviral encephalitides. *Vet J* 1999;157:123–38.

1207. Weaver SC, Anishchenko M, Bowen R, et al. Genetic determinants of Venezuelan equine encephalitis emergence. *Arch Virol Suppl* 2004;18:43–64.

1208. Weaver SC, Ferro C, Barrera R, et al. Venezuelan equine encephalitis. *Annu Rev Entomol* 2004;49:141–74.

1209. Webb HE, Rao RL. Kyasanur forest disease: a general clinical study in which some cases with neurological complications were observed. *Trans R Soc Trop Med Hyg* 1961;55:284–98.

1210. Weber B, Enders G, Schlosser R, et al. Congenital rubella syndrome after maternal reinfection. *Infection* 1993;21:118–21.

1211. Wechsler SL, Weiner HL, Fields BN. Immune response in subacute sclerosing panencephalitis: reduced antibody response to the matrix protein of measles virus. *J Immunol* 1979;123:884–9.

1212. Weigler BJ, Hird DW, Hilliard JK, et al. Epidemiology of cercopithecine herpesvirus 1 (B virus) infection and shedding in a large breeding cohort of rhesus macaques. *J Infect Dis* 1993;167:257–63.

1213. Weil ML, Itabashi H, Cremer NE, et al. Chronic progressive encephalitis due to rubella virus simulating subacute sclerosing panencephalitis. *N Engl J Med* 1975;292:994–8.

1214. Weiland F, Cox JH, Meyer S, et al. Rabies virus neuritic paralysis: immunopathogenesis of nonfatal paralytic rabies. *J Virol* 1992;66:5096–9.

1215. Weinstein L. Influence of age and sex on susceptibility and clinical manifestations in poliomyelitis. *N Engl J Med* 1957;257:47–52.

1216. Weissert R. Progressive multifocal leukoencephalopathy. *J Neuroimmunol* 2011;1–2:73–7.

1217. Wenger F. Venezuelan equine encephalitis. *Teratology* 1977;16:359–62.

1218. Westaway E, Brinton M, Gaidamovich S, et al. Flaviviridae. *Intervirology* 1985;24:183–92.

1219. Westmore GA, Pickard BH, Stern H. Isolation of mumps virus from the inner ear after sudden deafness. *Br Med J* 1979;i:14–15.

1220. White MK, Khalili K. Pathogenesis of progressive multifocal leukoencephalopathy – revisited. *J Infect Dis* 2011;5:578–86.

1221. White PD, Thomas JM, Amess J, et al. The existence of a fatigue syndrome after glandular fever. *Psychol Med* 1995;25:907–16.

1222. White PD, Thomas JM, Amess J, et al. Incidence, risk and prognosis of acute and chronic fatigue syndromes and psychiatric disorders after glandular fever. *Br J Psychiatry* 1998;173:475–81.

1223. Whitley R, Lakeman AD, Nahmias A, Roizman B. DNA restriction-enzyme analysis of herpes simplex virus isolates obtained from patients with encephalitis. *N Engl J Med* 1982;307:1060–62.

1224. Whitley RJ. Neonatal herpes simplex virus infections: pathogenesis and therapy. *Pathol Biol* 1992;40:729–34.

1225. Whitley RJ. Neonatal herpes simplex virus infections. *J Med Virol* 1993;1(Suppl):13–21.

1226. Whitley RJ, Lakeman F. Herpes simplex virus infections of the central nervous system: therapeutic and diagnostic considerations. *Clin Infect Dis* 1995;20:414–20.

1227. Whitley RJ, Soong SJ, Linneman C, Jr, et al. Herpes simplex encephalitis: clinical assessment. *J Am Med Assoc* 1982;247:317–20.

1228. Whitley RJ, Alford CA, Hirsch MS, et al. Factors indicative of outcome in a comparative trial of acyclovir and vidarabine for biopsy-proven herpes simplex encephalitis. *Infection* 1987;15:S3–8.

1229. Wiemers MA, Stallman ND. Immunoglobulin M in Murray Valley encephalitis. *Pathology* 1975;7:187–91.

1229a. Wigand R, Sabin AB. Properties of ECHO types 22, 23 and 24 viruses. *Arch Gesamte Virusforsch* 1961;11:224–47.

1230. Wiktor SZ, Piot P, Mann JM, et al. Human T cell lymphotropic virus type I (HTLV-I) among female prostitutes in Kinshasa, Zaire. *J Infect Dis* 1990;161:1073–7.

1231. Wiktor SZ, Pate EJ, Murphy EL, et al. Mother-to-child transmission of human T-cell lymphotropic virus type I (HTLV-I) in Jamaica: association with antibodies to envelope glycoprotein (gp46) epitopes. *J Acquir Immune Defic Syndr* 1993;6:1162–7.

1232. Wiley CA, VanPatten PD, Carpenter PM, et al. Acute ascending necrotizing myelopathy caused by herpes simplex virus type 2. *Neurology* 1987;37:1791–4.

1233. Wilfert CM, Buckley RH, Mohanakumar T, et al. Persistent and fatal central-nervous-system ECHOvirus infections in patients with agammaglobulinemia. *N Engl J Med* 1977;296:1485–9.

1234. Willems WR, Kaluza G, Boschek CB, et al. Semliki forest virus: cause of a fatal case of human encephalitis. *Science* 1979;203:1127–9.

1235. Winkler WG, Fashinell TR, Leffingwell L, et al. Airborne rabies transmission in a laboratory worker. *J Am Med Assoc* 1973;226:1219–21.

1236. Winter PM, Dung NM, Loan HT, et al. Proinflammatory cytokines and chemokines in humans with Japanese encephalitis. *J Infect Dis* 2004;190:1618–26.

1237. Wolinsky JS, Berg BO, Maitland CH. Progressive rubella panencephalitis. *Arch Neurol* 1976;33:722–3.

1238. Wolinsky JS, Dau PC, Buimovici KE, et al. Progressive rubella panencephalitis: immunovirological studies and results of isoprinosine therapy. *Clin Exp Immunol* 1979;35:397–404.

1239. Wolinsky JS, Waxham MN, Hess JL, et al. Immunochemical features of a case of progressive rubella panencephalitis. *Clin Exp Immunol* 1982;48:359–66.

1239a. Wolthers KC, Benschop KS, Schinkel J, et al. Human parechoviruses as an important viral cause of sepsislike illness and meningitis in young children. *Clin Infect Dis* 2008;47(3):358–63.

1240. Wong KT. Emerging and re-emerging epidemic encephalitis: a tale of two viruses. *Neuropathol Appl Neurobiol* 2000;26:313–18.

1241. Woo HH, Rezai AR, Knopp EA, et al. Contrast-enhancing progressive multifocal leukoencephalopathy: radiological and pathological correlations – case report. *Neurosurgery* 1996;39:1031–4.

1242. Woodman CB, Collins SI, Vavrusova N, et al. Role of sexual behavior in the acquisition of asymptomatic Epstein–Barr virus infection: a longitudinal study. *Pediatr Infect Dis J* 2005;24:498–502.

1243. World Health Organization. Two rabies cases following corneal transplantation. *Wkly Epidemiol Rec* 1994;69:330.

1244. World Health Organization. RABNET: strengthening international surveillance of human and animal rabies. *Wkly Epidemiol Rec* 1998;73:254–6.

1245. World Health Organization. Progress towards elimination of measles and prevention of congenital rubella infection in the WHO European Region, 1990–2004. *Wkly Epidemiol Rec* 2005;80:66–71.

1246. World Health Organization. Standardization of the nomenclature for genetic characteristics of wild-type rubella viruses. *Wkly Epidemiol Rec* 2005;80:126–32.

1247. Wu E, Dickson DW, Jacobson S, Raine CS. Neuroaxonal dystrophy in HTLV-1-associated myelopathy/tropical spastic paraparesis: neuropathologic and neuroimmunologic correlations. *Acta Neuropathol* 1993;86:224–35.

1248. Wuthrich C, Cheng YM, Joseph JT, et al. Frequent infection of cerebellar granule cell neurons by polyomavirus JC in progressive multifocal leukoencephalopathy. *J Neuropathol Exp Neurol* 2009;1:15–25.

1249. Wuthrich C, Dang X, Westmoreland S, et al. Fulminant JC virus encephalopathy with productive infection of cortical pyramidal neurons. *Ann Neurol* 2009;6:742–8.

1250. Xiao C, Bator CM, Bowman VD, et al. Interaction of coxsackievirus A21 with its cellular receptor, ICAM-1. *J Virol* 2001;75:2444–51.

1251. Yadav M, Nambiar S, Khoo SP, Yaacob HB. Detection of human herpesvirus 7 in salivary glands. *Arch Oral Biol* 1997;42:559–67.

1252. Yamamoto LJ, Tedder DG, Ashley R, Levin MJ. Herpes simplex virus type 1 DNA in cerebrospinal fluid of a patient with Mollaret's meningitis. *N Engl J Med* 1991;325:1082–5.

1253. Yamanishi K, Okuno T, Shiraki K, et al. Identification of human herpesvirus-6 as a causal agent for exanthem subitum. *Lancet* 1988;i:1065–7.

1254. Yamshchikov G, Borisevich V, Kwok CW, et al. The suitability of yellow fever and Japanese encephalitis vaccines for immunization against West Nile virus. *Vaccine* 2005;23:4785–92.

1255. Yanagi Y, Takeda M, Ohno S. Measles virus: cellular receptors, tropism and pathogenesis. *J Gen Virol* 2006;87:2767–79.

1256. Yanagi Y, Takeda M, Ohno S, Hashiguchi T. Measles virus receptors. *Curr Top Microbiol Immunol* 2009;**329**:13–30.

1257. Deleted in proof.

1258. Yanagihara N, Honda N, Hato N, Murakami S. Edematous swelling of the facial nerve in Bell's palsy. *Acta Otolaryngol* 2000;**120**:667–71.

1259. Yanagihara R. Human T-cell lymphotropic virus type I infection and disease in the Pacific basin. *Hum Biol* 1992;**64**:843–54.

1260. Yao K, Crawford JR, Komaroff AL, *et al.* Review part 2: human herpesvirus-6 in central nervous system diseases. *J Med Virol* 2010;**10**:1669–78.

1261. Yao QY, Rickinson AB, Epstein MA. A re-examination of the Epstein–Barr virus carrier state in healthy seropositive individuals. *Int J Cancer* 1985;**35**:35–42.

1262. Yoshioka A, Hirose G, Ueda Y, *et al.* Neuropathological studies of the spinal cord in early stage HTLV-I-associated myelopathy (HAM). *J Neurol Neurosurg Psychiatry* 1993;**56**:1004–7.

1263. Yu Y. Phenotypic and genotypic characteristics of Japanese encephalitis attenuated live vaccine virus SA14-14-2 and their stabilities. *Vaccine* 2010;**21**:3635–41.

1264. Yunis EJ, Atchison RW, Michaels RH, DeCicco FA. Adenovirus and ileocecal intussusception. *Lab Invest* 1975;**33**:347–51.

1265. Zaidman GW, Billingsley A. Corneal impression test for the diagnosis of acute rabies encephalitis. *Ophthalmology* 1998;**105**:249–51.

1266. Zanin MP, Webster DE, Martin JL, Wesselingh SL. Japanese encephalitis vaccines: moving away from the mouse brain. *Expert Rev Vaccines* 2003;**2**:407–16.

1267. Zarranz J, Rouco I, Gomez-Esteban JC, Corral J. Human T lymphotropic virus type I (HTLV-1) associated myelopathy acquired through a liver transplant. *J Neurol Neurosurg Psychiatry* 2001;**71**:818.

1268. Zarranz J, Gomez Esteban JC, Rouco Axpe I, *et al.* Post-transplantation HTLV-1 myelopathy in three recipients from a single donor. *J Neurol Neurosurg Psychiatry* 2003;**8**:1080–84.

1269. Zerr DM, Meier AS, Selke SS, *et al.* A population-based study of primary human herpesvirus 6 infection. *N Engl J Med* 2005;**352**:768–76.

1270. Zhang SY, Jouanguy E, Sancho-Shimizu V, *et al.* Human Toll-like receptor-dependent induction of interferons in protective immunity to viruses. *Immunol Rev* 2007;**220**:225–36.

1271. Zheng DP, Frey TK, Icenogle J, *et al.* Global distribution of rubella virus genotypes. *Emerg Infect Dis* 2003;**9**:1523–30.

1272. Ziebold C, von Kries R, Lang R, *et al.* Severe complications of varicella in previously healthy children in Germany: a 1-year survey. *Pediatrics* 2001;**108**:E79.

1273. Zimmer WM, Rogers RS, Reeve CM, Sheridan PJ. Orofacial manifestations of Melkersson-Rosenthal syndrome: a study of 42 patients and review of 220 cases from the literature. *Oral Surg Oral Med Oral Pathol* 1992;**74**:610–19.

1274. Zoubak S, Richardson JH, Rynditch A, *et al.* Regional specificity of HTLV-I proviral integration in the human genome. *Gene* 1994;**143**:155–63.

1275. Zu Rhein G, Chou SM. Particles resembling papova viruses in human cerebral demyelination disease. *Science* 1965;**148**:1477–9.

1276. Zwaagstra J, Ghiasi H, Slanina SM, *et al.* Activity of herpes simplex virus type 1 latency associated transcript (LAT) promoter in neuron-derived cells: evidence for neuron specificity and for a large LAT transcript. *J Virol* 1990;**64**:5019–28.

Bacterial Infections

Martina Deckert

INTRODUCTION TO CENTRAL NERVOUS SYSTEM INFECTIONS

Bacterial infections of the central nervous (CNS) are severe, life-threatening diseases. Although they are much rarer than bacterial infections of other organs, they are much more devastating, causing more severe morbidity with much higher morbidity rates. Despite modern antibiotic regimens, they still carry an unacceptably high death rate and permanent neurologic sequelae in surviving patients. Thus, bacterial infections of the CNS differ fundamentally from infections of other organs, even if initiated by the same pathogens. *Escherichia coli* mainly causes harmless, frequently asymptomatic urinary tract infections in adults; in contrast, in newborns, *E. coli* induces life-threatening bacterial meningitis. These clinical observations point to the crucial role of both host- and pathogen-associated parameters. In addition to the host immune system, specific features of the target organ also play an important role, particularly in the case of the CNS, which differs fundamentally from other organs because of its immunological privilege.

To protect the highly differentiated CNS, which compared to other organs has a limited regenerative capacity, organisms have evolved several important mechanisms. Specific anatomical features of the CNS provide unique features for protection against pathogens: the bony structures of the skull and vertebral column as well as the blood–brain barrier (BBB) prevent access of bacteria to the CNS. Even in exclusively extracerebral infections with pathogens that also have the capacity to invade the brain, complex mechanisms of immunosurveillance are activated to protect the CNS.[81] During exclusively systemic infections, antigen-specific T-cells patrol the CNS and specifically home to those CNS structures that would be targeted by the infectious pathogen should it achieve access to the CNS.[81] These well-tuned neuroimmune mechanisms and the pathogenesis of CNS infections have been deciphered in detail thanks to major progresses in neuroimmunology. Most of our current knowledge on the pathogenesis of CNS infections is derived from animal models, which parallel human CNS infections in many important aspects. Collectively, these models have unravelled complex interactions between the host and the offending pathogen, and have identified important host and pathogen parameters that determine the clinical course and outcome from bacterial CNS infections. Bacteria have also evolved elegant strategies to take advantage of physiologic host reactions and strategies using specific anatomic features and hijacking the host immune defense machinery.

CLASSIFICATION OF BACTERIAL CENTRAL NERVOUS SYSTEM INFECTIONS

Bacterial infections of the CNS can be classified based on their topography into:

- osteitis: infection of the bony structures of the skull and the vertebral column;
- epidural abscess: infection in the space between bone and dura;
- subdural empyema: inflammation in the space between dura and leptomeninges;

- meningitis: inflammation within the subarachnoid space between the arachnoid and the pia mater;
- encephalitis: inflammation of the brain parenchyma, which occurs in several forms:
- panencephalitis: encephalitis of both the grey and the white matter of the CNS parenchyma;
- polioencephalitis: inflammation of the grey matter of the CNS parenchyma;
- encephalitis of the white matter;
- ventriculitis: inflammation in the lumen and/or of the walls of the ventricular system;
- brain abscess: circumscribed, focally restricted inflammation of the brain parenchyma demarcated from the surrounding tissue by a capsule.

All of these types of bacterial infections are characterized by a specific pathogenesis, the characteristics of the causative pathogens and the clinical course, which may be acute, subacute, or chronic, and the outcome.

BACTERIAL MENINGITIS

Introduction and Aetiology

Bacterial meningitis still is a life-threatening, challenging disorder. It is the leading CNS infection[59] and the most frequent bacterial infection of the CNS. Worldwide, one to two million cases of bacterial meningitis are estimated to occur annually[111] causing 170 000 deaths per year,[132] thereby ranking in the top ten causes of infection-related deaths.[69]

Bacterial meningitis shows a geographic distribution and/or seasonal outbreaks. Although endemic meningitis is rare in developed countries, epidemics of meningococcal meningitis are common in the sub-Saharan African region (the 'meningitis belt') and have been observed every 5 to 10 years since 1905.[146] Thus, the incidence rate varies geographically and also depends on climatic factors as well as demographics of the population, including social and public healthcare standards.[129] According to the World Health Organization (WHO), 70 per cent of CNS infections occur in patients in Africa and South East Asia.[166] In the United States, the incidence of bacterial meningitis declined significantly from 2 to 1.38 cases per 100 000 population from 1998 to 2007.[152] However, among infants below the age of 2 months, the incidence did not decrease.[152] The median age of patients suffering from bacterial meningitis increased from 30.8 years in 1998/99 to 41.9 years in 2006/2007. Despite these overall alterations in disease incidence, case fatality rates did not change significantly, still being as high as 14.3 per cent and ranging from 15–25 per cent.[71] A major risk factor for fatal outcome is delay in diagnosis and therapy; time to initiation of appropriate therapy is a major determinant of prognosis and sequelae.[71] This is particularly important, because in surviving patients residual neurologic symptoms are severely disabling and a major socioeconomic burden.

Worldwide, *Streptococcus pneumoniae*, *Neisseria meningitidis* and *Haemophilus influenzae* are responsible for more than 80 per cent of all meningitis cases. In the United States and Europe, the introduction of pneumococcal

and *H. influenzae* type B conjugate vaccine programs has significantly reduced the frequency of bacterial meningitis caused by these pathogens. These highly efficient vaccination programmes have also had a strong impact on the relative frequency of bacteria genus responsible for meningitis. This enormous clinically important success is impressively illustrated for *H. influenzae* type B, the leading cause of bacterial meningitis accounting for 11 000 cases in the United States annually. Upon introduction of the vaccine program *H. influenzae* meningitis declined by 55 per cent. Now, *S. pneumoniae*, group B *streptococci*, *N. meningitidis*, *H. influenzae* and *Listeria monocytogenes* are the five most frequent pathogens responsible for meningitis in the United States, accounting for 58 per cent, 18.1 per cent, 13.9 per cent, 6.7 per cent and 3.4 per cent of bacterial meningitis, respectively.[152] In contrast to the Western world, non-typhoidal *Salmonella* species are a frequent cause of meningitis in Malawi, Tanzania and northern Uganda,[57,99,159,160] where they have emerged as the second most common cause of paediatric meningitis after the introduction of HiB vaccine. In Asia and Africa, *S. suis* is a frequent agent causing meningitis in adults.[55] These demographic data further demonstrate that, overall, extracellular bacteria are the most relevant cause responsible for bacterial meningitis. The spectrum of infectious agents likely to cause meningitis largely depends on host factors, including age and immune status. In the newborn period, *E. coli* K1, *S. agalactiae* (group B *streptococci*) and *L. monocytogenes*, a facultative intracellular pathogen, are important causes of meningitis, but these bacteria are unlikely to cause meningitis in adults. In developing countries, *Klebsiella*, *S. aureus* and non-typhoidal *Salmonella* species have frequently been isolated from neonates.[160] In bacterial meningitis, polymicrobial infections are unusual.

Thus, the risk for bacterial infections of the CNS is determined both by parameters of the host and the pathogen, and by their complex interactions. With regard to host factors, age (newborns and elderly), underlying diseases, diabetes, malnutrition, alcohol abuse, drug addiction and, particularly, immunodeficiencies are of major importance (Table 20.1). Even slight, but prolonged, immunosuppressive medication may render patients susceptible to meningitis. With respect to the pathogen, intrinsic virulence factors, geographical distribution and seasonal aspects are relevant.

Pathogenesis of Bacterial Meningitis

The pathogenesis of bacterial meningitis is a multistep process ultimately providing bacterial access to the subarachnoid space and subsequent inflammation (Figure 20.1).

In general, three pathways of bacterial CNS invasion can be distinguished, which are mutually not exclusive. Firstly, haematogenous spread from extracerebral infectious foci, mainly from the nasopharynx, lung, genitourinary tract, skin and other sites, may facilitate entry into the CNS. Most blood-borne pathogens are commensal inhabitants of the normal mucosal flora. Haematogenous dissemination is responsible for the majority of bacterial meningitis cases nowadays. Secondly, contiguous spread of bacteria from nearby foci (i.e. otitis media, mastoiditis, sinusitis and dental abscess) may cause meningitis. This mechanism was of

TABLE 20.1 Etiology of bacterial meningitis: dependency on patient's characteristics

Group of patients	Causative pathogens
Neonates (<1 month)	E. coli K1 Group B β-haemolytic streptococci L. monocytogenes S. aureus S. epidermidis Klebsiella spp. P. aeruginosa
Children (1 month–15 years)	S. pneumoniae N. meningitidis H. influenzae
Adults (>15 years), immunocompetent	S. pneumoniae N. meningitidis (Group B streptococci)
Patients with shunt infection	S. epidermidis S. aureus
Patients with preceding neurosurgery	S. aureus S. epidermidis P. aeruginosa Gram-negative bacteria
Patients with skull fracture	S. pneumoniae H. influenzae
Patients immunocompromised as a result of old age, diabetes, corticosteroids, alcoholism	L. monocytogenes Group B streptococci

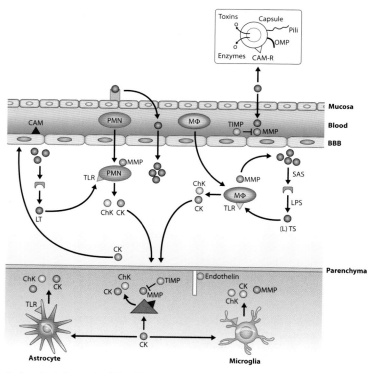

20.1 Pathophysiology of acute bacterial meningitis. CAM, cell adhesion molecules; BBB: blood-brain barrier; CAM-R, cell adhesion molecule receptor; ChK, chemokines; CK, cytokines (both pro-inflammatory and immunoregulatory); LPS, lipopolysaccharide; LT, lymphotoxin; (L)TA, (lipo)teichoic acid; PMN, polymorphonuclear leukocyte; MΦ, macrophage; MMP, matrix metalloproteinases; OMP, outer membrane proteins; SAS, subarachnoid space; TLR, toll-like receptors; TIMP, tissue inhibitors of MMP.

major importance in the past. Bone defects due to trauma or neurosurgical intervention may also facilitate bacterial access to the brain. Thirdly (and rarely), bacteria may use the axonal transport of peripheral and cranial nerves to reach the CNS. This elegant pathway, which is more frequently used by viruses, has been described for L. monocytogenes. The respective pathways used to gain access to the CNS also explain the topographical location of meningitis. In haematogenous spread, the meninges overlying the hemispheres are preferentially affected, whereas the base of the brain or circumscribed areas of the frontal and parietal lobes in the neighbourhood of ear, nose and teeth, respectively, are less frequently involved.

Thus, in order to reach the brain, blood-borne bacterial pathogens need to resist host defense mechanisms and to interact with the host in a specific manner at several distinct sites. Major challenges for all bacteria involve three major steps and sites of action: (i) mucosa: colonization; (ii) bloodstream: invasion and survival; and (iii) BBB and blood–cerobrospinal fluid (CSF) barrier: transversion. Extracellular bacteria are particularly well equipped to overcome these barriers, and hence most blood-borne infections are due to these organisms. Immunity to extracellular bacteria is mediated primarily by the innate immune system, although the immune response to intracellular bacteria also depends on the adaptive immune system.

Mucosal Colonization

Remarkably, most meningitis-inducing bacterial species, including N. meningitidis and S. pneumoniae, are commensals of the nasopharyngeal or the gastrointestinal mucosa. Asymptomatic colonization of the nasopharyngeal mucosa by S. pneumoniae occurs in up to 37 per cent and 58 per cent of young children and persons in day care centres and in up to 40 per cent of adults in hospitals and other long-term care facilities, including prisons and shelters.[100] Between 8 per cent and 25 per cent of healthy persons may carry N. meningitidis, the incidence being highest in adolescents.[132]

Under physiological conditions, the normal host defenses are sufficient to prevent bacterial binding to the mucosal surface. In the respiratory tract, mucus and lysozyme establish important barriers. Several virulence factors of bacteria target these protective mechanisms to enable their adherence to the mucosal surface. Mucus entrapment is prevented by an external polysaccharide capsule and bacterial enzymes. Accordingly, the polysaccharide capsule of S. pneumoniae and N. meningitidis interferes with mucus entrapment, supports mucosal colonization and protects from opsonization as well as from complement-mediated and phagocytic killing. The external polysaccharide capsule of S. pneumoniae repulses the sialic acid residues of mucus by its negative charges.[100] Outer membrane proteins of N. meningitidis include pili, which extend from the cell surface and facilitate initial attachment to cells and bacterial movement through mucus and over epithelial surfaces. The presence of these outer membrane components (i.e. capsular polysaccharide, outer membrane proteins as well as lipopolysaccharide [LPS]), is linked to the virulence of N. meningitidis.[146] Phosphorylcholine expressed on the surface of S. pneumoniae contributes to mucosal adhesion.[79] Bacterial enzymes also play a role in this scenario: pneumococcal enzymes including neuraminidase A and B and β-galactosidase enhance colonization by decreasing mucus viscosity, thereby preventing mucus entrapment. Furthermore, S. pneumoniae possesses deacetylating enzymes that render the bacterium resistant to lysozyme, a host enzyme that degrades the bacterial wall.[100]

Both S. pneumoniae and N. meningitidis produce immunoglobulin (Ig) A proteases that neutralize IgA antibodies. As IgA antibodies interfere with bacterial opsonization, these bacteria may inactivate the local antibody immune response in epithelial cells.[132] Pneumolysin of S. pneumoniae, a pore-forming toxin, decreases epithelial ciliary beating and facilitates bacterial binding to epithelial cells.

Epithelial Transmigration

Bacteria are able to bind specifically to epithelial cells. S. pneumoniae binds to carbohydrates on epithelial cells (GalNAc(β1–3)Gal, GalNAc(β1-4)Gal) and sialic acid.[79] The opacity-associated adhesion molecules Opa and Opc of N. meningitidis are important for adherence by binding to CECAM (CD66) expressed on the surface of nasopharyngeal epithelium and neutrophils.[132]

Following colonization of the nasopharyngeal mucosa, epithelial transmigration by endocytosis and transcytosis is required to gain access to the bloodstream. Bacterial binding to specific receptors mediates this process: S. pneumoniae may bind to the platelet-activating factor receptor on activated epithelial and endothelial cells via phosphorylcholine and also to the epithelial polymeric immunoglobulin receptor, allowing transcytosis. Epithelial permeability is regulated by cadherins and modulated by the innate immune system.[100] At the basal site of the epithelium or endothelium, bacterial hyaluran lyase degrades the extracellular matrix providing access to blood.[100]

In the Bloodstream

In order to reach the CNS, bacteria must survive in the blood in sufficient numbers. Therefore, they have to resist several further host defense mechanisms. The most important virulence factor to survive in the hostile microenvironment of the blood is the polysaccharide capsule that is present in important meningitis-inducing bacteria, (e.g. S. pneumoniae, N. meningitidis and E. coli K1).[69] In addition to its antiphagocytic properties,[79] the external capsule prevents activation of the host complement system, an important first-line defense in bacterial infections. Normally, the complement system becomes activated as soon as bacteria enter the blood; however, pneumococcal surface proteins prevent complement deposition and complement-dependent opsonophagocytosis. Bacterial toxins such as pneumococcal pneumolysin reduce the opsonic serum activity and cause the consumption of complement factors.[79,100] The complement system not only plays a role in the early phases of haematogenous spread of bacteria, but is also highly important at later stages when bacteria have reached the subarachnoid space (see p. 1196).

Bacteria in the blood also affect coagulation, because the rate of bacterial growth determines the magnitude of endotoxin release. High plasma concentrations of endotoxin excessively upregulate coagulation and downregulate fibrinolysis, ultimately resulting in disseminated intravascular coagulation.[146] Coagulation disturbances contribute significantly to mortality in bacterial meningitis. In fulminant septicaemia, a severe, often lethal complication of meningococcal infection, plasma concentrations of natural anticoagulants including antithrombin and protein C are low, whereas levels of the tissue factor pathway inhibitor are increased.[146] Large plasma amounts of plasminogen activator inhibitor type 1 (PAI-1), which is induced by interleukin

(IL)-1β and tumour necrosis factor (TNF)-α, cause a pro-coagulant state by limiting fibrinolysis.[100] This mechanism underlies the inhibition of fibrinolysis in meningococcal septicaemia; functionally important PAI-1 concentrations are a strong predictor of fatality in meningococcal infections.[146] Interestingly, PAI-1 polymorphisms affect the risk of disseminated intravascular coagulation. Patients with a genetic polymorphism of the PAI-1 gene have particularly high PAI-1 blood levels, which are directly correlated with increased fatality rates.[6] Thus, in addition to bacterial factors, host factors also determine the risk for disseminated intravascular coagulation.

In the CNS, rapidly fatal bacterial meningitis due to disseminated intravascular coagulation leads to severe brain oedema with ubiquitous petechiae within a few hours, mostly before purulent meningitis has developed.

Central Nervous System

Invasion

The magnitude of bacteraemia is an important determinant for subsequent development of meningitis. Generally, high numbers of bacteria are required to induce meningitis, further pointing to the existence of potent and highly effective protective host mechanisms and their central role in protection of the CNS. However, the magnitude of bacteraemia is not the only parameter determining CNS invasion, because bacteria need to traverse the BBB, or the blood–CSF barrier.[40] Invasion of the CNS via the blood–CSF barrier has been demonstrated experimentally for *S. suis*[150,151] and also for *L. monocytogenes*, which infects choroid plexus epithelial and ependymal cells.[133] Overall, the blood–CSF pathway is less often disrupted than the BBB, because most bacteria have developed sophisticated strategies to get across the BBB.

Bacteria may use four, not mutually exclusive, pathways to traverse the BBB: (i) the transcellular route (i.e. passive or adhesion-induced transcytosis); (ii) the paracellular route (i.e. passage through opened tight junctions); (iii) disruption of endothelial cells (e.g. resulting from cytotoxicity); and (iv) inside leukocytes (i.e. the Trojan horse mechanism).[59,69] Bacteria differ in their preferred mechanism of CNS entry; several bacteria (*S. pneumoniae*,[59,132] *S. agalactiae*,[59] *E. coli*[59] and *N. meningitidis*[132]) can use the transcytosis route. *N. meningitidis* may also cross the BBB via paracellular penetration.[132] There is little evidence that extracellular bacteria use the Trojan horse mechanism; in contrast, intracellular bacteria such as *L. monocytogenes* and *Mycobacterium tuberculosis*, which target macrophages in the CNS, may reach the brain within leukocytes. *M. tuberculosis* can also cross the BBB as a free pathogen.[69]

An elegant strategy of bacteria to cross the BBB is to bind to specific receptors expressed on the BBB, thereby taking advantage of mechanisms physiologically used by leukocytes to home to the CNS. Most bacteria possess several receptors to ensure binding to cerebral endothelium; *S. pneumoniae* and *H. influenzae* serotype B can bind to endothelial platelet-activating factor receptor.

Bacteria may also induce the expression of cell adhesion molecules on cerebral endothelial cells: *Borrelia* stimulate the expression of E-selectin, ICAM-1 (CD54) and VCAM-1 (CD106) and, thereby, facilitate invasion of brain tissue.[7,19,27] *Treponema pallidum* induces the induction of ICAM-1, VCAM-1 and E-selectin on vascular endothelial cells. Although data from studies with cerebral endothelium have not been reported so far, one might speculate that *T. pallidum* may use a similar mechanism at the BBB.[7]

The interaction of *N. meningitidis* with BBB endothelium induces localized cytoskeletal remodelling of endothelial cells and induces a dynamic redistribution of ICAM-1, VCAM-1 and CD44, which leads to the formation of 'endothelial docking structures' or 'transmigratory cups'. *N. meningitidis* therefore elegantly hijacks the cellular machinery used for leukocyte entry across the BBB into the CNS.[59]

Laminin receptors on cerebral endothelial cells provide binding opportunities for several bacteria, including pneumococci, meningococci and *H. influenzae*.[100,104] *E. coli* K1 fimbrial adhesin may bind to endothelial CD48.[69] Endothelial CD46 allows binding of *N. meningitidis* and is also used by measles virus, adenovirus and human herpesvirus 6 to enter the brain.[69,132] *N. meningitidis* as well as *S. agalactiae* interact with integrin receptors expressed on cerebral endothelial cells: *N. meningitidis* binds to fibronectin and anchors the bacterium to the integrin receptor α5β1;[69,132] *S. agalactiae* PilA protein as part of bacterial pili binds to collagen, promoting bacterial interaction with α2β1 integrin.[6] *N. meningitidis* as well as *T. pallidum* also bind to endothelial fibronectin.[13,117] A further mechanism to facilitate entry of the CNS is provided by bacterial toxins: pneumolysin is toxic to microvascular endothelial cells.[40] The meningitis-inducing capacity of bacteria correlates with their level of hyaluronidase activity; for example, meningitis-inducing *S. pneumoniae* strains exhibit significantly higher hyaluronidase activity when compared to strains that do not cause meningitis.[7,132] In addition, bacteria can also promote extracellular matrix degradation, as observed for *B. burgdorferi*.

The mechanisms that allow bacterial invasion of the CNS and activation of the host immune system are closely linked; for example streptococcal adhesion plays a dual role fostering bacterial entry into the CNS and concomitantly activating host chemokine expression and recruitment of neutrophils.[6] Vice versa, activation of the innate immune system also supports bacterial entrance into the CNS. During bacterial replication and autolysis, as occurs in bacteraemia, highly immunogenic bacterial components activate the innate immune system, which increases BBB permeability and facilitates bacterial invasion of the CNS.[59]

Immune Reactions in the CNS

Once bacteria have succeeded in entering the subarachnoid space, they have a growth advantage, because in the subarachnoid space there are low levels of complement and low numbers of resident leukocytes (i.e. meningeal, perivascular and plexus macrophages), although T and B-cells are largely absent. This situation facilitates bacterial replication.

Complement system The complement system provides the first arm of the innate immune system. It is activated once pathogens have invaded the bloodstream and is also required for bacterial defense in the subarachnoid space. Complement, together with opsonizing antibodies, kills bacteria. This is an important line of defense against bacteria such as meningococci and pneumococci, two highly relevant meningitis-inducing pathogens.

Although complement levels are generally low (or even undetectable) in the normal CSF, various components of the complement system are produced during bacterial meningitis from cellular sources including microglial cells and macrophages. However, compared to blood, CSF complement levels are still low, even under inflammatory conditions. All pathways of the complement system (i.e. the classical, the alternative and the lectin-mediated pathways) are involved in host defenses against meningitis-inducing bacteria.[132] Accordingly, persons with deficiencies in all of these complement pathways have an increased risk for meningitis.[132] Complement factors also contribute to bacterial elimination by supporting polymorphonuclear leukocyte recruitment to the CSF and fostering their phagocytic and bactericidal activity.[100]

The critical role of the complement system in the CNS for limiting bacterial growth has been demonstrated impressively in an experimental model of rabbit pneumococcal meningitis, in which C3 deficiency allowed enhanced bacterial replication, although numbers of leukocytes in the CSF were reduced, ultimately resulting in increased mortality rates.[157] Accordingly, bacteria have developed diverse strategies to escape the complement arm of the immune system.

Toll-like receptors Replicating bacteria require glucose, levels of which are low in the CSF. Thus, increasing bacterial numbers induces insufficient nutritional conditions, which results in bacterial autolysis. In this regard, it is of note that antibiotic therapy also causes bacterial degradation and autolysis. This observation underlies the rationale to include corticosteroids in the treatment regimen in patients with bacterial meningitis to control the magnitude of liberation of bacterial components and their release into the subarachnoid space. Bacterial components, in particular cell wall components, including LPS, teichoic acids (TA) and lipoteichoic acids (LTA) and peptidoglycan, strongly activate the innate immune system and exert potent pro-inflammatory effects.

In the subarachnoid space, bacterial components are recognized by pathogen-associated molecular patterns, including the family of Toll-like receptors (TLRs). TLRs are evolutionary conserved pattern-recognition transmembrane receptors[14] that detect microbial products irrespective of their life-cycle stage and immunological memory. In the CNS, TLRs are constitutively expressed on macrophages in the meninges, the choroid plexus and the perivascular spaces. Resident cell populations of the CNS parenchyma exhibit a cell-type specific TLR expression: microglial cells express all TLRs known so far,[14] whereas astrocytes express TLR1, TLR2, TLR4, TLR5, TLR6, TLR7 and TL9.[50] In contrast, TLR expression by oligodendrocytes and neurons is more restricted.[50]

TLR2 and TLR4 recognize peptidoglycan and lipoproteins as well as LPS. LPS, a product of Gram-negative bacteria, is the most potent inducer of TLR4 and also induces TLR2. Lipoproteins and peptidoglycan, components of both Gram-positive and Gram-negative bacteria, as well as LTA and TA mainly stimulate TLR2, whereas bacterial DNA is recognized by TLR9. *S. pneumoniae* and *N. meningitidis*

are recognized via TLR2, TLR4 and TLR9.[50] Astrocytes recognize *S. aureus* via TLR2.[50] The LTA and flagellin of *L. monocytogenes* are recognized by TLR2 and TLR5.[50] Most TLRs except for TLR3 sense through MyD88, the central adaptor molecule. TLR4 can signal through both the MyD88-dependent and the MyD88-independent pathways. Ultimately, activation of the TLR signalling cascades converges on nuclear factor (NF)-κB activation and induces the release of a plethora of pro-inflammatory mediators, including cytokines and chemokines.

With these characteristics, TLRs are an indispensable first-line defense for initiation of an effective immune response in bacterial meningitis to achieve control of bacterial growth and their elimination from the CNS. Their important role in bacterial meningitis has been illustrated in mouse mutants lacking individual TLRs, in which bacterial replication is significantly enhanced.[75,78] The functional role of TLR is not confined to their activation of the innate immune system, because TLR stimulation of antigen-presenting cells also stimulates adaptive immunity by priming cells for subsequent activation and expansion of antigen-specific T-cells. The severity and outcome of severe infections, including meningitis, are determined by polymorphisms in genes that regulate pathogen recognition, including TLR2 and TLR4.[146] Thus, host genetic factors that regulate non-specific immune reactions are important determinants of susceptibility for bacterial CNS infections, their course and prognosis.

Soluble mediators: cytokines, chemokines and matrix metalloproteinases In bacterial meningitis, the important early response cytokines TNF-α, IL-1β and IL-6 are produced. Cellular sources of these potent pro-inflammatory mediators are perivascular, meningeal and plexus macrophages, cerebral endothelial cells, microglia and astrocytes. IL-1β and TNF-α reach maximal CSF levels as early as within the first 18 and 24 hours, respectively.[100] They upregulate cell adhesion molecules, chemokines and their receptors on cerebral endothelial cells, fostering recruitment of polymorphonuclear leukocytes to the CSF. Furthermore, TNF exerts potent direct antibacterial effects. Genetically engineered mouse mutants lacking TNF impressively demonstrate the protective function of TNF in bacterial meningitis, as they succumb to fulminant necrotizing CNS infection with the inability to control bacterial growth.[161] The pleiotropic cytokine IL-6 potently activates acute phase proteins and the complement system.[54]

In addition to these early response cytokines, a plethora of pro-inflammatory cytokines and chemokines is released into the CSF during bacterial meningitis, including IL-12p70, MIF, IFN-γ and GRO-α (CXCL-1), MIP-1α (CCL3), MIP-1β (CCL4) and MCP1 (CCL2). IL-8 (CXCL-8), MIP-1α and MIP-1β, MIP-2, GRO-α (CXCL-1) potently attract polymorphonuclear leukocytes and macrophages/monocytes to the site of infection.[141] Furthermore, reactive nitrogen species such as inducible nitric oxide synthase (iNOS), nitric oxide (NO) and reactive oxygen species (ROS) are released into the CSF, which exert potent antimicrobial properties. Nevertheless, despite these essential protective functions, unwanted side effects of these mediators as well as of TNF disturbance the BBB mediate neurotoxicity, unfortunately contributing to long-term neurological sequelae. Therefore, the production of counterbalancing mediators is important to prevent over-reaction of the immune response.

The potent anti-inflammatory mediator IL-10 is also released into the CSF in bacterial meningitis.[35] IL-10 is produced by macrophages, T-lymphocytes and B-lymphocytes. IL-10 downregulates the immune response by reducing the number of immune cells and the level of pro-inflammatory cytokines without affecting bacterial elimination;[24] this specific immunosuppressive activity is important in the setting of a strong pro-inflammatory immune reaction directed against intracerebral bacteria in order to counterbalance the immune reaction.

Cytokines induce matrix metalloproteinases (MMPs).[87] MMPs are a large family of endopeptidases that are released on demand in an inactive form. Among cytokines that provide the stimulatory signal for MMP, IL-1β and TNF-α/β are the most potent inducers of MMP, but components of infectious pathogens may also promote MMP secretion.[87] Cells of the immune system are the main sources of MMPs, predominantly polymorphonuclear leukocytes and macrophages, as well as T-cells. In addition, various resident brain cell populations (i.e. astrocytes, microglia, endothelial cells, neurons and vascular smooth muscle cells) also contribute to MMP secretion. Generally, MMPs control tissue degradation and remodelling by regulating components of the extracellular matrix; specifically, MMPs help to maintain the structural integrity of the BBB. In bacterial meningitis, MMPs contribute to BBB opening and invasion of the brain parenchyma by immune cells. MMP induction is an early event in bacterial meningitis; elevated MMP9 levels in the CSF are detectable as early as 15 minutes after infection of rats with Pneumococcus.[85] MMP8 and MMP9 are also upregulated in the CSF of children with bacterial meningitis and the increase of MMP8 is regarded as being specific for bacterial meningitis.[87] High CSF levels of MMP9 have been identified as a risk factor for the subsequent development of the neuronal damage that underlies the long-term neurological sequelae of bacterial meningitis.[87]

In addition to their interaction with components of the extracellular matrix, MMPs also interact with cytokines and cell adhesion molecules, indicating a complex reciprocal interaction between these various components of the immune response. Selectins and ICAM-1 further amplify MMPs in activated endothelium, and also serve as substrate for MMPs. MMPs also induce the proteolytic release of membrane-bound cytokines; in order to regulate this pro-inflammatory activity, MMPs are counterbalanced by tissue inhibitors of MMPs (TIMPs), levels of which are also elevated in the CSF in bacterial meningitis. TIMPs are induced by pro-inflammatory cytokines IL-1β and TNF-α in astrocytes, microglia, cerebral endothelial cells[114,148] and neurons.[48] Their effect is protective and homeostatic through MMP inhibition, thereby preserving matrix components and maintaining the integrity of the BBB. Neuronal TIMP production aims at protection against glutamate-mediated neurotoxicity and thereby fosters neuronal survival and prevents cortical damage.[48]

Recruitment of immune cells to the central nervous system Following cytokine-mediated upregulation of cell adhesion molecules on cerebral endothelial cells, polymorphonuclear leukocytes are the first cell population recruited to the subarachnoid space.

Tethering of neutrophils is mediated by P-, E- and L-selectin, which are required for initial rolling of the cells at the endothelial surface.[45] Subsequently, integrins on neutrophils assure their tight adhesion to cerebral endothelial cells. Neutrophils bind predominantly through CD11b/CD18 to ICAM-1 expressed on cerebral endothelium.

Neutrophils enter the subarachnoid space mainly at the venous sites of the penetrating cerebral blood vessels.[100] From here, they invade the perivascular space. The formation of inflammatory cuffs of neutrophils occurs as rapidly as within 6 hours after infection. Polymorphonuclear cells exert direct antimicrobial activity by opsonizing, phagocytosing and destroying bacteria together with complement and antibody.[100] In addition, they contribute to the antibacterial immune response by their release of reactive nitric and oxygen species.[100]

Effects of the bacteria-induced immune response on the central nervous system parenchyma

Activation of resident brain cell populations: Following activation of the immune response in the subarachnoid space, some neutrophils may also invade the perivascular space within the adjacent cortex. TLRs and the pro-inflammatory cytokines TNF, IL-1 and IL-6 can activate microglial cells and astrocytes in the brain. Activation is evidenced by upregulation of cell adhesion molecules, including ICAM-1 and MHC class I and II molecules on microglia as well as MHC class I antigen on astrocytes.[25] In addition, microglia and astrocytes upregulate TLRs and produce TNF and iNOS, which contribute to bacterial elimination but also alter cerebral blood flow, thereby contributing to hypoxia and brain oedema, and may cause neuronal damage.

Cerebral blood flow: In bacterial meningitis, cerebral blood flow is altered at different stages of disease. Early in meningitis, cerebral blood flow is increased, whereas it is reduced in later phases with a global reduction in advanced meningitis.

Cerebral blood flow disturbances result from inflammation of both large and small arteries and veins, which narrows the lumen of the affected vessels and causes vasospasm (fostered by toxic mediators), ultimately resulting in ischaemic or haemorrhagic infarction of the brain parenchyma supplied. In early meningitis, NO has a vasodilatory effect on pial arterioles,[76] which may even protect against ischaemia, but it reduces cerebral blood flow in later stages. ROS produced by granulocytes, macrophages and endothelial cells also contribute to cerebral blood flow reduction. In addition to these mediators, endothelins derived from endothelial cells, glial cells and neurons cause vasoconstriction, thereby contributing to ischaemia.[77] Global reduction of cerebral blood flow in late stages is due to a loss of autoregulation,[158] which was also demonstrated in experimental pneumococcal meningitis,[76] causing increased intracranial pressure as well as systemic hypotension.

Brain oedema: Bacterial cell wall components, the release of pro-inflammatory mediators with toxic side effects and BBB disturbances may cause vasogenic, cytotoxic and interstitial brain oedema. Brain oedema may be severe enough to cause herniation and brain stem compression and, in the worse cases, cessation of cerebral perfusion.

Neuronal damage: Neuronal damage is a frequent and unwanted complication of bacterial meningitis, induced by neurotoxic mediators such as TNF, NO produced by endothelial nitric oxide synthase and iNOS as well as ROS. *S. pneumoniae* and *L. monocytogenes* meningitis is characterized by segmental apoptosis of hippocampal neurons, affecting the CA1–4 region.[41,105,134] In *S. pneumoniae*-induced experimental meningitis, pneumolysin and the pneumococcal toxin H_2O_2 cause pyknosis of neurons in the hippocampal dentate gyrus, followed by caspase-dependent apoptosis of immature neurons in the subgranular region of the dentate gyrus.[100] In addition to the hippocampus, cerebellar Purkinje cells are susceptible to apoptosis in *L. monocytogenes* meningitis.[134]

White matter damage: White matter damage may result from vasculitis leading to ischaemic changes in the brain tissue.[40] In addition to focal ischaemia, global ischaemia and cytotoxic oedema may contribute to white matter lesions, which differ considerably in their prominence and may be widespread in individual cases. The subcortical areas, deep white matter, thalamus, brain stem and cerebellum may show a focal loss of myelinated fibre and axonal damage.[1,104]

Regulatory pathways: The pro-inflammatory immune reaction must be finely tuned and tightly regulated to achieve an optimal immune response with rapid and complete bacterial elimination, however, not at cost of excessive inflammation that may cause secondary unwanted injury to the brain. This includes the expression of Fas/FasL and TRAIL, which induces removal of damaged cells including neutrophils from the CSF by apoptosis. In addition, multifunctional neuroimmunoregulatory molecules including exchange protein activated by cyclic AMP (EPAC1) that regulates cytokine synthesis and endothelial permeability, SOCS inhibiting macrophages/microglia, CD200 expressed by neurons and cerebral endothelial cells providing an antiphagocytic signal and downregulating microglial activation, CD47 downregulating pro-inflammatory cytokines and upregulating TGF-β to reduce neutrophil homing to the CNS and to prevent microglial phagocytosis, sialic acid-binding Ig-like lectins, and thrombomodulin all contribute to a well-balanced immune response in the CNS.[106] Regulatory components of the complement pathway expressed by glia, neurons and BBB endothelium reduce complement activation in the later phase of meningitis in order to finally reduce inflammatory cytokines, neutrophil infiltration and to clear apoptotic cells.[106]

Clinical Characteristics

Clinically, bacterial meningitis is an acute, life-threatening, often fulminant disease, which may complicate a preceding nasopharyngeal or other infection outside the CNS. Neurologically, the hallmarks of bacterial meningitis are headache (87 per cent of patients), neck stiffness (74 per cent of patients), fever (44 per cent of patients), and impaired consciousness.[71] However, patients do not necessarily manifest all of these symptoms. Only 44 per cent of patients with bacterial meningitis present with all four symptoms;[71] in 95 per cent of patients, at least two of these four major symptoms are present.[71] Furthermore, patients complain of nausea, vomiting and photophobia. Epileptic seizures occur in 5–10 per cent of patients,[71] and additional focal neurologic symptoms are present in one-third of patients.[71]

Rapid diagnosis and immediate initiation of appropriate treatment are of key importance and predict outcome. It is important to stress that delay in diagnosis and therapy is a major adverse prognostic factor responsible for poor outcome and long-term neurological sequelae, and accounts for the fact that despite the availability of appropriate modern antibiotics, fatality rates are still unacceptably high.

Newborns, Elderly and Immunocompromised Patients

Immunocompromised patients, including newborns and elderly persons, are at increased risk of bacterial meningitis. The clinical presentation of meningitis differs in these groups of patients, because they often present with milder neurological symptoms and may lack signs of meningeal irritation. This is because the clinical symptoms of meningeal irritation, such as neck stiffness, Kernig and Brudzinski's signs, develop as a consequence of the host immune response in the subarachnoid space. In patients with an impaired immune system that precludes generation of a strong immune response in the subarachnoid space, the absence of meningism does not exclude bacterial meningitis. Newborn infants with bacterial meningitis frequently lack nuchal rigidity and a bulging fontanelle; the presence of fever or hypothermia, lethargy, feeding problems and seizures should alert to the differential diagnosis of bacterial meningitis. In elderly persons with meningitis, confusion and impaired consciousness may be more prominent than in younger patients. Thus, bacterial meningitis needs to be excluded in febrile elderly patients who show alterations in their mental status and consciousness.

An increased risk for meningitis due to specific bacteria is determined by the nature of the underlying immunodeficiency (Table 20.2). Patients with defects in cell-mediated immunity have an increased risk for meningitis due to intracellular bacteria, because efficient control of infection caused by intracellular pathogens requires an interaction with antigen-specific T-lymphocytes and macrophages. *L. monocytogenes* infection is frequently observed in neonates who acquired the pathogen from a maternal infection (e.g. of the genitourinary tract), and in pregnant women, elderly persons, diabetics and alcohol addicts. HIV-infected patients are particularly susceptible to opportunistic infections due to parasites, fungi and bacteria, including *M. tuberculosis* and *T. pallidum*.

Patients with defects in humoral immunity show increased susceptibility to bacterial infections in which antibodies play a major protective role (i.e. infections with encapsulated bacteria). These patients are therefore at increased risk for *S. pneumoniae*, *N. meningitidis* and *H. influenzae* meningitis.

Patients with neutropenia due to either insufficient numbers of polymorphonuclear leukocytes or impaired neutrophil function are at increased risk of developing meningitis caused by *Pseudomonas aeruginosa* and members of the *Enterobacteriaceae* family.[4] Patients lacking neutrophils may also either lack these signs or may present with only minimal meningeal irritation because formation of inflammatory infiltrates in the subarachnoid space is impaired. Thus, in patients with neutropenia, the presence of fever

TABLE 20.2 Immune defects associated with increased risk for specific bacterial infections of the CNS

Immune defect	Causative pathogen
Neutropenia	P. aeruginosa Enterobacteriaceae
Splenectomy	S. pneumoniae H. influenzae type B N. meningitidis
Impairment of cell-mediated immunity (neonates, lymphoma, organ transplantation, prolonged corticosteroid therapy)	L. monocytogenes
Defects in humoral immunity (CLL, Hodgkin's disease, radiotherapy/chemotherapy)	S. pneumoniae H. influenzae type B N. meningitidis

with headache and alterations of consciousness should raise the suspicion of bacterial meningitis, even in the absence of meningeal signs.

Splenectomized patients are at increased risk for meningitis caused by encapsulated bacteria and are in danger of fulminant meningitis with uncontrolled bacterial replication leading to an extraordinarily high level of bacteraemia. Furthermore, the production of IgM antibodies is impaired in these patients, who consequently lack the opsonizing property of IgM antibodies.

Diagnosis

Following neurological examination, CSF analysis provides the most important diagnostic information (Figure 20.2 and Table 20.3). CSF cell counts usually exceed 10 000 cells/µL, with elevated protein levels, and low glucose levels due to glucose consumption by replicating bacteria. Polymorphonuclear granulocytes dominate in the early stage, when bacteria may be identified by Gram staining. At this time point, the identification of bacteria by Gram staining and bacterial culture reaches a sensitivity of up to 90 per cent.[71] Latex agglutination tests are highly sensitive for demonstration of H. influenzae (78–100 per cent), S. pneumoniae (67–100 per cent) and N. meningitidis (50–93 per cent) with 90–100 per cent specificity.[71] PCR analysis may be helpful in cases of negative Gram staining and antigen tests.

Although CSF analysis is of upmost importance, lumbar puncture should be restricted to patients without elevated brain pressure. In patients with elevated intracranial pressure in whom lumbar puncture is risky, blood cultures should be set up prior to the immediate application of antibiotic therapy. Neuroradiology should then be performed to exclude increased intracranial pressure; if increased intracranial pressure has been ruled out, lumbar puncture should be performed. It is important to recognize that a delay in the initiation of antibiotic therapy is a decisive parameter determining residual neurologic sequelae and outcome. The major role of neuroimaging in the diagnosis of bacterial meningitis is the exclusion of increased intracerebral pressure and co-existing local space-occupying mass lesions (brain abscess).

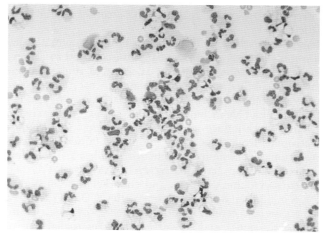

20.2 CSF in acute bacterial meningitis. Many polymorphonuclear granulocytes and a few monocytes in the highly cellular CSF. Note huge numbers of bacteria mainly residing within the cytoplasm of neutrophils. Pappenheim stain, original magnification x400.

Neuropathology

Infections caused by various pyogenic bacteria lead to common neuropathology, irrespective of the underlying bacterial strain. Only some minor differences may be noticed between infections caused by different pathogens. In H. influenzae meningitis, the purulent exudate may be particularly prominent and bulky in the basilar cisterns and cerebral sulci, whereas in S. pneumoniae meningitis, the convexities of the cerebral hemispheres are predominantly involved.

In autopsy cases, careful inspection should be performed to identify a primary focus of infection (i.e. inspection of the scalp, respiratory, teeth and gums, sinuses, heart valves, lungs, etc.).

Morphologically, cases with a hyperacute course leading to death within 24 hours are distinct from acute and subacute cases. In patients who succumb to fulminant disease, massive brain oedema and acute disseminated bleeding (multiple petechiae) due to coagulopathy are predominant, although pus formation is still absent. In these cases, the

TABLE 20.3 CSF findings in bacterial CNS infections

Disease	Opening pressure	WBC	Protein	Glucose	Microscopy	Specific tests
Bacterial meningitis, untreated	↑ >180 mm H$_2$O	↑ (10 000 cells/mm^3) polymorphonuclear granulocytes dominate	↑ >50–500 mg/dL	↓ <40 mg/dL	Gram stain + (60–90%)	Latex agglutination specific for *S. pneumoniae*, *N. meningitidis*, *H. influenzae* + (50–100%)
Bacterial meningitis, treated, regressing	normal	↑ ↓ neutrophils ↑ lymphocytes ↑ monocytes ↑ histiocytes ↑ plasma cells	↑ >50–500 mg/dL	↓ <40 mg/dL	Gram stain ±	
Brain abscess	normal or ↑	↑ ≤10 000 cells/mm^3	normal or ↑	normal or ↓	Gram stain −	
Tuberculosis	normal or ↑	↑ 50–300 cells/mm^3	↑ 100–200 mg/dL	↓ <40 mg/dL	Ziehl–Neelsen ± Fluorochrome stain ±	
Neurosyphilis[a]	normal	↑ 50–400 cells/mm^3 lymphocytes dominate	normal or ↑ up to 200 mg/dL	normal or slight ↓	−	VDRL+
Neuroborreliosis	normal or ↑ up to 500 mm H$_2$O	↑ 100–200 cells/mm^3 <500 cells/mm^3 >90% lymphocytes B-cells dominate immunoblasts plasma cells	↑ 100–300 mg/dL	normal slight ↓ possible	−	IgM+, IgG+, IgA+ oligoclonal IgG+

[a]Cerebrospinal fluid may be normal.

leptomeninges are congested. Microscopy usually reveals huge numbers of bacteria in the absence of an inflammatory host reaction. Bacteria cover the meninges and may also invade blood vessel walls and the perivascular spaces of leptomeningeal and cortical vessels.

Within the first 48 hours of bacterial meningitis, macroscopic detection of pus may be difficult. In these cases, comprehensive histopathological analyses of brain tissue, including meninges taken from multiple different areas, are required in association with microbacterial cultures, even if the meninges look normal on macroscopic inspection. Pus is usually first detectable in the basal cisterns. Beyond 48 hours, pus is usually easily detected: the meninges become cloudy as a result of pus formation. With time, the exudate may become yellow, greenish and creamy. The meninges of the cerebral convexity as well as the basal cisterns, where the subarachnoid space is most deep, are most prominently involved (Figures 20.3 and 20.4). The inflammatory exudate may spread over the whole surface of the brain to cerebellum, brain stem, cranial nerves and spinal cord. The exudate enlarges the subarachnoid space, but is confined to the subarachnoid space and does not encroach on the brain parenchyma (Figure 20.5).

Microscopically, in the early phases the composition of the leptomeningeal infiltrate is similar to the CSF. Neutrophils are intermingled with bacteria in the subarachnoid space and the leptomeningeal vessels, some containing phagocytosed bacteria. Bacteria may also reside extracellularly and can invade the upper cortical layers. At this time point, although inflammatory infiltrates are confined to the subarachnoid space, neuronal damage in the adjacent oedematous cortex is reflected in increased cytoplasmic eosinophilia. With time, inflammatory infiltrates also encroach on blood vessels in the leptomeninges and in the upper cortical layers. This may proceed to transmural inflammation, which may result in fibrinoid necrosis of the vessel wall and thrombosis, ultimately leading to cortical necrosis. Infection of the leptomeningeal veins may progress to thrombophlebitis and to thrombosis of sinus veins, with surrounding brain oedema.

At the end of the first week, the composition of the inflammatory infiltrate in the subarachnoid space changes. Numbers of neutrophils decline while macrophages, lymphocytes, monocytes, plasma cells and histiocytes increase in number. In the upper layers of the adjacent cortex, damaged neurons show increased cytoplasmic eosinophilia and pyknosis. In addition, astrocytes and microglial cells are activated, as with upregulation of GFAP and MHC class I and II antigens, respectively. Astrocytes exhibit swollen processes, and microglial cells show enlarged, rod-shaped nuclei and prominent, stellate cellular processes. White matter damage, similar to that observed with ischaemia,

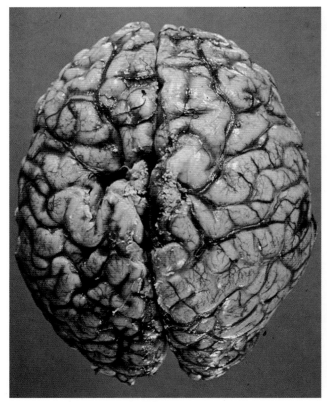

20.3 Acute bacterial meningitis. Pus overlying the convexities of the cerebral hemispheres. In addition, the brain is markedly swollen.

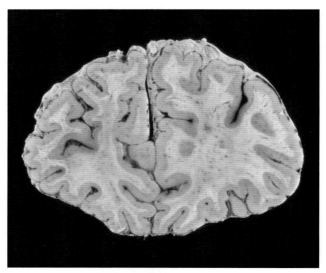

20.4 Acute bacterial meningitis. Purulent exudate in the subarachnoid space of the convexities also extending into the interhemispheric fissure.

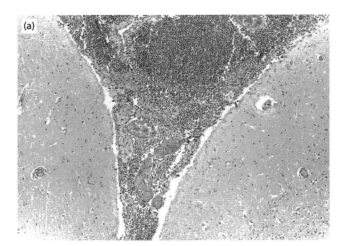

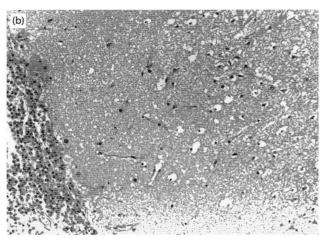

20.5 Acute bacterial meningitis. (a) Marked enlargement of the subarachnoid space by a purulent inflammatory infiltrate. Note the presence of inflammatory infiltrates in the Virchow-Robin space of cortical vessels and cortical oedema. H&E stain, original magnification ×100. **(b)** Oedema and neuronal damage in the cortex adjacent to inflamed leptomeninges infiltrated by predominantly neutrophils, macrophages and some lymphocytes. H&E stain, original magnification ×100.

becomes obvious with loss of myelinated fibres in the subcortical white matter as well as in other areas of the brain, including caudal regions (i.e. brain stem and cerebellum).

Because the subarachnoid space and the ventricular system are in continuity, purulent inflammation may spread to the ventricles. In severe cases, even pyocephalus may develop, with pus covering the choroid plexus and ependymal lining of the ventricular wall. Oedema of the ependymal and subependymal brain parenchyma may cause desquamation of the ependymal cell layer, subsequently stimulating activation of astrocytes and microglial cells. Destruction of the ependyma, adhesions and fibrous scarring may disturb CSF circulation, resulting in obstructive hydrocephalus. Impaired CSF resorption may lead to communicating hydrocephalus. Neurons in areas adjacent to the ventricles may be damaged and undergo apoptosis. These morphological alterations are particularly marked in neurons of the hippocampus and dentate gyrus and underlies subsequent learning disabilities in children who recover from purulent bacterial meningitis.[105] Inflammatory infiltrates of cranial nerves and their roots may lead to axonal degeneration, resulting in the deafness if the VIII nerve is involved.

At the end of the second week, the inflammatory purulent exudate increases in cases with progressive infection. At this time point, the infiltrate may show a bilayered appearance, with neutrophils composing the outer layer close to the arachnoid and a mixed inflammatory infiltrate consisting of macrophages, lymphocytes and plasma cells forming the inner layer close to the pia mater. However, in contrast to other CNS infections (e.g. tuberculosis and neurosyphilis), bacterial meningitis rarely runs a chronic course.

Complications and Prognosis

Complications that are major determinants of a poor prognosis include vascular alterations (vasculitis, vasospasm), hydrocephalus, sepsis, increased intracranial pressure as a result of oedema, which may eventually lead to herniation, seizures and ischaemic insults[46] (Figure 20.6). These complications, unfortunately, are not rare: among adult patients with pneumococcal meningitis, 22 per cent and 10 per cent developed arterial and venous vascular complications, respectively, 5 per cent had subarachnoid haemorrhage in the presence of vasculitis, and 1-9 per cent had intracranial bleeding.[62] Many important complications have been attributed to the host immune response rather to the bacteria. In this regard, pro-inflammatory cytokines, particularly TNF, iNOS and ROS, which exert prominent neurotoxic properties, play an important role. These observations further stress the importance of an optimally balanced immune reaction that efficiently eliminates bacteria while avoiding damage of the CNS.

Up to 30 per cent of surviving patients suffer from long-term neurological symptoms.[79] These include seizures (28 per cent),[72] sensorineural deafness (in 26 per cent and 31 per cent of adult and paediatric patients with pneumococcal meningitis, respectively),[62] focal neurological symptoms, including haemiplegia as well as cognitive, mental and behavioural abnormalities. In children, mental impairment and retardation, cognitive deficits, learning disabilities and behavioural abnormalities may result. In neonates, hydrocephalus, epilepsy, mental impairment and hypotonia may develop. Obstructive hydrocephalus may require the introduction of a ventriculoperitoneal shunt with the subsequent risk of catheter dysfunction and shunt infection. Development of a subdural effusion or hygroma occurs

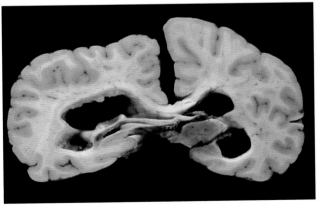

20.6 Ventriculitis. Purulent ventriculitis as complication of acute bacterial meningitis. The walls of the lateral ventricle are covered by a purulent exudate.

preferentially in children. In most cases, therapeutic intervention is not required.

In the special case of the Gram-positive facultative intracellular bacterium *L. monocytogenes*, encephalitis and brain abscess may complicate meningitis, particularly if antibiotic therapy was inadequate. This capacity of *L. monocytogenes*, which has a special affinity for the fourth ventricle and the brain stem, can be attributed at least in part to the infection not only of macrophages, ependymal cells, and choroid plexus epithelium, but also of neurons, which provide a safe harbour allowing the bacteria to escape from therapy.[133] The development of rhombencephalitis and brain stem abscess is a characteristic feature of *L. monocytogenes* infection of the CNS and is a serious complication of *L. monocytogenes*-induced meningitis. Thus, in suspected cases a careful search for *L. monocytogenes* is required (Gram staining, immunohistochemistry), which may demonstrate the bacteria both intracellularly and extracellularly in the CSF and in target cells, respectively.

Chronic meningitis may develop upon insufficient treatment with incomplete resolution of the inflammatory infiltrate, which may result in fibrotic, thickened meninges. The organized, fibrous infiltrate may lead to hydrocephalus as a result of disturbance of the arachnoid villi and blockade of the basal cisterns. In the spinal cord, such organized granulation tissue may compress the parenchyma of the spinal cord and may impair blood flow, sometimes resulting in spinal cord infarction or venous occlusion.

BRAIN ABSCESS

Introduction and Aetiology

Brain abscess is defined as space-occupying, focal infectious inflammation demarcated from the adjacent brain tissue. Brain abscess is the second most common infectious disorder of the CNS. In the United States, brain abscess accounts for one in every 10 000 hospital admissions.[64] In addition to bacteria, fungi and parasites may cause brain abscess and should therefore be considered in the differential diagnosis. As with meningitis, brain abscess may result from local extension of an extracerebral infectious focus (e.g. of teeth, ear [otitis, mastoiditis], frontal sinus). Nowadays, most cases are caused by haematogenous spread from a distant infectious focus, most commonly in the heart (endocarditis, congenital heart defect with shunt) or lung (bronchiectasis). In addition, penetrating head trauma may lead to brain abscess, and brain abscess may also develop after a neurosurgical intervention.

In contrast to bacterial meningitis, several pathogens may simultaneously underlie a brain abscess. In immunocompetent adult patients, most cases are due to streptococcal species, particularly *S. milleri* (approximately 50 per cent), *Bacteroides* species (20–40 per cent), Gram-negative enterobacterieae including *Proteus*, *E. coli*, *Klebsiella* and *Pseudomonas* (20–30 per cent) and *S. aureus* (10–15 per cent),[71] although many other bacteria may cause brain abscesses. In traumatic and postoperative brain abscess, *S. aureus* is the most frequent etiologic agent. In mixed infections, *Proteus* species are most frequent, particularly in abscess following dental infection. Otogenic brain abscess is particularly caused by *P. aeruginosa*, which may also cause abscess following a neurosurgical intervention or head trauma, as well as abscess resulting from haematogenous spread. Anaerobic bacteria are frequently isolated from mixed cultures.[63] The spectrum of bacteria in neonates differs from adult patients, with *Proteus mirabilis* accounting for 90 per cent, *E. coli* for 7 per cent, and *Serratia marcescens* in 3 per cent, respectively.[63,126]

The majority (75–90 per cent) manifests as a single brain abscess. The topography of the abscess depends on the underlying aetiology; sinusitis and otitis usually cause abscess in a frontal and temporal location, respectively. Abscesses resulting from septicaemia are frequently located in the territory supplied by the middle cerebral artery, whereas haematogenously induced abscesses may be multiple. Overall, abscesses are often located at the border of the grey to white matter and within the white matter. Abscesses are located in decreasing frequency in the following regions: frontal, temporal, parietal and occipital lobes. The midbrain, cerebellum and brain stem are less commonly affected.

Pathogenesis of Brain Abscess

Neuroimmunologically, brain abscess can be regarded as a controlled, focal immune response to an infectious pathogen. However, the immune response is not able to totally eradicate the pathogen and to achieve healing (i.e. complete resolution of the lesion). Thus, brain abscess represents a suboptimal immune reaction that is still able to control and to locally restrict the infection. Whenever the immunological balance between the host and the pathogen (which still may have persisted, even in low numbers) shifts (e.g. during immunosuppression), control may be lost with enlargement of the abscess, necrosis and rupture into the ventricular system, which carries a high mortality rate of 80 per cent.[64]

Immune Reactions in Brain Abscess

The intracerebral immune responses during brain abscess development have been elucidated in detail in a murine model of experimental *S. aureus*-induced brain abscess, which mimics human brain abscess in important aspects including both the kinetics of disease as well as its neuropathological characteristics.[33,65,145] These studies revealed interesting parallels in the immune reactions against the infectious pathogen in brain abscess and pyogenic bacterial meningitis, and indicated the common factors of the host immune system required for survival.

In experimental brain abscess, TLR-mediated activation of the innate immune system is required to initiate appropriate immune responses in the brain. In the absence of TLR2, TLR4 and MyD88, mice were unable to prevent a lethal course of disease because of unrestricted bacterial replication and spread throughout the CNS.[67,144] The presence of pyogenic bacteria in the brain parenchyma strongly activates the TLRs. In the brain adjacent, astrocytes rapidly respond to TLR2, and microglia appear to react particularly to MyD88 stimulation. In the acute phase of abscess formation, pro-inflammatory cytokines and chemokines are induced, including IL-1α, IL-1β, IL-6, TNF-α, MCP-1, MIP-1α, MIP-1β, MIP-2 and RANTES.[66,142,143] In

addition, cerebral endothelial cells are activated and upregulate ICAM-1 and platelet endothelial cell adhesion molecule.[65,66,68,143] The indispensable role for the early immune response cytokines IL-1 and TNF in bacterial clearance has been demonstrated impressively in respective mouse mutants, which succumb to unrestricted bacterial replication with overwhelming, necrotizing encephalitis and a failure to locally restrict inflammation.[145,143] Together, these immune factors stimulate the recruitment of leukocytes, at first of neutrophils and macrophages, to the infected brain parenchyma. Thereafter, CD4 and CD8 T-cells also home to the CNS. Immune cells surround the infectious, necrotic focus and efficiently eliminate bacteria from the abscess.[145] In addition to pro-inflammatory mediators, an important role was also identified for the immunosuppressive cytokine IL-10, which balances the immune response by limiting numbers of neutrophils, macrophages, and T-lymphocytes. IL-10 is also required for prevention of a necrotizing vasculitis, microvascular haemorrhage and severe brain oedema, as well as for restriction of abscess size.[142] The hallmark of brain abscess is the local confinement of inflammation in the brain parenchyma due to the formation of characteristic layers of immune cells and a capsule consisting of mixed glial and mesenchymal fibres. In experimental murine brain abscess, several factors relevant for capsule formation have been identified. Early in intracerebral infection, astrocytes are activated and their activation persists throughout disease into late chronic stages. Astrocyte activation leads to upregulation of GFAP, with increased production of glial fibres and gliosis. The important bordering function of astrocytic GFAP was impressively demonstrated in GFAP-deficient mice, which were unable to locally confine inflammation and which developed large, ill-defined inflammatory lesions with increased bacterial replication and lack of restriction of bacterial propagation. This scenario resulted in widespread dissemination of the inflammation into the contralateral hemisphere, purulent ventriculitis, vasculitis and severe brain oedema.[142] In addition to resident brain cells, mesenchymal elements also contribute to abscess wall formation to sequester the lesion. Both M1 macrophages, which exert potent inflammatory and microbicidal effects, and M2 macrophages, which contribute to resolution of inflammation and fibrosis, are present in brain abscesses.[3] Hypoxia-inducible factor-1α is also induced preceding the fibrotic and angiogenic response during which fibronectin and type I collagen are produced.[3] These specific neuroimmune reactions contribute to the characteristic neuropathology of brain abscess.

It is still an open and challenging question why the neuroimmune response achieves bacterial control and sequestration of pyogenic inflammation of the brain tissue, but does not achieve complete healing. The factors that limit effectiveness and prevent healing with complete eradication of the infectious pathogen and resolution of the inflammation still remain to be identified. In this regard, it is of note that brain abscess development requires pre-existing damage of the brain parenchyma. One predisposing factor is regional hypoxia, which facilitates subsequent development of brain tissue necrosis upon bacterial colonization. Interestingly, hypoxia-inducible factor-1α has been demonstrated in experimental brain abscess, which supports the hypothesis for a pathogenetic role of hypoxia.[3]

Clinical Characteristics

Neurological symptoms depend on abscess localization within the brain, because it is a space-occupying mass lesion. The onset of symptoms may be sudden or insidious. Frequently, patients present within two weeks; however, duration of disease may vary from a few hours up to several months.[71] There may be a clinical history of preceding infections (e.g. sinusitis, otitis, mastoiditis, dental abscess, lung disease, endocarditis). Symptoms and speed of their development depend on the topographical location of the lesion, bacterial virulence and the presence of associated disorders, again indicating that in addition to the offending pathogen, host factors of the CNS and the immune system influence the ensuing disease. Symptoms include headache (70–90 per cent), fever (50 per cent), focal neurological symptoms (20–50 per cent; including hemiparesis, ataxia, hemianopia, aphasia), nausea and vomiting (25–50 per cent), papilloedema (25–40 per cent), signs of meningeal irritation (25–30 per cent) and seizures (20–30 per cent).[71]

The mortality rate from brain abscess is nowadays below 10 per cent.[71] Old age, delay in diagnosis, insufficient treatment, ventricular rupture and coma influence prognosis adversely.[63] In surviving patients, long-term complications include epilepsy in 12 per cent of cases, focal neurological deficits, and, in children, cognitive impairment and behavioural abnormalities.[63]

Diagnosis

Routine blood studies and blood cultures are usually uninformative. The CSF often shows non-specific findings, including increased numbers of leukocytes (up to 100 000 cells/µL). CSF protein levels may be normal or increased, and glucose levels are variably normal or decreased. Attempts to identify the pathogen usually fail. In addition to the limited diagnostic value of CSF analysis, lumbar puncture is dangerous and may induce cerebral herniation in patients with cerebral abscesses.

Neuroimaging is valuable in establishing the diagnosis of brain abscess; in particular, magnetic resonance imaging (MRI) is highly sensitive in the detection of brain abscess. A similar 'ring-like structure' may be detected in patients with glioblastoma multiforme, which, in addition to other intracerebral tumours (e.g. CNS metastases), is an important differential diagnosis to be ruled out. A definite diagnosis can be achieved by stereotactic biopsy, which reveals the necrotic centre and parts of the abscess capsule and may also lead to the identification of the underlying pathogen. Stereotactic aspiration is also the therapy of choice and is superior to open neurosurgical excision, which has a mean mortality rate of 12.7 per cent.[124] If repeated aspirations and antibiotic therapy do not result in healing, an open neurosurgical approach may be required. If present, the primary focus of infections also needs to be treated.

Frequent complications of brain abscess are brain oedema, which may be pronounced, and hydrocephalus. Rupture of the abscess into the ventricular system is associated with a high mortality of 80 per cent of cases[63,64] and, because the ventricular system is contiguous with the subarachnoid space, meningitis, disturbance of CSF flow and a further increase in intracranial pressure may develop. Rarely, haemorrhage into the abscess cavity may occur.

Neuropathology

Brain abscess develops in a highly characteristic and sequential manner within a reasonably well-defined period of time. After 3–4 weeks, the typically layered composition is achieved.

Four stages of brain abscess development can be discerned (Table 20.4):

I. **Early cerebritis (day 1–3 after infection)**: This early stage is characterized by focal purulent encephalitis. The factors inducing brain abscess to develop from the focal encephalitic lesion in humans are still ill-defined. It is assumed that pre-existing focal brain parenchymal damage predisposes to development of brain abscess. As an initiating event, microvascular damage is considered important. Microvascular damage most frequently affects brain tissue at the border of the grey to the white matter. In these areas the collateral vascular supply is limited, which may result in local hypoxia, as with observations in the murine model of brain abscess. Bacteria damage small blood vessels, allowing invasion of the adjacent brain tissue. Here, they induce a small area of necrosis and initiate inflammation, which is locally confined, poorly demarcated and associated with prominent oedema and activation of microglial cells and astrocytes.

II. **Late cerebritis (day 4–9 after infection)**: This stage of disease is characterized by focal purulent encephalitis with confluent central necrosis. The necrotic centre of the lesion is now demarcated and surrounded by a slender rim of inflammatory cells (Figures 20.7 and 20.8). Within the necrotic centre, bacteria may be detectable and the surrounding inflammatory infiltrate predominantly consists of neutrophils with invading macrophages and monocytes. Activated microglia and astrocytes persist, as does oedema.

III. **Early capsule stage (day 10–13 after infection)**: This stage of the disease is characterized by the encapsulation of the inflamed area. The inflammatory infiltrate around the necrotic centre of the abscess has become more prominent. In addition to neutrophils, macrophages, monocytes, lymphocytes and plasma cells all contribute to the infiltrate. Leukocytes reside within many newly generated capillaries. Starting at day 10, fibroblasts proliferate, giving rise to collagen fibres, which together with glial fibres produced by reactive astrocytes form the abscess capsule. At this stage, the fibrous capsule is still subtle, and surrounding brain tissue is oedematous with persistent activation of astrocytes and microglial cells.

IV. **Late capsule stage (beyond day 14 after infection)**: At this stage of the infection, most abscesses show a well-delineated, layered structure with central necrosis surrounded by granulation tissue consisting of blood vessels intermingled with leukocytes. Inflammatory infiltrates consist of lymphocytes, monocytes, macrophages, plasma cells, and low numbers of neutrophils and eosinophils. The capsule now sequesters the lesion from the surrounding brain parenchyma; the thickening of the capsule results from increased collagen deposition, and collagen fibres are intermingled with glial fibres. The capsule is of irregular thickness, being more prominent and thickest at the cortical side, and less thick towards the white matter and the ventricular system. The overall size and shape of cerebral abscesses are markedly variable.

TABLE 20.4 Stage-specific characteristics of brain abscess

Stage	Designation	Time after infection	Morphological characteristics
I	Early cerebritis	1–3 days	Bacteria Focal necrosis Pus (some neutrophils) Oedema
II	Late cerebritis	4–9 days	Centre: demarcated necrosis (bacteria) neutrophils Border: inflammatory infiltrate • neutrophils • macrophages/monocytes activated microglia activated astrocytes Oedema
III	Early capsule stage	10–13 days	Centre: demarcated necrosis Border: inflammatory infiltrate ↑ • neutrophils • macrophages/monocytes • lymphocytes • plasma cells neovascularization • capillaries fibroblast proliferation activated astrocytes activated microglia Oedema
IV	Late capsule stage	≥14 days	Centre: demarcated necrosis ↓ Border: granulation tissue ↑ inflammatory infiltrates (neutrophils) • lymphocytes • macrophages/monocytes • plasma cells neovascularization fibrous capsule • collagen fibres • glial fibres[a] activated astrocytes activated microglia

↑ increase in size or number; ↓ decrease in size or number.
[a] Produced by activated astrocytes.

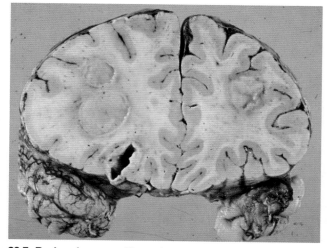

20.7 Brain abscess. Three large well-demarcated purulent, centrally necrotic lesions in the white matter; two lesions are close to the border of the grey matter. Frontobasally, the necrotic centre of an old abscess has been resorbed.

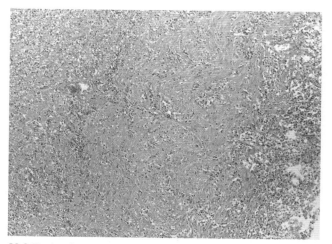

20.8 Brain abscess. Stage II of a brain abscess. The centre of the abscess is lined by a granulation tissue consisting of inflammatory cells and newly formed blood vessels. Prominent perivascular proliferation of fibroblasts is also present. H&E stain, original magnification x10.

SUBDURAL EMPYEMA

Introduction

Subdural empyema was reported to account for 20 per cent of all intracranial infections in the 1990s.[12,51,60]

Subdural empyema relates to an infection in the space between the dura and the arachnoid. Both intracranial as well as spinal forms may occur.

Cranial Subdural Empyema

Aetiology and Epidemiology

Intracranial subdural empyema may develop in young patients with local infections, most commonly secondary to paranasal sinusitis, otitis media and mastoiditis; subdural empyema is the most common sinusitis-associated intracranial infection. Subdural empyema may also develop after meningitis, particularly in infants (in whom subdural effusions complicating meningitis may become infected secondarily), following head trauma, as a postoperative complication with facial or scalp cellulitis, and as a result of infection of a previously sterile subdural haematoma.[127]

In addition to direct extension from a local infection, subdural empyema may develop indirectly. The latter mechanism is more common; here, thrombophlebitis of the mucosal veins spreads to the valveless diploe veins into the cavernous sinus and other sinuses, thereby providing a connection with the dural venous system and from here extending into the subdural space. Once infection has reached the subdural space, further spread is facilitated by the lack of anatomical barriers in the subdural space.[112] Complications of thrombophlebitis associated with subdural empyema include thrombosis, infarction and infection of the brain parenchyma. Haematogenous spread from a distant infectious focus is rare (less than 5 per cent of all cases).

In most cases, intracranial subdural empyema is caused by anaerobic Gram-positive cocci, *Streptococcus* and *Staphylococcus* species and anaerobic Gram-negative bacilli. Polymicrobial infections are frequent.[112]

Clinical Characteristics

Patients present with symptoms of meningeal irritation and increased intracranial pressure. The clinical course is variable; rapid deterioration is common, illustrating that subdural empyema is a neurosurgical emergency; however, a more indolent course may occur.[112]

Diagnosis

CSF analysis is not helpful in establishing the diagnosis. Lumbar puncture is contraindicated in patients with subdural empyema, particularly if patients present with signs and symptoms of increased intracranial pressure. The CSF shows pleocytosis, predominantly due to neutrophils with elevated protein and normal glucose levels. Isolation of the infectious pathogen from the CSF is unusual; Gram staining is usually negative, and CSF cultures are negative in more than 85 per cent of cases (76).

Neuropathology

The convexities of the cerebral hemispheres are more frequently affected than the base of the brain; infratentorial infections are infrequent, accounting for less than 10 per cent of all cases. In subdural empyema following sinusitis, purulent infection affects predominantly the anterior and parafalcine convexities. The base of the frontal lobe may also be covered by a purulent inflammatory infiltrate, which may also reach the falx and spread to the contralateral hemisphere. It is of note that the site of the primary infectious focus does not necessarily determine the site of subdural empyema location.[127] In addition to antibiotic treatment, surgical intervention may be required to ensure complete removal of purulent material and to decompress the brain.[112]

Spinal Subdural Empyema

Spinal subdural empyema is rare and represents the least common localized CNS infection.[162] *S. aureus* is the most frequent causative agent.[162] Direct spread from infected CSF, following spinal surgery or local interventions or indirect haematogenous spread from an infection at other sites may lead to subdural empyema.[162] Anatomical abnormalities of the vertebral column and the spinal cord have been identified as predisposing factors.[162] The lumbar region is most frequently affected.[162]

EPIDURAL ABSCESS

Introduction

Epidural abscess is defined as a purulent infection in the space between the dura and surrounding bony structures. This refers to the skull and the osseoligamentous confines of the vertebral column, respectively. It is a potentially life-threatening condition but relatively uncommon; most cases involve the vertebral column. Intracranially, where the dura adheres to the bony skull, epidural abscesses are extremely rare.

Intracranial Epidural Abscess

Aetiology

Intracranial epidural abscess mainly results from direct extension of an adjacent infection. Frontal sinusitis is the most important predisposing factor as 60–90 per cent of cases are associated with sinusitis or otitis. Rarely, dental infection may be complicated by intracranial epidural abscess. Intracranial epidural abscess is more frequent in young patients between the age of 7 and 20 years than in older patients.[10,120] Patients in this age group are likely have vascular diploic bone, which increases valveless bidirectional flow between the mucosa of the frontal sinus and the venous drainage of the dura emptying into the superior sagittal sinus. This drainage pathway may even lead to sinus thrombosis.[120] In addition, trauma and neurosurgical intervention may be complicated by intracranial epidural abscess.

Intracranial epidural abscesses are frequently polymicrobial including anaerobic cocci, *Staphylococcus* species and *Streptococcus* species.[120]

Clinical Characteristics

Clinically, upper respiratory tract infection or otitis has preceded an epidural abscess in 55 per cent of patients, and non-specific symptoms may have existed over preceding weeks or months.[10] Thereafter, intracranial epidural abscess develops over a period of several days with fever, headache and neck pain, nausea, vomiting, seizures, and mental status changes.[120] Periorbital cellulitis or frontal oedema is present in 45 per cent of patients.[120]

Neuropathology

The inflammatory reaction is similar to spinal epidural abscess (see below); the composition of the inflammatory infiltrate depends on the stage of infection. Characteristically, the brain parenchyma underlying the epidural abscess is not involved.

Spinal Epidural Abscess

Aetiology and Epidemiology

In 1975, the incidence of spinal epidural abscess ranged from 0.2 to 1.2 per 10 000 hospital admissions per year;[23,138] in the subsequent decades, the incidence has significantly increased and is now estimated to account for 2.5 to 3 cases per 10 000 hospital admissions.[138] This increased incidence is attributed to an ageing population in developed countries with increasing numbers of patients at risk. Most patients with spinal epidural abscess have at least one predisposing condition.[10,120] Although all age groups may be affected, spinal epidural abscess mostly manifests in patients between 50 and 70 years of age, with a male predominance.[138]

Pathogenesis

Spinal epidural abscess may develop from direct extension of an infectious focus (e.g. osteomyelitis of the vertebral column, discitis, retropharyngeal and psoas abscesses). Contiguous spread accounts for approximately one-third of cases; approximately 50 per cent of cases occur via haematogenous bacterial dissemination,[23] originating from the skin and soft tissues.[9] Iatrogenic inoculation can lead to spinal epidural abscess and is estimated to account for approximately 15 per cent of cases.[138] Abscesses develop preferentially in locations where the epidural space is wide and contains fat. The dura mater approaches the periosteum to create a true epidural space posterior and lateral to the spinal cord, in the thoracic and lumbosacral levels,[138] which are most often involved, although the cervical levels are less frequently involved. The abscess may extend over several (mostly 3 to 4) vertebral levels;[23,169] extension along the entire length of the spinal cord has been reported. Abscesses located anteriorly to the spinal cord are frequently, but not exclusively, associated with vertebral osteomyelitis.[138] Circumferential extension around the perimeter of the thecal sac is unusual.[9] The underlying infectious pathogens are those that have caused the primary infection, (i.e. most frequently staphylococci and streptococci, as well as many other bacteria species including *E. coli* and *P. aeruginosa*).[23] *S. aureus* and *Streptococcus* spp. account for approximately 66 per cent and 7 per cent of all cases, respectively.[23]

Spinal epidural abscesses may damage the spinal cord both directly as a result of mechanical compression and indirectly because of vascular complications, which involve veins and arteries. Inflammation and thrombosis of the veins draining the spinal cord may cause haemorrhagic infarction and oedema of the spinal cord, whereas arterial compression may lead to spinal cord infarction.

Clinical Characteristics

Clinically, only a minority of patients present with the classical triad of back pain (75 per cent), neurological deficits (30 per cent), and fever (50 per cent).[23] Pain is localized to the level of the affected spine, but may also radiate as a result of involvement of the nerve roots. With increasing abscess size, pareses, bladder and bowel dysfunction may progress to paraplegia.

The single most important prognostic parameter predicting outcome is the patient's neurological status immediately prior to surgery.[9,23] Mortality is approximately 5 per cent with a wide range of 2–20 per cent,[138] mostly as a result of sepsis, meningitis, or other underlying disorders.[23] Patients with concomitant sepsis have a particularly poor prognosis and usually succumb to disease.[9] In surviving patients, permanent neurological sequelae are common.[9] Neurological outcome is determined, at least in part, by the topography of the abscess; a non-cervical location carries a better prognosis.[9] Rapid establishment of the diagnosis and initiation of treatment are of upmost importance in minimising neurological sequelae.

Diagnosis

Epidural abscess may give rise to bacteraemia, which allows isolation and identification of the infectious agent in approximately 60 per cent of patients, particularly if caused by *S. aureus*.[23] The CSF shows the non-specific characteristics of parameningeal inflammation, with polymorphonuclear or mononuclear pleocytosis and high protein levels.[23] Aims to identify the causative agent by Gram staining usually fails and cultures yield a positive result in only 25 per cent of patients.[23] Interestingly, if the CSF culture is positive, generally, blood cultures are also positive.[23] Overall, CSF analysis is of limited diagnostic value and, therefore, routine lumbar puncture is not recommended, in particular, because it may be associated with the risk of inducing meningitis or subdural empyema.[23] Instead, spinal MRI, which carries a degree of high sensitivity, is the diagnostic tool of choice.[23]

Neuropathology

Microscopy reveals pus with inflammatory cells and granulation tissue in the extradural space between dura and the periosteum of the vertebral column. The composition of the inflammatory infiltrate is similar to that in pyogenic bacterial meningitis and depends on the age of the lesion. Most cases evaluated by neuropathology, are from a chronic stage, frequently after repeated orthopaedic injections. Biopsies show chronic inflammation with infiltrates consisting predominantly of lymphocytes and plasma cells within granulation tissue. Fibrosis and old haemorrhage may be prominent. In most of these cases, Gram staining is negative. Complete investigation of the biopsy material is required to exclude small foci of acute inflammation with pus and polymorphonuclear leukocytes.

SPONDYLODISCITIS

Spondylodiscitis is defined as inflammation of the intervertebral discs. From primary infection of the nucleus pulposus, the infection spreads to adjacent bony endplates.

Aetiology and Epidemiology

Spondylodiscitis is a rare disease with an incidence of 1:100 000–1:250 000 in developed countries and a mortality rate of 2 per cent.[169] Advanced age, previous spinal trauma, tumours, immunosuppression, diabetes mellitus, obesity, malnutrition, and long-term hospitalization increase the risk for spondylodiscitis.[42] Spondylodiscitis may result from haematogenous spread or iatrogenic spread by direct inoculation from a contagious nearby focus. The incidence following previous surgery ranges from 0.21–3.6 per cent,[42] being 1 per cent after discectomy. All levels of the spine may be affected, and infection may spread to epidural and paravertebral sites. The most frequent causative pathogens are *S. aureus* and *E. coli*, which account for 60 per cent and 30 per cent of all cases, respectively.[2]

Clinical Characteristics

Pain is the most characteristic symptom. Neurological symptoms are variable, but noticed. Paravertebral muscle spasm and tenderness occur in the affected area.

Diagnosis

The diagnosis is established by MRI scans.

Neuropathology

In the acute phase, inflammation is characterized by neutrophils, macrophages and bacteria; cartilage and bony endplates may be necrotic, and pus may be detected. With time, the inflammatory infiltrate changes to predominantly lymphocytes and plasma cells, and vascularized granulation tissue develops.

HYPERTROPHIC PACHYMENINGITIS

This is a rare inflammatory disorder characterized by hypertrophy of the dura mater and chronic inflammation. Most patients are in their sixth or seventh decade. Clinically, local pain may progress to radiculopathy and even myelopathy. Both the cranial and spinal dura may be involved; cranial disease mainly affects the base of the skull and the posterior fossa, whereas most spinal disease involves the cervical and thoracic levels, and may be solitary or multiple, diffuse or nodular.

Pathology is required to establish the diagnosis. Concentric layers of dense fibrous tissue underlie dural hypertrophy, mixed with inflammatory cells consisting of lymphocytes, polyclonal plasma cells and, occasionally, foreign body giant cells. The underlying pathogens usually cannot be identified. In the differential diagnosis, an underlying tumour should be considered that may have induced a strongly inflammatory fibrosing reaction. The aetiology of hypertrophic pachymeningitis is unknown, but autoimmune diseases (e.g. Wegener's granulomatosis, rheumatoid arthritis, polyarteritis nodosa, cholangitis, fibrosclerotic disorders, mediastinal or subcutaneous fibrosis and thyroiditis) have been implicated.

Recurrence after surgical decompression and immunosuppressive therapy has been reported in 12 per cent of patients with spinal hypertrophic pachymeningitis within a period ranging from 3 months to 2 years (mean 1.3 years) from treatment.[121]

MYCOBACTERIAL INFECTIONS

The acid-fast bacilli *M. tuberculosis* and non-tuberculous mycobacteria of the *M. avium intracellulare* complex (MAC) cause CNS infections in immunocompetent and immunodeficient patients, respectively.

Central Nervous System Tuberculosis

Aetiology and Epidemiology

Although the incidence of tuberculosis has declined over the last century, it still poses a serious medical problem in developing countries. CNS tuberculosis is a rare manifestation of tuberculosis caused by *M. tuberculosis* infection, and occurs in approximately 1 per cent of all patients with tuberculosis. However, it is clinically important and constitutes a serious, potentially devastating complication with high morbidity and high mortality. A large Taiwanese study conducted between 1997 and 2001 reported that 1.5 per cent of deaths from tuberculosis were due to CNS involvement.[128] Once tuberculous meningitis has developed, the mortality rate increases to between 20 per cent and 57 per cent.[128] Risk factors for CNS tuberculosis are young age, HIV infection, alcoholism, malnutrition, underlying tumours, and therapeutic iatrogenic immunosuppression. Approximately 4 per cent of children with tuberculosis will develop tuberculous meningitis.[29] In children, the overall mortality of CNS tuberculosis is as high as 13 per cent, and 47 per cent of surviving children develop permanent neurological sequelae.[29] In HIV-infected patients with tuberculosis, 22 per cent of extrapulmonary cases involved the CNS.[83]

Pathogenesis

M. tuberculosis is acquired through inhalation, thereafter interacting with alveolar macrophages, which initiate granuloma formation.[128] Early in this process (i.e. prior to containment of the infection) low-level bacteraemia allows the spread of *M. tuberculosis* throughout the body. During this process, acid-fast bacilli preferentially home to highly oxygenated organs, including the brain. In HIV-infected patients with tuberculosis, these two different pathogens reciprocally facilitate spread to the CNS, because both pathogens cause lymphocytic inflammation and both use lymphocytes/monocytes to enter the CNS via a 'Trojan horse' mechanism. CNS tuberculosis starts when a small tuberculous focus (Rich focus or Rich nodule) develops in the CNS. Meningeal foci evolve in nearly all cases of CNS tuberculosis and are important for the pathogen to enter the subarachnoid space. Thus, miliary tuberculosis is frequently associated with tuberculous meningitis,[128] and disseminated miliary tuberculosis increases the likelihood of development of Rich foci, which may rupture into the subarachnoid space to cause tuberculous meningitis. In the CNS, microglial cells are the target cell of *M. tuberculosis*.[128] *M. tuberculosis* is able to enter macrophages and to replicate within these cells.[128] Development of multinucleated cells results from the interaction of CD14, CD18, and TNF.[128] Infected microglia produce pro-inflammatory cytokines including TNF and IL-1β as well as chemokines, although their IL-10 production is suppressed.[128]

Clinical Characteristics

Patients with tuberculous meningitis usually develop slowly progressive symptoms with an insidious onset. However, the clinical symptoms may also resemble those of acute meningitis with rapid onset and dramatic course. Cranial nerve deficits account for most focal neurological signs, which are evident in 30 per cent of patients.[171] The abducens nerve is the most frequently affected cranial nerve, followed by the oculomotor, trochlear, and facial nerves; cranial nerves may be affected unilaterally and/or bilaterally. Signs of meningeal irritation are variable as are headache and confusional states. A clinical history of preceding extracerebral tuberculosis is frequently obtainable.

The duration of symptoms from the initial presentation, marked alterations of consciousness and coma at initial presentation, and an advanced stage of disease with major neurological symptoms are all risk factors indicating a poor prognosis in up to 72 per cent of patients.[128] Among survivors, 20–30 per cent suffer from permanent neurologic sequelae including cranial nerve palsies, ophthalmoplegia, seizures, ataxia, hemiparesis and psychiatric signs and symptoms.[128]

Diagnosis

Traditionally, CSF analysis establishes the diagnosis. Lymphocytic pleocytosis, moderately elevated protein, and reduced glucose levels are characteristic. In early stages, neutrophils may dominate, raising the differential diagnosis of bacterial meningitis. It is of note that the CSF in patients under antituberculous therapy may briefly switch to a neutrophil predominance ('paradoxical CSF response'), which is interpreted as a hypersensitivity reaction related to the release of proteins of the infectious pathogen following treatment.[128] Because the cellular alterations in the CSF are not specific for CNS tuberculosis, identification of the pathogen in the CSF is the most important diagnostic approach and a major challenge.[128] Culture and staining techniques are relatively insensitive, and hence, although culture formally is still regarded as a gold standard, negative results do not exclude tuberculosis, because CSF cultures have been reported to yield a positive result in only 10–20 per cent of cases.[135] Acid-fast bacilli cannot be detected by Gram staining. Ziehl–Neelsen, Knyoun, and fluorochrome

(auramine-rhodamine) stains are employed; however, a positive reaction requires a minimum of approximately 100 acid-fast bacilli/mL of CSF.[128] Acid-fast bacilli are identified in less than 10 per cent of cases;[135] it is of note that the number of pathogens is remarkably low in most cases of CNS tuberculosis, and intralaboratory and interlaboratory staining sensitivity is highly variable. A minimum volume of 6 mL of CSF for investigation as well as at least 30 minutes of careful microscopy have been shown to be required for identification of acid-fast bacilli, thereby confirming the diagnosis of CNS tuberculosis.[128] In order to increase diagnostic sensitivity and rapidity, several immunological and molecular diagnostic tools are now employed, including antibody detection, antigen detection and PCR. Assessment of antibodies in the CSF is rapid, but is limited by often poor sensitivity and specificity due to problems of cross-reactivity; furthermore, this technique does not distinguish between acute and previous infections.[128] ELISPOT assays have a degree of high sensitivity both in the early and later phases of the infection, reaching 100 per cent within four weeks of onset of tuberculous meningitis. PCR analysis amplifying mycobacterial DNA is a highly sensitive technique that recognizes 2-CFU/mL.[128] However, it is controversial whether the sensitivity and specificity of PCR assays is in fact superior to traditional smear and culture methods,[128] particularly for those cases in which formalin-fixed paraffin-embedded tissue is investigated instead of fresh CSF samples or unfixed tissue. Currently, it is recommended to use established diagnostic tools such as smear and culture and to apply PCR as supplement to these conventional approaches to monitor treatment.[128] Nevertheless, it must be borne in mind that a negative result in any of these diagnostic tests does not rule out the possibility of tuberculosis, confirming the importance of clinical judgement.[128]

Neuropathology of Central Nervous System Tuberculosis

CNS tuberculosis may manifest in various forms, for example as meningitis, tuberculoma, or brain abscess as well as osteomyelitis of adjacent bony structures.

Tuberculous Meningitis

Tuberculous meningitis affects predominantly the base of the brain, where bacteria induce caseating inflammation. Macroscopically, a gelatinous, viscous exudate of grey to white colour covers the subarachnoid space at the base of the brain, often extending into the suprasellar region anteriorly, the interpeduncular fossa and the prepontine cistern, encroaching on the brain stem, cranial nerves and spinal cord (Figure 20.9). The exudate may also be present within the lateral ventricles, involving the choroid plexus and leading to hydrocephalus. Rich foci, which may develop in an early phase, are usually located around the blood vessels and reside in the meninges as well as in the brain parenchyma.[128]

Arteries at the base of the brain are covered by the viscous exudate, which may severely impair cerebral blood flow. Vasculitis is a serious complication of tuberculous meningitis, occurring more frequently than in meningitis as a result of purulent bacteria. Vasculitis may affect the

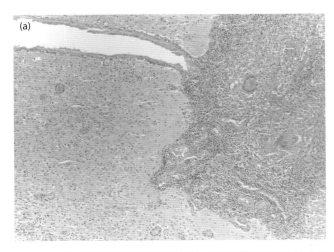

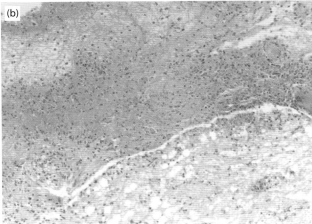

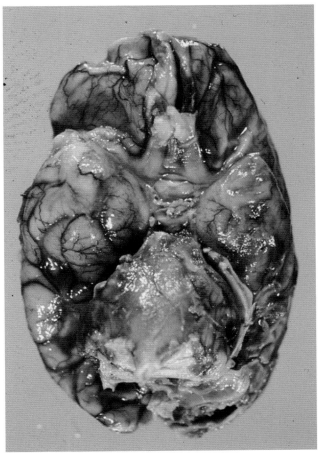

20.9 CNS tuberculosis. Greyish, gelatinous, viscous exudate covering the base of the brain in tuberculous meningitis. Note that the circle of Willis and the cranial nerves are engulfed by the exudate.

20.10 CNS tuberculosis. (a) Prominent lymphocytic inflammatory infiltrate in the subarachnoid space with giant cells of Langhans type. Some vessels in the adjacent cortex are surrounded by lymphocytic infiltrates. H&E stain, original magnification ×200. **(b)** Caseating inflammation in the subarachnoid space with focal encroachment on the adjacent markedly oedematous brain tissue. H&E stain, original magnification ×200.

vessels of the circle of Willis, the vertebrobasilar arteries and the perforating branches of the middle cerebral artery. The adventitia and intima of middle-sized and small arteries may be infiltrated and panarteritis may occur, resulting in thrombosis and subsequent ischaemic infarction in the territory of the affected arteries. Veins may also become inflamed and thrombosed. Meningitis may progress to invasion of the adjacent brain parenchyma resulting in tuberculous meningoencephalitis.

Microscopically, granulomatous inflammation is a diagnostic hallmark. The inflammatory infiltrate is composed predominantly of T-lymphocytes, macrophages, epithelioid cells and some plasma cells. In the very early phase of meningitis, some neutrophils may be present, but the main diagnostic features are the presence of multinucleated Langhans giant cells and caseous necrosis (Figure 20.10). Because a very low number of mycobacteria is sufficient to induce meningitis, the number of bacteria within the inflammatory infiltrate is variable and may be very low. Thus, if Ziehl–Neelsen staining fails to detect mycobacteria, PCR analysis is required. However, a negative PCR reaction does not exclude the diagnosis of tuberculous meningitis, as it is still unclear whether diagnostic sensitivity and specificity of PCR using formalin-fixed paraffin-embedded material is superior to standard diagnostic techniques.

In immunocompromised patients, the inflammatory reaction may lack the characteristic granulomatous pattern. Multinucleated giant cells are typically absent, in contrast to the large numbers of mycobacteria.

Tuberculoma

Tuberculoma is a space-occupying mass lesion resulting from haematogenous spread of acid-fast bacilli to the CNS, commonly seen in patients with miliary tuberculosis. Nowadays, in developed countries intracranial tuberculomas are rare, underlying only 0.1–0.2 per cent of all intracranial space-occupying masses.[44] In contrast, tuberculoma is much more frequent in developing countries, where it still accounts for as much as 30 per cent of intracranial space-occupying lesions.[44]

Tuberculomas may arise from enlargement of tubercles in the brain parenchyma without rupture into the subarachnoid space. They may occur both in the presence and the absence of tuberculous meningitis.[128] Ten per cent of tuberculomas have been reported to be associated with tuberculous meningitis.[44] Tuberculomas may be single or multiple;[128] in the majority of patients, they occur as single lesions, whereas in 15–34 per cent of cases, multiple lesions have been reported.[44]

Tuberculomas are greyish, circumscribed, encapsulated, enlarging space-occupying lesions. Although their size is usually less than 1 cm in diameter, they may eventually reach the size of an orange. Tuberculomas can reside in the subarachnoid space, subdural and epidural spaces, as well as in the brain parenchyma of the cerebrum and cerebellum. The location of tuberculomas differs in paediatric and adult patients, with children mostly harbouring infratentorial lesions, whereas in adults supratentorial tuberculomas occur more frequently, located at the border of the grey to the white matter of the brain.

In most cases, biopsy is required for diagnosis. Microscopically, a caseous necrotic centre consisting of lymphocytes, epithelioid cells and multinucleated Langhans type giant cells is surrounded by an outer layer of lymphocytes, monocytes, fibroblasts and collagen; this layering of the inflammatory reaction is a characteristic feature. Frequently, acid-fast bacilli cannot be identified by morphological techniques; the presence of granulomatous inflammation with giant cells of Langhans type and caseous necrosis together with a positive tuberculin skin test is indicative of tuberculoma and can be regarded sufficient for treatment initiation[44] (Figure 20.11). In the differential diagnosis, tuberculous abscess needs to be considered, which may develop from a tuberculoma, but is less frequent. In general, tuberculous abscesses contain multiple acid-fast bacilli (which are detectable morphologically) with surrounding oedema and a mass effect. Clinically, tuberculous abscess shows a more severe and accelerated course compared to tuberculoma.[44] Over time, tuberculomas may calcify, with intensive gliosis in the surrounding brain tissue. If a tuberculoma leads to increased intracranial pressure as a result of its space-occupying mass effect, neurosurgical intervention may become necessary.

Tuberculous Brain Abscess

This is a rare manifestation of CNS tuberculosis and may occur as single or multiple lesions.[128] Brain abscesses may develop from parenchymal granulomas, meningeal foci and tuberculoma.[128] The necrotic centre may contain acid-fast bacilli surrounded by a fibrous wall (Figure 20.12). The absence of a granulomatous reaction is characteristic and serves as a differential diagnostic criterion in the distinction of tuberculous abscess from caseating, liquefied granuloma.[128] Generally, the capsule of a tuberculous abscess is much thicker than in a pyogenic bacterial brain abscess and consists of vascular granulation tissue mixed with lymphocytes.[128]

Central Nervous System Infections Caused by Non-tuberculous *M. avium intracellulare* Complex

In addition to *M. tuberculosis*, clinically relevant non-tuberculous mycobacterial infections in immunocompromised patients (particularly in HIV-infected patients) are caused by atypical mycobacteria. Less frequently, MAC infections

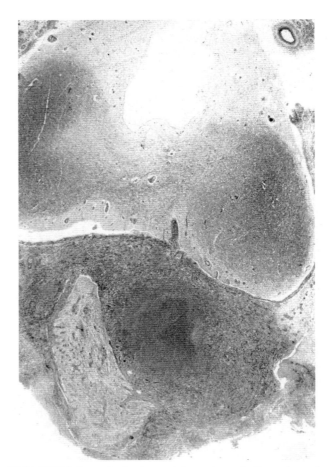

20.11 CNS tuberculosis. Large tuberculoma in the subarachnoid space with central necrosis and surrounding granulomatous inflammation. Cresyl violet stain.

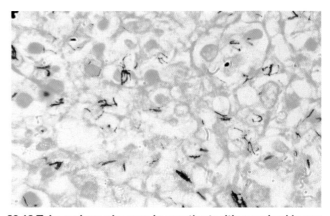

20.12 Tuberculous abscess in a patient with acquired immunodeficiency syndrome (AIDS). The necrotic centre contains numerous acid-fast bacilli. Ziehl–Neelsen.

Courtesy of Professor C Vedrenne, Hôpital Sainte Anne, Paris, France.

also occur in patients with tumours or prolonged steroid therapy and have also been observed in patients without obvious underlying disease.[16,167]

Atypical mycobacteria gain access to the CNS by haematogenous spread within histiocytes from an infectious focus in the gastrointestinal or respiratory tract, usually in patients with disseminated disease. Remarkably, many (18.3 per cent) HIV-infected patients with CNS involvement by MAC remain asymptomatic, with atypical mycobacteria not demonstrated before autopsy. Thus, the absence of neurological symptoms does not rule out CNS MAC infection.[53] The most common neurological symptoms are impaired cognitive function and psychomotor retardation together with fever, sweating and gastrointestinal symptoms. CSF analysis may reveal mild lymphocytic pleocytosis with normal or slightly elevated protein levels and normal glucose levels.

In patients with disseminated *M. avium* infection,[88] neuropathology demonstrates meningitis or subacute meningoencephalitis with mild to moderate meningeal inflammation. Parenchymal inflammation involves the grey and white matter with perivascular infiltrates, prominent microglial nodules, reactive astrocytes and small demyelinating foci, with inflammatory infiltrates around blood vessels. However, inflammatory infiltrates may be discrete or even absent.[139,164] Granuloma formation is sparse; in contrast to infection with tuberculous acid-fast bacilli, there is a lack of central necrosis in MAC infection. Acid-fast bacilli may be demonstrated by classical staining, with foamy histiocytes containing multiple bacilli[167] present in some, but not all patients (Figure 20.13).

WHIPPLE'S DISEASE

Aetiology and Epidemiology

Whipple's disease is a rare, multisystem chronic infectious disease with an estimated annual incidence rate of less than 1 per 1 000 000 population,[136] caused by the Gram-positive actinomycete rod *Tropheryma whipplei*. The pathogen is distributed ubiquitously, in contrast to the rarity of Whipple's disease and indicates that both host genetic and immune factors determine susceptibility. Specific HLA alleles (HLA-B27, HLA-DRB1*13, HLA-BDQ*01) have been observed more frequently in patients with Whipple's

disease; however, these observations could not be confirmed in other studies.[26] Although the disease occurs worldwide, the typical patient is male, middle aged and white.[26]

CNS involvement is the most serious complication of Whipple's disease, and occurs in three situations: (i) in classic Whipple's disease, which affects the gastrointestinal tract causing diarrheal disease, either isolated or in combination with involvement of other organs; (ii) in neurological relapse of previously treated Whipple's disease; and (iii) in isolated CNS disease.

Symptomatic involvement of the CNS in patients with classical duodenal Whipple's disease has been demonstrated by identifying *T. whipplei* DNA in the CSF by PCR.[26] Neurological involvement has been reported in 6–63 per cent of patients with classical Whipple's disease[31] and is considered to result from oral infection. In a small autopsy series including 11 cases, CNS lesions were detected in 10 patients (91 per cent).[28] In cases of dissemination, the brain is an organ preferentially targeted by *T. whipplei*. Isolated CNS manifestation is rare, and only incidental cases have been described. Without appropriate therapy, Whipple's disease is uniformly fatal. Spinal cord involvement was detected by MRI in exceptional patients.[21] Prognosis in CNS disease is less favourable than in extracerebral disease; more than 25 per cent of patients die within 4 years. In patients with neurologic recurrence prognosis is particularly poor.[31]

Pathogenesis

Our current knowledge on the pathogenesis of Whipple's disease stems from sophisticated studies of systemic (i.e. mucosa and peripheral blood) immune reactions in patients with Whipple's disease. They are impaired in their ability to mount a Th1 immune response against *T. whipplei*, which indicates a host immune defect at the T-cell and macrophage level.[93] Peripheral Th1 responses of CD4 T-cells are significantly reduced with a high production of IL-4, whereas IFN-γ production is low, resulting in a milieu fostering macrophages to differentiate into alternatively activated macrophages both locally in the duodenum as well as systemically, thereby favouring development of

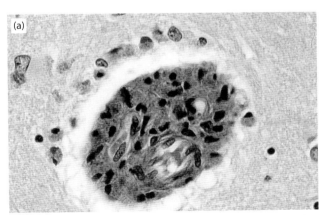 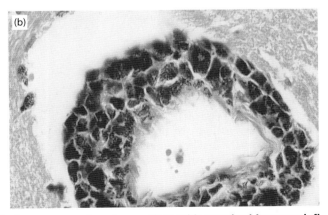

20.13 *Mycobacterium avium intracellulare* **infection of the central nervous system in a patient with acquired immunodeficiency syndrome (AIDS). (a)** Perivascular macrophages containing granular eosinophilic material. **(b)** A Ziehl–Neelsen stain shows the material to comprise numerous acid-fast bacilli.

Courtesy of Professor F Scaravilli, Institute of Neurology, London, UK.

Th2 responses.[26,101] Reduced levels of IL-12 also result in reduced IFN-γ levels, which contribute to impaired macrophage activation and function.[94] Macrophage dysfunction is evidenced by their impaired microbicidal function with an impaired oxidative burst. Although macrophages are able to phagocytose *T. whipplei*, bacterial degradation is impaired, thereby allowing further immunomodulation and *T. whipplei* replication. Interestingly, the pathogen itself contributes to its own multiplication by triggering alternatively activated macrophages favouring Th2 responses, which ultimately reduce the capacity to digest bacteria,[101] and also favour macrophage apoptosis, thereby facilitating bacterial dissemination.[26,93,101]

Thus, high macrophage numbers contrast with their functional inability to eliminate the pathogen. It is of note that after cessation of treatment, bacteria within macrophages disappear but the macrophages persist.[31]

Clinical Characteristics

Neurological symptoms are highly variable and include cognitive alterations (71 per cent) eventually progressing to dementia, changes of consciousness (50 per cent), psychiatric symptoms (44 per cent), seizures (23 per cent), myoclonus (25 per cent), upper motor neuron signs (37 per cent), hypothalamic manifestations (31 per cent), cranial nerve abnormalities (25 per cent), sensory deficits (12 per cent) and ataxia (20 per cent). Oculomotor symptoms, in particular supranuclear ophthalmoplegia (32–51 per cent), oculomasticatory or oculofacioskeletal myorhythmia (8–20 per cent) are regarded as pathognomonic.[26,31,136]

Diagnosis

At diagnosis, CSF abnormalities corresponding to lymphocytic meningitis (elevated white cell count with or without elevated protein) were identified in 38 per cent of patients, whereas in the remaining 62 per cent of patients, CSF was normal.[21] PCR detected *T. whipplei* DNA in 92 per cent of patients irrespective of CSF cytology.[21] During followup, CSF analysis may indicate persistent or *de novo* mild meningitis in patients with improved CNS disease without further evidence of ongoing infection, which may be rather indicative of an IRIS developing in the early months of treatment.[82]

Neuropathology

Macroscopically, small yellow-greyish nodules, 1–2 mm in size, are scattered diffusely throughout the cortical, subcortical, subependymal and cerebellar grey matter. Affected regions include the thalamus, hypothalamus, dentate nucleus of the cerebellum and periventricular regions. In addition to multifocal lesions, solitary space-occupying lesions may occur, mimicking a tumour.[34,90] In fact, localized CNS involvement seems to be the third major chronic manifestation.[26]

Biopsy of the affected tissue is required for diagnosis. Brain biopsy usually shows huge collections of enlarged macrophages, often in perivascular clusters, with subsequent reactive inflammation and oedema in the brain tissue. Astrocytes and microglial cells are prominently activated,

and microglial nodules may form. A PAS stain identifies diastase-resistant intracytoplasmic rods, which cluster in high numbers (Figure 20.14). PAS-positive cells may be detected in the CSF of patients with Whipple's disease; however, this is rare.[21,39] Although highly characteristic, PAS-positive inclusions are not specific for Whipple's disease because they may also be present in patients with MAC infection or may represent abnormal glycogen or polyglucosan bodies, which reside within neurons. In contrast to mycobacteria, the rods in Whipple's disease are negative on Ziehl–Neelsen staining. In addition, extracellular PAS-positive material may be observed. The identification of PAS-positive rods in macrophages should foster further diagnostic studies for pathogen identification (i.e. immunohistochemistry and PCR) (Figure 20.15). Immunohistochemistry is more

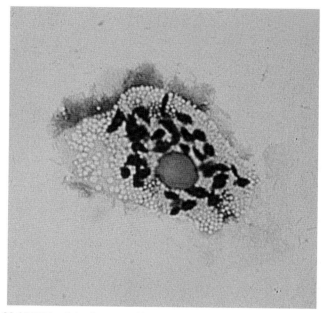

20.14 Whipple's disease. Characteristic sickle particle-containing cell in the cerebrospinal fluid. Periodic acid–Schiff reagent.

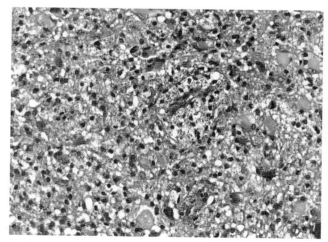

20.15 Whipple's disease. Many enlarged, foamy macrophages, preferentially clustering perivascularly, contain PAS-positive rodlike structures corresponding *to T. whipplei*. PAS reaction, original magnification ×400.

sensitive and more specific than PAS staining,[86] however, antibodies of sufficient quality are not readily commercially available. PCR analysis of formalin-fixed paraffin-embedded brain specimens can be employed. In addition to primers directed against the 16S rRNA of *T. whipplei*, a qRT-PCR assay with increased sensitivity and identical specificity has been developed.[125] Targeting of repeated sequences increased sensitivity without altering specificity.[30] However, PCR is not recommended as a screening method and should be reserved to patients with clinical suspicion of Whipple's disease.[136] Furthermore, use of formalin-fixed paraffin-embedded tissue may impede PCR analysis. At present, confirmation of a positive PCR result by sequencing of hybridization probes in a real-time PCR assay is recommended. Generally, one diagnostic tool with a positive result should be categorically confirmed by a second method to avoid false positive results. If only one approach gives a positive result, a tentative diagnosis of Whipple's disease can be made, although two positive tests yielded by two independent techniques allow a presumed diagnosis of Whipple's disease to be confirmed.[93]

SPIROCHETAL INFECTIONS

Among spirochetes affecting the CNS, *T. pallidum* and *Borrelia burgdorferi* cause clinically relevant neurologic symptoms.

Neurosyphilis

Aetiology and Epidemiology

Towards the end of the 20th century, the incidence of syphilis had decreased. In the United States, a minimum of 2.1 cases per 100 000 persons[170] was reached in the year of 2000. However, in the acquired immunodeficiency syndrome (AIDS) era, the incidence of syphilis has increased again, reaching 3.5 cases per 100 000 persons in 2005.[170] HIV-infected patients have an increased risk for neurosyphilis, particularly for early symptomatic neurosyphilis. HIV-infected patients with low CD4 T-cell counts ($\leq$350 cells/μL) are three times more likely to develop neurosyphilis.[92] They may present with asymptomatic or symptomatic neurosyphilis. Many of these patients had received prior treatment for early syphilis. It has been hypothesized that in these immunosuppressed patients, antibiotic therapy did not achieve complete eradication of *T. pallidum* from the CNS,[92] thereby, subsequently allowing neurosyphilis to develop. In addition to alterations in incidence rates, the pattern of neurosyphilis has also changed, with meningeal and vascular manifestations having become more frequent.[17] Neurosyphilis refers to any kind of CNS involvement at any stage of disease.

Most studies including large numbers of patients are historic and date back into the 1940s, because neurosyphilis is much rarer now than in the past; nowadays, only individual cases are incidentally reported. Our knowledge of the neuropathology of neurosyphilis therefore largely depends on historical, albeit pioneering, studies.[97]

T. pallidum, a spirochete of 5–15 μm length, may reach the CNS early during infection. Exposure of rabbits to *T. pallidum* results in spirochete dissemination into the CSF within hours.[20] This observation supports the hypothesis that the CNS already becomes infected early in *T. pallidum* infection of humans. *T. pallidum* is prone to invade blood vessels, and induces expression of cell adhesion molecules in cerebral endothelial cells. They can bind to fibronectin via an outer membrane protein,[7,13,117] which may facilitate brain invasion.

CNS involvement in syphilis is diverse and occurs through all stages of the infection, albeit with different neurological manifestations. Asymptomatic and symptomatic neurosyphilis have to be distinguished.

Diagnosis

CSF analysis is important to establish diagnosis of neurosyphilis. The CSF shows aseptic meningitis, irrespective of the stage of neurosyphilis and specific type of neurological manifestation. Lymphocytoid pleocytosis may be mild, with fewer than 50 leukocytes/μ, but may also reach levels of 400 leukocytes per microlitre.[91,92,97] CSF protein is moderately elevated (usually <75 mg/dL).[91,92,97] The CSF is normal in up to 4 per cent of all patients with symptomatic neurosyphilis, particularly in the more advanced stages of disease.[17] It has been reported that CSF abnormalities decline with the duration of disease. Nevertheless, CSF abnormalities may persist even after appropriate treatment.[170] A positive VDRL test is diagnostic of neurosyphilis and is considered the gold standard because it has a high degree of specificity. However, CSF VDRL is not very sensitive, being positive in only 22–70 per cent of cases.[52,95] The VDRL test may be falsely positive if the CSF has been contaminated by peripheral blood.[17]

Asymptomatic Neurosyphilis

Asymptomatic neurosyphilis may develop early in infection and refers to pathologic CSF with a positive VDRL and a slight leukocytic pleocytosis in the absence of neurological symptoms. Later, these patients may proceed to symptomatic neurosyphilis.

Symptomatic Neurosyphilis

Symptomatic neurosyphilis includes several manifestations (i.e. aseptic meningitis, meningovascular syphilis, parenchymal neurosyphilis, the latter including general paresis and tabes dorsalis).

Aseptic Meningitis

Meningitis provides the first evidence of CNS involvement in syphilis. It is an early event of neurosyphilis, occurring in approximately 12 per cent of patients in the primary stage and in 30 per cent of patients in the secondary stage.[47]

Aseptic meningitis shows CSF abnormalities, including a moderate lymphocytic pleocytosis with 200–400 leukocytes/μL[97] and moderately elevated protein. The meninges are diffusely inflamed. If these alterations persist beyond the early phase, meningovascular and parenchymatous syphilis may develop.

Meningovascular Syphilis

Meningovascular syphilis usually develops months or years after primary infection with an average duration of 7 years (range 5–12 years)[97] (i.e. during the secondary stage of disease). Its incidence has decreased in the antibiotic era from incidence rates reaching 15 per cent (range: 3–15 per cent) in the pre-antibiotic era.[43] Two Danish reports viewing the time period (1971–1997) identify meningovascular syphilis in approximately 10 per cent of neurosyphilis patients.[22,116] Partial and insufficient therapy of early systemic syphilis may allow *T. pallidum* to survive and persist in the CNS; after a latency period of months to years, persisting spirochetes may cause meningovascular syphilis.[17] Remarkably, in HIV-infected patients, meningovascular syphilis may occur as early as within a few months after infection.[17]

Morphologically, meningovascular syphilis is characterized by lymphocytic vasculitis in the course of syphilitic meningitis. Macroscopically, the inflamed meninges contain a cloudy exudate and may be fibrosed. Impairment of CSF circulation with hydrocephalus and cranial nerve palsies may result from thickening of the meninges. In the pre-antibiotic era, the spinal cord was less frequently affected than the brain and 'spinal arachnoiditis' was detected in 0.72 per cent of all patients with syphilis.[97] Arteries of all size and anywhere in the CNS may be affected. Arteritis of large and small vessels correspond to Heubner's arteritis (Figure 20.16) and Nissl-Alzheimer endarteritis, respectively. In larger vessels, the vasa vasorum are also affected. Obliterative endarteritis is characterized by concentric thickening of the intima due to fibroblast proliferation with increased collagen deposition and thinning of the media, whereas the elastic lamina remains intact, leading to blood vessel narrowing. Endothelial cells also proliferate and contribute to luminal narrowing. Inflammatory infiltrates consist of lymphocytes and some plasma cells. Complications of arteritis include thrombotic occlusion, ischaemia, and infarction. Consequently, patients present with symptoms of stroke of either acute or subacute onset.[43] As for all CNS infarcts, neurological symptoms of 'syphilitic stroke' depend on the topography of the ischaemic area. Most frequently, the middle cerebral artery or its branches are affected.[43] The spinal cord vessels may also be involved; infarction in the territory of the anterior spinal artery is more common than in the region of the posterior spinal artery.[43] Transverse myelitis may ensue.

Gummas, round lesions of various size ranging from 1 mm to 4 cm in diameter, are present and cause a mass effect. Their consistency is hard and their centre necrotic (Figure 20.17). They are in contact with both the dura and the brain and many become embedded in the brain parenchyma. Most frequently, they reside over the convexities of the cerebral hemispheres and may also occur in the hypothalamus, cerebral peduncles, and the spinal cord. Microscopically, the central gummatous necrosis (which may still contain spirochetes) is surrounded by an inflammatory infiltrate consisting of epithelioid cells, multinucleated cells of foreign body type[61] and fibroblasts (Figure 20.18). In the outer layer of the gumma wall, lymphocytes, plasma cells and multinucleated giant cells are lined by collagenous fibrous tissue. Pathogenetically, a hyperimmune reaction resulting in necrosis underlies gumma formation.

Parenchymal Neurosyphilis

Parenchymal neurosyphilis, which includes general paresis and tabes dorsalis, is less frequent now than in the

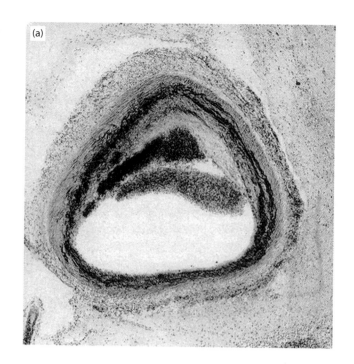

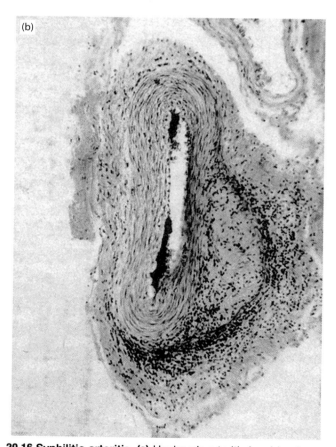

20.16 Syphilitic arteritis. (a) Heubner's arteritis in a blood vessel on the surface of the cerebellum. There is infiltration and thickening of the adventitia, thinning of the media, duplication of the elastica and proliferation of the intima. Elastin. **(b)** A small gumma in the wall of the anterior spinal artery. Haematoxylin/ van Gieson.

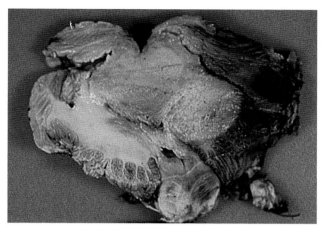

20.17 Cerebellar gumma in a patient with acquired immunodeficiency syndrome (AIDS). Round, red-tan-grey, rubbery lesion with a central area of softening.

Courtesy of Dr M Valsamis, New York Medical College, Valhalla, NY, USA.

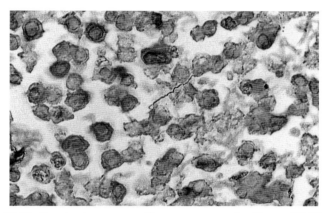

20.18 Cerebral gumma. Same case as in Figure 20.17. Spirochaete within a necrotic area. Modified Steiner stain.

Courtesy of Dr M Valsamis, New York Medical College, Valhalla, NY, USA.

pre-antibiotic era.[17] In rare cases, general paresis and tabes dorsalis may occur in the same patient.

General paresis   General paresis was rare, even in the pre-antibiotic era, occurring in 5 per cent of syphilis patients, and has further declined in the antibiotic era.[43,97] This form of neurological disease develops 5 to 25 years after infection.[43,97] Clinically, patients present with psychosis and dementia and may be erroneously misdiagnosed as suffering from a neuropsychiatric disease.

Neuropathologically, general paresis[43] presents as chronic progressive meningoencephalitis characterized by diffuse cortical atrophy, most prominently affecting the frontal and temporal lobes (Figure 20.19a). The basal ganglia and cerebellum may also be involved. The motor, sensory and occipital cortex are characteristically spared. The lateral ventricle is dilated and granular ependymitis is present. Chronic meningitis with thickening of the leptomeninges is accentuated over atrophic areas of the brain.

Microscopically, the meninges are thickened, overlying an atrophic cortex that has lost its normal laminar pattern (Figure 20.19b,c). Severe neuronal loss with shrinkage of remaining nerve cells causes marked atrophy. Subependymal hypertrophic astrocytes cluster and form irregular protrusions, which underlie granular ependymitis. Microglial activation is particularly prominent, with rod cells with enlarged nuclei and prominent stellate cellular processes (Figure 20.19d). Spirochetes are present in large number in the lesions, and *T. pallidum* has been identified in 50–100 per cent of brain specimens from patients with general paresis in the subcortical grey matter.[97,165] Endothelial cells and microglia have been identified as target cells of *T. pallidum* in the brain.[97] The presence of *T. pallidum* in the lesions is a characteristic feature distinguishing general paresis from other tertiary forms of syphilis.

Tabes dorsalis   Tabes dorsalis occurred in 9 per cent of syphilis patients in the pre-antibiotic era.[96,97] Neurological symptoms include pupillary abnormalities (Argyll-Robertson pupils), declining visual acuity as a result of atrophy of the optic nerve, lightning pains, ataxia, and bladder and bowel dysfunction. These symptoms are attributed to progressive inflammatory degeneration of the posterior spinal nerve roots and dorsal root ganglia, which undergo atrophy, leading to ascending degeneration of the posterior columns of the spinal cord.

Macroscopically, the posterior roots and posterior column of the spinal cord are shrunken. The lumbosacral spinal nerve roots are most frequently affected, but the cervical nerve roots may also be damaged. Microscopically, axons and myelin fibres are lost from the posterior columns of the spinal cord, which show prominent astrogliosis (Figure 20.20). Although the leptomeninges are thickened and show variable chronic inflammation, there is no inflammation in the spinal cord, and *T. pallidum* cannot be demonstrated.

Congenital Neurosyphilis

Congenital neurosyphilis may result from CNS infection during pregnancy or at birth in mothers infected with *T. pallidum*. Clinical manifestation, latency periods and course of disease are similar to the various forms of neurosyphilis in adult patients. Meningeal neurosyphilis manifests in infancy, meningovascular syphilis develops during the first years of life, and parenchymal neurosyphilis starts in puberty or early adulthood.[97]

Neuroborreliosis

Aetiology and Epidemiology

The spirochete *B. burgdorferi* has a marked tropism for the CNS.[49] Involvement of the nervous system occurs in 10–15 per cent of patients.[49] Neurological symptoms may develop some weeks to months after ixodid tick bite; *B. burgdorferi* sensu stricto causes disease in the United States, whereas *B. burgdorferi* sensu stricto has been isolated from only single patients in Europe, where *B. garinii* and *B. afzelii* are prevalent.[113] The likelihood of developing neuroborreliosis depends on geographical factors and the season.[113] The pathology of neuroborreliosis is considered to result from

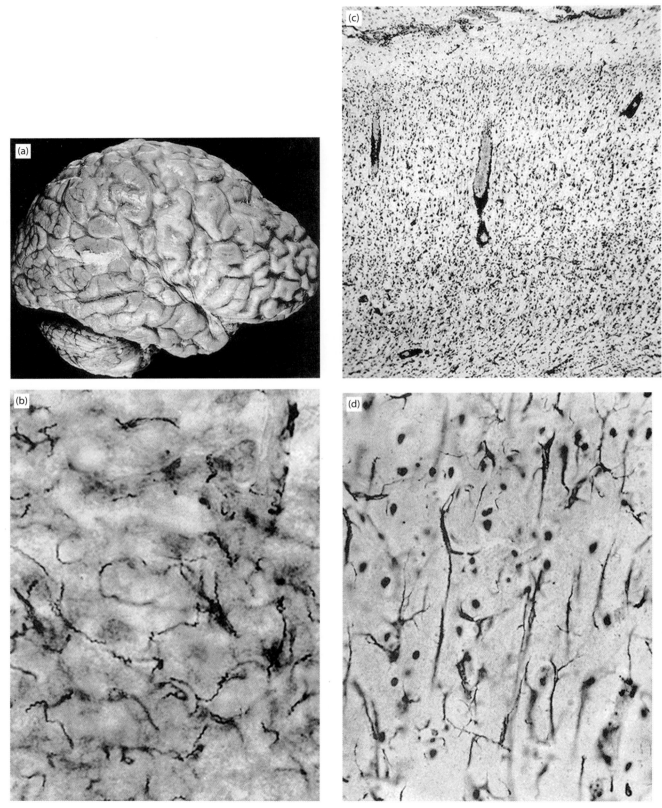

20.19 Paretic dementia. (a) External surface of the brain, showing thickening of the arachnoid and atrophy of the frontal gyri. **(b)** Treponemes in cortex. Jahnel's silver method. **(c)** The cortex shows loss of definition of the cell layers and perivascular infiltration. Nissl. **(d)** Rod-shaped microglia. Silver carbonate.

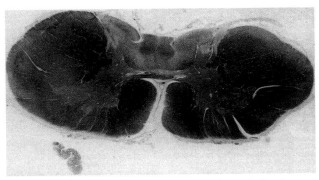

20.20 Tabes dorsalis. Horizontal section through the thoracic cord, showing severe degeneration of the posterior columns. Loyez.

spirochete invasion of the central and peripheral nervous system with resultant inflammation affecting meninges and perineural tissue.[113] In early stages, meningitis, cranial neuritis and radiculitis prevail, while in late stages patients may present with a subtle encephalopathy or mild peripheral neuropathy.[113]

Pathogenesis

Dissemination from the skin, the entry site of spirochetes, to the CNS is likely to be haematogenous. This event is considered to be frequent in patients with Lyme disease in the United States.[130] In addition, *Borrelia* may spread along peripheral nerves. It has been speculated that the mechanism of spread to the CNS may be different in Europe and the United States, with meningopolyradiculitis in Bannwarth's syndrome possibly resulting from passage along the nerves to the nerve roots, and with meningitis being due to haematogenous dissemination, respectively.[130] The spirochetes may bind to cerebral endothelial cells by inducing endothelial expression of the cell adhesion molecules E-selectin, ICAM-1 and VCAM-1 or by binding via integrins.[19,27] Whether *Borrelia* penetrates between cerebral endothelial cells or uses the transcellular route to pass the BBB is still controversial.[130] *Borrelia* can degrade extracellular matrix components and, accordingly, MMPs are considered essential for brain invasion by *Borrelia*.[7] Once in the CNS, meningitis is induced via activation of the innate immune system including TLR and production of pro-inflammatory cytokines (IL-6, IL-8, IL-12, IL-18, IFN-γ) and chemokines (CXCL12, CXCL13).[130] High CSF levels of CXCL12 and CXCL13 may account for the recruitment of high numbers of B-lymphocytes into the CNS; remarkably, in neuroborreliosis the CSF contains the highest amount of B-cells, exceeding other infections.[130] IgG, IgM and IgA antibodies to *B. burgdorferi* are elevated in the CSF, and oligoclonal IgG antibodies are detectable. In addition, a clonal accumulation of activated CD8 T-cells has been reported in early neuroborreliosis.[58] The precise mechanisms underlying CNS dysfunction in neuroborreliosis still remain to be elucidated. In addition to direct interactions between spirochetes and resident cells of the CNS, neurotoxic mediators have been hypothesized to be involved in the pathogenesis.[130] Autoimmune-mediated damage induced by spirochetes according to the concept of molecular mimicry has also been discussed to contribute to neural dysfunction.[130]

Clinical Characteristics

The symptoms of infection with American neuroborreliosis are those of subacute meningitis with or without facial palsy; this clinical presentation is characteristic.[113] European neuroborreliosis usually presents with painful radiculitis as part of Bannwarth's syndrome, which also includes lymphocytic meningitis.[113] In contrast to its high frequency in adults, Bannwarth's syndrome is rare in children (<5 per cent of the patients with neuroborreliosis).[118] Both in the American as well as in the European form, the peripheral nervous system may be affected.[113] Demyelinating and/or axonal neuropathies may occur, mostly axonal polyneuropathy.[118] Polyneuropathy frequently manifests as mononeuropathy multiplex due to perivascular lymphocytic infiltrates.[49]

Active encephalitis in neuroborreliosis is unusual, but encephalopathy has been described.[113] Cerebral vasculitis affecting the vertebrobasilar system and carrying a risk for ischaemic infarction of the brain stem and cerebellum[118] has been reported. However, this association is controversial, because many reports lack convincing evidence for concomitant vasculitis and borreliosis.[49] So far, reports providing definite neuropathological proof of vasculitis are lacking. Although it is generally accepted that the brain and spinal cord parenchyma can be involved in rare cases,[49] the question is still unresolved whether Lyme encephalopathy may be directly caused by *Borrelia*, or rather represents a toxic-metabolic encephalopathy due to circulating cytokines or other soluble neuro-immunomodulators that accompany active systemic inflammatory disorders irrespective of their precise etiology.[49]

Diagnosis

Diagnosis is established by combined serum ELISA and Western blot assays.[113,118] CSF shows lymphomonocytic pleocytosis (10–1000 cells/µL) and mildly to moderately elevated protein levels.[118] Detection of *Borrelia* in the CSF has been uneventful in chronic neuroborreliosis and was positive only in low numbers of patients with acute disease (10–15 per cent).[118] The yield of PCR or culture is low.[113] In European neuroborreliosis, *B. burgdorferi* antibodies are measured in serum and CSF to calculate the antibody index in order to determine production of intrathecal *Borrelia* antibodies (130). The antibody index is not commonly used in the United States.[113]

Neuropathology

Neuropathological studies of CNS borreliosis are very rare and confined to single autopsy case reports.[8,98] Macroscopically, brain atrophy or oedema with leptomeningeal fibrosis was described in individual patients. Microscopically, chronic meningitis with lymphocytic infiltrates and some plasma cells was evident. Medium- and small-sized arteries showed fibrous thickening of the intima with narrowing the vascular lumen and occasional reduplication of the interval elastic lamina. The adventitia harboured lymphocytic infiltrates and fibrous tissue. Some leptomeningeal vessels were totally occluded by organized thrombi; consequently, pale infarcts had developed. Using silver impregnation, a few coiled spirochetes similar to *B. burgdorferi* were identified in the leptomeninges.

Diffuse astrocytic hypertrophy with granular ependymitis, widespread microglial activation as well as microglial nodules, diffuse demyelination and spongiform changes of the white matter have all been observed.[8,98]

NEUROLOGICAL SYNDROMES INDUCED BY BACTERIAL TOXINS

Bacterial toxins are effective virulence factors that inactivate and reduce the host immune response. Some bacteria damage the nervous system by selecting their secretion of a toxin, whereas other bacteria use toxins among several other strategies to escape host immune responses.

In the nervous system, clostridial infections, predominantly *Clostridium tetani* and *C. botulinum*, are the most important sources of neurotoxins. Pathogenetically, neurotoxins interfere with release of neurotransmitters. Despite the severity of the life-threatening neurological disease caused by these pathogens, neuropathological findings in fatal tetanus cases are discrete and mostly reflect terminal hypoxia rather than specific toxin-induced alterations.[5] *C. perfringens* epsilon toxin damages cerebral endothelial cells and specifically accumulates in the brain.[102,103] Subsequently, vascular permeability increases, resulting in the rapid development of severe brain oedema and neuronal death.[32] Hippocampal neurons are the target cells. Neurological symptoms include head retraction, opisthotonus, convulsions, agonal struggling, and roaming. Most likely, this all results from excessive glutamate release.[119] In long-term survivors of tetanus, muscular hypercontraction may develop and, ultimately, lead to myositis ossificans.

NEUROSARCOIDOSIS

Aetiology and Epidemiology

Neurological manifestations are reported in 5–15 per cent of patients with sarcoidosis, a multisystem disorder of unknown origin.[56,147] However, it is estimated that the prevalence of subclinical neurosarcoidosis may be much higher, because post-mortem studies suggest that nervous system involvement is detected in only 50 per cent of affected patients during their lifetime.[56] The course of disease may be both acute and chronic,[56] and any part of the nervous system may be involved.

Although sarcoidosis is most common among North Americans of African heritage and North European white persons, all races, both sexes and all ages may be affected. Disease typically occurs in adults between 20 and 40 years of age, with a second peak in women older than 50 years in Scandinavian countries and Japan.[56]

Pathogenesis

An exaggerated Th1 immune reaction in response to infectious pathogens or environmental factors with the production of pro-inflammatory cytokines (IL-2, IL-6, IL-12, IL-16, TNF) has been suggested to underlie this disease.[108,109] In cases with a prolonged duration, a switch to a Th2 response may lead to fibrosis. A specific pathogen that might initiate this immune response has not so far been identified.

Clinical Characteristics

Neurologically, cranial neuropathy is the most common manifestation of neurosarcoidosis (50–75 per cent). Unilaterally or bilaterally peripheral facial palsy (25–50 per cent) is most frequent; the optic nerve is the second most frequently involved cranial nerve, but other cranial nerves may also be affected.[56]

Between 10 per cent and 20 per cent of patients develop aseptic meningitis, which may be acute or chronic. Chronic aseptic meningitis is commonly recurrent.[56] Hydrocephalus (10 per cent) and brain parenchymal disease (overall 50 per cent) occur with preferential involvement of the base of the brain, leading to hypothalamic dysfunction.[147] Brain parenchymal mass lesions have been noticed in 5–10 per cent of patients.[147] In the spinal cord, both intramedullary and extramedullary lesions as well as cauda equina syndromes have been reported.[147] Involvement of the peripheral nervous system manifests as neuropathy (15 per cent) including sensory, sensorimotor, motor, axonal and demyelinating forms, mononeuropathy, mononeuropathy multiplex, and Guillain–Barré syndrome (15 per cent). Skeletal muscle may be affected both symptomatically (1.4–2.3 per cent) as well as asymptomatically (50–80 per cent).[56]

Diagnosis

CSF analysis in patients with aseptic meningitis reveals sterile lymphomononuclear pleocytosis, normal or decreased (20 per cent) glucose levels and elevated protein levels. Oligoclonal bands may also be present. Normal CSF is noticed in one-third of patients.[56] Elevated ACE levels in CSF, however, are non-specific.[56]

MRI is the most sensitive diagnostic tool to detect granulomatous lesions in neurosarcoidosis; however, the findings are not specific and highly variable.[56]

Neuropathology

The preferential involvement of the base of the brain may be explained by the fact that leptomeningeal inflammation can spread easily along the Virchow-Robin spaces, which are especially large at the base of the brain, into the brain parenchyma.[109] From here, the hypothalamus and the pituitary gland may be readily reached by the exudate, resulting in formation of parenchymatous space-occupying mass lesions, which may cause endocrine disturbances. The third ventricle is also affected and periventricular white matter lesions may occur.[56]

Morphological characteristics of sarcoidosis are granulomas consisting of macrophages, epithelioid cells, lymphocytes and monocytes (Figure 20.21). Multinucleated giant cells of Langhans type are frequently present. The absence of caseating necrosis is a hallmark and helps to distinguish neurosarcoidosis from tuberculosis. Granulomas may show a perivascular distribution, and involved blood vessel walls may thicken considerably and become fibrotic. Although this histological pattern is characteristic, it is not specific for sarcoidosis. Careful examination should be directed at the

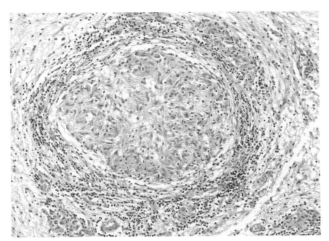

20.21 Neurosarcoidosis. Granuloma formation with central scarring bordered by a rim of lymphocytes. The surrounding brain tissue shows reactive astrocytic gliosis. H&E stain, original magnification ×200.

exclusion of focal caseating necrosis and pathogens including mycobacteria and fungi. The differential diagnosis includes a group of further infectious agents (*T. whipplei*, leprosy, *T. pallidum*, helminths), multiple sclerosis, ADEM, foreign body giant cell reaction, Behçet's disease, vasculitis of other origin and lymphocytic inflammation of the anterior pituitary gland.

Supratentorial granulomas are more frequent than infratentorial lesions, but cerebellar granulomas have been reported.[56] The blood vessels may also be affected, leading to granulomatous cerebral angiitis.[56] In the spinal cord, neurosarcoidosis may manifest as arachnoiditis, mass lesions in an extradural or intradural extramedullary location or in an intramedullary location, the latter being extremely rare.[56]

Granulomas of the cranial nerves may underlie cranial neuropathy, which may also be due to increased intracranial pressure or basal meningitis. In the peripheral nervous system, epineural and perineural lesions and granulomatous vasculitis may result in ischaemia or local pressure leading to axonal and demyelinating damage of peripheral nerves. Furthermore, small-fibre neuropathy appears to occur frequently.[56]

In skeletal muscle, most granulomas reside in the connective tissue,[56] but may also involve the muscle itself, making muscle biopsy a useful tool for diagnosis.

CENTRAL NERVOUS SYSTEM INFECTIOUS COMPLICATIONS

Infectious Endocarditis

CNS complications are frequent and a leading cause of death from infectious endocarditis.[11,107] Their mean incidence of 30 per cent (range: 20–40 per cent) has remained constant over the years.[15] CNS complications develop particularly with lesions of the left side of the heart, and the side of valve involvement (left) is important in determination of neurological complications.[15]

Neurological complications of infective endocarditis include meningitis, brain abscess and encephalopathy. *S. aureus* and streptococci are the most frequent causative pathogens.[15]

Pathogenetically, emboli residing within cerebral arteries may lead to their occlusion. Septic emboli as well as bacteria that have reached the CNS during bacteraemia may involve the meninges and the cerebral arteries. Ischaemic or haemorrhagic infarcts, intracerebral, subarachnoid or subdural haemorrhage, abscess and mycotic aneurysm may result.

Septic embolic encephalitis is distinct from septic metastatic encephalitis both clinically and neuropathologically.[149] Septic embolic encephalitis most frequently develops subsequent to an embolus infected by bacteria originating from the endocardium and, usually presents with stroke-like episodes. Septic metastatic encephalitis can be caused by any bacterial focus at any site in the organism and is dominated by inflammation instead of ischaemia.[149]

Intracranial Mycotic Aneurysm

A mycotic aneurysm is defined as localized dilation of the wall of an arterial blood vessel. It results from infectious arteritis with destruction of the muscular layer of the arterial wall and thus corresponds to a pseudoaneurysm instead of being a true aneurysm. Any infectious pathogen can cause a mycotic aneurysm and the term 'mycotic' is not restricted to fungal infections underlying the aneurysm, but designates infective aneurysms of any pathogen, including bacteria. Streptococci and staphylococci account for 89 per cent of bacterial aneurysms, in this regard being similar to bacterial endocarditis. Mycotic aneurysms are uncommon; they account for 2.6–6.4 per cent of all intracranial aneurysms and most frequently result from infectious endocarditis.[15] More than 80 per cent of mycotic aneurysms develop subsequent to infective endocarditis. Neuroradiology is important to establish the diagnosis. MRI with magnetic resonance angiography is highly sensitive and specific in detection as is DW MRI.[15] The decision in favour of medical antibiotic treatment versus or plus surgery or endovascular treatment depends on clinical and neuroradiological results.

Any artery irrespective of size and location may be affected. The aorta is the most frequently affected arterial vessel. Arteries of the CNS are the second most frequently involved blood vessels, preferentially in peripheral vessels at branching points. The middle cerebral artery is affected in more than 75 per cent of cases.[15] Mycotic aneurysms may be multiple, but several mycotic aneurysms do not necessarily manifest simultaneously. To initiate formation of mycotic aneurysms, septic emboli are required; simple bacteraemia apparently is insufficient. In addition to septic emboli, thrombophlebitis of the cavernous sinus and superinfection of a congenital aneurysm during infective endocarditis or bacteraemia may cause mycotic aneurysm. The latter usually affects arteries of the circle of Willis at the base of the brain in elderly persons.[15]

Neuropathology reveals small, either saccular or fusiform, aneurysms. Following inflammation of the adventitia, inward spread of the inflammation induces focal necrosis of the media of the blood vessel wall with destruction of the muscular layer. The vessel wall is infiltrated by leukocytes (predominantly neutrophils) and microabscesses may develop (Figure 20.22). In acute cases, bacteria may be demonstrated by Gram staining, but attempts to morphologically identify the pathogen may also fail. In chronic cases,

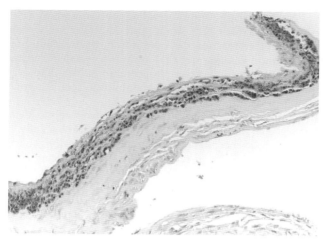

20.22 Mycotic aneurysm. Blood vessel wall infiltrated by neutrophilic granulocytes. Chloracetatesterase, original magnification ×200.

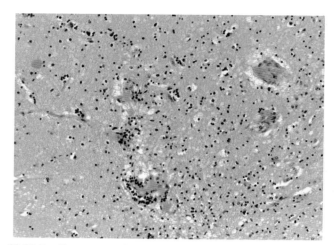

20.23 Septic metastatic encephalitis. Perivascular clusters of inflammatory cells, mainly lymphocytes, which are also diffusely scattered throughout the basal ganglia. Prominent activation of microglia is also present. H&E stain, original staining ×200.

the composition of the inflammatory infiltrate changes with a reduction of granulocytes in favour of lymphocytes and plasma cells. Granulation tissue develops with fibroblastic proliferation and scarring.

A severe complication is rupture of the inflamed vessel wall, resulting in acute subarachnoid haemorrhage. Clinical symptoms of subarachnoid haemorrhage may be the presenting features. However, preceding neurological symptoms may have been overlooked or misinterpreted (e.g. severe localized headache, seizures, focal neurologic symptoms due to ischaemia, and cranial nerve lesions).[15]

The risk of death from mycotic aneurysms is high, with an overall mortality rate of 46 per cent. Among this group, an 80 per cent mortality rate has been reported for patients with ruptured mycotic aneurysm, and a 30 per cent mortality rate for those patients without evidence for bleeding.[15]

Metastatic CNS Infections

Any bacterial focus in the body may give rise to metastatic infections that may manifest as meningitis, meningoencephalitis, brain abscess or infectious arteritis. In the spinal cord, an abscess may lead to mechanical compression of the CNS tissue.

Neuropathologically, microabscesses are frequently located at the white matter border of the neocortex and basal ganglia. In addition to granulocytic infiltrates, microglial nodules and reactive astrocytes with astrogliosis prevail. Diffuse axonal injury and secondary demyelination are characteristic features, although there is neither evidence for primary demyelination nor for ischaemic lesions, which helps to distinguish septic metastatic encephalitis from septic embolic encephalitis[149] (Figure 20.23). With resolution of the lesions, granulocytes are replaced by lymphocytes.

Iatrogenic CNS Infections

Surgery may cause iatrogenic bacterial infections of the brain and spinal cord, leading to meningitis, abscess, or epidural or subdural empyema. In addition, ventricular shunts may also become the targets of an infection.

Shunt Infections

A shunt may become infected either at its initial placement or at later time points. The rate of shunt infections is inversely related to the experience of neurosurgeons.[38] Children have a higher probability of developing shunt infections than adults.[172]

Early shunt infections usually arise from the patient's skin or a contaminated wound. Pathogens may reach the shunt as early as during implantation, and may spread from the distal end of the catheter or reach the shunt haematogenously from other foci.

Clinical symptoms include fever plus signs of catheter dysfunction (e.g. progressive hydrocephalus). CSF analysis is important in the diagnostic workup. Bacterial and also fungal cultures as well as blood cultures are required. Because CSF taken from the lumbar region may yield negative results, analysis of CSF taken from the shunt reservoir is required. Ommaya and Rickham reservoir infections may be caused by staphylococci, Corynebacterium, or Gram-negative bacteria, with S. aureus and S. epidermidis that are able to form biofilms on catheter surfaces being the most common cause.[36,74,140] Biofilm growth may attenuate the host immune response in favour of bacterial persistence.[140] Because treatment of catheter-associated infections is difficult, the infected catheter is removed.[156]

Gram staining identifies the infectious pathogen in 46 per cent of patients.[110] With time, reactive granulation tissue may develop consisting of fibrous tissue intermingled with some lymphocytes, monocytes and plasma cells, which may obstruct the tip of the catheter.

Differential diagnosis includes aseptic meningitis, which may occur with any neurosurgical intervention including shunt implantation. In aseptic meningitis, the CSF is sterile as demonstrated by negative Gram staining and negative CSF cultures. Infectious meningitis has been reported to complicate craniotomy in less than 5 per cent of cases;

however, the risk is increased in patients with repeated neurosurgical interventions.

Bacterial Infections after Neurosurgical Intervention

Meningitis following neurosurgery is mostly caused by Gram-negative bacteria,[84] but *S. aureus* infection may also occur in these patients. Patients who develop postoperative meningitis have mostly been operated for trauma or tumours. The incidence of bacterial meningitis after neurosurgical intervention is low (approximately 0.5 per cent). In the differential diagnosis of bacterial meningitis, aseptic meningitis has to be considered. Aseptic meningitis is much more frequent than bacterial meningitis and has been reported in up to 50 per cent of patients. Pathogenetically, blood and blood products in the subarachnoid space are suggested to stimulate a sterile inflammatory reaction. Clinically, distinction of bacterial from aseptic meningitis can be difficult, because signs of meningeal irritation as well as fever and headache are present under both conditions. Attempts to identify CSF parameters that reliably distinguish between these two entities, have so far failed.

Bacterial Infections after Trauma

In patients with preceding head trauma, bacterial meningitis may develop, becoming manifest either immediately or late after trauma. A trauma-induced fistula linking the subarachnoid space with an extracerebral non-sterile site, mainly the nasal cavity, paranasal sinuses and middle ear may allow easy spread of bacteria to the CNS. After skull fracture, dura fistulas mostly develop in the anterior fossa, where the bony structures of the cribriform plate and the dura are tightly attached. In these cases, CSF rhinorrhea results. CSF can be distinguished from nasal secretions by determination of glucose levels, which are very low in nasal secretions. However, in patients with bacterial meningitis, glucose levels may also be decreased as a result of glucose consumption of replicating bacteria, thereby yielding a false negative glucose test. Approximately 25 per cent of patients with CSF rhinorrhea subsequently develop meningitis.[155]

MISCELLANEOUS RARE BACTERIAL INFECTIONS OF THE CENTRAL NERVOUS SYSTEM

A plethora of bacteria may infect the CNS; however, many of these are rare. Some bacteria that rarely involve the CNS, but may be clinically important, are discussed later.

Nocardia Infection of the CNS

CNS infections are caused by *Nocardia asteroides*. After haematogenous or lymphatic dissemination from a pulmonary focus, the brain is the organ most commonly infected following systemic spread (Figure 20.24). Immunosuppressed patients (including organ-transplant recipients and HIV-infected patients) are at increased risk for *Nocardia* infection.

    N. asteroides may cause a suppurative brain abscess that is frequently multiloculate; 0.4 per cent of all brain abscesses are caused by *Nocardia*.[63] Rarely, meninges overlying the abscess may also be inflamed.

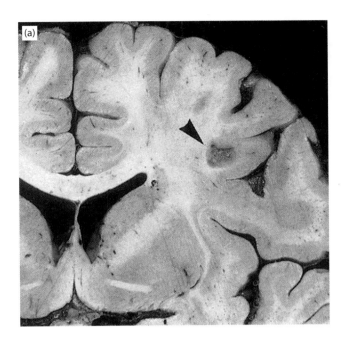

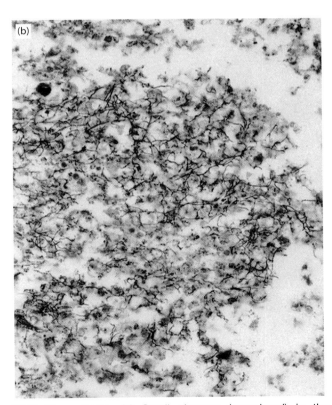

20.24 Nocardiosis. (a) Small abscess (arrowhead) in the brain. **(b)** Delicate branching hyphae are seen in the abscess. Methenamine silver.

Courtesy of Dr M Nilsson, London School of Hygiene and Tropical Medicine, London, UK.

Histological examination shows pus, necrosis with neutrophilic granulocytes and macrophages. *N. asteroides* can be identified by Gram and Gomori methenamine silver stains.

Actinomyces Infections of the Central Nervous System

Human actinomycosis is most frequently due to *Actinomyces israelii* (Figure 20.25). Among all brain abscesses, 0.6 per cent are due to *A. israelii*.[63]

Microscopically, a suppurative abscess is characterized by necrosis, which is lined by many foamy macrophages and bordered by epithelioid histiocytes as well as giant cells of both Langhans type and foreign body type. The lesion contains eosinophilic granules, which consist of *Actinomyces* filaments that lie in an amorphous, eosinophilic matrix. *Actinomyces* stain positively with a modified Gram stain and are also detectable by the Gomori methenamine silver stain. This morphology of the pathogenetic agent raises the differential diagnosis of a fungal abscess.

Brucella Infection of the Central Nervous System

Brucella, a facultative intracellular, Gram-negative coccobacillus, may cause acute or chronic meningitis, encephalitis, meningoencephalitis and abscess.[137] However, involvement of the CNS is rare and has been reported in 4-13 per cent of cases.[73] In *Brucella* meningitis, the CSF is abnormal and may show lymphocytosis, increased protein and decreased glucose levels. Gram staining is usually negative and CSF culture is positive in less than 25 per cent of cases.[168] The diagnosis is established by serology or PCR.

Neuropathology may reveal inflammatory lymphocytic infiltrates. It has also been suggested that CNS pathology may be immune mediated, because incidental cases revealed diffuse white matter with excessive infiltration of CD8 T-cells, prominent astrogliosis and concomitant microglial activation in the absence of demonstrable pathogens.[137]

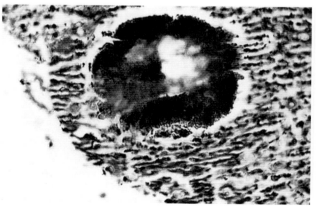

20.25 Actinomycotic abscess. 'Sulphur granule' in a necrotic inflammatory exudate in a brain abscess due to *Actinomyces israelii*. H&E stain.

Rickettsiosis

The CNS may be affected in infections with several rickettsiae. Rickettsiae are obligatory intracellular Gram-negative bacteria that require the presence of living eukaryotic cells. Rickettsiae are transmitted by the bites of ticks, which serve as vectors and transmit bacteria to humans. In rare cases, infections resulting from faeces and blood transfusion have been reported.[123] Although in the past, typhus was a clinically relevant infection worldwide, diseases caused by rickettsiae are rare today and do not play a major role in neuropathological diagnostic practice. Most cases reported occur as a result of Rocky Mountain spotted fever.

Rocky Mountain Spotted Fever

Aetiology and Epidemiology

Rocky Mountain spotted fever is the most severe rickettsiosis resulting from infection with *Rickettsia rickettsii*. It occurs in the United States as well as in Central and South America. Seasonal variations are characteristic, and the majority of cases occur from April to September. Approximately 500 to 1000 cases per year are reported. Children below the age of 10 years have an increased risk for Rocky Mountain spotted fever.[122]

Pathogenesis

Rickettsiae invade endothelial cells of cerebral blood vessels and may also injure smooth muscle cells.[122] This leads to inflammation with the formation of perivascular leukocytic cuffs and thrombosis of arteries, resulting in cerebral infarction.

Clinical Characteristics

After a tick bite, fever and rash develop. CNS involvement usually occurs in the more severe forms of Rocky Mountain spotted fever. Neurological symptoms are diverse, depending on the CNS territory involved. Focal neurologic deficits (hemiplegia, ataxia, cranial nerve palsies) as well as headache, sensitivity to light and alterations of consciousness potentially progressing to coma have been described.[70] Twenty per cent of patients present with signs of meningeal irritation, suggesting the differential diagnosis of pyogenic or viral meningitis.[70]

Neurological complications of Rocky Mountain spotted fever are frequently the ultimate cause of death.[122] Fulminant Rocky Mountain spotted fever may be fatal within 5 days.[163] The majority of surviving patients exhibit permanent neurological disabilities.[122]

Diagnosis

CSF abnormalities have been reported in 30 per cent of patients. The CSF shows moderate lymphocytosis, usually not exceeding 100 cells/mm³ (38 per cent), elevated protein levels (35 per cent) and moderately decreased glucose levels (8 per cent).[122]

Neuropathology

Macroscopically, the major findings are brain oedema and petechial haemorrhages. Microscopy demonstrates inflamed blood vessels with or without thrombosis, with subsequent ischaemic infarction of the brain territory supplied. Fibrinoid blood vessel necrosis is usually absent. The leptomeninges may be mildly inflamed and contain perivascular mononuclear cells in association with haemorrhage. Microglial cell activation with formation of microglial nodules is a hallmark. To detect rickettsiae, immunofluorescence, Giemsa and Gimenez staining techniques as well as immunohistochemistry are applied. As a result of their capacity to infect and to invade cerebral endothelial cells, rickettsiae are detectable in the cytoplasm of cerebral endothelium.

Epidemic Typhus

Typhus is caused by *R. prowazekii*, which is transmitted through inhalation of aerosols derived from infected faeces. Neurological involvement is common. Patients complain of headache of sudden onset, and altered consciousness is frequent and may rapidly progress to coma. The diagnosis is established by serology, but PCR analysis may detect rickettsiae in the peripheral blood. Neuropathology reveals inflammatory foci composed of lymphocytes and macrophages in the brain.

Q Fever

Coxiella burnetti, an obligate intracellular rickettsial organism, transmitted to humans from pets (cats) via aerosols causes Q fever. In the majority of patients, *C. burnetti* infection remains asymptomatic. Only 1 per cent of patients who have developed Q fever progress to CNS involvement, which may manifest as meningoencephalitis, encephalitis, encephalomyelitis and optic neuritis.[80] The most frequent neurological symptom is headache. In addition, toxic confusional states may result. Patients with meningoencephalitis show seizures and disturbed consciousness, which may progress to coma. Serological analysis establishes the diagnosis of *C. burnetti* infection. Most patients recover from Q fever, even in the absence of therapy. Neuropathological alterations have not been reported.

Bartonella Infections

Bartonella species are alphaproteobacteria that may cause CNS disease.

Oroya Fever

Oroya fever is an acute infection caused by *Bartonella bacilliformis* with meningoencephalitis occurring in 10 per cent of patients. Patients present with severe headache of acute onset, fever, altered consciousness that may rapidly progress to coma, and signs of meningeal irritation. However, clinical symptoms of meningeal irritation do not necessarily correlate with the presence of meningoencephalitis and vice versa. The CSF may show a mild mononuclear pleocytosis with elevated protein levels. The leukocytes harbour bacteria in their cytoplasm.

In Oroya fever, endothelial cells of cerebral blood vessels are damaged.[154] Endothelial cells contain intracytoplasmic inclusions (Rocha-Lima inclusions), corresponding to large phagosomes that contain many degenerating bacteria.[37] Leptomeningeal veins are congested and may be

thrombosed, which results in haemorrhages and oedema. Further ischaemic damage may develop in the course of the severe haemolytic anaemia. A rare observation is the presence of 'verrucomas', granuloma-like nodules of microglial cells and histiocytes, in the brain parenchyma, the choroid plexus and the ependyma.

Trench Fever

Trench fever is due to *B. quintana*. Only incidental cases of CNS infection have been described. Usually, headache is not associated with morphological alterations. In an HIV-infected patient, necrotizing granulomatous inflammation of the brain tissue was reported in the intracerebral presence of *B. quintana* DNA.[115]

Cat-Scratch Disease

Cats are the major reservoir of *B. henselae*, a worldwide distributed Gram-negative coccobacillus, the causative pathogen of cat-scratch disease that is transferred through an unrecognized scratch or a bite. Neurologic manifestations are diverse and include encephalopathy, neuroretinitis, cranial and peripheral neuropathies, and transverse myelitis.[18,89,131,153] The incidence rate for encephalopathy to occur in cat-scratch disease has been estimated to be 2–4 per cent. The latency time between acquirement of *B. henselae* and onset of encephalopathy is variable. In most cases, CNS affection follows lymphadenopathy, but CNS symptoms may manifest without or prior to lymphadenopathy. Headache, seizures, focal neurological deficits, and intellectual impairment have all been reported.

Microscopically, meningoencephalitis is characterized by perivascular lymphocytes or granulomatous inflammation. In the CNS as well as in affected lymph nodes rod-shaped *B. henselae* can be identified by Warthin-Starry stain and Gram staining. Immunohistochemical identification may be tried; however, because of the rarity of CNS infection, experience with commercially available antibodies is limited and they may be of low sensitivity. Negative immunohistochemistry does not exclude *B. henselae* infection of the CNS, but should be followed by PCR analysis to identify *B. henselae* DNA. Although it has been a matter of debate for a long time whether neurological symptoms in patients with cat-scratch disease are due to direct invasion of *B. henselae* into the CNS, *B. henselae* DNA has recently been demonstrated in a CNS biopsy obtained from a patient with encephalitis (unpublished observation). CSF data are variable and non-specific; lymphocytic pleocytosis and elevated protein levels may occur, but are not correlated.

Mycoplasma pneumoniae Infection of the Central Nervous System

Mycoplasma pneumoniae may involve the CNS, mostly with ongoing or previous infection of the respiratory tract. CNS infection may manifest as meningitis, encephalitis, meningoencephalitis, myelitis, cranial neuropathies and polyradiculitis. In addition to direct infection of the CNS, *M. pneumoniae* may cause autoimmune inflammation manifesting as postinfectious leukoencephalopathy. The exact pathogenesis of CNS disease, however, still remains to be elucidated.

REFERENCES

1. Adams RD, Kubik CS, Bonner FJ. The clinical and pathological aspects of influenzal meningitis. *Arch Pediatr* 1948;**65**:408–41.
2. Ahlhelm FJ, Lieb JM, Ulmer S, Sprenger T, Stippich C, Kelm J. [Inflammatory diseases of the spinal column and the myelon]. *Radiologe* 2011;**51**:763–71.
3. Aldrich A, Kielian T. Central nervous system fibrosis is associated with fibrocyte-like infiltrates. *Am J Pathol* 2011;**179**:2952–62.
4. Armstrong D, Wong B. Central nervous system infections in immunocompromised hosts. *Annu Rev Med* 1982;**33**:293–308.
5. Baker AB. The central nervous system in tetanus. *J Neuropathol Exp Neurol* 1942;**1**:394–405.
6. Banerjee A, Van Sorge NM, Sheen TR, Uchiyama S, Mitchell TJ, Doran KS. Activation of brain endothelium by pneumococcal neuraminidase NanA promotes bacterial internalization. *Cell Microbiol* 2010;**12**:1576–88.
7. Bencurova E, Mlynarcik P, Bhide M. An insight into the ligand-receptor interactions involved in the translocation of pathogens across blood-brain barrier. *FEMS Immunol Med Microbiol* 2011;**63**:297–318.
8. Bertrand E, Szpak GM, Pilkowska E, Habib N, Lipczynska-Lojkowska W, Rudnicka A, et al. Central nervous system infection caused by *Borrelia burgdorferi*. Clinico-pathological correlation of three post-mortem cases. *Folia Neuropathol* 1999;**37**:43–51.
9. Bluman EM, Palumbo MA, Lucas PR. Spinal epidural abscess in adults. *J Am Acad Orthop Surg* 2004;**12**:155–63.
10. Bockova J, Rigamonti D. Intracranial empyema. *Pediatr Infect Dis J* 2000;**19**:735–7.
11. Bohmfalk GL, Story JL, Wissinger JP, Brown WE, Jr. Bacterial intracranial aneurysm. *J Neurosurg* 1978;**48**:369–82.
12. Bradley PJ, Shaw MD. Subdural empyema management of the primary source. *Br J Clin Pract* 1984;**38**:85–8.
13. Brinkman MB, McGill MA, Pettersson J, Rogers A, Matejkova P, Smajs D, et al. A novel *Treponema pallidum* antigen, TP0136, is an outer membrane protein that binds human fibronectin. *Infect Immun* 2008;**76**:1848–57.
14. Bsibsi M, Ravid R, Gveric D, van Noort JM. Broad expression of Toll-like receptors in the human central nervous system. *J Neuropathol Exp Neurol* 2002;**61**:1013–21.
15. Cavassini M. Complications of infective endocarditis. In: Scheld WM, Whitley RJ, Marra CM, editors. *Infections of the central nervous system*. Philadelphia: Lippincott Williams & Wilkins; 2004.
16. Cegielski JP, Wallace RJ, Jr. Central nervous system infections with nontuberculous mycobacteria. *Clin Infect Dis* 1997;**25**:1496–7.
17. Chahine LM, Khoriaty RN, Tomford WJ, Hussain MS. The changing face of neurosyphilis. *Int J Stroke* 2011;**6**:136–43.
18. Chrousos GA, Drack AV, Young M, Kattah J, Sirdofsky M. Neuroretinitis in cat-scratch disease. *J Clin Neuroophthalmol* 1990;**10**:92–4.
19. Coburn J, Magoun L, Bodary SC, Leong JM. Integrins alpha(v) beta3 and alpha5

20. beta1 mediate attachment of lyme disease spirochetes to human cells. *Infect Immun* 1998;**66**:1946–52.
20. Collart P, Franceschini P, Durel P. Experimental rabbit syphilis. *Br J Vener Dis* 1971;**47**:389–400.
21. Compain C, Sacre K, Puechal X, Klein I, Vital-Durand D, Houeto JL, et al. Central nervous system involvement in Whipple disease: clinical study of 18 patients and long-term follow-up. *Medicine (Baltimore)* 2013;**92**:324–30.
22. Danielsen AG, Weismann K, Jorgensen BB, Heidenheim M, Fugleholm AM. Incidence, clinical presentation and treatment of neurosyphilis in Denmark 1980–1997. *Acta Derm Venereol* 2004;**84**:459–62.
23. Darouiche RO. Spinal epidural abscess. *N Engl J Med* 2006;**355**:2012–20.
24. Deckert M, Soltek S, Geginat G, Lutjen S, Montesinos-Rongen M, Hof H, et al. Endogenous interleukin-10 is required for prevention of a hyperinflammatory intracerebral immune response in *Listeria monocytogenes* meningoencephalitis. *Infect Immun* 2001;**69**:4561–71.
25. Deckert-Schluter M, Schluter D, Hof H, Wiestler OD, Lassmann H. Differential expression of ICAM-1, VCAM-1 and their ligands LFA-1, Mac-1, CD43, VLA-4, and MHC class II antigens in murine Toxoplasma encephalitis: a light microscopic and ultrastructural immunohistochemical study. *J Neuropathol Exp Neurol* 1994;**53**:457–68.
26. Desnues B, Al Moussawi K, Fenollar F. New insights into Whipple's disease and *Tropheryma whipplei* infections. *Microb Infect* 2010;**12**:1102–10.
27. Ebnet K, Brown KD, Siebenlist UK, Simon MM, Shaw S. *Borrelia burgdorferi* activates nuclear factor-kappa B and is a potent inducer of chemokine and adhesion molecule gene expression in endothelial cells and fibroblasts. *J Immunol* 1997;**158**:3285–92.
28. Enzinger FM, Helwig EB. Whipple's disease: a review of the literature and report of fifteen patients. *Virch Archiv Pathol Anat Physiol Klin Med* 1963;**336**:238–69.
29. Farinha NJ, Razali KA, Holzel H, Morgan G, Novelli VM. Tuberculosis of the central nervous system in children: a 20-year survey. *J Infect* 2000;**41**:61–8.
30. Fenollar F, Fournier PE, Robert C, Raoult D. Use of genome selected repeated sequences increases the sensitivity of PCR detection of *Tropheryma whipplei*. *J Clin Microbiol* 2004;**42**:401–3.
31. Fenollar F, Puechal X, Raoult D. Whipple's disease. *N Engl J Med* 2007;**356**:55–66.
32. Finnie JW, Blumbergs PC, Manavis J. Neuronal damage produced in rat brains by *Clostridium perfringens* type D epsilon toxin. *J Comp Pathol* 1999;**120**:415–20.
33. Flaris NA, Hickey WF. Development and characterization of an experimental model of brain abscess in the rat. *Am J Pathol* 1992;**141**:1299–307.
34. Frazier JL, Quinones-Hinojosa A. Isolated Whipple disease of the brain resembling a tumour. *Acta Neurochir (Wien)* 2009;**151**:173–5.
35. Frei K, Nadal D, Pfister HW, Fontana A. Listeria meningitis: identification of a cerebrospinal fluid inhibitor

36. of macrophage listericidal function as interleukin 10. *J Exp Med* 1993;**178**:1255–61.
36. Fux CA, Quigley M, Worel AM, Post C, Zimmerli S, Ehrlich G, et al. Biofilm-related infections of cerebrospinal fluid shunts. *Clin Microbiol Infect* 2006;**12**:331–7.
37. Garcia FU, Wojta J, Hoover RL. Interactions between live *Bartonella bacilliformis* and endothelial cells. *J Infect Dis* 1992;**165**:1138–41.
38. George R, Leibrock L, Epstein M. Long-term analysis of cerebrospinal fluid shunt infections. A 25-year experience. *J Neurosurg* 1979;**51**:804–11.
39. Gerard A, Sarrot-Reynauld F, Liozon E, Cathebras P, Besson G, Robin C, et al. Neurologic presentation of Whipple disease: report of 12 cases and review of the literature. *Medicine (Baltimore)* 2002;**81**:443–57.
40. Gerber J, Nau R. Mechanisms of injury in bacterial meningitis. *Curr Opin Neurol* 2010;**23**:312–8.
41. Gerber J, Bruck W, Stadelmann C, Bunkowski S, Lassmann H, Nau R. Expression of death-related proteins in dentate granule cells in human bacterial meningitis. *Brain Pathol* 2001;**11**:422–31.
42. Gerometta A, Bittan F, Rodriguez Olaverri JC. Postoperative spondilodiscitis. *Int Orthop* 2012;**36**:433–8.
43. Ghanem KG. REVIEW: Neurosyphilis: a historical perspective and review. *CNS Neurosci Ther* 2010;**16**:e157–68.
44. Giese A, Kucinski T, Hagel C, Lohmann F. Intracranial tuberculomas mimicking a malignant disease in an immunocompetent patient. *Acta Neurochir (Wien)* 2003;**145**:513–7; discussion 7.
45. Granert C, Raud J, Xie X, Lindquist L, Lindbom L. Inhibition of leukocyte rolling with polysaccharide fucoidin prevents pleocytosis in experimental meningitis in the rabbit. *J Clin Invest* 1994;**93**:929–36.
46. Greenberg BM. Central nervous system infections in the intensive care unit. *Semin Neurol* 2008;**28**:682–9.
47. Hahn RD, Clark EG. Asymptomatic neurosyphilis; a review of the literature. *Am J Syph Gonorrhea Vener Dis* 1946;**30**:305–16.
48. Haldorsen IS, Krossnes BK, Aarseth JH, Scheie D, Johannesen TB, Mella O, et al. Increasing incidence and continued dismal outcome of primary central nervous system lymphoma in Norway 1989–2003: time trends in a 15-year national survey. *Cancer* 2007;**110**:1803–14.
49. Halperin JJ. Nervous system lyme disease: is there a controversy? *Semin Neurol* 2011;**31**:317–24.
50. Hanke ML, Kielian T. Toll-like receptors in health and disease in the brain: mechanisms and therapeutic potential. *Clin Sci (Lond)* 2011;**121**:367–87.
51. Harris LF, Haws FP, Triplett JN, Jr., Maccubbin DA. Subdural empyema and epidural abscess: recent experience in a community hospital. *South Med J* 1987;**80**:1254–8.
52. Hart G. Syphilis tests in diagnostic and therapeutic decision making. *Ann Intern Med* 1986;**104**:368–76.
53. Hawkins CC, Gold JW, Whimbey E, Kiehn TE, Brannon P, Cammarata R,

et al. *Mycobacterium avium* complex infections in patients with the acquired immunodeficiency syndrome. *Ann Intern Med* 1986;**105**:184–8.

54. Hirano T, Akira S, Taga T, Kishimoto T. Biological and clinical aspects of interleukin 6. *Immunol Today* 1990;**11**:443–9.

55. Ho Dang Trung N, Le Thi Phuong T, Wolbers M, Nguyen Van Minh H, Nguyen Thanh V, Van MP, et al. Aetiologies of central nervous system infection in Viet Nam: a prospective provincial hospital-based descriptive surveillance study. *PLoS One* 2012;**7**:e37825.

56. Hoitsma E, Faber CG, Drent M, Sharma OP. Neurosarcoidosis: a clinical dilemma. *Lancet Neurol* 2004;**3**:397–407.

57. Iriso R, Ocakacon R, Acayo JA, Mawanda MA, Kisayke A. Bacterial meningitis following introduction of Hib conjugate vaccine in northern Uganda. *Ann Trop Paediatr* 2008;**28**:211–6.

58. Jacobsen M, Zhou D, Cepok S, Nessler S, Happel M, Stei S, et al. Clonal accumulation of activated CD8+ T-cells in the central nervous system during the early phase of neuroborreliosis. *J Infect Dis* 2003;**187**:963–73.

59. Join-Lambert O, Morand PC, Carbonnelle E, Coureuil M, Bille E, Bourdoulous S, et al. Mechanisms of meningeal invasion by a bacterial extracellular pathogen, the example of *Neisseria meningitidis*. *Prog Neurobiol* 2010;**91**:130–9.

60. Joubert MJ, Stephanov S. Computerized tomography and surgical treatment in intracranial suppuration. Report of 30 consecutive unselected cases of brain abscess and subdural empyema. *J Neurosurg* 1977;**47**:73–8.

61. Kaplan JG, Sterman AB, Horoupian D, Leeds NE, Zimmerman RD, Gade R. Luetic meningitis with gumma: clinical, radiographic, and neuropathologic features. *Neurology* 1981;**31**:464–7.

62. Kastenbauer S, Pfister HW. Pneumococcal meningitis in adults: spectrum of complications and prognostic factors in a series of 87 cases. *Brain* 2003;**126**:1015–25.

63. Kastenbauer S, Pfister HW, Wispelwey B, Scheld WM. Brain abscess. In: Scheld WM, Whitley RJ, Marra CM, editors. *Infections of the central nervous system*. 3rd ed. Philadelphia: Lippincott Williams & Wilkins; 2004; p. 479–508.

64. Kielian T. Immunopathogenesis of brain abscess. *J Neuroinflamm* 2004;**1**:16.

65. Kielian T, Hickey WF. Proinflammatory cytokine, chemokine, and cellular adhesion molecule expression during the acute phase of experimental brain abscess development. *Am J Pathol* 2000;**157**:647–58.

66. Kielian T, Bearden ED, Baldwin AC, Esen N. IL-1 and TNF-alpha play a pivotal role in the host immune response in a mouse model of *Staphylococcus aureus*-induced experimental brain abscess. *J Neuropathol Exp Neurol* 2004;**63**:381–96.

67. Kielian T, Phulwani NK, Esen N, Syed MM, Haney AC, McCastlain K, et al. MyD88-dependent signals are essential for the host immune response in experimental brain abscess. *J Immunol* 2007;**178**:4528–37.

68. Kielian T, van Rooijen N, Hickey WF. MCP-1 expression in CNS-1 astrocytoma cells: implications for macrophage infiltration into tumors in vivo. *J Neurooncol* 2002;**56**:1–12.

69. Kim KS. Mechanisms of microbial traversal of the blood-brain barrier. *Nat Rev Microbiol* 2008;**6**:625–34.

70. Kirk JL, Fine DP, Sexton DJ, Muchmore HG. Rocky Mountain spotted fever. A clinical review based on 48 confirmed cases, 1943–1986. *Medicine (Baltimore)* 1990;**69**:35–45.

71. Klein M, Pfister HW. [Bacterial infections of the central nervous system]. *Nervenarzt* 2010;**81**:150–61.

72. Klein M, Koedel U, Pfister HW, Kastenbauer S. Meningitis-associated hearing loss: protection by adjunctive antioxidant therapy. Ann Neurol 2003;**54**:451–8.

73. Kochar DK, Agarwal N, Jain N, Sharma BV, Rastogi A, Meena CB. Clinical profile of neurobrucellosis: a report on 12 cases from Bikaner (northwest India). *J Assoc Physicians India* 2000;**48**:376–80.

74. Kockro RA, Hampl JA, Jansen B, Peters G, Scheihing M, Giacomelli R, et al. Use of scanning electron microscopy to investigate the prophylactic efficacy of rifampin-impregnated CSF shunt catheters. *J Med Microbiol* 2000;**49**:441–50.

75. Koedel U. Toll-like receptors in bacterial meningitis. *Curr Top Microbiol Immunol* 2009;**336**:15–40.

76. Koedel U, Bernatowicz A, Paul R, Frei K, Fontana A, Pfister HW. Experimental pneumococcal meningitis: cerebrovascular alterations, brain edema, and meningeal inflammation are linked to the production of nitric oxide. *Ann Neurol* 1995;**37**:313–23.

77. Koedel U, Gorriz C, Lorenzl S, Pfister HW. Increased endothelin levels in cerebrospinal fluid samples from adults with bacterial meningitis. *Clin Infect Dis* 1997;**25**:329–30.

78. Koedel U, Rupprecht T, Angele B, Heesemann J, Wagner H, Pfister HW, et al. MyD88 is required for mounting a robust host immune response to *Streptococcus pneumoniae* in the CNS. *Brain* 2004;**127**:1437–45.

79. Koedel U, Scheld WM, Pfister HW. Pathogenesis and pathophysiology of pneumococcal meningitis. *Lancet Infect Dis* 2002;**2**:721–36.

80. Kofteridis DP, Mazokopakis EE, Tselentis Y, Gikas A. Neurological complications of acute Q fever infection. *Eur J Epidemiol* 2004;**19**:1051–4.

81. Kwok LY, Miletic H, Lutjen S, Soltek S, Deckert M, Schluter D. Protective immunosurveillance of the central nervous system by *Listeria*-specific CD4 and CD8 T-cells in systemic listeriosis in the absence of intracerebral Listeria. *J Immunol* 2002;**169**:2010–9.

82. Lagier JC, Fenollar F, Lepidi H, Liozon E, Raoult D. Successful treatment of immune reconstitution inflammatory syndrome in Whipple's disease using thalidomide. *J Infect* 2010;**60**:79–82.

83. Leeds IL, Magee MJ, Kurbatova EV, Del Rio C, Blumberg HM, Leonard MK, et al. Site of extrapulmonary tuberculosis is associated with HIV infection. *Clin Infect Dis* 2012;**55**:75–81.

84. Lefrock JL, Smith BR. Gram-negative bacillary meningitis in adults. In: *Handbook of clinical neurology*. Amsterdam: Elsevier; 1998.

85. Leib SL, Clements JM, Lindberg RL, Heimgartner C, Loeffler JM, Pfister LA, et al. Inhibition of matrix metalloproteinases and tumour necrosis factor alpha converting enzyme as adjuvant therapy in pneumococcal meningitis. *Brain* 2001;**124**:1734–42.

86. Lepidi H, Fenollar F, Gerolami R, Mege JL, Bonzi MF, Chappuis M, et al. Whipple's disease: immunospecific and quantitative immunohistochemical study of intestinal biopsy specimens. *Hum Pathol* 2003;**34**:589–96.

87. Leppert D, Lindberg RL, Kappos L, Leib SL. Matrix metalloproteinases: multifunctional effectors of inflammation in multiple sclerosis and bacterial meningitis. *Brain Res Brain Res Rev* 2001;**36**:249–57.

88. Levy RM. Central nervous system dysfunction in acquired immunodeficiency syndrome. In: Rosenblum ML, Levy RM, Bredesen DE, editors. *AIDS and the nervous system*. New York: Raven Press; 1988; p. 29–63.

89. Lewis DW, Tucker SH. Central nervous system involvement in cat-scratch disease. *Pediatrics* 1986;**77**:714–21.

90. Lohr M, Stenzel W, Plum G, Gross WP, Deckert M, Klug N. Whipple disease confined to the central nervous system presenting as a solitary frontal tumor. Case report. *J Neurosurg* 2004;**101**:336–9.

91. Marra CM. Neurosyphilis. In: Scheld WM, Whitley RJ, Marra CM, editors. *Infections of the central nervous system*. 3rd ed. Philadelphia: Lippincott Williams & Wilkins; 2004; p. 649–58.

92. Marra CM, Maxwell CL, Smith SL, Lukehart SA, Rompalo AM, Eaton M, et al. Cerebrospinal fluid abnormalities in patients with syphilis: association with clinical and laboratory features. *J Infect Dis* 2004;**189**:369–76.

93. Marth T, Schneider T. Whipple disease. *Curr Opin Gastroenterol* 2008;**24**:141–8.

94. Marth T, Neurath M, Cuccherini BA, Strober W. Defects of monocyte interleukin 12 production and humoral immunity in Whipple's disease. *Gastroenterology* 1997;**113**:442–8.

95. Matlow AG, Rachlis AR. Syphilis serology in human immunodeficiency virus-infected patients with symptomatic neurosyphilis: case report and review. *Rev Infect Dis* 1990;**12**:703–7.

96. Merritt HH. The early clinical and laboratory manifestations of syphilis of the central nervous system. *N Engl J Med* 1940;**223**:446–50.

97. Merritt HH, Adams RD, Solomon HC. *Neurosyphilis*. Oxford: New York; 1946.

98. Miklossy J, Kuntzer T, Bogousslavsky J, Regli F, Janzer RC. Meningovascular form of neuroborreliosis: similarities between neuropathological findings in a case of Lyme disease and those occurring in tertiary neurosyphilis. *Acta Neuropathol* 1990;**80**:568–72.

99. Molyneux EM, Mankhambo LA, Phiri A, Graham SM, Forsyth H, Phiri A, et al. The outcome of non-typhoidal salmonella meningitis in Malawian children, 1997–2006. *Ann Trop Paediatr* 2009;**29**:13–22.

100. Mook-Kanamori BB, Geldhoff M, van der Poll T, van de Beek D. Pathogenesis and pathophysiology of pneumococcal meningitis. *Clin Microbiol Rev* 2011;24:557–91.

101. Moos V, Schmidt C, Geelhaar A, Kunkel D, Allers K, Schinnerling K, et al. Impaired immune functions of monocytes and macrophages in Whipple's disease. *Gastroenterology* 2010;138:210–20.

102. Nagahama M, Sakurai J. Distribution of labeled *Clostridium perfringens* epsilon toxin in mice. *Toxicon* 1991;29:211–7.

103. Nagahama M, Sakurai J. High-affinity binding of *Clostridium perfringens* epsilon-toxin to rat brain. *Infect Immun* 1992;60:1237–40.

104. Nau R, Gerber J, Bunkowski S, Bruck W. Axonal injury, a neglected cause of CNS damage in bacterial meningitis. *Neurology* 2004;62:509–11.

105. Nau R, Soto A, Bruck W. Apoptosis of neurons in the dentate gyrus in humans suffering from bacterial meningitis. *J Neuropathol Exp Neurol* 1999;58:265–74.

106. Neal JW, Gasque P. How does the brain limit the severity of inflammation and tissue injury during bacterial meningitis? *J Neuropathol Exp Neurol* 2013;72: 370–85.

107. Netzer RO, Zollinger E, Seiler C, Cerny A. Infective endocarditis: clinical spectrum, presentation and outcome. An analysis of 212 cases 1980–1995. *Heart* 2000;84:25–30.

108. Newman LS, Rose CS, Maier LA. Sarcoidosis. *N Engl J Med* 1997;336:1224–34.

109. Nowak DA, Widenka DC. Neurosarcoidosis: a review of its intracranial manifestation. *J Neurol* 2001;248:363–72.

110. Odio C, McCracken GH, Jr., Nelson JD. CSF shunt infections in pediatrics. A seven-year experience. *Am J Dis Child* 1984;138:1103–8.

111. World Health Organization. Epidemic meningococcal disease. WHO Fact Sheet 105. Geneva: World Health Organization; 1998.

112. Osborn MK, Steinberg JP. Subdural empyema and other suppurative complications of paranasal sinusitis. *Lancet Infect Dis* 2007;7:62–7.

113. Pachner AR, Steiner I. Lyme neuroborreliosis: infection, immunity, and inflammation. *Lancet Neurol* 2007;6:544–52.

114. Pagenstecher A, Stalder AK, Kincaid CL, Shapiro SD, Campbell IL. Differential expression of matrix metalloproteinase and tissue inhibitor of matrix metalloproteinase genes in the mouse central nervous system in normal and inflammatory states. *Am J Pathol* 1998;152:729–41.

115. Parrott JH, Dure L, Sullender W, Buraphacheep W, Frye TA, Galliani CA, et al. Central nervous system infection associated with *Bartonella quintana*: a report of two cases. *Pediatrics* 1997;100:403–8.

116. Perdrup A, Jorgensen BB, Pedersen NS. The profile of neurosyphilis in Denmark A clinical and serological study of all patients in Denmark with neurosyphilis disclosed in the years 1971–1979 incl. by Wassermann reaction (CWRM) in the cerebrospinal fluid. *Acta Derm Venereol Suppl (Stockh)* 1981;96:1–14.

117. Peterson KM, Baseman JB, Alderete JF. *Treponema pallidum* receptor binding proteins interact with fibronectin. *J Exp Med* 1983;157:1958–70.

118. Pfister HW, Rupprecht TA. Clinical aspects of neuroborreliosis and post-Lyme disease syndrome in adult patients. *Int J Med Microbiol* 2006;296(Suppl 40):11–6.

119. Popoff MR, Poulain B. Bacterial toxins and the nervous system: neurotoxins and multipotential toxins interacting with neuronal cells. *Toxins* 2010;2:683–737.

120. Pradilla G, Ardila GP, Hsu W, Rigamonti D. Epidural abscesses of the CNS. *Lancet Neurol* 2009;8:292–300.

121. Ranasinghe MG, Zalatimo O, Rizk E, Specht CS, Reiter GT, Harbaugh RE, et al. Idiopathic hypertrophic spinal pachymeningitis. *J Neurosurg Spine* 2011;15:195–201.

122. Raoult D. Rickettsiosis, ehrlichiosis, and Q fever. In: Scheld WM, Whitley RJ, Marra CM, editors. *Infections of the central nervous system*. Philadelphia: Lippincott Williams & Wilkins; 2004. p. 423–39.

123. Raoult D, Roux V. Rickettsioses as paradigms of new or emerging infectious diseases. *Clin Microbiol Rev* 1997;10:694–719.

124. Ratnaike TE, Das S, Gregson BA, Mendelow AD. A review of brain abscess surgical treatment--78 years: aspiration versus excision. *World Neurosurg* 2011;76:431–6.

125. Relman DA, Schmidt TM, MacDermott RP, Falkow S. Identification of the uncultured bacillus of Whipple's disease. *N Engl J Med* 1992;327:293–301.

126. Renier D, Flandin C, Hirsch E, Hirsch JF. Brain abscesses in neonates. A study of 30 cases. *J Neurosurg* 1988;69:877–82.

127. Rich PM, Deasy NP, Jarosz JM. Intracranial dural empyema. *Br J Radiol* 2000;73:1329–36.

128. Rock RB, Olin M, Baker CA, Molitor TW, Peterson PK. Central nervous system tuberculosis: pathogenesis and clinical aspects. *Clin Microbiol Rev* 2008;21: 243–61, table of contents.

129. Roos KL, Tunkel AR, Scheld, WM . Acute bacterial meningitis. In: Scheld WM, Whitley RJ, Marra, CM, editor. *Infections of the central nervous system*. Philadelphia: Lippincott Williams & Wilkins; 2004; p. 347–422.

130. Rupprecht TA, Koedel U, Fingerle V, Pfister HW. The pathogenesis of lyme neuroborreliosis: from infection to inflammation. *Mol Med* 2008;14:205–12.

131. Salgado CD, Weisse ME. Transverse myelitis associated with probable cat-scratch disease in a previously healthy pediatric patient. *Clin Infect Dis* 2000;31:609–11.

132. Sanders MS, van Well GT, Ouburg S, Morre SA, van Furth AM. Genetic variation of innate immune response genes in invasive pneumococcal and meningococcal disease applied to the pathogenesis of meningitis. *Genes Immun* 2011;12:321–34.

133. Schluter D, Chahoud S, Lassmann H, Schumann A, Hof H, Deckert-Schluter M. Intracerebral targets and immunomodulation of murine *Listeria monocytogenes* meningoencephalitis. *J Neuropathol Exp Neurol* 1996;55:14–24.

134. Schluter D, Domann E, Buck C, Hain T, Hof H, Chakraborty T, et al. Phosphatidylcholine-specific phospholipase C from *Listeria monocytogenes* is an important virulence factor in murine cerebral listeriosis. *Infect Immun* 1998;66:5930–8.

135. Schmutzhardt E. ZNS-Tuberkulose und ZNS-Kryptokokkose. In: Schmutzhardt E, editor. Entzündliche Erkrankungen des Nervensystems. Stuttgart: Thieme; 2000; p. 87–101.

136. Schneider T, Moos V, Loddenkemper C, Marth T, Fenollar F, Raoult D. Whipple's disease: new aspects of pathogenesis and treatment. *Lancet Infect Dis* 2008;8: 179–90.

137. Seidel G, Pardo CA, Newman-Toker D, Olivi A, Eberhart CG. Neurobrucellosis presenting as leukoencephalopathy: the role of cytotoxic T lymphocytes. *Arch Pathol Lab Med* 2003;127:e374–7.

138. Sendi P, Bregenzer T, Zimmerli W. Spinal epidural abscess in clinical practice. *QJM* 2008;101:1–12.

139. Snider WD, Simpson DM, Nielsen S, Gold JW, Metroka CE, Posner JB. Neurological complications of acquired immune deficiency syndrome: analysis of 50 patients. *Ann Neurol* 1983;14:403–18.

140. Snowden JN, Beaver M, Beenken K, Smeltzer M, Horswill AR, Kielian T. *Staphylococcus aureus* sarA regulates inflammation and colonization during central nervous system biofilm formation. *PLoS One* 2013;8:e84089.

141. Sprenger H, Rosler A, Tonn P, Braune HJ, Huffmann G, Gemsa D. Chemokines in the cerebrospinal fluid of patients with meningitis. *Clin Immunol Immunopathol* 1996;80:155–61.

142. Stenzel W, Dahm J, Sanchez-Ruiz M, Miletic H, Hermann M, Courts C, et al. Regulation of the inflammatory response to *Staphylococcus aureus*-induced brain abscess by interleukin-10. *J Neuropathol Exp Neurol* 2005;64:1046–57.

143. Stenzel W, Soltek S, Miletic H, Hermann MM, Korner H, Sedgwick JD, et al. An essential role for tumor necrosis factor in the formation of experimental murine *Staphylococcus aureus*-induced brain abscess and clearance. *J Neuropathol Exp Neurol* 2005;64:27–36.

144. Stenzel W, Soltek S, Sanchez-Ruiz M, Akira S, Miletic H, Schluter D, et al. Both TLR2 and TLR4 are required for the effective immune response in *Staphylococcus aureus*-induced experimental murine brain abscess. *Am J Pathol* 2008;172:132–45.

145. Stenzel W, Soltek S, Schluter D, Deckert M. The intermediate filament GFAP is important for the control of experimental murine *Staphylococcus aureus*-induced brain abscess and Toxoplasma encephalitis. *J Neuropathol Exp Neurol* 2004;63:631–40.

146. Stephens DS, Greenwood B, Brandtzaeg P. Epidemic meningitis, meningococcaemia, and *Neisseria meningitidis*. *Lancet* 2007;369:2196–210.

147. Stern BJ. Neurological complications of sarcoidosis. *Curr Opin Neurol* 2004;17:311–6.

148. Suryadevara R, Holter S, Borgmann K, Persidsky R, Labenz-Zink C, Persidsky Y, et al. Regulation of tissue inhibitor of metalloproteinase-1 by astrocytes: links to HIV-1 dementia. *Glia* 2003;44:47–56.

149. Tauber SC, Bunkowski S, Bruck W, Nau R. Septic metastatic encephalitis:

coexistence of brain damage and repair. *Neuropathol Appl Neurobiol* 2011;**37**:768–76.

150. Tenenbaum T, Adam R, Eggelnpohler I, Matalon D, Seibt A, GE KN, et al. Strain-dependent disruption of blood-cerebrospinal fluid barrier by *Streptoccocus suis* in vitro. *FEMS Immunol Med Microbiol* 2005;**44**: 25–34.

151. Tenenbaum T, Papandreou T, Gellrich D, Friedrichs U, Seibt A, Adam R, et al. Polar bacterial invasion and translocation of *Streptococcus suis* across the blood-cerebrospinal fluid barrier in vitro. *Cell Microbiol* 2009;**11**:323–36.

152. Thigpen MC, Whitney CG, Messonnier NE, Zell ER, Lynfield R, Hadler JL, et al. Bacterial meningitis in the United States, 1998–2007. *N Engl J Med* 2011;**364**:2016–25.

153. Thompson PK, Vaphiades MS, Saccente M. Cat-scratch disease presenting as neuroretinitis and peripheral facial palsy. *J Neuroophthalmol* 1999;**19**:240–1.

154. Trelles JO, Palomino L, Trelles L. [Neurologic form of Carrion's disease. Clinical-anatomical study of 9 cases]. *Rev Neuropsiquiatr* 1969;**32**:245–306.

155. Tunkel AR, Scheld WM. Acute infectious complications of head injury. In: Brackman R, editor. *Handbook of clinical neurology - head injury*. Amsterdam: Elsevier; 1990; p. 317–26.

156. Tunkel AR, Hartman BJ, Kaplan SL, Kaufman BA, Roos KL, Scheld WM, et al. Practice guidelines for the management of bacterial meningitis. *Clin Infect Dis* 2004;**39**:1267–84.

157. Tuomanen E, Hengstler B, Zak O, Tomasz A. The role of complement in inflammation during experimental pneumococcal meningitis. *Microb Pathog* 1986;**1**:15–32.

158. Tureen JH, Dworkin RJ, Kennedy SL, Sachdeva M, Sande MA. Loss of cerebrovascular autoregulation in experimental meningitis in rabbits. *J Clin Invest* 1990;**85**:577–81.

159. Vaagland H, Blomberg B, Kruger C, Naman N, Jureen R, Langeland N. Nosocomial outbreak of neonatal *Salmonella enterica* serotype *Enteritidis* meningitis in a rural hospital in northern Tanzania. *BMC Infect Dis* 2004;**4**:35.

160. van Sorge NM, Doran KS. Defense at the border: the blood-brain barrier versus bacterial foreigners. *Future Microbiol* 2012;**7**:383–94.

161. Virna S, Deckert M, Lutjen S, Soltek S, Foulds KE, Shen H, et al. TNF is important for pathogen control and limits brain damage in murine cerebral listeriosis. *J Immunol* 2006;**177**:3972–82.

162. Vural M, Arslantas A, Adapinar B, Kiremitci A, Usluer G, Cuong B, et al. Spinal subdural *Staphylococcus aureus* abscess: case report and review of the literature. *Acta Neurol Scand* 2005;**112**:343–6.

163. Walker DH, Dumler SJ. Rickettsial infections. In: Connor DH, Chandler FW, Schwartz DA, Manz HJ, Lack EE, editors. *Pathology of infectious diseses*. Stamford, Connecticut: Appleton & Lange; 1997; p. 789–99.

164. Wallace JR, Jr. Infections due to nontuberculous mycobacteria. In: Scheld WM, Whitley RJ, Marra CM, editors. *Infections of the central nervous system*. Philadelphia: Lippincott Williams & Wilkins; 2004; p. 461–77.

165. Walton J. Syphilis of the nervous system. In: Walton J, editor. *Brain's diseases of the nervous system*. New York: Oxford University Press; 1985; p. 263–73.

166. WHO. The global burden of diseases: 2004 update. Geneva, Switzerland: World Health Organization, 2008.

167. Wu HS, Kolonoski P, Chang YY, Bermudez LE. Invasion of the brain and chronic central nervous system infection after systemic *Mycobacterium avium* complex infection in mice. *Infect Immun* 2000;**68**:2979–84.

168. Young EJ. Brucellosis. In: Connor DH, Chandler FW, Schwartz DA, Manz HJ, Lack EE, editors. *Pathology of infectious diseases*. Stamford, Connecticut: Appleton & Lange; 1997; p. 447–52.

169. Zarghooni K, Rollinghoff M, Sobottke R, Eysel P. Treatment of spondylodiscitis. *Int Orthop* 2012;**36**:405–11.

170. Zetola NM, Klausner JD. Syphilis and HIV infection: an update. *Clin Infect Dis* 2007;**44**:1222–8.

171. Zuger A. Tuberculosis. In: Scheld WM, Whitley RJ, Marra CM, editors. *Infections of the central nervous system*. 3rd ed. Philadelphia: Lippincott Williams & Wilkins; 2004.

172. Zunt JR. Iatrogenic infections of the central nervous system. In: Scheld WM, Whitley RJ, Marra CM, editors. *Infections of the central nervous system*. 3rd ed. Philadelphia: Lippincott Williams & Wilkins; 2004; p. 569–81.

Parasitic Infections

Sebastian Lucas

INTRODUCTION

A wide range of parasitic infections can affect the central and, to a lesser extent, the peripheral nervous and muscle systems of man and cause clinical disease. Some of them latently infect the nervous system, and only if immunosuppression supervenes do they become clinically evident, so only a minority of those infected actually develop disease (so-called opportunistic infections).

Epidemiologically, there are great differences in the frequencies of these infections in different populations around the world. Many of the parasitic infections are geographically restricted for reasons of climate and availability of intermediate hosts to transmit them to man. The frequency of immunosuppression in populations is highly variable, depending on medical practice (damaged immunity is a consequence of much modern medical therapy) and, most importantly, on the local prevalence of HIV infection. Thus, neuropathological practice varies greatly according to location.

Routes of Infection and Pathogenesis

Parasitic infections include single cell protozoa, multicellular metazoa, and some higher invertebrates, such as insect larvae. Their life cycles may be complex, involving one or more intermediate hosts in the environment. The routes of infection to the central nervous system (CNS) are limited to:

- via the skin and bone of the skull, through trauma or surgery;
- haematogenous spread, either in blood fluid or within blood cells;
- retrograde spread up nerves–peripheral and cranial nerves.

How and why infectious agents cause disease is complicated. Not all of the parasitic infections necessarily cause disease when presented to the nervous system. Disease is the result of interactions between the infectious agent and the host through resistance factors, when the host either fails to overcome the infection, or does so but causes tissue damage in the process. The resistance factors include natural immunity (i.e. polymorphonuclear leukocytes, macrophages, many serum factors), as well as acquired or allergic factors that include all the functions of the immune system. Genetic polymorphisms are increasingly recognised as factors accounting for variation in disease frequency and presentation between individuals.

In the following account, the parasites are considered in standard sequence of epidemiology, life cycle and transmission, clinical features, pathology, pathogenesis, diagnosis and treatment. The diagnostic methods for CNS infections continue to expand:

- clinical features;
- neuroimaging–with increasing refinement of computed tomography (CT) and magnetic resonance (MR) scanning modes;
- classical histopathology and cytology, with application of immunohistochemistry;
- serological studies of cerebrospinal fluid (CSF) and blood for antigens and antibodies;
- molecular diagnostics, e.g. polymerase chain reaction (PCR) detection of infective agent DNA, in samples of CSF and tissue;
- electron microscopy of tissue samples.

The proportion of CNS parasitic diagnoses made with imaging, serology and PCR studies augments constantly, in part because of the problems inherent in a brain biopsy for tissue. The key to successful diagnosis in infrequently encountered infections is knowledge of the range of what can happen and what they can do to the CNS, and collaboration with clinical and radiology colleagues in addressing the optimum diagnostic approach. Throughout the chapter, correlation is between the clinical, imaging and pathological features. A comprehensive review of parasite infection neuroimaging was published in 2011.[192]

In addition to the CNS, many parasites also affect the conjunctiva or interior of the eye, and skeletal muscle (Tables 21.1 and 21.2) and these are described in the appropriate sections.

Information Resources on Parasitic Infections and their Agents

A general textbook of the clinical pathology of all infectious diseases in man, including those affecting the CNS, is that edited by Connor and Chandler.[41] Guttierez' comprehensive monograph (second edition published in 2000) on the pathology of parasitic infections contains a lifetime of experience.[87] The now-defunct USA Armed Forces Institute of Pathology published a comprehensive illustrated text on the pathology of helminths (worms).[146] The related Defense Technical Information Center has recently issued, online only, a parallel text on the pathology of protozoa and arthropods.[147] The standard comprehensive textbook – regularly updated – on clinical, taxonomic, diagnostic and treatment aspects of infectious disease is that by edited by Mandell, Bennett and Dolin.[131] The World Health Organization (www.who.int) also provides up to date epidemiological data on the major parasitic infections.

Parasite life cycles, and well as much relevant epidemiology, are published online by the USA Centers for Disease Control and Prevention (CDC), and are used in this chapter (www.cdc.gov).

PROTOZOAL INFECTIONS

Protozoa are single-cell organisms and are widely distributed in nature. The major protozoal infections of man are malaria, trypanosomiasis, amoebiasis, toxoplasmosis and

TABLE 21.1 Parasitic infections of the CNS

Parasite	Disease
The major protozoal infections	
Plasmodium spp.	Malaria
Toxoplasma gondii	Toxoplasmosis
Balamuthia and *Acanthamoeba* spp.	Granulomatous amoebic encephalitis
Naegleria spp.	Primary amoebic encephalitis
Trypanosoma brucei spp.	African trypanosomiasis
Trypanosoma cruzi	South American trypanosomiasis
The major helminth infections	
Cestodes	
Taenia solium	Neurocysticercosis*
Echinococcus granulosus	Hydatid cyst†
Taenia multiceps	Coenurosis†
Spirometra spp.	Sparganosis‡
Trematodes	
Schistosoma spp.	Schistosomiasis*
Paragonimus spp.	Paragonimiasis*
Nematodes	
Strongyloides stercoralis	Strongyloidiasis*
Trichinella spiralis	Trichinosis†
Loa loa	Loiasis*
Onchocerca volvulus	Onchocerciasis*
Toxocara canis	Visceral larva migrans‡
Angiostrongylus cantonensis	Angiostrongyliasis, larva migrans‡
Gnathostoma spinigerum	Gnathostomiasis, larva migrans‡

Key to biological behaviour of the helminth infections:
*Specific helminths to human hosts.
†Animal helminth infections, man accidentally infected, normal migration and development pattern.
‡Animal helminth infections, man accidentally infected, limited maturation and aberrant migration.

TABLE 21.2 Parasitic infections of the eye and muscle	
Eye	*Acanthamoeba* spp.
	Microsporidians
	Toxplasma gondii
	Plasmodium falciparum
	Trypanosoma cruzi
	Loa loa
	Onchocerca volvulus
	Wuchereria bancrofti
	Toxocara canis
	Fasciola hepatica
	Taenia solium
	Gnathostoma spp.
	Angiostrongylus cantonensis
	Halicephalobus spp.
	Myiasis (fly maggot larvae)
Skeletal muscle (not all the rarities are covered in this chapter)	Microsporidians
	Toxoplasma gondii
	Trypanosoma cruzi
	Acanthamoeba spp.
	Sarcocystis spp.
	Toxocara spp.
	Trichinella spiralis
	Dracunculus medinensis
	Gnathostoma spp.
	Taenia solium
	Taenia multiceps
	Echinococcus granulosus
	Sparganosis
	Myiasis (fly maggot larvae)

leishmaniasis. All can affect the CNS, although leishmaniasis is exceedingly rare there. Also considered in this section are the microsporidial infections, which have become apparent as significant human CNS diseases only in the last two decades.

Falciparum Malaria (*Plasmodium falciparum*)

Two related genera–*Plasmodium* and *Babesia*–are intra-erythrocytic parasites in man, but only one species, *Plasmodium falciparum*, causes clinical brain disease. The other malarias (*P. vivax, P. malariae, P. ovale, P. knowlesi*), although variably debilitating, involve less complex

interactions between red blood cells and endothelium; with the exception of *P. knowlesi*,[46] they do not result in the sequestration of parasitized erythrocytes in the small vessels of the brain, which is the essential aetiopathogenesis of cerebral malaria. Rare cases of *P. vivax* infection resulting in clinical cerebral malaria are published, but without pathology are difficult to evaluate.[11] *Babesia* spp. blood infections do not result in CNS disease.[131]

Epidemiology

One third of the world's population is exposed to *P. falciparum* infection, the largest number being in Africa; but south east Asia, India, central and south America are also endemic zones. WHO estimates about 216 million clinical cases per year. It was only in the twentieth century that Europe was cleared of malaria. The impact of malaria in a community and area depends on the intensity of transmission of infection by mosquitoes and whether the infection is constant (holo-endemic) or seasonal.

The drugs available for treating clinical malaria and for prophylaxis are limited by the development of drug resistance. A vaccine is theoretically feasible, but none studied have as yet been so effective as to be taken up and used outside clinical trials. A powerful measure that is being increasingly applied across endemic areas is the use of anti-mosquito bed nets at night, especially when impregnated with a chemical insecticide. More than clinical medicine, this may reverse the toll of severe malaria in Africa and elsewhere in the tropics.

WHO estimated that malaria causes about 665 000 deaths a year, mostly of young children in Africa. Other patient groups significantly affected are:

* pregnant women–particularly first pregnancy;
* people who grew up in endemic areas for malaria but have lost their acquired immunity by migration, and then return to the endemic zone;
* non-immune travellers from non-endemic zones, e.g. tourists, military, business.

Life Cycle

The parasite has two life cycles, the first involving sexual reproduction in an anopheline mosquito vector, and the second asexual reproduction and multiplication in the intermediate human host (Figure 21.1). An infected mosquito injects sporozoites into the bloodstream where they are taken up into hepatocytes.[147] Multiplication there results in each hepatocyte rupturing and releasing thousands of merozoites after 7–10 days. In the blood, these invade red blood cells and undergo the intra-erythrocytic development: ring forms, later trophozoites and then schizonts (Figure 21.2). The parasites ingest and catabolise host haemoglobin as nutrition, and release the breakdown product haemozoin, a dark brown refractile pigment (this haemozoin is essentially similar to the breakdown product of schistosome worms, which also feed on haemoglobin).

The red cells with schizonts rupture (i.e. haemolyse) and release 24–32 newly infective merozoites, which reinvade uninfected red cells. Some merozoites mature

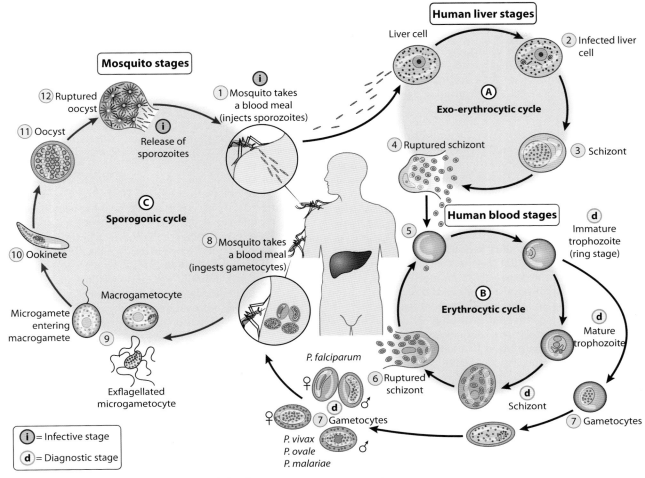

21.1 Life cycle of *Plasmodium falciparum* infection.

Figure courtesy of United States Centers for Disease Control and Prevention, Division of Parasitic Diseases.

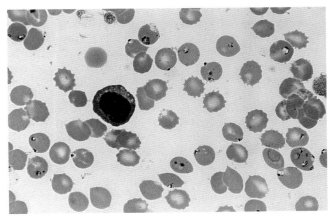

21.2 Falciparum malaria. Blood film showing a high proportion of erythrocytes parasitized by ring forms and trophozoites. Giemsa.

into gametocytes (male and female), which can be taken up by a biting mosquito, to initiate the sexual phase of the life cycle in the gut and salivary glands of the mosquito.

The cycle of red cell invasion, parasite multiplication and release occurs every 48 hours with *P. falciparum*, and the release phase coincides with the spikes of fever so characteristic of malaria.

Clinical Manifestation of Cerebral Malaria

Severe falciparum malaria has many clinical signs and symptoms.[131] In children, the common triad is:

- anaemia;
- cerebral malaria;
- metabolic acidosis and respiratory distress.

In adults, it is more protean, and includes:

- anaemia;
- cerebral malaria;
- acidosis;
- hypoglycaemia;
- renal failure and blackwater fever (hyper-haemolysis);
- shock, jaundice and disseminated intravascular coagulation;

- non-specific symptoms: fever, diarrhoea, malaise, headache, nausea and vomiting, myalgia.

Thus recognition of severe malaria by clinical criteria alone may be difficult, and malaria enters into the differential diagnosis of travellers with these features. The progression to cerebral malaria, coma and death may be rapid, within 1–2 days of the start of symptoms.

The most important complication of severe malaria, and the most baffling to understand, is cerebral malaria (CM). This is a diffuse but potentially reversible encephalopathy, associated with loss of consciousness, fitting and sometimes focal neurological signs. The decreased consciousness can range from confusion to stupor to coma. Seizures can be prolonged, particularly in children, as status epilepticus. The overall global mortality of CM is variable, depending on medical facilities, and may be 20 per cent or more. In the UK, the average mortality rate from imported malaria is 2.6 per cent, but is highest (8.4 per cent) in areas with the least experience of the disease.[31] Spontaneous recovery can also occur. Remarkably, most patients who recover on therapy do so speedily and without permanent loss of cerebral function. However, permanent neurological complications may persist in about 10 per cent – more in children than adults – and include learning difficulties, cognitive impairment, quadriplegia, epilepsy, cerebellar syndromes and cortical blindness.[94,230]

There is also an uncommon post-treatment brain syndrome in adults termed 'post-malaria neurological syndrome' (PMNS). The clinical signs include delirium, cerebellar ataxia, and ophthalmoparesis; there is abnormal imaging on MRI. Blood smears are negative and full recovery with steroid therapy is usual.[80,140,203] Because no pathological studies have been performed on PMNS, it will not be considered further.

Imaging in Cerebral Malaria

CT and MRI scans of brains of adults and children with CM usually show mild cerebral swelling but not parenchymal oedema, which is usually an agonal phenomenon. The swelling is usually interpreted as due to engorgement of cerebral vessels.[143] A few patients with CM have been imaged using single photon emission computed tomography (SPECT) and near-infrared spectroscopy (NIRS) during coma and after recovery on treatment. There is focal cerebral blood hypoperfusion and decreased oxygen saturation, correlating with the focal neurological signs and returning to normal.[108] Crucially, there is controversy over whether there is consistent breakdown of the blood–brain barrier and cerebral oedema in CM.[80,127,143,145] Some but not all studies have demonstrated a reduction in total cerebral blood flow in comatose patients.

Neuropathology of Cerebral Malaria

The original descriptions of the pathology of cerebral malaria were made over 100 years ago in Italy, and in some respects have not been modified.[133,219] Our understanding of why infected patients develop cerebral malaria, how some recover, and why some die is still imperfect, despite much comparative morphological, radiological, physiological and molecular analytical work.

One issue is the comparability of patient groups. There is no doubt that the clinical features and pathology, and implicitly the pathophysiology, of paediatric cerebral malaria differs from that in adults. Moreover, it appears that the pathology differs subtly in populations in South East Asia compared with those in Africa.[25,219] This suggests that, although the parasite is the same, there are differences in host immune response and their underlying genetic polymorphisms, which may account for the different clinico-pathological features.

CM cannot be morphologically studied in life (brain biopsies are not performed) but only after death. What is seen after death may not represent what was happening when the patient developed CM. Treatment and survival in intensive care settings further affect brain morphology. Certainly in patients treated in modern medical care settings, there is often an overlay of secondary pathologies, such as hypoxic encephalopathy, cerebral swelling and sometimes intracranial haemorrhages, which are not directly related to the CM process but to the management of it. Not surprisingly, the observed neuropathology is variable.

Macroscopic Findings

At autopsy, the brain weight may be increased by cerebral swelling but is often within the normal range.[41,219] The degree of swelling is variable but usually mild, and coning of the cerebellar tonsils through the foramen magnum is rare, in both adults and children. The meninges are congested and the external colour of the brain is often a characteristic dusky dark red; this can become dark grey after fixation (Figure 21.3). In severe cases, petechial haemorrhages are seen on the cortical surfaces.

On slicing, there may be obliteration of the sulci and flattening of the gyri. The mammillary bodies can be displaced below Greenhall's line and some compression of the ventricular system can be seen.[127] Any swelling is usually symmetrical. The colour of the cut brain varies. In patients with co-existent severe anaemia, the surface can be pale, whereas in a heavily parasitized brain, the deposition of malaria pigment can give a slate-grey appearance, particularly to the grey matter. This colour is similar to that imparted to any brain where there is hydrogen sulphide production, from post-mortem decomposition or toxic intake.

Petechial haemorrhages are a well-described macroscopic feature of malarial encephalopathy[219] and their presence depends greatly on the cadence of the disease in the individual patient. They are prominent in the subcortical white matter, corpus callosum, cerebellum, and brain stem (Figure 21.3); they are also seen in the cerebellar grey matter in children. They are frequent in those whose disease evolves over several days and who have been kept alive in medical care; they are less common and frequently absent in those who have died acutely of cerebral malaria, without medical attention.

Microscopic Findings

Fixation of the brain is obviously desirable to neuropathologists but not essential in making the diagnosis of cerebral malaria. Overnight fixation of samples, and immediate brain smears (see later), are sufficient for diagnostic purposes. To make the diagnosis of CM, it is not always necessary to remove the brain. Sampling of brain tissue via supraorbital needle puncture provides material for brain smears.[226]

In acute CM, the most common feature is *sequestration* of parasitized red blood cells (PRBCs) within cerebral microvessels (Figure 21.4).[50,147] Non-parasitized RBC contribute to the severe congestion.[186] There is packing of capillaries and post-capillary venules, but it may also be reflected in margination of PRBC in larger calibre vessels.[207,219] PRBCs can most easily be recognised under high dry lens or oil immersion, as small ring-forms, or later and larger trophozoites and schizonts. They are also recognised by the intra-erythrocytic pigment (haemozoin) body in the later trophozite or schizont stages. Electron microscopy

also demonstrates the intravascular packing of infected erythrocytes, which are attached to endothelial cells via dense 'knob' proteins on the PRBC surface (Figure 21.5).[185]

If the brain is examined after 3–4 days of standard quinine or artemisinin therapy,[230] few sequestered PRBCs may be seen. In this case, the presence of residual malarial pigment is a diagnostic clue. Ultrastructurally, all antimalarial drugs induce degenerative changes in the parasites and reduce haemozoin production.[198] The haemozoin pigment may obscure the parasites in the trophozoite stage, and can appear similar to formalin pigment, although usually forming smaller and darker granules. Pigment deposition occurs microscopically in the lining of the blood vessels, especially in the meninges and choroid plexus. Circulating monocytes also phagocytose the pigment. The granules lining blood vessels are often associated with ruptured erythrocyte ghosts.

In addition to sequestration, a characteristic *microvascular pathology* is common.[217]

Petechial haemorrhages are variable in frequency (see earlier) and are of several types. They occur in the white

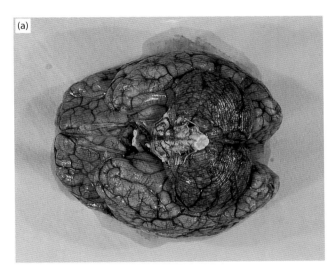

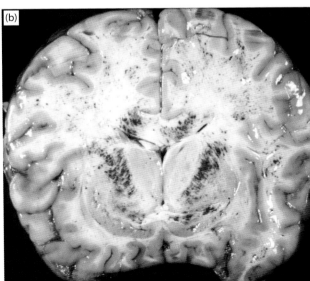

21.3 Malaria (a) Paediatric patient. Marked congestion and duskiness of the meninges, particularly over the cerebellum. **(b)** Adult patient. The brain is swollen, the ventricles compressed and there are small haemorrhages throughout the white matter.

Image (b) courtesy of F Scaravilli, Institute of Neurology, London, UK and G Turner, John Radcliffe Hospital, Oxford, UK.

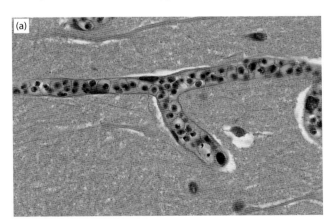

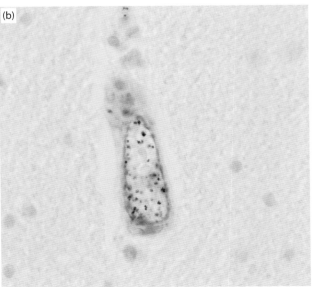

21.4 Malaria. Microvascular sequestration of parasitized red blood cells (PRBCs). **(a)** The PRBCs fill the capillary. **(b)** ICAM-1 immunolabelling reveals upregulation of the adhesion molecule on the endothelial cell. Numerous parasites are visible adhering to the endothelium.

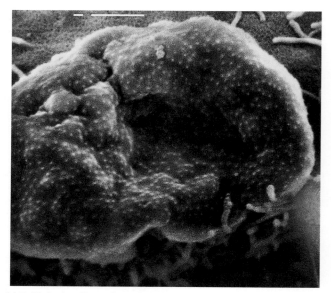

21.5 Malaria. Scanning electron micrograph of a parasitized erythrocyte showing the numerous small knobs in the cell surface.

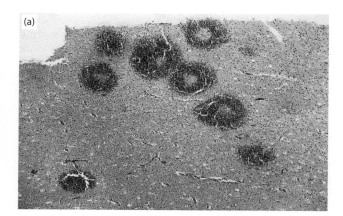

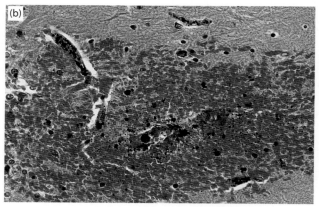

21.6 Malaria. (a) Ring haemorrhages in the white matter of paediatric patient, low-power view. **(b)** Rupture of a capillary with heavy parasite load and much haemozoin pigment, with formation of a ring haemorrhage. Microthrombus is present in the centre.

matter at all levels of the brain and in the cerebellar grey matter. Simple parenchymal haemorrhages are associated with ruptured small vessels. More common is the ring haemorrhage, consisting of concentric zones of PRBCs and some lymphocytes, uninfected erythrocytes, and a central necrosed blood vessel. The central vessel may or may not contain a fibrin thrombus and there are monocytes laden with haemozoin pigment–features more commonly seen in paediatric cases (Figure 21.6).[84,185,217] Typically, the red blood cells in the outer rim of the haemorrhage have a low parasite density compared with the red cells within adjacent vessels.

Retinal haemorrhages, particularly well studied in children with CM,[228] correlate in severity with the degree of cerebral haemorrhages in those who die.

These brain haemorrhages are not unique to CM, because they can also occur in:

- barotrauma;
- fat and air embolism;
- carbon monoxide poisoning;
- systemic septic infections, e.g. rickettsiosis;
- acute haemorrhagic leukoencephalitis.

Focal necrosis of the brain parenchyma also occurs in the white matter. This is ischaemic in origin or follows the petechial haemorrhage. It elicits a focal cellular reaction and is termed the Dürck granuloma (Figure 21.7). There is a rim of reactive astrocytes, microglial cells and some lymphocytes, surrounding a focus of necrotic parenchyma. Evidence of previous haemorrhage, as haemosiderin granules, may be present.

Cerebral oedema is problematic in its evaluation in CM, in part because of a lack of a straightforward neuropathological case definition, and from fixation artefact. When cerebral oedema is evident in CM, it may be perivascular, perineuronal or parenchymal, represented by round, fluid holes in the neuropil. Several studies have noted

more significant cerebral oedema in autopsy material from African children than in Vietnamese adults.[157]

Widespread ischaemic neuronal changes are rare as a primary event in CM and are usually the consequence of cardiorespiratory arrest (i.e. near death and resuscitation);[185] less commonly from secondary neuropathology such as haemorrhage or brain stem displacement. Widespread demyelination is not a feature of CM; focal demyelinated patches in the white matter are associated with haemorrhages. Axonal damage, using β-amyloid precursor protein staining, is well described in CM, and is associated with the microvascular pathology. Its distribution is either diffuse or focal in the basal ganglia and pons.[144]

CM is not an encephalitis, in that cellular inflammation around vessels and in the parenchyma is not a usual feature. However perivascular lymphocytes and activated macrophages are documented in some series, and leukocyte intravascular sequestration is also variably reported.[80,167] If a patient has died after some days of treatment, haemozoin-laden monocytes and neutrophils can be seen in some blood vessels, which phagocytose erythrocyte ghosts adherent to vascular endothelial cells.

Immunocytochemical and molecular biological studies have confirmed that there is a parenchymal inflammatory response in CM. Widespread astroglial activation is seen both surrounding blood vessels and as glial nodules

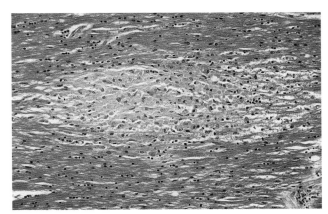

21.7 Malaria. Dürck granuloma in the white matter. An ovoid mass of enlarged microglial cells/macrophages replacing a previous ring haemorrhage with necrosis.

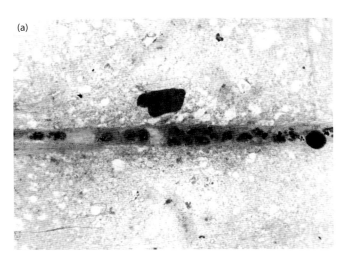

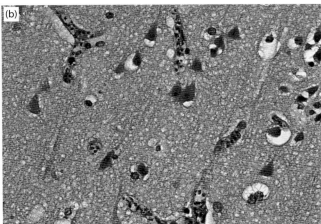

21.8 Falciparum malaria. Smear **(a)** of brain tissue and paraffin section **(b)** from adult patient with severe sequestration of parasitized erythrocytes in cerebral vessels, but who did not have clinical cerebral malaria.

within the brain stem.[19] Markers of microglial cells activation, such as CD68, HLA-II antigens and scavenger receptors, are upregulated in the brain in CM.[207] Endothelial cell activation is also evident by the increased expression (upregulation) of ICAM-1 and related molecules (Figure 21.4c).

Diagnosis

Cerebral malaria remains a clinical rather than a pathological diagnosis: coma or other appropriate neurological abnormalities in a patient with *P. falciparum* parasites in the blood, and other common causes of diffuse cerebral disease excluded (meningitis, hypoglycaemic coma).[230] The pathologist faced with an autopsy to confirm or refute the clinical suspicion of CM will usually find the diagnosis easy. It may be more difficult to assess the proportionate mortality of the cerebral versus the other systemic processes in malaria. The possible presentations are:

1. Acute death from untreated (or unsuspected) CM: the gross and microscopic findings will be typical as described, with abundant parasites, sequestration may or may not be accompanied by secondary microvascular pathology.
2. Death following prolonged treatment or illness, the diagnosis having been established on blood films. The appearances can be variable, and the parasites are cleared quite rapidly. After 3–4 days of treatment, the sequestered PRBCs can be difficult to find in the brain. The presence of petechial haemorrhages (some maturing into Dürck granulomas), pigment deposition and pigment-laden monocytes in vessels are all clues.
3. Death with parasitaemic infection, and sequestration in the brain without microvascular pathology, but the cause of death is not the cerebral infection (Figure 21.8).[217] This also occurs with *P. knowlesi* infection. In these cases, there is no upregulation of endothelial cell ICAM-1.[46]

Oil immersion examination can identify scanty parasites. Picric acid digestion removes pigment (formalin more than haemozoin) to aid clarification of parasites. Correlation with the other organs' pathologies is obviously important: haemozoin pigment remains in the liver, spleen and bone marrow for days to weeks after therapy.

In most cases where the brain is examined, the diagnosis of *P. falciparum* infection will have already been made on blood smears or is suspected. However, a small proportion of cases are only suspected and diagnosed at autopsy, from the characteristic brain and other organs' appearances. The technique of brain smear is valuable in providing a rapid, sensitive and specific means of identifying significant cerebral malaria in these cases (Box 21.1).

In active cerebral malaria cases, the capillaries will contain abundant parasitized red cells. The forms of the parasites can vary, from mid to late trophozoites, and schizonts

BOX 21.1. Technique of brain smear in cerebral malaria

- Take a 2–3mm cube of cerebral cortical grey matter
- Place on a slide
- Appose a blank slide on top, press gently and pull apart the slides to make smears on both
- Air dry
- Fix in methanol
- Stain with Giemsa and coverslip

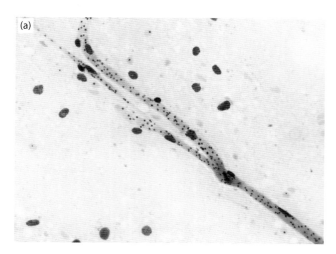

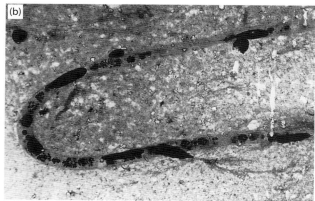

21.9 Malaria. Brain smears from adult patients. **(a)** Capillary containing mature trophozoites. Giemsa. **(b)** Capillary loop containing schizonts with visible haemozoin brown pigment. Giemsa.

may also be seen, according to the time of death in relation to the parasite replication cycle (Figure 21.9). The cytology technique is useful in diagnosing cerebral malaria in decomposing cadavers also: the red cells may have disappeared or be blurred, but the endovascular parasites remain visible.

Immunohistochemistry and molecular diagnostics (PCR) can demonstrate *Plasmodium* infections[46,74] in formalin-fixed paraffin-embedded sections. Antibody to *P. falciparum* histidine rich protein-2 (HRP-2) has proven useful in clinically obscure cases, staining the cytoplasm and membranes of parasites.

Pathogenesis

Few diseases have generated as much controversy over pathogenesis as CM. Until the 1980s, the theses of parasite sequestration and abnormal vascular permeability that had held sway since the 1890s were unchallenged.[20,230] Because the parasites stick to endothelial cells in small vessels in the brain, there is reduced blood flow, local hypoxia and local nutrient deprivation,[222] which leads to coma and death. Factors such as parasite consumption of local glucose, and a possible toxic role for haemozoin pigment may contribute. Brain swelling represents cerebral oedema, a consequence of breakdown of the blood–brain barrier because of increased vascular permeability. The swelling contributes

to reduced blood supply and causes internal herniation and brain stem compression. Many studies showed close correlation between the intensity of PRBC sequestration and clinically pure cerebral malaria (as opposed to mortality from malaria anaemia or respiratory distress and acidosis, or secondary bacterial infection).

Then it was suggested that some or all the features of severe malaria could be accounted for by the systemic release host cytokines in response to malaria infection; the analogy was with organ dysfunction in septic shock.[37,38] Tumour necrosis factor-α (TNF-α) is released from host leukocytes, with high blood levels in severe malaria. Nitric oxide synthase induction in endothelial cells, with release of the neuroactive mediator nitric oxide (NO), is another process that occurs in malaria.[132] From multiple subsequent case and series studies of acutely ill patients, it is generally agreed that cytokine-related phenomena are part of the explanation of CM but the core process is sequestration.

Animal Models

Animal models have proved of limited use because there is no natural comparable malarial disease outside man. *P. burghei* infection in mice is a standard model. There are about 10 times more studies of this infection than there are of human falciparum malaria. Investigation of adjunctive therapeutic interventions in experimental malaria often prove successful; in contrast, few trials of interventions in human disease seem to improve outcomes.[182,227]

Case Definition and Cause of Death

A fundamental problem in clinical studies, and thus of contributions of pre-mortem investigations to pathogenesis, is that of case definition. A notable paediatric study in Malawi, with autopsy follow-up, diagnosed clinical CM stringently as a syndrome of unrousable coma not attributable to convulsions, hypoglycaemia or meningitis in a patient with *P. falciparum* parasitaemia.[217] However, nearly one quarter of children dying with CM by clinical definition actually died of something else, as identified at autopsy. All those with sequestration plus microvascular pathology (see earlier) fulfilled the case definition; but many non-CM deaths did have pure sequestration in the brain (see Figure 21.8). Ultrastructural studies have found more concentrated sequestration in the vessels of adults and children who suffered coma as opposed to other lethal manifestations of falciparum malaria.[50,185] There is a descending gradient of severity of sequestration from cerebrum to brain stem.

Endothelial Cell Immunopathology

Parasitized erythrocyte sequestration is a specific receptor-mediated process, caused by adhesion to host receptors expressed on the endothelial cell (EC) surface. The most characterized molecule on the PRBC is PfEMP-1 (*Plasmodium falciparum* erythrocyte membrane protein-1), a parasite protein product that forms the knobs on the surfaces of PRBCs (Figure 21.5). The knob proteins bind to cell adhesion molecules on EC surfaces; these include intercellular adhesion molecule-1 (ICAM-1) and vascular cell adhesion molecule-1 (VCAM-1), among others. Cerebral ECs show marked activation in CM, as part of systemic EC activation, and there is upregulation of expression of ICAM-1, CD36 and VCAM-1 on ECs.[230] As well as aiding sticking of PRBCs, this also causes structural changes to cerebral ECs, including disruption of intercellular junctional protein complexes and consequent activation of perivascular monocytes and astrocytes. TNF-α is a factor that induces such upregulation.

Blood–Brain Barrier

There is also increasing evidence to support a role for structural and functional disturbances of the blood–brain barrier (BBB) function in CM.[80] The parasite never enters the brain parenchyma and yet can cause severe neurological dysfunction and death.[143] Gaps between endothelial cells are seen, red cells escape through the gaps, there is demonstrable fibrin leakage and oedema fluid around damaged vessels, along with perivascular haemorrhage–in some but not all cases. Where there is breakdown of the BBB and microvascular pathology, the patient has a poor prognosis; but patients also die of CM with intact BBB and no haemorrhages. Further, the fact that most people do recover fully, when treated, from CM suggests that BBB dysfunction is not bound to cause a pathological injury in itself.[143] It may be an epiphenomenon.

In summary, the pathological phenomena that are consistently associated with coma due to falciparum malaria are:

1. Intensity of parasite sequestration
2. Congestion of the vessels with infected and uninfected erythrocytes
3. Axonal injury in the white matter
4. Retinopathy in children

Non-associations or inconsistent associations with coma are:

1. Cerebral oedema
2. Damage to the blood–brain barrier
3. Ring-haemorrhages (i.e. microvascular pathology)
4. Glial reaction
5. Myelin disruption

There are evidently variant pathogenetic pathways in CM. Sequestration is an essential feature but not sufficient to explain everything; but the contributions of immunological phenomena at the endothelial cell level and damage to the blood–brain barrier are still uncertain. Finally, different genetically controlled host reactions to injury must also be important in determining how and why some infected patients go on to develop CM and die, where others do not.

Toxoplasmosis

Toxoplasmosis is caused by infection with coccidian parasite *Toxoplasma gondii*. It is distributed globally, with the cat as the definitive host, but any warm-blooded animal, including man, can be an intermediate host.[131] Infection can be acquired *in utero*, with severe damage to the developing brain and eye, but most people become infected after childhood and the primary infection is usually clinically silent

and latent. Significant disease, of which CNS pathology is the most common and important, happens if the latent infection reactivates. HIV infection and immunosuppression is now by far the most common underlying cause of reactivation, and cerebral toxoplasmosis is a major syndrome in HIV disease progression.

Epidemiology

The proportion of a population that is infected with *T. gondii*–and therefore liable to develop disease–varies widely, mainly because of climate and dietary practices. The prevalence ranges from 5 per cent (Zambia[235]) to 90 per cent (e.g. Paris and francophone West Africa[126]). In the UK and USA, the average is 10–40 per cent prevalence.[131] This is quantified by serology for IgG antibodies in the blood. Without antimicrobial prophylaxis, the proportion of those with HIV infection and latently infected with *T. gondii* who go on to develop toxoplasmic encephalitis before death ranges from 25 to 50 per cent.[39]

Life Cycle

The sexual phase of the life cycle of *T. gondii* is in the enterocytes of cats (Figure 21.10). People become infected either by ingesting oocysts shed in cat faeces (directly or via contaminated water) or through eating raw or undercooked meat that contains tissue cysts (this is probably the more frequent route). Such meat is from intermediate hosts such as pig, sheep and cattle that have become directly and chronically infected by eating oocysts.[91]

Following ingestion of tissue cysts, the parasite invades through the gut wall and enters the circulation where it undergoes an acute phase of rapid division of the tachyzoite stage within many types of host cells, predominantly macrophages. *T. gondii* is a member of the group of protozoa called the apicomplexa, which also includes malaria, in which the crescent-shaped infective stages are characterized by an apical complex of organelles involved in host cell invasion (Figure 21.11a). It is an obligate intracellular parasite capable of infecting any nucleated host cell; this is done in about 10–20 seconds via parasite proteases and a unique gliding motility locomotion.[26] The internalized tachyzoite undergoes division by internal budding–termed 'endodyogeny'. Repeated division can occur before the cell ruptures and releases the parasites. Tachyzoites spread through the circulation to many organs including skeletal muscle, eye and brain, but also cardiac and smooth muscle. The development of an effective cellular immune response suppresses replication and eradicates most of the tachyzoites, thus ending the acute phase of infection.

In brain and muscle, acute phase tachyzoites can undergo stage conversion into bradyzoites. These divide slowly within special parasitophagous vacuoles, where homogenous parasite material precipitate under the limiting membrane of the vacuole to form a cyst wall (Figure 21.11b). In murine models of the disease, tissue cysts are retained within viable host cells that can be identified as neurons. Under conditions of stress *in vitro*, parasites can form cysts in many types of host cells, including astrocytes. In the murine model, cyst rupture occurs rarely, probably associated with host cell death, but in immunocompetent individuals, a rapid immune response limits

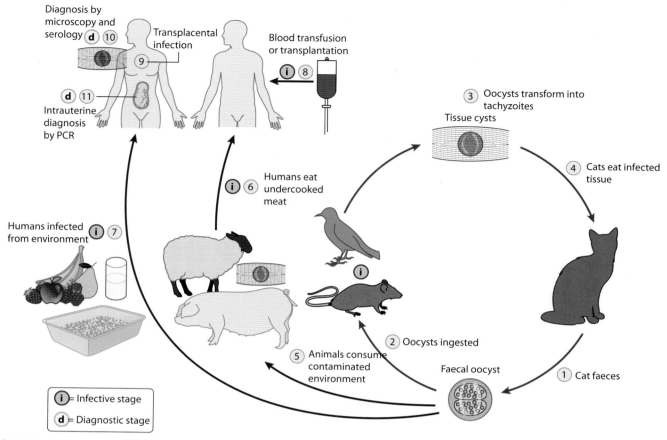

Diagnosis by microscopy and serology **d** ⑩

Transplacental infection

⑨

Blood transfusion or transplantation

i ⑧

③ Oocysts transform into tachyzoites

Tissue cysts

④ Cats eat infected tissue

d ⑪

Intrauterine diagnosis by PCR

Humans eat undercooked meat

i ⑥

Humans infected from environment **i** ⑦

i

② Oocysts ingested

Faecal oocyst

① Cat faeces

⑤ Animals consume contaminated environment

i = Infective stage

d = Diagnostic stage

21.10 *Toxoplasma gondii* **life cycle.**

Figure courtesy of United States Centers for Disease Control and Prevention, Division of Parasitic Diseases.

damage to small inflammatory foci. Cysts are latent in CNS, skeletal and cardiac muscle, and the eye. They vary in size between 12–14 μm (containing a few organisms) and 100 μm (containing thousands of zoites).

Clinical Syndromes of Toxoplasmosis

Most patients with toxoplasmosis disease have underlying HIV infection. However, the complete list of clinicopathological syndromes is:

- primary toxoplasmosis in immunocompetent individuals;
- toxoplasmosis in immunosuppressed patients;
  - HIV disease;
  - post-transplantation immunosuppression;
  - congenital immunodeficiency syndromes.
- congenital toxoplasmosis;
- controversially, there may be an association with schizophrenia and epilepsy.[47]

Development of toxoplasmosis in man depends on host susceptibility and immune status. Circulating antibody constitute the initial immune response; this limits extracellular dissemination of infection. Cell-mediated immune responses limit the capacity of latent infection, once established, to reactivate and redisseminate. Thus there are different patterns of disease severity depending on whether infection occurs in an immune-intact individual, or one who is immunocompromised, or in a foetus or young child before the development of fully effective immune competence. There are also variations in virulence of *T. gondii* strains.

Primary Acquired Toxoplasmosis in the Immunocompetent Host

From the sero-epidemiological data, this is obviously a common occurrence, but uncommonly results in clinical disease. The manifestations are variable and usually subside spontaneously. There may be an infectious mononucleosis-like febrile illness, lymphadenopathy (typical cervical nodes), a rash and an encephalitic syndrome.

The primary encephalitic syndrome is rare.[89] It may present as a non-specific encephalopathy or a diffuse meningo-encephalitis or with a space-occupying lesion. Pathologically, the features are identical to those of toxoplasmosis in HIV disease, described later.

Foci of asymptomatic toxoplasmosis are occasionally detected in the brains of people dying of unrelated causes.[189] These are the potential sources of reactivation. In the eye, toxoplasmosis may attack the choroid, the ciliary body or the retina, producing small foci of granulomatous inflammation and scarring.

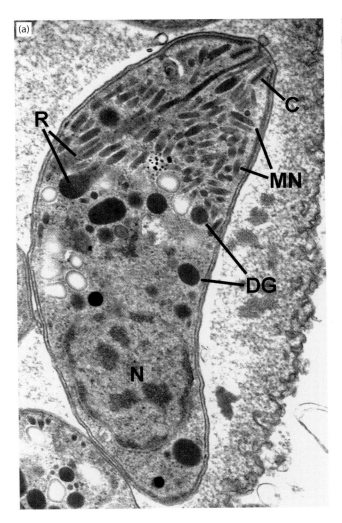

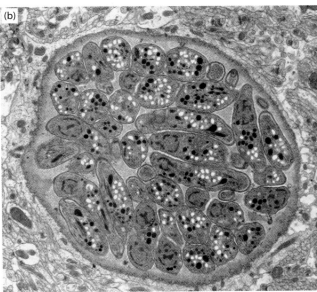

21.11 Toxoplasmosis. (a) Transmission electron micrograph (TEM) showing a tachyzoite form of *Toxoplasma gondii*, from murine central nervous system (CNS). The ultrastructural details of the apical complex are seen, including the conoid body **(C)**, rhoptry **(R)** and micronemes **(MN)**. Within the cytoplasm, dense granules **(DG)** and the nucleus **(N)** can be identified. The tachyzoite form takes up a bow-like configuration. **(b)** TEM of a *T. gondii* cyst within murine CNS, containing bradyzoites within a well-demarcated cyst wall.

(a) Reproduced by permission from Biologist and Professor David Ferguson, Oxford University.
(b) Reproduced by permission from Parasitology Today and Professor David Ferguson, Oxford University.

Toxoplasmosis in Immunocompromised Individuals

The massive increase in the prevalence of cerebral toxoplasmosis since the 1980s is almost solely due to the HIV pandemic (Table 21.3). Cerebral toxoplasmosis is the most common opportunistic CNS infection. From a range of autopsy studies, the prevalence of CNS toxoplasmosis in HIV varies from 4 per cent in African children[12] to 35 per cent in France and Brazil.[34] In HIV-infected adults in Africa, it is far more common than cerebral lymphoma; thus focal neurological lesions can be empirically treated without specific diagnosis.[126] The majority of HIV+ patients presenting with toxoplasma encephalitis have a blood CD4+ T-cell count <50/μL.

The disease is less common in certain HIV infection risk groups, including children and haemophiliacs. Among non-HIV infected immunocompromised patients (e.g. post-transplantation and treated leukaemia), CNS disease is less common at around 5 per cent in several series. Infection occurs when a serologically negative recipient receives an organ (e.g. heart, kidney) from a seropositive latently infected donor.

Clinical and Radiological Features

The clinical presentation of CNS toxoplasmosis in association with HIV disease varies, and is often the first

TABLE 21.3 Differential diagnosis of CNS mass lesions in HIV disease (see Figure 21.37)
Toxoplasmosis
Tuberculosis
American trypanosomiasis
Granulomatous amoebic encephalitis
Microsporidiosis
Cryptococcoma (*Cryptococcus neoformans*)
Aspergillosis
Herpes simplex encephalitis
Progressive multifocal leukoencephalopathy (JC virus encephalitis)
Lymphoma

presentation of advanced disease. The most common is the effects of a mass lesion, including seizures and focal neurological signs. The three main clinicopathological patterns are:

- mass effect, simulating a neoplasm;
- diffuse nodular encephalitis;[85]
- ependymitis (ventriculitis) and periventricular necrosis, associated with obstructive hydrocephalus.[202]

The mass lesion has a differential diagnosis including lymphoma, tuberculoma, herpes encephalitis, granulomatous amoebic encephalitis, bacterial abscess and infarction. Progressive multifocal leukoencephalopathy can also simulate toxoplasmosis. The periventricular pattern presents non-specifically as fever, confusion and headache, and simulates CMV ventriculitis. CNS toxoplasmosis can also, of course, be one of several opportunistic diseases within the cranium presenting at the same time. Spinal cord involvement, with a myelopathy, is uncommon (as is myopathy).[116]

After clinical suspicion, imaging and immunodiagnostics are the main diagnostic methods. In mass lesions, contrast-enhanced CT scanning demonstrates one or more ring-enhancing lesions (Figure 21.12). The most common sites are basal ganglia, cortical grey-white matter junction zones and the thalamus.[159] MRI is more sensitive in detecting multiple lesions and permits more accurate differentiation from other focal lesions.

Pathology

In man, the acute phase of infection may be asymptomatic, or present as a febrile illness, and uncommonly as lymphadenopathy, typically cervical node swelling, biopsy of which shows granulomatous lymphadenitis but rarely visible parasites.

CNS toxoplasmosis in HIV disease causes a number of different pathological lesions.[147] The basic process is cell infection and associated inflammation, forming a microglial nodule with surrounding astrocytosis (Figure 21.13). Infected cell necrosis and necrosis of surrounding tissues is usual, with expansion of lesions into the mass lesions that are most usually seen. Blood vessels are involved with parasites in their walls, associated with vasculitis and thrombotic occlusion. Haemorrhage results from rupture of vessels.

The mass lesions are sited both above and below the tentorium, with the basal ganglia and the grey-white matter cortical junctions being characteristic locations (Figure 21.14). The pathology evolves if the patient survives the effects of the toxoplasma foci, which act as space-occupying lesions:

1. First, there are necrotizing abscesses consisting of poorly circumscribed areas of necrosis, with variable haemorrhage. Microscopically, the necrosis is typically coagulative and 'dirty', with abundant nuclear debris (some of which are actually toxoplasma tachyzoites) (Figure 21.15). As well as vasculitis, endarteritis obliterans is a characteristic feature (Figure 21.16). Around the necrosis is oedema, reactive microgliosis and astrocytosis. The parasites are usually abundant, both as 2-μm haematoxyphilic extracellular tachyzoites within the necrosis and, around the periphery of the lesion, bradyzoites (Figure 21.17 and Table 21.4). The latter may be scanty in treated lesions. Immunocytochemistry with anti-*T. gondii* antibodies is a sensitive means to identify parasites, and particularly useful when bradyzoites are not visible.

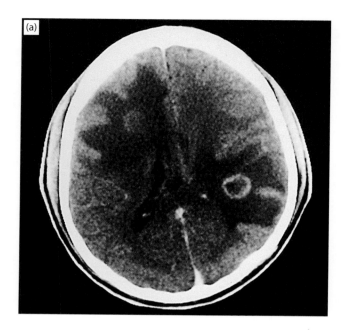

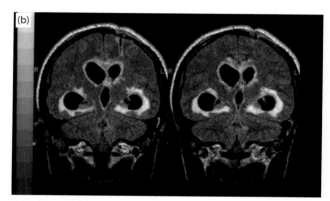

21.12 Toxoplasmosis. (a) CT scan of typical cerebral mass lesion with ring-enhancing lesion and surrounding oedema. **(b)** MR scan showing less common periventricular pattern of infection; histopathology showed necrosis to a depth of 1 cm, with abundant zoites.

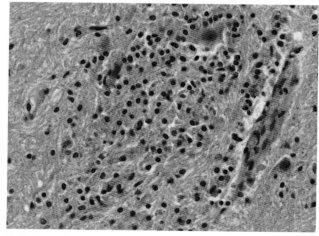

21.13 Toxoplasmosis. A microglial nodule in the pons, with a cluster of tachyzoites.

2. In more chronic lesions, the central area of coagulative necrosis is surrounded by macrophages, and organisms are more scanty, but still detectable by immunocytochemistry.

3. In chronic, treated lesions, the necrosis is well demarcated and may become cystic, with a macrophage fringe and peripheral microglial nodules with astrocytosis (Figure 21.18). Immunolabelling may or may not identify residual antigen in these lesions.

In the diffuse encephalitic pattern, there is little or no necrosis, but microglial nodules including parasites throughout the cerebral white and grey matter. In the periventricular pattern, there is a rim of necrosis up to 1 cm thick along the lateral and third ventricles, and abundant parasites visible.

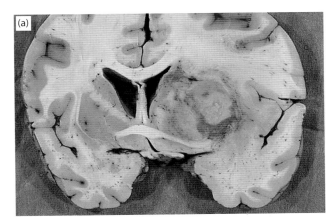

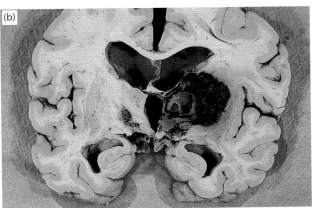

21.14 Toxoplasmosis in HIV disease. (a) Mass lesion with necrosis and cerebral swelling. **(b)** Mass lesion with haemorrhage.

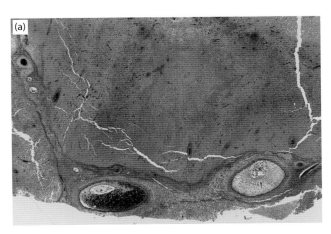

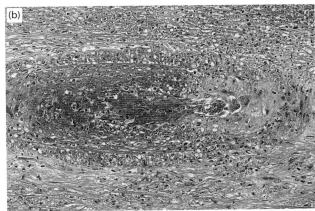

21.16 Toxoplasmosis. (a) Necrotic zone with adjacent endarteritis obliterans. **(b)** Vasculitis (immunolabelling showed zoites within the artery muscle layer).

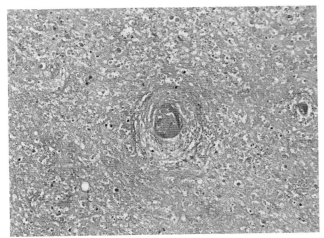

21.15 Toxplasmosis. Typical infarcted pattern of necrosis, with a central vessel showing 'onion-skinning' and containing thrombus.

TABLE 21.4 Differential diagnosis of small haematoxyphilic bodies in the context of suspected infection in central nervous system material

Toxoplasma gondii	
Leishmania	
Trypanosoma cruzi	
Microsporidians	
Histoplasma capsulatum	
Helminth larval nuclei	*Loa*
	Toxoxara canis
	Strongyloides
	Halicephalobus
Apoptotic nuclear debris	

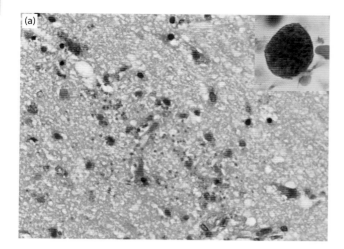

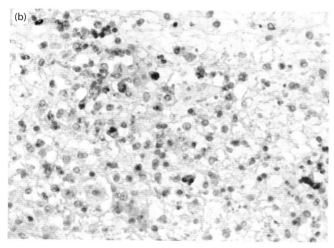

21.17 Toxoplasmosis. (a) Numerous small haematoxyphilic bodies (tachyzoites) in the neuropil, with a mild microglial reaction. Inset: bradycyst—an infected host cell containing hundreds of zoites. **(b)** Immunolabelled toxoplasma zoites within lesion (anti-*T. gondii*).

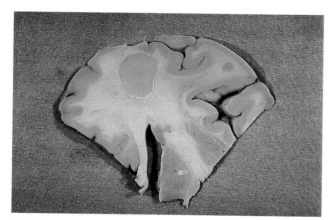

21.18 Toxoplasmosis. Chronic treated lesion showing a well-defined rim and a necrotic centre.

In reality, there is much heterogeneity of CNS toxoplasma lesions, with overlapping patterns and sometimes temporal heterogeneity. The brain stem may be more involved than supratentorial zones. A predominantly vascular pattern of infection is described, considered to represent primary haematogenous invasive disease rather than reactivation of latent cerebral infection.[97]

Immune Constitution Inflammatory Syndrome

With anti-HIV treatment, the blood viral load drops and the CD4+ T-cell count rises. This can lead to reactive inflammatory lesions at sites of infection, reflecting a rise in cell-mediated immunity. These immune constitution inflammatory syndrome (IRIS) lesions are either paradoxical (i.e., worsening despite treatment of a known lesion) or unmasking (a new lesion developing at a site of previously silent infection—see Chapter 19). The time interval between the start of combination antiretroviral therapy (cART) and IRIS is 1–6 months. In HIV-associated cerebral toxoplasmosis, unmasking IRIS lesions are mainly described,[135] with rare paradoxical types.[21] Thus, a new neurological syndrome with inflammatory swelling develops in the brain, on imaging similar to lesions in untreated HIV disease, or in paradoxical IRIS an increase in size and signal intensity. The histopathology of IRIS lesions indicates a major perivascular influx of CD8+ T-cells, a feature common to many IRIS lesions.

Ocular and Other Organ Toxoplasmosis

Ocular toxoplasmosis occurs in 2–3 per cent of patients (not immunosuppressed) with symptomatic acquired toxoplasmosis.[172] In HIV-infected people, concomitant eye involvement from toxoplasmosis is less common than with CMV infection. The eye lesions are only studied at end-stage. Histologically, there is retinochoroiditis and, in severe cases, retinal necrosis associated with parasites. In less destructive lesions, there is a granulomatous reaction with scanty parasites.[147,166] Other visceral lesions occur in a minority of patients, usually immunosuppressed with HIV disease, including heart and skeletal muscle infection,[75,116] and lung disease with miliary necrotizing pneumonitis.[64]

Congenital Toxoplasmosis

Congenital toxoplasmosis is a rare condition with an estimated incidence of 3.4 cases per 100 000 live births in England and Wales, but is likely to be more common among all pregnancies.[77] However, the risk of maternal exposure, and therefore of transmission to the foetus, is geographically variable.[125] Pregnant women encounter *Toxoplasma gondii* either through ingestion of undercooked, infected meat or through contact with domestic cats.[91]

Women who acquire a primary *T. gondii* infection during pregnancy and who become seropositive may develop a mild illness characterized by lymphadenopathy, fever and headache. Alternatively, the infection may be clinically silent.[91] Parasitaemia occurs during the primary infection and blood-borne organisms are able not only to infect the placenta, causing focal lesions, but also to cross to the fetus.[9] Different strains of *Toxoplasma* vary in their ability in this regard.[9] In one large study of mothers who seroconverted during pregnancy, 32 per cent of the offspring were found subsequently to have acquired congenital toxoplasmosis.[153]

The introduction of screening programmes to detect congenitally affected individuals has been debated, but not universally advocated, because *Toxoplasma gondii* is most readily transmitted late in pregnancy and the effects of congenital toxoplasmosis are relatively mild at this stage of development.[77,91] Not all children presenting with toxoplasma-associated chorioretinitis have acquired their infection before birth. Some cases may result from a postnatal primary infection.[77] Even those children who are themselves infected with HIV do not appear to be at particular risk of developing toxoplasmosis when they become immune suppressed and the prevalence of toxoplasmosis is low in paediatric AIDS.[12,117]

Clinical Features

The clinical presentation of congenital toxoplasmosis is variable. The CNS and the eyes are the principal targets of disease in the fetus.[2] The mildest manifestation of prenatal infection involves only the eyes, causing chorioretinitis. In contrast, the most severely affected infants display microcephaly, hydrocephalus and cerebral calcifications in addition to chorioretinitis.[2] Systemic organs may be involved, including the skin and the liver. At birth, it may be difficult to distinguish the effects of congenital toxoplasmosis from those caused by other fetal infections that together constitute the TORCH syndrome (*Toxoplasma*, Rubella, Cytomegalovirus and Herpes Simplex I and II).[62] The diagnosis of congenital toxoplasmosis is based on the detection of specific antibodies including immunoglobulins A and M,[62,153] but now also includes PCR for *T. gondii* DNA.[2,15] PCR analysis of amniotic fluid for *Toxoplasma* has also been reported recently.[154]

The single most important factor in determining whether a foetus is infected or not is the timing of maternal infection.[54,91] Gestational age also determines the severity of the outcome. The risk of *Toxoplasma* transmission from mother to foetus is lowest in the first trimester and rises during the course of pregnancy. Although the risk is comparatively low early in pregnancy, a fetal *Toxoplasma* infection at this stage is likely to cause major disruption of CNS organogenesis with resulting severe abnormality. Severity and patterns of disease are also influenced by genetic polymorphisms in mother and child.[105]

Fetal death or hydrops may occur and microphthalmia, hydrocephalus and widespread cerebral calcifications are not uncommon.[2,91] If the foetus survives, microcephaly is an inevitable result. During the second trimester, the risk of maternal transmission rises to about 30 per cent, and late in the third trimester the risk is as high as 100 per cent.[54] Conversely, the severity of the complications of congenital toxoplasmosis declines with advancing pregnancy, although premature delivery and fetal death may still result from late infection. More commonly, the effect of congenital toxoplasmosis acquired late in pregnancy may be subclinical and benign, characterized only by chorioretinitis and minor brain calcifications.[91] The chorioretinitis may be detected soon after birth or may become apparent only later in childhood or adolescence.[15] This is because the involvement of the choroid and retina is usually patchy and focal and generally spares the macula.

Pathogenesis and Pathology of Congenital Toxoplasmosis

T. gondii is not usually a virulent pathogen for the human host. The foetus is at risk in the context of maternal *Toxoplasma* infection because immune responses are not yet fully developed. Particularly in the first half of gestation, the effects of congenital toxoplasmosis are different from those seen in the adult because the infective process involves developing organs that have not yet achieved final differentiation. *T. gondii* is an intracellular pathogen that affects ependyma and glial cells particularly in the periventricular and periaqueductal region, causing cell death and necrosis directly. The resulting acute inflammatory response is facilitated by the action of maternal antibody, leading to thrombosis and secondary ischaemic necrosis that further disrupt organogenesis. Leptomeningeal spread and hydrocephalus may occur; periaqueductal infection and secondary stenosis lead to hydrocephalus. If fetal death and miscarriage do not follow, the inflammation within the brain resolves and focal calcification may supervene.

The gross pathology of fatal congenital toxoplasmosis is typically a hydrocephalic brain with calcification (Figure 21.19). There may be bilateral cortical cysts.[86] Histologically, *Toxoplasma* organisms are hard to detect within frankly necrotic areas and are generally best seen at the reactive margins.

Pathogenesis of Toxoplasmosis: Overview

As an obligate intracellular parasite, *T. gondii* has evolved immune evasion tools, and the control of *T. gondii* infection in the human host is cell-mediated.[47] This is T-cell mediated, via both CD8+ and CD4+ types, and both interferon-γ and perforin-mediated immune.[72,100,150,213] Interferon-γ and interleukin-2 activate macrophages that secrete IL-12 and TNF-α, and kill parasites or inhibit their replication.[194] It is presumed that periodically the latent bradycysts rupture and release tachyzoites locally; the immune response then acts to eliminate the parasites and the process is clinically silent. However, if the host is immunodeficient the infection can progress and disseminate. Antibodies may lyse extracellular tachyzoites, but cannot protect against live parasites within cells.

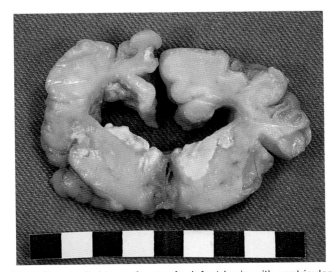

21.19 Congenital toxoplasmosis. Infant brain with ventricular dilatation, necrosis and calcification of several parts of the grey and white matter.

The pathogenesis of the tissue lesions and necrosis in toxoplasmosis is not clear. The likely mechanisms include:

1. Direct cytotoxicity and apoptosis induction through cell-to-cell contact with the parasite[60]
2. Direct infection vasculitis, vascular obstruction and local infarction[60]
3. Cytokine-induced necrosis, as a bystander effect of the immunopathological response to infection[72,99,100]

Diagnosis and Treatment of Toxoplasmosis

CNS infection is suspected on clinical grounds supported by consistent imaging. Proving the infection is more difficult and treatment is often empirical, particularly in patients with HIV. CSF examination rarely identifies parasites in lumbar fluid (although ventricular fluid is more productive),[164] but positive antibodies may be present. PCR is increasingly used on CSF and tissue samples. Serology is usually, but not always, positive in patients with CNS toxoplasmosis, with IgG or IgM present.[131] Similarly, CSF antibody detection and PCR DNA detection are sensitive, but not 100 per cent so. The issue is compounded by the widespread prevalence of latent infection, which results in a low IgG titre.

Brain biopsy may be undertaken to prove cerebral toxoplasmosis. The main differential diagnosis, in HIV disease, is cerebral lymphoma, from which it can be difficult to distinguish on clinical or imaging criteria–they both produce multifocal haemorrhagic lesions (see Fig. 21.37). In addition, even when an autopsy brain is examined, the gross examination may be non-specific and the final diagnosis only confirmed microscopically. In South America, Chagas' disease causes similar gross CNS lesions to toxoplasmosis.

Pyrimethamine is the main drug used for treatment, which kills the tachyzoites but does not act against the bradycyst (latent) forms. Co-trimoxazole is used as prophylaxis in HIV disease against pneumocystosis, and it is also reduces the likelihood of reactivation of latent toxoplasmosis. In HIV+ patients on cART, once the blood CD4+ T-cell count exceeds 200/μL, anti-toxoplasma prophylaxis can be stopped.

Sarcocystosis

Sarcocystis spp. are globally distributed as intestinal infections of carnivores, and are taxonomically related to *Toxoplasma gondii*.[147] Man becomes infected by accidentally eating oocysts in faeces, and the parasite passes to heart and skeletal muscle (including tongue muscle). Most identifications are made incidentally, when muscle biopsy or autopsy material is being examined. There are a few reported outbreaks of myositis attributable to *Sarcocystis* infection.[131]

Morphologically, there are several patterns of muscle infection with slightly different muscle cyst and zoite dimensions. The infected myofibre has an expansion filled with tightly packed parasites about $2 \times 10\,\mu m$ in size (Figure 21.20). The cyst is up to 400 μm long.[147] In the rare myositis cases, there is associated eosinophilic inflammation.[7]

Trypanosomiasis

There are three species of *Trypanosoma* protozoa that affect man, all transmitted by blood-feeding insects. Though morphologically similar in their trypomastigote blood form (Figure 21.21), they give rise to quite different diseases in South America and Africa, respectively.[131]

Human African Trypanosomiasis (African Sleeping Sickness)

Epidemiology, Transmission and Life Cycle

Human African trypanosomiasis (HAT) is caused by two blood parasites, *Trypanosoma brucei rhodesiense* and *Trypanosoma brucei gambiense*. Morphologically identical but causing significantly different clinical syndromes, they are found in west Africa (*T.b. gambiense*) and in eastern and southern Africa (*T.b. rhodesiense*), separated geographically by the Rift Valley (Figure 21.22).[169,224] Uganda uniquely is home to both infections. *T.b. rhodesiense* is a zoonosis with cattle as the reservoir (with significant veterinary consequences); *T.b. gambiense* has man as the sole host. HAT is transmitted from man to man or cattle to man by *Glossina* spp. tsetse flies. The two parasites are differentiated by their ability to survive in human serum (serum resistance assay) and now by DNA analysis.

Both infections cause a systemic and CNS encephalitic syndrome in man with high mortality when untreated. Currently about 60 million people are at risk of infection with HAT. New recorded annual cases vary according to

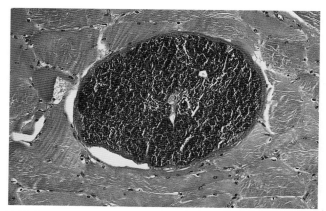

21.20 Sarcocystosis. Skeletal muscle cell containing a cyst of compacted zoites. There is no inflammation.

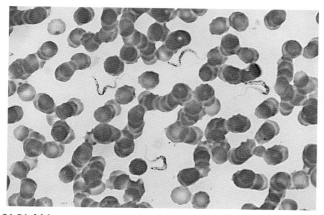

21.21 African trypanosomiasis. Blood film showing the flagellate trypomastigotes. *T.b. rhodesiense* and *T.b. gambiense* are morphologically indistinguishable. Giemsa.

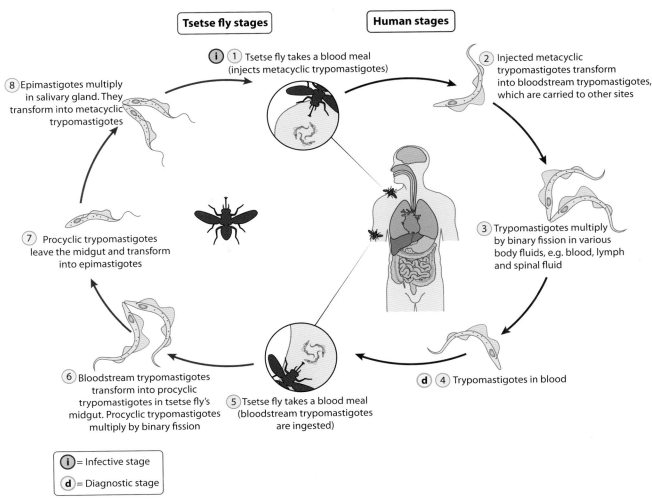

21.22 Life cycle of human African trypanosomes.

Figure courtesy of United States Centers for Disease Control and Prevention, Division of Parasitic Diseases.

intensity of disease surveillance, civil war and access to treatment; it has been as bad as 500 000, but currently fewer than 10 000 new cases are diagnosed. Angola, DR Congo, Chad and Sudan are the worst affected countries (www.who.int). Co-infection with HIV has not affected the epidemiology or virulence of these infections.[142,169,170]

An infected bite causes a local skin inflammatory lesion—the chancre—in which trypanosomes can be seen. This heals completely within weeks. There may later be a generalized allergic rash. The parasite invades the bloodstream and infects the lymphoreticular system, with chronic lymphadenopathy and hepatosplenomegaly. This is the haemolymphatic stage of HAT. Constitutional symptoms, including fever, fluctuate.

The infection passes into the brain and spinal cord across the blood–brain barrier after a few weeks, and there is infection of the choroid plexus. This sets up the second, meningoencephalitic stage of HAT.[112,131] It takes place within weeks in the case of *T.b. rhodesiense* infection and months with *T.b. gambiense*.

Disease from *T.b. rhodesiense* has a rapid onset with more than 80 per cent mortality within 6 months when untreated. The haemolymphatic stage blends into the CNS stage without clear distinction, and death is from carditis, encephalitis, inanition and secondary bacterial infections (e.g. pneumonia) (Table 21.5).

TABLE 21.5 Clinical and pathological features of HAT[147]

	Trypanosoma brucei gambiense	*Trypanosoma brucei rhodesiense*
Duration of illness	Months to years	<9 months
Haemolymphatic and meningoencephalitic stage	Distinct	Run together
Parasitaemia	Low	High
Parasites found in cerebrospinal fluid	+	++
Parasites found in brain	No	Sometimes in meninges
Carditis	No	Yes
Lymphadenopathy	Prominent	Minimal

Infection with *T.b. gambiense* produces a chronic condition with long, symptom-free periods, which may last years. Lymphadenopathy is more prominent (large nodes in the posterior cervical triangle in HAT constitute Winterbottom's sign). The CNS manifestations are protean, non-focal and easily misdiagnosed when the patient is out of context, as in migrants to non-endemic countries. Irritability, personality change, headache and somnolence are typical. Extrapyramidal signs with chorea, ataxia and muscle fasciculation lead to coma and death. In children, the disease course may be more rapid than in adults. Electroencephalogram (EEG) findings are slow delta wave oscillations mimicking those of normal sleep. MR imaging shows diffuse hyperintensity in the basal ganglia and internal capsule (Figure 21.23). After successful chemotherapy, imaging may demonstrate cerebral atrophy.[78]

Neuropathology

The brain may have cloudy meninges and be swollen. The histopathological changes are uniform throughout the CNS white matter,[147] but also involve deep subcortical regions of the thalamus, hypothalamus and periventricular regions. Demyelination is uncommon and neurons are not directly damaged. The meninges show chronic inflammation with lymphocytes and plasma cells. There is a true arteritis, the vessel walls being inflamed but not necrotic. In the parenchyma, there is intense perivascular inflammation, including the 'morula cells of Mott', which are plasma cells stuffed with eosinophilic Russell bodies (i.e. non-secreted immunoglobulins) (Figure 21.24). Microglial activation is universal and nodules are variable; there is always a diffuse astrocytosis. Crucially, no parasites are evident on light microscopy in the neuropil, and rarely in the meningeal spaces (except in acute *T.b. rhodesiense* infections).

Pathogenesis

The parasite does not invade cells in any organ, but causes pathology indirectly. The lymph nodes show reactive follicular hyperplasia and medullary plasmacytosis, and with *T.b. rhodesiense* infection parasites may be visible. In this infection also, the heart may be involved with a chronic pancarditis and, in severe cases, a true myocarditis,[147] which results in fibrosis in survivors.

The parasites cross the blood–brain barrier and induce immunopathology, which has been more studied experimentally. Polyclonal activation of B-cells is characteristic, with large amounts of immunoglobulins in CSF and blood. Constant antigenic variation of the surface glycoprotein (i.e. at frequency higher than random mutation rates) is a feature of HAT infection, which means that the immune system cannot eliminate the infection through production of neutralizing antibody. Also, by entering the perivascular spaces of the brain, the parasite escapes the host immune system and lysis.

Autoantibodies are released in HAT, including to host components such as DNA, smooth muscle and red cell membranes. In animal models, antibody to myelin basic protein correlates with the degree of CNS pathology.[131] Immune complexes of HAT antigen plus antibody are found; they may trigger complement activation, so causing endothelial cell damage and the endarteritis noted.

Breakdown of the blood–brain barrier is evident with vasogenic oedema.[175]

Recent focus has been on the balance of production and effect of pro-inflammatory cytokines (e.g. TNF-α, IL-1) versus counter-inflammatory cytokines (e.g. IL-10), and production of the somnogenic prostaglandin PGD2.[115]

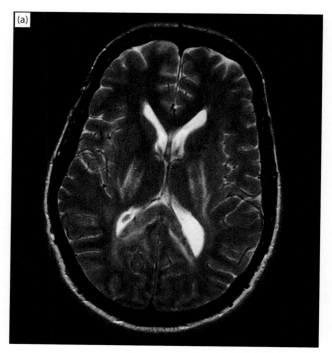

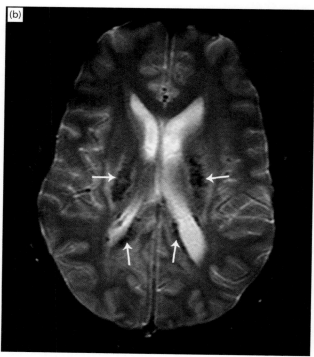

21.23 African trypanosomiasis. MR scans of patient with *T.b. rhodesiense* acute infection. **(a)** Encephalitis with inflammation in the basal ganglia, occipital and frontal lobe white matter. **(b)** Same patient following treatment with melarsoprol and development of reactive encephalopathy. Note the extensive abnormal signal in the basal ganglia and periventricular zones.

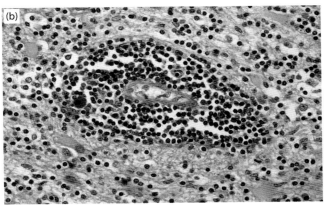

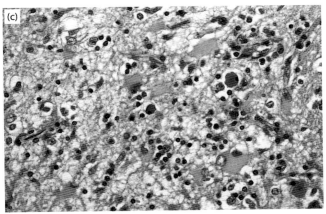

21.24 African trypanosomiasis. Encephalitis in a fatal case of *T.b. gambiense* infection. **(a)** Low power view of severe white matter encephalitis. **(b)** Marked perivascular lymphocytosis, characteristic of the infection. **(c)** Astrocytosis, microgliosis and two morula cells of Mott (plasma cells with eosinophilic globules).

There is also genetic polymorphism of the parasites which, coupled with evident variation in host inflammatory response genes, makes our understanding of this classical tropical disease only rudimentary at present.[112]

Diagnosis and Treatment

Diagnosis of HAT is made by finding the parasites and antibodies in samples of blood and CSF, and parasites in lymph node aspirate. In *T.b. rhodesiense* parasites are usually present in blood and node, but parasites more difficult to find in patients with *T.b. gambiense* infection because of low parasite load. Similarly, the CSF is more likely to test positive for parasites in *T.b. rhodesiense* infection.

Distinction of the haemolymphatic from the cerebral stage is critical, because the toxic drugs necessary for the invasive disease are not needed for the earlier stage. A CSF leukocyte count of >5cells/μL is characteristic of the meningoencephalitic stage, and plasma cells may be present (including the morula cell of Mott).[119] CSF protein is raised through synthesis of IgM, and the finding of IgM concentrations higher than those of IgA and IgG. Similarly, blood IgM is raised. Trypanosome-specific IgM can also be quantified. CSF examination can also indicate structural damage to the brain in second stage (CNS) disease by detection of glial fibrillary acidic protein and light subunit neurofilament.[131]

Treatment of HAT is not optimal. Pentamidine is used for the haemolymphatic stage of infection, but is ineffective in the meningoencephalitic stage because it does not cross the blood–brain barrier. Eflornithine plus nifurtimox is effective in *T.b. gambiense* infection in both stages and, apart from sometimes causing seizures and hearing loss, is not toxic.[113,196] For the treatment of *T.b. rhodesiense* second-stage sleeping sickness, melarsoprol ('Mel B'), an organo-arsenical drug, is still the first choice. It is toxic and can provoke severe adverse reactions. The most important is a reactive encephalitic syndrome that occurs in 5–10 per cent of treated patients and is fatal in about half of these (Figure 21.23).[112] Pathologically, this ranges from an acute exacerbation of the CNS disease with enhanced perivascular inflammation and microglial activation; the most severe form is a haemorrhagic leukoencephalitis. Steroids can ameliorate these reactions.[171] Pathogenetically, an immune restoration phenomenon is probable, with reduced parasite loads in conjunction with a post-treatment enhanced immune reactivity that produces an immune overreaction.

American Trypanosomiasis – Chagas' Disease
Epidemiology and Life Cycle

Chagas' disease is caused by the protozoan *Trypanosoma cruzi*, which can take up the undulating, bloodstream flagellate trypomastigote form, or the *Leishmania*-like amastigote form (Figure 21.25). Discovered in 1909 in Brazil by Carlos Chagas,[29] Chagas' disease or American trypanosomiasis is widespread throughout Latin America, particularly in rural areas. Despite a substantial reduction in its incidence, about 25 million people are still at risk, with about 10 million infective cases per year and 10 000 deaths (www.who.int), emphasizing the need to sustain and extend control strategies, because its morbidity and mortality remain high.[131]

The main control strategy relies on prevention of transmission by eliminating the domestic insect vectors especially *Triatoma infestans*, and control of accidental transmission by blood transfusion. The HIV pandemic has altered the epidemiology of Chagas' disease somewhat, because reactivation of infection is more likely in immunocompromised people.[43]

Its life cycle involves obligatory passage through vertebrate (mammals, including man) and invertebrate

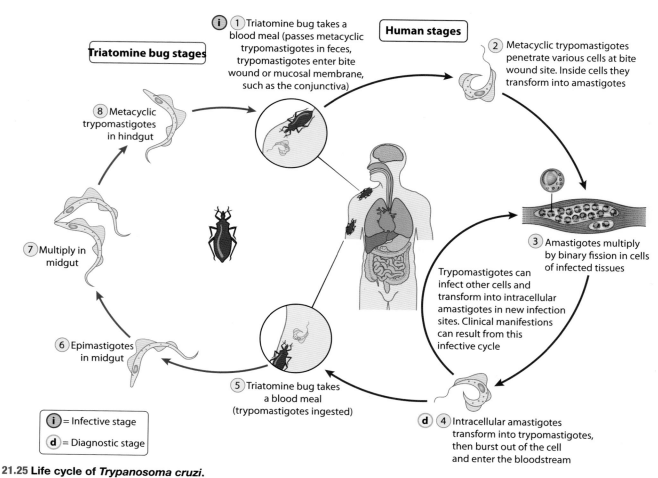

21.25 Life cycle of *Trypanosoma cruzi*.

Figure courtesy of United States Centers for Disease Control and Prevention, Division of Parasitic Diseases.

(haematophagous triatomine bugs) hosts. Bugs inhabit the roofs of mud houses, carry the parasites in the posterior intestine, in the form of trypomastigotes which are eliminated in the faeces when they bite, and enter at the site of the bite because of itching and scratching. Following invasion of vertebrate host cells, particularly smooth or striated muscle, macrophages, fibroblasts, Schwann cells, Langerhans' and parafollicular cells in lymphoid organs, trypomastigotes undergo differentiation into amastigotes, the proliferating intracellular form. This parasite evades host immune surveillance by coating its surface with microvesicles released from blood cells early during infection.[28] After several reproductive cycles and rupture of infected cells, amastigotes transform to trypomastigotes, the form responsible for the dissemination of the infection through the blood or lymphatic circulation, when autonomic ganglia and nerve fibres of the cardiac and superficial plexus of Meissner and Auerbach, cardiac muscle and microglia may also become infected.[33]

The transmission occurs mainly by the insect vector (80–90 per cent), but also by blood transfusion (5–20 per cent), congenital routes (0.5–8 per cent), through organ transplants, and accidental laboratory infection.

Clinical Features

The disease has a variable clinical course, ranging from asymptomatic infection to severe chronic disease with cardiovascular or gastrointestinal involvement or, occasionally, overwhelming acute episodes. After infection and a subsequent incubation period, the acute phase begins. It is directly related to the parasitaemia, may be asymptomatic or course with fever, swollen eyelids, hepatosplenomegaly and enlarged lymph nodes.[131] In the absence of specific treatment, the symptoms persist for about 2 months. About 10 per cent of the patients, especially children, develop a severe acute illness with encephalitis and myocarditis, death ensuing in virtually all cases.

After recovery, patients enter an intermediate stage, when circulating parasites disappear. However, scanty parasitized cells persist as a latent infection, remaining as inflammatory foci in cardiac and extracardiac tissues. During this phase, the host immune response is assumed to suppress both recrudescence of infection and the autoimmune reactions that may characterize the chronic disease. It is believed that 20–40 per cent of patients who suffer acute Chagas' disease progress to the chronic form. This is mainly extracranial disease affecting gut and heart, but with some brain syndromes, including stroke, encephalopathy and reactivated acute lesions.

Whether or not there is a chronic encephalopathy in Chagas' disease, there is no debate that CNS vascular associated lesions (ischaemic or haemorrhagic) are frequently found in patients with the chronic disease. Chagas' myocardiopathy leads to congestive heart failure, dysrhythmia and thromboembolic phenomena, causing strokes.[160]

The factors influencing the clinical variability of acute infection have not been completely elucidated. Soon after the first rounds of replication in the vertebrate host tissues, parasites are thought to trigger the synthesis of proinflammatory cytokines that initiate the production of IFN-γ by natural killer cells, CD4+CD8–β+ and CD4–CD8+β+ T lymphocytes. In addition to these, tumour necrosis factor, interleukin and nitric oxide have crucial roles in host resistance to infection with *T. cruzi*.[82,148] It is likely that the genetic variability of both the host and the parasite are also important.

Pathology

CNS involvement may occur in the acute infective stage, possibly in the chronic stage, because of autoimmune damage or parasite persistence, and in reactivation of latent infection in the chronic phase in immunosuppressed patients. In this context, new pathological presentations of the disease have been recorded in HIV-infected patients.[34]

Severe encephalitis in the acute stage presents with brain oedema, congestion and scattered petechial haemorrhages. Perivascular infiltrates of lymphocytes, some polymorphs, multiple foci of microglial proliferation, and microglial nodules are scattered within the brain parenchyma. Amastigote forms of the parasite are present in glial cells, or less frequently, in microglia at the centre of nodules, macrophages and endothelial cells (Figure 21.26). Lesions can also be seen in the meninges and choroid plexus. Case reports have also described individual cases where the pathological picture included a diffuse granulomatous process or tumour-like mass, such as an acute Chagas' disease presenting with a suprasellar mass and panhypopituitarism diagnosed by biopsy of the hypothalamus that revealed marked inflammation and macrophages containing amastigotes.[35] Amastigote forms can be detected by conventional histology, by immunohistochemistry, *in situ* hybridization and PCR.

Pathogenesis

Parasites most probably penetrate the blood vessel walls, invade the endothelium of cerebral vessels and subsequently pass into astrocytes and microglia, but access via the CSF, perhaps through a damaged choroid plexus, is another possibility.[168] The presence of *T. cruzi* in the CSF is a frequent finding in the acute phase, even in patients without neurological symptoms.[93]

Patients with the milder or asymptomatic acute form, probably have no CNS infection or, in some cases, mild encephalitis that may totally regress, or small paucicellular inflammatory nodules without parasites may persist, either to be eventually cleared, or possibly to be reactivated in the chronic stage of the disease.

In the chronic phase, although Chagas admitted the existence of a chronic form affecting the CNS, which included a range of unexplained clinical presentations,

this has not been well documented. Various neurological syndromes have been reported, including spastic paralysis, dementia, involuntary movements and cerebellar ataxia. These are relatively rare and some authors do not feel there is a distinct, separate chronic chagasic encephalopathy in non-immunocompromised patients. CT brain studies do not show focal lesions but cerebral atrophy, more marked than that expected for the age of the patients, is well documented and is not necessarily due to microemboli from the heart.[161,176]

Neuropathologically, in a study of 22 patients with the chronic chagasic encephalopathy, three patients showed multifocal encephalitis, involving some deep grey nuclei, and parasites were found in one case.[107] Neuronal depletion due to cellular destruction has been considered as the main pathogenetic mechanism to explain the chronic forms of the CNS involvement. However, it is also possible that neuronal loss and focal inflammatory changes may be due both to chronic hypoxia secondary to the cardiomyopathy accompanying chronic Chagas' disease and to microemboli from thrombi within chagasic hearts.[106]

The whole genome sequencing of the *T. cruzi* has been concluded.[61] Genomic and proteomic approaches will lead to the identification of crucial genes and proteins directly associated with the disease, and these advances will certainly bring about major developments in our understanding of *T. cruzi* biology.

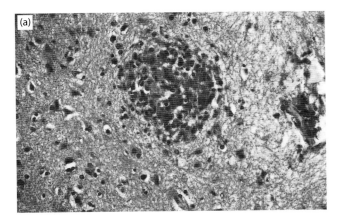

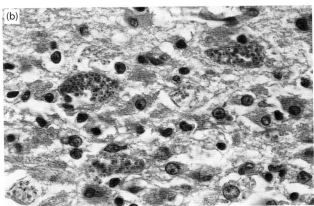

21.26 American trypanosomiasis. (a) Encephalitic microglial nodule without visible parasites. **(b)** Heavily parasitized cells containing many amastigote forms. The kinetoplast rod is visible in some of the parasites.

Immunodeficiency and Chagasic Encephalitis

With HIV-related immunodeficiency, chronically infected patients develop extensive necrotizing encephalitis and space-occupying, tumour-like lesions probably reflecting reactivation of dormant infection (Figure 21.27).[34,195] This is an acute necrohaemorrhagic encephalitis characterized pathologically by nodules of microglial reaction, with associated haemorrhage and necrosis, and numerous amastigote forms of the parasite within macrophages and astrocytes (Figure 21.28).[163] Fatal acute Chagas' encephalitis associated with HIV infection is also reported.[67] Cerebral mass lesions may mimic tumour or toxoplasmosis. Astrocytes are the main target of the parasites, and neurons are spared in spite of their proximity to both parasites and nodular reaction containing macrophages. The cellular immunodeficiency may allow free *T. cruzi* multiplication in tissues and liberation of the parasite into circulating blood, indicating the presence of parasites in chronic cases.

The outcome of HIV-*Trypanosoma cruzi* co-infection when it presents clinically is poor.[3]

Ocular myositis may accompany meningoencephalitis in reactivation of infection in HIV+ patients.[51] Heart transplant recipients who already have Chagas' disease are also at risk of reactivating a cerebral mass lesion.[43]

Peripheral Nervous System

Although lesions in the CNS in the absence of immunosuppression are not prominent, the peripheral nerve, particularly the autonomic nervous system, is frequently involved in the chronic phase. The conduction systems of the heart and autonomic plexi in the wall of the oesophagus and gut are particularly affected leading to dysfunction in peristalsis, which culminates in the development of mega-oesophagus and/or megacolon. The pathogenetic mechanisms responsible for the lesion in the cardiac autonomic nervous system are multiple, but all contribute to the final result: denervation of the organ and subsequent cardiomegaly, cardiomyopathy, arrhythmias and death.[6] Vagal dysfunction is thought to be an early, primary and specific abnormality of chronic Chagas' disease,[48] although the vagus nerve studied in autopsies of patients with chronic chagasic cardiomyopathy, did not show significant morphological abnormalities.[130]

The peripheral somatosensory neuropathies including involvement of dorsal root ganglia, anterior horn neurons and peripheral sensory and motor nerve fibres are less frequent than the autonomic neuropathy, but have been well documented, clinically and electrophysiologically in chronic cases, some of them supported by morphological reports in humans.[223,229] Both axonal and demyelinating, predominantly axonal neuropathy have been diagnosed, but most probably both types of lesions are combined. No clinical evidence of spinal motor neuron damage is found, although their involvement was suggested by the presence of some polyphasic enlarged amplitude motor unit potentials. It is likely that the number of motor neurons involved does not reach the levels needed to give overt clinical manifestations. Muscle biopsies show denervation atrophy.[215]

Peripheral neuropathies are postulated to result from several autoimmune mechanisms, including the loss of protective immunosuppression, which may be mediated

in part by specific CD8+ T-cells.[216] In addition, surface proteins on the parasite, such as flagellar proteins, induce

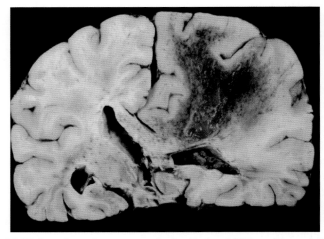

21.27 American trypanosomiasis. Brain of HIV-positive adult with necrotic haemorrhagic lesions in the occipital lobe and corpus callosum, following reactivation of infection.

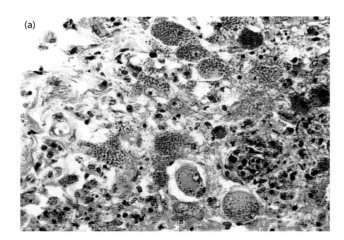

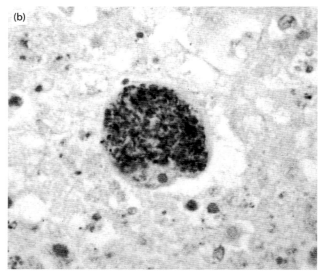

21.28 American trypanosomiasis. HIV-positive reactivation lesion. **(a)** Abundant parasites in cells. **(b)** Immunohistochemistry confirms the parasite species (anti-*T. cruzi*).

antibodies that cross-react with host epitopes, such as neurons and myelinated nerve sheaths, a process of molecular mimicry.[174] There is a high prevalence of antibodies reacting with nervous system antigens in the sera of patients and infected animals, suggesting that autoantibodies triggered as a consequence of *T. cruzi* infection are able to mediate, at least in part, the electrophysiological abnormalities observed in peripheral nerves during the course of Chagas' disease.[218] Delayed-type hypersensitivity may be induced by the presence of the parasites, because they were observed in the sciatic nerve of infected mice during the acute phase, but not in the chronic phase, whereas the permanence of *T. cruzi* antigens in the inflammatory infiltrate was detected with immunological methods and could be responsible for maintaining the immune reaction.

Chronic Chagas' Disease Pathogenesis

Chronic Chagas' neuropathy and carditis has been considered a paradigm of infection-induced autoimmune disease. This view is supported particularly because of the apparent discrepancy between the intensity of inflammatory reaction and scarce number of parasites in chronic chagasic myocarditis.[55,82] Antigen-specific and antigen-non-specific mechanisms have been described by which *T. cruzi* infection might activate T- and B-cells, leading to autoimmunity. Among the first mechanisms, molecular mimicry may be responsible for misdirecting immune responses originally elicited by parasite antigens toward cross-reactive host tissue antigens, in this way playing an accidental role in the pathogenesis of Chagas' disease.[79] However, with modern molecular methods, the parasite is increasingly detected in chronically infected hosts and may also be the cause of pathology either directly or through parasite-specific mediated inflammatory responses. A consensus is emerging that *T. cruzi* bears primary direct responsibility for producing chagasic pathology.[114]

Congenital Infection

Congenital cases of Chagas' disease are well recognized.[71] The trophoblast acts as a barrier to *T. cruzi*, although parasitization of trophoblastic cells can occur with associated necrosis and inflammation, which may allow breaks in the placental barrier and transplacental spread.[14] Placental involvement is not always accompanied by fetal infection, but there are cases of stillbirth or a mild meningoencephalitis with epithelioid and giant cells, and inflammation of the heart, skeletal muscle, oesophagus and intestine. The risk of infected mothers (chronic phase) transmitting the disease to their foetus during pregnancy is probably <1 per cent.[191]

Treatment

Chemotherapy for Chagas' disease is unsatisfactory. The two main drugs are nifurtimox and benznidazole,[131] but cure even in acute infection is only in about 70 per cent of cases.

Amoebiasis

There are four clinicopathologically distinct amoebic infections of the CNS:

1. Cerebral amoebiasis (*Entamoeba histolytica* infection)
2. Primary amoebic meningoencephalitis (*Naegleria fowleri* infection)
3. Granulomatous amoebic encephalitis (*Acanthamoeba* and *Balamuthia* spp. infections)
4. Encephalitis due to *Sappinia diploidea*

Acanthamoeba, *Balamuthia* and *Naegleria* spp. are free-living amoebae, and man is an accidental host.[131,147] *Entamoeba histolytica* is essentially a human colonic infection and spread to the brain is rare. *Sappinia* infection is even rarer (see later). The HIV pandemic has altered the epidemiology in that granulomatous amoebic encephalitis (but not the other three patterns of disease) is associated with this immunodeficiency syndrome and has thus become more commonly seen. In addition, *Acanthamoeba* spp. can cause corneal infection, termed *Acanthamoeba* keratitis.

Cerebral Amoebiasis

Entamoeba histolytica infection is a global disease that causes protocolitis with bloody dysentery and liver abscesses.[131] Transmission is by ingestion of cysts in infected faeces. Cerebral abscess is a fortunately rare occurrence. It enters the brain through haematogenous spread from liver.

Clinically, its onset is abrupt with a rapid progression to death within 72 hours if not treated. It starts as a focal neurological lesion with local meningitis, and may mimic bacterial meningitis. CT scans show an irregular lesion without a capsule or surrounding enhancement.

Most cases are diagnosed at autopsy, where it appears as a necrotic mass in the grey and white matter, up to 4 cm or larger. Histopathologically, the necrosis is featureless (but lacks polymorphs) and there are characteristic amoebic trophozoites by vessels, in the necrosis, and at the advancing edge of the lesion. The parasites are 10–60 µm in size, with granular eosinophilic cytoplasm and a round nucleus with a small central karyosome, and many have phagocytosed erythrocytes (Figure 21.29). The amoebae are intensely periodic acid–Schiff (PAS) positive, which helps distinguish them from macrophages.[137] Specific antisera can also be used to identify them by immunocytochemistry.

Pathogenetically, amoebiasis is necrotizing because the parasites:

- secrete lytic enzymes;
- secrete an ionophore (amoebapore) that, when contact is made causes a hole to be made in the host cell membrane, so the cell dies;
- actively phagocytose cellular dead host cells.[190]

If a diagnosis can be made in time and the cerebral lesion excised, followed by treatment with metronidazole, recovery is possible.[212] Patients with systemic amoebiasis are usually seropositive for specific antibodies to *E. histolytica*. Molecular diagnostics now includes PCR identification of this infection in CSF.[209]

Primary Amoebic Meningoencephalitis

The free living *Naegleria fowleri* is endemic globally in soil, fresh water and hot springs. Exposure is therefore probably

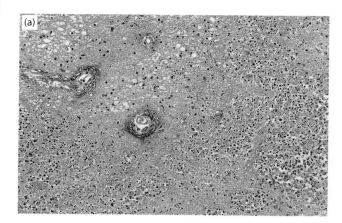

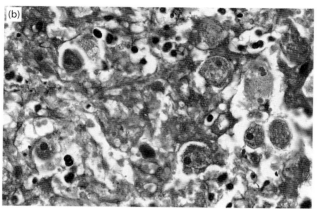

21.29 Cerebral amoebiasis. (a) White matter necrosis following spread of infection from an *E. histolytica* liver abscess. The parasites are centred on the vessels and there is peripheral mononuclear and neutrophil inflammation. **(b)** The amoebic trophozoites have a round purple nucleus and several contain phagocytosed red blood cells.

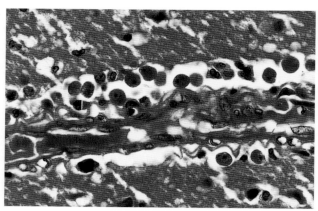

21.30 Primary amoebic encephalitis. Trophozoites of *Naegleria fowleri* infiltrating outside a vessel. They have pale vesicular nuclei and prominent nucleoli.

very common, but infection uncommon. The organism invades the nasal mucosa and enters the brain by travelling along the olfactory nerves.[131]

The incubation period is 1–14 days, followed by a rapidly progressive course that is usually fatal. There is meningitis, with headache, fever and vomiting. Seizures, coma and death follow. CT scans show diffuse contrast enhancement of grey matter and obliterated cisterns.

Grossly, there is a fulminant acute meningoencephalitis, with cerebral swelling.[147] Characteristically, there is haemorrhagic necrosis affecting the orbital surface of the frontal lobes (where the brain is first affected) and necrosis of the olfactory bulbs.[137] Histologically, the inflammatory reaction is polymorphonuclear, with variable mononuclear cell infiltrate; there are no granulomas. The trophozoites are small, up to 10 µm in diameter in fixed tissues. The cytoplasm is vacuolated and the nucleus contains a prominent nucleolus (Figure 21.30). This inflammation and infection can be seen extending along the Virchow–Robin spaces, associated with haemorrhagic necrosis of the brain grey and white matter, and some reactive astrocytosis if the patient has lived long enough. If the nasal mucosa is examined, there is inflammation of the epithelium extending through the cribriform plate.

The diagnosis is difficult to make in life. CSF examination shows a purulent inflammation without bacteria, and a high protein. A Gram stain destroys the parasites, so a wet mount with phase contrast illumination is required; in wet preparations, the parasites appear larger at 10–20 µm diameter.[136] More recently, PCR techniques have been used to diagnose the infection. Treatment is with amphotericin B, but the overall mortality is 95 per cent.

Granulomatous Amoebic Encephalitis

The free living amoebae that cause this pattern of disease, less fulminant than *Naegleria* infection but still with high mortality, are present all around the world in soil. *Acanthamoeba castellanii*, *A. polyphaga* and, particularly, *Balamuthia mandrillaris* (Figure 21.31) are increasingly recognized infections; they cause identical clinical disease and have similar morphology when seen in CNS pathological specimens. The differentiation is made by *in vivo* culture, specific immunocytochemistry and molecular diagnostic methods.[134,141]

The infection is acquired via the upper respiratory tract, the conjunctiva, or injury to the skin with environmental contamination.[152] An organ donor with an active skin infection has also transmitted *Balamuthia* to several recipients.[27] Immunocompetent people usually have limited disease, i.e. skin, ear, bone and eye. However, immunodeficient people may develop a fulminant CNS disease. The main risk factors are:

* HIV disease;
* lymphoma;
* malnutrition;
* cirrhosis;
* diabetes;
* solid organ transplant recipient.

The infection reaches the CNS via the bloodstream; this is usually from a skin lesion and not from conjunctival infection. It causes a vasculitis, local necrosis and a mixed inflammatory reaction. Clinically, the presenting features include headache, seizures, focal neurological signs and

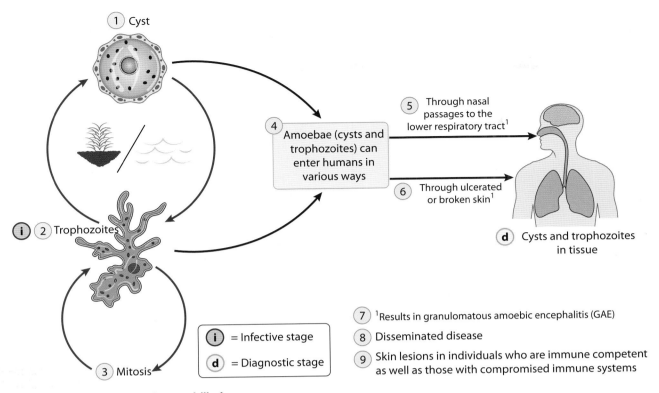

21.31 Life cycle of *Balamuthia mandrillaris*.

Figure courtesy of United States Centers for Disease Control and Prevention, Division of Parasitic Diseases.

meningism. It is important to note that the time from infection to developing CNS disease can be very prolonged, e.g. several months. Once CNS disease has developed, then the progression is more rapid with death between 1 week and 6 months later (average about a month).

CT imaging of the brain shows multifocal non-enhancing lucent lesions, and the differential diagnosis includes bacterial abscess, tuberculosis, toxoplasmosis and infarction.[200] Grossly, the lesions are haemorrhagic and necrotic (Figure 21.32).[147] All parts of the brain are equally affected and there is marked oedema and cerebral swelling.

Histopathologically, the lesions are often seen to be angiocentric, with the parasites clustered around vessels that are inflamed and showing fibrinoid necrosis.[103] In contrast to *Naegleria* infection, both trophozoites and cysts are observed. The trophozoites are 14–40 μm in size, and cysts slightly smaller (Figure 21.33). Trophozoites have a pale eosinophilic granular cytoplasm and a prominent nucleus. Cysts have a thicker cell wall; PAS stain highlights them. The surrounding brain tissue is necrotic and shows marked astrocytosis and microgliosis. The cell reaction is combined acute and chronic. True tuberculoid granulomas are not usually seen, but characteristically there are many foreign body and Langhans type giant cells in the inflamed areas.

Diagnosis in life is difficult because lumbar puncture is often contraindicated. CSF may show polymorphs and lymphocytes and a raised protein. A clue may be the presence of a chronic skin ulcer or nodule, and biopsy can provide

the diagnostic clue to the brain lesion.[225] The skin pathology is a mixed acute and granulomatous dermatitis and the trophozoites are rather scanty, but look the same as in the brain.[152] The specific diagnosis, in biopsy or autopsy specimens, should be confirmed by *in vivo* culture or by immunocytochemistry in a specialist centre. Drug treatment, if the disease is suspected, is empirical, and many agents have been used (including amphotericin B and fluconazole), usually with little positive effect. The mortality is >95 per cent even with treatment.[141]

The pathogenesis of granulomatous amoebic encephalitis is poorly understood, but includes active phagocytosis of host cells, induction of apoptosis,[208] and secretion of toxic enzymes.

Acanthamoeba Keratitis

This is a rare sight-threatening corneal keratitis that is particularly associated with the wearing of contact lenses and with infected corneal transplants.[131,210] Direct trauma to the cornea with soil containing cysts is another factor. It causes pain, conjunctivitis, photophobia, and corneal ulceration that is recurrent and relapsing.

The diagnosis is made by scraping the cornea and examining for cysts and trophozoites, or by corneal biopsy. Microscopically, there are sequential stages.[147,211] First, progressive inflammation, oedema, and loss of epithelium, with trophozoites and cysts; then convalescence, with stromal necrosis, hyperaemia, neovascularization, repair of the

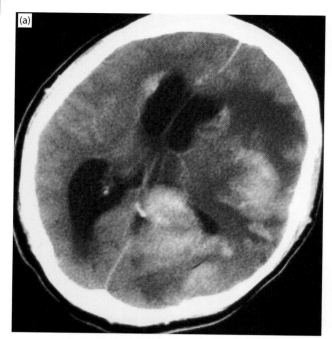

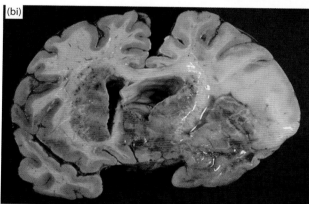

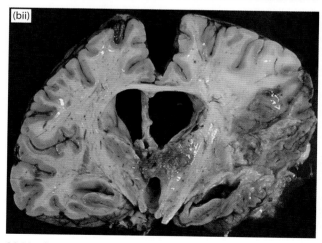

21.32 Granulomatous amoebic encephalitis. *Balamuthia mandrillaris* infection that spread to brain from a cutaneous traumatic lesion. **(a)** CT scan showing enhancing lesions, obstructive hydrocephalus and oedema. **(b)** Brain slice showing multiple necrotic lesions and associated oedema.

Courtesy of Dr I Bodi, King's College Hospital, London, UK.

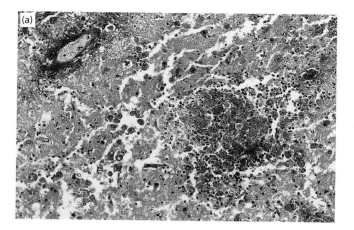

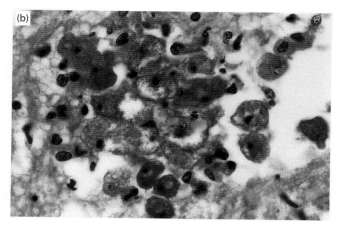

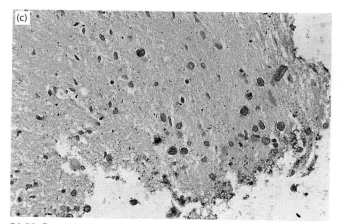

21.33 Granulomatous amoebic encephalitis. *Acanthamoeba castellani* infection in an HIV-positive person. **(a)** Fibrinoid necrosis of a vessel, acute and chronic inflammation of the neuropil and many trophozoites. **(b)** Trophozoites of *Acanthamoeba*. They have eosinophilic cytoplasm, pale vesicular nucleus and a prominent nucleolus. **(c)** Immunostain to confirm genus and species identity of *Acanthamoeba* infection (anti-*A. castellani*).

epithelial defect, and shrunken cysts; finally, in the scarring stage, resolving inflammation and shrunken cysts. PAS stain highlights the parasites (Figure 21.34). Early diagnosis is important to retain sight, and treatment includes debridement of necrotic areas and application of conazole antibiotic agents.

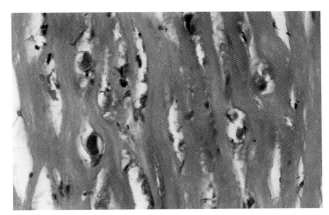

21.34 *Acanthamoeba* **keratitis.** Cysts and trophozoites in the corneal stroma. The cysts have a well-defined wall with retracted cytoplasm. There is little associated inflammation. Periodic acid–Schiff.

Encephalitis due to Sappinia diploidea

This is a rare amoebic encephalitis that causes necrotic haemorrhagic lesions in the brain.[146] The inflammation does not include eosinophils or granulomas. The distinctive features are (1) the nucleus of the large (40–70 μm) trophozoites, which have two nuclei attached to each other by connecting filaments as seen with electron microscopy and (2) erythrophagocytosis.[73]

Microsporidiosis

The phylum *Microsporidia* comprises a large group of obligate intracellular protozoa that are common parasites of invertebrates (insects) and non-human vertebrates (e.g. fish), with significant disease impact. Hence the associated diseases are well known to veterinary pathologists.[131] However, human infection is uncommon and only with increased prevalence of immunosuppression among transplant recipients and HIV infection have numbers of cases emerged.[147] Transmission to man is from the environment.

The most common risk group is those patients, children and adults, with advanced HIV disease, followed by renal transplant patients and leukaemic patients. Cerebral microsporidiosis is always part of disseminated disease, with virtually all organs infected including gut, kidney, liver, heart and cornea.[45]

Microsporidians are unique in their life cycle, by having an internal coiled tube through which sporoplasm is extruded when the tube is externalized to infect a host cell. They are small 1–3 μm obligate intracellular parasites that have a unique structure. The identification of species requires electron microscopy, although molecular diagnostics are increasingly used.[147] Within four families, there are 170 genera and >1300 species. Some affect mainly conjunctiva, producing a keratoconjunctivitis – in normal as well as immunocompromised hosts. Others can cause disseminated inflammatory and necrotic lesions in all organs, including the brain, and some affect mainly skeletal muscle. New species are being described. For brain

infection, the main species involved are *Encephalitozoon cuniculi* and *Trachipleistophora anthropophthera*. In the eye, *Enc. cuniculi*, *Enc. hellem* and *Enc. intestinalis* are recorded.[45]

Pathology

The CNS pathology is a diffuse, nodular encephalitis, sometimes with necrotic inflammatory foci, throughout the brain. Clinically and radiologically, it can mimic cerebral toxoplasmosis. Microscopically, astrocytes are parasitized (but not neurons) and there is localized microglial proliferation. The parasites are seen in clusters as haematoxyphilic nuclear dots within refractive clear cytoplasm. They are Brown–Hopps Gram-positive and variably PAS and Ziehl–Neelsen positive (Figure 21.35). Eye infection results in corneal ulceration. The parasites are seen in the epithelium (Figure 21.36).

Treatment is variably effective, albendazole usually being used.

Leishmaniasis

Although visceral leishmaniasis (*Leishmania donovani*) is a relatively common infection in all continents except Australasia, and spreads haematogenously in the body, CNS involvement virtually does not occur. Experimentally, *L. amazonensis* can cause encephalitis with parasites in the cerebral parenchyma,[1] but there is only one recorded case of CNS infection by *L. donovani* in man. A child with drug-refractory visceral leishmaniasis had meningitis associated with parasites in the CSF, and this was cured by treatment with amphotericin B, which crosses the blood–brain barrier.[187] Ocular infection rarely occurs in transplant recipients. The neurological manifestations of leishmaniasis have been recently reviewed.[173]

METAZOAL INFECTIONS

The major worm (helminth) infections that affect the nervous system of man are listed in Table 21.6. Traditionally, they are grouped into nematodes (roundworms) and flatworms, which comprise trematodes and cestodes. Biologically, there are three patterns of infection in man, which relate to the specificity of the human as host and how the worms mature and develop during infection.

A final notable variant of biological behaviour is where host immunosuppression induces hyperinfection and abnormal migration of the worm infection; the best described is the *Strongyloides* hyperinfection syndrome in people immunocompromised by chemotherapy or HTLV-1 infection.

There is a wide range of other, rarer worm infections that occasionally affect man, often in single case reports only. Many are animal infections and man is an accidental host. These are summarized at the end of each section. A comprehensively illustrated textbook of helminth infections is by Meyers *et al.*[146]

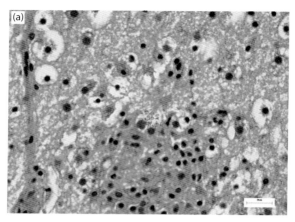

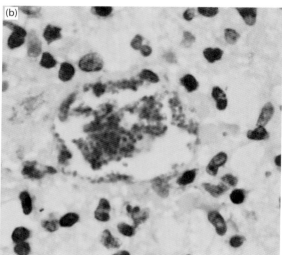

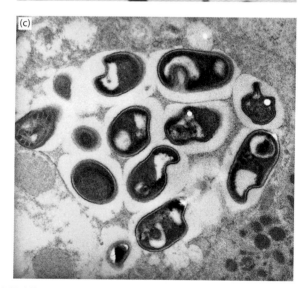

21.35 Microsporidiosis. A cerebral lesion. **(a)** Microglial nodule with the parasites as small haematoxyphilic dots. **(b)** A Gram stain demonstrates the Gram-positive spore walls of the microsporidia. **(c)** Transmission electron micrograph showing intracellular spores of *Enc. intestinalis*. In some, the cross-sections of the polar tube can be seen under the cell membrane.

(a) and (b) courtesy of Dr S Smith, University of Edinburgh, Edinburgh, UK.

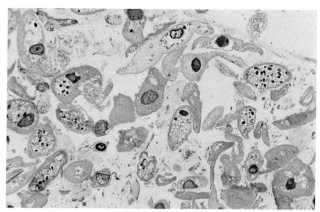

21.36 Microsporidiosis. Corneal scraping showing numerous parasites (*Enc. intestinalis*) within epithelial cells. In some, the nucleus is clearly seen within the cytoplasm. (semi-thin section, toluidine blue).

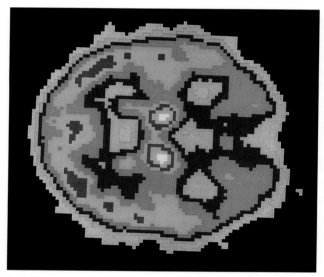

21.37 Single photon-emission computed tomography (SPECT) showing basal ganglia lesions in a human immunodeficiency virus (HIV)-positive patient. It is impossible to differentiate between, for example, toxoplasmosis and lymphoma: autopsy proved the lesions to be B-cell lymphoma.

TABLE 21.6 Major worm (helminth) infections that affect the nervous system of humans

1.	Infection by a larval form that develops into the adult, and this produces eggs or other forms of immature worm that can be transmitted to the environment (sometimes via a vector) and so complete the infection cycle. Man is the definitive host.
2.	Zoonotic (animal) disease and man gets infected accidentally, although the migration and development pattern of the parasites is comparable to that in animals. Man is the intermediate host.
3.	An animal helminth infection accidentally infects man and cannot mature or develop (paratenic) – these result in aberrant migration, prominent eosinophilia and are sometimes termed the 'visceral larva migrans syndromes'.

NEMATODE INFECTIONS

Nematodes are 'roundworms' and include a large variety of intestinal worms and filarial worms whose adults and/or larvae may uncommonly invade into the CNS.

Toxocariasis

Toxocara canis is a zoonotic worm infection, the definitive host being dogs. The syndrome of infection and larval migration in man, with CNS involvement, has only been recognized since 1951.[131] It is distributed worldwide and is a common cause of the visceral larva migrans (VLM) syndrome.

The adult worms reside in the dog intestine and release eggs in the faeces. These are accidentally ingested, usually by children, and hatch into larvae in the gut. Following penetration into the portal venous system, the larvae migrate to the liver, causing a granulomatous hepatitis, or pass into the lungs and thence to any organ, including the CNS.[128] In man, toxocariasis is a paratenic infection, i.e. the larvae do not mature and adult worms do not develop.

Epidemiology

Although VLM is typically a disease of children, CNS involvement is also seen in adults. This is not common, with only 20 neurotoxocariasis cases published between 1956 and 2004. In one highly endemic zone in Brazil, where 30 per cent of children admitted to hospital have antibodies to *T. canis*, 0.7 per cent of autopsied brains had subclinical brain lesions due to larva migrans.[151]

Clinical Features

Clinically, the initial infection may be accompanied by fever, cough and malaise; abdominal pain, hepatomegaly and pneumonitis with wheezing also occur. Eosinophilia is characteristic. The neurological features are heterogeneous: headache, mental confusion, Jacksonian or generalized seizures, meningoencephalitis, ataxia, paresis, ADEM-like syndrome, and diabetes insipidus result from cerebral invasion.[138] The association of *Toxocara* VLM with epilepsy in childhood is still debated.[8]

Imaging with MR scans may show focal irregular hyperintense lesion[104] or abscesses.[149] Eye infection is often the sole manifestation, with chorioretinitis and an inflammatory mass lesion within the eye that is a differential diagnosis with retinoblastoma.

Pathology

Pathologically, the lesions are giant cell and epithelioid cell granulomas around fragments of disintegrating larva, which are small, $400 \times 25 \mu m$ (Figure 21.38). There is eosinophilia and surrounding fibroplasia. Vasculitis is also recorded. The lesions are in any part of the CNS, involving the leptomeninges, cerebrum and subtentorial brain and spinal cord.[131,146]

The essential pathogenesis is an allergic reaction to the larva with formation of inflammatory tracks as it enters tissues, blood eosinophilia and a granulomatous reaction about the larva as it dies.

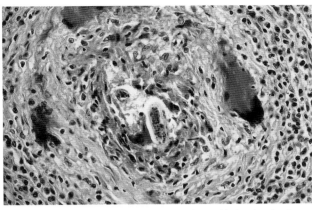

21.38 Visceral larva migrans. Disseminated infection by larvae of *Toxocara canis*. The larvae have a thick pale cuticle and have induced a giant cell granulomatous reaction in the neuropil.

The diagnosis is supported by positive serology in an appropriate clinical setting, and eosinophilia in the blood and CSF; most cases are diagnosed without CNS histopathology. Antihelminthic treatment is with albendazole, usually plus steroid anti-inflammatory cover.

Ocular Toxocariasis

Children present with reduced vision, strabismus, uveitis or leukocoria.[131] The larvae migrate into the retina and vitreous humour.[146] As they die, they excite a florid eosinophilic inflammatory response. Granulomas and fibrosis may be seen, but larvae are not always identified in the specimens.

Other Neurological and Ocular Larva Migrans Syndromes

The differential diagnosis of toxocariasis includes strongyloidiasis, angiostrongyliais, and other, rarer, visceral larva migrans syndromes, such as caused by *Ascaris lumbricoides*, other *Toxocara* species, *Halicephalobus*[165] and *Baylisacaris*[98] infections[41] (see Other Rare Nematode Infections, later in chapter).

Strongyloidiasis

Strongyloides stercoralis is an intestinal infection with man as the definitive host. It distributed widely in the tropics and subtropics, but not in northwestern Europe. Adult female worms in the small bowel mucosa lay eggs that rapidly transform into larvae. These are excreted and develop further in the soil, so that infection to another person is via penetration of bare skin. *Strongyloides* in virtually unique in that it also has an autoinfection cycle: larvae in the bowel reinvade the host, perpetuating the infection for decades after initial exposure.[131]

This autoinfection cycle is important because it underlies the potential for severe systemic infection and subsequent CNS lesions. Immunosuppression permits the autoinfection cycle to accelerate and produce rapidly overwhelming infection (hyperinfection syndrome) that disseminates to all organs. The main causes of this include HTLV-1 infection, old age and steroid therapy; HIV is a less common association.[131] However, occasional cases of

CNS strongyloidiasis are recorded in non-immunocompromised people.[118]

Hyperinfection causes eosinophilia and often Gram-negative septicaemia, with meningitis (the bacteria are thought to travel, from the host intestine, within the larval gut). Even with treatment, this syndrome has a fatality rate of about 75 per cent.

Clinically, the most common CNS manifestation is purulent meningitis. There may also be focal neurological syndromes from small vessel obstruction. Pathologically, the purulent meningitis may also manifest with filariform larvae of *S. strongyloides* in the meninges. The larvae also obstruct small vessels and cause microinfarction with local inflammation (Figure 21.39). A granulomatous reaction may occur, and sometimes small cerebral abscesses – *E. coli* being the most common associated bacterium.[146] Usually, clinical CNS involvement is part of the generalized systemic infection, but may be the presenting feature.

Eosinophilic Meningoencephalitis

The term usually refers to aberrant infection with the rat lungworm, *Angiostrongylus cantonensis*. However, there are other worm infections,[83] as well as other

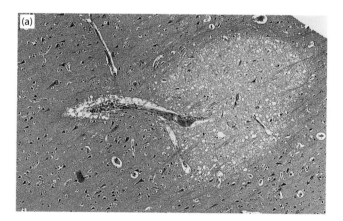

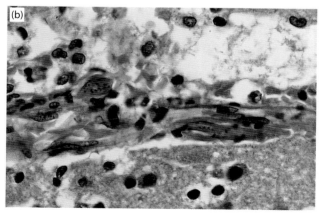

21.39 Strongyloidiasis. Disseminated *Strongyloides stercoralis* infection in an HIV-positive patient. **(a)** Cerebral cortical microinfarct associated with obstruction of an arteriole. **(b)** Two filariform larva of *S. stercoralis* associated with thrombotic microangiopathy. The larvae are seen in longitudinal and tangential section, with small nuclei within the parasite.

pathologies, that result in similar clinicopathological syndromes (Table 21.7). The diagnosis of this group of infections is unsatisfactory because, beyond clinical suspicion, confirmation can only be made by tissue biopsy (unusual), positive antibody or antigen tests on blood and CSF (which are not widely available or standardized), or at autopsy. Treatment of these syndromes is often empirical.

Angiostrongyliasis

The definitive host of *Angiostrongylus cantonensis* is the rat where the worm adults reside in the lung. Eggs are excreted in the faeces; these are taken up by molluscs (snails), prawns and crabs. Upon ingestion of these intermediate hosts (by rat or, accidentally, man) the larvae migrate to lung, then brain for maturation, and back to the lung. In man, the migration stops at the brain, causing local inflammatory syndromes. The infection is widespread in the South Pacific, South East Asia, and has been recognized in the Caribbean area, southern United States and Egypt.[131,221]

Clinical manifestations are usually mild. The incubation period is 1–6 days after exposure, followed by headache, stiff neck, nausea and vomiting. Neurological impairment ranges from nothing, to paraesthesiae, cranial nerve palsy (4th and 6th particularly), radiculitis and weakness (simulating Guillain–Barré syndrome), and focal neurological signs. Coma and death are uncommon. Affected patients are not as ill as those with bacterial meningitis. Examination of the CSF shows an eosinophil leukocytosis (up to 3000 per

TABLE 21.7 Causes of eosinophilic meningitis and encephalitis	
Parasites	*Angistrongylus cantonensis*
	Gnathostoma spp.
	Paragonimus spp.
	Strongyloides stercoralis
	Toxocara canis
	Loa loa
	Schistosoma spp.
	Fasciola hepatica
	Trichinella spiralis
	Baylisascaris spp.
	Halicephalobus spp.
	Sparganosis
	Cysticercosis
Fungi	*Coccidioides immitis, Aspergillus* spp.
Tumours	Lymphoma, glioblastoma, carcinomatosis
Drug	Post-myelography, antibiotics
	Ventriculoperitoneal shunt
Other	Vasculitis, primary eosinophilic meningitis

After Wang *et al.*[221]

mm³) and occasionally a larva. Imaging with MR shows meningeal enhancement and subcortical lesions in heavy infections; hyperintense basal ganglia abnormalities are also noted. The eye may also be infected.[221]

Pathologically, the lesions include specific and non-specific phenomena. Grossly, the brain in fatal cases may be oedematous or normal externally; haemorrhagic is uncommon. Microscopically, larvae (often degenerate) may be seen with a granulomatous surround and eosinophilia; in an appropriate plane of section, tracks made by migrating larvae comprise eosinophilic necrosis surrounded by degenerate axons and myelin, and macrophages (Figure 21.40). The larvae are 120 μm width by up to 12 mm long. Non-specific features are an eosinophilic meningitis, with Charcot–Leyden crystals (from eosinophil proteins) and plasma cells.[146] Sometimes, there is endarteritis obliterans or vascular necrosis, with secondary occlusion and local infarction. In the eye, there is retinitis and vitritis.

Specific antihelminth infection is controversial and not usually recommended because premature death of the larvae releases more antigens, generates larger inflammatory lesions, and so worsens the clinical disease. Steroid therapy can reduce the inflammation. Recovery is usual within 2 months.

Gnathostomiasis

Gnathostomiasis is a visceral larva migrans syndrome whereby a helminth that cannot mature in man wanders around until it dies. Usually this occurs in the subcutaneous tissues, any organ can be involved and the brain is occasionally so parasitized. There are various species within the *Gnathostoma* genus, the most common being *G. spinigerum*. Most infections are described from South East Asia, but Mexico, Spain and Japan have also reported infections.[131]

The adult worm resides in the stomach of many types of mammals. Eggs in the faeces are taken up by *Cyclops* copepods, which in turn are consumed by fishes, amphibians and reptiles; and the maturing larvae in these intermediate hosts are eaten by a definitive host and make their way to the stomach wall. In man, the larvae may go to

the brain and cause an eosinophilic meningoencephalitis; it is less common than the similar syndrome caused by *Angiostrongylus*.

Clinically, there is meningitis and, because the larva is more invasive than *Angiostronglyus*, more frequently focal neurological signs. Cranial nerve palsies, characteristically painful radiculitis, paraplegia and quadriplegia–from tumour-like lesions in the cord–can occur. The eye is also a site of infection. Subarachnoid haemorrhage, subdural, and superficial cerebral haemorrhage are typical. Histologically, there is haemorrhagic necrosis in the cerebral hemispheres and spinal cord with oedema and reactive astrocytosis. Eosinophils are common. The parasitic larvae (third stage) are usually difficult to identify in biopsy material (they wander and cause lesions much greater than their physical volume), and are quite large at 2 mm in length. Their cross-section appearance is characteristic with the cuticle covered in short spines (Figure 21.41).[146]

Diagnosis is suspected on clinical, imaging and epidemiological criteria, supported by blood and or xanthochromia in the CSF and eosinophilia. Specific antibodies can be identified in specialist centres to prove the diagnosis. Occasionally, biopsy may make the diagnosis, or the infection is identified at autopsy. Compared with angiostrongyliasis, CNS gnathostomiasis involves the cord more often and causes more haemorrhage.[111] Like the parasite in sparganosis, it migrates in the neuroaxis.

Trichinosis
Epidemiology and Life Cycle

Of the many *Trichinella* species, *T. spiralis* is the most common to affect man. They are globally distributed,[131] and the normal hosts are carnivores, such as foxes and pigs. The adult worm lives in the gut of carnivores and produces first-stage larvae that enter the portal system and disseminate around the body (including the brain), and then invade skeletal muscle cells. There they encyst and can survive for years. The muscle is eaten by another host, and the larvae migrate to the intestine to repeat the cycle. Man is infected usually by eating undercooked pork or horse meat, and there may be outbreaks.

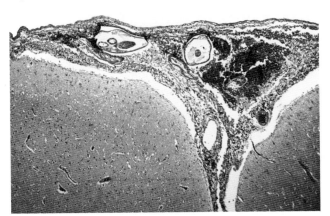

21.40 Eosinophilic meningoencephalitis caused by *Angiostrongylus*. The parasite is in the meninges, eliciting an eosinophilic reaction.

Courtesy of AIFP, Washington, DC, USA.

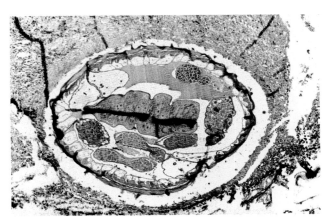

21.41 Gnathostomiasis. Cross-section of a *Gnathostoma* larva in brain. The spines are evident on the cuticle.

Courtesy of AIFP, Washington, DC, USA.

Clinical Features

The main symptoms and signs of disseminated infection are fever, myalgia, weakness and malaise, periorbital oedema and headache. Death is very uncommon and is usually from myocarditis, encephalitis or pneumonia.[131] In severe infections, a larval meningoencephalitis can occur during the early infection stage, but this probably occurs in <1 per cent of infections.[5,58] Symptoms include dizziness and seizures. CSF and blood examination shows eosinophilia, and there may be CSF xanthochromia.

Pathology

The muscle infection is pathologically characteristic. One of more first-stage larvae, which encyst only in skeletal muscle, are coiled within the myofibre. The larva is 1 mm–40 μm. The sarcomeres disappear and the myofibre becomes amorphous. Around this 'nurse cell', there are oedema and acute and chronic inflammation (Figure 21.42).

In the rarely seen brain infection, there is microglial nodular encephalitis with small larvae or fragments visible.[146]

The diagnosis of trichinosis is usually on clinical grounds and confirmed by serology and muscle biopsy. Treatment is not satisfactory, but mebendazole is used with steroid cover to reduce inflammation.[131]

Filarial Infections (Filariasis)

The major filariases of man are onchocerciasis, lymphatic filariasis, loiasis, dirofilariasis and mansonelliasis.[131] The brain and cord are not infected by the adult worms. The only significant neurological problems are infections of the eye, in the case of *Onchocerca volvulus* and *Loa loa*, and rare encephalopathies that may occur with the chemotherapy of both infections.

Onchocerciasis

Onchocerca volvulus is the cause of 'river blindness', and is endemic in west and central Africa, and in Central America. It is transmitted by simuliid blackflies, and the adult worms form fibrotic inflammatory nodules in the subcutis. Vast numbers of microfilariae (larvae) are released and migrate locally, causing inflammation and fibrosis as they die.

The eye is involved if there are nodules about the neck and head. The microfilariae migrate into the conjunctiva, cornea and anterior chamber of the eye. Chronic infection results in sclerosing keratitis, and iridocyclitis with posterior synechiae and glaucoma. The degree of damage is highly variable across individual patients, reflecting the fact that the reaction against the microfilariae is immunopathological: some patients are more allergic than others and suffer proportionately more eye damage. Slit lamp examination shows the microfilariae in the anterior chamber and on the surface of the lens.

Histological examination of affected eyes is not commonly performed, but the microfilariae are seen, alive and dead, in all parts and layers of the eye.[146] The inflammatory reaction is eosinophilic and fibrosing; with progressive inflammation, there is disorganization and degeneration of the eye. The microfilariae are 350 × 6 μm and have identifiable morphological characteristics for specialist laboratories (Figure 21.43).

Rarely, microfilariae have been identified in the CSF, and there is a case report of a transient encephalopathy following treatment of onchocerciasis with diethylcarbamazine (DEC).[53] Epidemiologically, there is a possible association between onchocerciasis and epilepsy.[52] A clinicopathological mechanism is, at present, obscure.

Loiasis

Loa loa is endemic in West and Central Africa.[131] It is transmitted by *Chrysops* flies and the adult worms migrate through the subcutaneous tissues. The microfilariae circulate in the blood. The adults may wander across the conjunctiva and cornea of the eye, but do not seem to cause significant permanent eye damage. Occasional observations of subcorneal fibrosis around a worm are made.

One standard therapy for loiasis is DEC. This can cause adverse reactions because of the death of microfilariae in the blood, and an ensuing immunopathological reaction. Clinically, it is an encephalopathy commencing soon after treatment with DEC, mainly in those patients with high

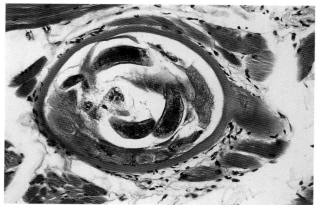

21.42 Trichinosis. Larvae of *Trichinella spiralis* within an expanded skeletal myofibre–'nurse cell'. There is mild chronic inflammation in the endomysium.

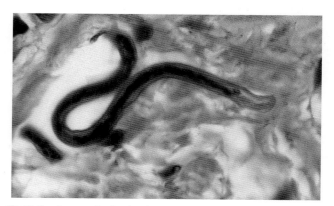

21.43 Onchocerciasis. A microfilaria of *Onchocerca volvulus* in the cornea. The nuclei are arranged in narrow lines along its length, and the pale sheath at the end is characteristic.

microfilaraemias. The same syndrome occurs with ivermectin therapy.[17] Pathologically, there are mild oedema and petechial haemorrhages in the brain. Histologically, in the small blood vessels are thrombi enmeshing the microfilariae and filling the vessels (Figure 21.44).[146] The brain shows secondary perivascular petechial haemorrhage, microglial reaction and astrocytosis.

Other Rare Filarial Infections of the CNS

Meningonema Spp.

This is a parasite of the subarachnoid spaces in the CNS of monkeys in Africa. There is a case record of asymptomatic infection with the parasite seen in CSF.[16]

Mansonella perstans

This filarial worm resides in the serous cavities of man in Africa and South America.[131] Microfilariae are sometimes found in the CSF, but association with any particular clinical syndrome is not proven. Infection of the eye with visual impairment is documented.[18]

Wuchereria bancrofti

Lymphatic filariasis caused by *Wuchereria* is highly prevalent across the tropics.[131] Microfilariae travel in the blood and occasionally can cause intraocular disease. There is abnormal vision and the microfilariae can be seen in the anterior chamber (Figure 21.45), as well as evidence of chorioretinitis.[139]

Other Rare Nematode Infections

These two disseminating larval infections, described later, have tropism to the brain and eye. In the brain, they cause meningoencephalitis with or without eosinophilia, much necrosis and haemorrhage. Nearly all cases are fatal, usually diagnosed at autopsy.

Halicephalobus (Ex-Micronema) Spp.

This is a group of free-living nematodes, like *Strongyloides stercoralis*. All recorded human infections are fatal and involve the brain. Uniquely, the infecting worms, which are transmitted through skin trauma or solid organ transplantation (personal observation), can reproduce parthenogenetically in human tissues, so building up a colossal infection load (Figure 21.46a,b).[165]

Baylisascaris

There are several *Baylisascaris* spp. that infect the intestine lumen of raccoons and bears in North America. There is an intermediate host stage involving smaller mammals. Human infection is accidental from eating eggs, and the larvae mature and migrate as they would in the normal intermediate host (i.e. it is not a paratenic infection).[146] The larvae are often encapsulated within fibrous tissue.[70,98]

In some cases, it may be possible to definitively identify these infections histomorphologically;[146] parasite culture and, increasingly, molecular diagnostics are helpful.

Trematode Infections

Trematode flukes include the two common genera of *Paragonimus* and *Schistosoma*. Like other trematode infections, they have complex life cycles involving snails and sometimes other intermediate hosts in water; man is the definitive host for these two most common trematode infections that affect the brain.[131,146]

Schistosomiasis

There are five species of *Schistosoma* that affect man; *S. mansoni*, *S. haematobium* and *S. japonicum* cause well-documented CNS disease in brain or spinal cord.[155] The most common species affecting the brain is *S. japonicum*, whereas *S. haematobium* and *S. mansoni* are the usual causes of spinal cord lesions.[65] *S. mekongi* is a rare documented agent in cerebral disease,[96] and there are no reports of *S. intercalatum* affecting the CNS.

Epidemiology

Schistosomiasis is endemic in 74 resource-poor countries in the world, affecting more than 230 million people. *S. mansoni* is prevalent throughout Africa and eastern Latin America; *S. haematobium* is prevalent in Africa and the Middle East; *S. japonicum* is restricted to the Pacific

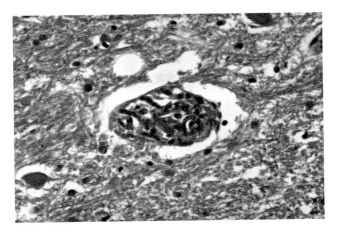

21.44 Loiasis. Tangle of *Loa* microfilariae in a cerebral vessels with thrombosis.

Courtesy of AIFP, Washington, DC, USA.

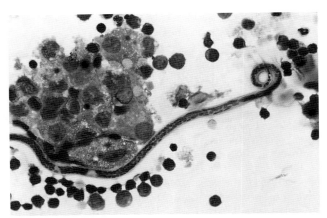

21.45 *Wuchereria bancrofti* microfilaria (unsheathed). Giemsa.

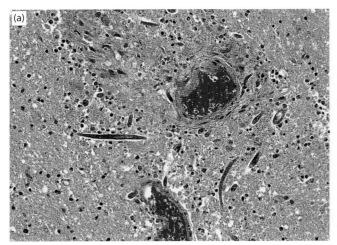 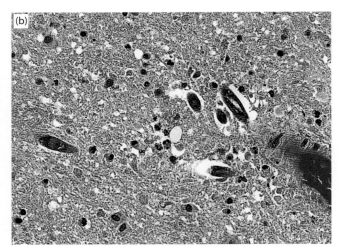

21.46 *Halicephalobus* **in the brain of renal transplant patient.** There is a mixture of larvae and adults, proliferating and causing a necrotizing encephalitis. The adults are up to 460 μm long, and in cross-section the gut lumen is visible.

region, distributed in China, Thailand, Indonesia and the Philippines. *S. mekongi* is found in Laos and Cambodia. Infection is most common among the rural poor who lack modern sanitation and water supply, and are therefore exposed to infected water. In some areas, e.g. southern Malawi, infection rates with *S. haematobium* can exceed 50 per cent of the population.

Life Cycle and Transmission

The paired adult worms (measuring 1 cm × 0.5 mm) reside in deep veins of the human host, but elicit no reaction as they coat themselves with ABO antigens. Eggs are secreted daily from the female worms into the small veins and attempt to pass out into the environment via urine or faeces; about half of all eggs are retained in the body and so cause disease (Figure 21.47). *S. mansoni* and *S. haematobium* females produce 300 eggs per day; *S. japonicum* about 3000 eggs per day. Once in water, the eggs hatch into miracidia and penetrate aquatic snails. Further multiplication within the snails results in vast numbers of cercariae released into water. These attach to human skin and rapidly penetrate into the dermis, enter dermal veins, lose the tail to become schistosomulae, access the lungs and mature. The skin penetration may cause a local inflammatory reaction and 'swimmers' itch'. Within the lung system, maturation to adults takes about 6 weeks, and thence the adults seek their definitive vascular location, by haematogenous passage. Then egg laying commences.[131]

Pathogenesis

At the time of the start of egg laying, 4 weeks post-infection, some people are very allergic to the new egg antigens and develop a systemic transient syndrome of acute toxic schistosomiasis (Katayama fever) with eosinophilia, fever, cough, diarrhoea and hepatosplenomegaly.[131] The CNS syndrome at this stage is described later.

The disease depends on the species of *Schistosoma* and the location of the worms. Most *S. mansoni* and *S. japonicum* adult worms reside in the venous plexuses of large and small bowel, so releasing eggs into the portal venous system. Most *S. haematobium* adults reside in pelvic veins

around the bladder. Focal disease results when a large number of eggs are deposited in one site by worms that do not move about locally.

Worms can migrate to ectopic (i.e. unusual) sites, including the CNS vasculature. Occasionally, adult schistosome worms are found in the spinal cord arteries and veins or in the choroid plexus. In addition to ectopic initial vascular migration, worms may gain access to CNS vessels through the arteriovenous shunts in the lungs, the porto-pulmonary connections via the azygos veins,[22] and retrogradely through the valveless epidural venous plexus of Batson.[10]

The essential lesion of schistosomiasis arises from an immune reaction to secreted egg antigens. The eggs are viable for only 3–4 weeks after being laid, and then die and degenerate, with the central miracidium often scooped out by invading macrophages. The egg shell persists, often for years. The immune response is initially a Gell and Coombs type 3 immune complex phenomenon, followed by a type 4 cell-mediated granulomatous process. Acute toxic schistosomiasis and encephalitis (see later) may involve acute cellular reactions to new eggs, but it is also likely that a systemic vasculopathy with eosinophil-mediated vasculitis and small vessel thrombosis is important.

Clinical Disease

Three neurological syndromes are described.[65]

1. Acute schistosomal encephalopathy (ASE). Occurring shortly after infection (usually first infection), it comprises headache, focal weakness, visual disturbances and a variable dementia, but without meningism. Imaging shows multifocal small contrast enhancing lesions throughout the brain.
2. Pseudotumoural encephalic schistosomiasis (PES). These comprise usually single tumour-like lesions in the brain, including the cerebellum.[66,181] The eggs laid locally induce a florid inflammatory reaction, often with much local necrosis, that is a space-occupying lesion. Cerebral and cerebellar foci present as focal neurological defects. Seizures, visual disturbances and ataxia may also be presenting signs.

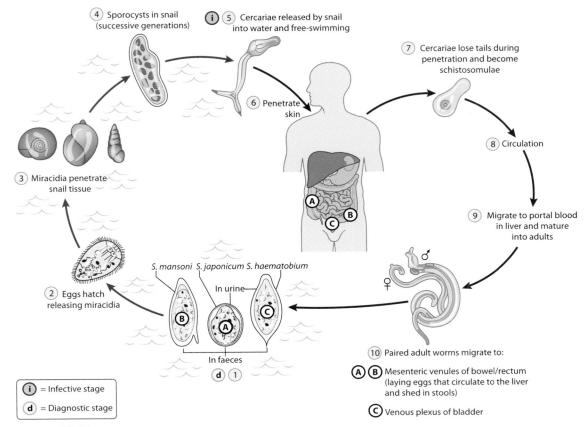

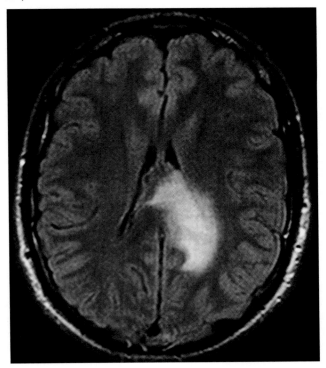

21.47 Life cycle of *Schistosoma* spp.

Figure courtesy of United States Centers for Disease Control and Prevention, Division of Parasitic Diseases.

3. Spinal cord schistosomiasis (SCS). This is less common than PES, and is mostly due to *S. mansoni*. Within the spinal canal, infection may be mainly in the cord *per se*, myeloradicular with nerve root involvement, or conus-cauda equina. There is spinal cord compression and sometimes transverse myelitis.[44,201] Clinically, SCS presents as acute or subacute back and limb pain, and sphincter disturbances and sometimes paraplegia.[57] A minority of patients have a local subarachnoid haemorrhage from vasculitis.

CT MR imaging may be characteristic and suggest the diagnosis. In cord lesions, there is expansion of the cord and intramedullary nodular enhancement, and linear radicular enhancement.[199] In the brain, there are irregular ring-enhancing lesions and surrounding oedema (Figure 21.48).[131]

Patients with these CNS lesions are usually, but not necessarily, those chronically infected with established disease in liver, gut or bladder; visitors from non-endemic areas can acquire schistosomiasis for the first time and present as acute neuroschistosomiasis with a CNS focus.

Pathology

There are no pathological descriptions of the transient acute schistosomal encephalitis. In PES and SCS, the gross appearances of clinically significant lesions are

21.48 Schistosomiasis. Magnetic resonance image of enhancing cerebral lesions affecting grey and white matter.

Courtesy of Dr A Dean, Addenbrooke's Hospital, Cambridge, UK.

non-specific, appearing only necrotic, and sometimes haemorrhagic. Histologically, the schistosome lesion evolves through three stages, and all may be seen in a chronic lesion.[146] Acutely, live eggs are surrounded by eosinophils (intact and degranulating), oedema and variable necrosis. Immunocytochemistry reveals immune complexes with IgM. Peripherally there is lymphoplasmacytic infiltration, gliosis and astrocytosis.[178] After the acute phase, when the egg has died, epithelioid and giant cell granulomas form around the egg shells, frequently with central coagulative necrosis in the centre (Figure 21.49). Finally, this declines, leaving necrosis and peripheral fibrosis. In very chronic lesions, the inflammation effectively subsides, leaving an egg shell and surrounding fibrillary astrocytosis only.[180] Cytological smears (Figure 21.50) show eosinophilic necrosis, epithelioid cells, eosinophils and worm eggs – sometimes with diagnostic specific morphology.

The schistosome egg shells are characteristically brown in colour. The internal nuclear detail and nuclear corona of the miracidium are only appreciated in live eggs. The species of *Schistosoma* may be assessed by the shape and size of the egg shell: *S. haematobium* are about $150 \times 55\,\mu m$ with a terminal spine; *S. mansoni* are similar in size but with a lateral tangential spine; *S. japonicum* has no really visible spine and is the smallest ($80 \times 60\,\mu m$).[146] Ziehl–Neelsen stain is helpful, because the egg morphology is often distorted by disintegration and the trauma of microtomy: *S. mansoni* and *S. japonicum* shells retain carbol fuchsin, whereas those of *S. haematobium* do not (Figure 21.51). Occasionally, an adult worm or pair may be seen in a blood vessel in the tissue sample.

Because schistosomiasis is an intravascular infection, vasculitis is often seen as an involvement of the vessel wall in the inflammatory reaction to the egg. There may be erosion of the wall and disruption of the elastic lamina; mycotic aneurysm and rupture of small vessels is well recognized, with secondary subarachnoid, cerebral and cerebellar haemorrhage.[184]

In patients with advanced hepatosplenic schistosomiasis, eggs are carried in the bloodstream to all parts of the body including the brain. Scattered microscopic egg granulomas with local vascular dilatation may be seen at autopsy, which had little or no clinical significance prior to death.[177]

Diagnosis

ASE is diagnosed clinically and radiologically, with serological or parasitological evidence of acute schistosomiasis. Many PES and SCS lesions are diagnosed on biopsy (histology and/or cytology), which requires invasive and potentially destructive neurosurgery. Schistosome infection induces a long-lived antibody response, detectable in blood and CSF.[131] Imaging reveals an inflammatory space-occupying lesion, and in the context of appropriate geographical history with positive serology and, perhaps, egg excretion identified in urine of faeces, a diagnosis of CNS schistosomiasis can sometimes be made without biopsy.[155] Molecular diagnostics, as with all infections, is increasingly applied, and the schistosoma species can be confirmed by PCR analysis.[101]

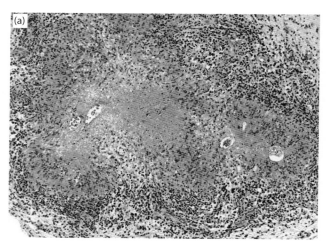

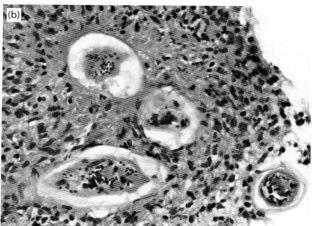

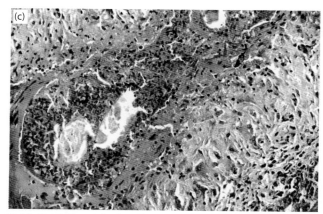

21.49 Schistosomiasis. Same patient as in Figure 21.48. **(a)** Brain biopsy showing necrotic granuloma with disintegrating schistosoma eggs. **(b)** The eggs contain nuclei but the shells are not well preserved. **(c)** A spinal cord lesion that caused paraplegia. The dead (anuclear) eggs of *S. haematobium* elicit a necrotizing, eosinophilic and granulomatous reaction.

Treatment

The standard chemotherapy for schistosomiasis is praziquantel,[131] with steroid cover to dampen the inflammation and reduce the space-occupying lesion.[69,183] Surgical decompression will also have played a role in most cases for diagnosis.

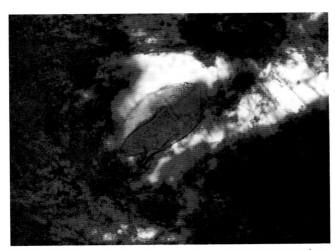

21.50 Schistosomiasis. Perioperative cytology smear from CNS schistosomiasis. The inferior lateral spine indicates this is *S. mansoni*.

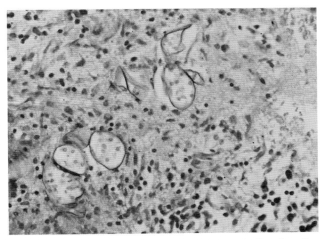

21.51 The egg shells retain carbol fuchsin, indicating they are S. mansoni. Ziehl–Neelsen.

Paragonimiasis

There are several species of the lung fluke *Paragonimus* endemic in South and Central America, Central and West Africa, South East Asia, the Philippines and India. The most common is *P. westermani*. The usual clinical pathology is chest infection that simulates pulmonary tuberculosis.[131]

The life cycle involves crayfish and crabs as intermediate hosts and infection is acquired by eating these. The larvae exit the gut into the peritoneal cavity, cross the diaphragm and enter the lung, where they settle in a fibrous-walled cavity. Excreted eggs pass into the airways and are coughed up. Adults live for several years in the lung, and measure up to 13×6mm in size. CNS infection occurs if the larvae migrate aberrantly and end up in ectopic sites in the brain or spinal cord; this could be from direct invasion of the foramina at the base of the brain or via the bloodstream. Favouring the former is the most common location of the worms in the posterior part of the brain.

The frequency of clinical CNS disease in those with pulmonary paragonimiasis is probably <1 per cent.[36] In the CNS, the adults excrete eggs that cannot escape, so enhancing the inflammatory reaction to the infection. The clinical manifestations are headache, meningitis, focal neurological signs such as hemiplegia, and seizures–features of a space-occupying lesion. There may be papilloedema. The temporal and occipital lobes are most frequently affected. Spinal cord compression can occur, but is much less common than is seen in schistosomiasis. Skull X-rays may show cysts in the brain with calcified worms and eggs, that resemble soap bubbles, and CT and MRI scans show ring-enhancing lesions with surrounding oedema (like schistosomiasis). Rapid presentation with intracerebral and subarachnoid haemorrhage can occur.[32,36] Chronic infections (>30 years) are also recorded.[109]

The CNS lesions are chronic and so the pathology is varied. In old, healed cases, there is a fibrous scar and calcification. In younger lesions, there are nodules 2–4cm in diameter with a central worm surrounded by inflammation and peripheral fibrosis. In acute cases, the lesion resembles a haemorrhagic abscess. There may be significant tissue eosinophilia. The worms are seen in various stages of viability or disintegration and may show the characteristic trematode cuticle and internal disposition of organs; in chronic lesions, the worms may have disappeared, leaving only dead eggs.[36] The easier diagnostic feature is the characteristic morphology of the eggs: they have an operculum, a relatively thick golden brown shell (like *Schistosoma* eggs), do not possess a spine and measure 80–120µm long by 50–60µm wide (Figure 21.52). The eggs may elicit a granulomatous reaction.

Apart from direct observation of worm or eggs, the diagnosis in suspected cases is supported by positive serology.[131] Treatment is with praziquantel and corticosteroid cover.

Other Rare Trematode Infections of the Central Nervous System
Fasciola hepatica

A globally common human parasite that burrows into the liver and lives in the biliary tree.[131,146] Aberrant migration can lead to cerebral infection. This is an abscess with adult worm and eggs present and a markedly eosinophilic reaction; secondary haemorrhages can mimic a cerebral aneurysm.[234]

Heterophyes heterophyes

A parasite of the human intestinal lumen, aberrant migration can produce cerebral lesions.[146,186] These are cystic, containing the adult worm and eggs.[40]

Cestode Infections

The main cestode infections of man are cysticercosis and hydatid disease. In the former, the adult tapeworm lives in

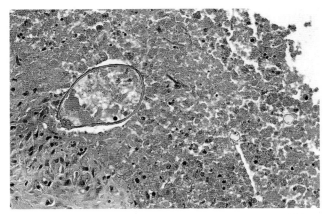

21.52 Paragonimiasis. A dead *Paragonimus* egg within a necrotic focus. The large size and thick brown shell are characteristic, but the operculum is not seen.

the human gut, i.e. we are the definitive host, but pigs are the usual intermediate hosts for the larval cysts. In hydatid disease, dogs are the definitive host, and the usual intermediate hosts are sheep. Thus, in both these diseases, man is an abnormal intermediate host. The rarer coenurosis and sparganosis are also described.

Cysticercosis

Infection with cysticerci – larvae of the tapeworm *Taenia solium* – is the most common of all worm infections to cause CNS disease. The infection is endemic in all parts of the world, though more common in the tropics, related to poverty and lack of hygiene, and where man and pigs live closely. It is sporadic in Europe and Australia. The prevalence of clinical neurocysticercosis can be up to 4 per cent, the highest rates being in South America. In Mexico, Brazil and India, neurocysticercosis is the most common space-occupying lesion in the brain and also the most common identifiable cause of epilepsy.[24,179] It is unusual in peoples who do not eat pig meat, e.g. Jews and Muslims, but not unknown.[131] Asymptomatic neurocysticercosis – estimated from clinical, imaging and serology – in a pig-farming community in India was estimated at 15 per cent.[188]

Life Cycle

The *Taenia solium* tapeworm has man as the definitive host and resides in the gut (Figure 21.53). Excreted eggs are ingested by pigs, in which they hatch and disseminate to the skeletal muscles. There the eggs develop into larval cysts, each of which contains one scolex, the head of a future tapeworm. When this infected meat is eaten, under-cooked so that the larva are not killed, the cyst wall disintegrates, and the scolex everts and attaches to the small bowel mucosa. Over several months it grows into the adult tape, which has 1000 or more segments (proglottids). The worm is hermaphroditic and each proglottid excretes eggs onto the soil, via faeces. The tapeworms can remain in the bowel for more than 20 years.

Human cysticercosis happens when man ingests eggs in food or water or via faecal contamination. The eggs are usually from others, but self-infection is also common (oro-faecal, rather than by reverse peristalsis). The egg hatches in the gut (with exposure to bile) into oncospheres, which burrow into the gut wall and enter the vessels and disseminate to internal organs within 2 hours. They migrate to any organ, but preferentially to skeletal muscle, heart, subcutaneous tissue, eye and brain.[146] Within 2–3 months, the oncosphere develops into a cysticercus, and it lives for a few years before dying. The clinical pathology of cysticercosis in the CNS is usually caused by the death of the parasite rather than by its presence *per se* when alive. Cysts mature and then degenerate and resolve into calcified nodules.

Clinical Features

The disease can occur from 2 months to 30 years after infection.[23] The most common sign is subcutaneous nodules (each nodule being a cysticercus as a 1–2 cm space-occupying lesion). Radiology may reveal multiple calcified dead cysticerci in major muscles, such as the quadriceps. The most important locations are the brain and eye because they are most likely to produce symptoms and pathology. Spinal disease is uncommon. Heart infection can also occur. Why there is this organ tropism is not understood.

The clinical presentation depends on the location, the number of cysts, their stage of development and degeneration, the host inflammatory reaction, and the age of the patient. In the majority of those with CNS infection, infection is actually asymptomatic. Seizures are the most common presenting sign at around 80 per cent, children being more affected than adults.[23,90] About one third of patients have headache, and intracranial hypertension is diagnosed in one fifth (more commonly in adults).

The different clinicopathological forms are:[179]

1. Seizures, the presenting form in about 50–80 per cent, from parenchymal cysts.
2. Leptomeningitis, often basal with hydrocephalus. It may be eosinophilic.
3. Intraventricular, the fourth ventricle being the most common, and the cysts may be attached or floating free. When the aqueduct is obstructed, acute raised intracranial pressure results.
4. Cerebrovascular, with endarteritis obliterans and thrombosis due to inflammation from an adjacent cyst and host reaction.
5. Encephalitic, due to inflammation around multiple degenerating cysts.
6. Spinal localization, which is rare, but may lead to arachnoiditis, with transverse myelitis or signs of a local mass lesion.
7. Dementing.
8. Sudden death, from seizures or a cyst blocking the third ventricle.

There are several other classifications of neurocysticercosis, which relate to the cysticercus stage, location and

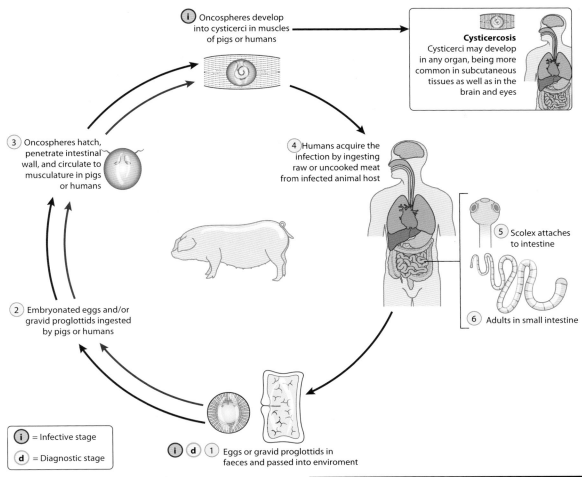

21.53 Life cycle of *Taenia solium* infection.

Figure courtesy of United States Centers for Disease Control and Prevention, Division of Parasitic Diseases.

also to CT imaging (Figure 21.54): as CT and MR have become the major diagnostic methods for the disease, these are relevant.[192,233] Morphologically, a cyst is also termed 'active' while it is viable, 'transitional' when it is degenerating, and 'inactive' when it is dead.[24] The location within the CNS is either parenchymal or extraparenchymal (meningeal). The four CT phases are:

1. Vesicular: no surrounding parenchymal reaction around a viable cysticercus (indicating tolerance), non-enhancing.
2. Colloidal: annular enhancement, when the cyst starts degenerating.
3. Granular-nodular: irregular perilesional oedema, the fluid content of the cyst being isodense with the parenchyma, and a capsule. This stage correlates with the florid inflammatory response to a degenerating cyst, and is associated with seizures.[156]
4. Calcified: homogeneous high density image on CT–a dead cysticercus.

Neuropsychological tests suggest that neurocysticercosis also contributes to abnormal behavioural function.[120] Hypothalamic lesions have been associated with obesity, possibly through the hypothalamic hyperphagic syndrome.[123]

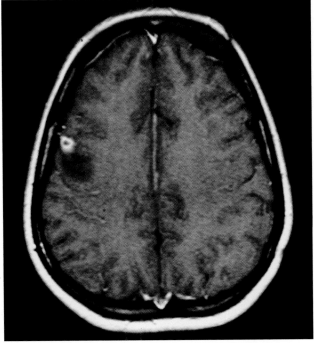

21.54 Cysticercosis. Computed tomography scan of a patient with epilepsy. There is a superficial cyst with local oedema.

Image courtesy of Dr A Checkley, Hospital for Tropical Diseases, London, UK.

Pathogenesis

The host immune response to cysticerci is both humoral and cellular. Antibody responses in blood and CSF indicate immune reactivity to viable cysts (but no significant host reaction). The major inflammatory reaction to cysts is mainly Th2 mediated; antibody levels correlate with disease severity.[30] However, whether this immune response initiates the degeneration of the cysticercus or occurs as a result of natural degeneration is uncertain.

As with falciparum cerebral malaria, neurocysticercosis research throws up ever more complexities in our understanding of the pathogenesis because the clinical heterogeneity results from complex interactions among parasite, host and environmental factors.[68]

Pathology

The gross pathology of cerebral cysticercosis varies greatly according to the number and site of the cysts. The cysts are about 0.5–2 cm in diameter. They may be located in the ventricle, the cortical parenchyma (70 per cent) or in the meningeal spaces.[124] The number present in a patient can vary from a single cyst to hundreds (Figure 21.55).

The cysticercus is a bladder containing fluid and an inverted head, or protoscolex. The wall is 100–200 μm thick and has an outer tegument, with microvilli on the surface. Beneath are smooth muscle cells haphazardly arranged and tegumental cells. These merge into a loose parenchyma that characteristically contains many haematoxyphilic calcareous bodies (corpuscles)—a typical feature of several cestode larvae.[146] The protoscolex has four 300 μm suckers and a rostellum with protruding hooklets, numbering between 22 and 36. These hooklets are about 110 μm long, birefringent, visible on haematoxylin and eosin (H&E) staining and particularly well stained red with the Ziehl–Neelsen method. They are shaped rather like a scimitar (Figure 21.56).

Viable cysts evoke virtually no inflammatory response, and if brain is examined, there may only be a minimal fibrous capsule around, and no inflammatory cells. When the cysts degenerate, the inflammatory response is initially neutrophilic, with varying amounts of eosinophils, granulation tissue and surrounding fibrosis (Figure 21.57). The cysticercus structure becomes less distinct, and the whole lesion may resemble an abscess. As the cysticercus dies, it calcifies and the inflammation becomes more mononuclear and less marked. The intramuscular cysticercus shows a similar morphology and host reaction sequence to those in the brain (Figure 21.58). A large autopsy study in Brazil found that one quarter of cysts contained viable larvae.[124]

Racemose and HIV-Associated Cysticercosis

In the subarachnoid space, a cysticercus may develop a different morphology and become a 'racemose cyst'.[76] The cyst forms connecting multiple grape-like bladders and the scolex disappears (Figure 21.59). This form of cysticercus has been considered to be a different species of *Taenia*, but DNA analysis indicates identity to *T. solium*, and the morphological variation is a result of local physical space factors and perhaps immune response.[92]

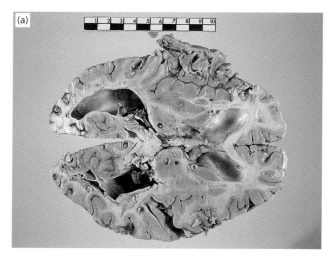

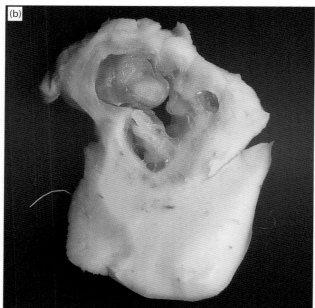

21.55 Cysticercosis. (a) Brain of a patient who died of epilepsy due to heavy infection by *Taenia solium* larvae. There is hydrocephalus from obstruction of the ventricles and numerous cysticerci are scattered throughout the parenchyma and ventricles. **(b)** A single cortical cysticercus, about 2 cm in diameter. The solid part is the scolex.

Although cases of co-infection are few, it appears that in those with HIV, parenchymal lesions are more multiple than in HIV –ve patients, are associated with co-infections such as tuberculosis and toxoplasmosis, and can present as immune reconstitution inflammatory syndrome (IRIS) on commencing antiretroviral therapy.[204] The racemose form is described as more frequent among HIV-infected patients.[49]

Diagnosis and Treatment

The diagnosis is usually based on clinical suspicion and imaging. Serology may have a role, but is complicated by the fact that antibodies indicate previous infection as well as possibly present active disease. The sensitivity of serology in single cyst disease is <50 per cent, but approaches

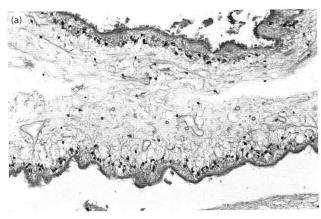

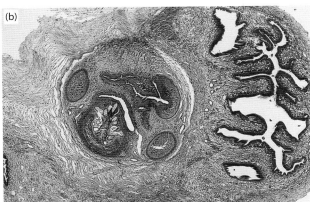

21.56 Cysticercosis. (a) Cysticercus wall with microvilli on the tegument surface, a layer of tegument cells and, beneath, a loose stroma with excretory channels (the holes). **(b)** Invaginated scolex showing three of the four suckers and several hooklets. The tegument is seen adjacent.

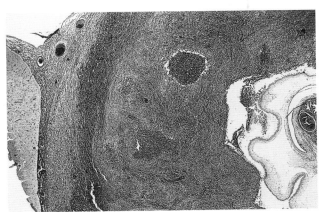

21.57 Cysticercosis. A submeningeal cysticercus with an unusual amount of inflammation. The larva is still intact.

100 per cent when there are multiple parenchymal cysts.[90] In patients who are not from endemic areas, however, seropositivity is more significant. Differential detection of *T. solium* antigen and antibody in paired serum and CSF samples is becoming helpful,[197] and DNA detection in biopsy samples is now available.[90] The differential diagnosis, from clinical and imaging studies, includes tumours and tuberculosis.

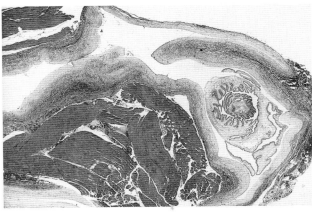

21.58 Cysticercosis. Skeletal muscle with a cysticercus. The invaginated scolex is clearly seen, and the rim of fibrous tissue around the cyst.

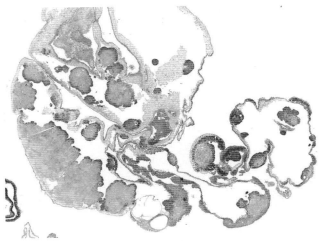

21.59 Racemose cysticercosis. Low power photograph of the complex cyst. Within the convoluted cysticercus there are multiple degenerate solid nodules.

Courtesy of Dr Leslie Bridges, London, UK.

Antihelminth drugs, such as albendazole (or praziquantel) plus steroidal anti-inflammatory cover, are commonly used for live-appearing cysts, but there is no certain evidence base that they are effective in reducing the likelihood of developing seizure or hydrocephalus.[81] Dead cysts may not require chemotherapy. Surgery is used diagnostically, for accessible cysts in basal cisterns, and neuroendoscopy can remove intraventricular cysts; and a ventriculoperitoneal shunt may be required for hydrocephalus.

There is a case report of reactivation of CNS disease years after praziquantel therapy and when the lesions were calcified and apparently inactive. CT scan showed oedema and pathogenetically this may be a local immune reconstitution phenomenon.[206]

Coenurosis

Coenurosis is a rare zoonotic disease, similar to cysticercosis but caused by *Taenia multiceps* and related species.[131] The definitive host is not man, but dogs that harbour the adults in their intestine. It is present in Africa, Europe and the Americas. Infection is via the eggs in the faeces; when ingested, they pass into the circulation and develop into coenurus cysts in the brain and meninges, subcutaneous tissue, skeletal muscle, the eye and around the spinal cord.[102]

The clinical features are headache and raised intracranial pressure, as hydrocephalus is common from ventricle outlet compression and basal meningitis. Cranial nerve palsies also occur. Imaging shows one or more cysts in the subarachnoid space or in a ventricle.

The characteristic feature is the cyst. It is thin, like a *T. solium* cysticercus, but larger (2–10 cm) and contains not one but hundreds of scolices (Figure 21.60). The rest of the cyst contents are watery fluid. Each scolex has a rostellum with rows of hooklets.[146] The surrounding reaction is gliosis within the brain, and meningeal fibrosis if the cysts are located there. There may be associated endarteritis and thrombosis of vessels.

The diagnosis is made on surgical removal of the coenurus. Some cases can be mistaken for a hydatid cyst until tissue diagnosis upon removal.[129]

Hydatid Disease

In man, there are two different hydatid infection syndromes, caused respectively by

- *Echinococcus granulosus*: classical hydatid cyst disease;
- *Echinococcus multilocularis*: less common alveolar hydatid disease.

Echinococcus granulosus Hydatid Disease

Life Cycle and Epidemiology   The more common *E. granulosus* hydatid disease is endemic worldwide – particularly the Middle East and east Africa – including Australasia and Latin America (and it is still present in the UK).[131,146,158] The definitive host is the dog and other canines, in whose intestine the adult 5 mm-long tapeworm resides. These release eggs into the faeces, which are ingested by sheep, cattle, goats, camels and other herbivores. In the duodenum of these intermediate hosts, the egg hatches and the oncosphere burrows through the gut wall and reaches the

liver. Over years it grows into the hydatid cyst, and may spread to other parts of the body. The life cycle is complete when a canine eats offal containing a cyst (Figure 21.61). The scolices in the cyst become the head segments of future adult tapeworms in the host intestine.

Man acquires hydatid cyst disease by accidentally ingesting canine faeces containing eggs. Thus it is a rural disease for the most part. In areas of high endemicity (e.g. Iraq, northern Kenya), the cyst is so common that consideration of a tumour in any part of the body has to include hydatid cyst in the diagnosis. Children are affected as well as adults.

The cyst grows at about 1 cm diameter per year. Although more than three quarters of cysts are in the liver, 1–2 per cent of patients have CNS or paravertebral disease via bloodstream spread. The cyst behaves as a space-occupying lesion, exciting usually little host inflammatory reaction and a little fibrosis. If a cyst ruptures, it spreads locally and sets up new cysts.

Clinical Features   Within the brain or head, the order of frequency of site is the brain parenchyma, the ventricles,[88] extradural location, the cerebellum and the orbit.[42,63,214] The skull may also have a cyst. Clinical presentation is with focal neurological signs, seizures, hemiparesis, chorea and speech disorders.[122] There is raised intracranial pressure. CT scan of cerebral cysts shows a smooth cystic lesion with no rim enhancement and no peripheral oedema.[131]

Brain hydatids can also present as both haemorrhagic stroke and ischaemic stroke – the latter as an embolic obstruction to the middle cerebral artery.[13,110] Like liver hydatid cysts, occasional cranial cases may be associated with the nephrotic syndrome.[205]

Pathology   The CNS cysts can be up to 10 cm in diameter and are associated with hydrocephalus (Figure 21.62). Grossly, the cyst wall is white, flimsy and satin-like to touch. Internally there may be just one cyst or several daughter cysts.[146] Old degenerate cysts are collapsed and infolded. They are much larger than the cysts of neurocysticercosis.

Histopathologically, the outer wall is 2–3 mm thick and comprises a laminated membrane (Figure 21.63); this is PAS-positive. Within this are the germinal membrane and flattened cellular nucleated layer. This gives rise to the scolices either directly or from smaller internal brood capsules. The scolices are characteristic: 200 μm long ovoid cellular structures with four spherical suckers, a rostellum and two rows of hooklets. These features are better appreciated on cytology preparations than in histopathological slides. The hooklets retain carbol fuchsin, so are highlighted by a Ziehl–Neelsen stain; this is useful if the scolices have degenerated and died, because the hooklets remain in the cyst.

Around a viable unruptured cyst, the host inflammatory reaction is usually minimal, with little astrocytosis. How the cyst evades immune detection and attack is unclear. However, as the cyst dies, it generates a more marked, allergic, inflammatory reaction, with polymorphs, eosinophils and granulomas, and fibrosis. In the brain around this, there are astrocytosis and microgliosis.

Spinal cord involvement is not uncommon, and develops from extradural or bone infection.[122] The cyst expansion causes spinal cord compression. Presentation is with

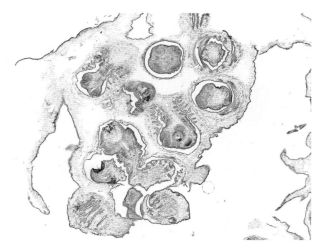

21.60 Coenurosis. An excised cyst containing numerous scolices.

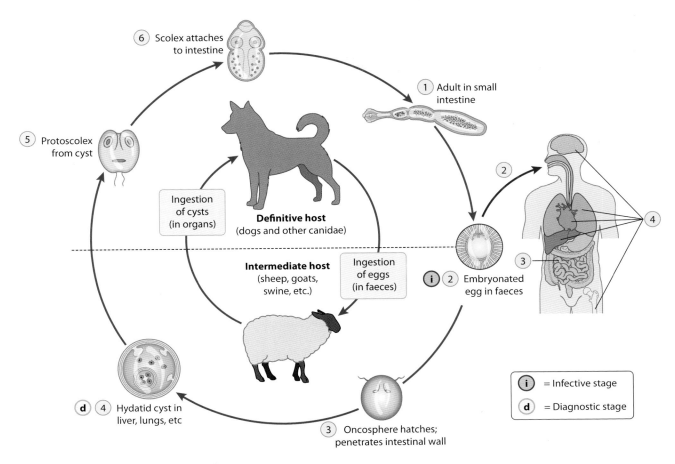

6 Scolex attaches to intestine

1 Adult in small intestine

5 Protoscolex from cyst

2

Ingestion of cysts (in organs)

Definitive host (dogs and other canidae)

3

4

Intermediate host (sheep, goats, swine, etc.)

Ingestion of eggs (in faeces)

i 2 Embryonated egg in faeces

i = Infective stage

d = Diagnostic stage

d 4 Hydatid cyst in liver, lungs, etc

3 Oncosphere hatches; penetrates intestinal wall

21.61 Life cycle of *Echinococcus granulosus*.

Figure courtesy of United States Centers for Disease Control and Prevention, Division of Parasitic Diseases.

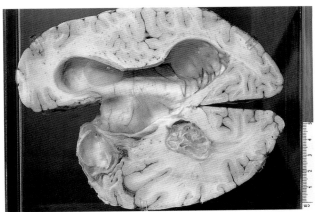

21.62 Hydatid disease. Brain with several hydatid cysts of *Echinococcus granulosus*. The live ones are translucent, lying within the ventricles. The collapsed and condensed cyst is dead. There is hydrocephalus from obstruction to the third ventricle.

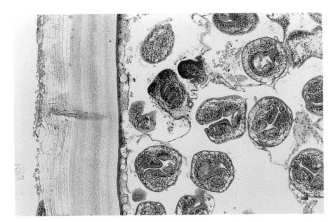

21.63 Hydatid cyst. Wall of an *E. granulosus* hydatid cyst: at left, the pale laminated membrane on which lies the unicellular germinal layer; many scolices are present within the cyst. Inverted eosinophilic suckers and some hooklets are visible. H&E.

radicular pain, limb weakness and progressive paralysis.[59] Skull bone disease is rare. Within the bone in most surgical specimens, there are fragments of degenerate laminated membrane associated with a chronic osteomyelitis reaction.

Diagnosis and Treatment The diagnosis of CNS hydatid disease is usually suggested by the known presence of a liver cyst and characteristic imaging findings. About 70 per cent of those with a cyst have antibodies in the blood; CSF also has positive serology in some but not all infected patients. Tissue biopsy may be done for diagnostic purposes, but aspiration of cyst contents can show scolices, hooklets and positive serology. Molecular diagnostics are now also applied in case work-up.[232]

The treatment is part surgery and part chemotherapy.[131] If the cyst can be completely and safely removed intact (the Dowling procedure), that is optimal. The risk of anaphylactic shock from accidental spillage of hydatid antigen during surgery is low.[122] Albendazole is the chemotherapy, and occasionally patients may be cured with chemotherapy alone.[4] Unfortunately, many patients with paravertebral cysts continue with active infection despite this; repeat biopsies of material from sinuses or bone biopsies show degenerate hydatid material that is continuing to proliferate despite appearing dead.

Alveolar Hydatid Cyst

E. multilocularis infection is restricted geographically to the forest areas of northern USA and Canada, Russia, China, Turkey and Central Europe, including Germany and Switzerland.[56,146] The definitive host is the fox. It is less common than *E. granulosus* and behaves more aggressively. Cerebral infections are rare and represent spread from intra-abdominal disease.[231] They present as a space-occupying lesion, mimicking a cerebral tumour or metastasis. Imaging shows a multiseptate irregular mass, partly solid, partly cystic, with incomplete rim enhancement. Diagnosis is made on biopsy or at autopsy.

The pathology is of an invasive cyst with thin laminated membrane; protoscolices may be scanty or absent. Instead of a smooth outline as with *E. granulosus*, the cyst wall penetrates into the parenchyma, like a cancer, with islands of small cyst material separate from the main body (Figure 21.64). The host reaction is florid with much necrosis, granulomas and fibrosis.[146] There is no agreed therapy and the prognosis is very poor, despite surgery.[220]

Sparganosis

This is a zoonotic larval cestode infection caused by *Spirometra* spp.[131] It occurs mainly in South East Asia, but also in Africa. The life cycle is one of the more bizarre encountered in parasitology. The adult worms reside in dog and cat intestines. Eggs pass in water to copepods and mature to the next procercoid stage. This is eaten by frogs and snakes and some mammals and a plerocercoid larva (the sparganum) develops. When these second intermediate hosts are eaten by dogs or cats, the cycle is completed. Man becomes accidentally infected by drinking water contaminated by copepods, or eating undercooked meat of the second intermediate host; or rarely by using poultices of infected animal flesh on skin lesions.

In man, the larvae cannot mature, and wander while growing to a size of up to 40 cm by 3 mm wide. Subcutaneous tissue, eye and CNS involvement are the most common clinical presentations. Children and adults are affected. In the brain, as it migrates, the larva causes headache seizures, focal neurological signs and focal haemorrhage.[95] The disease may be indolent over years. CT and MR imaging is characteristic, with hyperintense foci and perilesional oedema – mimicking tuberculoma, which is the main imaging differential diagnosis,[193] or cysticercosis. Migration through the brain is a key diagnostic feature on imaging in cerebral sparganosis.[121]

The larva itself resembles spaghetti, white and solid (Figure 21.65).[146] Grossly, there appear to be multiple lesions because the sparganum is long and not straight. Histologically, the worm has small smooth muscle bundles through the length, excretory ducts and calcareous corpuscles within the mesenchyme, and a typical cestode cuticle. As with all cestode larvae, there is no intestine; sparagana also do not have hooklets. The host inflammatory reaction is usually granulomatous and necrotic. There may be eosinophilia, but if the worm is not captured on biopsy, it all looks very like tuberculosis (Figure 21.66).

Treatment, ideally, is complete neurosurgical excision. However, usually some of the worm remains and long-term albendazole is given.

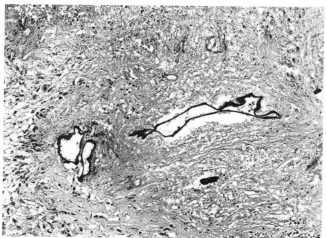

21.64 Alveolar hydatid cyst. The parasite membrane is thin, without scolices, and is invading the local tissue with much necrosis. PAS stain.

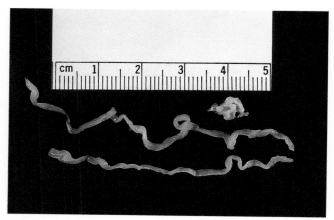

21.65 Sparganosis. A sparganum – elongated spaghetti-like larva.

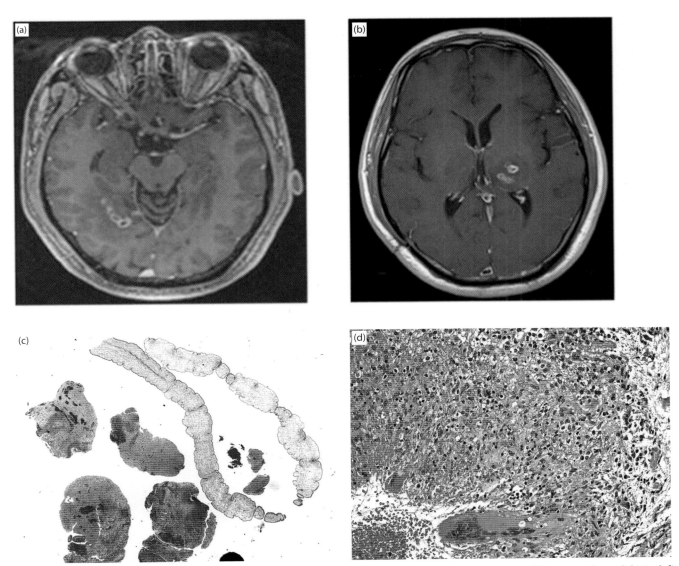

21.66 Sparganosis. (a, b) Magnetic resonance images taken 4 years apart, indicating the migration of the worm from right to left cerebral hemisphere. **(c)** The biopsied worm–low power view. **(d)** The host reaction around the worm–granulomatous and similar to that of tuberculosis.

Courtesy of Dr A Dean, Addenbrooke's Hospital, Cambridge, UK. First published by Biomed Central in Bennett HM, et al. The genome of the sparganosis tapeworm Spirometra erinaceieuropaei isolated from the biopsy of a migrating brain lesion. Genome Biol 2014;15:510.

ARTHROPOD INFECTIONS

Myiasis

Myiasis results from infection by larvae (maggots) of dipteran flies. It is most prevalent in the tropics and thus many cases are imported to industrialized countries following travel.[131] The most common flies that cause this disease are *Dermatobia*, *Oestrus* (botfly) and *Cordylobia* spp. For pathologists, it is impossible to differentiate the genera as microscopically, in sections, they look similar. Precise identification comes from the examination of a gross specimen of maggot when extracted. Also, the maggot is often dead at presentation, rendering identification difficult. These larvae elicit a brisk immune response and (in veterinary work at least) serology could aid diagnosis.[162] Rarely, a maggot invades through the skull into the brain, to produce an abscess.[147]

Ophthalmomyiasis

Eggs from a gravid female fly are laid on the conjunctiva and burrow inside, affecting all parts. There is inflammation and abscess formation and often the eye is removed because it has failed, or on suspicion of tumour. Pathologically, the maggot has a thick corrugated cuticle, sometimes pigmented. Internally, there are large foamy cytoplasm cells and striated muscle (this helps distinction from metazoan parasites, which do not have striated muscle) (Figure 21.67).[147]

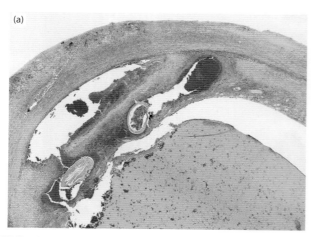 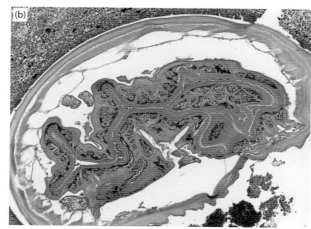

21.67 Oculomyiasis. (a) A maggot within the eye, associated with much inflammation and subscleral fibrosis. **(b)** Thick cuticle, internal large vacuolated cells, pigment, and the racemose internal tubes are characteristic of these larvae.

Courtesy of Dr H Mudhar, Department of Pathology, Royal Hallamshire Hospital, Sheffield, UK.

ACKNOWLEDGEMENTS

The author acknowledges the contributions in the 8th edition by Leila Chimelli (American trypanosomiasis) and Jeanne Bell (congenital toxoplasmosis), which have been updated in this 9th edition.

REFERENCES

1. Abreu-Silva AL, Calabrese KS, Tedesco RC, Mortara RA, da Costa SC. Central nervous system involvement in experimental infection with *Leishmania amazonensis*. *Am J Trop Med Hyg* 2003;**68**:661–5.
2. Ajzenberg D, Cogne N, Paris L, *et al.* *Toxoplasma gondii* isolates associated with human congenital toxoplasmosis, and correlation with clinical findings. *J Infect Dis* 2002;**186**:684–689.
3. Almeida EA, Lima JN, Lages-Silva E, *et al.* Chagas' disease and HIV co-infection in patients without effective antiretroviral therapy: prevalence, clinical presentation and natural history. *Trans R Soc Trop Med Hyg* 2010;**104**:447–52.
4. Altas M, Serarslan Y, Davran R, Evirgen O, Yilmaz N. A medically treated multiple cerebral hydatid cyst. *J Neurosurg* 2010;**54**:79–82.
5. Ancelle T, Dupouy-Camet J, Bougnoux ME, *et al.* Two outbreaks of trichinosis caused by horsemeat in France in 1985. *Am J Epidemiol* 1988;**127**:1302–11.
6. Andrade ZA. Pathogenesis of Chagas' disease. *Res Immunol* 1991;**142**:126–9.
7. Arness MK, Brown JD, Dubey JP, Neafie RC, Granstrom DE. An outbreak of acute eosinophilic myositis attributed to human *Sarcocystis* infection. *Am J Trop Med Hyg* 1999;**61**:548–53.
8. Bachli H, Minet JC, Gratzl O. Cerebral toxocariasis: a possible cause of epileptic seizure in children. *Childs Nerv Syst* 2004;**20**:468–72.
9. Barragan A, Sibley LD. Migration of *Toxoplasma gondii* across biological barriers. *Trends Microbiol* 2003;**11**:426–30.
10. Batson OV. The function of the vertebral veins and their role in the spread of metastases. *Ann Surg* 1940;**112**:138–49.
11. Beg MA, Khan R, Baig SM, *et al.* Cerebral involvement in benign tertian malaria. *Am J Trop Med Hyg* 2002;**67**:230–2.
12. Bell JE, Lowrie, S, Koffi K, *et al.* The neuropathology of HIV-infected African children in Abidjan, Côte d'Ivoire. *J Neuropathol Exp Neurol* 1997;**56**:686–92.
13. Benomar A, Yahyaoui M, Birok N, Vidailhet M, Chkili T. Middle cerebral artery occlusion due to hydatid cysts of myocardial and intraventricular cavity origin. *Stroke* 1994;**25**:886–8.
14. Bittencourt AL. Congenital Chagas' disease. *Am J Dis Child* 1976;**130**:97–103.
15. Bonfioli AA, Orefice F. Toxoplasmosis. *Semin Ophthalmol* 2005;**20**:129–41.
16. Boussinesq M, Bain O, Chabaud AG, *et al.* A new zoonosis of the cerebrospinal fluid of man probably caused by *Meningonema peruzzii*. *Parasite* 1995;**2**:173–6.
17. Boussinesq M, Gardon J, Gardon-Wendel N, *et al.* Three probable cases of *Loa loa* encephalopathy following ivermectin treatment for onchocerciasis. *Am J Trop Med Hyg* 1998;**58**:461–9.
18. Bregani ER, Ceraldi T, Rovellini A, Ghiringhelli C. Case report: intraocular localization of *Mansonella perstans* in a patient from south Chad. *Trans R Soc Trop Med Hyg* 2002;**96**:654.
19. Brown H, Hien TT, Day N, *et al.* Evidence of blood–brain barrier dysfunction in human cerebral malaria. *Neuropathol Appl Neurobiol* 1999;**25**:331–40.
20. Brown H, Rogerson S, Taylor TE, *et al.* Blood–brain barrier function in cerebral malaria in Malawian children. *Am J Trop Med Hyg* 2001;**64**:207–13.
21. Cabral RF, Valle Bahia PR, Gasparetto EL, Chimelli L. Immune reconstitution inflammatory syndrome and cerebral toxoplasmosis. *AJNR Am J Neuroradiol* 2010;**31**:E65–6.
22. Calabresi P, Abelmann WH. Porto-caval and porto-pulmonary anastomoses in Laennec's cirrhosis and in heart failure. *J Clin Invest* 1957;**36**:1257–65.
23. Carabin H, Ndimubanzi PC, Budke CM, *et al.* Clinical manifestations associated with neurocysticercosis: a systematic review. *PLoS Neglec Trop Dis* 2011;**5**:e1152.
24. Carpio A. Neurocysticercosis: an update. *Lancet Infect Dis* 2002;**2**:751–62.
25. Carr RA, Molyneux ME, Mwenechanya JJ, *et al.* Macroscopic evidence of moderate brain swelling in paediatric cerebral malaria: an autopsy study. *Proc Am Soc Trop Med Hyg* 1998;**58**(Suppl):239.
26. Carruthers VB. Proteolysis and *Toxoplasma* invasion. *Int J Parasitol* Morb Mortal Wkly Rep 2006;**36**:595–600.
27. Centers for Disease Control and Prevention. Notes from the field: transplant-transmitted *Balamuthia mandrillaris* – Arizona, 2010. *MMWR Morb Mortal Wkly Rep* 2010;**59**:1182.
28. Cestari I, Ansa-Addo E, Deolindo P, Inal JM, Ramirez MI. *Trypanosoma cruzi* immune evasion mediated by host cell-derived microvesicles. *J Immunol* 2012;**188**:1942–52.
29. Chagas C. Nova tripanosomiase humana. *Mem Inst Osw Cruz* 1909;**1**:218.
30. Chavarria A, Fleury A, Garcia E, *et al.* Relationship between the clinical heterogeneity of neurocysticercosis and the immune-inflammatory profiles. *Clin Immunol* 2005;**116**:271–8.
31. Checkley AM, Smith A, Smith V, *et al.* Risk factors for mortality from imported falciparum malaria in the UK over 20

years: an observational study. *Br Med J* 2012;344:e2116.

32. Chen Z, Zhu G, Lin J, Wu N, Feng H. Acute cerebral paragonimiasis presenting as hemorrhagic stroke in a child. *Pediat Neurol* 2008;39:133–6.

33. Chimelli L, Scaravilli F. Trypanosomiasis. *Brain Pathol* 1997;7:599–611.

34. Chimelli L, Rosemberg S, Hahn MD, Lopes MBS, Netto MB. Pathology of the central nervous system in patients infected with the human immunodeficiency virus (HIV): a report of 252 autopsy cases from Brazil. *Neuropathol Appl Neurobiol* 1992;18:478–88.

35. Choi JH, Cornford M, Wang L, Sun J, Friedman TC. Acute Chagas' disease presenting with a suprasellar mass and panhypopituitism. *Pituitary* 2004;7:111–14.

36. Choo J-D, Suh B-S, Lee H-S, et al. Chronic cerebral paragonimiasis combined with aneurysmal subarachnoid hemorrhage. *Am J Trop Med Hyg* 2003;69:466–9.

37. Clark IA, Cowden WB. Why is the pathology of falciparum worse than that of vivax malaria? *Parasitol Today* 1999;15:458–61.

38. Clark IA, Schofield L. Pathogenesis of malaria. *Parasitol Today* 2000;16:451–4.

39. Cohen BA. Neurologic manifestations of toxoplasmosis in AIDS. *Semin Neurol* 1999;19:201–11.

40. Collomb H, Deschies R, Demmarchi J. Sur deux cas de diastomose cerebrale a *Heterophyes heterophyes*. *Bull Soc Path Exot* 1960;53:144–7.

41. Connor DH, Chandler FW. *Pathology of infectious diseases*. Appleton & Lange, Stanford, 1997.

42. Copley IB, Fripp PJ, Erasmus AM, Otto DD. Unusual presentations of cerebral hydatid disease in children. *Br J Neurosurg* 1992;6:203–10.

43. Cordova E, Boschi A, Ambrosini J, Cudos C, Corti M. Reactivation of Chagas disease with CNS involvement in HIV-infected patients in Argentina, 1992–2007. *Int J Infect Dis* 2008;12:587–92.

44. Cosnett JE, van Dellen JR. Schistosomiasis (bilharzia) of the spinal cord: case report and clinical profile. *Q J Med* 1986;61:1131–9.

45. Cowley GP, Miller RF, Papadaki L, Canning EU, Lucas SB. Disseminated microsporidiosis (*Encephalitozoon intestinalis*) in a patient with AIDS. *Histopathology* 1997;30:386–9.

46. Cox-Singh J, Hiu J, Lucas SB, et al. Severe malaria – a case of fatal *Plasmodium knowlesi* infection with post-mortem findings: a case report. *Malar J* 2010;9:10.

47. da Silva RC, Langoni H. *Toxoplasma gondii*: host-parasite interaction and behaviour manipulation. *Parasitol Res* 2009;105:893–8.

48. Davila DF, Santiago JJ, Odreman WA. Vagal dysfunction and the pathogenesis of chronic Chagas' disease. *Int J Cardiol* 2005;103:227–9.

49. Delobel P, Signate A, El Guedj M, et al. An unusual form of neurocysticercosis associated with HIV infection. *Eur J Neurol* 2004;11:55–8.

50. Dorovini-Zis K, Schmidt K, Huynh H, et al. The neuropathology of fatal cerebral malaria in Malawian children. *Am J Pathol* 2011;178:2146–58.

51. dos Santos S, Almeida GHD, Monteiro MLR, et al. Ocular myositis and diffuse meningoencephalitis from *Trypanosoma cruzi* in an AIDS patient. *Trans R Soc Trop Med Hyg* 1999;93:535–6.

52. Druet-Cabanac M, Boussinesq M, Dongmo L, et al. Review of epidemiological studies searching for a relationship between onchocerciasis and epilepsy. *Neuroepidemiology* 2004;23:144–9.

53. Duke BO, Vincette J, Moore PJ. Microfilariae in the CSF, and neurological complications, during treatment of onchocerciasis with diethlycarbamazine. *Tropenmed Parasitol* 1976;27:123–32.

54. Dunn D, Wallon M, Peyron F, et al. Mother-to-child transmission of toxoplasmosis: risk estimates for clinical counselling. *Lancet* 1999;353:1829–33.

55. Dutra WO, Rocha MO, Teixeira MM. The clinical immunology of human Chagas' disease. *Trends Parasitol* 2005;21:581–7.

56. Eckert J, Deplazes P. Alveolar echinococcosis in humans: the current situation in central Europe and the need for countermeasures. *Parasitol Today* 1999;15:315–19.

57. Elkliayal RA, Girgis M. Bilharzial granuloma of the conus: case report. *Neurosurgery* 1993;32:1022–4.

58. Ellrodt A, Halfon P, Le Bras P, et al. Multifocal central nervous system lesions of three patients with trichinosis. *Arch Neurol* 1987;44:432–4.

59. El-On J, Ben-Noun L, Galitza Z, Ohana N. Case report: clinical and serological evaluation of echinococcosis of the spine. *Trans R Soc Trop Med Hyg* 2003;97:567–9.

60. el-Sagaff S, Salem HS, Nichols W, Tonkel AK, Abo-Zenadah NY. Cell death pattern in cerebellum neurons infected with *Toxoplasma gondii*. *J Egypt Soc Parasitol* 2005;35:809–18.

61. El-Sayed NM, Myler PJ, Bartholomeu DC, et al. The genome sequence of *Trypanosoma cruzi*, etiologic agent of Chagas' disease. *Science* 2005;309:409–15.

62. Epps RE, Pittelkow MR, Su WP. TORCH syndrome. *Semin Dermatol* 1995;14:179–86.

63. Ergun R, Okten AI, Yuksel M, et al. Orbital hydatid cyst: report of four cases. *Neurosurg Rev* 1997;20:33–7.

64. Eza DE, Lucas SB. Fulminant toxoplasmosis causing fatal pneumonitis and myocarditis. *HIV Med* 2006;7:1–6.

65. Ferrari TCA, Moreira PR. Neuroschistosomiasis: clinical symptoms and pathogenesis. *Lancet Neurol* 2011;10:853–64.

66. Ferreira LA, Lima FL, dos Anjos Mdo R, Costa JM. Tumor form of encephalic schistosomiasis: presentation of a case surgically treated. *Rev Soc Bras Med Trop* 1998;31:89–93.

67. Ferreira MS, de Nishioka S, Rocha A, et al. Acute fatal *Trypanosoma cruzi* meningoencephalitis in an human immunodeficiency virus-positive hemophiliac patient. *Am J Trop Med Hyg* 1991;45:723–7.

68. Fleury A, Escobar A, Fragoso G, Sciutto E, Larralde C. Clinical heterogeneity of human neurocysticercosis results from complex interactions among parasite, host and environmental factors. *Trans R Soc Trop Med Hyg* 2010;104:243–50.

69. Fowler R, Lee C, Keystone J. The role of corticosteroids in the treatment of cerebral schistosomiasis caused by *Schistosoma mansoni*: case report and discussion. *Am J Trop Med Hyg* 1999;61:47–50.

70. Fox AS, Kazacos KR, Gould NS, et al. Fatal eosinophilic meningoencephalitis and visceral larva migrans caused by the racoon ascarid *Baylisascaris procyonis*. *N Engl J Med* 1985;312:1619–23.

71. Freilij H, Altcheh J. Congenital Chagas' disease: diagnostic and clinical aspects. *Clin Infect Dis* 1995;21:551–5.

72. Gazzinelli RT, Amichay D, Sharton-Kersten T, et al. Role of macrophage-derived cytokines in the induction and regulation of cell-mediated immunity to *Toxoplasma gondii*. *Curr Top Immunol* 1996;219:127–40.

73. Gelman BB, Popov V, Chaljub B, et al. Neuropathological and ultrastructural features of amebic encephalitis caused by *Sappinia diploidea*. *J Neuropathol Exp Neurol* 2003;62:990–8.

74. Genrich GL, Guarner J, Paddock C, et al. Fatal malaria infection in travellers: novel immunohistochemical assays for the detection of *Plasmodium falciparum* in tissues and implications for pathogenesis. *Am J Trop Med Hyg* 2007;76:251–9.

75. Gherardi R, Baudrimont M, Lionnet F, et al. Skeletal muscle toxoplasmosis in patients with acquired immunodeficiency syndrome: a clinical and pathological study. *Ann Neurol* 1992;32:535–42.

76. Ghosh D, Dubey TN, Prabhakar S. Brain parenchymal, subarachnoid racemose, and intraventricular cysticercosis in an Indian man. *Postgrad Med J* 1999;75:164–7.

77. Gilbert R, Tan HK, Cliffe S, Stanford M, Guy E. Symptomatic toxoplasma infection due to congenitally and postnatally acquired infection. *Arch Dis Child* 2006;91:625.

78. Gill DS, Chatha DS, del Carpio-O'Donovan R. MR imaging findings in African trypanosomiasis. *Am J Neuroradiol* 2003;24:1383–5.

79. Girones N, Cuervo H, Fresno M. *Trypanosoma cruzi*-induced molecular mimicry and Chagas' disease. *Curr Top Microbiol Immunol* 2005;296:89–123.

80. Gitau EN, Newton CRJ. Blood–brain barrier in falciparum malaria. *Trop Med Int Health* 2005;10:285–92.

81. Gogia S, Talukdar B, Choudhoury V, Arora BS. Neurocysticercosis in children: clinical findings and response to albendazole therapy in a randomized. double-blind, placebo-controlled trial in newly diagnosed cases. *Trans R Soc Trop Med Hyg* 2003;97:416–21.

82. Golgher D, Gazzinelli RT. Innate and acquired immunity in the pathogenesis of Chagas' disease. *Autoimmunity* 2004;37:399–409.

83. Graeff-Teixeira C, da Silva AC, Yoshimura K. Update on eosinophilic meningoencephalitis and its clinical relevance. *Clin Microbiol Rev* 2009;22:322–48.

84. Grau GE, MacKenzie CD, Carr RA, et al. Platelet accumulation in brain microvessels in fatal pediatric cerebral malaria. *J Infect Dis* 2003;187:461–6.

85. Gray F, Gherardi RK, Wingate E, et al. Diffuse 'encephalitic' cerebral toxoplasmosis in AIDS. *J Neurol* 1989;236:273–7.

86. Gupta K, Vasishta RK, Bansal A, et al. Cortical cysts with hydrocephalus and ventriculitis: an unusual presentation of congenital toxoplasmosis at autopsy. *J Clin Pathol* 2011;64:272–4.

87. Gutierrez Y. *Diagnostic pathology of parasitic infections with clinical correlations.* Oxford University Press, Oxford, 2000.
88. Guzel A, Tatli M, Maciaczk J, Altinors N. Primary cerebral intraventricular hydatid cyst: a case report and review of the literature. *J Child Neurol* 2008;23:585–8.
89. Habek M, Ozretic D, Zarkovic K, Djakovic V, Mubrin Z. Unusual cause of dementia in an immunocompetent host: toxoplasmic encephalitis. *Neurol Sci* 2009;30:45–9.
90. Harrington AT, Creutzfeldt CJ, Sengupta DJ, et al. Diagnosis of neurocysticercosis by detection of *Taenia solium* DNA using a global DNA screening platform. *Clin Infect Dis* 2009;48:86–90.
91. Hill D, Dubey JP. *Toxoplasma gondii:* transmission, diagnosis and prevention. *Clin Microbiol Infect Dis* 2002;8:634–40.
92. Hinojosa-Juarez AC, Sandoval-Balanzario M, McManus DP, Monroy-Ostria A. Genetic similarity between cysticerci of *Taenia solium* isolated from human brain and from pigs. *Infect Genet Evol* 2008;8:653–6.
93. Hoff R, Teixeira RS, Carvalho JS, Mott BH. *Trypanosoma cruzi* in the cerebrospinal fluid during the acute phase of Chagas disease. *N Engl J Med* 1978;298:604–6.
94. Holding PA, Stevenson J, Peshu N, Marsh K. Cognitive sequelae of severe malaria with impaired consciousness. *Trans R Soc Trop Med Hyg* 1999;93: 529–34.
95. Holodniy M, Almenoff J, Loutit J, Steinberg GK. Cerebral sparganosis: case report and review. *Rev Infect Dis* 1991;13:155–9.
96. Houston S, Kowalewska-Grochowska K, Naik S, et al. First report of *Schistosoma mekongi* infection with brain involvement. *Clin Infect Dis* 2004;38:e1–6.
97. Huang TE, Chou SM. Occlusive hypertrophic arteritis as the cause of discrete necrosis in CNS toxoplasmosis in the acquired immunodeficiency syndrome. *Hum Pathol* 1988;19:1210–14.
98. Hung T, Neafie RC, McKenzie IA. *Baylisacaris procyonis* infection in elderly person, British Columbia, Canada. *Emerg Infect Dis* 2012;18:341–2.
99. Hunter CA, Remington JS. Immunopathogenesis of toxoplasmic encephalitis. *Infect Dis* 1994;170:1057–67.
100. Hunter CA, Suzuki Y, Subauste CS, Remington JS. Cells and cytokines in resistance to *Toxoplasma gondii.* *Curr Top Immunol* 1996;219:113–26.
101. Imai K, Koibuchi T, Kumagai T, et al. Cerebral schistosomiasis due to *S.haematobium* confirmed by PCR analysis of brain specimen. *J Clin Microbiol* 2011;49:3703–6.
102. Ing MB, Schantz PM, Turner JA. Human coenurosis in North America: case report and review. *Clin Infect Dis* 1998;27:519–23.
103. Intalapaporn P, Sunakratay S, Shuangshoti S, et al. *Balamuthia mandrillaris* meningoencephalitis: the first case in southeast Asia. *Am J Trop Med Hyg* 2004;70:666–9.
104. Jabbour RA, Kanj SS, Sawaya RA, et al. *Toxocara canis* myelitis: clinical features, magnetic resonance imaging (MRI) findings, and treatment outcome in 17 patients. *Medicine (Baltimore)* 2011;90:337–43.
105. Jamieson SE, de Roubaix LA, Cortina-Borja M, et al. Genetic and epigenetic factors at COL2A1 and ABCA4 influence clinical outcome in congenital toxoplasmosis. *PLoS One* 2008;3:e2285.
106. Jesus PA, Neville I, Cincura C, et al. Stroke history and Chagas disease are independent predictors of silent cerebral microembolism in patients with congestive cardiac failure. *Cerebrovasc Dis* 2011;31:19–23.
107. Jorg ME, Azader A, Brocheriou J, Bessola T. Encefalitis cronica por *Trypanosoma cruzi. Prensa Med Argentina* 1981;68:85–93.
108. Kampfl A, Pfausler B, Haring H.-P, et al. Impaired microcirculation and tissue oxygenation in human cerebral malaria: a SPECT and NIRS study. *Am J Trop Med Hyg* 1997;56:585–7.
109. Kang SY, Kim TK, Kim TY, et al. A case of chronic cerebral paragonimiasis westermanii. *Korean J Parasitol* 2000;38:167–71.
110. Kanj AH, Fares YH, Yehya RR, Hamzeh FF. Unusual appearance of a cerebral hydatid cyst as a haemorrhagic infarct. *Neurosciences (Riyadh)* 2010;15:275–6.
111. Kanpittaya J, Sawanyawisuth K, Intapan PM, et al. A comparative study of neuroimaging features between human neuro-gnathostomiasis and angiostrongyliasis. *Neurol Sci* 2012;33:893–8.
112. Kennedy PGE. Diagnostic and neuropathogenesis issues in human African trypanosomiasis. *Int J Parasitol* 2006;36:505–12.
113. Kennedy PGE. The continuing problem of human African trypanosomiasis (sleeping sickness). *Ann Neurol* 2008;64:116–26.
114. Kierszenbaum F. Where do we stand on the autoimmunity hypothesis of Chagas' disease? *Trends Parasitol* 2005;21:513–16.
115. Kristnensson K, Nygard M, Bertini G, Bentivoglio M. African trypanosome infections of the nervous system: parasite entry and effects on sleep and synaptic functions. *Prog Neurobiol* 2010;91:152–71.
116. Kung DH, Hubenthal EA, Kwan JY, et al. Toxoplasmosis myelopathy and myopathy in an AIDS patient. *Neurologist* 2011;17:49–51.
117. Lacroix C, Vazeux R, Brousse N, et al. Étude neuropathologique de 10 enfants infectés par le VIH. *Rev Neurol* 1993;149:37–45.
118. Lahn MM, Staub-Schmidt T, Himy R, et al. *Strongyloides stercoralis* infection in a non-immunosuppressed tourist with involvement of the CNS. *Trop Geogr Med* 1994;46:368–70.
119. Lejon V, Buscher P. Cerebrospinal fluid in human African trypanosomiasis: a key to diagnosis, therapeutic decision and post-treatment follow up. *Trop Med Int Health* 2005;10:395–403.
120. Levav M, Mirsky AF, Cruz ME, Cruz I. Neurocysticercosis and performance on neuropsychologic tests: a family study in Ecuador. *Am J Trop Med Hyg* 1995;53:552–7.
121. Li YX, Ramashye H, Yin B, et al. Migration: a notable feature of cerebral sparganosis on follow-up MR imaging. *AJNR Am J Neuroradiol* 2013;34:327–33.
122. Limaien F, Bellil S, Bellil K, et al. Primary hydatidosis of the CNS: a retrospective study of 39 Tunisian cases. *Clin Neurol Neurosurg* 2010;112:23–8.
123. Lino RS, Reis LC, Reis MA, Gobbi H, Teixeira VPA. Hypothalamic neurocysticercosis as a possible cause of obesity. *Trans R Soc Trop Med Hyg* 2000;94:294.
124. Lino-Junior RS, Faleiros AC, Vinaud MC, et al. Anatomopathological aspects of neurocysticercosis in autopsied patients. *Arq Neuropsiquiatr* 2007;65:87–91.
125. Lowichik A, Siegel JD. Parasitic infections of the central nervous system in children. Part I: Congenital infections and meningoencephalitis. *J Child Neurol* 1995;10:4–17.
126. Lucas SB, Hounnou A, Peacock CS, et al. The mortality and pathology of HIV disease in a West African city. *AIDS* 1993;7:1569–79.
127. Lucas SB, Hounnou A, Bell JE, et al. Severe cerebral swelling is not observed in children dying with malaria. *Q J Med* 1996;89:351–3.
128. Magnaval JF, Galindo V, Glickman LT, Clanet M. Human *Toxocara* infection of the central nervous system and neurological disorders: a case control study. *Parasitology* 1997;115:537–43.
129. Mahadevan A, Dwarakanath S, Pai S, et al. Cerebral coenurosis mimicking hydatid disease – report of two cases from South India. *Clin Neuropathol* 2011;30:28–32.
130. Mahler-Araújo MB, Chimelli L. Automonic dysfunction in Chagas' disease: lack of participation of the vagus nerve. *Trans R Soc Trop Med Hyg* 2000;94:408.
131. Mandell GL, Bennet JE, Dolin R. *Mandell, Douglas & Bennet's principles and practice of infectious diseases.* Churchill Livingstone Elsevier, Philadelphia, 2009.
132. Maneerat Y, Viriyavejakul P, Punpoowong B, et al. Inducible nitric oxide synthase expression is increased in the brain in fatal cerebral malaria. *Histopathology* 2000;37:269–77.
133. Marchiafava E, Bignami A. On summer-autumnal malaria fevers. In: *Malaria and the parasites of malarial fevers*, Vol. 150. The Syndenham Society, London, 1894: 1–234.
134. Marciano-Cabral F, Cabral G. *Acanthamoeba* spp as agents of disease in humans. *Clin Microbiol Rev* 2003;16:273–307.
135. Martin-Blondel G, Alvarez M, Delobel P, et al. Toxoplasma encephalitis IRIS in HIV-infected patients: a case series and review of the literature. *J Neurol Neurosurg Psychiatry* 2012;82:691–3.
136. Martinez AJ, Visvesvara GS. Laboratory diagnosis of pathogenic free-living amoebas: Naegleria, Acanthamoeba, and Leptomyxid. *Clin Lab Med* 1991;11:861–72.
137. Martinez AJ, Visvesvara GS. Free-living, amphizoic and opportunistic amebas. *Brain Pathol* 1997;7:583–98.
138. Marx C, Lin J, Masruha MR, et al. Toxocariasis of the CNS simulating acute disseminated encephalomyelitis. *Neurology* 2007;69:806–7.
139. Mathai E, David S. Intraocular filariasis due to *Wuchereria bancrofti. Trans R Soc Trop Med Hyg* 2000;94:317–18.
140. Matias G, Canas N, Antunes I, Vale J. Post-malaria neurologic syndrome. *Acta Med Port* 2008;21:387–90.
141. Matin A, Siddiqui R, Jayasekera S, Khan NA. Increasing importance of *Balamuthia mandrillaris. Clin Microbiol Rev* 2008;21:435–48.

142. Meda HA, Doua F, Laveissiere C, *et al.* HIV infection and human African trypanosomiasis: a case-control study in Côte d'Ivoire *Trans R Soc Trop Med Hyg* 1995;**89**:639–43.

143. Medana IM, Turner GD. Human cerebral malaria and the blood-brain barrier. *Int J Parasitol* 2006;**36**:555–68.

144. Medana IM, Day NP, Hien TT, *et al.* Axonal injury in cerebral malaria. *Am J Pathol* 2002;**160**:655–60.

145. Medana IM, Day NP, Sachanonta N, *et al.* Coma in fatal adult human malaria is not caused by cerebral oedema. *Malar J* 2011;**10**:267.

146. Meyers WM, Neafie RC, Marty AM. *Pathology of infectious diseases*, Vol 1. Helminthiases. Armed Forces Institute of Pathology, Washington, DC 2000.

147. Meyers WM, Firpo A, Wear DJ. *Topics on the pathology of protozoan and invasive arthopod diseases.* Armed Forces Institute of Pathology, Washington DC; Defense Technical Information Center, VA, USA, 2012.

148. Michailovsky V, Silva NM, Rocha CD, *et al.* Pivotal role of IL-12 and interferon axis in controlling tissue parasitism and inflammation in the heart and central nervous system during *Trypanosoma cruzi* infection. *Am J Pathol* 2001;**159**:1723–33.

149. Moiyadi A, Mahadevan A, Anandh B, *et al.* Visceral larva migrans presenting as multiple intracranial and intraspinal abscesses. *Neuropathology* 2007;**27**:3712–74.

150. Mordue DG, Monroy F, La Regina M, Dinarello CA, Sibley LD. Acute toxoplasmosis leads to lethal overproduction of Th1 cytokines. *J Immunol* 2001;**167**:4574–84.

151. Moreira-Silva SF, Rodrigues MG, Pimenta JL, *et al.* Toxocariasis of the central nervous system: with report of two cases. *Rev Soc Bras Med Trop* 2004;**37**:169–74.

152. Murakawa GJ, McCalmont T, Altman J, *et al.* Disseminated Acanthamebiasis in patients with AIDS. A report of five cases and a review of the literature. *Arch Dermatol* 1995;**131**:1291–6.

153. Naessens A, Jenum PA, Pollak A, *et al.* Diagnosis of congenital toxoplasmosis in the neonatal period: a multicenter evaluation. *J Pediatr* 1999;**135**: 714–19.

154. Nagy N, Ban Z, Beke A, *et al.* Detection of *Toxoplasma gondii* from amniotic fluid; a comparison of four different molecular biological methods. *Clin Chim Acta* 2006;**368**:131–7.

155. Nascimento-Carvalho CM, Moreno-Carvalho OA. Neuroschistosomiasis due to *Schistosoma mansoni*: a review of pathogenesis, clinical syndromes and diagnostic approaches. *Rev Inst Med Trop Sao Paulo* 2005;**47**:179–84.

156. Nash TE, Pretell EJ, Lescano AJ, *et al.* Perilesional brain oedema and seizure activity in patients with calcified neurocysticercosis: a prospective cohort and nested case-control study. *Lancet Neurol* 2011;**7**:1099–105.

157. Newton CR, Warrell DA. Neurological manifestations of falciparum malaria. *Ann Neurol* 1998;**43**:695–702.

158. Nourbakhsh A, Vannemreddy P, Minagar A, *et al.* Hydatid disease of the central nervous system: a review of literature with an emphasis on Latin American countries. *Neurol Res* 2010;**32**:245–51.

159. Offiah CE, Turnbull IW. The imaging appearances of intracranial CNS infections in adult HIV and AIDS patients. *Clin Radiol* 2006;**61**:393–401.

160. Oliveira-Filho J, Viana LC, Viera-de-Melo RM, *et al.* Chagas' disease is an independent risk factor for stroke: baseline characteristics of a Chagas' disease cohort. *Stroke* 2005;**36**:2015–17.

161. Oliveira-Filho J, Viera-de-Melo RM, Reis PS, *et al.* Chagas disease is independently associated with brain atrophy. *J Neurol* 2009;**256**:1363–5.

162. Ottranto D. The immunology of myiasis: parasite survival and host defence strategies. *Trends Parasitol* 2001;**17**:176–82.

163. Pagano MA, Segura MJ, Di Lorenzo GA, *et al.* Cerebral tumor-like American trypanosomiasis in acquired immunodeficiency syndrome. *Ann Neurol* 1999;**45**:403–6.

164. Palm C, Tumani H, Pietzcker T, Bengel D. Diagnosis of cerebral toxoplasmosis by detection of *T.gondii* tachzoites in CSF. *J Neurol* 2008;**255**:939–41.

165. Papadi B, Boudreaux C, Tucker JA, *et al.* Case report: *Halicephalobus gingivalis*: a rare cause of fatal meningoencephalitis in humans. *Am J Trop Med Hyg* 2013;**88**:1062–4.

166. Parke DW, Font RL. Diffuse toxoplasmic retinochoroiditis in a patient with AIDS. *Arch Ophthalmol* 1986;**104**:571–5.

167. Patnaik J, Das B, Miskra S, *et al.* Vascular clogging, mononuclear cell margination, and enhanced vascular permeability in the pathogenesis of human cerebral malaria. *Am J Trop Med Hyg* 1994;**51**:642–7.

168. Pentreath VW. Trypanosomiasis and the nervous system. *Trans R Soc Trop Med Hyg* 1995;**89**:9–15.

169. Pepin J, Meda HA. The epidemiology and control of human African trypanosomiasis. *Adv Parasitol* 2001;**49**:71–132.

170. Pepin J, Ethier L, Kazadi C, Milord F, Ryder RW. The impact of human immunodeficiency virus infection on the epidemiology of *Trypanosoma brucei gambiense* sleeping sickness in Nioki, Zaire. *Am J Trop Med Hyg* 1992;**47**:133–40.

171. Pepin J, Milord F, Khonde N, *et al.* Risk factors for encephalopathy and mortality during melarsoprol treatment of *Trypanosoma brucei gambiense* sleeping sickness. *Trans R Soc Trop Med Hyg* 1995;**89**:92–97.

172. Perkins ES. Ocular toxoplasmosis. *Br J Ophthalmol* 1973;**57**:1–17.

173. Petersen CA, Greenlee MHW. Neurologic manifestations of *Leishmania spp.* infection. *J Neuroparasitol* 2011;**2**:pii N110401.

174. Petry K, Van Voorhis WC. Antigens of *Trypanosoma cruzi* that mimic mammalian nervous tissues: investigations of their role in the autoimmune pathophysiology of chronic Chagas' disease. *Res Immunol* 1991;**142**:151–6.

175. Philip KA, Dascombe MJ, Fraser PA, Pentreath VW. Blood–brain barrier damage in experimental African trypanosomiasis. *Ann Trop Med Parasitol* 1994;**88**:607–16.

176. Pittella JE. Brain involvement in the chronic cardiac form of Chagas' disease. *J Trop Med Hyg* 1985;**88**:313–17.

177. Pittella JE. Vascular changes in cerebral *Schistosomiasis mansoni*: a histopathological study of fifteen cases. *Am J Trop Med Hyg* 1985;**34**:898–902.

178. Pittella JE. Neuroschistosomiasis. *Brain Pathol* 1997;**7**:649–62.

179. Pittella JE. Neurocysticercosis. *Brain Pathol* 1997;**7**:681–93.

180. Pittella JE, Lana-Peixoto MA. Brain involvement in hepatosplenic *Schistosomiasis mansoni*. *Brain* 1981;**104**:621–32.

181. Pittella JHE, Gusmão SNS, Carvalho GTC, da Silveira RL, Campos GF. Tumoral form of cerebral Schistosomiasis mansoni, A report of four cases and a review of the literature. *Clin Neurol Neurosurg* 1996;**98**:15–20.

182. Planche T, Krishna S. The relevance of malaria pathophysiology to strategies of clinical management. *Curr Opinion Infect Dis* 2005;**18**:369–75.

183. Pollner JH, Schwartz A, Kobrine A, Parenti DM. Cerebral schistosomiasis caused by *Schistosoma haematobium*: case report. *Clin Infect Dis* 1994;**18**:354–7.

184. Pompeu F, Sampaio de Lacerda PR. Subarachnoid hemorrhage due to *Schistosoma mansoni*: a rare etiology. *J Neurol* 1979;**221**: 203–7.

185. Pongponratn E, Turner GD, Day NP, *et al.* An ultrastructural study of the brain in fatal *Plasmodium falciparum* malaria. *Am J Trop Med Hyg* 2033;**69**:345–359.

186. Ponsford MJ, Medana IM, Prapanslip P, *et al.* Sequestration and microvascular congestion are associated with coma in cerebral malaria. *J Infect Dis* 2012;**205**:663–71.

187. Prasad LSN, Sen S. Migration of *Leishmania donovani* amastigotes in the cerebrospinal fluid. *Am J Trop Med Hyg* 1996;**55**:652–4.

188. Prasad KN, Verma A, Srivastava S, *et al.* An epidemiological study of asymptomatic neurocysticercosis in a pig farming community in northern India. *Trans R Soc Trop Med Hyg* 2011;**105**:531–6.

189. Pusch L, Romeleike B, Deckert M, Marwin C. Persistent toxoplasma bradyzoite cysts in the brain: incidental finding in an immunocompetent patient without evidence of toxoplasmosis. *Clin Neuropathol* 2009;**28**:210–12.

190. Ramakrishnan G, Petri WA. Pathogenesis and molecular biology. In: Ravdin JI ed. *Amebiasis*. Imperial College Press, London, 2000: 91–112.

191. Rassi A, Amato Neto V, Rassi GG, *et al.* A retrospective search for maternal transmission of Chagas' infection from patients in the chronic phase. *Rev Soc Bras Med Trop* 2004;**37**:485–9.

192. Razek A, Watcharakom A, Castillo M. Parasitic diseases of the central nervous system. *Neuroimaging Clin N Am* 2011;**21**:815–41.

193. Rengarajan S, Nanjegowda N, Bhat D, *et al.* Cerebral sparganosis: a diagnostic challenge. *Br J Neurosurg* 2008;**22**:784–6.

194. Roberts F, McLeod R. Pathogenesis of toxoplasmic retinochoroiditis. *Parasitol Today* 1999;**15**:51–7.

195. Rocha A, De Meneses ACO, Da Silva AM, *et al.* Pathology of patient with Chagas' disease and acquired immunodeficiency syndrome. *Am J Trop Med Hyg* 1994;**50**:261–8.

196. Rodgers J. Human African trypanosomiasis, chemotherapy and CNS disease. *J Neuroimmunol* 2009;211:16–22.
197. Rodriguez S, Dorny P, Tsang VC, *et al.* Detection of *Taenia solium* antigens and anti-*T.solium* antibodies in paired serum and SCF samples from patients with intraparenchyma or extraparenchymal neurocysticercosis. *J Infect Dis* 2009;199:1345–52.
198. Sachanonta N, Chotivanich K, Chaisri U, *et al.* Ultrastructural and real-time microscopic changes in *P.falciparum*-infected red blood cells following treatment with antimalarial drugs. *Ultrastruct Pathol* 2011;35:214–225.
199. Saleem S, Belal AI, el-Ghandour NM. Spinal cord schistosomiasis: MRI imaging appearance with surgical and clinical correlation. *Am J Neuroradiol* 2005;26:1646–54.
200. Schumacher DJ, Tein RD, Lane K. Neuroimaging findings in rare amebic infection of the central nervous system. *Am J Neuroradiol* 1995;16:930–5.
201. Scrimgeour EM, Gajdusek DC. Involvement of the central nervous system in *Schistosoma mansoni* and *S. haematobium* infection. *Brain* 1985;108:1023–38.
202. Sell M, Klingebiel R, Di Iorio G, Sampaolo S. Primary cerebral toxoplasmosis: a rare case of ventriculitis and hydrocephalus in AIDS. *Clin Neuropathol* 2005; 24:106–11.
203. Senanayake N, de Silva HJ. Delayed cerebellar ataxia complicating falciparum malaria: a clinical study of 74 patients. *J Neurol* 1994;241: 456–9.
204. Serpa JA, Moran A, Goodman JC, Giordano TP, White AC. Neurocysticercosis in the HIV era: a case report and review of the literature. *Am J Trop Med Hyg* 2007;77:113–17.
205. Sharma T, Khosla VK, Brar R. Primary extradural hydatid cyst associated with nephrotic syndrome in a pediatric patient. *Child Nerv Syst* 2010;26:1247–9.
206. Sheth TN, Lee C, Kucharczyk W, Keystone J. Reactivation of neurocysticercosis: case report. *Am J Trop Med Hyg* 1999;60:664–7.
207. Silamut K, Phu NH, Whitty C, *et al.* A quantitative analysis of the microvascular sequestration of malaria parasites in the human brain. *Am J Pathol* 1999;155:395–410.
208. Sissons J, Kim KS, Stins M, *et al.* *Acanthamoeba castellani* induces host cell death via a phosphatidylinositol

3-kinase-dependent mechanism. *Infect Immun* 2005;73:2704–8.
209. Solaymani-Mohammadi S, Lam MM, Zunt JR, Petri WA. *Entamoeba histolytica* encephalitis diagnosed by PCR of cerebrospinal fluid. *Trans R Soc Trop Med Hyg* 2007;101:311–13.
210. Stehr-Green JK, Bailey TM, Visvesvara GS. The epidemiology of Acanthoemeba keratitis in the United States. *Am J Ophthalmol* 1989;107:331–6.
211. Sun Y, Hong J, Zhang P, Peng R, Xiao G. Pathological characteristics of the different stages of *Acanthamoeba* keratitis. *Histopathology* 2013;63:862–8.
212. Sundaram C, Prasad BC, Bhaskar G, Lakshmi V, Murthy JM. Brain abscess due to *Entamoeba histolytica. J Assoc Physicians India* 2004;52:251–2.
213. Suzuki Y, Sa Q, Gehman M, Ochiai E. Interferon-gamma and perforin-mediated immune responses for resistance against *T. gondii* in the brain. *Expert Rev Mol Med* 2011;13:e31.
214. Taratuto AL, Venturiello SM. Echinococcosis. *Brain Pathol* 1997;7:673–9.
215. Taratuto AL, Pagano M, Fumo T, Sanz O, Sica REP. Histological and histochemical changes of the skeletal muscle in human chronic Chagas' disease. *Arq Neuropsiquatr* 1978;36:328–30.
216. Tarleton RL, Koller BH, Latour A, Ponstan M. Susceptibility of b2-microglobulin deficient mice to *Trypanosoma cruzi* infection. *Nature* 1992;356:338–40.
217. Taylor TE, Fu WJ, Carr RA, *et al.* Differentiating the pathologies of cerebral malaria by postmortem parasite counts. *Nat Med* 2004;10:143–5.
218. Tekiel V, Losavio A, Jones M, Muchnik S, Gonzalez-Cappa SM. Changes in the mouse sciatic nerve action potential after epineural injection of sera from *Trypanosoma cruzi*-infected mice. *Parasit Immunol* 2001;23:533–9.
219. Turner GD, Mai NTH, Phu NH, *et al.* The neuropathology of fatal malaria in Vietnam. *Trans R Soc Trop Med Hyg* 1995;89:138A.
220. Wang J, Cai B, You C. Surgical treatment options for cerebral alveolar echinococcosis: experience of six patients. *Neurol India* 2009;57:157–61.
221. Wang Q-P, Lai D-H, Zhu X-Q, Chen X-G, Lun Z-R. Human angiostrongyliasis. *Lancet Infect Dis* 2008;8:621–30.
222. Warrell DA, White NJ, Veall N, *et al.* Cerebral anaerobic glycolysis and

reduced cerebral oxygen transport in human cerebral malaria. *Lancet* 1988;2:534–538.
223. Weffort JL. Clinico-neurologic, electroneuromyographic and pathologic aspects of predominantly somato-sensitive peripheral neuropathy associated with chronic Chagas' disease. *Arq Neuropsiquiatr* 1995;53:54–5.
224. Welburn SC, Fevre EM, Coleman PG, Odit M, Maudlin I. Sleeping sickness: a tale of two diseases. *Trends Parasitol* 2001;17:19–24.
225. White JML, Barker RD, Salisbury JR, *et al.* Granulomatous amoebic encephalitis. *Lancet* 2004;364:220.
226. White NJ, Silamut K. Postmortem brain smear assessment of fatal malaria. *J Infect Dis* 2005;192:547.
227. White NJ, Turner GD, Medana IM, Dondorp AM, Day NP. The murine cerebral malaria phenomenon. *Trends Parasitol* 2010;26:11.
228. White VA, Lewallen S, Beare N, *et al.* Correlation of retinal haemorrhages with brain haemorrhages in children dying of cerebral malaria in Malawi. *Trans R Soc Trop Med Hyg* 2001;95: 618–21.
229. Woodhouse JIJA. The prevalence of clinical peripheral neuropathies in human chronic Chagas' disease. *J Army Med Corps* 1993;139:54–5.
230. World Health Organization. Severe falciparum malaria. *Trans R Soc Trop Med Hyg* 2000;94:1–90.
231. Yang YR, Vuitton DA, Jones MK, Criag PS, McManus DP. Brain metastasis of alveolar echinococcosis in a hyperendemic focus of *Echinococcus multilocularis* infection. *Trans R Soc Trop Med Hyg* 2005;99:937–41.
232. Yang YR, Sun T, Zhang J, McManus DP. Molecular confirmation of a case of multiorgan cystic echinococcosis. *J Parasitol* 2006;92:206–8.
233. Zee CS, Go JL, Kim PE, DiGiorgio CM. Imaging of neurocysticercosis. *Neuroimaging Clin N Am* 2000;10:391–407.
234. Zhou L, Luo L, You C, *et al.* Multiple brain haemorrhages and haematomas associated with ectopic fascioliasis in brain and eye. *Surg Neurol* 2008;69:516–21.
235. Zumla A, Savva D, Wheeler RB, *et al.* Toxoplasma serology in Zambian and Ugandan patients infected with the immunodeficiency virus. *Trans R Soc Trop Med Hyg* 1991;85:227–9.

Fungal Infections

Sebastian Lucas

INTRODUCTION

Fungal infections (mycoses) of the central nervous system (CNS) are more common than hitherto thought because of ever-increasing populations with compromised immune status and host defences. This is due to the pandemic of HIV disease and, ironically, to advances in medical care.

Fungi are generally saprophytic organisms that live in the soil and buildings. Man is constantly exposed to them, through aerosol and percutaneous implantation, but can usually mount a defence that prevents disease. A few fungi, such as *Candida*, have become commensals in the mucosae and gut. A larger group cause a primary infection in the lung, which is often non-symptomatic, and induce a latent infection that may reactivate later to cause systemic infection including CNS disease, or remain dormant for the lifetime of the individual.[45]

LOCATIONS AND ROUTES OF INFECTION

Fungal infections (also termed mycoses) are most easily classified by genus, route and location of infection in man. Considering the latter, there are

- superficial fungal infection – e.g. dermatophytes;
- cutaneous infection – e.g. the tineas;
- subcutaneous infection – e.g. mycetoma;
- systemic infection – e.g. histoplasmosis, acquired via the respiratory tract.

For the CNS, the majority of fungal infections are part of systemic infection; the routes are listed in Box 22.1.

EPIDEMIOLOGY

Fungal infections of the CNS were relatively uncommon until recent decades. In part this is due to improved diagnostics and case recognition. However, four other trends are more important, including healthcare-associated infection transmission:[12,15]

1. More people with haematological malignancy, solid organ cancers and organ transplants are being treated and surviving longer.
2. Similarly, there are more patients with debilitating chronic diseases, such as diabetes, systemic lupus, renal failure, and liver failure.
3. HIV disease emerged as a major factor, causing suppression of the cell-mediated immunity that happens to be the major defence against many fungal infections.
4. There is a rise in injection drug abuse and infections from contaminated syringes and needles.

In haematological malignancy, aspergillosis is the main problem. Because of the association with pandemic HIV, CNS cryptococcosis is the most important of all these infections.

BOX 22.1. The routes of fungal infection into the meninges, brain and spinal canal

- Systemic infection from initial primary pulmonary infection, including reactivation of a latent primary infection
- Systemic infection from cutaneous and visceral mycosis (particularly in immunocompromised hosts)
- Systemic infection from mycosis implanted from the environment – including direct spread from scalp skin
- Direct spread from nasal sinus or mastoid cavity
- Systemic spread from infected heart valve
- Acquired as a healthcare-associated infection (HCAI)
  - during neurosurgery
  - from contaminated paraspinal steroid injections

The newer immunosuppressive therapies, such as drugs active against tumour necrosis factor-α (TNF-α), are increasingly reported as risk factors for systemic mycoses such as aspergillosis.[69] In 2012, an outbreak of fungal meningitis occurred in the United States, causing hundreds of cases and many deaths. It resulted from the contamination during manufacture of methylprednisone injectable solutions by *Aspergillus* spp. and an unusual black mould *Exserohilum* spp.[30]

CENTRAL NERVOUS SYSTEM CLINICAL PATHOLOGY

The clinicopathological patterns of CNS mycotic infections are varied and include:

- diffuse encephalitis;
- meningitis;
- focal mycetoma of the meninges;
- space-occupying lesion in CNS parenchyma – granulomas and abscesses;
- infarction from vascular invasion and thrombosis causing stroke;
- haemorrhage from mycotic aneurysm and rupture;
- myelopathy;
- epilepsy.

Many of the mycoses can produce several of these disease patterns at the same time.

CLASSIFICATION

The taxonomy of the vast number of fungus species is changing as new entities are recognized in man and other animals, aided by the explosion of molecular DNA technology; it is a confusing area, as names change and genera relationships are reorganized. This is particularly true with the hyphal fungi and moulds; the yeasts are more straightforward. Many species are dimorphic (both yeast and hyphal form) in that they have different forms in nature and in pathological lesions. Confusingly, although *Candida* is known to all pathologists to be dimorphic in tissues, a few other classic visceral yeast infections may occasionally produce hyphae as well (*Histoplasma capsulatum* and *Coccidioides*). There is also a rapidly evolving literature on the pathogenesis of mycotic infections, particularly in terms of fungal secretions and host responses.

The most common fungal infection to affect the CNS in man is cryptococcosis (because of the HIV pandemic). A list of the most frequently encountered agents is in Box 22.2.

TABLE 22.1 Neurotropic fungi	
Neurotropic colourless fungi	**Neurotropic dematiaceous (brown)**
Cryptococcus neoformans	*Cladophialophora bantiana* (ex-*Cladosporium*)
Pseudallescheria/ Scedosporium spp.	*Exophilia dermatitidis*
	Rhinocladiella mackenziei (ex-*Ramichlodium*)
	Ochroconis gallopava

Some fungi are especially neurotropic, and the CNS can be the only location of disease (irrespective of how the agent arrived there). Visually for pathologists, most fungi are colourless or haematoxyphilic on staining, and known as 'pale-grain' if they are moulds; but some are pigmented brown (dematiaceous or melanized).[31] The neurotropic colourless and dematiaceous genera are listed in Table 22.1.

DIAGNOSTIC TECHNIQUES AND RESOURCES FOR MYCOTIC INFECTIONS

Historically, morphological diagnosis – fixed-tissue histopathology and direct microbiological examination – has dominated the identification of fungus infections, with fungal culture as desirable confirmation. The standard special stains – PAS and Grocott silver stains – are usually more definitive than haematoxylin and eosin (H&E) evaluation alone. In fact, comparative evaluation of biopsies with formal culture has demonstrated that histomorphology is not totally reliable, even in experienced hands. *Candida/Cryptococcus/Histoplasma* can be confused, as can *Cryptococcus/Coccidioides*; *Aspergillus* versus Mucorales genera is a standard confusion; and there are many non-pigmented mould hyphae in human disease that are not *Aspergillus*.[58] These diagnoses matter because drug sensitivities vary between genera, and many fungal infections are virulent and require rapid diagnostic confirmation.

Specification of the yeast infections is aided by their relative sizes – see Box 22.3.

BOX 22.2. The most frequent fungal infections of the central nervous system

- *Aspergillus* spp.
- *Blastomyces dermatitidis*
- *Candida* spp.
- *Cryptococcus neoformans*
- *Histoplasma capsulatum*
- Mucorales genera (including *Rhizopus*, ex-*Mucor*)
- Chromomycotic (pigmented) fungi
- Other mould infections (e.g. *Scedosporium*)

BOX 22.3. Relative size of yeast infections in the brain, as an aid to diagnosis[23]

- Small yeasts (3–5 μm diameter) – *Candida* spp., *Histoplasma capsulatum*, *Pneumocystis jiroveci*, *Penicillium marneffei*
- Medium-sized yeasts (5–15 μm diameter) – *Cryptococcus neoformans*, *Blastomyces dermatitidis*, *Paracoccidioides brasiliensis*, *Sporothrix schenckii*
- Large yeasts (15–100 μm diameter) – *Coccidioides immitis*, *Rhinosporidium seeberi*

Under treatment, some fungi alter their shape and shrink, e.g. *Cryptococcus* can lose its capsule and appear smaller.

Immunohistochemistry for fungus infections has a limited role because the reagents are not widely available or standardized – the exception here is *Pneumocystis*, where the labelled antibodies used for cytological confirmation in bronchial aspirates work well on formalin-fixed paraffin-embedded tissue (FFPE).

Serological antibody and antigen detection has a major role in diagnostic pathways;[17,23] however, apart from cryptococcal antigen body fluid tests, they are not widely available. The major growth area is in fungal molecular diagnostics with polymerase chain reaction (PCR).[26,64] This is becoming the gold standard alongside culture. The test systems, originally for fresh tissue analysis of yeasts and moulds, increasingly reliably work with FFPE. Central public health institutes include PCR in the repertoire for reference diagnostics (e.g. in the UK, the Bristol Mycology Reference Centre).

There is no current comprehensive clinical pathology text for fungus infections. Mandell's classic infectious disease text contains much clinical and diagnostic information.[45] A good, illustrated review of most aspects of the histopathological differential diagnosis of mycoses can be found in Guarner and Brandt.[23] This also includes a comparative overview of the relative diagnostic powers of histopathology, immunohistochemistry, *in situ* hybridization and PCR technology in the assessment of fungal infection.

Diagnostically, most patients with CNS mycoses will have neuroimaging; the radiological differential diagnosis of brain tumour, tuberculosis, pyogenic abscess and meningitis, and mycosis is often not specific, but contributes to the multimodality work-up of patients.[28] The fungal causes of intracerebral haemorrhage are those that destroy blood vessels: *Aspergillus*, *Candida* and *Coccidioides*.

In the following sections, the more common CNS fungi are considered alphabetically and in clinicopathological groups. Because antifungal chemotherapy is now specialized and complicated,[17] references to drug treatment are minimized.

SPECIFIC FUNGAL INFECTIONS

Aspergillosis

Aspergillus spp. are ubiquitous globally. Of the hundreds of known species, the most common pathogens in man are *A. fumigatus* (the majority of cases), *A. flavus*, *A. terreus* and *A. niger*. The organisms are found in soil and decaying vegetation and the infective conidia are inhaled into the lung.[45]

People with intact immunity and host defences rarely acquire aspergillosis,[37] although occasional cases of isolated CNS infection are recorded in intravenous drug injectors. The major risk factors for infection are:

- neutropenia (<100 neutrophils/μL of blood);
- haematological malignancies;[53]
- solid organ and bone marrow transplantation, with immunosuppressive treatment;
- corticosteroid therapy;
- HIV disease;
- alcoholism;
- collagen diseases and their treatment;
- chronic granulomatous disease in childhood.[3]

Aspergillus spreads haematogenously and locally. The most common origin site is lung infection, but maxillary sinusitis can be the source: this is noted particularly in India where working in a 'mouldy environment' is considered the root cause.[48] The fungus typically invades through vessel walls and obliterates vascular lumens, so contributing to the necrosis. Cerebral aspergillosis has the highest mortality (90 per cent) of the invasive aspergillosis syndromes, and is usually associated with concomitant pulmonary infection. The risk of cerebral infection depends on the underlying condition of the patient, and is overall 10–20 per cent of all cases with invasive aspergillosis. Patients with leukaemia and organ transplants have the highest risk. In contrast with cryptococcosis, it is less common in HIV-infected patients. In transplantation, it often develops months after the transplant and is associated with extensive immunosuppression, such as treatment for graft-versus-host disease.

Other sources of CNS infection are the gastrointestinal tract, ear and orbit, and skin following head injury. Diffuse myelitis is also recorded as an indirect immunopathological consequence of treated dural aspergillosis.[46]

Pathology

Brain infection usually presents as a single or multiple abscesses, but may also be granulomatous and solid. Grossly the abscess lesions are necrotic haemorrhagic lesions, with much surrounding oedema. They are located usually in the territories of the anterior and middle cerebral arteries, but cases of subdural location around the thoracic cord are noted.

Histologically, the abscess lesions depend on the underlying immune status of the patient and the chronicity of the lesion. There may just be proliferating pale (hyaline) fungal septate hyphae, about 5 μm in diameter, branching typically at 45 degrees, arranged in a star-burst pattern from a vessel with local necrosis and no inflammation (Figure 22.1); or neutrophils may be present and the lesion is more purulent.

Granulomatous lesions with large giant cells, fibrosis and no necrosis are seen in more chronic lesions and in immunocompetent people, when cell-mediated immunity is more preserved; the hyphae are more scanty and broken up, and the histology is parallel to that of chronic fibrosing paranasal aspergillosis. Eosinophils may also be present in these lesions. Mycotic aneurysms can develop from disseminated aspergillus infection, with thrombosis and subarachnoid haemorrhage.

Importantly, *Aspergillus* spp. are *not* the only pale fungal hyphae that infect the brain.[58] The differential diagnosis includes *Pseudallescheria/Scedosporium* (see later), *Paecilomyces* and *Fusarium* species – all of which can look similar to *Aspergillus*. It is here that PCR diagnostics plays an increasing role. The distinction morphologically from the Mucorales (see later) is vital since the treatment is different; the latter are much wider than the other hyphae, with thinner walls and more bizarre morphology and without septa.

Blastomycosis

Blastomyces dermatitidis is endemic in the southern United States, Africa, India, the Middle East, and Central

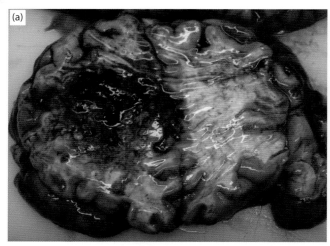

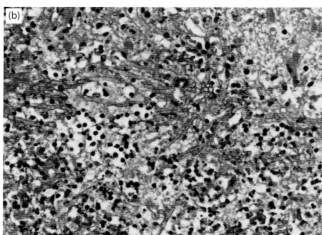

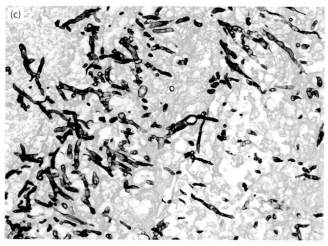

22.1 Aspergillosis. (a) Necrotic and haemorrhagic cerebral lesion, with oedema. **(b)** Typically radiating septate hyphae, with associated necrosis. **(c)** Septate hyphae, with angular branching and typical variation in width of hypha. Grocott stain.

and South America. It is not indigenous to Europe, but can be imported in travellers. The fungus resides in the soil. Infection is via the lung, with dissemination to many organs, including the CNS.[45]

In the normal host, CNS disease is uncommon, reported in less than 5 per cent of cases.[14] HIV is a particular

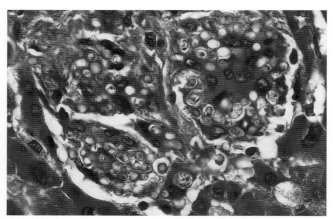

22.2 Blastomycosis. Granulomatous lesion with many yeasts of *Blastomyces dermatitidis*. The yeasts have thick walls, evident nuclear material and broad-based budding.

predisposing factor, with 40 per cent of those with advanced HIV disease and blastomycosis having CNS lesions.[54] The presentation is with meningitis, meningoencephalitis, single or multiple abscesses, or dural abscess. The spinal cord may also be affected with radiculopathy. Hydrocephalus resulting from cranial osteomyelitis and obstructive meningeal infection are also recorded, as is hypopituitism.[1]

Histopathologically, the reaction is primarily granulomatous but may also include acute inflammatory cells.[23] In abscesses, the centre is caseous, and in the brain and elsewhere blastomycosis and tuberculosis may be indistinguishable clinicopathologically.[57] Sometimes, blastomycotic meningitis is very suppurative, mimicking pyogenic infection.[25] The fungi are medium-sized yeasts 8–15 µm in diameter, with a thick refractile cell wall. In contrast to *Cryptococcus*, the yeasts have a more solid-appearing body, and cell division is by budding with a typically broad base (Figure 22.2). The fungi are seen within macrophages.

Candidiasis

There are more than 150 species of *Candida* genus, but only nine are regarded as frequent human pathogens, the most common being C. *albicans*. C. *veronae* is also noted as a CNS infection. As well as living in soil, food and hospital environments, *Candida* is a normal commensal on skin, in the gut and airways and in the vagina. The infection is globally distributed.[45]

CNS infection is very uncommon unless the host defences are abnormal. The major risk factors for this are:

- neonatal intensive care,[47] particularly in premature babies;
- HIV infection;
- diabetes;
- haematological malignancy and lymphoma;
- intravenous drug injection;
- ventricular shunt infection, neurosurgery and lumbar puncture.[39]

Clinically, the signs are those of meningitis and single or multiple parenchymal lesions. Usually, patients with CNS candidiasis also have other organ infection, including kidney and heart, from candidaemia. Grossly, the lesions may resemble those of aspergillosis, being haemorrhagic necroses (Figure 22.3). In more chronic cases, they are solid and granulomatous.

Diagnosis in life is made by lumbar puncture and direct examination of cerebrospinal fluid (CSF) and culture. Histopathologically, there is a very variable mixture of necrosis, acute inflammation, granulomas and vasculitis with thrombotic obstruction. The fungi are characteristically dimorphic in tissues: there are budding yeasts (3–5 µm diameter) and pseudohyphae (strings of budding cells, often elongated and thus resembling true tubular hyphae) together (Figure 22.3). On H&E, the fungi are rather basophilic, and they stain well with PAS and silver stains.[23]

Untreated, the mortality is very high, in part because of multiorgan disease.

Coccidioidomycosis

Coccidioides immitis is endemic in the semi-arid soils of the southern United States, central America and many countries in South America. Travellers visiting these regions can bring the infection to anywhere in the world and present clinically. In endemic areas, up to 50 per cent of people may be infected, mostly subclinically, but the lung lesion is a latent infection that can reactivate.[45]

Coccidioidomycosis is primarily a pulmonary infection, and the common lesion is a pulmonary granulomatous fibronecrotic nodule that resembles tuberculosis. In about 0.5 per cent of those infected, there is extrapulmonary spread, of which meningeal infection is the most serious. The risk of such spread is greatly augmented by certain risk factors:

- HIV infection;
- transplantation and associated immunosuppression;[36]
- lymphoma;
- steroid therapy;
- pregnancy.

The main CNS diseases are basal meningitis, spinal cord compression by a paravertebral abscess, and intracerebral lesions including cerebellar abscess; one third of cases do not have meningitis.[7] The meningitis may cause hydrocephalus and is fatal unless treated.

The histological reaction to *Coccidioides* is typical of many fungal infections: mixed granulomatous with acute inflammatory foci, and a surprising amount of eosinophilia. More chronic lesions are nodular with a caseous-type necrosis with surrounding granulomas and fibrosis. In HIV-positive patients, the reaction is less granulomatous.[23] A vasculitis is frequent, causing arterial obstruction and infarctive necrosis. Occasionally, it causes dural and cerebral venous thrombosis resulting in haemorrhagic infarction.[35]

Coccidioides immitis is a dimorphic fungus, with mycelial hyphae in the soil, but in man the yeast form is seen. The fungi are highly characteristic histologically because they can be large yeasts 10 µm up to 100 µm in diameter (the largest common yeast infection seen in man). When they also contain numerous tiny 2–5 µm endospores (Figure 22.4), there is no differential diagnosis. Special centres may have specific antibodies that can support the diagnosis. Rarely, hyphae are also encountered as a reversion to the saprophytic form. This appears to be associated with inserted plastic CNS

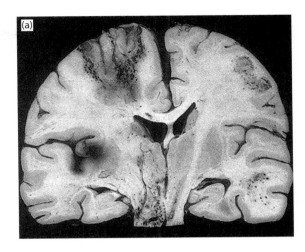

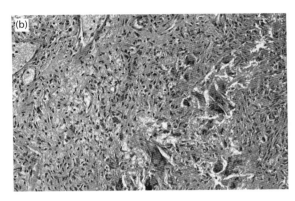

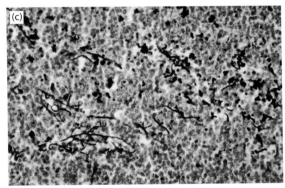

22.3 Candidiasis. (a) Brain showing numerous necrotic and haemorrhagic areas in grey and white matter. **(b,c)** Chronic cerebral lesion from a patient with leukaemia. **(b)** Granulomatous reaction. **(c)** Dimorphic fungal morphology typical of *Candida*: both yeasts and hyphae are seen. Grocott stain.

Panel (a) courtesy of F Scaravilli, Institute of Neurology, London, UK and G Turner, John Radcliffe Hospital, Oxford, UK.

devices, and has obvious implications for diagnosis of the infection. Culture is diagnostic in these cases.[24]

Cryptococcosis

Cryptococcus neoformans and the less common *C. gattii*[10] are fungi harboured in the soil and the faeces of birds. The distribution is global.[45] CNS infection follows infection via

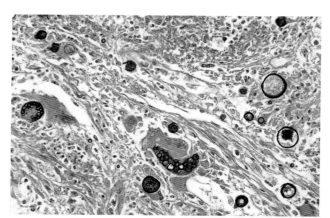

22.4 Coccidioidomycosis. Characteristic large yeast forms of *Coccidioides immitis*, two of which contain numerous endospores. Combined Grocott/haematoxylin and eosin (H&E).

the respiratory tract (i.e. systemic infection), although the initial lung focus is not usually apparent and may have resolved long before the CNS becomes involved. The infection is borne haematogenously to the brain and cord.

The great majority of patients with CNS *C. neoformans* are immunocompromised. The HIV pandemic currently accounts for most such cases. *C. gattii* can infect both immunocompetent and compromised hosts. The other associations are:

- cirrhosis;
- lymphoproliferative diseases;
- transplantation;
- immunosuppressive steroid and cancer chemotherapy;
- sarcoidosis;
- malnutrition.

Early on, cryptococcal meningoencephalitis was made an AIDS-defining condition, and without treatment is always fatal in such patients. However, with treatment, the mortality of cryptococcal meningitis is similar in both HIV-infected and non-infected people, at about 30 per cent.[40] The proportion of HIV-infected patients developing the infection varies according to geography and the availability of antiretroviral therapy. It usually develops only after the blood CD4+ T-cell count has dropped below 100/μL. Globally, 5–10 per cent of patients with HIV will have cryptococcal CNS infection at some time in their disease course, and it is frequently the first specific disease to present clinically. In some African countries in the era before anti-retroviral therapy, 15–45 per cent of HIV patients succumbed to cryptococcosis. It affects both adults and children. After mucosal candidiasis, this infection is the most common mycosis in HIV-positive patients. However, immunocompetent individuals are also affected by cryptococcal CNS infection, in whom it has a more benign course. The syndrome of HIV-negative idiopathic CD4+ T-cell lymphopenia can also present with CNS cryptococcosis.[51]

Clinically, CNS cryptococcosis presents with headache, confusion and dementia, cranial nerve palsies, coma and sometimes focal neurological signs. Imaging abnormalities are often subtle: because of lack of meningeal inflammation, the infiltration may not be very evident on computed tomography (CT) or magnetic resonance (MR) imaging (Figure 22.5). Cryptococcal masses in the parenchyma show as non-enhancing hypodensities or hypointensities on CT and MR.[52]

Pathogenesis

Because of its importance in HIV/AIDS, much work continues on the pathogenesis of this infection.[43] From a cryptococcemia, the fungus appears to cross the blood-brain barrier by passing through endothelial cells.[13,56] The unique cryptococcal capsular material, composed of glucuronoxylomannan, is the major virulence factor and can inhibit host defence responses.[49] It is striking, histologically, how in severe immunodepression there is essentially no host reaction to the fungus; whereas in the immunocompetent and in HIV-positive people who are reconstituting their cell-mediated immunity on antiretroviral treatment (see below), the host reaction is granulomatous. CD4+ T-cells are critical in determining this outcome.

Pathology

The location of infection is usually a meningitis, affecting brain and spinal cord together. Sometimes purely spinal infection or a lumbosacral polyradiculitis may develop. The gross pathology is characteristic in fatal untreated cases. In the immunosuppressed, there is a granular milky texture to the meninges over the brain surface. The brain may be swollen, related to hydrocephalus from blockage of the arachnoid villi by infection.

On cutting the brain, the meninges are perceptibly thickened by pale exudates. The parenchyma is usually also involved, although this may only be evident microscopically. In gross cases, there is a 'Swiss cheese'–like appearance, often around the basal ganglia, caused by gelatinous accumulations of fungi (Figure 22.5).

Microscopically, the fungi are characteristic. They are budding oval yeasts, sized 5–10 μm with typically empty cell contents (Figure 22.5). The walls stain well with H&E, Grocott and PAS stains. The yeast cells are surrounded by a polysaccharide capsule up to 5 μm thick, which does not stain with H&E, although it is coloured by mucicarmine and, to a lesser extent, by Alcian blue stains. Thus, on H&E, the infection often appears rather hypocellular, in a sea of pale vacuoles (Figure 22.5). As well as the meninges, the fungus infiltrates along the Virchow–Robin spaces and spreads laterally into the parenchyma. In advanced HIV disease, there is virtually no cellular reaction in the meninges; only a few macrophages are seen containing yeasts. There is also little astrocytic or microgliotic reaction.

In immunocompetent patients, the meningeal reaction may be granulomatous, simulating tuberculosis, both grossly and microscopically, with Langhans giant cells containing the yeasts. The infection load is markedly lighter than in the non-reactive pattern. This inflammatory reaction is also seen in some HIV patients with usual non-reactive cryptococcal meningitis, who have recovered cellular immunity through treatment with antiretroviral therapy – the so-called IRIS phenomenon (immune reconstitution inflammatory syndrome).[42,61] In such patients,

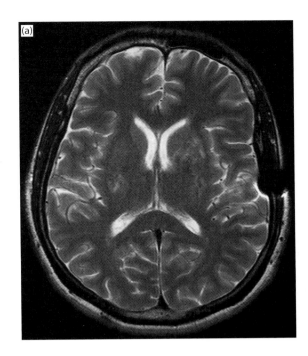

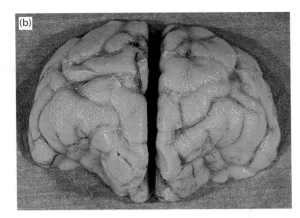

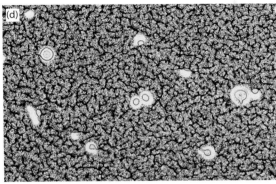

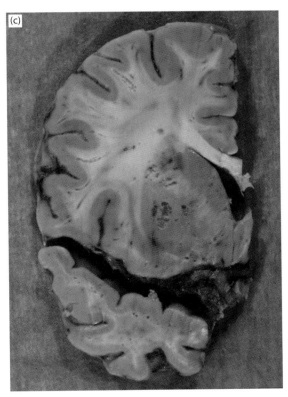

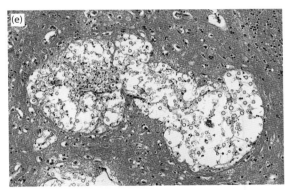

22.5 Cryptococcosis. (a) Human immunodeficiency virus (HIV)–positive patient with cryptococcal meningoencephalitis. Magnetic resonance scan showing no meningeal enhancement, some basal ganglia infiltration, and mild ventricular compression. **(b,c)** Meningoencephalitis in a patient with HIV disease. **(b)** Frontal lobes, showing granular, milky meninges. **(c)** Thickened pale meninges and several clear cystic lesions in the white matter and basal ganglia – 'Swiss cheese' effect of masses of cryptococcal yeasts with minimal inflammation. **(d)** CSF counterstained by India ink, highlighting the encapsulated yeasts. **(e)** Parenchymal aggregates of yeasts, producing the 'Swiss cheese' effect. H&E.

the presentation can be abrupt with seizures, neurological signs, increased intracranial pressure and even rapid death (Figure 22.6). The differential diagnosis between IRIS and progressive infection may be difficult, but quantification of infection load and assessment of the cellular response assist the distinction.

Localized granulomatous lesions – cryptococcomas – were described in the brain in the pre-HIV era, often with no associated meningitis or fungi detectable in the CSF.

Intramedullary and intraspinal cord location of a cryptococcoma is even more rare.[62]

Diagnosis and Treatment

The diagnosis is usually made on CSF samples by direct vision using, classically, India ink background contrast (Figure 22.5). Cryptococcal antigen detection methods (the CrAg test) are supplanting this, in both CSF and

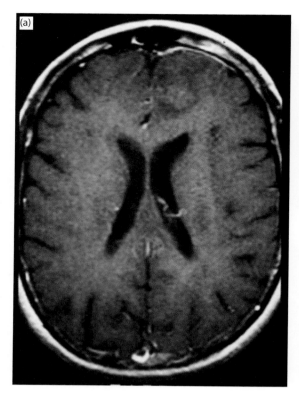

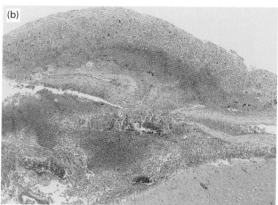

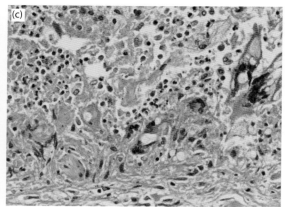

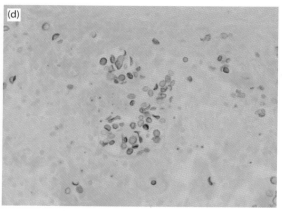

22.6 Cryptococcosis and immune reconstitution inflammatory syndrome (IRIS). A human immunodeficiency virus (HIV)–positive patient with cryptococcal meningitis who developed an immune reconstitution reaction on receiving anti-HIV therapy. **(a)** Magnetic resonance scan showing irregular meningeal enhancement and ventricular dilation. **(b)** Granulomatous meningitis. **(c)** Giant cell granulomatous reaction, with yeasts visible in the macrophages. **(d)** *Cryptococcus* yeasts, varying in size and including some crenated, collapsed forms. Untoned Grocott silver impregnation.

blood samples, because they are more sensitive.[45] Culture of CSF or biopsy material provides further confirmation. Morphologically, the diagnosis is usually straightforward because of the capsule, unique to this fungus. Corpora amylaceae can be mistaken for cryptococci, being of similar size and staining characteristics, and also perivascular, although usually more solid and haematoxyphilic in appearance, and without a capsule. CSF cytological preparations may lack an inflammatory component, and sometimes abundant yeasts may be mistaken to be washed-out erythrocytes.

CNS cryptococcosis is treated with antifungal agents and, in HIV patients, antiretroviral therapy. HIV patients require long-term chemoprophylaxis against recurrence or reactivation of infection unless their blood CD4+ count rises >200/μL, at which point the prophylaxis can usually be stopped.

Ocular Cryptococcosis

Eye involvement by *Cryptococcus* is frequent in HIV patients, causing loss of vision.[34] The fungi can infiltrate the retina and under the cornea. Infiltration of the optic nerve is probably the main pathogenesis of blindness.[45]

Histoplasmosis

There are two species of *Histoplasma* that affect man. The smaller yeast form, *Histoplasma capsulatum*, is the more frequent and important; the African form, *Histoplasma duboisii* infection, has not been recorded to affect the CNS.

Histoplasma capsulatum is widely distributed globally in the soil of all continents, but not in northwestern Europe.[45] It is associated with bird and bat guano. Cases of histoplasmosis in the U.K. are all imported. In highly endemic areas, up to 25 per cent of the population will acquire a primary pulmonary infection, asymptomatic in >90 per cent, which leaves a lung lesion as latent infection.[22]

The risk factors for progressive disseminated infection or later reactivation with dissemination are:

- HIV infection;
- haematological malignancies and lymphoma;
- old age *per se*.

Between 10 and 20 per cent of those with disseminated infection develop CNS disease. However, even in HIV disease, only 1–2 per cent of those with histoplasmosis develop CNS lesions.

The CNS manifestations of disseminated infection are meningitis, mass cerebral lesions and diffuse encephalitis; chronic basal meningitis is the most frequent. Clinically, there is headache, cranial nerve palsy, altered mentation and focal neurological signs. Hydrocephalus is frequently a feature, particularly in those who are not immunocompromised.[59]

Grossly, the meningitis is a grey-yellow exudate. The histopathology of histoplasmosis is determined by its pathogenesis, which is cell-mediated immunity. Granulomas, with giant cells, are typical. In the larger intracerebral lesions, there is caseous necrosis and surrounding fibrosis. Occasionally, a lesion may be so large as to mimic a tumour. As with tuberculous meningitis, there is endarteritis obliterans, with local ischaemic necrosis of brain in severe cases; and with treatment and resolution, there is fibrosis. In immunosuppressed patients, the reaction may be less granulomatous and more of diffuse macrophage infiltration.

The fungi are obligatory intramacrophage infections. They are small ovoid yeasts 2–4 μm in diameter, which divide by budding.[23] On H&E, they appear as small fried eggs, the grey nucleus occupying much of the cell. PAS stains highlight the cell wall, and they appear larger and most distinctive with silver stains (Figure 22.7). The differential diagnosis lies with penicilliosis and pneumocystis, both of which are uncommon in the CNS. Occasionally, *Histoplasma capsulatum* can present with rather larger yeast forms and so cause confusion with *Cryptococcus* and *Blastomyces*.

Paracoccidioidomycosis

Paracoccidioides brasiliensis is endemic in Latin America from Mexico to Argentina.[45] It is primarily a lung infection, with dissemination to other organs, including uncommonly to the CNS. It causes intracerebral mass lesions, most commonly meningitis, and eye infections, and it is associated with HIV infection.[19,20] The organism is histologically characteristic, with multiple small yeasts, 4–5 μm in diameter, budding from a central medium-sized yeast (up to 60 μm), so resembling 'Mickey Mouse ears' (Figure 22.8).[23]

Penicilliosis

Of the many species of *Penicillium* genus, *P. marneffei* has become clinically important because it is an opportunistic infection associated with HIV infection. It is restricted geographically to Southeast Asia and China, but will be encountered in people who have acquired the infection there and travelled to anywhere else.[45] Visceral infection (all organs)

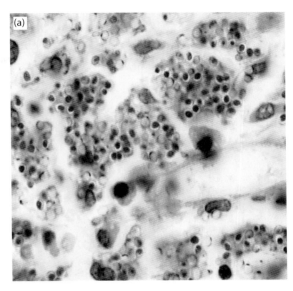

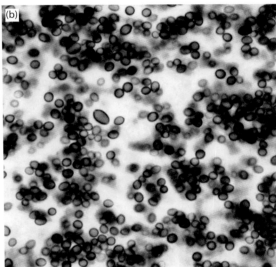

22.7 Histoplasmosis. The organisms appear as oval bodies when stained with either **(a)** periodic acid–Schiff (PAS) or **(b)** methenamine silver. PAS and methenamine silver stains show the real size of the organisms; they are much smaller in H&E stains, which reveal only their central part.

Images courtesy of F Scaravilli, Institute of Neurology, London, UK and G Turner, John Radcliffe Hospital, Oxford, UK.

and meningitis are reported in HIV-infected patients. The small fungus is very similar to *Histoplasma capsulatum* in size and shape, but divides by splitting instead of budding (Figure 22.9).

There are case reports of other *Pencillium* spp. causing brain abscess in HIV-negative people.[50]

Pneumocystosis

Pneumocystis jirovecii (ex-*carinii*) infection is one of the prototypical opportunistic diseases that became clinically prominent with the HIV pandemic.[45] Normally it affects just the lungs, but about 2 per cent of patients in the era

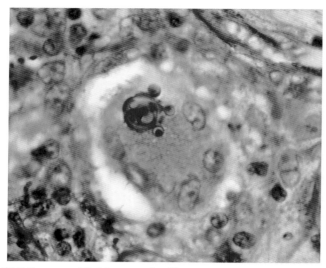

22.8 Paracoccidioidomycosis. Characteristic yeast with small satellites, resembling a ship's steering wheel. Periodic acid–Schiff (PAS) stain.

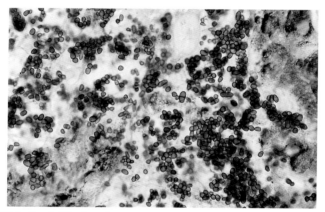

22.9 Penicilliosis. Small fungal yeasts, closely resembling *Histoplasma capsulatum*, but they show splitting as well as budding. Grocott stain.

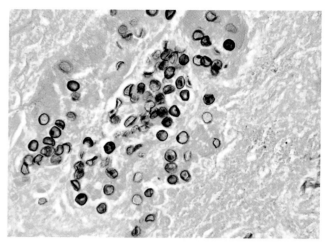

22.10 Pneumocystosis. *Pneumocystis* yeasts with characteristic shape (some crenated) and the dense dot on the cell wall. Grocott stain.

Infection occurs by inhalation, contamination of nasal mucosa and inoculation through the skin. Risk factors for infection include HIV infection with low CD4+ T-cell count,[65] transplantation, diabetes, ventriculoperitoneal shunt and intravenous drug injection. CNS infection is a noted feature: for example, half of solid-organ transplant recipients with pseudallescheriasis had CNS involvement.[11] Another particular clinical subset includes the survivors of drowning.[33] CNS infection is via the lung or nose and the clinical course is prolonged, but with a 70 per cent mortality even in the immunocompetent. The brain is the main organ affected, with multiple abscesses, but there is often visceral dissemination as well.

The cerebral disease is meningitis and cerebral abscess. Pathologically, around the septate non-pigmented hyphae and necrosis is a mixed neutrophilic and granulomatous reaction. Vascular obstruction and local cerebral infarction is common. Another pathological form of CNS pseudallescheriasis is the intraspinal mycetoma (see later).

Sporotrichosis

Sporothrix schenckii infection is global, from the soil[45] and mainly a cutaneous infection that can slowly extend proximally via lymphatics to cause so-called 'sporotrichoid' nodules. Less commonly, there is pulmonary infection that can spread to all parts of the body, including the CNS. Risk factors for such dissemination include HIV infection and organ transplantation with immunosuppression.[18]

This infection causes a chronic meningitis and sometimes encephalitis with small abscesses and granulomas. Histologically, the fungi are 3–6 μm ovoid yeasts that bud. Formal diagnosis requires culture or PCR proof.

MUCORACEOUS MOULD INFECTIONS ('MUCORMYCOSIS'; EX-'ZYGOMYCOSIS')

The causative agents are several members of the order Mucorales; the genera most often encountered are *Rhizopus, Rhizomucor, Mucor, Cunninghamella, Absidia*

before modern antiretroviral therapy developed extrapulmonary pneumocystosis as a late complication. Rarely, it spreads haematogenously to the brain.[8]

Clinically, it causes focal neurological signs, and all cases were diagnosed only post mortem. The sites infected include the cerebral cortex, the meninges, the basal ganglia and the pituitary. The organisms cluster around blood vessels, and are small yeasts similar to *Histoplasma capsulatum* in size; but they are characteristically often crenated and have a silver-positive dot-like thickening on the cell wall (Figure 22.10). Unlike for most other fungi, there are available specific monoclonal antibodies for confirmatory immunocytochemistry.

Pseudallescheriasis/Scedosporiosis

The hyphal mycoses caused by *Pseudallescheria boydii* (anamorph: *Scedosporium angiospermum*) have clinical pathology similar to that of phaeohyphomycosis (see later under Chromomycosis), but are not dematiaceous.

and *Apophysomyces*, with *Rhizopus* the most common.[17,45] The fungi are ubiquitous, being found in the soil, manure and decaying vegetable matter. Morphologically, they are distinctive in being the largest hyphal fungal forms to affect man. They can affect all organs of the body, including the CNS, and are angioinvasive and angio-obstructive, thus causing considerable tissue destruction.

Although CNS infection is reported in previously healthy people,[60] the great majority of those affected have compromised host defences, from various underlying conditions.[45] The most important ones are:

- diabetic ketoacidosis – strongly associated with rhino-orbito-cerebral disease;
- haematological malignancies;
- transplantation and associated immunosuppression;
- intravenous drug injection;
- HIV disease;
- head trauma (particularly noted with *Apophysomyces* infection).[41]

The two distinct clinicopathological patterns of infection are rhino-orbito-cerebral mucormycosis and CNS mucormycosis.

Rhino-orbito-cerebral infection commences with invasion of the palate and orbital cellulitis, then invasion across bone into the basal meninges and brain (Figure 22.11). Cranial nerve palsies are frequent. Grossly, there is black necrotic ulceration of mucosa and bone below the brain. Because the infection causes carotid artery and cavernous sinus thrombosis, there is regional infarction of brain, as well as meningitis.[6]

Cerebral mucormycosis usually develops from a pre-existing focus, most frequently a skin or visceral infection, or following open head injury. Multiple focal neurological signs and cranial nerve palsies are the clinical manifestations. Occasionally, cerebral mucormycosis can develop without any apparent extracerebral focus.[21]

Histopathologically, the inflammatory reaction to the fungi is neutrophilic and necrotizing, and there is invasion through the vessels with secondary thrombosis.[23] Sometimes numerous giant cells, but not true granulomas, are observed. The hyphae are broad and twisted, about 10 μm thick, irregularly branching and non-septate. On H&E, they may be seen only as ill-defined empty holes in the tissues, but silver stains highlight them well (Figure 22.11).

The outcome of these infections is usually rapidly progressive and poor. Surgical debridement of necrotic tissue,

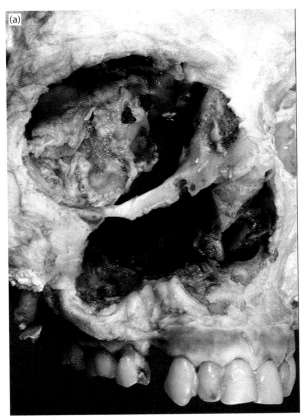

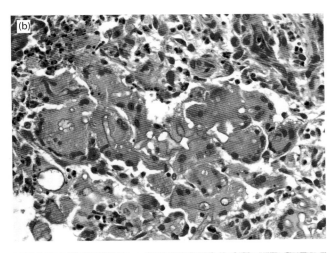

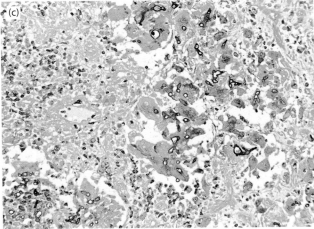

22.11 Mucormycosis. (a) The invasiveness of these fungi. Autopsy skull showing necrosis and destruction of maxilla and orbit in a diabetic patient. **(b)** Bizarre distended thin-walled hyphae. This case has giant cells, which is unusual in the brain. **(c)** The shape of the hyphae is well seen in the Grocott stain. The main differential diagnosis is *Aspergillus* spp., which are not so wide or abnormally shaped (compare this with Figure 22.1c). Grocott stain.

treatment of the underlying condition and amphotericin B are employed, but the overall mortality is 50 per cent or more, depending on the severity of the underlying condition.

Chromomycoses and Mycetoma

Chromomycosis is a term encompassing infections caused by a heterogeneous group of dematiaceous fungi, i.e. those producing a brown melanin pigment, which is distinctive under the microscope as well as grossly if the fungus produces grain colonies. They are globally distributed in soil and decomposing plant material. The genera are numerous and include *Alternaria, Bipolaris, Cladophialophora, Curvularia, Exophilia, Fonsecaea, Madurella, Ochroconis, Phialophora, Rhinocladiella* and *Wangiella* spp.[9,68] Histologically, some of these are yeast infections (e.g. classical chromoblastomycosis caused by, *inter alia, Cladophialophora* spp.), but most are morphologically hyphae, resembling *Aspergillus* in structure. Within these descriptions, the infections look similar microscopically, so to precisely diagnose the infection, culture or PCR is necessary; histopathology alone cannot do this.

Clinicopathologically, they cause a wide range of subcutaneous and visceral diseases, in both immunosuppressed and immunocompetent people, the main patterns being:

- phaeohyphomycosis;
- chromoblastomycosis;
- eumycotic mycetoma.

Phaeohyphomycosis and Chromoblastomycosis

Phaeohyphomycosis indicates the presence of pigmented hyphae in tissue, both extracellular and within macrophages; however, yeast-forming fungi are sometimes also included within this description.[31] Strictly speaking, chromoblastomycosis means the presence of the sclerotic muriform brown yeast forms that divide by splitting, not budding; these are seen within macrophages. Chromoblastomycosis, by this definition, is rarely encountered in CNS infection,[32] because it is mainly a subcutaneous disease. Thus, the majority of the non-mycetoma chromomycoses are phaeohyphomycotic.[16,63]

Infection is usually from implantation through the skin. The CNS infections can develop in immunocompetent people, with no evidence of extraneural infection,[16] presumably by haematogenous spread. Debilitating conditions associated with CNS infections include:

- fungal endocarditis;
- intravenous drug injection;
- HIV infection;
- renal failure with transplantation or peritoneal dialysis catheterization.

The CNS clinical pathology includes meningitis, cerebral abscess in any part of the brain and diffuse encephalitis. Grossly, the meningitis and abscess lesions are no different from their counterparts caused by bacterial infections. Histologically, the reaction is mixed acute inflammation and granulomas, with surrounding reactive gliosis and

fibrosis. Vascular occlusion may also occur with secondary ischaemic lesions. In the diffuse encephalitis pattern, there is cerebral swelling without a visible focal lesion (Figure 22.12). Microscopically, the fungal hyphae are seen around vessels eliciting a variably granulomatous macrophage reaction with giant cells. Acute inflammation is also present (the 'mixed granulomatous' inflammatory reaction typical of many mycoses).

Intracranial and Intraspinal Mycetoma

Mycetoma – a disease process where the infective agent forms large, often visible clumps or colonies in the tissue – is

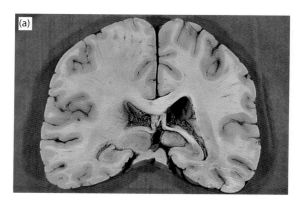

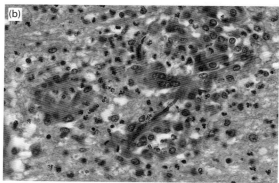

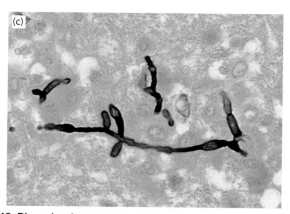

22.12 Phaeohyphomycosis. Human immunodeficiency virus (HIV)–positive patient who died from increased intracranial pressure. **(a)** Brain showing asymmetrical white matter expansion but no visible focal lesion. **(b)** Encephalitis, with a mixed inflammatory infiltrate surrounding pigmented, septate fungal hyphae. **(c)** Irregular septate branching hyphae, consistent with *Cladosporium* spp. Grocott stain.

a chronic granulomatous slowly progressive infection of the skin and subcutis that can spread locally to involve muscle and bone. It is caused by both true fungi of many genera ('eumycetoma') and certain Gram-positive bacilli; the latter includes *Actinomyces*, *Nocardia* and *Streptomyces* spp. and is commonly termed 'actinomycetoma'. Both types can rarely cause intraspinal infection and very rarely intracranial mycetoma.

The pathogenesis of such fungal infections is often obscure in individual cases. Mycetoma infection is typically implanted through the skin, the saprophytic agent being on a sharp plant or other contaminated object. Local progressive spread is usual, and metastatic spread, e.g. to lymph nodes, is uncommon. Intracranial mycetoma following infection of facial or scalp skin and invasion through skull bones is recorded. Intraspinal mycetoma is noted following spinal surgery and intrathecal injections, and episodes of near-drowning in contaminated fresh waters.[38] The former implies contamination during medical interventions, and the latter suggests infection via the oropharyngeal mucosal route. However, many patients with intraspinal mycetoma have no such history[5] and the infection is exclusively intraspinal.

Clinical presentation is usually with paraplegia, sphincter malfunction and paraesthesia. At surgery, the infection may be extradural or involve the dura, which is grossly thickened, and can be local to a few vertebrae or extend the length of many. Grains of the infectious agent may be seen, especially if it is caused by a black-grain fungus (e.g. *Madurella mycetomatis*).

Histologically, the mycetoma colonies are surrounded by acute inflammation within a granulomatous reaction, and there is much local fibroplasia. If it is a eumycetoma, the colonies or grain is pigmented dark brown or may be non-pigmented, depending on the genus (Figure 22.13). Hyphae comprise the grain, with often expanded club-shaped forms (chlamydospores) at the periphery. The fungi that cause this include *Madurella mycetomatis* (black-grain) and *Pseudallescheria boydii* (anamorph: *Scedosporium angiospermum* – pale-grain).[45]

'Actinomycetoma' infections have a similar presentation. Pathologically, they differ because the infection grain is not a fungus but a bacterium. *Streptomyces somaliensis* has been described.[45] The bacteria are Gram-positive filamentous bacilli. A Grocott silver method will stain both eumycetoma and actinomycetoma, but fungal hyphae are >5 μm thick and are usually septate, whereas the bacilli are 1 μm thick and often beaded.

Other CNS Mycoses

There are thousands of other fungal species in nature and, not surprisingly, almost any of them can rarely affect the CNS of man under special conditions of exposure,

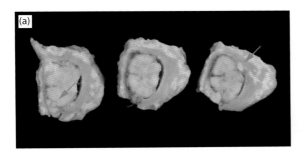

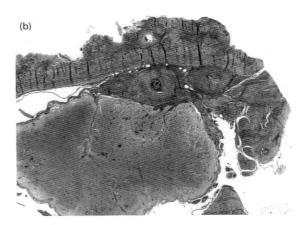

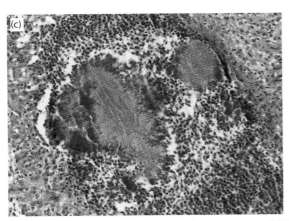

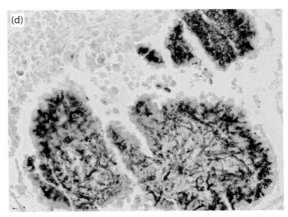

22.13 Mycetoma. Patient with spinal cord compression. **(a)** Horizontal slices through cervical cord. The dura is markedly thickened and contains multiple white mycetoma nodules. Further nodules (arrows to some) are present in the leptomeninges. **(b)** Inflammation and thickening of the dura with fungal colonies on both sides, but no invasion of the cord. **(c)** Colony of non-pigmented hyphae, surrounded by an eosinophilic Hoeppli–Splendore reaction, and a polymorphonuclear reaction. **(d)** The colony contains irregular septate hyphae and some bulbous peripheral expansions (chlamydospores). Grocott stain.

medical interventions (e.g. infected intravascular cannulae), infective endocarditis or abnormal host defences. When CNS mycoses are encountered diagnostically, most are categorizable to the genus level (e.g. cryptococcosis) or to the disease level (e.g. pigmented mycetoma) on histopathology alone; however, culture, PCR or serological diagnostic support is always recommended, because treatment and other management options vary according to the genus.

When the fungus is not readily identifiable morphologically, then it is either an abnormal form of a common infection (e.g. hyphae in coccidioidomycosis or histoplasmosis) or an unusual fungus, in which case culture and/or molecular diagnostics are the only means of making the true diagnosis. Some examples of these rarer brain infections include *Nodulisporium* spp.,[67] *Fonsecaea pedrosi*[44] and *Rhinocladiella mackenziei* – the latter appears to be geographically limited to the Middle East, and CNS disease has been diagnosed on cytology.[2,4] The skin infection *Trichosporon asahii* can cause a meningitis following burns.[27]

Fungal Infections of the Eye and Orbit

The most important part of the eye to be infected with fungi is the surface: conjunctiva and cornea. Fungal infections of the eye can happen to anyone, although a particular risk factor is the wearing of contact lenses.[29] Internal vitreous and choroid mycosis may be part of disseminated infection in the immunosuppressed (e.g. cryptococcosis and paracoccidioidomycosis; see earlier). Aspergillosis and Mucorales fungi may involve the eye as part of orbital invasion. Table 22.2 lists the eye mycotic infections.

Fungal keratitis is the most important pathology, with ulceration caused by the fungi. There appears to be an increase in keratitis, presumably associated with increased usage of therapeutic and non-therapeutic soft contact lenses[66] and also more eye surgery, such as penetrating keratoplasty, and application of topical steroids. Over time, the proportion of hyphal infections compared with yeast infections has risen. Non-iatrogenic risk factors include trauma with vegetable matter contamination and agricultural employment.

The pathology is a suppurative ulcerating keratitis, and the diagnosis is usually made on cytology from direct scrape

TABLE 22.2 Fungus infections of the eye

Yeast infections	Hyphal (filamentous) infections
Candida spp.	*Alternaria* spp.
Cryptococcus neoformans	*Aspergillus* spp.
Paracoccidioides brasiliensis	*Curvularia* spp.
Rhinosporidium seeberi	*Fusarium* spp.
	Trichosporon asahii

smears and culture. Identification of the genus of fungus is important to determine the best antifungal agent.

Rhinosporidiosis

Rhinosporidium seeberi is a chronic infection of mucus membranes in cattle and man. Most cases occur in the Indian subcontinent. Previously considered to be fungus, following DNA analysis, it is now known to be a protistan parasite.[45] As well as in the nose, polyps form on the conjunctiva, containing large numbers of the infectious agent.[55] The histopathology is pathognomonic, with large sporangia containing numerous endospores (Figure 22.14).

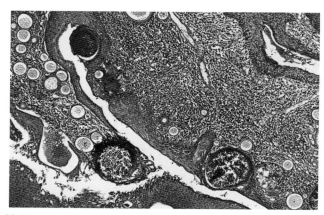

22.14 Rhinosporidiosis. Conjunctival polyp, with numerous small and large sporangia pathognomonic of *Rhinosporidium seeberi*. The large sporangia contain myriad spores.

REFERENCES

1. Abrams E, Dean HJ, Bunge MK, *et al.* Blastomycosis of the CNS in a child: a rare cause of hypopituitarism. *J Pediatr Endocrinol Metab* 2011;24:775–7.
2. Al-Tawfiq JA, Boukhamseen A. Cerebral phaeohyphomycosis due to *Rhinocladiella mackenziei* (formerly *Ramichloridium mackenziei*): case presentation and literature review. *J Infect Public Health* 2011;4:96–102.
3. Alsultan A, Williams MS, Lubner S, Goldman FD. Chronic granulomatous disease presenting with disseminated intracranial aspergillosis. *Pediatr Blood Cancer* 2006;47:107–10.

4. Amr SS, Al-Tawfiq JA. Aspiration cytology of brain abscess from a fatal case of cerebral phaeohyphomycosis due to *Ramichloridium mackenziei*. *Diagn Cytopathol* 2007;35:695–9.
5. Arbab MAR, El Hag IA, Gadir AFGA, Siddik H el R. Intraspinal mycetoma: report of two cases. *Am J Trop Med Hyg* 1997;56:27–9.
6. Bae MS, Kim EJ, Lee KM, Choi WS. Rapidly progressive rhino-orbito-cerebral mucormycosis complicated with unilateral carotid artery occlusion: a case report. *Neurointervention* 2012;7:45–9.

7. Banuelos AF, Williams PL, Johnson RH, *et al.* Central nervous system abscesses due to *Coccidioides immitis*. *Clin Infect Dis* 1996;22:240–50.
8. Bartlett JA, Hulette C. Central nervous system pneumocystosis in a patient with AIDS. *Clin Infect Dis* 1997;25:82–5.
9. Brandt ME, Warnock DW. Epidemiology, clinical manifestations, therapy of infections caused by dematiaceous fungi. *J Chemother* 2003;15:36–47.
10. Byrnes EJ, Bartlett KH, Perfect JR, Heitman J. *Cryptococcus gattii*: an emerging fungal pathogen infecting

humans and animals. *Microbes Infect* 2011;**13**:895–907.

11. Castiglioni B, Dutton DA, Rinaldi MG, *et al. Pseudoallescheria boydii* (anamorph *Scedosporium apiospermum*): infection in solid organ transplant recipients in a tertiary medical center and review of the literature. *Medicine* 2002;**81**:333–48.

12. Chakrabarti A. Epidemiology of central nervous system mycoses. *Neurol India* 2007;**55**:191–7.

13. Chang Y, Stins MF, McCaffery MJ, *et al.* Cryptococcal yeast cells invade the CNS via transcellular penetration of the blood-brain barrier. *Infect Immun* 2004;**72**:4985–95.

14. Chapman SW, Lin AC, Hendricks KA, *et al.* Endemic blastomycosis in Mississippi: epidemiological and clinical studies. *Semin Respir Infect* 1997;219–28.

15. Cunha BA. Central nervous system infections in the compromised host: a diagnostic approach. *Infect Dis Clin North Am* 2001;**15**:567–90.

16. Deb S, Khan SK, Debasish B, Subroto B. Intracranial necrotizing granuloma caused by *Cladophialophora bantiana*. *Neurol India* 2005;**53**:335–6.

17. Denning DW, Kibbler CC, Barnes RA, *et al.* British Society for Medical Mycology proposed standards of care for patients with invasive fungal infections. *Lancet Infect Dis* 2003;**3**:230–40.

18. Donabedian H, O'Donnell E, Olszewski C, *et al.* Disseminated cutaneous and meningeal sporotrichosis in an AIDS patient. *Diag Microbiol Infect Dis* 1994;**18**:111–15.

19. Elias J, dos Santos AC, Carlotti CG, *et al.* Central nervous system paracoccidioidomycosis: diagnosis and treatment. *Surg Neurol* 2005;**63**:S13–S21.

20. Finamor LP, Muccioli C, Martins MC, *et al.* Ocular and central nervous system paracoccidioidomycosis in a pregnant woman with AIDS. *Am J Ophthalmol* 2002;**134**:456–69.

21. Gollard R, Rabb C, Larsen R, Chandrasoma P. Isolated cerebral mucormycosis: case report and therapeutic considerations. *Neurosurgery* 1994;**34**:174–7.

22. Goodwin RA, Lloyd JE, Des Peres RM. Histoplasmosis in normal hosts. *Medicine (Baltimore)* 1981;**60**:231–66.

23. Guarner J, Brandt ME. Histopathologic diagnosis of fungal infections in the 21st century. *Clin Microbiol Rev* 2011;**24**:247–80.

24. Hagman HM, Madnick EG, D'Agostino AN, *et al.* Hyphal forms in the central nervous system of patients with coccidioidomycosis. *Clin Infect Dis* 2000;**30**:349–53.

25. Harley W, Lomis M, Haas DW. Marked polymorphonuclear pleocytosis due to blastomycotic meningitis: case report and review. *Clin Infect Dis* 1994;**18**:816–18.

26. Hay RJ, Morris Jones R. New molecular tools in the diagnosis of superficial fungal infections. *Clin Dermatol* 2010;**28**:190–6.

27. Heslop OD, Nyi Nyi MP, Abbott SP, *et al.* Disseminated trichosporonosis in a burn patient: meningitis and cerebral abscess due to *Trichosporon asahii*. *J Clin Microbiol* 2011;**49**:4405–8.

28. Jain KK, Mittal SK, Kumar S, Gupta RK. Imaging features of central nervous system fungal infections. *Neurol India* 2007;**55**:241–50.

29. Jurkunas U, Behlau I, Colby K. Fungal keratitis: changing pathogens and risk factors. *Cornea* 2009;**28**:638–43.

30. Kainer M, Wiese AD, Benedict K, *et al.* Multistate outbreak of fungal infections associated with injection of methylprednisolone acetate solution from a single compounding pharmacy – United States 2012. *MMWR* 2012;**61**:839–42.

31. Kantacioglu AS, De Hoog GS. Infections of the CNS by melanized fungi: a review of cases presented between 1999 and 2004. *Mycoses* 2004;**47**:4–13.

32. Kasantikul V, Shuangshoti S, Sampatanukul P. Primary chromoblastomycosis of the medulla oblongata: complication of heroin addiction. *Surg Neurol* 1988;**29**:319–21.

33. Katragkou A, Dotis J, Kotsiu M, *et al. Scedosporium apiospermum* infection after near-drowning. *Mycoses* 2007;**50**:412–21.

34. Kestelyn P, Taelman H, Bogaerts J, *et al.* Ophthalmic manifestations of infections with *Cryptococcus neoformans* in patients with AIDS. *Am J Ophthalmol* 1993;**116**:721–7.

35. Kleinschmidt-DeMasters BK, Mazowiecki M, Bonds LA, *et al.* Coccidioidomycosis meningitis with massive dural and cerebral venous thrombosis and tissue arthroconidia. *Arch Pathol Lab Med* 2000;**124**:310–4.

36. Kokseng SL, Blair JE. Subclinical disssemination of coccidioidomycosis in a liver transplant patient. *Mycopathologia* 2012;**172**:223–6.

37. Kose S, Cavdar G, Senger SS, Akkoclu G. CNS aspergillosis in an immunocompetent patient. *J Infect Dis Ctries* 2011;**5**:313–5.

38. Kowacs PA, Soares Sivado CE, Monteiro de Almeida S, *et al.* Infection of the CNS by *Scedosporium apiospermum* after near drowning. Report of a fatal case and analysis of its confounding factors. *J Clin Pathol* 2004;**57**:205–7.

39. Kulkova N, Spanik S, Demitrovicova A, *et al.* Neuroinfections after neurosurgery caused by pathogenic fungi. *Neuro Endocrinol Lett* 2012;**33**:47–50.

40. Lee YC, Wang JT, Sun HY, Chen YC. Comparisons of clinical features and mortality of cryptococcal meningitis between patients with and without HIV infection. *J Microbiol Immunol Infect* 2011;**44**:338–45.

41. Liang KP, Tieyjeh IM, Wilson WR, *et al.* Rhino-orbitocerebral mucormycosis caused by *Apophysomyces elegans*. *J Clin Microbiol* 2006;**44**:892–8.

42. Lipman M, Breen R. Immune reconstitution inflammatory syndrome in HIV. *Curr Opin Infect Dis* 2006;**19**:20–5.

43. Liu TB, Perlin D, Xue C. Molecular mechanisms of cryptococcal meningitis. *Virulence* 2012;**3**:173–81.

44. Madhugiri VS, Bhagavatula ID, Mahadevan A, Siddaiah N. An unusual infection, an unusual outcome - *Fonsecaea pedreosi* cerebral granuloma. *J Neurosurg Pediatr* 2011;**8**:229–32.

45. Mandell GL, Bennet JE, Dolin R. *Mandell, Douglas & Bennet's principles and practice of infectious diseases*. Philadelphia: Elsevier, 2009.

46. Mollahoseini R, Nikoobakht M. Diffuse myelitis after treatment of cerebral aspergillosis in an immune competent patient. *Acta Med Iran* 2011;**49**:402–6.

47. Moylett EH. Neonatal *Candida* meningitis. *Semin Pediatr Infect Dis* 2003;**14**:115–22.

48. Murthy JM, Sundaram C, Prasad VS, *et al.* Sinonasal aspergillosis: a form of CNS aspergillosis in India. *Mycoses* 2001;**44**:141–5.

49. Neuville S, Dromer F, Chretien F, *et al.* Physiopathology of meningoencephalitis caused by *Cryptococcus neoformans*. *Ann Med Intern* 2002;**153**:323–8.

50. Noritomi DT, Bub GL, Beer I, *et al.* Multiple brain abscesses due to *Penicillium* spp infection. *Rev Inst Med Trop Sao Paulo* 2005;**47**:167–70.

51. Nunez MJ, de Lis JM, Rodriguez JR, *et al.* Disseminated encephalic cryptococcosis as a form of presentation of idiopathic T-CD4 lymphocytopenia. *Rev Neurol* 1999;**28**:390–3.

52. Offiah CE, Turnbull IW. The imaging appearances of intracranial CNS infections in adult HIV and AIDS patients. *Clin Radiol* 2006;**61**:393–401.

53. Pagano L, Caira M, Falcucci P, Fianchi L. Fungal CNS infections in patients with hematologic malignancy. *Expert Rev Anti Infect Ther* 2005;**3**:775–85.

54. Pappas PG, Pollage JC, Powderly WG, *et al.* Blastomycosis in patients with the acquired immunodeficiency syndrome. *Ann Intern Med* 1992;**116**:847–53.

55. Reidy JJ, Sudesh S, Klafter AB, *et al.* Infection of the conjunctiva by *Rhinosporidium seeberi*. *Surv Ophthalmol* 1997;**41**:409–13.

56. Sabiiti W, May RC. Capsule independent uptake of the fungal pathogen *Cryptococcus neoformans* into the brain microvascular endothelial cells. *PLoS One* 2012;**7**:e35455.

57. Saccente M, Woods GL. Clinical and laboratory update on blastomycosis. *Clin Microbiol Rev* 2010;**23**:367–81.

58. Sangoi AR, Rogers WM, Longacre TA, *et al.* Challenges and pitfalls of morphologic identification of fungal infections in histologic and cytologic specimens. *Am J Clin Pathol* 2009;**131**:364–75.

59. Schestatsky P, Chedid MF, Amaral OB, *et al.* Isolated central nervous system histoplasmosis in immunocompetent hosts: a series of 11 cases. *Scand J Infect Dis* 2006;**38**:43–8.

60. Sharma PR, Pawar SJ, Delmendo A, *et al.* Fatal rhino-orbito-cerebral mucormycosis in an apparently normal host: case report and literature review. *J Clin Neurosci* 2001;**8**:583–6.

61. Skiest DJ, Hester LJ, Hardy RD. Cryptococcal immune reconstitution inflammatory syndrome: report of 4 cases in three patients and a review of the literature. *J Infect* 2005;**51**:e289–e297.

62. Su MC, Ho WL, Chen JH. Intramedullary cryptococcal granuloma of spinal cord: a case report. *Chung Yuan (Taipei)* 1994;**53**:58–61.

63. Surash S, Tyagi A, De Hoog GS, *et al.* Cerebral phaeohyphomycosis caused by *Fonseca monophora*. *Med Mycol* 2005;**43**:465–72.

64. Susever S, Yegenoglu Y. Evaluation of the significance of molecular methods in the diagnosis of invasive fungal infections: comparison with conventional methods. *Mikrobiyol Bul* 2011;**45**:325–35.

65. Tammer I, Tintelnot K, Braun-Dullaeus RC, *et al.* Infections due to *Pseudoallescheria/Scedosporium* species in patients with advanced HIV disease – a diagnostic and therapeutic challenge. *Int J Infect Dis* 2011;**15**:429.

66. Tuli SS, Iyer SA, Driebe WT. Fungal keratitis and contact lenses: an old enemy unrecognized or a new nemesis on the block? *Eye Contact Lens* 2007;**33**: 415–17.

67. Umabala P, Lakshmi V, Murthy AR, *et al.* Isolation of a *Nodulisporium* species from

a case of cerebral phaeohyphomycosis. *J Clin Microbiol* 2001;**39**:4213–18.

68. Wang TK, Chiu W, Chim S, *et al.* Disseminated *Ochroconis galloparvum* infection in a renal transplant recipient: the first reported case and a review of the literature. *Clin Nephrol* 2003;**60**:415–23.

69. Warris A, Bjorneklett A, Gaustad P. Invasive pulmonary aspergillosis associated with infliximab therapy. *N Engl J Med* 2001;**344**:1099–100.

Demyelinating Diseases

G R Wayne Moore and Christine Stadelmann-Nessler

INTRODUCTION

Demyelinating diseases of the central nervous system (CNS) traditionally have been defined as acquired disorders in which myelin and oligodendrocytes are the principal targets of injury. In conditions with 'primary demyelination', myelin exhibits the initial and most marked damage, and axons are relatively preserved. Because of this selectivity, the heavily myelinated central white matter manifests the most extensive and recognizable abnormalities. The term 'secondary demyelination' is often used to refer to degeneration of myelin as a consequence of axonal or neuronal injury, for example in long tracts following trauma or infarction. Demyelination and axon injury are often concurrent, however, and they can have common pathogenetic mechanisms and physiological effects.

Multiple sclerosis (MS) is the most prevalent human primary demyelinating disease. However, demyelination is a major feature of a broad range of paediatric and adult neurological diseases with multiple aetiologies and is associated with diverse clinical presentations and syndromes (Table 23.1). Conversely, because of their wide range of neurological manifestations, demyelinating diseases are often included in the differential diagnosis of patients who present with unexplained CNS dysfunction or in whom neuroimaging abnormalities predominantly affect the white matter. The major CNS demyelinating diseases, particularly the various forms of MS and acute disseminated encephalomyelitis (ADEM), can be diagnosed only when genetic, metabolic, infectious and other causes (Table 23.2) have been excluded.

Demyelinating diseases are diagnosed on the basis of a complete clinical history and neurological examination and objective data from cerebrospinal fluid (CSF), neuroimaging and neurophysiological studies. The diagnosis of MS often requires long-term and repeated observation and testing to

TABLE 23.1 Clinical syndromes associated with central nervous system (CNS) demyelination

Disease pattern	Examples
Diffuse or multifocal CNS dysfunction	MS, ADEM, leukodystrophies, other inborn metabolic disorders, intoxication (e.g. carbon monoxide)
CNS and PNS dysfunction	MS, GBS, MLD, GLD
Focal mass lesion mimicking neoplasm or infection	Solitary demyelinating lesion
Co-existing pathological processes	
Infarct, trauma, compression	Secondary demyelination/tract degeneration
Infection	SSPE, PML, varicella zoster
Neoplasm	Primary CNS lymphoma or glioma
Systemic disease	SLE, haemophagocytic lymphohistiocytosis
Complication of previous treatment	Treated CNS lymphoma, high-dose MTX or other chemotherapy, X-irradiation injury

ADEM, acute disseminated encephalomyelitis; CNS, central nervous system; GBS, Guillain-Barré syndrome; GLD, globoid cell leukodystrophy; MLD, metachromatic leukodystrophy; MS, multiple sclerosis; MTX, methotrexate; PML, progressive multifocal leukoencephalopathy; PNS, peripheral nervous system; SLE, systemic lupus erythematosus; SSPE, subacute sclerosing panencephalitis.

demonstrate the requisite dissemination of lesions in both time and space.[481,586,587,592] Biopsy of a brain or, even more rarely, spinal cord lesion in cases of possible demyelinating disease is usually undertaken only when there is clinical suspicion of another type of disorder, such as neoplasm or

TABLE 23.2 Central white matter diseases in humans in which myelin loss may exceed axonal loss

Autoimmune and suspected autoimmune (demyelinating diseases)
Acute and chronic MS and variants
ADEM (perivenous encephalomyelitis, post-infectious and post-vaccinal encephalomyelitis)
Rabies post-vaccinal encephalomyelitis
Acute haemorrhagic leukoencephalitis (Hurst disease)

Viral/infectious
Progressive multifocal leukoencephalopathy
Subacute sclerosing pan-encephalitis
HIV encephalopathy
HIV vacuolar myelopathy
HTLV type I- and II-associated myelopathy (tropical spastic paraplegia)
Whipple's disease

Genetic
Adrenoleukodystrophy, adrenomyeloneuropathy
Metachromatic leukodystrophies (sulphatide lipidoses)
Globoid cell leukodystrophy (Krabbe disease, galactosylceramide lipidosis)
Pelizaeus–Merzbacher disease and related *PLP1* mutations
Spongiform leukodystrophy (Canavan disease)
Dysmyelinogenetic leukodystrophy (Alexander disease)
Membranous lipodystrophy (Nasu–Hakola disease)
Neuroaxonal leukodystrophy
Leukoencephalopathy with vanishing white matter and related disorders
Adult-onset autosomal dominant and other genetically defined and familial leukodystrophies
Phenylketonuria
CADASIL
Mitochondrial leukoencephalopathies
Leber's hereditary optic neuropathy with MS-like syndrome

Nutritional/metabolic
Marchiafava–Bignami disease
Vitamin B12 deficiency (subacute combined degeneration)
Central pontine myelinolysis
Hereditary coproporphyria

Toxic
Hexachlorophene intoxication
Solvent vapour leukoencephalopathy
Leukoencephalopathy associated with combined antimitotic medication and radiotherapy
Chemotherapeutic agents, e.g. 5-fluorouracil, amphotericin B, amphotericin B methyl ester
Carbon monoxide poisoning
Heroin leukoencephalopathy

Disorders with varied and overlapping pathogenesis
Prolonged cerebral oedema
Hypoxic–ischaemic leukoencephalopathy (anoxic and ischaemic anoxia)
Cerebrospinal fluid exchange
Multifocal necrotizing leukoencephalopathy
Focal demyelination associated with compression in trigeminal neuralgia
Leukoencephalopathy in patients with AIDS on antiretroviral therapy
Small vessel ischaemia
Vasculitis/arteritis
Congophilic angiopathy with leukoencephalopathy
Solitary focal demyelination associated with paraneoplastic syndrome

ADEM, acute disseminated encephalomyelitis; AIDS, acquired immunodeficiency syndrome; CADASIL, cerebral autosomal dominant arteriopathy with subcortical infarcts and leukoencephalopathy; HIV, human immunodeficiency virus; HTLV, human T-cell lymphotropic virus; MS, multiple sclerosis.

infection, and in cases with atypical clinical or neuroimaging features.

The principal pathological features that in combination define the CNS demyelinating diseases and distinguish them from other predominantly white matter diseases are summarized as follows:

- multiple focal lesions of varying sizes are found virtually anywhere in the CNS, with a particular predisposition to perivenous, subpial or subependymal locations;
- the lesions exhibit perivascular inflammation and destruction of myelin, which is largely converted to sudanophilic neutral lipids;
- there is relative sparing of axons and neurons.

Of these features, perivenous demyelination identified by microscopy is the most specific. Criteria for evaluating the histopathological features of demyelinating diseases in CNS biopsy samples are described in Table 23.3 and discussed in detail later (see Tumefactive Multiple Sclerosis and Biopsy Diagnosis of Multiple Sclerosis, p. 1343).

MULTIPLE SCLEROSIS

Introduction

The first detailed descriptions of MS in the medical literature were by Carswell[133a] and Cruveilhier[171a] in the early nineteenth century.[162] They demonstrated the characteristic MS plaques, the hallmarks of the disease visible on examination of brain and spinal cord tissue. These discrete areas of discolouration and myelin loss are to the naked eye located predominantly in the brain and spinal cord white matter. Later, Charcot synthesized the clinical and pathological features of the disease and defined it as a distinct entity.[141,162]

The cardinal clinical and anatomical features of MS, although highly variable in individual patients, have been consistent since the early descriptions. Advances in diagnostic technologies and in the basic sciences have, however, aided clinical assessment and have promoted progress towards an understanding of the pathobiology of the disease.[411,412,572,758] Neuroimaging of live patients in particular has had a major impact not only on early diagnosis and management, but also in the evolving recognition of the effects of the disease on the entire CNS.[644,757] Consequently, MS is now no longer considered to be a disease limited to readily recognized classic CNS white matter plaques that can be identified either radiologically or at autopsy. Despite this progress in appreciating the scope of MS, however, many fundamental concepts remain unclear. In particular, questions concerning whether MS is one disease or the manifestation of many diseases, and how genetic and toxic/metabolic factors and infectious agents may contribute to its pathogenesis and clinical and pathological heterogeneity, are critical and as yet unanswered.

Clinical Manifestations

The classic clinical presentation of MS is that of a relapsing–remitting disease with dissemination of lesions in time

TABLE 23.3 Histopathological assessment of central nervous system (CNS) tissue biopsies of demyelinating lesions

Method	Histopathological features	Diagnostic considerations
Essential positive findings		
H&E stain	Hypercellularity, vacuolation	Rule out neoplasm, metabolic processes
	Perivascular and parenchymal lipid-containing macrophages	Characteristic of demyelination, but need to rule out infarct and infection
Myelin stain (e.g. LFB–PAS, Klüver–Barrera)	Demyelination, especially if sharply demarcated from intact white matter	Pathognomonic for demyelination
Axon method (Bielschowsky, Bodian or immunohistochemistry for neurofilament, or other axon protein)	Acute axonal injury with relative preservation compared with myelin loss	Axon loss commensurate with myelin loss suggests infarct or necrosis due to the cause
Essential negative findings		
Gram, acid-fast bacilli, fungal (e.g. silver methenamine) stains (also Dieterle, other organism stains)	No organisms	Rule out infectious process
H&E stain	Viral inclusions	Absence militates against PML
	Blood vessel abnormalities (e.g. microthrombi, vasculitis)	Rule out vasculopathic and other vasculocentric processes
Immunohistochemistry for toxoplasmosis, PML, herpesviruses, other organisms	No organisms or evidence of infection	Rule out infectious process
Findings often observed in acute inflammatory/demyelinating lesions		
H&E stain	Perivascular lymphocytic cuffs (variable)	Characteristic of demyelinating conditions, but not pathognomonic
	Mitotic figures	Consistent with neoplasm and demyelination
	Astrocytosis, atypical astrocytes	Reactive 'Creutzfeldt cells' versus neoplastic
	Oligodendrocyte increase or loss	Regional variations in biopsy
Additional studies		
Immunohistochemistry for:		
GFAP	Astrocytosis	Additional lesion characterization
	Astrocyte loss	Consistent with NMO
Aquaporin-4	Aquaporin-4 loss	Consistent with NMO
CD4, CD8, CD20, other	Lymphocyte subsets	Additional lesion characterization
CD68, CD163, HAM-56, MHC class II	Microglia/macrophages	Additional lesion characterization
β-APP	Acutely injured axons	Additional lesion characterization
C3d, C9-neo, myelin proteins	Demyelination patterns	Additional lesion characterization
IDH1 mutation	Negative	Rule out glioma
Lymphoma markers	No neoplastic markers	Rule out lymphoma
Electron microscopy	Variable	Rule out metabolic, other processes
Studies requiring frozen tissue:		
Oil red O stain	Lipid in macrophages	Additional lesion characterization
Additional immunohistochemistry		Additional lesion characterization
Biochemical, molecular analyses		Additional lesion characterization Rule out other processes

APP, amyloid precursor protein; GFAP, glial fibrillary acidic protein; H&E, haematoxylin and eosin; IDH1, isocitrate dehydrogenase 1; LFB, Luxol fast blue; MHC, major histocompatibility complex; PAS, periodic acid-Schiff; PML, progressive multifocal leukoencephalopathy; NMO, neuromyelitis optica.

and space. Unfortunately, many patients at some point in their disease develop a progressive phase of neurological deterioration.

Despite the diversity in the specific symptoms and signs of MS, there are several recognized patterns of clinical presentation and evolution in most patients with typical chronic MS and in the broader clinicopathological spectrum of MS variants (Table 23.4). This clinicopathologic spectrum is evolving, particularly with the emergence of neuromyelitis optica and its variants, as nosologic entities that appear to be distinct from MS.

The mean age of onset of MS is approximately 30 years, but the disease may first be manifest in patients over the age of 50 years and under the age of 15 years. Women are affected more often than men and this gender predisposition has been increasing and currently approaches 3.2:1.[550] Gender also effects many clinical aspects. For example, males more frequently develop progressive disease than do females.[167]

The type and severity of neurological impairment in individual patients are highly variable. The most common initial symptoms relate to sites of lesion predilection and include the visual system (optic neuritis)[691] and spinal cord, the latter resulting in limb paraesthesias and paralysis and bowel and bladder disturbances. Incoordination and gait abnormalities due to brain stem and cerebellar lesions are also common initial manifestations. Cognitive impairment is more common than previously appreciated and has been detected in 43–65 per cent of patients and is frequently present early in the disease course;[26] the degree of impairment correlates with the amount of brain structural damage.[499] Trigeminal neuralgia[433] and other forms of central pain are also common.[551]

Myriad clinical manifestations have been associated with lesions in other distinct CNS anatomical sites in MS, but specific correlations are often difficult to make at the time of autopsy because of the typically long course of MS. Newer neuroimaging techniques (see under Magnetic Resonance Imaging and Its Pathological Correlates in Multiple Sclerosis, p. 1365) have provided additional insight and correlations. For example, lesions in the temporal limbic system have been associated with depression,[71] and lesions in the hypothalamus may be associated with impaired hypothalamic–pituitary–adrenal axis and a worse disease course.[324]

Transient symptoms characteristic of MS include thermal lability (deterioration with a rise in body temperature, exercise, heat exposure or eating a hot meal – Uhthoff's phenomenon), paraesthesias induced by neck flexion (Lhermitte's symptom) and myokymia (especially affecting the facial muscles). Other features include spontaneous episodes of paroxysmal dysarthria, ataxia or muscle spasm, lasting for seconds or minutes and repeated many times in the course of a day, and impairment or distortion of the senses of smell, taste and hearing. Muscle wasting and manifestations of cortical involvement such as dysphasia and epilepsy may also occur. It is often not possible to correlate specific lesions identified either radiologically or even at autopsy with specific symptoms or signs. Moreover, MS may be discovered at autopsy without any documented clinical manifestations.[263,489]

Diagnostic Criteria

The initial clinical presentation of MS is often referable to involvement of only one focal area of the CNS. However, the clinical diagnosis of MS requires the demonstration of multiple lesions separated in time and space. The occurrence of a first clinical episode suggestive of an inflammatory CNS disorder, such as MS, without evidence of other lesions disseminated in time and space is referred to as a clinically isolated syndrome (CIS).[495,737] The subsequent 'conversion' to a diagnosis of MS is largely dependent on the anatomical location of the lesion responsible for the CIS.[495] For example, in the case of optic neuritis, a very common presentation of CIS, the figure varies from 10 to 85 per cent, depending on the study, but generally the conversion rate is quite high.[495] On the other hand, spinal cord CIS and brain stem CIS show conversion rates between 41 and 61 and between 53 and 60 per cent, respectively.[495]

Formal diagnostic criteria to demonstrate dissemination in space and time have undergone a number of iterations,[659] the most recent versions of which are referred to as the 'McDonald criteria'. Initially, they were based purely on clinical assessment, with laboratory data, i.e. evidence of intrathecal immunoglobulin synthesis and delayed evoked potentials, providing supportive evidence.[592] Because of its exquisite sensitivity, brain magnetic resonance imaging (MRI) has been substituted for detecting focal lesions when clinical assessment does not identify more than one lesion (Figure 23.1). Initially, MR imaging was used to demonstrate dissemination in space[481] and subsequently to determine dissemination in time when new lesions are shown to appear on follow-up scans.[586] The latest version, however, allows the determination of dissemination in time on the basis of a single MRI scan if gadolinium-enhancing and non-enhancing lesions are present, simplifying the approach to CIS significantly.[587] The brain MR imaging features used in these assessments are characteristic of MS, but there are no MR imaging findings that are pathognomonic for MS. Current diagnostic criteria have also incorporated MR

TABLE 23.4 Clinical and pathological variants of MS and related conditions
Acute and subacute MS variants
Marburg type (acute MS)
Baló type (concentric sclerosis)
Concentric lacunar leukoencephalopathy
Schilder's type
Chronic MS variants
Relapsing and remitting
Secondary progressive
Progressive-relapsing
Primary progressive
Monosymptomatic and asymptomatic (benign MS)
Disseminated subpial demyelination
Large single or multiple demyelinating lesions (mass lesions, cystic lesions) diagnosed by biopsy that evolve into MS
MS associated with CIPD
MS associated with hypertrophic polyradiculoneuropathy
Optico-spinal MS

CIPD, chronic inflammatory demyelinating polyradiculoneuropathy.

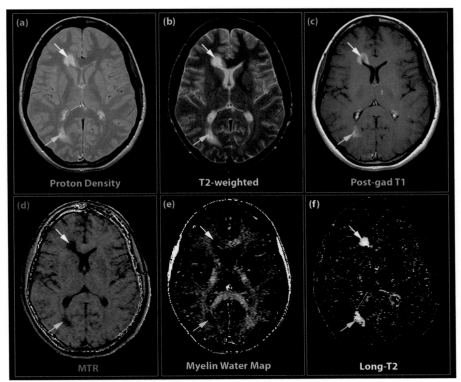

23.1 Magnetic resonance imaging (MRI) in multiple sclerosis (MS). *In vivo* MRI of the same axial slice of brain in a patient with relapsing-remitting MS. Periventricular frontal (white arrows) and occipital (blue arrows) plaques appear as regions of hyperintensity on the proton density **(a)** and T2-weighted **(b)** scans. T1-weighted imaging enhancement with gadolinium-diethylenetriamine penta-acetic acid (gad) indicates breakdown of the blood–brain barrier in both plaques **(c)**. The magnetization transfer ratio is reduced in both **(d)**. Demyelination is evident as a loss or absence of signal within both lesions on the myelin water map (short-T2 component) **(e)**. Both also have a long-T2 component **(f)**, the histopathological basis of which is not yet defined but has been postulated to originate from extracellular fluid. Adjacent to both plaques is diffusely abnormal white matter (DAWM), characterized by an intermediate signal intensity in the proton density **(a)** and T2-weighted **(b)** scans. The remaining white matter not affected by plaque or DAWM is referred to as normal appearing white matter (NAWM).

Reproduced from Moore GR, Laule C. Neuropathological correlates of magnetic resonance imaging in multiple sclerosis. J Neuropathol Exp Neurol 2012;71(9):762–78. With permission from Lippincott Williams & Wilkins/Wolters Kluwer Health.

imaging of spinal cord lesions (Figure 23.2).[587] The diagnosis of primary progressive MS is more difficult, however, because of the lack of dissemination of clinical attacks, and sometimes even of MR lesions, in time and space (see Primary Progressive Multiple Sclerosis, p. 1356). Thus, current diagnostic criteria for MS are based on combinations of clinical attacks and objective demonstration of CNS lesions by MRI. Multiplicity, gadolinium enhancement and anatomical localization of lesions contribute to the assessment.

However, it is important to realise many other conditions may mimic MS.[104] Table 23.5 lists some of these disorders, but despite its length, it is incomplete, because the differential diagnosis of MS encompasses multiple categories of disease and isolated examples of disorders that can produce clinical and/or radiological features that are disseminated in time and space or mimic the clinical progression of MS continue to be recognized.[643] Thus, the consideration of 'no better explanation' to explain the clinical and paraclinical manifestations in a given patient should always apply before rendering a diagnosis of MS.[143] 'Red flags' that suggest that MS may not be the best explanation (but by no means rule out MS) include a gradually progressive clinical course without relapses and remissions from a young age, a family history of a similar disease, early cognitive involvement, sites, shape and extent of lesions that are unusual for MS, involvement of the peripheral nervous system (PNS), constitutional symptoms and indications that other organ systems are also affected.[494,630]

Disease Patterns and Course

Based on an international survey assessing the opinions of many neurologists involved in patient care and research in MS, uniform criteria for the clinical courses of typical chronic MS were defined (Table 23.6).[436] The terms 'chronic progressive MS' and 'relapsing progressive MS' that were used in the past were no longer recommended.

Multiple sclerosis is most often characterized by relapses and remissions of neurological dysfunction, often with a subsequent gradual accumulation of residual impairment following incomplete remissions. Usually, episodes have an acute or subacute onset, with symptoms increasing over days to a few weeks followed by a period of a few weeks with little change and then a period of recovery over 1–2 months. This relapsing–remitting form of MS (RRMS)

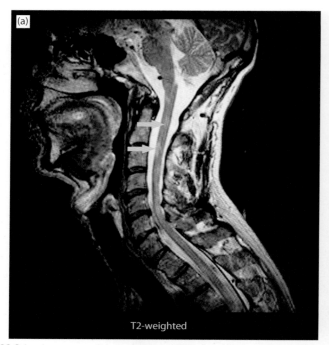
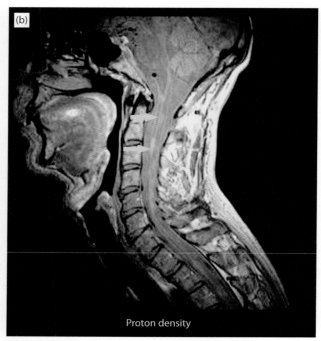

23.2 *In vivo* **magnetic resonance (MR) imaging of cervical spinal cord.** Multiple sclerosis (MS) plaques (arrows) are indicated on **(a)** T2-weighted and **(b)** proton density MR images.

Courtesy of Dr DKB Li, University of British Columbia, Vancouver, BC, Canada.

occurs in approximately 55–70 per cent of patients.[435] The next most prevalent form occurs in 15–30 per cent of patients and begins similarly, but evolves with an unremitting progressive course (secondary progressive MS [SPMS]). Smaller numbers of patients (approximately 10 per cent) have a steadily progressive course from the outset (primary progressive MS [PPMS]), and others have a progressive course with intermittent relapses (progressive–relapsing MS [PRMS]). The latter is the least common of these forms, occurring in approximately 5 per cent of patients. These course patterns are illustrated in Figure 23.3. The temporal progression and accumulation of disability in MS are, however, unpredictable, and although there are favourable and unfavourable indicators, at present there are no clinical or laboratory parameters that can reliably predict the course of an individual patient. With respect to clinical severity, the terms 'benign' and 'malignant' MS are used, with the caveat that their use should not imply that the future disease course progression is known.[436] Moreover, the definition and determination of a benign course over time may be difficult.[669]

Very recently the categorization of MS clinical course subtypes has been revisited and it has been recommended that patients be assessed at least on an annual basis.[436a] Those with relapsing forms of the disease would then be also designated as 'active' or 'not active' depending on whether there is clinical and/or imaging evidence of new lesions, and those with progressive forms be designated as 'progressing' or 'not progressing' based on clinical evaluations.[436a] This would then essentially eliminate the category of 'progressive relapsing MS' since such patents would be designated 'PPMS - active, with/without progression'.[436a]

Acute MS has a distinct clinical temporal profile of an acute monophasic illness, in contrast to the relapsing–remitting clinical course of classic MS. Acute MS is frequently referred to as 'Marburg's disease' and is discussed in more detail under Pathology of the Acute Multiple Sclerosis Plaque, p. 1334.

Survival in patients with chronic MS is highly variable. The length of the illness can vary; in some patients there may be an asymptomatic or minimally symptomatic period of survival until death from another cause many years after the initial manifestation. Many patients with significant neurological deficits survive to die of other diseases, and when MS is a contributing factor it is usually through infectious complications of paralysis and bladder dysfunction. Death in patients with MS can, however, be due to an acute lower brain stem or upper cervical spinal cord lesion occurring either early in otherwise typical RRMS or during the course of acute MS with extensive CNS lesions.[54,609] Overall, in MS the median expectation of life from onset is approximately 31 years, a reduction of 5–10 years compared to the general population.[163]

Epidemiology

Multiple sclerosis is the most common cause of acquired neurological dysfunction in early and mid-adulthood in temperate climates. The incidence is approximately 5–12 per 100 000 in the United States, Canada and northern Europe[201] and the prevalence rate is greater than 100 per 100 00 in these high-risk areas.[376] There are many regional variations in this determination; case ascertainment is

TABLE 23.5 Selected disorders that mimic MS clinically and/or radiologically

Disorder	Representative reference/review
Autoimmune/inflammatory disorders	
Acute disseminated encephalomyelitis (ADEM)	Krupp et al.[393]
Antiphospholid syndrome	Mayer et al.[478]
Behçet's disease	Ashjazadeh et al.[39]
Neuromyelitis optica (NMO)	Sellner et al.[685]
Paraneoplastic cerebellar degeneration	Gracien et al.[275]
Sarcoidosis	Pawate et al.[567]
Sjogren's syndrome	Massara A et al.[469]
Susac's syndrome	Pawate et al.[566]
Systemic lupus erythematosus (SLE)	Kurne et al.[401]
Vasculitis	Ropper et al.[646]
Wegener's granulomatosis	Brinar et al.[106]
Congenital anomalies	
Arnold–Chiari malformation Type I	Wurm et al.[834]
Neuroenteric cysts	Vinters and Gilbert[792]
Indeterminate nosology	
Cervical spondylotic myelopathy	Brinar[104]
Midbrain cleft	Ahmad et al.[13]
Migraine	Absinta et al.[6]
Superficial siderosis	Papadimas et al.[557]
Transverse myelitis	Brinar[104]
Infectious diseases	
AIDS (HIV encephalopathy or myelopathy)	Brinar and Habek[105]
Brucellosis	Karaoglan et al.[355]
Cat scratch disease (*Bartonella hensellae*)	Brinar and Habek[105]
Coxsackie B viral meningoencephalitis	Berger et al.[72]
HAM/TSP	Beeravolu et al.[64]
Hepatitis C	Brinar and Habek[105]
Human Herpes Virus 6 (HHV-6)	Brinar and Habek[105]
Leptospirosis	Brinar and Habek[105]
Lyme disease	Brinar and Habek[105]
Mediterranean spotted fever (*Rickettsia conorii*)	Brinar and Habek[105]
Mycoplasma	Brinar and Habek[105]
Progressive multifocal leukoencephalopathy	Boster et al.[95]
Syphilis	Brinar and Habek[105]
Toxoplasmosis	Brinar[104]
Whipple's disease	Brinar and Habek[105]

Continued

TABLE 23.5 Selected disorders that mimic MS clinically and/or radiologically (*Continued*)

Disorder	Representative reference/review
Inherited diseases	
Autosomal-dominant optic atrophy	Verny et al.[790]
CADASIL	Andreadou et al.[32]
Fabry's disease	Saip et al.[664]
Methionine synthase deficiency	Watkins and Rosenblatt[802]
Methylenetetrahydrofolate reductase mutations	Mavragani et al.[477]
Mitochondrial disorders	Cawley et al.[135]
Leber's optic atrophy	Palace[555]
Leigh's disease	Malojcic et al.[460]
Polyglucosan body disease	Kohler[378]
Tumour necrosis factor receptor-associated periodic syndrome	Hoffmann et al.[313]
Spinocerebellar ataxia	Ratchford and Calabresi[630]
Leukodystrophies	
Adrenoleukodystrophy	Kumar et al.[400]
Alexander's disease	Johnson and Brenner[344]
Autosomal-dominant leukodystrophy	Padiath and Fu[554]
Krabbe's disease	Ratchford and Calabresi[630]
Leukoencephalopathy with neuroaxonal spheroids	Keegan et al.[360]
Metachromatic leukodystrophy	Chebel et al.[146]
Vanishing white matter disease	Lucas et al.[437]
Neoplastic	
CNS lymphoma	Brecher et al.[99]
Glioma	Roytta and Latvala[657]
Gliomatosis cerebri	Taipa et al.[739]
Intravascular lymphoma	Liew et al.[429]
Xanthoma disseminatum	Beard et al.[63]
Prion disorders	
Creutzfeldt–Jakob disease	Brinar and Habek[105]
Neurodegenerative	
Motor neuron disease	Rolak and Fleming[643]
Trauma	
Craniocerebral trauma	Brinar[104]
Toxic/metabolic	
Toxic leukoencephalopathy	Al-Hasani and Smith[16]
Vitamin B12 deficiency	Miller et al.[491]
Vascular disorders	
Carotid artery dissection	Hart and Ahmed[296]
Cavernous angioma	Vrethem et al.[798]
Cerebrovascular disease	Bot et al.[96]

TABLE 23.5 Selected disorders that mimic MS clinically and/or radiologically (*Continued*)

Disorder	Representative reference/review
Obliterating intracranial vasculopathy	Boentert *et al.*[91]
Ischaemic optic neuropathy	Cawley *et al.*[135]
Spinal dural arterio-venous fistula	Wityk[822]

AIDS, acquired immunodeficiency syndrome; CADASIL, cerebral autosomal dominant arteriopathy with subcortical infarcts and leukoencephalopathy; CNS, central nervous system; HAM/TSP, human T-cell lymphotropic virus type 1 (HTLV1)-associated myelopathy/tropical spastic paraparesis; HIV, human immunodeficiency virus.

highly variable, and data from many countries are incomplete. Accumulating evidence suggests that the incidence in different regions is dynamic and may be influenced by migration patterns, seasonal variations and diverse genetic and environmental factors in different populations.[160]

It has long been held that in populations of northern European origin, MS prevalence increases with increasing latitude from the equator in both the northern and the southern hemispheres. Studies have, however, identified exceptions to this generalization.[647] The patterns have become less clear as a result of methodological reassessments and an increasing appreciation of the multifaceted effects of genetic determinants on disease. Moreover, increasingly complex global migration patterns have complicated these analyses further and additional studies point to intraregional variations.

The effect of migration has long attracted interest by suggesting that exposure to an environmental factor or infectious agent in early life affects the subsequent development of MS in later adulthood.[124,403] It was noted that MS has a relatively low prevalence among individuals of northern European descent born in South Africa. For those who emigrated after adolescence from high-prevalence areas in northern Europe, the risk was high, whereas in those emigrating in childhood, the risk was low. Similarly, in Asian and African Caribbean populations migrating to the UK, the prevalence in adult migrants is low, whereas in their offspring it is comparable to that of the European residents.[200a] The nature of the hypothesized environmental factor or factors is uncertain. Most likely, they are an infectious agent or agents (see under Virology and Microbiology, p. 1307), but other factors, including immunizations, diet and occupational exposure, could be involved.[467] To date, however, there has been no unequivocal demonstration that an infection causes MS or affects its course. It is possible that an infection predisposes to the development of MS by sensitizing the immune system of an individual to the infectious agent, and that the subsequent disease is not associated with an active infection, but is nevertheless an indirect consequence of the earlier infection.

More recent studies have implicated sun exposure as the important factor in the explanation of the north–south gradient. There is evidence to suggest this may be linked to low levels of vitamin D, the synthesis of which is linked to ultraviolet light exposure.[295] Moreover, it has been determined that a vitamin D response element (that responds to vitamin D receptor) is found within the HLA DRB1 promoter region of the genome and the haplotype that is involved in this association is HLA-DRB1*15, the very haplotype that has a strong association with MS (see Genetics, following).[295]

Genetics

Considerable epidemiological and molecular evidence supports significant roles for genetic factors in susceptibility to MS.[198,541] Family members of patients with MS have a greater risk than the general population of developing MS: monozygotic twins have approximately 30 per cent concordance; dizygotic twins have approximately 5 per cent concordance; half-siblings have roughly half the risk of full siblings; and adopted siblings have the same risk as the general population.[534,663] The genetic effects are complex, however, and MS susceptibility may result from the contributions of multiple interacting polymorphic genes, each of which exerts some effect on the overall risk, clinical severity and phenotype in an individual.

It has been known since the 1970s that there are human leukocyte antigen (HLA) associations with MS. In most populations, the disease is associated with *HLA-DR2* (for example, *DRB1*1501*, *DQA1*0102*, *DQB1*0602* in northern Europeans).[161,625] To date, class II and, to a lesser extent, class I major histocompatibility complex (MHC) gene regions correlate most strongly with susceptibility and may in part determine clinical course.[282,541,815] Genome-wide association studies (GWAS) have shown the contributions of other genes,[564] particularly those associated with immune responses but these associations are not as strong as HLA-DR2.[542] Given that vitamin D is implicated in MS (see Epidemiology, p. 1302), it is interesting that the gene for 25-hydroxyvitamin D-1α-hydroxylase (CYP27B1) has been associated with MS in a recent study,[627] but not in another.[52] Genetic associations are under investigation worldwide and their effects may vary in different populations. Moreover, there are relatively rare but increasingly recognized genetic disorders, such as those affecting the formation or maintenance of CNS myelin, that can mimic MS.[349,387,800] Patients with such alternative causes for MS-like syndromes could potentially complicate case ascertainment and genetic analyses of MS populations.

The elucidation of mechanisms by which the associated genes contribute to MS susceptibility remains a considerable challenge, as there are multiple potential epigenetic and post-translational interactions that may greatly add to the complexity and heterogeneity of the disease. Moreover, because the majority of monozygotic twins are discordant for MS, genetic factors alone are insufficient to explain the disease, and other (presumably environmental)

TABLE 23.6 Clinical course patterns of chronic multiple sclerosis (MS)

Type	Abbreviation	Definition
Relapsing-remitting MS	RRMS	Clearly defined disease relapses with full recovery or with sequelae and residual deficit upon recovery; periods between disease relapses characterized by lack of disease progression
Secondary progressive MS	SPMS	Initial RRMS disease course followed by progression, with or without occasional relapses, minor remissions and plateaus
Primary progressive MS	PPMS	Disease progression from onset with occasional plateaus and temporary minor improvements allowed
Progressive-relapsing MS	PRMS	Progressive disease from onset, with clear acute relapses, with or without full recovery; periods between relapses characterized by continuing progression
Benign MS		Patient remains fully functional in all neurological systems 15 years after disease onset
Malignant MS		Disease with a rapid progressive course, leading to significant disability in multiple neurological systems or death in a relatively short time after disease onset

From Lublin and Reingold.[436] With permission from Lippincott Williams & Wilkins/Wolters Kluwer Health.

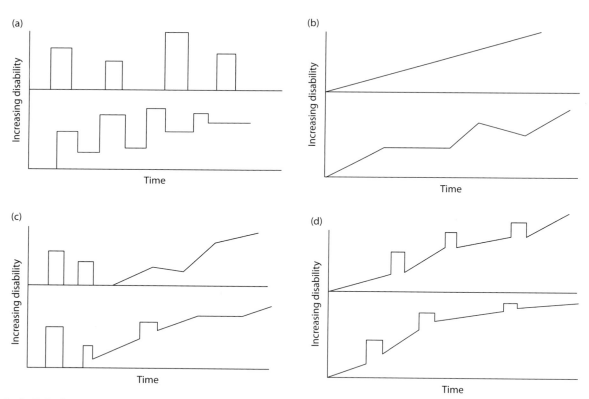

23.3 Typical clinical courses in patients with multiple sclerosis (MS). **(a)** Relapsing-remitting MS; **(b)** primary progressive MS; **(c)** secondary progressive MS; **(d)** progressive-relapsing MS.

Adapted from Lublin,[435] with permission from Elsevier.

factors, as discussed under Epidemiology (p. 1302), are also likely to contribute to the disease.[663] The genes that are currently implicated are involved in the regulation of immune responses, but their effects might not be direct. It is, for example, possible that any one of a number of infectious agents might interact with a genetically primed immune system to produce abnormal responses that result in focal or mild immune-mediated CNS injury. Thus, an initial, otherwise innocuous insult might in turn result in certain individuals becoming prone to further ongoing or episodic immune-mediated damage as a consequence of expansion of their immune response repertoire and auto-sensitization to additional CNS tissue antigens.

Virology and Microbiology

The epidemiology of MS has long been touted as evidence for an environmental factor important in the aetiology and pathogenesis of MS (Box 23.1). Over the years, a variety of viruses have been implicated as the environmental agent responsible for the disease. These include measles, rabies, scrapie-like agent, carp agent, paramyxovirus, coronavirus, rubella, measles, mumps, chimpanzee cytomegalovirus, tick-borne encephalitis flavivirus, canine distemper, Marek's Semliki forest virus, animal and human retroviruses, human T-cell lymphoma virus type 1, parainfluenza virus 1, varicella zoster, human T-lymphotropic virus 1 (HTLV-1), simian virus 5, herpes simplex types 1 and 2, human herpesviruses (HHV) 6 and 7, Epstein–Barr virus (EBV), Torque Teno virus, and Kaposi's sarcoma-associated virus.[348,594] However, despite many studies, to date none of these viruses have unequivocally been shown to be the causal agent of MS.

A number of mechanisms may be invoked to explain the role of viruses in MS. These include non-specific activation of antigen-presenting cells via pathogen-associated molecular patterns (PAMP), molecular mimicry wherein the epitope recognized on the virus is identical or similar to one in the host tissues, epitope spreading caused by unmasking of normally sequestered antigens during the immune attack on the virus, and maintenance or stimulation of immune cells by the virus.[348]

Recently, a few viruses have had a relatively high profile in MS research. These are the herpesviruses HHV-6 and EBV. HHV-6, a lymphotropic virus, has been implicated because of increased viral load during relapses; it has also been isolated from MS tissue, but also from controls.[348]

A great deal of excitement, but associated with the inevitable controversy surrounding the role of viruses in MS, has centred on EBV (also known as HHV-4). EBV, responsible for a very common often asymptomatic infection in young children or infectious mononucleosis in older individuals, is serologically demonstrable in over 99 per cent of MS patients (compared to 85–95 per cent in healthy controls). The association is particularly strong for the EBV nuclear antigens (EBNA), occurring 15–20 years before the onset of clinically evident MS and showing a dose–reponse relationship.[438] Moreover, there is a significantly higher incidence of infectious mononucleosis in MS patients compared to other viral infections.[626] The notion that EBV was important in the pathogenesis of MS was further fueled by the demonstration of the virus in B-cells in MS tissue.[690] However, these findings could not be confirmed and the role of EBV in MS remains controversial.[414]

Human endogenous retroviruses (HERVs) comprise part of the human genome. One, MS-associated retrovirus (MSRV), has been frequently isolated from MS CSF and serum and has been implicated in the pathogenesis of MS. However, it has also been found in other inflammatory disorders but less frequently in controls.[35] It is of interest that RNA of two HERV families (MSRV/HERV-W

and HERV-H) have proviral copies inserted in chromosome region 7q21-22, and another HERV-W sequence is in 14q11.2 within the gene encoding T-cell receptor α/δ chains–both these regions having been implicated in MS susceptibility.[570] The determination of the relationship of HERVs to MS requires much more work.

BOX 23.1. Evolving concepts: MS as an infectious/autoimmune disease

Despite extensive neuropathological analyses and major advances in the understanding of the pathobiology of MS, the earliest manifestations and precise mechanisms of CNS injury in MS and its variants are matters of considerable controversy and the subjects of intense investigation. Cellular inflammatory responses in the CNS have long been widely regarded as the earliest morphologically identifiable and most likely initiating events.[175,609] Using standard gadolinium-enhanced MR imaging, the earliest detectable change in most lesions is an increase in the permeability of the blood–brain barrier associated with inflammation. Indeed, typical early MS lesions in patients who have died when the disease is clinically active or who have undergone diagnostic CNS tissue biopsies[582,774] show multiple foci of inflammation and demyelination. An inflammatory/immune pathogenesis of MS is also strongly, although circumstantially, supported by the known contributions of immune response-related genes to susceptibility and the clinical expression of MS (see Genetics section) and by numerous studies that implicate both cellular and humoral immunity in its pathogenesis.[57,306,612a,721]

Many concepts of the pathogenesis of early lesions have been extrapolated from studies of autoimmune and other inflammatory animal CNS disease models. In these models, immune responses to defined antigens, usually peptides of either a myelin protein or a virus, are induced by immunization or infection. In these models, the passage of leukocytes from the circulation into otherwise intact CNS parenchyma is associated with breakdown of the blood–brain barrier and a cascade of immunopathological processes that culminate in demyelination and axonal injury. Inasmuch as immune responses to many of these molecules can induce experimental autoimmune encephalomyelitis (EAE) in laboratory animals, including non-human primates (see Experimental Autoimmune [Allergic] Encephalomyelitis), they also represent potential autoantigens in MS (Table 23.7). Furthermore, once the disease is initiated, it might progress as a consequence of additional sensitization and increased pathogenetic responses to these potential autoantigens, i.e. 'epitope spreading'.[484] Advances in gene and proteomic array technology have elucidated involvement of many additional potential autoantigens.[19,351]

Unlike the animal models, however, the initiators of an immune response in patients with MS are not known. Early inflammatory responses might represent true autoimmunity, direct responses to as yet unidentified infectious agents (as suggested by epidemiological studies; see Epidemiology, p. 1302), or immune cross-recognition of commonly recognized epitopes of self and foreign antigens, i.e. 'molecular mimicry'.[246] In view of the clinical and pathological heterogeneity of MS, it seems likely that immune responses to diverse self or environmental antigens could initiate the disease and contribute to its progression in different patients or in an individual patient at different times. Multiple responses might also expand, contract and evolve in a single patient over time, thereby obscuring the distinction between autoimmune and infectious aetiologies. The clinical and pathological disease may, therefore, result from a combination of multiple distinct immunopathogenetic mechanisms.

The paradigms of a primary immunopathogenesis of early MS lesions have long been controversial.

Organisms other than viruses may also be implicated in the aetiology and pathogenesis of MS. The occurrence of autoimmune demyelination induced by a bacterium is not without precedence, as evidenced by the involvement of *Campylobacter jejuni* in Guillain-Barré syndrome in the PNS. In this regard, the role of bacterial organisms, particularly the flora of the gastrointestinal tract, in the pathogenesis of MS is being increasingly scrutinized.[537] The role of helminths in MS, particularly from a protective point of view, is also being explored.[203]

Immunology

As will be evident in the discussion of the neuropathology of the MS lesion, virtually all components of the innate and adaptive immune systems figure prominently in its active state. This represents a compelling argument that the pathogenesis of the MS plaque is at the very least immunologic and, in the opinion of many, autoimmune in origin (see Box 23.1). There are many CNS antigens that have been proposed as the offending antigen, but none have been proven (Table 23.7). However, morphology does not necessarily directly translate into pathophysiology. So employing a histopathologic approach alone, it is not sufficient to determine with certainty the relative contributions of components of the immune system to the genesis of MS.

In situ tissue considerations aside, there are many aberrations of immune function demonstrable in the blood and CSF in MS. Although these studies provide *in vivo* data, it is often difficult to say how relevant they are to what is occurring in the CNS target organ. In any event, immunological studies of MS have shown that there is predominately a proinflammatory cytokine response, a relative reduction of cell types that downregulate immune responses, and in the CSF oligoclonal immunoglobulin, all of which again provide strong evidence of an immune pathogenesis.[92]

Experimental immunology has had an important role in moulding the concepts of the immunopathogenesis of the MS lesion. This is particularly so of experimental autoimmune

BOX 23.2. Evolving concepts: MS as a neurodegenerative disease

The more recently emphasized axonal loss in MS has spawned the notion that MS may be a primary neurodegenerative disease. Certainly, there seems little doubt that much of the axonal loss in MS is a secondary neurodegenerative phenomenon, caused by multiple factors generated directly or indirectly by the inflammatory infiltrates and the associated breakdown of the blood–brain barrier in the MS plaque (see Axonal Injury and Loss, p. 1331). However, a very important and fundamental question is whether MS is a primary neurodegenerative disorder and the inflammatory and/or autoimmune features, although obviously very important in the pathogenesis of tissue destruction and its clinical expression, are simply secondary phenomena, possibly due to an immunological response to epitopes unmasked during such a neurodegenerative process. Although such a notion would be considered heretical only a few years ago, there is increasing evidence that this concept should be given proper attention and investigation.[734,758] In this regard, it is noteworthy that in the early stages of the disease, even when the patient presents as a clinically isolated syndrome and the demonstration of dissemination in time and space has not yet been established to make a definite diagnosis of MS, there is evidence of significant axonal loss in normal-appearing white matter on MRI.[493,803] Such widespread changes may also be seen in patients with very few plaques,[181] suggesting that they are not secondary to the plaques in these individuals. From a histopathologic point of view, the earliest changes described in the MS plaque to date, whether it be oligodendrocyte apotosis[54] or degeneration of perivascular astrocytic end-feet[560] occur in the absence of inflammation, again raising the possibility that early events in MS are not due to inflammatory cells. Thus, the possibility that MS is a primary neurodegenerative condition will be receiving increasing attention in the coming years.

(or allergic) encephalomyelitis (EAE), an inflammatory autoimmune disorder of the CNS that is induced by the inoculation of myelin or myelin proteins, or by the passive transfer of T-cells sensitized to these proteins, into animals with the appropriate immune response haplotype (see later under Experimental Autoimmune [Allergic] Encephalomyelitis, in Animal Models of Human Demyelinating Diseases, p. 1387). There are also viruses that induce an autoimmune demyelinating in animals of predisposing genetic background (see under Pathogen-induced Models, in Animal Models of Human Demyelinating Diseases, p. 1389). There is considerable controversy as to the significance of these animal models to MS because they do not absolutely recapitulate the clinical features or histopathology of the human disease. The fact that a given immunological phenomenon can occur in experimental autoimmune demyelination does not necessarily imply that it occurs in the MS lesion. Nevertheless, these experimental models have provided us with a considerable body of knowledge of the immunological reactions of the CNS.

The literature on the immunology of MS and its experimental models is extensive and it is not the purpose of this textbook to review it in detail here. However, here we will translate the histopathological changes of MS into possible immunopathogenetic mechanisms that may be relevant to understanding the overall pathogenesis of the disease. For more detailed information on the immunology of MS, the reader is referred to recent excellent reviews on the subject.[92,156,188,247,536,794,832]

TABLE 23.7 Candidate autoantigens in MS

Myelin and oligodendrocyte molecules:
Myelin proteolipid protein (PLP)
Myelin basic protein (MBP)
Myelin oligodendrocyte glycoprotein (MOG)
Myelin-associated glycoprotein (MAG)
2′,3′-cyclic nucleotide 3′-phosphodiesterase (CNPase)
Myelin-associated oligodendrocyte basic protein (MOBP)
Oligodendrocyte-specific protein (OSP)
Transaldolase
Nogo-A
NG2 and other oligodendrocyte precursor molecules

Other molecules:
α-B crystallin (α-B-C)
Heat-shock proteins
S100β protein
Gangliosides, e.g. GM3
Glycolipids
Aquaporin-4 water channel
? Immunoglobulins
? Other neuronal and axonal protein and lipid antigens
? Other glial ion channel proteins

Aetiological Considerations

The aetiology of MS is unknown. As could be deduced from the earlier discussions, there are two main schools of thought, namely immunological/autoimmunological and infectious (see Box 23.1). More recently, the thought that MS is a neurodegenerative disorder has also emerged (Box 23.2). Still more recently, a vascular aetiology has received considerable attention.

The notion that MS is an autoimmune disease receives support from the finding of many components of the immune system in the CNS, the immunologic perturbations in the peripheral blood and CSF, the strong association with the HLA complex that controls antigen presentation in the adaptive immune response, and the fact that autoimmune demyelination can be induced experimentally.[92]

Of the various infectious agents, viruses take centre stage as candidates for the aetiology of MS.[348] As noted earlier, there have been many such candidates, and whereas serological studies for various viruses have shown increased titres in MS, no such agent has been convincingly and consistently isolated from or demonstrated in the CNS to date.

Many are of the opinion that these two possibilities are not at all mutually exclusive, and that MS is an autoimmune disease induced by a virus that had been acquired earlier in life. Figuring prominently in this scenario is the concept of molecular mimicry, wherein cross-reactivity between a viral epitope and a self-antigen results in an immune response orchestrated by an MS-susceptible HLA haplotype that allows and facilitates the presentation of that particular antigen.[145]

The recognition that there is a significant neurodegenerative component that underpins much of the clinical progression of the disease has spawned the concept that MS is a primary neurodegenerative disease and the immune-mediated events, which are particularly evident in the early stage of the disease, are simply secondary phenomena (see Box 23.2).[734]

Over the last several years, there has been considerable controversy of the role of venous obstruction in the pathogenesis of MS. This revolves around the concept of chronic cerebrospinal venous insufficiency (CCSVI), which holds that MS is due to an obstruction of the internal jugular and/or azygous veins.[844] This had origin in the observation of reflux into the jugular vein of a patient who was undergoing angiography and some apparent similarities in the histopathology of chronic cutaneous venous stasis ulcers and MS, both of which had been reported to show venous thrombosis and perivasular iron deposition.[844] This subsequently led to the study of a series of patients who showed constrictions in the jugular or azygous systems in MS but not in individuals without MS, constrictions in the azygous vein or lumbar venous plexus being particularly associated with PPMS.[846] A clinical study of venous angioplasty on the internal jugular and azygous veins in MS reported an improvement in clinical parameters.[845] This received a great deal of coverage in the media, particularly in some countries, and a lively debate, both in the public and scientific forum, ensued.[631] The histopathology underlying the radiographic venous abnormalities has not yet been reported. Several professional societies, clinicians and radiologists have weighed in on the issue and have expressed caution in the use of these invasive interventions.[51,230,364,632] Nevertheless, these procedures have been carried out in many centres throughout the world, and some of these interventions have been associated with complications.[122] To date, there is no incontrovertible evidence that CCSVI is important in the aetiology of MS.[42] At present, there are comprehensive rigorous scientific studies underway to resolve this highly controversial and high-profile issue,[58] the results of which to date have not supported a relationship between CCSVI and MS.[59,757a,856]

Neuropathology: General Considerations

There are a number of molecular and histopathologic features that are common to all MS lesions and these will be discussed in general terms before the pathology of individual types of MS plaques are presented.

Some of the terms used to characterize histopathological reactions and types of MS lesions are often applied rather loosely and this may be confusing, particularly if being interpreted by individuals from different academic disciplines. This is particularly so of the terms 'acute' and 'active'. In the context of MS, the term 'acute' refers to a short temporal profile of the disease or of a lesion, and not to the types of inflammatory cell involved. Thus, even though it refers to circumstances where there may be a considerable degree of inflammation, it is not to be confused with 'acute inflammation' routinely employed in histopathology to refer to the presence of polymorphonuclear leukocytes (or neutrophils). In fact, polymorphonuclear leukocytes are quite rare in MS lesions, even in the very early stages of their genesis. 'Active' refers to an on-going pathological process in the MS lesion. It may refer to the presence of inflammatory infiltrates or to the presence of ongoing demyelination, but because inflammation and demyelination are virtually inseparable pathogenetically, it usually implies both. 'Active' lesions are in contradistinction to 'inactive' or 'silent' lesions, where these processes are quiescent. 'Early' and 'late' simply refer to the stage in the temporal development of a lesion. As for the term 'lesion', this refers to a focal parenchymal abnormality and, therefore, in MS is usually synonymous with 'plaque'. Although the term 'lesion' is usually not used to refer to a histological abnormality in the parenchyma not involved with plaques, it is now becoming increasingly apparent that there are significant diffuse abnormalities in the 'non-plaque' parenchyma in MS.

Molecular and Cellular Components in Multiple Sclerosis Lesions

The fundamental histopathologic components of an acute MS plaque are inflammation demyelination, remyelination, gliosis, and axonal loss and injury. Each of these will be discussed in turn from the point of their cellular composition and relationship to the pathogenesis of the MS plaque.

Inflammation

Peripheral immune activation probably occurs in patients with MS outside the CNS,[57] but permeability of the blood–brain barrier associated with *in situ* immune activation of endothelial cells and initial infiltration by lymphocytes are currently the earliest recognizable inflammatory abnormalities within

CNS tissue. The precise temporal sequence of these events and the extent of inflammatory cell infiltration necessary for initiating them are, however, unclear.

Lymphocytes are usually recognizable in perivascular inflammatory cell cuffs in early MS lesions, although macrophages can be more numerous. Small numbers of plasma cells may also be seen, but they are generally more abundant in chronic lesions. Neutrophils and eosinophils are observed only very rarely in typical acute lesions, but are more characteristic of neuromyelitis optica (NMO) (see Neuromyelitis Optica, p. 1373). The early inflammatory events and the specific interacting cell types in the inflammatory process in typical lesions are now considered.

Peripheral Immune Organs

The instigating antigen in the presumed autoimmune response underlying the pathogenesis of the MS plaque is unknown. It is generally assumed that the initial antigen presentation with activation of antigen-specific T-cells, as would occur in the molecular mimicry paradigm with cross-reacting epitopes from an antecedent viral infection, occurs in the peripheral immune system. When this event occurs, the activated lymphocyte acquires its functional phenotype (Th1, Th2, Th17 or T reg), downregulates molecules required for lymph node entry and upregulates those that allow it to enter the systemic circulation and interact with endothelial cells.[596]

Endothelial Cells

The egress of activated T-cells across the blood–brain barrier (BBB) is a multi-step process, illustrated in Figure 23.4.[461] The BBB is comprised of endothelial cells that have relatively few pinocytotic vesicles, are joined by tight junctions between adjacent cells and interact with astrocytes in the adjacent parenchyma.[1] These tight junctions are not encountered in the vascular beds of other organs. In order to reach their CNS target, inflammatory cells must attach themselves to and then traverse this tightly regulated barrier. Much of the knowledge in this area has been gleaned from *in vitro* studies or in animal models, examining particularly T-cells. The immunohistochemical demonstration of some of the molecules involved in these processes in MS tissue is supportive evidence that these mechanisms are operative in the MS lesion.

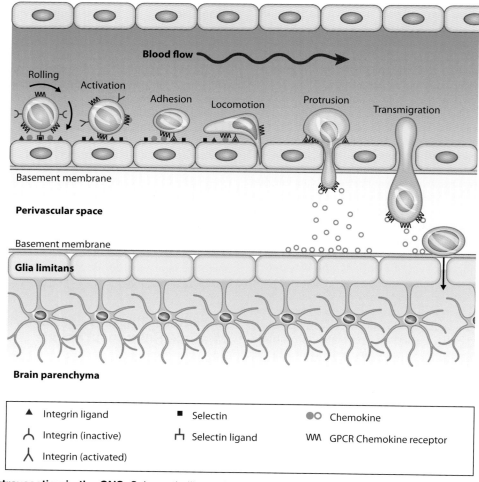

23.4 Leukocyte extravasation in the CNS. Schematic illustration of the mechanisms involved in extravasation of leukocytes from the vasculature through the blood–brain barrier into the perivascular space, and thence into the parenchyma.

From Man S, Ubogu EE, Ransohoff RM. Inflammatory cell migration into the central nervous system: a few new twists on an old tale. Brain Pathol 2007;2:243–50. With permission from John Wiley and Sons. © International Society of Neuropathology.

The first interaction of activated T-cells with endothelial cells of most vascular beds is via glycoprotein ligands on the lymphocyte surface binding to selectins on the endothelial cell surface. This binding slows the transit of the lymphocyte and induces rolling (Figure 23.4). E-selectin has been shown in endothelia in MS,[801] but the role of selectins in MS is unclear as it appears that the capture of circulating activated lymphocytes is an immediate arrest without a preliminary rolling stage in deep CNS vessels, whereas selectins may be more important in leptomeningeal vessels.[317] Such findings illustrate the heterogeneity of the vasculature in the CNS. In the early phases of the interaction of lymphocyte and endothelium, chemokine receptors on the lymphocyte interact with chemokines on the endothelial surface. This initiates, via G-protein signalling, configurational changes in integrins on the lymphocyte such that they have a much greater avidity for their respective endothelial adhesion molecule receptors. Of interest, lymphocytes seem to scan the vessels preferentially against the blood flow.[60] A number of chemokines have been found to be upregulated in MS lesions, including CCL5 (also referred to as RANTES) and its receptor CCR5,[700,720] and CXCL10 and its receptor CXCR3.[48,699] However, these chemokines were not found on endothelial cells. Dendritic cells in inflammatory MS lesions express CCR7.[373] CCL19, which is found in normal brain and is a receptor for CCR7, which is also found on T-cells and B-cells, is upregulated in active MS lesions,[392] as are CXCL12 and CXCL13.[391] CXCL12 has been found on endothelial cells and as such has been implicated in lymphocyte recruitment to the endothelium as described earlier.[317]

The binding of the integrin very late antigen-4 (VLA-4) to its ligand vascular cell adhesion molecule-1 (VCAM-1) mediates the adhesion of the lymphocyte to the endothelial cell (Figure 23.4).[461] VCAM-1 and VLA-4 have been immunohistochemically demonstrated in MS.[130] Antibodies blocking VLA-4 are used for the treatment of patients with MS.[635]

Intercellular adhesion molecule-1 (ICAM-1), which is constitutively expressed on some CNS blood vessels, is significantly upregulated on vessels in MS lesions and there are large numbers of cells positive for its receptor, leukocyte function antigen -1(LFA-1) in these lesion.[84,716] LFA-1/ICAM-1 interactions are important in lymphocyte locomotion and protrusion through the tight junctions between adjacent endothelial cells that constitute a major component of the BBB (Figure 23.4).These events appear to be restricted to the post-capillary venule,[317] again pointing out the heterogeneity within the CNS vasculature. This chemotactic process is mediated by chemokine gradients, because of positioning of chemokines on the abluminal aspect of the vessel.[461] In addition to this paracellular route, lymphocytes traverse the BBB by penetrating through the cell body of the endothelial cell, the transcellular route.

A further adhesion molecule, activated leukocyte cell adhesion molecule (ALCAM), is also important in the interaction of lymphocytes and endothelial cells in the breach of the BBB, and this molecule is also significantly upregulated in active MS lesions.[136] Platelet endothelial cell molecule-1 (PECAM-1) or CD31, is expressed at interendothelial cell junctions and is thought to help guide inflammatory cells to that locale.[317] Recently, Ninjurin-1 (Ninj1) was identified as a key adhesion molecule for activated T-cells to the CNS microvasculature, whose blockade effectively prevents EAE induction.[329,540]

Certain cytokines, which have been demonstrated in MS lesions (see under T-lymphocytes, p. 1313) are also thought to play an important role in the egress of lymphocytes across the BBB,[409] inasmuch as several of these upregulate VCAM[829] and ICAM[828] on endothelial cells.

Although most of the work on leukocyte migration across the BBB summarized earlier is in reference to T-cells, *in vitro* studies have shown that B-cell migration is highly dependent on LFA-4/ICAM interactions and the CCL2 (MCP-1) chemokine.[22] It appears that different inflammatory cell types may employ different arrays of molecules to direct their journey through the BBB. For example, it has been recently shown that monocytes preferentially utilize CXCL12 in adhesion to the BBB when compared to lymphocytes.[462]

It should also be noted that whereas much of the population and expansion of the MS perivascular inflammatory infiltrate is modulated at the level of the endothelial cell of the BBB, it is thought the first entry of antigen-specific lymphocytes that populate the parenchyma to initiate the early plaque may have been via the choroid plexus during immune surveillance sorties (see later under Choroid Plexus, Cerebrospinal Fluid and Periventricular White Matter, p. 1354).

Aside from a variable degree of swelling, by routine light microscopy endothelial cells in MS plaques usually appear normal. At the ultrastructural level in areas with active disease, they show increased numbers of pinocytotic vesicles[110] and reduced numbers of mitochondria in more chronic stages.[153] There is, however, both neuroimaging evidence of significant dysfunction and immunohistochemical evidence of functional disruption of microvascular endothelial cells in early MS lesions.[498] Indeed, the resulting oedematous loosening of the tissue has long been recognized as a major histological hallmark of MS lesions.[609] Alterations of endothelial cell tight junctional integrity leading to increased barrier permeability are reflected in beading, interruption, absence or diffuse cytoplasmic localization of tight junctional proteins, and the perivascular leakage of serum components normally excluded from the CNS parenchyma (Figure 23.5)[250,584] and the expression of cytokines and chemokines that mediate leukocyte–endothelial cell adhesion and transmigration.[24,697] Endothelial cells of capillaries and small venules concurrently exhibit alterations that indicate immune activation, including

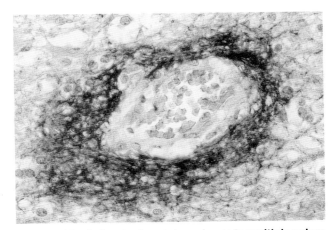

23.5 Blood-brain barrier breakdown in acute multiple sclerosis (MS). Perivascular extravasation of fibrinogen into the adjacent parenchyma. Immunohistochemistry without counterstain.

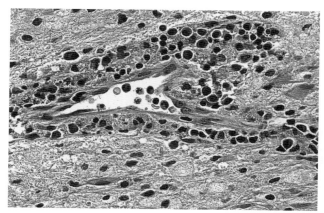

23.6 Perivascular inflammation in acute multiple sclerosis (MS). Brain biopsy from male aged 35 years with a 3-month history. Perivascular mononuclear cells include lymphocytes, macrophages and plasma cells. Haematoxylin and eosin.

the upregulation of class II MHC molecules.[774] The coincident microvascular basement membrane protein alterations resulting from the destruction of the extracellular matrix may facilitate leukocyte transmigration into the perivascular space and parenchyma.[713,779] It is generally assumed that the alterations in endothelial permeability are secondary to the vascular inflammatory infiltrates (Figure 23.6), but the possibility that a BBB abnormality initiates and antedates the inflammation cannot be completely excluded.

Perivascular Space

Lymphocytes that have crossed the endothelium have now arrived in the perivascular space, which is bounded by a basement membrane on the abluminal side of the endothelium and a basement membrane resting on the glia limitans of the adjacent parenchyma (Figure 23.4). Inflammatory cuffs within the perivascular space can be prominent in MS lesions (Figures 23.4, 23.6 and 23.7). In addition to T-cells, these comprise B-cells and microglia/macrophages. Experimental data involving 2-photon *in vivo* imaging indicate that the perivascular space is constantly scanned by T-cells in the search for antigen.[60] Intriguingly, under normal circumstances, the CXCL12 chemokine is located on the parenchymal side of the endothelium, and it is thought this polarity confines lymphocytes to the perivascular space and prevents them from entering the parenchyma. In MS, this polarity is abolished and CXCL12 is redistributed to both the parenchymal and the luminal sides of the endothelium, allowing egress of activated CXCR4-positive lymphocytes not only across the endothelium, but also into the adjacent parenchyma.[479] This entry into the parenchyma is facilitated by the secretion of matrix metalloproteinases by macrophages, which degrade components of the extracellular matrix (see under Extracellular Matrix, p. 1319).[839]

The perivascular space is the last stop for the numerous amoeboid macrophages, laden with myelin breakdown products (Figure 23.7 and Figure 23.8), before they exit the endothelium into the venous circulation. Perivascular microglia have a ramified morphology and upregulate MHC Class II and co-stimulatory molecules for T-cells (Figure 23.9).[83,214] Therefore, they may process and present antigens to activated antigen-specific T-cells that have

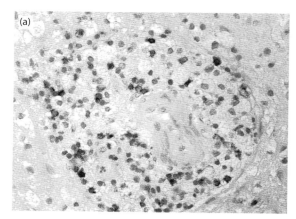

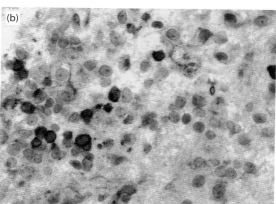

23.7 Acute inflammatory/demyelinating lesions. (a) Brain biopsy from a male aged 48 years with a 2-year history. Numerous leukocyte common antigen-(CD45)-positive cells are mixed with foamy macrophages in a perivenous inflammatory cell cuff. Immunoperoxidase with haematoxylin. **(b)** Brain biopsy from a female aged 65 years with a several-week history and a solitary demyelinating lesion. CD4+ lymphocytes are mixed with foamy macrophages in the parenchyma. Immunoperoxidase stain with haematoxylin.

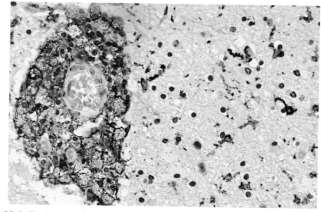

23.8 Perivascular foamy macrophages in multiple sclerosis (MS). Brain biopsy of acute multiple sclerosis (MS) lesion. Same case as shown in Figure 23.6. Human leukocyte antigen (HLA)-DR+ foamy macrophages are present in the perivascular inflammatory cell cuff on the left side of the field. Prominent HLA-DR expression is seen on parenchymal microglia in the right side of the field. Immunoperoxidase stain with haematoxylin.

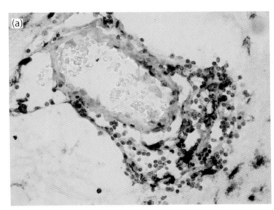

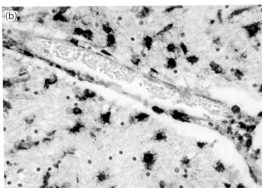

23.9 Perivascular microglia in multiple sclerosis (MS). Immunohistochemistry for class II MHC (HLA-DR) shows activated microglia within **(a)** and adjacent to **(b)** the edge of a chronic active multiple sclerosis plaque. Note activated microglia, which retain their ramified appearance (in contrast to the amoeboid form when they have become macrophages as illustrated in Figure 23.8), are evident in the lesional perivascular space where they are intimately associated with lymphocytes **(a)**, but are also seen in the perivascular space and the parenchyma in the adjacent white matter **(b)** where some have taken on a more rounded appearance in the process of transforming to macrophages. Counterstained with haematoxylin.

entered through the endothelial barrier and accumulated in perivascular inflammatory cell cuffs (Figure 23.6). The close approximation of the inflammatory cells (Figure 23.7a) additionally allows leukocyte–leukocyte interactions that require direct cell contacts. Dendritic cells, which are professional antigen-presenting cells of myeloid origin, also populate the perivascular inflammatory cuffs where they are in close proximity to individual T-cells, a physical relationship that would facilitate early events in the immune response.[689] Through their release of vasoactive molecules, perivascular mast cells may facilitate T-cell migration through the vessel walls.[390,847] Eventually perivascular fibrosis may accompany the chronic vessel damage as a consequence of the destructive effects of products of the inflammatory infiltrates. Thus, the perivascular space is a critical way-station in the initiation and progression of CNS immune responses, in which key immune activation steps that result in subsequent acute and chronic parenchymal injury are likely to occur. The perivascular space is also continuous with draining lymphatic channels from which CNS antigens are transported to the periphery,[809] where they have been detected in lymph nodes.[786] This may result in autosensitization and expansion

of a potential autoimmune repertoire (see earlier under Peripheral Immune Organs, p. 1310, and later under Animal Models of Human Demyelinating Diseases, p. 1387).

Leptomeninges

The perivascular space is continuous with the subarachnoid space. Thus, it is not surprising that leptomeningeal inflammation is a feature of MS pathology. In fact, B-cells in the leptomeninges have been found to form follicle-like structures similar to those found normally in peripheral lymph nodes—again consistent with an on-going immunological response in the CNS.[322,688] Moreover, it has been postulated that the inflammatory response in the leptomeninges is important in the pathogenesis of changes in the underlying cortex (see later under Cortical Plaques, p. 1348).[322] As noted earlier, these vessels may employ different means to capture activated lymphocytes than those of the parenchyma (see earlier under Endothelial Cells, p. 1310).

T-lymphocytes

Early immunohistochemical analyses demonstrated the presence of perivascular and parenchymal CD3+ (pan T-cell), CD4+ (helper T-cell) (Figure 23.7) and CD8+ (cytotoxic T-cell) markers in active MS lesions.[761] One school of thought holds that CD4+ T-cells proliferate and akin to a delayed-type hypersensitivity reaction initiate the formation of lesions through recruited macrophages following presentation of the processed antigen. What the critical antigen(s) are in the initiation of the lesion is unknown.[482] Moreover, it is possible these may increase and change over time, so-called 'epitope spreading'.[174] CD4+ T-helper 1 (Th1) cells produce, among other molecules, the pro-inflammatory cytokines interleukin 1 (IL-1), interleukin 2 (IL-2), tumour necrosis factor-α (TNF-α) and interferon-γ (IFN-γ) that have all been demonstrated by immunohistochemistry in active MS lesions[76,130] and generally enhance immune reponses.[154] Th2-type cytokines interleukin 4 (IL-4), interleukin 10 (IL-10) and transforming growth factor β (TGF-β) are also found in MS lesions of different ages.[130,325] The latter[154] tend to down-regulate the immune response and promote B-cells to produce antibodies and to counteract the activation of macrophages induced by IFN-γ. Their activities, therefore, generally dampen the cell-mediated immunopathological processes. More recently, interest has focused on the Th17 T-cell subtype, which is regulated by interleukin 23 (IL-23), expresses, among other markers, interleukin 17 (IL-17), and has been shown to be important in the pathogenesis of experimental autoimmune demyelination.[154] This cell type has been found in significant numbers in active areas of MS plaques[766] and its receptor has been demonstrated on endothelial cells in these lesions;[359] it is thought to initially enter the CNS via the choroid plexus (see later under Choroid Plexus, Cerebrospinal Fluid and Periventricular White Matter, p. 1354).[628]

Th9 cells, which produce IL-9 and stimulate mast cells, are also thought to be capable of demyelination,[92] but have not yet been reported in MS lesions.

Although to date they have been investigated to a lesser extent, CD8+ T-lymphocytes are as or more numerous than CD4+ T-cells in active lesions and may mediate antigen-specific cytotoxic tissue injury.[240,274] In fact, brain-infiltrating

CD8+ T-cell clones expand and persist over time.[704] Overall, however, the precise and likely overlapping contributions of different T-cell subpopulations to the various injury mechanisms in active MS lesions are not understood. Moreover, T-cell accumulations may be secondary or 'reactive'; they may not necessarily represent antigen-specific responses,[221] and they could also be neuroprotective (rather than destructive) as has been postulated for some other constituents of the immune response.[268,723] The finding of HLA-E (a MHC Class 1b marker that induces an immunoregulatory phenotype in CD8+ cells) on endothelial cells and astrocytes in active MS lesions might indicate one means by which CD8+ cells may downregulate the immune response.[193] Downregulation of the autoimmune response may result from a number of other mechanisms, such as the emergence of FoxP3+ CD4+ and FoxP3+ CD8+ cells that suppress the immune response, referred to as CD4+ Tregs and CD8+ Tregs, respectively. However, in MS, a subset of CD4+ Tregs appears to be defective and this has been thought to be responsible for increasing levels of IL-17. Furthermore, relapsing MS patients have fewer circulating CD8+ Tregs than those in remission. Both these scenarios would result in a continuation of the autoimmune attack in the MS lesion.[92] However, very few if any FoxP3+ cells are found in active MS lesions,[241,766] but are frequent in the CSF, this discrepancy being attributed to their susceptibility to apoptosis.[241] The disappearance of T-cell infiltrates that occurs as the lesion becomes inactive probably involves apoptotic cell death-related protein pathways in many of the inflammatory cell types.[500,667]

In terms of numbers, the main lymphocyte populations in active lesions are CD4+ and CD8+ T-cells, but other T-cell populations may respond to different antigens and have particular roles in antigen presentation and co-stimulation, in defining the specific cytokine micro-environments, and in mediating injury.[109,721] For example, T-cell receptor γ/δ cells that recognize lipid antigens[94] are present in MS lesions,[686] where they may lyse oligodendrocytes through their secretion of perforin,[850] whereas NK T-cells, also important mediators of lipid immunity, are not very numerous in MS lesions.[332] These are not to be confused with another cell type the natural killer (NK) cells found in MS peripheral blood that probably have immunoregulatory functions.[740]

B-lymphocytes, Plasma Cells and Immunoglobulins

Under normal conditions, B-lymphocytes are excluded from the CNS parenchyma; in early MS lesions, they are less numerous than T-lymphocytes, but nevertheless present.[302] B-cells undergo clonal expansion in the intrathecal compartment early in the course of MS, and as noted earlier may form follicle-like structures in the leptomeninges.[322] The significance of B-cells in the pathogenesis of MS has been a matter of controversy but there is increasing evidence that they do have an important role, particularly in view of the marked reduction in clinical relapses after treatment with a monoclonal antibody directed against them.[186] The B-cells mature to plasma cells, which may be quite numerous in long-standing lesions.[601] The most abundant immunoglobulin they produce is IgG.[208] The IgG that diffuses into the CSF from the parenchymal and leptomeningeal B-cell/plasma cell sources is predominantly of the IgG$_1$ and IgG$_3$ isotypes. CSF oligoclonal bands, the restricted

immunoglobulin banding patterns that result from the clonal proliferations, are characteristic of MS but not diagnostic, and specific antibody band patterns may persist in individual patients over the disease course.[121,305] Other immunoglobulins are detected in MS plaques, with small amounts of IgA and IgM also being present. Intrathecal oligoclonal IgM against myelin lipids, particularly phosphatidyl choline, has been documented in MS and this appears to reflect a more aggressive clinical course.[791]

However, B-cells may also have an immunomodulatory function mediated by contact with T-cells through CD154–CD40 and CD28–B7 complexes to cause the production of inhibitory cytokines such as IL-10 and TGF-β.[92]

Complement and Other Innate Immunity Components

As for adaptive immunity, so the components of the innate immune system figure prominently in the immunopathology of active MS lesions. Various components of the complement cascade have been immunohistochemically detected in MS lesions. C3d has been found to be associated with myelin sheaths.[608] C3b on microglia adjacent to MS lesions has been reported as a sign of microglial priming in anticipation of demyelination.[624] The deposition of the terminal membrane attack complex (C9 neoantigen) in regions of ongoing demyelination indicates that the complement cascade had gone to completion (Figures 23.10 and 23.11).[440] Although complement does indeed induce demyelination,[486] its absence on myelin in other studies[252] questions the importance of complement as an absolute pre-requisite for the pathogenesis of the MS lesion or may indicate it is not present at certain stages of the genesis of

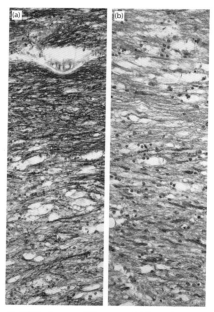

23.10 Acute MS plaque. 20-year-old female with a 6-week history. **(a)** Luxol fast blue (LFB)–periodic acid-Schiff (PAS) stain showing the ill-defined edge of an acute MS plaque with vacuolated myelin sheaths. **(b)** The same area immunohistochemically stained for activated complement (C9 neoantigen) shows positively stained myelin sheaths.

Courtesy of Professor JW Prineas and Dr M Barnett, University of Sydney, Sydney, Australia.

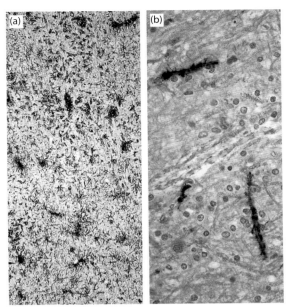

23.11 Secondary progressive multiple sclerosis (MS). Male aged 43 years with a 13-year history. **(a)** Numerous microglia in periplaque white matter are immunostained for leukocyte common antigen. **(b)** A corresponding area immunostained for activated complement.

Courtesy of Professor JW Prineas, University of Sydney, Sydney, Australia.

the plaque. The reduced CSF levels of the terminal component of complement (C9) is consistent with its consumption in the formation of membrane attack complexes in MS.[517] In addition, complement receptors are expressed widely on neurons,[56] and complement activation could, therefore, be a partially neuroprotective mechanism.[661]

Toll-like receptors (TLRs) are types of pattern recognition receptors on dendritic cells and macrophages that, on ligand binding, can prime these cells for antigen presentation and cytokine production.[613] TLRs are upregulated in MS lesions[118] and their ligands exist in the MS lesion in the form of fibrin, as a result of blood–brain barrier breakdown, and oxidized lipids.[413] It is possible that TLR, functioning as mediators of the innate immune system, smay be important in the immunopathogenesis of MS.[613]

Microglia/Macrophages and Monocytes

Microglia and macrophages have pivotal roles in the pathogenesis of the MS plaque by virtue of the fact that they can present antigen and macrophages are the effector cells in demyelination. In addition to microglia, monocytes from the peripheral blood contribute to the pool of macrophages in the MS lesion. Monocytes are attracted from the circulation to endothelial cell luminal surfaces and then migrate through micro-vessel walls and accumulate in perivascular inflammatory cuffs. These processes result from an array of specific adhesion molecule- and chemokine-mediated recognition mechanisms.[317] There is evidence to suggest that these haematogenous macrophages are responsible for on-going immune-mediated demyelination, whereas their microglial-derived counterparts may have an effect on dampening this process.[623]

Furthermore, recent studies indicate that these two pools of macrophages respond in different ways when subjected to conditions that drive them toward either an M1 or an M2 phenotype.[192] M1-cells are immunostimulatory and are neurotoxic, whereas M2 cells are said to downregulate immune responses and have regenerative effects.[368] In this context, it is of interest that in the MS lesion lipid-laden macrophages that have degraded myelin demonstrate an immunomodulatory cytokine and chemokine profile characteristic of M2 cells, whereas those that are actively involved in ingesting myelin at the outer demyelinating lesion edge express these markers to a lesser degree.[97] This is in agreement with experimental work that shows lipid-laden macrophages are immunosuppressive.[97] A further correlate of this is that they also express CD163, a marker associated with the M2 phenotype that is also found on perivascular macrophages in the MS plaque.[214]

Morphology

Macrophages are found throughout MS plaques. They are the most numerous cells in active lesions and have proliferative capacity.[719] Whether of haematogenous or microglial origin, they have a rounded appearance indicative of their amoeboid properties (Figures 23.7, 23.8, 23.12 and 23.13). Microglial cells that have not transformed into macrophages retain their ramified morphology. However, their activated state is evident in the upregulation of various activation markers, most notably HLA-DR (Figures 23.8 and 23.14). The latter is an exquisitely sensitive immunohistochemical marker for microglial activation and it persists when they transform into macrophages. In non-plaque white matter, macrophages are relatively rare, but ramified activated microglia are numerous (Figure 23.14).[18]

Pathological Roles

Activation of monocyte- and microglia-derived macrophages within the parenchyma involves gene expression programmes initiated by extracellular signals from the pro-inflammatory environment, i.e. from cytokines,[69,76] lipid and lipopolysaccharide mediators[675] and growth factors. The latter are likely to include macrophage colony-stimulating factor,[810] insulin-like growth factors[287] and nerve growth factor (NGF).[769] These extracellular activation stimuli trigger nuclear factor κB (NFκB) transcription factor[286] and other intracellular signalling pathways.[70,527,623] Among the key consequences of this activation are elevated levels of the inducible form of nitric oxide synthase (iNOS) and the production of nitric oxide (NO), one of the major effectors of myelin and oligodendrocyte damage[310] and of action potential conduction block (see later under Neurophysiology of Multiple Sclerosis, p. 1362). Macrophages also express cyclooxygenase-2 (COX-2), which produces reactive oxygen species in the synthesis of prostanoids such as prostaglandins.[648] The activated macrophage phenotype is also manifested by enhanced immunoreactivity for CD45 antigen, IgG (see later Figure 23.26), osteopontin, components of activated complement, the receptor for the Fc part of IgG and certain chemokine receptors.[137,252,456,608,695,762]

As indicated by their expression of HLA-DR, a major function of activated microglia and macrophages within

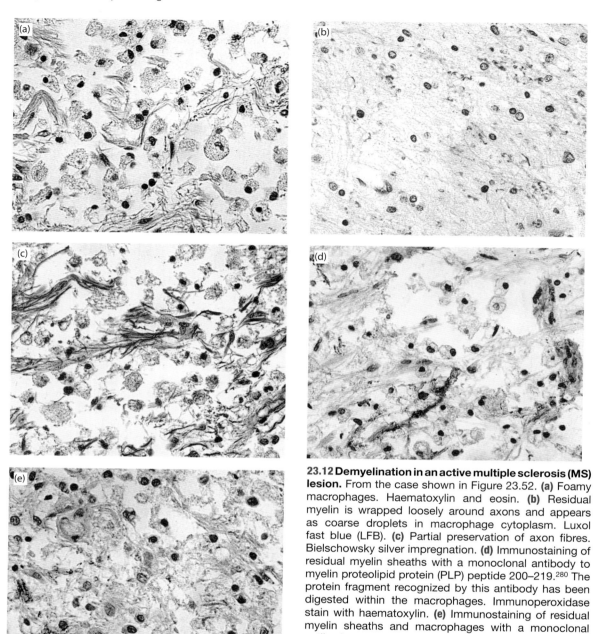

23.12 Demyelination in an active multiple sclerosis (MS) lesion. From the case shown in Figure 23.52. **(a)** Foamy macrophages. Haematoxylin and eosin. **(b)** Residual myelin is wrapped loosely around axons and appears as coarse droplets in macrophage cytoplasm. Luxol fast blue (LFB). **(c)** Partial preservation of axon fibres. Bielschowsky silver impregnation. **(d)** Immunostaining of residual myelin sheaths with a monoclonal antibody to myelin proteolipid protein (PLP) peptide 200–219.[280] The protein fragment recognized by this antibody has been digested within the macrophages. Immunoperoxidase stain with haematoxylin. **(e)** Immunostaining of residual myelin sheaths and macrophages with a monoclonal antibody to myelin PLP peptide 100–123.[280] In contrast to (d), there is more particulate macrophage staining for this portion of the PLP molecule, indicating that at this stage it is only partially digested in the macrophages.

the MS lesion is antigen presentation to activated T-cells that routinely traffic through the CNS to carry out immune surveillance.[552] An early T-cell-microglial interaction in the CNS probably occurs at the level of the perivascular microglial cell just after the activated T-cell has transgressed the blood–brain barrier.[768] An immune response will be initiated if the antigen recognized by the T-cell (presumably a CNS antigen) is the one being presented. Through their interactions with other infiltrating inflammatory cells and CNS resident cells, microglia have many additional critical immune, neural and regulatory roles in MS. They express cytokine and chemokine receptors.[218] Because they express potassium channels, mobilize calcium, respond to neuronal activity, and have glutamate and γ-aminobutyric acid

(GABA) receptors, microglia have many neurophysiological effects.[218] They may sense astrocyte activity through purinergic receptors.[218] They may also be effector cells of neuronal excitatory injury.[741]

Macrophages are the principal cells that mediate demyelination, i.e. the stripping of myelin lamellae and the phagocytosis and intracellular catabolism of myelin.[598,603,609] Myelin lamellae in close proximity to a macrophage may show an ultrastructural change referred to as 'vesicular demyelination', whereby the lamellar pattern is replaced by a vacuolar or vesicular appearance, very reminiscent of that seen in experimental proteolysis (Figure 23.15). Thus, this change has been interpreted as due to the effect of enzymes or other myelinotoxic species produced by the macrophage. However,

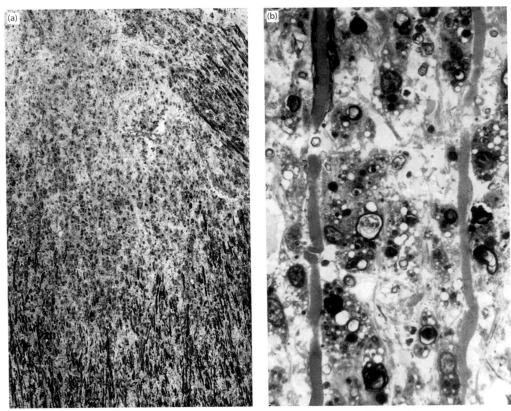

23.13 Demyelination in acute multiple sclerosis (MS). Female aged 29 years with a 10-month history. A newly forming spinal cord lesion shows macrophages containing phagocytosed myelin particles aligned alongside demyelinated and partially demyelinated axons. **(a)** 6 µm epoxy section of osmicated tissue. Unstained. **(b)** 1 µm thick section. Toluidine blue.

it is possible that in many instances this is a fixation arte-fact as it is rarely seen in optimally fixed human material.[602] However, macrophage processes do insinuate themselves between myelin lamellae and engage in removal of fragments of myelin from the myelin sheath (Figures 23.15–23.17).[616] Macrophages recognize and phagocytose myelin through their Fc, complement and scavenger receptors.[654,710] It is unclear whether this involves the binding of a myelin-specific ligand, such as an immunoglobulin[600] directed against and bound to myelin *in situ* or whether this is a non-specific phe-nomenon on the part of the macrophage simply ingesting myelin debris previously lysed from the myelin sheath prior to its arrival. The determination of which scenario applies is obviously fundamental to understanding the pathogenesis, and probably the aetiology, of immune-mediated demyelin-ation in MS. In any event, myelin lamellae become attached to clathrin-coated pits on the macrophage surfaces and are then ingested (Figures 23.16 and 23.17).[598] Following inter-nalization, particulate myelin fragments are digested by lipases and proteases in lysosomes (Figure 23.13).[623] These biochemical processes are reflected in progressive disintegra-tion of the lamellar pattern of the ingested myelin.[408]

The tempo of the biochemical degradation of myelin protein constituents in macrophages has been employed to determine the relative duration of MS plaques.[773,776] Thus, myelin-associated glycoprotein (MAG) and myelin-oligodendrocyte protein (MOG) are degraded earlier than

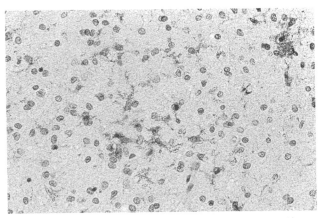

23.14 Activated microglia. Reactive microglia express human leukocyte antigen (HLA)-DR in the parenchyma adjacent to an acute inflammatory demyelinating lesion. Biopsy sample from a 35-year-old female with a 5-week history. Immunoperoxidase with haematoxylin.

myelin basic protein (MBP) (Figure 23.18) and proteolipid protein (PLP).[773,776] The retention of Luxol fast blue (LFB)-positivity in myelin fragments is thought to indicate that frag-ment was recently phagocyosed (Figure 23.19), but eventually the myelin lipids in the lysosome are degraded to neutral lipids in the form of esterified cholesterol, the major lipid component

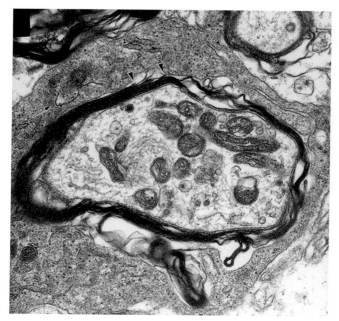

23.15 Demyelination in multiple sclerosis (MS). The edge of a chronic multiple sclerosis (MS) lesion shows lysis (arrowheads) and endocytosis (arrow) of superficial myelin lamellae by macrophage processes enveloping a partially vesiculated but still largely compact sheath. Electron micrograph.

Courtesy of Professor JW Prineas, University of Sydney, Sydney, Australia.

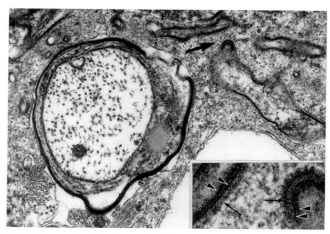

23.17 Demyelination in multiple sclerosis (MS). Enlargement of Figure 23.16. Insert of the area indicated by the arrow shows myelin entering the cell in the form of two major dense lines (arrowheads) that are separated by a constant gap from the plasma membrane of the macrophage (small arrows). The membrane on the right exhibits the electron-dense undercoat of a coated pit. Electron micrograph.

Reproduced from Prineas and Connell.[598] With permission from Lippincott Williams & Wilkins/Wolters Kluwer Health.

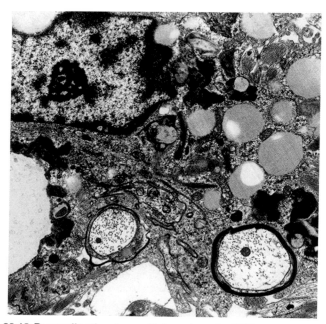

23.16 Demyelination in multiple sclerosis (MS). Active multiple sclerosis (MS) lesion. A macrophage closely invests two myelinated fibres in periplaque white matter. The sheath on the left is loose and has been partly taken up by the macrophage. Electron micrograph.

Reproduced from Prineas and Connell.[598] With permission from Lippincott Williams & Wilkins/Wolters Kluwer Health.

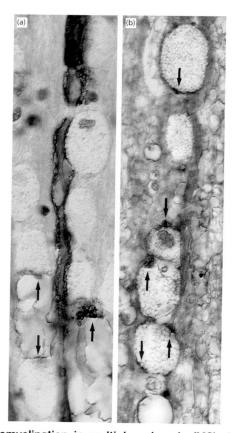

23.18 Demyelination in multiple sclerosis (MS). (a) At the edge of a plaque, there are fibres immunostained for myelin basic protein (MBP) and stained debris (arrows) at the poles of closely apposed macrophages. **(b)** Immunoglobulin G (IgG) caps (arrows) are seen at one or both poles of macrophages engaged in active myelin destruction.

Reproduced from Prineas et al.[603] With permission from Elsevier.

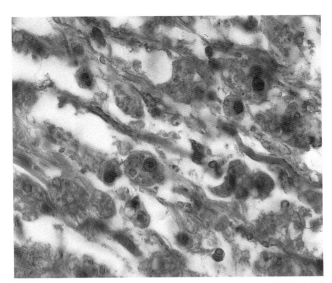

23.19 Macrophages in acute multiple sclerosis (MS). Male aged 25 years with a 24-day history. Macrophages containing Luxol fast blue (LFB)-positive particles of myelin, indicating relatively recent myelin phagocytosis, are present among partially demyelinated axons. The periodic-acid Schiff (PAS)-positive granules represent residual glycoprotein from myelin that was previously degraded in lysosomes. Cells resembling oligodendrocytes are absent. LFB–PAS.

Courtesy of Professor JW Prineas, University of Sydney, Sydney, Australia.

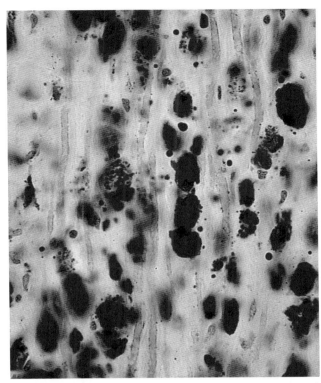

23.20 Macrophages and remyelination in multiple sclerosis (MS). Lipid-containing macrophages surround thinly myelinated remyelinating axon fibres in a resolving spinal cord multiple sclerosis (MS) plaque in which there was no evidence of active demyelination. Frozen section stained with oil red O.

Courtesy of Professor JW Prineas, University of Sydney, Sydney, Australia.

of lipid-laden macrophages, also referred to as 'foamy macrophages' or 'gitterzellen' (Figures 23.7, 23.8, 23.12 and 23.13). The neutral lipids can be identified with sudanophilic dyes, such as oil red O or Sudan black, in tissue that has not been treated with alcohol (Figure 23.20). Residual glycoprotein in macrophage lysosomes can be demonstrated by the periodic acid-Schiff (PAS) stain (Figure 23.19). Macrophages have been show to express markers in a specific temporal sequence and this has also been used to date lesions;[113a] for example, MRP14 and 27E10 are expressed earlier than 25F9.[113]

Extracellular Matrix

Given the inflammatory nature of active MS lesions, it would follow that there would be significant alterations of the extracellular matrix (ECM). Indeed, in active MS lesions, there is reduction of the ECM components tenascin-C and –R,[285] lecticans and dermatan sulphate proteoglycan, with upregulation of the latter at the plaque edge.[715] Thus, matrix metalloproteinases (MMP), which are normally utilized to remodel the extracellular matrix,[447] are upregulated in MS plaques[795] as is one of their antagonists, tissue inhibitors of metalloproteinase 1 (TIMP1).[503] This is associated with significant increase in the perivascular expression of components of collagens I, III and V, some of which inhibit the production of CCL1 chemokine, important in the recruitment of inflammatory cells. The temporal and spatial distribution of MMPs and TIMP1 in the MS lesion are likely to influence the degree and structure of focal perivascular fibrosis and the inflammatory milieu of the ECM.[447] The same is true of other ECM remodellers, such as ADAMTS (a disintegrin and metalloproteinase with thrombospondin motifs) and the inhibitor TIMP3.[291]

ECM alterations in MS plaques are a consequence of immune activity, myelin breakdown, chronically increased BBB permeability, release and activation of extracellular proteases, and altered turnover of synthesis of ECM components.[407,715] In particular, a pathologically altered ECM may present a barrier to migrating OPCs at lesion edges and preclude cell–cell contacts necessary for remyelination. Extracellular myelin debris also inhibits remyelination.[385] The release and activation of certain key ECM proteases, such as matrix metalloproteinase 9 (MMP-9), may promote injury by enhancing parenchymal invasion by inflammatory cells through ECM breakdown and facilitate remyelination by digesting endogenous myelination inhibitors.[410]

Astrocytes and Gliosis

Morphology

Hypertrophic astrocytes are conspicuous within and surrounding early white matter MS lesions (Figure 23.21), whereas dense fibrillary gliosis is a feature of chronicity (Figure 23.22). Astrocytes may have multiple, giant or bizarre convoluted nuclei, cells referred to as 'Creutzfeldt cells' and normal or granular mitotic figures, i.e. large rod-like centrioles and chromatin-containing particles in the cytoplasm (Figure 23.23).[533] Their bizarre appearances can result in the erroneous diagnosis of astrocytic neoplasm, particularly in biopsy samples. The altered morphology of

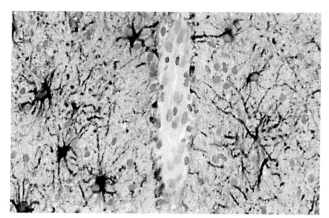

23.21 Reactive astrocytes within an early multiple sclerosis (MS) lesion. Female aged 37 years. Brain biopsy, demonstrating an acute inflammatory/demyelinating lesion. Prominent reactive astrocytes are immunostained for glial fibrillary acidic protein (GFAP). Immunoperoxidase with haematoxylin.

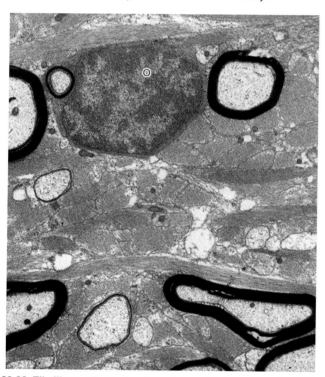

23.22 Fibrillary gliosis in chronic multiple sclerosis (MS). Thinly myelinated axons at the edge of a chronic multiple sclerosis (MS) lesion are separated by densely packed, fibrillary astrocytic processes. Sectioned longitudinally, such fibres have been shown to consist of a mixture of remyelinating and partially demyelinated axons. Electron micrograph. O, oligodendrocyte.

Reproduced from Prineas and Connell.[598] With permission from Lippincott Williams & Wilkins/Wolters Kluwer Health.

astrocytes is due in large part to dynamic changes in their major cytoskeletal proteins, i.e. glial fibrillary acidic protein (GFAP) (Figure 23.24) and vimentin.[205,532,666]

Pathological Roles

As in other disorders of the CNS, the astrocyte produces the glial scar of the MS plaque. The resulting sclerotic nature of

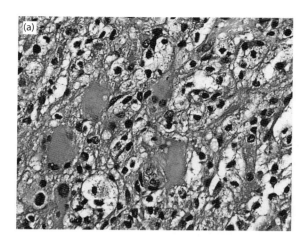

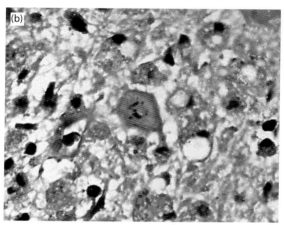

23.23 Abnormal astrocytes in acute inflammatory/demyelinating multiple sclerosis (MS) lesions. (a) Multinucleated astrocytes; **(b)** abnormal chromatin pattern in mitosis. Both are stained with Luxol fast blue (LFB)–haematoxylin and eosin.

Courtesy of Dr T Sangruchi, Mahidol University, Bangkok, Thailand.

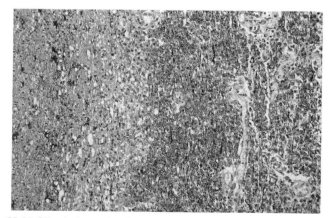

23.24 Gliosis in multiple sclerosis (MS). Prominent glial fibrillary acidic protein (GFAP)-positive astrocytes at the edge of a chronic active multiple sclerosis (MS) plaque. Female aged 69 years with a 4-month history. Intact white matter with scattered reactive astrocytes is on the left side of the field; the active plaque centre is to the right side of the field. There is a dense band of fibrillary gliosis at the plaque border. Immunoperoxidase with haematoxylin.

the multiple lesions is responsible for the disorder's name. In the advanced stage of the plaque, numerous sinuous processes of fibrillary astrocytes separate the demyelinated axons (Figure 23.25). These 'scar astrocytes', however, are by no means inert, for they produce nestin and embryonic neural cell adhesion molecule, as well as growth factors and receptors such as fibroblast growth factor receptor 4, epidermal growth factor receptor, basic fibroblast growth factor, and nerve growth factor.[315]

Reactive astrocytes also contribute to the immunopathogenesis of MS lesions. They produce and respond to NO[431] and may regulate its production by microglia.[497] They produce tenascins, and thus may be important in the remodelling of the ECM in MS.[285] They express chemokine receptors, and their production of chemokines may promote macrophage recruitment to lesions and thus may be important in inducing neuronal death.[27,129,134,777] The heat shock protein αB crystallin is also produced by astrocytes.[782] Their expression of NGF receptors within active lesions probably reflects their regulation by NGF.[769]

Whether and to what extent astrocytes present peptide antigens to T-cells in MS lesions has long been controversial.[165,189,388,768] Astrocyte β2-adrenergic receptor expression is decreased in MS lesions, and the resultant loss of adrenergic influence might permit their expression of class II MHC molecules, thereby enhancing their antigen presentation capacity.[177] Indeed, astrocytes in active MS lesions may express the co-stimulatory molecules required for efficient antigen presentation.[851] Furthermore, although they may not process whole proteins, they can present myelin peptides to T-cells.[383] Thus, astrocytes may act as facultative antigen-presenting cells once myelin proteins have undergone initial degradation.

Astrocytes also secrete proteases that catabolize myelin and regulate microglial myelin phagocytosis.[711] Because they possess Fc-receptors, astrocytes are capable of binding and internalizing immunoglobulins (Figure 23.26). Astrocytes themselves have been shown to act as phagocytes in MS lesions, in that they may phagocytose myelin, axonal and cellular debris.[422,516] They also internalize oligodendrocytes (Figure 23.27); it is unclear whether this phenomenon, not exclusive to MS, has a destructive or protective effect.[516, 605,831]

The morphological alterations of reactive astrocytes indicate disruption of their numerous physiological functions, particularly maintenance of the BBB and extracellular fluid balance, glutamate metabolism and glio-transmission (see later under Glial Alterations, p. 1364).[36,65,258,793] The normal network of intercellular astrocyte connections may be disrupted as their processes change shape and their gap junction proteins are decreased.[98] It is becoming increasingly evident that astrocytes have many more roles in the MS plaque than merely forming a scar.[490]

Neovascularization

There is evidence that the blood vessel density in the CNS is increased in MS, both in lesions and non-lesional white

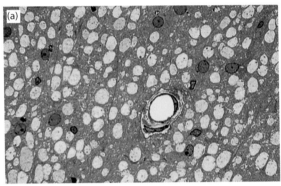

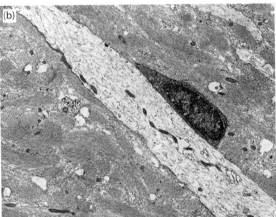

23.25 Fibrillary gliosis in chronic multiple sclerosis (MS). **(a)** Centre of a chronic plaque showing demyelinated axons embedded in a dense gliotic matrix. Toluidine blue and safranin. **(b)** Fibrillary gliosis with impaired remyelination. An oligodendrocyte contacts a demyelinated axon within a chronic plaque in which there is no widening of the extracellular compartment. Evidence of new myelin formation was not seen in this lesion. Electron micrograph.

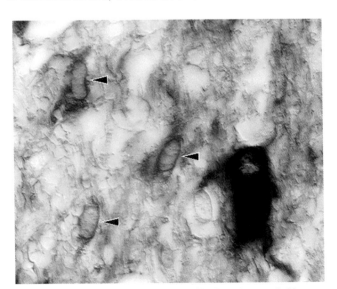

23.26 Acute multiple sclerosis (MS). Female aged 40 years with a 10-week history. An area in a newly forming lesion shows microglia/macrophages (arrowheads) that stain for immunoglobulin G (IgG). A reactive astrocyte (lower right) is also stained. Immunohistochemistry without counterstain.

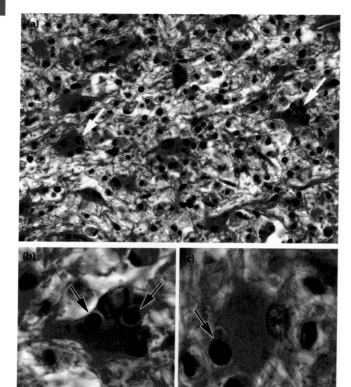

23.27 Envelopment of oligodendroglia by astrocytes in an acute (MS) plaque. (a) There is oligodendroglial hyperplasia; most of the cells with small round nuclei are oligodendrocyes in this acute MS plaque. Many are being enveloped by astocytes (white arrows). **(b)** High magnification of the astrocyte indicated by the right white arrow in **(a)**, showing the eosinophilic processes of the reactive astrocyte enveloping two oligodendroglial perikarya (black arrows). **(c)** Another hyperplastic reactive astrocyte is engulfing an oligodendrocyte (black arrow). Haematoxylin-eosin–periodic acid-Schiff (H&E–PAS).

Courtesy of Dr K G Warren, University of Alberta, Canada.

matter; this is particularly true of lesions that are subacute.[316] This is accompanied by, and probably secondary to, the increased production of vascular endothelial growth factor (VEGF) by glial cells and its receptor by glial and endothelial cells.[680] These phenomena may be important factors either in the extension of the MS lesion or as a response to tissue injury, or both.

Demyelination

Multiple distinct cellular and molecular mechanisms result in the injury of oligodendrocytes and compact myelin in active inflammatory demyelinating lesions. These processes progress and ultimately culminate in oligodendrocyte depletion (Figure 23.19) and the failure of remyelination in chronic lesions. They probably involve specific antigen targeting through adaptive immunity (T-cell and antibody responses), innate immunity through toll-like receptor (TLR) recognition and complement deposition, and so-called 'bystander injury'. The interrelationships and extent

of overlap among these injury pathways and how they may evolve over time in lesions and in individual patients are unclear. As noted earlier, the major effector cell of myelin phagocytosis is the macrophage, but whether this is specifically directed by an autoimmune reaction to myelin dictated by antigen-specific T-cells (analogous to a delayed type hypersensitivity reaction) or the macrophage is simply scavenging myelin destroyed by another autoimmune or non-immune process is not entirely clear.

Whereas the most obvious consequence of demyelination is loss of the myelin sheath, demyelination is also associated with a number of changes that occur in the axonal cell membrane (axolemma), particularly in regions near the node of Ranvier.[180] The molecular anatomy of the node of Ranvier and its adjacent apparatus is shown schematically in Figure 23.28.[180] The nodes of Ranvier, being the short unmyelinated segments of the axolemma, are the site of the voltage-gated sodium channels that mediate the influx of sodium ions responsible for the inwardly directed current of the action potential. Also embedded in the nodal axolemma are contactin and the neuronal isoform of neurofascin, Nfasc186, which dictates the clustering of sodium channels at that site. On either side of the node of Ranvier is the paranode, where together with contactin, the major molecular constituents are the oligodendroglial isoform of neurofascin, Nfascin 155, and Caspr (sometimes referred to as paranodin). Immediately adjacent to the paranode is the juxtaparanode, which possesses voltage-gated potassium channels associated with caspr2 and Tag1. The scaffolding proteins in the node and paranode region are ankyrins and spectrins, which link to the axonal cytoskeleton. The paranode forms glioaxonal junctions which effectively isolate the sodium channel-rich nodal axolemma from the potassium channel-rich juxtaparanode – an arrangement critical to efficient saltatory conduction of the action potential.[694]

The fate of these nodal and paranodal structures has been studied immunohistochemically in demyelinated MS plaques. Many axons in acute MS lesions demonstrate diffuse, more or less continuous redistribution (or reinsertion) of sodium channels along the demyelinated axolemma and these are thought to be responsible for continuous action potential conduction through this segment (see later under Neurophysiology of Multiple Sclerosis, p. 1362). There are many isoforms of the voltage-gated sodium channel. The voltage-gated sodium channel that mediates the action potential and is normally expressed at nodes of Ranvier is $Na_v1.6$, and that in unmyelinated axons (of which there are some in the human CNS) is $Na_v1.2$. However, both of these isoforms are present in the demyelinated regions of axons in MS (Figure 23.29a).[168] The occurrence of sodium channels in the axolemma of the demyelinated axon appears to be related to lesion duration and activity, as this is a relatively rare finding in older inactive lesions.[168]

Multifocal clusters (as opposed to diffuse distribution) of $Na_v1.6$ channels have been demonstrated in demyelinated axons in chronic MS lesions.[82] Whether such clusters can support saltatory conduction in the absence of insulating myelin is unclear. However, sodium channel clusters, referred to as 'phi nodes', have also been reported in experimental PNS demyelination where they have been shown to mediate saltatory conduction.[708] Furthermore, they are thought to dictate the location of future nodes of Ranvier

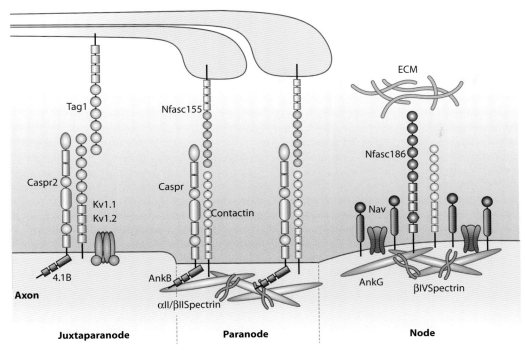

23.28 Molecular constituents of the node of Ranvier, paranode and juxtaparanode. ECM, extracellular matrix; Ank, ankyrin; Kv, voltage-gated potassium channels; Nav, voltage-gated sodium channels; Nfasc, neurofascin.

From Desmazieres A, Sol-Foulon N., Lubetzki C. Changes at the nodal and perinodal axonal domains: a basis for multiple sclerosis pathology? Mult Scler 2012;18(2):133–7. Copyright © 2012, SAGE Publications. Reprinted by permission of SAGE.

during the remyelinating process. There is evidence that this is also the case in MS plaques and that sodium channel insertion followed by nodal and then paranodal molecules antedate the myelin ensheathment of what will later be the remyelinated internode.[158] Thus, the existence of sodium channel clusters in demyelinated axons in MS raises the possibility of functional saltatory conduction resulting in clinical recovery before remyelination.[707]

Immunohistochemistry has shown that the distribution of representative nodal, paranodal and juxtaparanodal molecules in the MS periplaque region is similar to that in controls (Figure 23.29b, A and B).[158] The nodal molecule Caspr has been reported to be either absent[827] or distributed diffusely[158] along demyelinated axons in MS plaques. These discrepant findings are probably related to differences in techniques used to study the tissue, and the latter finding is illustrated in Figure 23.29b, C.[158] In fact, diffuse distribution of the juxtaparanodal protein Caspr2 and potassium channels along demyelinated axolemma has also been found in the lesion centre[158] and at the plaque edge (Figure 23.29b, D–G).[827] An early change prior to demyelination is the abnormal spread of neurofascin 155 into the adjacent juxtaparanode and the spread of potassium channels from the juxtaparanode into the paranode, thus bringing them closer to the sodium channels in the node of Ranvier and resulting in an overlap of the paranode and juxtaparanode (Figure 23.29c, A–G).[320] Overlap of potassium channels with the node of Ranvier also occurs (Figure 23.29c, H). The subsequent complete loss of oligodendroglial neurofascin 155 that occurs with demyelination allows the spread of potassium channels along the demyelinated axolemma (Figure 23.29b, D).[320]

The physiological consequences of these changes will be discussed later under Neurophysiology of Multiple Sclerosis section, p. 1362. The specific mechanisms that mediate demyelination are now considered.

Mechanisms of Demyelination

B-Cells, Antibodies and Complement
Anti-myelin antibodies have been implicated in experimental demyelination. For example, sera and CSF from patients with MS and from animals with EAE can cause demyelination in CNS organotypic cultures *in vitro*.[609,619] These antibodies in some MS patients are complement dependent and are directed against a variety of myelin and axolemmal molecules.[202] Furthermore, although autoreactive T-cells are necessary for the development of inflammation in EAE, antibodies directed against both protein and lipid myelin components enhance the clinical disease and the extent of demyelination.[351,511,621] In particular, in MOG-induced EAE immune responses, T-cell- and antibody-mediated mechanisms can mediate a disease spectrum that parallels the spectrum of human demyelinating diseases.[731]

In vitro and experimental *in vivo* studies suggest that anti-myelin antibodies combined with activated complement may mediate CNS demyelination by binding to Fc-receptors and complement receptors on the macrophage surface.[709] That immunoglobulins are deposited in MS lesions is well established.[208,440,600] IgG-capping of macrophages has been observed in active MS lesions (Figure 23.18), an appearance that would be consistent with its being a ligand for receptor-mediated phagocytosis.[600] However, immunoglobulin staining of myelin sheaths has only been equivocal. This, coupled with the observation that macrophages with IgG and complement are not specific for MS,[55] suggests that immunoglobulins in the MS lesion may not be important in the demyelinating process. Moreover, oligoclonal bands in the CSF do not react with any known protein component of myelin. However, the recent finding of CSF immunoglobulins recognizing lipids may indicate the importance of anti-lipid antibodies in the pathogenesis of autoimmune demyelination.[101] MS patients have increased levels of serum antibodies to components of CNS myelin,[794] but again the relationship of this finding to demyelination is unclear.

The autoantibody repertoire in patients with MS may, like that of T-cell responses, increase over the course of the disease as a result of autosensitization following tissue injury. The exposure and targeting of additional epitopes, referred to as 'epitope spreading', could, based on experimental work, contribute to progression of demyelination.[538] Antibodies in patients with MS are, however, not limited to recognition of myelin components and, indeed, antibodies to non-myelin targets, including heat shock proteins, axonal, retinal, node of Ranvier and paranodal proteins and other antigens, probably have major pathological effects [150,272,487,853] With breaches of the BBB associated with inflammation and vascular damage, antibodies from the systemic circulation readily enter the CNS parenchyma.

If they target neural tissue components, they might also mediate further damage.

Therefore, the role of B-cells and their products in the pathogenesis of demyelination is not clear. However, the improvement of some patients with plasma exchange[361] and the therapeutic response to an antibody directed at CD20, a major B-cell marker,[169] indicates that B-cell biology does play a role in the pathogenesis of MS, but what this role is remains uncertain at present.

Lymphocyte-Mediated Injury

The presence of large numbers of T-lymphocytes in early MS lesions suggests that oligodendrocytes may be specific targets of cytolytic T-cells. Although most Class II MHC-restricted CD4+ T-cells deploy a cellular intermediary (usually a macrophage) to destroy a particulate or molecular target, Class I MHC-restricted CD8+ cytotoxic T-cells recognize cell membrane antigens and lyse the target cell directly. Oligodendrocytes can express MHC class I molecules in MS lesions and could, therefore, be antigen targets for CD8+ cytotoxic T-cells,[274,314] but this scenario was not verified experimentally.[267] Because oligodendrocytes do not express MHC class II molecules, they would probably not be recognized by cytolytic CD4+ T-cells. Oligodendrocytes do, however, express the CD56 molecule, and CD4+ CD56+ T-cells and CD56+ natural killer

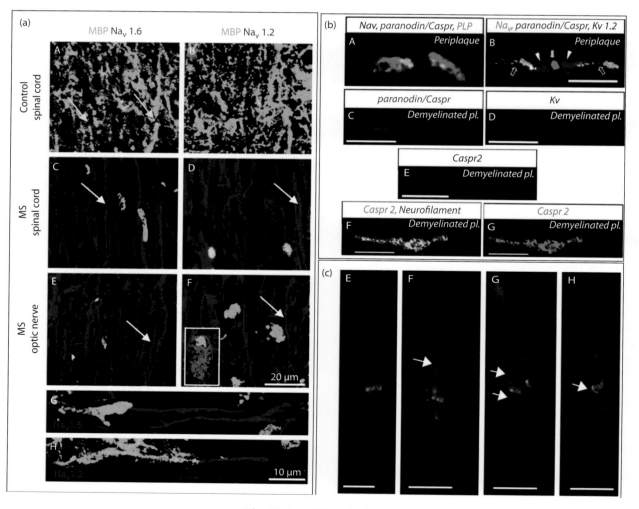

Nfasc155 (green), Kv1.2 (red)   *See legend on next page.*

(c)

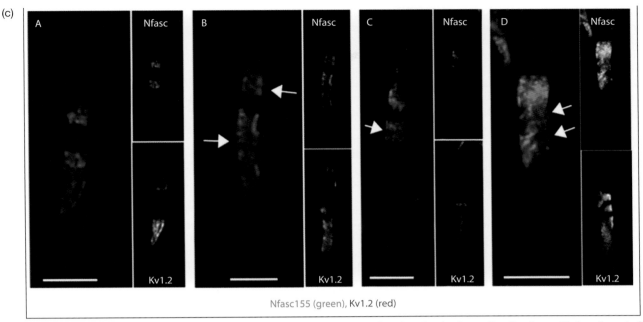

Nfasc155 (green), Kv1.2 (red)

23.29 Ion channels, and nodal, paranodal and juxtaparanodal axolemmal molecules in demyelination in multiple sclerosis (MS).
(a) Sodium channels. Confocal immunofluorescence micrographs of normal spinal cord (A and B), MS spinal cord (C and D, G and H) and MS optic nerve (E and F) white matter stained for myelin basic protein (MBP) (green), $Na_v1.6$ (red in A, C, E and G) and $Na_v1.2$ (red in B, D, F and H). In normal spinal cord white matter, $Na_v1.6$ channels are confined to nodes of Ranvier (A, yellow arrows), which do not possess $Na_v1.2$ channels (B). In MS spinal cord (C and D) and optic nerve (E and F), there are demyelinated axons, the only MBP (green) present being within macrophages (F inset, blue fluorescence for *Ricinus communis* agglutinin 1, a macrophage marker). Demyelinated axons express $Na_v1.6$ (red, examples indicated with white arrows) in C and E and $Na_v1.2$ (red, examples indicated with white arrows) in D and F. At the border of an active spinal cord plaque (G and H) are focally demyelinated axons with $Na_v1.6$ and $Na_v1.2$ expressed in the demyelinated region. **(b)** Nodal, paranodal and juxtaparanodal molecules. Confocal immunofluorescence micrographs show that the periplaque region (A and B) has a normal distribution of voltage-gated sodium channels (demonstrated with a pan Na_v antibody) (blue in A, green in B) localized to the node of Ranvier (arrow in B) between myelinated internodes (labelled for proteolipid protein, PLP, green, in A). Paranodin/Caspr (red in A and B) is confined to the paranode (arrowheads in B) and voltage-gated potassium channels ($K_v1.2$) (blue in B) are localized to the juxtaparanode (open arrows in B), as is also seen in the normal state. However, in the demyelinated plaque (C–G) paranodin/Caspr (red in C) (normally confined to the paranode), voltage-gated potassium channels (K_v) (blue in D) and Caspr 2 (blue in E) (normally confined to the juxtaparanode) are now distributed diffusely over the axon. Caspr 2 (green in F and G) is distributed diffusely along a dystrophic axon stained for neurofilament SMI (red in F; co-localization with Caspr2 is yellow). **(c)** Further nodal, paranodal and juxtaparanodal molecules. Normally (A), $K_v1.2$ channels (red) are located in the juxtaparanode, lateral to the neurofascin 155-positive (green) paranode. In demyelinated lesions (B–D) $K_v1.2$ channels (red in B–D) overlap (arrows in B–D) neurofascin (NFasc) 155 (green in B–D), a paranodal molecule, which has an elongated, abnormal distribution. Bottom right, previous page: Nodal Nfasc186-positive domains (green in E–G) associate with $K_v1.2$ channels (red in E–G) that are now displaced to the paranode where they form bands (arrows in F and G). The $K_v1.2$ channels (red in H) are also seen to overlap with Nfasc186 (green in H) at the node of Ranvier (arrow).

(a) Reproduced with permission from Craner et al.[168] Copyright (2004) National Academy of Sciences, U.S.A. (b) Modified from Coman et al.[158] With permission of Oxford University Press on behalf of The Guarantors of Brain. (c) Modified from Howell et al.[320] With permission of Oxford University Press on behalf of The Guarantors of Brain.

T-cells are capable of lysing CD56+ target cells through homotypic CD56–CD56 interactions that do not require antigen presentation.[593a] Moreover, γδ T-cell recognition of oligodendrocytes[593a] through recognition of heat-shock proteins[622] and NK T-cell recognition of oligodendroglial cell membrane lipid antigens[332] might be the basis for other scenarios of oligodendroglial demise in MS. Thus, multiple T-lymphocyte populations may specifically target and lyse oligodendrocytes. How such mechanisms directed against the myelin sheath, which is an extension of the oligodendrocyte cell membrane, would be operative is unclear, because the inflicted damage would, at the most, only involve a focal segment of the targeted oligodendrocyte-myelin unit.

It would seem the most efficient means would be to target the cell body, as discussed later, with consequent disintegration of its dependent myelin sheaths (see Oligodendrocyte Cell Body Destruction, p. 1326).

Macrophage/Microglia-Mediated Injury

Different expression patterns of chemokines and other markers among macrophage populations in MS lesions suggest that the lesions are heterogeneous.[455] The distinct roles of different pathogenetic processes in different lesion stages and micro-environments are probably influenced by many factors, including the number of T-cells recruited, the anatomical location, and the extent and mechanisms of myelin damage.[5]

As noted previously, a major function of macrophages is the removal of myelin, whether this is a primary or a secondary process in the initiation of the demyelinating process.

However, there are a number of other ways the macrophage can be implicated in the attack on myelin. Activated macrophages produce NO, diffusible reactive oxygen and nitrogen species (such as peroxynitrite), extracellular proteolytic enzymes, and cytokines such as TNF that either alone or in combination can cause damage to myelin and oligodendrocyte membranes.[130,170,310,339,523,695,772,795] This relatively indiscriminate 'bystander' damage is probably a major mechanism of injury of not only myelin and oligodendrocytes but other cell types in the affected field as well.

Microglia/macrophages are also integral components of adaptive (antigen-specific) immunity, by virtue of their ability to present antigens. In addition, it is probable that macrophage-mediated myelin degradation enhances the susceptibility of the CNS to the action of anti-myelin antibodies, by exposing previously untargeted epitopes to antigen-presenting cells.

Microglia/macrophages also function as part of the innate immune system. Complement-decorated myelin could act as a ligand for their complement-receptors and initiate myelin stripping. However, as discussed earlier, it is unclear to what degree or what stage this is operative in the MS lesion. The widespread expression of TLR by microglia/macrophages probably also provides an important mechanism by which they can recognize and interact with both exogenous, i.e. infectious, and endogenous ligands, such as heat-shock proteins, within the CNS.[339] Engagement of these receptors also results in the production of NO and TNF.[118,331] Thus, the use of common effector molecules, particularly NO and TNF, in overlapping pathogenetic pathways suggests that these pathways may be closely, and perhaps inextricably, linked in the pathogenesis of demyelination in MS lesions.[706]

Mechanisms of Oligodendrocyte Depletion

In addition to demyelination, the progressive overall loss of oligodendrocytes that precludes adequate remyelination of remaining axons is a hallmark of MS pathology (Figure 23.19). Although damage to myelin and depletion of oligodendrocytes are inseparable processes *in vivo*, for the purposes of discussion the preceding sections have addressed cellular and molecular mechanisms that principally mediate damage to myelin membranes; the following sections focus on the processes by which oligodendrocytes are depleted.

The rate of progression of overall oligodendrocyte loss is probably influenced by the contributions of diverse injury mechanisms and by concurrent proliferation of immature oligodendrocytes, particularly at plaque edges and in early lesions (Figures 23.30–23.32).[138,604,620,719] There may also be differences in oligodendrocyte susceptibility to injury in different anatomical regions. Moreover, the simultaneous degeneration and loss of axons add further to the complexity and dynamic nature of the pathological processes that result in oligodendrocyte loss. Making clear distinctions among the simultaneous processes in human biopsy and autopsy tissue samples is particularly difficult, and the relative contributions of each mechanism are controversial.[244]

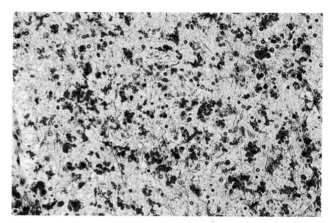

23.30 Oligodendroglial hyperplasia and macrophages in multiple sclerosis (MS). The border of a multiple sclerosis (MS) plaque shows numerous oligodendrocytes (small round nuclei) in an area with residual myelin lipid-containing macrophages. Frozen section, oil red O and haematoxylin.

Courtesy of Professor JW Prineas, University of Sydney, Sydney, Australia.

Oligodendrocyte Cell Body Destruction

There is morphologic evidence to suggest that the initial insult in the genesis of an MS plaque may be oligodendroglial death. In a study of lesions responsible for a very rapid clinical course, it was noted that the only significant cellular change in the immediately adjacent white matter (the 'pre-phagocytic zone') was oligodendroglial apoptosis associated with microglial activation.[54] There were no inflammatory infiltrates associated in this area, making it difficult to invoke the products of the immune response as being responsible for this early change. What is responsible for this early oligodendroglial apoptosis is not known.[54] A number of possible immunologic mechanisms may be considered.[120] Of note is the recent finding of oxidized DNA and oxidized lipid in oligodendrocytes in this area, suggesting that free radicals were important in their demise.[292] Free radical formation in MS lesions originates from the actions of microglial/macrophage enzymes, such as myeloperoxidase, xanthine oxidase and nicotinamide adenine dinucleotide phosphate (NADPH) oxidase and from mitochondrial dysfunction.[781] There is evidence to indicate that the oxidative burst, with upregulation of NADPH oxidase, in microglia may be responsible for generating these reactive molecular species in the MS lesion.[233] In addition, in some MS lesions, oligodendroglia show mitochondrial defects (as demonstrated by immunohistochemistry for cytochrome *c* oxidase-1 [COX-I]), which is thought to be due to their susceptibility to oxidative stress.[457]

However, in areas of myelin breakdown and phagocytosis, evidence for apoptosis of oligodendrocytes is variable,[112] sometimes associated with the expression of p53, and in some cases negligble[131] compared to controls, even though receptors associated with the apoptotic cascade are demonstrable on these cells.[131] This may in part be due to their expression of the anti-apoptotic protein bcl-2.[394]

Oligodendrocytes express glutamate receptors and are very susceptible to glutamate toxicity, which may be

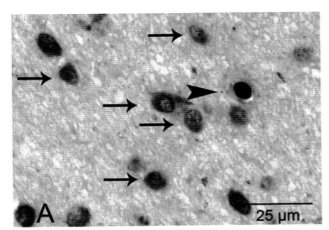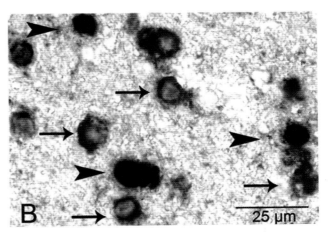

23.31 Oligodendroglial precursors in chronic (MS). (a) Non-MS white matter with oligodendrocyte precursor cells expressing OLIG 2 (arrowhead) and mature oligodendrocytes expressing low levels of OLIG2 and Nogo A (arrows). Nogo A indicates differentiation commitment on the part of the cell expressing it. **(b)** MS periplaque white matter with mature oligodendrocytes (arrows) expressing OLIG 2 and Nogo A and increased numbers of oligodendrocyte precursor cells staining strongly for OLIG2 (arrowheads). Double-staining immunohistochemistry for OLIG2 in black and Nogo A in red.

Reproduced fom Kuhlmann T, Miron V, Cuo Q, et al. Differentiation block of oligodendroglial progenitor cells as a cause for remyelination failure in chronic multiple sclerosis. Brain 2008;131:1749–58. With permission of Oxford University Press on behalf of The Guarantors of Brain.

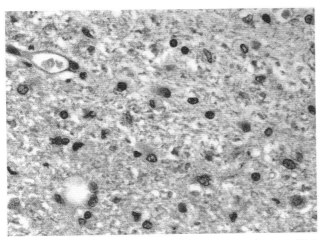

23.32 Oligodendroglial hyperplasia in an active multiple sclerosis (MS) lesion. Same case as shown in Figure 23.52. Immunostaining of cells expressing the oligodendrocyte differentiation antigen 2′,3′-cyclic nucleotide 3′-phosphodiesterase (CNPase). Immunoperoxidase with haematoxylin.

operative in the MS lesion because of release of glutamate by microglia and cells undergoing oxidative stress, among other sources.[476,556] This is compounded by the impaired ability of the oligodendrocyte to handle glutamate in MS.[811]

Oligodendrocytes in MS lesions also express the highly immunogenic heat shock protein αB-crystallin and this has been postulated to be an antigen in MS that will result in oligodendroglial elimination.[782] The interaction of components of the innate immune system with microglia to produce oligodendrocyte destruction has been discussed earlier under Demyelination Macrophage/Microglia-Mediated Injury, p. 1325.

Dying Back Oligodendrogliopathy

Oligodendrocytes may also succumb to degeneration as a result of pathology in their distal processes. This has been shown experimentally.[444,445] The same degeneration of inner myelin loops has been seen in biopsy material of acute MS lesions.[639] These lesions also show widening of inner myelin lamellae.[639] These phenomena are consistent with an injury to the oligodendrocyte cell body that results in its inability to maintain myelin integrity in its most distal processes–a 'dying-back gliopathy'.[444] Indeed, in some lesions, loss of immunoreactivity of periaxonal MAG precedes that of the other major myelin proteins, such as myelin basic protein (MBP) and PLP.[336,440,442] Supporting the notion that demyelination is secondary to oligodendrocyte death in MS is the same observation in progressive multifocal leukoencephalopathy (see Chapter 1315), in which myelin breakdown is preceded by virus infection of oligodendrocytes.

Remyelination

Remyelination of demyelinated axons in MS lesions is necessary for restoring saltatory conduction, and protecting them from further injury. Remyelination occurs spontaneously in the human CNS, but is often structurally and functionally incomplete. The extent of remyelination of acute MS lesions is variable and in some lesions appears to be transient and aberrant (Figures 23.33 and 23.34).[609,618] It is generally much less evident in chronic lesions,[271] and when present is at lesion borders with ongoing inflammatory demyelination (Figure 23.34) and is associated with increased numbers of oligodendroglial cells (Figures 23.30–23.33).[609,620,825] However, extensive sampling has shown that remyelination may be more widespread in chronic disease than previously appreciated (Figure 23.22).[562] The degree of remyelination

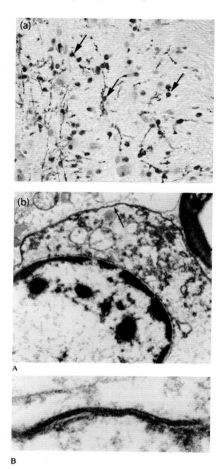

23.33 Oligodendroglial hyperplasia and aberrant remyelination in multiple sclerosis (MS). (a) Immunohistochemical stain for 2′3′-cyclic nucleotide 3′-phophosdiesterase (CNP) at the edge of a chronic active MS plaque shows that numerous oligodendroglia have upregulated CNP (arrows), indicative of remyelination; these are often in pairs (right arrow) or clusters. Many of the oligodendroglia have long, expansive CNP-positive process (middle arrow). **(b)** Electron micrographs of autopsy material from a band of myelin in a Baló's concentric sclerosis lesion showing aberrant myelination of the perikaryon of an oligodendrocyte (A). Higher magnification of the region indicated by the arrow in A shows a few lamellae of myelin on the surface of the oligodendrocyte (B).

(b) From Moore et al.[512] With permission of John Wiley and Sons. Copyright © 1985 The American Neurological Association.

is quite variable from patient to patient and is dependent on the lesion location, periventricular plaques tending to show less extensive remyelination.[563]

Morphology

Newly formed myelin sheaths are thinner and have shorter internodal distances than the original sheaths (Figures 23.20, 23.22, 23.34–23.36). In fact, these parameters reflect a major difference between the process of myelination during development and remyelination.[217] During myelination, there is a relationship between axonal diameter and myelin sheath thickness, such that the greater the axonal diameter the thicker the myelin sheath and the longer the internodal

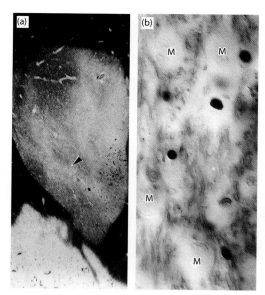

23.34 Shadow plaque. Large remyelinating multiple sclerosis (MS) shadow plaque located in cerebellar white matter. **(a)** Grey and white areas indicate partial reduction in myelin densities. **(b)** Enlargement of the area indicated by an arrowhead in **(a)** shows a lattice arrangement of the smoothly contoured new thin myelin sheaths in the presence of unstained foamy macrophages (M) that are present throughout the tissue. Heidenhain.

Reproduced from Prineas et al.[607] By permission of Oxford University Press on behalf of The Guarantors of Brain.

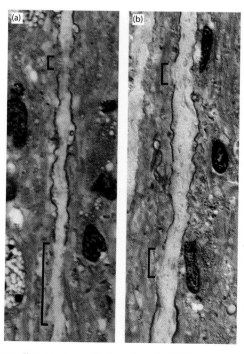

23.35 Remyelination in multiple sclerosis (MS). (a,b) Longitudinal sections of thinly myelinated fibres in a remyelinating shadow plaque, showing short, thin internodes of uniform thickness separated by gaps that may represent regenerating nodes of Ranvier (bars). Toluidine blue.

Reproduced by permission from Prineas et al.[602] Copyright © 2006, John Wiley and Sons.

distance, whereas in remyelination both the regenerated sheath thickness and the internodal length are constant irrespective of axonal diameter. Moreover, neither of these parameters reaches the same values as in the normal state, although in the case of small diameter axons this can be very difficult to discern by routine microscopy.[217] Partially remyelinated lesions may contain redundant whorls of myelin close to or around oligodendrocyte perikarya, oligodendrocytes that are abnormally clumped together in pairs or groups, some of which are non-myelinating or 'demyelinated' (Figure 23.33). There may also be uncompacted oligodendroglial cytoplasm, and gradually tapering of the myelin sheath as it approaches the node of Ranvier with the formation of junctional complexes and paranodal-like periodic densities between adjacent oligodendroglial cytoplasmic loops.[609,615,736]

In partially remyelinated lesions, the distribution length of sodium channels at the new nodes of Ranvier and their adjacent paranode (as indicated by Caspr and neurofascin 155 staining) is increased, but the juxtaparanode length is normal.[158,320] The occurrence of very short distances between some of the aggregates of Caspr in these regions is consistent with exceedingly short remyelinated internodes.[827] It has been hypothesized that some remyelinated internodes at the plaque edge may arise from lengthening of the node of Ranvier, in addition to the well-accepted response to internodal axonal demyelination.[827] In addition, the occurrence of paranodes in triplicate in remyelination suggests that these may be a transient phenomenon in the subsequent fusion of two nodes that they temporarily demarcate.[320]

Shadow Plaques

In the earlier MS literature, the term 'shadow plaque' referred to any area of partial reduction in myelin density.[609] More recent analyses have shown that these are remyelinating or remyelinated areas in which there are thin, short, smoothly contoured myelin internodes, usually of similar thicknesses (Figures 23.34 and 23.36). Many shadow plaques remain permanently remyelinated, but others may become sites of new demyelinating activity, either within or overlapping previously remyelinated areas (Figure 23.37).[606,607] Shadow plaques may, therefore, represent the less common occurrence of a single episode of focal demyelination that has been remyelinated.[607] Variable degrees of axon abnormalities in shadow plaques have been reported.[381,535] The distribution of sodium channels, paranodal and juxtaparanodal makers and potassium channels in shadow plaques is no different from controls.[158,320] However, as noted previously, in zones of other MS plaques that are only partially remyelinated the node and paranode are lengthened.[158,320]

Remyelination by Oligodendroglia and Their Precursors

Survival of oligodendrocytes in MS lesions is quite variable.[439,604] However, experimental evidence to date would indicate that these mature oligodendrocytes are not capable of remyelination.[238] On the other hand, there are robust data to indicate that remyelination in MS is accomplished by oligodendrocyte precursor cells (OPCs), which abound in the

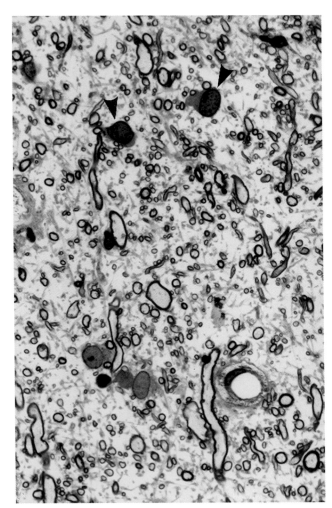

23.36 Remyelination in multiple sclerosis (MS). Epoxy-embedded section of remyelinating multiple sclerosis (MS) shadow plaque showing thinly myelinated axons. The two darkly staining cells (arrowheads) are probably oligodendrocytes, and the lightly staining cells are small fibrous astrocytes. Toluidine blue.

Courtesy of Professor JW Prineas, University of Sydney, Sydney, Australia.

adult CNS and are present even in chronic MS lesions.[138] OPCs express a number of markers, particularly the proteoglycan NG2,[138] platelet-derived growth factor receptor-α (PDGFRα)[237,817] and Golli proteins,[226] and less frequently the transcription factors OLIG1, ACSL1 and MYT1.[237] They also express OLIG2 (Figure 23.31) and O4 (Figure 23.38),[825] markers that are also shared by oligodendroglial lineage cells later in differentiation.[237] Interestingly, OPC may also generate neurons and astrocytes.[237] They respond to neurotrophins.[23] They also express glutamate receptors and are electrophysiologically active,[46] suggesting that they are communicating with neurons.[237]

The observation that remyelination in MS is frequently accompanied by inflammation suggests that the inflammatory response plays a role in driving the OPC-mediated remyelinating process.[238,620,826] Indeed, experimentally, it has been shown that inflammation stimulates

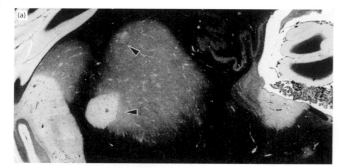

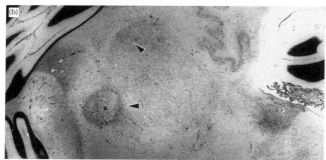

23.37 Recurrent demyelination in multiple sclerosis (MS) shadow plaques. The figure shows cerebellar white matter with three remyelinated shadow plaques, each overlapped by additional lesions. The shadow plaque in the centre is the site of two newly forming perivascular lesions (arrowheads). The remyelinated shadow plaque bordering the demyelinated plaque on the left shows evidence of commencing perivascular demyelination. The remyelinated lesion on the right is overlapped by a fresh periventricular lesion. **(a)** Heidenhain. **(b)** Nissl.

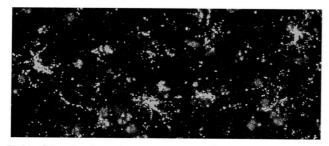

23.38 Oligodendrocyte precursor cells in multiple sclerosis (MS). Process-bearing O4-positive oligodendrocyte precursors (green) are present among autofluorescent lipid-containing macrophages (orange) in demyelinated tissue in a female aged 57 years with a 19-year history of multiple sclerosis (MS). Immunostained for O4 antigen. Green fluorescein isothiocyanate (FITC).

remyelination[236] and depletion of macrophages or T-cells dampens remyelination.[385a,386]

However, although remyelination may be evident during active disease, this remyelinated myelin is also subject to demyelination[602] and by the time the lesion has reached a chronic stage, the demyelinated zone is usually devoid of any remyelinated myelin despite the presence of OPC, which although reduced in number in comparison to more active lesions, are nevertheless present.[397] Thus, the OPC seems incapable of remyelination in the chronic lesion.

Effective remyelination normally proceeds along a specific sequence. The first step is the activation of OPC, which is associated with upregulation of transcription factors such as OLIG2, NKX2.2, MYT1 and SOX2, modulated by the cell cycle regulatory protein p27Kip1 and induced by PDGF and fibroblast growth factor (FGF).[237,245,830] After activation, OPCs are recruited to the axons requiring remyelination, a process that is less efficient in aged individuals,[142] and undergo differentiation into myelin-generating cells. FGF and IGF1 figure prominently in both recruitment and differentiation.[237] CXC chemokine receptors are expressed on cells of oligodendrocyte lineage in MS, indicating these molecules may also be involved in these processes.[545]

The bulk of current evidence suggests that the remyelination failure in MS is due to a failure of differentiation by OPC, rather than any deficiencies in activation or recruitment, and this phenomenon becomes progressively worse with ageing, but is enhanced by female hormones, such as oestrogen[386] – factors that may be pertinent in the pathogenesis of PPMS, which is particularly prevalent in older males (see later under Primary Progressive Multiple Sclerosis, p. 1356). Supportive of this is an immunohistochemical study of OLIG 2 and NKX2.2 in chronic MS lesions that showed features consistent with an arrest in OPC differentiation.[397]

The reason for this differentiation failure is unclear but a number of mechanisms, either individually or in combination, have been proposed as culprits. One is the accumulation of hyaluran, a known inhibitor of OPC differentiation, synthesized by astrocytes.[44] Another is the expression of the polysialylated form of neural cell adhesion molecule (PAS-NCAM),[144,157] and other not-yet-recognized inhibitors of remyelination, by demyelinated axons.[237] Further, semaphorins, which can have a chemorepulsive effect (semaphorin 3A) or a chemo-attractant effect (semaphorin 3F), may, in the case of semaphorin 3A, also delay differentiation. The finding of both these molecules in MS active lesions suggests that their expression at different stages in the evolution of the early lesion may involve a delicate balancing act between positive and negative effects on OPC.[155,386,816] Notch 1, a negative differentiation regulator (but probably not an absolutely necessary one in the case of remyelination), is found on immature cells of oligodendroglial lineage in MS lesions without remyelination, and its ligand, Jagged 1, is present on neighbouring astrocytes.[343] On the other hand, non-canonical activation of the notch pathway by FC3/Contactin ligands via signalling through the Notch intracellular domain (NICD)–Deltex complex can induce OPC differentiation, but this appears to be overridden in MS by the OCP expression of TIP30, an antagonist of contacin-mediated differentiation.[386,520] Canonical activation of Wnt ('wingless') signalling pathway, known to delay OPC differentiation, has also been implicated, because its transcription factor Tcf4 (also known as Tcf712), which acts by forming a nucleoprotein complex with dephosphorylated β-catenin, is also expressed by O4-positive oligodendroglial cells in MS lesions.[216] Moreover, sonic hedgehog and its cleavage product, which is important in oligodendrocyte maturation, are reduced in MS.[471]

The effect of such factors that delay differentiation and retain the OPC in the activation/recruitment state may be very important and this has been referred to as the 'dysregulation hypothesis', whereby the timing of events, rather than the presence or absence of their effects, is the critical variable.[237] Thus, a delay in the timing of differentiation may be sufficient to cause the OPC to 'miss out' on the effect of potent molecules that favourably interact with cells at a more advanced stage of their differentiation. Another pertinent hypothesis is that in chronic MS there is misguided differentiation that directs OPC to differentiate into astrocytes rather than oligodendrocytes–hence the astrocytic scar of chronic MS.[386]

Important in the consideration of OPC differentiation failure in MS is the observation that myelin itself is an important contributor to this.[738] Thus, in addition to the positive effects of macrophages in inducing remyelination, they also serve the important function of removal of the inhibitory effects of myelin debris.[386]

What the inhibiting component in myelin is, is not known; however, the well-known myelin-associated inhibitors of CNS axonal regeneration, such as NogoA (which is expressed on oligodendroglia at the edge of chronic active MS lesions[668]), MAG and oligodendrocyte myelin glycoprotein do not negatively affect OPCs.[386,738]

Remyelination by Schwann Cells

Remyelination of demyelinated axons by Schwann cells near the entry zones of posterior spinal roots can occur in MS in lesional areas with no astrocytes, suggesting that astrocytes are inhibitory to PNS remyelination within the CNS (Figure 23.39)[337] or favour oligodendroglial remyelination.[742] Peripheral-type myelin is identifiable in these areas by its darker blue staining compared with that of central myelin on the Luxol fast blue stain and by electron microscopy, where the remyelinated myelin is associated with cells with a basement membrane (characteristic of Schwann cells, but not oligodendrocytes[260]). It is generally held that

Schwann cells invade the demyelinated tissue from nearby spinal roots. However, a recent experimental study has provided evidence to suggest that these Schwann cells may be of OPC origin.[848]

Axonal Injury and Loss
History and Significance

Axonal injury was documented in the earliest descriptions of MS lesions.[162] Because of the more overt involvement of white matter and relative neuron and axonal preservation in active lesions (Figures 23.40 and 23.41), however, MS research focused in large part on immune mechanisms and demyelination for most of the twentieth century. Since the late 1990s, the extent and clinical importance of axonal injury in acute MS lesions have become better appreciated.[222,261,395,760] Axon injury within MS lesions results in both wallerian degeneration of the axon and retrograde degeneration of the cell body.[571] Although it is not possible to determine the precise age of injury in human biopsy or autopsy samples, it is now generally accepted that axonal damage and concomitant neuronal dysfunction are intrinsic to MS pathophysiology from its early stages. Moreover, progressive axonal loss is considered the major determinant of clinical progression and permanent disability in the later stages of the disease.[178,571,572,576,744] Despite the loss of myelinated and demyelinated axons, it appears that unmyelinated axons, such as subcortical white matter interneurons, are able to regenerate in MS lesions.[139]

Morphology

Axons in active lesions are frequently irregularly swollen, giving them a beaded appearance; they are also interrupted, forming so-called retraction bulbs (axonal end bulbs). These alterations are most abundant in areas with maximal ongoing demyelination and are demonstrable using

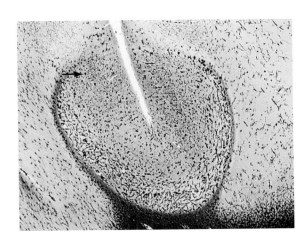

23.40 Leukocortical plaque. A multiple sclerosis (MS) plaque centred on a sulcus extends into the subcortical white matter. Neurons within the demyelinated cortex appear normal. The area indicated by an arrow is in the upper left of the plaque. Golgi silver technique.

Courtesy of Dr TH Moss, Frenchay Hospital, Bristol, UK.

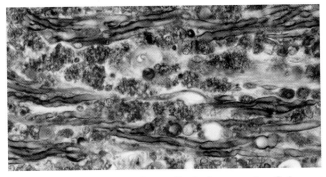

23.39 Remyelination of demyelinated axons by Schwann cells. Recent multiple sclerosis (MS) spinal cord lesion. There was no evidence of ongoing demyelination in this resolving lesion. 6-μm epoxy section of osmicated tissue.

Reproduced from Prineas et al.[607] By permission of Oxford University Press on behalf of The Guarantors of Brain.

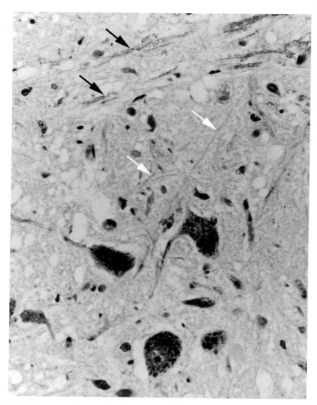

23.41 Neuronal sparing in a multiple sclerosis (MS) plaque. Intact pyramidal neurons in a chronic inactive MS plaque involving the nucleus ambiguus. A few myelinated axons are seen in the lesion edge (black arrows), and faint profiles of demyelinated axons (white arrows) in close proximity to the surviving neurons are evident within the plaque. Luxol fast blue–cresyl violet (LFB–CV).

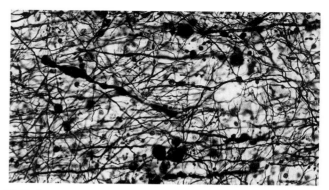

23.42 Axonal injury in acute multiple sclerosis (MS). Lesion in a 44-year-old male with a 27-day history. Irregularly swollen axons are visible within a newly forming cerebral plaque. Bodian silver impregnation.

Courtesy of Professor JW Prineas, University of Sydney, Sydney, Australia.

standard silver impregnation techniques (Figure 23.42). Swollen axons with evenly dispersed neurofilaments associated with reduced argentophilia have also been observed in some plaques. As in other disease processes where there is acute transection of the axon, there is an accumulation of amyloid precursor protein (APP) in the axon such that it can be detected immunohistochemically (Figure 23.43).[222] Quantitative studies show frequent damaged axons in acute lesions[222] and to a lesser degree in chronic lesions.[760]

Mechanisms

The molecular pathways that result in axonal and neuronal injury in patients with MS are not understood. Our understanding of the failure of subsequent CNS axonal regeneration in most conditions, including MS, is also rudimentary.[404,465] Numerous simultaneous processes in inflammatory demyelinating lesions are likely to act in concert, proceed at different rates and probably contribute to heterogeneous injury and axonal loss in different anatomical sites and types of lesion. The discussion that follows will outline some of the mechanisms that may underlie axonal loss and degeneration in the MS lesion.

The Inflammatory/Immune Response

Axonal transection in MS is frequently associated with inflammation.[194] The range of antigens that can be demonstrated in swollen axons and end bulbs in active lesions is likely to reflect multiple injury mechanisms and secondary abnormalities. Molecules that have been detected include vitronectin,[717] amyloid β-precursor protein (APP) (Figure 23.43),[222] the α1B pore-forming subunit of N-type calcium channels,[382] osteopontin[185] and ephrin A and EphA receptors (Figure 23.44)[714] - ephrins being inhibitors of neurite outgrowth.[68] The ubiquitination of axons in NAWM adjacent to plaques, possibly mediated by the proteosomal pathway,[265] is also consistent with axonal degeneration. Enhanced immunoreactivity for non-phosphorylated neurofilaments is typical of demyelinated axons. Axonal swellings are frequently spatially related to microglia and macrophages;[760] chronic and recurrent inflammation may result in impaired axonal transport and amputations of axons.[14] Cytotoxic enzymes, pro-inflammatory cytokines, chemokines, glutamate, MMP, free radicals and NO produced by the infiltrating leukocytes and microglia/macrophages may mediate these effects.[194,307,391] Free radicals produced by microglia/macrophages can result in mitochondrial, DNA and lipid damage in neurons.[233,292] Impaired fibrinolysis may also lead to axon damage,[288] and neuritic beading induced by activated microglia. Based on experimental data, it has been proposed that neurodegeneration in MS is mediated by multimolecular nanocomplexes in the internodal axolemma; these nanocomplexes comprise a variety of molecules including glutamate receptors, $Ca_v1.2$ L-type calcium channels and neuronal nitric oxide synthetase (nNOS).[729] In addition to macrophages/microglia, CD4+ and CD8+ T-cells are capable of destroying neurons in an antigen-independent Class I MHC-independent manner.[267,593a] The finding that α-synuclein, a protein marker of neurodegenerative synucleinopathies (see Chapters 12, Extrapyramidal Diseases of Movement, and 16, Dementia), in MS lesions was linked to inflammatory activity suggests yet another neurodegenerative process mediated by inflammation.[434] Thus, it is very likely that inflammation is a major contributor to axonal damage in MS and many of the mechanisms by which this is mediated are potential therapeutic targets.[77,243,353,553]

Aside from these non-specific effects of inflammation on the axon, there is evidence to suggest that a specific

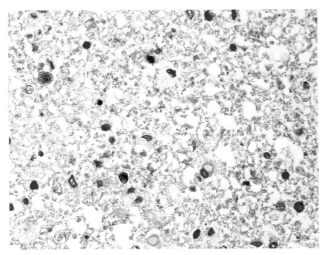

23.43 Amyloid precursor protein (APP) in multiple sclerosis (MS). APP accumulates in recently injured and transected axons (seen in cross-section) in an active multiple sclerosis (MS) lesion. Same case as shown in Figure 23.24. Immunoperoxidase with haematoxylin.

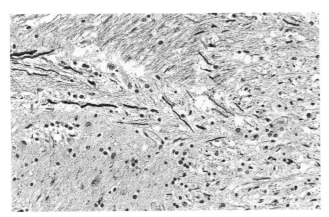

23.44 Ephrin A1 in multiple sclerosis (MS). Swollen injured axons within and at the edge of an acute multiple sclerosis (MS) plaque show immunolabelling for ephrin A1. Same case as shown in Figure 23.21. Immunoperoxidase with haematoxylin.

immune-mediated attack on the axon may be operative in the MS. Immunoglobulins are localized on axons in MS lesions and that may, therefore, represent binding to specific antibody targets.[407,853] Anti-neuronal antibodies are detected in the sera and CSF of patients with MS and may correlate with the extent of brain atrophy.[184,200] Some MS patients have antibodies with the capacity to destroy axons in tissue culture.[202] Antibody cross-recognition, for example the recognition of shared myelin and non-myelin epitopes by a single antibody, could also have pathophysiological consequences.[280] As in paraneoplastic and other disorders, anti-neuronal or anti-axonal antibodies might perturb cellular functions in the absence of florid morphological alterations.

Blood–Brain Barrier Breakdown

As noted earlier (see Endothelial Cells, p. 1310), the disruption of the BBB is readily apparent in MS lesions in immunohistochemical studies demonstrating serum components, normally confined to the blood vessel lumen, in the perivascular parenchyma. This occurrence would imply the presence of any number of circulating compounds that could disrupt neuronal and glial homeostasis.[485]

Demyelination

There is an intimate functional and trophic relationship between the myelin sheath and the axon. Thus, for the demyelinated axon, the absence of myelin represents more than just a loss of its insulating sheath. This is reflected in neurofilament dephosphorylation[760] and a reduction in axonal diameter.[598] The insertion of sodium channels in the demyelinated axolemma (Figure 23.29a) (see earlier under Demyelination, p. 1322, and later under Neurophysiology of Multiple Sclerosis, p. 1362) results in excessive intra-axonal sodium. The $Na_v1.6$ channels also produce, in addition to rapidly activating and inactivating current, a persistent current resulting in a constant influx of sodium into the axon.[168] The reduction in Na^+/K^+ ATPase[840] also contributes to the intra-axonal sodium accumulation. The sodium is substituted for calcium by the sodium-calcium exchanger,[168,382] which has been co-localized with sodium channels in demyelinated degenerating axons (manifested by their expression of amyloid precursor protein) (Figure 23.45).[168] This situation is further compounded by the insertion of calcium channels in the demyelinated axolemma (Figure 23.46).[382] The increase in calcium results in axonal degeneration or death by activating neutral proteases, such as calpains.[733] The changes in the axon have been likened to a state of chronic relative hypoxia with the energy demands of the various changes outlined earlier outstripping its supply.[759] Thus, the remodelling of the demyelinated axolemma may contribute significantly to neurodegeneration in the acute MS lesion.

Based on the finding of excessive citrullination of myelin basic protein (MBP) in MS, it has also been proposed that the degenerative process occurs initially in the myelin sheath, rather than only secondarily in the axon.[470]

Mitochondrial Dysfunction

As is the case with oligodendroglia, axons in some MS lesion show mitochondrial abnormalities. This takes the form of reduced mitochondrial complex IV in axons within regions of ongoing demyelination.[457,458] The association of these changes with inflammation would suggest that they are secondary phenomena. As noted above, it has been hypothesized that mitochondrial defects are the basis for a mismatch between energy supply and demand, resulting in calcium-mediated axon death.[195] The effect is compounded by increased neuronal firing due to a reduction in inhibitory GABAergic neurotransmission in the MS cortex.[195]

Types of White Matter Plaques in Multiple Sclerosis

These molecular and cellular features may be found in various permutations and combinations in the white matter plaques of MS. The classification of these plaques is often based on the presence or absence of some of these features, particularly inflammation and ongoing demyelination. The classification schemes that have been employed usually attempt to categorise plaques to reflect their duration and

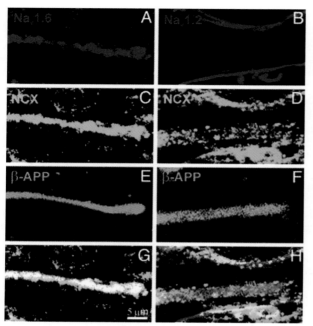

23.45 Sodium–calcium exchanger in demyelinated axons in acute multiple sclerosis (MS) lesions. Amyloid-β precursor protein (β-APP)-positive axons (blue in E, F, G and H) express $Na_v1.6$ (red in A and G) and $Na_v1.2$ (red in B and H). There is co-expression of the sodium–calcium exchanger (NCX) (green in C, D, G and H) in β-APP-positive axons that possess $Na_v1.6$ channels (G) but not in those with $Na_v1.2$ channels (H). However NCX is evident in $Na_v1.2$-positive axons that are negative for β-APP (H). G is a merged image of A, C and E (white represents co-localization of red, green and blue). H is a merged image of B, D and F (yellow represents co-localization of green and red). A, immunofluorecence (red) for $Na_v1.6$; B, immunofluorescence (red) for $Na_v1.2$; C and D, immunofluorescence for NCX (green); E and F, immunofluorescence for β-APP (blue); G, merged images of A, C and E; H, merged image B, D and F.

whether or not they are continuing to show active disease and expansion.

A number of systems for plaque classification have been used, each of which has advantages and shortcomings.[776] Most of the common schemes that have been or are currently being used are summarized and compared in Table 23.8. Traditionally, MS plaques have been classified into acute, chronic active and chronic silent (inactive) plaques. This is the approach that will be followed in this chapter, not because it is necessarily superior to any of the others but because it is the most straightforward and has been in use for the longest period. As such for the purposes of presentation, other classification schemes can usually be translated into its three categories. However, it should be noted that this is by no means always possible, and frequently what one scientific article is describing cannot be readily transposed or compared with data from another that has employed a different classification system.

Pathology of the Acute Multiple Sclerosis Plaque

The traditional concept of the acute MS plaque is that it is the lesion that characterizes acute MS. Acute MS has a distinct clinical temporal profile of an acute monophasic illness, as opposed to the relapsing-remitting clinical course of the classic early clinical presentation. Acute MS is also frequently referred to as 'Marburg's disease'. Marburg described three cases of a fulminant disease in which there were symptoms, such as acute paraplegia that improved dramatically after a brief neurological illness.[466] In most acute cases of acute MS reported subsequently, the illness followed a rapidly progressive or stepwise downhill course, with focal neurological signs similar to those seen in chronic MS, except at a much brisker tempo and accompanied by diffuse signs such as confusion and seizures. In contrast to acute disseminated encephalomyelitis (ADEM), which can have a similar acute onset (see later under Acute Disseminated Encephalomyelitis and Related Disorders, p. 1379), fever and meningeal signs are usually absent. Also unlike ADEM, often there is no history of preceding infection or immunization. The CSF protein level and lymphocyte count are normal or moderately elevated, and elevated IgG levels and oligoclonal bands are present less often than in chronic MS. Neuroimaging studies can demonstrate one or more lesions that may not be distinguishable from other disorders, including chronic MS. Whereas death early in the course of typical MS is uncommon, most deaths in cases of acute MS occur 1–6 months after clinical onset. Cases of even shorter duration have been reported.[609] Thus, abrupt onset and rapid temporal progression are the most distinct clinical features in acute MS.

The freshly sectioned brain and spinal cord of acute MS reveal numerous opaque white or yellow areas ranging from approximately 2 mm to 5 cm in diameter. Their distribution is similar to that in chronic MS, with the brain, spinal cord and optic nerves usually involved, and with a predilection for periventricular areas and the cortical grey matter–white matter junction. In fact, very early lesions in chronic MS are indistinguishable from those of acute MS.

By microscopy, acute MS lesions have a more or less uniform appearance throughout their extent, which is also similar from one lesion to the next, correlating with the monophasic clinical profile. However, even in acute MS, there is often indication of dissemination in time, as evidenced by a subtle variability in the morphology of lesions.[604] The acute MS plaque is characterized by a focal area of demyelination that is hypercellular, often with ill-defined boundaries (Figures 23.47 and 23.48). There is macrophage-mediated demyelination, with relative preservation of axons (Figure 23.13), and perivascular mononuclear cell infiltrates (Figures 23.6 and 23.47) comprising lymphocytes and monocytes (Figure 23.7). Reactive astrocytes, with prominent cell bodies, abound (Figures 23.23, 23.26 and 23.27). Numerous demyelinated axons are evident (Figure 23.13). There may be oligodendrocyte loss (Figure 23.19), or proliferation and remyelination.[604,618]

Axons within the acute lesion retain their Na^+/K^+ ATPase pumps at internodes (as is the normal situation).[840] There are frequent acutely transected axons, immunoreactive for amyloid precursor protein (APP) indicative of disruption of axon transport, that will subsequently undergo wallerian degeneration.[222,395,760] As noted previously, many axons within the acute MS lesion demonstrate redistribution (or reinsertion)

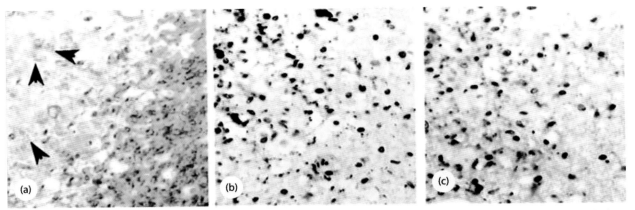

23.46 Calcium channels in axons in multiple sclerosis (MS). (a) Luxol fast blue (LFB) stain showing myelin fragments within macrophages (arrowheads) in an actively demyelinating MS plaque. **(b)** Amyloid-β precursor protein (APP)-positive axons are seen within the plaque. **(c)** Axons expressing α_{1B}, the pore-forming subunit of N-type voltage-gated calcium channels, are evident in the plaque and, in smaller numbers, in the periplaque white matter.

Reproduced from Kornek B, Storch MK, Bauer J, et al. Distribution of a calcium channel subunit in dystrophic axons in multiple sclerosis and experimental autoimmune encephalomyelitis. Brain 2001;Pt 6:1114–24. With permission of Oxford University Press on behalf of The Guarantors of Brain.

TABLE 23.8 Classification schemes of MS plaques

Classification system	Traditional	Sanders–Conrad-Tourtellotte	Bö–Trapp	van der Valk–De Groot modification	Brück–Lassmann	The Vienna Consensus 1997	UK MS Tissue Bank	Lucchinetti et al.
Plaque types		Type 1 (pre-plaque)		Preactive			Preactive	
	Acute	Type 2	Active	Active demyelinating	Early active	Acute–Inflammatory + demyelinating	Early active	Type 1 Type 2 Type 3 Type 4
					Active			
				Active non-demyelinating		Acute–Inflammatory	Late active	
	Chronic active	Type 3	Chronic active	Chronic active	Early active	Chronic active, Inflammatory + demyelinating	Chronic active	
					Active	Chronic active, Inflammatory		
					Early remyelinating			
	Chronic inactive (silent)	Type 4	Chronic inactive	Chronic inactive	Late remyelinating	Chronic inactive	Shadow	
					Inactive		Chronic inactive	
Parameters	Inflammation, demyelination	Oil red 0-positive macrophages, Class II MHC	Class II MHC	Class II MHC	Macrophage markers, myelin degradation products in macrophages	Inflammation, demyelination	Inflammation, myelin degradation products in macrophages, Class II MHC	Complement and IgG, oligodendrocyte loss pattern, MAG loss
Reference	Raine[616]	Sanders and Conrad[665]	Bö et al.[83]	van der Valk and De Groot[776]	Brück et al.[113a]	Lassmann et al.[413a]	Reynolds et al.[634]	Lucchinetti et al.[440]

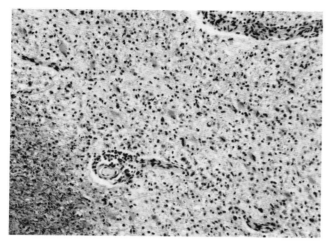

23.47 Acute multiple sclerosis (MS) plaque. The plaque is hypercellular and has a rather ill-defined edge (towards bottom left corner of figure). There are sheets of macrophages, some containing luxophilic granules of myelin debris, and perivascular accumulations of lymphocytes, particularly around blood vessels. Luxol fast blue and cresyl violet stain.

Courtesy of Professor Seth Love, Institute of Clinical Neurosciences, Frenchay Hospital, Bristol, UK.

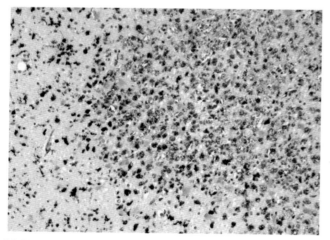

23.48 Acute multiple sclerosis (MS) plaque. This section, from the same area of acute demyelination as illustrated in Figure 23.47, has been immunolabelled with antibody to CD68, which highlights the numerous macrophages within the plaque, as well as scattered macrophages and microglia in the adjacent white matter.

Courtesy of Professor Seth Love, Institute of Clinical Neurosciences, Frenchay Hospital, Bristol, UK.

of sodium channels along the demyelinated axolemma and these are thought to be responsible for continuous axon potential conduction through this segment (see later under Neurophysiology of Multiple Sclerosis, p. 1362) and, along with associated other changes in axolemmal ionic channels and pumps, may contribute significantly to axonal degeneration and death (see earlier under Demyelination, in Axonal Injury and Loss, p. 1333).

In the acute plaque, there are few features that denote chronicity, such as hypocellular areas and prominent fibrillary gliosis. Cases in which there are multiple lesions that appear older should be considered as chronic MS. In these cases, even though there is an abrupt onset of a monophasic clinical profile, the presence of older lesions suggests previous subclinical involvement, the acute lesions being the substrate for the acute clinical deficit. Thus, although the acute plaque is characteristic of acute MS (Marburg's disease), as noted previously, it is also found in the more chronic forms of the disease (Figure 23.49), where presumably, if located in a clinically eloquent area, it is responsible for a new relapse. In the chronic forms of the disease, these lesions also represent the early changes of what will eventually mature into a chronic active MS plaque. The very earliest event in the genesis of an MS lesion, be it an acute lesion or one that will become a chronic plaque, is unknown, but very early changes have been detected by MRI studies and the underlying pathogenesis and histopathology of these findings is unclear (Box 23.3).

Acute plaques have been referred to as 'active' by other classification systems (Table 23.8).[83,634,776,784] The term still implies a lesion showing uniform histopathologic features and changes indicative of a short duration. They can be further subdivided into 'early active' and 'late active',[634] and also classified as to the degree of demyelination[776] that they manifest. The fact that the myelin debris within lysosomes[112] shows a predictable course of loss of staining for myelin components over time allowing for temporal staging of the active (or acute) lesion.[634] For example, LFB staining of myelin debris (Figure 23.19) is eventually replaced by the oil red O staining of neutral lipid and the PAS staining of residual glycoprotein (Figure 23.19), and macrophage digestion of the myelin proteins MOG and CNP occurs before that of MBP and PLP (Figure 23.12d and e).[112]

Immunohistochemistry for Class II MHC has also been used to demonstrate the active/acute lesion with[665] or without[83] staining for neutral lipid with oil red O. Just as the uniform picture of histopathology characterizes the active plaque, so too does the uniform distribution of Class II-immunoreactive microglia/macrophages throughout the lesion (Figures 23.49 and 23.50).[83] This again is indicative of the short and monophasic temporal profile of the clinical course of acute MS.

The most recent classification scheme has categorized actively demyelinating plaques into four patterns.[440,442] Two of these show macrophage-mediated demyelination: pattern II lesions show IgG and C9 neoantigen deposition, which are absent from pattern I lesions. The other two show pathology consistent with an oligodendrogliopathy: pattern III is a distal dying back oligodendrogliopathy with extensive loss of MAG, which is normally located in the distal oligodendroglial process in the adaxonal area and in uncompacted myelin. Pattern IV is due to primary oligodendroglial degeneration and has rarely been documented—only in a few patients with PPMS. The authors of this classification system feel that each of the patterns is patient-specific, only one pattern being evident in all the lesions of a given patient.[440] This interpretation has been controversial (Box 23.4).

The cellular and molecular mechanisms occurring in acute MS lesions, based on the material presented in Molecular and Cellular Components of Multiple Sclerosis Lesions (see p. 1309), are summarized diagrammatically in Figure 23.51.

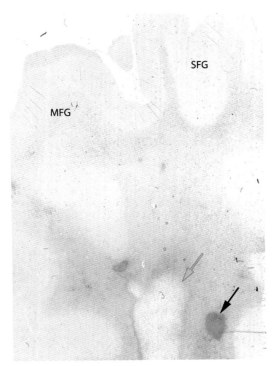

23.49 Acute multiple sclerosis (MS) plaque in chronic MS. Immunohistochemistry for Class II MHC showing an acute MS plaque, with uniform staining for Class II MHC (black arrow), medial to a large periventricular chronic active plaque, with Class II MHC staining concentrated at its border (grey arrow). Note that in MS there is diffuse upregulation of Class II MHC in the non-lesional white matter as well. MFG, middle frontal gyrus; SFG, superior frontal gyrus.

Pathology of the Chronic Active Multiple Sclerosis Plaque

The pathology of the chronic active MS plaque is a reflection of the chronicity of the classic relapsing-remitting presentation of the disease with which it is associated. It is difficult to assess the stage of evolution of individual plaques based on macroscopic appearances; chronic plaques tend to have sharper borders, more brownish discolouration and a more sunken appearance, reflecting tissue loss over time. Ongoing activity at the lesion edge may sometimes be apparent as an indistinct irregular border (Figure 23.52).

The chronic active plaque shows a topography of older changes in its centre and increasing more recent changes centrifugally up to its border with the adjacent normal-appearing white matter (NAWM) (Figure 23.53). The morphological features of inflammatory demyelination in the advancing borders of chronic active plaques are indistinguishable from those in early lesions. A centrifugal gradient of decreasing oedema, inflammation, microglial/macrophage infiltration and astrocytosis may extend from the edges of active white matter plaques into adjacent areas with intact myelin. Concurrently, progressive neurodegeneration culminates in marked white matter atrophy in chronic MS. The relationships between the focal pathological processes that occur in plaques and diffuse NAWM atrophy, i.e. whether they are independent processes, and whether and how they may be inextricably interwoven, are unclear. The neuroimaging correlates of these processes,

BOX 23.3. Evolving concepts: the initial MS lesion

The initial event in the pathogenesis of an MS plaque is unknown. Early changes on unconventional MR include the reduction of magnetization transfer ratio,[228,415] an increase in choline,[747] increases in cerebral blood volume and flow,[833] and changes on diffusion imaging.[812] The histopathologic basis of these changes is unknown. One of the earliest histopathologic changes in the pathogenesis of the MS plaque documented to date is apoptosis of oligodendrocytes in lesions of very short duration.[54] This finding in this 'pre-phagocytic' region of the plaque occurred in the absence of any inflammatory infiltrates, and suggests that inflammation is not important in the early pathogenesis of the plaque. More recently, degeneration of foot processes of perivascular astrocytes has been described as the earliest morphologic change in the plaque that even antedates oligodendrocyte apoptosis, and thus it has been postulated that MS is a disorder of the perivascular astrocyte with inflammatory demyelination being a secondary event.[560] Another focal change that is seen in MS white matter in the absence of inflammation is the upregulation of HLA-DR on clusters of microglia.[775] Such lesions are referred to as 'preactive' lesions and again it is not clear what is inducing this reactive change in microglia. In the context of the autoimmune hypothesis of MS pathogenesis, this could be considered to be the site of initial antigen presentation in what will later be an MS plaque. However, there is evidence that these microglia are responding to oligodendroglial stress and by production of alpha B-crystallin, the preactive lesion actually represents a phase where there is oligogodendroglial protection and prevention of evolution into a demyelinative inflammatory plaque.[783] Evidence for the disappearance of many preactive lesions is consistent with such a concept.[783] Thus, it is possible that the initial pathogenetic events in the MS lesion could be halted by targeted therapy, once these events are elucidated.[783] Finally, some thought should be given to the possibility that the initial event in the pathogenesis of MS may not reside in the plaque but may be a widespread primary neurodegenerative process and the early events in the plaque may be focal phenomena secondary to this process (see Box 23.2: Evolving concepts: MS as a neurodegenerative disease, p. 1308).

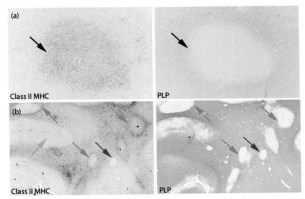

23.50 Class II MHC (HLA-DR) in multiple sclerosis (MS) plaques. (a) Acute MS plaque (black arrows) with intense uniform Class II MHC staining (left panel) in a region of acute demyelination shown as a region of absence of staining for proteolipid protein (PLP) (right panel). **(b)** In contrast, chronic active MS plaques (blue arrows) shown at lower magnification as focal areas of loss of PLP staining (right panel), with intense staining of Class II MHC (left panel) at their edges. A chronic inactive plaque (red arrows) shows uniformly reduced Class II MHC staining. The cortical plaques (green arrows) show similar features, indicating in this case they are also chronic inactive plaques. Immunohistochemical stains on thick (10 μm) sections, without counterstain.

particularly on non-conventional MR imaging, are discussed later under Magnetic Resonance Imaging and Its Pathological Correlates in Multiple Sclerosis, p. 1365.

The centre of the chronic active plaque represents the oldest part of the lesion and is the decimated battlefield left behind after the destruction by microglia/macrophages and their cellular and molecular compatriots and commanders (see Molecular and Cellular Components in Multiple Sclerosis Lesions, p. 1309). Thus there are numerous demyelinated axons separated by astrocytic processes. These tend to be more fibrillar than the reactive astrocytes evident in more peripheral recent regions of the lesion (Figure 23.53). There is also a gradient of lipid-laden macrophages, being relatively sparse in the central regions of older-duration lesions, where if present they have now made their way to the perivascular spaces, and are increasingly numerous the closer the region is to the edge of active demyelination (Figure 23.53). In the more peripheral regions of the chronic active plaque, the demyelinated axons are separated by a somewhat oedematous extracellular space containing numerous lipid-laden macrophages and reactive astrocytes. There is a reduction of axons and neurofilament dephosphorylation in these plaques.[671] Evidence of neurodegeneration is also seen in the form of loss of Na$^+$/K$^+$-ATPase in many, but not all lesions.[840]

The ongoing demyelination in the chronic active lesion occurs at its edge, bordering the adjacent NAWM (Figure 23.53). In this relatively narrow zone, one appreciates the same activity that is seen throughout the active/acute plaque, with myelin stripping and demyelination by macrophages accompanied, and probably directed, by lymphocytes and their cytokine-chemokine and free radical armamentarium. These lymphocytes (see earlier under T-lymphocytes, p. 1313, and B-lymphocytes, Plasma Cells and Immunoglobulins, p. 1314) are particularly evident in perivascular chronic inflammatory cuffs, but some penetrate the glia limitans to reside in the lesion parenchyma. Prominent reactive astrocytes further contribute to the hypercellularity of the lesion edge (Figures 23.24 and 23.53) and are also responsible for the dense gliosis in the immediately adjacent white matter (Figures 23.53 and 23.54). Oligodendrocytes may also be seen in increased numbers in this region.[439,620] This is associated with remyelination. In fact, there appears to be a cycle of regeneration of new myelin followed by its demyelination occurring in this zone (Figure 23.55).[602]

The plaque edge also shows a marked increase in microglia immunoreactive for Class II MHC (Figure 23.49 and Figure 23.50). This feature has been employed in some classification systems to define the chronic active plaque (see Table 23.8).[83,634,776] Again, this reflects the shift from the uniformly diffuse immune-mediated demyelination of the active/acute plaque to the border of the more chronic expanding lesion.

The expansion of the chronic active plaque into the periplaque white matter occurs by centrifugal advancement of the demyelination zone into the adjacent NAWM. It also occurs as finger-like projections of demyelination around perivenular inflammatory cuffs that extend from the plaque edge into the NAWM. These are frequently referred to as 'Dawson's fingers' (Figure 23.53), named after the pathologist who initially described them in his classic monograph on the neuropathology of MS.[175] The

BOX 23.4. Evolving concepts: the spectrum of pathogenetic mechanisms

Increasing understanding of biochemistry, developmental and cellular neurobiology, and immunology have elucidated the complexities of multiple pathogenetic mechanisms in MS; neuroimaging technologies have revealed the previously unappreciated extent of alterations that occur in the CNS of patients with MS over time; and experience with MR imaging-directed diagnostic brain biopsies and the therapeutic effects on the disease have expanded clinical perspectives on MS. The advances and new data require continued reassessment and integration with traditional morphologic data. For example, evidence that new lesions in acute and chronic MS are qualitatively similar is provided by biopsy findings in patients presenting with one or more cerebral lesions and in whom the disease subsequently follows a typical chronic MS course.[582] Newly forming lesions in patients with the relapsing–remitting form of MS (RRMS) show the same stereotyped changes in enhanced MR imaging both early and late in the course, suggesting that their pathogenesis remains unchanged over time. Therefore, a contemporary discussion of MS and its variants requires an integrated approach encompassing historical precedents, i.e. the morphology of well-established distinct clinicopathological entities, such as Marburg disease and Baló sclerosis, with recent relevant advances in the basic and clinical sciences.

Distinct clinical and pathological variants of MS have been described and well characterized for many years (see Table 23.4, p. 1300), and even cases of typical chronic MS are pathologically and clinically heterogeneous. At any point in the disease, and including in patients whose disease has been present for decades, multiple lesions often exhibit different degrees of inflammation, demyelination, remyelination, and oligodendrocyte and axonal loss, indicating that they are in different stages of pathological evolution. Studies of a large collection of MS biopsies and autopsies[411,439,440,442] have described distinct pathological/immunopathological patterns of early/active MS lesions (see Pathology of the Acute MS Plaque, p. 1334). These investigators have proposed a working classification system of four types of early MS lesion pathology in which the predominant lesion pattern is a consequence of distinct mechanisms (see Pathology of the Acute MS Plaque, p. 1334). These studies have provided a useful framework for determining how different pathogenetic mechanisms may be reflected in distinct neuropathological features in different patients. This ongoing work suggests that distinct injury pathways, such as oligodendrogliopathy versus antibody-mediated myelin or axonal injury in different patients, may converge into the final clinicopathological entity of MS. The authors of this classification system feel that each of the patterns is patient-specific, only one pattern being evident in all the lesions of a given patient.[440] This interpretation has been controversial, because others have found differing results in this regard and feel either that MS lesional pathogenesis is not uniform within a patient[54] or that IgG-complement complexes underlie lesion pathogenesis in all cases.[100] There are a number of arguments put forth by both sides of the issue (reviewed in Ref. 509) and the discrepancies can be resolved, in part but not completely, if a number of factors such as timepoints in the lesion sampling process, vagaries of immunohistochemistry in formalin-fixed paraffin-embedded tissue and the use of autopsy material versus biopsy material are considered.[209] The resolution of these issues in the understanding of the pathogenesis of the MS plaque has important therapeutic implications, particularly if it leads to specifically tailored treatment in subsets of patients.[115,361] Thus, currently evolving concepts of MS lesion pathogenesis potentially have a direct impact on clinical management.

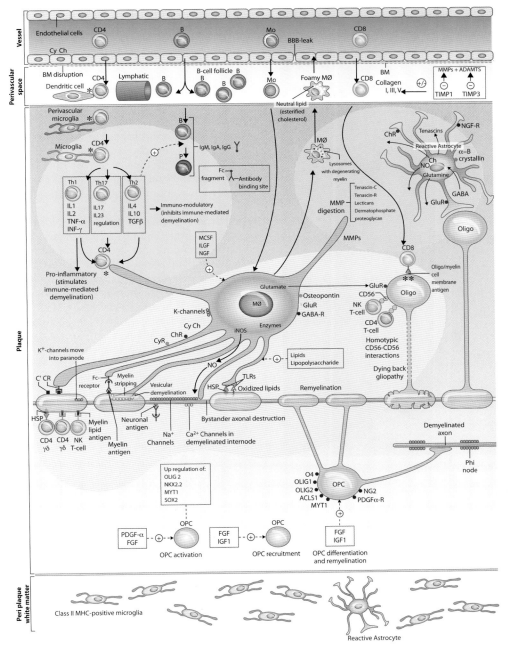

23.51 Pathogenesis of an early multiple sclerosis lesion. Events in the blood vessel are shown in the red area, in the perivascular space in the adjacent yellow area (see also schematic in Figure 23.4 for details of events at these two locales), lymphocyte interactions in the green area, demyelination in the beige area, remyelination in the white area, and gliosis and changes in the extracellular matrix in the blue area. Antigen presentation to CD4-positive T-cells by Class II major histocompatibility complex (MHC)-positive cells (microglia or macrophages) is indicated by a single asterisk (*). Class I MHC-restricted cytotoxicity by CD8-positve cells is indicated by double asterisks (**). Dashed lines with arrowheads and a plus (+) sign indicate a positive (or stimulatory effect), those with a minus (–) sign indicate a negative (or inhibitory) effect, and those with both (±) indicate a positive or negative effect depending on the interaction of the molecules indicated and their antagonists. ADAMTS, a disintegrin and metalloproteinase with thrombospondin motifs; B, B-cell; CD4, helper T-cell; C′, complement; Ca²⁺-channel, calcium channel; CD4-γδ, helper T-cell with T-cell receptor with gamma delta chains; CD8, cytotoxic T-cell; Ch, chemokines; ChR, chemokine receptors; CR, complement receptors; Cy, cytokines; CyR, cytokine receptors; FGF, fibroblast growth factor; GABA, gamma-amino butyric acid; GABA-R, receptor for gamma-amino butyric acid; GluR, glutamate receptors; HSP, heat shock proteins; Ig, immunoglobulin; IFN-γ, interferon-gamma; IL, interleukin; IGF1, insulin growth factor 1; ILGF, insulin-like growth factors; iNOS, inducible nitric oxide synthase; K-channel, voltage-gated potassium channel; P, plasma cell; MCSF, macrophage colony-stimulating factor; Mo, monocyte; MØ, macrophage; MMPs, matrix metalloproteinases; Na⁺-channel, voltage-gated sodium channel; NCX, sodium-calcium exchanger; NG2, NG2 proteoglycan; NGF, nerve growth factor; NGF-R, nerve growth factor receptor; NO, nitric oxide; OPC, oligodendroglial precursor cell; PDGF-α, platelet-derived growth factor-alpha; PDGFα-R, receptor for PDGFα; TGF-β, transforming growth factor-beta; TIMP, tissue inhibitors of metalloproteinase; TLRs, toll-like receptors; TNF, tumour necrosis factor.

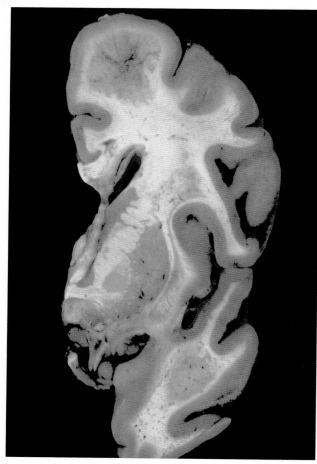

23.52 Chronic multiple sclerosis (MS). Freshly sectioned brain of a 12-year-old female with chronic multiple sclerosis (MS). Chronic plaques (superior frontal and temporal lobe white matter) have sharp borders. More recent plaques (e.g. in corpus callosum and adjacent to the claustrum) are paler and have indistinct and ragged borders.

Courtesy of Dr C Greco, University of California Davis, Sacramento, CA, USA.

Pathology of the Chronic Inactive (Silent) Multiple Sclerosis Plaque

Chronic inactive plaques, the classic hallmark of MS, are the most prevalent lesions in patients with MS, particularly in those who have had the disease for decades. Unlike acute/active and chronic active plaques, these lesions are no longer the sites of inflammatory demyelination and, therefore, represent the end stages of immunopathological injury. These features are reflected in all the plaque classification systems where the inactive lesion figures.

Chronic plaques can be seen on the exterior white matter portions of the brain stem and spinal cord as discrete areas of brown discolouration and indentation (see Figure 23.56). Following sectioning, they appear as multiple well-demarcated depressed areas of varying sizes located predominantly in white matter (Figure 23.57a, Figure 23.57b), but occasionally extending into deep cortical and other grey matter structures. Plaques may become more visible in the cut sections after exposure to air for some time. In cases of long duration, extensive confluent plaques may encompass most of the cut section area of the white matter (Figure 23.57b). As noted previously, on gross inspection, chronic inactive and chronic active plaques cannot usually be distinguished, but the borders of the former may appear more distinct (Figures 23.52, 23.57 and 23.58).

Inactive plaques appear as sharply demarcated areas (see Figures 23.57, 23.59–23.63) that are hypocellular and pale on haematoxylin and eosin-stained sections (Figure 23.62) and show absence of staining for myelin components (Figures 23.58–23.65). The size and anatomical location of a lesion and the intensity of the preceding inflammatory process are likely to be among the factors that contribute to variability in temporal evolution of lesions; it has been estimated that it takes 18 months or longer for an active plaque to acquire this appearance.[609] Myelin protein components are not detectable in any foamy macrophages that may be present. Because myelin lipid components are only slowly and partially catabolized in macrophages, foamy macrophages may persist in them for long periods. In general, mature oligodendrocytes are most often completely lost in inactive plaques.

There may be many demyelinated but otherwise intact axons and astrocytic glial processes filling the spaces previously occupied by the myelin in these lesions (Figures 23.25 and 23.65). There is considerable variation in different plaques, but axon densities are often significantly reduced in chronic inactive plaques (Figures 23.58 and 23.65).[432] Of the remaining axons, fewer are swollen in chronic inactive plaques than in active/acute and chronic active lesions,[760] and some may have reduced diameters.[432] There may also be a reduction in staining intensity with silver impregnation methods and neurofilament abnormalities.[432] The fact that few axons in these inactive lesions are positive for amyloid β-precursor protein suggests that fewer axons are undergoing acute degeneration with attendant interruption of axonal transport.[82] Rather, it is thought that most axons in these old lesions may be degenerating slowly (the so-called 'slow burn') and this may be very important in the progressive neurodegenerative phase of the disease. The mechanisms of neurodegeneration in these chronic inactive lesions may be different from those operative in acute lesions, in as much as

myelinated periplaque white matter region immediately adjacent to the plaque also shows reactive astrocytes (Figure 23.53) and inflammatory cuffs around veins unassociated with demyelination. Interestingly, the perivascular cuffs in the periplaque white matter contain almost exclusively lymphocytes, whereas in the plaque the cuffs contain lymphocytes and cells of histiocytic origin, a fact that implicates the lymphocyte as being important in the early pathogenesis of the lesion.[7]

In keeping with the epidemiological and genetic studies implicating a role for vitamin D deficiency in the pathogenesis of MS, a recent study of chronic active MS lesions showed upregulation of vitamin D receptor and two enzymes important in vitamin D metabolism, 25-hydroxyvitamin D-1α-hydroxylase (CYP27B1) and 1,25-dihydroxyvitamin D24-hydroxylase (CYP24A1), in chronic active MS plaques,[712] CYP27B1 having also been variably associated with MS in molecular genetics studies (see earlier under Genetics, p. 1305).[52,627]

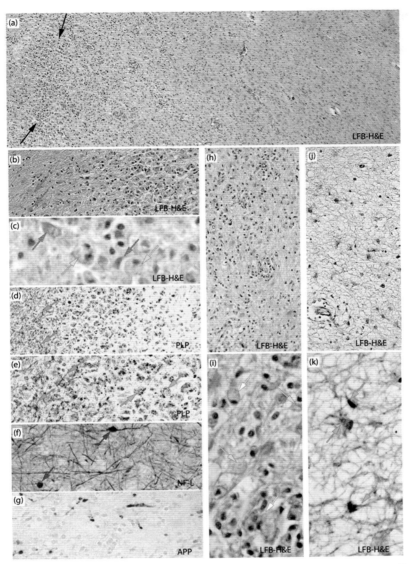

23.53 Chronic active multiple sclerosis (MS) plaque. Representative sections of chronic active plaques illustrating peri-plaque white matter **(a,b)**, the demyelinating plaque edge **(a–g)**, the intermediate zone between the plaque edge and centre **(h,i)** and the plaque centre **(j,k)**. The regional histology reflects the temporal topography of the lesion. **(a)** Low magnification of a chronic active MS plaque stained with Luxol fast blue–haematoxylin and eosin (LFB–H&E) showing the immediately adjacent (not yet demyelinated) peri-plaque white matter (far left). The central region of the plaque (far right) is much less cellular, and the degree of cellularity progressively increases centrifugally up to the plaque edge. The plaque edge (black arrows) is markedly hypercellular. A finger-like extension ('Dawson's finger') of the lesion into the adjacent white matter is evident in the upper left. **(b)** Intermediate magnification of the adjacent white matter (left) and the active edge of demyelination (right) shows that much of the hypercellularity at the edge is due to the presence of macrophages and other less frequent inflammatory and glial cells. **(c)** High magnification shows that many of these macrophages contain recently phagocytosed LFB-positive myelin debris (yellow arrows) and there are frequent reactive astrocytes with prominent eosinophilic cell bodies (red arrows), which are also seen in the immediate peri-plaque white matter (red arrows in panel b). **(d)** Immunohistochemistry for proteolipid protein (PLP) shows intact PLP-positive myelin sheaths (blue arrows) in the peri-plaque white matter (left) but none in the plaque (right). Again, the hypercellularity of the plaque edge (centre) is evident with many macrophages containing PLP-positive myelin debris. **(e)** Higher magnification of the peri-plaque white matter and plaque edge in **(d)**, showing macrophages with PLP-positive myelin debris (green arrows) at the plaque edge (indicating on-going demyelination) and preseved PLP-positive myelin sheaths in the periplaque white matter (blue arrows). **(f)** Immunohistochemistry for light neurofilaments (NF-L) showing intact axons in the hypercellular area at the plaque edge where active demyelination is occurring. Scattered swollen dystrophic axons are also evident (purple arrows). **(g)** Immunohistochemistry for amyloid precursor protein (APP) shows positive axons in the demyelinating edge, indicative of acute/subacute injury to these axons at that location. **(h)** Intermediate magnification of LFB–H&E stain of the plaque region between the demyelinating edge and the plaque centre. Note the complete absence of myelin and the gradient of increasing hypercellularity from the area closest to the plaque centre (below) to that nearest the plaque edge (above). **(i)** High magnification of **(h)** shows there are foamy macrophages (white arrows) containing droplets of neutral lipid indicative of advanced myelin breakdown; some of these have made their way to the perivascular space (lower white arrow). Very few macrophages with LFB-positive myelin debris (yellow arrows) indicative of early myelin phagocytosis are seen in this region. **(j)** Intermediate magnification of LFB–H&E stain of a hypocellular plaque centre, the most chronic region in the plaque, with very few inflammatory cells including macrophages. **(k)** High magnification of **(j)** showing the astrocytes are taking on a more fibrillary form (grey arrows), indicative of chronicity, compared to the large hypertrophic ones seen at the demyelinating edge and peri-plaque white matter.

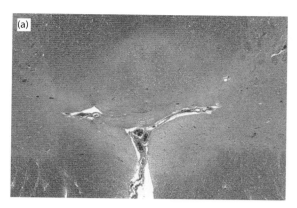

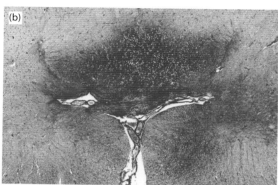

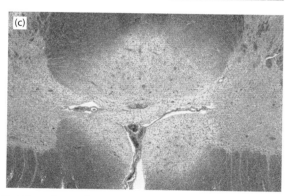

23.54 Chronic active multiple sclerosis (MS) plaque. A chronic active plaque in the spinal cord is centred around the central canal from the same case as shown in Figure 23.21. Dense gliosis extends beyond the demyelinated plaque borders. **(a)** Haematoxylin and eosin; **(b)** Holzer for glial fibres; **(c)** Klüver–Barrera for myelin.

persistent sodium influx probably plays less of a role because very few axons expressing $Na_v1.6$ are present. There are also no $Na_v1.2$ channels and no sodium-calcium exchangers in the axons of these lesions, but these are demonstrable on astrocytes.[82] Some axons in these old lesions, however, do possess voltage-gated calcium channels, but in far fewer numbers than in acute plaques and chronic active plaques;[382] nevertheless, this would provide a means of influx of calcium into the axoplasm with its attendant destructive effects. Moreover, the loss of Na^+/K^+-ATPase in the internodal axolemma in chronic plaques (both active and inactive), which is not a feature of the acute lesion, would imply that these axons are now not functional and may be subject to fluid shifts across the axolemma that could eventually lead to

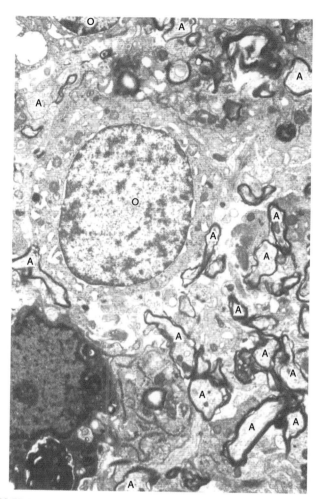

23.55 Demyelination of remyelinated myelin in MS. Electron micrograph showing two oligodendrocytes (O) associated with axons (A) with thin (probably remyelinated) myelin sheaths. Processes from myelin debris-containing macrophages (lower left and upper right) are approaching and appear to be demyelinating some of these myelin sheaths.

Reproduced with permission from Prineas JW, Kwon EE, Cho ES, Sharer LR. Continual breakdown and regeneration of myelin in progressive multiple sclerosis plaques. Ann NY Acad Sci 1984;436: 11–32, Fig. 11. Copyright © 2006, John Wiley and Sons.

their degeneration.[840] This, together with the loss of sodium channels in chronic lesions compared to acute lesions, also suggests that loss of axonal functionality may antedate, rather than necessarily be a result of, neurodegeneration.[840] The clinical implication of progressive loss of neurological function would apply to either scenario, but if functional loss does indeed precede structural neurodegeneration, this may indicate the possibility of halting or reversing this progressive process, if intervention occurs early in its course.

Unless it is also a shadow plaque, the edge of a chronic inactive plaque is usually quite sharp. Interestingly, the myelinated axons in the plaque edge, even in the chronic inactive state, may still include long areas of redistribution of caspr from the paranode, as in the active state.[827]

Chronic silent plaques contain fibrillary astrocytes, having transformed into long sinuous cells from the reactive prominent cell bodies of reactive astrocytes evident in of circulating high-molecular weight compounds, normally excluded from the parenchyma.[407] This residual blood–brain barrier breakdown in inactive plaques probably impairs reparative processes as it allows continuous leakage of serum components into the extracellular space/matrix, resulting in exposure of demyelinated axons and glia to cytokines, antibodies and other factors in the circulation that may inhibit oligodendrocyte regeneration and new myelin formation.[407] Both densely gliotic and hypocellular plaques with large volumes of extracellular fluid may also present physical barriers to repopulating OPCs and preclude the cell–cell contact interactions necessary for normal myelination of the remaining axons (see earlier under Remyelination, p. 1327). Nevertheless, remyelinated axons may be found in chronic inactive MS plaques (Figure 23.67).

Infiltrating inflammatory cells are usually inconspicuous in inactive lesions. There are variable numbers of persistent lipid-laden macrophages, particularly in perivascular spaces. Light- and electron-microscopic studies of perivascular spaces in chronic lesions show that these spaces are organized in a manner resembling that of a lymph node sinus, with lymphocytes and resident macrophages located within smooth-walled channels formed by reticular cells and with plasma cells that may be located outside the channels (Figures 23.68 and 23.69).[597] The proportionally high number of perivascular and parenchymal plasma cells in chronic plaques suggests sustained antibody production.[609,853]

Over time, macrophage numbers decrease in the centre of lesions, but they remain numerous at the edges of chronic active lesions, where their demyelinating activity results in centrifugal expansion of plaques. As myelin is depleted, immune activation, as well as phagocytosis decrease, and the foamy macrophages themselves may contribute to a dampening of the immune response.[97] The precise pathways by which macrophages disappear from lesions are unclear and may include returning to the blood directly through vessel walls (as suggested by their perivascular accumulation) and exiting via perivascular spaces or other CNS outflow pathways. Myelin phagocytes also appear around small blood vessels in relatively preserved tissue, i.e. NAWM, suggesting proximity to (and spread from) an active lesion or that a lower level of demyelination or other injury occurs in areas with otherwise intact-appearing myelin (see later under Normal-Appearing White Matter, p. 1368).

The major histopathological components of chronic inactive lesions are shown in Figure 23.70.

Tumefactive Multiple Sclerosis and Biopsy Diagnosis of Multiple Sclerosis

The diagnosis of demyelinating diseases does not routinely require biopsy. Nevertheless, it is not uncommon for patients who present with monophasic symptoms and signs of a solitary space-occupying lesion that by conventional computed tomography (CT) and MR imaging studies appears to be a primary or metastatic neoplasm to undergo a diagnostic biopsy procedure that demonstrates that the lesion is due to an acute demyelinating process. Such lesions are often large and can be located away from the ventricles; they may show ring enhancement or cystic change and may or may not cause mass

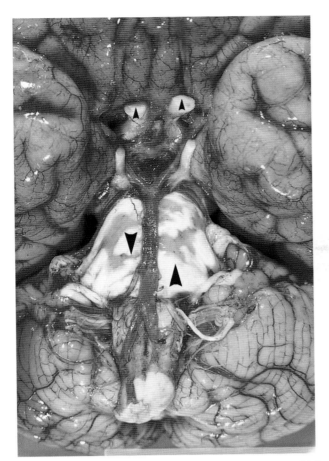

23.56 Macroscopic external appearance of brain in multiple sclerosis (MS). Several MS plaques are seen on the surface of the pons (large arrowheads). Small plaques are evident in both optic nerves (small arrowheads).

Reproduced with permission from Esiri M, Perl D. Multiple sclerosis. In: Oppenheimer's diagnostic neuropathology: a practical manual, 3rd ed. London: Hodder Arnold, 2006:211–222.

active inflammatory demyelination. In some lesions, astroglial processes filled with closely packed intermediate filaments of GFAP occupy most of the space created by myelin loss (Figure 23.25). In other lesions, the tissue has a looser texture, with astroglial processes and reduced numbers of axons lying in a markedly expanded extracellular space (Figure 23.66).[53] Plaques containing numerous Rosenthal fibres have also been reported.[308a] By electron microscopy, astrocyte processes are attached to the surface of demyelinated axons by desmosomes and gap junctions.[614]

Veins inside plaques often have thicker walls and wider perivascular spaces than veins in the surrounding tissue. Haemosiderin and fibrin deposits associated with plaque blood vessels and prominent amyloid deposition in plaque blood vessels have also been observed in rare cases.[609,676] Microvascular endothelial cells in chronic plaques show abnormalities, such as increase of pinocytotic vesicles, a reduced number of mitochondria, tight junction alterations and expression of laminin receptors, that indicate persistent blood–brain barrier breakdown in the absence of ongoing inflammation.[153,371,718] This is also supported by the immunohistochemical demonstration of extravasation

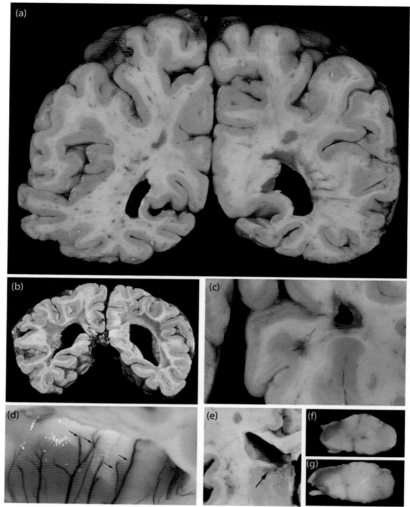

23.57 Macroscopic appearance of chronic multiple sclerosis (MS). Chronic MS plaques appear as focal areas of grey discolouration of the white matter, situated particularly in the periventricular region **(a–c)**. They are also evident as isolated lesions in the deep white matter **(a, e)**. The more recent lesions have less well defined borders and more of a brown hue and are not depressed, whereas the older lesions are well demarcated, greyer and depressed. Plaques are often seen to extend around veins (Dawson's fingers), e.g. radiating out from the right periventricular plaque in **(a)**. This is evident as pale brown perivenular extensions of a plaque involving the wall of the lateral ventricle in **(d)** (small arrows). In very chronic cases periventricular white matter plaques may be quite prominent, extending deep into the hemispheric white matter **(b)**. MS plaques, in contrast to most leukodystrophies, do not completely spare subcortical U-fibres and often extend through them to the cortex (b, right hemisphere). In fact, U-fibre lesions are a characteristic location of MS (open arrow in c). In addition to the obvious white matter plaques, occasionally grey matter plaques, such as the one in **(e)** (arrow), can be appreciated on gross examination. Spinal cord plaques may also be evident macroscopically, as shown at two levels in the left lateral funiculus of the cervical cord in **(f)** and **(g)**.

effect. Advanced imaging techniques and repeated examinations may provide information more suggestive of inflammatory/demyelination,[123,206] but biopsy sampling for diagnosis may be essential to determine the nature of the lesion. In the majority of cases, these tumefactive lesions are solitary and located in the cerebrum. They can, however, also be multiple and may be in other sites, such as the cervical spinal cord, and associated with a clinically isolated syndrome.[61] Patients who are known to have MS and develop lesions with atypical clinical or neuroimaging features may require a biopsy to rule out a concurrent disease process such as glioma.[123]

The major features useful for diagnosing demyelinating lesions in biopsy material include hypercellularity, ongoing demyelination, relative axonal preservation and inflammation (Figure 23.71). To the extent that the tissue sample size permits, it is important to perform studies that rule out other pathological processes, particularly infection, infarction and neoplasia (see Table 23.3), and to be aware of non-specific features, especially in frozen section diagnosis. Reactive features, including inflammation and astrocytosis, may be seen adjacent to lesions with an entirely different aetiology, for example abscesses and infarcts, the diagnostic components of which may not be included in the sample.

A number of histological features can help in the distinction of inflammatory demyelination from other pathological processes.[396,843] Hypercellularity of the tissue is usually due to the presence of many lipid-containing foamy macrophages that are typically aligned along axons and may contain PAS-positive material and LFB-positive myelin debris, depending on the duration of the lesion (see earlier under Pathology

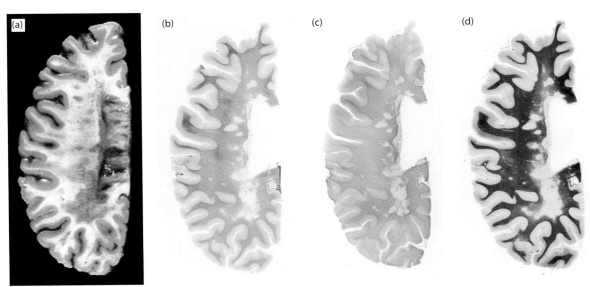

23.58 Chronic multiple sclerosis (MS). Serial sections of a cerebral hemisphere from a patient with chronic multiple sclerosis (MS). **(a)** Multiple plaques appear as focal, often depressed areas of grey discolouration of the white matter. Many plaques are periventricular, but some are more peripheral in the corona radiata. The plaques show absence of myelin staining with **(b)** Luxol fast blue (LFB) and **(c)** myelin basic protein (MBP) immunohistochemistry stains. **(d)** There is also pallor in the Bielschowsky preparation, indicating axonal loss. Macroscopically and on inspection of the myelin and axon preparations, much of the white matter appears normal, but histopathological abnormalities can be identified in 'normal-appearing white matter' (NAWM) on higher magnification, particularly when morphometric methods are used; NAWM abnormalities can also be detected using non-conventional magnetic resonance (MR) imaging.

Reproduced in part and modified from Moore et al.[513] With permission from Lippincott Williams & Wilkins/Wolters Kluwer Health.

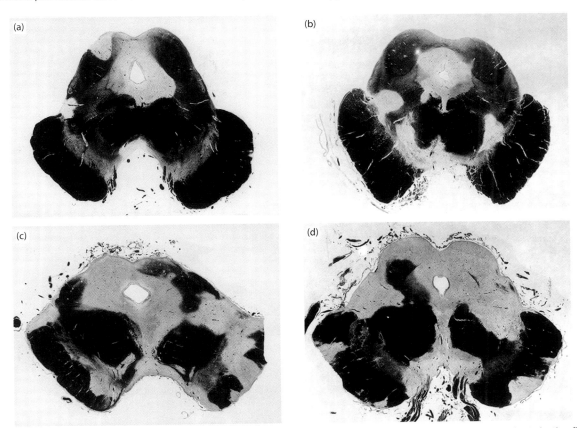

23.59 Midbrain sections from four patients with multiple sclerosis (MS). (a–d) Lesions around the aqueduct, in the floor of the interpeduncular fossa and beneath the pia. Heidenhain.

Courtesy of Professor JW Prineas, University of Sydney, Sydney, Australia.

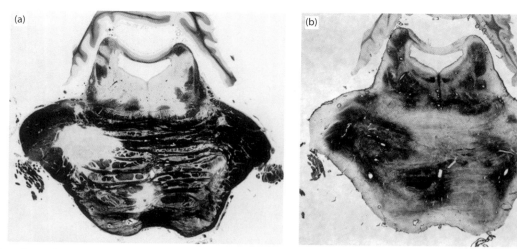

23.60 Chronic multiple sclerosis (MS) lesions in the pons. 56-year-old female with a 27-year history. **(a)** Heidenhain; **(b)** Holzer stain for glial fibres.

Courtesy of Professor JW Prineas, University of Sydney, Sydney, Australia.

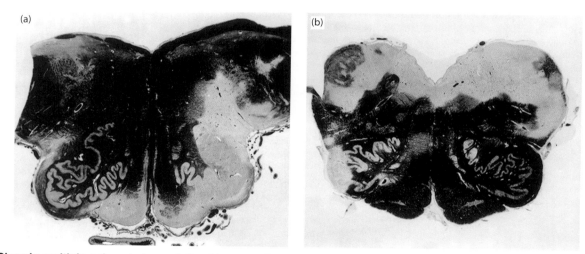

23.61 Chronic multiple sclerosis in medulla oblongata. Sharply demarcated chronic MS plaques in subventricular and subpial areas of the medulla oblongata demonstrated with Heidenhain stain. **(a)** 41-year-old female with a 20-year history; **(b)** 42-year-old female with an 8-year history.

Courtesy of Professor JW Prineas, University of Sydney, Sydney, Australia.

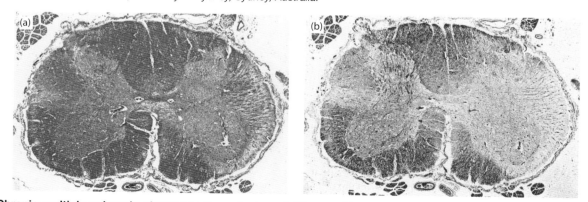

23.62 Chronic multiple sclerosis plaques in the spinal cord. 59-year-old male with chronic multiple sclerosis (MS). The large plaque on the right encompasses approximately one-third of the cross-sectional area of the cord, including grey matter, at this level. A second subpial lesion is present in the white matter on the left side. There is additional myelin pallor beyond the boundaries of the plaques that may represent tract degeneration and/or ongoing disease activity. Note the sparing of the peripheral nervous system myelin in the nerve roots. **(a)** Haematoxylin and eosin; **(b)** Luxol fast blue (LFB)–periodic acid-Schiff (PAS).

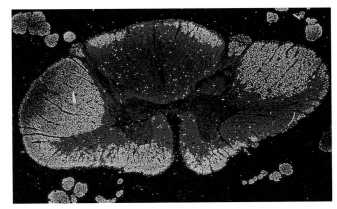

23.63 Spinal cord multiple sclerosis (MS) plaque. 70-year-old female with a 32-year history of multiple sclerosis (MS). There is axonal preservation throughout the demyelinated tissue. Note the immunostaining of spinal nerve roots in addition to intact myelin in the cord. Immunocytochemistry for neurofilament (red, Cy3) and myelin basic protein (green, fluorescein isothiocyanate [FITC]).

Courtesy of Dr G Wolswijk, Netherlands Institute for Brain Research, Amsterdam, the Netherlands.

of the Acute MS Plaque, p. 1334). Although foamy macrophages are characteristic of inflammatory demyelinating lesions and most often indicate non-neoplastic processes, they are not specific, because they are also characteristic of resolving infarcts and necrosis due to a variety of other causes. They can also be found in gliomas and other neoplasms. The demonstration of myelin loss, using myelin stains, and relative preservation of axons, usually by silver impregnation techniques or neurofilament immunohistochemistry, is essential for the diagnosis of a demyelinating process. Some axons appear injured and axonal numbers may be partially depleted, but their loss should be comparatively less than that of myelin. Axonal damage as demonstrated by amyloid precursor protein (APP) staining occurs in early lesions and may also prove useful in assessing biopsy samples. If axons are depleted to the same extent as myelin, or if grey matter with hypoxic–ischaemic neurons is present in the sample, the lesion is more likely to be an infarct or other necrotizing process than demyelination. Vacuolation or oedema of the tissue is often prominent, although not specific.

Perivascular inflammatory cuffs consisting predominantly of CD3+ T-lymphocytes are often present, but are not essential for the diagnosis of a demyelinating lesion. A predominance of B-cells is unusual and raises the possibility of a lymphoproliferative disorder. Large numbers of neutrophils, fibrinoid necrosis of vessels and intravascular thrombi also suggest alternative disease processes such as infection and vasculitis. Astrocytes may be relatively inconspicuous in early lesions, but reactive astrocytes with nuclear atypia, mitotic figures and 'granular mitoses' (Creutzfeldt cells) are often seen in acute inflammatory demyelinating lesions; their presence should not result in the incorrect interpretation of an astrocytic neoplasm.

In the absence of clinical and neuroimaging data and, in particular, knowledge of the temporal evolution of the lesion, a precise diagnosis based on the findings of an acute inflammatory demyelinating lesion may not be possible. The majority of cases diagnosed by biopsy in an initial clinical episode

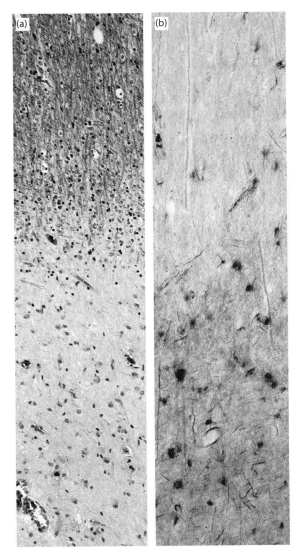

23.64 Immunoglobulin G (IgG) in a multiple sclerosis plaque. The edge of a chronic inactive multiple sclerosis (MS) plaque shows IgG positive astrocytes and axons in the demyelinated zone (lower portions), with an abrupt decrease in IgG immunoreactivity at the plaque margin (upper portions). **(a)** Luxol fast blue (LFB)–periodic acid-Schiff (PAS); **(b)** immunohistochemistry for IgG without counterstain.

Reproduced from Kwon and Prineas.[407] With permission from Lippincott Wiliams & Wilkins/Wolters Kluwer Health.

progress to clinically definite MS.[582] A wide spectrum of pathological features may be found in biopsies of acute inflammatory demyelinating lesions, in the numerous acute and chronic forms of MS and ADEM.[33,444,582] In view of the sample size limitations (Figure 23.71) and lesion heterogeneity, prognostication based on histopathological features in a biopsy may be difficult. In patients with previously undiagnosed CNS lymphomas who have been treated with corticosteroids or other immunosuppressive agents, the tumour cells may undergo lysis and may not be evident in the biopsy sample; the tissues remaining can have features that mimic acute demyelinating lesions. Another caveat is that in rare instances, demyelination can be observed adjacent to a non-demyelinating lesion, such as a neoplasm[641] or may herald a lymphoma.[327]

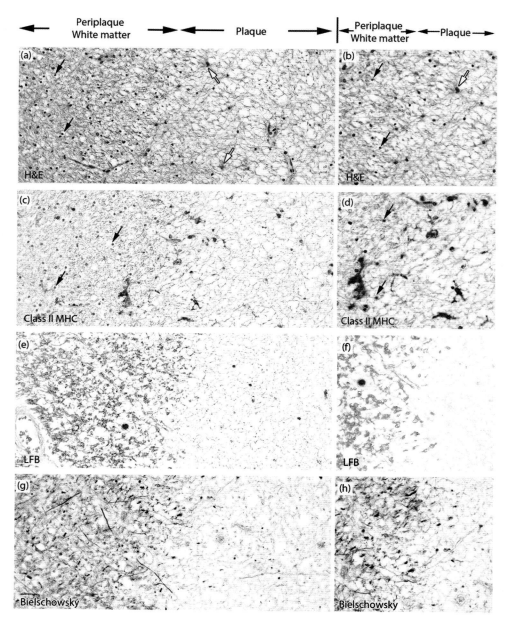

23.65 Edge of a chronic inactive multiple sclerosis (MS) plaque. Low **(a,c,e,g)** and higher **(b,d,f,h)** magnification images of the edge of a chronic inactive plaque, stained with haematoxylin and eosin (H&E) **(a,b)**, immunostained for Class II MHC and counterstained with haematoxylin **(c,d)**, stained with Luxol fast blue (LFB) **(e,f)**, and with Bielschowsky silver impregnation **(g,h)**. In each of the panels, the plaque is on the right and the adjacent white matter on the left. The plaque shows pallor on H&E staining **(a,b)**. There is a relative reduction in the numbers of oligodendrocytes, which are abundant in the adjacent white matter (a–d, black arrows). Gliosis is manifest in the plaque by astrocytes with fibrillary processes (a,b, white arrows). The plaque, which has a relatively sharp border, shows almost complete loss of LFB-positive myelin sheaths **(e,f)**. The Bielschowsky stain demonstrates lesional axonal loss **(g,h)**; the surviving axons are less intensely impregnated with the silver salt than their counterparts in the adjacent white matter **(g,h)**. Although Class II MHC-positive microglia are present **(c,d)**, these have a predominantly ramified morphology, indicative of an activated state. However, ongoing demyelination by round amoeboid macrophages is not present.

Grey Matter Plaques in Multiple Sclerosis

Cortical Plaques

Traditionally, MS was regarded as a predominantly white matter disorder. At least as early as 1916, however, cortical lesions were discussed in MS,[175] but they were subsequently documented only occasionally.[609] However, with recognition of their poor detection rate by conventional MR imaging, their unique neuropathological features and their possible relationship to some clinical manifestations of MS, cortical plaques are receiving increased attention.[88] They have been reported to be particularly associated with primary progressive MS and secondary progressive MS,[405] are less frequent in clinically benign MS,[125] increase in size and number over time[126] and appear to be independent of white matter pathology in their pathogenesis.[89] In fact, there is MRI evidence to indicate that some MS patients may initially present with cortical plaques without evidence of white matter involvement.[127]

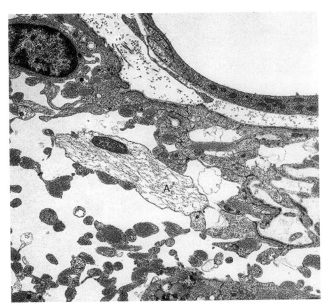

23.66 Prominent extracellular space in a chronic multiple sclerosis (MS) plaque. Electron micrograph of a chronic periventricular multiple sclerosis (MS) lesion, showing widening of the extracellular space and a paucity of axons. A, axon.

Courtesy of Dr D Barnes, Institute of Neurology, National Hospital for Neurology and Neurosurgery, London, UK.

Cortical lesions are rarely visualized by routine MR imaging, but the yield is increased with the use of contrast agents or fluid-associated inversion recovery (FLAIR),[257,365] double inversion recovery (DIR)[683] and phase-sensitive inversion recovery (PSIR),[530] three-dimensional magnetization-prepared rapid acquisition with gradient echo (3D MPRAGE)[529] and high-field strength MRI.[674] On neuropathological examination, these lesions often go undetected when LFB is used as the myelin stain. They are better visualized with the Heidenhain stain, but they are best delineated by immunohistochemistry for myelin proteins such as myelin basic protein (MBP), proteolipid protein (PLP) and 2′, 3′-cyclic nucleotide 3′-phosphodiesterase (CNP) (Figure 23.72).[86] With the latter, they appear as focal areas with absence of staining and are quite common.[725] However, remyelination is also a frequent finding.[15] There is relative neuronal cell body (Figure 23.40) and axonal (Figure 23.72) sparing. Cortical plaques are most commonly subpial (Figure 23.72a, Figure 23.72b) in location and generally do not extend deeper than layer 4 or 5. These lesions can, however, be quite extensive, involving large areas of the cortex.[86] The demyelination may extend through the cortex and yet not involve the subcortical U fibres.[86] They can also occur as focal plaques of myelin loss completely within central cortical layers. Cortical plaques are not an exclusively MS phenomenon, as they are also seen in progressive multifocal leukoencephalopthy (PML). However, in the latter condition they show an anatomical distribution opposite to that in MS, with most plaques being deeper in the cortex and no subpial involvement.[505] The subpial predilection for cortical lesions in MS suggests the adjacent CSF is important in their pathogenesis. In this regard, leptomeningeal inflammatory infiltrates have been

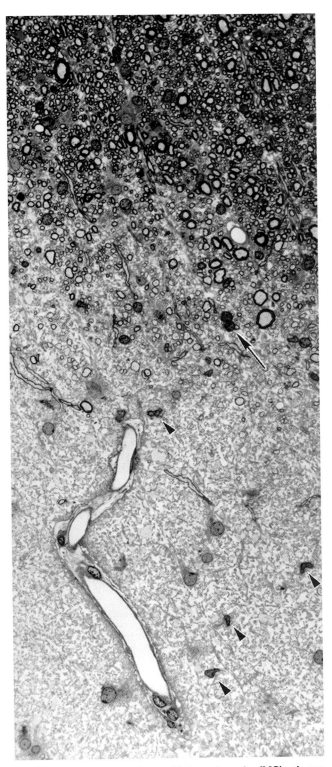

23.67 Edge of a chronic multiple sclerosis (MS) plaque. Note the thinly myelinated axons at the plaque border (centre of figure), fibrous astrocytes and microglia (arrowheads). Oligodendrocytes (arrow) are depleted in the demyelinated tissue. Toluidine blue.

Courtesy of Professor JW Prineas, University of Sydney, Sydney, Australia.

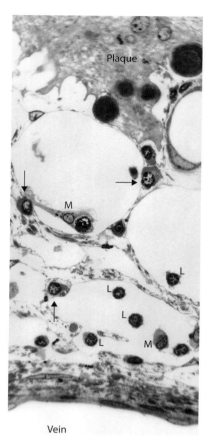

23.68 Organization of an inflammatory cell cuff in a chronic multiple sclerosis (MS) plaque. The perivascular space contains many thin-walled channels in which there are lymphocytes (L) and macrophages (M); plasma cells (arrows) are located outside the channels. Toluidine blue.

Reproduced from Prineas.[597] With permission of the American Association for the Advancement of Science.

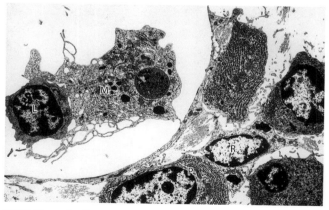

23.69 Organization of an inflammatory cell cuff in a chronic multiple sclerosis (MS) plaque. A channel within a perivascular space in a chronic multiple sclerosis (MS) plaque contains a macrophage (M) intimately contacting a lymphocyte (L). Surface contacts of lymphocytes with macrophages may result in antigen presentation. Plasma cells (P) are clustered around a cell (R) outside the channel. Electron micrograph.

Reproduced from Prineas.[597] With permission of the American Association for the Advancement of Science.

variably correlated with subpial inflammation.[322,380,443] In MS and PML, some cortical plaques extend into the subcortical white matter (see Figures 23.40 and 23.73); cortical involvement can also be due to extension of a lesion localized primarily in the subcortical U-fibres.[86,365] These plaques involving cortex and adjacent white matter are referred to as 'leuko-cortical plaques'. Cortical plaques have been classified depending on their locations[85,365] and on their activity based on Class II MHC staining of microglia/macrophages at the lesion edge (Figure 23.50).[85] The topography of cortical plaques is such that a cortical venule located in the centre of the lesion may be important in the genesis of the deeper intracortical lesions.[365] It would seem, however, that cortical veins would be unlikely epicentres of lesions in the superficial cortical ribbon, which may be related to leptomeningeal inflammation.[85,322,443] Cases of 'general cortical subpial demyelination' may represent cases of MS without major deep white matter involvement but with extensive cortical plaques.[86]

Most reports indicate that the histopathological features of purely cortical MS lesions usually differ significantly from those of white matter plaques. Cortical lesions were described as hypocellular, with very few inflammatory cells,[365] the numbers of T- and B-lymphocytes being no different in nondemyelinated and control normal cortices.[85] Furthermore, no immunohistochemical evidence of break down of the BBB, vascular basement membrane remodelling or gliosis was found.[780] Plaques that involve the deeper cortex, as well as the underlying white matter ('leukocortical' lesions), show typical features of white matter plaques in the white matter component of the lesion but significantly fewer inflammatory cells in the cortical component.[573] Complement components are demonstrable less frequently in cortical plaques than white matter plaques,[107] but oligodendrocytes have been shown to immunostain for C4d in cortical lesions.[677] Class II MHC-positive microglia are present in cortical lesions but are not nearly as numerous as in white matter plaques. They are present in increased numbers throughout and at the borders of active lesions, but not in chronic silent cortical lesions or normal cortex. Although this pattern is similar to that in white matter plaques, microglia in cortical plaques retain their rod-like shapes, whereas in white matter plaques most have matured into round phagocytic macrophages. Nevertheless, the activated microglia, that have been shown to produce myeloperoxidase[277] could still be capable of inflicting damage on myelin and neurons, as their processes are intimately associated with neuron cell bodies and neurites.[573]

In contradistinction to previous assessments of cortical plaques as being relatively inert from the point of view of inflammation, a recent study of cortical plaques in biopsies from patients with a relatively short clinical course showed inflammation in the form of T-cell infiltrates in these lesions. Moreover, the cortical plaques also included macrophages that contained lipid or myelin breakdown products.[443] The reasons for the discrepancies between these findings and previous studies are unclear but may have to do with the fact that the more recent series comprised surgical material: the cortical lesions in the more recent study were probably earlier than those in the previous autopsy studies of patients with disease of longer duration. There is evidence of neurodegeneration in cortical plaques. Transected neurites are identifiable in these lesions, and their abundance

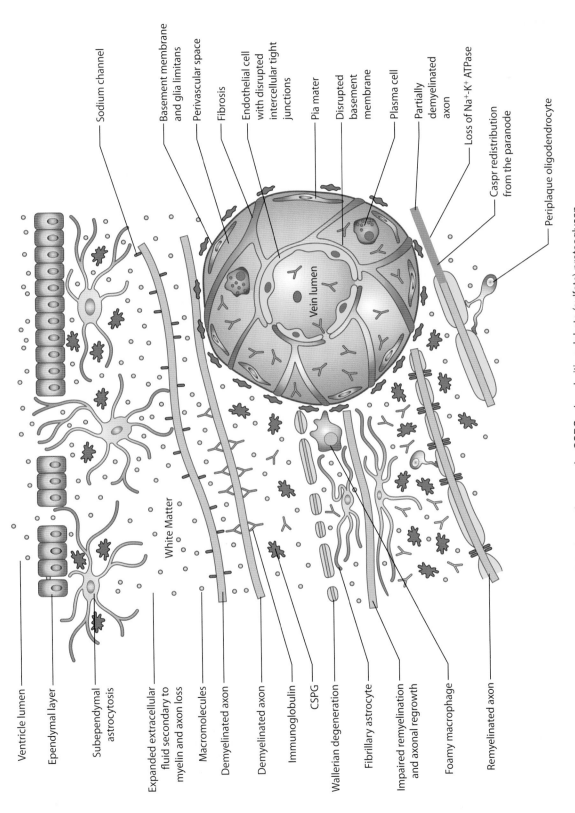

Ventricle lumen

Ependymal layer

Subependymal astrocytosis

Expanded extracellular fluid secondary to myelin and axon loss

Macromolecules

Demyelinated axon

Demyelinated axon

Immunoglobulin

CSPG

Wallerian degeneration

Fibrillary astrocyte

Impaired remyelination and axonal regrowth

Foamy macrophage

Remyelinated axon

Sodium channel

Basement membrane and glia limitans

Perivascular space

Fibrosis

Endothelial cell with disrupted intercellular tight junctions

Pia mater

Disrupted basement membrane

Plasma cell

Partially demyelinated axon

Loss of Na⁺-K⁺ ATPase

Caspr redistribution from the paranode

Periplaque oligodendrocyte

White Matter

Vein lumen

23.70 Late stages of multiple sclerosis (MS) lesion pathogenesis. CSPG, chondroitin sulphate (sulfate) proteoglycan.

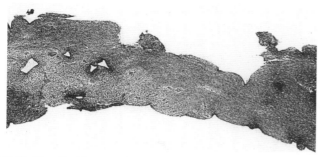

correlates with the degree of microglial activation. Neurons undergoing apoptosis are also a feature of cortical plaques, and this may contribute to neuronal loss and reduced synaptic density in chronic MS.[573,808] MMP-9-mediated degradation of perineuronal nests, the specialized extracellular matrix around some GABA-producing neurons and pyramidal cells, has also been reported in cortical plaques.[278]

Deep Grey Matter Plaques

Plaques often involve subcortical grey matter structures in MS (Figures 23.57 and 23.74), but there have been few studies of these using the techniques that have been applied to cortical plaques. One study reported that the hypothalamus can show quite active lesions.[323] These lesions appear

23.71 Needle biopsy of acute inflammatory/demyelinating lesion. Same case as shown in Figure 23.21. Despite the limited size of the sample, the myelin stain demonstrates both perivascular and confluent areas of inflammatory demyelination. Luxol fast blue (LFB)–periodic acid-Schiff (PAS).

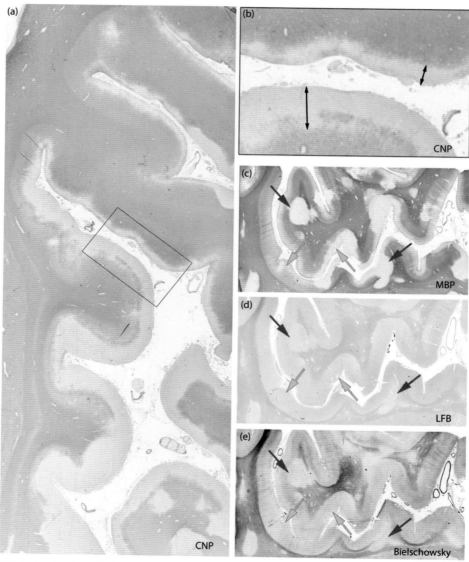

23.72 Cortical and leukocortical multiple sclerosis (MS) plaques. (a) On the immunohistochemical stain for 2',3'-cyclic nucleotide 3'-phosphodiesterase (CNP) extensive subpial cortical demyelination is evident. The area in the black rectangle is shown at higher magnification in **(b)**, where the demyelination is seen to extend for variable depths (double-headed arrows) into the cortex. The immunohistochemical stain for myelin basic protein (MBP) **(c)** shows focal cortical (green arrows) and leukocortical (red arrows) plaques. Note that cortical myelin loss is evident on MBP immunohistochemistry **(c)**, but not Luxol fast blue (LFB) staining **(d)**, although the white matter component of the leukocortical plaques is seen with both stains. Bielschowsky silver impregnation **(e)** shows axonal loss in the regions of white matter demyelination but not in the cortex; however, higher magnification would show evidence of transected neurites in cortical plaques.

to be more active than those elsewhere in the deep grey matter,[789] but it is unclear whether this is simply related to different patient populations in the two studies. Deep grey matter plaques tend be periventricular in those nuclei that are adjacent to the ventricular system (such as the thalamus, hypothalamus and caudate nucleus), whereas other deeper grey matter structures (such as the globus pallidus and the putamen) tend to have perivenular plaques.[789] Most deep grey matter plaques involve both the grey matter neuropil and myelinated tracts, whereas a minority demyelinate only the grey matter component of the structure. As in the case of cortical plaques, gliosis is usually not obvious. Both 'active' deep grey matter lesions, with uniform immunoreactivity for Class II MHC, and 'chronic active' lesions, with Class II MHC labelling at lesion borders, are relatively rare in deep grey matter structures.[789] Akin to the leukocortical plaque, macrophages with lipid and/or myelin protein breakdown products are very sparse in the grey matter component, where there are numerous activated ramified microglia, but are more apparent in the myelinated fibre bundles in deep grey nuclei. Infiltrates of lymphocytes may be present but are more obvious in the grey matter component. Of interest is the fact that there may be a distinct boundary between the demyelinated grey matter component and an adjacent component of white matter, but the reverse is not true when white matter tracts are involved in the lesion.[789] This is also the case for spinal lesions.[264]

Clinical Significance of Grey Matter Plaques

The clinical significance of cortical and other grey matter plaques is not well defined. However, in RRMS the accumulation of cortical plaques is associated with the occurrence of epilepsy, faster cognitive decline and greater diasblity.[128] Hypothalamic plaques may account for some of the autonomic and endocrine perturbations seen in MS patients.[323] Hippocampal pathology appears to be important in the memory loss and depressive symptoms often documented in MS.[374] Hippocampal demyelination has been well documented.[259] It is associated with reduction of mRNA and protein levels of genes important in axonal transport, memory function, and glutamate neurotransmission and homeostasis, as well as reduced synaptic density with relative preservation of neurons.[196] Affected hippocampi also show increased levels of miRNAs, which impair translation of mRNA, suggesting that demyelination, at least in the hippocampus, may have a significant effect on neuronal protein synthesis and memory function via miRNAs.[197] Grey matter plaques in the cerebellar cortex and spinal cord (Figure 23.62) with histological features similar to those of cortical plaques have also been reported, and these could presumably also have a clinical effect in addition to their white matter counterparts.[264,406]

Specific Lesion Localization Patterns

Although MS pathology may occur anywhere in the CNS, certain sites tend to be involved more frequently. There are also other areas of involvement that one would not necessarily expect. Considerable data from EAE models suggest that differences in immune responses to distinct encephalitogenic epitopes may result in differential tropism of T-cells

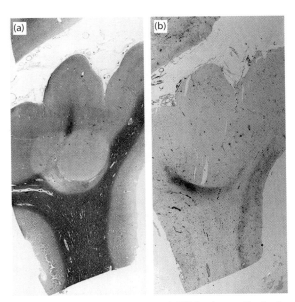

23.73 Chronic multiple sclerosis (MS) leukocortical plaque. A chronic inactive plaque overlaps the cortex and subcortical white matter and stains positively for extravascular immunoglobulin M (IgM). **(a)** Luxol fast blue (LFB)–periodic acid-Schiff (PAS); **(b)** immunohistochemistry for IgM without counterstain.

Reproduced by permission from Kwon and Prineas.[407]

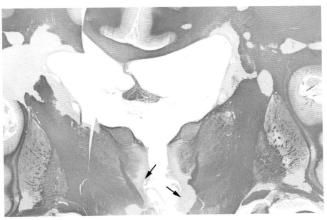

23.74 Deep grey matter multiple sclerosis (MS) plaques. In addition to the prominent white matter plaques adjacent to the lateral ventricles, deep grey matter plaques are seen in the thalamus (black arrows) abutting the third ventricle and in the putamen bilaterally (blue arrows). Immunohistochemical stain for myelin oligodendrocyte glycoprotein (MOG), without counterstain.

to specific CNS regions; these lesion localization predilections may result in distinct clinical phenotypes in affected animals.[518] Similarly, in patients with MS, heterogeneous composition of myelin or other antigens targeted by specific immune responses in different regions could contribute to distinct lesion localizations. Although differences in viral tropisms for different CNS anatomic regions have not been correlated with lesion topography in MS,[764] such differences could possibly affect an aetiopathogenic virus or other infectious agent and hence influence the distribution of lesions.

Choroid Plexus, Cerebrospinal Fluid and Periventricular White Matter

The most obvious region of predilection for MS plaques is the periventricular white matter.[111] The preferential periventricular (and periaqueductal) lesion localization in patients with MS (Figures 23.57–23.61) may reflect the contribution of circulating factors in the CSF to the initiation or promotion of plaques.[67,609] An association has been found between the occurrence of periventricular lesions and CSF oligoclonal bands in Japanese patients with MS.[524] Because ependymal cells do not have a major barrier function, the blood–CSF barrier is located in the choroid plexus. Unlike CNS parenchymal micro-vessels, however, choroid plexus endothelial cells do not have functional tight junctions, the barrier to entry into the CSF being junctional complexes between epithelial cells.[823]

Choroid plexus epithelium is involved in neural–immune regulation and immunosurveillance.[823] It also regulates CSF concentrations of bioactive organic anions[342] and may be a source of matrix metalloproteinases that facilitate leukocyte migration.[732] Therefore, proximity to higher CSF concentrations of inflammatory mediators or toxic substances originating in, or not cleared efficiently by, the choroid plexus may contribute to enhanced periventricular inflammatory lesion formation and growth. In this regard, a detailed immunopathological study of early MS lesions has suggested that a diffusing, complement-fixing, myelinolytic substance in the CSF may contribute to early development of periventricular lesions.[251]

It has been postulated that the choroid plexus, rather than the parenchymal endothelium, may be the site of entry of circulating T-cells engaged in immune surveillance of the CNS.[596] The mechanisms by which inflammatory cells cross the choroid plexus to the CSF and thus gain access to the CNS parenchyma by this route are unclear. However, E-selectin and P-selectin are constitutively expressed on the endothelium of large choroid plexus veins, ICAM-1 is normally expressed on small and large vessels in the stroma of the choroid plexus,[372] and VCAM-1 is also evident at that location in MS.[788] These findings suggest that lymphocytic recruitment and migration mechanisms may be, at least in part, similar to those in the parenchymal endothelium described earlier (see Endothelial Cells, p. 1310). Scattered T-cells have been demonstrated in the stroma in normal individuals indicating transendothelial migration does occur in the choroid plexus.[372] Furthermore, immunohistochemical studies have shown inflammatory infiltrates (comprised of T-cells and monocytes/macrophages with upregulation of Class II MHC) in choroid plexus stroma and blood vessels in MS.[788] There is strong immunoreactivity for CCL21 in the epithelium both in MS and in controls,[373] suggesting that this process may involve interactions between this cytokine and lymphocytes expressing its CCR7 receptor. However, it is now thought that the first wave of inflammation into the CNS may be CCR6-bearing Th17 memory cells that interact with CCL20 on choroid plexus epithelium, allowing these cells to traverse the tight junctions of the epithelium.[628] Once within the CSF of the subarachnoid space, these T-cells, when they encounter the appropriate antigen, are restimulated, leading to the cascade of events that allows T-cells to now enter through the

BBB at the level of the endothelial cell utilizing mechanisms that are discussed earlier (see Endothelial Cells, p. 1310).

Alternatively, it has been suggested that the early stage of the periventricular plaque is the formation of a lesion around a subependymal vein and that adjacent lesions later coalesce and that CSF does not play a role in initial lesion development.[8]

Subpial

The subpial preferential location of plaques in the brain stem and spinal cord (Figures 23.56, 23.57 and 23.62) again bespeaks of CSF being important in their pathogenesis. This is also true of the subpial location of most cortical plaques (see earlier under Cortical Plaques, p. 1348).

Subcortical U-Fibres

It is also not at all clear why plaques tend to occur in the subcortical U-fibres at the junction of cortex and white matter (Figures 23.57c and 23.75),[111] the very area spared in the inherited leukodystrophies (see Chapter 6, Lysosomal Diseases, and Chapter 8, Peroxisomal Diseases).

Spinal Cord

Why the cervical spinal cord (Figure 23.57f) tends to have more plaques than other spinal levels is unknown, although the effects of trauma mediated via the denticulate ligaments has been postulated.[548]

Optic Nerve

Plaques within the optic nerve are very common in MS. In fact, in some earlier pathology series this was an invariant finding.[448] The initial presentation of MS is often optic neuritis. For these reasons, it will be presented in more detail here.

Clinical Features

Optic neuritis is the initial clinical event in up to 20 per cent of patients with MS.[691] Although optic neuritis is not always associated with MS, it is one of the more common clinically isolated syndromes. Optic neuritis can present with loss of visual acuity, visual field defects, mild pain particularly upon eye movement, and loss of colour vision.[691] As with MS plaques in other locations, symptoms may be worsened by heat (Utthof's phenomenon) and may be produced by local deformation/traction, analogous to Lhermitte's sign, but in this case related to eye movement.[691] The clinical syndrome is associated with delayed visual evoked responses (VERs), but these may be present without a previous clinical history of optic neuritis.[294] Improvement of vision by a few weeks, along with improvement of VERs,[294] is generally the rule but recurrences are possible.[691] Approximately 50 per cent of patients with optic neuritis will develop further CNS involvement to qualify for the diagnosis of MS over the ensuing 15 years.[549]

Neuroimaging Features

Even at the time of monophasic presentation of visual system abnormality, MR imaging often shows one or more cerebral lesions, in addition to the optic nerve plaque; the presence of such lesions is associated with a higher risk of subsequently converting to MS.[549] Analogous to the diffuse atrophy in the brain and spinal cord in MS (see later under Atrophy, p. 1370), optic neuritis is often followed by progressive atrophy of the optic nerve that is probably due to axonal damage and/or loss.[309] This is also reflected in atrophy of the nerve fibre layer in the retina, demonstrable *in vivo* by optical coherence tomography (OCT)[577] and by scanning laser polarimetry.[763]

Pathology

Even though acute optic neuritis is a well-established clinical entity,[763] the neuropathological features of the acute

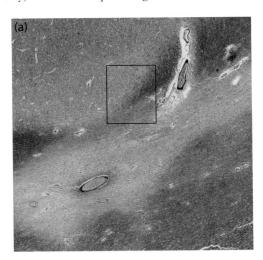

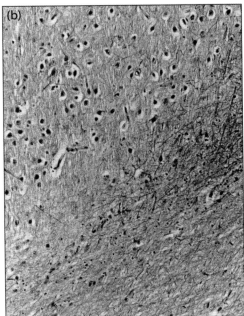

23.75 Multiple sclerosis (MS) plaque in subcortical U-fibres. **(a)** Luxol fast blue (LFB)–Bielschowsky stain of a MS plaque in the subcortical U-fibres. **(b)** Higher magnification of the region shown in the rectangle in **(a)**. The demyelinated axons, without LFB-positive myelin sheaths, are evident in the plaque, which also extends into the deeper layers of the overlying cortex (upper half of panels [a] and [b]). Thus, this plaque may be classified as a leukocortical plaque.

optic neuritis lesion are not well documented. By contrast, atrophy and established chronic plaques similar to those seen elsewhere in the CNS are common findings in the optic nerves at autopsy in patients with MS (Figures 23.56 and 23.76).

Retina

The changes in the optic nerve are frequently reflected in the optic disc as atrophy. Atrophy of the optic nerve head has been confirmed histopathologically[362,755] and is associated with cupping, often with a fibrovascular membrane and perivenular fibrosis and gliosis.[279] In keeping with the findings on OCT, this is also associated with degeneration of the retinal nerve fibre layer,[279,362,755] reflecting loss of the same axons that form the retinal nerve fibre layer and optic nerve: as a manifestation of a primary neurodegenerative process, neurodegeneration secondary to inflammation, or wallerian degeneration from axonal transection in optic nerve plaques. Any of these scenarios would also explain the well-documented degeneration of their cell bodies in the ganglion cell layer.[279,755] In addition, a recent histopathologic and immunohistochemical study of a large number of eyes in MS has shown degeneration of the inner nuclear layer (comprising bipolar and horizontal cells) as well.[279] Retrograde trans-synaptic degeneration was felt to be the most likely explanation for this finding, similar to the anterograde trans-synaptic degeneration that has been documented in the lateral geniculate nucleus.[213]

Vascular inflammation in the form of perivenous sheathing and extravasation of fluorescein have been well documented in patients with MS.[430] This 'periphlebitis retinae' has been confirmed in pathology studies, which have shown retinal perivascular chronic inflammatory infiltrates.[279,693,755] that are sometimes granulomatous.[37] Some of the cells are positive for Class II MHC and are sometimes seen outside the perivascular space infiltrating the retinal nerve, ganglion cell and inner nuclear layers.[279] Only occasional blood vessels in the retina show abnormalities of endothelial tight juctions.[279]

Questions concerning the contributions of primary neurodegenerative and primary inflammatory processes

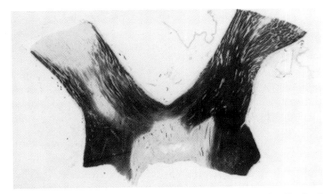

23.76 Optic nerve plaques in multiple sclerosis (MS). Optic nerve and chiasm plaques in a male aged 42 years with a 12-year history of multiple sclerosis (MS). Heidenhain.

Courtesy of Professor JW Prineas, University of Sydney, Sydney, Australia.

to the MS plaque in the brain are also applicable to the retinal pathology. The diffuse nature of the neuronal changes and the fact that the inflammatory changes are relatively focal raises the possibility of a primary neurodegenerative process that is independent of inflammation.[279] Another issue raised by the retinal involvement in MS is that (at least in the majority of humans) it is an unmyelinated structure, suggesting that myelin antigens may not be important in any immunopathogenic process occurring at this location (and possibly, by inference, in MS in general).[480]

Uvea

In the clinical sphere, the occurrence of uveitis in MS has been somewhat controversial, but there appears to be an association, albeit relatively minor.[425] However, from the histopathological point of view, inflammation, fibrosis or neovascularization involving the anterior uvea, particularly the iris, is seen in a large majority of cases.[279] indicating that this may be subclinical in many cases.

Peripheral Nervous System

The selectivity of CNS demyelination in MS is evident in subpial plaques located at the junctions of spinal nerve roots and cranial nerves with the parenchyma. In these areas, demyelination often appears to end abruptly at the point where central myelin gives way to intact peripheral myelin (see Figures 23.62 and 23.63). Thus, MS is primarily a CNS disease. The incidence of clinical peripheral neuropathy is usually low but is variable in different reports. A retrospective review of the records of 150 MS patients showed an incidence of 8 per cent of focal radiculopathy and peripheral neuropathy of only 3 per cent.[849] Subclinical radiculopathy, mononeuropathy and polyneuropathy detected by electrophysiology have been reported in patients with MS,[585] and myelin reduction has been identified in nerve biopsies.[187] Earlier autopsy studies also reported cases in which proximal and distal nerves showed myelin breakdown and axonal loss,[301] but peripheral neuropathies in patients with advanced MS may be attributable to additional factors, including metabolic causes, malnutrition, cytotoxic drugs, entrapment neuropathies, pressure palsies and cachexia. However, more recent clinical studies suggest that the association may be more than just an epiphenomenon.[849]

The most obvious pathogenetic association would be the concomitant involvement of CNS and PNS in autoimmune/immune-mediated demyelination. There are only rare reports of coincident chronic inflammatory demyelinating polyradiculoneuropathy (CIDP) and MS.[350,692] The PNS signs and symptoms may either antedate or follow the clinical diagnosis of MS,[215] but usually the CNS disorder presents first.[350] In some patients with CIDP, CNS lesions have been found by neuroimaging,[421] rather than by the clinical expression of CNS signs and symptoms. These observations suggest the existence of overlap syndromes with a common pathogenesis, such as autoimmune responses to common CNS and PNS antigens.[350] In view of the atypical nature of the CNS and PNS features of some of these cases with evidence of concomitant CNS and PNS involvement, such as lack of CSF oligoclonal bands and

absence of PNS conduction block despite demyelination, it has been suggested that they may represent a separate clinical entity rather than a concurrence of MS and CIDP.[350,852]

There are a few reports of Schwann cell onion-bulb formations surrounding thinly myelinated axons in nerve roots close to the spinal cord in MS,[599,609] but there are more striking cases of patients with the clinical and/or pathological diagnosis of MS who have associated hypertrophic neuropathies.[611] Co-existent CIDP with onion bulbs and MS has also been reported.[610] These cases have been considered examples of a distinct MS variant, although their rarity suggests that some of the individuals so affected might have hypertrophic polyneuropathy due to other (e.g. genetic) causes co-existing with MS.[20,650]

Cranial Nerves

Optic neuritis has been discussed earlier (see Optic Nerve, p. 1354). The optic nerve has CNS myelin of oligodendroglial origin. Of the remaining cranial nerves with PNS myelin of Schwann cell origin, the trigeminal nerve is relatively commonly involved and its demyelination is responsible for trigeminal neuralgia in MS.[2] The lesion responsible is, however, usually at the nerve root entry zone and is characterized by demyelination of the CNS axons (oligodendrocyte-myelinated) in that region.[433] Although vascular compression is often the basis of demyelination as a cause of trigeminal neuralgia in patients without MS, it is not necessarily a prerequisite in the clinical setting of MS.[2] The enhancement of the trigeminal nerve as it traverses the subarachnoid space, evident on MRI scans, suggests that the PNS component of the nerve may also be involved.[173] One study has shown that an isolated cranial nerve palsy (including trigeminal neuralgia and/or a trigeminal sensory deficit) occurred as the presenting sign or CIS in 7.3 per cent and as part of a relapse in 3.1 per cent of MS patients.[842] Other than the trigeminal, the oculomotor, trochlear, abducens, facial and cochlear nerves may be involved and the clinical deficit is not necessarily attributable to a brain stem lesion demonstrable by MRI.[749,842] The latter observation may imply involvement of the PNS or the lack of sensitivity of the MRI scanner to very small demyelinative lesions in the brain stem.

Autonomic Nervous System

Autonomic dysfunction in patients with MS may be due to involvement at any level from the hypothalamus,[323] or brain stem[308] to the spinal cord, involvement of the latter being related to focal plaques[398] or diffuse axonal loss,[179] and may have distinct immune, physiological, pathogenetic and pharmacological consequences.[242,727]

Primary Progressive Multiple Sclerosis
Clinical and Imaging Features

Patients with PPMS exhibit relentless progression from the disease onset without distinct relapses (Table 23.6 and Figure 23.3b). Although mild periodic fluctuations in disease severity without definite relapses or remissions are permitted according to the international consensus definition,[436] the term 'transitional' is sometimes applied to the clinical course of patients who show such minor deviations from the relentlessly progressive clinical course (Figure 23.3).[750] Patients with PPMS represent a minority of MS patients, with varying proportions reported depending on the criteria used to define them.[435,507] PPMS usually affects older patients, tends to be more frequent in males, and manifests as progressive dysfunction in a single system, most commonly as spastic paraparesis. Progression of cerebellar dysfunction, hemiplegia, visual loss, brain stem dysfunction and cognitive abnormalities have also been described.[507] The MR imaging findings differ from those in SPMS in that there are fewer cerebral lesions and new lesions rarely enhance.[507] Despite the frequent clinical presentation of a spastic paraparesis, focal spinal cord lesions are seen on MR imaging no more frequently than in other forms of MS. Nevertheless, newer MRI data indicate that the lesion location in the brain is an important determinant of progression.[90] Furthermore, MR spectroscopy and MTI have failed to show consistent differences in the abnormalities in NAWM between PPMS and SPMS.[507] There is also no distinct immunological profile that distinguishes PPMS from other forms of the disease. However, increased T-cell reactivity to GM3 and GQ1b gangliosides has been reported in PPMS compared to other neurological diseases, suggesting a primary or secondary immune attack on the axon.[569]

The reluctance to attribute a purely progressive neurological syndrome to MS without evidence of intrathecal synthesis of IgG or oligoclonal banding,[824] even when the MR imaging appearance would otherwise be considered characteristic of PPMS, may previously have artefactually excluded cases that are biologically the same disease.[658] It was proposed, therefore, to include cases in which CSF oligoclonal bands are absent but that would otherwise fulfil the criteria, as 'probable' PPMS.[751] This issue has been addressed in the more recent iterations of MS diagnostic criteria in which a positive CSF is no longer an absolute requirement for the diagnosis of PPMS[586,587] MR images of patients with PPMS with evidence of intrathecal IgG synthesis in the CNS, however, show more evidence of enhancement, more lesions, larger lesions and more tissue destruction within lesions than do patients with negative CSF findings.[824] Currently, there is no specific treatment for PPMS.

Neuropathology

The neuropathology of PPMS has received little attention as it has been the primary subject of only a few studies. This is probably in part a reflection of the fact that until recently PPMS was not distinguished from SPMS. Both disorders were previously designated as 'chronic progressive MS', a term no longer recommended.[436] Correlating with the comparatively small numbers of contrast-enhancing lesions on MR imaging, there is less inflammation (perivascular cuffing in lesions and parenchymal hypercellularity) compared with SPMS.[633] However, although there are fewer T-lymphocytes in lesions of PPMS, a greater proportion of these cells are immunopositive for the anti-apoptotic marker bcl-2. This suggests that T-cells may survive longer and hence induce prolonged immune-mediated damage in PPMS. There is also a trend towards decreased numbers of oligodendrocytes,

with those present exhibiting decreased expression of bcl-2, suggesting a greater vulnerability to apoptosis and a lesser capacity for remyelination by the remaining oligodendrocytes in PPMS lesions.[116] Consistent with this, an unusual pattern of demyelination with periplaque oligodendroglial death in the absence of deposition of IgG and complement was reported to be unique to PPMS and was not found in other forms of the disease.[440] A greater degree of diffuse axonal injury than in acute MS and RRMS is presumed to account for clinical progression in PPMS and SPMS.[405] The finding that the degree of reduction of axons in the lateral corticospinal tract of PPMS patients correlated with their disability grade just prior to death supports this.[744] Moreover, in PPMS the axonal loss in focal plaques is greater than in those of SPMS.[743] As noted earlier, the reasons for this neurodegeneration in MS are unknown and may be multiple. It has been proposed that the neurodegeneration in the progressive forms of MS is due to the persistence of inflammatory cells in the leptomeninges, perivascular spaces and parenchyma.[412] A further factor to be considered is based on the observation that in both SPMS[29] and PPMS,[31] there is accumulation of insoluble hyperphosphorylated tau in glia and axons, in contrast to early MS in which only soluble tau is demonstrable.[30] This suggests that insoluble hyperphosphorylated tau may be important in the pathogenesis of MS neurodegeneration, as it is in several neurodegenerative diseases.

Understanding of PPMS is currently rudimentary, and further investigations into its clinical, imaging, immunological and neuropathological facets are needed to define its position within the MS spectrum. Such studies should shed light on whether this variant has the same pathophysiological basis as secondary progression in the more familiar forms of the disease. Moreover, unravelling its pathogenesis should shed light on the fundamental question, which is being increasingly raised, as to whether the neurodegeneration in MS is a primary or secondary phenomenon.

Opticospinal Multiple Sclerosis

This is reviewed in the context of its occurrence in Asia, where it has been extensively studied (see later under Asian 'Optico-spinal' MS, p. 1375), and the reader is referred to the section later on Neuromyelitis Optica, p. 1373, for a discussion of the relationship of this disorder(s) to NMO and classic (or 'Western') MS. Although this form of 'Asian', 'non-Western' or 'optico-spinal' MS has been reported and investigated extensively in Japan, it has also been described in other Asian countries, in South America and in African American people.[559,579,609] All of these non-Caucasian demographic groups have a relatively low incidence of classic MS.

Baló's Concentric Sclerosis

This spectacular pattern of demyelination was first described by Marburg in 1906[466] and subsequently by Barré in 1926. However, the eponym eventually bore Baló's name after his case description published shortly thereafter.[49]

Clinical Features and Diagnosis

Previously, when Baló's sclerosis was diagnosable only at autopsy, the condition was thought to be invariably associated with a rapid monophasic neurological course resembling acute MS. It was usually seen in young people and often initially presented with a disorder of mentation or signs of increased intracranial pressure; focal signs may have supervened later.

More recently, several cases showing the characteristic rings on MR imaging were confirmed histopathologically to be Baló's concentric sclerosis, and many further, non-fatal cases have been described in the neuroradiology literature.[354] The circumferential concentric pattern is considered diagnostic of this condition (Figure 23.77).[132] MR imaging of some patients showed that the lesions became smaller or did not progress.[354] and were not necessarily always associated with an aggressive clinical course.[140] Thus, the poor prognosis originally ascribed to concentric sclerosis arose from the fact that before the MR imaging era, the diagnosis could be made only at autopsy. Indeed, by MR imaging, some of the lesions evolve into established non-concentric lesions typical of MS. Moreover, it is common

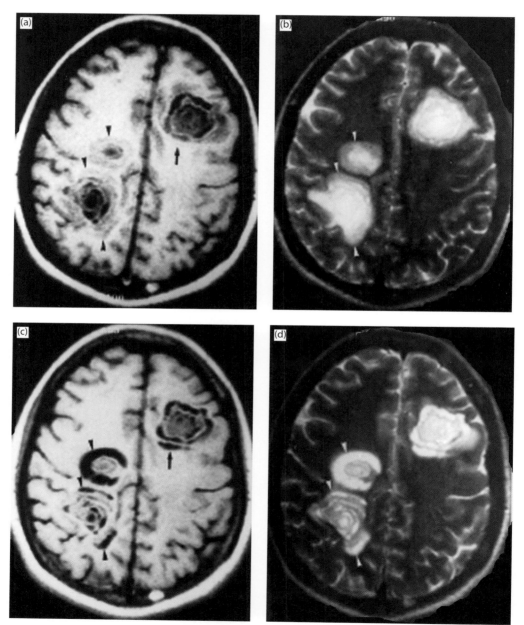

23.77 Magnetic resonance (MR) imaging of Baló's concentric sclerosis. Three concentric lesions are seen on T1-weighted **(a,c)** and T2-weighted **(b,d)** imaging, both on the initial scans **(a,b)** and on scans 1 month later. Note the evolving peripheral bands of demyelination (arrowheads) and the appearance of a new band on the later scans (arrow).

to find MS plaques in the CNS of patients with concentric sclerosis at autopsy[338,512] or by MRI during life.[140] There is, therefore, a prevailing consensus that Baló's sclerosis is a variant of MS.[338,512,514] Furthermore, the association of Baló lesions with large areas of non-concentric hemispheric demyelination and diffuse myelinoclastic sclerosis (see later under Schilder's Disease [Myelinoclastic Diffuse Sclerosis], p. 1361),[745] both of which may also have typical MS plaques, supports the view that these conditions are all variants within the spectrum of MS.[514] This notion is reinforced further by the finding of a similar concentric pattern at the periphery of some MS plaques.[724]

Neuropathology

The classic lesion of Baló's concentric sclerosis is that of circumferential rings or bands of myelin loss alternating with rings or bands with relative myelin preservation centred on a perivenular zone of myelin loss (Figure 23.78). The histological features suggest that the centre of the lesion is oldest and that the peripheral rims of demyelination have developed more recently, so that there is a gradient from the centre to the periphery (Figure 23.78). The lesions may also take on geographic patterns (Figure 23.79a) or complex floral shapes. Baló lesions are characteristically in the cerebral hemispheres but have also been found in the cerebellum, pons, medulla oblongata and spinal cord (Figure 23.79b) at autopsy.[514] They have also been demonstrated in the thalamus by MRI in vivo.[45] The band or ring pattern has a stereotypic appearance, i.e. the myelinated bands are narrower than the demyelinated bands and their inner margins are sharp, whereas their outer margins are less well defined.[609] Microscopically, the bands of myelin have been found to possess normal myelin sheaths,[514] myelin undergoing early demyelination,[838] or thin myelin sheaths with ultrastructural evidence of remyelination (Figure 23.33b).[512] These apparently contradictory observations may be related to the timing of sampling of lesions in different patients. Cases with remyelinated myelin show numerous oligodendrocytes,[512] whereas those with degenerating myelin show reduced numbers of oligodendrocytes.[838] The bands of myelin loss include varying numbers of gemistocytic and fibrillary astrocytes and macrophages with myelin degradation products. There is also axonal loss in these rings of demyelination. In addition, perivascular chronic inflammatory infiltrates with variable composition are common.[724]

Pathogenesis

The reasons for the concentric arrangement of the lesions have been the subject of considerable conjecture.[166a,401a,514,609] For example, the ring formation has been likened to a colloid physicochemical process, with the precipitation of a toxin or lecithinolytic factor in so-called 'Liesegang rings'. It has also been noted that a similar pattern of concentric ring pathology could be induced experimentally in rats by potassium cyanide injection. Others have suggested an ischaemic aetiology, pointing out that concentric patterns have also been described at the edge of infarcts.

In an immunohistochemical study of myelin proteins and of markers induced by hypoxia in Baló's sclerosis, it

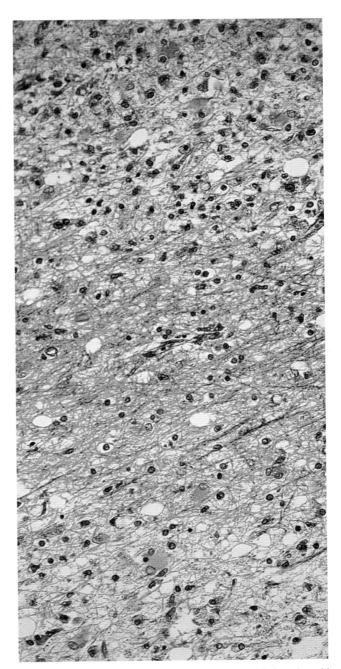

23.78 Baló's concentric sclerosis. 48-year-old female with symptoms present for 18 days. A band of preserved myelin separates two demyelinated zones of different histological age (upper and lower portions). The older, more centrally located zone at the bottom of the figure is less cellular and contains fewer macrophages than the more recently formed zone at the top of the figure. Luxol fast blue (LFB)–periodic acid-Schiff (PAS).

Courtesy of Professor JW Prineas, University of Sydney, Sydney, Australia.

was suggested that the relative preservation of myelin in the myelinated bands could be due to preconditioning of the areas at the edge of the expanding concentric lesion.[724] Their finding of the absence of MAG along with the presence of other myelin proteins in the peripheral actively

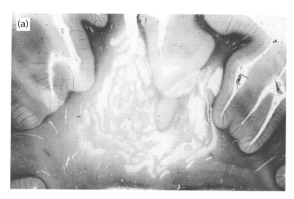

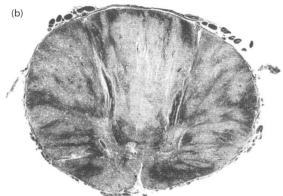

23.79 Baló's concentric sclerosis. Cerebral hemisphere **(a)** and spinal cord **(b)** with typical lesions of Baló's concentric sclerosis. Luxol fast blue (LFB).

Courtesy of Dr DL Yao, National Institutes of Health, Bethesda, MD, USA.

demyelinating band of the lesion indicates relatively recent demyelination and is consistent with the central to peripheral temporal gradient. This is similar to that observed in some ischaemic lesions, some inflammatory disorders, and MS lesions with apoptotic oligodendrocyte destruction.[4,440] Moreover, the neuroprotective factors hypoxia-inducible factor 1α and heat-shock protein 70, which are expressed in many of these conditions, were found at the edge of the Baló lesions, suggesting a 'hypoxic' cause for the progressive expansion of the lesions.[724] Because vascular occlusion has been described in MS lesions only rarely, these findings probably do not indicate a hypoxic–ischaemic insult resulting from vascular occlusion as occurs in cerebral infarcts. More likely, the free radical products of the exuberant immune response, i.e. NO and reactive oxygen species, have a toxic effect on mitochondria and induce focal histotoxic anoxia.[3] In these lesions, the upregulation of the protective factors at the lesion edge might prevent tissue destruction locally, but this protection may be overcome by the demyelinating process, resulting in the formation of the next band of demyelination peripheral to the neuroprotected zone.[724] In a similar fashion, sparing of myelin might also be due to immunomodulation in that zone, resulting in relative protection from immune-mediated demyelination;[512] to date, however, these mechanisms have not been proven. Recent studies of Baló's concentric sclerosis have demonstrated that both the bands of demyelination and the bands of myelin

sparing show an absence of the water-channel marker aquaporin 4 in astrocytes that still express GFAP.[370] Yet these patients do not have aquaporin 4-antibodies.[370] This is in contrast to neuromyelitis optica lesions, where aquaporin-4 antibodies are quite frequent and there is an ablation of astrocytes as evidenced by the absence of both these makers (see later under Neuromyelitis Optica, p. 1373). Thus, it has also been postulated that Baló's concentric sclerosis is an astrocytopathy that produces the peculiar ring formations in the setting of tissue preconditioning.[370]

Neuroimaging

With the advent of MR imaging, there has been an unprecedented opportunity to observe the evolution of the concentric lesion. Enhancement may be seen in all the abnormal bands (Figure 23.80), suggesting that there may not be a progressive layering of the lesion but that all demyelinating rings are being formed simultaneously.[147,354,357] Because enhancement may persist for some time, however, it is possible that the rings are of different ages and that the more central ones, although older, show persistent enhancement. On the other hand, newly enhancing layers have been documented at the outer border of the concentric lesion as enhancement in the more central rings fades away; the areas of enhancement correspond to the areas of T1-weighed hypointensity and T2-weighted hyperintensity that alternate with bands of isointensity. As the lesion progresses, additional bands of abnormal signal are added to the periphery of the lesion in a centrifugal stepwise fashion (Figure 23.77).[148] By MR spectroscopy, the N-acetyl aspartate/creatine (NAA/Cr) ratio decreases over time, consistent with axonal loss noted in histological studies, although this is reversible to some degree. A reverse trend is noted for the choline/creatine (Cho/Cr) ratio and lactate, and fluctuating lipid peaks are also evident.[147] As the lesion regresses, the lamellar pattern becomes ill defined and the abnormal-appearing bands thicken to become a central non-laminated region.[703] In as much as established MS plaques

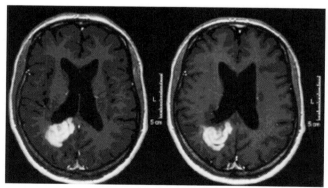

23.80 Magnetic resonance (MR) imaging of Baló's concentric sclerosis. T1-weighted magnetic resonance (MR) image with gadolinium–diethylenetriamine penta-acetic acid (DTPA), showing simultaneous contrast enhancement of several bands of a concentric lesion.

Reproduced from Kastrup et al.[357] With kind permission of Springer Science and Business Media.

have been documented at the site of previous concentric lesions,[283] this process may proceed to completion, with the eventual dissolution of the myelin bands, probably in a centrifugal fashion.

Based on the association of concentric lesions with acute MS plaques, the varied composition of the myelin bands, the radiological and histological evidence of a centrifugal temporal gradient of formation of the demyelinated bands,[514] and the radiological evidence for the subsequent centrifugal demyelination of the myelinated bands, a schema of the pathogenesis of the Baló's lesion can be constructed (Figure 23.81).

Concentric Lacunar Leukoencephalopathy

Concentric lacunar leukoencephalopathy is a very rare disorder with a concentric layering pattern similar to Baló's sclerosis. However, there is extensive axonal loss, and the banding pattern consists of bands of necrosis alternating with bands in which there is little or no surviving myelin.[171, 609] The exact nosological position of this condition and its relationship to Baló's sclerosis is unclear.[171] It seems possible that these cases represent advanced Baló's concentric sclerosis in which the inflammation or hypoxic damage in the bands of myelin was so severe that it resulted in necrosis and cavitation.

Schilder's Disease (Myelinoclastic Diffuse Sclerosis)

This condition has also been the subject of controversy since its first description.[591] In 1912, Schilder described a 12-year-old girl with rapid neurological deterioration and who showed extensive bilateral hemispheric demyelination, for which he used the term 'encephalitis periaxialis diffusa'. The patients he described subsequently under this designation in 1913 and 1924 did not, however, have what is now termed 'Schilder's disease'; the first of these patients had a leukodystrophy and the second had subacute sclerosing pan-encephalitis. Further confusion resulted from the use of the term 'diffuse sclerosis' for both Schilder's disease and various other entities. Most of the patients with diffuse hemispheric demyelination that had been referred to as 'Schilder's disease' were subsequently identified to have adrenoleukodystrophy, which, like many other leukodystrophies, shows diffuse hemispheric demyelination (see Chapter 6, Lysosomal Diseases, Chapter 7, Mitochondrial Diseases, and Chapter 8, Peroxisomal Diseases).[609,669a,669b]

To characterize Schilder's disease, which is now also referred to as 'myelinoclastic diffuse sclerosis', and to distinguish it from leukodystrophies, specific criteria have been developed for its diagnosis.[593] With the advent of MR imaging, these criteria have since been extended (Table 23.9).[12]

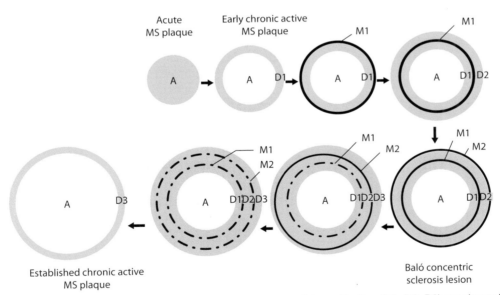

23.81 Postulated pathogenesis of Baló's concentric sclerosis. Regions of demyelination (D1, D2, D3) are shown in grey; bands of myelin preservation in which there is downregulation of immune-mediated demyelination are shown in black (M1, M2). The arrows indicate the sequence of postulated events. The lesion begins as a confluent area of active demyelination as an acute multiple sclerosis (MS) plaque A. The demyelination will eventually be confined to the edge (D1) of the plaque, which is now an early chronic active plaque. A band of suppression of demyelination (M1) eventually develops in the periphery of this region of demyelination. However, the protection affects only a narrow rim, and the active demyelination begins again adjacent to it in zone D2. Demyelination zone D2, in turn, develops a band of suppression of demyelination at its periphery (M2). Demyelination begins again in zone D3. This continues for any number of cycles, resulting in an equivalent number of bands of myelin sparing. At some point, the suppression of demyelination is no longer effective and the bands of myelin preservation are destroyed by the demyelinating process. This begins at the centre and spreads centrifugally, leaving the outermost active border of what was the Baló's concentric lesion (in this case, D3) as the active demyelinating border of the now established chronic active MS plaque, with the areas occupied by the previous zones D2, D1 and A showing progressively fewer recent changes.

TABLE 23.9 Criteria for the diagnosis of myelinoclastic diffuse sclerosis (Schilder's disease)

Symmetric bilateral plaques measuring at least 3 × 2 cm involving the centrum semiovale*
No other lesions demonstrable by clinical, para-clinical or imaging methods
No involvement of the peripheral nervous system
Normal adrenal function
Normal very-long-chain fatty acids
Histology identical to multiple sclerosis

*Subsequently it was suggested that this be extended to include cases with multiple lesions in the same hemisphere, cases with unilateral single lesions, and cases with diffuse involvement of one hemisphere.

Because of the application of these strict criteria, several cases of Schilder's disease have been documented, although it remains a rare condition,[12] difficult to diagnose. The patients are usually children or young adults who present with mentation or psychiatric symptoms, focal deficits, including aphasia, hemiplegia, ataxia, cortical blindness or optic neuritis, or signs of increased intracranial pressure.[12] Some patients remit clinically, particularly when treated with corticosteroids;[12,249,384] other patients are left with a permanent deficit;[593] some progress;[249] and still others have a relapsing–remitting course.[426] Occasional patients are adults.[367,609] Imaging reveals the large centrum ovale lesion(s), which may have a mass effect and be mistaken for a neoplasm or abscess.[249,367,609] Therefore, patients often present to a neurosurgeon. However, the spontaneous reduction in lesion size over time favours the diagnosis of a demyelinating lesion.[43] Moreover, the lack of significant mass effect can be quite remarkable, particularly in view of the magnitude of the lesion(s).[43]

The neuropathology of Schilder's disease is that of inflammatory demyelination as seen in classic active MS, except there is extensive confluent hemispheric involvement. Although perivascular lymphocytic inflammation is also evident in adrenoleukodystrophy, it is found exclusively within the demyelinated zone, in contrast to MS, in which inflammatory cell cuffs are also located at the periphery of and outside of the area of demyelination. This has been interpreted to indicate that in adrenoleukodystrophy the inflammation is a reaction to myelin breakdown, whereas in MS it may be an initiating mechanism.[595] Also in contrast to leukodystrophies, demyelination may spread focally into the subcortical U-fibres, and oligodendrocyte loss is usually evident in all demyelinated regions in most leukodystrophies. There is axonal loss in lesions, but this is not as marked as the myelin loss.[591] The inflammatory process may be so pronounced as to cause necrosis and cyst formation, the latter frequently noted in biopsies.[249,384] Reactive astrocytes are numerous and some take on bizarre multinucleate forms,[591] a common feature of many acutely demyelinating inflammatory lesions. Perivascular lymphocytic cuffs may be absent in older lesions.[591]

As in other rare forms of inflammatory demyelination, the relationship of Schilder's disease to MS is not clear. There are cases with diffuse hemispheric demyelination characteristic of Schilder's disease that also have MS plaques located elsewhere in the CNS. Such cases have been termed 'transitional sclerosis' and also have been documented by MR imaging to have developed focal plaques after the diffuse hemispheric myelinoclastic event.[334] Furthermore, as in MS the CSF can contain oligoclonal bands,[593] but unlike in MS periventricular areas are typically not involved in Schilder's disease. It is possible that myelinoclastic diffuse sclerosis is syndromic and that some cases are a manifestation of MS and others represent a distinct entity. Further studies must be undertaken to resolve these issues.

Neurophysiology of Multiple Sclerosis

In experimental animal models, the predominant histopathological features of MS plaques, i.e. demyelination, remyelination, inflammation and gliosis, can affect axonal physiology, and these results have been extrapolated to human diseases. Inferences on the mechanisms of dysfunction in MS have also been made from clinical neurophysiological studies.[705,707,804–806]

Specific deficits can result from focal demyelinated lesions within an eloquent pathway in the CNS (e.g. paresis from a lesion in the lateral corticospinal tract, sensory loss from a lesion in the lateral spinothalamic tract, internuclear ophthalmoplegia from disruption of the medial longitudinal fasciculus). The potential complexity of neurological dysfunction in patients with MS results from the multifocality and widespread distribution of plaques. Moreover, the cumulative effects of multiple focal lesions are also important, particularly with respect to hemispheric plaques; it appears, for example, that dementia can ensue once a critical threshold of burden of white matter disease is exceeded.[629]

In the following sections, the physiological aspects of each of the histopathological features found in MS plaques are discussed separately, although many of the resulting symptoms and focal deficits are likely to be a consequence of their combined effects. The neurophysiology of non-lesional white matter and cortex is largely unexplored at present.

Demyelination

The myelin sheath is a structure of high electrical resistance and low conductance that is admirably suited for saltatory conduction of the action potential. This contrasts with the much slower continuous conduction of the unmyelinated axons that are present only in comparatively smaller numbers in the mammalian CNS. Action potentials are initiated by voltage-gated sodium channels that allow the influx of extracellular sodium ions into the axon, producing the membrane depolarization characteristic of the initial upswing of the action potential.[377] Sodium channels are distributed throughout the axolemma of the unmyelinated axon but in the myelinated axon are in high concentration only in the initial axon segment and at the node of Ranvier, which is flanked by the paranode, adjacent to which is the juxtaparanodal region (see earlier under Demyelination, p. 1322) (see Figure 23.28).[180,806]

Loss of the myelin sheath can have a number of adverse physiological effects. Conduction block has the greatest clinical importance because it results in focal negative symptoms and signs, i.e. loss of function.[707] Conduction block can be a consequence of either segmental or paranodal demyelination, which results in the inability of the exposed internodal axolemma to conduct action potentials. Furthermore, in MS, disruption of the paranode may occur without loss of the myelin sheath and the loss of this barrier that separates nodal sodium channels from juxtaparanodal potassium channels is sufficient to produce action potential conduction failure.[320]

Symptom fluctuations in patients with MS, such as worsening with increased temperature, known as Uhthoff's phenomenon, must have underlying pathophysiological explanations. The temperature effect has been explained by the fact that at lower body temperatures, the action potential is prolonged, increasing the likelihood that the demyelinated axon membrane may be depolarized to a threshold for the ensuing action potential.[707] On the other hand, the often remarkable recovery from focal deficits of patients with RRMS implies that conduction blocks can be overcome spontaneously. Similarly, the localization in eloquent areas of some demyelinated plaques that do not cause neurological deficits also suggests that conduction of action potentials can occur within these lesions.[707] Early recovery of function and dissolution of conduction block are probably due to the redistribution of sodium channels throughout the axolemma of the demyelinated segment that allows continuous conduction through the segment.[707] Both the $Na_v1.6$ channels and the $Na_v1.2$ channels that have been demonstrated on demyelinated axons in MS lesions[168] produce rapidly activating and inactivating currents that could allow the conduction of action potential along the demyelinated axolemma, but at the expense of increasing the intra-axonal sodium concentration in this region (Figure 23.29a).

There are several other types of sodium channels, each encoded by a different gene and with significant differences in behaviour with respect to threshold of firing, voltage dependence, kinetic characteristics and pharmacological responses.[804] A study of patients with MS with clinically evident cerebellar dysfunction and cerebellar plaques showed that the Purkinje cells synthesized the mRNA and transcribed the protein for a sodium channel normally not expressed by these cells.[80] Thus, the sodium channels in remodelled demyelinated axolemma are not necessarily of the original type, and the admixture of different types manifesting from such 'transcriptional channelopathies' may result in different patterns of neuronal activity and desynchronized function.[805] The diversity of sodium channels, particularly those that are normally not functional but may be upregulated in MS, raises the possibility that they could be selectively targeted pharmacologically.[806] The demyelinated axon also shows a reduction of Na^+/K^+ ATPase, which results in a reduced exchange of intracellular sodium for extracellular potassium.[840]

As discussed previously (see earlier under Demyelination, in Axonal Injury and Loss, p. 1333), the accumulation of intracellular sodium drives the sodium–calcium exchanger, causing rises in intracellular calcium concentration[806] that might lead to axonal degeneration or death by activating neutral proteases.[382,733] Co-localization of the sodium–calcium exchanger with Nav1.6, but not Nav1.2, has been demonstrated in degenerating demyelinated axons (Figure 23.45).[168] Moreover, intracellular calcium influx could also be mediated by newly inserted axolemmal calcium channels that have been demonstrated in dystrophic axons in active MS lesions

and appear to be associated with the disruption of axonal transport (Figure 23.46).[382] Thus, sodium and calcium channel perturbations are likely to be important mechanisms for progressive axonal loss in MS.

As noted previously (see earlier under Demyelination, in Cellular and Molecular Components in Multiple Sclerosis Lesions, p. 1322), clusters of $Na_v1.6$ channels have been demonstrated in demyelinated axons in chronic MS lesions,[82] and whether such clusters can support saltatory conduction in the absence of insulating myelin, is unclear. However, sodium channel clusters, referred to as 'phi nodes' have been reported in experimental PNS demyelination where they have been shown to mediate saltatory conduction.[708] The existence of sodium channel clusters in demyelinated axons in MS raises the possibility of functional saltatory conduction resulting in clinical recovery before remyelination.[707]

In addition to loss-of-function (negative) symptoms, patients with MS may also experience positive symptoms even early in the disease course.[765] These symptoms, such as the radiating shock-like dysaesthesias produced by neck flexion with cervical spinal cord lesions (Lhermitte's sign) and spontaneous or stimulus-induced motor spasms, are usually paroxysmal, of short duration and stereotyped. They are postulated to be manifestations of spontaneous electrical activity in demyelinated axons with increased or altered expression patterns of sodium channels.[705] Experimentally, mechanical deformation of demyelinated spinal cord can produce trains of action potentials. Lhermitte's sign may also be due to mechanical sensitivity of demyelinated axons that may have acquired the ion channel characteristics of peripheral mechanoreceptors.[707]

Although difficult to substantiate *in vivo*, ephaptic transmission (the transmission of a spontaneously generated impulse from a demyelinated axon to an adjacent axon or neuron) has also been invoked as a mechanism of positive symptoms in patients with MS.[705,707] In support of this concept, transmission directly from the auditory system to trigeminal pathways appeared to occur in a lesion in the dorsolateral pons.[298] It has also been proposed, based on computer simulation, that continuous activation of nodes of Ranvier demarcating the demyelinated segment ('persistent reflection') may also be the physiological basis for positive symptoms in MS.[857]

Remyelination

The clinical significance of remyelination is difficult to assess, but remyelinated internodes can conduct action potentials.[707] Recovery due to remyelination is probably not as early as sodium channel redistribution, which may occur in a matter of days.[806] In optic neuritis, for example, an early period of improvement in visual-evoked responses was attributed to sodium channel distribution and late recovery of function to remyelination.[345] Moreover, computer simulations suggest that insertion of just two short (corresponding to remyelinated) internodes at the junction between a normally myelinated axon and a demyelinated zone can allow entry of the action potential into the demyelinated zone.[707] Once in an MS lesion, the action potential could be propagated by continuous conduction if sodium channel redistribution had occurred. Thus, it is possible that modest remyelination, such as occurs at the edges of chronic MS plaques, may contribute to some recovery.

Inflammation

The abundance of cytokines, chemokines, free radicals and other molecules with potential electrophysiological effects in active MS plaques suggests that inflammation itself may contribute to neurological dysfunction. Indeed, in an EAE model in which there is CNS inflammation but little or no demyelination, affected animals may show significant neurological signs.[621] Similarly, in MS, clinical recovery frequently occurs when Gd-DTPA-enhancement on MR imaging has resolved, suggesting that resolution of inflammation played a role in the recovery.[707]

Earlier studies showed that introduction of MS serum into the CNS had neurophysiological effects that appeared to be due to the IgG fraction. Subsequent studies of antibody effects on neuronal physiology have produced conflicting results, and at present the relationship of these so-called 'neuroelectric blocking factors' to an expanding list of molecules associated with the immune response in the CNS is unclear.[705]

Numerous inflammatory cell products affect neuronal function. In concentrations that would be anticipated in an inflammatory lesion, NO rapidly and reversibly blocks axonal conduction.[706] Several pro-inflammatory cytokines slow visual-evoked responses (TNF-α, IFN-γ, IL-1) and decrease neural activity in dorsal nerve roots (IL-1β, interleukin 6 (IL-6), TNF) *in vivo* in experimental animals; TNF-α and IFN-γ may also be associated with conduction block in patients with MS, although an effect mediated by NO cannot be excluded[705] and TNF may play a role in the genesis of ectopic discharges in MS.[707] An endogenously produced pentapeptide with local anaesthetic properties ('endocaine' or 'QYNAD') has been found in MS CSF. This potent sodium channel blocker appears to be released during inflammation and/or myelin breakdown in the CNS and PNS and might, therefore, have an important role in rapid changes in symptoms.[108] A transcranial magnetic stimulation study has shown that high intrathecal levels of IL-13 are associated with increased GABA-mediated cortical inhibition.[652] CSF of MS patients with active MRI lesions inhibits GABA transmission *in vitro*, and this has been attributed to IL-1β.[653]

Inflammation and breakdown of the blood–brain barrier are associated with vasogenic oedema, the extension of which can cause a mass effect to the point of simulating a neoplasm (see earlier under Tumefactive MS and Biopsy Diagnosis of MS, p. 1343); the resolution of oedema is thought to explain shrinkage of plaques after the disappearance of lesion enhancement. Oedema might also contribute to the extent of tissue injury in lesions with specific anatomical localizations (e.g. spinal cord, optic nerves) by expansion in a non-yielding compartment. The contribution of oedema *per se* to neurophysiological alterations in MS is not certain, but changes in ion concentration and osmolarity are likely to have important effects[707] as is the direct introduction of circulating serum components through the damaged BBB.

Glial Alterations

Astrocytes and microglia also produce several cytokines and NO, with the potential neurophysiological effects described earlier. Astrocytes form a syncytium connected by gap junctions that function as aqueous pores between adjacent cells. This syncytial arrangement mediates the spread of electrical and chemical signals throughout the astroglial network.[65] In the presence of the inflammatory mediators, these junctions are markedly attenuated, compromising astrocytic syncytial functions and their interactions with neurons.[366]

Astrocytes provide glutamine for glutamate synthesis by neurons, release and take up glutamate, and participate in the uptake of GABA. They also possess glutamate receptors,[65] including metabotropic glutamate receptors that are upregulated in MS lesions.[256] Thus, astrocytes prevent extracellular glutamate overload and the ensuing neurotoxicity. In this regard, reactive astrocytes have been implicated in the induction of experimental seizures, regardless of the underlying disease process,[752] raising the possibility of their involvement in seizures in MS patients. The intimate association of astrocytic processes with the nodes of Ranvier and demyelinated axons also raises the possibility of an astrocytic contribution to neurophysiological disturbances in gliotic white matter plaques.[807] Oligodendrocytes also remove extracellular glutamate, and their loss in MS lesions predisposes existing neural structures to the same fate.[581]

Axonal Loss in Lesions and Non-lesional White Matter

Axonal loss due to injury within plaques[571] and to wallerian degeneration in the NAWM[212] contributes to progressive neurological deficits. Other factors that may be operative in the pathogenesis of neurodegeneration in MS are discussed earlier (see Axonal Injury and Loss, p. 1331). Whatever the mechanism, the loss of the axon implies permanent loss of neurological function. Although a significant degree of functional plasticity has been demonstrated by functional MRI (see later under Grey Matter, in Magnetic Resonance Imaging and Its Pathological Correlates in Multiple Sclerosis, p. 1370), there is a limit to these compensatory mechanisms[475] and as a result permanent disability ensues.

Grey Matter

Little is known about the pathophysiology of focal grey matter plaques and normal appearing grey matter (NAGM). However, the extensive demyelination that can be present in the cortex would be expected to have a significant clinical effect. The occurrence of cortical clinical phenomena such as epilepsy would be anticipated to be the result of cortical involvement in MS. Indeed, it has been shown that RRMS patients with epilepsy have more cortical plaques on MRI, and these lesions evolve rapidly and are accompanied by cortical atrophy.[128] Cognitive decline and disability measures are also more severe in this group of patients.[128] Furthermore, white matter damage cannot account for all cognitive abnormalities in MS, and deep grey matter pathology, in particular atrophy and neurodegeneration (see under Grey Matter, under Magnetic

Resonance Imaging and Its Pathological Correlates in Multiple Sclerosis, p. 1370), may also contribute to cognitive and physical disability.[318] Hippocampal demyelination may be important in memory deficits and depression and may mediate these effects by interference with neuronal protein synthesis (see earlier under Clinical Significance of Grey Matter Plaques, p. 1353).[197]

In view of their differing pathology and physiological and biochemical milieu, it is probable that different combinations of factors contribute to dysfunction in grey matter and white matter. Because astrocytes regulate extracellular pH and potassium ion concentration and participate in glutamate and GABA homeostasis, changes in their density and metabolism in MS grey matter could affect the extracellular environment of the neuron cell body, contributing to disturbed neuronal function.[65] No doubt the neurite damage and synaptic loss in grey matter lesions[808] have a pivotal role in the pathophysiology of these lesions. As in other CNS diseases with neurodegeneration, microglia are likely to be important in the disturbed electrophysiology of grey matter, particularly in view of their close proximity to transected cortical neurites.[573]

Magnetic Resonance Imaging and Its Pathological Correlates in Multiple Sclerosis

Magnetic resonance (MR) imaging is a sensitive technique for the detection of MS plaques and the understanding of how tissue changes correlate with these images is an area of active research.[510] Therefore, imaging assessments are incorporated into the criteria for the diagnosis of MS and are used routinely to determine outcomes in therapeutic trials and other longitudinal studies.[587] Magnetic resonance relaxation techniques, which are employed routinely in clinical practice, measure relaxation phenomena of hydrogen protons subjected to a radio-frequency pulse in a magnetic field; the scanning parameters can be set such that the scan is T1-weighted (Figure 23.1c) or T2-weighted (Figure 23.1b). T2-weighted imaging and proton density (Figure 23.1a) scanning are used widely for the demonstration and follow up of MS plaques.[757] However, because similar findings may be seen in other demyelinating and non-demyelinating conditions, and as MS may manifest with unusual MR features, the MR imaging appearances, although characteristic, are not diagnostic of MS. The MR imaging must, therefore, be interpreted in the context of clinical and other findings. This is highlighted by the fact that not infrequently patients who have been scanned for other reasons have the MRI findings that are characteristic of MS.[543] This so-called 'radiologically isolated syndrome' (RIS) is reminiscent of the finding of asymptomatic incidental MS at autopsy.[263] Approximately 35 per cent of patients with RIS will convert to CIS or MS,[722] and this conversion rate is higher if there is a lesion in the spinal cord[544] or if there are cortical lesions.[266] The clinical approach to RIS and its relationship to the diagnosis of MS is currently evolving.

Magnetic resonance imaging–pathological correlative studies in MS have confirmed that large focal abnormalities on routine clinical scans (proton density, T2-weighted and T1-weighted modalities) (Figure 23.1a–c) are indeed MS plaques (Figure 23.82).[565] A multiplicity of focal periventricular, brain stem, corpus callosal and spinal lesions on MR imaging and the presence of lesions that are greater than 3 mm in diameter suggest the diagnosis. The lesions are often more numerous than would be predicted on clinical grounds, indicating that clinical observations alone are relatively insensitive for detecting disease activity in MS.[757] There is also a relatively poor correlation between fluctuations of T-cell reactivity to myelin antigens and MRI findings.[303] Moreover, the total lesion load detected on brain MR scanning correlates poorly with disability.[103] These discrepancies have been attributed to localization of lesions in 'clinically silent areas', functional cortical adaptation, spinal involvement and abnormalities in the seemingly normal-appearing white and grey matter. However, when analysis of tissue intensity is correlated with specific anatomical regions, this 'clinical–radiological' paradox is no longer apparent for a variety of neurological deficits.[290] Magnetic resonance imaging also demonstrates clearly the dynamic nature of the disease in that focal lesions may appear and disappear or undergo progressive expansion or involution over a few weeks.[757]

Neuroimaging – Post-mortem Correlations

The exquisite sensitivity of MR scans for the focal lesions in MS is also reflected in post-mortem studies in which lesions that are not evident on gross examination of the brain are readily visualized by MR imaging. Interestingly, these are usually acutely demyelinating lesions and lesions with inflammation without demyelination (the so-called '(p)reactive lesions', see Box 23.3), whereas grossly visible lesions are frequently chronic inactive lesions.[176] Thus, MR imaging is very useful in post-mortem examination to detect active and early lesions that would otherwise be overlooked.[87] In this manner, it has also been used with stereotaxis for co-registration in lesion sampling.[672] There a number of other protocols that have been developed for MRI–pathologic correlative studies. These include imaging of the brain *in situ* as well as unfixed brain slices.[176,234,681]

However, important technical issues confound MR imaging–pathological correlative studies, particularly in MS. Tissue autolysis is the first consideration. Compared with autopsy tissue, rapidly acquired biopsy material will show less autolysis and will more closely resemble what is occurring *in vivo*. On the other hand, a biopsy is a limited sample of a lesion that could be histologically heterogeneous, and it is usually obtained in a clinical setting in which demyelinating disease is not necessarily the first diagnostic consideration.[508] Autopsy provides the entire CNS for sampling, but autolysis is inevitable. However, surprisingly, within a 24-hour period or even longer, MR relaxation parameters are affected only minimally.[508] After formalin fixation, there is a shortening of both T1 and T2.[508] Nevertheless, because the relative relationships of lesions and normal anatomical structures are similar to those in the unfixed state, formalin-fixed tissue can be used for MR imaging–pathological correlation studies (Figure 23.82).[519]

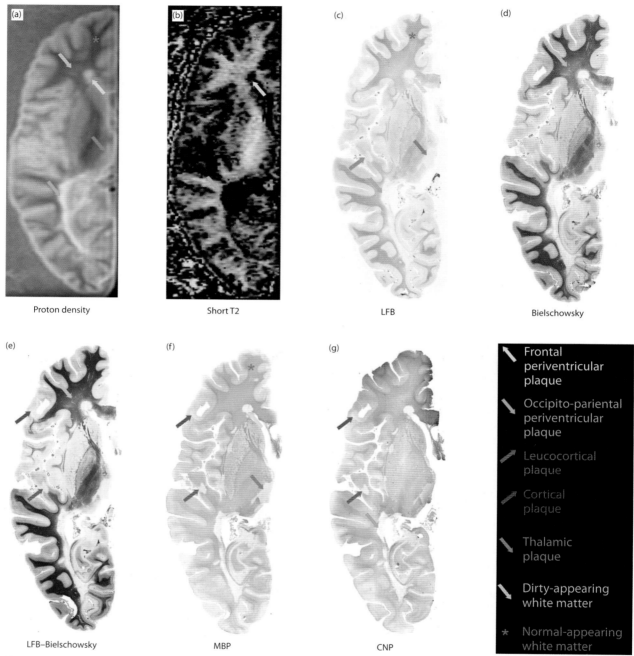

23.82 Magnetic resonance (MR) imaging–pathology correlation in multiple sclerosis (MS). Magnetic resonance images and histological sections are from the same slice of formalin-fixed cerebral hemisphere. Note the periventricular plaque in the frontal white matter (yellow arrows) and the much larger periventricular plaque in the occipito-parietal white matter (green arrows), which are evident as increased areas of signal intensity on the proton density scan **(a)** and as absence of signal on the short T2 component distribution (myelin water fraction) **(b)**. The short T2 component distribution corresponds to the distribution of myelin. The plaques show loss of myelin as demonstrated by absence of staining in the Luxol fast blue (LFB) stain **(c)** and myelin basic protein (MBP) **(f)** and 2',3'-cyclic nucleotide 3'-phosphodiesterase (CNP) **(g)** immunostains. They also show severe axonal loss, as indicated by decreased colouration in the Bielschowsky preparation **(d)**. A plaque in the thalamus (blue arrow) shows similar imaging and staining characteristics. A cortical plaque (red arrow) best seen in the MBP and CNP stains is not detected by MR imaging. A leukocortical plaque (purple arrow) is more evident than the cortical plaque in the LFB stain, probably because of demyelination of the subcortical U-fibres; it is also not evident on the MR scans. Diffusely abnormal white matter, or dirty-appearing white matter (DAWM; gold arrow), located peripheral to the periventricular plaques and deep to the normal-appearing white matter (NAWM; orange asterisk), is characterized by a signal intensity intermediate between that of plaque and NAWM. DAWM is seen as pallor on the LFB and Bielschowsky preparations, and on their combination stain **(e)**. It is not as distinct in the MBP and CNP stains.

Magnetic resonance images courtesy of Dr AL MacKay, University of British Columbia, Vancouver, BC, Canada. Histological sections courtesy of Ms E Leung, University of British Columbia, Vancouver, BC, Canada.

Volume averaging is another issue in correlations of MR imaging with histopathology. Magnetic resonance scanners average signals over a given voxel area through a slice that usually ranges from 3 to 5 mm in thickness. By contrast, the histological section taken from the slice to represent it is usually only 3–10 μm thick. This difference is particularly important for small lesions and irregular borders of larger plaques that may be averaged with normal-appearing or other tissue above or below the lesion. It is possible, therefore, that a lesion, or a portion of it, may not appear in the tissue section depending on the level taken from within the slice; conversely, a small lesion signal may be obscured and the lesion overlooked as a result.[508]

Focal Lesions

Earlier studies attempted to equate changes on the MR scan with specific histological features of the MS plaque. A variety of pathological features, including demyelination, macrophage infiltrates, vascular permeability, oedema, expansion of the extracellular space, and gliosis, were found to correspond to the focal MR imaging abnormalities.[508] Consequently, it became clear that routine MR imaging does not show histological specificity and that a variety of histopathological changes may correlate with the same change in the scan. In T1-weighted images, the chronic 'black holes' seen with this technique were found to correspond to areas of severe tissue destruction and presumably irreversible axonal loss.[784] Subsequently, in a study following patients after biopsy, it was determined that some black holes are reversible and that some of the biopsy samples showed remyelination. In addition, the reversibility of some of these 'acute black holes' was attributed to decreased extracellular free water as a result of resolving oedema and inflammation.[78]

The MR imaging appearance of patterns within certain MS lesions does appear to correlate with the geographical variation in the microscopic appearance of certain lesions, particularly in Baló's Concentric Sclerosis (see earlier under Neuroimaging, in Baló's Concentric Sclerosis, p. 1360)[132,354] and in the signal change at the periphery of some lesions that may be due to the presence of numerous macrophages at the borders of chronic active plaques.[114]

Several newer imaging techniques offer the promise of greater histopathological specificity. One is based on the short T2 component, sometimes referred to as the 'myelin water map' (Figure 23.1e), which is derived from a non-negative least-squares algorithm employed to decompose the T2 decay curve into an arbitrary number of exponential components.[452] Three components are manifest with this paradigm. The longest, greater than 1 s in duration, represents CSF; the intermediate, 70–95 ms in duration, is thought to emanate from intra- and extracellular water; the distribution of the short component, 10–50 ms in duration, correlates with the anatomical distribution of myelin.[513] The short-T2 component intensity correlates with the intensity of LFB staining of myelin (see Figure 23.82).[417] That the short-T2 component recognizes water associated with myelin sheaths is also supported by its absence in chronic inactive lesions that lack myelin but have some surviving axons.[513] Thus, this technique offers promise for following demyelination and possibly remyelination[787] in MS lesions.

The origin of the intermediate T2 component has been unexplored, but it is believed to originate from both extracellular and intracellular water. More recently, a long T2 component has been described in MS patients, particularly those with a long disease duration (Figure 23.1f).[418] In some of these lesions there are also diffusion tensor imaging (DTI) changes to indicate the presence of elongated processes, which has been postulated to be caused by isomorphic fibrillary gliosis.[379]

Magnetization transfer imaging (MTI) detects protons interacting with macromolecular structures and thus assesses the structural integrity of tissue components such as myelin[673] and axons.[784] Multiple sclerosis plaques show a reduction in the magnetization transfer ratio (MTR) (Figure 23.1d),[655] and the degree of magnetization transfer effect is dependent on the age of the lesion.[753]

Diffusion tensor imaging (DTI) assesses the degree of random motion of protons expressed as an apparent diffusion coefficient (ADC) or mean diffusivity.[656] The latter is increased in MS lesions, and fractional anisotropy, the determination of directionally dependent restricted diffusion, is reduced. Fractional anisotropy allows for the elegant depiction of fibre tracts in the brain by tensor imaging, and eventually this may be applied to the determination of direct or secondary tract involvement in MS. Up to recently, it has been difficult to do this on postmortem human brain, but this has now been achieved with excellent tractography images.[496]

Proton MR spectroscopy (MRS) allows for the *in vivo* evaluation of the presence of certain molecules in selected areas. The presence, absence or reduction of a molecule specific for a given cell type reflects the fate of that particular cell type. One such molecule is *N*-acetyl aspartate (NAA), a marker of neurons and axons.[79] Magnetic resonance spectroscopy shows that NAA is reduced in MS plaques[38] and that this reduction may be partially reversible. Magnetic resonance spectroscopy also detects abnormal lipid peaks in MS plaques that are attributed to myelin breakdown.[525] Choline, which is thought to be a component of cell membranes in inflammatory demyelinating lesions, is increased in enhancing lesions.[525] Choline is, however, also increased in chronic lesions with fibrillary gliosis, suggesting that astrocytes may also be a source of choline in abnormal MR spectroscopic spectra.[75] Increases in lesional myoinositol[102] and creatine[304] are thought to reflect gliosis. Elevated lactate correlates with the presence of activated macrophages,[75] and MR spectroscopy for phosphorus shows reduced levels of phospholipids in MS plaques.[328]

Susceptibility-weighted imaging (SWI) is influenced by iron deposition and shows the iron accumulation in the MS basal ganglia and thalamus,[289] which also appears as hypointensity on T2-weighted imaging.[47] SWI also demonstrates MS plaques quite well and it is possible this may not be necessarily a function of iron content, but it may also delineate structure.[837]

Perfusion MRI tracks a contrast dye or blood to measure cerebral perfusion and has shown reductions in perfusion in MS that correlate with disability and cognition.[319]

Clearly of great importance in understanding the pathogenesis of MS is the histopathological correlate of the earliest detectable change at the site of what will later be an established plaque (see Box 23.3). One of the earliest changes seen with routine MR imaging is focal enhancement after the infusion of gadolinium–diethylenetriamine penta-acetic acid (Gd-DTPA) (Figure 23.1c). It is generally accepted that this represents a breakdown of the BBB associated with infiltration of lymphocytes[358] and, particularly, macrophages.[531] The presence of newly formed blood vessels may also correlate with enhancement.[446] However, even the earliest changes seen on routine MR scans are preceded by abnormalities on unconventional MR imaging that antedate the former by weeks to months.[228,415] The histological correlate of these MR findings has not been determined, but there has been much speculation about their underlying causes. The earliest change is probably a focal reduction in the MTR in white matter.[228,415] Oedema, gliosis, demyelination, remyelination or early immune attack on myelin before recruitment of nonspecific lymphocytes have all been proposed as candidates for the cause of this very early abnormality.[228,415] Additional early changes at these 'pre-lesional' sites detected by other techniques include an increase in choline,[747] increases in cerebral blood volume and flow,[833] and changes on DTI.[812]

Magnetic resonance imaging–clinicopathological correlation studies focusing on individual MS cases can provide insights into lesion pathogenesis. For example, the biopsy of a patient with high titres of anti-MOG and anti-MBP serum antibodies showed deposition of immunoglobulins and complement C9neo on oligodendrocytes and myelin at the actively demyelinating edge of an enhancing lesion, suggesting that this is an antibody-mediated form of demyelination and that the patient would respond favourably to plasmapheresis.[115] The unusual situation in which serial biopsies are performed on an individual patient during the acute phases of the disease offers the opportunity to correlate the evolution of the disease process with changes on MR images. These studies are limited, however, by the small sizes of biopsy samples and the likelihood that each lesion is histologically heterogeneous.

Routine MR imaging underestimates pathological features in the spinal cord,[74] but focal completely demyelinated plaques do appear as areas of high signal intensity on high-resolution proton density imaging (Figure 23.2).[450] The latter technique also shows regions of mildly increased signal in the spinal cord that correspond to areas of relative axonal preservation and mild reduction of LFB staining, interpreted as partial demyelination.[450]

Normal-Appearing White Matter

Biochemical, histochemical and morphological abnormalities have been documented in MS NAWM, but these had been attributed in part to the presence of small focal lesions in macroscopically normal-appearing tissue. Early MR imaging studies of MS focused on plaques,[565] and the NAWM was regarded as 'normal' tissue. Later studies of NAWM utilizing non-conventional MR imaging techniques have shown widespread abnormalities in areas that appear normal on routine imaging. These findings have contributed to considerable renewed interest in the clinical and pathological importance of the NAWM in MS.[229,493]

Earlier work described microscopic changes in MS NAWM that included diffuse gliosis, cells with increased numbers of lysosomes, perivascular inflammation, perivascular deposition of lipofuscin, and occasional demyelination.[17] More recently, microglial activation (Figure 23.83),[18] upregulation of transcription factors involved in MHC expression[269] and expression of peripheral benzodiazepine binding sites[50] and upregulation of osteopontin and αB-crystallin[701] have been described in MS NAWM. Moreover, activated microglia and perivascular inflammatory cuffs in NAWM express matrix metalloproteinases that can degrade the extracellular matrix and facilitate inflammatory cell transmigration.[528,649] There is also evidence of BBB dysfunction in NAWM, characterized by abnormal endothelial tight junctions and extravasation of permeability markers into the CNS parenchyma.[371,584] These latter findings probably correlate with subtle increased enhancement in NAWM detected in quantitative contrast-enhanced MR scans.[698] Axonal abnormalities in perilesional NAWM include upregulation of certain ephrin A1 and ephrin receptors Eph A3, -A4 and -A7 and APP expression (Figure 23.84).[199,714]

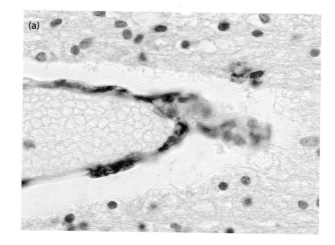

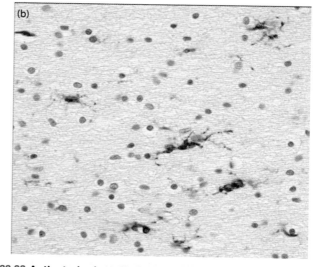

23.83 Activated microglia in normal-appearing white matter (NAWM) in multiple sclerosis (MS). Immunohistochemistry for Class II MHC shows positive activated microglia, with their characteristic ramified morphology, in the perivascular space **(a)** and parenchyma **(b)** of NAWM. Haematoxylin counterstain.

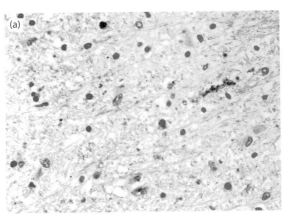
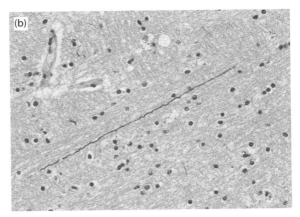

23.84 Axon abnormalities in normal-appearing cerebral white matter in chronic multiple sclerosis (MS). (a) Axon swellings are highlighted with a stain for β-amyloid precursor protein. **(b)** A single dystrophic axon in longitudinal section expresses Ephrin receptor A7. Immunoperoxidase with haematoxylin.

There is also evidence to indicate that ischemic preconditioning may be an important neuroprotective mechanism in NAWM.[276]

Of particular clinical interest, and correlating with MR spectroscopy studies (see later), is the finding of wallerian degeneration and axonal loss in corpus callosal NAWM that is likely to be a result of axonal destruction within plaques.[211,212] The presence of low levels of inflammation throughout the CNS and meninges in chronic MS probably also contributes to the degeneration.[405] In general, by MRI the neurodegeneration does not appear to correlate with the plaque burden and, therefore, may involve pathogenetic mechanisms in addition to wallerian degeneration.[493] In this regard, it is noteworthy that an immunohistochemical study of Caspr and neurofascin 155 in NAWM implicated microglia in the induction of early axonal changes by showing disruption of the paranode, which correlated directly with microglial activation (as shown by HLA-DR- or iNOS-positivity) and damaged axons (as evidenced by axonal neurofilament dephosphorylation), some of which were even devoid of sodium channels at their nodes of Ranvier.[321]

Axonal loss in MS NAWM has been documented in MR spectroscopic studies of NAA.[493,757] Magnetic resonance spectroscopy has also shown reduced phospholipid,[328] prominent lipid peaks,[526] and increased myoinositol,[223] creatine and choline in NAWM.[333] Further evidence of a diffuse abnormality in NAWM is found in the reduced MTR,[229] higher ADC[813] and reduced fractional anisotropy.[284] Relaxation studies have also shown NAWM abnormalities in the form of prolongation of T1,[785] prolongation of T2,[814] a reduction in the short T2 component and an increase in the total water content.[416] Studies of the histopathologic correlates of NAWM are very few. A recent study reported that the changes in NAWM, as defined by the MTR abnormality, correlate with different histopathologic features depending on the distance from a plaque. NAWM close to the plaque shows a correlation with microglial activation and axonal pathology, the latter presumably secondary to axonal damage inflicted in the plaque. In contrast, MTR reduction in NAWM remote from the plaque correlates with microglial activation but not axonal changes.[506]

The widespread abnormalities in MS NAWM are clinically relevant and, in contrast to plaque load, correlate with disability[756] and cognitive impairment.[493] Therefore, they may be the major basis for clinical progression in patients with chronic MS. In as much as they are demonstrable even at the time of first clinical presentation as CIS, these changes occur very early in the disease.[493] Not unexpectedly, changes in NAWM are also apparent in regions other than the cerebral hemispheres, i.e. the spinal cord and the optic nerve.[451] Axons with small diameters are predominantly affected in the non-lesional white matter in these areas.[213,248]

Diffusely Abnormal White Matter

Subsequent to the discovery of MR imaging abnormalities in MS NAWM, reports emerged of non-lesional white matter with subtle abnormalities that had not been appreciated previously in routine T2-weighted and proton density imaging.[854] In these regions, there is an intermediate signal between that of a plaque and of NAWM, i.e. essentially with the intensity of grey matter but occurring in white matter. The areas have been referred to as 'dirty-appearing white matter' or more recently as 'diffusely abnormal white matter' (DAWM) (see Figures 23.1 and 23.82). Because DAWM was recognized after the MR imaging abnormalities were documented in NAWM, it is possible that some previous studies on 'NAWM' may have included DAWM in their sampling.

DAWM shows poorly defined boundaries and generally is adjacent to plaque, particularly in the periventricular and occipital regions (see Figure 23.1). It has a reduced MTR,[253] an increase in water content (T1$_{free}$),[645] and reduction of the short-T2 component.[419] Pathological correlative studies have shown evidence of BBB breakdown in DAWM attributed to the presence of perivascular inflammation.[796] Some studies show a reduction in myelin and axonal loss in DAWM.[682] Other studies have shown reduced staining of DAWM with Luxol fast blue, Weil's and axonal stains, yet with normal myelin protein immunohistochemistry. Because Luxol fast blue and Weil's stains demonstrate phospholipids, these findings suggest that in DAWM there is an early myelin phospholipid abnormality that does not involve myelin proteins and is associated with neurodegeration.[419,420,515] The relation of DAWM to the pathogenesis of plaque formation and the changes in NAWM is not clear.[149] However, its MRI appearance in SPMS is different from that in PPMS.[797]

Grey Matter

As noted previously, cortical lesions are rarely detected by routine MR imaging, but are with the use of contrast agents or fluid-associated inversion recovery (FLAIR),[257,365] double inversion recovery (DIR)[683] and phase-sensitive inversion recovery (PSIR),[530] three-dimensional magnetization-prepared rapid acquisition with gradient echo (3D MPRAGE)[529] and high-field strength MRI.[674] In addition to the focal lesions in the cortex, there are abnormalities detected by non-conventional MRI in the 'normal-appearing grey matter' (NAGM). These include abnormalities detected by MTI and DWI and a reduction in NAA by MR spectroscopy, some of which may be present at the time of first clinical presentation.[493] The pathological basis of cortical NAGM abnormalities in MS is unknown. Postulated possibilities include the presence of cortical plaques, neurodegeneration including wallerian degeneration secondary to the cortical plaques, diffuse abnormality in grey matter not related to focal lesions, degeneration of the grey matter secondary to focal or diffuse white matter pathology, and combinations of these processes.[493]

Functional MR (fMR) imaging has demonstrated considerable plasticity of the cerebral cortex in the face of the diffuse and focal abnormalities of MS.[475] This applies to motor as well as cognitive function and may even increase with rehabilitation.[231] As the degree of disability in a specific modality increases, there is an increased recruitment of cortical regions removed from the normal functional area for that modality. The capacity for recruitment appears to decrease with advanced disability, particularly in the motor system.[475]

Aside from the accumulation of iron commented on previously, the deep grey matter structures show atrophy. For instance, the thalamus[152] shows a significant degree of neuronal loss correlating with reduction in volume and reduction of NAA by MRI. Similarly, the caudate nucleus volume is reduced and shows changes in DTI parameters.[300] These findings are felt to be indicative of significant neurodegeneration in the deep grey matter.

Atrophy

In view of the extensive focal and diffuse pathological abnormalities, it is not surprising that neuroimaging studies detect considerable cerebral atrophy that correlates with physical and neuropsychological disability in patients with RRMS, SPMS and PPMS.[492] Cerebral atrophy, like many of the diffuse changes in MS, begins early in the course of the illness, but opinions vary as to the most appropriate method for measuring it *in vivo*.[66] Particularly early in the disease, atrophy may sometimes be more apparent than real, simply reflecting the baseline cerebral volume after resolution of oedema (so-called 'pseudo-atrophy').[492] It is generally believed that axonal loss is a significant factor in the progressive cerebral atrophy in patients with MS, but the degree to which other histopathological features, such as demyelination and fibrillary gliosis, are responsible is uncertain.[449] Atrophy is progressive and affects grey matter to a greater extent than white

matter, and the grey matter atrophy has a greater impact on disability.[235] Moreover, MRI shows that in the early stages of the disease, grey matter atrophy is already evident, when it involves particularly the limbic structures and the deep grey matter,[41] a finding that correlated with a quantitative neuropathology study that showed substantial neuronal loss and size reduction of the hippocampus in MS,[558] possibly underlying memory deficits and depression.

The MS spinal cord also shows atrophy that correlates with disability.[73] Axonal loss is evident both in lesions and in non-lesional white matter;[248] its presence in the latter appears to be independent of the focal lesions,[73] suggesting a progressive degenerative process unrelated to wallerian degeneration. Similarly, optic nerves in patients with MS show progressive atrophy and, as noted earlier, reduced numbers of axons.[213,637]

Radiological and Pathological Correlates of the Clinical Expression of Multiple Sclerosis

Focal Multiple Sclerosis Lesions

The development of specific symptoms and signs concurrent with the detection of new MR lesions in relevant central pathways has led to the conclusion that acute MR changes correlate with acute deficits and altered neurophysiology. For obvious reasons, however, the clinical and radiological manifestations in living patients cannot be correlated directly with cellular neurophysiological and histological alterations. The schema in Figure 23.85 postulates how neuroimaging data may be integrated with current understanding of the pathophysiological processes that result in clinical manifestations in patients with MS.

The initial event in the formation of a focal MS plaque is indicated by a focal change in MTR[228,415] and other changes detected by MR spectroscopy,[747] DTI[812] and perfusion studies[833] before the appearance of focal Gd-DTPA enhancement. Early transgression of the blood–brain barrier by activated antigen-specific T-lymphocytes may not result in blood–brain barrier changes that are of sufficient magnitude to be detectable by routine imaging and enhancement techniques. Antigen presentation to a few antigen-specific T-cells *in situ* may, however, induce activation and initiate a pro-inflammatory cytokine, and particularly chemokine, environment that promotes recruitment of additional antigen-non-specific inflammatory cells to the site. Additional histological changes, such as astrocyte swelling and expansion of the extracellular fluid space, probably also occur and contribute to the early MR findings.[415] As the inflammatory focus expands, both in numbers of accumulated cells and in micro-vessels involved, BBB dysfunction increases and affects sufficient tissue volume for leakage of Gd-DTPA into the parenchyma to be detected as an area of uniform enhancement by routine T1-weighted imaging. At this point, demyelination by recruited macrophages has probably begun and astrocytes exhibit reactive features. A uniform lesion at this stage would correspond to an acute MS plaque and could be associated with clinical dysfunction (either a CIS or a relapse), or could be subclinical or a lesion in RIS if not located in an eloquent region.

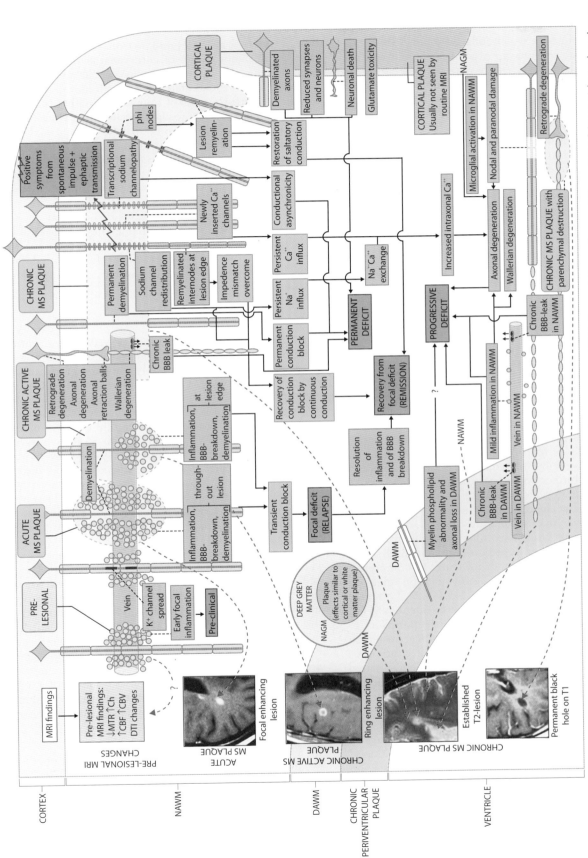

23.85 Clinical, physiological, radiological and histopathological correlates in multiple sclerosis (MS). A correlation scheme of the cellular (blue text boxes) and neurophysiological (green text boxes) changes with their clinical (red text boxes) and MRI manifestations in MS. Text boxes joined with arrows indicate the postulated flow of events. Interrupted orange arrows link a given lesion or area to the corresponding MRI finding. The term 'chronic', unless otherwise indicated, refers to both chronic active and chronic silent plaques. BBB, blood-brain barrier; Ca++, calcium; CBF, cerebral blood flow; CBV, cerebral blood volume; Ch, choline; DAWM, diffusely-abnormal white matter; DTI, diffusion tensor imaging; MRI, magnetic resonance imaging; MS, multiple sclerosis; MTR, magnetization transfer ratio; Na+, sodium; NAWM, normal-appearing white matter.

Lesions continue to expand with a centrifugal gradient of inflammation, neovascularization[446] and active demyelination occurring at the edges; these areas show extensive BBB breakdown evident as a rim of enhancement on the MR images. Plaques in which inflammation in the centre declines, but that continue to expand at the borders, are chronic active plaques that can be detected as focal lesions on T2-weighted imaging.[565] Some plaques may progress through an intermediary stage of a Baló's concentric sclerosis-like lesion in the transition from acute to chronic active stage.[512,514]

As discussed earlier, the products of inflammatory infiltrates and other factors may induce axonal death,[571] followed by wallerian degeneration, the basis of a permanent deficit attributable to the lesion. Moreover, persistent BBB impairment may contribute to permanent dysfunction by the introduction of systemic circulating neurotoxic substances and ionic and osmolarity imbalances in the tissue. Permanent demyelination may also be responsible for persistent conduction block, with attendant irreversible focal deficit.[707] The decline in the inflammatory processes, particularly reduction of neurophysiologically potent inflammatory mediators and resolution of oedema, probably contribute to recovery of function in early stages of clinical remissions.[707]

When inflammation-associated BBB breakdown is no longer detectable in the plaque edge as enhancement, the plaque has probably entered the inactive stage; most T2 abnormalities that do not expand further over time probably represent chronic inactive plaques. Despite non-enhancement, however, some plaques continue to grow, suggesting that lesser degrees of inflammatory demyelination and BBB breakdown continue, but that they cannot be detected with currently available techniques. Chronic plaques can also exhibit new enhancement at their borders and a period of further centrifugal growth after a period of quiescence, suggesting recrudescence of the inflammation, which may result in clinical progression.

Axonal demyelination manifesting as dysfunction (negative signs and symptoms) due to conduction block or as positive or temperature-sensitive signs and symptoms is evident as a reduction of the short T2 component and the MTR on MR imaging. Remyelination might be indicated by the disappearance of a black hole,[78] a return of the short T2 component[787] or an improvement in MTR. Even a small degree of remyelination at the periphery of a chronic plaque may overcome impedance mismatch and introduce the action potential to the continuous conduction provided by the remodelled demyelinated axolemma. These mechanisms may be important in late functional recovery in remissions,[345] whereas reduction of inflammation and axolemmal channel remodelling probably affect earlier time points in remissions.[806]

A reduction in MTR, indicating decreased tissue integrity at the macromolecular level, may reflect demyelination[673] or axonal loss,[784] or both. Severe parenchymal destruction can result in a permanent black hole on T1-weighted imaging.[784] A lesion of this type may result in a permanent deficit if it is located in an eloquent area.

Cortical plaques are generally not visualized and are unappreciated by routine MR imaging (see Figure 23.82).[257,365] The mechanisms by which they may contribute to seizures and intellectual deficits have not been determined, but the impact of demyelination and axonal loss is probably physiologically similar to that in white matter plaques. Additionally, however, reduction of neurites, synapses and neuronal cell bodies[808] are likely to be major causes of permanent cortical dysfunction. The neuron destruction may be due to glutamate excitotoxicity exacerbated by reductions in oligodendroglia;[581] perturbations of potassium and pH buffering of the perineuronal extracellular environment by changes in astrocytes probably also contribute to neuronal dysfunction.[65] Functional MR studies demonstrate that the remaining intact, as well as possibly damaged, cortical structures may be responsible for modifications of neuronal circuitry following white and grey matter injuries in MS.[475]

Deep grey matter plaques are also evident in MS and although it is highly probable they contribute to the clinical picture in MS, they have not been studied extensively. However, plaques within the hypothalamus have been associated with endocrine and autonomic dysfunction.[323]

Non-lesional White Matter

Despite the relative preservation of NAWM on routine MR imaging, wallerian degeneration resulting from axon transection in plaques probably contributes to abnormalities seen in NAWM on non-conventional MR imaging techniques.[493] Presumably, they detect the absence or degeneration of axons that formerly traversed the NAWM from these lesions.[212] The mild chronic inflammatory infiltrates, activated microglia, altered extracellular matrix and continuous BBB leakage in NAWM may contribute to further destruction of axons. This degeneration is, however, less localized and may proceed at a slower rate than in plaques. Gradual reduction in axonal numbers in NAWM, in addition to the progressive loss of axons in focal lesions, probably contributes to gradual clinical progression.

Further abnormalities are detected in non-lesional white matter on routine T2-weighted MR images as intermediate signal intensity between lesion and NAWM, i.e. DAWM;[854] this region also shows axonal loss. In addition, however, studies suggest that there may be a reduction of myelin phospholipid,[419,420,515] the importance of which is unknown. Because this reduction affects the myelin sheath, it is possible that it impairs electrical resistance and thereby interferes with conduction of action potentials of remaining myelinated axons. DAWM also shows evidence of axonal abnormalities,[419,420,515,682] indicating that it also contributes to neurodegeneration and thus permanent and progressive clinical deficits.

Non-lesional Grey Matter

In addition to plaques, there are diffuse neurodegenerative changes, associated with atrophy, in the cortex and deep grey matter that will contribute to the patient's disability.[835] The deep grey matter structures also contain iron,[47] a finding that is enigmatic in the pathogenesis of MS, but nevertheless probably clinically relevant.

In summary, the clinical expression and neuroimaging findings depend on numerous microscopic, molecular and electrophysiological alterations that occur not only in classic focal MS lesions but also in the relatively intact white and grey matter. Many investigations are shedding light on these phenomena, and the information yielded will continue to impact on the diagnosis, treatment and management of MS. Although MS was previously regarded as a single disease that was primarily inflammatory in its initial genesis, this research has already and will continue to alter fundamental concepts of MS.

Implications of Multiple Sclerosis Pathology for Treatment Strategies

The fundamental features of the pathology of MS are well characterized, but the cellular and molecular pathophysiology of the disease remains incompletely understood. The major pathogenetic processes, i.e. inflammation, demyelination, neurodegeneration and the failure of endogenous repair, are all potential targets for therapeutic intervention.[159,190] In addition to the complex patterns of injury that occur in typical white matter plaques, those in non-classic lesions and in normal-appearing areas are now delineated more precisely and are the subjects of considerable current research. In conjunction with advances in neuroimaging, patients in whom specific mechanisms and lesion locations predominate may be identified, allowing future therapies to be individually tailored and optimized.

Current widely used therapies focus primarily on pathological immune responses, i.e. by immunomodulation and immunosuppression. Starting with the use of interferon-β in the treatment of MS in the late 1980s, there have been significant strides in the use of immunosuppressive or immunomodulatory medications in MS, most of which have an effect on the inflammatory aspects of the disease (i.e. relapses), but whether these disease-modifying therapies have any effect on the progressive phase of the disease is not clear at this time. The list of these agents currently available and to be released in the future continues to expand (Box 23.5). The precise effects and mechanisms of action of some agents are not understood completely, and unanticipated adverse reactions may occur, particularly with the use of newer pleiotropic agents.[244] Examples include the occurrence of progressive multifocal leukoencephalopathy in some patients treated with natalizumab[375] and the immune reconstitution inflammatory syndrome (IRIS) in these patients when it is discontinued (see Chapter 19, Viral Infections).[488]

The manipulation of key mediators and signalling pathways in lymphocytes, macrophages, glia and the blood–brain barrier may prove useful in future strategies[151] and in targeting specific stages of the evolution of the plaque.[34] The promotion of remyelination, by stimulating oligodendrocytes and their precursors, and overcoming its inhibition would also be of considerable benefit.[237,386]

The attribution of clinical progression and disability to neuroaxonal degeneration indicates that preserving and repairing neurons and axons holds the greatest promise for restoring neurological function in patients with chronic

---

BOX 23.5. MS treatment modalities currently available or under study

Immune suppression and immune modulation:
- Immunomodulation by unknown mechanism: Interferon-β[817a]
- Induction of Th2 cells and T-regulatory cells: Glatiramer acetate[817a]
- Generalized immunosuppression: Mitoxantrone[817a]
- Binding to very late antigen 4 (VLA4), preventing lymphocyte and monocyte entry across the blood–brain barrier (BBB): Natalizumab[817a]
- Prevention of lymphocyte exit from lymph nodes: Fingolimod[236a,817a]
- Broad-based immunomodulation: Laquinimod[236a,817a]
- Monoclonal antibody-mediated B-cell depletion: Anti-CD20 (rituximab, ocrelizumab, ofatumumab)[236a,817a]
- Monoclonal antibody-mediated B-cell, T-cell and monocyte/macrophage depletion (Anti-CD52): Alemtuzumab[236a,817a]
- Monoclonal antibody-mediated Interleukin-2 receptor blockade: Anti-CD25 (daclizumab)[236a,817a]
- DNA repair interference-mediated B-cell and T-cell depletion: Cladribine[236a]
- Immunomodulation: Dimethyl fumarate[236a,817a]
- Inhibition of pyrimidine synthesis in proliferating B-cells and T-cells: Teriflunomide[236a,817a]
- Immunomodulation, anti-inflammatory and neuroprotective: Minocycline[149a]
- Immunomodulation, anti-inflammatory and neuroprotective: Statins[152a]
- Selective co-stimulation modulation of CTLA-4: Abatacept[790a]

Vitamin D[726]
Plasma exchange[454]
Transplantation
- Bone marrow transplantation[239,662]
- Mesenchymal stem cell transplantation[164]

Natural antibodies to induce remyelination (? future clinical trials)[799]

MS. Therefore, neuroprotection, i.e. preventing ongoing axon injury and degeneration and promoting neuronal regrowth, is a major current therapeutic goal.[574] The mechanisms of neuroaxonal loss, the intrinsic inability of mature neurons to regenerate, and the critical factors in the distinct pathological milieu that may prevent neuronal regrowth in patients with MS need to be further elucidated. At present, stem cell therapies for myelin and axonal replacement are in the early stages of investigation for their potential application to MS.[164]

NEUROMYELITIS OPTICA

History and Nosology

The coincidental occurrence of bilateral visual loss and a myelopathy was first described by Allbutt in 1870 as a case of 'acute myelitis' associated with an 'eye disorder'. Literature on the syndrome was reviewed by Gault, with encouragement by his teacher Dévic,[182] whose name has been associated with the condition, which has been variously termed 'Dévic's disease', 'Dévic's syndrome' or neuromyelitis optica (NMO).

Based on purely clinical manifestations there had been considerable controversy as to whether NMO was a variant of MS, a separate distinct clinicopathological entity, or a clinical syndrome that can be manifested by a variety of disorders. Indeed, the simultaneous occurrence of an optic neuropathy or neuritis and a myelopathy had been described in a variety of conditions, including infections, endocrinopathies, connective tissue diseases and gluten sensitivity.[340] Rare familial cases have also been described.[836] Thus, it was frequently unclear whether a patient with the syndrome was manifesting an optic–spinal presentation of MS, a form of ADEM or a distinct disease. However, over the last several years, an emerging body of clinical, radiological, laboratory and neuropathological data is providing strong evidence that NMO is a distinct entity and not a variant of MS. For this reason, in this edition of this textbook, NMO is being discussed in a section on its own (Box 23.6).

Neuromyelitis Optica

Up to 2004, it was generally assumed that most cases of NMO were a variant of MS with optic nerve and spinal cord involvement that curiously was not associated with CSF OCBs.[220] However, reports of necrosis, rather than pure demyelination, in NMO lesions and the associated poor prognosis strongly suggested that this was a different disorder from MS.[463] Diagnostic criteria for NMO included the absolute requirement for both optic neuritis and myelitis, that could occur simultaneously or at different times and as a monophasic or relapsing-remitting course.[820] Major criteria recognized the fact that the spinal lesions of NMO extended over more than three vertebral

levels (Figure 23.86) and that there was usually a CSF pleocytosis (>50 cells/mm³) or polymorphonuclear leukocytes in the CSF,[820] all these features being exceedingly unusual in MS. In addition, an absence of cerebral lesions at clinical onset was, at that point, also felt to be a feature of NMO.[820]

A pivotal milestone in the understanding of the pathogenesis of NMO in 2004 was the discovery that it was associated with a circulating immunoglobulin that bound to cerebral microvessels, perivascular regions, the pia and subpial regions.[423] This highly specific antibody was called 'NMO-IgG' and was subsequently found to recognize aquaporin 4,[424] a water channel concentrated in the foot processes of astrocytes adjacent to pia and blood vessels

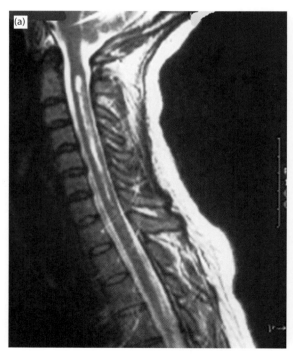
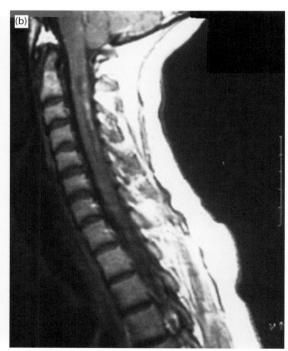

23.86 Magnetic resonance (MR) imaging of neuromyelitis optica (NMO). Spinal cord swelling and hyperintensity extend over several segments in the T2-weighted scan **(a)**. There is linear enhancement in the lesion on the T1-weighted scan with gadolinium–diethylenetriamine penta-acetic acid (Gd-DTPA) **(b)**.

and in the basolateral cell membrane of ependymal cells.[28] In view of this, the diagnostic criteria were subsequently modified to include the detection of aquaporin 4 antibody as a supportive criterion,[821] which was also reflected in the slightly modified versions that were to follow.[494,685] There is a variety of assays for NMO-IgG and no one method has been universally accepted. At present, indirect immunofluorescence is the preferred technique. The significance of patients with clinical NMO who are negative for NMO-IgG is uncertain. Possible explanations include the use of a relatively insensitive assay to detect the antibody or the existence of a subset of NMO patients in whom the autoimmunity is directed toward a different as yet undiscovered antigen.[341]

NMO Spectrum

It soon became apparent that in addition to the classic presentation of optic nerve and spinal cord involvement, the presence of circulating aquaporin 4 antibody was also associated with a variety of other presentations, some of which reflected involvement of either the optic nerve or spinal cord alone and some of which did not involve either of these sites. Thus, the concept of 'NMO spectrum' disorders was born, of which there are four general categories,[472] as follows.

Spatially Limited NMO-Spectrum Disorders

These are instances where only optic nerves or only longitudinally extensive myelitis is present with detection of NMO-IgG. Many, but not all, may go on to show signs and symptoms at the site that was not initially affected.[472] Thus, NMO-spectrum (as well as MS) enters into the differential diagnosis of what clinically has been termed 'transverse myelitis'[93] or 'transverse myelopathy', i.e. an acute or subacute isolated non-compressive intramedullary spinal cord syndrome. Most of these patients who have longitudinally extensive involvement are NMO-IgG-positive and thus considered to have a NMO-spectrum disorder.[93] However, at least 35 per cent with an extensive longitudinal myelopathy are not NMO-IgG-positive;[93] these presumably, at least for now, are idiopathic and cannot be classified as part of the NMO spectrum.

Asian 'Optico–spinal MS'

'Optico–spinal MS' (OSMS) is much more common in non-Caucasian than Caucasian patients and has been extensively studied in Japan. It too, as the name indicates, presents with optic neuritis and spinal cord involvement. It is now felt that those patients with longitudinally extensive myelitis have NMO and indeed many do have the NMO antibody.[93] However, there is a group of Asian OSMS patients whose spinal lesions are not extensive and who are NMO-IgG negative, and who are therefore felt to have MS with optic and spinal plaques, rather than NMO.[746] A third group of Asian OSMS patients are positive for NMO-IgG and have longitudinally extensive spinal lesions characteristic of NMO/NMO spectrum,

but also have periventricular brain lesions characteristic of MS.[473] This has led to the suggestion that there may be an overlap in the MRI appearance in classic MS (also referred to as 'Western' MS as it is seen predominately in Caucasian populations) without NMO-IgG positivity and those with NMO with NMO-IgG positivity, and may indicate a common mechanism for the formation of periventricular plaques in both of these settings.[473] In any event, it appears that the distinction between NMO and the various clinical expressions of 'Asian' OSMS is not as clear cut as between NMO and 'Western' MS. Why this is so is not clear, and is fertile ground for future studies.

Atypical NMO

Although the initial diagnostic criteria for NMO excluded the possibility of brain lesions, it is now known that the brain MRI may show lesions in up to 60 per cent of longstanding cases that fulfil current diagnostic criteria for NMO.[583] These brain lesions comprise nonspecific lesions that are often asymptomatic, in a minority of cases lesions that are typical of MS, or in some cases (particularly paediatric), cerebral, diencephalic and brain stem lesions in locations that are atypical of MS but where aquaporin 4 channels are concentrated (Figure 23.87).[583] These lesions that are atypical for MS are now believed to be typical for NMO/NMO spectrum. Thus, hypothalamic lesions are thought to be responsible for the endocrinopathies sometimes seen in NMO, and have also been recognized as the basis for narcolepsy and coma secondary to reduced production of hypocretin (orexin).[133] Persistent nausea and hiccoughs, which occasionally may be the presenting symptoms and frequently abate, are due to lesions in the area postrema and associated chemoreceptor trigger zone in the floor of the fourth ventricle.[589] The corpus callosal lesions in NMO/NMO spectrum are large and oedematous–again different from MS plaques at that location.[521] A further atypical white matter lesion associated with NMO/NMO spectrum is that of posterior reversible encephalopathy syndrome (PRES), thought to be vasogenic oedema secondary to disturbance of water handling as a result of an aquaporin 4 channel abnormality in the setting of hypertension or sudden fluid shifts.[453]

Association with Other Disorders and Other Antibodies

Aquaporin 4 autoimmunity may coexist with other autoimmune conditions such as myasthenia gravis, Graves' disease, Hashimoto's thyroiditis,[472] pernicious anaemia, ulcerative colitis, primary sclerosing cholangitis, idiopathic thrombocytopenic purpura,[685] and coeliac disease.[819] Patients with NMO may also have a high prevalence of anti-neuronal antibodies, such as anti-glutamic acid decarboxylase and anti-collapsin response mediator protein-5 (CRMP-5).[472] NMO has been associated with systemic lupus erythematosus (SLE) and Sjögren's syndrome, neither of which, however, shows NMO-IgG positivity in the absence of a myelopathy or optic neuritis.[819] This has led to the notion that these two rheumatological diseases and NMO are separate entities coexisting in patients with

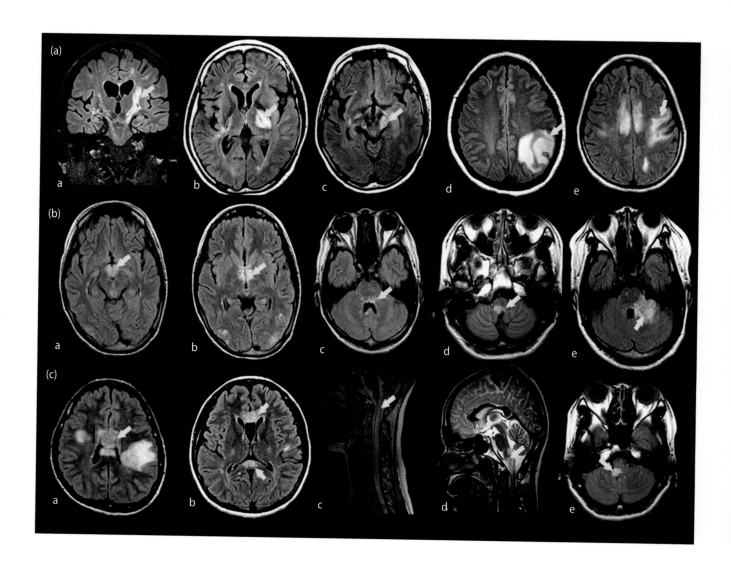

23.87 Cerebral lesions in atypical neuromyelitis optica (NMO). NMO lesions are indicated by yellow arrows. **(a)** Longitudinal corticospinal tract lesions involving internal capsule (a and b) and cerebral peduncle (c) and extensive hemispheric lesions that are tumefactive (d) or spindle-like (e). **(b)** Periependymal lesions in the diencephalon abutting the third ventricle (a and b) and in the brain stem abutting the fourth ventricle (c-e). **(c)** Periependymal lesions abutting the lateral ventricles (a), which with involvement of the full thickness of the corpus callosum may produce an arch-bridge sign (b), and longitudinal medulla oblongata lesions that are contiguous with cervical spinal cord lesions (c-e).

From Huh S-Y, Min JH, Kim W, et al. The usefulness of brain MRI at onset in the differentiation of multiple sclerosis and seropositive neuromyelitis optica spectrum disorders. Mult Scler 2014;20:695–704. © 2014, SAGE Publications. Reprinted by permission of SAGE.

a propensity to autoimmunity. Thus, it is now thought that the myelopathy and optic nerve involvement that may be evident in SLE and Sjogren's syndrome is not due to involvement of those structures by these connective tissue diseases but rather due to co-existing NMO.[819] In addition to autoimmune disorders, NMO has also been described as a paraneoplastic syndrome, where the relationship is also probably an autoimmune phenomenon.[311]

Clinical Features and Imaging

NMO may present as a monophasic or relapsing disorder, and the level of NMO-IgG correlates with clinical outcome and reflects disease activity.[341] The optic neuritis may be unilateral or bilateral and may affect the chiasm and optic tract. The visual deficits, although similar in kind to those in MS, tend to be more severe in NMO and often permanent, in contrast to the usual recovery from optic neuritis in MS. The same is true of the myelopathy, which produces symptoms and signs referable to the spinal level of its most rostral extent. Thus, the acquisition of progressive neurologic deficit in NMO is quite different from MS. In NMO, it is stepwise and due to the accumulated residua from individual relapses, whereas in MS it is gradual and generally independent of relapses.[685] The spinal cord lesions tend to involve the cervical and upper thoracic cord, and they may also extend into the medulla oblongata. As such, they are frequently associated with respiratory failure, rarely seen in MS, and this can be a cause of death.[820] The spinal lesions of NMO produce a complete transverse myelopathy with symmetrical neurological signs, as opposed to the asymmetrical and milder spinal involvement of the MS relapse.[685] Clinical cerebral involvement is relatively unusual but certainly may occur, particularly in children, manifesting as the clinical syndromes of the atypical forms of NMO/NMO spectrum discussed earlier. As noted previously, the finding of a CSF pleocytosis, particularly if polymorphonuclear leukocytes and/or eosinophils are present, also distinguishes NMO from MS.[820] The massive increase in GFAP in the CSF during relapses is no doubt due to the destruction of astrocytes in the NMO lesions (see later under Neuropathology, this page).[502]

The single most useful MRI feature of NMO is the longitudinally extensive myelopathy spanning three or more vertebral levels (Figure 23.86).[820] These lesions often show irregular enhancement during a relapse.[685] In addition to its longitudinal extent, the myelitis of NMO also differs in its cross-sectional appearance from the spinal MS plaque, being central and often associated with spinal cord swelling in contrast to the more peripheral, posterior and lateral locations of the MS plaque. The optic nerve(s) often show enhancement and the abnormality may extend to the chiasm.[685] In addition to abnormalities seen in the brain by routine imaging described earlier, diffuse abnormalities in normal-appearing grey matter[227] and in the normal-appearing white matter in NMO[660] can be demonstrated by non-routine MRI techniques.

Intravenous corticosteroids have been used in the treatment of relapses.[818] Plasmapheresis or intravenous immunoglobulin has also been employed.[472,818] The response to the latter treatment and to rituximab, a monoclonal antibody directed against CD20 on the surface of the B-cell,[472,818] is further evidence of the importance of humoral immunity in the pathogenesis of this disorder. Non-specific immunotherapy has also been used in NMO.[818] Interferon-β, frequently used in the treatment of MS, is less effective in NMO and in some cases may worsen the clinical manifestations.[472]

It should also be noted that some patients presenting with optic neuritis and a myelopathy will not necessarily have NMO or an NMO-spectrum disorder, as defined earlier, and that other conditions such as MS (see earlier under Asian 'Optico–spinal MS', p. 1375), ADEM and some systemic diseases may present in this fashion. To encompass such conditions and in an attempt to reverse the nosological confusion that has plagued the terms 'Dévic's disease' and 'neuromyelitis optica' in the past, it has been suggested that these be referred to as 'Dévic syndrome' whereas the pure form of NMO with distinct clinical and pathological features be termed 'Dévic disease',[679] now referred to as NMO/NMO-spectrum disorders. Alternatively, it may be best to designate a patient with an optic–spinal clinical syndrome who fulfils the NMO diagnostic criteria as NMO, and for the cases in whom the underlying condition has been determined to be a condition other than NMO to simply indicate the disorder (MS, ADEM, etc.) presented as an optico–spinal syndrome. Those cases in whom the underlying condition has not been determined could be designated as an optico–spinal syndrome of undetermined classification. These distinctions are clearly important, because treatment for these groups of patients is different.

Neuropathology

NMO lesions may show heterogeneity of histopathological features. Thus lesions may show demyelination and/or necrosis, which may progress to cystic cavitation (Figure 23.88a,b).[441,463] The spinal cord lesions involve grey and white matter and are usually centrally located (Figure 23.88a). Optic nerves show demyelination, which in most studies is inactive,[441,560] or necrosis with cyst formation.[501] These findings probably reflect the sampling time rather than an indication of the early features of the optic nerve lesion. Necrosis is associated with axon end-bulbs.

In contrast to MS, the perivascular inflammatory infiltrates contain very few T-lymphocytes but many eosinophils and neutrophils (Figure 23.88c,d); the degranulation of these leukocytes is thought to be the cause of the necrosis.[441] The presence of CCR3, a receptor for the eosinophil chemotactic cytokine eotaxin, may be responsible for the recruitment of eosinophils. In addition, there is deposition of immunoglobulins M (IgM) and G (IgG) (Figure 23.88e), particularly the former, and complement C9 neoantigen around the thickened hyalinized blood vessels (Figure 23.88f).[441] In these regions, there is also loss of immunoreactivity for aquaporin 4 and often GFAP (Figure 23.89).[501] Moreover, in NMO lesions, C9 neoantigen is also evident on astrocytic foot processes where aquaporin 4 molecules are concentrated.[501,640] Some lesions show demyelination, whereas others do not (Figure 23.90), but aquaporin 4 loss is evident in all NMO lesions, despite the degree of demyelination.[501,640] Of particular note are lesions in the floor of the fourth ventricle, where there is intense inflammation and aquaporin loss, with reactive GFAP-positive astrocytes and preserved myelin, indicating that aquaporin 4 loss antedates loss of astrocytes and myelin; these

23.88 Neuromyelitis optica (NMO). Spinal cord lesion in NMO. There is extensive destruction of the parenchyma **(a,b)**, with perivascular infiltrates of eosinophils **(c)** and polymorphonuclear leukocytes **(d)**, and perivascular deposition of immunoglobulin **(e)** and C9 neoantigen **(f)**. (a,b) Luxol fast blue (LFB)–periodic acid-Schiff (PAS); (c,d) haematoxylin and eosin; (e) immunohistochemistry for immunoglobulin; (f) immunohistochemistry for C9 neoantigen.

Adapted from Lucchinetti et al.[441] By permission of Oxford University Press on behalf of The Guarantors of Brain.

medullary lesions have been surmised to be reversible and the underlying cause of transient nausea and hiccoughing in NMO (Figure 23.91).[589,640] The loss of aquaporin 4 in astrocytes in early NMO lesions is in contrast to the early MS plaque, where aquaporin 4 is upregulated in reactive astrocytes[702] and is then expressed in a lesional stage-related manner, being absent only in chronically demyelinated MS plaques.[640]

Examination of lesions of different ages explains the heterogeneity of the lesions in NMO. In early lesions, myelin is still present[501] and axons are intact but apoptotic oligodendrocytes and expansion of the extracellular space or vacuolation consistent with intramyelinic edema may be evident.[560] These early lesions show fragmenting

GFAP-positive astrocytes and macrophage phagocytosis of GFAP-positive debris.[560] The demyelination that follows is characterized by macrophages that now no longer contain GFAP-positive debris but rather LFB-positive myelin debris and neutral lipid.[560] Within these lesions, which are eventually depleted of stellate astrocytes, emerges a population of small unipolar or bipolar GFAP-positive aquaporin 4-negative cells thought to be astrocyte precursors (Figure 23.90c).[560] As the lesion matures and demyelination goes to completion, astrocytes form elongated processes that are again positive for GFAP and negative for aquaporin 4. These astrocytes tend to be in bundles running between demyelinated axons and macrophages; the tendency to form bundles of astrocytic processes appears

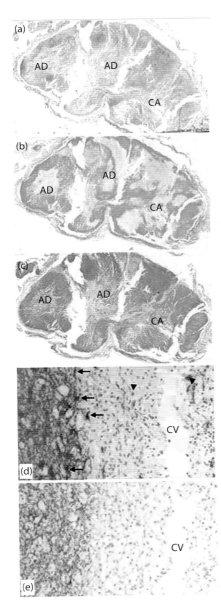

23.89 Astrocytes and myelin in neuromyelitis optica (NMO). Glial fibrillary acidic protein (GFAP) **(a)** and aquaporin 4 (AQP4) **(b)** are absent in NMO lesions, whether they are actively demyelinating (AD) or chronic active (CA), but myelin basic protein (MBP) **(c)** is variably spared. At higher magnifications, GFAP-positive reactive astrocytes **(d,** arrows) are seen at the lesion edge and perilesional parenchyma. Only fragments of GFAP-positive debris (d, arrowheads) remain in the cavitating lesion (CV). No AQP4-positivity is seen in the lesion **(e)**. (a,d) Immunohistochemistry for GFAP; (b,e) immunohistochemistry for AQP4; (c) immunohistochemistry for MBP.

From Misu T, Fujihara K, Kakita A, et al. Loss of aquaporin 4 in lesions of neuromyelitis optica: distinction from multiple sclerosis. Brain 2007;130 (Pt 5):1224–34.[501] With permission of Oxford University Press on behalf of The Guarantors of Brain.

represents the end-stage of the tissue destruction mediated by the products of inflammatory cells and the immune response.[441] It is of interest that, unlike in MS, cortical demyelination is not a feature of NMO.[588]

The histopathologic features of these aquaporin 4-depleted lesions, with localization of immunoglobulin and complement to perivascular regions where this molecule is normally concentrated in astrocytic foot processes, is consistent with the current prevailing concept that humoral autoimmunity to aquaporin 4 is the basis of this disorder that is distinct from MS. Despite this progress, however, it is presently unclear as to why the NMO lesions have a particular predilection for the optic nerves and spinal cord. Hypotheses include oedema within the non-yielding confines of the spinal cord pia mater and the optic canal and possible peculiarities of the microvasculature at these sites.[441,609]

OTHER CENTRAL NERVOUS SYSTEM INFLAMMATORY DEMYELINATING DISEASES

Acute Disseminated Encephalomyelitis and Related Disorders

History and Nosology

Acute disseminated encephalomyelitis (ADEM), an inflammatory demyelinative disorder of the CNS with a presumed autoimmune pathogenesis, has been referred to by a variety of terms in the literature that emphasize its triggering events, histopathology, pattern of lesion distribution or immunopathogenesis.[748] Such terms include post-infectious encephalomyelitis, post-vaccinal encephalomyelitis, post-infectious multifocal encephalitis, perivenous encephalomyelitis, acute perivascular myelinoclasis, disseminated vasculomyelinopathy, acute demyelinating encephalomyelitis, hyperergic encephalomyelitis, post-vaccinal perivenous encephalomyelitis, and post-encephalitis demyelination.[748] The first reports of the disorder emerged as descriptions of post-infectious and post-vaccinal perivenous encephalomyelitis in the early 1920s.[609]

Epidemiology

The incidence of ADEM is estimated to be approximately 0.2–0.8/100 000 per year.[561] It appears to be somewhat more frequent in males and is more frequent in young children and adolescents than in adults, 80 per cent of cases occurring before 10 years of age.[561,678] ADEM has been reported following a large number of viral, bacterial, spirochetal, rickettsial[561] and protozoan[464] infections and after vaccinations[561] and the disorder tends to occur more in the winter and spring months.[172,748] It has also been reported as a paraneoplastic syndrome.[561,735]

Clinical Features and Neuroimaging

Acute disseminated encephalomyelitis usually presents with an abrupt onset of a neurological syndrome, the differential diagnosis of which is quite broad and

to be characteristic of NMO and is a further characteristic that distinguishes it from MS. It appears that necrosis, although usually a prominent feature in NMO, occurs relatively late, as it is evident in old lesions.[560] It presumably

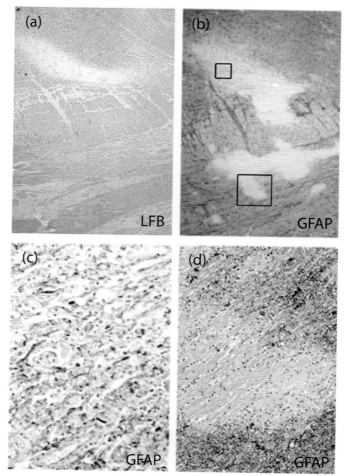

23.90 Astrocytic loss and astrocytic progenitors in neuromyelitis optica (NMO). An NMO lesion shows an absence of myelin on Luxol fast blue (LFB) staining **(a)**. However, immunohistochemistry for glial fibrillary acidic protein (GFAP) shows astrocytic loss well beyond the area of demyelination **(b)**. High magnification of the area indicated by the upper box in B shows there are elongated GFAP-positive astrocytic progenitors in this region **(c)**. A more recently involved area **(d)**, indicated by the lower box in B, is GFAP-negative in the absence of macrophages and GFAP-positive debris, indicating astrocytic pathology antedates demyelination in NMO.

From Parratt JD, Prineas JW. Neuromyelitis optica: a demyelinating disease characterized by acute destruction and regeneration of perivascular astrocytes. Mult Scler 2010;16:1156–1172.[560] *© 2010, SAGE Publications. Reprinted by permission of SAGE.*

includes various infectious diseases.[748] There is often a history of infection, or rarely vaccination, in the preceding few weeks. The clinical presentation, which may involve the motor, sensory, cerebellar, brain stem and spinal systems in any combination, tends to be polysymptomatic, as opposed to the monosymptomatic presentation that usually characterizes an MS relapse.[172,561] Some patients present with optic neuritis, which is usually bilateral, unilateral involvement being very unusual in ADEM, and if present, should raise the possibility of MS or NMO.[172] However, particularly characteristic of ADEM is the occurrence of encephalopathic symptoms and signs, including seizures, alterations in mental status and/or reduced level of consciousness.[172] Fever with pleocytosis in peripheral blood and CSF are common.[172] Headache, nausea, vomiting and meningismus may also be manifest.[172,748] Elevated CSF protein is a common finding whereas oligoclonal bands are unusual,[172]

being more frequent in older individuals.[561] Rarely concomitant involvement of the peripheral nervous system has been reported, and this appears to be a more likely occurrence in adults.[748]

The clinical distinction of ADEM from MS is often difficult. Criteria have been developed by the International Pediatric MS Study Group (IPMSSG) for the diagnosis of ADEM and its distinction from paediatric MS on an operational basis and, no doubt, will be modified as future research unravels these two closely related entities.[393] These criteria require the clinical syndrome to be polysymptomatic and encephalopathic with no other aetiologies to explain its occurrence, followed by clinical or MRI improvement, although there may be fluctuating symptoms, signs and MRI findings over a 3-month period.[393] However, it has been shown that not all patients with ADEM necessarily have encephalopathy,[21] and depressed level of consciousness appears

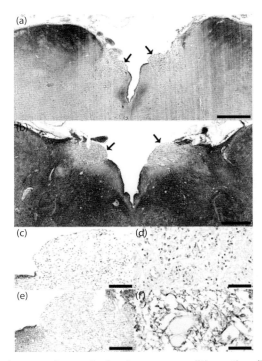

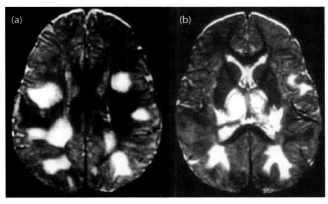

23.92 Acute disseminated encephalomyelitis (ADEM) magnetic resonance imaging (MRI). T2-weighted MRI shows bilateral hyperintense poorly-marginated lesions in central, periventricular and juxtacortical white matter **(a)**, internal capsules and thalami **(b)**.

From Tenembaum S, Chitnis T, Ness J, Hahn JS. Acute disseminated encephalomyelitis. Neurology 2007;68(Suppl 2):S23–36.[748] With permission from Lippincott Williams & Wilkins/Wolters Kluwer Health.

23.91 Area postrema lesion in neuromyelitis optica (NMO). **(a)** Area postrema lesion in a patient with NMO (**a**, arrows), who presented with an episode of nausea and intractable vomiting shows loss of aquaporin 4 (AQP4), compared to the control area postrema (**b**, arrows) in a patient with acute MS **(b)**. High magnification of the region indicated by the right arrow in **(a)**, **(c)** shows depletion of AQP4, with sparing of the immediate subependymal region. The AQP4 loss is particularly perivascular **(d)**. Note the contrast to the control **(e)** and **(f)**, which shows preservation of AQP4-positive astrocytic perivascular processes in a comparable area (indicated by the left arrow in **(b)**). Immunohistochemistry for AQP4. Scale bars: (a), (b), 1 mm; (c), 100 μm; (d), (f), 50 μm; (e), 200 μm.

From Popescu BF, Lennon VA, Parisi JE, et al. Neuromyelitis optica unique area postrema lesions: nausea, vomiting, and pathogenic implications. Neurology 2011;76:1229–37.[589] With permission from Lippincott Williams & Wilkins/Wolters Kluwer Health.

to correlate better with the characteristic neuropathology of ADEM than does encephalopathy.[841] Moreover, occasional patients with MS may have encephalopathy at their first presentation.[363] IPMSSG MRI criteria for the diagnosis of ADEM (Figure 23.92) include multifocal (or rarely a single) lesion(s) greater than 1 cm in size in the supratentorial and infratentorial white matter or in the spinal cord; grey matter, particularly the basal ganglia and thalamus, is frequently involved.[393] Periventricular and corpus callosal lesions are less common than in MS, but may be more common in adults than children with ADEM.[561,748] The incidence of gadolinium-enhancing lesions is quite variable, having been described in 30 to 100 per cent of patients in various studies.[748] MRS shows reduction of NAA and elevated lactate, without elevation of choline, in the lesions; these changes reverse after normalization of the clinical status and T2-weighted abnormalities.[748] Diffusion-weighted imaging and perfusion-weighted imaging show variable results.[748]

The disease is usually monophasic, with good recovery, both clinically and by imaging, even in the absence of treatment.[748] However, death during the illness and residual neurological deficits may occur, more commonly in adults than children.[363] Despite the overall good prognosis, it is becoming apparent that patients with ADEM may be left with mild cognitive impairment.[363,561,748]

Treatment is directed against the inflammatory/immune response and consists of corticosteroids as a first line of defence and usually IVIg therapy or plasmapheresis as alternatives, should the disease be steroid unresponsive.[561,748]

Recurrent and Multiphasic ADEM and Their Relationship to MS

Although most patients with ADEM experience a single episode of inflammatory demyelination, there are a minority of patients that go on to have one or more further attacks of the disease. As would be anticipated, the number of such patients varies from study to study, depending on the criteria used for the diagnosis of ADEM and for relapse and the duration of the follow up. The figures vary from 5 to 21 per cent.[561,748] The IPMSSG has defined 'recurrent ADEM' as a recurrence of the same symptoms and signs as the initial event without any new involvement by clinical and MRI parameters and without a better explanation than disease relapse, occurring at least 3 months after the initial episode and/or 1 month after cessation of steroid treatment.[393] 'Multiphasic ADEM' is defined as a new clinical event, with the same temporal restrictions just noted, still fulfilling the criteria for ADEM diagnosis but now with evidence of new anatomic regions of involvement by clinical and MRI assessment and partial or complete resolution of the original lesions on MRI.[393] The latter scenario, because there is now evidence of dissemination in time and space, makes the distinction from MS problematic and controversial. However, current

IPMSSG recommendations state that the initial ADEM event should not be used for the determination of space and time dissemination and the distinction from MS can be made on the basis of the fulfilment of diagnostic criteria for an ADEM event (as discussed earlier) applied to the second event;[393] but as also noted earlier, these diagnostic criteria do not capture nor distinguish all cases of MS and ADEM. The issue becomes particularly troubling when more than two distinct events occur in a patient with the diagnosis of ADEM. IPMSSG suggests that such cases should be considered extremely suspicious for MS.[393] The distinction between ADEM and MS is important, because the former is short-lived and is treated with anti-inflammatory agents, whereas the latter is a lifelong disease that can be treated with long-term immune suppression or immunomodulation.

Although it is clear some patients with ADEM, both adults[678] and children,[748] subsequently fulfil the diagnostic criteria for and 'convert to' MS, the exact risk for this is not yet clear, variously reported as 0 to 29 per cent.[561,748] Risk factors that have been reported to be operative include initial presentation with optic neuritis or brain stem syndrome, older age at presentation, family history of MS, periventricular lesions, fulfilment of 2005 McDonald criteria for MS at the first ADEM presentation, elevated CSF albumin, female gender, peripheral nervous system involvement, absence of encephalopathy, and absence of seizures, but by no means are any of these absolute.[428,561,748]

Thus, it is clear from the earlier discussion that the boundaries between ADEM and MS are ill-defined. Hopefully, future research will help clarify whether these are two separate entities or are varied temporal and pathogenetic manifestations of the same underlying disease process. The pathologic features of the two are distinct, but even here there are occasional cases that show histopathologic features of both.

Pathology

In patients who die during the acute phase of the disease, the brain may appear swollen and congested, with evidence of transtentorial and cerebellar tonsillar herniation. Swelling of the brain stem or spinal cord is seen in cases in which lesions are concentrated in these regions (Figure 23.93). In contrast to cases of MS of comparable duration in which newly forming lesions may be evident macroscopically in the freshly sliced brain, in cases of ADEM there is usually little to see, apart from swelling.[609] Some petechial haemorrhages may sometimes be seen in the corona radiata, brain stem and cerebral cortex.[297]

In most cases, numerous microscopic perivenous lesions are present throughout the CNS, but they can be limited to a single region. Although they are most numerous in white matter (Figure 23.94), the lesions frequently involve deeper layers of the cerebral cortex and other grey matter regions. Involvement of periventricular blood vessels is also common. Narrow zones of subpial demyelination in the spinal cord and brain stem, and rarely in the cerebral and cerebellar cortex, may also

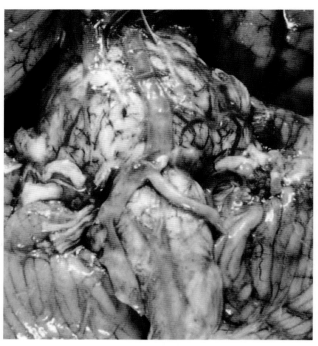

23.93 Acute disseminated encephalomyelitis (ADEM). Fatal ADEM in a 70-year-old male with a 7-week history. Lesions were located predominantly in the brain stem and cerebellar white matter. The pons and medulla were swollen and were softened.

Courtesy of Dr LS Forno, Veterans Affairs Health Care System, Palo Alto, CA, USA.

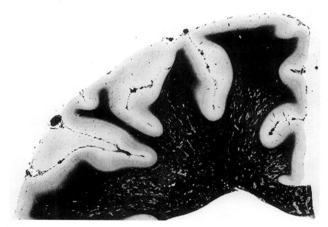

23.94 Acute disseminated encephalomyelitis (ADEM). 34-year-old male who died on the sixth day of a neurological illness. There was no preceding febrile illness or vaccination. Necropsy revealed a swollen brain, with numerous small perivascular foci of demyelination throughout the cerebrum. Heidenhain.

Courtesy of Dr CJ Bruton, formerly of Runwell Hospital, Wickford, Essex, UK.

be seen.[183,468] Marginal demyelination may involve the circumference of the cord or may be especially prominent along the anterior median fissure and more laterally dorsal to the anterior horns. Mild lymphocytic meningitis is invariably present. Occasionally, inflammatory demyelination may be present in the spinal ganglia and nerve roots, peripheral nerves and cranial nerves (Figure 23.95).[468]

The characteristic lesions of ADEM consist of small veins that are often engorged and are surrounded by foamy macrophages (Figures 23.96 and 23.97), with or without a minor lymphocytic/mononuclear cell component.[183,281] The vascular inflammatory infiltrates are sometimes associated with necrosis of the blood vessel wall and fibrinous exudates.[297] The immediately adjacent parenchyma appears pale and is undergoing active demyelination and sometimes even necrosis.[297] The occasional occurrence of necrosis in the vasculature and the parenchyma in this otherwise demyelinating condition highlights the overlap of ADEM and acute haemorrhagic leukoencephalitis (see later under Acute Haemorrhagic Leukoencephalitis, p. 1386). Occasionally, neutrophils are seen in the perivascular cuffs and, as do lymphocytes, sometimes accompany the macrophages in the perivascular parenchyma.[609]

Macrophages typically contain LFB-positive myelin fragments and neutral lipids (Figure 23.98). Mitotic figures and pyknotic nuclei are relatively common among the perivascular and infiltrating cells.[10] Reactive astrocytes are usually relatively inconspicuous. Demyelination remains restricted to extended serpentiginous perivenular sleeve-like hypercellular zones (Figures 23.96 and 23.99), but the size of these zones is variable. In cases preceded by viral illnesses, occasionally microglial nodules are observed.[297] In patients who die within a few days of onset, there may be minimal or no apparent changes in myelin but leptomeningeal and perivascular inflammatory infiltrates are usually present,[297] whereas in patients dying later, the lesions may encompass larger volumes around the vessels with innumerable foamy macrophages and more extensive myelin loss. Although they are preserved relative to myelin loss, axons show typical features of acute injury (Figure 23.99).[261]

In typical ADEM, the foci appear to be of similar histological age.[183] Some patients may have focal lesions with features that overlap with those in acute haemorrhagic leukoencephalitis.[297] Some patients have an associated necrotic myelopathy.[312] Patients dying months or years after clinical recovery have shown either no evidence of the earlier illness or variable degrees of perivascular gliosis, fibrosis of perivascular spaces, perivascular rarefaction of myelinated tissue, or more diffuse myelin loss.[210,459]

A recent report has documented cortical lesions in ADEM consisting of perivenous demyelination, subpial demyelination, and aggregates of activated microglia that were not necessarily associated with demyelination or were adjacent to pyramidal neurons in cortical layer III.[841]

Although the occurrence of non-confluent perivenous lesions are characteristic of ADEM and are distinguishable from the large confluent perivenous lesions of MS, there are occasional cases in which the clinical history or pathology overlap. Thus, there are rare cases with a protracted history thought to be MS that at autopsy have the characteristic lesions of ADEM.[25,547] Whether such cases would be

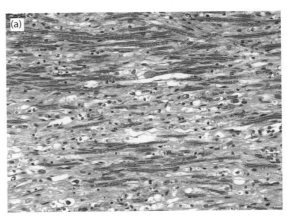
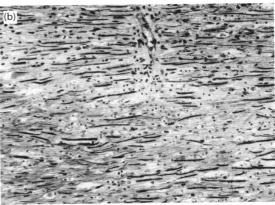

23.95 Cranial nerve involvement in acute disseminated encephalomyelitis (ADEM). Same case as shown in Figure 23.93. The third cranial nerve shows diffuse mononuclear cell infiltration, demyelination and some axonal injury. Note the axonal spheroids **(a)** and the loss of myelin **(b)**. (a) Haematoxylin and eosin; (b) Luxol fast blue (LFB)–Bielschowsky.

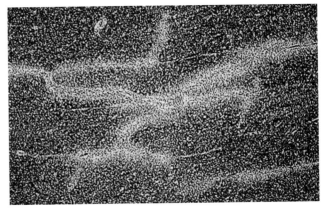

23.96 Acute disseminated encephalomyelitis (ADEM). Same case as shown in Figure 23.94, showing a sleeve-like perivascular demyelination in central white matter. Mallory.

Courtesy of Professor JW Prineas, University of Sydney, Sydney, Australia.

diagnosed as ADEM now using current clinical criteria is unclear. There are also cases in the older literature labelled as acute MS that have had an antecedent infectious exanthematous illness.[166,330,771]

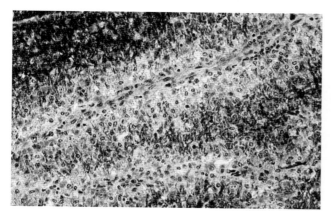

23.97 Acute disseminated encephalomyelitis (ADEM). Enlarged view of lesion illustrated in Figure 23.96, showing a perivascular cellular infiltrate composed largely of macrophages and other mononuclear cells. Mallory.

Courtesy of Professor JW Prineas, University of Sydney, Sydney, Australia.

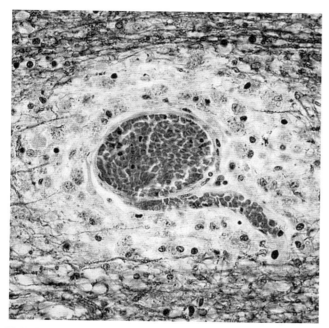

23.98 Acute disseminated encephalomyelitis (ADEM). Same case as shown in Figure 23.94. Higher magnification of a small perivenous demyelinating lesion, showing myelin loss associated with a perivascular macrophage infiltrate. Luxol fast blue (LFB)–Nissl.

Pathogenesis

The pathogenesis of ADEM is uncertain. Attempts to recover virus from the brain and to demonstrate viral antigens and viral nucleic acid in affected CNS tissues in ADEM have, for the most part, been negative. This, together with the fact that the pathological changes are unlike those seen in known viral and other pathogen infections, argues against direct invasion of the CNS by an infectious agent as the cause of ADEM. Moreover,

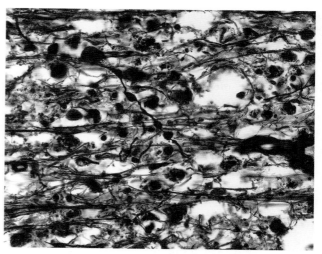

23.99 Acute disseminated encephalomyelitis (ADEM). Same case as shown in Figure 23.93. A high-power magnification demonstrates acute axonal injury as beading in a demyelinated focus. Note the absence of blue staining of myelin. Combined Luxol fast blue (LFB)–Bielschowsky.

the clinical and pathological uniformity among most cases following infection or vaccination argues in favour of a common autoimmune pathogenesis. The immune response has been postulated to be directed against inoculated CNS tissue components in the post-vaccination cases and possibly involving molecular mimicry between the pathogen and CNS tissues in post-infectious cases. Alternatively, it has also been proposed that the disorder is due to non-specific activation of a pre-existing anti-myelin immune response during an inflammatory process.[748] As MS, ADEM is also associated with Class II MHC alleles; in the case of ADEM, these include HLA-DRB1*01, HLA-DRB*03, HLA-DRB1*1501 and HLA-DRB5*0101.[748] Also consistent with an autoimmune reaction is the observation that the usual time periods between infection or immunization and onset of the neurological illness are similar to those observed in acute EAE models (see later under Experimental Autoimmune [Allergic] Encephalomyelitis, p. 1387). Moreover, there are several studies in which MBP-reactive lymphocytes have been detected in the peripheral blood and CSF in patients with post-infectious ADEM.[291a] Serum antibodies to MOG have also been found in ADEM.[539,687] In addition to the neuropathological similarities between ADEM and EAE lesions, in both conditions recovery from acute clinical disease appears to correlate with widespread T-cell apoptosis.[62,568] Further, autoimmune demyelination after a viral infection has experimental counterparts (see later under Pathogen-induced Models, p. 1389).

Rabies Post-vaccinal Encephalomyelitis

History

Neuroparalytic accidents from ADEM complicating rabies vaccination were first recognized within a few years of the introduction by Louis Pasteur of an attenuated virus vaccine prepared from desiccated infected rabbit spinal cord. Vaccines of this type were replaced in the early 1900s by Semple-type vaccines prepared using formalin- or phenol-treated infected neural tissue from a variety of animal species. In the 1930s, it was shown that inoculation of neural tissue into experimental animals produced perivenous demyelination.[636] Subsequent vaccines prepared using suckling mouse brain, duck embryo and human diploid cell lines have reduced the incidence of neurological complications. The incidence of ADEM associated with neural rabies vaccines is 1:7000 to 1:300, but with non-neural rabies vaccines this incidence drops to 1:15 000.[399]

Clinical and Pathological Features

Clinically, the disorder presents as a transverse myelitis, encephalomyelitis, optic neuritis or polyradiculitis closely resembling the Guillain-Barré syndrome, the last with lesions restricted to the PNS. In other respects, the clinical, neuroimaging and pathological features resemble those of other forms of ADEM, but spinal cord clinical presentations are the most common. In addition to the known nature of the inciting stimulus and the close pathological resemblance to EAE in animals, an autoimmune pathogenesis has been proposed, particularly in patients with chronic neurological complications. Rare cases of rabies post-vaccinal encephalomyelitis have also shown changes resembling those seen in acute MS.[609]

Transitional Cases

The concomitant occurrence of the histopathologic features of non-confluent thin perivenous sheaths of inflammatory demyelination of ADEM and the larger confluent plaques of MS, although quite rare, is well established both in patients with a clinical presentation compatible with ADEM and those clinically felt to have acute MS.[10,224,232,389,547,575,684,767,770,771,841] This observation again points out the ill-defined boundary between ADEM and MS. The controversy as to whether this observation indicates ADEM and MS are related diseases[9] or these are just two superimposed diseases[546] is not resolved.[299,841]

Human Experimental Autoimmune (Allergic) Encephalomyelitis

The inadvertent or vaccinational inoculation of CNS tissue in humans can produce an 'allergic encephalomyelitis'. The most common such occurrence is evident after neural rabies vaccines (see earlier under Rabies Post-vaccinal Encephalomyelitis, p. 1384). As noted, the vast majority of cases with neuroparalytic instances after rabies vaccine show the histopathology of ADEM. Similarly, ADEM may be seen after inoculation of CNS tissue for reasons other than rabies vaccination. Among such cases are that of a woman who had been given repeated injections of xenogeneic CNS tissue as 'fresh cell therapy' and who developed a fatal coma with CNS lesions suggestive of ADEM.[270] Therapeutic immunization trials have occasionally led to unexpected adverse effects that suggest EAE-like mechanisms.[225]

In the 1950s, a monophasic form of rabies post-vaccinal encephalomyelitis with prominent cerebral symptoms, especially memory loss and personality change, was described in Japan.[767] Fever, meningeal signs and impaired consciousness were present at the onset of the illness, and the patients who survived improved without recurrences.[696] This disease had been relatively common in Japan, but subsequently disappeared for unknown reasons. Nine autopsied cases had lesions that closely resembled those seen in acute MS, i.e. large, sharply circumscribed, inflammatory demyelinating lesions with hypercellular borders that were often located adjacent to lateral ventricles (Figure 23.100). Unlike acute MS, however, there were also microscopic perivascular demyelinating and inflammatory lesions disseminated throughout the brain and spinal cord. All lesions appeared to be of the same histological age. These cases, therefore, exhibited clinical features of ADEM, but had neuropathological features in common with both ADEM and MS, i.e. they may also be considered to be 'transitional cases', as discussed earlier.

Other cases have been reported of patients inoculated with neural tissue who subsequently developed MS-like plaques: one was a patient with rabies post-vaccinal

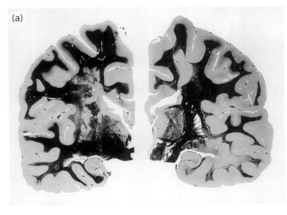

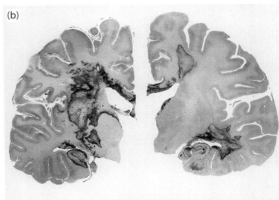

23.100 Rabies post-vaccinal encephalomyelitis. Cerebral form in a 41-year-old Japanese male. The patient died 90 days after the first inoculation of Calmette vaccine. Confluent and perivascular foci of demyelination are apparent adjacent to the lateral and third ventricles. **(a)** Woelcke; **(b)** thionine.

Reproduced from Uchimura and Shiraki.[767] With permission from Lippincott Williams & Wilkins/Wolters Kluwer Health.

encephalomyelitis who later developed a progressive neurological illness and who died 6 years after vaccination with changes typical of longstanding MS present at autopsy.[754] Another developed MS-like lesions acutely after receiving multiple injections of a preparation containing neural tissue as treatment for Parkinson's disease (Figure 23.101).[684]

These rare cases again illustrate the unresolved relationship between ADEM and MS.

The clinical and pathological features of disseminated encephalomyelitis and acute MS are compared in Table 23.10.

Acute Haemorrhagic Leukoencephalitis

Clinical Features and Neuroimaging

First recognized as a discrete entity by Weston Hurst in 1941[326] and hence sometimes referred to as 'Weston Hurst disease', acute haemorrhagic leukoencephalitis (AHLE) is a usually fatal disease characterized clinically by an abrupt onset of fever, neck stiffness and neurological deficits, often progressing rapidly to seizures and coma. In most fatal cases, death occurs within 1–5 days.[11,326] The CSF pressure is usually elevated, with an increase in protein content and a pleocytosis chiefly of neutrophils, often with red blood cells. An elevated erythrocyte sedimentation rate and a peripheral neutrophil leukocytosis are common.[609] The presenting clinical picture is, therefore, similar to that of ADEM, but the course of AHLE is usually more fulminant and ADEM is rarely fatal.

The disease has been seen in most age groups, including infant siblings.[483] It appears to be rare in elderly people. In approximately 50 per cent of cases there is a prodromal febrile illness, almost always an upper respiratory tract infection, 1–13 days before onset. Usually the offending pathogen cannot be documented, but AHLE has occasionally been associated with herpes simplex, varicella zoster, human herpes virus 6, measles, mumps and Epstein–Barr viruses. Rare cases have also been associated with *Mycoplasma pneumoniae*, laparotomy and gastrointestinal disturbances.[578,609]

Morbidity is usually high in surviving patients, but patients with recovery following early treatment have been reported. Treatment modalities have included various combinations of corticosteroids, immunoglobulin, cyclophosphamide and plasma exchange.[748]

The CT and MR imaging features of ADEM and AHLE are similar, but the latter has larger lesions, more oedema and mass effect and punctate haemorrhages. The distinction between the two is difficult. However, early in the course of AHLE, there are hyperintense areas in diffusion-weighted images and low signal intensity in maps of the apparent diffusion coefficient.[580] The use of 2D gradient recalled echo T_2^*-weighted imaging and susceptibility-weighted imaging to detect haemorrhage may also be helpful in the diagnosis of AHLE.[352,580]

Macroscopic Pathology

At autopsy, the brain appears congested and swollen, sometimes asymmetrically in patients with unilateral signs. Cingulate, parahippocampal and tonsillar herniations are frequent. Multiple petechial haemorrhages affect the central part of the centrum ovale, internal capsule, subcortical white matter and corpus callosum and involve grey and white matter in the midbrain, pons, medulla, and cerebellar peduncles (Figure 23.102). Confluent haemorrhages or large asymmetrical foci of necrosis with cavitation may be present. The spinal cord may also be affected, and rare cases have been restricted to the brain stem, cerebellum or cord.[117,580,609] Affected grey matter areas are discoloured and oedematous.

Microscopic Pathology

Histologically, perivascular lesions consist of ball or ring haemorrhages surrounding necrotic venules, sometimes with fibrinoid exudates within the blood vessel wall or extending into adjacent tissue. There are cuffs of mononuclear cells and neutrophils (Figures 23.103 and 23.104), but to a lesser degree in cases in which the duration of the illness has been brief. There is also substantial axonal injury in these areas,[261] and oedema is usually conspicuous. The extent of microvascular damage and consequent haemorrhage is greater in AHLE than ADEM (Figure 23.105). Neutrophils are also frequently present in the leptomeninges. Many of these features have been reported in stereotactic biopsy samples.[262] Demyelination *per se* is not usually evident in these haemorrhagic lesions and when it is present is usually associated with necrosis.[297] However, it should be noted that some perivascular demyelinative lesions of the type seen in ADEM may be also seen in AHLE, but apparently not in the first 4 days.[273]

Pathogenesis

Most authors conclude that AHLE represents a hyperacute form of ADEM, and that the two disorders represent a spectrum of the same disease process. This is supported by the fact that in ADEM, there are instances where the haemorrhagic lesions similar to those of AHLE are also present, and vice versa. As in ADEM an allergic mechanism is suggested by the appearance of the lesions, which in the case of AHLE

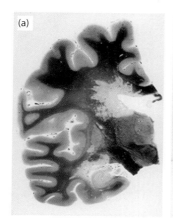
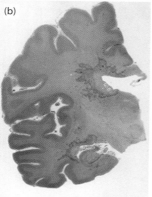

23.101 Human experimental autoimmune encephalomyelitis (EAE). Case of a 51-year-old man who had received seven injections of calf neural tissue over 18 months as a treatment for Parkinson's disease. He developed an encephalitis that resulted in death after 10 weeks. The resemblance to acute multiple sclerosis (MS) is striking. **(a)** Heidenhain. **(b)** Cresyl violet.

Reproduced from Seitelberger et al.[684] With kind permission of Springer Science and Business Media.

TABLE 23.10 Clinical pathological features of acute disseminated encephalomyelitis and acute multiple sclerosis

	Acute disseminated encephalomyelitis	Acute multiple sclerosis
Stimulus	Antecedent infection, immunization, vaccines in most cases	No recognized preceding infection or immunization
Prodromal illness	Headache, fever	None
Neurological illness	Meningism, stupor, focal signs	Focal signs
	Course usually non-progressive	Variably progressive course
	Recovery rapid and often complete	Recovery variable; may be rapid and complete
	Relapses rare	Relapses common
	Often does not progress to MS	Progresses to chronic MS
Macroscopic features	Diffuse vascular congestion and swelling	Vascular congestion and swelling limited to lesions
	Lesions usually not visible or appear as narrow rings of discoloured tissue around small blood vessels	Lesions several millimetres to several centimetres in diameter
Lesion number and location	Innumerable small perivascular lesions throughout central nervous system grey and white matter; may be restricted to a particular region	Variable number of lesions in grey and white matter of the brain, spinal cord and optic nerves
	Subpial and subependymal demyelination common	Subpial and subependymal demyelination common
Microscopic features	Narrow perivenous sleeves of demyelination that retain same shape and size throughout illness	Within days, individual lesions appear as large, irregularly shaped plaques
	Margins sharp	Margins sharp; growth by radial extension or by confluence of periplaque perivascular lesions or concentric bands of demyelination
	Age of lesions uniform	Lesions of different ages
	Demyelination associated with appearance of macrophages	Demyelination associated with appearance of macrophages
	Astrocytic reaction inconspicuous	Astrocytes numerous and enlarged, with mitoses and multinucleate and giant forms
	Perivascular and parenchymal lymphocytic infiltration and appearance of neutrophils	Perivascular and parenchymal lymphocytic infiltration; blood vessel wall destruction and granulocytic infiltration usually absent
	Axonal injury present	Axonal injury present

resembles those seen in 'hyperacute' EAE where a modified adjuvant containing pertussis vaccine is administered[427] with the immunogenic CNS tissue.

ANIMAL MODELS OF HUMAN DEMYELINATING DISEASES

Animal models contribute indispensable insight into human CNS demyelinating diseases. They elucidate complex mechanisms of CNS immunity, tissue injury, chronic degeneration, regeneration, and the failure of spontaneous repair. They are also employed for advances in the management of patients, for example through testing therapies and neuroimaging techniques. Representative models are listed in Table 23.11.

Experimental Autoimmune (Allergic) Encephalomyelitis

In 1935, it was discovered that the repeated inoculation of normal rabbit brain into non-human primates over several months resulted in a neurological illness that resembled ADEM.[636] It was subsequently shown that the latency to disease onset could be markedly reduced by inoculation of the neural tissue in complete Freund's adjuvant (comprised of an emulsion of killed *Mycobacterium tuberculosis* in oil)[347] and that the disease could be induced in small laboratory animals.[427] Later chronic EAE was introduced, some with a relapsing-remitting course and with large demyelinative lesions that resembled those of MS (Figures 23.106 and

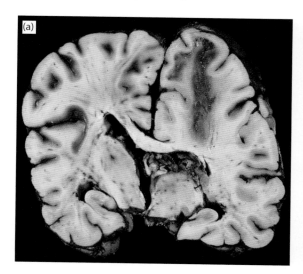

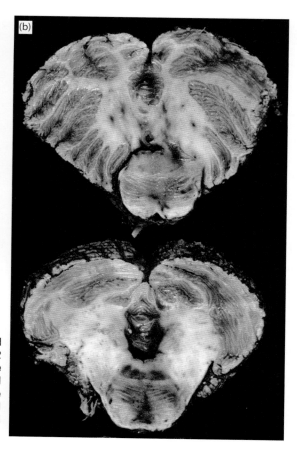

23.102 Acute haemorrhagic leukoencephalitis. 22-year-old male who developed a rapidly fatal neurological disease 2 weeks following an upper respiratory tract infection. **(a)** There are multiple scattered petechial haemorrhages, oedema and focal diffuse haemorrhage in the cerebral hemispheric white matter. The patient was on a respirator, and there is additional cortical hypoxic–ischaemic damage. **(b)** Multiple petechial haemorrhages in the cerebellar white matter and basis pontis.

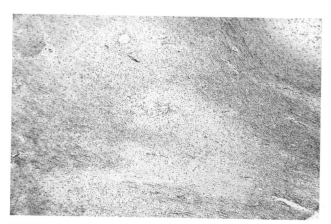

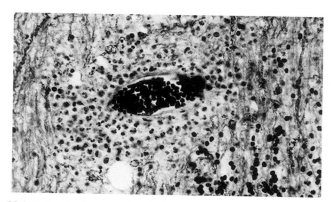

23.103 Acute haemorrhagic leukoencephalitis. Same case as shown in Figure 23.102. The subcortical white matter shows multiple foci of inflammatory demyelination, with diffuse oedema in the adjacent, more intact white matter. Klüver–Barrera.

23.104 Acute haemorrhagic leukoencephalitis. 42-year-old male with a 3-day history following pneumonia. Perivascular neutrophil infiltrates in cerebral white matter. Luxol fast blue (LFB)–Nissl.

Courtesy of Dr CJ Bruton, formerly of Runwell Hospital, Wickford, Essex, UK.

23.107).[617] The evolution of EAE models in the second half of the twentieth century paralleled the discovery and biochemical characterization of diverse myelin and other CNS tissue components and advances in understanding molecular and cellular immunology and neurobiology, particularly the mechanisms of demyelination (Figures 23.108 and 23.109). Immunization protocols progressed from the use of whole CNS tissue homogenates to purified myelin protein components for EAE induction. Following the identification of encephalitogenic epitopes, synthetic peptide immunogens and protocols involving cell transfer of antigen-specific T-cell lines and clones have been employed widely. Although T-cell-mediated autoimmunity was thought to be the basis for most forms of EAE, more recently the marmoset model with MOG as the encephalitogen appears to be antibody-mediated (Figure 23.110).

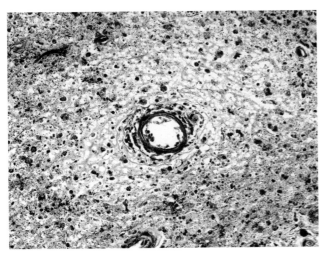

23.105 Acute haemorrhagic leukoencephalitis. Acute haemorrhagic demyelinating lesion. There is marked destruction of both myelin and axons, with prominent fibrin leakage into the parenchyma. Luxol fast blue (LFB)–Bielschowsky preparation.

As in human demyelinating diseases, susceptibility to EAE, its clinical manifestations, and its pathological and immunopathological mechanisms are heterogeneous and are influenced by genetic and epigenetic factors.[204, 206a,207,731,855] The range of clinical EAE phenotypes now includes hyperacute, acute monophasic, chronic progressive and relapsing-remitting forms; CNS lesion features generally correlate with the disease duration and clinical severity. In addition to inflammatory demyelination, axonal damage is also recognized as a feature of EAE (Figure 23.109),[617] but the progressive neurodegenerative phase of MS has not yet been addressed to any significant extent in EAE models, but some emerging models may offer some promise in this area.[402] In this regard, it would be of great interest to determine if the autoimmune process in these experimental models can induce progressive axonal degeneration.

Recently, transgenic mice have been developed with transgenes for T-cell receptors that recognize specific myelin encephalitogenic epitopes or MHC alleles that are associated with autoimmune demyelination and these animals spontaneously (i.e. without inoculation of the encephalitogen) develop EAE.[402] Transgenic mice with transgenes for cytokines and chemokines have also been developed.[670] In several T-cell receptor transgenic mouse models, there are distinct CNS lesion localization patterns that correspond to those in human disease subtypes, such as opticospinal.[402] Knockout mice have also been used in the study of autoimmune demyelination, such as the studies showing the importance of IL17 in its pathogenesis.[402] Also the utilization of 'humanized' mice, wherein the pertinent human transgene is inserted into murine DNA, will lead to further insights into the pathogenesis and immunopathogenesis of experimental demyelination and its relationship to MS.[40,612]

EAE is used extensively worldwide as a demyelinating disease model, as a paradigm for organ-specific autoimmunity and for determining efficacy of potential therapies of MS and other demyelinating diseases.[293]

Pathogen-Induced Models

Several CNS virus infections address the possible viral aetiology of MS. In these models, demyelination may be a result of oligodendrocyte infection and death, persistent infection that impairs oligodendrocyte functions, a virus-specific immune response that mediates so-called 'bystander damage' of myelin and oligodendrocytes (i.e. by elaboration of toxic molecules such as TNF and NO), or cross-reactive immunity.[609,730]

Theiler's Murine Encephalomyelitis Virus

Virulent strains of Theiler's murine encephalomyelitis virus (TMEV), a non-enveloped, single-stranded RNA picornavirus, induce lethal encephalitis following intracerebral injection into mice. Avirulent strains first cause mild, transient encephalitis due to neuronal infection, followed by a persistent infection that results in demyelination secondary to both lytic infection of oligodendrocytes and immune-mediated mechanisms.[638] Oligodendrocytes proliferate in recent lesions, and there is both remyelination and local recurrent inflammatory demyelinating activity in chronic infections (Figure 23.111).[484,522,637a]

Mouse Hepatitis Virus

The A-59 strain of mouse hepatitis virus (MHV), an enveloped single-stranded mRNA coronavirus, produces multifocal demyelination following intracranial injection into C57Bl/6 mice. Demyelination due to lytic infection of glial cells, and motor signs appear early in the infection; when the virus is cleared, there is widespread remyelination and corresponding functional recovery. The JHM strain of MHV is also toxic to oligodendrocytes and can produce a persistent and recurrent demyelinating disease.[474]

Semliki Forest Virus

Semliki forest virus (SFV) is an alphavirus of the Togavirus family. Following systemic infection, the avirulent A7 strain produces small perivascular foci of demyelination associated with the site of entry into the CNS. Focal demyelination is thought to result from activities of cytotoxic CD8+ T-cells on virus-infected oligodendrocytes and from production of antibodies that recognize myelin components.[219,504]

Canine Distemper Virus

Canine distemper virus (CDV) is an enveloped paramyxovirus closely related to human measles virus that causes immunosuppression and a demyelinating neurological disease in dogs.[821a] In the early stage, there is disseminated encephalomyelitis with demyelination that is associated with viral replication in the white matter, restricted infection of oligodendrocytes and microglial activation. A progressive or relapsing disease course associated with chronic inflammatory demyelination may be

TABLE 23.11 Selected animal models of demyelinating diseases

Type	Examples	Representative reference/review
Autoimmune	Acute and chronic EAE induced by active sensitization or adoptive transfer of T-cells sensitized for myelin and other CNS antigen epitopes	Kurschus et al.[402]
		Raine and Genain[617]
Viral	Theiler's murine encephalomyelitis virus (TMEV) infection	Rodriguez et al.[638]
	Mouse hepatitis virus (JHM) encephalomyelitis	Matthews et al.[474]
	Semliki forest virus (SFV) encephalitis	Mokhtarian et al.[504]
	Canine distemper encephalomyelitis	Vandevelde and Zurbriggen[778]
	Visna	Georgsson[254]
	Herpes simplex virus (HSV) Type I	Kastrukoff et al.[352]
	Herpes simplex virus (HSV) Type II	Georgsson et al.[255]
Genetic	Naturally occurring and inbred myelin-deficient and dysmyelinating mouse mutants: Jimpy, Twitcher, Quaking, Shiverer mice	Duncan et al.[191]
	Myelin-deficient and dysmyelinating rats	Duncan et al.[191]
	Myelin antigen-specific T-cell receptor transgenic mice that develop spontaneous EAE	Kurschus et al.[402]
	Transgenic mice with transgenes for cytokines and chemokines	Scheikl et al.[670]
	'Humanized' mice	Attfield et al.[40]
Toxic	Lysolecithin Kotter et al.[385a]	
	Ethidium bromide	Black et al.[81]
	Cuprizone	Kipp et al.[369]
	Triethyl tin	Aleu et al.[15a]
	Hexachlorophene	Lampert et al.[408a]
	6-aminonicotinamide	Schneider and Cervos-Navarro[674a]
	Hypocholesterolaemic agents	Suzuki and Zagoren[736a]
	Cyanide	Brierley et al.[103a]
Nutritional/metabolic	Electrolyte-induced demyelination	Rojiani et al.[642]
	Swayback (copper deficiency)	Innes and Shearer[335]
Physical manipulations	Spinal cord compression	Jones et al.[346,583a]
	Cerebrospinal fluid exchange	Bunge et al.[119]
	Heat injury	Sasaki and Ide[665a]
	X-irradiation in young animals	Blakemore and Patterson[82a]
	X-irradiation in adult animals	Mastaglia et al.[469a]

CNS, central nervous system; EAE, experimental autoimmune encephalomyelitis.

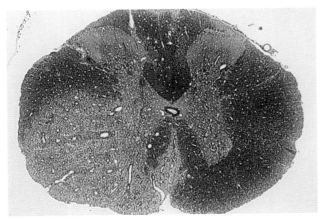

23.106 Experimental autoimmune encephalomyelitis (EAE). Large demyelinating lesion in the spinal cord of a juvenile Hartley guinea pig 7 weeks after sensitization for EAE. Toluidine blue.

Courtesy of Drs Y Maeda and R Maeda, University of Medicine and Dentistry of New Jersey, Newark, NJ, USA.

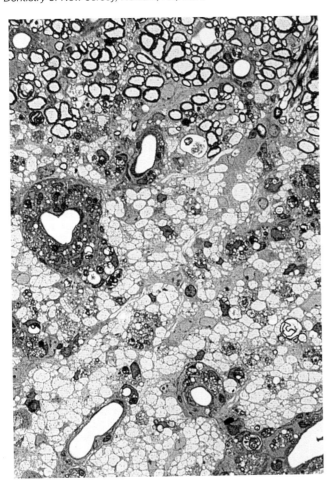

23.107 Experimental autoimmune encephalomyelitis (EAE). Large demyelinated lesion in the spinal cord of a juvenile Hartley guinea pig 10 weeks after sensitization with guinea pig central nervous system white matter for induction of EAE. Toluidine blue.

Courtesy of Drs Y Maeda and R Maeda, University of Medicine and Dentistry of New Jersey, Newark, NJ, USA.

due to interactions between macrophages and antiviral antibodies. Non-cytolytic selective spread of the virus and restricted infection may permit viral persistence and escape from immune surveillance (Figure 23.112).[778]

Visna

Visna is a naturally occurring retroviral infection of the nervous system in ruminants that can manifest demyelinative lesions,[254] thought to be due to a bystander effect of the inflammation.[609]

Herpes Simplex Virus

Herpes simplex virus (HSV) Type I inoculation into the trigeminal ganglion of mice results in demyelinative white matter lesions.[356] The virus is present in a variety of cell types in the lesions and the pathogenesis of tissue damage appears to be related to inflammation, a viral cytopathic effect and immune-mediated mechanisms.[356,609] Intracerebral or genital introduction of HSV Type II in mice leads to a necrotizing encephalitis or predominately white matter disease with viral-induced oligodendrocyte death.[255,609]

Genetic Models

Dysmyelinating animal mutants are important models for investigating the physiology and development of myelin constituents and elucidating the pathogenesis of inherited human diseases of CNS myelin. Models with counterparts in human leukodystrophies include twitcher mice and canine globoid leukodystrophy (see Chapter 6, Lysosomal Diseases). Despite having a primary genetic basis, these models provide critical insights into CNS pathophysiology that are highly relevant to human demyelinating diseases.[191] Various clinically and pathologically distinct phenotypes of spontaneous mutants, such as Jimpy and Shiverer mice and myelin-deficient rats, are due to mutations of myelin genes. These animals have been particularly useful for testing cell transfer therapies.[191] Recombinant technology has also produced transgenic mouse models that elucidate the roles of specific antibodies, cytokines and other molecular mediators of inflammatory demyelination (see also under Experimental Autoimmune [Allergic] Encephalomyelitis, p. 1387).[402]

Toxic and Other Chemical Models of Demyelination

Chemicals that are toxic to oligodendrocytes or myelin sheaths are often used to create experimental demyelination. In many cases, the precise mechanisms of the demyelination, i.e. whether due to oligodendrocyte dysfunction or death, myelin sheath injury or a combination of these mechanisms, are not clear. The chemical models are sometimes referred to as 'gliotoxin models' and are induced either by systemic delivery, such as in drinking water, or by injecting directly into the CNS white matter or another site. Because the induced injury is generally limited to either a fixed time period or a single injection, it is monophasic and the resulting demyelination is frequently followed by remyelination.

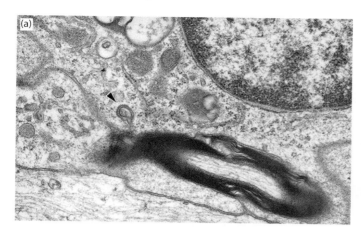
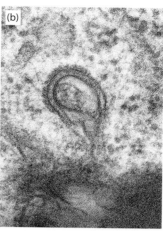

23.108 Experimental autoimmune encephalomyelitis (EAE). Rabbit 14 days after immunization with bovine central nervous system white matter. Electron micrographs. **(a)** Obliquely sectioned myelinated fibre is enveloped by a macrophage. Early demyelination involves the attachment of myelin to a coated pit on the macrophage surface (arrowhead). **(b)** Enlarged view of the area indicated by the arrowhead in **(a)**.

Reproduced from Epstein LG, Prineas JW, Raine CS. Attachment of myelin to coated pits on macrophages in experimental allergic encephalomyelitis. J Neurol Sci 1983;61:341–8.[206a] With permission from Elsevier.

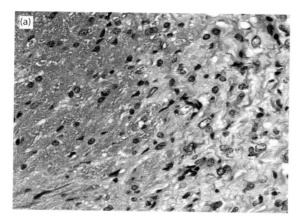
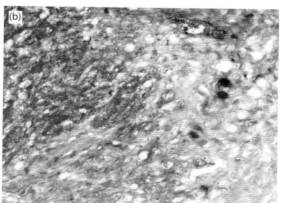
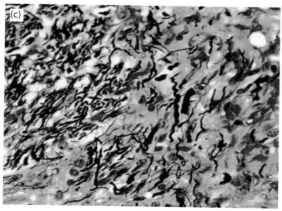

23.109 Experimental autoimmune encephalomyelitis (EAE). Border of chronic EAE lesion (right side of fields), with intact white matter in the brain of a C57Bl/6 mouse 3 months after immunization with an encephalitogenic peptide of myelin oligodendrocyte glycoprotein. At this late stage, the lesion shows scant inflammation but there is marked demyelination **(a,b)**. Axonal injury and depletion are evident in **(c)**. (a) Haematoxylin and eosin; (b) Luxol fast blue (LFB)–periodic acid-Schiff (PAS); (c) Bielschowsky.

Systemically Administered Agents

The most widely used systemic chemical model involves feeding mice with a diet containing cuprizone, a copper-chelating agent that causes demyelination in particular brain regions in mice. This lesion has been used widely in remyelination studies[444] and as a means of studying demyelination and remyelination in transgenic and knock-out mice.[369,728] Other, less frequently used models involve the systemic administration of triethyl tin,[15a] 6-aminonicotinamide,[674a] hexachlorophene,[408a] cyanide,[103a] and hypocholesterolaemic drugs in young animals[736a] (see Table 23.11).[609]

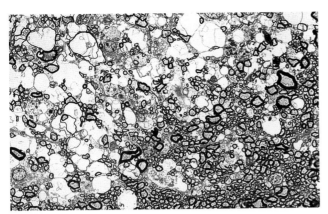

23.110 Experimental autoimmune encephalomyelitis (EAE). Evolving spinal cord lesion in a marmoset with myelin oligodendrocyte glycoprotein (MOG)-induced EAE. Intramyelinic oedema is the dominant pathological alteration in this animal examined 28 days after sensitization. Toluidine blue.

Courtesy of Dr CS Raine, Albert Einstein College of Medicine, Bronx, NY, USA.

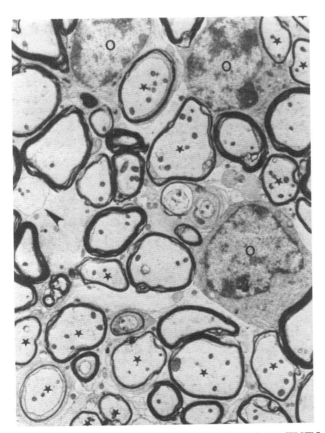

23.111 Theiler's murine encephalomyelitis virus (TMEV). Remyelination by oligodendrocytes (O) is seen in the spinal cord of a SJL/J mouse infected with the DA strain of TMEV and treated with serum from a mouse hyperimmunized with spinal cord homogenate. The remyelination is characterized by myelin sheaths that are inappropriately thin for the diameter of the axons they ensheath (stars). A demyelinated axon is present (arrowhead).

Reproduced with permission from Rodriguez.[637a] Copyright © 2006, John Wiley and Sons.

Focally Administered Agents

Two frequently used chemicals that induce demyelination following local administration into the CNS are lysolecithin[385a] and ethidium bromide.[81] Lysolecithin (Figure 23.113) is a phospholipid that acts by solubilizing myelin membranes via a general detergent effect. Ethidium bromide is a DNA-intercalating agent that prevents DNA replication and disrupts RNA and thus protein synthesis, leading to cell death. A particular advantage of these models is that there is precise control over anatomical localization of the lesion, and it is thus easily sampled or manipulated by, for example, cell transplantation.[81] Other chemicals that have been used to induce demyelination by direct injection are 6-aminonicotinamide, diphtheria toxin, calcium ionophores, and zymosan.[590] Focal areas of demyelination can also be created by direct injection of antibodies against myelin components or antibody-producing cells.[651]

Nutritional/Metabolic Models

Demyelination has been produced by an electrolyte disturbance resulting from hypertonic saline.[642] Although this is a primary demyelinating disorder, its mechanism of induction is particularly pertinent to central pontine myelinolysis (see Chapter 9, Nutritional and Toxic Diseases).

Copper deficiency has been associated with a demyelinating disease in animals referred to as 'swayback'.[335]

Physical Injury

Central nervous system myelin fibres are particularly susceptible to physical injury, a property that has been exploited in several experimental models of demyelination. A technique of historical importance, although used rarely now, is that of CSF barbotage, in which small volumes of CSF are injected forcibly on to the surface of the spinal cord. It was with this technique that the process of remyelination following superficial demyelination was first described.[119] In spinal cord injury models, acute compression or concussion of the cord induces inflammation and demyelination, which are common features of human spinal cord injury.[346,583a] Other CNS injury models, such as chronic cord compression, X-irradiation in young and adult animals,[82a,469a] and thermal injury,[665a] also result in demyelination, whereas cold probe injury tends to induce more axonal damage (see Table 23.11).[609]

Limitations of Demyelinating Disease Models and Their Relevance to Human Diseases

The scientific value of animal models of human demyelinating diseases cannot be overestimated and, indeed, they often provide impetus for analogous studies of human diseases. It should be emphasized, however, that although EAE models closely replicate most features of human ADEM, no naturally occurring animal CNS disease corresponds to MS. The nosological distinction between ADEM and acute MS is, therefore, particularly important in this context. Because of the strong

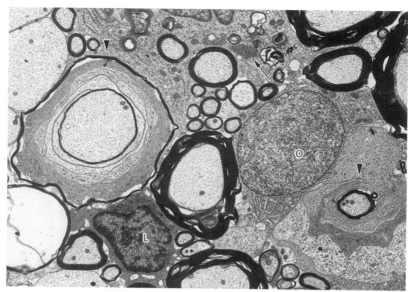

23.112 Canine distemper. 10 days after onset, nerve fibres are seen to undergo active demyelination by encircling macrophage processes (arrowheads). Distemper virus can be seen in the macrophage cytoplasm (arrow). There is a denuded axon at the upper left. Electron micrograph. L, lymphocyte; O, oligodendrocyte.

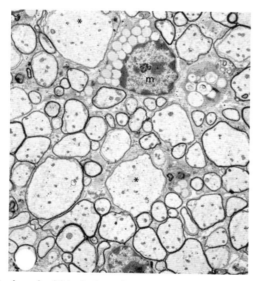

23.113 Lysolecithin-induced remyelination. The demyelination that follows lysolecithin is followed by remyelination, shown here 21 days after its injection. Macrophages (m) contain droplets of neutral lipid. Many axons (asterisks) have thin remyelinated myelin sheaths.

similarities between EAE models and ADEM, a close relationship between MS and ADEM would support the widely held view that EAE is a relevant laboratory model for MS. Morphological and other evidence, based on the existence of 'transitional' or overlapping cases with features of both MS and ADEM, and of findings in cases of rabies post-vaccinal encephalomyelitis and of 'human EAE', provide further conceptual support for a close relationship.

There are, however, numerous factors intrinsic to animal disease models that preclude their faithful recapitulation of human diseases. The models are generally induced in uniform, genetically homogeneous test groups, either by an artificial induction process (sensitization, infection) or through genetic manipulation. Therefore, they contrast dramatically with the spontaneous diseases that develop in outbred human populations. Often overlooked, furthermore, are the large disparities in lesion size between typical MS plaques and microscopic inflammatory demyelinating foci in small animal models.

In particular, EAE is by definition an autoimmune disease. The view that the human demyelinating diseases are also autoimmune diseases (with the possible exception of post-infectious and post-vaccination encephalomyelitides; see earlier under Other Central Nervous System Inflammatory Demyelinating Diseases, p. 1379) continues to rest largely on circumstantial, although strongly suggestive, evidence that implicates CNS myelin, oligodendrocytes or other antigen(s) as autoimmune targets in MS. Thus, despite multiple common pathological features and pathogenetic mechanisms, the relationships of human diseases (particularly MS) to EAE (and to other currently used models) remain approximate. As a further precaution, the therapies that may be successful in treatment trials in animal models may not be beneficial and can be harmful in MS. Table 23.12 compares features of MS and major types of animal demyelinating disease models currently employed.

TABLE 23.12 Features of multiple sclerosis and experimental demyelinating diseases

	MS	EAE models	Viral-induced models	Chemical/toxic models	Genetic models (spontaneous and induced)
Inflammation	Yes	Yes	Yes	Not usually	Variable
Demyelination	Yes	Yes	Yes	Yes	Yes
Acute axonal injury	Yes	Yes	Yes	Variable	Often
Chronic neurodegeneration	Yes	Yes	Yes	Usually minimal	Often
Known aetiology or pathogenetic agent	No	Yes	Yes	Yes	Yes
Autoimmune mechanisms	Presumed but unproven	Yes	Some	No	Variable
Peripheral nervous system involvement	Variable	Variable	Variable	Variable	Variable

EAE, experimental autoimmune encephalomyelitis; MS, multiple sclerosis.

ACKNOWLEDGEMENTS

The authors wish to record their gratitude to Professor John W Prineas for permission to reprint many of his illustrations in this chapter, and to Dr Raymond A Sobel for his contributions to portions of the text that have been retained from the previous edition. Dr Moore's research is supported by grants from the Multiple Sclerosis Society of Canada.

REFERENCES

1. Abbott NJ, Ronnback L, Hansson E. Astrocyte–endothelial interactions at the blood–brain barrier. *Nat Rev Neurosci* 2006;7:41–53.
2. Abhinav K, Love S, Kalantzis G, et al. Clinicopathological review of patients with and without multiple sclerosis treated by partial sensory rhizotomy for medically refractory trigeminal neuralgia: a 12-year retrospective study. *Clin Neurol Neurosurg* 2012;114:361–5.
3. Aboul-Enein F, Lassmann H. Mitochondrial damage and histotoxic hypoxia: a pathway of tissue injury in inflammatory brain disease? *Acta Neuropathol (Berl)* 2005;109:49–55.
4. Aboul-Enein F, Rauschka H, Kornek B, et al. Preferential loss of myelin-associated glycoprotein reflects hypoxia-like white matter damage in stroke and inflammatory brain diseases. *J Neuropathol Exp Neurol* 2003;62:25–33.
5. Aboul-Enein F, Bauer J, Klein M, et al. Selective and antigen-dependent effects of myelin degeneration on central nervous system inflammation. *J Neuropathol Exp Neurol* 2004;63:1284–96.
6. Absinta M, Rocca MA, Colombo B, et al. Patients with migraine do not have MRI-visible cortical lesions. *J Neurol* 2012;259:2695–8.
7. Adams CW. Pathology of multiple sclerosis: progression of the lesion. *Br Med Bull* 1977;33:15–20.
8. Adams CW, Abdulla YH, Torres EM, Poston RN. Periventricular lesions in multiple sclerosis: their perivenous origin and relationship to granular ependymitis.

Neuropathol Appl Neurobiol 1987;13:141–52.
9. Adams RD. A comparison of the morphology of the human demyelinating diseases and experimental 'allergic' encephalomyelitis. In: Kies MW, Alvord EC Jr eds. *Allergic encephalomyelitis.* Springfield, IL: Charles C Thomas, 1959:183–209.
10. Adams RD, Kubik CS. The morbid anatomy of the demyelinative disease. *Am J Med* 1952;12:510–46.
11. Adams RD, Cammermeyer J, Denny-Brown D. Acute necrotizing hemorrhagic encephalopathy. *J Neuropathol Exp Neurol* 1949;8:1–29.
12. Afifi AK, Follett KA, Greenlee J, et al. Optic neuritis: a novel presentation of Schilder's disease. *J Child Neurol* 2001;16:693–6.
13. Ahmad O, Reddel S, Lueck CJ. Midbrain cleft as a cause of chronic internuclear ophthalmoplegia, progressive ataxia, and facial weakness. *J Neuroophthalmol* 2010;30:145–9.
14. Ahmed Z, Gveric D, Pryce G, et al. Myelin/axonal pathology in interleukin-12 induced serial relapses of experimental allergic encephalomyelitis in the Lewis rat. *Am J Pathol* 2001;158:2127–38.
15. Albert M, Antel J, Bruck W, Stadelmann C. Extensive cortical remyelination in patients with chronic multiple sclerosis. *Brain Pathol* 2007;17:129–38.
15a. Aleu FP, Katzman R, Terry RD. Fine structure and electrolyte analyses of cerebral edema induced by alkyl tin intoxication. *J Neuropathol Exp Neurol* 1963;22:403–13.

16. Al-Hasani OH, Smith C. Traumatic white matter injury and toxic leukoencephalopathies. *Expert Rev Neurother* 2011;11:1315–24.
17. Allen IV. Demyelinating diseases. In: Adams JH, Corsellis JAN, Duchen LW eds. *Greenfield's neuropathology.* New York: John Wiley & Sons, 1984:338–84.
18. Allen IV, McQuaid S, Mirakhur M, Nevin G. Pathological abnormalities in the normal-appearing white matter in multiple sclerosis. *Neurol Sci* 2001;22:141–4.
19. Almeras L, Lefranc D, Drobecq H, et al. New antigenic candidates in multiple sclerosis: identification by serological proteome analysis. *Proteomics* 2004;4:2184–94.
20. Almsaddi M, Bertorini TE, Seltzer WK. Demyelinating neuropathy in a patient with multiple sclerosis and genotypical HMSN-1. *Neuromuscul Disord* 1998;8:87–9.
21. Alper G, Heyman R, Wang L. Multiple sclerosis and acute disseminated encephalomyelitis diagnosed in children after long-term follow-up: comparison of presenting features. *Dev Med Child Neurol* 2009;51:480–6.
22. Alter A, Duddy M, Hebert S, et al. Determinants of human B cell migration across brain endothelial cells. *J Immunol* 2003;170:4497–505.
23. Althaus HH. Remyelination in multiple sclerosis: a new role for neurotrophins? *Prog Brain Res* 2004;146:415–32.
24. Alvarez JI, Cayrol R, Prat A. Disruption of central nervous system barriers in multiple sclerosis. *Biochim Biophys Acta* 2011;1812:252–64.

25. Alvord EC Jr. Disseminated encephalomyelitis: its variations in form and their relationships to other diseases of the nervous system. In: Vinken PJ, Bruyn GW, Klawans HL eds. *Handbook of clinical neurology, Vol 47. Demyelinating diseases.* Amsterdam: Elsevier, 1985:467–502.

26. Amato MP, Portaccio E, Goretti B, *et al.* Cognitive impairment in early stages of multiple sclerosis. *Neurol Sci* 2010;**31**(Suppl 2):S211–14.

27. Ambrosini E, Remoli ME, Giacomini E, *et al.* Astrocytes produce dendritic cell-attracting chemokines in vitro and in multiple sclerosis lesions. *J Neuropathol Exp Neurol* 2005;**64**:706–15.

28. Amiry-Moghaddam M, Ottersen OP. The molecular basis of water transport in the brain. *Nat Rev Neurosci* 2003;**4**:991–1001.

29. Anderson JM, Hampton DW, Patani R, *et al.* Abnormally phosphorylated tau is associated with neuronal and axonal loss in experimental autoimmune encephalomyelitis and multiple sclerosis. *Brain* 2008;**131**(Part 7):1736–48.

30. Anderson JM, Patani R, Reynolds R, *et al.* Evidence for abnormal tau phosphorylation in early aggressive multiple sclerosis. *Acta Neuropathol* 2009;**117**:583–9.

31. Anderson JM, Patani R, Reynolds R, *et al.* Abnormal tau phosphorylation in primary progressive multiple sclerosis. *Acta Neuropathol* 2010;**119**:591–600.

32. Andreadou E, Papadimas G, Sfagos C. A novel heterozygous mutation in the NOTCH3 gene causing CADASIL. *Swiss Med Wkly* 2008;**138**:614–17.

33. Annesley-Williams D, Farrell MA, Staunton H, Brett FM. Acute demyelination, neuropathological diagnosis, and clinical evolution. *J Neuropathol Exp Neurol* 2000;**59**:477–89.

34. Antel J. New directions in multiple sclerosis therapy: matching therapy with pathogenesis. *Can J Neurol Sci* 2010;**37**(Suppl 2):42–8.

35. Antony JM, Deslauriers AM, Bhat RK, *et al.* Human endogenous retroviruses and multiple sclerosis: innocent bystanders or disease determinants? *Biochim Biophys Acta* 2011;**1812**:162–76.

36. Aoki-Yoshino K, Uchihara T, Duyckaerts C, *et al.* Enhanced expression of aquaporin 4 in human brain with inflammatory diseases. *Acta Neuropathol (Berl)* 2005;**110**:281–8.

37. Arnold AC, Pepose JS, Hepler RS, Foos RY. Retinal periphlebitis and retinitis in multiple sclerosis: I. Pathologic characteristics. *Ophthalmology* 1984;**91**:255–62.

38. Arnold DL, Matthews PM, Francis GS, *et al.* Proton magnetic resonance spectroscopic imaging for metabolic characterization of demyelinating plaques. *Ann Neurol* 1992;**31**:235–41.

39. Ashjazadeh N, Borhani Haghighi A, Samangooie Sh, Moosavi H. Neuro-Behcet's disease: a masquerader of multiple sclerosis. A prospective study of neurologic manifestations of Behcet's disease in 96 Iranian patients. *Exp Mol Pathol* 2003;**74**:17–22.

40. Attfield KE, Dendrou CA, Fugger L. Bridging the gap from genetic association to functional understanding: the next generation of mouse models of multiple sclerosis. *Immunol Rev* 2012;**248**:10–22.

41. Audoin B, Zaaraoui W, Reuter F, *et al.* Atrophy mainly affects the limbic system and the deep grey matter at the first stage of multiple sclerosis. *J Neurol Neurosurg Psychiatry* 2010;**81**:690–5.

42. Awad AM, Marder E, Milo R, Stuve O. Multiple sclerosis and chronic cerebrospinal venous insufficiency: a critical review. *Ther Adv Neurol Disord* 2011;**4**:231–5.

43. Bacigaluppi S, Polonara G, Zavanone ML, *et al.* Schilder's disease: non-invasive diagnosis? A case report and review. *Neurol Sci* 2009;**33**:421–30.

44. Back SA, Tuohy TM, Chen H, *et al.* Hyaluronan accumulates in demyelinated lesions and inhibits oligodendrocyte progenitor maturation. *Nat Med* 2005;**11**:966–72.

45. Badar F, Azfar SF, Ahmad I, *et al.* Balo's concentric sclerosis involving bilateral thalami. *Neurol India* 2011;**59**:597–600.

46. Bakiri Y, Burzomato V, Frugier G, *et al.* Glutamatergic signaling in the brain's white matter. *Neuroscience* 2009;**158**:266–74.

47. Bakshi R, Benedict RH, Bermel RA, *et al.* T2 hypointensity in the deep gray matter of patients with multiple sclerosis: a quantitative magnetic resonance imaging study. *Arch Neurol* 2002;**59**:62–8.

48. Balashov KE, Rottman JB, Weiner HL, Hancock WW. CCR5(+) and CXCR3(+) T cells are increased in multiple sclerosis and their ligands MIP-1alpha and IP-10 are expressed in demyelinating brain lesions. *Proc Natl Acad Sci U S A* 1999;**96**:6873–8.

49. Baló J. Encephalitis periaxialis concentrica. *Arch Neurol Psychiatry* 1928;**19**:242–64.

50. Banati RB, Newcombe J, Gunn RN, *et al.* The peripheral benzodiazepine binding site in the brain in multiple sclerosis: quantitative in vivo imaging of microglia as a measure of disease activity. *Brain* 2000;**123**(Part 11):2321–37.

51. Baracchini C, Valdueza JM, Del Sette M, *et al.* CCSVI and MS: a statement from the European Society of Neurosonology and Cerebral Hemodynamics. *J Neurol* 2012;**259**:2585–9.

52. Barizzone N, Pauwels I, Luciano B, *et al.* No evidence for a role of rare CYP27B1 functional variations in multiple sclerosis. *Ann Neurol* 2013;**73**:433–7.

53. Barnes D, Munro PM, Youl BD, *et al.* The longstanding MS lesion. A quantitative MRI and electron microscopic study. *Brain* 1991;**114**(pt 3):1271–80.

54. Barnett MH, Prineas JW. Relapsing and remitting multiple sclerosis: pathology of the newly forming lesion. *Ann Neurol* 2004;**55**:458–68.

55. Barnett MH, Parratt JD, Cho ES, Prineas JW. Immunoglobulins and complement in postmortem multiple sclerosis tissue. *Ann Neurol* 2009;**65**:32–46.

56. Barnum SR. Complement in central nervous system inflammation. *Immunol Res* 2002;**26**:7–13.

57. Bar-Or A. Immunology of multiple sclerosis. *Neurol Clin* 2005;**23**:149–75.

58. Barreto AD. Time to reevaluate the role of venous hemodynamics in MS pathophysiology? Controversy mounts. *Neurology* 2011;**77**:1218–19.

59. Barreto AD, Brod SA, Bui TT, *et al.* Chronic cerebrospinal venous insufficiency: case-control neurosonography results. *Ann Neurol* 2013;**73**:721–8.

60. Bartholomaus I, Kawakami N, Odoardi F, *et al.* Effector T cell interactions with meningeal vascular structures in nascent autoimmune CNS lesions. *Nature* 2009;**462**:94–8.

61. Bashir K, Whitaker JN. Importance of paraclinical and CSF studies in the diagnosis of MS in patients presenting with partial cervical transverse myelopathy and negative cranial MRI. *Mult Scler* 2000;**6**:312–16.

62. Bauer J, Stadelmann C, Bancher C, *et al.* Apoptosis of T lymphocytes in acute disseminated encephalomyelitis. *Acta Neuropathol (Berl)* 1999;**97**:543–6.

63. Beard W, Foster DB, Kepes JJ, Guillan RA. Xanthomatosis of the central nervous system. Clinical and pathological observations of a case with a posterior fossa syndrome. *Neurology* 1970;**20**:305–14.

64. Beeravolu LR, Frohman EM, Frohman TC, *et al.* Pearls & Oysters: 'Not multiple sclerosis' and the changing face of HTLV-1: a case report of downbeat nystagmus. *Neurology* 2009;**72**:e119–20.

65. Benarroch EE. Neuron–astrocyte interactions: partnership for normal function and disease in the central nervous system. *Mayo Clin Proc* 2005;**80**:1326–38.

66. Benedict RH, Bakshi R, Simon JH, *et al.* Frontal cortex atrophy predicts cognitive impairment in multiple sclerosis. *J Neuropsychiatry Clin Neurosci* 2002;**14**:44–51.

67. Benjelloun N, Charriaut-Marlangue C, Hantaz-Ambroise D, *et al.* Induction of cell death in rat brain by a gliotoxic factor from cerebrospinal fluid in multiple sclerosis. *Cell Mol Biol (Noisy-le-grand)* 2002;**48**:205–12.

68. Benson MD, Romero MI, Lush ME, et al. Ephrin-B3 is a myelin-based inhibitor of neurite outgrowth. *Proc Natl Acad Sci U S A* 2005;**102**:10694–9.

69. Benveniste EN. Cytokine actions in the central nervous system. *Cytokine Growth Factor Rev* 1998;**9**:259–75.

70. Benveniste EN, Nguyen VT, Wesemann DR. Molecular regulation of CD40 gene expression in macrophages and microglia. *Brain Behav Immun* 2004;**18**:7–12.

71. Berg D, Supprian T, Thomae J, *et al.* Lesion pattern in patients with multiple sclerosis and depression. *Mult Scler* 2000;**6**:156–62.

72. Berger JR, Fee DB, Nelson P, Nuovo G. Coxsackie B meningoencephalitis in a patient with acquired immunodeficiency syndrome and a multiple sclerosis-like illness. *J Neurovirol* 2009;**15**:282–7.

73. Bergers E, Bot JC, De Groot CJ, *et al.* Axonal damage in the spinal cord of MS patients occurs largely independent of T2 MRI lesions. *Neurology* 2002;**59**:1766–71.

74. Bergers E, Bot JC, van der Valk P, *et al.* Diffuse signal abnormalities in the spinal cord in multiple sclerosis: direct postmortem in situ magnetic resonance imaging correlated with in vitro high-resolution magnetic resonance imaging

and histopathology. *Ann Neurol* 2002;51:652–6.

75. Bitsch A, Bruhn H, Vougioukas V, *et al.* Inflammatory CNS demyelination: histopathologic correlation with in vivo quantitative proton MR spectroscopy. *AJNR Am J Neuroradiol* 1999;20: 1619–27.

76. Bitsch A, Kuhlmann T, Da Costa C, *et al.* Tumour necrosis factor alpha mRNA expression in early multiple sclerosis lesions: correlation with demyelinating activity and oligodendrocyte pathology. *Glia* 2000;29:366–75.

77. Bitsch A, Schuchardt J, Bunkowski S, *et al.* Acute axonal injury in multiple sclerosis. Correlation with demyelination and inflammation. *Brain* 2000;123(Part 6): 1174–83.

78. Bitsch A, Kuhlmann T, Stadelmann C, *et al.* A longitudinal MRI study of histopathologically defined hypointense multiple sclerosis lesions. *Ann Neurol* 2001;49:793–6.

79. Bjartmar C, Battistuta J, Terada N, *et al.* N-acetylaspartate is an axon-specific marker of mature white matter in vivo: a biochemical and immunohistochemical study on the rat optic nerve. *Ann Neurol* 2002;51:51–8.

80. Black JA, Dib-Hajj S, Baker D, *et al.* Sensory neuron-specific sodium channel SNS is abnormally expressed in the brains of mice with experimental allergic encephalomyelitis and humans with multiple sclerosis. *Proc Natl Acad Sci U S A* 2000;97:11598–602.

81. Black JA, Waxman SG, Smith KJ. Remyelination of dorsal column axons by endogenous Schwann cells restores the normal pattern of Nav1.6 and Kv1.2 at nodes of Ranvier. *Brain* 2006;129 (Part 5):1319–29.

82. Black JA, Newcombe J, Trapp BD, Waxman SG. Sodium channel expression within chronic multiple sclerosis plaques. *J Neuropathol Exp Neurol* 2007;66: 828–37.

82a. Blakemore WF, Patterson RC. Observations on the interaction of Schwann cells and astrocytes following X-irradiation of neonatal rat spinal cord. *J Neurocytol* 1975;4:573–85.

83. Bö L, Mörk S, Kong PA, *et al.* Detection of MHC class II-antigens on macrophages and microglia, but not on astrocytes and endothelia in active multiple sclerosis lesions. *J Neuroimmunol* 1994;51:135–46.

84. Bö L, Peterson JW, Mörk S, *et al.* Distribution of immunoglobulin superfamily members ICAM-1, -2, -3, and the beta 2 integrin LFA-1 in multiple sclerosis lesions. *J Neuropathol Exp Neurol* 1996;55:1060–72.

85. Bö L, Vedeler CA, Nyland H, *et al.* Intracortical multiple sclerosis lesions are not associated with increased lymphocyte infiltration. *Mult Scler* 2003;9: 323–31.

86. Bö L, Vedeler CA, Nyland HI, *et al.* Subpial demyelination in the cerebral cortex of multiple sclerosis patients. *J Neuropathol Exp Neurol* 2003;62: 723–32.

87. Bö L, Geurts JJ, Ravid R, Barkhof F. Magnetic resonance imaging as a tool to examine the neuropathology of multiple sclerosis. *Neuropathol Appl Neurobiol* 2004;30:106–17.

88. Bö L, Geurts JJ, Mörk SJ, van der Valk P. Grey matter pathology in multiple sclerosis. *Acta Neurol Scand Suppl* 2006;183:48–50.

89. Bo L, Geurts JJ, van der Valk P, *et al.* Lack of correlation between cortical demyelination and white matter pathologic changes in multiple sclerosis. *Arch Neurol* 2007;64:76–80.

90. Bodini B, Battaglini M, De Stefano N, *et al.* T2 lesion location really matters: a 10 year follow-up study in primary progressive multiple sclerosis. *J Neurol Neurosurg Psychiatry* 2011;82:72–7.

91. Boentert M, Kraus J, Kloska S, *et al.* Obliterating intracranial vasculopathy mimicking multiple sclerosis. *Acta Neurol Scand* 2009;120:68–71.

92. Boppana S, Huang H, Ito K, Dhib-Jalbut S. Immunologic aspects of multiple sclerosis. *Mt Sinai J Med* 2011;78:207–20.

93. Borchers AT, Gershwin ME. Transverse myelitis. *Autoimmun Rev* 2012;11: 231–48.

94. Borsellino G, Koul O, Placido R, *et al.* Evidence for a role of gamma delta T cells in demyelinating diseases as determined by activation states and responses to lipid antigens. *J Neuroimmunol* 2000;107:124–9.

95. Boster A, Hreha S, Berger JR, *et al.* Progressive multifocal leukoencephalopathy and relapsing-remitting multiple sclerosis: a comparative study. *Arch Neurol* 2009;66:593–9.

96. Bot JC, Barkhof F, Lycklama à Nijeholt G. *et al.* Differentiation of multiple sclerosis from other inflammatory disorders and cerebrovascular disease: value of spinal MR imaging. *Radiology* 2002;223:46–56.

97. Boven LA, Van Meurs M, Van Zwam M, *et al.* Myelin-laden macrophages are anti-inflammatory, consistent with foam cells in multiple sclerosis. *Brain* 2006;129 (Part 2):517–26.

98. Brand-Schieber E, Werner P, Iacobas DA, *et al.* Connexin43, the major gap junction protein of astrocytes, is down-regulated in inflamed white matter in an animal model of multiple sclerosis. *J Neurosci Res* 2005;80:798–808.

99. Brecher K, Hochberg FH, Louis DN, *et al.* Case report of unusual leukoencephalopathy preceding primary CNS lymphoma. *J Neurol Neurosurg Psychiatry* 1998;65:917–20.

100. Breij EC, Brink BP, Veerhuis R, *et al.* Homogeneity of active demyelinating lesions in established multiple sclerosis. *Ann Neurol* 2008;63:16–25.

101. Brennan KM, Galban-Horcajo F, Rinaldi S, *et al.* Lipid arrays identify myelin-derived lipids and lipid complexes as prominent targets for oligoclonal band antibodies in multiple sclerosis. *J Neuroimmunol* 2011;238:87–95.

102. Brex PA, Parker GJ, Leary SM, *et al.* Lesion heterogeneity in multiple sclerosis: a study of the relations between appearances on T1 weighted images, T1 relaxation times, and metabolite concentrations. *J Neurol Neurosurg Psychiatry* 2000;68:627–32.

103. Brex PA, Ciccarelli O, O'Riordan JI, *et al.* A longitudinal study of abnormalities on MRI and disability from multiple sclerosis. *N Engl J Med* 2002;346:158–64.

103a. Brierley JB, Brown AW, Calverley J. Cyanide intoxication in the rat: physiological and neuropathological aspects. *J Neurol Neurosurg Psychiatry* 1976;39:129–40.

104. Brinar VV. The differential diagnosis of multiple sclerosis. *Clin Neurol Neurosurg* 2002;104:211–20.

105. Brinar VV, Habek M. Rare infections mimicking MS. *Clin Neurol Neurosurg* 2010;112:625–8.

106. Brinar VV, Cikes N, Petelin Z, *et al.* Cerebral demyelination in Wegener's granulomatosis. *Clin Neurol Neurosurg* 2004;106:233–6.

107. Brink BP, Veerhuis R, Breij EC, *et al.* The pathology of multiple sclerosis is location-dependent: no significant complement activation is detected in purely cortical lesions. *J Neuropathol Exp Neurol* 2005;64:147–55.

108. Brinkmeier H, Aulkemeyer P, Wollinsky KH, Rudel R. An endogenous pentapeptide acting as a sodium channel blocker in inflammatory autoimmune disorders of the central nervous system. *Nat Med* 2000;6:808–11.

109. Brosnan CF, Raine CS. Mechanisms of immune injury in multiple sclerosis. *Brain Pathol* 1996;6:243–57.

110. Brown WJ. The capillaries in acute and subacute multiple sclerosis plaques: a morphometric analysis. *Neurology* 1978;28 (9 Pt 2):84–92.

111. Brownell B, Hughes JT. The distribution of plaques in the cerebrum in multiple sclerosis. *J Neurol Neurosurg Psychiatry* 1962;25:315–20.

112. Brück W, Schmied M, Suchanek G, *et al.* Oligodendrocytes in the early course of multiple sclerosis. *Ann Neurol* 1994;35:65–73.

113. Brück W, Sommermeier N, Bergmann M, *et al.* Macrophages in multiple sclerosis. *Immunobiology* 1996;195:588–600.

113a. Brück W, Porada P, Poser S, *et al.* Monocyte/macrophage differentiation in early multiple sclerosis lesions. *Ann Neurol* 1995;38:788–96.

114. Brück W, Bitsch A, Kolenda H, *et al.* Inflammatory central nervous system demyelination: correlation of magnetic resonance imaging findings with lesion pathology. *Ann Neurol* 1997;42:783–93.

115. Brück W, Neubert K, Berger T, Weber JR. Clinical, radiological, immunological and pathological findings in inflammatory CNS demyelination – possible markers for an antibody-mediated process. *Mult Scler* 2001;7:173–7.

116. Brück W, Lucchinetti C, Lassmann H. The pathology of primary progressive multiple sclerosis. *Mult Scler* 2002;8:93–7.

117. Brunn A, Nacimiento W, Sellhaus B, *et al.* Acute onset of hemorrhagic leukoencephalomyelitis (Hurst) in the spinal cord. *Clin Neuropathol* 2002;21:214–19.

118. Bsibsi M, Ravid R, Gveric D, van Noort JM. Broad expression of Toll-like receptors in the human central nervous system. *J Neuropathol Exp Neurol* 2002;61:1013–21.

119. Bunge MB, Bunge RP, Ris H. Ultrastructural study of remyelination in an experimental lesion in adult cat spinal cord. *J Biophys Biochem Cytol* 1961;10:67–94.

120. Buntinx M, Stinissen P, Steels P, *et al.* Immune-mediated oligodendrocyte

injury in multiple sclerosis: molecular mechanisms and therapeutic interventions. *Crit Rev Immunol* 2002;**22**:391–424.

121. Burgoon MP, Gilden DH, Owens GP. B cells in multiple sclerosis. *Front Biosci* 2004;**9**:786–96.

122. Burton JM, Alikhani K, Goyal M, *et al.* Complications in MS patients after CCSVI procedures abroad (Calgary, AB). *Can J Neurol Sci* 2011;**38**: 741–6.

123. Butteriss DJ, Ismail A, Ellison DW, Birchall D. Use of serial proton magnetic resonance spectroscopy to differentiate low grade glioma from tumefactive plaque in a patient with multiple sclerosis. *Br J Radiol* 2003;**76**:662–5.

124. Cabre P, Signate A, Olindo S, *et al.* Role of return migration in the emergence of multiple sclerosis in the French West Indies. *Brain* 2005;**128**(Part 12): 2899–910.

125. Calabrese M, Filippi M, Rovaris M, *et al.* Evidence for relative cortical sparing in benign multiple sclerosis: a longitudinal magnetic resonance imaging study. *Mult Scler* 2009;**15**:36–41.

126. Calabrese M, Filippi M, Rovaris M, *et al.* Morphology and evolution of cortical lesions in multiple sclerosis. A longitudinal MRI study. *Neuroimage* 2008;**42**:1324–8.

127. Calabrese M, Gallo P. Magnetic resonance evidence of cortical onset of multiple sclerosis. *Mult Scler* 2009;**15**:933–41.

128. Calabrese M, Grossi P, Favaretto A, *et al.* Cortical pathology in multiple sclerosis patients with epilepsy: a 3 year longitudinal study. *J Neurol Neurosurg Psychiatry* 2012;**83**:49–54.

129. Calderon TM, Eugenin EA, Lopez L, *et al.* A role for CXCL12 (SDF-1alpha) in the pathogenesis of multiple sclerosis: regulation of CXCL12 expression in astrocytes by soluble myelin basic protein. *J Neuroimmunol* 2006;**177**: 27–39.

130. Cannella B, Raine CS. The adhesion molecule and cytokine profile of multiple sclerosis lesions. *Ann Neurol* 1995;**37**:424–35.

131. Cannella B, Gaupp S, Omari KM, Raine CS. Multiple sclerosis: death receptor expression and oligodendrocyte apoptosis in established lesions. *J Neuroimmunol* 2007;**188**:128–37.

132. Caracciolo JT, Murtagh RD, Rojiani AM, Murtagh FR. Pathognomonic MR imaging findings in Balo concentric sclerosis. *AJNR Am J Neuroradiol* 2001;**22**:292–3.

133. Carlander B, Vincent T, Le Floch A, *et al.* Hypocretinergic dysfunction in neuromyelitis optica with coma-like episodes. *J Neurol Neurosurg Psychiatry* 2005;**79**:333–4.

133a. Carswell R. *Pathological anatomy: illustrations of the elementary forms of disease.* London: Orme, Brown, Green & Longman, 1838.

134. Cartier L, Hartley O, Dubois-Dauphin M, Krause KH. Chemokine receptors in the central nervous system: role in brain inflammation and neurodegenerative diseases. *Brain Res Brain Res Rev* 2005;**48**:16–42.

135. Cawley N, Molloy A, Cassidy L, Tubridy N. Late-onset progressive visual loss in a man with unusual MRI findings: MS,

Harding's, Leber's or Leber's Plus? *Ir J Med Sci* 2010;**179**:599–601.

136. Cayrol R, Wosik K, Berard JL, *et al.* Activated leukocyte cell adhesion molecule promotes leukocyte trafficking into the central nervous system. *Nat Immunol* 2008;**9**:137–45.

137. Chabas D, Baranzini SE, Mitchell D, *et al.* The influence of the proinflammatory cytokine, osteopontin, on autoimmune demyelinating disease. *Science* 2001;**294**:1731–5.

138. Chang A, Tourtellotte WW, Rudick R, Trapp BD. Premyelinating oligodendrocytes in chronic lesions of multiple sclerosis. *N Engl J Med* 2002;**346**:165–73.

139. Chang A, Smith MC, Yin X, *et al.* Neurogenesis in the chronic lesions of multiple sclerosis. *Brain* 2008;**131** (Part 9): 2366–75.

140. Chaodong W, Zhang KN, Wu XM, *et al.* Balo's disease showing benign clinical course and co-existence with multiple sclerosis-like lesions in Chinese. *Mult Scler* 2008;**14**:418–24.

141. Charcot JM. Histologie de le sclérose en plaques. *Gazette Hôpitaux* 1868;**41**:554,557–558,566.

142. Chari DM, Crang AJ, Blakemore WF. Decline in rate of colonization of oligodendrocyte progenitor cell (OPC)-depleted tissue by adult OPCs with age. *J Neuropathol Exp Neurol* 2003;**62**: 908–16.

143. Charil A, Yousry TA, Rovaris M, *et al.* MRI and the diagnosis of multiple sclerosis: expanding the concept of 'no better explanation'. *Lancet Neurol* 2006;**5**:841–52.

144. Charles P, Reynolds R, Seilhean D, *et al.* Re-expression of PSA-NCAM by demyelinated axons: an inhibitor of remyelination in multiple sclerosis? *Brain* 2002;**125**(Part 9):1972–9.

145. Chastain EM, Miller SD. Molecular mimicry as an inducing trigger for CNS autoimmune demyelinating disease. *Immunol Rev* 2012;**245**:227–38.

146. Chebel S, Barboura I, Boughammoura-Bouatay A, *et al.* Adult-type metachromatic leukodystrophy mimicking multiple sclerosis. *Can J Neurol Sci* 2009;**36**:521–3.

147. Chen CJ. Serial proton magnetic resonance spectroscopy in lesions of Baló concentric sclerosis. *J Comput Assist Tomogr* 2001;**25**:713–18.

148. Chen CJ, Chu NS, Lu CS, Sung CY. Serial magnetic resonance imaging in patients with Baló's concentric sclerosis: natural history of lesion development. *Ann Neurol* 1999;**46**:651–6.

149. Chen SC, Chung HW, Liou M. Measurement of volumetric lesion load in multiple sclerosis: moving from normal- to dirty-appearing white matter. *AJNR Am J Neuroradiol* 2003;**24**:1929–30.

149a. Chen X, Ma X, Jiang Y, Pi R, Liu Y, Mal. The prospects for minocycline in multiple sclerosis. *J Neuroimmunol* 2011;**235**:1–8.

150. Chiba S, Yokota S, Yonekura K, *et al.* Autoantibodies against HSP70 family proteins were detected in the cerebrospinal fluid from patients with multiple sclerosis. *J Neurol Sci* 2006;**241**:39–43.

151. Chofflon M. Mechanisms of action for treatments in multiple sclerosis: does a

heterogeneous disease demand a multi-targeted therapeutic approach? *BioDrugs* 2005;**19**:299–308.

152. Cifelli A, Arridge M, Jezzard P, *et al.* Thalamic neurodegeneration in multiple sclerosis. *Ann Neurol* 2002;**52**:650–3.

152a. Ciurleo R, Bramanti P, Marino S. Role of statins in the treatment of MS. *Pharmacol Res* 2014;**87**:133-43.

153. Claudio L, Raine CS, Brosnan CF. Evidence of persistent blood–brain barrier abnormalities in chronic-progressive multiple sclerosis. *Acta Neuropathol (Berl)* 1995;**90**:228–38.

154. Codarri L, Fontana A, Becher B. Cytokine networks in multiple sclerosis: lost in translation. *Curr Opin Neurol* 2010;**23**:205–11.

155. Cohen RI. Exploring oligodendrocyte guidance: 'to boldly go where no cell has gone before'. *Cell Mol Life Sci* 2005;**62**:505–10.

156. Comabella M, Khoury SJ. Immunopathogenesis of multiple sclerosis. *Clin Immunol* 2012;**142**:2–8.

157. Coman I, Barbin G, Charles P, *et al.* Axonal signals in central nervous system myelination, demyelination and remyelination. *J Neurol Sci* 2005;**233**: 67–71.

158. Coman I, Aigrot MS, Seilhean D, *et al.* Nodal, paranodal and juxtaparanodal axonal proteins during demyelination and remyelination in multiple sclerosis. *Brain* 2006;**129**(Part 12):3186–95.

159. Compston A. The pathogenesis and basis for treatment in multiple sclerosis. *Clin Neurol Neurosurg* 2004;**106**:246–8.

160. Compston A, Confavreux C. The distribution of multiple sclerosis. In: Compston A, Confavreux C, Lassmann H, *et al.* eds. *McAlpine's multiple sclerosis.* Amsterdam: Churchill Livingstone, 2006:71–112.

161. Compston A, Wekerle H. The genetics of multiple sclerosis. In: Compston A, Confavreux C, Lassmann H, *et al.* eds. *McAlpine's multiple sclerosis.* Amsterdam: Churchill Livingstone, 2006:113–81.

162. Compston A, Lassmann H, McDonald WI. The story of multiple sclerosis. In: Compston A, Confavreux C, Lassmann H, *et al.* eds. *McAlpine's multiple sclerosis.* Amsterdam: Churchill Livingstone, 2006:3–68.

163. Confavreux C, Compston A. The natural history of multiple sclerosis. In: Compston A, Confavreux C, Lassmann H, *et al.* eds. *McAlpine's multiple sclerosis.* Amsterdam: Churchill Livingstone, 2006:183–272.

164. Connick P, Kolappan M, Patani R, *et al.* The mesenchymal stem cells in multiple sclerosis (MSCIMS) trial protocol and baseline cohort characteristics: an open-label pre-test: post-test study with blinded outcome assessments. *Trials* 2011;**12**:62.

165. Constantinescu CS, Tani M, Ransohoff RM, *et al.* Astrocytes as antigen-presenting cells: expression of IL-12/IL-23. *J Neurochem* 2005;**95**:331–40.

166. Courville CB. Studies on the pathogenesis of multiple sclerosis. IV. Post-infectious (measles) encephalitis. *Bull Los Angeles Neurol Soc* 1965;**30**:131–41.

166a. Courville CB. Concentric Sclerosis. In: Vinken PJ, Bruyn GW, eds. Handbook of Clinical Neurology, Vol 9. *Multiple sclerosis and other demyelinating diseases*. Amsterdam: North-Holland; 1970:437–51.

167. Coyle PK. Gender issues. *Neurol Clin* 2005;**23**:39–60, v–vi.

168. Craner MJ, Newcombe J, Black JA, *et al.* Molecular changes in neurons in multiple sclerosis: altered axonal expression of Na$_v$1.2 and Na$_v$1.6 sodium channels and Na$^+$/Ca2+ exchanger. *Proc Natl Acad Sci U S A* 2004;**101**:8168–73.

169. Cross AH, Waubant E. MS and the B cell controversy. *Biochim Biophys Acta* 2011;**1812**:231–8.

170. Cross AH, Manning PT, Keeling RM, *et al.* Peroxynitrite formation within the central nervous system in active multiple sclerosis. *J Neuroimmunol* 1998;**88**:45–56.

171. Currie S, Roberts AH, Urich H. The nosological position of concentric lacunar leucoencephalopathy. *J Neurol Neurosurg Psychiatry* 1970;**33**:131–7.

171a. Cruveilhier J. *Anatomie pathologique du corps humain; descriptions avec figures lithographiées et coloriees; des diverses alterations morbides dont le corps humain est susceptible.* Paris: J.B. Baillière, 40 livraisons, 1829–42.

172. Dale RC, de Sousa C, Chong WK, *et al.* Acute disseminated encephalomyelitis, multiphasic disseminated encephalomyelitis and multiple sclerosis in children. *Brain* 2000;**123**(Part 12): 2407–22.

173. da Silva CJ, da Rocha AJ, Mendes MF, *et al.* Trigeminal involvement in multiple sclerosis: magnetic resonance imaging findings with clinical correlation in a series of patients. *Mult Scler* 2005;**11**:282–5.

174. Davies S, Nicholson T, Laura M, *et al.* Spread of T lymphocyte immune responses to myelin epitopes with duration of multiple sclerosis. *J Neuropathol Exp Neurol* 2005;**64**: 371–7.

175. Dawson JW. The histology of disseminated sclerosis. *Trans R Soc Edin* 1916;**50**:517–740 (with plates). Reproduced by the Montreal Neurological Institute, Montreal, 1973.

176. De Groot CJ, Bergers E, Kamphorst W, *et al.* Post-mortem MRI-guided sampling of multiple sclerosis brain lesions: increased yield of active demyelinating and (p) reactive lesions. *Brain* 2001;**124**(Part 8): 1635–45.

177. De Keyser J, Zeinstra E, Frohman E. Are astrocytes central players in the pathophysiology of multiple sclerosis? *Arch Neurol* 2003;**60**:132–6.

178. DeLuca GC, Ebers GC, Esiri MM. Axonal loss in multiple sclerosis: a pathological survey of the corticospinal and sensory tracts. *Brain* 2004;**127**(Part 5): 1009–18.

179. De Seze J, Stojkovic T, Gauvrit JY, *et al.* Autonomic dysfunction in multiple sclerosis: cervical spinal cord atrophy correlates. *J Neurol* 2001;**248**:297–303.

180. Desmazieres A, Sol-Foulon N, Lubetzki C. Changes at the nodal and perinodal axonal domains: a basis for multiple sclerosis pathology? *Mult Scler* 2012;**18**:133–7.

181. De Stefano N, Narayanan S, Francis SJ, *et al.* Diffuse axonal and tissue injury in patients with multiple sclerosis with low cerebral lesion load and no disability. *Arch Neurol* 2002;**59**:1565–71.

182. Dévic E. Myélite subaigué compliquée de névrite optique. *Le Bulletin Medical (Paris)* 1894;**8**:1033–4.

183. DeVries E. *Postvaccinial perivenous encephalomyelitis.* Amsterdam: Elsevier, 1960.

184. DeVries GH. Cryptic axonal antigens and axonal loss in multiple sclerosis. *Neurochem Res* 2004;**29**:1999–2006.

185. Diaz-Sanchez M, Williams K, Deluca GC, Esiri MM. Protein co-expression with axonal injury in multiple sclerosis plaques. *Acta Neuropathol (Berl)* 2006;**111**:289–99.

186. Disanto G, Morahan JM, Barnett MH, *et al.* The evidence for a role of B cells in multiple sclerosis. *Neurology* 2012;**78**:823–32.

187. Di Trapani G, Carnevale A, Cioffi RP, *et al.* Multiple sclerosis associated with peripheral demyelinating neuropathy. *Clin Neuropathol* 1996;**15**:135–8.

188. Dobson R, Meier UC, Giovannoni G. More to come: humoral immune responses in MS. *J Neuroimmunol* 2011;**240-241**:13–21.

189. Dong Y, Benveniste EN. Immune function of astrocytes. *Glia* 2001;**36**:180–90.

190. Dubois-Dalcq M, Ffrench-Constant C, Franklin RJ. Enhancing central nervous system remyelination in multiple sclerosis. *Neuron* 2005;**48**:9–12.

191. Duncan ID, Kondo Y, Zhang SC. The myelin mutants as models to study myelin repair in the leukodystrophies. *Neurotherapeutics* 2011;**8**:607–24.

192. Durafour BA, Moore CS, Zammit DA, *et al.* Comparison of polarization properties of human adult microglia and blood-derived macrophages. *Glia* 2012;**60**:717–27.

193. Durrenberger PF, Webb LV, Sim MJ, *et al.* Increased HLA-E expression in white matter lesions in multiple sclerosis. *Immunology* 2012;**137**:317–25.

194. Dutta R, Trapp BD. Mechanisms of neuronal dysfunction and degeneration in multiple sclerosis. *Prog Neurobiol* 2011;**93**:1–12.

195. Dutta R, McDonough J, Yin X, *et al.* Mitochondrial dysfunction as a cause of axonal degeneration in multiple sclerosis patients. *Ann Neurol* 2006;**59**:478–89.

196. Dutta R, Chang A, Doud MK, *et al.* Demyelination causes synaptic alterations in hippocampi from multiple sclerosis patients. *Ann Neurol* 2011;**69**:445–54.

197. Dutta R, Chomyk AM, Chang A, *et al.* Hippocampal demyelination and memory dysfunction are associated with increased levels of the neuronal microRNA miR-124 and reduced AMPA receptors. *Ann Neurol* 2013;**73**:637–45.

198. Dyment DA, Herrera BM, Cader MZ, *et al.* Complex interactions among MHC haplotypes in multiple sclerosis: susceptibility and resistance. *Hum Mol Genet* 2005;**14**:2019–26.

199. Dziedzic T, Metz I, Dallenga T, *et al.* Wallerian degeneration: a major component of early axonal pathology in multiple sclerosis. *Brain Pathol* 2010;**20**:976–85.

200. Eikelenboom MJ, Petzold A, Lazeron RH, *et al.* Multiple sclerosis: neurofilament light chain antibodies are correlated to cerebral atrophy. *Neurology* 2003;**60**:219–23.

200a. Elian M, Nightingale S, Dean G. Multiple sclerosis among United Kingdom-born children of immigrants from the Indian subcontinent, Africa and the West Indies. *J Neurol Neurosurg Psychiatry* 1990;**53**:906–11.

201. Eliasdottir OJ, Olafsson E, Kjartansson O. Incidence of multiple sclerosis in Iceland, 2002-2007: a population-based study. *Mult Scler* 2011;**17**:909–13.

202. Elliott C, Lindner M, Arthur A, *et al.* Functional identification of pathogenic autoantibody responses in patients with multiple sclerosis. *Brain* 2012;**135** (Part 6):1819–33.

203. Elliott DE, Weinstock JV. Helminth-host immunological interactions: prevention and control of immune-mediated diseases. *Ann N Y Acad Sci* 2012;**1247**:83–96.

204. Encinas JA, Lees MB, Sobel RA, *et al.* Identification of genetic loci associated with paralysis, inflammation and weight loss in mouse experimental autoimmune encephalomyelitis. *Int Immunol* 2001;**13**:257–64.

205. Eng LF, Ghirnikar RS, Lee YL. Glial fibrillary acidic protein: GFAP-thirty-one years (1969–2000). *Neurochem Res* 2000;**25**:1439–51.

206. Enzinger C, Strasser–Fuchs S, Ropele S, *et al.* Tumefactive demyelinating lesions: conventional and advanced magnetic resonance imaging. *Mult Scler* 2005;**11**:135–9.

206a. Epstein LG, Prineas JW, Raine CS. Attachment of myelin to coated pits on macrophages in experimental allergic encephalomyelitis. *J Neurol Sci* 1983;**61**:341–8.

207. Ercolini AM, Miller SD. Mechanisms of immunopathology in murine models of central nervous system demyelinating disease. *J Immunol* 2006;**176**:3293–8.

208. Esiri MM. Immunoglobulin-containing cells in multiple-sclerosis plaques. *Lancet* 1977;**2**:478–480.

209. Esiri MM. MS: is it one disease? *Int MS J* 2009;**16**:39–41.

210. Esiri M, Perl D. *Oppenheimer's diagnostic neuropathology: a practical manual.* London: Hodder Arnold, 2006.

211. Evangelou N, Esiri MM, Smith S, *et al.* Quantitative pathological evidence for axonal loss in normal appearing white matter in multiple sclerosis. *Ann Neurol* 2000;**47**:391–5.

212. Evangelou N, Konz D, Esiri MM, *et al.* Regional axonal loss in the corpus callosum correlates with cerebral white matter lesion volume and distribution in multiple sclerosis. *Brain* 2000;**123** (Part 9): 1845–9.

213. Evangelou N, Konz D, Esiri MM, *et al.* Size-selective neuronal changes in the anterior optic pathways suggest a differential susceptibility to injury in multiple sclerosis. *Brain* 2001;**124** (Part 9):1813–20.

214. Fabriek BO, Van Haastert ES, Galea I, *et al.* CD163-positive perivascular macrophages in the human CNS express molecules for antigen recognition and presentation. *Glia* 2005;**51**:297–305.

215. Falcone M, Scalise A, Minisci C. *et al.* Spreading of autoimmunity from central to peripheral myelin: two cases of clinical association between multiple sclerosis and chronic inflammatory demyelinating polyneuropathy. *Neurol Sci* 2006;**27**: 58–62.

216. Fancy SP, Baranzini SE, Zhao C, *et al.* Dysregulation of the Wnt pathway

inhibits timely myelination and remyelination in the mammalian CNS. *Genes Dev* 2009;**23**:1571–85.

217. Fancy SP, Chan JR, Baranzini SE, et al. Myelin regeneration: a recapitulation of development? *Annu Rev Neurosci* 2011;**34**:21–43.

218. Farber K, Kettenmann H. Physiology of microglial cells. *Brain Res Brain Res Rev* 2005;**48**:133–43.

219. Fazakerley JK. Pathogenesis of Semliki Forest virus encephalitis. *J Neurovirol* 2002;**8**(Suppl 2):66–74.

220. Fazio R, Radaelli M, Furlan R. Neuromyelitis optica: concepts in evolution. *J Neuroimmunol* 2011;**231**:100–4.

221. Felts PA, Woolston AM, Fernando HB, et al. Inflammation and primary demyelination induced by the intraspinal injection of lipopolysaccharide. *Brain* 2005;**128**(Part 7):1649–66.

222. Ferguson B, Matyszak MK, Esiri MM, Perry VH. Axonal damage in acute multiple sclerosis lesions. *Brain* 1997;**120**(Part 3):393–9.

223. Fernando KT, McLean MA, Chard DT, et al. Elevated white matter myo-inositol in clinically isolated syndromes suggestive of multiple sclerosis. *Brain* 2004;**127** (Part 6):1361–9.

224. Ferraro a. Studies on multiple sclerosis. I. Multiple sclerosis viewed as a chronic disseminated encephalomyelitis. II. Etio-pathogenesis of multiple sclerosis (infectious allergic or toxic allergic). *J Neuropathol Exp Neurol* 1958;**17**:278–97.

225. Ferrer I, Boada Rovira M, Sanchez Guerra ML, et al. Neuropathology and pathogenesis of encephalitis following amyloid-beta immunization in Alzheimer's disease. *Brain Pathol* 2004;**14**:11–20.

226. Filipovic R, Rakic S, Zecevic N. Expression of Golli proteins in adult human brain and multiple sclerosis lesions. *J Neuroimmunol* 2002;**127**:1–12.

227. Filippi M, Rocca MA. MR imaging of Dévic's neuromyelitis optica. *Neurol Sci* 2004;**25**(Suppl 4):371–3.

228. Filippi M, Rocca MA, Martino G, et al. Magnetization transfer changes in the normal appearing white matter precede the appearance of enhancing lesions in patients with multiple sclerosis. *Ann Neurol* 1998;**43**:809–14.

229. Filippi M, Comi C, Rovaris M eds. *Normal-appearing white and grey matter damage in multiple sclerosis.* Milan: Springer, 2004.

230. Filippi M, Rocca MA, Barkhof F, et al. Multiple sclerosis and chronic cerebrospinal venous insufficiency: the neuroimaging perspective. *AJNR Am J Neuroradiol* 2011;**32**:424–7.

231. Filippi M, Riccitelli G, Mattioli F, et al. Multiple sclerosis: effects of cognitive rehabilitation on structural and functional MR imaging measures – an explorative study. *Radiology* 2012;**262**:932–40.

232. Finley KH. Discussion of the interrelationships of demyelinating diseases. In: Kies MW, Alvord EC eds. *Allergic encephalomyelitis.* Springfield, IL: Charles C Thomas, 1959:210–228.

233. Fischer MT, Sharma R, Lim JL, et al. NADPH oxidase expression in active multiple sclerosis lesions in relation to oxidative tissue damage and mitochondrial injury. *Brain* 2012;**135**(Part 3):886–99.

234. Fisher E, Chang A, Fox RJ, et al. Imaging correlates of axonal swelling in chronic multiple sclerosis brains. *Ann Neurol* 2007;**62**:219–28.

235. Fisher E, Lee JC, Nakamura K, Rudick Ra. Gray matter atrophy in multiple sclerosis: a longitudinal study. *Ann Neurol* 2008;**64**:255–65.

236. Foote AK, Blakemore WF. Inflammation stimulates remyelination in areas of chronic demyelination. *Brain* 2005;**128**(Part 3):528–39.

236a. Fox EJ, Rhoades RW. New treatments and treatment goals for patients with relapsing-remitting multiple sclerosis. *Curr Opin Neurol* 2012;**25**(suppl 1): S11–S19.

237. Franklin RJ, ffrench-Constant C. Remyelination in the CNS: from biology to therapy. *Nat Rev Neurosci* 2008;**9**:839–55.

238. Franklin RJ, Kotter MR. The biology of CNS remyelination: the key to therapeutic advances. *J Neurol* 2008;**255**(Suppl 1):19–25.

239. Freedman MS, Cohen JA. Meta-analysis of bone marrow transplantation treatment studies: mixing 'apples and oranges'. *Mult Scler* 2011;**17**:131–2.

240. Friese MA, Fugger L. Autoreactive CD8+ T cells in multiple sclerosis: a new target for therapy? *Brain* 2005;**128**(Part 8):1747–63.

241. Fritzsching B, Haas J, Konig F, et al. Intracerebral human regulatory T cells: analysis of CD4+ CD25+ FOXP3+ T cells in brain lesions and cerebrospinal fluid of multiple sclerosis patients. *PLoS One* 2011;**6**:e17988.

242. Frohman EM, Monson NL, Lovett-Racke AE, Racke MK. Autonomic regulation of neuroimmunological responses: implications for multiple sclerosis. *J Clin Immunol* 2001;**21**:61–73.

243. Frohman EM, Filippi M, Stuve O, et al. Characterizing the mechanisms of progression in multiple sclerosis: evidence and new hypotheses for future directions. *Arch Neurol* 2005;**62**:1345–56.

244. Frohman EM, Racke MK, Raine CS. Multiple sclerosis–the plaque and its pathogenesis. *N Engl J Med* 2006;**354**:942–55.

245. Frost EE, Nielsen JA, Le TQ, Armstrong RC. PDGF and FGF2 regulate oligodendrocyte progenitor responses to demyelination. *J Neurobiol* 2003;**54**:457–72.

246. Fujinami RS. Molecular mimicry that primes for autoimmunity which is triggered by infection. *Mol Psychiatry* 2002;**7**(Suppl 2):S32–3.

247. Gandhi R, Laroni A, Weiner HL. Role of the innate immune system in the pathogenesis of multiple sclerosis. *J Neuroimmunol* 2010;**221**:7–14.

248. Ganter P, Prince C, Esiri MM. Spinal cord axonal loss in multiple sclerosis: a post-mortem study. *Neuropathol Appl Neurobiol* 1999;**25**:459–67.

249. Garell PC, Menezes AH, Baumbach G, et al. Presentation, management and follow-up of Schilder's disease. *Pediatr Neurosurg* 1998;**29**:86–91.

250. Gay D, Esiri M. Blood–brain barrier damage in acute multiple sclerosis plaques. An immunocytological study. *Brain* 1991;**114**(Part 18):557–72.

251. Gay FW. Early cellular events in multiple sclerosis. Intimations of an extrinsic myelinolytic antigen. *Clin Neurol Neurosurg* 2006;**108**:234–40.

252. Gay FW, Drye TJ, Dick GW, Esiri MM. The application of multifactorial cluster analysis in the staging of plaques in early multiple sclerosis. Identification and characterization of the primary demyelinating lesion. *Brain* 1997;**120** (Part 8):1461–83.

253. Ge Y, Grossman RI, Babb JS, et al. Dirty-appearing white matter in multiple sclerosis: volumetric MR imaging and magnetization transfer ratio histogram analysis. *AJNR Am J Neuroradiol* 2003;**24**:1935–40.

254. Georgsson G. Neuropathologic aspects of lentiviral infections. *Ann N Y Acad Sci* 1994;**724**:50–67.

255. Georgsson G, Martin JR, Stoner GL, Webster HF. Virus spread and initial pathological changes in the nervous system in genital herpes simplex virus type 2 infection in mice. A correlative immunohistochemical, light and electron microscopic study. *Acta Neuropathol* 1987;**72**:377–88.

256. Geurts JJ, Wolswijk G, Bö L, et al. Altered expression patterns of group I and II metabotropic glutamate receptors in multiple sclerosis. *Brain* 2003;**126** (Part 8):1755–66.

257. Geurts JJ, Bö L, Pouwels PJ, et al. Cortical lesions in multiple sclerosis: combined postmortem MR imaging and histopathology. *AJNR Am J Neuroradiol* 2005;**26**:572–7.

258. Geurts JJ, Wolswijk G, Bö L, et al. Expression patterns of Group III metabotropic glutamate receptors mGluR4 and mGluR8 in multiple sclerosis lesions. *J Neuroimmunol* 2005;**158**:182–90.

259. Geurts JJ, Bo L, Roosendaal SD, et al. Extensive hippocampal demyelination in multiple sclerosis. *J Neuropathol Exp Neurol* 2007;**66**:819–27.

260. Ghatak NR, Hirano A, Doron Y, Zimmerman HM. Remyelination in multiple sclerosis with peripheral type myelin. *Arch Neurol* 1973;**29**:262–7.

261. Ghosh N, DeLuca GC, Esiri MM. Evidence of axonal damage in human acute demyelinating diseases. *J Neurol Sci* 2004;**222**:29–34.

262. Gibbs WN, Kreidie MA, Kim RC, Hasso AN. Acute hemorrhagic leukoencephalitis: neuroimaging features and neuropathologic diagnosis. *J Comput Assist Tomogr* 2005;**29**:689–93.

263. Gilbert JJ, Sadler M. Unsuspected multiple sclerosis. *Arch Neurol* 1983;**40**:533–6.

264. Gilmore CP, Bo L, Owens T. et al. Spinal cord gray matter demyelination in multiple sclerosis-a novel pattern of residual plaque morphology. *Brain Pathol* 2006;**16**:202–8.

265. Giordana MT, Richiardi P, Trevisan E, et al. Abnormal ubiquitination of axons in normally myelinated white matter in multiple sclerosis brain. *Neuropathol Appl Neurobiol* 2002;**28**:35–41.

266. Giorgio A, Stromillo ML, Rossi F, et al. Cortical lesions in radiologically isolated syndrome. *Neurology* 2011;**77**:1896–9.

267. Giuliani F, Goodyer CG, Antel JP, Yong VW. Vulnerability of human neurons to

T cell-mediated cytotoxicity. *J Immunol* 2003;**171**:368–79.

268. Glezer I, Lapointe A, Rivest S. Innate immunity triggers oligodendrocyte progenitor reactivity and confines damages to brain injuries. *FASEB J* 2006;**20**:750–2.

269. Gobin SJ, Montagne L, Van Zutphen M, *et al.* Upregulation of transcription factors controlling MHC expression in multiple sclerosis lesions. *Glia* 2001;**36**:68–77.

270. Goebel HH, Walther G, Meuth M. Fresh cell therapy followed by fatal coma. *J Neurol* 1986;**233**:242–7.

271. Goldschmidt T, Antel J, Konig FB, *et al.* Remyelination capacity of the MS brain decreases with disease chronicity. *Neurology* 2009;**72**:1914–21.

272. Gorczyca WA, Ejma M, Witkowska D, *et al.* Retinal antigens are recognized by antibodies present in sera of patients with multiple sclerosis. *Ophthalmic Res* 2004;**36**:120–3.

273. Gosztonyi G. Acute haemorrhagic leucoencephalitis (Hurst's disease). In: Vinken PJ, Bruyn GW, Klawans HL eds. *Handbook of clinical neurology, Vol 34. Infections of the nervous system, Part II.* Amsterdam: North-Holland, 1978:**34** 587–604.

274. Goverman J, Perchellet A, Huseby ES. The role of CD8+ T cells in multiple sclerosis and its animal models. *Curr Drug Targets Inflamm Allergy* 2005;**4**:239–45.

275. Gracien R, Kordulla M, Ziemann U. Paraneoplastic cerebellar degeneration mimicking development of secondary progressive multiple sclerosis in a patient with relapsing-remitting multiple sclerosis. *Mult Scler* 2011;**17**:498–500.

276. Graumann U, Reynolds R, Steck AJ, Schaeren-Wiemers N. Molecular changes in normal appearing white matter in multiple sclerosis are characteristic of neuroprotective mechanisms against hypoxic insult. *Brain Pathol* 2003;**13**:554–73.

277. Gray E, Thomas TL, Betmouni S, *et al.* Elevated activity and microglial expression of myeloperoxidase in demyelinated cerebral cortex in multiple sclerosis. *Brain Pathol* 2008;**18**:86–95.

278. Gray E, Thomas TL, Betmouni S, *et al.* Elevated matrix metalloproteinase-9 and degradation of perineuronal nets in cerebrocortical multiple sclerosis plaques. *J Neuropathol Exp Neurol* 2008;**67**:888–99.

279. Green AJ, McQuaid S, Hauser SL, *et al.* Ocular pathology in multiple sclerosis: retinal atrophy and inflammation irrespective of disease duration. *Brain* 2010;**133**(Part 6):1591–601.

280. Greenfield EA, Reddy J, Lees A, *et al.* Monoclonal antibodies to distinct regions of human myelin proteolipid protein simultaneously recognize central nervous system myelin and neurons of many vertebrate species. *J Neurosci Res* 2006;**83**:415–31.

281. Greenfield JG. The pathology of measles encephalomyelitis. *Brain* 1929;**52**:171–195.

282. Greer JM, Pender MP. The presence of glutamic acid at positions 71 or 74 in pocket 4 of the HLA-DRbeta1 chain is associated with the clinical course of multiple sclerosis. *J Neurol Neurosurg Psychiatry* 2005;**76**:656–62.

283. Gu J, Wang R, Lin J, Fang S. Concentric sclerosis: imaging diagnosis and clinical analysis of 3 cases. *Neurol India* 2003;**51**:528–30.

284. Guo AC, Jewells VL, Provenzale JM. Analysis of normal-appearing white matter in multiple sclerosis: comparison of diffusion tensor MR imaging and magnetization transfer imaging. *AJNR Am J Neuroradiol* 2001;**22**:1893–900.

285. Gutowski NJ, Newcombe J, Cuzner ML. Tenascin-R and C in multiple sclerosis lesions: relevance to extracellular matrix remodelling. *Neuropathol Appl Neurobiol* 1999;**25**:207–14.

286. Gveric D, Kaltschmidt C, Cuzner ML, Newcombe J. Transcription factor NF-kappaB and inhibitor I kappaB alpha are localized in macrophages in active multiple sclerosis lesions. *J Neuropathol Exp Neurol* 1998;**57**:168–78.

287. Gveric D, Cuzner ML, Newcombe J. Insulin-like growth factors and binding proteins in multiple sclerosis plaques. *Neuropathol Appl Neurobiol* 1999;**25**:215–25.

288. Gveric D, Herrera BM, Cuzner ML. tPA receptors and the fibrinolytic response in multiple sclerosis lesions. *Am J Pathol* 2005;**166**:1143–51.

289. Haacke EM, Makki M, Ge Y, *et al.* Characterizing iron deposition in multiple sclerosis lesions using susceptibility weighted imaging. *J Magn Reson Imaging* 2009;**29**:537–44.

290. Hackmack K, Weygandt M, Wuerfel J, *et al.* Can we overcome the 'clinico-radiological paradox' in multiple sclerosis? *J Neurol* 2012;**259**:2151–60.

291. Haddock G, Cross AK, Plumb J, *et al.* Expression of ADAMTS-1, -4, -5 and TIMP-3 in normal and multiple sclerosis CNS white matter. *Mult Scler* 2006;**12**:386–96.

291a. Hafler DA, Benjamin DS, Burks J, Weiner HL. Myelin basic protein and proteolipid protein reactivity of brain- and cerebrospinal fluid-derived T cell clones in multiple sclerosis and postinfectious encephalomyelitis. *J Immunol* 1987;**139**:68–72.

292. Haider L, Fischer MT, Frischer JM, *et al.* Oxidative damage in multiple sclerosis lesions. *Brain* 2011;**134**(Part 7): 1914–24.

293. Hall SW, Cooke A. Autoimmunity and inflammation: murine models and translational studies. *Mamm Genome* 2011;**7–8**:377–89.

294. Halliday AM, McDonald WI. Pathophysiology of demyelinating disease. *Br Med Bull* 1977;**33**:21–7.

295. Handunnetthi L, Ramagopalan SV, Ebers GC. Multiple sclerosis, vitamin D, and HLA-DRB1*15. *Neurology* 2010;**74**:1905–10.

296. Hart G, Ahmed I. Carotid dissection presenting as demyelinating disease on magnetic resonance imaging. *Mo Med* 2003;**100**:605–8.

297. Hart MN, Earle KM. Haemorrhagic and perivenous encephalitis: a clinical-pathological review of 38 cases. *J Neurol Neurosurg Psychiatry* 1975;**38**: 585–91.

298. Hartmann M, Rottach KG, Wohlgemuth WA, Pfadenhauer K. Trigeminal neuralgia triggered by auditory stimuli in multiple sclerosis. *Arch Neurol* 1999;**56**:731–3.

299. Hartung HP, Grossman RI. ADEM: distinct disease or part of the MS spectrum? *Neurology* 2001;**56**:1257–60.

300. Hasan KM, Halphen C, Kamali A, *et al.* Caudate nuclei volume, diffusion tensor metrics, and T(2) relaxation in healthy adults and relapsing-remitting multiple sclerosis patients: implications for understanding gray matter degeneration. *J Magn Reson Imaging* 2009;**29**:70–7.

301. Hasson J, Terry RD, Zimmerman HM. Peripheral neuropathy in multiple sclerosis. *Neurology* 1958;**8**:503–10.

302. Hauser SL, Bhan AK, Gilles F, *et al.* Immunohistochemical analysis of the cellular infiltrate in multiple sclerosis lesions. *Ann Neurol* 1986;**19**:578–87.

303. Hellings N, Gelin G, Medaer R, *et al.* Longitudinal study of antimyelin T-cell reactivity in relapsing-remitting multiple sclerosis: association with clinical and MRI activity. *J Neuroimmunol* 2002;**126**:143–60.

304. Helms G, Stawiarz L, Kivisakk P, Link H. Regression analysis of metabolite concentrations estimated from localized proton MR spectra of active and chronic multiple sclerosis lesions. *Magn Reson Med* 2000;**43**:102–10.

305. Hemmer B, Archelos JJ, Hartung HP. New concepts in the immunopathogenesis of multiple sclerosis. *Nat Rev Neurosci* 2002;**3**:291–301.

306. Hemmer B, Kieseier B, Cepok S, Hartung HP. New immunopathologic insights into multiple sclerosis. *Curr Neurol Neurosci Rep* 2003;**3**:246–55.

307. Hendriks JJ, Teunissen CE, de Vries HE, Dijkstra CD. Macrophages and neurodegeneration. *Brain Res Brain Res Rev* 2005;**48**:185–95.

308. Hengstman GJ, Kusters B. Sudden cardiac death in multiple sclerosis caused by active demyelination of the medulla oblongata. *Mult Scler* 2011;**17**:1146–8.

308a. Herndon RM, Rubinstein LJ, Freeman JM, Mathieson G. Light and electron microscopic observations on Rosenthal fibres in Alexander's disease and in multiple sclerosis. *J Neuropathol Exp Neurol* 1970;**29**:524–51.

309. Hickman SJ, Brierley CM, Brex PA, *et al.* Continuing optic nerve atrophy following optic neuritis: a serial MRI study. *Mult Scler* 2002;**8**:339–42.

310. Hill KE, Zollinger LV, Watt HE, *et al.* Inducible nitric oxide synthase in chronic active multiple sclerosis plaques: distribution, cellular expression and association with myelin damage. *J Neuroimmunol* 2004;**151**:171–9.

311. Hinson SR, McKeon A, Lennon VA. Neurological autoimmunity targeting aquaporin-4. *Neuroscience* 2010;**168**: 1009–18.

312. Hoffman HL, Norman RM. Acute necrotic myelopathy associated with perivenous encephalomyelitis. *J Neurol Neurosurg Psychiatry* 1964;**27**:116–24.

313. Hoffmann LA, Lohse P, Konig FB, *et al.* TNFRSF1A R92Q mutation in association with a multiple sclerosis-like demyelinating syndrome. *Neurology* 2008;**13**(Part 2):1155–6.

314. Höftberger R, Aboul-Enein F, Brueck W, *et al.* Expression of major histocompatibility complex class I molecules on the different cell types in multiple sclerosis lesions. *Brain Pathol* 2004;**14**:43–50.

315. Holley JE, Gveric D, Newcombe J, *et al*. Astrocyte characterization in the multiple sclerosis glial scar. *Neuropathol Appl Neurobiol* 2003;**29**:434–44.

316. Holley JE, Newcombe J, Whatmore JL, Gutowski NJ. Increased blood vessel density and endothelial cell proliferation in multiple sclerosis cerebral white matter. *Neurosci Lett* 2010;**470**:65–70.

317. Holman DW, Klein RS, Ransohoff RM. The blood-brain barrier, chemokines and multiple sclerosis. *Biochim Biophys Acta* 2011;**1812**:220–30.

318. Horakova D, Kalincik T, Blahova Dusankova J, Dolezal O. Clinical correlates of grey matter pathology in multiple sclerosis. *BMC Neurol* 2012;**12**:10.

319. Horsfield MA. MR image postprocessing for multiple sclerosis research. *Neuroimaging Clin N Am* 2008;**18**:637–49.

320. Howell OW, Palser A, Polito A, *et al*. Disruption of neurofascin localization reveals early changes preceding demyelination and remyelination in multiple sclerosis. *Brain* 2006;**129** (Part 12):3173–85.

321. Howell OW, Rundle JL, Garg A, *et al*. Activated microglia mediate axoglial disruption that contributes to axonal injury in multiple sclerosis. *J Neuropathol Exp Neurol* 2010;**69**:1017–33.

322. Howell OW, Reeves CA, Nicholas R, *et al*. Meningeal inflammation is widespread and linked to cortical pathology in multiple sclerosis. *Brain* 2011;**134**(Part 9):2755–71.

322a. Huh S-Y, *et al*. The usefulness of brain MRI at onset in the differentiation of multiple sclerosis and seropositive neuromyelitis optica spectrum disorders. *Multiple Sclerosis* 2014;**20**:695–704.

323. Huitinga I, De Groot CJ, Van der Valk P, *et al*. Hypothalamic lesions in multiple sclerosis. *J Neuropathol Exp Neurol* 2001;**60**:1208–18.

324. Huitinga I, Erkut ZA, van Beurden D, Swaab DF. Impaired hypothalamus–pituitary–adrenal axis activity and more severe multiple sclerosis with hypothalamic lesions. *Ann Neurol* 2004;**55**:37–45.

325. Hulshof S, Montagne L, De Groot CJ, Van Der Valk P. Cellular localization and expression patterns of interleukin-10, interleukin-4, and their receptors in multiple sclerosis lesions. *Glia* 2002;**38**: 24–35.

326. Hurst EW. Acute hemorrhagic leucoencephalitis: a previously undefined entity. *Med J Aust* 1941;**2**:1–6.

327. Husseini L, Saleh A, Reifenberger G, *et al*. Inflammatory demyelinating brain lesions heralding primary CNS lymphoma. *Can J Neurol Sci* 2012;**39**:6–10.

328. Husted CA, Goodin DS, Hugg JW, *et al*. Biochemical alterations in multiple sclerosis lesions and normal-appearing white matter detected by in vivo 31P and 1H spectroscopic imaging. *Ann Neurol* 1994;**36**:157–65.

329. Ifergan I, Kebir H, Terouz S, *et al*. Role of Ninjurin-1 in the migration of myeloid cells to central nervous system inflammatory lesions. *Ann Neurol* 2011;**70**:751–63.

330. Iizuka R, Jacob H, Solcher H. Multiple sclerosis plaques in rubella. *J Neurol Sci* 1972;**15**:327–38.

331. Iliev AI, Stringaris AK, Nau R, Neumann H. Neuronal injury mediated via stimulation of microglial toll-like receptor-9 (TLR9). *FASEB J* 2004;**18**:412–14.

332. Illes Z, Kondo T, Newcombe J, *et al*. Differential expression of NK T cell V alpha 24J alpha Q invariant TCR chain in the lesions of multiple sclerosis and chronic inflammatory demyelinating polyneuropathy. *J Immunol* 2000;**164**:4375–81.

333. Inglese M, Li BS, Rusinek H, *et al*. Diffusely elevated cerebral choline and creatine in relapsing-remitting multiple sclerosis. *Magn Reson Med* 2003;**50**:190–5.

334. Iniguez C, Pascual LF, Ramon y Cajal S, *et al*. Transitional multiple sclerosis (Schilder's disease): a case report. *J Neurol* 2000;**247**:974–6.

335. Innes JRM, Shearer GD. 'Swayback': a demyelinating disease of lambs with affinities to Schilder's encephalitis in man. *J Comp Pathol* 1940;**53**:1–39.

336. Itoyama Y, Sternberger NH, Webster HD, *et al*. Immunocytochemical observations on the distribution of myelin-associated glycoprotein and myelin basic protein in multiple sclerosis lesions. *Ann Neurol* 1980;**7**:167–77.

337. Itoyama Y, Ohnishi A, Tateishi J, *et al*. Spinal cord multiple sclerosis lesions in Japanese patients: Schwann cell remyelination occurs in areas that lack glial fibrillary acidic protein (GFAP). *Acta Neuropathol (Berl)* 1985;**65**: 217–23.

338. Itoyama Y, Tateishi J, Kuroiwa Y. Atypical multiple sclerosis with concentric or lamellar demyelinated lesions: two Japanese patients studied post mortem. *Ann Neurol* 1985;**17**: 481–7.

339. Jack C, Ruffini F, Bar-Or A, Antel JP. Microglia and multiple sclerosis. *J Neurosci Res* 2005;**81**:363–73.

340. Jacob S, Zarei M, Kenton A, Allroggen H. Gluten sensitivity and neuromyelitis optica: two case reports. *J Neurol Neurosurg Psychiatry* 2005;**76**: 1028–30.

341. Jarius S, Wildemann B. AQP4 antibodies in neuromyelitis optica: diagnostic and pathogenetic relevance. *Nat Rev Neurol* 2010;**6**:383–92.

342. Johanson C, Stopa E, McMillan P, *et al*. The distributional nexus of choroid plexus to cerebrospinal fluid, ependyma and brain: toxicologic/pathologic phenomena, periventricular destabilization, and lesion spread. *Toxicol Pathol* 2011;**39**:186–212.

343. John GR, Shankar SL, Shafit-Zagardo B, *et al*. Multiple sclerosis: re-expression of a developmental pathway that restricts oligodendrocyte maturation. *Nat Med* 2002;**8**:1115–21.

344. Johnson AB, Brenner M. Alexander's disease: clinical, pathologic, and genetic features. *J Child Neurol* 2003;**18**:625–32.

345. Jones SJ, Brusa A. Neurophysiological evidence for long-term repair of MS lesions: implications for axon protection. *J Neurol Sci* 2003;**206**:193–8.

346. Jones TB, McDaniel EE, Popovich PG. Inflammatory-mediated injury and repair in the traumatically injured spinal cord. *Curr Pharm Des* 2005;**11**:1223–36.

347. Kabat EA, Wolf A, Bezer AE. The rapid production of acute disseminated encephalomyelitis in rhesus monkeys by injection of heterologous and homologous brain tissue with adjuvant. *J Exp Med* 1947;**85**:117–130.

348. Kakalacheva K, Munz C, Lunemann JD. Viral triggers of multiple sclerosis. *Biochim Biophys Acta* 2011;**1812**:132–40.

349. Kalman B, Leist TP. Familial multiple sclerosis and other inherited disorders of the white matter. *Neurologist* 2004;**10**:201–15.

350. Kamm C, Zettl UK. Autoimmune disorders affecting both the central and peripheral nervous system. *Autoimmun Rev* 2012;**11**:196–202.

351. Kanter JL, Narayana S, Ho PP, *et al*. Lipid microarrays identify key mediators of autoimmune brain inflammation. *Nat Med* 2006;**12**:138–143.

352. Kao HW, Alexandru D, Kim R, *et al*. Value of susceptibility-weighted imaging in acute hemorrhagic leukoencephalitis. *J Clin Neurosci* 2012;**19**:1740–1.

353. Kapoor R, Davies M, Blaker PA, *et al*. Blockers of sodium and calcium entry protect axons from nitric oxide-mediated degeneration. *Ann Neurol* 2003;**53**:174–80.

354. Karaarslan E, Altintas A, Senol U, *et al*. Balo's concentric sclerosis: clinical and radiologic features of five cases. *AJNR Am J Neuroradiol* 2001;**22**:1362–7.

355. Karaoglan I, Akcali A, Ozkur A, Namydurua M. Neurobrucellosis mimicking demyelinizating disorders. *Ann Saudi Med* 2008;**28**:148–9.

356. Kastrukoff LF, Lau AS, Kim SU. Multifocal CNS demyelination following peripheral inoculation with herpes simplex virus type 1. *Ann Neurol* 1987;**22**:52–9.

357. Kastrup O, Stude P, Limmroth V. Balo's concentric sclerosis. Evolution of active demyelination demonstrated by serial contrast-enhanced MRI. *J Neurol* 2002;**249**:811–14.

358. Katz D, Taubenberger JK, Cannella B, *et al*. Correlation between magnetic resonance imaging findings and lesion development in chronic, active multiple sclerosis. *Ann Neurol* 1993;**34**:661–9.

359. Kebir H, Kreymborg K, Ifergan I, *et al*. Human T_H17 lymphocytes promote blood-brain barrier disruption and central nervous system inflammation. *Nat Med* 2007;**13**:1173–5.

360. Keegan BM, Giannini C, Parisi JE, *et al*. Sporadic adult-onset leukoencephalopathy with neuroaxonal spheroids mimicking cerebral MS. *Neurology* 2008;**70**;**13(Pt 2)**: 1128–33.

361. Keegan M, Konig F, McClelland R, *et al*. Relation between humoral pathological changes in multiple sclerosis and response to therapeutic plasma exchange. *Lancet* 2005;**366**:579–82.

362. Kerrison JB, Flynn T, Green WR. Retinal pathologic changes in multiple sclerosis. *Retina* 1994;**14**:445–51.

363. Ketelslegers IA, Visser IE, Neuteboom RF, *et al*. Disease course and outcome of acute disseminated encephalomyelitis is more severe in adults than in children. *Mult Scler* 2011;**17**:441–8.

364. Khan O, Filippi M, Freedman MS, *et al*. Chronic cerebrospinal venous insufficiency and multiple sclerosis. *Ann Neurol* 2010;**67**: 286–90.

365. Kidd D, Barkhof F, McConnell R, *et al*. Cortical lesions in multiple sclerosis. *Brain* 1999;**122**(Part 1):17–26.

366. Kielian T, Esen N. Effects of neuroinflammation on glia–glia gap

junctional intercellular communication: a perspective. *Neurochem Int* 2004;**45**:429–36.

367. Kiernan MC, Vonau M, Bullpitt PR, *et al*. Butterfly lesion of the corpus callosum due to Schilder's disease. *J Clin Neurosci* 2001;**8**:367–9.

368. Kigerl KA, Gensel JC, Ankeny DP, *et al*. Identification of two distinct macrophage subsets with divergent effects causing either neurotoxicity or regeneration in the injured mouse spinal cord. *J Neurosci* 2009;**29**:13435–44.

369. Kipp M, Clarner T, Dang J, *et al*. The cuprizone animal model: new insights into an old story. *Acta Neuropathol* 2009;**118**:723–36.

370. Kira J. Astrocytopathy in Balo's disease. *Mult Scler* 2011;**7**:771–9.

371. Kirk J, Plumb J, Mirakhur M, McQuaid S. Tight junctional abnormality in multiple sclerosis white matter affects all calibres of vessel and is associated with blood–brain barrier leakage and active demyelination. *J Pathol* 2003;**201**: 319–27.

372. Kivisakk P, Mahad DJ, Callahan MK, *et al*. Human cerebrospinal fluid central memory CD4+ T cells: evidence for trafficking through choroid plexus and meninges via P-selectin. *Proc Natl Acad Sci U S A* 2003;**100**:8389–94.

373. Kivisakk P, Mahad DJ, Callahan MK, *et al*. Expression of CCR7 in multiple sclerosis: implications for CNS immunity. *Ann Neurol* 2004;**55**:627–38.

374. Kiy G, Lehmann P, Hahn HK, *et al*. Decreased hippocampal volume, indirectly measured, is associated with depressive symptoms and consolidation deficits in multiple sclerosis. *Mult Scler* 2011;**17**:1088–97.

375. Kleinschmidt-DeMasters BK, Tyler KL. Progressive multifocal leukoencephalopathy complicating treatment with natalizumab and interferon beta-1a for multiple sclerosis. *N Engl J Med* 2005;**353**:369–74.

376. Koch-Henriksen N, Stenager E, Bronnum-Hansen H. Studies based on the Danish Multiple Sclerosis Registry. *Scand J Public Health* 2011;**39**(7 Suppl):180–4.

377. Koester J, Siegelbaum SA. Propagated signaling: the action potential. In: Kandel ER, Schwartz JH, Jessell TM eds. *Principles of neural science*. New York: McGraw-Hill, 2000:150–70.

378. Kohler W. Diagnostic algorithm for the differentiation of leukodystrophies in early MS. *J Neurol* 2008;**255** (Suppl 6):123–6.

379. Kolind SH, Laule C, Vavasour IM *et al*. Complementary information from multi-exponential T2 relaxation and diffusion tensor imaging reveals differences between multiple sclerosis lesions. *Neuroimage* 2008;**40**:77–85.

380. Kooi EJ, Geurts JJ, van Horssen J, *et al*. Meningeal inflammation is not associated with cortical demyelination in chronic multiple sclerosis. *J Neuropathol Exp Neurol* 2009;**68**:1021–8.

381. Kornek B, Storch MK, Weissert R, *et al*. Multiple sclerosis and chronic autoimmune encephalomyelitis: a comparative quantitative study of axonal injury in active, inactive, and remyelinated lesions. *Am J Pathol* 2000;**157**:267–76.

382. Kornek B, Storch MK, Bauer J, *et al*. Distribution of a calcium channel subunit in dystrophic axons in multiple sclerosis and experimental autoimmune encephalomyelitis. *Brain* 2001;**124** (Part 6):1114–24.

383. Kort JJ, Kawamura K, Fugger L, *et al*. Efficient presentation of myelin oligodendrocyte glycoprotein peptides but not protein by astrocytes from HLA-DR2 and HLA-DR4 transgenic mice. *J Neuroimmunol* 2006;**173**:23–34.

384. Kotil K, Kalayci M, Koseoglu T, Tugrul A. Myelinoclastic diffuse sclerosis (Schilder's disease): report of a case and review of the literature. *Br J Neurosurg* 2002;**16**: 516–19.

385. Kotter MR, Li WW, Zhao C, Franklin RJ. Myelin impairs CNS remyelination by inhibiting oligodendrocyte precursor cell differentiation. *J Neurosci* 2006;**26**: 328–32.

385a. Kotter MR, Setzu A, Sim FJ, et al. Macrophage depletion impairs oligodendrocyte remyelination following lysolecithin-induced demyelination. *Glia* 2001;**35**:204–12.

386. Kotter MR, Stadelmann C, Hartung HP. Enhancing remyelination in disease–can we wrap it up? *Brain* 2011;**134**(Part 7): 1882–900.

387. Kovács GG, Höftberger R, Majtényi K, *et al*. Neuropathology of white matter disease in Leber's hereditary optic neuropathy. *Brain* 2005;**128**(Part 1): 35–41.

388. Krogsgaard M, Wucherpfennig KW, Cannella B, *et al*. Visualization of myelin basic protein (MBP) T cell epitopes in multiple sclerosis lesions using a monoclonal antibody specific for the human histocompatibility leukocyte antigen (HLA)-DR2-MBP 85–99 complex. *J Exp Med* 2000;**191**: 1395–412.

389. Krucke W. On the histopathology of acute haemorrhagic leukoencephalitis, acute disseminated encephalitis and concentric sclerosis. In: Shiraki H, Yonezawa T, Kuroiwa Y eds. *The aetiology and pathogenesis of the demyelinating diseases*. Tokyo: Japanese Society of Neuropathology, 1976: 11–27.

390. Kruger PG. Mast cells and multiple sclerosis: a quantitative analysis. *Neuropathol Appl Neurobiol* 2001;**27**:275–80.

391. Krumbholz M, Theil D, Cepok S, *et al*. Chemokines in multiple sclerosis: CXCL12 and CXCL13 up-regulation is differentially linked to CNS immune cell recruitment. *Brain* 2006;**129**: 200–11.

392. Krumbholz M, Theil D, Steinmeyer F, *et al*. CCL19 is constitutively expressed in the CNS, up-regulated in neuroinflammation, active and also inactive multiple sclerosis lesions. *J Neuroimmunol* 2007;**190**:72–9.

393. Krupp LB, Banwell B, Tenembaum S. Consensus definitions proposed for pediatric multiple sclerosis and related disorders. *Neurology* 2007;**68**(Suppl 2): S7–12.

394. Kuhlmann T, Lucchinetti C, Zettl UK, *et al*. Bcl-2-expressing oligodendrocytes in multiple sclerosis lesions. *Glia* 1999;**28**: 34–9.

395. Kuhlmann T, Lingfeld G, Bitsch A, *et al*. Acute axonal damage in multiple sclerosis is most extensive in early disease stages and decreases over time. *Brain* 2002;**125**(Part 10):2202–12.

396. Kuhlmann T, Lassmann H, Bruck W. Diagnosis of inflammatory demyelination in biopsy specimens: a practical approach. *Acta Neuropathol* 2008;**115**:275–87.

397. Kuhlmann T, Miron V, Cuo Q, *et al*. Differentiation block of oligodendroglial progenitor cells as a cause for remyelination failure in chronic multiple sclerosis. *Brain* 2008;**131**(Part 7): 1749–58.

398. Kulcu DG, Akbas B, Citci B, Cihangiroglu M. Autonomic dysreflexia in a man with multiple sclerosis. *J Spinal Cord Med* 2009;**32**:198–203.

399. Kulkarni V, Nadgir D, Tapiawala S, *et al*. Biphasic demyelination of the nervous system following anti-rabies vaccination. *Neurol India* 2004;**52**:106–8.

400. Kumar AJ, Kohler W, Kruse B, *et al*. MR findings in adult-onset adrenoleukodystrophy. *AJNR Am J Neuroradiol* 1995;**16**:1227–37.

401. Kurne A, Isikay IC, Karlioguz K, *et al*. A clinically isolated syndrome: a challenging entity: multiple sclerosis or collagen tissue disorders: clues for differentiation. *J Neurol* 2008;**255**: 1625–35.

401a. Kuroiwa Y: Concentric sclerosis. In: Koetsier JC, ed. Demyelinating diseases. *Handbook of Clinical neurology*, Vol 3 (47). Amsterdam: Elsevier; 1985: 409–17.

402. Kurschus FC, Wortge S, Waisman a. Modeling a complex disease: multiple sclerosis. *Adv Immunol* 2011;**110**: 111–37.

403. Kurtzke JF. Epidemiology and etiology of multiple sclerosis. *Phys Med Rehabil Clin N Am* 2005;**16**:327–49.

404. Kury P, Abankwa D, Kruse F, et al. Gene expression profiling reveals multiple novel intrinsic and extrinsic factors associated with axonal regeneration failure. *Eur J Neurosci* 2004;**19**:32–42.

405. Kutzelnigg A, Lucchinetti CF, Stadelmann C, *et al*. Cortical demyelination and diffuse white matter injury in multiple sclerosis. *Brain* 2005;**128**(Part 11):2705–12.

406. Kutzelnigg A, Faber-Rod JC, Bauer J, *et al*. Widespread demyelination in the cerebellar cortex in multiple sclerosis. *Brain Pathol* 2007;**17**:38–44.

407. Kwon EE, Prineas JW. Blood–brain barrier abnormalities in longstanding multiple sclerosis lesions. An immuno-histochemical study. *J Neuropathol Exp Neurol* 1994;**53**:625–36.

408. Lampert PW. Fine stucture of the demyelinating process. In: Hallpike JF, Adams CWM, Tourtellotte WW eds. *Multiple sclerosis: pathology, diagnosis and management*. Baltimore: Williams & Wilkins, 1983:29–46.

408a. Lampert PW, O'Brien J, Garrett R. Hexachlorophene encephalopathy. *Acta Neuropathol* 1973;**23**:326–33.

409. Larochelle C, Alvarez JI, Prat A. How do immune cells overcome the blood-brain barrier in multiple sclerosis? *FEBS Lett* 2011;**585**:3770–80.

410. Larsen PH, Wells JE, Stallcup WB, *et al*. Matrix metalloproteinase-9 facilitates remyelination in part by processing the inhibitory NG2 proteoglycan. *J Neurosci* 2003;**23**:11127–35.

411. Lassmann H. Multiple sclerosis pathology: evolution of pathogenetic concepts. *Brain Pathol* 2005;**15**:217–22.

412. Lassmann H. New concepts on progressive multiple sclerosis. *Curr Neurol Neurosci Rep* 2007;7:239–44.

413. Lassmann H. Mechanisms of inflammation induced tissue injury in multiple sclerosis. *J Neurol Sci* 2008;274:45–7.

413a. Lassmann H, Raine CS, Antel J, Prineas JW. Immunopathology of multiple sclerosis. *J Neuroimmunol* 1998;86:213–17.

414. Lassmann H, Niedobitek G, Aloisi F, Middeldorp JM. Epstein–Barr virus in the multiple sclerosis brain: a controversial issue--report on a focused workshop held in the Centre for Brain Research of the Medical University of Vienna, Austria. *Brain* 2011;134(Part 9):2772–86.

415. Laule C, Vavasour IM, Whittall KP, et al. Evolution of focal and diffuse magnetisation transfer abnormalities in multiple sclerosis. *J Neurol* 2003;250:924–31.

416. Laule C, Vavasour IM, Moore GR, et al. Water content and myelin water fraction in multiple sclerosis. A T2 relaxation study. *J Neurol* 2004;251:284–93.

417. Laule C, Leung E, Lis DK, et al. Myelin water imaging in multiple sclerosis: quantitative correlation with histopathology. *Mult. Scler* 2006;12:747–53.

418. Laule C, Vavasour IM, Kolind SH, et al. Long T2 water in multiple sclerosis: what else can we learn from multi-echo T2 relaxation? *J Neurol* 2007;254:1579–87.

419. Laule C, Vavasour IM, Leung E, et al. Pathological basis of diffusely abnormal white matter: insights from magnetic resonance imaging and histology. *Mult Scler* 2011;17:144–50.

420. Laule C, Pavlova V, Leung E, et al. Diffusely abnormal white matter in multiple sclerosis: further histologic studies provide evidence for a primary lipid abnormality with neurodegeneration. *J Neuropathol Exp Neurol* 2013;72:42–52.

421. Laura M, Leong W, Murray NM, et al. Chronic inflammatory demyelinating polyradiculoneuropathy: MRI study of brain and spinal cord. *Neurology* 2005;64:914–16.

422. Lee SC, Moore GR, Golenwsky G, Raine CS. Multiple sclerosis: a role for astroglia in active demyelination suggested by class II MHC expression and ultrastructural study. *J Neuropathol Exp Neurol* 1990;49:122–36.

423. Lennon VA, Wingerchuk DM, Kryzer TJ, et al. A serum autoantibody marker of neuromyelitis optica: distinction from multiple sclerosis. *Lancet* 2004;364:2106–12.

424. Lennon VA, Kryzer TJ, Pittock SJ, et al. IgG marker of optic-spinal multiple sclerosis binds to the aquaporin-4 water channel. *J Exp Med* 2005;202:473–7.

425. Le Scanff J, Seve P, Renoux C, et al. Uveitis associated with multiple sclerosis. *Mult Scler* 2008;14:415–17.

426. Leuzzi V, Lyon G, Cilio MR, et al. Childhood demyelinating diseases with a prolonged remitting course and their relation to Schilder's disease: report of two cases. *J Neurol Neurosurg Psychiatry* 1999;66:407–8.

427. Levine S. Hyperacute, neutrophilic, and localized forms of experimental allergic encephalomyelitis: a review. *Acta Neuropathol* 1974;28:179–89.

428. Liao MF, Huang CC, Lyu RK, et al. Acute disseminated encephalomyelitis that meets modified McDonald criteria for dissemination in space is associated with a high probability of conversion to multiple sclerosis in Taiwanese patients. *Eur J Neurol* 2011;18:252–9.

429. Liew CL, Shyu WC, Tsao WL, Li H. Intravascular lymphomatosis mimicks a cerebral demyelinating disorder. *Acta Neurol Taiwan* 2006;15:264–8.

430. Lightman S, McDonald WI, Bird AC, et al. Retinal venous sheathing in optic neuritis. Its significance for the pathogenesis of multiple sclerosis. *Brain* 1987;110(pt2):405–14.

431. Liu JS, Zhao ML, Brosnan CF, Lee SC. Expression of inducible nitric oxide synthase and nitrotyrosine in multiple sclerosis lesions. *Am J Pathol* 2001;158:2057–66.

432. Lovas G, Szilagyi N, Majtenyi K, et al. Axonal changes in chronic demyelinated cervical spinal cord plaques. *Brain* 2000;123(Part 2):308–17.

433. Love S, Gradidge T, Coakham HB. Trigeminal neuralgia due to multiple sclerosis: ultrastructural findings in trigeminal rhizotomy specimens. *Neuropathol Appl Neurobiol* 2001;27:238–44.

434. Lu JQ, Fan Y, Mitha AP, et al. Association of alpha-synuclein immunoreactivity with inflammatory activity in multiple sclerosis lesions. *J Neuropathol Exp Neurol* 2009;68:179–89.

435. Lublin FD. Clinical features and diagnosis of multiple sclerosis. *Neurol Clin* 2005;23:1–15, v.

436. Lublin FD, Reingold SC. Defining the clinical course of multiple sclerosis: results of an international survey. National Multiple Sclerosis Society (USA) Advisory Committee on Clinical Trials of New Agents in Multiple Sclerosis. *Neurology* 1996;46:907–11.

436a. Lublin FD, Reingold SC, Cohen JA, et al. Defining the clinical course of multiple sclerosis: the 2013 revisions. *Neurology* 2014;83:278-86.

437. Lucas M, Suarez R, Marcos A, et al. Arg113His mutation of vanishing white matter is not present in multiple sclerosis. *Mult Scler* 2007;13:442–7.

438. Lucas RM, Hughes AM, Lay ML, et al. Epstein-Barr virus and multiple sclerosis. *J Neurol Neurosurg Psychiatry* 2011;82:1142–8.

439. Lucchinetti C, Brück W, Parisi J, et al. A quantitative analysis of oligodendrocytes in multiple sclerosis lesions. A study of 113 cases. *Brain* 1999;122(Part 12):2279–95.

440. Lucchinetti C, Brück W, Parisi J, et al. Heterogeneity of multiple sclerosis lesions: implications for the pathogenesis of demyelination. *Ann Neurol* 2000;47:707–17.

441. Lucchinetti CF, Mandler RN, McGavern D, et al. A role for humoral mechanisms in the pathogenesis of Dévic's neuromyelitis optica. *Brain* 2002;125(Part 7):1450–61.

442. Lucchinetti CF, Parisi J, Brück W. The pathology of multiple sclerosis. *Neurol Clin* 2005;23:77–105, vi.

443. Lucchinetti CF, Popescu BF, Bunyan RF, et al. Inflammatory cortical demyelination in early multiple sclerosis. *N Engl J Med* 2011;365:2188–97.

444. Ludwin SK. The pathogenesis of multiple sclerosis: relating human pathology to experimental studies. *J Neuropathol Exp Neurol* 2006;65:305–18.

445. Ludwin SK, Johnson ES. Evidence for a 'dying-back' gliopathy in demyelinating disease. *Ann Neurol* 1981;9:301–5.

446. Ludwin SK, Henry JM, McFarland H. Vascular proliferation and angiogenesis in multiple sclerosis: clinical and pathogenetic implications. *J Neuropathol Exp Neurol* 2001;60:505.

447. Lukes A, Mun-Bryce S, Lukes M, Rosenberg GA. Extracellular matrix degradation by metalloproteinases and central nervous system diseases. *Mol Neurobiol* 1999;19:267–84.

448. Lumsden C. The neuropathology of multiple sclerosis. In: Vinken PJ, Bruyn GW, eds. Handbook of Clinical Neurology, Vol 9. *Multiple Sclerosis and other demyelinating diseases.* Amsterdam: North Holland Publishing; 1970:217-309.

449. Lycklama à Nijeholt GJ. Reduction of brain volume in MS. MRI and pathology findings. *J Neurol Sci* 2005;233:199–202.

450. Lycklama à Nijeholt GJ, Bergers E, Kamphorst W, et al. Post-mortem high-resolution MRI of the spinal cord in multiple sclerosis: a correlative study with conventional MRI, histopathology and clinical phenotype. *Brain* 2001;124 (Part 1):154–66.

451. Lycklama G, Thompson A, Filippi M, et al. Spinal-cord MRI in multiple sclerosis. *Lancet Neurol* 2003;2:555–62.

452. MacKay A, Whittall K, Adler J, et al. In vivo visualization of myelin water in brain by magnetic resonance. *Magn Reson Med* 1994;31:673–7.

453. Magana SM, Matiello M, Pittock SJ, et al. Posterior reversible encephalopathy syndrome in neuromyelitis optica spectrum disorders. *Neurology* 2009;72:712–17.

454. Magana SM, Keegan BM, Weinshenker BG, et al. Beneficial plasma exchange response in central nervous system inflammatory demyelination. *Arch Neurol* 2011;68:870–8.

455. Mahad D, Trebst C, Kivisakk P, et al. Expression of chemokine receptors CCR1 and CCR5 reflects differential activation of mononuclear phagocytes in pattern II and pattern III multiple sclerosis lesions. *J Neuropathol Exp Neurol* 2004;63:262–73.

456. Mahad D, Callahan MK, Williams KA, et al. Modulating CCR2 and CCL2 at the blood–brain barrier: relevance for multiple sclerosis pathogenesis. *Brain* 2006;129(Part 1):212–23.

457. Mahad D, Ziabreva I, Lassmann H, Turnbull D. Mitochondrial defects in acute multiple sclerosis lesions. *Brain* 2008;131(Part 7):1722–35.

458. Mahad DJ, Ziabreva I, Campbell G, et al. Mitochondrial changes within axons in multiple sclerosis. *Brain* 2009;132 (Part 5):1161–74.

459. Malamud N. Sequelae of post measles encephalo-myelitis; a clinico-pathologic study. *Arch Neurol Psychiatry* 1939;41:943–54.

460. Malojcic B, Brinar V, Poser C, Djakovic V. An adult case of Leigh disease. *Clin Neurol Neurosurg* 2004;106:237–40.

461. Man S, Ubogu EE, Ransohoff R. M. Inflammatory cell migration into the central nervous system: a few new twists on an old tale. *Brain Pathol* 2007;17:243–50.

462. Man S, Tucky B, Cotleur A, et al. CXCL12-induced monocyte-endothelial

interactions promote lymphocyte transmigration across an in vitro blood-brain barrier. *Sci Transl Med* 2012;**4**:119ra14.

463. Mandler RN, Davis LE, Jeffery DR, Kornfeld M. Devic's neuromyelitis optica: a clinicopathological study of 8 patients. *Ann Neurol* 1993;**34**:162–8.

464. Mani S, Mondal SS, Guha G, et al. Acute disseminated encephalomyelitis after mixed malaria infection (*Plasmodium falciparum* and *Plasmodium vivax*) with MRI closely simulating multiple sclerosis. *Neurologist* 2011;**17**:276–8.

465. Manitt C, Kennedy TE. Where the rubber meets the road: netrin expression and function in developing and adult nervous systems. *Prog Brain Res* 2002;**137**: 425–42.

466. Marburg O. Die sogenannte 'akute multiple Sklerose' (Encephalomyelitis periaxialis scleroticans). *Jahrbücher für Psychiatrie und Neurologie (Leipzig)* 1906;**27**:213–311.

467. Marrie RA. Environmental risk factors in multiple sclerosis aetiology. *Lancet Neurol* 2004;**3**:709–18.

468. Marsden JP, Hurst EW. Acute perivascular myeloclasis ('acute disseminated encephalomyelitis') in smallpox. *Brain* 1932;**56**:181–225.

469. Massara A, Bonazza S, Castellino G, et al. Central nervous system involvement in Sjogren's syndrome: unusual, but not unremarkable-clinical, serological characteristics and outcomes in a large cohort of Italian patients. *Rheumatology (Oxford)* 2010;**49**:1540–9.

469a. Mastaglia FL, McDonald WI, Watson JV, Yogendran K. Effects of x-radiation on the spinal cord: an experimental study of the morphological changes in central nerve fibres. *Brain* 1976;**99**: 101–22.

470. Mastronardi FG, Moscarello MA. Molecules affecting myelin stability: a novel hypothesis regarding the pathogenesis of multiple sclerosis. *J Neurosci Res* 2005;**80**:301–8.

471. Mastronardi FG, daCruz LA, Wang H, et al. The amount of sonic hedgehog in multiple sclerosis white matter is decreased and cleavage to the signaling peptide is deficient. *Mult Scler* 2003;**9**:362–71.

472. Mata S, Lolli F. Neuromyelitis optica: an update. *J Neurol Sci* 2011;**303**: 13–21.

473. Matsushita T, Isobe N, Piao H, et al. Reappraisal of brain MRI features in patients with multiple sclerosis and neuromyelitis optica according to anti-aquaporin-4 antibody status. *J Neurol Sci* 2010;**291**:37–43.

474. Matthews AE, Weiss SR, Paterson Y. Murine hepatitis virus – a model for virus-induced CNS demyelination. *J Neurovirol* 2002;**8**:76–85.

475. Matthews PM. An update on neuroimaging of multiple sclerosis. *Curr Opin Neurol* 2004;**17**:453–8.

476. Matute C, Domercq M, Sanchez-Gomez MV. Glutamate-mediated glial injury: mechanisms and clinical importance. *Glia* 2006;**53**:212–24.

477. Mavragani CP, Patronas N, Dalakas M, Moutsopoulos HM. Ill-defined neurological syndromes with autoimmune background: a diagnostic challenge. *J Rheumatol* 2007;**34**:341–5.

478. Mayer M, Cerovec M, Rados M, Cikes N. Antiphospholipid syndrome and central nervous system. *Clin Neurol Neurosurg* 2010;**112**:602–8.

479. McCandless EE, Piccio L, Woerner BM, et al. Pathological expression of CXCL12 at the blood-brain barrier correlates with severity of multiple sclerosis. *Am J Pathol* 2008;**172**:799–808.

480. McDonald I, Compston A. The symptoms and signs of mutiple sclerosis. In: Compston A, Confavreux C, Lassmann H, et al. eds. *McAlpine's mutiple sclerosis*. Philadelphia: Churchill Livingstone Elsevier, 2006:287–346.

481. McDonald WI, Compston A, Edan G, et al. Recommended diagnostic criteria for multiple sclerosis: guidelines from the International Panel on the Diagnosis of Multiple Sclerosis. *Ann Neurol* 2001;**50**:121–7.

482. McFarland HF, Martin R. Multiple sclerosis: a complicated picture of autoimmunity. *Nat Immunol* 2007;**8**:913–19.

483. McLeod DR, Snyder F, Bridge P, Pinto a. Acute hemorrhagic leukoencephalitis in male sibs. *Am J Med Genet* 2002;**107**:325–9.

484. McMahon EJ, Bailey SL, Castenada CV, et al. Epitope spreading initiates in the CNS in two mouse models of multiple sclerosis. *Nat Med* 2005;**11**:335–9.

485. McQuaid S, Cunnea P, McMahon J, Fitzgerald U. The effects of blood-brain barrier disruption on glial cell function in multiple sclerosis. *Biochem Soc Trans* 2009;**37**(Part 1):329–31.

486. Mead RJ, Singhrao SK, Neal JW, et al. The membrane attack complex of complement causes severe demyelination associated with acute axonal injury. *J Immunol* 2002;**168**:458–65.

487. Meinl E, Derfuss T, Krumbholz M, et al. Humoral autoimmunity in multiple sclerosis. *J Neurol Sci* 2011;**306**:180–2.

488. Metz I, Radue EW, Oterino A, et al. Pathology of immune reconstitution inflammatory syndrome in multiple sclerosis with natalizumab-associated progressive multifocal leukoencephalopathy. *Acta Neuropathol* 2012;**123**:235–45.

489. Mews I, Bergmann M, Bunkowski S, et al. Oligodendrocyte and axon pathology in clinically silent multiple sclerosis lesions. *Mult Scler* 1998;**4**: 55–62.

490. Miljkovic D, Timotijevic G, Mostarica Stojkovic M. Astrocytes in the tempest of multiple sclerosis. *FEBS Lett* 2011;**23**:3781–8.

491. Miller A, Korem M, Almog R, Galboiz Y. Vitamin B12, demyelination, remyelination and repair in multiple sclerosis. *J Neurol Sci* 2005;**233**: 93–7.

492. Miller DH, Barkhof F, Frank JA, et al. Measurement of atrophy in multiple sclerosis: pathological basis, methodological aspects and clinical relevance. *Brain* 2002;**125**(Part 8): 1676–95.

493. Miller DH, Thompson AJ, Filippi M. Magnetic resonance studies of abnormalities in the normal appearing white matter and grey matter in multiple sclerosis. *J Neurol* 2003;**250**:1407–19.

494. Miller DH, Weinshenker BG, Filippi M, et al. Differential diagnosis of suspected multiple sclerosis: a consensus approach. *Mult Scler* 2008;**14**:1157–74.

495. Miller DH, Chard DT, Ciccarelli O. Clinically isolated syndromes. *Lancet Neurol* 2012;**11**:157–69.

496. Miller KL, Stagg CJ, Douaud G, et al. Diffusion imaging of whole, post-mortem human brains on a clinical MRI scanner. *Neuroimage* 2011;**57**:167–81.

497. Min KJ, Yang MS, Kim SU, et al. Astrocytes induce hemeoxygenase-1 expression in microglia: a feasible mechanism for preventing excessive brain inflammation. *J Neurosci* 2006;**26**: 1880–7.

498. Minagar A, Alexander JS. Blood–brain barrier disruption in multiple sclerosis. *Mult Scler* 2003;**9**:540–9.

499. Mineev KK, Prakhova LN, Il'ves AG, et al. Characteristics of neurological and cognitive status in patients with multiple sclerosis in relation to the location and volumes of demyelination foci and the severity of brain atrophy. *Neurosci Behav Physiol* 2009;**39**:35–8.

500. Ming X, Li W, Maeda Y, et al. Caspase-1 expression in multiple sclerosis plaques and cultured glial cells. *J Neurol Sci* 2002;**197**:9–18.

501. Misu T, Fujihara K, Kakita A, et al. Loss of aquaporin 4 in lesions of neuromyelitis optica: distinction from multiple sclerosis. *Brain* 2007;**130**(Part 5):1224–34.

502. Misu T, Takano R, Fujihara K, et al. Marked increase in cerebrospinal fluid glial fibrillar acidic protein in neuromyelitis optica: an astrocytic damage marker. *J Neurol Neurosurg Psychiatry* 2009;**80**:575–7.

503. Mohan H, Krumbholz M, Sharma R, et al. Extracellular matrix in multiple sclerosis lesions: fibrillar collagens, biglycan and decorin are upregulated and associated with infiltrating immune cells. *Brain Pathol* 2010;**20**:966–75.

504. Mokhtarian F, Huan CM, Roman C, Raine CS. Semliki Forest virus-induced demyelination and remyelination – involvement of B cells and anti-myelin antibodies. *J Neuroimmunol* 2003;**137**:19–31.

505. Moll NM, Rietsch AM, Ransohoff AJ, et al. Cortical demyelination in PML and MS: Similarities and differences. *Neurology* 2008;**70**:336–43.

506. Moll NM, Rietsch AM, Thomas S, et al. Multiple sclerosis normal-appearing white matter: pathology-imaging correlations. *Ann Neurol* 2011;**70**:764–73.

507. Montalban X. Primary progressive multiple sclerosis. *Curr Opin Neurol* 2005;**18**:261–6.

508. Moore GR. MRI-clinical correlations: more than inflammation alone – what can MRI contribute to improve the understanding of pathological processes in MS? *J Neurol Sci* 2003;**206**: 175–9.

509. Moore GR. Current concepts in the neuropathology and pathogenesis of multiple sclerosis. *Can J Neurol Sci* 2010;**37**(Suppl 2):S5–15.

510. Moore GR, Laule C. Neuropathologic correlates of magnetic resonance imaging in multiple sclerosis. *J Neuropathol Exp Neurol* 2012;**71**:762–78.

511. Moore GR, Traugott U, Farooq M, et al. Experimental autoimmune encephalomyelitis. Augmentation of

demyelination by different myelin lipids. *Lab Invest* 1984;51:416–24.

512. Moore GR, Neumann PE, Suzuki K, *et al.* Baló's concentric sclerosis: new observations on lesion development. *Ann Neurol* 1985;17:604–11.

513. Moore GR, Leung E, MacKay AL, *et al.* A pathology-MRI study of the short-T2 component in formalin-fixed multiple sclerosis brain. *Neurology* 2000;55:506–10.

514. Moore GR, Berry K, Oger JJ, *et al.* Baló's concentric sclerosis: surviving normal myelin in a patient with a relapsing-remitting clinical course. *Mult Scler* 2001;7:375–82.

515. Moore GR, Laule C, Mackay A, *et al.* Dirty-appearing white matter in multiple sclerosis: preliminary observations of myelin phospholipid and axonal loss. *J Neurol* 2008;255:1802–11, discussion 1812.

516. Morcos Y, Lee SM, Levin MC. A role for hypertrophic astrocytes and astrocyte precursors in a case of rapidly progressive multiple sclerosis. *Mult Scler* 2003;9:332–41.

517. Morgan BP, Campbell AK, Compston DA. Terminal component of complement (C9) in cerebrospinal fluid of patients with multiple sclerosis. *Lancet* 1984;2:251–4.

518. Muller DM, Pender MP, Greer JM. Blood–brain barrier disruption and lesion localisation in experimental autoimmune encephalomyelitis with predominant cerebellar and brainstem involvement. *J Neuroimmunol* 2005;160:162–9.

519. Nagara H, Inoue T, Koga T, *et al.* Formalin fixed brains are useful for magnetic resonance imaging (MRI) study. *J Neurol Sci* 1987;81:67–77.

520. Nakahara J, Kanekura K, Nawa M, *et al.* Abnormal expression of TIP30 and arrested nucleocytoplasmic transport within oligodendrocyte precursor cells in multiple sclerosis. *J Clin Invest* 2009;119:169–81.

521. Nakamura M, Misu T, Fujihara K, *et al.* Occurrence of acute large and edematous callosal lesions in neuromyelitis optica. *Mult Scler* 2009;15:695–700.

522. Nakane S, Zoecklein LJ, Gamez JD, *et al.* A 40-cM region on chromosome 14 plays a critical role in the development of virus persistence, demyelination, brain pathology and neurologic deficits in a murine viral model of multiple sclerosis. *Brain Pathol* 2003;13:519–33.

523. Nakanishi H. Microglial functions and proteases. *Mol Neurobiol* 2003;27:163–76.

524. Nakashima I, Fujihara K, Miyazawa H, *et al.* Relevance of callosal and periventricular MRI lesions to oligoclonal bands in multiple sclerosis. *Acta Neurol Scand* 2006;113:125–31.

525. Narayana PA, Doyle TJ, Lai D, Wolinsky JS. Serial proton magnetic resonance spectroscopic imaging, contrast-enhanced magnetic resonance imaging, and quantitative lesion volumetry in multiple sclerosis. *Ann Neurol* 1998;43:56–71.

526. Narayana PA, Wolinsky JS, Rao SB, *et al.* Multicentre proton magnetic resonance spectroscopy imaging of primary progressive multiple sclerosis. *Mult Scler* 2004;10(Suppl 1):S73–8.

527. Natarajan C, Sriram S, Muthian G, Bright JJ. Signaling through JAK2-

STAT5 pathway is essential for IL-3-induced activation of microglia. *Glia* 2004;45:188–96.

528. Nelissen I, Gveric D, van Noort JM, *et al.* PECAM-1 and gelatinase B coexist in vascular cuffs of multiple sclerosis lesions. *Neuropathol Appl Neurobiol* 2006;32:15–22.

529. Nelson F, Poonawalla A, Hou P, *et al.* 3D MPRAGE improves classification of cortical lesions in multiple sclerosis. *Mult Scler* 2008;14:1214–19.

530. Nelson F, Datta S, Garcia N, *et al.* Intracortical lesions by 3T magnetic resonance imaging and correlation with cognitive impairment in multiple sclerosis. *Mult Scler* 2011;17:1122–9.

531. Nesbit GM, Forbes GS, Scheithauer BW, *et al.* Multiple sclerosis: histopathologic and MR and/or CT correlation in 37 cases at biopsy and three cases at autopsy. *Radiology* 1991;180:467–74.

532. Nicholas AP, Sambandam T, Echols JD, Tourtellotte WW. Increased citrullinated glial fibrillary acidic protein in secondary progressive multiple sclerosis. *J Comp Neurol* 2004;473:128–36.

533. Nishie M, Mori F, Ogawa M, *et al.* Multinucleated astrocytes in old demyelinated plaques in a patient with multiple sclerosis. *Neuropathology* 2004;24:248–53.

534. Noseworthy JH, Lucchinetti C, Rodriguez M, Weinshenker BG. Multiple sclerosis. *N Engl J Med* 2000;343:938–52.

535. Nowacki P, Potemkowski A, Korwin-Piotrowska T, Nocon D. Morphometric analysis of axons in the minute multiple sclerosis lesions and shadow plaques in patients with multiple sclerosis. *Folia Neuropathol* 2000;38:104–10.

536. Nylander A, Hafler DA. Multiple sclerosis. *J Clin Invest* 2012;122:1180–8.

537. Ochoa-Reparaz J, Mielcarz DW, Begum-Haque S, Kasper LH. Gut, bugs, and brain: role of commensal bacteria in the control of central nervous system disease. *Ann Neurol* 2011;69:240–7.

538. O'Connor KC, Appel H, Bregoli L, *et al.* Antibodies from inflamed central nervous system tissue recognize myelin oligodendrocyte glycoprotein. *J Immunol* 2005;175:1974–1982.

539. O'Connor KC, McLaughlin KA, De Jager PL, *et al.* Self-antigen tetramers discriminate between myelin autoantibodies to native or denatured protein. *Nat Med* 2007;13:211–17.

540. Odoardi F, Sie C, Streyl K, *et al.* T cells become licensed in the lung to enter the central nervous system. *Nature* 2012;488:675–9.

541. Oksenberg JR, Hauser SL. Genetics of multiple sclerosis. *Neurol Clin* 2005;23:61–75, vi.

542. Oksenberg JR, Hauser SL. Decoding multiple sclerosis. *Ann Neurol* 2011;70:A5–7.

543. Okuda DT, Mowry EM, Beheshtian A, *et al.* Incidental MRI anomalies suggestive of multiple sclerosis: the radiologically isolated syndrome. *Neurology* 2009;72:800–5.

544. Okuda DT, Mowry EM, Cree BA, *et al.* Asymptomatic spinal cord lesions predict disease progression in radiologically isolated syndrome. *Neurology* 2011;76:686–92.

545. Omari KM, John GR, Sealfon SC, Raine CS. CXC chemokine receptors on human oligodendrocytes: implications for multiple sclerosis. *Brain* 2005;128 (Part 5):1003–15.

546. Oppenheimer DR. *Observations on the pathology of demyelinating diseases.* Oxford: University of Oxford, 1962.

547. Oppenheimer DR. Demyelinating diseases. In: Blackwood W, Corsellis JAN eds. *Greenfield's neuropathology.* London: Edward Arnold, 1976:470–499.

548. Oppenheimer DR. The cervical cord in multiple sclerosis. *Neuropathol Appl Neurobiol* 1978;4:151–62.

549. Optic Neuritis Study Group. Multiple sclerosis risk after optic neuritis: final optic neuritis treatment trial follow-up. *Arch Neurol* 2008;65:727–32.

550. Orton SM, Herrera BM, Yee IM, *et al.* Sex ratio of multiple sclerosis in Canada: a longitudinal study. *Lancet Neurol* 2006;5:932–6.

551. Osterberg A, Boivie J, Thuomas KA. Central pain in multiple sclerosis – prevalence and clinical characteristics. *Eur J Pain* 2005;9:531–42.

552. Ousman SS, Kubes P. Immune surveillance in the central nervous system. *Nat Neurosci* 2012;15:1096–101.

553. Owens T. The enigma of multiple sclerosis: inflammation and neurodegeneration cause heterogeneous dysfunction and damage. *Curr Opin Neurol* 2003;16:259–65.

554. Padiath QS, Fu YH. Autosomal dominant leukodystrophy caused by lamin B1 duplications a clinical and molecular case study of altered nuclear function and disease. *Methods Cell Biol* 2010;98:337–57.

555. Palace J. Multiple sclerosis associated with Leber's hereditary optic neuropathy. *J Neurol Sci* 2009;286:24–7.

556. Pampliega O, Domercq M, Soria FN, *et al.* Increased expression of cystine/glutamate antiporter in multiple sclerosis. *J Neuroinflammation* 2011; 8:63.

557. Papadimas GK, Rentzos M, Zouvelou V, *et al.* Superficial siderosis of central nervous system mimicking multiple sclerosis. *Neurologist* 2009;15:153–5.

558. Papadopoulos D, Dukes S, Patel R, *et al.* Substantial archaeocortical atrophy and neuronal loss in multiple sclerosis. *Brain Pathol* 2008;19:238–53.

559. Papais-Alvarenga RM, Miranda-Santos CM, Puccioni-Sohler M, *et al.* Optic neuromyelitis syndrome in Brazilian patients. *J Neurol Neurosurg Psychiatry* 2002;73:429–35.

560. Parratt JD, Prineas JW. Neuromyelitis optica: a demyelinating disease characterized by acute destruction and regeneration of perivascular astrocytes. *Mult Scler* 2010;16:1156–72.

561. Parrish JB, Yeh Ea. Acute disseminated encephalomyelitis. *Adv Exp Med Biol* 2012;724:1–14.

562. Patani R, Balaratnam M, Vora A, Reynolds R. Remyelination can be extensive in multiple sclerosis despite a long disease course. *Neuropathol Appl Neurobiol* 2007;33:277–87.

563. Patrikios P, Stadelmann C, Kutzelnigg A, *et al.* Remyelination is extensive in a subset of multiple sclerosis patients. *Brain* 2006;129(Part 12):3165–72.

564. Patsopoulos NA, Esposito F, Reischl J, *et al.* Genome-wide meta-analysis

identifies novel multiple sclerosis susceptibility loci. *Ann Neurol* 2011;70:897–912.

565. Paty DW, Moore GRW. Magnetic resonance imaging changes as living pathology in multiple sclerosis. In: Paty DW, Ebers GC eds. *Multiple sclerosis*. Philadelphia: FA Davis, 1998:328–69.

566. Pawate S, Agarwal A, Moses H, Sriram S. The spectrum of Susac's syndrome. *Neurol Sci* 2009;30:59–64.

567. Pawate S, Moses H, Sriram S. Presentations and outcomes of neurosarcoidosis: a study of 54 cases. *QJM* 2009;102:449–60.

568. Pender MP, Rist MJ. Apoptosis of inflammatory cells in immune control of the nervous system: role of glia. *Glia* 2001;36:137–44.

569. Pender MP, Csurhes PA, Wolfe NP, et al. Increased circulating T cell reactivity to GM3 and GQ1b gangliosides in primary progressive multiple sclerosis. *J Clin Neurosci* 2003;10:63–6.

570. Perron H, Perin JP, Rieger F, Alliel PM. Particle-associated retroviral RNA and tandem RGH/HERV-W copies on human chromosome 7q: possible components of a 'chain-reaction' triggered by infectious agents in multiple sclerosis? *J Neurovirol* 2000;6(Suppl 2):S67–75.

571. Perry VH. Inflammation and axonal degeneration. In: Waxman SG ed. *Multiple sclerosis as a neuronal disease*. Amsterdam: Elsevier Academic Press, 2005:241–53.

572. Peterson JW, Trapp BD. Neuropathobiology of multiple sclerosis. *Neurol Clin* 2005;23:107–29, vi–vii.

573. Peterson JW, Bö L, Mörk S, et al. Transected neurites, apoptotic neurons, and reduced inflammation in cortical multiple sclerosis lesions. *Ann Neurol* 2001;50:389–400.

574. Petratos S, Azari MF, Ozturk E, et al. Novel therapeutic targets for axonal degeneration in multiple sclerosis. *J Neuropathol Exp Neurol* 2010;69:323–34.

575. Pette H. *Die akut entzundlichen Erkrankungen des Nervensystems. (Virus-krankheiten, Entmarkungsenzephalomyelitiden, Neuritiden.)*. Leipzig: Thieme, 1942.

576. Petzold A, Eikelenboom MJ, Keir G, et al. Axonal damage accumulates in the progressive phase of multiple sclerosis: three year follow up study. *J Neurol Neurosurg Psychiatry* 2005;76:206–11.

577. Petzold A, de Boer JF, Schippling S, et al. Optical coherence tomography in multiple sclerosis: a systematic review and meta-analysis. *Lancet Neurol* 2010;9:921–32.

578. Pfausler B, Engelhardt K, Kampfl A, et al. Post-infectious central and peripheral nervous system diseases complicating *Mycoplasma pneumoniae* infection. Report of three cases and review of the literature. *Eur J Neurol* 2002;9:93–6.

579. Phillips PH, Newman NJ, Lynn MJ. Optic neuritis in African Americans. *Arch Neurol* 1998;55:186–92.

580. Pinto PS, Taipa R, Moreira B, et al. Acute hemorrhagic leukoencephalitis with severe brainstem and spinal cord involvement: MRI features with neuropathological confirmation. *J Magn Reson Imaging* 2011;33:957–61.

581. Pitt D, Nagelmeier IE, Wilson HC, Raine CS. Glutamate uptake by oligodendrocytes: implications for excitotoxicity in multiple sclerosis. *Neurology* 2003;61:1113–20.

582. Pittock SJ, McClelland RL, Achenbach SJ, et al. Clinical course, pathological correlations, and outcome of biopsy proved inflammatory demyelinating disease. *J Neurol Neurosurg Psychiatry* 2005;76:1693–7.

583. Pittock SJ, Lennon VA, Krecke K, et al. Brain abnormalities in neuromyelitis optica. *Arch Neurol* 2006;63:390–6.

583a. Plemel JR, Keough MB, Duncan GJ, et al. Remyelination after spinal cord injury: is it a target for repair? *Prog Neurobiol* 2014;117:54-72.

584. Plumb J, McQuaid S, Mirakhur M, Kirk J. Abnormal endothelial tight junctions in active lesions and normal-appearing white matter in multiple sclerosis. *Brain Pathol* 2002;12:154–69.

585. Pogorzelski R, Baniukiewicz E, Drozdowski W. [Subclinical lesions of peripheral nervous system in multiple sclerosis patients]. *Neurol Neurochir Pol* 2004;38:257–64.

586. Polman CH, Reingold SC, Edan G, et al. Diagnostic criteria for multiple sclerosis: 2005 revisions to the McDonald criteria. *Ann Neurol* 2005;58:840–6.

587. Polman CH, Reingold SC, Banwell B, et al. Diagnostic criteria for multiple sclerosis: 2010 revisions to the McDonald criteria. *Ann Neurol* 2011;69:292–302.

588. Popescu BF, Parisi JE, Cabrera-Gomez JA, et al. Absence of cortical demyelination in neuromyelitis optica. *Neurology* 2010;75:2103–9.

589. Popescu BF, Lennon VA, Parisi JE et al. Neuromyelitis optica unique area postrema lesions: nausea, vomiting, and pathogenic implications. *Neurology* 2011;76:1229–37.

590. Popovich PG, Guan Z, McGaughy V, et al. The neuropathological and behavioral consequences of intraspinal microglial/macrophage activation. *J Neuropathol Exp Neurol* 2002;61:623–33.

591. Poser CM. Myelinoclastic diffuse sclerosis. In: Koetsier JC ed. Handbook of clinical neurology, Vol 3 (47). *Demyelinating diseases*. Amsterdam: Elsevier, 1985:419–28.

592. Poser CM, Paty DW, Scheinberg L, et al. New diagnostic criteria for multiple sclerosis: guidelines for research protocols. *Ann Neurol* 1983;13:227–31.

593. Poser CM, Goutieres F, Carpentier MA, Aicardi J. Schilder's myelinoclastic diffuse sclerosis. *Pediatrics* 1986;77:107–12.

593a. Pouly S, Antel JP. Multiple sclerosis and central nervous system demyelination. *J Autoimmun* 1999;13:297–306.

594. Power C, Antony JM, Ellestad KK, et al. The human microbiome in multiple sclerosis: pathogenic or protective constituents? *Can J Neurol Sci* 2010;37(Suppl 2):S24–33.

595. Powers JM, Liu Y, Moser AB, Moser HW. The inflammatory myelinopathy of adreno-leukodystrophy: cells, effector molecules, and pathogenetic implications. *J Neuropathol Exp Neurol* 1992;51:630–43.

596. Prendergast CT, Anderton SM. Immune cell entry to central nervous system--current understanding and prospective therapeutic targets. *Endocr*

Metab Immune Disord Drug Targets 2009;9:315–27.

597. Prineas JW. Multiple sclerosis: presence of lymphatic capillaries and lymphoid tissue in the brain and spinal cord. *Science* 1979;203:1123–5.

598. Prineas JW, Connell F. The fine structure of chronically active multiple sclerosis plaques. *Neurology* 1978;28(9 Part 2):68–75.

599. Prineas JW, Connell F. Remyelination in multiple sclerosis. *Ann Neurol* 1979;5:22–31.

600. Prineas JW, Graham JS. Multiple sclerosis: capping of surface immunoglobulin G on macrophages engaged in myelin breakdown. *Ann Neurol* 1981;10:149–58.

601. Prineas JW, Wright RG. Macrophages, lymphocytes, and plasma cells in the perivascular compartment in chronic multiple sclerosis. *Lab Invest* 1978;38:409–21.

602. Prineas JW, Kwon EE, Cho ES, Sharer LR. Continual breakdown and regeneration of myelin in progressive multiple sclerosis plaques. *Ann N Y Acad Sci* 1984;436:11–32.

603. Prineas JW, Kwon EE, Sternberger NH, Lennon VA. The distribution of myelin-associated glycoprotein and myelin basic protein in actively demyelinating multiple sclerosis lesions. *J Neuroimmunol* 1984;6:251–64.

604. Prineas JW, Kwon EE, Goldenberg PZ, et al. Multiple sclerosis. Oligodendrocyte proliferation and differentiation in fresh lesions. *Lab Invest* 1989;61:489–503.

605. Prineas JW, Kwon EE, Goldenberg PZ, et al. Interaction of astrocytes and newly formed oligodendrocytes in resolving multiple sclerosis lesions. *Lab Invest* 1990;63:624–36.

606. Prineas JW, Barnard RO, Kwon EE, et al. Multiple sclerosis: remyelination of nascent lesions. *Ann Neurol* 1993;33:137–51.

607. Prineas JW, Barnard RO, Revesz T, et al. Multiple sclerosis. Pathology of recurrent lesions. *Brain* 1993;116(Part 3):681–93.

608. Prineas JW, Kwon EE, Cho ES, et al. Immunopathology of secondary-progressive multiple sclerosis. *Ann Neurol* 2001;50:646–57.

609. Prineas JW, McDonald WI, Franklin RJM. Demyelinating diseases. In: Graham DI, Lantos PL eds. *Greenfield's neuropathology*. London: Arnold, 2002:471–550.

610. Quan D, Kleinschmidt-DeMasters BK. A 71-year-old male with 4 decades of symptoms referable to both central and peripheral nervous system. *Brain Pathol* 2005;15:369–70, 373.

611. Quan D, Pelak V, Tanabe J, et al. Spinal and cranial hypertrophic neuropathy in multiple sclerosis. *Muscle Nerve* 2005;31:772–9.

612. Quandt JA, Baig M, Yao K, et al. Unique clinical and pathological features in HLA-DRB1*0401-restricted MBP 111-129-specific humanized TCR transgenic mice. *J Exp Med* 2004;200:223–34.

612a. Qin Y, Duquette P. B-cell immunity in MS. *Int MS J* 2003;10:110–20.

613. Racke MK, Drew PD. Toll-like receptors in multiple sclerosis. *Curr Top Microbiol Immunol* 2009;336:155–68.

614. Raine CS. Membrane specialisations between demyelinated axons and

astroglia in chronic EAE lesions and multiple sclerosis plaques. *Nature* 1978;**275**:326–7.

615. Raine CS. Multiple sclerosis and chronic relapsing EAE: comparative ultrastructural neuropathology. In: Hallpike JF, Adams CWM, Tourtellotte WW eds. *Multiple sclerosis: pathology, diagnosis and management.* Baltimore: Williams & Wilkins, 1983:413–60.

616. Raine CS. Demyelinating disease. In: Davis RL, Robertson DM eds. *Textbook of neuropathology.* Baltimore: Williams & Wilkins 1997:627–714.

617. Raine CS, Genain CP. Models of chronic relapsing experimental autoimmune encephalomyelitis. In: Raine CS, Mcfarland HF, Hohlfeld R eds. *Multiple sclerosis: a comprehensive text.* Edinburgh: Saunders Elsevier, 2008:237–59.

618. Raine CS, Wu E. Multiple sclerosis: remyelination in acute lesions. *J Neuropathol Exp Neurol* 1993;**52**:199–204.

619. Raine CS, Johnson AB, Marcus DM, et al. Demyelination in vitro. Absorption studies demonstrate that galactocerebroside is a major target. *J Neurol Sci* 1981;**52**:117–31.

620. Raine CS, Scheinberg L, Waltz JM. Multiple sclerosis. Oligodendrocyte survival and proliferation in an active established lesion. *Lab Invest* 1981;**45**:534–46.

621. Raine CS, Traugott U, Farooq M, et al. Augmentation of immune-mediated demyelination by lipid haptens. *Lab Invest* 1981;**45**:174–82.

622. Raine CS, Wu E, Ivanyi J, et al. Multiple sclerosis: a protective or a pathogenic role for heat shock protein 60 in the central nervous system? *Lab Invest* 1996;**75**:109–23.

623. Raivich G, Banati R. Brain microglia and blood-derived macrophages: molecular profiles and functional roles in multiple sclerosis and animal models of autoimmune demyelinating disease. *Brain Res Brain Res Rev* 2004;**46**:261–81.

624. Ramaglia V, Hughes TR, Donev RM, et al. C3-dependent mechanism of microglial priming relevant to multiple sclerosis. *Proc Natl Acad Sci U S A* 2012;**109**:965–70.

625. Ramagopalan SV, Knight JC, Ebers GC. Multiple sclerosis and the major histocompatibility complex. *Curr Opin Neurol* 2009;**22**:219–25.

626. Ramagopalan SV, Valdar W, Dyment DA, et al. Association of infectious mononucleosis with multiple sclerosis. A population-based study. *Neuroepidemiology* 2009;**32**:257–62.

627. Ramagopalan SV, Dyment DA, Cader MZ, et al. Rare variants in the CYP27B1 gene are associated with multiple sclerosis. *Ann Neurol* 2011;**70**:881–6.

628. Ransohoff RM. Immunology: In the beginning. *Nature* 2009;**462**:41–2.

629. Rao SM. White matter disease and dementia. *Brain Cogn* 1996;**31**:250–68.

630. Ratchford JN, Calabresi PA. The diagnosis of MS: white spots and red flags. *Neurology* 2008;**70**(13 Part 2):1071–2.

631. Reekers JA. CCSVI and MS: a never-ending story. *Eur J Vasc Endovasc Surg* 2012;**43**:127–8.

632. Reekers JA, Lee MJ, Belli AM, Barkhof F. Cardiovascular and Interventional Radiological Society of Europe commentary on the treatment of chronic cerebrospinal venous insufficiency. *Cardiovasc Intervent Radiol* 2011:**34**:1–2.

633. Revesz T, Kidd D, Thompson AJ, et al. A comparison of the pathology of primary and secondary progressive multiple sclerosis. *Brain* 1994;**117**(Part 4):759–65.

634. Reynolds R, Roncaroli F, Nicholas R, et al. The neuropathological basis of clinical progression in multiple sclerosis. *Acta Neuropathol* 2011;**122**:155–70.

635. Rice GP, Hartung HP, Calabresi PA. Anti-alpha4 integrin therapy for multiple sclerosis: mechanisms and rationale. *Neurology* 2005;**26**:1336–42.

636. Rivers TM, Schwentker FF. Encepahalomyelitis accompanied by myelin destruction experimentally produced in monkeys. *J Exp Med* 1935;**61**:689–702.

637. Rocca MA, Hickman SJ, Bo L, et al. Imaging the optic nerve in multiple sclerosis. *Mult Scler* 2005;**11**:537–41.

637a. Rodriguez M. Mechanisms of virus-induced demyelination and remyelination. *Ann N Y Acad Sci* 1988;**540**:240–51.

638. Rodriguez M, Oleszak E, Leibowitz J. Theiler's murine encephalomyelitis: a model of demyelination and persistence of virus. *Crit Rev Immunol* 1987;**7**:325–65.

639. Rodriguez M, Scheithauer BW, Forbes G, Kelly PJ. Oligodendrocyte injury is an early event in lesions of multiple sclerosis. *Mayo Clin Proc* 1993;**68**:627–36.

640. Roemer SF, Parisi JE, Lennon VA, et al. Pattern-specific loss of aquaporin-4 immunoreactivity distinguishes neuromyelitis optica from multiple sclerosis. *Brain* 2007;**130**(Part 5):1194–205.

641. Roemer SF, Scheithauer BW, Varnavas GG, Lucchinetti CF. Tumefactive demyelination and glioblastoma: a rare collision lesion. *Clin Neuropathol* 2011;**30**:186–91.

642. Rojiani AM, Cho ES, Sharer L, Prineas JW. Electrolyte-induced demyelination in rats. 2. Ultrastructural evolution. *Acta Neuropathol* 1994;**88**:293–9.

643. Rolak LA, Fleming JO. The differential diagnosis of multiple sclerosis. *Neurologist* 2007;**13**:57–72.

644. Rooney WD, Coyle PK. Recent advances in the neuroimaging of multiple sclerosis. *Curr Neurol Neurosci Rep* 2005;**5**:217–24.

645. Ropele S, Strasser-Fuchs S, Augustin M, et al. A comparison of magnetization transfer ratio, magnetization transfer rate, and the native relaxation time of water protons related to relapsing-remitting multiple sclerosis. *AJNR Am J Neuroradiol* 2000;**21**:1885–91.

646. Ropper AH, Ayata C, Adelman L. Vasculitis of the spinal cord. *Arch Neurol* 2003;**60**:1791–4.

647. Rosati G. The prevalence of multiple sclerosis in the world: an update. *Neurol Sci* 2001;**22**:117–39.

648. Rose JW, Hill KE, Watt HE, Carlson NG. Inflammatory cell expression of cyclooxygenase-2 in the multiple sclerosis lesion. *J Neuroimmunol* 2004;**149**:40–9.

649. Rosenberg GA. Matrix metalloproteinases and neuroinflammation in multiple sclerosis. *Neuroscientist* 2002;**8**:586–95.

650. Rosenberg NL, Bourdette D. Hypertrophic neuropathy and multiple sclerosis. *Neurology* 1983;**33**:1361–4.

651. Rosenbluth J, Schiff R, Liang WL, Dou W. Antibody-mediated CNS demyelination II. Focal spinal cord lesions induced by implantation of an IgM antisulfatide-secreting hybridoma. *J Neurocytol* 2003;**32**:265–76.

652. Rossi S, Mancino R, Bergami A, et al. Potential role of IL-13 in neuroprotection and cortical excitability regulation in multiple sclerosis. *Mult Scler* 2011;**17**:1301–12.

653. Rossi S, Studer V, Motta C, et al. Inflammation inhibits GABA transmission in multiple sclerosis. *Mult Scler* 2012;**18**:163–5.

654. Rotshenker S. Microglia and macrophage activation and the regulation of complement-receptor-3 (CR3/MAC-1)-mediated myelin phagocytosis in injury and disease. *J Mol Neurosci* 2003;**21**:65–72.

655. Rovaris M, Rocca MA, Filippi M. Magnetic resonance-based techniques for the study and management of multiple sclerosis. *Br Med Bull* 2003;**65**:133–44.

656. Rovaris M, Gass A, Bammer R, et al. Diffusion MRI in multiple sclerosis. *Neurology* 2005;**65**:1526–32.

657. Röyttä M, Latvala M. Diagnostic problems in multiple sclerosis. Two cases with clinical diagnosis of MS showing only a diffusely growing malignant astrocytoma. *Eur Neurol* 1986;**25**:197–207.

658. Rudick R. Mechanisms of disability progression in primary progressive multiple sclerosis: are they different from secondary progressive multiple sclerosis? *Mult Scler* 2003;**9**:210–12.

659. Rudick RA. Diagnostic criteria in multiple sclerosis: headed in the right direction but still a ways to go. *Ann Neurol* 2011;**69**:234–6.

660. Rueda Lopes FC, Doring T, Martins C, et al. The role of demyelination in neuromyelitis optica damage: diffusion-tensor MR imaging study. *Radiology* 2012;**263**:235–42.

661. Rus H, Cudrici C, Niculescu F. C5b-9 complement complex in autoimmune demyelination and multiple sclerosis: dual role in neuroinflammation and neuroprotection. *Ann Med* 2005;**37**:97–104.

662. Saccardi R, Freedman M, Sormani M, et al. A prospective, randomized, controlled trial of autologous haematopoietic stem cell transplantation for aggressive multiple sclerosis: a position paper. *Mult Scler* 2012;**18**:825–34.

663. Sadovnick AD. The genetics and genetic epidemiology of multiple sclerosis: the 'hard facts'. *Adv Neurol* 2006;**98**:17–25.

664. Saip S, Uluduz D, Erkol G. Fabry disease mimicking multiple sclerosis. *Clin Neurol Neurosurg* 2007;**109**:361–3.

665. Sanders V, Conrad AJ, Tourtellotte WW. On classification of post-mortem multiple sclerosis plaques for neuroscientists. *J Neuroimmunol* 1993;**46**:207–16.

665a. Sasaki M, Ide C. Demyelination and remyelination in the dorsal funiculus of the rat spinal cord after heat injury. *J Neurocytol* 1989;**18**:225–39.

666. Satoh J, Yamamura T, Arima K. The 14-3-3 protein epsilon isoform expressed in reactive astrocytes in demyelinating lesions of multiple sclerosis binds to vimentin and glial fibrillary acidic protein

in cultured human astrocytes. *Am J Pathol* 2004;**165**:577–92.

667. Satoh J, Nakanishi M, Koike F, *et al*. Microarray analysis identifies an aberrant expression of apoptosis and DNA damage-regulatory genes in multiple sclerosis. *Neurobiol Dis* 2005;**18**:537–50.

668. Satoh J, Onoue H, Arima K, Yamamura T. Nogo-A and nogo receptor expression in demyelinating lesions of multiple sclerosis. *J Neuropathol Exp Neurol* 2005;**64**:129–38.

669. Sayao AL, Devonshire V, Tremlett H. Longitudinal follow-up of 'benign' multiple sclerosis at 20 years. *Neurology* 2007;**68**:496–500.

669a. Schaumburg HH, Powers JM, Raine CS, et al. Adrenoleukodystrophy: a clinical and pathological study of 17 cases. *Arch Neurol* 1975;**32**:577–91.

669b. Schaumburg HH, Richardson EP, Johnson PC, et al. Schilder's disease: sex-linked recessive transmission with specific adrenal changes. *Arch Neurol* 1972;**27**:458–60.

670. Scheikl T, Pignolet B, Mars LT, Liblau RS. Transgenic mouse models of multiple sclerosis. *Cell Mol Life Sci* 2010;**67**:4011–34.

671. Schirmer L, Antel JP, Bruck W, Stadelmann C. Axonal loss and neurofilament phosphorylation changes accompany lesion development and clinical progression in multiple sclerosis. *Brain Pathol* 2011;**21**:428–40.

672. Schmierer K, Scaravilli F, Barker GJ, *et al*. Stereotactic co-registration of magnetic resonance imaging and histopathology in post-mortem multiple sclerosis brain. *Neuropathol Appl Neurobiol* 2003;**29**:596–601.

673. Schmierer K, Scaravilli F, Altmann DR, *et al*. Magnetization transfer ratio and myelin in postmortem multiple sclerosis brain. *Ann Neurol* 2004;**56**:407–15.

674. Schmierer K, Parkes HG, So PW, *et al*. High field (9.4 Tesla) magnetic resonance imaging of cortical grey matter lesions in multiple sclerosis. *Brain* 2010;**133** (Part 3):858–67.

674a. Schneider H, Cervos-Navarro J. Acute gliopathy in spinal cord and brain stem induced by 6-aminonicotinamide. *Acta Neuropathol* 1974;**27**:11–23.

675. Schrijver IA, van Meurs M, Melief MJ, *et al*. Bacterial peptidoglycan and immune reactivity in the central nervous system in multiple sclerosis. *Brain* 2001;**124**(Part 8):1544–54.

676. Schröder R, Nennesmo I, Linke RP. Amyloid in a multiple sclerosis lesion is clearly of A-lambda type. *Acta Neuropathol (Berl)* 2000;**100**:709–11.

677. Schwab C, McGeer PL. Complement activated C4d immunoreactive oligodendrocytes delineate small cortical plaques in multiple sclerosis. *Exp Neurol* 2002;**174**:81–8.

678. Schwarz S, Mohr A, Knauth M, *et al*. Acute disseminated encephalomyelitis: a follow-up study of 40 adult patients. *Neurology* 2001;**56**:1313–18.

679. Scolding N. Dévic disease and autoantibodies. *Lancet Neurol* 2005;**4**:136–7.

680. Seabrook TJ, Littlewood-Evans A, Brinkmann V, *et al*. Angiogenesis is present in experimental autoimmune encephalomyelitis and pro-angiogenic factors are increased in multiple sclerosis lesions. *J Neuroinflammation* 2010;**7**:95.

681. Seewann A, Kooi EJ, Roosendaal SD, *et al*. Translating pathology in multiple sclerosis: the combination of postmortem imaging, histopathology and clinical findings. *Acta Neurol Scand* 2009;**119**:349–55.

682. Seewann A, Vrenken H, van der Valk P, *et al*. Diffusely abnormal white matter in chronic multiple sclerosis: imaging and histopathologic analysis. *Arch Neurol* 2009;**66**:601–9.

683. Seewann A, Kooi EJ, Roosendaal SD, *et al*. Postmortem verification of MS cortical lesion detection with 3D DIR. *Neurology* 2012;**78**:302–8.

684. Seitelberger F, Jellinger K, Tschabitscher H. Zur Genese der akuten Entmarkungsencephalitis. *Wien Klin Wochenschr* 1958;**70**:453–9.

685. Sellner J, Boggild M, Clanet M, *et al*. EFNS guidelines on diagnosis and management of neuromyelitis optica. *Eur J Neurol* 2010;**17**:1019–32.

686. Selmaj K, Brosnan CF, Raine CS. Colocalization of lymphocytes bearing gamma delta T-cell receptor and heat shock protein hsp65+ oligodendrocytes in multiple sclerosis. *Proc Natl Acad Sci U S A* 1991;**88**:6452–6.

687. Selter RC, Brilot F, Grummel V, *et al*. Antibody responses to EBV and native MOG in pediatric inflammatory demyelinating CNS diseases. *Neurology* 2010;**74**:1711–15.

688. Serafini B, Rosicarelli B, Magliozzi R, *et al*. Detection of ectopic B-cell follicles with germinal centers in the meninges of patients with secondary progressive multiple sclerosis. *Brain Pathol* 2004;**14**:164–74.

689. Serafini B, Rosicarelli B, Magliozzi R, *et al*. Dendritic cells in multiple sclerosis lesions: maturation stage, myelin uptake, and interaction with proliferating T cells. *J Neuropathol Exp Neurol* 2006;**65**:124–41.

690. Serafini B, Severa M, Columba-Cabezas S, *et al*. Epstein-Barr virus latent infection and BAFF expression in B cells in the multiple sclerosis brain: implications for viral persistence and intrathecal B-cell activation. *J Neuropathol Exp Neurol* 2010;**69**:677–93.

691. Shams PN, Plant GT. Optic neuritis: a review. *Int MS J* 2009;**16**:82–9.

692. Sharma KR, Saadia D, Facca AG, *et al*. Chronic inflammatory demyelinating polyradiculoneuropathy associated with multiple sclerosis. *J Clin Neuromuscul Dis* 2008;**9**:385–96.

693. Shaw PJ, Smith NM, Ince PG, Bates D. Chronic periphlebitis retinae in multiple sclerosis. A histopathological study. *J Neurol Sci* 1987;**77**:147–52.

694. Sherman DL, Tait S, Melrose S, *et al*. Neurofascins are required to establish axonal domains for saltatory conduction. *Neuron* 2005;**48**:737–42.

695. Shields DC, Avgeropoulos NG, Banik NL, Tyor WR. Acute multiple sclerosis characterized by extensive mononuclear phagocyte infiltration. *Neurochem Res* 2000;**25**:1517–20.

696. Shiraki H. Etiopathogenesis of multiple sclerosis mainly from the neuropathological viewpoint. In: Kuroiwa Y ed. *Multiple sclerosis in Asia*. Baltimore, MD: University Park Press, 1976:161–93.

697. Shukaliak JA, Dorovini-Zis K. Expression of the beta-chemokines RANTES and MIP-1 beta by human brain microvessel endothelial cells in primary culture. *J Neuropathol Exp Neurol* 2000;**59**:339–52.

698. Silver NC, Tofts PS, Symms MR, *et al*. Quantitative contrast-enhanced magnetic resonance imaging to evaluate blood–brain barrier integrity in multiple sclerosis: a preliminary study. *Mult Scler* 2001;**7**:75–82.

699. Simpson JE, Newcombe J, Cuzner ML, Woodroofe MN. Expression of the interferon-gamma-inducible chemokines IP-10 and Mig and their receptor, CXCR3, in multiple sclerosis lesions. *Neuropathol Appl Neurobiol* 2000;**26**:133–42.

700. Simpson JE, Rezaie P, Newcombe J, *et al*. Expression of the beta-chemokine receptors CCR2, CCR3 and CCR5 in multiple sclerosis central nervous system tissue. *J Neuroimmunol* 2000;**108**:192–200.

701. Sinclair C, Mirakhur M, Kirk J, *et al*. Up-regulation of osteopontin and alphaBeta-crystallin in the normal-appearing white matter of multiple sclerosis: an immunohistochemical study utilizing tissue microarrays. *Neuropathol Appl Neurobiol* 2005;**31**:292–303.

702. Sinclair C, Kirk J, Herron B, *et al*. Absence of aquaporin-4 expression in lesions of neuromyelitis optica but increased expression in multiple sclerosis lesions and normal-appearing white matter. *Acta Neuropathol (Berl)* 2007;**113**:187–94.

703. Singh S, Kuruvilla A, Alexander M, Korah IP. Balo's concentric sclerosis: value of magnetic resonance imaging in diagnosis. *Australas Radiol* 1999;**43**:400–4.

704. Skulina C, Schmidt S, Dornmair K, *et al*. Multiple sclerosis: brain-infiltrating CD8+ T cells persist as clonal expansions in the cerebrospinal fluid and blood. *Proc Natl Acad Sci USA* 2004;**101**:2428–33.

705. Smith KJ, Hall SM. Factors directly affecting impulse transmission in inflammatory demyelinating disease: recent advances in our understanding. *Curr Opin Neurol* 2001;**14**:289–98.

706. Smith KJ, Lassmann H. The role of nitric oxide in multiple sclerosis. *Lancet Neurol* 2002;**1**:232–41.

707. Smith KJ, McDonald WI. The pathophysiology of multiple sclerosis: the mechanisms underlying the production of symptoms and the natural history of the disease. *Philos Trans R Soc Lond B Biol Sci* 1999;**354**:1649–73.

708. Smith KJ, Bostock H, Hall SM. Saltatory conduction precedes remyelination in axons demyelinated with lysophosphatidyl choline. *J Neurol Sci* 1982;**54**:13–31.

709. Smith ME. Phagocytosis of myelin in demyelinative disease: a review. *Neurochem Res* 1999;**24**:261–8.

710. Smith ME. Phagocytic properties of microglia in vitro: implications for a role in multiple sclerosis and EAE. *Microsc Res Tech* 2001;**54**:81–94.

711. Smith ME, Hoerner MT. Astrocytes modulate macrophage phagocytosis of myelin in vitro. *J Neuroimmunol* 2000;**102**:154–62.

712. Smolders J, Schuurman KG, van Strien ME, et al. Expression of vitamin D receptor and metabolizing enzymes in multiple sclerosis-affected brain tissue. *J Neuropathol Exp Neurol* 2013;72: 91–105.

713. Sobel RA. The extracellular matrix in multiple sclerosis lesions. *J Neuropathol Exp Neurol* 1998;57:205–17.

714. Sobel RA. Ephrin A receptors and ligands in lesions and normal-appearing white matter in multiple sclerosis. *Brain Pathol* 2005;15:35–45.

715. Sobel RA, Ahmed AS. White matter extracellular matrix chondroitin sulfate/ dermatan sulfate proteoglycans in multiple sclerosis. *J Neuropathol Exp Neurol* 2001;60:1198–207.

716. Sobel RA, Mitchell ME, Fondren G. Intercellular adhesion molecule-1 (ICAM-1) in cellular immune reactions in the human central nervous system. *Am J Pathol* 1990;136:1309–16.

717. Sobel RA, Chen M, Maeda A, Hinojoza JR. Vitronectin and integrin vitronectin receptor localization in multiple sclerosis lesions. *J Neuropathol Exp Neurol* 1995;54:202–13.

718. Sobel RA, Hinojoza JR, Maeda A, Chen M. Endothelial cell integrin laminin receptor expression in multiple sclerosis lesions. *Am J Pathol* 1998;153:405–15.

719. Solanky M, Maeda Y, Ming X, et al. Proliferating oligodendrocytes are present in both active and chronic inactive multiple sclerosis plaques. *J Neurosci Res* 2001;65:308–17.

720. Sorensen TL, Tani M, Jensen J, et al. Expression of specific chemokines and chemokine receptors in the central nervous system of multiple sclerosis patients. *J Clin Invest* 1999;103:807–15.

721. Sospedra M, Martin R. Immunology of multiple sclerosis. *Annu Rev Immunol* 2005;23:683–747.

722. Spain R, Bourdette D. The radiologically isolated syndrome: look (again) before you treat. *Curr Neurol Neurosci Rep* 2011;11:498–506.

723. Stadelmann C, Kerschensteiner M, Misgeld T, et al. BDNF and gp145trkB in multiple sclerosis brain lesions: neuroprotective interactions between immune and neuronal cells? *Brain* 2002;125(Part 1):75–85.

724. Stadelmann C, Ludwin S, Tabira T, et al. Tissue preconditioning may explain concentric lesions in Balò's type of multiple sclerosis. *Brain* 2005;128(Part 5): 979–87.

725. Stadelmann C, Albert M, Wegner C, Brück W. Cortical pathology in multiple sclerosis. *Curr Opin Neurol* 2008;21: 229–34.

726. Stein MS, Liu Y, Gray OM, et al. A randomized trial of high-dose vitamin D2 in relapsing-remitting multiple sclerosis. *Neurology* 2011;77:1611–18.

727. Sternberg Z. Sympathetic nervous system dysfunction in multiple sclerosis, linking neurodegeneration to a reduced response to therapy. *Curr Pharm Des* 2012;18:1635–44.

728. Stidworthy MF, Genoud S, Li WW, et al. Notch1 and Jagged1 are expressed after CNS demyelination, but are not a major rate-determining factor during remyelination. *Brain* 2004;127 (Part 9):1928–41.

729. Stirling DP, Stys PK. Mechanisms of axonal injury: internodal nanocomplexes and calcium deregulation. *Trends Mol Med* 2010;16:160–70.

730. Stohlman SA, Hinton DR. Viral induced demyelination. *Brain Pathol* 2001;11: 92–106.

731. Storch MK, Stefferl A, Brehm U, et al. Autoimmunity to myelin oligodendrocyte glycoprotein in rats mimics the spectrum of multiple sclerosis pathology. *Brain Pathol* 1998;8:681–94.

732. Strazielle N, Khuth ST, Murat A, et al. Pro-inflammatory cytokines modulate matrix metalloproteinase secretion and organic anion transport at the blood-cerebrospinal fluid barrier. *J Neuropathol Exp Neurol* 2003;62:1254–64.

733. Stys PK, Jiang Q. Calpain-dependent neurofilament breakdown in anoxic and ischemic rat central axons. *Neurosci Lett* 2002;328:150–4.

734. Stys PK, Zamponi GW, van Minnen J, Geurts JJ. Will the real multiple sclerosis please stand up? *Nat Rev Neurosci* 2012;13:507–14.

735. Summerfield R, Al-Saleh A, Robbins SE. Small cell lung carcinoma presenting with acute disseminated encephalomyelitis. *Br J Radiol* 2010;83:e54–7.

736. Suzuki K, Andrews JM, Waltz JM, Terry RD. Ultrastructural studies of multiple sclerosis. *Lab Invest* 1969;20:444–54.

736a. Suzuki K, Zagoren JC. Degeneration of oligodendroglia in the central nervous system of rats treated with AY9944 or triparanol. *Lab Invest* 1974;31:503–15.

737. Swanton JK, Fernando K, Dalton CM, et al. Modification of MRI criteria for multiple sclerosis in patients with clinically isolated syndromes. *J Neurol Neurosurg Psychiatry* 2006;77:830–3.

738. Syed YA, Baer AS, Lubec G, et al. Inhibition of oligodendrocyte precursor cell differentiation by myelin-associated proteins. *Neurosurg Focus* 2008;24:E5.

739. Taipa R, da Silva AM, Santos E, et al. Gliomatosis cerebri diagnostic challenge: two case reports. *Neurologist* 2011;17:269–72.

740. Takahashi K, Aranami T, Endoh M, et al. The regulatory role of natural killer cells in multiple sclerosis. *Brain* 2004;127 (Part 9):1917–27.

741. Takeuchi H, Mizuno T, Zhang G, et al. Neuritic beading induced by activated microglia is an early feature of neuronal dysfunction toward neuronal death by inhibition of mitochondrial respiration and axonal transport. *J Biol Chem* 2005;280:10444–54.

742. Talbott JF, Loy DN, Liu Y, et al. Endogenous Nkx2.21/Olig21 oligodendrocyte precursor cells fail to remyelinate the demyelinated adult rat spinal cord in the absence of astrocytes. *Exp Neurol* 2005;192:11–24.

743. Tallantyre EC, Bo L, Al-Rawashdeh O, et al. Greater loss of axons in primary progressive multiple sclerosis plaques compared to secondary progressive disease. *Brain* 2009;132(Part 5):1190–9.

744. Tallantyre EC, Bo L, Al-Rawashdeh O, et al. Clinico-pathological evidence that axonal loss underlies disability in progressive multiple sclerosis. *Mult Scler* 2010;16:406–11.

745. Tanaka J, Garcia JH, Khurana R, et al. Unusual demyelinating disease. A form of diffuse-disseminated sclerosis. *Neurology* 1975;25:588–93.

746. Tanaka M, Tanaka K, Komori M, Saida T. Anti-aquaporin 4 antibody in Japanese multiple sclerosis: the presence of optic spinal multiple sclerosis without long spinal cord lesions and anti-aquaporin 4 antibody. *J Neurol Neurosurg Psychiatry* 2007;78: 990–2.

747. Tartaglia MC, Narayanan S, De Stefano N, et al. Choline is increased in pre-lesional normal appearing white matter in multiple sclerosis. *J Neurol* 2002;249:1382–90.

748. Tenembaum S, Chitnis T, Ness J, Hahn JS. Acute disseminated encephalomyelitis. *Neurology* 2007;68(16 Suppl 2):S23–36.

749. Thomke F, Lensch E, Ringel K, Hopf HC. Isolated cranial nerve palsies in multiple sclerosis. *J Neurol Neurosurg Psychiatry* 1997;63:682–5.

750. Thompson AJ, Polman CH, Miller DH, et al. Primary progressive multiple sclerosis. *Brain* 1997;120(Part 6):1085–96.

751. Thompson AJ, Montalban X, Barkhof F, et al. Diagnostic criteria for primary progressive multiple sclerosis: a position paper. *Ann Neurol* 2000;47:831–5.

752. Tian GF, Azmi H, Takano T, et al. An astrocytic basis of epilepsy. *Nat Med* 2005;11:973–81.

753. Tomiak MM, Rosenblum JD, Prager JM, Metz CE. Magnetization transfer: a potential method to determine the age of multiple sclerosis lesions. *AJNR Am J Neuroradiol* 1994;15:1569–74.

754. Toro G, Vergara I, Roman G. Neuroparalytic accidents of antirabies vaccination with suckling mouse brain vaccine. Clinical and pathologic study of 21 cases. *Arch Neurol* 1977;34:694–700.

755. Toussaint D, Perier O, Verstappen A, Bervoets S. Clinicopathological study of the visual pathways, eyes, and cerebral hemispheres in 32 cases of disseminated sclerosis. *J Clin Neuroophthalmol* 1983;3:211–20.

756. Traboulsee A, Dehmeshki J, Peters KR, et al. Disability in multiple sclerosis is related to normal appearing brain tissue MTR histogram abnormalities. *Mult Scler* 2003;9:566–73.

757. Traboulsee A, Zhao G, Li DK. Neuroimaging in multiple sclerosis. *Neurol Clin* 2005;23:131–48.

757a. Traboulsee AL, Knox KB, Machan L, et al. Prevalence of extracranial venous narrowing on catheter venography in people with multiple sclerosis, their siblings, and unrelated healthy controls: a blinded, case-control study. *Lancet* 2014;383:138–45.

758. Trapp BD, Nave KA. Multiple sclerosis: an immune or neurodegenerative disorder? *Annu Rev Neurosci* 2008;31:247–69.

759. Trapp BD, Stys PK. Virtual hypoxia and chronic necrosis of demyelinated axons in multiple sclerosis. *Lancet Neurol* 2009;8:280–91.

760. Trapp BD, Peterson J, Ransohoff RM, et al. Axonal transection in the lesions of multiple sclerosis. *N Engl J Med* 1998;338:278–85.

761. Traugott U, Reinherz EL, Raine CS. Multiple sclerosis. Distribution of T cells, T cell subsets and Ia-positive macrophages in lesions of different ages. *J Neuroimmunol* 1983;4:201–21.

762. Trebst C, Staugaitis SM, Kivisakk P, et al. CC chemokine receptor 8 in the central nervous system is associated with phagocytic macrophages. *Am J Pathol* 2003;**162**:427–38.

763. Trip SA, Schlottmann PG, Jones SJ, et al. Scanning laser polarimetry quantification of retinal nerve fiber layer thinning following optic neuritis. *J Neuroophthalmol* 2010;**30**:235–42.

764. Tuke PW, Hawke S, Griffiths PD, Clark DA. Distribution and quantification of human herpesvirus 6 in multiple sclerosis and control brains. *Mult Scler* 2004;**10**:355–9.

765. Tuzun E, Akman-Demir G, Eraksoy M. Paroxysmal attacks in multiple sclerosis. *Mult Scler* 2001;**7**:402–4.

766. Tzartos JS, Friese MA, Craner MJ, et al. Interleukin-17 production in central nervous system-infiltrating T cells and glial cells is associated with active disease in multiple sclerosis. *Am J Pathol* 2008;**172**:146–55.

767. Uchimura I, Shiraki H. A contribution to the classification and the pathogenesis of demyelinating encephalomyelitis; with special reference to the central nervous system lesions caused by preventive inoculation against rabies. *J Neuropathol Exp Neurol* 1957;**16**:139–203; discussion, 203–8.

768. Ulvestad E, Williams K, Bø L, et al. HLA class II molecules (HLA-DR, -DP, -DQ) on cells in the human CNS studied in situ and in vitro. *Immunology* 1994;**82**: 535–41.

769. Valdo P, Stegagno C, Mazzucco S, et al. Enhanced expression of NGF receptors in multiple sclerosis lesions. *J Neuropathol Exp Neurol* 2002;**61**:91–8.

770. van Bogaert L. Histopathologische Studie uber die Encephalitis nach windpocken. *Z Gesamte Neurol Psychiatrie* 1932;**140**:201–17.

771. Van Bogaert L. Post-infectious encephalomyelitis and multiple sclerosis; the significance of perivenous encephalomyelitis. *J Neuropathol Exp Neurol* 1950;**9**:219–49.

772. Van der Goes A, Brouwer J, Hoekstra K, et al. Reactive oxygen species are required for the phagocytosis of myelin by macrophages. *J Neuroimmunol* 1998;**92**:67–75.

773. van der Goes A, Boorsma W, Hoekstra K, et al. Determination of the sequential degradation of myelin proteins by macrophages. *J Neuroimmunol* 2005;**161**:12–20.

774. van der Maesen K, Hinojoza JR, Sobel RA. Endothelial cell class II major histocompatibility complex molecule expression in stereotactic brain biopsies of patients with acute inflammatory/demyelinating conditions. *J Neuropathol Exp Neurol* 1999;**58**:346–58.

775. van der Valk P, Amor S. Preactive lesions in multiple sclerosis. *Curr Opin Neurol* 2009;**22**:207–13.

776. van der Valk P, De Groot CJ. Staging of multiple sclerosis (MS) lesions: pathology of the time frame of MS. *Neuropathol Appl Neurobiol* 2000;**26**:2–10.

777. Van Der Voorn P, Tekstra J, Beelen RH, et al. Expression of MCP-1 by reactive astrocytes in demyelinating multiple sclerosis lesions. *Am J Pathol* 1999;**154**:45–51.

778. Vandevelde M, Zurbriggen A. Demyelination in canine distemper virus infection: a review. *Acta Neuropathol (Berl)* 2005;**109**:56–68.

779. van Horssen J, Bö L, Vos CM, et al. Basement membrane proteins in multiple sclerosis-associated inflammatory cuffs: potential role in influx and transport of leukocytes. *J Neuropathol Exp Neurol* 2005;**64**:722–9.

780. van Horssen J, Brink BP, de Vries HE, et al. The blood-brain barrier in cortical multiple sclerosis lesions. *J Neuropathol Exp Neurol* 2007;**66**: 321–8.

781. van Horssen J, Witte ME, Schreibelt G, de Vries HE. Radical changes in multiple sclerosis pathogenesis. *Biochim Biophys Acta* 2011;**1812**:141–50.

782. van Noort JM, van Sechel AC, Bajramovic JJ, et al. The small heat-shock protein alpha B-crystallin as candidate autoantigen in multiple sclerosis. *Nature* 1995;**375**:798–801.

783. van Noort JM, van den Elsen PJ, van Horssen J, et al. Preactive multiple sclerosis lesions offer novel clues for neuroprotective therapeutic strategies. *CNS Neurol Disord Drug Targets* 2011;**10**:68–81.

784. van Waesberghe JH, Kamphorst W, De Groot CJ, et al. Axonal loss in multiple sclerosis lesions: magnetic resonance imaging insights into substrates of disability. *Ann Neurol* 1999;**46**:747–54.

785. van Walderveen MA, van Schijndel RA, Pouwels PJ, et al. Multislice T1 relaxation time measurements in the brain using IR-EPI: reproducibility, normal values, and histogram analysis in patients with multiple sclerosis. *J Magn Reson Imaging* 2003;**18**:656–64.

786. van Zwam M, Huizinga R, Melief MJ, et al. Brain antigens in functionally distinct antigen-presenting cell populations in cervical lymph nodes in MS and EAE. *J Mol Med* 2009;**87**:273–86.

787. Vavasour IM, Laule C, Li DK, et al. Longitudinal changes in myelin water fraction in two MS patients with active disease. *J Neurol Sci* 2009;**276**:49–53.

788. Vercellino M, Votta B, Condello C, et al. Involvement of the choroid plexus in multiple sclerosis autoimmune inflammation: a neuropathological study. *J Neuroimmunol* 2008;**199**:133–41.

789. Vercellino M, Masera S, Lorenzatti M, et al. Demyelination, inflammation, and neurodegeneration in multiple sclerosis deep gray matter. *J Neuropathol Exp Neurol* 2009;**68**:489–502.

790. Verny C, Loiseau D, Scherer C, et al. Multiple sclerosis-like disorder in OPA1-related autosomal dominant optic atrophy. *Neurology* 2008;**70**(13 Part 2):1152–3.

790a. Viglietta V, Bourcier K, Buckle GJ, et al. CTLA4Ig treatment in patients with multiple sclerosis. An open-label, phase 1 trial. *Neurology* 2008;**71**:917–24.

791. Villar LM, Sadaba MC, Roldan E, et al. Intrathecal synthesis of oligoclonal IgM against myelin lipids predicts an aggressive disease course in MS. *J Clin Invest* 2005;**115**:187–94.

792. Vinters HV, Gilbert JJ. Neurenteric cysts of the spinal cord mimicking multiple sclerosis. *Can J Neurol Sci* 1981;**8**: 159–61.

793. Volterra A, Meldolesi J. Astrocytes, from brain glue to communication elements: the revolution continues. *Nat Rev Neurosci* 2005;**6**:626–40.

794. von Budingen HC, Bar-Or A, Zamvil SS. B cells in multiple sclerosis: connecting the dots. *Curr Opin Immunol* 2011;**23**:713–20.

795. Vos CM, van Haastert ES, de Groot CJ, et al. Matrix metalloproteinase-12 is expressed in phagocytotic macrophages in active multiple sclerosis lesions. *J Neuroimmunol* 2003;**138**:106–14.

796. Vos CM, Geurts JJ, Montagne L, et al. Blood–brain barrier alterations in both focal and diffuse abnormalities on postmortem MRI in multiple sclerosis. *Neurobiol Dis* 2005;**20**:953–960.

797. Vrenken H, Seewann A, Knol DL, et al. Diffusely abnormal white matter in progressive multiple sclerosis: in vivo quantitative MR imaging characterization and comparison between disease types. *AJNR Am J Neuroradiol* 2010;**31**:541–8.

798. Vrethem M, Thuomas KA, Hillman J. Cavernous angioma of the brain stem mimicking multiple sclerosis. *N Engl J Med* 1997;**336**:875–6.

799. Warrington AE, Rodriguez M. Method of identifying natural antibodies for remyelination. *J Clin Immunol* 2010;**30**(Suppl 1):S50–5.

800. Warshawsky I, Rudick RA, Staugaitis SM, Natowicz MR. Primary progressive multiple sclerosis as a phenotype of a PLP1 gene mutation. *Ann Neurol* 2005;**58**:470–3.

801. Washington R, Burton J, Todd RF 3rd, et al. Expression of immunologically relevant endothelial cell activation antigens on isolated central nervous system microvessels from patients with multiple sclerosis. *Ann Neurol* 1994;**35**:89–97.

802. Watkins D, Rosenblatt DS. Functional methionine synthase deficiency (cblE and cblG): clinical and biochemical heterogeneity. *Am J Med Genet* 1989;**34**:427–34.

803. Wattjes MP, Harzheim M, Lutterbey GG, et al. Prognostic value of high-field proton magnetic resonance spectroscopy in patients presenting with clinically isolated syndromes suggestive of multiple sclerosis. *Neuroradiology* 2008;**50**:123–9.

804. Waxman SG. Transcriptional channelopathies: an emerging class of disorders. *Nat Rev Neurosci* 2001;**2**:652–9.

805. Waxman SG. Ion channels and neuronal dysfunction in multiple sclerosis. *Arch Neurol* 2002;**59**:1377–80.

806. Waxman SG. Sodium channels as molecular targets in multiple sclerosis. *J Rehabil Res Dev* 2002;**39**:233–42.

807. Waxman SG, Black JA, Sontheimer H, Kocsis JD. Glial cells and axo–glial interactions: implications for demyelinating disorders. *Clin Neurosci* 1994;**2**:202–10.

808. Wegner C, Esiri MM, Chance SA, et al. Neocortical, neuronal, synaptic and glial loss in multiple sclerosis. *Neurology* 2006;**67**:960–7.

809. Weller RO, Engelhardt B, Phillips MJ. Lymphocyte targeting of the central nervous system: a review of afferent and efferent CNS-immune pathways. *Brain Pathol* 1996;**6**:275–88.

810. Werner K, Bitsch A, Bunkowski S, et al. The relative number of macrophages/microglia expressing macrophage colony-stimulating factor and its receptor decreases in multiple sclerosis lesions. *Glia* 2002;**40**:121–9.

811. Werner P, Pitt D, Raine CS. Multiple sclerosis: altered glutamate homeostasis in lesions correlates with oligodendrocyte and axonal damage. *Ann Neurol* 2001;**50**:169–80.

812. Werring DJ, Brassat D, Droogan AG, et al. The pathogenesis of lesions and normal-appearing white matter changes in multiple sclerosis: a serial diffusion MRI study. *Brain* 2000;**123** (Part 8):1667–76.

813. Werring DJ, Clark CA, Droogan AG, et al. Water diffusion is elevated in widespread regions of normal-appearing white matter in multiple sclerosis and correlates with diffusion in focal lesions. *Mult Scler* 2001;**7**:83–9.

814. Whittall KP, MacKay AL, Li DK, et al. Normal-appearing white matter in multiple sclerosis has heterogeneous, diffusely prolonged T_2. *Magn Reson Med* 2002;**47**:403–8.

815. Wiendl H, Feger U, Mittelbronn M, et al. Expression of the immune-tolerogenic major histocompatibility molecule HLA-G in multiple sclerosis: implications for CNS immunity. *Brain* 2005;**128** (Part 11):2689–704.

816. Williams A, Piaton G, Aigrot MS, et al. Semaphorin 3A and 3F: key players in myelin repair in multiple sclerosis? *Brain* 2007;**130**(Part 10):2554–65.

817. Wilson HC, Onischke C, Raine CS. Human oligodendrocyte precursor cells in vitro: phenotypic analysis and differential response to growth factors. *Glia* 2003;**44**:153–65.

817a. Wingerchuk DM, Carter JL. Multiple Sclerosis; current and emerging disease-modifying therapies and treatment strategies. *Mayo Clin Proc* 2014;**89**:225–40.

818. Wingerchuk DM, Weinshenker BG. Neuromyelitis optica. *Curr Treat Options Neurol* 2005;**7**:173–182.

819. Wingerchuk DM, Weinshenker BG. The emerging relationship between neuromyelitis optica and systemic rheumatologic autoimmune disease. *Mult Scler* 2012;**18**:5–10.

820. Wingerchuk DM, Hogancamp WF, O'Brien PC, Weinshenker BG. The clinical course of neuromyelitis optica (Dévic's syndrome). *Neurology* 1999;**53**:1107–14.

821. Wingerchuk DM, Lennon VA, Pittock SJ, et al. Revised diagnostic criteria for neuromyelitis optica. *Neurology* 2006;**66**:1485–9.

821a. Wisniewski H, Raine CS, Kay WJ. Observations on viral demyelinating encephalomyelitis. Canine distemper. *Lab Invest* 1972;**26**:589–99.

822. Wityk RJ. Dural arteriovenous fistula of the spinal cord: an uncommon cause of myelopathy. *Semin Neurol* 1996;**16**:27–32.

823. Wolburg H, Paulus W. Choroid plexus: biology and pathology. *Acta Neuropathol* 2010;**119**:75–88.

824. Wolinsky JS. The diagnosis of primary progressive multiple sclerosis. *J Neurol Sci* 2003;**206**:145–52.

825. Wolswijk G. Oligodendrocyte survival, loss and birth in lesions of chronic-stage multiple sclerosis. *Brain* 2000;**123** (Part 1):105–15.

826. Wolswijk G. Oligodendrocyte precursor cells in the demyelinated multiple sclerosis spinal cord. *Brain* 2002;**125**(Part 2):338–49.

827. Wolswijk G, Balesar R. Changes in the expression and localization of the paranodal protein Caspr on axons in chronic multiple sclerosis. *Brain* 2003;**126**(Part 7):1638–49.

828. Wong D, Dorovini-Zis K. Upregulation of intercellular adhesion molecule-1 (ICAM-1) expression in primary cultures of human brain microvessel endothelial cells by cytokines and lipopolysaccharide. *J Neuroimmunol* 1992;**39**:11–21.

829. Wong D, Dorovini-Zis K. Expression of vascular cell adhesion molecule-1 (VCAM-1) by human brain microvessel endothelial cells in primary culture. *Microvasc Res* 1995;**49**:325–39.

830. Woodruff RH, Fruttiger M, Richardson WD, Franklin RJ. Platelet-derived growth factor regulates oligodendrocyte progenitor numbers in adult CNS and their response following CNS demyelination. *Mol Cell Neurosci* 2004;**25**:252–62.

831. Wu E, Raine CS. Multiple sclerosis. Interactions between oligodendrocytes and hypertrophic astrocytes and their occurrence in other, nondemyelinating conditions. *Lab Invest* 1992;**67**:88–99.

832. Wu GF, Alvarez E. The immunopathophysiology of multiple sclerosis. *Neurol Clin* 2011;**29**:257–78.

833. Wuerfel J, Bellmann-Strobl J, Brunecker P, et al. Changes in cerebral perfusion precede plaque formation in multiple sclerosis: a longitudinal perfusion MRI study. *Brain* 2004;**127**(Part 1):111–19.

834. Wurm G, Pogady P, Markut H, Fischer J. Three cases of hindbrain herniation in adults with comments on some diagnostic difficulties. *Br J Neurosurg* 1996;**10**:137–42.

835. Wylezinska M, Cifelli A, Jezzard P, et al. Thalamic neurodegeneration in relapsing-remitting multiple sclerosis. *Neurology* 2003;**60**:1949–54.

836. Yamakawa K, Kuroda H, Fujihara K, et al. Familial neuromyelitis optica (Dévic's syndrome) with late onset in Japan. *Neurology* 2000;**55**:318–20.

837. Yao B, Bagnato F, Matsuura E, et al. Chronic multiple sclerosis lesions: characterization with high-field-strength MR imaging. *Radiology* 2012;**262**:206–15.

838. Yao DL, Webster HD, Hudson LD, et al. Concentric sclerosis (Baló): morphometric and in situ hybridization study of lesions in six patients. *Ann Neurol* 1994;**35**:18–30.

839. Yong VW, Zabad RK, Agrawal S, et al. Elevation of matrix metalloproteinases (MMPs) in multiple sclerosis and impact of immunomodulators. *J Neurol Sci* 2007; **259**:79–84.

840. Young EA, Fowler CD, Kidd GJ, et al. Imaging correlates of decreased axonal Na+/K+ ATPase in chronic multiple sclerosis lesions. *Ann Neurol* 2008;**63**:428–35.

841. Young NP, Weinshenker BG, Parisi JE, et al. Perivenous demyelination: association with clinically defined acute disseminated encephalomyelitis and comparison with pathologically confirmed multiple sclerosis. *Brain* 2010;**133**(Part 2):333–48.

842. Zadro I, Barun B, Habek M, Brinar VV. Isolated cranial nerve palsies in multiple sclerosis. *Clin Neurol Neurosurg* 2008;**110**:886–8.

843. Zagzag D, Miller DC, Kleinman GM, et al. Demyelinating disease versus tumor in surgical neuropathology. Clues to a correct pathological diagnosis. *Am J Surg Pathol* 1993;**17**:537–45.

844. Zamboni P. The big idea: iron-dependent inflammation in venous disease and proposed parallels in multiple sclerosis. *J R Soc Med* 2006;**99**:589–93.

845. Zamboni P, Galeotti R, Menegatti E, et al. A prospective open-label study of endovascular treatment of chronic cerebrospinal venous insufficiency. *J Vasc Surg* 2009;**50**:1348–58.

846. Zamboni P, Galeotti R, Menegatti E, et al. Chronic cerebrospinal venous insufficiency in patients with multiple sclerosis. *J Neurol Neurosurg Psychiatry* 2009;**80**:392–9.

847. Zappulla JP, Arock M, Mars LT, Liblau RS. Mast cells: new targets for multiple sclerosis therapy? *J Neuroimmunol* 2002;**131**:5–20.

848. Zawadzka M, Rivers LE, Fancy SP, et al. CNS-resident glial progenitor/stem cells produce Schwann cells as well as oligodendrocytes during repair of CNS demyelination. *Cell Stem Cell* 2010;**6**:578–90.

849. Zee PC, Cohen BA, Walczak T, Jubelt B. Peripheral nervous system involvement in multiple sclerosis. *Neurology* 1991;**41**:457–60.

850. Zeine R, Cammer W, Barbarese E, et al. Structural dynamics of oligodendrocyte lysis by perforin in culture: relevance to multiple sclerosis. *J Neurosci Res* 2001;**64**:380–91.

851. Zeinstra E, Wilczak N, De Keyser J. Reactive astrocytes in chronic active lesions of multiple sclerosis express co-stimulatory molecules B7-1 and B7-2. *J Neuroimmunol* 2003;**135**:166–71.

852. Zephir H, Stojkovic T, Latour P, et al. Relapsing demyelinating disease affecting both the central and peripheral nervous systems. *J Neurol Neurosurg Psychiatry* 2008;**79**:1032–9.

853. Zhang Y, Da RR, Hilgenberg LG, et al. Clonal expansion of IgA-positive plasma cells and axon-reactive antibodies in MS lesions. *J Neuroimmunol* 2005;**167**:120–30.

854. Zhao GJ, Li DKB, Cheng Y, et al. MRI dirty-appearing white matter in MS (abstract). *Neurology* 2000;**54**(Suppl 3):A121.

855. Zhu B, Luo L, Moore GR, et al. Dendritic and synaptic pathology in experimental autoimmune encephalomyelitis. *Am J Pathol* 2003;**162**:1639–50.

856. Zivadinov R, Lopez-Soriano A, Weinstock-Guttman B, et al. Use of MR venography for characterization of the extracranial venous system in patients with multiple sclerosis and healthy control subjects. *Radiology* 2011;**528**:562–70.

857. Zlochiver S. Persistent reflection underlies ectopic activity in multiple sclerosis: a numerical study. *Biol Cybern* 2010;**102**:181–96.

Diseases of Peripheral Nerves

Robert E Schmidt and Juan M Bilbao

INTRODUCTION

The axons and dendrites of peripheral nerves arise from ganglion cells lying within the ventral grey matter of the spinal cord, from brain stem nuclei, and from neurons situated within the sensory ganglia of cranial and spinal nerves and the ganglia of the autonomic nervous system and enteric plexuses. They end in synaptic contact with other neurons in the dorsal horns of the spinal cord or other sensory nuclei in the central nervous system (CNS), with autonomic ganglia or with secretory or muscular effector cells; alternatively, in the case of sensory axons, they end as free terminal arborizations or specialized terminals within a variety of encapsulated sense organs.[504]

Nerve trunks, their branches and distal twigs are composite structures of nerve fibres, Schwann cells, layers of connective tissue and perineurial cells and vessels. This unique arrangement of tissues derived from the CNS, the neural crest and mesenchyme constitutes the peripheral nervous system (PNS). The PNS comprises the ten lower cranial nerves, nerve roots of the spinal cord, spinal ganglia, plexuses, nerve trunks and their terminations in skin and muscle, as well as the autonomic ganglia and nerves. At any level, this system may be affected by a variety of multifocal and systemic disorders. Because nerves travel through subcutaneous tissues and narrow anatomical channels, they are often involved in lacerations, blunt trauma and repetitive injuries leading to entrapment neuropathies and pressure palsies.

The traditional pathological classification of peripheral nerve disorders emphasized the component of the PNS most likely to be affected, thus:[504]

- neuronopathies consist of conditions affecting loss of neurons (lower motor neurons and/or sensory and autonomic neurons) that contribute nerve fibres to peripheral nerves;
- axonopathies occur when there is axonal degeneration, with preservation of the cell body. More often, in generalized axonopathy, the degeneration commences distally and advances proximally towards the cell body in a 'dying back' manner. Rarely, the axonal degenerative process begins proximally and progresses downstream. Axonopathies may also be focal;
- disorders that directly affect the Schwann cell or myelin lead to primary segmental demyelination. When demyelination occurs as a consequence of axonal influences, it is termed 'secondary demyelination';
- Conditions that primarily affect connective tissue and vasculature often have secondary effects on the nerve fibre and Schwann cells.

It is this biological interdependence of the ganglion cell, the axon or dendrites, the Schwann cell and the supporting connective vascular tissue that explains the stereotyped response of the nerve fibre to a variety of different pathological insults.

CLINICOPATHOLOGICAL FEATURES OF NEUROPATHY

Three fundamental features characterize a neuropathy clinically:

- spatial distribution;
- time course;
- fibre type involvement.[325]

A fourth feature, axonal versus demyelinating, is largely an electrophysiological determination.

Spatial Distribution

Polyneuropathies may occur diffusely or in a multifocal manner. The most common pattern is a length-dependent process in which the distal parts of extremities are affected first, symmetrically, with progression evolving from toes to ankles and from fingertips to wrist, and into the classic glove–stocking pattern. Many aetiologies can cause this 'distal axonopathy', including toxic and metabolic conditions, genetic disorders and inflammatory and paraneoplastic diseases. At the other extreme are focal and multifocal neuropathies, which in classic form are designated clinically as 'mononeuritis multiplex' (Table 24.1).

However, the progression of multifocal peripheral nerve disease with summation of insults affecting contiguous nerves on both sides of the body, as may occur in polyarteritis nodosa (PAN), blurs the clinical distinction between multiple mononeuropathy and symmetrical polyneuropathy, thus setting the stage for misdiagnosis.

Time Course

Consideration of time course is helpful in assessing a patient with peripheral neuropathy. Subacute processes evolving over days to a month are usually inflammatory, such as Guillain–Barré syndrome (GBS), hyperacute vasculitic syndrome and paraneoplastic sensory neuropathy, although some toxic neuropathies can evolve rapidly as well. Processes developing over a period of 3–5 years often have a genetic basis, even when there is no family history of a neuromuscular disorder. Paraproteinaemic neuropathy and some metabolic conditions may also have a slow, indolent course. Neuropathies that evolve over many years without causing major disability often elude diagnosis despite extensive testing (cryptogenic neuropathies) and are particularly common in elderly patients.

Fibre Type Involvement

Most neuropathies affect sensory and motor function. In many cases, sensory symptoms and signs tend to dominate initially, because the longest axons are those supplying the feet and toes, whereas motor involvement necessitates progression of the disease to involvement of more proximal segments of nerve serving major muscle groups. Commonly, sensory involvement affects both large and small fibres. Dysfunction of large fibres produces deficits in vibration and joint position sensation, and impairment of deep tendon reflexes that are transmitted by 1A afferent sensory axons. This pattern is non-specific. There is a narrow range of diagnoses for polyneuropathies affecting small fibres (Table 24.2). Pure sensory neuropathies other than small-fibre neuropathy are uncommon; aetiologies include paraneoplasia, paraproteinaemia, sensory chronic inflammatory demyelinating polyneuropathy (CIDP) and genetic causes. The diagnosis of pure motor neuropathy is fraught with difficulty because of the overlapping clinical features of peripheral nerve motor dysfunction with diseases of the lower motor neuron. Known causes of pure motor neuropathy include multifocal motor neuropathy (MMN) and CIDP. When nerve conduction and electromyographic (EMG) studies suggest demyelination in the pathogenesis of a neuropathy, the differential diagnosis is restricted to GBS, CIDP, Charcot–Marie–Tooth (CMT) disease, leukodystrophies, a few toxins and, rarely, mitochondrial disease. However, there is frequent discordance between electrophysiological and histological characterization of a neuropathic process.[325]

Compounding the problem of diagnosing a polyneuropathy is the patient who presents with concurrent medical conditions such as cancer, and subsequent therapy, and underlying diabetes. Such conditions may result in clinical and electrophysiological changes of their own that hinder attempts to arrive at a diagnosis. Furthermore, patients with generalized peripheral neuropathy appear more susceptible to compression neuropathies.

Although histological assessment of a peripheral nerve trunk may provide important clues for the diagnosis of a polyneuropathy and occasionally may unmask amyloid deposits or vasculitis as the cause of a cryptogenic polyneuropathy, it is obvious that nerve biopsy is not a screening test for neuropathy.[62] The current clinical approach to a patient with peripheral neuropathy comprises:

- history and clinical examination;
- examination of kindred even without a phenotype suggestive of a familial neuromuscular disorder;
- nerve conduction, EMG and sensory studies;
- autonomic testing;

TABLE 24.1 Multifocal neuropathies

Hereditary neuropathy with liability to pressure palsies
Neuritic leprosy
Sarcoidosis
Necrotizing vasculitis
Multiple entrapments
Multifocal motor neuropathy
Diabetic neuropathy
Multifocal chronic inflammatory and demyelinating
  polyneuropathy
Multiple intraneural deposits of amyloid

TABLE 24.2 Small fibre neuropathy

Diabetes (most common)
Amyloid neuropathy
Alcoholic neuropathy
Fabry disease
Pseudo-syringomyelic form of Tangier disease (extremely rare)
Hereditary sensory and autonomic neuropathy
Acute pandysautonomia
Idiopathic distal sensory neuropathy (common)

- laboratory testing, including blood glucose testing, assessment for monoclonal gammopathy and, in the appropriate clinical setting, specific antibody assays, including anti-glycolipid antibody and anti-Hu antibody;
- examination of spinal fluid (which rarely provides a specific diagnosis); adipose tissue, salivary gland, nerve, muscle or skin biopsy.

In patients with symptoms of peripheral nerve dysfunction, clinical examination and electrophysiological studies may be normal or borderline abnormal; in such cases, it is likely that the microscopic examination of a subcutaneous nerve will not result in a specific diagnosis. Limitations of nerve biopsy relate to the small size of tissue removed, the great susceptibility of peripheral nerve to artefacts when a strict method for handling and processing is not followed and the absence of ganglion cells in the sample. Because some subcutaneous nerves contain nerve fibres that are far removed from their parent ganglion cell (the separation may exceed 1 metre in nerves to the lower limb), any estimate of disease affecting the perikaryon is a prediction made by inference of abnormalities in distal dendrites and axons. When compared with the dimension of the cell body, axons and dendrites in peripheral nerve may constitute the largest component of the total mass of the neuron; however, only small segments of nerve bundles are visualized in a nerve biopsy. Since the 1990s, the indication for nerve biopsy has decreased considerably because genetic testing can now identify the majority of neuropathies of CMT-1, CMT-X, hereditary neuropathy with liability to pressure palsies (HNPP), familial amyloidosis, spinocerebellar ataxias (SCAs) and many of the genetically determined metabolic conditions that produce peripheral neuropathy.

Detailed information on biopsy site, technique of tissue removal, complications of the procedure, specimen handling, and the methods used for tissue preparation, which comprise paraffin embedding, histostains and immunostains, plastic-resin embedding and transmission electron microscopy, post-fixation maceration and 'teasing' and 'snap freezing', are found in a number of texts.[34,324,325,447]

The diagnostic yield of the peripheral nerve biopsy varies considerably but it remains a necessary part of the analysis of peripheral neuropathy.[91,113,324,325,516] In many specimens the morphological abnormality is non-specific, without providing clues as to a definite aetiology. Furthermore, in some instances, autopsy studies have shown that histological change, however specific, proximal to the biopsy site, may be associated with 'downstream' (at biopsy site) non-specific axonal degeneration. For example, in a large series of subcutaneous nerve biopsies performed over a 33-year period and comprising nearly 1000 consecutive cases at the University of Toronto, a specific diagnosis was established only in about 29 per cent of cases.[34]

Although in many patients with peripheral neuropathy all types of nerve fibre are involved, some neuropathic processes affect only small-diameter fibres. This syndrome of small-fibre neuropathy is a source of frustration for the clinician, because the search for a specific diagnosis with physical examination, electrodiagnostic studies and even subcutaneous nerve biopsy often results in an absence of objective findings. The implementation of skin biopsy for the demonstration of depletion of dermal and intra-epidermal nerve fibres (IENFs) provides the rationale for a morphological–quantitative diagnosis for a neuropathy.[239] Patients with neuropathies involving small-diameter fibres (a category that includes some cases of distal, painful peripheral neuropathy) experience reduced sensitivity to pain and temperature, and dysaesthetic burning and searing pains that are more troublesome at night. The mechanisms underlying painful neuropathies are complex and may involve contribution by multiple levels of the CNS and PNS.[343,564] Muscle strength, myotendinous reflexes, and motor and sensory nerve conduction velocities (which measure large-fibre function) are typically normal; as a result, no objective evidence for peripheral nerve dysfunction has been documented. The differential diagnosis of predominantly small-fibre neuropathy is limited (Table 24.2). In these cases, skin biopsy has a number of advantages over conventional nerve biopsy because IENF density can be decreased significantly, despite normal sural nerve morphometry.

The fine innervation of the human epidermis was originally described in 1868 by Paul Langerhans, then a medical student.[263] Using gold chloride impregnation (0.5 per cent solution) of skin obtained from surgical and autopsy specimens, he observed, and illustrated with a drawing, free nerve endings in the epidermis between keratinocytes. In 1928, working with methylene blue staining and metallic (both gold and silver) techniques, Kadanoff published detailed drawings of human IENFs and their mode of termination as free endings.[295] In 1959, Arthur and Shelley demonstrated IENFs using intra vital and *in vitro* techniques of methylene blue staining and examining sections 50 µm thick under oil immersion,[15] providing the first quantification of IENFs in humans at different sites. They estimated the number of nerve endings per unit area and found a range of individual variation and a rostral to caudal gradient of innervation. However, this method was cumbersome and time-consuming; in addition, because the results could not be photographed, there was a paucity of convincing illustrations. Arthur and Shelley's findings were confirmed more than 30 years later by the discovery that the antibody to neuropeptide protein gene product (PGP) 9.5 can be used to visualize almost any nerve fibre. Combined with the advances provided by the confocal microscope, which allows the three-dimensional reconstruction of thick sections of skin, this stimulated research into the cutaneous innervation and the study of patients with small-fibre neuropathies.[239,265]

Because the small-diameter nerve fibres traverse the skin perpendicular to the epidermis, the number of epidermal neurites per millimetre can be quantitated in punch skin biopsies, and normative reference ranges for nerve fibre densities are being reported. Punch biopsy of non-glabrous skin of limbs is preferred. The fresh sample is immediately immersed in a chilled paraformaldehyde-based fixative, cryosectioned at 50 µm and immunostained for PGP 9.5. Additional immunolabelling for other neuropeptides allows assessment of the innervation of sweat glands, arterioles, papilla and hair follicles. One of the limitations of this technique is the need to have an adequate bank of control specimens from the different parts of the body to correlate with the biopsy sites used. In addition, the normal sample has to be obtained from age-matched controls that have been subjected to rigorous neurological and electrophysiological studies to rule out subclinical disease. Furthermore, the distribution density of epidermal nerve fibres differs in various parts of the body: studies have shown the density of epidermal fibres to be lower in men and to decrease with age (range 4.5–26.5/mm).

NORMAL STRUCTURE OF PERIPHERAL NERVE

The basic architecture of a peripheral nerve trunk is illustrated in Figure 24.1 and the micro-anatomy is shown in Figure 24.2 (see also Figure 24.3 and 24.5 for normal ultrastructural appearance of peripheral nerve components). Normal peripheral nerves consist of a bundle of fascicles encased in a fibrovascular stroma termed the epineurium. Individual peripheral and autonomic nerve fascicles are further ensheathed by perineurium, a specialized structure

functionally akin to the arachnoid membrane. Contained within the perineurium is the endoneurium, consisting of a collagenous matrix housing the axons, Schwann cells, fibroblasts, macrophages, mast cells and capillaries.

The Epineurium

The epineurium consists of massed collagen fibrils (types 1 and 3) interspersed with occasional elastin fibres, fibroblasts, mast cells, and the small arterial and venous blood vessels that supply the capillary plexus of the underlying nerve. Superficially, the epineurium merges with the surrounding areolar connective tissue of the deep fascia, and on its deep surface with the outermost layer of the perineurium. It is distinguishable as a separate sheath only in the largest nerves and nerve trunks; its thickness diminishes as the nerves pass distally, and a distinct epineurial layer cannot usually be identified around the smaller peripheral branches in most species.

The Perineurium

The perineurium, or sheath of Henle, consists of layers of flattened cells, interspersed by thin layers of fine collagen fibrils aligned parallel to the axis of the nerve. The number of layers is highest proximally, progressively diminishing to a single layer at the finest distal cutaneous and intramuscular nerve branches. In larger nerves, septa composed of two or three layers of perineurial cells arising from the inner aspect of the sheath may subdivide individual funiculi into

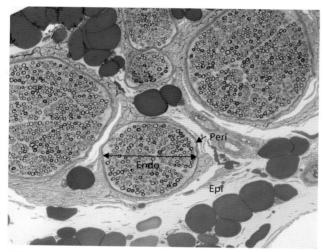

24.1 Architecture of normal peripheral nerve. Five individual fascicles are shown, with surrounding epineurium (Epi). Endo, endoneurium; Peri, perineurium.

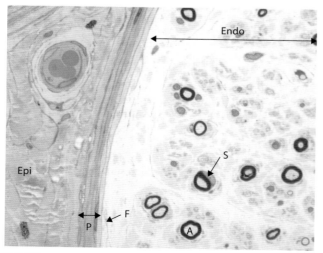

24.2 Micro-anatomy of peripheral nerve. A, axon; Endo, endoneurium; Epi, epineurium; F, fibroblast; P, perineurium; S, Schwann cell.

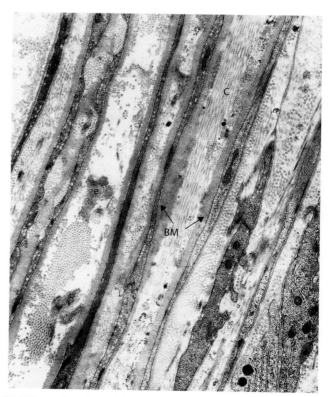

24.3 Normal perineurial ultrastructural appearance. Note the thin perineurial cells, both faces of which are covered by a thick basement membrane (BM). The connective tissue between the layers shows collagen fibrils (C) and elaunin (e).

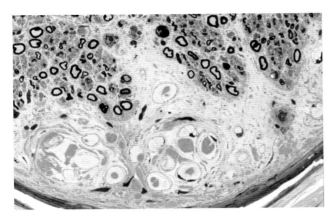

24.4 Renaut body.

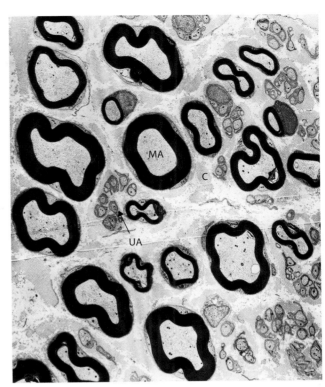

24.5 Normal endoneurial ultrastructural appearance. Note abundant collagen fibrils **(C)** within the matrix running in parallel with the axons. MA, myelinated axon; UA, unmyelinated axon.

two or more subsidiary fascicles. Blood vessels penetrating the perineurium to supply the endoneurial capillary plexus also carry sleeves of perineurial cells with them into the endoneurium for short distances.

In sections, the individual perineurial cells appear as thin sheets of cytoplasm, often no more than 0.1 μm thick, that contain occasional small cisterns of endoplasmic reticulum and numerous pinocytotic vesicles that open on to both the external and the internal surfaces of the cell (see Figure 24.3). The cells are somewhat thicker in their central zones (1.0–1.5 μm), where two equally thin layers of cytoplasm enclose a thin discoid nucleus. Both faces of the perineurial cells are covered by basal lamina, which may become thickened when compared with the basal laminae of other cells, even in quite young subjects, and to which the cell membrane may be anchored by scattered hemi-desmosomes. The connective tissue between these layers of cells consists of collagen fibrils (40–80 nm) and occasional elastic fibrils. The outer layers may also contain occasional fibroblasts and mast cells. At their margins, the individual perineurial cells overlap and interdigitate and are linked by tight junctions between their apposed membranes. Renaut bodies (see Figure 24.4) are normal subperineurial structures that may be better shown in epon-embedded sections than in tissue embedded in paraffin. They are thought to be perineurial in origin, with constituent cells being epithelial membrane antigen (EMA)-positive and sometimes being mistaken for pathological structures.

The Endoneurium

The interstices between the fibres of peripheral nerves are packed with collagen fibrils in a mucopolysaccharide ground substance. This inter-fibre matrix constitutes the endoneurium. The great majority of the collagen fibrils run longitudinally in parallel with the nerve fibres (see Figure 24.5) and have a relatively uniform diameter in the range 30–65 nm. In addition, each nerve fibre is surrounded immediately outside the Schwann cell basal lamina by a thin sleeve of much finer, more irregularly disposed reticulin fibres. The principal cellular constituents of the endoneurium are fibroblasts. These are angular cells lacking a basal lamina that lie free between the endoneurial collagen fibrils. The endoneurial fibroblast population

has been reported to range from 5 per cent to 25 per cent of the nuclear profiles visible in transversely sectioned peripheral nerves, and it is believed to be responsible for the production of the major part of the extracellular endoneurial connective tissue.

Other cells that may be found within the endoneurium are mast cells and macrophages. Resident macrophages are a normal constituent of the endoneurium, contributing some 2–5 per cent of the population. They are situated predominantly near blood vessels or the inner aspect of the perineurium, and they tend to have a dendritic morphology, with their processes oriented along the longitudinal axis of the nerve. These CD68 immunoreactive cells are the principal intrinsic antigen-presenting cells of the PNS and express many of the antigens common to other tissue macrophages, including major histocompatibility complex (MHC) class I and class II antigens (see review[181]). Injury to, or disease of, peripheral nerves results in a rapid influx of a further haematogenously derived population of macrophages at the site of the lesion, the trigger for recruitment being the presence of degenerating axons. These cells play the predominant role in myelin phagocytosis, probably aided by the Schwann cells.

Function of Peripheral Nerve Sheaths

A primary function of the connective tissue that contributes to the structure of the peripheral nerve sheath is a mechanical one. The massed array of collagen in parallel with the nerve fibres has considerable mechanical strength and resilience, which may serve to protect the nerve fibres from the stresses imposed by movement of the bodily parts through which they run. The sheaths of peripheral nerves are also resistant to penetration by foreign materials and infective agents. A considerable body of experimental work has demonstrated that the principal barrier to the entry of materials into the peripheral nerve is the perineurial sheath, particularly its innermost layers in which the constituent cells are linked by a continuous series of tight junctional complexes. Such material that does enter the endoneurium appears to be transported actively across the perineurial cells *via* pinocytotic vesicles. The perineurial barrier may be disrupted by mechanical trauma or osmotic shock. The perineurial barrier may be circumvented at the sites of penetration of the perineurium by blood vessels and at the peripheral open ends of the perineurial tubes, particularly at the neuromuscular junction; the latter has been suggested to be an important portal of entry for viruses and toxins into the PNS.

Vasculature of Peripheral Nerves

Peripheral nerves are supplied by branches from their local regional blood vessels that ramify and branch within the epineurium. Pre-capillary vessels penetrate the perineurium at an oblique angle and are ensheathed for a short distance within the endoneurial compartment by internal prolongations of the innermost layers of the perineurial sheath. They then divide to supply the endoneurial plexus, which appears to consist nearly exclusively of capillaries. The plexus has a predominantly longitudinal orientation and drains directly to collecting blood vessels situated outside the perineurium, with few smooth muscle containing venules being found within the endoneurium.

The contacts between the edges of adjacent capillary endothelial cells of the endoneurial circulation are completely sealed by tight junctions, and, in most species, this arrangement provides a second and effective barrier to the penetration of higher-molecular-weight materials into the endoneurial compartment. This blood–nerve barrier is, however, much less effective in the spinal nerve roots and in the dorsal root and autonomic ganglia, to which plasma proteins and exogenous tracer molecules such as horseradish peroxidase have relatively unimpeded access. The anatomical basis for this difference has been attributed to a lack of tight junctions between the capillary endothelial cells of the endoneurial compartment at these sites and the presence of 'fenestrated' capillaries within the dorsal root ganglia of some species.

Nerve Fibres

The nerve fibres are readily distinguishable into two classes, myelinated and unmyelinated, according to the presence or absence of a densely staining sheath of myelin around the axon. All axons of the PNS are ensheathed by chains of satellite or Schwann cells along the greater part of their length; the term 'Remak cell' is used occasionally to distinguish Schwann cells that surround unmyelinated axons. Myelin is a proteophospholipid material produced by Schwann cells enclosing the axon. Myelinated fibres are distinguished further by their generally much larger calibre, having diameters in the range 2–20 μm in human peripheral nerves. Unmyelinated axons are always of small diameter and pass through the nerve trunk in groups of 8–15 within a common chain of Schwann cells. Nerve fibres have been classified according to their calibre into three groups: A, B and C (Table 24.3).

Transmission of the Nerve Impulse

The most significant axonal function is its capacity to transmit signals over considerable distances in the form of propagated action potentials. The basis of this property lies in the polarization of the axolemma, the internal surface of which is maintained at a negative potential of around 70 mV by energy-dependent adenosine triphosphate (ATP)-utilizing, ionic-pumps that are integral components of the membrane. The principal partitioned ion is sodium, and this is pumped outwards into the extracellular space. Electrical or mechanical disturbance of the axolemma at any point along

TABLE 24.3 Classification of mammalian peripheral nerve fibre types					
Type	Subtype	Myelinated	Function	Diameter (μm)	Conduction velocity (m/s)
A	α	Yes	Proprioception, somatic motor	12–20	70–120
	β	Yes	Touch, pressure, motor	5–12	30–70
	γ	Yes	Motor to muscle spindles	3–6	15–30
	δ	Yes	Pain, cold, touch	2–5	12–30
B		Yes	Preganglionic autonomic	<3	3–15
C	Dorsal root	No	Pain, temperature, some mechano-reception, reflex responses	0.4–1.2	0.5–2
	Sympathetic	No	Postganglionic sympathetics	0.3–1.3	0.7–2.3

its course results in a transient increase in permeability to sodium ions, which then flow into the cell down concentration and voltage gradients. The advance of current through the axoplasm causes depolarization of adjacent segments of the axolemma, resulting in a continuously propagated wave of depolarization, which spreads along the axon. In unmyelinated fibres, the large capacitance of the axon membrane attenuates forward axial flow of current within the axoplasm and limits conduction to a speed of around 1 m/s. In myelinated fibres, on the other hand, electrical activity is restricted to the narrow spaces between the myelin segments, the nodes of Ranvier (The Internode and Node of Ranvier, see p. 1423), with the myelin insulating the much more extensive intervening internodal segments of the axon membrane from depolarization; the effect of this localized activity is that ionic activity leaps from one node to the next in series, a process termed 'saltatory conduction'. The principal functional implication of this saltatory activity is a considerable enhancement of conduction velocity in myelinated fibres over that achieved by nonmyelinated fibres, i.e. to between 20 m/s and 70 m/s, depending upon fibre diameter and myelin sheath thickness, as well as to improve the metabolic efficiency of impulse transmission. Loss of one or more myelin segments from a myelinated axon, as a consequence of either naturally occurring pathology or localized experimental injury, results acutely in conduction block, but the axon subsequently develops the capacity to sustain continuous conduction, in a manner comparable to that seen in normal unmyelinated fibres.

The Axon

The axon of a peripheral nerve is a more or less cylindrical extension of the nerve cell body bounded externally by a prolongation of its cell membrane, the axolemma. Because of its great length (which may exceed 1 m in nerves to and from the human lower limb), when compared with the dimensions of the cell soma, the axonal cytoplasm, in most instances, contributes by far the largest component to the total mass of the neuron. Furthermore, this cytoplasm, termed 'axoplasm', lacks the cellular structures usually associated with protein synthetic activity or assembly (ribosomes, rough endoplasmic reticulum, Golgi membranes); this feature, in conjunction with the length of peripheral nerve axons, has important consequences for their growth, long-term maintenance and mechanisms of intracellular communication.

Axoplasm

The axoplasm of a peripheral nerve has a somewhat simple structure and internal organization when compared with the cytoplasm of its parent neuron (Figure 24.6). Neurofilaments, microtubules, mitochondria and smooth endoplasmic reticulum are present, but there is no rough endoplasmic reticulum or Golgi apparatus. All protein synthesis occurs in the cell body or locally at the nerve terminal. The smallest of the axoplasmic constituents that can be distinguished morphologically are microfilaments 5–7 nm in diameter, each of which is thought to be composed of paired helical chains of actin. They appear to be homologous with the thin filaments of muscle cells and contribute approximately 10 per cent to the total complement of

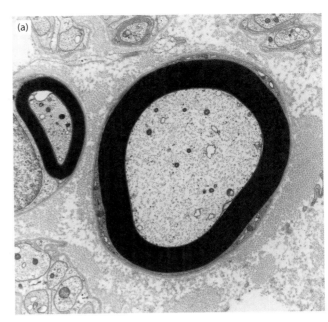

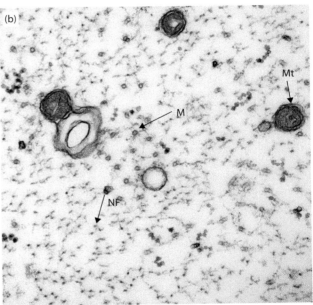

24.6 Normal axonal ultrastructural appearance. (a) Myelinated axon (×12 000); **(b)** high-power view of the axonal structures (×80 000). Note the neurofilaments (NF), microtubules (M), mitochondria (Mt) and the absence of rough endoplasmic reticulum and Golgi apparatus.

axonal protein. They are most conspicuous in the growth cones of actively elongating neurites and are less evident in unmyelinated axons and in the internodal portions of myelinated axons, where they appear to be confined to the cortical zone of axoplasm immediately subjacent to the axolemma. They may have contractile function and play a part in the mechanisms responsible for intra-axonal transport, growth cone motility and axon guidance.[112,187]

Neurofilaments are far more obvious and ubiquitous components of axoplasm (see review[269]). These are longitudinally oriented filaments of 8–11 nm in diameter, linked by ill-defined lateral interconnections of a less dense axoplasmic component into an irregular polygonal lattice. Neurofilaments have a packing density of the order of 100–300/μm^2 of axon cross-sectional area; this density remains constant along the length of individual axons and is not affected by changes in axon diameter. Biochemical studies indicate that neurofilaments are composed of four or five chains of globular protein subunits and are akin, but not identical, to the 10-nm 'intermediate filaments' of other cell types. The three principal constituent proteins have been identified and have molecular masses of 70 kDa (L), 160 kDa (M) and 200 kD (H). The L, M and H proteins are the products of separate genes and are immunocyto-chemically distinct. All contain α-helical, coiled-coil core domains with highly homologous amino acid sequences, and all are phosphorylated *in vivo* on both amino-terminal head and carboxy-terminal tail regions, with numerous isoforms. The degree of phosphorylation is an important determinant of their functional and immunological properties. Phosphorylation of the carboxy-terminal domain may play a part in stabilizing the axonal cytoskeleton by promoting cross-linking between the individual filaments. The degree of phosphorylation of the amino-terminal head regions of the subunits may be of importance in controlling their assembly into filaments and the stability of such filaments once formed.

The axoplasm also contains microtubules, an additional class of larger-diameter filamentous structures, sometimes referred to by the specific term 'neurotubules'. They play a major role in axonal transport (see Axoplasmic Flow and Intra-axonal Transport, below). They are oriented longitudinally and occur singly or in parallel arrays. In cross-section, the microtubular walls can be seen to be composed of 13 globular, 4-nm subunits of the protein tubulin, arranged in a simple 4 nm by 5 nm lattice. The greater part of this material exists in two distinct monomeric forms, α and β, having molecular weights of 57 kDa and 54 kD, respectively. Each microtubule is composed of helically arranged chains of alternating α and β monomers.

Cross-linking between individual microtubules to form arrays, and between microtubules and adjacent neurofilaments, is a function of a range of microtubule-associated proteins (MAPs) of high relative molecular mass. These include MAP1, MAP2, found predominantly in dendrites, and tau, a rod-like molecule of 55–70 kD, which is the predominant MAP in axons. Microtubules in neurites are usually much more stable than those in most interphase cells, owing to the presence of neuronal MAPs. The axoplasm also contains a variety of types of membranous organelle, including mitochondria, smooth endoplasmic reticulum, lysosomes and empty and dense-cored vesicles of a range of sizes.

Axoplasmic Flow and Intra-axonal Transport

The problems of maintenance and communication presented to a cell such as the neuron, in which most of the cytoplasm is at a considerable distance from the cell soma and its nuclear-controlled metabolic systems have been much investigated (see review[187]). There are well-organized transport mechanisms within axons capable of moving material both towards and away from the cell body concurrently and at a variety of rates. Most of the proteins that are needed in the axon and synaptic terminals are synthesized in the cell body and transported along the axon in membranous organelles or protein complexes. In the axon and dendrites, microtubules run in a longitudinal orientation and serve as rails along which membranous organelles and macromolecular complexes can be transported. Microtubules have intrinsic polarity, with a fast-growing 'plus end' and an opposite, slow-growing 'minus end'. Microtubules in axons and distal dendrites are unipolar, with the plus end pointing away from the cell body. However, the microtubules in proximal dendrites are of mixed polarity. Molecular motors of the kinesin and dynein super-families move along microtubules. Many kinesin super-family proteins move towards the plus end of microtubules ('plus end-directed motors') and participate in anterograde transport, selectively transporting molecules from the cell body to axons and dendrites. By contrast, retrograde transport, from the axonal or dendritic terminals to the cell body, is carried out mostly by cytoplasmic dyneins, which are minus end-directed motors. The anterograde transport mechanisms have been found to operate at a minimum of two and probably in excess of five different rates. For the purposes of description, these are usually divided into a slow transport component, moving at 0.25–4 mm/day, and a fast transport component, which may reach speeds in excess of 400 mm/day.

Unmyelinated Nerve Fibres

The principal structural features of a typical unmyelinated nerve fibre are illustrated in Figure 24.7. Each small-diameter axon lies recessed within a separate cleft in the surface of the Schwann cell, itself one of a chain of similar cells arranged end-to-end with some overlap and

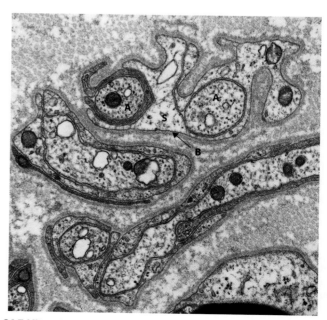

24.7 Ultrastructural appearance of unmyelinated axons. The axons **(A)** lie recessed within the surface of the Schwann cell **(S)**. A single basal lamina **(B)** surrounds the entire fibre.

interdigitation of the terminal processes at their points of junction. The apposed cell membranes that form the wall of the cleft contain the axon and connect it to the surface of the Schwann cell are known as the 'mesaxon'. A single basal lamina surrounds the entire fibre. A not uncommon feature of unmyelinated fibres is the enclosure of bundles of endoneurial collagen fibrils within a longitudinal furrow in the surface of the Schwann cell. Such collagen pockets appear to be formed only by the Schwann cells of unmyelinated fibres, and it has been suggested that they may serve to anchor the unmyelinated fibre to the adjacent endoneurial connective tissue.

Unmyelinated axons are small, ranging in diameter from 0.2 μm to 3.0 μm in humans, with a unimodal size distribution having its peak at around 1.5 μm. Even smaller diameter axons (i.e. <0.1 μm) may be seen in pathological material, and such small profiles are usually considered to represent regrowing axonal sprouts. The axoplasm of unmyelinated fibres shows no evidence of regional specialization and contains representatives of all of the subcellular components listed in the aforementioned general description of axoplasm. The only general features that distinguish them from the axons of myelinated fibres are the much higher proportion of axonal microtubules compared with neurofilaments, the frequent presence of dense-cored vesicles in autonomic efferent fibres, and a higher density of sodium channels; unmyelinated fibres possesses sodium channels at a density of around $110/\mu m^2$ compared with $25/\mu m^2$ in the internodal axolemma of myelinated fibres.

Myelinated Fibres

The features of myelinated axons that distinguish them from their unmyelinated neighbours are their large diameter (which may occasionally exceed 20 μm), the enclosure of each within its own individual chain of Schwann cells, and the presence of a myelin sheath, which is a proteophospholipid multilayered spiral derived from the apposed and compacted membranes of a greatly elaborated Schwann cell mesaxon. Ultrastructurally, a radially repeating structure of alternately dense and less dense lines is seen. The dense lines are derived from the cytoplasmic aspect of each pair of membranes, and the less dense lines from the apposed outer surfaces of each pair of membranes.

The thickness of the myelin sheath varies in fibres of differing axonal diameters, large fibres having thicker sheaths than smaller diameter fibres. The relationship between axon diameter, d, and fibre diameter, D (i.e. d + twice the myelin sheath thickness; Figure 24.8), is usually expressed as the ratio d/D, or the g-ratio. In the human sural nerve, the g-ratio normally has a mean of about 0.65. An abnormally thin myelin sheath has a g-ratio greater than 0.7 and an abnormally thick sheath has a g-ratio less than 0.4.

Structure and Chemical Composition of Myelin

Myelins of the CNS and PNS are broadly similar in their constitution, but consistent differences can be found. For example, peripheral and central myelin have only one protein in common. PNS and CNS myelin lipid compositions differ with PNS myelin containing a much larger proportion of sphingomyelin and glycoprotein. Differential extraction

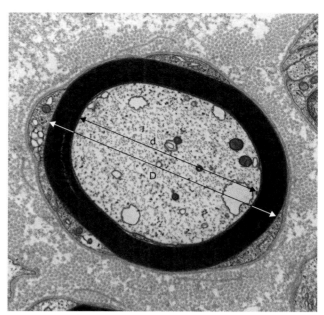

24.8 Calculation of g-ratio: g-ratio = d/D, where d is axon diameter and D is fibre diameter.

of myelin glycolipid content during processing accounts for variation in staining (i.e. PNS-purple, CNS blue-green) with Luxol fast blue-periodic acid Schiff (LFB-PAS).

The principal PNS myelin protein is P_0, a type I transmembrane glycoprotein, which contributes 50 per cent of the total myelin protein and is thought to play an important role in myelin compaction and in stabilizing the major dense line. Autoantibodies against P_0 have been associated with a severe childhood hypertrophic neuropathy, and mutations in the P_0 gene have been implicated in the inherited neuropathies hereditary motor and sensory neuropathy 1B (HMSN-1B) and Dejerine–Sottas Disease (DSD; see p. 1438).

A further 15–20 per cent of the protein content of PNS myelin is provided by a series of myelin basic proteins (MBPs) of 12–22 kDa. These are highly charged molecules, located in the major dense line; deletions in the genes responsible for their production, although causing major changes in the CNS, have only minor effects on PNS myelin. Peripheral myelin protein 22 (PMP22) is a 22-kDa membrane-associated protein that contributes a further 2–5 per cent of PNS myelin protein. Its exact function is unknown, but mutations in the PMP22 gene are responsible for CMT disease type IA.[439] A further 15-kDa protein, P2, is located in the myelin major dense line in concentrations ranging from less than 1 per cent to 14 per cent, depending upon the species studied. It has a single structural domain and appears to have lipid-binding properties.

The other major component of peripheral nerve myelin is myelin-associated glycoprotein (MAG), which consists of five extensively glycosylated extracellular immunoglobulin-like domains and is localized to the external and periaxonal layers of the myelin sheath and to non-compact myelin at the Schmidt–Lanterman incisures and paranodal terminal. Myelin-associated glycoprotein may be involved in Schwann cell–axon interactions and is one of the glycoproteins expressing a carbohydrate epitope that is the target antigen for immunoglobulin M (IgM) monoclonal antibodies in patients with a demyelinative neuropathy that may develop in association with gammopathy (see Neuropathy of Dysproteinaemia, p. 1480). An additional protein associated with non-compact myelin, gap junction protein β1 (GJB1, also known as connexin 32), is localized to the paranodes and the Schmidt–Lanterman incisures and may participate in a 'short-cut' transmyelin connection for ions and low-molecular-weight compounds between the adaxonal and abaxonal Schwann cell cytoplasm. Mutations in the *GJB1* gene are the second most common mutations in CMT. The molecular anatomy and genetics of myelin proteins in the PNS were reviewed by Snipes and Suter.[475]

The Schwann Cell

Schwann cells are derived during development from the neural crest and, to a lesser extent, the neural tube. They accompany, or possibly precede, the outgrowing neurites of the primitive peripheral nerves. The factors that lead to the selection of some axons but not others for myelination are still largely unknown, but experimental studies have shown that all Schwann cells, including those of normally wholly unmyelinated autonomic nerve trunks, are competent to produce myelin. The axon provides the stimulus (probably neuregulin-1)[377] necessary for the initiation of myelin formation, the signalling being related to axon calibre.[400] The processes that lead to the final mature pattern of axon calibre and ensheathment by satellite cells[331] also involve the spontaneous loss of some axons and Schwann cells. Schwann cells respond acutely to loss of their contained axon by proliferation within the pre-existing basal lamina tube to form the 'bands of Büngner' characteristic of wallerian and axonal degeneration (see Axonal Degeneration, p. 1424; but in chronically denervated nerve trunks, the Schwann cells dwindle in number and are replaced by connective tissue, indicating their trophic dependence on innervation in the longer term.

The gap between the innermost Schwann cell membrane and the axolemma is known as the periaxonal space. Over the greater part of the internode, this space is represented by a uniform interval of 20–25 nm between the two membranes; the gap is obliterated at either end of the myelin segment by close attachment of the proximal and distal margins of the myelin spiral to the axolemma immediately adjacent to each node. Apart from this specialized myelin attachment zone, specific contacts have not been described between the axolemma and the adaxonal Schwann plasma membrane. The external compartment of the Schwann cell is more substantial and more complex in its arrangement. Major accumulations of material occur adjacent to both poles of the longitudinally oriented ellipsoidal nucleus, which generally lies slightly distal to the midpoint of the internodal segment. This perinuclear cytoplasm contains conspicuous accumulations of rough endoplasmic reticulum, Golgi membrane systems and mitochondria and is clearly the site of considerable metabolic activity (Figure 24.9). Two other organelles that may be found within the external Schwann cell compartment in the fibres of larger mammals and humans are (i) the Reich or pi granule (Figure 24.10), a metachromatic rod-shaped body about 1 μm long and containing fine granular material stacked in regular lamellae with a spacing of 5–6 nm; and (ii) the Marchi-positive globular Elzholz body

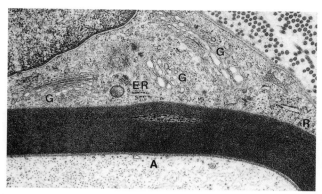

24.9 Ultrastructural appearance of the perinuclear region of the Schwann cell. A, axon; ER, endoplasmic reticulum; G, Golgi apparatus; R, ribosome.

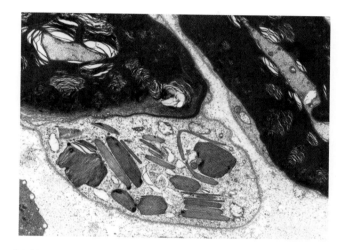

24.10 Reich or pi granules are seen within the cytoplasm of this myelinating Schwann cell.

containing unsaturated lipid. Both occur most frequently in the perinuclear zone of the Schwann cell, and both are probably forms of secondary lysosomes.

Schmidt–Lanterman Incisures

In small-diameter fibres, the only connection between the inner and outer Schwann cell compartment is *via* the continuous spiral of Schwann cytoplasm within the expanded end of each layer of the myelin sheath, where these make contact with the axolemma at the margins of the nodes of Ranvier. In larger-diameter fibres, the compact myelin is interrupted at intervals by the presence of oblique clefts at an angle of about 9° to the long axis of the sheath, the incisures of Schmidt–Lanterman, with the result that the sheath is divided into a series of interlocking cylindricoconical segments. Electron microscopy (Figure 24.11) shows the incisures to be narrow oblique zones at which the myelin lamellae are compacted less tightly than elsewhere along the sheath. Lamellar continuity is maintained, but the major dense line, the fused cytoplasmic surfaces of the paired membranes that constitute each lamella, is replaced by a continuous spiral of Schwann cytoplasm, which thus

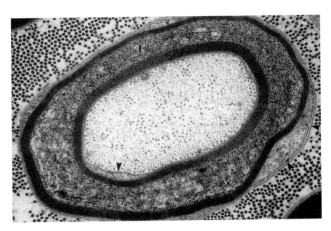

24.11 Ultrastructural appearance of a Schmidt–Lanterman incisure (I). Arrowheads mark the inner and outer mesaxons.

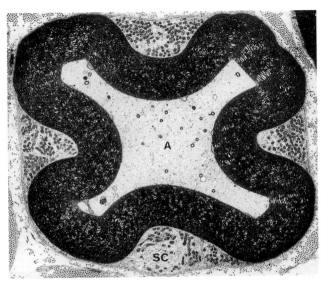

24.12 Paranodal region. A, axon; SC, Schwann cell.

connects the outer, nuclear and inner adaxonal, Schwann cell compartments, the 'spiral of Golgi–Rezzonico' of light microscopy. The intraperiod line of the myelin to either side of the cytoplasmic spiral also separates at the incisure, creating potential paired spiral extracellular connections between the endoneurium and the periaxonal space beneath the myelin sheath. The functional significance of the Schmidt–Lanterman incisures is still an open question. They provide a pathway for protoplasmic connections between the inner and outer compartments of the Schwann cell, and this may be the route by which metabolic materials may pass between these two parts of the cell, and possibly onwards to the axon–a transport function that is supported by the near-universal presence of one or more microtubules within the cytoplasmic spiral of the incisures. The adjacent extracellular spirals at the intraperiod line to either side of the cytoplasmic component may also permit interchange of ions between the periaxonal space and the exterior of the fibre, although it is claimed that both the outer and the inner ends of this cleft are sealed by tight junctions. Equally little is known for certain about the role of the incisures in the normal metabolism of myelin sheaths, their growth in length or thickness during development, or to what extent the presence or absence of incisures may influence the electrical properties of myelinated nerve fibres. Mechanical damage to nerves results in dilation of the incisures, and where nerve degeneration occurs distal to a nerve section (i.e. in wallerian degeneration), the fragmentation of the myelin sheath into primary ovoids appears to be initiated at the sites of the swollen incisures, which have been shown to be rich in acid phosphatase and esterases.

The Internode and Node of Ranvier

At the point along the axon where two Schwann cells meet, the myelin sheath formed by each one ends and the two Schwann cells extend cytoplasmic processes that interdigitate with one another and separate the axolemma from the extracellular space. This region is termed the 'node of Ranvier' (Figures 24.12–24.14). An internode is the distance covered by one Schwann cell (usually 200–1500 μm in length, see review[442]). A fairly close and direct relationship exists between axon diameter and internodal length,

small fibres having short internodes and large fibres longer internodes. During development, the total number of Schwann cells along the length of an axon is fixed, and subsequent growth in fibre length is accommodated by elongation of this finite population of Schwann cells and their contained myelin segments. Internode length can be evaluated diagnostically if individual fibres are teased out and examined longitudinally. Excessively short myelin segments occur, representing a manifestation of previous Schwann cell damage with subsequent regeneration.

The Schwann cell basal lamina is continuous across the node of Ranvier. Histochemical studies at a fine structural level have demonstrated that the gap substance filling the space between the Schwann cell nodal processes and the basal lamina contains glycosaminoglycans with cation-binding and -exchange properties. The gap substance may act as an ion-exchange buffer with a capacity to concentrate and maintain a high but osmotically inactive concentration of sodium ions immediately adjacent to the axolemma, and to limit diffusion away from the axolemma of potassium ions, which have passed outwards through the membrane during the passage of an action potential. The axolemma underlying the nodal region is rich in sodium channels important for impulse propagation (see Transmission of the Nerve Impulse, p. 1418); these are seen as a patchy electron-dense 'undercoating' of amorphous osmiophilic material some 20–30 nm thick on electron microscopy (see Figures 24.13–24.14). In contrast, the normal internodal sodium channel concentration is insufficient to maintain a propagated impulse. Both the arrangement and the content of organelles within the nodal and juxtanodal axon show consistent differences from those seen elsewhere along the internode. The vesicle content of the nodal axoplasm is increased, and elements of the axonal smooth endoplasmic reticulum, microtubules, lamellated autophagic vesicles, dense lysosome-like granules of varying size and glycogen granules are also found in greater numbers in the nodal

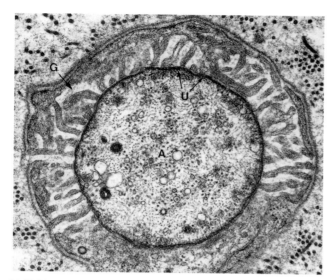

24.13 Node of Ranvier. A, axon; G, gap substance; U, 'under-coating'.

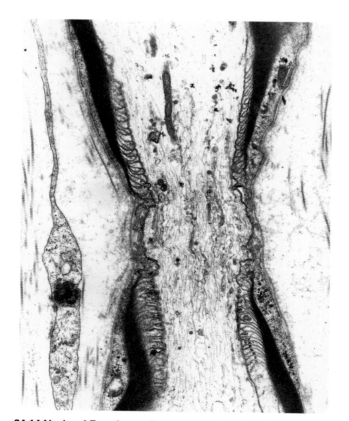

24.14 Node of Ranvier and paranodal region, longitudinal.

axon (see Figure 24.13). Relatively few neurofilaments are evident in transverse sections of the nodal axon, and these retain the same packing density as in the internodal regions. Mitochondria are approximately five times more numerous in the paranode, reflecting the existence of continuous energy-consuming activity in this region of the Schwann cell. Schwann cell mitochondria help maintain the axoglial interactions required for the long-term support of

unmyelinated and myelinated axons as shown by the results from the selective deletion of TFAM, a mitochondrial transcription factor, in Schwann cells.[524] The paranodal portion of adjacent Schwann cells at each node, including their nodal microvilli and gap substance, forms a functional unit, the paranodal apparatus; this may function to provide a source of energy-rich compounds to fuel the ion-translocation mechanisms necessary to maintain the polarization of the nodal axolemma, either directly or by controlling the ionic milieu within the nodal gap.

BASIC PATHOLOGICAL MECHANISMS

Although there are several hundred experimental, veterinary and clinical conditions that result in dysfunction of peripheral nerves, their pathological substrates can be classified into a few patterns of injury. These important processes can be divided into axonal degeneration, segmental demyelination, secondary demyelination, axonal atrophy and axonal dystrophy, each of which is discussed subsequently in this section. In a number of conditions, several of these patterns occur simultaneously or sequentially, for example sublethal degenerative axonal changes or axonal atrophy resulting in secondary demyelination. Although the current focus in this chapter is the axon, Schwann cell and myelin sheath, the cell body ('neuronopathy') may represent an early and critical target that induces secondary changes in peripheral nerves.

Axonal Degeneration

Axonal degeneration, by far the most common form of axonopathy, is produced by a myriad of disease entities, toxins and drugs. The process by which nerves are damaged and reconstituted is a complex ballet of degeneration and regeneration in which multiple cellular elements play a role (Figure 24.15) (reviewed[122]). The structural and molecular events associated with axonal injury have been studied most extensively in nerve damaged by mechanical crush injury, i.e. the paradigm initially used by Waller–'wallerian degeneration'[540]–a process that shares many features with axonal degeneration.

Axonal Events

Although the ability to conduct impulses is maintained for as long as 48 hours distal to a site of axonal transection,[61] a variety of structural and biochemical changes begins almost immediately. Within hours, organelles in transit within the distal axon accumulate in paranodal regions and in the perilesional parts of the proximal and distal stumps, where they distend the axon and thin the overlying myelin sheath (Figure 24.16). Disorganization of axonal microtubules and the endoplasmic reticulum occurs within 12–24 hours.[324] The neurofilamentous cytoskeleton is degraded shortly thereafter as the result of Ca2+ influx *via* ion-specific channels and subsequent activation of the protease calpain,[542] with contribution by the proteosome–ubiquitin system,[134] producing watery unstructured axoplasm (Figure 24.17).[324] These changes may occur even more quickly in small axons, which are engulfed by Schwann cells and macrophages. Axonal degeneration

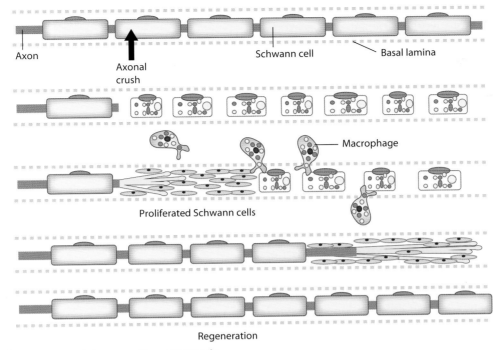

Axon

Axonal
crush

Schwann cell

Basal lamina

Macrophage

Proliferated Schwann cells

Regeneration

24.15 Peripheral nerve: axonal degeneration schematic.

Based on Poirier J, Chevreau J. Feuillets d'histologie humaine. Paris: Maloine, 1970.

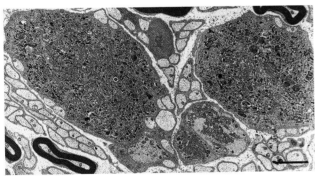

24.16 Wallerian degeneration 48 hours after nerve section. Dilated expansions of unmyelinated axons close to the site of transection are filled with numerous subcellular organelles. ×9500.

occurs independently of classic apoptotic cascades.[152] These degenerative changes have been variously reported to develop simultaneously along the entire nerve fibre or, conversely, in a proximodistal gradient, with differences depending on the focus on axonal or Schwann cell/myelin changes, respectively.[504]

Studies of the *Wld^s* (*wallerian degeneration slow*) mutant mouse, in which a striking post-transection maintenance of axonal function and integrity may delay wallerian degeneration for up to 3 weeks, suggest that degeneration of the distal axonal segment is an active process rather than simply a loss of synthetic support normally provided by the perikaryon.[402,541,565] The delay results from increased expression of the *Wld^s* fusion protein, resulting in increased expression of nicotinamide mononucleotide adenylyltransferase, increased nuclear nicotine adenine

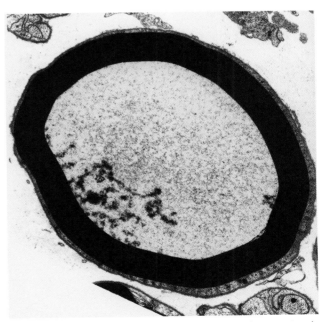

24.17 Early axonal degeneration. The axon shows granular disintegration of its cytoskeleton (microtubules and neurofilaments) in the presence of an intact myelin sheath. ×1250.

dinucleotide (NAD) levels and, subsequently, increased activity of the NAD-dependent deacetylase SIRT1.[13] *Wld^s* protein not only saves axons from wallerian degeneration but also preserves the integrity and function of synaptic connections and confers resistance to experimental toxic neuropathies.[170] The dual leucine kinase (DLK) has been shown to promote degeneration of severed axons in

Drosophila and mice, and its target JNK promotes degeneration locally in axons as they commit to degenerate. Similar mechanisms promote axonal degeneration after exposure to chemotherapy, evidence for participation in a general axon self-destruction program.[326] Several lines of evidence (see review[402]) suggest that both wallerian degeneration and axonal degeneration are molecularly distinct from apoptosis and that both processes may operate within a single neuron. Differences between protection of sensory and motor axons and their endings in *Wld^s* mice may be accounted for by variation in the overall amount of expression of Wld^s protein expressed in sensory and motor neurones and their axonal branches.[366] Although wallerian degeneration is greatly slowed in Wld^s neurons, neuronal apoptosis is not. Cultured Wld^s sympathetic neurons deprived of nerve growth factor (NGF) undergo rapid neuronal apoptosis (within 36 hours), whereas the axon survives for 6 days or more.[110] If the distal part of an axon of a wild-type cultured sympathetic neuron is locally deprived of NGF, that part degenerates while the rest of the cell body and proximal portions of the axon survive.[72] Predictably, wallerian degeneration and axonal degeneration induced by local NGF withdrawal are insensitive to caspase inhibitors.[402] Additionally, in Wld^s mice, transected axonal neurofilaments are degraded slowly, recruitment of macrophages is delayed, downregulation of myelin gene expression occurs more slowly, and the dramatic increases in NGF, p75 and tenascin-C mRNA levels that normally occur distal to the injury site in nerve do not occur.[484]

The distal portion of the longest axons may be preferentially involved in a wide variety of chronic neuropathies (e.g. those associated with acrylamide, diabetes, acquired immunodeficiency syndrome (AIDS), alcohol, arsenic, thallium, uraemia, isoniazid and many others)[76,402] each characterized by axonal degeneration that appears to spread from the distal part of the axon towards the cell body ('central–peripheral distal axonopathy' or 'dying-back neuropathy').[76] Although, intuitively, the distal axon would appear to be at the greatest risk because it is furthest from the neuron's synthetic source (the cell body), nerve terminals may be preferentially served by rapid axonal transport rather than representing the last stop on the slower forms of axonal transport. Accumulation of mitochondrial pathology, possibly reflecting injury secondary to local oxidative stress to the mitochondrial genome or difficulty with mitochondrial calcium homeostasis, may underlie distal axonopathy. Raff and colleagues proposed that dying-back axonal degeneration results from the activation of a self-destruct programme in the distal parts of an axon in response to a neuronal insult.[402] Specifically, the nature, extent and time course of an insult present a neuron with the choice of activating its caspase-dependent death programme and undergoing apoptosis or activating its caspase-independent, terminal axonal self-destruct programme while preserving its cell body and proximal axon segment.[402] Thus, the loss of the terminal axon may represent a controlled self-protective reaction to a metabolic burden, which allows the neuron to conserve its resources so that the preterminal axon and axon terminals can be regenerated at a later time when the neuropathic stress has abated.[402]

Schwann Cells, Macrophages and Myelin Catabolism

The initial destruction and early catabolism of myelin and axons are mediated by Schwann cells in a process that is probably triggered by a positive signal from the injured axon.[201,268] As axonal integrity is lost over the first 2 days after injury, degeneration of the myelin sheath begins. The first structural changes begin with paranodal myelin retraction and widening of Schmidt–Lanterman clefts, the site at which myelin begins to be degraded into short stretches ('myelin ovoids'; Figure 24.18),[324] resulting in Schwann cells containing an admixture of axonal and myelin debris (Figure 24.19). Within 2 days of injury, formerly myelinating Schwann cells have already downregulated steady-state mRNA levels of myelin-directed proteins.[268,402] Subsequently, they dedifferentiate and acquire a phenotype with features similar to pre-/non-myelinating Schwann cells, i.e. exhibiting increased expression of p75, GFAP, glial maturation factor β, cell adhesion molecules L1 and nerve cell adhesion molecule (NCAM), re-expressing Pax3 (a myelin gene repressor) and c-jun, and downregulating Krox-2.[63,226,246,402,586] Almost immediately following transection injury, mitotically quiescent Schwann cells in the

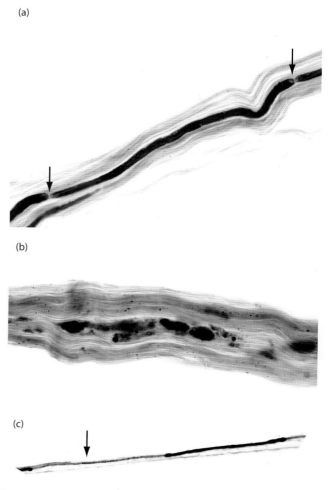

(a)

(b)

(c)

24.18 Teased fibre preparations of sural nerves. (a) Individual teased fibres show the appearance of normal axons (arrows, nodes of Ranvier); **(b)** those undergoing axonal degeneration; **(c)** segmental demyelination (arrow, demyelinated segment). ×150.

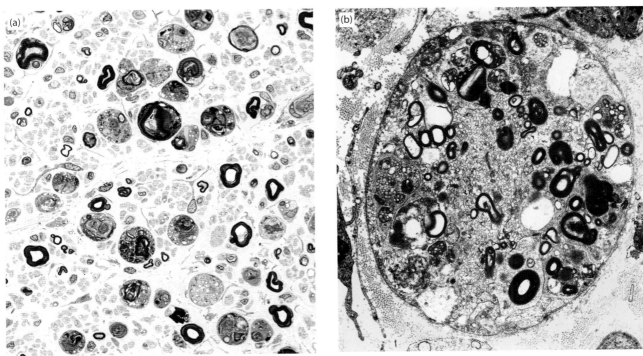

24.19 Axonal degeneration. Initial digestion of the axon and its myelin sheath occurs within the Schwann cell: **(a)** 1-μm plastic section, ×600; **(b)** electron micrograph, ×7500.

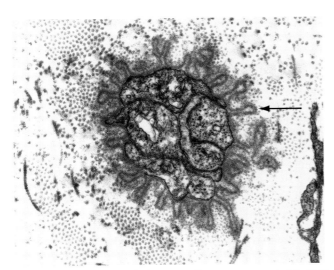

24.20 Band of Büngner. Schwann cell processes are held within the corrugated remnants of the original basal membrane (arrow) that enclosed the Schwann cell–axon unit. Electron micrograph, ×15 300.

distal stump proliferate to form aggregates of Schwann cell processes ('bands of Büngner') within the original basal lamina of the axon–Schwann cell unit (Figure 24.20). Schwann cell proliferation is greater in nerves with large myelinated axons than in those containing mostly small fibres. These changes involve the axonal growth cone and Schwann cell-derived neuregulin-1, functioning as a dedifferentiation factor, and upregulation of Schwann cell erbB2 and erbB3 neuregulin receptors, 3–7 days post-axotomy.[73] Neuregulin has a role in regulation of Schwann

cell apoptosis during the first postnatal week; later, the Schwann cell survival switches from neuregulin dependence (presumably an axonal factor) to dependence on endogenously produced non-neuregulin factors. Schwann cells not associated with axons will, in time, undergo apoptosis, whereas those in contact with axons will proliferate and migrate along the axon as needed, not synthesizing myelin until a proper numerical relationship is established.[73] Axonal neuregulin signals information about axon size to Schwann cells; hypomyelination and hypermyelination result from reduced expression and overexpression of neuregulin, respectively.[323] Schwann cell proliferation, derived from both myelinated and unmyelinated axons, peaks 3–4 days after injury and tapers off.

Macrophages are an important part of wallerian degeneration (Figure 24.21).[56] After 3–4 days, activated endogenous endoneurial macrophages are joined by haematogenously derived macrophages. Schwann cells actively participate in recruitment of macrophages by releasing a variety of mediators, such as interleukin 1β (IL-1β), stromal cell-derived factor 1 (SDF-1), leukaemia inhibitory factor, tumour necrosis factor α (TNF-α) and monocyte chemoattractant protein 1 (MCP-1).[147] In addition, mast cells release histamine and serotonin, enhancing capillary permeability and facilitating macrophage migration.[61] However, there is little evidence of substantive T-cell or more than transient neutrophil infiltration. Myelin phagocytosis differs in Schwann cells and macrophages; specifically, Schwann cell myelin catabolism is thought to be lectin-mediated and opsonin-independent, and macrophage-mediated myelin phagocytosis is opsonin-dependent, requiring complement receptor type 3 (CR3) expression on macrophages and complement component

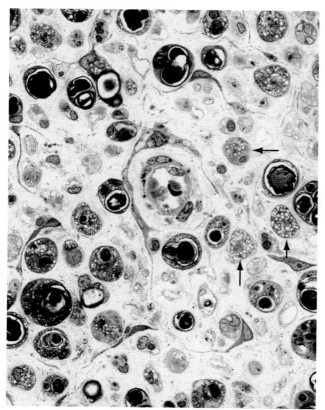

24.21 Axonal degeneration. Foamy macrophages (arrows), swollen with partially degraded axonal and myelin debris, accumulate near an endoneurial venule during axonal degeneration. 1-μm plastic section, ×600.

C3 on degenerating myelin sheaths.[57] Schwann cell myelin debris can be engulfed by macrophages as it is released into the extracellular space,[202,280] directly removed from the Schwann cell in an intimate, poorly understood process (Figure 24.22), or degraded *in situ* with residua maintained in the Schwann cell. Macrophages also participate in the synthesis and secretion of apolipoprotein E for reutilizing lipids.[476] Macrophages subsequently migrate to local lymph nodes and spleen. Lipid may accumulate in macrophages, fibroblasts, Schwann and perineurial cells and endothelial cells, and this material may persist for months.[324]

Axonal Regeneration

Within a few days of axonal injury, a series of changes in the distal segment begins to contribute to the formation of a micro-environment that is supportive of axonal regeneration.[147] Denervated Schwann cells are induced by macrophage-derived IL-1 and possibly transforming growth factor β (TGF-β)[278] to express NGF and its receptor p75,[20,495] which presumably entice and guide regenerating axons, serving both trophic and tropic roles.[495] Also increased are other neurotrophic substances, including glial cell-derived neurotrophic factor (GDNF) and its receptor GFRα,[192,509] brain-derived neurotrophic factor (BDNF),[2] fibroblast growth factor 2 (FGF-2), LIF[217] and insulin-like growth factor-1 (IGF-1) (produced by Schwann cells and

macrophages)[89] and its receptor. In contrast, the production of ciliary neurotrophic factor (CNTF), which is present in non-injured nerve, requires intact axon–Schwann cell interactions and, consequently, CNTF expression is reduced in the distal nerve stump.[458] A variety of cytokines (interleukins 6 [IL-6], 10 [IL-10] and 12 [IL-12], interferon γ [IFN-γ]), cell-surface molecules (NCAM, L1, ninjurin 1, ninjurin 2),[12] tenascin and N-cadherin, integrins that interact with type 2 laminin, and types IV and VI collagen contribute to the extracellular matrix of the regenerative milieu.[131,307]

Axon growth occurs along the surface of Schwann cells within the proliferated Schwann cell processes comprising the bands of Büngner and/or the inner surface of the original basal lamina of the Schwann cell–axon unit. It can be difficult to distinguish reinnervated bands of Büngner from Schwann processes alone, although this is often simplified by the demonstration of significant aggregates of ribosomes in Schwann cell processes, increased Schwann cell cytoplasmic osmiophilia, prominence of cytoplasmic filaments in Schwann cells, and microtubules in axonal processes. Depletion of Schwann cells does not influence axonal elongation when the basal lamina remains in continuity, which suggests a critical role of extracellular matrix proteins in axon regeneration.[157] Loss of growth-permissive Schwann cells in the denervated distal nerve pathways accounts for the progressive decline in the capacity of injured axons to regenerate back to their original targets.[487]

The outgrowth of initial, typically abortive, axonal sprouting may begin within a day of transection. By 5 days after injury, large numbers (as many as 25 from a single parent axon) of regenerating axon sprouts originate from the most distal part of the axon proximal to a crush injury site (Figure 24.23) or from nearby nodes of Ranvier.[504] Neuronal perikaryal synthesis of growth-associated protein 43 (GAP-43, a growth cone constituent) and cytoskeletal proteins peripherin and β-tubulin increases and neurofilament gene expression decreases.[484] However, growth cone initiation and guidance may also involve local protein synthesis,[556] particularly of cytoskeletal elements, and proteosome-dependent degradation.[521] Growth cones, the tips of regenerating axons (Figure 24.24), are rich in actin and tubulovesicular membrane elements and, when secondarily frustrated in their regenerative effort, may become engorged with organelles. In experimental and clinical crush injuries, a wave of axonal degeneration may precede regeneration; however, in most clinical cases, axonal degenerative and regenerative processes may occur simultaneously. Axonal regeneration is partially dependent on the reutilization of cholesterol within the endoneurium.[174] Regenerating axons are thought to receive polyribosomes from their accompanying Schwann cells.[106] Reported rates of regeneration, which vary widely from 0.5 mm/day to 9 mm/day (most typically 3–5 mm/day), decrease with increasing distance from the cell body.[61,73] Multiple axons begin to mature within a single Schwann cell tube, giving rise to small groups of thinly myelinated axons ('regenerative clusters'; red arrows, Figure 24.25a) held within the basal lamina of the original Schwann cell (arrow, Figure 24.25b), although, with time, the original basal lamina may disappear. One dominant axon emerges and the others regress, leaving behind a myelinated axon

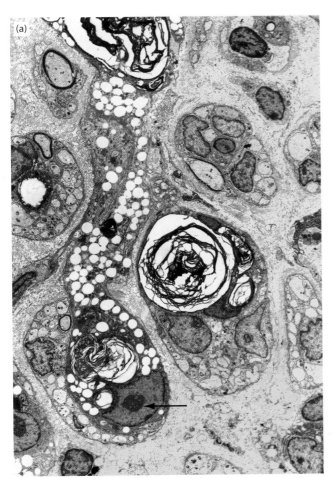 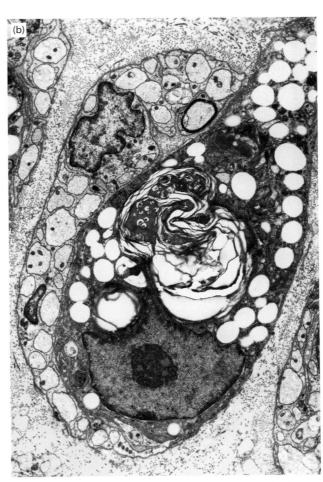

24.22 Macrophage phagocytosis in axonal degeneration/regeneration. A macrophage (arrow) is shown that has finished removing axonal and myelin debris from one Schwann cell containing regenerating axonal sprouts and is sending a process to a second Schwann cell at the upper margin of the micrograph. Electron micrographs: **(a)** ×1600; **(b)** ×3300.

with a myelin sheath that is relatively thin for its axon calibre (blue arrows, Figure 24.25a) but that may recover to nearly normal thickness with time.

As denervated Schwann cells are contacted by regrowing axons, the myelin-gene repressing transcription factor Pax3 and c-jun are downregulated, whereas SCIP (a transcription factor) is transiently upregulated, indicating a premyelinating Schwann cell stage.[246] Downregulation of SCIP is followed by reinduction of myelin-specific genes[268] and persistent expression of the transcription factor Krox-20, which is implicated in myelination.[268] Functional recovery eventually may occur, although reconstitution of the original complement of axons is uncommon. Failure of regeneration/reconnection results in loss of axon diameter proximal to the injury site[61] and relatively thick myelin for axon calibre. Large clusters of frustrated regenerating axons composing a traumatic neuroma suggest the failure to eliminate supernumerary axons. Regenerating unmyelinated axons have a more loose arrangement of axonal sprouts with basal lamina and Schwann cell processes and may persist as groups not associated with Schwann cell processes.

The mechanisms by which regenerating axons result in precise matching of the original axon with its Schwann cell tube are unknown. Experimental freeze injury, in which

regenerating axons are typically contained by their original basal lamina, favours regeneration.[61] Individual axons bearing a fluorescent reporter respond to crush injury by retracing their original pathway to form neuromuscular junctions on the same muscle fibres originally innervated.[341] Brushart showed that motor axons preferentially reinnervate motor pathways as a result of guidance molecules of the L2/HNK-1 family,[308] a carbohydrate epitope common to a family of recognition molecules. L2/HNK-1 is detectable in ventral root and motor axon-related Schwann cells of intramuscular nerves, but not in dorsal roots and sensory cutaneous nerves.[308] After nerve transection, myelinating Schwann cells previously associated with motor neurons differ from those that previously myelinated sensory axons by their ability to express L2/HNK-1 when contacted by motor axons. Regenerating rat femoral motor axons send out collateral branches into both appropriate and inappropriate nerve branches, the latter of which are pruned, perhaps as the result of deficient neurotrophic signals.[402] If regenerating axons reach a functionally unrelated end organ, then further maturation may not occur.

A chronic severe neuropathic process may result in an end-stage nerve in which only rare preserved axons are accompanied by scattered fibroblasts and diminished

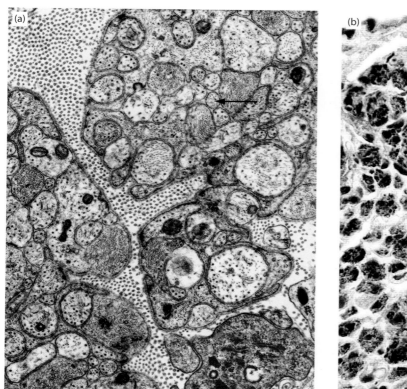

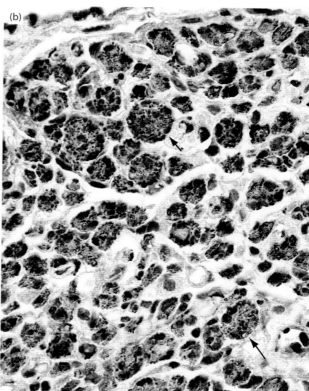

24.23 Early regenerating axonal sprouts. (a) Numerous tiny axonal sprouts (arrow) are shown admixed with Schwann cell processes following axotomy of a visceral nerve. Electron micrograph, ×16 000. **(b)** Neurofilament immunohistochemistry, ×450.

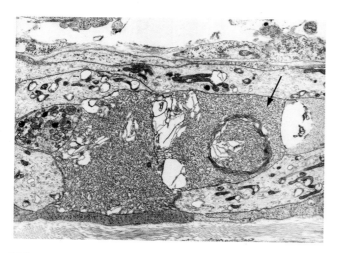

24.24 Growth cones regenerating in crushed rat sciatic nerve. A growth cone (arrow) containing large numbers of tubulovesicular elements is enveloped by Schwann cell processes. Electron micrograph, ×10 250.

numbers of Schwann cells, providing little information concerning the process that preceded it. Loss of unmyelinated axons may result in the formation of numerous 'collagen pockets' (Figure 24.26), in which longitudinal bundles of collagen are held by Schwann cells in lieu of axons, a process that may be deceptively unimpressive by light microscopy.

Teased fibre preparations may contribute to understanding the pathological history of individual axons in which axonal degeneration has previously occurred. Specifically,

morphometric plots of internodal length versus axonal diameter in normal nerves show a linear relationship; however, axons that have previously degenerated and regenerated have a uniform internodal length (200–400 μm) despite varying considerably in their diameter.

Wallerian Degeneration Versus Axonal Degeneration

Although the terms 'axonal degeneration' and 'wallerian degeneration' are used interchangeably, strictly speaking, wallerian degeneration refers to the microscopic reactions of a nerve segment distal to a site of crush or transection injury.[540] Clinical presentations resulting in wallerian degeneration include transection secondary to trauma, vertebral collapse with compression due to tumour or infection and vasculitis with ischaemia involving proximal nerve segments. Although there are similarities between the biochemical and pathological processes occurring in axonal degeneration and wallerian degeneration, in the latter the histological changes appear stereotyped and synchronized (i.e. most axons and Schwann cells in any given fascicle are at the same stage of reaction; Figure 24.27) whereas in chronic neuropathies axonal degeneration and regeneration often coexist in the same nerve fascicle. The histological appearance of wallerian degeneration is also stereotyped in contrast to axonal degenerations, in which distinctive pathological signatures differ between specific axonal degenerations. Pathological signatures include neurofilamentous aggregates (acrylamide, hexacarbon,

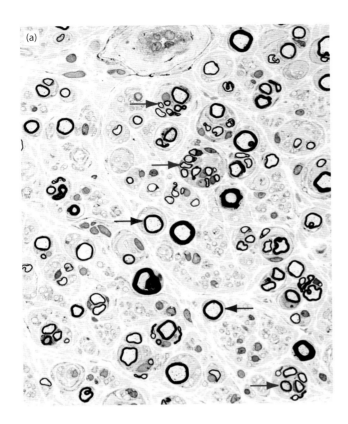

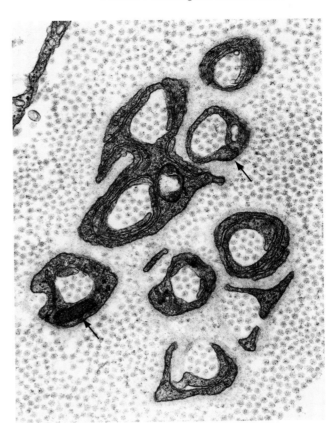

24.26 Collagen pockets surrounded by Schwann cell processes (arrows) may mimic intact unmyelinated axons when examined by light microscopy. Electron micrograph, ×23 200.

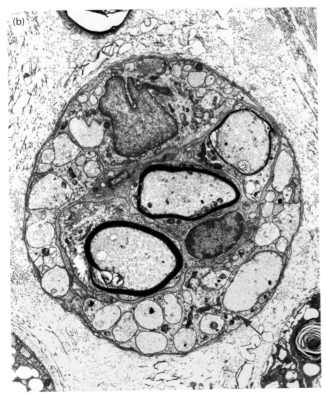

24.25 Regenerating axonal clusters. Groups of small thinly myelinated axons (red arrows), which represent maturing sprouts from a single parent axon, are visible by light microscopy **(a)** and ultrastructure **(b)**. Occasional regenerated axons have myelin sheaths too thin for axon calibre (blue arrows). (a) 1-μm plastic section, ×600; (b) electron micrograph, ×1750.

disulfiram), tubulovesicular aggregates (zinc pyridine-thione, tri-orthocresylphosphate), mitochondrial abnormalities (thallium) and neuroaxonal dystrophy. In some chronic neuropathies, an unusual Schwann cell response is evident in which adaxonal processes grow into the subjacent axon to form multiple compartments ('honeycombs'; Figure 24.28) that contain axonal organelles; this response presumably represents a mechanism to remove accumulated or dysfunctional intra-axonal organelles.[481] This unusual morphological change is seen most commonly in the axonal degenerations that accompany isoniazid treatment, thiamine deficiency, uraemia, porphyria, and intoxication with hexacarbon, acrylamide, thallium and cisplatin,[324] and is absent in wallerian degeneration.

Axonal Atrophy

Axonal atrophy is suggested by the demonstration of an axon inappropriately small for its surrounding myelin sheath, or separated from it by lucent adaxonal Schwann cell cytoplasm, as well as myelin wrinkles, bubbles and loops (Figure 24.29). The most definitive proof of axonal atrophy requires morphometric determinations in which the plot of the ratio of axonal diameter to axon 1 myelin thickness (i.e. the g-ratio) is altered. There are normal variations in axon diameter and myelin thickness near the node of Ranvier. Demonstration of atrophy has been accomplished

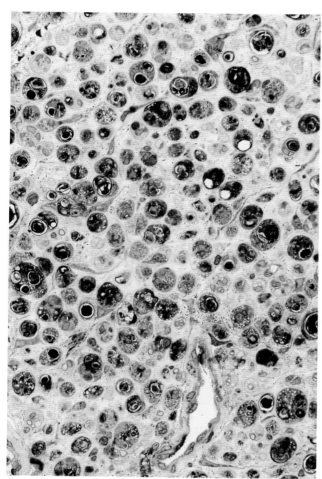

24.27 Wallerian degeneration. All visible myelinated fibres are degenerating synchronously in this patient with traumatic avulsion of the brachial plexus. 1-µm plastic section, ×600.

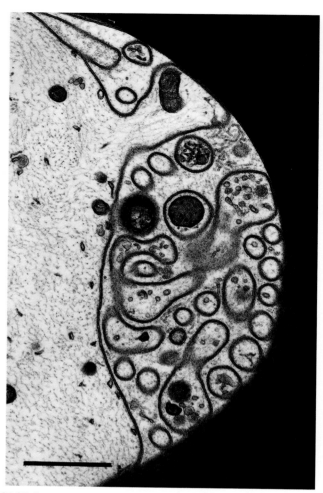

24.28 Axonal–Schwann cell network. Axonal debris may be sequestered by an adaxonal Schwann cell process, leading to 'honeycomb' formation. ×28 600.

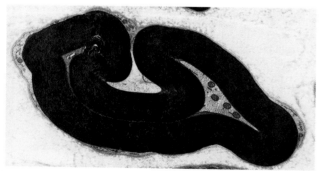

24.29 Axonal atrophy. The axon of this myelinated axon in a solvent-abusing patient is shrunken and atrophic and is enclosed by a collapsed and folded myelin sheath. Electron micrograph, ×11 000.

for neuropathies associated with uraemia, Friedreich's ataxia and permanent axotomy and, less definitively, for neuropathies associated with cisplatin and with human immunodeficiency virus (HIV), HMSN-I and HMSN-II, hereditary sensory and autonomic neuropathies (HSANs), and neuropathies associated with ethylene oxide.[324] Determination of axonal neurofilament density, which is similar between normal myelinated axons of different sizes, suggests atrophy if the axon is smaller but the neurofilament density is unchanged from that of normal axons in comparison with artefactual shrinkage in which axonal neurofilament density is increased.[324]

Axonal Dystrophy

A number of clinical and experimental processes appear to involve a specialized form of axonopathy, (neuro)axonal dystrophy, in which distal axons and nerve terminals balloon to an enormous size and have distinctive ultrastructural changes (Figure 24.30, Table 24.4).[444] Although often considered a form of axonal degeneration, dystrophic axonal segments are rarely seen to degenerate actively or be engulfed by macrophages/microglia and may, in some cases, represent a long-lived pathological structure. Dystrophic segments may not always represent termini and have been demonstrated as multifocal expansions along individual axons. Portions of axons distal to dystrophic axons may or may not degenerate. The continued supply of membranous elements may result in complex, occasionally crystalline membranous aggregates. Studies of gad (gracile axonal dystrophy) mutant mice identified an inactivation of the ubiquitin carboxy-terminal hydrolase, UCH-L1, a member of the ubiquitin–proteosome system, suggesting that the accumulation of organelles at the nerve terminal results from failure of their degradation.[256] Proposed pathogenetic mechanisms for axonal dystrophy include 'synaptic dysplasia' (an abnormal outcome of normal cycles of synaptic degeneration and regeneration), frustrated axonal regeneration and/or imbalance of orthograde, retrograde and turnaround axonal transport.[446]

Segmental Demyelination

The symbiotic relationship between the axon and the Schwann cell is only now being defined.[133] Localization of sodium and potassium channels at the node and juxtaparanode requires the presence of the Schwann cell[14,225] and sulphatide (sulfatide), a myelin constituent.[215] The Schwann cell locally influences the phosphorylation of neurofilaments, resulting in changes in axonal diameter,[115] and influences slow anterograde axonal transport.

Segmental demyelination represents preferential damage to one or several internodes of the myelin sheath with relative preservation of axonal integrity (Figure 24.31) and is the result of processes directed against the Schwann cell or the myelin sheath. Initial myelinopathy may be subtle, with vesicular degeneration, splitting of myelin lamellae, widening of the nodal gap or unusual folding of the myelin sheath. Vesicular demyelination represents splitting at the major dense line and can be seen in a variety of experimental and clinical diseases (diabetes, injection of GBS sera into animal nerves, radiation injury, intoxication with lead or tellurium)[324] and as an artefact of delayed fixation. Treatment of Schwann cell cultures with the calcium ionophore A23187 increases Ca2+ leakage into Schwann cell cytoplasm, activates endogenous phospholipase A2 and results in demyelination. Mechanical compression of nerve also produces myelinopathy. If sustained or of appropriate severity, a pathological process involving the Schwann cell or the myelin sheath results in the degeneration of the myelin sheath and, if the original Schwann cell survives

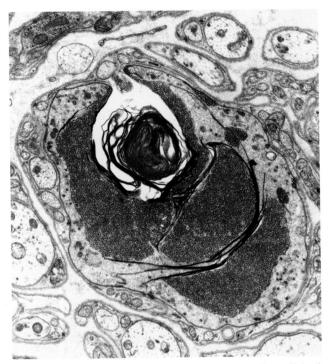

24.30 Axonal dystrophy. An unmyelinated axon in a diabetic sympathetic ganglion is swollen by unusual membranous collections. Electron micrograph, ×12 300.

TABLE 24.4 Conditions associated with neuroaxonal dystrophy (NAD)

Human	Experimental rodent models
Infantile neuroaxonal dystrophy (Seitelberger's disease)	Gracile axonal dystrophy (gad) mouse
Pantothenate kinase-associated neurodegeneration (formerly Hallervorden–Spatz disease)	Boggler deer mouse
Nasu–Hakola disease	Paraplegin-deficient mouse
Neuroaxonal leukodystrophy	Aged rat and mouse
Ageing (sensory and sympathetic)	BB/Wor and STZ diabetic rat
Schindler's disease (α-N-acetylgalactosaminidase deficiency, type I)	Glycosylasparaginase knockout mouse
	Rabbit inherited C6 deficiency
Diabetes (sympathetic ganglia)	Swainsonine intoxication
Vitamin E deficiency	Lumbosacral NAD (LND) mouse
Niemann–Pick disease, type C	Giant axonopathy mouse (gaxp) mouse
	Generalized NAD (gnd) mouse
Veterinary	Vestibulomotor degeneration (vmd) mouse
Equine grass sickness	Niemann–Pick type C mouse
Rottweiler inherited sensory ataxia	Rat bromophenylacetylurea (BPAU) toxicity
Feline inherited disease	Rat zinc pyridinethione toxicity

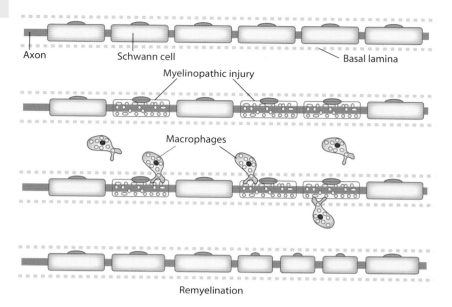

24.31 Peripheral nerve: segmental demyelination schematic.

Based on Poirier J, Chevreau J. Feuillets d'histologie humaine. Paris: Maloine, 1970.

the insult, myelin degradation typically begins within the Schwann cell cytoplasm. As in axonal degeneration, haematogenous and intrinsic macrophages engulf the debris provided by the Schwann cell. Myelin debris is usually cleared rapidly, and the presence of macrophages containing this debris after several weeks is evidence for ongoing demyelination. Macrophages can be the primary effector cells of active demyelination, as in GBS syndrome and chronic inflammatory demyelinating polyradiculoneuropathy (CIDP, see p. 1457), where they strip otherwise normal-appearing myelin or secondarily engulf myelin damaged by other processes, such as intraneural injection of lysolecithin. Schwann cell proliferation results in the eventual remyelination of individual internodes, typically replacing each lost myelin internode with several shorter intercalated internodes. Remyelination requires Schwann cell proliferation from demyelinated segments as well as adjacent unmyelinated axons. After remyelination, surplus Schwann cells are displaced peripherally, undergo atrophy and, with time, decrease in number,[324] unless cycles of demyelination occur before the elimination of supernumerary Schwann cells, which culminate in the formation of hypertrophic 'onion bulbs'.[504] Onion bulbs are characteristically seen in CMT-I (HMSN-I), Dejerine–Sottas disease (HMSN-III), Refsum's disease, CIDP, experimental allergic neuritis, lead neuropathy and recurrent external compression. The presence of onion bulbs suggests a cyclical demyelinative/remyelinative process active for several months or more. Although experimental insults may produce acute demyelination followed by remyelination, in nearly all demyelinative neuropathies, demyelination and remyelination occur concurrently.

Teased fibre analysis is particularly useful for establishing that a neuropathic process has a demyelinating component. Plotting axonal diameter versus internodal length in teased fibre preparations shows marked variation from node to node in previously demyelinated and remyelinated nerves compared with normal nerves; this pattern corresponds to the replacement of myelin originally lost from the domain of a single Schwann cell by several proliferated Schwann cells with smaller territories.

Secondary Demyelination

The concept of secondary demyelination integrates axonopathy and demyelination. In contrast to segmental demyelination, in which foci of demyelination are located randomly on individual axons, secondary demyelination preferentially involves selected axons, which may show atrophic or other degenerative axonopathic changes, while entirely sparing other axons. The mechanism appears to involve an abnormality in the relationship of the Schwann cell to its ensheathed axon, resulting sequentially in axonal atrophy and myelin wrinkling, followed by paranodal demyelination and segmental demyelination, and remyelination that may be cyclical.[127,131] The best-studied example is uraemic neuropathy, although the process may occur in a number of other diseases (e.g. acute intermittent porphyria, diabetes, Friedreich's ataxia, giant axonal neuropathy, thiamine deficiency, paraproteinaemic neuropathy, hexacarbon intoxication, Tangier disease)[324] and, in small numbers, in almost any axonal process. The presence of onion bulbs is most typically associated with primary segmental demyelination rather than secondary demyelination.

Hypermyelination

Most neuropathic processes reduce myelin thickness, either directly or as a result of regeneration; however, a few produce increased myelin thickness. Although focal areas of apparent increased myelin thickness (Figure 24.32) are encountered not uncommonly in a variety of neuropathic processes (e.g. IgM paraproteinaemic neuropathy, CMT (HMSN)-Ib, familial recurrent brachial plexus neuropathy), patients with 'hereditary neuropathy with pressure palsies' (HNPP) have focal thickening of the myelin sheath, forming 'tomaculi' ('sausages'). These are best seen with teased fibre analysis and result from an increased number of myelin lamellae produced by redundant folds, myelin loops ('jelly rolls') and reversals of myelin spiral direction.

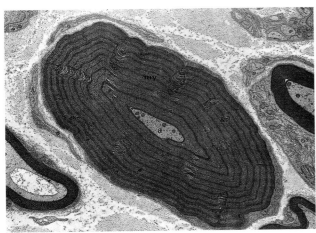

24.32 Hypermyelinated axon. This compressed axon is surrounded by markedly thickened redundant loops of myelin. Electron micrograph, ×10 600.

INHERITED NEUROPATHY

Neuropathy may occur as the salient manifestation of a variety of inherited disorders, in association with involvement of the CNS, or as part of a complex multisystem disorder. Primary inherited peripheral neuropathies are the most common monogenetically inherited diseases of the nervous system, with a prevalence between 1 and 4 per 10 000.[258,504] Many of these diseases have a relatively benign and slowly progressive course, with most patients leading a nearly normal life. In this section, we concentrate on some morphological and molecular-genetic aspects of CMT disease and related disorders, the hereditary sensory and autonomic neuropathies, the neuropathy of sphingolipidosis and the peripheral nerve changes of some rare inherited conditions (Table 24.5).

A short note on the morphogenesis of the 'onion bulb' is relevant from the outset because this histological abnormality is a common feature in many of the inherited polyneuropathies. Repeated episodes of primary segmental demyelination and remyelination lead to the formation of onion bulbs, a term that refers to imbricated layers of supernumerary Schwann cell processes arranged in rings around the long axis of nerve fibres separated by collagen fibres. Onion bulbs, the pathological hallmark of hypertrophic neuropathy, can be confidently detected only in cross-sections (Figure 24.33). In advanced cases, the added accumulation of extracellular matrix and collagen in the endoneurium results in distension of the fascicles by expansion of the intrafascicular area, which is easily recognizable by light microscopy (Figure 24.34). Although hypertrophic neuropathy is a prominent feature of several of the genetically determined neuropathies, onion bulbs can also occur in CIDP and, to a lesser extent, in diabetic neuropathy and other acquired polyneuropathies.

Charcot–Marie–Tooth Diseases

The syndrome of hereditary motor and sensory neuropathy (HMSN) or peroneal muscular dystrophy covers a heterogeneous group of inherited polyneuropathies[406] that have a

TABLE 24.5 Inherited neuropathies

Hereditary motor sensory neuropathy (Charcot-Marie-Tooth, CMT disease spectrum)
Hereditary focal recurrent neuropathies
Hereditary sensory and autonomic neuropathies
Neuropathy of sphingolipidosis
    Krabbe disease
    Metachromatic leukodystrophy
    Fabry disease
    Farber disease
    Gangliosidosis
    Niemann–Pick disease
    Neuronal ceroid lipofuscinosis
Other hereditary neuropathies
    Tangier disease
    Bassen–Kornsweig disease
    Adult polyglucosan body neuropathy
    Giant axonal neuropathy
    Neuroaxonal dystrophy
    Glycogen storage diseases
    Peroxisomal disorders
    Cerebrotendinous xanthomatosis
    Mitochondrial encephalomyopathies
    Chediak–Higashi disease
    Neuropathy in hereditary ataxia
    CADASIL

CADASIL, cerebral autosomal dominant arteriopathy with subcortical infarcts and leukoencephalopathy.

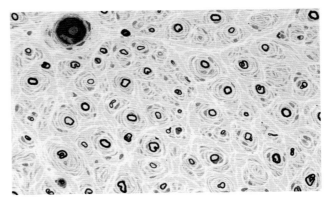

24.33 Charcot–Marie–Tooth disease, type 1. Transverse section of sural nerve, showing 'onion bulbs'. Epon-araldite, Thionin and acridine orange. ×600.

similar clinical phenotype: the development, during childhood or adolescence, of distal weakness predominantly in the lower limbs and often associated with foot deformities, with ensuing sensory loss of variable severity. Patients with pure motor involvement can be separated as examples of distal muscular atrophy. Because of the success of chromosomal linkage studies and gene identification in the separation of similar phenotypes, the designation of CMT disease is now the summary term[29] for the most frequent forms of inherited peripheral neuropathies that affect motor and sensory neurons and nerve fibres and have a complex pathogenesis.[443] Charcot– Marie–Tooth disease historically has been divided into the neuronal forms (characterized by normal or slightly slowed nerve conduction velocity) and the demyelinating or hypertrophic forms (in which nerve conduction velocity is markedly and diffusely reduced).[465] Patients who exhibit a peroneal muscular dystrophy syndrome without

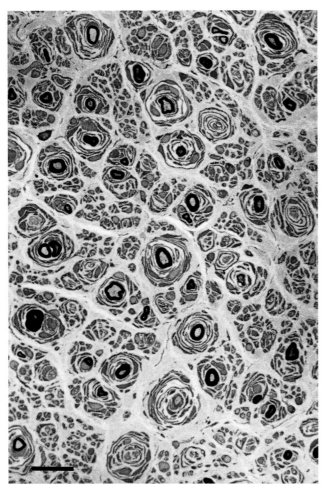

24.34 Hypertrophic neuropathy. Myelinated axons surrounded by concentrically proliferated Schwann cells. Plastic resin, ×1500.

clinical or electrophysiological evidence of sensory impairment are separated into the group of hereditary motor neuropathies or spinal muscular atrophy, including the distal hereditary motor neuropathies.[321]

Charcot–Marie–Tooth Disease Type 1

The most common variant of CMT disease is type 1 (formerly HMSN-I). The condition has a prevalence of 1 in 2500 and is characterized by motor nerve conduction velocity (MNCV) slowing (<38m/s) and autosomal dominant inheritance. Autosomal recessive forms[26,365] are classified as CMT-4 (see Charcot–Marie–Tooth Disease Type 4). Clinical onset in CMT-1 is during the first to fourth decades of life, and the course is protracted. Twenty per cent of patients have no family history and represent new mutations. Patients develop weakness and wasting distally in the lower extremities, associated with areflexia and sensory loss. The upper extremities are involved at a later stage. Pes cavus, hammer toes and scoliosis may be present as early manifestations from childhood. Distal weakness of upper limbs occurs in about 70 per cent of patients. Visible and palpable hypertrophy of peripheral nerves, especially the

greater auricular nerve, can be found. Some patients exhibit ataxia and postural tremor of the upper limbs; this has been designated the Roussy–Levy syndrome, but these patients are not genetically distinct from those with other CMT-1 variants. Marked slowing of nerve conduction is always demonstrated. Histology reveals expanded fascicular areas because of increased matrix and collagen; there are reduced numbers of myelinated nerve fibres, with a deficiency of both large- and small-diameter elements and evidence of extensive segmental demyelination and remyelination. Hypertrophic onion-bulb changes with concentric Schwann cell proliferation are frequent (Figure 24.34) and constitute the benchmark example of hypertrophic neuropathy.[160] Although estimation of nerve fibre density is obscured by the hypertrophic features, nerve fibre loss is variable and not uncommonly significant. Many thinly myelinated fibres are seen. Increased myelin spiral length in relation to axon diameter, which has been interpreted as evidence of axonal atrophy, possibly reflects overexpression of PMP22, leading to myelin thickening before demyelination occurs. Variable amounts of chronic inflammation can be found in some cases.[504] Histological assessment of muscle in patients with CMT-1 reveals chronic denervation with wide-ranging fibre type grouping and large group atrophy of myofibres.

Charcot–Marie–Tooth disease type 1 has several discrete genetic loci. The most common variant, accounting for 70–80 per cent of all patients, is due to a defect in expression of PMP22 protein that is caused by a tandem duplication of the PMP22 gene (on chromosome 17p11.2–p12).[207] Messenger RNA for PMP22 is significantly elevated in nerve biopsies of patients with CMT-1A.[569] DNA testing for CMT-1A is available, and it is an accepted part of the evaluation of any patient suspected to have hereditary neuropathy.[81] In CMT-1B, the defect is in another peripheral myelin protein, the P_0 protein (myelin protein zero, MPZ), whose gene is located on chromosome 1. Patients with CMT-1B are clinically indistinguishable from patients with CMT-1A. The light-microscopic features are also indistinguishable, but an ultrastructural finding that suggests the diagnosis of the myelin P_0 (MPZ) mutation (CMT-1B) is the presence of uncompacted myelin.[161] Charcot–Marie–Tooth disease type 1D, due to a mutation of *EGR2* (*early growth response 2* gene), has been described. EGR2 influences the transcription of other myelin protein genes and is most likely an important regulator of myelination. Other families with the CMT-1 phenotype do not appear to link to any of these genes, implying further genetic heterogeneity. For a complete and updated list of CMT genes, CMT loci and mutations, see www.molgen.ua.ac.be/CMTMutations.

Charcot–Marie–Tooth Disease Type 2

A less common condition is CMT-2 (formerly HMSN-II), which is the autosomal dominant neuronal form of the disease showing motor nerve conduction velocities of 38m/s or greater. The prevalence of CMT-2 is about one-third that of CMT-1. In seven large pedigrees, a missense mutation of *MFN2* (*mitochondrial fusion protein 2* gene) has been found to be the cause of CMT-2A.[588] Mitofusin 2 (Mfn2) is a mitochondrial membrane protein that participates in mitochondrial fusion in mammalian cells. Mfn2 loss of function inhibits pyruvate, glucose and fatty acid oxidation and reduces mitochondrial membrane potential. Experimental data support the notion that Mfn2 loss of function causes axonopathy by impairing energy production along the axon, which may reflect abnormal tethering of mitochondria to ER.[385] Data suggest that approximately 20 per cent of cases of CMT-2 are associated with MFN2 mutations. Type 2A CMT is clinically similar to CMT-1, although on average the phenotype is milder (peripheral nerves are not enlarged) and the disease develops later (mean age of onset 20 years), there is less prominent involvement of upper limbs (particularly the hands), and less ataxia, tendon areflexia and sensory loss. Histologically, this disorder displays ventral horn and spinal ganglia neuronal loss, maximal in the lumbosacral region, and tract degeneration in the gracilis fasciculi. In peripheral nerves there is mostly chronic axonal loss affecting large myelinated fibres, axonal atrophy as evidenced by an increase in the axon calibre/myelin thickness ratio, abundant regenerating clusters, and no hypertrophy (Figure 24.35).[30,74,189] That two inherited conditions of widely different pathogenesis would have a similar clinical phenotype is a source of confusion. In both the demyelinating (type 1) and the axonal (type 2) forms of CMT disease, patients have tapering of the legs below the knees, weakness and sensory loss in the distal extremities, and high arched feet and hammer toes. However, CMT-2 has a wider range of onset and disability than CMT-1. The different forms of CMT-2 are not distinguishable electrophysiologically, although some phenotypic characteristics are described for the subtypes. Mutations in the *RAB7* (*small GTPase late endosomal protein*) gene cause CMT-2B, a predominantly sensory neuropathy complicated by chronic foot ulcers and amputations.[267] Type 2D is associated with mutations of the *GARS* (*glycil tRNA synthetase*) gene and consists of upper extremity wasting and weakness, with corresponding sensory impairment; lower extremities are involved to a lesser degree.[267] Other mutations are likely to be discovered for other types of autosomal dominant CMT-2. Autosomal recessive forms of CMT-2 are called autosomal recessive CMT (AR-CMT). Recessive mutations of the LMNA (lamin A/C) gene are the cause of the axonal neuropathy in AR-CMT-2 (formerly known as CMT-4C

and CMT-2B1). The onset of this form of the disease is in the second decade, with rapid progression involving upper limbs and proximal muscles, leading to severe disability. Motor nerve conduction velocities are slowed slightly. Biopsies reveal a reduction of myelinated axons and clusters of regenerating units.[83] Other histological studies have found little regenerative activity and widespread depletion of large myelinated fibres in the absence of active degeneration, suggesting a maturation disturbance. Of interest is that particular LMNA mutations are associated with a number of other inherited diseases, including limb-girdle muscular dystrophy type 1B, autosomal dominant Emery–Dreifuss muscular dystrophy, dilated cardiomyopathy type 1A, and autosomal dominant partial lipodystrophy. This suggests the existence of distinct functional domains in lamin A/C that are essential for different cell types. All the recessive forms of CMT-2 are exceedingly rare.[571]

X-Linked Charcot–Marie–Tooth Disease

This type of CMT disease, which is probably the second most common form of the disease, is a genetically separate, X-linked condition. More than 250 mutations of the *CX32* (*connexin 32, gap junction protein β1*) gene have been found to be the cause of this syndrome. Males with CMTX display a more severe clinical, electrophysiological and histopathological disease than heterozygous females, befitting the notion that having two X chromosomes confers some protection. The pathological changes are somewhat non-specific, but just as the condition is often considered 'intermediate' between CMT-1 and CMT-2, so too are its nerve conduction velocities and histopathological findings (Figure 24.36).[437,532,539] Classic onion bulbs are not very frequent, but 'pseudo-onion bulbs' are common. In these formations, a regenerating cluster is centred by a myelinated fibre and surrounded by several unmyelinated axons and their associated Schwann cells (Figure 24.37). Axon numbers are often relatively preserved in CMTX, because large myelinated fibres degenerate or atrophy, but regenerative clustering activity provides numerical compensation. As is typical for genetic processes, the histopathological picture appears chronic, with no active

24.35 Charcot–Marie–Tooth disease type 2. Regenerating clusters of nerve fibres and no features of hypertrophy. Epon-araldite, toluidine blue.

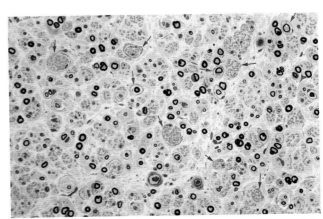

24.36 X-linked Charcot–Marie–Tooth disease. 'Intermediate' pathological changes: onion bulbs (red arrows), pseudo-onion bulbs and clusters of regenerating fibres (blue arrows). Epon-araldite, toluidine blue.

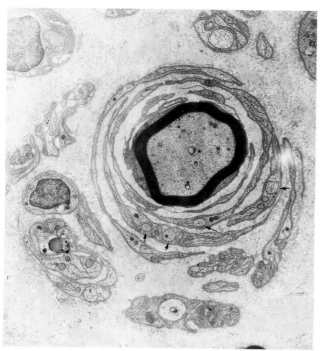

24.37 Pseudo-onion bulb. Note small axons incorporated in Schwann cell processes (arrows). ×2400.

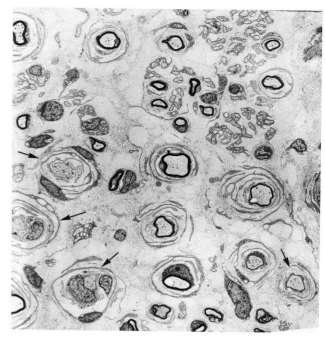

24.38 Dejerine–Sottas disease. Onion bulbs containing hypomyelinated or demyelinated (arrows) fibres. ×900.

axonal loss (i.e. wallerian degeneration) or active demyelination visible on cross-sections, although teased fibres may show some ongoing axonal degeneration.

Dejerine–Sottas Disease

Formerly designated HMSN-III, Dejerine–Sottas disease (DSD or CMT-3) is a severe hypertrophic polyneuropathy of early onset with delayed milestones. The mode of inheritance can be autosomal dominant or recessive, but many cases are sporadic. In some patients with a seemingly recessive mode of inheritance, dominant de novo mutations have been identified. The clinical features include sensory motor neuropathy with an aggressive course, ataxia, skeletal abnormalities and markedly enlarged nerves. The cerebrospinal fluid (CSF) protein content is elevated, presumably because the spinal roots are involved. A progressive and debilitating clinical course is the rule. Electrophysiological studies disclose very slow conduction velocities (<12 m/s). Nerve biopsy shows large numbers of onion bulbs, endoneurial fibrosis, loss of axons and specifically hypomyelination: many fibres that for axon diameter should be myelinated lack myelin or show disproportionately thin myelin sheaths (Figure 24.38 and 24.39).[188] The concept of CMT-3/DSD as a separate entity is becoming progressively eroded;[159] furthermore, it is occasionally difficult to distinguish CIDP starting in infancy from inherited neuropathy with DSD phenotype. Dejerine–Sottas disease is a genetically complex syndrome caused in some patients by point mutations of the PMP22 (peripheral myelin protein 22) gene and in other patients by mutations in the MPZ gene encoding P₀ myelin protein; these are dominantly inherited. Thus, some authors consider CMT-1 and DSD as variants of the same CMT group caused by mutations of the same

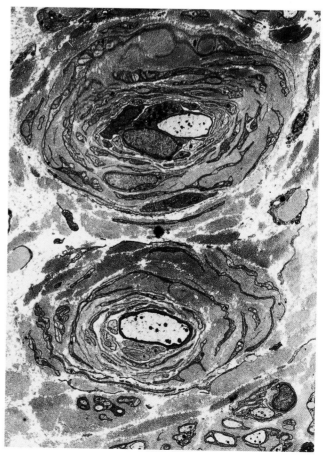

24.39 Dejerine–Sottas disease. Transverse section through two 'onion bulbs'. The lower axon is thinly myelinated and the upper devoid of a myelin sheath. ×3000.

group of genes. To complete the spectrum, the newest member of this group with the same mutations is congenital hypomyelinating neuropathy (CHN), which is characterized by hypotonia and muscle weakness at birth, resulting in slow development. Nerve biopsy shows marked reduction or even absence of myelin and onion bulbs composed of basal lamina reduplication.[159] Congenital hypomyelinating neuropathy is not a distinct genetic entity and the modes of inheritance may be autosomal dominant or recessive. A subset of patients with congenital amyelination manifest a most severe syndrome exhibiting flaccidity at birth, often with arthrogryposis, respiratory distress and swallowing difficulties, leading to death within days or months. The motor nerve conduction velocities are extremely reduced. Mutations of the *PMP22* and *MPZ*, *PRX* and *EGR2* genes have been reported.[258]

Charcot–Marie–Tooth Disease Type 4

The designation CMT-4 includes rare neuropathies exclusively inherited as autosomal recessive disorders that are more prevalent in North Africa, particularly Tunisia and Algeria.[26,369] In CMT-4A, the disease begins before the age of 2 years, with delayed motor milestones. This condition is caused by a mutation in the *GDAP1* (*ganglioside-induced differentiation-associated protein 1*) gene. The encoded protein is probably localized in the cell membrane and may be involved in development of the PNS. Muscle weakness starts distally and then progresses proximally. There are associated skeletal abnormalities. The gait deteriorates, and the patient becomes wheelchair-bound, with mild sensory and hearing loss. Death occurs in the fourth to fifth decade. Motor nerve conduction velocities are in the demyelinating range but not to the degree seen in DSD. Nerve biopsy shows features of severe reduction of myelinated fibre density and hypomyelination. Although some reports indicate the presence of onion bulbs with redundant layers of basal lamina referred to as 'basal lamina onion bulbs', other studies document less specific changes, with a paucity of onion bulbs.

The designation CMT-4B is a heterogeneous group called autosomal recessive hereditary motor and sensory neuropathy with focally folded myelin, which emphasizes the salient pathological feature (Figure 24.40). The *MTMR2* (*myotubularin-related protein 2*) gene has been shown to be mutated in patients with CMT-4B1, who show normal early motor milestones and an MNCV usually less than 12 m/s. Onset of symptoms is in the second or third year of life, with a relatively severe neuropathy, both distal and proximal, followed by a relentlessly progressive course culminating in wheelchair dependency and early death.[159] Mutation in the *SBF2* (*set binding factor 2/ myotubularin-related protein-13*) gene leads to disease in CMT-4B2.[571]

In CMT-4C, disabling scoliosis and childhood onset of a demyelinating sensorimotor neuropathy is the presenting manifestation in children. The condition is linked to mutations in an uncharacterized transcript *K1AA1985* (chromosome 5q23–q33). This gene is expressed widely in peripheral nerve. Nerve biopsy shows loss of large myelinated fibres; few fibres have a diameter larger than 8 μm. Unusual ultrastructural findings are basal lamina onion bulbs and extended Schwann cell processes (Figure 24.41).[162]

Mutation in the *NDRG1* (*N-Myc-downstream-regulated gene 1*) gene has been found to be responsible for CMT-4D, also called HMSN-Lom. This rare recessive demyelinating syndrome also includes hearing loss and dysmorphism and affects individuals of the Romany population settled near the town of Lom in Bulgaria. The histological features include demyelination, remyelination, onion bulbs and axonal regenerative clusters.[245]

The designation CMT-4E is caused by mutations in the *EGR2* gene and is therefore allelic to CMT-1D.[546] Patients present with floppy infant syndrome at birth. Motor milestones are delayed, but the two patients described by Warner and colleagues eventually learned to walk with crutches.[546] Weakness and atrophy are distally accentuated, but proximal weakness is also present. Motor nerve conduction velocities are extremely reduced to 3–8 m/s, and sural nerve biopsies show virtual absence of myelin.

Patients with CMT-4F have a mutation in the *PRX* (periaxin, chromosome 19q13) gene that leads to a severe CMT phenotype with marked sensory impairment.[493] Periaxin is a membrane-associated protein that is exclusively expressed in myelinated Schwann cells. The clinical picture of severe infantile axonal neuropathy with respiratory failure is striking. Most infants exhibit intrauterine growth retardation. Respiratory failure develops within days, weeks or months after birth. Muscle weakness is predominantly distal. Study of nerve biopsies reveals demyelination, onion bulbs and occasional tomacula formation, with focal myelin thickening, abnormalities of the paranodal myelin loops and focal absence of paranodal septate-like junctions between the terminal loops and axon.[493]

Hereditary Recurrent Focal Neuropathies

Hereditary Neuropathy with Liability to Pressure Palsies

A deletion affecting the region of chromosome 17 harbouring the *PMP22* gene has been documented in 85 per cent of patients with a polyneuropathy called HNPP, also known as 'tomaculous neuropathy'.[82,296] The allelic relationship of HNPP and CMT-1 was unexpected in the premolecular era. The term 'tomaculous' refers to the sausage-like configuration of the pathological abnormality as viewed on teased nerve preparations (Figure 24.42). Myelin 'tomaculae' appear in other conditions such as CIDP and in the spectrum of CMT. Thus, the term 'tomaculous neuropathy' should be used only in a descriptive sense. Hereditary neuropathy with liability to pressure palsies is inherited as an autosomal dominant trait, with onset in the second or third decade. Patients typically experience recurrent episodes of paralytic mononeuropathy, often precipitated by trivial trauma or compression load to the nerve, the dysfunction usually lasting days to weeks. The most commonly affected nerves are the ulnar nerve at the elbow, the peroneal nerve at the head of the fibula, and the median nerve at the wrist. Some patients with the same molecular abnormality and without a history of pressure-sensitive recurrent neuropathy have a syndrome of mild sensorimotor polyneuropathy similar to CMT-1. Painless brachial plexopathy may accompany HNPP. Nerve conduction studies reveal focal slowing of conduction velocities in direct relation to sites of entrapment. Nerve

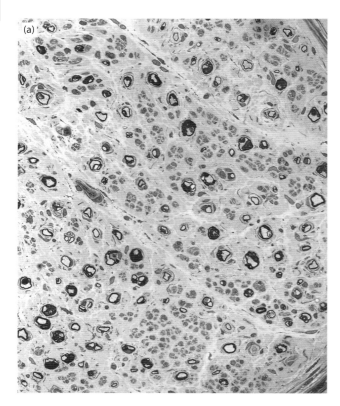

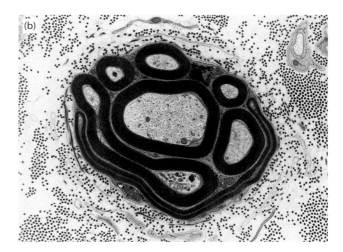

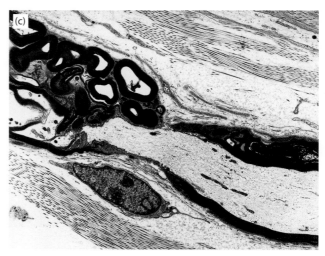

24.40 Hereditary neuropathy with excessively folded myelin.
(a) Transverse section showing irregular myelin sheaths. Thionin and acridine orange. ×370. **(b)** Central axon surrounded by profiles of myelin and axonal outpouchings. ×8000. **(c)** Longitudinal section at a node of Ranvier, showing that the myelin outpouchings are not spread evenly along the internode. ×3600.

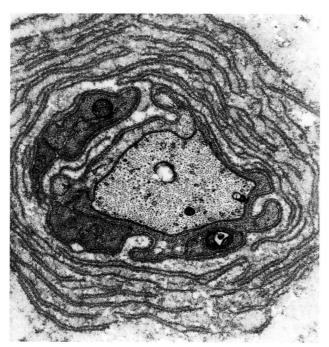

24.41 Transverse section through an 'onion bulb' largely composed of concentrically arranged paired basal laminae not associated with Schwann cell processes. ×15 000.

biopsy shows a background of almost normal fibre density, some segmental demyelination, occasional regenerating clusters, rare onion bulbs and, most characteristically, segmental thickening of myelin with a 'jelly roll' (Figure 24.43) appearance on cross-sections that on electron microscopy corresponds to the wrapping of redundant loops of myelin around itself and the axon (Figure 24.44). The configuration of hypermyelinated segments of the nerve fibre are better defined by ultrastructural examination as a double folded redundant myelin loop that wraps around the axon to varying degrees, up to three or four tightly packed turns. Most often the redundant loops of myelin adhere to the contour of the axon in the paranodal region. Additional myelin abnormalities include the presence of uncompacted myelin in the inner layers of the myelin sheath.

Hereditary Neuralgic Amyotrophy

Hereditary neuralgic amyotrophy is a recurrrent brachial plexopathy inherited with autosomal dominantly high penetrance. The age of onset is usually in the first to third decades. Typically, days to weeks after a triggering event, such as a 'flu-like' illness, childbirth, trauma or strenuous exercise of the arm, the patient develops pain in the area of the shoulder girdle and arm, followed days later by paralysis of muscle groups of the shoulder and upper arm and

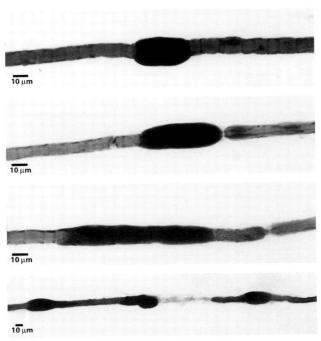

24.42 Hereditary neuropathy with liability to pressure palsies. Portions of isolated nerve fibres stained with osmium tetroxide, showing sausage-shaped expansions. The lowermost fibre possesses a short region of demyelination. ×50.

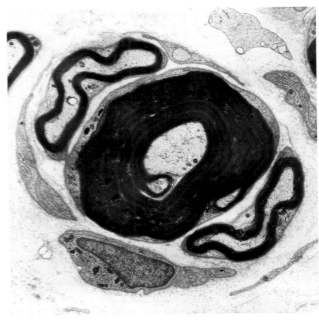

24.44 Cross-section through tomaculum forming part of a cluster. Redundant myelin loop is spiralled about itself and compacted. ×4400.

also the forearm and hand. Pain recedes after a few weeks, but paresis persists for weeks and up to 2 years after the attack.[558] Concomitant sensory deficit is common but not dominant. Some patients display minor dysmorphic features. During the attack, EMG unveils evidence of brachial plexus involvement, but signs of a generalized polyneuropathy are lacking. There are no pathological studies for this unusual condition. The HNA locus has been mapped to chromosome 17q25,[258] likely involving *septin 9 (SEPT9)*.

Hereditary Sensory and Autonomic Neuropathies

The polyneuropathies reported under the rubric of HSAN consist of at least five clinicopathological entities[129,418] that have in common the following: they are inherited and the primary sensory neurons of spinal ganglia and the autonomic system either fail to develop or undergo insidious atrophy and degeneration. Except for HSAN-I, all HSANs manifest symptoms in early life. Although particular syndromes are rare, as a group HSANs constitute an important cause of chronic peripheral neuropathies. With the discovery of a molecular defect involving the *tyrosine kinase receptor* gene for NGF in HSAN-IV, a new tabulation for these neuropathies is emerging based on the identification of the genetic abnormality. In the evaluation of these cases, it is important to exclude patients who have signs and symptoms of spinal cord pathology, specifically syringomyelia.

Hereditary Sensory and Autonomic Neuropathy Type I

The most common form of HSAN is the disorder first adequately described by Denny-Brown under the title 'hereditary sensory radicular neuropathy'; this corresponds to 'HSAN-I' of Dyck and colleagues;[129] other names for this entity have included mal perforans du pied and familial symmetrical gangrene with arthropathy (Hils). Type I can

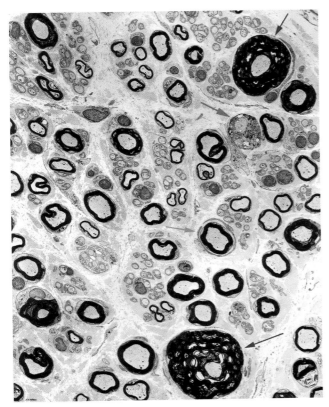

24.43 Hereditary neuropathy with liability to pressure palsies. Range of findings on low power examination: demyelination, onion bulbs and 'jelly rolls'. ×1740.

be identified by its late onset: symptoms develop in the second to fourth decades of life, with acrodistal sensory impairment, especially for pain and temperature, spontaneous pain, neuropathic ulcers, decreased reflexes, atrophy and distal anhydrosis. The condition is slowly progressive, and motor nerve conduction remains normal or borderline. One form of this disease is caused by a point mutation in the *SPLTLC1* (*serine-palmitoyltransferase 1*) gene.[258] Nerve biopsy shows preservation of the size of fascicles, notwithstanding severe loss of small myelinated and unmyelinated fibres (Figure 24.45) and lingering axonal disintegration with occasional myelin ovoids (degeneration in a previously fully developed nerve trunk). Large myelinated fibres are less affected. Spinal ganglia neurons are lost, and there is significant reduction in the number of fibres entering the dorsal columns of the spinal cord.

Hereditary Sensory and Autonomic Neuropathy Type II

This is a rare disorder often referred to as congenital sensory neuropathy, Morvan disease or syringomyelia of infancy. This condition occurs sporadically or with autosomal recessive inheritance.[129] The abnormality is present from birth, but medical attention is not sought until childhood, when painless mutilating injuries affecting both upper and lower extremities, fractures of the feet, Charcot joints, and ulcers on pressure areas of the feet develop. Motor strength is

preserved, and stretch reflexes are depressed. Distal sweating is impaired and patients may experience swallowing difficulties, severe constipation and tonic pupils. There is decreased sensation to all modalities in the extremities, and to a lesser degree in the trunk and face. In contrast to HSAN-I, sural nerve biopsy has shown hypoplasia of fascicles, with significant decreases in the number of myelinated nerve fibres, relative preservation of unmyelinated fibres and no evidence of active degeneration. In cross-section, the nerve appears to be composed of miniature fascicles (failure to develop) (Figure 24.46). Consequently, HSAN-II can be identified not only by a mutilating acropathy with deformed distal phalanges but also by a severe, distally pronounced impairment of all sensory qualities mediated by myelinated nerve fibres: light touch sensation, position sense and vibratory perception. Sensory qualities mediated by unmyelinated fibres are affected less severely. Investigations have demonstrated that mutations in *FAM134B*, the nervous system-specific HSN2 exon of *WNK1*, or *KIF1A*, with subsequent defects in off-loading axonal cargos at nerve terminals, are rare causes of HSAN II.[411]

Hereditary Sensory and Autonomic Neuropathy Type III

The Riley–Day syndrome, or familial dysautonomia (now designated HSAN-III), is an autosomal recessive illness that starts at birth, affects almost exclusively Ashkenazi (Eastern European) Jewish people,[18] and is the most common of the HSANs. The clinical features include recurrent vomiting, pulmonary infections, dysphagia, fractures of the bones of feet, corneal ulcers because of insensitivity, diminished lacrimation, defective temperature regulation, labile blood pressure, excessive sweating and skin blotching following emotional stimuli, and absence of fungiform papillae of the tongue and of axon flare response following histamine injection. Muscle strength is normal, and tendon reflexes are absent. Loss of pain sensibility is universal, with preservation of touch, vibration and position sensations. The disorder maps to chromosome 9q31 and arises from mutations to the IKBKAP (inhibitor of κ light polypeptide) gene in 99.5 per cent of cases. The exact function of the gene and the pathogenesis of HSAN-III remain to be elucidated. The genetic defect affects prenatal neuronal development, so that

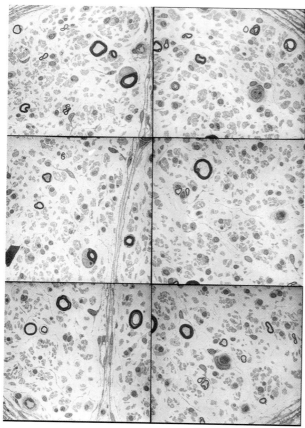

24.45 Hereditary sensory and autonomic neuropathy type I. Low-power collage showing preservation of fascicular volume and severe reduction in the number of small myelinated fibres. ×800.

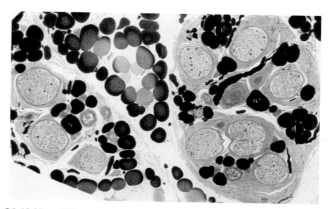

24.46 Hereditary sensory and autonomic neuropathy type II. Low-power view, showing hypoplasia of fascicles and reduction in the number of small myelinated fibres. Epon-araldite, toluidine blue.

symptoms are present from birth, but individual expression varies widely.[18] In the sural nerve, although the number of myelinated fibres is low, normally there is marked reduction in the number of unmyelinated fibres associated with denervated bands in the absence of axonal breakdown. Autopsy studies have shown a marked decrease in the number of neurons in sympathetic and spinal ganglia.[372,373] Decreased numbers of neurons in the intermediolateral grey column of the spinal cord suggest involvement of preganglionic neurons. Autonomic nerve fibre terminals cannot be demonstrated on peripheral blood vessels. These findings have been interpreted as evidence of developmental failure.

Hereditary Sensory and Autonomic Neuropathy Type IV

Congenital insensitivity to pain with anhydrosis or hereditary anhydrotic sensory neuropathy is also known as HSAN-IV. The first clinical manifestation of this disease is unexplained pyrexia in infancy caused by the patient's inability to sweat under high environmental temperatures. Although patients with HSAN-III have preserved sweat production, HSAN-IV is characterized by lack of sweat production. These patients have normal lacrimation. Affected children fail to respond normally to painful stimuli from birth, which results in cutaneous ulcerations and mutilations and neurogenic arthropathy. These children display self-mutilating behaviour and mental retardation.[129] Autopsy studies have reported an absence of small neurons in spinal ganglia, of small fibres in dorsal roots and of the Lissauer tract in the length of the spinal cord. Although autopsy data on sympathetic ganglia are lacking, absence of small fibres in peripheral nerves, skin and sweat glands suggests corresponding loss of sympathetic ganglion cells. Hereditary anhydrotic sensory neuropathy is inherited in an autosomal recessive manner. A variety of mutations of the NTRK1 (neurotrophin receptor tyrosine kinase 1 receptor on 1q21–22) gene have been demonstrated in these patients. NTRK1 is expressed not only by peripheral sensory neurons but also by certain brain cells, such as cholinergic neurons of the basal forebrain, which suggests potential pathomechanisms for the moderate mental retardation seen in patients.

Hereditary Sensory and Autonomic Neuropathy Type V

This is the least common of this group of neuropathies. The inheritance is probably autosomal recessive and the molecular abnormality is identical to that in HSAN-IV.[209] The clinical onset is in infancy or childhood, with absence of pain and temperature over limbs, but with preservation of other modalities of sensation. Although muscle strength and reflexes remain normal, acral ulcers, fractures and neurogenic arthropathy ensue. Histological studies have shown a significant reduction in the number of small myelinated and better preserved unmyelinated nerve fibres.

Neuropathy of the Sphingolipidoses

Krabbe Disease

Peripheral nerves are often involved in Krabbe globoid cell leukodystrophy (galactosyl ceramide lipidosis; see also Chapter 7, Mitochondrial diseases).[36] This autosomal recessive disease is caused by a deficiency of galactocerebroside β-galactosidase, resulting in the accumulation of psychosine (galactosylceramide) in oligodendrocytes and Schwann cells that activate a caspase 3 apoptotic death program. Most cases have an onset in infancy (80 per cent), but late infantile, juvenile and even adult-onset cases are encountered occasionally. Late infantile and juvenile cases usually present with gait disturbances, hemiplegia and visual loss, with or without peripheral neuropathy. About 50 per cent of adult patients have peripheral neuropathy, some as a presenting feature. Of histiocytic origin, multinucleated 'globoid' cells in the cerebral white matter constitute the morphologic hallmark of diagnosis. Although nerves show histiocytic infiltration, typical globoid cells are rare. Peripheral nerve lesions include thinly myelinated nerve fibres, axonal degeneration and segmental demyelination–remyelination, with hypertrophic features. Ultrastructurally, pathognomonic inclusions in Schwann cell cytoplasm and macrophages consist of straight or curved prismatic or tubular inclusions (Figure 24.47).[491] Depending on the plane of section, they may appear as empty clefts or as hollow, needle-like structures (Figure 24.48).

Metachromatic Leukodystrophy

Metachromatic leukodystrophy (MLD; see also Chapter 7, Mitochondrial Diseases) is a group of disorders transmitted as an autosomal recessive trait and characterized by demyelination and the accumulation of galactosyl sulphatide in the white matter of brain and in peripheral nerves. Late infantile, juvenile and adult-onset forms are recognized; most cases are due to a deficiency of arylsulphatase (arylsulfatase) A, which results in the accumulation of sulphatide in many tissues, particularly in the CNS, PNS and kidneys, except for the AB variant, where arylsulphatase activity is normal, the disorder being due to a deficiency of the sphingolipid activator protein B. A genetically distinct condition is multiple sulphatase deficiency, which combines features of both late infantile MLD and mucopolysaccharidosis. Regardless of the age of onset of MLD, CNS involvement predominates but most

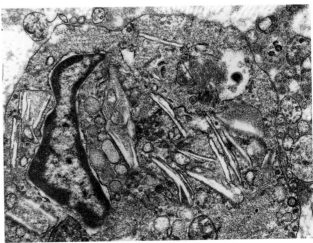

24.47 Krabbe disease. Endoneurial macrophage showing non-oriented straight or curved prismatic or hollow inclusions in a clear matrix. ×12 000.

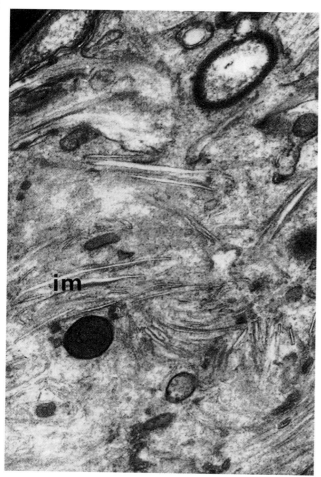

24.48 Krabbe disease. There is inclusion material (im) in Schwann cell cytoplasm. ×45 000.

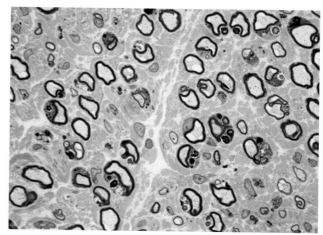

24.49 Metachromatic leukodystrophy, sural nerve. Deposits of osmiophilic material distend Schwann cells. Epon-araldite, toluidine blue.

patients show clinical or electrophysiological evidence of a demyelinating polyneuropathy. The peripheral nerves in the most common form, the late infantile variety, show a reduction in myelinated fibre numbers and evidence of demyelination. Fibre loss is usually less obvious in juvenile and adult-onset cases, but demyelination and remyelination ultimately become greater, and hypertrophic features may be more obtrusive. A characteristic histological feature of the neuropathy is the accumulation of granules in Schwann cell cytoplasm (Schwann cells associated with myelinated and unmyelinated axons) and endoneurial macrophages (Figure 24.49). Such lipid deposits give a brown metachromasia when a frozen section is treated with a solution of acidified cresyl violet or when stained with toluidine blue or thionine; with pseudo-isocyanine, the stored material develops a red–violet metachromasia.[28] Pretreatment of the section with lipid solvents abolishes the metachromatic reaction. These granules are associated with acid phosphatase and therefore are classifiable as lysosomes. By electron microscopy, many lysosomal lamellated inclusions can be seen, the most characteristic being the 'tuffstone' bodies (Figure 24.50a), prismatic stacks (Figure 24.50b)[503] and striated 'zebra bodies'. The pathogenesis of the demyelination is uncertain; it does not correlate clearly with the presence of metachromatic inclusions in Schwann cells.

Schwann cells associated with myelinated axons tolerate significant amounts of stored material without evidence of myelin damage (Figure 24.50a). These inclusions are not derived from myelin breakdown, because they are present in Schwann cells associated with myelinated and unmyelinated axons and in fetal nerves before demyelination is evident.

Fabry Disease

With an incidence of 1 in 40 000, Fabry disease (see also Chapter 7, Mitochondrial Diseases) is a sex-linked inborn error of glycosphingolipid catabolism, resulting from the deficiency of the lysosomal hydrolase α-galactosidase A in tissues.[114,165] Hundreds of mutations of the *GLA* (α-galactosidase A) gene have been identified. Approximately 75 per cent of the mutations causing Fabry disease are missense or nonsense mutations. Hemizygous males have extensive deposition of globotriaosylceramide (Gb Ose3 Cer) in the lysosomes of endothelium, pericytes and smooth muscle cells of blood vessels. There is also deposition in the ganglion cells, heart, kidneys, cornea and most other tissues. Clinical manifestations vary according to the severity of the phenotype but include corneal whorl dystrophy, renal failure, cutaneous angiokeratomata, and cardiac and cerebral vascular disease.[114] An important component of the disease is a mild sensory and autonomic neuropathy that manifests before the age of 20 years. Peripheral nerve dysfunction is accompanied by severe paroxysmal pain in the extremities (Fabry crises), but signs of neuropathy are absent in most patients. Carrier females may display minor manifestations but do not usually develop neuropathic symptoms. Nerve biopsies often show a normal population of fibres or some loss of myelinated and unmyelinated axons; all cases have massive accumulation of globotriaosylceramide in perineurium (Figure 24.51 and 24.52), endothelial cells and smooth muscle cells (Figure 24.53), but not in Schwann cells[375] or axons. The lipid accumulation is easily detected in semi-thin sections because of its osmiophilia. Frozen sections examined under polarized light disclose birefringent 'Maltese

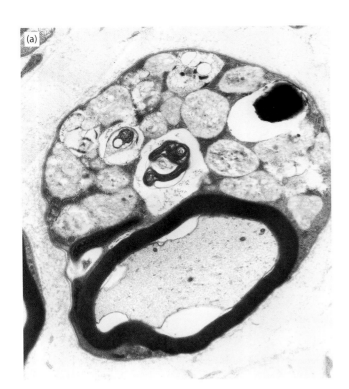

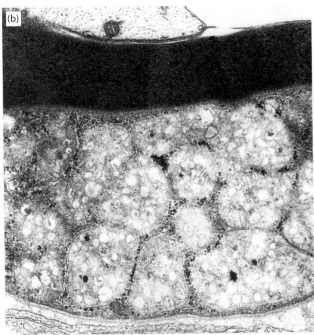

24.50 Metachromatic leukodystrophy. Schwann cell associated with myelinated axon containing **(a)** membrane-bound lamellated inclusions and tuffstone bodies. ×6400. **(b)** Prismatic stacks and tuffstone bodies. ×29 000.

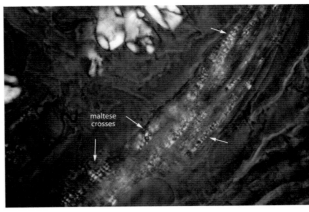

24.51 Fabry disease. Maltese crosses in perineurium are unveiled by polarized light on fresh frozen section of sural nerve.

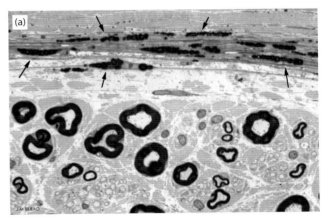

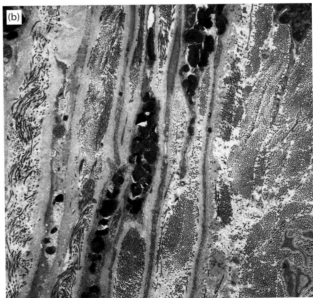

24.52 Fabry disease. (a) Lipid in perineurium (arrows) is demonstrated with osmium tetroxide impregnation and staining with toluidine blue. Epon-araldite. **(b)** Perineurium, showing multiple lamellar osmiophilic inclusions. ×2400.

crosses' (Figure 24.51) that co-localize with perineurium. The material stains in frozen section with lipid-soluble dyes and in paraffin sections with periodic acid–Schiff (PAS) and Luxol fast blue (LFB). Treatment of formalin-fixed tissue with 3 per cent potassium chromate helps preserve the lipid. Ultrastructurally, the lipid inclusions display a typical pattern of concentric lamellar inclusions with alternating light- and dark-staining bands with a periodicity of 6.3 nm. In some areas, the deposit has a spiral configuration. Assays for α-galactosidase A in serum or leukocytes typically demonstrate 10 per cent or less of the normal value in affected males, and 50 per cent of the normal value in heterozygous females. Autopsy studies have shown that the storage material is present in spinal ganglion cells. The number of these cells is reduced, particularly those of small size. Heterozygous females show a similar distribution of lipid deposits in peripheral nerves. Recombinant α-galactosidase protein therapy has shown positive results in clinical trials.

Farber Disease

Farber disease (see also Chapter 7, Mitochondrial Diseases) is an autosomal recessive disorder caused by a mutation in the gene encoding acid ceramidase, an enzyme required for the metabolism of the sphingolipid ceramide.[252] Clinical features include disseminated nodular subcutaneous and articular swellings and vocal cord thickening resulting in hoarseness. Biopsy of the skin lesions reveals granulomas containing macrophages with the lipid cytoplasmic inclusions. However, storage material may be found histologically in a variety of tissues, including Schwann cells. A few nerve biopsies have been studied in detail and show hypomyelination, with preservation of myelinated fibre density.[60,376] Ultrastructurally, characteristic 'banana bodies' are found in myelinating Schwann cells, with membrane-bound elongated bodies containing a central longitudinal striated region surrounded by amorphous electron-dense material (Figure 24.54).[324]

Gangliosidoses

Gangliosidoses (see also Chapter 7, Mitochondrial Diseases) are autosomal recessive inherited disorders characterized by accumulation of gangliosides, primarily in neurons, due to a deficiency in the enzymatic degradation of these lipids. There are two types of gangliosidosis: GM1, deficient in acid β-galactosidase; and GM2, deficient in either β-hexosaminidase (α- or β-subunit) or GM2 activator protein. Peripheral neuropathy is not a significant part of these diseases, but motor neuropathy may be seen in late-onset cases of GM2. Nerve biopsy has shown a reduction in myelinated fibre density and evidence of axonal regenerative activity.[146,329,330] Ultrastructural findings were not described in these case reports, but intra-axonal membranous lamellar inclusions have been noted in myelinated and unmyelinated nerve terminals in skin, rectal mucosa and muscle in GM2.[1,120,452]

Niemann–Pick Disease

Niemann–Pick disease (see also Chapter 7, Mitochondrial Diseases) is subdivided on the basis of biochemical and molecular criteria into two separate classes: types A and B are deficient in acid sphingomyelinase, and types C and D are deficient in the NPC-1 protein, with type D representing an allelic variant of type C. Foam cell infiltration and visceromegaly are common features in all cases, whereas severe neurological involvement occurs only in types A and C and not in type B. Nerve biopsy findings in Niemann–Pick disease are limited to case reports.[190,579] In both

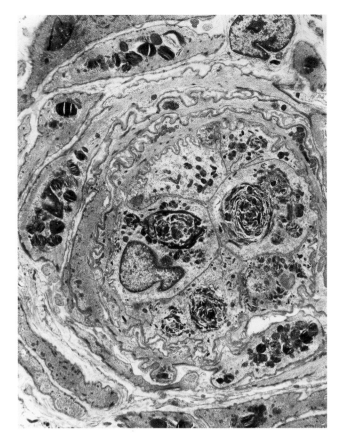

24.53 Fabry disease. Epineurial vessel, showing aggregates of lipid deposits in endothelial cells and smooth muscle cells. ×6240.

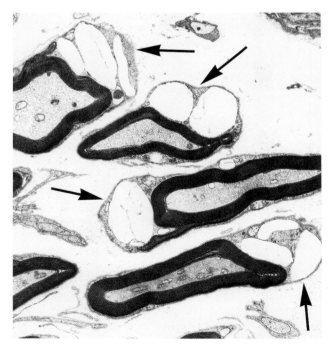

24.54 Farber disease. Schwann cells associated with myelinated axons, showing banana bodies (arrows). ×3200.

types A and C, electrodiagnostic studies reveal changes of a predominantly demyelinating motor and sensory polyneuropathy. On light microscopy, myelin sheaths are disproportionately thin, and there is evidence of chronic demyelination (onion bulbs) but usually no active demyelination. The majority of axons are preserved. In type C, axonal spheroids and cytoskeletal abnormalities akin to neuroaxonal dystrophy have been noted.[190] Membrane-bound lobulated lysosomal inclusions of electron-dense material similar to lipofuscin are present in Schwann cells, endoneurial fibroblasts, macrophages, pericytes and endothelial cells. In type C, Schwann cells of myelinated fibres can be filled with whorls of concentric osmiophilic membranous profiles and electrolucent material.[190]

Neuronal Ceroid Lipofuscinoses

Neuronal ceroid lipofuscinoses (NCL) (see also Chapter 7, Mitochondrial Diseases) are the most common lysosomal storage diseases of childhood and infancy. They are inherited in an autosomal recessive fashion, with the exception of the rare adult-onset form, which shows autosomal dominant inheritance.[172] The current classification is based on genetics and recognizes eight different diseases (NCL-1–8), each of which encompasses a spectrum of clinical phenotypes.[172] Although the storage material is present in various tissues, only the CNS and the retina show damage. Currently the diagnosis of NCL is based on clinical, pathological, biochemical and genetic findings. Tissues that may be biopsied for diagnosis include rectum, conjunctiva and skin. Blood lymphocytes may also be used. Nerve biopsies are performed only rarely in the diagnostic work-up of these diseases. Isolated case reports of peripheral nerve biopsies have described ultrastructural storage material (curvilinear bodies, fingerprint bodies or granular osmiophilic deposits) in Schwann cells (Figure 24.55), endothelial cells, perineurial cells and smooth muscle cells, with the exception of NCL-4, which is usually normal.

Other Hereditary Neuropathies

Tangier Disease

Tangier disease (hereditary high-density lipoprotein deficiency), named after an island in the Chesapeake Bay, is a rare autosomal recessive disorder of lipid metabolism characterized by a low serum cholesterol level, a normal or elevated triglyceride level, and almost absent high-density lipoprotein (HDL) and apolipoprotein A1 and A2. In 1999, several reports established that the disease is caused by a mutation of the *ABCA1* gene (*ATP-binding cassette transporter 1* gene on chromosome 9q31).[37,349] An *ABCA1* defect was also demonstrated in the original Tangier disease kindred. The clinical manifestations result from the deposition of cholesterol esters in various tissues, particularly in the tonsils (which become enlarged and yellowish), spleen, bone marrow, lymph nodes, intestinal submucosa and skin. In about one-third of patients with Tangier disease, the presenting symptoms are those of peripheral neuropathy, which may be of three different patterns: relapsing multifocal neuropathy, which can affect oculomotor and limb nerves; a distal symmetrical sensorimotor polyneuropathy; and a syringomyelia-like syndrome, with features including facial diplegia, bilateral wasting of hand muscles and loss of pain and temperature sensation over the trunk and limbs. Autopsy studies from patients with pseudo-syringomyelia show loss of neurons in the cervical spinal cord and in the facial nerve nucleus; in nerve biopsies,[251] there is a severe depletion of unmyelinated and myelinated fibres, particularly those of smaller size. Demyelination is not a feature. In addition, a striking abnormality is the accumulation of abundant lipid droplets and pleomorphic inclusions in the cytoplasm of Schwann cells (Figure 24.56); the inclusions are dissolved during paraffin processing, resulting in vacuolation of Schwann cells, pericytes and endothelium. In fresh-frozen sections, the material stains bright red with oil red O. Nerve biopsies from cases with multifocal neuropathy show demyelination and remyelination, and a restriction of the lipid droplets to those Schwann cells

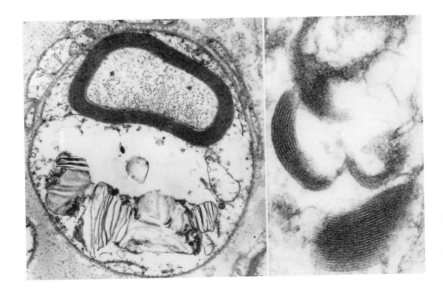

24.55 Neuronal ceroid lipofuscinosis. Schwann cell associated with myelinated axon, showing lipid accumulation as well as adjacent pi granules. Inset shows fingerprint profiles at higher magnification. ×16 640 and ×126 040.

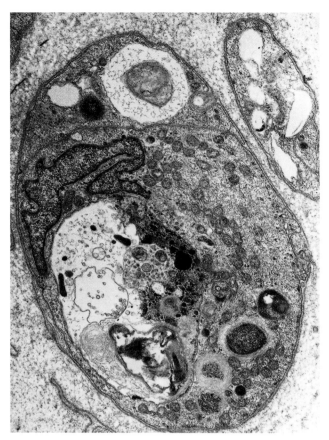

24.56 Tangier disease. Schwann cell, showing pleomorphic inclusion. ×8800.

associated with unmyelinated axons. Ultrastructurally, round or elliptic cytoplasmic electron-empty storage vacuoles, 0.5–3 μm in diameter, are seen in both myelinated and non-myelinated Schwann cells, perineurial cells, endothelial cells and pericytes.[143]

Bassen–Kornzweig Disease (Abetalipoproteinaemia)

In 1950, Bassen and Kornzweig described the first case of abetalipoproteinaemia in an 18-year-old girl with abnormal (thorny-appearing) erythrocytes associated with retinitis pigmentosa, chronic diarrhoea and an atypical form of Friedreich's ataxia. In the subsequent reported case, the erythrocyte abnormality was named 'acanthocytes' and ultimately 'acanthocytosis'. The term 'abetalipoproteinaemia' was used because of the lipoprotein pattern. Although abetalipoproteinaemia is autosomal recessive, a similar clinical disorder–familial hypobetalipoproteinaemia–is autosomal dominant but requires homozygosity for neurological manifestations. The gastrointestinal onset of symptoms is in infancy; neurological features develop after the age of 5 years, with progressive weakness, loss of vibration sense and proprioception, intentional tremor, dysarthria, ptosis, pes cavus and kyphoscoliosis; not surprisingly, these features have a similarity to those of Friedrich ataxia. The eye manifestations comprise pigment retinopathy, with night blindness and loss of colour vision, with macular sparing. Acanthocytes can be demonstrated

by blood smear and make up about 50 per cent of the circulating red blood cells. Patients have steatorrhoea and malabsorption of vitamin E, to which all neurological and ocular manifestations are attributed. Changes in peripheral nerves are non-specific and consist of reduced numbers of large myelinated fibres and myelin remodelling secondary to axonal influences. The molecular defect in abetalipoproteinaemia resides in the absence of microsomal triglyceride transfer protein,[554] which maps to chromosome 4q22–24. In patients with abetalipoproteinaemia, vitamin E is not assembled in chylomicrons for absorption from the intestine and transfer to the liver. Vitamin E secretion and transfer from the liver to peripheral tissues is also affected. In patients with familial hypobetalipoproteinaemia the molecular defect lies in apolipoprotein B truncation, which also interferes with vitamin E absorption and transfer from the intestine. Vitamin E deficiency produces dystrophic changes in sensory projections to the medullary gracile nuclei and loss of dorsal column axons. Vitamin E therapy can alter the natural course of the disease.

Adult Polyglucosan Body Disease

This rare disorder is characterized by urinary dysfunction, cognitive impairment and sensorimotor polyneuropathy. Most patients with adult polyglucosan body disease (APGBD) have no positive family history. However, familial clustering involving siblings has been reported in Israeli Jews. The constellation of neurological symptoms and signs may simulate a myelopathy or amyotrophic lateral sclerosis.[249] However, electrophysiological studies reveal a predominantly axonal sensory motor neuropathy, with normal cranial nerve function. Paraventricular and subcortical white matter changes may be demonstrated by magnetic resonance (MR) imaging; signal abnormality may also involve the brain stem, cerebellum and spinal cord. Reduced glycogen branching enzyme (GBE) activity is found in APGBD. In some families, genetic analysis of the *GBE* gene has shown a missense mutation. In nerve biopsy, polyglucosan bodies are typically intra-axonal and round, with a diameter in the range 5–70 μm. They occur in myelinated axons (Figure 24.57) and rarely in unmyelinated fibres and Schwann cells. They vary in number from one to many per fascicle in cross-sections and can be identified easily in plastic resin sections. Polyglucosan bodies are PAS-positive and consist almost entirely of glucose polymers, with only a small amount of protein. Under the electron microscope, polyglucosan bodies have no limiting membrane and an amorphous core surrounded by a corona of 6- to 8-nm-diameter branched filaments (Figure 24.57b). Polyglucosan bodies in peripheral nerve may also occur in glycogen storage disease type IV, phosphofructokinase deficiency, progressive myoclonic epilepsy and double athetosis (Bielschowsky bodies), and in normal older people.[77] In our experience, polyglucosan bodies are found in about 3 per cent of sural nerve biopsies. The incidence of polyglucosan bodies in nerves rises with age. Although nerve biopsy is commonly employed for the diagnosis of APGBD, skin biopsy may prove a reliable and less invasive procedure, showing an abundance of polyglucosan bodies in the myoepithelial cells of apocrine glands.

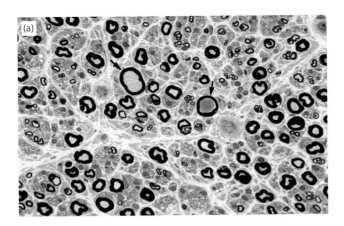

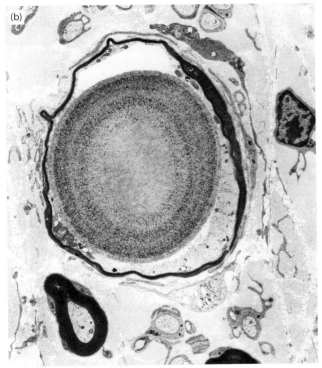

24.57 (a) Polyglucosan body, sural nerve. Distended myelinated axons containing round structures. Epon-araldite, toluidine blue. **(b)** Polyglucosan body disease, sural nerve. Tightly packed, randomly oriented, short-branched filaments distend a thinly myelinated axon. ×2400.

Giant Axonal Neuropathy

Berg and associates reported this rare autosomal recessive disorder involving both the CNS and the PNS in 1972. Sporadic cases have been reported. A generalized disorder of intermediate filament organization has been postulated as the cause of the disease.[184] Clinical onset is before the age of 7 years. Neonatal respiratory and feeding problems develop and milestones are delayed. The gait is described as 'clumsy', and there is weakness of the musculature of the lower limbs. Upper limbs are involved later and dysfunction of cranial nerves is variable. Central manifestations include pyramidal signs, dysarthric speech, tremors and mental retardation. Patients have tightly curled hair and skeletal abnormalities. The disorder is progressive, with death occurring by the third decade. By light microscopy, nerve sections show massively dilated axons, usually surrounded by thinned or no myelin (Figure 24.58a). The axons may reach a size of 50 μm in diameter, but typically are in the range of 20–30 μm. Several giant axons occur per fascicle. Axonal loss of variable severity is demonstrable. On teased nerve fibre preparations, axonal swellings are fusiform, are 100–200 μm in length and have no consistent relation to the nodes. The abnormal swelling may be present in up to 50 per cent of the teased fibres. Ultrastructural examination reveals axons distended with filaments that swirl and stream in haphazard configurations, marginating mitochondria, tubules and other organelles under the cell membrane (Figure 24.58b). In longitudinal sections, the abnormal accumulation of filaments is distributed focally along the length of the axon, interposed with more normal axoplasm. Distinctive of giant axonal neuropathy are focal osmiophilic condensations that are interspersed among the masses of filaments; this abnormality is not seen in the filamentous axonopathies of the toxic neuropathies of hexacarbons, carbon disulphide (disulfide) and acrylamide. In giant axonal neuropathy, filamentous accumulation has also been demonstrated in the Schwann cells, fibroblasts, perineurial cells and endothelial cells. Similar accumulations occur in Langerhans cells, mast cells and melanocytes from skin biopsy, thus permitting a diagnosis without nerve biopsy. Mutations have been documented in the GAN gene encoding the protein gigaxonin, a new member of the cytoskeletal BTP/kelch repeat family.[39]

Infantile Neuroaxonal Dystrophy

With an age of onset of 6–24 months, infantile neuroaxonal dystrophy is an inherited autosomal recessive disease characterized by weakness, hypotonia, areflexia, rigidity, incoordination, deafness, blindness and mental deterioration.[337] The condition is relentlessly progressive, leading to tetraparesis and death between the ages of 6 and 12 years. The disorder is both sporadic and hereditary, with a male preponderance. After a normal pregnancy and delivery and early development, patients present with delayed milestones followed by rapid motor and psychomotor deterioration. Findings on imaging point to cerebral and cerebellar atrophy (inferior vermis), atrophy of the optic chiasm and pallidonigral hypointensity. Dystrophic axonal swellings are found in the CNS, peripheral nerves (Figure 24.59), intramuscular nerve twigs and autonomic nerves. Axonal spheroids range in diameter from atrophic to swollen several-fold, and nerve fibre density may be normal or slightly reduced. Abnormal axons may appear irregular in contour, and granular or inhomogeneous, with their myelin thinned. Dystrophic axons may be infrequent, often with no more than two per fascicle, and are PAS-positive and argentophilic. Accumulations of randomly oriented tubulovesicular profiles associated with aggregates of mitochondria, filaments, glycogen and vacuoles are visualized on ultrastructural examination. Pleomorphic mitochondria may be prominent in some nerve fibres.

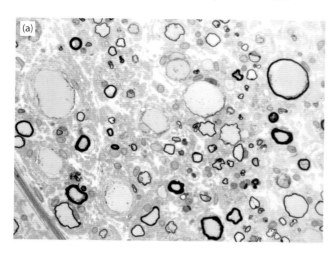

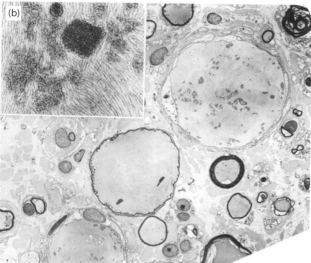

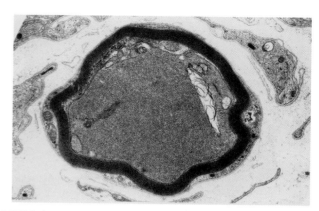

24.59 Infantile neuroaxonal dystrophy. Peripheral nerve axon, showing mild distension and accumulation of tubulovesicular elements. ×15 620.

24.58 Giant axonal neuropathy (a) Many axons are distended and display attenuated myelin. Epon-araldite, toluidine blue. ×100. **(b)** Axons massively enlarged by neurofilaments that swirl and stream in different configurations, seen at higher magnification in inset. **(b)** ×1980. Inset magnification is ×52 700.

Glycogen Storage Diseases

Peripheral neuropathy is not a common feature of most glycogen storage diseases. Ultrastructural examination may show glycogen accumulation in endoneurial and Schwann cells in Pompe's disease (glycogen storage disease type II)[306] and McArdle's disease (glycogen storage disease type V).[66] In type IV glycogen storage disease (Andersen's disease), polyglucosan bodies accumulate in various cells, including axons.[456] Peripheral neuropathy may occur in glycogen storage disease type III (Cori–Forbes disease); in addition to glycogen accumulation in endoneurial and Schwann cells,[511] severe axonal dropout and axons swollen with glycogen may be found.[511]

Peroxisomal Disorders

Peroxisomal disorders (see also Chapter 8, Peroxisomal Diseases) are rare systemic diseases resulting from either complete dysfunction of the peroxisome or single peroxisomal enzyme deficiencies. Peroxisomal disorders involving the PNS include hyperpipecolic acidaemia, adrenoleukodystrophy (ALD) and adrenomyeloneuropathy (AMN).[395] Hyperpipecolic acidaemia is one of the disorders of peroxisomal biogenesis inherited in an autosomal recessive fashion, but peripheral nerve biopsy findings have not been reported in this disorder. Both ALD and AMN are X-linked disorders of very-long-chain fatty acid (VLCFA) metabolism. They variably involve the nervous system, adrenal cortex and testis.[334,396] In childhood ALD, onset is before 10 years of age, with progressive behavioural and cognitive neurological deficits, inflammatory brain demyelination, and often total disability within 3 years. Both adolescent and adult variants of this cerebral type occur, with a similar clinical course to that of the childhood variant, but with a later onset. Adrenomyeloneuropathy typically starts with stiffness or clumsiness in the legs in the third or fourth decade, progressing slowly over the next several decades to severe spastic paresis. The gene maps to Xq28[334] and codes for a peroxisomal membrane protein, ALDP, which is a member of the ATP-binding cassette (ABC) transporter superfamily. Nerve biopsy does not play a role in the diagnosis of these disorders, which depends on the demonstration of increased levels of VLCFAs and mutation analysis. A number of patients have been studied, although in the older literature a distinction between ALD and AMN is not always made. On light microscopy, there may be no abnormality or a non-specific combination of chronic axonal loss, affecting both large and small myelinated fibres, and demyelinating changes with onion bulb formation.[324,396,442] In one study, morphometric analysis of the sural nerve from a patient with AMN revealed a more specific reduction of large myelinated fibres.[494] The lymphocytic infiltrate seen in the CNS is not a feature in the PNS. In both disorders, characteristic ultrastructural inclusions are seen but are much more difficult to detect in the peripheral nerve than in the CNS. When present, the storage material occurs in Schwann cells and macrophages, may be single-membrane bound and consists of randomly disposed or regularly arrayed aggregates of bilaminar linear profiles (Figure 24.60).[324]

Cerebrotendinous Xanthomatosis

Cerebrotendinous xanthomatosis is a rare autosomal recessive lipid storage disease, characterized by abnormal bile synthesis. There is a deficiency of the mitochondrial enzyme sterol 27-hydroxylase,[356] leading to a reduction in cholic acid and almost complete absence of chenodeoxycholic acid. The latter results in increased enzyme activity of 7α-hydroxylase, leading to increased production of cholestanol and cholesterol. The clinical spectrum includes the presence of premature cataracts, neurological signs and symptoms, tendon xanthomas, premature atherosclerosis and peripheral neuropathy. There is controversy regarding the peripheral nerve pathology: both demyelinating and axonal neuropathies have been reported.[523] A study of ten patients with the disease, in which three were examined histologically, revealed axonal degeneration with regenerative clusters and decreased density of large-diameter myelinated fibres, with sparing of unmyelinated fibres in two cases and onion bulbs and large bands of Büngner in the third case.[523] These findings suggest that, although axonal degeneration may be the predominant process, chronic demyelination and remyelination are also found. The mechanism underlying the peripheral nerve injury has not been elucidated.

Mitochondrial Encephalomyopathies

Peripheral neuropathy in association with mitochondrial disease has been well described, although the true

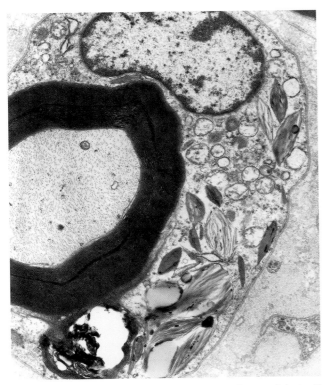

24.60 Adrenomyeloneuropathy. Schwann cell associated with myelinated axon, showing pi-like cytosomes composed of bilaminar subunits and lipid. ×10 400.

incidence is difficult to determine because no large prospective series of these patients have been reported. In addition to mitochondrial syndromes in which peripheral neuropathy is a defining feature of the disorder, neuropathy has also been described in a variety of other mitochondrial syndromes, including mitochondrial encephalomyopathy, lactic acidosis and stroke-like episodes (MELAS); myoclonus epilepsy with ragged-red fibres (MERRF); Leigh syndrome; progressive external ophthalmoplegia (PEO); and Kearns–Sayre syndrome (KSS).[336] As well as a primary peripheral neuropathy, patients with mitochondrial disease are frequently affected by other disorders that may secondarily involve the PNS, including diabetes, renal insufficiency and thyroid dysfunction. In a retrospective study of 108 patients with mitochondrial disease and polyneuropathy, 35 per cent of patients had the polyneuropathy attributed to their mitochondrial disease rather than to a secondary associated condition.[153] Supporting the hypothesis of direct involvement of peripheral nerve in mitochondrial disease is the finding of a similar proportion of mutant mitochondrial DNA in peripheral nerve as in involved muscle.[140]

Patients usually present with a mild sensorimotor polyneuropathy with sensory predominating over motor disturbances. Autonomic problems have also been described.[137] Nerve conduction studies show axonal neuropathy, but demyelinating features have also been reported.[153] Sural nerve biopsies (for review, see Finsterer[153]) demonstrate loss predominantly of large myelinated fibres, with less severe involvement of small myelinated and unmyelinated fibres. Thinly myelinated fibres, demyelinated axons and onion bulbs are also noted. Ultrastructural examination reveals abnormal enlarged mitochondria in Schwann cells, axons, perineurial cells and endothelial cells. The majority of descriptions of peripheral nerve pathology in these conditions, however, are based on only one or two cases; even in larger series, peripheral nerve biopsies have been performed only infrequently.

Peripheral neuropathy is a defining feature of three mitochondrial syndromes: sensory ataxic neuropathy, dysarthria and ophthalmoparesis (SANDO); mitochondrial neuro-gastrointestinal encephalomyopathy (MNGIE); and neuropathy, ataxia and retinitis pigmentosa (NARP).

Sensory Ataxic Neuropathy, Dysarthria and Ophthalmoparesis

Patients with SANDO present with a predominantly sensory ataxic neuropathy, with loss of vibratory and joint position sense in the distal lower extremities and areflexia, with or without loss of pinprick and temperature sensation. Patients then develop progressive external ophthalmoplegia and ataxia.[140] Mutations in the mitochondrial polymerase γ (POLG) gene are present in some patients, and the disorder may fall within the spectrum of progressive external ophthalmoplegia.[519] Sural nerve biopsies show severe loss of both large and small myelinated fibres, with endoneurial fibrosis.[140]

Mitochondrial Neuro-gastrointestinal Encephalomyopathy

This is an autosomal recessive disorder due to mutations in the *endothelial cell growth factor 1* (platelet-derived) gene (*ECGF1*), also called thymidine phosphorylase or gliostatin, on chromosome 22.[200,346] Defects in this nuclear-encoded protein result in depletion, point mutations and multiple deletions of mitochondrial DNA (mtDNA) with mtDNA alterations. The disease is characterized by ptosis, progressive external ophthalmoparesis, gastrointestinal dysmotility, cachexia, peripheral neuropathy and leukoencephalopathy.[200] The peripheral neuropathy is a mild to moderate sensorimotor polyneuropathy that can mimic CMT disease[434] or CIDP.[23] Electrophysiological studies may show either reduced motor and sensory response amplitudes or marked slowing of conduction velocity.[336] Similarly, nerve biopsies have demonstrated loss of myelinated fibres, segmental demyelination and remyelination, onion bulbs and axonal degeneration.[23,434] Abnormal mitochondria have also been noted in Schwann cells.[434]

Neuropathy, Ataxia and Retinitis Pigmentosa

This disorder results from a missense mutation in the mitochondrial *ATPase* gene (ATP6)[206] at a mutational burden of 70–90 per cent; patients with higher mutational burdens develop Leigh syndrome (see Chapter 8, Peroxisomal Diseases). Clinical presentation is characterized by sensory neuropathy, neurogenic proximal muscle weakness, seizures, dementia, ataxia and retinal pigmentary changes.[336] Nerve biopsy findings in this syndrome have not been reported.

Chediak–Higashi Disease

Chediak–Higashi disease is a rare autosomal recessive disorder characterized by severe immune deficiency, albinism, bleeding tendencies, recurrent pyogenic infections, progressive neurological deficits and a lymphoproliferative syndrome.[545] The disease results from mutations in the *CHS1* or *LYST* gene on chromosome 1q. Neurological symptoms include weakness, sensory deficits and gait problems. The few reported nerve biopsies[327] have shown myelinated fibre loss, with relative sparing of small myelinated fibres. Unmyelinated fibres are also affected. Ultrastructurally, giant lysosomes are seen in Schwann cells, endothelial cells and fibroblasts.

Neuropathy in Hereditary Ataxia

There are two groups of hereditary ataxias: the autosomal recessive ataxias and the autosomal dominant spinocerebellar ataxias (SCAs). Recessive ataxias are multisystem disorders characterized by inactivating mutations that result in loss of protein function. In SCA, cell death is mostly limited to the CNS, and cellular control of protein folding and processing is affected by an expansion of CAG-triplet repeats in the coding region of the disease gene, resulting in a toxic gain of function of the aberrant protein (for review, see Taroni and DiDonato[496]). However, peripheral neuropathy is a feature in SCA1, SCA2, SCA3, SCA4, SCA8, SCA18 and SCA25.[303] Neurophysiological findings in these disorders are compatible with a dying-back axonopathy and/or a neuronopathy.[518]

The rarer recessive ataxias can also be clinically classified as sensory and spinocerebellar ataxias, cerebellar ataxia with sensorimotor polyneuropathy, and purely cerebellar ataxias.[253] Ataxia with isolated vitamin E deficiency, abetalipoproteinaemia, Refsum's disease, infantile-onset spinocerebellar ataxia and ataxia with blindness and deafness fall into the first category. Examples of ataxia with sensorimotor polyneuropathy include ataxia with oculomotor apraxia 1 and 2 and spinocerebellar ataxia with neuropathy 1. For most of these disorders, detailed histological findings on nerve biopsy are not available; exceptions are Friedreich's ataxia, abetalipoproteinaemia and ataxia telangiectasia. Friedreich's ataxia is the most frequent early-onset autosomal recessive inherited ataxia and has received the most extensive pathological study of peripheral nerve. The majority of cases feature axonal degeneration involving large myelinated fibres.[429] Involvement of cutaneous unmyelinated sensory and autonomic nerve fibres has also been reported.[350] Peripheral nerve biopsies in abetalipoproteinaemia show evidence of a mild axonopathy, with depletion of large myelinating fibres and a slight increase in regenerating clusters, similar to findings in other causes of vitamin E deficiency.[555] Ataxia telangiectasia also shows loss of large myelinated fibres, with sparing of unmyelinated axons;[298] also characteristic are Schwann cells with large bizarre hyperchromatic nuclei with highly irregular outlines.

Cerebral Autosomal Dominant Arteriopathy with Subcortical Infarcts and Leukoencephalopathy

Cerebral autosomal dominant arteriopathy with subcortical infarcts and leukoencephalopathy (CADASIL) (see Chapter 2, Vascular Disease, Hypoxia and Related Conditions) is an inherited cerebral micro-angiopathy associated with mutations in the *NOTCH3* (*Notch homolog 3*) gene. In adults, *Notch 3* is expressed in vascular smooth muscle cells throughout the body; mutant *Notch 3* is associated with progressive vascular smooth muscle cell deterioration, with vascular mural thickening and luminal narrowing.[421] The CNS is predominantly affected, with subcortical infarcts resulting in progressive neurological deterioration, psychiatric changes and cognitive impairment. The presence of granular osmiophilic material in small arterioles of the CNS, peripheral nerves and other tissues is the pathological hallmark of the disease (Figure 24.61).[421] In addition to the microvascular changes, peripheral nerve damage has been reported in 7 of 11 examined patients.[466] Three of these patients had peripheral nerve biopsies that showed slight to moderate reduction in myelinated fibre density and ultrastructural evidence of unmyelinated fibre degeneration (groups of flat Schwann cell processes and collagen pockets).

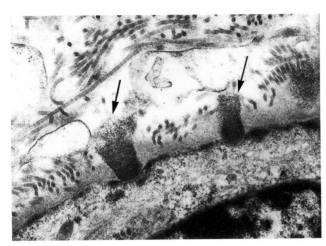

24.61 CADASIL, muscle biopsy. Smooth muscle cell, showing characteristic granular osmiophilic material (arrows) on cell surface. ×6400.

Photograph courtesy of Dr William Halliday, University of Toronto, Toronto, ON, Canada.

INFLAMMATORY AND INFECTIOUS NEUROPATHIES

Immune-Mediated Neuropathies

Immune-mediated neuropathies, once simply classified as either cell- or antibody-mediated, are complex processes with cellular elements recruited from the host as well as locally synthesized or haematogenously derived humoral antibodies, cytokines and reactive oxygen species (see Box 24.1).

Guillain–Barré Syndrome

Guillain–Barré syndrome, which occurs at a frequency of 1.5 cases per 100 000, is characterized by the development of a rapidly progressive paralytic syndrome with several patterns of PNS involvement.[179,211,241,461] Although often considered a motor disease, sensory and autonomic symptoms may actually anticipate motor dysfunction. Classically, patients exhibit increased CSF protein with a normal cell count (albuminocytological dissociation), particularly later in the course. Reaching a nadir within 1 month, patients typically recover, although residual disability is not uncommon, especially in older patients. Modern mortality rates are 1–2.5 per cent. Plasmapheresis and intravenous immunoglobulin reduce morbidity, but glucocorticoids are not an effective treatment. Clinical GBS may be subdivided into several clinicopathological categories.[561]

Acute Inflammatory Demyelinating Polyneuropathy

This pattern, most common in Europe and the USA, may involve ventral (and dorsal) roots, proximal spinal nerves, even distal sensory nerves (e.g. sural) and (in some patients) lower cranial nerves, resulting in patchy myelin loss with relative axonal sparing (Figure 24.62).

BOX 24.1. Experimental allergic neuritis

Experimental allergic neuritis (EAN) is produced by injection of animals with homogenized peripheral nerve, myelin or a variety of myelin proteins or peptide sequences–P_0, P_2, myelin basic protein, peripheral myelin protein 22 (PMP22) and myelin-associated glycoprotein (MAG)–typically in combination with adjuvant.[310] Additionally, EAN may be induced passively by injection of CD4+ T-cell lines directed against peripheral myelin proteins or foreign proteins injected into the nerve. Endoneurial perivenular lymphocytes and macrophages are associated with patches of demyelinated axons. Macrophages actively strip myelin lamellae from axons, induce vesicular disruption of the myelin sheath and phagocytose both intact and damaged myelin in the distinctive macrophage-mediated demyelination pattern shared with acute inflammatory demyelinating polyneuropathy (AIDP) and chronic inflammatory demyelinating polyneuropathy (CIDP). Studies of passively transmitted EAN have shown that differences in the extent of demyelination versus axonal degeneration may reflect the number of injected T-cells. The adoptive transfer of pure P2 protein-specific CD4+ T-cells derived from rats with EAN into recipient naive rats results in axonal degeneration with mild demyelination; however, if the inoculum includes anti-myelin antibodies, then a more demyelinating pattern of injury is produced, which may reflect opening the blood–nerve barrier to circulating antibodies.[497] Somatic nerves containing both sensory and motor axons are targeted, as well as myelin-rich portions of the autonomic nervous system (e.g. vagus and sympathetic preganglionic splanchnic nerves) and unmyelinated axons, the latter as a bystander effect.

T-cells must be activated in the periphery in order to cross the blood–nerve barrier. Homing and transmigration depend on a complex interaction of adhesion molecules, chemokines and matrix metalloproteinases. With the dissolution of the blood–nerve barrier, neural antigen-specific T-lymphocytes are locally reactivated by interacting with macrophages, expand clonally and release cytokines, especially interferon γ (IFN-γ) and tumour necrosis factor α (TNF-α). Macrophages are activated, generating reactive oxygen, nitric oxide metabolites, complement and proteases. Antibodies damage myelin by antibody-dependent cellular cytotoxicity, opsonizing targets to promote ingestion by macrophages, and/or activating complement to create the terminal complement attack complex (C5b-9) to induce myelin destruction via calcium-stimulated proteases. Complement also recruits macrophages into the nerve.

In a similar paradigm, rabbits immunized with human sympathetic ganglia develop vasomotor dysfunction and perivascular lymphocytes and mononuclear cells in the sympathetic ganglia and autonomic nerves.[11] Passive transfer of antisera directed against acetylcholinesterase produces a complement-mediated loss of cholinergic innervation of sympathetic ganglia, which eventually results in the loss of preganglionic sympathetic neurons in the intermediolateral nucleus.[50]

Active lesions are characterized by prominent perivascular epineurial and endoneurial lymphocytes, consisting mostly of several populations of CD4+ T-cells, and endoneurial macrophages, some intimately apposed to axons with intact myelin sheaths. Resin sections demonstrate patchy demyelination and remyelination (Figure 24.63a), often adjacent to macrophages containing myelin debris (Figure 24.63b). Macrophages characteristically strip otherwise normal-appearing myelin sheaths (Figure 24.64), displacing Schwann cells (Figure 24.64b), which generally remain free of myelin debris, a pattern

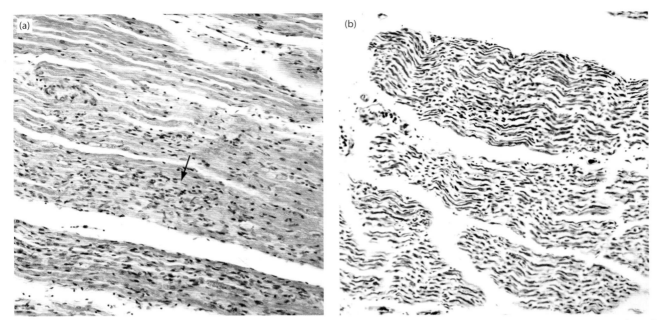

24.62 Guillain–Barré syndrome: acute inflammatory demyelinating polyneuropathy (AIDP) subtype. Peripheral nerves show **(a)** patchy myelin loss (arrow) and variable inflammation (Luxol fast blue–periodic acid–Schiff myelin stain); and **(b)** relative axonal sparing (Bodian axon stain, ×90).

unlike typical demyelination (e.g. following diphtheria), in which Schwann cells represent the initial degradative site. Some myelin sheaths may show initial vesicular myelin breakdown followed by macrophage-mediated stripping. Complement deposition and C5b-9 membrane attack complexes have been described on Schwann cell surfaces, although this is inconsistent and may simply reflect increased permeability of the endoneurial

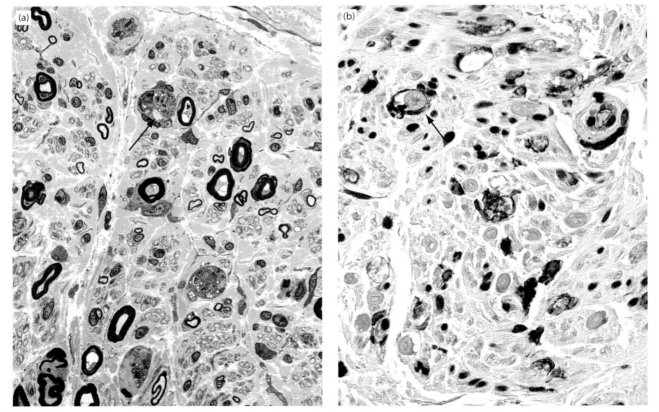

24.63 Guillain–Barré syndrome: acute inflammatory demyelinating polyneuropathy (AIDP) subtype. (a) Plastic sections of nerve show demyelination, often with a spared axon (arrow) as well as a degree of axon loss (1-μm plastic section **(b)** The intimate association of macrophages with the myelin sheath (arrow) is seen with CD45 immunolocalization. ×600.

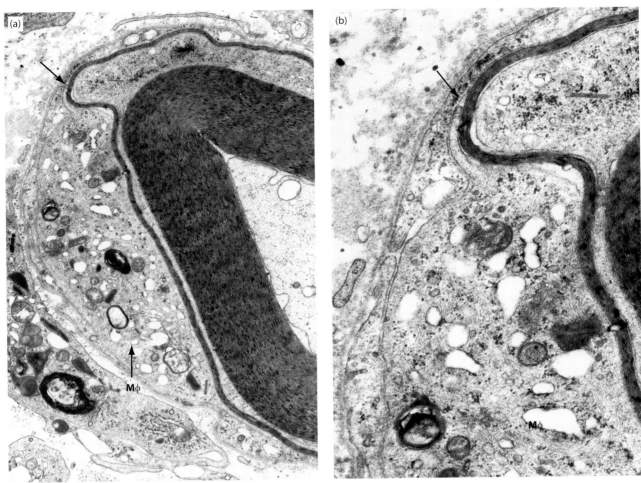

24.64 Macrophage-mediated demyelination: Guillain–Barré syndrome, acute inflammatory demyelinating polyneuropathy (AIDP) subtype. (a) Electron micrograph, ×3700. **(b)** A portion of a macrophage containing myelin debris, intercalated between the myelin sheath and Schwann cell cytoplasm, directly peels off a portion of the myelin sheath using delicate processes (arrow). Electron micrograph, ×9500.

microvasculature. Bound complement may result in pore formation, Ca2+ entry and vesicular disruption of myelin, a pattern mimicking autolysis. Schwann cells rarely degenerate; rather, they separate from their myelin sheaths, re-enter the cell cycle, produce daughter Schwann cells outside the original basal lamina and re-enter and remyelinate the denuded internode in the presence of ongoing demyelination in adjacent fibres and a persistent inflammatory infiltrate. Naked demyelinated axons may appear atrophic, perhaps reflecting the loss of Schwann cell-derived trophic support. Axonal loss or axonopathy may represent a 'bystander effect' due to endoneurial toxic cytokines (e.g. TNF-α) or oedema-induced local ischaemia and compression. Autonomic ganglia also show perivascular inflammatory infiltrates and inflammatory demyelination of preganglionic myelinated axons.

The pathogenesis of acute inflammatory demyelinating polyneuropathy (AIDP) involves significant immune system abnormalities. Circulating T-cells are activated in patients with GBS, as demonstrated by enhanced antigen expression, increased MHC class II and co-stimulatory molecules, and pro-inflammatory cytokines IFN-γ and TNF-α.[193] Perivascular epineurial and endoneurial lymphocytes,

mostly subpopulations of T-cells, contain γδT-lymphocytes and increased usage of Vβ15 T-cell receptor, suggesting a restricted T-cell response to a common antigen or defective regulation of γδT-cells permitting autoimmune attack on ganglioside-like epitopes.[102] Studies have also established a significant role for intraneural CD8+ T-lymphocytes in GBS.[544] Specific chemokine receptors on macrophages (CCR-1, CCR-5) and T-lymphocytes (CCR-2, CCR-3, CCR-4), a differential expression pattern of matrix metalloproteinases (MMP-7, MMP-9) and upregulation of macrophage nuclear factor κB (NF-κB)[241] are also thought to contribute (see reviews[270,289]). The self-limited nature of GBS has been proposed to reflect the effect of anti-inflammatory cytokines IL-10 and TGF-β on shifting the systemic T-cell population to Th2-type T-lymphocytes and induction of T-cell apoptosis.

A role for humoral factors,[544] either systemic entering the endoneurium or synthesized locally, is suggested by the beneficial effects of plasmapheresis and intravenous immunoglobulin administration, the presence of nerve-targeting circulating antibody from patients with GBS and immunoglobulin and complement identification on some myelinated fibres.[179] Antibodies against gangliosides GM1, GM1b,

GalNAc-GD1a, GM2, basal lamina components and several myelin proteins have also been identified;[179] however, no characteristic pattern of antiganglioside antibodies has been established in AIDP (compared with acute motor axonal neuropathy (AMAN)). Antibody against GM1 correlates with prominent motor involvement and a slower rate of recovery.

Not uncommonly, AIDP follows antecedent events, including immunizations and infection with Epstein–Barr virus, cytomegalovirus (CMV), HIV, *Haemophilus influenzae*, *Mycoplasma pneumoniae* and *Campylobacter jejuni*, which produce GBS of differing severity and more motor (following *C. jejuni*) versus sensory symptoms.[179,241] T-cells are thought to recognize an autoantigen, perhaps an epitope on an infectious agent ('molecular mimicry'), in the presence of MHC class II and co-stimulatory molecules on the surface of an antigen-presenting cell.[241] Activated T-cells cross the blood–nerve barrier and stimulate macrophages to release cytokines and toxic mediators, such as nitric oxide, that interfere with the integrity of the blood–nerve barrier and, locally or systemically, instruct B-cells to proliferate and secrete myelin-directed antibodies or cytokines, increasing the endoneurial influx of recruited monocytes and macrophages. Endoneurial cytokines further stimulate MHC class II expression on antigen-presenting cells (e.g. macrophages, Schwann cells), resulting in proliferation of T-cells and macrophages and release of additional cytokines, proteases and reactive oxygen species into the milieu; this combination ultimately results in myelinopathy. AIDP may share pathogenetic mechanisms with experimental allergic neuritis (EAN) (Box 24.1).

Acute Motor Axonal Neuropathy

Acute motor axonal neuropathy (an 'axonal' form of GBS) exhibits prominent electrophysiological and pathological evidence of axon loss with little demyelination[144] and, frequently, a more aggressive course than AIDP. Acute motor axonal neuropathy has been described predominantly in Japan and China, where it may occur in summertime epidemics. It is proposed that antigenic epitopes of infectious agents, such as the lipopolysaccharides of *C. jejuni*, a Gram-negative poultry-associated organism causing gastroenteritis, are shared with peripheral nerve antigens.[9,204] The association of *C. jejuni* with AMAN is more established than with AIDP and differs in different parts of the world. In China, serological evidence of *C. jejuni* infection was described in 76 per cent of cases of AMAN and 42 per cent of cases of AIDP.[204] There are differences in the distribution of HLA-DQB epitopes in patients with AMAN and AIDP from northern China, suggesting an immunogenetic component.[297] The presence of immunoglobulin IgG1 and IgG3 subclasses of anti-GM1 antibody is associated with slow and rapid recovery, respectively.[254] Different serotypes of ganglioside-like polysaccharide antigens in *C. jejuni* (e.g. HS/O:19) may be overrepresented in infections in patients with AMAN compared with patients with gastroenteritis but without GBS and may contribute to clinical and pathological variations in presentation.

The most striking differences between AIDP and AMAN are the paucity of lymphocytic inflammation, the lack of demyelination and a variable increase in the number of degenerating axons in AMAN (Figure 24.65). Activation products of IgG and complement are found exclusively on motor axons in AMAN.[179] Macrophages are found adjacent to or within the periaxonal space at the node of Ranvier, accompanied by swelling of adaxonal Schwann cell cytoplasm and, variably, axonal degeneration. Axonopathy ranges from diffuse axonal degeneration to distal axonal damage, with denervated neuromuscular junctions; the latter may be reversed rapidly. Predictably, sensory axon degeneration is mild in AMAN but may be extensive in acute motor sensory axonal neuropathy (AMSAN) (see Acute Motor Sensory Axonal Neuropathy, p. 1457). Correlation of functional changes with pathology is often imprecise.

In AMAN, the primary target of the immune attack is the axon rather than the Schwann cell or myelin. The condition has been associated with serum IgG binding to GM1, GD1a and GalNAc-GD1a gangliosides. GalNAc-GD1a ganglioside has been identified along the inner part of compact myelin and, in addition, involving the periaxonal axolemma in the ventral root, small-diameter dorsal root and motor axons.[229] The selectivity of AMAN for motor axons may reflect the different affinities of anti-GD1a antibodies for sensory GD1a and motor GD1a; experimental studies have shown that monoclonal anti-GD1a antibody preferentially stained motor axons and a subpopulation of small sensory axons[293] and that GalNAc-GD1a may be expressed only on motor axons.

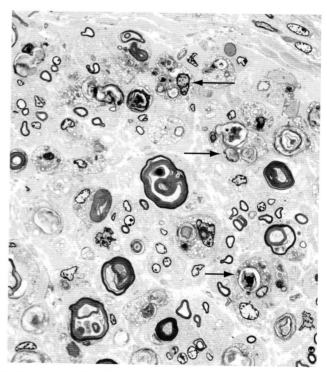

24.65 Guillain–Barré syndrome: acute motor axonal neuropathy (AMAN) subtype. In this form, axonal degeneration (arrows) may be prominent in the absence of inflammation and demyelination. 1-µm plastic section, ×600.

Immunoglobulin G anti-GD1a antibodies were found in 60 per cent of Chinese patients with GBS but in only 4 per cent of patients with AIDP, whereas anti-GM1 antibodies were frequent in both variants.[205]

The pathogenesis of AMAN may initially involve antibody targeting of a constituent of the node of Ranvier or paranodal axolemma, most likely a ganglioside, to which it binds, fixes complement and secondarily recruits macrophages; these events would culminate in axonal dysfunction or, in some cases, axonal degeneration. In support of this hypothesis, rabbits immunized with gangliosides or GM1 may develop weakness, high titres of anti-GM1 antibodies and pathological changes similar to human AMAN, with axonal degeneration confined to motor roots largely in the absence of inflammation.[578] Some people immunized with gangliosides have developed axonal forms of GBS.

Acute Motor Sensory Axonal Neuropathy

Sensory axon degeneration is mild in AMAN but may be extensive in AMSAN. Activation products of IgG and complement are also found in AMSAN, predominantly on motor axons, reflecting a primary axonal target.[179] In rare cases of GBS, electrophysiological studies showed decreased muscle and sensory nerve action potentials initially designated as an 'axonal variant of GBS'[145] and, more recently, as AMSAN.[182] Both AMAN and AMSAN are thought to be a part of the spectrum of a single type of immune attack on the axon,[182] a contention supported by the presence in both entities of anti-GM1 (64 per cent), anti-GM1b (66 per cent) and anti-GalNAc-GD1a (33 per cent) IgG antibodies[211,577] and the association of both conditions with *C. jejuni* enteritis.[182] Cases of AMSAN differ from AMAN in terms of slow clinical recovery.

Pathological changes include lengthening of nodes of Ranvier, distortion of paranodal myelin and degeneration of outermost myelin terminal loops, followed by intercalation of macrophage processes into the periaxonal space at the paranode, separating the axon from the adaxonal Schwann cell plasmalemma and eventually causing degeneration of Schwann cell cytoplasm but not loss of the internodal myelin sheath. Macrophages are found within the periaxonal spaces of myelinated nerve fibres and the axon. It has been proposed that AMSAN and AMAN may represent severe manifestations of the same immunopathological process, differing in severity, immunological presentation or distribution of a critical epitope.[182]

Miller Fisher Syndrome

The Miller Fisher syndrome (MFS) manifests as a triad of ataxia, areflexia and ophthalmoplegia.[557] Many patients with MFS have serum IgG binding to GQ1b ganglioside or antibodies cross-reactive with GT1a,[92] which appear to be concentrated at the nodes of Ranvier, particularly those of the oculomotor nerves.[92] Patients with Bickerstaff's brain stem encephalitis also show antibodies to GQ1b, and occasional patients with both CNS and PNS findings have been described. GQ1b epitopes are present in *C. jejuni* isolated from patients with MFS and anti-GQ1b autoantibodies.[9] Selected serotypes of *C. jejuni* are overrepresented in patients with MFS. A similar association is seen in patients seropositive for *H. influenzae* and with autoantibodies against GQ1b.[383] In patients with MFS, ophthalmoplegia correlates with the presence of anti-GQ1b antibody and with oropharyngeal weakness with anti-GT1a antibody. Serum or purified IgG from patients with MFS has been shown to reversibly inhibit presynaptic quantal release and reduce postsynaptic amplitudes in neuromuscular preparations *in vitro*,[59] but this effect was not dependent on GQ1b antibodies or complement.

Acute Pan-autonomic Neuropathy (Pan-dysautonomia)

Patients with this syndrome present acutely with diffuse parasympathetic and sympathetic failure in the absence of somatic nerve motor or sensory dysfunction.[55] Pure cholinergic failure, with urinary retention, sweating abnormality, blurred vision and constipation, is also described. There is a viral prodrome in 59 per cent, especially an upper respiratory or 'flu-like' syndrome. A monophasic course is typical. Neuropathological studies have demonstrated peripheral postganglionic epineurial mononuclear inflammation, involvement of preganglionic nerves, evidence of axonal regeneration, and a decrease in unmyelinated and small myelinated axon populations.[10] Antibodies against neuronal nicotinic (α3) acetylcholine receptor subunits have been reported in 30 per cent of cases.[522] Some patients have a recent history of Epstein–Barr virus infection. Pan-dysautonomia can also be part of a paraneoplastic syndrome, especially with small cell lung cancer, and probably occurs with increased frequency in diabetic people.

Chronic Inflammatory Demyelinating Polyradiculoneuropathy

Chronic inflammatory demyelinating polyradiculoneuropathy, or 'chronic GBS', is a chronic polyneuropathy characterized by symmetrical proximal and distal muscle weakness that worsens progressively or in relapsing fashion for at least 2 months.[241,255] Sensory loss, predominantly distal, is present in all patients but is rarely disabling. Electrophysiology shows features of a demyelinating neuropathy. Other laboratory changes can include enlargement or gadolinium enhancement of spinal roots on MR imaging and increased CSF protein without cells. The condition occurs with somewhat increased frequency in patients with diabetes, HIV, inflammatory bowel disease, lymphoma, melanoma, Sjögren's syndrome, hepatitis C, and IgG or immunoglobulin A (IgA) monoclonal gammopathy of unknown significance (MGUS). In diabetic individuals, CIDP is reported to be more severe, but with a significantly better response to intravenous immunoglobulin and fewer relapses.[221] There is evidence of both primary segmental demyelination and superimposed secondary demyelination initiated by axonal atrophy. Occasional patients with CIDP also have clinical or laboratory evidence of CNS demyelination. HLA-B8 is overrepresented in CIDP. The condition responds well to several treatment modalities, including steroids, plasma exchange, intravenous immunoglobulin and immunosuppressant drugs.[255] A potentially related condition, chronic immune sensory polyradiculopathy (CISP; sensory CIDP), preferentially affecting large myelinated fibres of the posterior roots, may be a restricted form of CIDP.[357] Other CIDP variants have been described, including Lewis–Sumner multifocal CIDP with predilection for the upper extremities.[274]

The value of nerve biopsy in CIDP has been debated, in part because pathology is most prominent in the roots and proximal nerve segments and because CIDP is not excluded by negative biopsy. The pathological findings in CIDP reflect ongoing cycles of demyelination (Figure 24.66a) and remyelination. Onion bulbs are seen in a minority (15–40 per cent) of cases (Figure 24.66b), some with intercalated inflammatory cells and others admixed with myelinated axons without onion bulbs, providing a differential separation from other hereditary onion bulb neuropathies. There are often prominent differences in the extent of fascicular involvement. Fewer than 50 per cent of cases have significant inflammation; those that do show monocytes, macrophages and lymphocytes within the endoneurium and epineurium (usually in the absence of perineuritis), few plasma cells, and increased subperineurial space containing deposits of amorphous non-amyloid material. As in AIDP, macrophage-mediated demyelination represents the pathological hallmark (see Figure 24.67), although it may be only sparsely represented. Both myelinated and unmyelinated axons are lost (Figure 24.66a), which may determine long-term prognosis. The condition typically results in only minor autonomic symptomatology; however, sympathetic trunks and axons constituting distal visceral innervation show enlargement and hypertrophic changes that may result in autonomic dysfunction.

Both CD4+ and CD8+ T-cells are found in the infiltrate, along with activated macrophages but without B-cells; the function of CD4+ Treg subpopulations, which mediate the suppression of effector T-cell function, is reportedly impaired.[477] Studies have also demonstrated natural killer (NK) T-cells and T-lymphocytes of a γδ71 TCR phenotype, consistent with a possible role of a cellular immune response against non-protein antigens.[562] Nerves contain soluble adhesion molecules, chemokines, matrix metalloproteinases, TNF-α, IFN-γ or interleukin 2 (IL-2) as evidence of T-cell activation.[576] T-cells are thought to activate resident endoneurial or passenger macrophages, which then discharge an array of neurotoxic and immunopotentiating molecules (i.e. oxygen radicals, nitric oxide metabolites, arachidonic acid metabolites, proteases, complement components) or engage in increased phagocytic and cytotoxic activity against myelin or Schwann cells. Early changes involve widening of the node of Ranvier. No dominant T-cell receptor (TCR) Vα utilization has been detected in CIDP nerve biopsies, suggesting that there are no clonally expanded T-cells in these biopsies.[41] Mice deficient in B7-2 co-stimulation develop a spontaneous autoimmune polyneuropathy, transferable by T-cells to SCID mice, similar clinically, electrophysiologically and pathologically to human CIDP.[436] Macrophages expressing MHC class I and

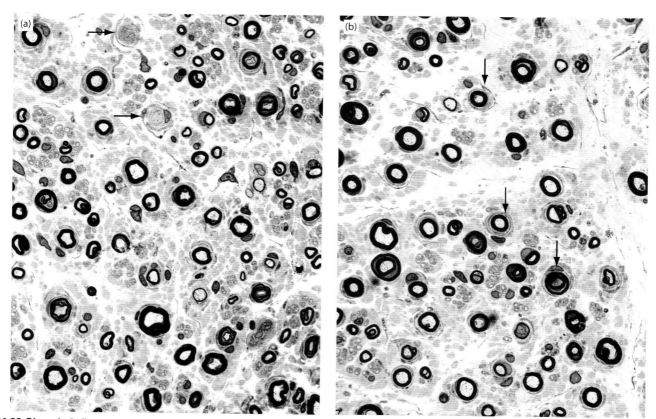

24.66 Chronic inflammatory demyelinating polyneuropathy (CIDP). (a) Sections of sural nerve demonstrate scattered demyelinated axons (arrows) and variably thinned myelin sheaths. **(b)** Onion bulbs (arrows) may be frequent in some cases, but rarely cause confusion with inherited onion-bulb neuropathies. 1-μm plastic sections. ×600.

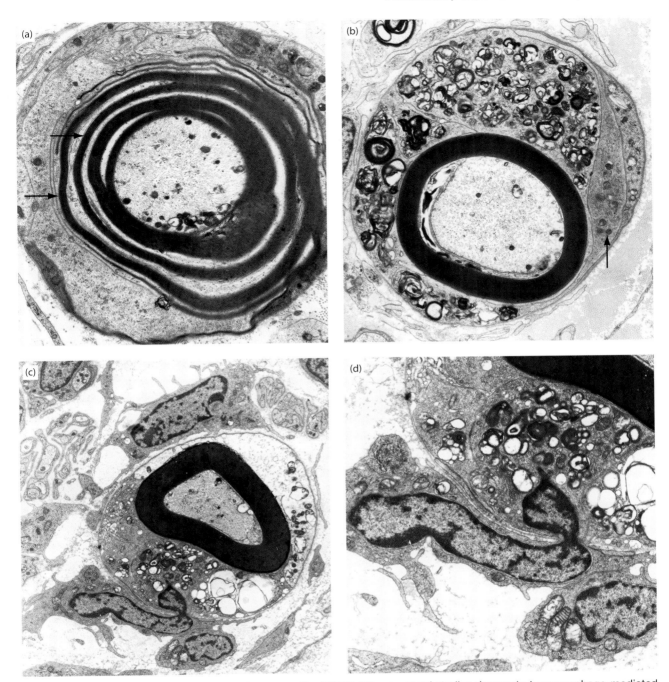

24.67 Chronic inflammatory demyelinating polyneuropathy (CIDP). Ultrastructural studies demonstrate macrophage-mediated demyelination similar to the acute inflammatory demyelinating polyneuropathy (AIDP) pattern of Guillain–Barré syndrome. **(a)** Removal of broad bands of otherwise normal myelin (arrows) results in complete loss of myelin present in the macrophage cytoplasm but not in the Schwann cell (arrow) cytoplasm **(b)**. **(c,d)** A particularly fortuitous section demonstrates a macrophage actively penetrating the Schwann cell basement membrane and displacing its cytoplasm. Note the intimate relationship of processes from adjacent lymphoid cells and macrophages in **(d)**. Electron micrographs: (a) ×6900; (b) ×5700; (c) ×5500; (d) ×10 900.

II molecules and CD1a serve as antigen-presenting cells in CIDP. Elevated serum and CSF levels of soluble adhesion molecules, chemokines and matrix metalloproteinases indicate active T-cell migration across the blood–nerve barrier.[240] The recovering endoneurial milieu also contains T-cell-derived downregulatory cytokines such as interleukin 4 (IL-4) and IL-10, or TGF-β, IL-6 mRNA, NGF, leukaemia inhibitory factor (LIF) and GDNF and their receptors,[566] as well as evidence of apoptosis of T-cells.

Despite the pathological similarities with GBS and a not infrequent history of premonitory viral syndrome, a role for molecular mimicry with agents producing GBS has not been established in CIDP. Nonetheless, the association of CIDP with melanoma[552] suggests the possibility of shared antigens, supported by the cross-reactivity of monoclonal anti-melanoma antibodies with several myelin-associated glycoproteins and glycolipids. The beneficial effects of plasmapheresis in some cases of CIDP also suggest a humoral component. The presence of immunoglobulin and complement deposition on axons in CIDP has been debated.[413]

Electrophysiological defects and demyelination have, however, been produced *in vitro* and *in vivo* by serum from patients with CIDP.[568] Upregulation of the chemokine receptor CXCR3 and other chemokines attracting T_h1 cells are found in biopsied sural nerves.[240] Intravenous immunoglobulin may be useful by the correction of the pathogenetic T_h1 shift but is not effective in patients with markedly depressed CSF T_h2 cells.[315] Serum in patients with CIDP may also have IgG or IgM antibodies directed against β2 tubulin, heparan sulphate (sulfate) or IgG, which binds cultured Schwann cell processes or neurites and may correlate with an atypical clinical picture.

Multifocal Motor Neuropathy

Multifocal motor neuropathy (MMN) is characterized by adult-onset, male-predominant (>2:1), slowly progressive, asymmetrical weakness with muscle wasting, cramps and fasciculations, without sensory dysfunction (reviewed[538]). The process often starts in the distal arm muscles and involves individual nerve territories (resembling mononeuritis multiplex).[348] Partial motor-conduction block at multiple sites is a characteristic but inconstant electrophysiological feature. Most patients have circulating high-titre antiganglioside GM1[382] or NP-9 IgM antibodies and, to a lesser extent, other glycolipids. These antibodies, which are not specific for MMN, are not seen in amyotrophic lateral sclerosis/motor neuron disease, which is often in the differential diagnosis. Patients have a higher frequency of homozygous SMN2 deletion than controls.[416] Although corticosteroids are ineffective and may produce dramatic worsening in some patients, MMN improves with intravenous immunoglobulin, cyclophosphamide, rituximab and plasmapheresis (in some cases with anti-GM1 antibodies), although plasma exchange has, conversely, been reported to be ineffective or deleterious.[379] Multifocal motor neuropathy resembles the CIDP variant known as Lewis–Sumner syndrome, which is an acquired demyelinating sensory and motor neuropathy. The major distinguishing features are the clinical and electrophysiological sensory involvement in Lewis–Sumner syndrome, its more restricted motor pattern[359] and the lack of anti-GM1 antibodies in Lewis–Sumner syndrome (whereas IgM anti-GM1 were found in 40 per cent of patients with MMN). Moreover, some patients with CIDP and Lewis–Sumner syndrome respond to steroid therapy, whereas this is ineffective in MMN. For these reasons, Lewis–Sumner syndrome can be considered intermediate between CIDP and MMN.

The pathology of MMN has not been studied extensively. In some cases, nerves exhibit multifocal demyelination, epineurial and endoneurial perivascular inflammation, onion bulbs in the area of conduction block and motor axon degeneration and loss (especially larger axons). These findings differ from CIDP in the absence of macrophage-mediated demyelination.[324] Immunoglobulin

deposition and inflammatory demyelination were found in motor roots in an autopsy case.[358]

The pathogenesis of MMN is not understood. Focal conduction block has been induced *in vivo* and *in vitro* after intraneural injection of sera from patients with high IgM anti-GM1 antibodies and MMN, but not with purified anti-GM1 antibodies.[194] Anti-GM1 antibodies react with the lipopolysaccharide of *C. jejuni*, but only 5 per cent of patients with MMN had high levels of antibodies to *C. jejuni*.[499]

Idiopathic Perineuritis

Patients with idiopathic perineuritis often present with a sensory neuropathy in a mononeuritis multiplex or CIDP pattern. Nerve biopsy shows infiltration of the perineurium by lymphocytes and macrophages, some of which are epithelioid and may form granulomas, with superimposed degenerating perineurial cells, proliferating fibroblasts, collagen deposition and proliferation of small perineurial vessels (Figure 24.68). The diagnosis of idiopathic perineuritis is made after exclusion of secondary perineuritis induced by cryoglobulinaemia, sarcoid, leprosy, lymphoma, Lyme disease, ulcerative colitis, rapeseed oil or L-tryptophan ingestion.[324] Fascicles exhibiting perineuritis frequently feature loss of myelinated axons and actively degenerating axons, demyelination and remyelination.

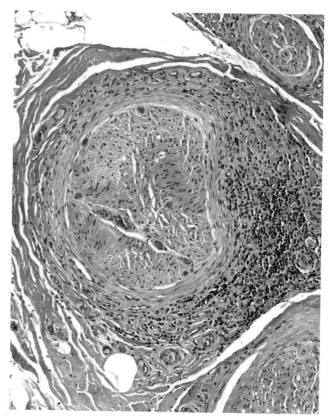

24.68 Idiopathic perineuritis. This fascicle shows perifascicular inflammation and thickening of the perineurium by increased numbers of perineurial cells and collagen. ×130.

Sarcoidosis

Sarcoidosis is a worldwide disease with ethnic predilections that differ between regions, involving African American people in the USA and white people in Europe, with an especially high frequency in Sweden.[432] A polygenic mode of inheritance is seen in some families, but little is known definitively about its pathogenesis.

Although somatic peripheral nerves may be involved by sarcoid, facial nerve palsy is the most common neurological manifestation of sarcoidosis.[432] The characteristic pathological changes of sarcoidosis are non-caseating granulomas (Figure 24.69), although they are not seen frequently in biopsied peripheral nerve. When present, they involve the epineurium and, less frequently, endoneurium; in the epineurium, they are relatively innocuous, usually occurring in the presence of a nearly normal complement of axons. Granulomas, when found, frequently occur adjacent to blood vessels and, in some cases, in the presence of a lymphocytic angiitis involving epineurial and perineurial vessels; the angiitis may result in ischaemia-induced axonal degeneration,[432] which frequently varies from fascicle to fascicle. The lymphocytic population is dominated by CD4+ rather than CD8+ T-cells. The differential diagnosis of sarcoidosis includes the tuberculoid form of leprosy (see Leprous Neuritis, p. 1466), Wegener's granulomatosis, Churg–Strauss disease, PAN, giant cell arteritis and lymphomatoid granulomatosis.[324] The clinical setting of neuropathy with fever, uveitis, parotid gland involvement, lymphadenopathy and granulomatous inflammation in a muscle biopsy (leprous granulomas do not involve muscle) favours the diagnosis of sarcoidosis. Treatment with steroids is typically helpful.

NEUROPATHIES ASSOCIATED WITH INFECTIOUS DISEASES

Herpes Zoster

Herpes zoster (see Chapter 19, Viral Infections) is characterized by the painful development of a vesicular cutaneous rash corresponding to the dermatomal distribution of an involved (typically thoracic) dorsal root ganglion or trigeminal ganglion. Varicella infecting the dorsal root ganglia during childhood becomes latent within individual neurons (demonstrable by *in situ* hybridization but not ultrastructurally). At poorly understood times of altered immune status, the virus may emerge from latency and undergo orthograde axonal transport to sensory nerve termini in the skin, where it results in a cutaneous eruption of herpes zoster, or shingles. During this period, the dorsal root ganglion typically shows haemorrhagic ganglioradiculitis, in which infected neurons and satellite cells are admixed with angionecrosis

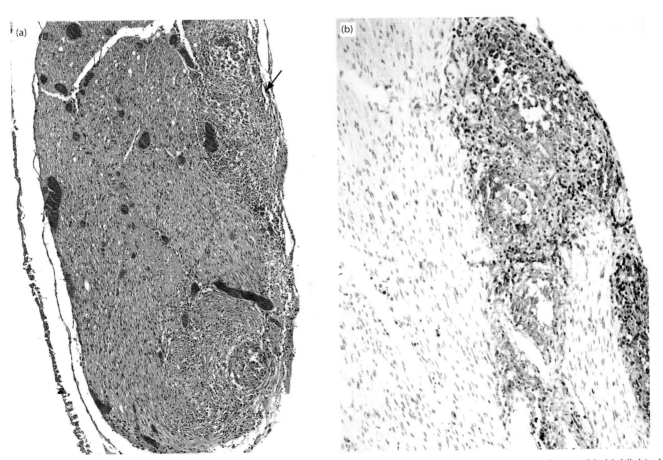

24.69 Sarcoid neuropathy. (a) Granulomatous inflammation (arrow) involves the endoneurium and perineurium and is highlighted by **(b)** CD45 immunostain. (a) ×80; (b) ×160.

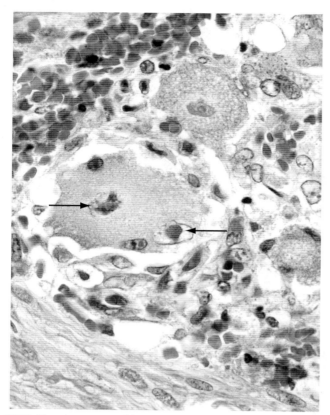

24.70 Herpes zoster. Varicella viral inclusions are found in degenerating dorsal root ganglia neurons and in satellite cells (arrows). ×600.

(Figure 24.70), haemorrhage and an inflammatory mononuclear cell infiltrate. Cowdry type A inclusions are seen in neurons and, more frequently, within satellite cell nuclei (arrows, Figure 24.70). Rarely, activated virus may spread centrally along dorsal roots to the spinal cord, producing myelitis.

Human Immunodeficiency Virus-Related Neuropathies

A number of types of peripheral neuropathy are associated with HIV infection (see Chapter 19, Viral Infections).[48,51,183,290] Although early studies suggested a direct effect of the HIV-1 agent in the pathogenesis of HIV-1-associated neuropathies, this point remains unestablished. Brew has proposed that the focus of the era before combined antiretroviral therapy (cART)/highly active antiretroviral therapy (HAART) on the duration of HIV disease as a measure of its severity should be replaced by current classifications that are more dependent on the CD4 cell count, a classification scheme adopted in the following text.[48]

Early Human Immunodeficiency Virus Disease (CD4 Cell Count >500 Cells/μL)

Seroconversion Neuropathies

Very early after the acute febrile illness characteristic of primary HIV infection, patients may develop a facial nerve palsy, the pathological basis of which is unknown.[389]

Guillain–Barré Syndrome

Early in seroconversion patients may develop a paralytic syndrome clinically indistinguishable from the typical AIDP type of GBS and, very rarely, its axonal form. This presentation differs from typical GBS by the predominance of CD8+ lymphocytes in the infiltrate and by the development (in half of the patients) of increased CSF protein and a mild mononuclear pleocytosis, even in those with normal CD4+ counts.[104]

Moderately Advanced Human Immunodeficiency Virus Disease (CD4 Cell Count 200–500 Cells/μL)

The neuropathies at this stage reflect immune dysregulation and/or co-infecting agents.[48]

Vasculitis

Vasculitides resulting in the clinical syndrome of mononeuritis multiplex have been described.[90] Pathologically, the process is vasocentric, ranging from an endoneurial perivascular inflammatory infiltration (proposed to reflect immune dysregulation) to necrotizing vasculitis (in which deposition of HIV antigens, cryoglobulins or immune complexes of HIV or hepatitis B or C may be the inciting agent).[45,277] In more advanced mononeuritis multiplex, CMV inclusions have been described in endothelial cells accompanied by focal demyelination and axonal degeneration.[419] In addition, a neuropathy associated with an angiocentric proliferation of predominantly CD8+ lymphocytes with vessel necrosis can be seen in HIV.[69]

Chronic Inflammatory Demyelinating Polyneuropathy

Chronic inflammatory demyelinating polyneuropathy may occur in early or moderately advanced HIV disease. A mononuclear pleocytosis is found in the CSF in HIV-associated CIDP. Disease associated with HIV shows increased macrophages and lymphocytic infiltrates rich in CD8+ lymphocytes and more significant axon loss than non-HIV CIDP.[51] Patients often receive intravenous globulin treatment, which spares overall immune function.

Superimposed Infections

Superimposed infections with hepatitis C (symmetrical distal sensory or mononeuritis multiplex neuropathy), syphilis, human T-cell lymphotropic virus I (HTLV-I; sensory neuropathy with axonal degeneration and demyelination) and varicella zoster (sensory ganglionitis) have been described.[48]

Diffuse Infiltrative Lymphocytosis Syndrome

A relatively rare syndrome, diffuse infiltrative lymphocytosis syndrome (DILS) presents as a subacute symmetrical painful sensorimotor neuropathy characterized by an intense perivascular epineurial and endoneurial CD8+ T-lymphocyte infiltration and markedly elevated HIV proviral load compared with other forms of HIV neuropathy.[167] The syndrome is responsive to cART.

Advanced Human Immunodeficiency Virus Disease (CD4 Cell Count <200 Cells/μL)

Diffuse Sensory Polyneuropathy

Diffuse sensory polyneuropathy (DSPN) is a subacutely developing distal neuropathy that can produce pain, selective vibration perception defects and paraesthesias in later stages of the disease. Pathologically, there is axonal degeneration and loss of both small and large myelinated fibres and, particularly, unmyelinated fibres. These changes are accompanied by macrophage infiltration in nerve and dorsal root ganglia (Figure 24.71) and minimal perivascular T-cell infiltrates.[181] The severity of the neuropathy tends to parallel plasma viral load.[181] Inflammatory cells contain HIV, as do dorsal root ganglion satellite cells, but neurons do not.[570] Activated macrophages, together with satellite cells, are part of the effector arm, expressing MHC class I and II molecules, TNF-α, IL-1, IL-6 and nitric oxide,[462] as well as the viral product gp120. Degeneration of dorsal root ganglion neurons with a resultant increase in nodules of Nageotte may be primary or secondary to axonal damage.[412] Infection with CMV may occur but is not obligatory for the development of DSPN. Skin biopsies of patients with DSPN have demonstrated an inverse correlation between neuropathic pain intensity and epidermal nerve fibre density.[412] Infection with HIV may be associated with the loss of cutaneous innervation even before the onset of sensory symptomatology.[312]

Treatment is symptomatic with clonazepam, carbamazepine, tricyclic antidepressants, valproic acid, gabapentin and topical capsaicin. A trial of NGF in DSPN significantly improved pain symptoms; however, there was no improvement of neuropathy severity as assessed by neurological examination, quantitative sensory testing and epidermal nerve fibre density.[311]

Cytomegalovirus Infection-Related Neuropathy

Polyradiculopathy

In approximately 2 per cent of patients with advanced HIV disease (CD4 cell count <50 cells/μL), and often in the presence of CMV myelopathy, patients develop distal lower limb areflexic paraparesis, distal sensory loss and, in the majority of cases, bladder dysfunction. Thickened nerve roots may be demonstrable by MR imaging. Analysis of the CSF shows a polymorphonuclear pleocytosis in at least 90 per cent of patients and CMV DNA demonstrable by polymerase chain reaction (PCR). The pathological findings consist of CMV infection of Schwann cells (Figure 24.72), a predominantly polymorphonuclear inflammatory infiltrate in the nerve roots (frequently more ventral rather than dorsal) or cranial nerves, and occasional mild myelitis. Some pathological analyses have shown both demyelinating and necrotizing features.[419] Treatment involves anti-CMV therapy with ganciclovir or foscarnet.[7] Intravenous immunoglobulin may also help.

Mononeuritis Multiplex

Infection with CMV may lead to mononeuritis multiplex in patients with very advanced HIV disease (CD4 cell count <50 cells/μL), presenting as an asymmetrical sensorimotor neuropathy of all extremities, with associated pain and variable progression. The most commonly involved nerves are the peroneal nerve; the lateral cutaneous nerve of the thigh; the radial, intercostal and recurrent laryngeal nerves; and dorsal root ganglion neurons. Cerebrospinal fluid polymorphonuclear leukocyte pleocytosis is significantly less frequent than in polyradiculopathy; however, CMV DNA is typically present, as are CMV virions in macrophages, fibroblasts and endoneurial cells in the superficial peroneal nerves[431] and spinal ganglia.

Polyneuropathy

Infection with CMV has also been demonstrated within venular endothelial cells of the epineurium of the sural nerve and in brachial and tibial nerves.[414]

Antiretroviral Drugs: Didanosine, Stavudine And Zalcitabine

Various therapeutic agents (e.g. dideoxycytosine, dideoxyinosine) may contribute to the neuropathic environment of HIV and produce a pattern of peripheral nerve injury

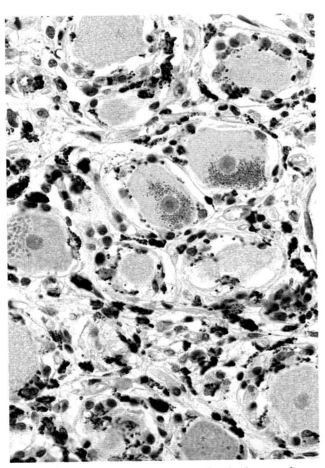

24.71 Diffuse sensory polyneuropathy in human immunodeficiency virus (HIV). Numerous CD68 immunoreactive macrophages may be found in nerve or, in this case, dorsal root ganglia. ×400.

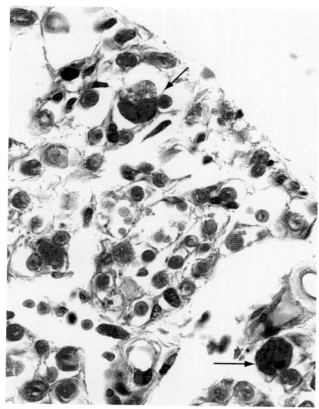

24.72 Cytomegalovirus (CMV) polyradiculopathy. CMV infection of Schwann cells (arrows) in spinal cord roots may occur in association with myelitis. ×600.

('nucleoside neuropathy') clinically indistinguishable from DSPN.[332] These agents are thought to interfere with mitochondrial DNA synthesis or repair by inhibiting γDNA polymerase activity.[275] The incidence ranges from 15 per cent to 40 per cent and requires a mean of 16–20 weeks of treatment before appearing. Pathological studies reveal axonal degeneration and prominent loss of unmyelinated fibres, with mitochondrial disruption and structural changes in cristae.[335] Myelin changes, including splitting and oedema, have been observed in animal models of dideoxyinosine peripheral neurotoxicity.[370]

Autonomic Neuropathy

Late in the course of HIV, a number of autonomic symptoms have been reported, including orthostatic hypotension, cardiovascular abnormalities, impotence, diarrhoea, anhydrosis and bladder dysfunction,[156] often in HIV-infected patients with dementia, myelopathy and distal neuropathy. Pathological findings in peripheral nerve include subtle axonopathy, dilated endoplasmic reticulum in Schwann cells, and immunohistochemical evidence of axon loss. Axonal loss involves the jejunal lamina propria or autonomic axons within somatic nerves affected by one of the HIV neuropathies.[22] Sympathetic ganglia exhibit mild inflammation associated with the presence of viral antigens and increased expression of MHC class II antigens.[138]

Lyme Disease

Lyme disease (see Chapter 20, Bacterial Infections) infection requires prolonged (>24–48 hours) attachment of the Ixodes sp. tick, during which time ingested blood triggers *Borrelia burgdorferi* proliferation in the tick gut, followed by dissemination within the tick and ultimately injection into the host.[427] Spirochaetaemia results in infection of the meninges, heart and peripheral nerve and may be accompanied by erythema migrans, a distinctive rash. Serological tests represent the most definitive diagnostic test.

Mononeuritis multiplex of cranial nerves (80 per cent of which involve the VII nerve), radiculoneuropathies (Bannwarth's syndrome) and, less frequently, diffuse neuropathies represent the most typical patterns of involvement in Lyme disease, usually during its secondary phase 1–2 months after infection.[427] All forms show patchy epineurial, perineurial or endoneurial perivascular lymphocytic/plasmacytic infiltrates, which, although often designated 'perivasculitis', are not necrotizing (Figure 24.73). Cases in the USA are reported to show milder loss of myelinated and unmyelinated axons than European cases.

Detailed neurophysiological and histopathological experimental studies have demonstrated that almost all infected immune-competent animals develop a mononeuropathy multiplex that is remarkably similar to the human disease.[415] As in humans, epineurial perivascular inflammatory infiltrates are evident, without demonstrable spirochaetes, immune complexes or other clear evidence for an underlying mechanism.[427] Inflammation can be meningeal around spinal roots and cranial nerves. A monkey model is characterized by marked mononuclear cell infiltrates surrounding intraneural blood vessels, with macrophages and B-lymphocytes, axonal degeneration and demyelination. *Borrelia burgdorferi* antigens are immunolocalized to macrophages and disappear with time. Axonal degeneration may reflect molecular mimicry between an axonal antigen and the organism. Although no organisms are typically seen in the nerve, they can be identified by PCR. A monoclonal antibody directed against *B. burgdorferi* flagellin binds to axonal cytoplasm and *in vitro* slows neurite outgrowth from cultured neuroblastoma cells by interacting with a heat-shock protein.[468] Damage to nerves may also reflect deposition of membrane attack complexes in the perineurium and epineurial blood vessels. Other studies have demonstrated[164] not only that *B. burgdorferi* binds to gangliosides, but also that animals immunized with this organism produce antiganglioside (primarily GM1) antibodies, which can bind antigens at the nodes of Ranvier. Early in the disease, oral regimens consisting of doxycycline and amoxicillin for 10–30 days are highly effective.[427]

Chagas' Disease

Chagas' disease (American trypanosomiasis) (see Chapter 20, Parasitic Infections) results from infection by the intracellular protozoan *Trypanosoma cruzi*, an organism found only in North and South America. The neurological sequelae become manifest during the chronic phase of the disease

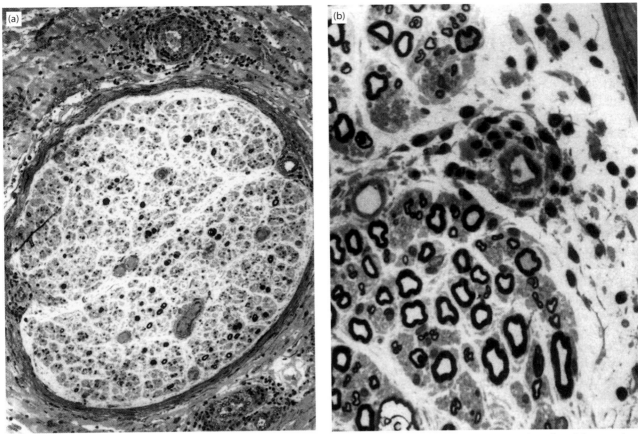

24.73 Lyme disease. Severe loss of myelinated fibres and perivascular inflammatory infiltrates in the epineurium **(a)** may also be accompanied by pericapillary and subperineurial inflammatory infiltrates consisting mainly of plasma cells and histiocytes **(b)**. (a) ×110; (b) ×450.

and are characterized by destruction of individual nerves, most often those affecting the heart and gastrointestinal tract. Autonomic dysfunction involves the parasympathetic, sympathetic and enteric nervous systems. Abnormalities in baroreceptor response and orthostatic hypotension may be accompanied by decreased plasma norepinephrine levels.[55] In addition, chronic cholinergic neuropathy and enteric ganglion involvement result in mega-oesophagus, megaduodenum and megacolon, producing symptoms of dysphagia and constipation.[151]

Peripheral nerve and ganglia (including cardiac and enteric ganglia) show inflammation, demyelination and ganglionic neuron loss.[492] Experimental studies have shown parasitization of supporting cells (Schwann cells and satellite cells), which, upon degeneration, are thought to produce an acute ganglionitis and periganglionitis, with resulting bystander effect on neighbouring neurons and axons.[492] There is no clear consensus regarding the precise biochemical and/or molecular basis of the nerve injury.

Diphtheria

Neuropathic symptoms appear 1–2 weeks after onset of infection with *Corynebacterium diphtheriae*, initially with cranial nerve dysfunction, especially involving the III nerve with resultant blurred vision, as well as innervation of the pharynx and larynx. Later (5–8 weeks), sensory and motor deficits appear in the limbs.[392] Spinal ganglia and nerve roots (sites of a leaky blood–nerve barrier) show collections of macrophages and mononuclear cells with little lymphocytic infiltrate that produce focal segmental demyelination and almost complete axonal sparing. Schwann cells phagocytose myelin, which is subsequently passed to macrophages, followed by Schwann cell proliferation and remyelination of denuded internodes, usually with several Schwann cells maintaining internodes initially served by one cell. Neuropathic changes reflect diphtheria toxin exposure, not active infection, inhibiting Schwann cell synthesis of proteolipid and myelin basic proteins as the result of inactivating eukaryotic elongation factor 2, needed for polypeptide synthesis.

Diphtheria toxin produces an almost pure demyelinative insult with little direct axonopathy and, as a result, has been used to produce myelinopathy in experimental models. Experimental animals (e.g. guinea pigs, rabbits, rats, chickens) develop a similar demyelinative neuropathy, but sensitivity to diphtheria toxin varies in dosage by orders of magnitude.[317] Toxin endocytosis is facilitated by a ligand for plasma membrane heparin-binding epidermal growth factor (HB-EGF) receptors[328] and a second substance that allows endosomal penetration into cytosol. Subsequently, the A chain catalyses transfer of adenosine diphosphate (ADP) ribose from oxidized nicotinamide adenine dinucleotide (NAD+) to polypeptide elongation factor 2, which blocks protein synthesis and results in cell death. The predilection of the process for Schwann cells may reflect the presence of increased HB-EGF receptors, which are needed to transduce neuregulin effects.[392]

Human T-Cell Lymphotropic Virus Type I

Infection by HTLV-1 (see Chapter 19, Viral Infections) is linked to adult T-cell leukaemia and tropical spastic paraparesis, which occur in Japan, India, the Seychelles and Jamaica. Peripheral nerves show variable segmental demyelination/remyelination, redundant folding of myelin, axonal degeneration and, in some cases, inflammation.[271]

Leprous Neuritis

Mycobacterium leprae is a Gram-positive, acid-fast, slightly curved bacillus measuring 1–8 μm in length and 0.2–0.5 μm in diameter. The organism proliferates preferentially in cool tissues, 30°C being optimal. Infection with *M. leprae* produces a chronic granulomatous disease predominantly in the skin, mucous membranes, anterior chamber of the eye, testes and peripheral nerves.[53] Prolonged exposure to an infected individual with nasal discharge is necessary for the organism to gain entry into the respiratory tract of a susceptible person. Acid-fast mycobacteria and *M. leprae* DNA are found in the nasal secretions of patients with lepromatous leprosy. *Mycobacterium leprae* cannot traverse the intact dermis in either direction, and the infection is not spread by skin-to-skin contact. The incubation period is estimated to be 2–7 years or more. Although leprosy was once distributed widely in Europe and Asia, it now occurs mainly in resource-poor countries in tropical and warm temperate regions. However, patients may present with the disease long after leaving an endemic area.[53] More than 90 per cent of individuals infected with *M. leprae* develop effective immunity without clinical evidence of disease.[171] A well-documented but unusual form of leprosy transmission is direct dermal implantation during tattooing.

Mycobacterium leprae is an obligate intracellular parasite with tropism for macrophages and Schwann cells. The organism can replicate in the mouse footpad and the nine-banded armadillo,[247] which have provided bacteria for study. Of note, more than half of the functional genes in the *Mycobacterium tuberculosis* genome are absent in *M. leprae* and have been replaced by inactivated genes and pseudo-genes. For unclear reasons, *M. leprae* seems to have jettisoned genes normally required for replication *ex vivo* and has apparently assumed a unique ecological niche with very limited host range and the need to grow within cells.[53]

Peripheral nerves are affected in all forms and stages of leprosy,[224,233,374,504] primarily nerve trunks near the surface of the skin and small dermal sensory and autonomic nerves. The unique predilection of *M. leprae* for Schwann cells is probably determined by the binding of the organism to the G domain of the α2 chain of laminin 2, which is a component of the Schwann cell basal lamina. This form of laminin is restricted to peripheral nerves, which explains the

specific tropism of *M. leprae*.[404] In addition, not only does *M. leprae* target Schwann cells, but also the immunologically mediated reactions seen during antimicrobial therapy of leprous neuropathy cause significant damage to the PNS and contribute substantially to disability.[362]

In a patient with leprosy, biopsy of a subcutaneous nerve may reveal pathological changes that are greater than (or at variance with) those suggested by skin biopsy or clinical examination.[191,410] The tissue response to *M. leprae* infection is determined largely by the natural resistance of the host, the bacillus itself being of low pathogenicity.[233] A two-stage model for genetic control of innate susceptibility to leprosy has been proposed. The expression of a single recessive autosomal gene may determine the susceptibility to disease, whereas the progression of the disease and the histological reaction that ultimately develops are associated with genes of the major histocompatibility complex; HLA-DR2 and -DR3 alleles are associated with tuberculoid disease and HLA-DQ1 is linked to lepromatous leprosy.[53,101,463]

The initial manifestations of leprosy are generally cutaneous lesions or, less commonly, peripheral neuropathy. The initial clinical stage of leprosy infection is referred to as 'indeterminate leprosy', a transitional form of the early infection with subtle clinical manifestations–usually a solitary hypopigmented macule with impaired sensation. This skin lesion may resolve spontaneously. If persistent, indeterminate leprosy progresses to one of the five major clinical types of the Ridley–Jopling classification,[409] which covers the spectrum from individuals with little cellular immunity to individuals with high cellular immunity. The histological lesions of leprosy are placed within the two poles of the pure tuberculoid (paucibacillary) and the pure lepromatous (pluribacillary) forms. The true borderline type is most unstable, with downgrading (towards the lepromatous form) in the absence of treatment, or upgrading (towards the tuberculoid form) with treatment.

Tuberculoid (paucibacillary) leprosy tends to pursue a more benign and less progressive course; mucosal, ocular and testicular involvement is absent. Localized, asymmetrical, anaesthetic and anhydrotic skin lesions associated with hair loss occur on the trunk, buttocks and face. Nerve enlargement develops in the regions showing skin lesions; the pattern can simulate a multiple mononeuropathy. In paucibacillary leprosy, there is a florid inflammatory response; lesions occur early during the disease and may be confined to a single nerve trunk. The subcutaneous nerve is irregularly thickened, with obliteration of the fascicular anatomy by confluent granulomas composed of epithelioid histiocytes, multinucleated giant cells and scattered lymphocytes (Figure 24.74). This may affect the whole cross-section of nerve, to the point that the neural architecture becomes unrecognizable. In this instance, immunohistochemical studies for EMA and S-100 protein may help to detect residual perineurium and Schwann cells. Caseating necrosis centred in nerves may occur (Figure 24.75). The finding of normal or marginally affected nerve bundles within a granuloma almost excludes the possibility of leprosy. In tuberculoid leprosy, bacilli are demonstrable only rarely with conventional stains, but *M. leprae*

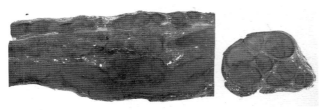

24.74 Tuberculoid leprosy. Multiple granulomas altering the microscopic anatomy of nerve fascicles. Whole mount preparation.

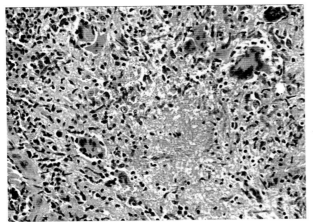

24.75 Tuberculoid leprosy. Epithelioid and giant cell granuloma with necrosis.

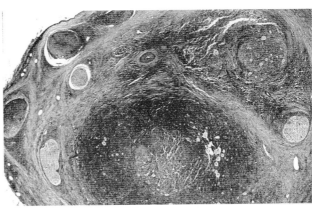

24.76 Pluribacillary leprosy. Transverse section through sural nerve biopsy specimen, showing variation in cellular infiltrates between fascicles with focal perineurial involvement.

antigens can be detected using cross-reacting anti-BCG antisera in epithelioid cells, Schwann cells and endothelium. A specific DNA probe and PCR for the detection of picogram quantities of *M. leprae* in tissues has been developed.[344]

Lepromatous (pluribacillary) leprosy is characterized by a selective anergy to *M. leprae* and its antigens. After entry of bacillus through the mucosa, a defect in cell-mediated immunity associated with decreased IFN-γ production leads to unchecked bacillary proliferation in mucocutaneous macrophages; this is followed by haematogenous spread and, eventually, colonization of subcutaneous nerves. Lepromatous patients have multiple symmetrical skin lesions distributed over the face, limbs and buttocks. The precise route the organism uses to enter the nerve is not clear. After haematogenous spread, *M. leprae* may bind directly to Schwann cells and dermal nerves of superficial skin in the cooler parts of the body. Other studies favour an initial colonization of the bacillus in perineurium and epineurium, followed by extension into endoneurium. Scollard and colleagues demonstrated that the endoneurial micro-vessels in the armadillo serve as the route of entry into the nerve, by demonstrating extensive infection of endothelial cells in perineurium and epineurium.[457]

A symmetrical polyneuropathy develops late in the course of lepromatous leprosy, with a peculiar pattern of sensory loss involving the legs (sparing the soles of the feet), dorsal aspect of the forearms, pinnae of the ears, nose and supraorbital regions. This distribution depends on

temperature gradients, as *M. leprae* proliferates more freely in cooler areas. Superficial nerves are enlarged, often with an abrupt transition with normal deeper segments. Nerve thickening may be uniform or nodular and palpation can be painful. Characteristic is preferential involvement of the greater auricular nerve in the neck, the supraorbital branch of the fifth cranial nerve and the ulnar nerve. In transverse sections, there appears to be an uneven involvement of fascicles (Figure 24.76), with some being infiltrated heavily by foamy histiocytes and a variable number of plasma cells. In nerve biopsies from presymptomatic patients with enlarged nerves, there is a predominant involvement of epineurium and perineurium, with later spread to endoneurium.[510] The perineurium is involved extensively, with lamination by foamy macrophages and separation of the perineurial leaves (Figure 24.77) but maintaining preservation of fascicular architecture. Perivascular lymphocytes may increase after treatment. Large numbers of bacilli are demonstrable in macrophages, Schwann cells, perineurial cells, endothelium (Figures 24.78–24.81) and, perhaps, axons. The number of bacilli in the endoneurial area not infrequently exceeds 1000 per single oil immersion field.[374] The bacilli are found mainly in the cytoplasm of macrophages (Figure 24.82) and Schwann cells in the configuration of 'globi' that contain dozens, or even hundreds, of organisms (Figure 24.78 and 24.79). Such cells in paraffin-embedded preparations acquire a typical foamy appearance and are termed 'lepra cells' (Figure 24.78). In Schwann cells and macrophages, the bacilli are located in vacuoles surrounded by a clear space (Figures 24.80–24.83). Both demyelination and axon loss occur in varying proportions from case to case. The mechanism of the nerve fibre damage is not understood. Demyelination may result from infection (Figure 24.83) and degeneration of Schwann cells.

Although initially the endoneurium is oedematous, the widespread bacillary multiplication and progress of disease may induce fibrosis and atrophy of nerve bundles. Bacilli may persist in nerves even after years of apparently successful treatment. Following treatment and even as part of the natural history of the disease, the subsiding inflammation unveils the devastation of the nerve: although fascicular anatomy is still discernible, the endoneurium is devoid of native elements (axons and Schwann cells)

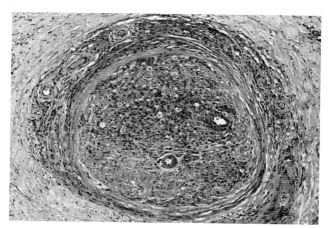

24.77 Pluribacillary leprosy. Perineurial and epineurial concentric inflammation.

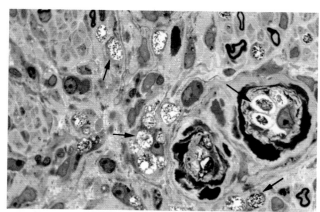

24.80 Pluribacilllary leprosy. Bacilli are readily demonstrable in endoneurium on a semi-thin section stained with toluidine blue. Organisms are present in histiocytes, Schwann cells and endothelium. Plastic resin, oil immersion.

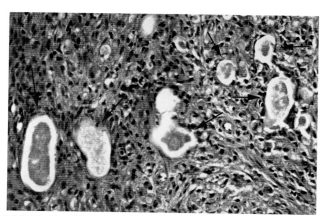

24.78 Pluribacillary leprosy. Heavy histiocytic endoneurial infiltrate with 'lepra cells'.

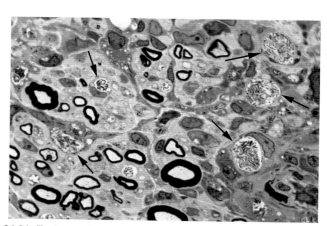

24.81 Endoneurium in pluribacillary leprosy. Arrows mark cytoplasmic aggregate of bacilli. Plastic resin, oil immersion.

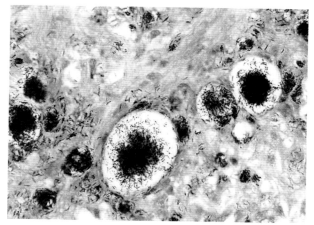

24.79 Pluribacillary leprosy. Large numbers of organisms in endoneurium are shown with Fite preparation.

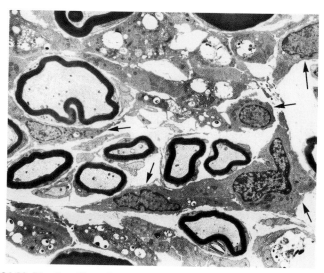

24.82 Pluribacillary leprosy. Endoneurial macrophages containing bacilli. Electrophotomicrograph, ×12 600.

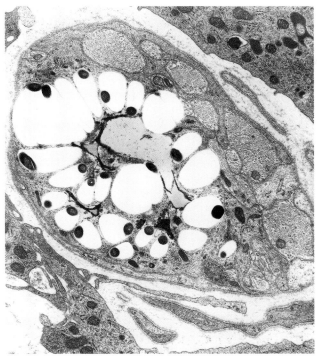

24.83 Pluribacillary leprosy. Schwann cell associated with unmyelinated axons, containing multiple bacilli. Electrophotomicrograph, ×21 000.

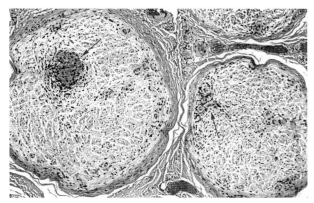

24.84 Scattered micro-granulomas (arrows) in primary neuritic leprosy.

and nerve bundles consist of cords of hyalinized connective tissue. Regressive changes include large vacuolated cells that contain much lipid and sometimes remnants of bacilli. Both axonal loss and demyelination are prominent in lepromatous leprosy, but the mechanism of damage is not understood well. Perineurial and endoneurial fibrosis contributes to nerve entrapment and hinders regeneration of nerve fibres. The selective pain and temperature loss and anhydrosis suggest that small myelinated and unmyelinated fibres are also affected significantly.

In borderline leprosy, where the immunological polarity is expressed only partially, the lesions are often early, widespread and severe. Small dermal sensory and autonomic nerves are affected, producing patches of hypoaesthesia and anhydrosis. Histological features of this form of leprous neuropathy may have an incongruous appearance, with both lepromatous and tuberculoid patterns present in the same specimen. Lymphocytes are most abundant in borderline leprosy; in nerve fascicles, they may appear densely packed in the epineurium or in the endoneurium adjacent to granulomas, or they may infiltrate the perineurium. Bacilli are almost always found in borderline lesions.

Painful erythematous cutaneous papules accompanied by painful focal nerve lesions announce the development of erythema nodosum leprosum (type 2 leprosy reaction). This is caused by the death of large numbers of bacilli during the first or second year after the initiation of treatment and can relapse intermittently. Patients are febrile and develop constitutional reactions, including iritis, orchitis, lymphadenitis and proteinuria. Vasculitic lesions and neutrophilic infiltrates occur within cutaneous nerves. Typically, arterioles in the vicinity of perineurium are involved; they can show fibrinoid necrosis and acute inflammation indistinguishable from those of hypersensitivity vasculitis. The condition resembles the Arthus reaction. Erythema nodosum leprosum is accompanied by high circulating concentrations of TNF-α and striking systemic toxicity.

Reversal reactions (type 1 leprosy reaction) are important in the production of neural damage. An 'upgrading' reaction may occur in one-third of borderline lepromatous cases during the first year of treatment. The peak time for this reaction to occur is in the first 2 months of treatment. It is characterized by a heightened T-cell reactivity to mycobacterial antigens and the infiltration of IFN-γ- and TNF-α-secreting CD4+ lymphocytes into skin lesions and nerves.[53] Upgrading lesions can also occur in untreated borderline tuberculoid cases. Swelling and reddening of existing skin lesions develop and new lesions appear. There is accompanying fever and malaise. Pain and swelling of nerve trunks occur with the appearance of sensory and motor deficits in the territory of affected nerves; loss of nerve function can be dramatic. Endoneurial granulomas, lymphocytic infiltration, vasculitis and perineuritis are observed. Bacilli are not seen. Tissue necrosis may result in the formation of nerve abscesses. The reaction subsides after some months, when many but not all patients are found to have moved towards the tuberculoid form in terms of classification. A 'downgrading' reaction occurs rarely in untreated or ineffectually treated borderline patients, involving a change in the lepromatous direction.

Patients with pure neuritic leprosy present with asymmetrical involvement of peripheral nerve trunks, display no skin lesions and are skin smear-negative for acid-fast bacilli. This form is seen most frequently, but not exclusively, in India and Nepal. Mononeuropathy multiplex is a common clinical pattern of nerve dysfunction in primary neuritic leprosy.[319] The diagnosis of this type of leprosy depends exclusively on nerve biopsy (Figure 24.84),[93,224] in which the entire spectrum of leprosy lesions can be observed. In a nerve biopsy study of 39 such patients, a significant proportion showed lepromatous histology and nearly two-thirds had a moderate to heavy bacterial load within the nerves. Whenever possible, a cutaneous sensory nerve such as greater auricular, medial antebrachial, superficial peroneal or sural should be chosen for biopsy. One report documents characteristic histological changes of leprosy in the normal-appearing sensory-altered skin in 31 per cent of patients clinically diagnosed with primary neuritic leprosy.[319] Additional studies using PCR on nerve biopsy tissue and enzyme-linked immunosorbent assay (ELISA) for the detection of anti-phenolic glycolipid I IgM antibodies may be useful to diagnose primary neuritic leprosy.[222]

VASCULITIC NEUROPATHY

Peripheral neuropathy, typically in the form of mononeuritis multiplex, is a major clinical feature of primary and secondary systemic vasculitides. Neuropathy often occurs early in the disease and is therefore of important diagnostic value. The vasculitic process usually affects the epineurial vessels, resulting in axonal ischaemia or, less commonly, frank infarction. Primary systemic vasculitides commonly affecting the PNS include PAN (50–75 per cent of cases), Wegener granulomatosis (11–67 per cent of cases), Churg–Strauss syndrome (50–78 per cent of cases) and microscopic polyangiitis (10–58 per cent of cases). A non-systemic vasculitic neuropathy has also been described.[231] Secondary causes of PNS vasculitis can be paraneoplastic, infectious, drug-related or connective tissue disease-related. Table 24.6 lists the causes of peripheral neuropathy due to vasculitis. A general description of the clinical, pathologic and pathogenetic features of PNS vasculitis follows, after which features of specific systemic vasculopathies affecting the PNS are discussed.

TABLE 24.6 Peripheral neuropathy due to vasculitis
Primary systemic necrotizing vasculitides affecting peripheral nervous system
Polyarteritis nodosa (PAN)
Churg–Strauss syndrome
Microscopic polyangiitis
Wegener's granulomatosis
Isolated peripheral nervous system vasculitis
Leukocytoclastic vasculitis
Hypersensitivity vasculitis
Henoch–Schönlein purpura
Cryoglobulinaemia
Connective tissue disorders associated with vasculitis
Systemic lupus erythematosus
Scleroderma
Rheumatoid arthritis
Sjögren syndrome
Mixed connective tissue disease
Behçet disease
Inflammatory diabetic vasculopathy
Vasculitis associated with infection
Lyme disease
Arthropod stings
Tuberculosis
Leprosy
Human immunodeficiency virus I
Cytomegalovirus
Paraneoplastic vasculitis
Paraprotein associated
Haematological or solid malignancy
Other
Eosinophilia myalgia syndrome
Toxic oil syndrome

Clinical Manifestations

Peripheral neuropathy is the initial symptom of systemic vasculitis in 36–56 per cent of patients.[42] Males are affected more frequently than females (ratio 2:1). Eighty per cent of presenting patients are over 50 years of age, and prognosis worsens with increasing age. The disease is quite rare in the paediatric age group. The onset is usually acute but may be more slowly progressive in elderly people.[367,428] The anatomical pattern is typically that of a mononeuritis multiplex, but asymmetrical multifocal neuropathy and distal symmetrical sensorimotor polyneuropathy patterns are also seen.[142] Pain, in particular burning dysaesthesias, is present in about 50 per cent of patients. Systemic features include fever, weight loss, arthralgias and fatigue, which may be related to an associated connective tissue disease. The most commonly affected nerves, in descending order, are the peroneal (60 per cent), popliteal (30 per cent) and ulnar (25 per cent) nerves.[428]

Diagnostic Investigations

Electromyography with nerve conduction studies typically reveals an axonal neuropathy and may show extensive denervation.[367] Both motor and sensory nerve action potentials demonstrate a marked decrease in amplitude and may even be absent. However, motor nerve conduction velocities are often normal or reduced only slightly.[367] Electrophysiological involvement can often be more profound than is clinically apparent. If systemic vasculitis is suspected to be the cause of a peripheral neuropathy and other investigations (e.g. antineutrophil cytoplasmic autoantibody (ANCA) testing, renal biopsy, arteriography) fail, then a neuromuscular biopsy is warranted. This is particularly relevant, because in approximately 20–30 per cent of patients with a muscle–nerve biopsy positive for vasculitis, the disease is restricted to the PNS.[98] Combined muscle–nerve biopsy is recommended because, in the hands of an experienced neuropathologist, it has the highest diagnostic sensitivity (about 60 per cent) and may be positive even in the face of normal EMG.[97] Muscle or nerve biopsy alone reduces the sensitivity to 38 per cent and 35 per cent respectively.[430] Serial sections of the entire sample must be examined, because the lesions are often focal and distributed randomly along the nerve. Furthermore, because it is the epineurial vessels that are involved, full-thickness rather than fascicular biopsies are required.

Pathological Findings

The epineurial vessels affected are usually small, with a diameter in the range of 45–210 µm. The histological hallmark of vasculitis is inflammation across the vessel wall, with associated mural necrosis or karyorrhexis (Figures 24.85–24.87). Martius scarlet blue (MSB) (Figure 24.88) or phosphotungstic acid haematoxylin (PTAH) staining may bring out fibrinoid change that is inconspicuous in standard haematoxylin and eosin (H&E) preparations. Disruption of the internal elastic lamina is a useful finding and can be highlighted with elastin stains (Figure 24.89), as is the finding of perivascular iron deposits, suggesting old vascular

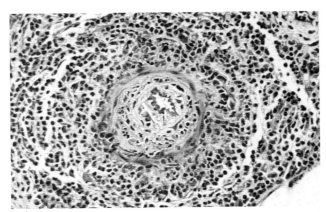

24.85 Transmural vascular inflammation is seen in this example of a Churg–Strauss vasculitis stained with haematoxylin–phloxin–saffron (HPS).

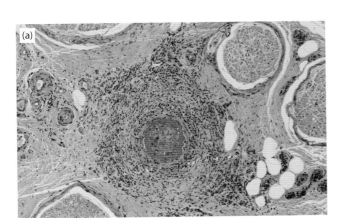

(a)

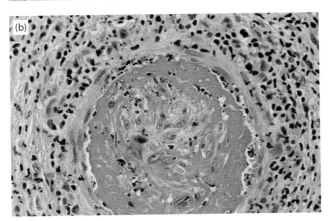

(b)

24.86 Vasculitis. (a,b) Fibrinoid necrosis of the vessel wall with associated inflammation is demonstrated on haematoxylin and eosin.

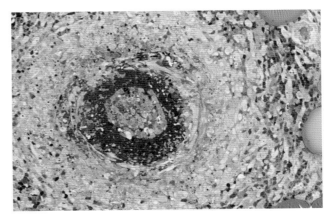

24.87 Vasculitis. Fibrinoid necrosis of the vessel wall may also be demonstrated on toluidine blue-stained semi-thin sections.

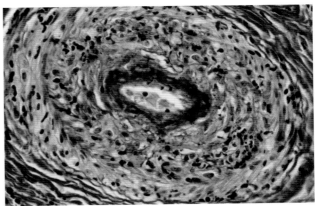

24.88 Vasculitis. Martius scarlet blue (MSB) staining highlights fibrinoid necrosis.

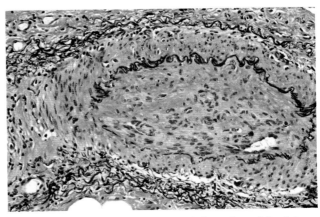

24.89 Vasculitis. Elastin stains reveal disruption of the internal elastic lamina, evidence of previous injury to the vessel wall.

injury and haemorrhage (Figure 24.90). Usually T-cells predominate over macrophages, with polymorphonuclear leukocytes present only in acute disease (Figure 24.91). Nerve biopsies with extravasation of neutrophils should be considered suspicious for vasculitis, with the caveat that this can be seen normally if the biopsy procedure takes more than 30 minutes.

Perivascular inflammatory infiltrates are an abnormal but non-specific finding. A definitive diagnosis of necrotizing vasculitis cannot be made in this case, but the degree of suspicion can be raised by finding one or more other pathological features that reflect angiopathic nerve injury. These include ischaemic changes (see later), regional necrosis of the perineurium and new vessel formation. The last represents a more chronic change, with luminal narrowing and vessel recanalization associated with an increased number of epineurial vessels and, in some cases, focal mural

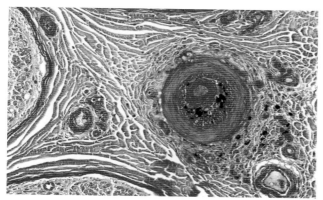

24.90 Vasculitis. Iron staining reveals the presence of intramural and perivascular iron, suggesting previous vascular injury and haemorrhage.

calcifications. These changes, however, can be seen in other types of small vessel disease such as diabetes, and therefore correlation with clinical history is important.

Necrosis of the perineurium is unusual except in vasculitis and in some cases perineurial cell loss with replacement by epineurial collagen is seen. The location of the involved vessels may also sometimes be of help as epineurial involvement is more common in vasculitis whereas endoneurial lymphocytes may suggest GBS or CIDP. In addition, immunophenotyping of the lymphocytes can be of use as B-cells are not found in CIDP or GBS.

Ischaemic neuropathy is an indirect sign of vasculitis. This is usually characterized by axonal degeneration, which is generally patchy and varies from fascicle to fascicle (Figure 24.92). The fascicular centres are predominantly involved, because this is the least vascularized part of the nerve and thus is most vulnerable to ischaemia.[333] Wedge-shaped or centrofascicular areas of infarct may be seen occasionally. Haemosiderin deposition, when present, is also suggestive of vasculitic neuropathy.

Differential Diagnosis

Although one can seldom be specific about the underlying cause of the vasculitis, certain features favour some diseases over others (Table 24.7). The differential diagnosis of granulomatous vasculitis includes leprosy, sarcoidosis and lymphomatoid granulomatosis. Non-vasculitic neural haemorrhage can occur in haemorrhagic diathesis, which can present as mononeuritis multiplex. Primary PNS vasculitis can be difficult to distinguish from CIDP in the absence of vessel necrosis. Acute axonal degeneration or a predominance of epineurial inflammation favours the former, whereas prominent segmental demyelination and an even distribution of epineurial and endoneurial inflammatory cells characterizes the latter. Infectious diseases causing neural vasculitis include hepatitis B and C, acute leprosy, CMV and Lyme disease. In addition, a neuropathy associated with an angiocentric proliferation of predominantly CD8+ lymphocytes with vessel necrosis can be seen in HIV (see Advanced Human Immunodeficiency Virus Disease, p. 1463).[69] Clinical history can often help to distinguish these entities and ancillary tests such as histochemistry, immunostaining, *in situ* hybridization and

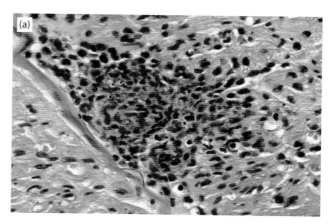

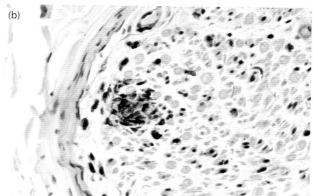

24.91 Vasculitis. Vasculitic involvement of an endoneurial blood vessel showing both lymphocytes and neutrophils invading the vessel wall **(a)**. **(b)** Immunohistochemical staining for CD45.

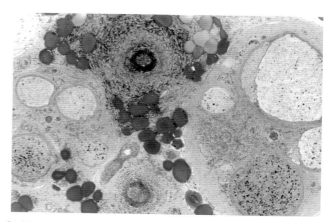

24.92 Vasculitis. Toluidine blue-stained semi-thin section, showing peripheral nerve affected by vasculitis. Note the variability in axonal loss from fascicle to fascicle.

PCR may also be helpful. A lymphocytic vasculitis of perineurial vessels, thought to be a secondary inflammatory response, also occurs in multifocal diabetic neuropathy.[428]

Pathogenesis

The normal PNS is protected from immunological attack by the blood–nerve barrier, with the exception of spinal ganglia. However, the PNS is affected far more

Characteristic	Type of Vasculitis
TABLE 24.7 Clues to the type of vasculitis	
Size of involved vessels	
Epineurial vessels (75–250 μm)	PAN, Churg–Strauss angiitis, Wegener's granulomatosis, isolated PNS vasculitis
Endoneurial vessels (<30 μm)	Hypersensitivity vasculitis
Either	Collagen vascular disease, overlap syndromes, cryoglobulinemia, malignancy
Type of vessel involved	
Veins	Wegener's granulomatosis, Churg–Strauss angiitis, PAN
Inflammatory cell types	
Marked eosinophil infiltration	Churg–Strauss, eosinophilia myalgia syndrome
Granulomata	PAN, SLE, RA, Wegener's granulomatosis, Churg–Strauss

PAN, polyarteritis nodosa; PNS, peripheral nervous system; RA, rheumatoid arthritis; SLE, systemic lupus erythematosus.

frequently than the CNS in systemic vasculitides; this may be related to differences in the blood–nerve and blood–brain barriers. Endothelial cells play an important role in the pathobiology of vascular inflammation along the blood–nerve barriers, because of their interactions with the systemic immune system. Endothelial cells of the PNS are distinct from those of the CNS; in the PNS, endothelial cells express MHC class I molecules and thus are involved in antigen presentation and interaction with cytotoxic T-cells; therefore, they are potentially active participants in vasculitis and not simply passive targets of injury. T-lymphocyte and macrophage infiltration is enhanced further by dysfunction of the blood–nerve barrier. Matrix metalloproteinases, which are able to degrade the subendothelial basement membrane, resulting in vessel destruction, are produced by invading macrophages and T-lymphocytes. Pro-inflammatory cytokines and oxidative stress-derived molecules may also play a role early in the disease. Involvement of the PNS in systemic vasculitis would thus result from blood–nerve barrier breakdown, followed by, or concomitant with, an abnormally upregulated immune response, with inflammatory cell infiltration, vessel destruction and subsequent ischaemic neuropathy. (For a more detailed discussion, see Pagnoux and Guillevin[367] and Younger.)[572,573] However, the exact mechanisms and the underlying triggering factors are still unclear and are probably disease-specific.

Specific Systemic Vasculopathies Affecting the Peripheral Nervous System

There are many proposed classifications of vasculitis based on aetiology, pathological characteristics, size of vessels involved and clinical presentation. The two schemes in most common use are those of the American College of Rheumatology and the Chapel Hill Consensus Conference.[214,223] The latter is used for the discussion in this chapter.

Medium-Sized Vessel Vasculitis: Polyarteritis Nodosa

This condition is commonly accompanied by peripheral nerve involvement, with 40–75 per cent of patients with PAN having a clinical neuropathy[185,276,428] and about 25 per cent of patients having necrotizing vasculitis demonstrated by peripheral nerve biopsy.[428] The disorder has been associated with hepatitis B surface antigen (HBsAg)-positive hepatitis in up to 70 per cent of cases.[472] The characteristic clinical picture is the occurrence of progressive multifocal peripheral nerve lesions ('mononeuritis multiplex') affecting both motor and sensory function and often accompanied by pain. The onset of individual lesions can be abrupt or gradual, and their eventual combination tends to produce symmetrical dysfunction. The lesions are those of a necrotizing arteritis of the vasa nervorum and resemble those that occur in other parts of the body. The predominant lesion is axonal degeneration; this affects myelinated nerve fibres of all sizes and also unmyelinated axons,[528] with larger myelinated nerve fibres being especially vulnerable.[158]

Small Vessel Vasculitis

The main vasculitides in this group causing a peripheral neuropathy are Churg–Strauss syndrome (63–92 per cent of patients), Wegener's granulomatosis (10–22 per cent of patients) and microscopic polyangiitis (14–58 per cent of patients).[276] In Churg–Strauss syndrome, distinguishing clinical features are a marked eosinophilic leukocytosis, pulmonary involvement with late-onset asthma or allergy history, and extravascular granulomas. Similar to PAN, the neuropathy is usually a mononeuritis multiplex and can be painful.[472] Involvement of the PNS is related to an eosinophil-rich necrotizing granulomatous vasculitis affecting the small epineurial vessels. Wegener's granulomatosis is an inflammatory multisystem disorder characterized by respiratory tract granulomas, glomerulonephritis and a systemic necrotizing vasculitis. Involvement of the PNS is typically a mononeuritis multiplex followed by distal symmetrical sensorimotor neuropathy.[345,472] In Wegener's granulomatosis, as with Churg–Strauss syndrome, the vasculitis is necrotizing granulomatous, with a mixed inflammatory cell population but without the prominent eosinophils seen in Churg–Strauss syndrome. In contrast, microscopic polyangiitis is a necrotizing non-granulomatous vasculitis. It is distinguished from PAN based on the size of the involved vessels, but it is often grouped with PAN in case series.

Connective Tissue Disorders

Rheumatoid Arthritis

A variety of different peripheral nerve abnormalities are encountered in this disorder. Median nerve compression in the carpal tunnel, secondary to tenosynovitis and arthritis of the carpal bones, is common, and other nerve entrapments related to joint involvement may be observed. Digital mononeuropathies are also well recognized, as is a relatively benign distal sensory neuropathy predominantly affecting the lower limbs.[368] The digital mononeuropathies may have a vasculitic basis; the explanation of the symmetrical sensory neuropathy is unclear, but it is probably also related to vasculitis. The most devastating type of neuropathy is a progressive multifocal neuropathy, with features similar to those of PAN. It is not necessarily associated with severe or active joint disease. Pathological studies have largely been confined to severe cases. A spectrum of vascular lesions can be defined, ranging from acute necrotizing lesions indistinguishable from those of PAN[195] to a bland intimal proliferation with preservation of the internal elastic lamina leading to partial or total occlusion of the vascular lumen.[67] Other blood vessels show mild inflammatory infiltration, with some deposition of fibrinoid material.

Systemic Lupus Erythematosus

Systemic lupus erythematosus (SLE) may be associated with peripheral neuropathy, although the PNS is affected less commonly than in rheumatoid disease.[212] A progressive multifocal neuropathy[212] or a sensorimotor or predominantly sensory neuropathy[313] may occur. Nerve biopsy shows axonal loss and vasculitis, and tuboreticular inclusions (Figure 24.93) may be seen within endothelial cells on ultrastructural examination.

Scleroderma

Involvement of the PNS in scleroderma is generally thought to be rare, with most series reporting a frequency of less than 5 per cent.[17] A study using nerve conduction and detailed sensory examination suggested that sensory neuropathy, particularly of the upper limbs, may be more common,[394] but this is unlikely to be secondary to vasculitis.

Sjögren's Syndrome

This syndrome comprises the combination of keratoconjunctivitis sicca and/or xerostomia with rheumatoid arthritis, SLE or other connective tissue disorder. A symmetrical

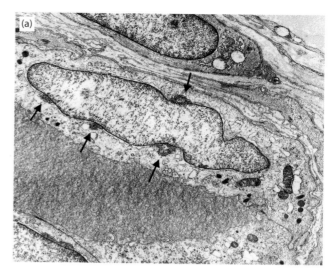

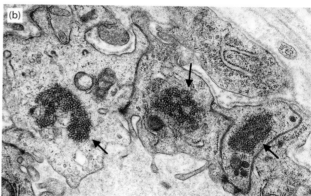

24.93 Ultrastructural appearance of tubular reticular inclusions (arrows) in the endothelial cells from a patient with systemic lupus erythematosus (SLE). (a) Low power; **(b)** high power.

sensorimotor or sensory neuropathy may occur, which may be associated with a trigeminal or autonomic neuropathy. Nerve biopsies show axonal degeneration and perivascular inflammatory infiltrates.[316] In cases with an ataxic sensory and autonomic neuropathy, biopsy of dorsal root ganglia has shown neuronal loss and lymphocytic T-cell infiltration, with focal clusters around neurons.[180]

Cranial (Giant Cell) Arteritis

Peripheral nerve disturbances have been described in patients with giant cell arteritis. Most commonly, these disturbances are mononeuropathies or multifocal neuropathies. These may represent inflammatory disease affecting larger arteries.[75]

AMYLOID NEUROPATHY

Endoneurial deposition of amyloid resulting in peripheral neuropathy can be divided into hereditary and acquired forms. Systemic acquired amyloid neuropathy is due primarily to accumulation of immunoglobulin light chains in the setting of lymphoproliferative disorders. Carpal tunnel syndrome may occur as a complication of amyloid composed of β2 microglobulin deposited in the flexor reticulatum in patients undergoing haemodialysis, but this is not a true amyloid neuropathy. Neuropathy does not occur in secondary amyloidosis, where there is deposition of AA amyloid as a complication of chronic inflammatory or infectious disease.[141] In the vast majority of cases, hereditary or familial amyloid polyneuropathy (FAP) is caused by a mutation in the *transthyretin (TTR)* gene; however, mutations in gelsolin and apolipoprotein A1 (Apo A1) have also been reported[342] (Table 24.8; for reviews, see Adams,[3] Reilly and Staunton[407] and Buxbaum[64]).

Systemic Acquired Amyloid Neuropathy

Systemic amyloid light chain (AL) amyloidosis, the most common systemic amyloidosis,[64] is a plasma cell disorder in which deposits of the N-terminal region of light chains cause progressive organ failure. In AL amyloid, the ratio of κ to λ light chains (1:3) is the reverse of that in both the normal state and in myeloma, in which the ratio is 3:2.[141] Sequence analysis of amyloidogenic light chains reveals specific amino acid substitutions compared with other immunoglobulin light chains. The amyloidosis is a dynamic process, and measures that reduce the supply of the amyloid fibril precursor protein can result in a major regression of the deposits.[459]

The prognosis of primary amyloidosis is generally poor, with a median survival of 1–2 years.[259] The underlying plasma cell dyscrasias are often difficult to detect or are unquantifiable, with fewer than 20 per cent of patients having classic multiple myeloma or Waldenström's macroglobulinaemia. Patients with features of amyloidosis and multiple myeloma have a survival similar to that of patients with amyloidosis alone. Clinical manifestations are varied and depend on where the amyloid deposition occurs. In a series of 474 patients with AL amyloidosis, 28 per cent of patients had nephrotic syndrome or renal failure, 17 per cent had congestive heart failure, 24 per cent had hepatomegaly, 17 per cent had peripheral neuropathy, 11 per cent had orthostatic hypotension, 21 per cent had carpal tunnel syndrome and 9 per cent had macroglossia.[259] Among patients with dominant neuropathy, the most common symptoms leading to the diagnosis of primary amyloid neuropathy are paraesthesias (81 per cent), muscle weakness (65 per cent) and numbness (58 per cent).[403]

Familial Amyloid Polyneuropathies

Transthyretin-Related Familial Amyloid Polyneuropathy

Transthyretin amyloidosis is the most common form of familial amyloid polyneuropathy (FAP). It is caused by mutations in the gene encoding the plasma protein TTR (previously called pre-albumin). Transthyretin is produced primarily in the liver and functions to transport thyroid hormone and vitamin A through a retinol binding protein. A point mutation in the TTR gene resulting in an amino acid substitution (Val30Met) and subsequent structural change in the protein is the most common TTR mutation and occurs in all major endemic populations: Portuguese, Swedish, French and Japanese. More than 100 other mutations have been described, usually limited to one family or to single cases; 13 of these are non-pathogenic.[8,100]

Clinically, there is heterogeneity of symptoms, even for patients with the same mutation. Usually a positive family history can be elicited, because there is an autosomal dominant inheritance pattern with high penetrance. Several phenotypes, including polyneuropathic, oculoleptomeningeal and cardiac types, have been described. In the leptomeningeal type, cerebral amyloid angiopathy and ocular amyloidosis predominate, leading to cerebral infarction and haemorrhage, with hydrocephalus, ataxia, spastic paralysis, convulsions and dementia.[175] Most cases are classified as the

TABLE 24.8 Features of familial amyloid polyneuropathy

Amyloidogenic protein	TTR	Gelsolin	Apolipoprotein A1
Mutations	Most common Val30Met; >100 others	Asp187Asn Asp187Tyr	Most common Gly26Arg and Lue90Pro; >7 others
Neuropathy	Distal symmetrical sensorimotor polyneuropathy Autonomic dysfunction	Sensory polyneuropathy Bulbar/facial neuropathy	Sensory polyneuropathy Autonomic neuropathy
Most common non-PNS clinical manifestations	Cardiac dysfunction Leptomeninges/CNS Renal dysfunction Vitreous opacity/ ⇒ loss of visual acuity	Corneal lattice dystrophy Cutis laxa	Nephropathy Cardiomyopathy Peptic ulcer disease
Common geographical locations	Portugal Sweden Japan France Also USA, Africa, Europe, Australia	Finland Holland USA Japan Czech Republic Denmark	USA (Iowa) France Canada

CNS, central nervous system; PNS, peripheral nervous system.

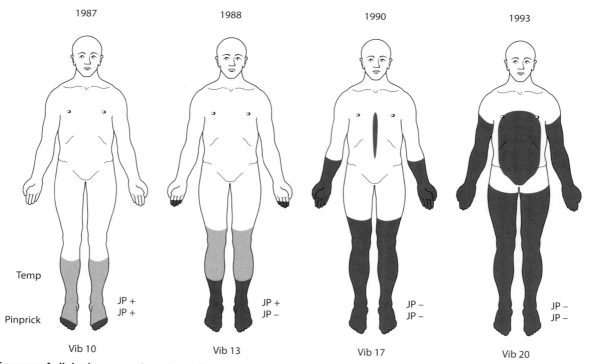

24.94 Diagram of clinical progression of peripheral nerve symptoms in a patient with transthyretin (TTR) gene-related familial amyloid polyneuropathy (FAP). Note that the lower limbs were involved before the upper limbs and the severe loss of pain and temperature (temp) sensation. JP, joint position sense; Vib, vibration sense threshold.

neuropathic type; these patients usually have the Val30Met mutation and typically present with a distal symmetrical sensory or sensorimotor polyneuropathy, with or without autonomic dysfunction. The combination of polyneuropathy and autonomic dysfunction is strongly suggestive of amyloid neuropathy in the absence of diabetes mellitus. Lower limbs are usually affected before upper limbs, sensory involvement occurs before motor involvement, and pain and temperature sensation are the most severely affected (Figure 24.94). Autonomic nervous system involvement leads to dyshydrosis, sexual impotence, diarrhoea alternating with constipation, orthostatic hypotension and urinary disturbances.[8] Constitutional symptoms such as weight loss and anaemia are also common. The heart is frequently affected, and other systems that can be involved include the vitreous humour, kidney, lung and bone.[407] Age of onset varies somewhat, depending on the endemic area (e.g. the third decade in Portugal versus the sixth or seventh decade in Sweden). The disease is slowly progressive and reaches the terminal stage in approximately 10 years.

Familial Amyloid Polyneuropathy Unrelated to Transthyretin

Gelsolin-related FAP, also known as familial amyloidosis of the Finnish type (FAF) or FAP type IV, was first described in a Finnish kindred[320] but has since been described in other areas, including Dutch, Japanese, Irish American and Portuguese families.[99,407] All cases have been secondary to a base mutation at nucleotide 654 of the *gelsolin* (*GSN*) gene on chromosome 9q34, resulting in an asparagine or tyrosine

substitution for aspartic acid at residue 187 (position 15 of the amyloid protein).[99,407] The gelsolin super-family of proteins control actin organization by severing filaments, capping filament ends and nucleating actin assembly.[469] The main clinical manifestations include corneal lattice dystrophy, progressive cranial and peripheral neuropathy, and skin changes (cutis laxa).[248] Symptoms related to renal, cardiac, spinal and cerebral amyloid deposition have also been reported. The onset of neuropathy is usually in the fifth decade, with slow progression marked by facial and minor sensory peripheral nerve signs and occasional carpal tunnel syndrome.[248] Older patients may develop bulbar signs, loss of vibration sense, areflexia, unsteady gait and manual clumsiness. Autonomic dysfunction is mild.

Apolipoprotein A1 is the main protein in HDL and is secreted by the liver and intestine. The *APOA1* gene (on chromosome 11) encodes a 267-amino-acid pro-peptide that is cleaved after secretion to leave the native 243-amino-acid protein. Most Apo A1 variants are associated with decreased plasma HDL or hypertriglyceridaemia. The first Apo A1-related FAP was described in an Iowa kindred;[517] the condition was subsequently attributed to a point mutation in the *APOA1* gene, resulting in an amino acid substitution at position 26 (Gly26Arg).[350] The clinical features in this kindred included peripheral neuropathy, peptic ulcer disease, nephropathy and death from renal failure. A number of other families have now been reported with the same or variant mutations, although the majority of kindreds do not present with peripheral neuropathy. Death in these cases is usually due to cardiomyopathy, renal failure or hepatic failure.

Pathogenesis

Amyloidosis refers to the deposition in organs of collections of β-pleated sheet-structured protein, leading to disruption of normal tissue structure and function. With respect to light-chain amyloid, the primary structure of the light chain appears to be the critical feature, with some light chains being highly amyloidogenic and others not.[483] An increase in the amount of the precursor, determined by expansion of the light-chain-producing clone, is also required. Both intact and cleaved proteins are found in the deposits, but it is not clear whether cleavage is required for deposition.[64]

Transthyretin is the most common constituent fibril in FAP, and most research has been done on this protein. Amyloid misfolding of a monomer subunit of the circulating tetramer generates the amyloidogenic precursor.[237] There does not appear to be a requirement for increased synthesis, but it is thought that inherited mutations in the molecule lead to changes in the primary structure, which increase its amyloidogenicity. This leads to an earlier age of onset and more severe disease[27] than is seen with normal ageing: in 20–25 per cent of people over the age of 80 years, deposition of wild-type TTR because amyloid can also occur, predominantly in the heart, lung and vessel walls.[33,553]

Apolipoprotein A1, on the other hand, normally has an extensive α-helical structure; mutations may result in incomplete degradation of the protein and β-pleated sheet structure formation in the remnant amino- or carboxy-terminal fragments. A similar non-degradable fragment may be responsible for amyloid formation in gelsolin mutations.[27]

Aside from the fibrils, amyloid deposits contain subsets of heparan and dermatan sulphated glycosaminoglycans and proteoglycans, which associate non-covalently with the fibrils and are thought to play a role in amyloidogenesis, possibly by influencing protein folding and/or promoting fibril stability.[203] The other universal constituent of amyloid deposits is the non-fibrillar normal plasma glycoprotein serum amyloid P (SAP) component, which is thought to be important in the pathogenesis and persistence of amyloid.[203] The use of radiolabelled SAP scintigraphy as a means of non-invasively imaging and monitoring amyloid deposits has enhanced diagnosis and management.[196]

Several hypotheses have been proposed to explain the neuropathy associated with amyloid deposition.[3] An ischaemic mechanism has been postulated because of the finding of mural deposition of amyloid in the peripheral nerve blood vessels; however, the preferential involvement of small fibres in amyloid neuropathy makes this unlikely, because these fibres are usually less sensitive to ischaemia. Another hypothesis is a direct mechanical compression of the nerve fibres by the amyloid, with larger myelinated fibres relatively protected by their myelin sheaths. Other hypotheses include a direct toxic or metabolic effect on the endoneurium.

Histopathology

Amyloid deposits can occur in any part of the PNS, including nerve trunks, plexuses and sensory and autonomic ganglia. Absence of the blood–nerve barrier in spinal ganglia allows intrusion of amyloid protein into the endoneurium and explains the massive deposits in this area compared with other peripheral nerves (Figure 24.95). In all types of systemic amyloidosis, amyloid appears as extracellular, amorphous deposits in the epineurium, perineurium or endoneurium (Figure 24.96). It is eosinophilic on H&E staining and blue on toluidine blue staining. It may be closely apposed to Schwann cells or collagen fibrils in the endoneurium, but it is found most commonly around blood vessels. The nerve fibres show axonal degeneration, with the degree of fibre loss dependent on the stage of disease (Figure 24.96). Morphometric studies show that, in the early stages, there is a preferential loss of small myelinated and unmyelinated axons.[125] Later, a diffuse loss occurs. Teased fibre studies demonstrate predominant axonal degeneration, with some segmental demyelination and remyelination, although the presence of the latter is controversial.[324]

The characteristic staining properties of amyloid, the most important of which is lime-green birefringence when viewed in polarized light after staining with Congo red (Figure 24.97), is conferred by the β-pleated molecular structure. At an ultrastructural level, the deposits in all types of amyloidosis consist of 7- to 10-nm unbranched 'rigid' fibrils, either in an irregular array or organized into parallel or fan-shaped bundles or sometimes radiating stellate clusters (Figure 24.98). The deposits regularly contain small quantities of a second component corresponding to SAP. Ultrastructurally, this consists of thick 9-nm pentagonal discs when examined in extracts from amyloid deposits. A potential pitfall of ultrastructural identification is misinterpretation of endoneurial deposits of oxytalan (Figure 24.98) and acid mucopolysaccharides, seen in many chronic neuropathies, as amyloid deposits. Diagnostically, distinguishing the underlying fibril protein composing the amyloid can be ascertained using immunohistochemical (Figure 24.99) or immunogold methods.

Studies investigating nerve biopsy features of a particular FAP have been published.[391] A retrospective study of 35 amyloid-containing peripheral nerve biopsies by Vital and colleagues,[537] 25 of which were TTR-related FAP, showed a dramatic myelinated fibre loss in the majority of patients. The distribution of fibre loss was bimodal in 15 cases, predominantly large fibre in 15 cases and predominantly small fibre in 4 cases. This myelinated fibre loss was associated with ovoids in six cases, regenerative clusters in five cases and both in six cases. Ultrastructurally, a

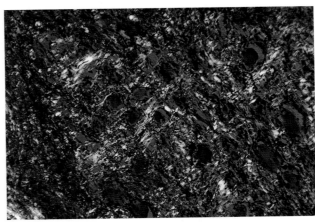

24.95 Amyloid neuropathy. Amyloid deposition in dorsal root ganglion. Congo red, polarized.

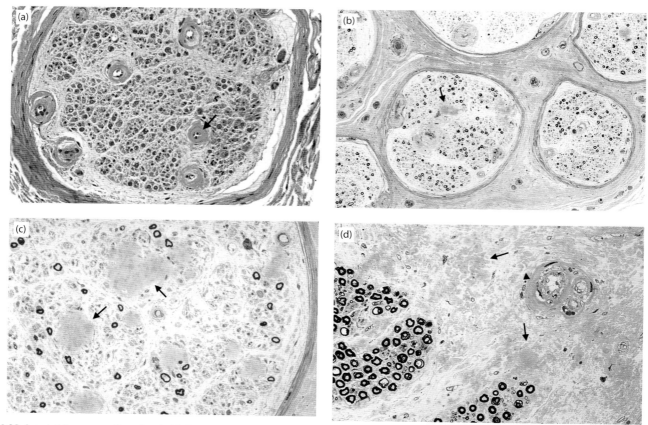

24.96 Amyloid neuropathy. Amyloid deposits in the **(a)** epineurium, **(b)** perineurium and **(c,d)** endoneurium. **(a)** Haematoxylin and eosin (H&E)-stained cross-section of peripheral nerve, demonstrating perivascular amyloid deposition (arrow). **(b-d)** Toluidine blue-stained semi-thin sections, showing endoneurial (b-d, arrows) and perivascular (d, arrowhead) amyloid deposition. **(c)** Extensive fibre loss is evident.

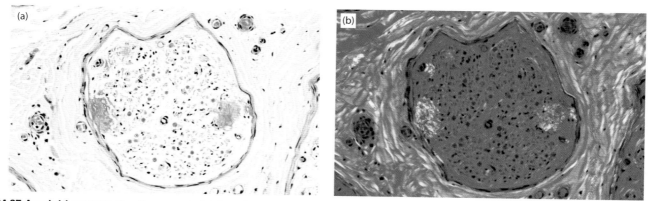

24.97 Amyloid neuropathy. Congo red staining of endoneurial amyloid without **(a)** and with **(b)** polarization.

few fibres showed features of subacute axonal degeneration, with severe damage to myelinated fibres in all cases. Another review of pathological findings in sural nerve biopsies from 14 patients with gelsolin FAP[248] revealed a significant reduction in density of myelinated and unmyelinated fibres when compared with controls. Further, biopsies of the patients with FAP had higher g-ratios and fewer large myelinated fibres. Histologically, hyaline thickening of the perineurium and blood vessel walls, increased endoneurial connective tissue and predominant large myelinated fibre loss with degenerating axons were noted in all 14 biopsies and regenerating

clusters in most. Onion bulbs were present in 6 patients and teased fibre preparations showed evidence of segmental demyelination. Congophilic amyloid deposition was seen in all cases in the perineurium or in the media of small vessels.

Differential Diagnosis/Pitfalls

The finding of amyloid deposits in a peripheral nerve biopsy is always abnormal and indicates the diagnosis of amyloid neuropathy. The underlying cause of the amyloid deposition then becomes an issue. Immunohistochemical

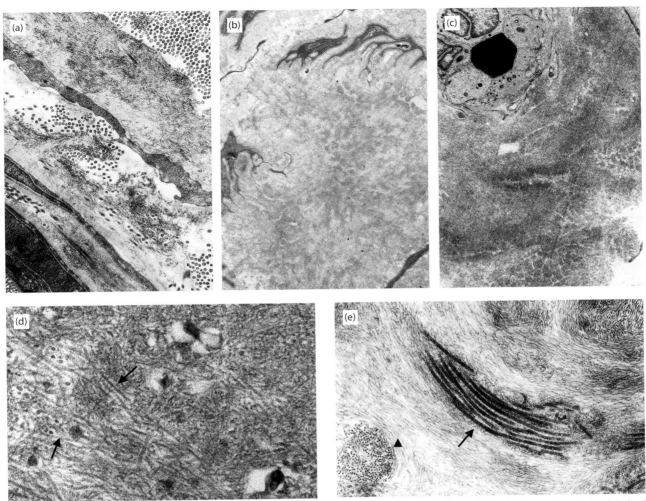

24.98 Amyloid neuropathy: ultrastructural appearance of amyloid. Amyloid deposits are shown in the perineurium **(a)**, in the endoneurium **(b)** and in a blood vessel wall **(c)**. **(d)** High-power ultrastructural appearance of the 7- to 10-nm amyloid fibrils; the larger fibrils in this image (arrows) represent collagen. **(e)** Ultrastructural appearance of oxytalan, a potential mimicker of amyloid; again, here the larger fibrils (arrow) represent collagen. Oxytalan fibrils in cross-section can be seen in the bottom left of the figure (arrowhead).

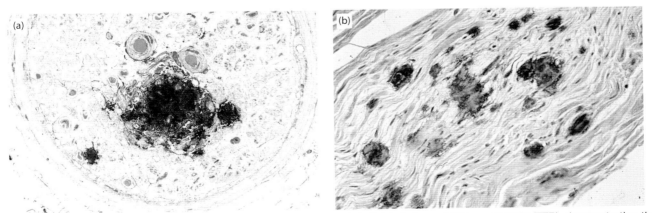

24.99 Amyloid neuropathy: immunohistochemical staining. (a) Lambda light chain; and **(b)** transthyretin (TTR), demonstrating the protein composing the amyloid deposits.

characterization of the protein deposited can be of help, as can ancillary testing. The latter can include serum and urine electrophoresis for detection of light chains or genetic testing for FAP (Figure 24.100). It should be noted, however, that detection of light chains in the urine is not always sufficient to categorize amyloid deposits, because cases of

24.100 Algorithm for management of patient with suspected amyloid neuropathy. FAP, familial amyloid polyneuropathy.

FAP with low-grade monoclonal gammopathies or urine positive for Bence Jones proteins have been reported.[63,262] On the other hand, a small number of patients with light-chain amyloidosis have no monoclonal gammopathy in serum or urine.

It should also be noted that a negative peripheral nerve biopsy does not rule out the disease. A whole-nerve biopsy with muscle, if possible, is recommended and Congo red and/or thioflavin stainings should be performed. Ultrastructural examination may also reveal amyloid deposits not recognized at the light-microscopy level. If clinical suspicion is high, then biopsy of another organ, such as rectum or periumbilical fat, should be considered in the event of a negative nerve biopsy.

NEUROPATHY OF DYSPROTEINAEMIA

The association of monoclonal gammopathy or paraproteinaemia with polyneuropathy is well known, and a search for a monoclonal protein in serum is essential in the evaluation of adult patients with chronic polyneuropathy.[228,236,417] The spectrum of diseases associated with paraproteinaemic neuropathies is shown in Table 24.9 and discussed later. Specific dysproteinaemic polyneuropathies (Table 24.10) may be a presenting feature of disease, before an underlying plasma cell dyscrasia becomes detectable (particularly in patients with light-chain amyloidosis and osteosclerotic myeloma) or, more often, neuropathy may develop in the setting of established multiple myeloma,[119] solitary plasmacytoma or Waldenström's macroglobulinaemia. The peripheral nerve deficit may be sensory, motor or mixed sensorimotor. The mechanism of nerve damage in the setting of monoclonal gammopathy is not invariably caused by amyloidosis: lymphocytic infiltration of nerve and damage on an immunological–inflammatory basis are also important. Studies have demonstrated binding to normal peripheral nerve structures of paraproteins from the patient's serum.

Monoclonal Gammopathy of Unknown Significance

Monoclonal gammopathy of unknown significance (recently reviewed)[210,347,405] results when a clonal transformation of plasma cells is associated with production

TABLE 24.9 Clinical diagnoses associated with monoclonal gammopathy

Multiple myeloma
Plasmacytoma–osteosclerotic myeloma
Indolent (smouldering) myeloma
Light-chain amyloidosis
Waldenström macroglobulinaemia
Lymphoma
Chonic lymphocytic leukaemia
Monoclonal gammopathy of unknown significance (MGUS)

Based on Kyle and Rajkumar[260] and Ropper and Gorson.[417]

TABLE 24.10 Specific paraprotein-associated neuropathies

Autoantibody-associated polyneuropathy syndromes
Chronic inflammatory demyelinating polyneuropathy associated with paraproteinaemia
Light-chain amyloid neuropathy
Immunoglobulin deposition disease
Cryoglobulinaemic neuropathy
POEMS syndrome and neuropathy in osteosclerotic myeloma

POEMS, polyneuropathy, organomegaly, endocrinopathy, M-protein and skin changes.

of a monoclonal protein consisting of two heavy polypeptide chains of the same subclass and two light polypeptide chains of the same type emerge (IgM is a pentamer of the four-chain basic structure). Sixty per cent of patients with paraproteinaemia have an MGUS, which denotes a serum protein value of less than 3g/L (IgM or IgG, κ), less than 5 per cent of plasma cells in the bone marrow, no proteinuria, normal haematology, no skeletal lesions and absence of systemic signs and symptoms.[260,261] About 5 per cent of patients with peripheral neuropathy are found to have MGUS.[474] Conversely, about one-third of patients with MGUS display peripheral neuropathy. Although IgG is the most common class of protein in patients with benign paraproteinaemia, IgM is more common in those with neuropathy (60 per cent), followed by IgG (30 per cent) and IgA (10 per cent). In some patients with plasma cell dyscrasias, only light chains are produced; these are secreted in the urine and referred to as 'Bence Jones proteins'.[261] Approximately 17 per cent of patients with MGUS develop a malignant lymphoproliferative disorder in 10 years and 33 per cent by 20 years, including multiple myeloma, plasmacytoma, Waldenström's macroglobulinaemia and lymphoma.

Among the syndromes of autoantibody-associated polyneuropathy, IgM anti-MAG paraproteinaemic neuropathy is the most common. Approximately half of patients with peripheral neuropathy and IgM monoclonal gammopathy have antibodies that bind to myelin. The most prevalent antibody activity among these IgM proteins is directed against MAG (a glycoprotein that constitutes about 1 per cent of peripheral nerve myelin)[318] and/or sulphate-3-glucuronyl paragloboside. Anti-MAG antibodies may also cross-react weakly to P_0 (myelin protein zero, a 28 000-kDa glycoprotein that makes up approximately 60 per cent of peripheral nerve protein). There is no correlation between the size of the M-protein and the anti-MAG titres, but high titres are more likely to be associated with peripheral neuropathy.[119] Patients whose IgM binds to MAG (mostly κ light chain) form a major and well-characterized subgroup associated with a distinct clinical picture: elderly male individuals are usually affected, and the onset of the neuropathy is insidious and progressive. The condition initially has predominantly demyelinating features affecting large sensory fibres, which translates to loss of joint and position sense, with gait ataxia and intentional tremor; distal limb weakness, with wasting and foot-drop, develops later. Sensory symptoms can extend to the upper limbs. Electromyography and nerve conduction show the classic findings of a demyelinating polyneuropathy, with marked slowing of nerve conduction velocities, prolonged distal latencies and areas of conduction block. The disease in some patients progresses slowly but inexorably over decades, mimicking a genetically determined condition. The majority of patients with anti-MAG antibody have no associated malignancy. Nerve conduction tracing discloses low velocities, and CSF levels of protein are commonly elevated. In a prospective study of patients with IgM paraproteinaemia, the presence of anti-MAG activity correlated with the presence of subclinical neuropathy and the development of neuropathy.[322,534] Rare cases have polyclonal IgM paraproteinaemia with anti-MAG reactivity. The neuropathy associated with IgG or IgA is more likely to show axonal changes.

In classic anti-MAG paraprotein-associated neuropathy, both axonal degeneration and segmental demyelination with occasional hypertrophic changes have been amply documented in nerve biopsies. The pathological abnormality in the early stages lacks uniformity on cross-section of nerve biopsy specimens: although some nerve fascicles are severely involved, others are well preserved (Figure 24.101 and 24.102). Inflammatory changes are not a feature of this neuropathy. By immunofluorescence, specific changes can be visualized: anti-MAG antibody can be localized to areas of myelin splitting[318] (Figure 24.103) and affects a significant number of myelinated fibres, as seen on cross-section.

Ultrastructurally, this is termed 'widely spaced myelin' (WSM) (Figures 24.104a and 24.105) and indicates focal separation of the intraperiod line. This abnormality is

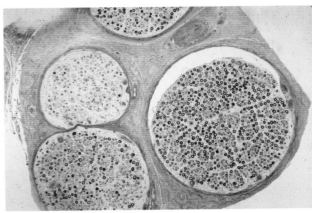

24.101 Nerve biopsy specimen from a case of neuropathy associated with Waldenström macroglobulinaemia. Uneven involvement of fascicles. Plastic resin.

barely discernible by light microscopy. The intraperiod line represents a virtual extracellular space composed of two thin leaflets 2–4 nm apart. The focal separation is brought about by the intrusion of anti-MAG antibodies that 'open up' the intraperiod line, giving a characteristic wide space between the myelin lamellae (20–30 nm) that leads to myelin breakdown and remodelling.[234] This is considered to be a unique feature of dysglobulinaemic neuropathy[529] and has been proven convincingly by immunohistochemistry at the ultrastructural level (Figure 24.106). By contrast, a superficially similar abnormality, uncompacted myelin (Fig 24.104b), consists of widening of the major dense line and is an uncommon finding in diverse neuropathies (see Osteo-sclerotic Myeloma, POEMS Syndrome and Castleman Disease, p. 1484).[535] Other abnormalities detected at the ultrastructural level include tomaculum formations (Figure 24.107a), redundant myelin folds (Figure 24.107b) and axonal atrophy. The mechanism of myelin breakdown in anti-MAG-associated polyneuropathy has not been elucidated; although macrophage-mediated demyelination is demonstrable (Figure 24.108), it does not occur to the same degree as in the inflammatory demyelinating neuropathies. The intensity of immunolabelling of antibody to MAG does not correlate well with the clinical severity of the neuropathy or with the pace of histological change (Figure 24.102). Lombardi and colleagues demonstrated IgM deposits on dermal myelinated fibres in all their patients with anti-MAG neuropathy.[283]

The differentiation of paraproteinaemic (anti-MAG) neuropathy from CIDP is difficult sometimes because (i) about 20 per cent of patients with CIDP also have a paraproteinaemia; (ii) both neuropathies respond to immunosuppressants; and (iii) both conditions have increased CSF protein. Electrophysiological studies are of some help in that CIDP shows a focal block of conduction in motor nerves, whereas in the anti-MAG paraprotein-associated neuropathy sensory fibres are severely affected and conduction slowing (without block) is more diffuse and distally predominant. Vital and colleagues have reported a peripheral nerve morphological study of 18 patients who had the co-existence of CIDP and monoclonal gammopathy; in 11 patients, ultrastructural examination revealed the classic features of macrophage-mediated

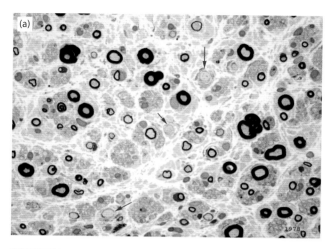

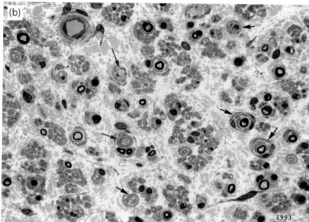

24.102 Transverse sections through nerve biopsy specimens, taken 16 years apart, from a case of neuropathy associated with immunoglobulin M (IgM) paraproteinaemia. **(a)** Year 1978: shows decreased number of myelinated fibres, segmental demyelination and myelin outfolds. **(b)** Year 1993: shows depletion of large myelinated fibres and onion bulbs. ×400.

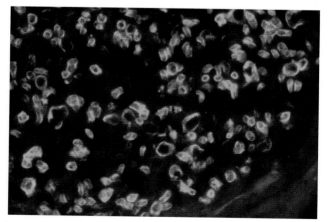

24.103 Transverse section through a nerve biopsy specimen from a case of neuropathy associated with immunoglobulin M (IgM) paraproteinaemia. Fluorescent IgM antibodies give a positive reaction on a large number of myelin sheaths. Frozen section.

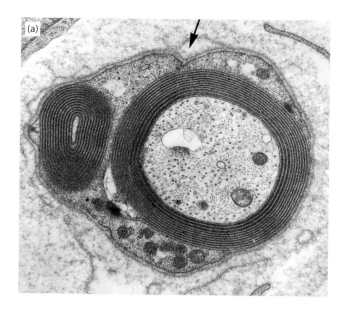

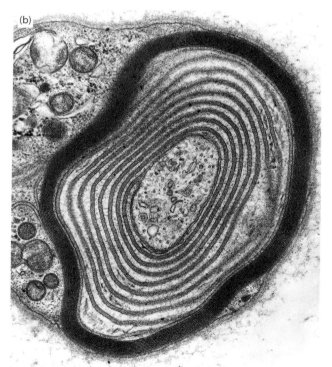

24.104 Neuropathy associated with immunoglobulin M (IgM) paraproteinaemia. **(a)** Cross-section, showing myelin sheath with abnormally wide periodicity; arrow points to widened external mesaxon. **(b)** Uncompacted myelin is a non-specific abnormality that occurs when the cytoplasmic aspect of the Schwann cell membrane fails to appose, leaving considerable amounts of cytoplasm between the two halves of the major dense line. (a) ×21 000; (b) ×7100.

demyelination, and of these 6 had WSM. The authors infer that, in some patients, a seamless transition between CIDP and paraproteinaemic neuropathy is possible.[531]

Patients with GALOP (gait disorder, antibody, late-age onset, polyneuropathy) syndrome have serum IgM directed against galopin (membrane-bound sulphatide) and typically

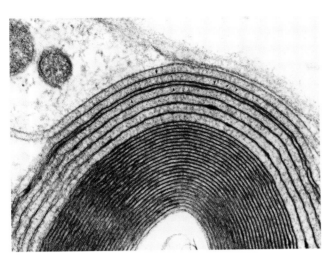

24.105 Neuropathy associated with immunoglobulin M (IgM) paraproteinaemia. Widely spaced myelin relates to separation of the intraperiod line. Same case as shown in Figure 24.104a. ×69 000.

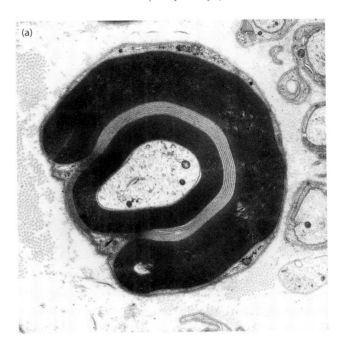

(a)

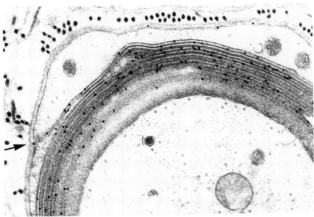

24.106 Transverse section of myelinated nerve fibre. Biopsy from a case of neuropathy associated with immunoglobulin M (IgM) paraproteinaemia. Anti-IgM immunogold preparation shows co-localization with widely spaced myelin; arrow, external mesaxon. ×7100.

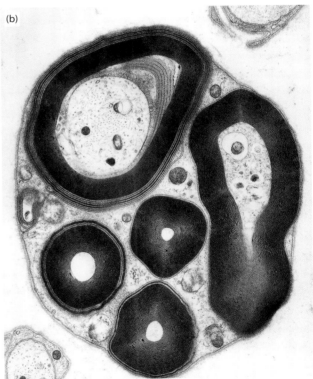

(b)

24.107 Neuropathy associated with immunoglobulin M (IgM) paraproteinaemia. (a) Tomaculum containing a portion of myelin sheath with widely spaced myelin abnormality. ×7100. **(b)** Redundant myelin loops and outfoldings of myelin sheaths with partial widely spaced configuration. ×7100.

a serum M-protein. Clinical presentation is late onset of gait ataxia and a sensorimotor (sensory-motor) polyneuropathy, with mild, if any, weakness.[381] Immunomodulation with intravenous immunoglobulin or cyclophosphamide results in functional improvement. Sural nerve biopsy discloses a moderately severe loss of large and small myelinated nerve fibres, lack of inflammation, segmental demyelination and axonal degeneration.

Sensory neuropathies with IgM or M-proteins against GD1b and Galnac-GD1a, and patients with GM2 with a monoclonal IgM antibody against GD1b without binding to GM1 ganglioside, develop a chronic, slowly progressive ataxic neuropathy syndrome,[489] which preferentially involves the distal loss of large-fibre sensory modalities in the extremities as well as cranial nerve disorders (ophthalmoplegia, bulbar dysfunction, perioral dysaesthesias) with preserved strength. Electrodiagnostic studies show axonal loss or demyelination, but sural nerve pathology has not been defined. Improvement may follow intravenous immunoglobulin therapy.[383] Patients with M-proteins against GalNAc-GD1a and GM2 present with large-fibre

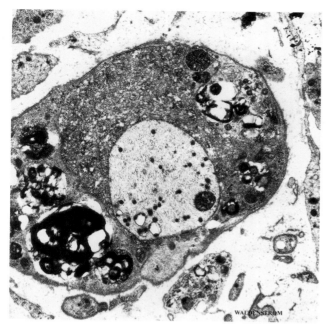

24.108 Macrophage-mediated demyelination in a case of paraproteinaemic neuropathy. ×6400.

sensory loss and sensory ataxia that responds to intravenous immunoglobulin but not steroids. It is thought that complement-mediated nodal disruption is a common mechanism in anti-ganglioside antibody mediated neuropathies.[490]

Patients with motor axonopathy with IgM anti-GM1 or -Galnac-GD1a develop weakness similar to MMN, preserved deep tendon reflexes and pathological findings of axon loss without demyelination. Electromyography separates motor neuron disorders from motor neuropathies, which show abnormal or normal paraspinous muscles respectively. Patients with distal motor neuropathies and serum IgM antibodies may improve after treatment with intravenous immunoglobulin or cyclophosphamide.[364]

Adult patients with CANOMAD (chronic ataxic neuropathy, ophthalmoplegia, M-protein agglutination, disialosyl antibodies) syndrome develop a progressive large- and small-fibre sensory neuropathy, with variable ataxia and weakness and polyclonal IgG or monoclonal IgM anti-GD1b (disialosyl) antibodies and an M-protein.[489] Cranial nerve symptoms may be prominent, including ophthalmoplegia and perioral paraesthesias. The autoantibody is directed against disialosyl groups found in GD3, GD2, GT1b, GQ1b (but not GM1), GM3 and GD1a and binds to dorsal root ganglion cells and nerve terminals. Electrophysiological studies demonstrate loss of sensory nerve amplitude, with mild, if any, motor findings. Pathological findings in one autopsied case included loss of large myelinated axons and dorsal root ganglion neurons, and demyelination of nerve roots.[353]

Other syndromes of autoantibody-associated polyneuropathy include the following:

- a sensory neuropathy of older patients presenting with pan-modal sensory loss and mild motor symptoms is associated with anti-neurofilament H antibodies;

- a syndrome of axonal sensory neuropathy with IgM binding to trisulphated heparin disaccharide (TS-HDS), which interferes with FGF-2 binding to its receptor, involves older, mostly female patients, who present with progressive distal symmetrical painful sensory loss involving all modalities except proprioception.[384] Pathological studies of TS-HDS show loss of unmyelinated axons and perivascular IgM deposition.

Immunoglobulin Deposition Disease

This is a rare condition in which monoclonal light and/or heavy chains deposit diffusely in tissue without the amyloid configuration. Non-amyloid light chain deposition may occur in the setting of myeloma, Waldenström's macroglobulinaemia and MGUS. The deposits appear as coalescent amorphous eosinophilic pools within the endoneurium, associated with blood vessels, and appear as hyaline bluish deposits in toluidine blue-stained semi-thin plastic sections (Figure 24.109a). This material is PAS-positive and resistant to diastase digestion, and is Congo red-negative. Most cases exhibit positive immunoreactivity for kappa light chain (Figure 24.109b). Ultrastructurally, non-amyloid deposits are amorphous granular or finely reticulated, lacking the characteristic fibrillary appearance of amyloid.

Cryoglobulinaemia

Curved tubular structures arranged in a fingerprint pattern may be seen in the endoneurium adjacent to Schwann cells and in the cytoplasm of endothelial cells and pericytes in cases of IgG myeloma with cryoglobulinaemia. A vasculitis involving peripheral nerves resulting in ischaemic neuropathy has been described in mixed cryoglobulinaemia. Ischaemia of nerve may also be caused by intravascular cryoglobulin deposition in the absence of inflammation. Hepatitis C virus infection is a common cause of chronic liver disease and appears to be the most common cause of mixed cryoglobulinaemia.[166,340] The disorder is characterized by cryoprecipitable immunocomplexes in serum and by involvement of one or more organs or systems (liver, kidney, peripheral nerve).[6,530] In a large series of patients with mixed cryoglobulinaemia, the prevalence of peripheral neuropathy was 74 per cent.[6,530] Peripheral nerve involvement was severe and progressive in 25 per cent of patients. Nemmi and colleagues reported the detection of epineurial vasculitis in sural nerve biopsies in 8 of 25 cases of hepatitis C virus-associated cryoglobulinaemia;[340] this was associated with axonal loss in a non-uniform asymmetrical pattern. An occlusive micro-angiopathy by immunoglobulin precipitation has been proposed as the mechanism for paraneoplastic cryoglobulinaemia neuropathy.[398] Evidence suggests that endothelial cells of peripheral nerve micro-vessels may be the target of viral infection and that viral-related proteins expressed on the cell surface attract immunocomplexes.

Osteosclerotic Myeloma, POEMS Syndrome and Castleman Disease

Peripheral neuropathy is often the initial manifestation of a rare form of malignant plasma cell dyscrasia: osteosclerotic

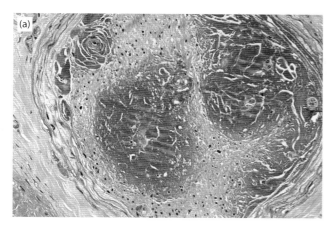

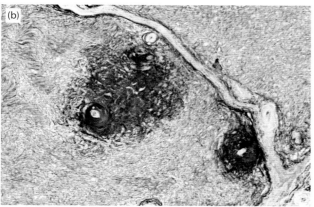

24.109 Immunoglobulin M (IgM) paraproteinaemic neuropathy. **(a)** Abundant amorphous material accumulated under the perineurium and about endoneurial micro-vessels; nerve fibres are depleted. Material is Congo red-negative. **(b)** Positive immunolabelling for kappa light chain. (a) Periodic acid–Schiff; (b) immunoperoxidase.

myeloma. The unchecked proliferation of plasma cells occurs as discrete bony lesions that result in a radiological appearance that is sclerotic or mixed lytic–sclerotic, as opposed to the purely lytic lesions encountered in multiple myeloma and solitary plasmacytoma. The diagnosis of osteosclerotic myeloma relies on the demonstration of monoclonal plasma cells in the biopsy of a sclerotic lesion, which characteristically involves the spine, pelvis or ribs. Skull lesions rarely develop.

Patients with osteosclerotic myeloma may display a variety of systemic changes affecting many organs and systems, which together constitute the POEMS (polyneuropathy, organomegaly, endocrinopathy, M-protein, skin changes) syndrome or Crow–Fukase syndrome.[479] Of note, POEMS syndrome can also occur in patients without osteosclerotic myeloma but with Castleman disease (see later), extramedullary myeloma or MGUS. Despite the acronym, not all five features are observed in all patients or occur at the same time in every patient. Research has shown that an elevation of serum vascular endothelial growth factor (VEGF) levels is a consistent feature of the POEMS syndrome.[440] Peripheral nerves are one of the principal targets in POEMS syndrome.[536] The neuropathy of osteosclerotic myeloma resembles CIDP; autonomic fibres are spared and there is no involvement of cranial

nerves, although papilloedema may occur. A chronic slowly progressive course is typical, beginning in the feet and manifesting as tingling, paraesthesias and coldness. Motor involvement follows the sensory symptoms. The electrophysiological features of POEMS syndrome resemble those of severe CIDP, which may be predominantly axonal or, more commonly, in the demyelinating range with prolonged distal latencies. Cytoalbuminological dissociation may be present in the CSF. The M-protein in this rare variant of multiple myeloma is usually of the IgG or IgA heavy chain class; most are λ light chain type. In specimens from these patients, ultrastructural examination demonstrates uncompacted myelin lamellae (Figure 24.104b).[536] Although suggestive of POEMS syndrome, this finding is non-specific, because it has been observed in other conditions, such as hereditary neuropathy with pressure palsies, CMT-1 and inflammatory demyelinating polyradiculoneuritis. However, in the appropriate clinical setting, the demonstration of uncompacted myelin around many axons is highly suggestive of the neuropathy associated with POEMS. Endoneurial deposits of immunoglobulin are exceptional and inflammation has not been reported. The pathogenesis of nerve damage in POEMS remains undetermined; endoneurial microvascular endothelial injury caused by overexpression of VEGF leading to hyperpermeability has been proposed as a possible mechanism.

Angiofolicular lymph node hyperplasia (Castleman disease) is an uncommon non-malignant disorder that occurs as either a localized or a multicentric form. Patients have a monoclonal lambda IgA gammopathy and may have other systemic signs with features of POEMS. Two histological varieties of Castleman disease are recognized: the vast majority consists of the hyaline vascular form, and the plasma cell form accounts for the remainder. The multicentric plasma cell variant is more likely to be associated with a chronic demyelinating polyneuropathy with predominant and severe motor dysfunction. A report documents PCR evidence of human herpes virus 8 (HHV-8) infection in Castleman disease associated with POEMS.[243]

DIABETIC NEUROPATHIES

The prevalence of diabetic neuropathy, currently the most common neuropathy in Europe and North America, is expected to increase substantially as the result of the looming epidemic of type 2 diabetes. Diabetic neuropathy is not a single neuropathy; rather, it is a complex spectrum of neuropathies (Table 24.11), including symmetrical sensorimotor, asymmetrical (involving cranial and somatic nerves) and autonomic (reviewed in Llewelyn *et al.*)[281] types, the pathogenesis of which is being unravelled in human and experimental animal studies.[281] Clinical presentations include sensory loss, occasionally complicated by disabling neuropathic pain, autonomic insufficiency involving many modalities and distributions, and weakness.[35] Practical concerns may prompt nerve biopsy in a patient with recognized diabetes (Box 24.2). Patients may develop neuropathy as adults or children, and after years of diabetes or at initial presentation. The frequency of diabetic neuropathy, which develops in both type 1 and type

TABLE 24.11 Classification of diabetic neuropathies

Impaired glucose tolerance and hyperglycaemic neuropathy
Generalized (symmetrical) neuropathies
    Sensorimotor
    Acute painful (including treatment-induced)
    Autonomic
    Acute motor
Focal and multifocal neuropathies
    Cranial
    Thoracolumbar
    Lumbosacral radioplexus (Bruns–Garland syndrome)
Superimposed chronic inflammatory demyelinating
    polyneuropathy (CIDP)
Hypoglycaemic neuropathy

Based on Llewelyn et al.[281]

2 diabetes, is a function of the criteria selected, ranging from 10 per cent of diabetic individuals who are clinically symptomatic[309] to 48–90 per cent of diabetic people with electrophysiologically detectable dysfunction.[130] Diabetic neuropathy is commonly associated with other diabetic complications, including retinopathy and nephropathy, and increases with duration of diabetes, age, hypertension and smoking (in people with type 1 diabetes), patient height, alcohol consumption and worsening degree of glycaemic control.[116,281,309]

Neuropathy with Impaired Glucose Tolerance

A number of patients may present with idiopathic, typically painful neuropathy in the absence of elevated HbA1c or fasting hyperglycaemia but in the presence of an impaired glucose tolerance test.[351] Research suggests that small axons, including those comprising the epidermal innervation, are prominently affected and their involvement may be the earliest detectable sign of neuropathy in glucose dysmetabolism.[473,488] A syndrome of paraesthesias and pain in newly diagnosed diabetes ('hyperglycaemic neuropathy')[548] or increased resistance to intentionally induced ischaemia may be particularly sensitive to normalization of blood glucose values.

Symmetrical Sensorimotor Polyneuropathy

Symmetrical sensorimotor polyneuropathy is the best known of the neuropathies of diabetes, ranging from trivial electrophysiological alterations to distal 'stocking–glove' anaesthesia that may increase the risk of amputation. Pathological findings are dominated by variable degrees of myelinated and unmyelinated axon loss (Figure 24.110), particularly in the distal aspects of the lower limbs. Axonal degeneration is accompanied by the formation of numerous bands of Büngner and regenerative axonal clusters, which may disappear with severe or sustained neuropathy.[324] Pathological findings are frequently patchy, with foci of degeneration and regeneration that occasionally form a mini-neuroma with interruption of the perineurium.[324] Some patients, including a number with chronic involvement or mild symptoms, show demyelination (both primary and secondary forms),

BOX 24.2. Diabetes

Diabetes is a common disease that is threatening to increase to near-epidemic proportions in the future. It is not true that all patients with diabetes and peripheral nerve dysfunction have 'diabetic neuropathy'; rather, neuropathy in some diabetic patients may represent a second superimposed process rather than diabetes itself. Therefore, the initial work-up of a diabetic patient requires a careful history (including duration and severity of diabetes, degree of control), laboratory data (e.g. glycosylated haemoglobin (HbA1c) levels, presence of a paraprotein, autoantibodies) and electrophysiological data. Although neuropathy may be the presenting symptom of patients with unrecognized diabetes leading to a first-time diagnosis, patients with otherwise idiopathic neuropathy may have only impaired glucose tolerance and, thus, an uncertain pathogenesis. Patients with recognized diabetes and neuropathic symptoms are infrequently biopsied if their neuropathic presentation is consistent with the classic findings in symmetrical sensory neuropathy (i.e. chronic symmetrical sensory neuropathy with a predilection for the lower extremities). However, these patients may be biopsied if their presentation is dominated by motor symptoms, severe sensory loss (particularly joint and vibration sense) out of proportion to the severity of diabetes, asymmetry of involvement or an acute, rapidly worsening course. Such issues are more than academic, because an atypical presentation or course may reflect the superimposition of other neuropathic processes including, but not limited to, vasculitis and chronic inflammatory demyelinating polyneuropathy (CIDP), which can be treated successfully if recognized. The identification of the pathological substrate of diabetic lumbosacral radioplexus neuropathy and similar pathological features in the sural nerve of some patients has suggested a possible immune pathogenesis and the therapeutic possibility of immune suppression. Patients with autonomic symptoms are rarely biopsied in life, although new studies using skin biopsies may permit the practical identification of autonomic pathology in living diabetic patients.[294] The possibility exists, therefore, that diabetic neuropathies have different pathogenetic mechanisms and different therapies.

remyelination and occasional onion bulbs,[19] although the association of CIDP with diabetes suggests possible coexistence. Discrimination of thinly myelinated regenerating axons from true demyelination is difficult in the absence of teased fibre analysis; however, the presence of active axonal degeneration, numerous bands of Büngner and regenerative clusters suggests that most are regenerative. Axonal atrophy has not been demonstrated consistently in human diabetic neuropathy.[486] Thickened basement membranes, which may reflect failure in the turnover of biochemically altered basal laminae, involve the endoneurial microvasculature (Figure 24.111), Schwann cells and, particularly, perineurial cells (Figure 24.112) and may result in the persistence of circular basement membranes following nerve fibre loss (Figure 24.113).[244] The diabetic endoneurial microvasculature is often surrounded by multiple concentric layers of basal laminae and collagen, which markedly thicken its walls (Figure 24.111); however, this characteristic pattern is not specific for diabetes. Studies of 'early' diabetic neuropathy have reported normal myelinated fibre density, axonal area and g-ratio in the presence of teased fibre studies showing paranodal abnormalities, segmental demyelination and remyelination without active degeneration of myelinated axons.[301] In this study, Schwann cells lacking associated axons and unmyelinated

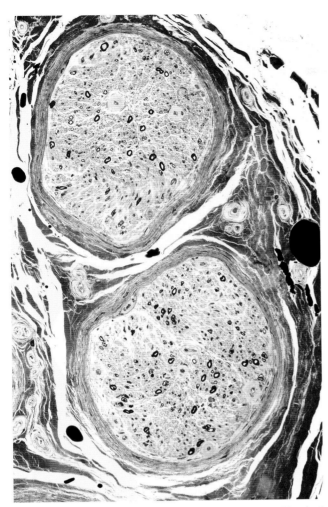

24.110 Diabetic symmetrical sensory neuropathy. The hall-mark of diabetic sensory neuropathy is axon loss, which may be extensive. 1-μm plastic section. ×200.

axon density were increased in the presence of a decrease in unmyelinated axon diameter.

Differences between type 1 and type 2 diabetes in the neuropathology of diabetic somatic nerves have been described in animals and humans. People with type 1 diabetes are reported to develop fewer foci of patchy axonal degeneration and more evidence of myelinopathy than those with type 2 diabetes, in which axonal degeneration is prominent. Axoglial dysjunction, an unusual and debated ultrastructural and molecular alteration of the perinodal junctional apparatus, has been advanced as the explanation for paranodal demyelination and conduction defects, especially in type 1 diabetes in rats and humans.[470] Somatic neuropathy in type 1 diabetic BB/Wor rats is characterized by severe nerve conduction defects, axonal atrophy, node of Ranvier-based pathology with molecular alterations of nodal proteins, defects in axonal regeneration[132] and, eventually, significant loss of myelinated axons.[470] In comparison, diabetic somatic neuropathy in the type 2 diabetic BBZDR/Wor rat is associated with only mild atrophy of myelinated axons, minimal nodal pathology with no molecular changes, segmental demyelination and active wallerian degeneration in the

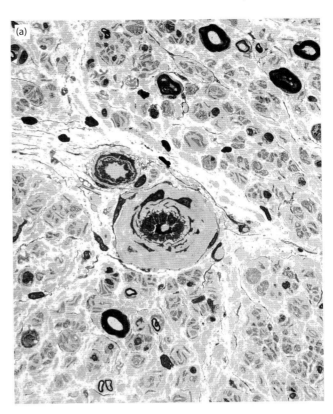

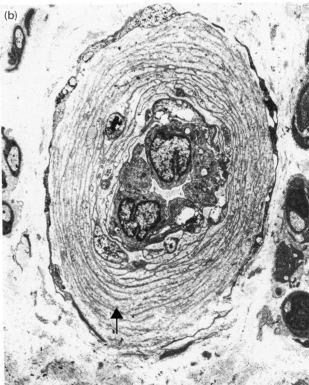

24.111 Diabetic symmetrical sensory neuropathy. Marked thickening of endoneurial venules and capillaries is produced by accumulation of concentric multilamellar collections of basal laminae (arrow, b). **(a)** ×600; **(b)** ×2950.

absence of axon loss, which may reflect increased axonal regeneration.[470]

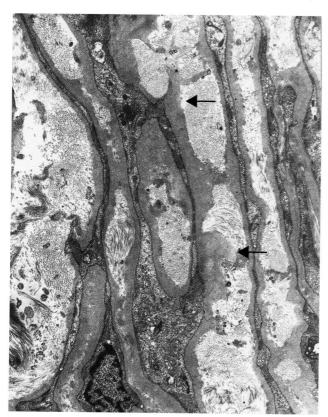

24.112 Diabetic perineurium. Diabetes increases the thickness of the perineurial basal laminae (arrows). ×4000.

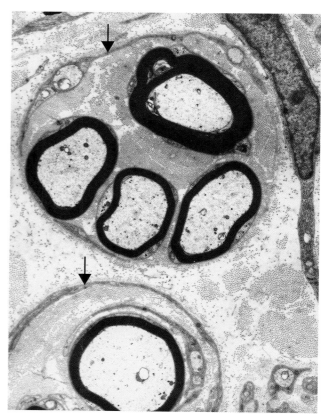

24.113 Diabetic neuropathy. Circular rigid preservation of basal laminae (arrows) surrounding regenerative axonal clusters suggests biochemical changes in basal lamina. ×5650.

Studies showing multifocal axon loss in the development of human diabetic neuropathy have been interpreted as evidence for an ischaemic pathogenesis. The diffuse symmetrical nature of the neuropathy distally has been explained as the result of summation of ischaemic foci along the course of the nerve.[128] However, multifocal loss of axons is not pathognomonic of vasculopathy or ischaemia and is typical in some forms of inherited neuropathy. Endothelial cell and pericyte degeneration, endothelial cell hyperplasia/hypertrophy,[548] decreased luminal area and altered blood–nerve barrier permeability are seen in endoneurial microvasculature,[168,300] findings that correlated with electrophysiological measures of the severity of the neuropathy.[299] Microvasculopathy may anticipate the development of significant neuropathy in humans. Theriault and colleagues measured nerve blood flow using laser Doppler flowmetry in diabetic patients with early polyneuropathy and determined that local blood flow was not decreased, even in the presence of definitive evidence of decreased sensory nerve action potential (SNAP) amplitudes and decreased numbers of axons.[500] Microvascular pathology has been variously interpreted as critical evidence for an ischaemic pathogenesis in diabetic neuropathy and as an unrelated but parallel change.[582] The epineurial vasculature is typically less severely involved, although vasculopathy has been reported.

Painful neuropathy, initially suspected to reflect a predilection for small-fibre damage, has not been correlated consistently with active fibre degeneration or regeneration in sural nerve,[52] but examination of intra-epidermal sensory nerve fibre density suggests such a correlation.[378] Ectopic discharges related to pain perception have been demonstrated to arise from dorsal root ganglion neurons and accompany changes in sensory neuron sodium channels.[107] The dorsal root ganglia of autopsied diabetic patients contain neurofilament-laden, calcitonin gene-related peptide (CGRP)-, trkA- and substance P-immunoreactive dystrophic swellings involving recurrent collateral axons that terminate on adjacent perikarya,[450] but there is no proven association with painful neuropathy. The mechanisms underlying painful neuropathies are complex and may involve contribution by multiple levels of the CNS and PNS.[343,564]

Skin biopsies have been recently used in the analysis of diabetic symmetrical sensory polyneuropathy and autonomic neuropathy.[265,266,294,312,378] Fibre loss demonstrable in skin biopsies has been reported in the absence of axon loss in the sural nerve in diabetic sensory neuropathy, which reflects loss of the most distal sensory complement of axons. The ability to perform multiple skin biopsies in the essential absence of neuropathic residua is one of the assets of skin biopsy and can be used to follow the progress of treatment. After capsaicin-induced sensory skin denervation, diabetic patients show a slower rate of IENF regeneration compared with healthy subjects, suggesting the ability to identify incipient neuropathy by regenerative stress at the earliest stages, in which it may be most amenable to therapy. The demonstration of distal pre-terminal nerve-fiber swellings in diabetes may represent

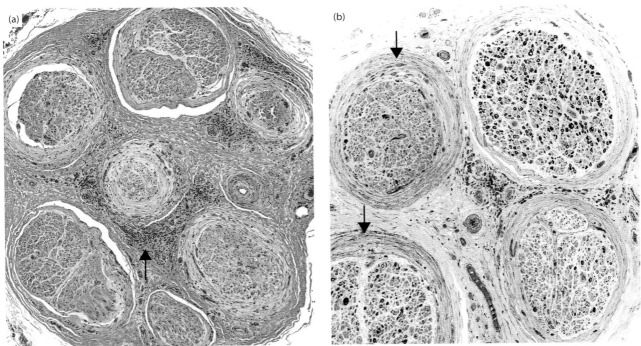

24.114 Diabetic lumbosacral radioplexus neuropathy. Characteristic pathological findings include **(a)** perivascular inflammation involving the epineurium (arrow), and **(b)** differential fascicular axon loss and proliferation of perineurial cells (arrows). (a) ×60; (b) ×100.

a 'pre-degenerative' change. Skin biopsies may also help distinguish neuropathies from radiculopathies, which typically do not produce epidermal nerve changes because the root damage is proximal to the DRG. Small, thinly myelinated Aδ (A-delta) axons, which subserve cutaneous mechanoreceptors and thermal receptors, can also be identified in skin biopsies.

Another recent novel approach is the examination of corneal nerves by non-invasive *in vivo* confocal microscopy.[4] Findings using this technique have been correlated with the presence and severity of diabetic autonomic neuropathy and its improvement following combined pancreas/kidney transplantation. Similar changes have been described in idiopathic small fibre neuropathy and Fabry disease.

Asymmetrical Diabetic Neuropathies

This category includes diabetic lumbosacral radioplexus neuropathy (LRPN; also known as 'diabetic amyotrophy', 'Bruns–Garland syndrome', 'femoral neuropathy of diabetes' and 'proximal diabetic neuropathy'), truncal radiculopathy, upper limb mononeuropathy and cranial nerve palsies (usually cranial nerves III, IV and VI) (recently reviewed).[573] Occasional diabetic patients, often early in diabetes, following institution of insulin therapy or associated with significant weight loss, experience sudden or subacute onset of motor dysfunction with muscle wasting, involving large nerves to the lower limb or cranial nerves. Lumbosacral radioplexus neuropathy develops more commonly in middle-aged and elderly men with type 2 diabetes and typically involves more than the proximal musculature;[281] rarely, upper limb involvement occurs.

The pathological characterization of this group of neuropathies may involve an autoimmune component resulting in an inflammatory micro-vasculitis with T-cell infiltrates,[575] although not typically angionecrosis (Figure 24.114), involving the epineurial vasa nervorum with endoneurial and perineurial haemosiderin deposition. Vascular changes are also accompanied by perineuritis and an axonopathy, which ranges from scattered degenerating axons to the formation of an 'injury neuroma'.[282,433] At least some 'infarcts' described in early studies may have represented Renaut bodies. Loss of intra-epidermal nerve fibres has also been described in biopsies taken from symptomatic areas.[266] The pathological findings in diabetic LRPN are identical to those seen in patients with non-diabetic LRPN, although it has been suggested that 'non-diabetic' patients with LRPN may also have abnormal glucose tolerance.[235] The usual course results in spontaneous recovery over several months.

Diabetic Autonomic Neuropathy

Both sympathetic and parasympathetic dysfunction occurs in diabetes[25] and may be accompanied and exaggerated by superimposed enteric or visceral sensory dysfunction. Myriad autonomic functions may be targeted individually or in groups (reviewed[423]): R-R interval may be abnormal early on, cardiac reflexes may be lost and orthostatic hypotension represents a later complication. Impotence occurs in 35 per cent of diabetic men. Other symptoms include gastrointestinal dysfunction, such as oesophageal dysmotility, gastroparesis and chronic diarrhoea or constipation; bladder distension and infection; and pupillomotor or sweating abnormalities. The presence of symptomatic diabetic autonomic neuropathy significantly increases morbidity and mortality, which may reflect the development of cardiac arrhythmias, superimposition of nephropathy, stroke, or increased perioperative mortality.[139,281] Visceral dysfunction in diabetes also involves the enteric nervous system,[547] the non-adrenergic non-cholinergic pathway in the pylorus[363] and, particularly for urinary bladder function, the visceral sensory nervous system. The development of autonomic and peripheral somatic neuropathies may be divergent in diabetic patients, suggesting the possibility that different pathophysiological processes or targeted subpopulations of autonomic neurons/axons underlie these neuropathies.[498]

The examination of the innervation of sweat glands, arrector pili and arterioles extends the usefulness of skin biopsies to the analysis of autonomic nerves in diabetic autonomic neuropathy,[239] Parkinson's disease and familial dysautonomia. Sweat glands are innervated by different populations of autonomic fibers expressing multiple different neurotransmitters and may be differentially susceptible to experimental and clinical insults. Skin biopsy correlates with sweat gland nerve fiber density, neuropathic symptoms, neurological deficits and sweat production in diabetic patients. Similar approaches have been used to demonstrate abnormal innervation of the gastric mucosa in diabetic patients.

Systematic autopsy studies of diabetic patients have demonstrated the development of markedly swollen neurofilament-laden axons and synapses (neuroaxonal dystrophy; Figure 24.115) in the relative absence of neuron loss in diabetic prevertebral sympathetic autonomic ganglia that serve the bowel and viscera.[449] Similar development of neuroaxonal dystrophy involves preterminal axons and synapses of sympathetic prevertebral and lumbosacral chain ganglia, while largely sparing the superior cervical ganglion.[445] The presence of lymphocytic infiltrates in a widely quoted study of the sympathetic ganglia of diabetic patients with symptomatic autonomic neuropathy[123] has been interpreted as evidence for its possible autoimmune pathogenesis.[401] However, lymphocytic infiltration was neither more frequent nor of greater intensity in diabetic subjects compared with non-diabetic subjects in one large series.[446] Significant loss of myelinated axons in the greater splanchnic nerves (i.e. the preganglionic axons to prevertebral sympathetic ganglia)[288] and the abdominal vagus nerve in diabetic gastroparesis[288] has also been described. Studies of parasympathetic ganglia suggest the selective loss of nitrergic innervation of the stomach and penis of diabetic mice.[80] In other diabetic animal models, subpopulations of autonomic fibres within the gut, bladder, penis and other end organs may show preferential damage (reviewed in Schmidt).[448]

Proposed Pathogenetic Mechanisms of Diabetic Neuropathy

The detailed pathogenesis of PNS dysfunction in experimental and clinical diabetes is unknown; however, a variety of pathogenetic mechanisms have been proposed and tested in experimental animal models of diabetic neuropathy (Table 24.12), which have been recently

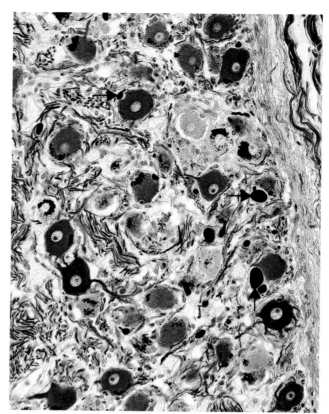

24.115 Diabetic autonomic neuropathy. Numerous dystrophic swellings (arrows) involve terminal axons and synapses in prevertebral sympathetic ganglia. Bielschowsky stain, ×300.

reviewed.[281,355,527] Although there is currently no consensus regarding which mechanisms are operative, multiple mechanisms may participate interactively and, indeed, may vary between different forms of diabetic neuropathy. Although it is generally believed that tight glucose control does delay the development of somatic and autonomic neuropathy, it does not prevent it, and even intensive diabetic treatment of type 2 diabetics produced minimal improvement in established neuropathy.[512] The following mechanisms have been suggested to play a role in its pathogenesis:

Oxidative Stress

Both increased production of oxidant stressors and reduction in antioxidant defences may contribute to the pathogenesis of diabetic neuropathy,[354] possibly by increasing production of lipid peroxides, DNA damage, mitochondrial injury, and damage to intracellular and extracellular proteins. Antioxidants may produce a salutary effect on biochemical and physiological defects of diabetic nerves.[354] Recent investigation has shown that hyperglycaemia inactivates neuronal acetylcholine receptors in autonomic ganglia through a mechanism involving an elevation in reactive oxygen species and an interaction with highly conserved cysteine residues located near the intracellular mouth of the nAChR channel.[71] Diabetic mice have depressed ganglionic transmission and reduced sympathetic reflexes, whereas diabetic mice expressing mutant postsynaptic nAChRs that lack the conserved cysteine residues on the a3 subunit have

TABLE 24.12 Diabetic neuropathies: proposed pathogenetic mechanisms

Increased oxidative stress (Schwann cells, axon, cell bodies)
Mitochondriopathy
Impaired neurotrophic support (NGF, BDNF, NT-3, IGF-I)
Enhanced polyol pathway activity
Accumulation of AGEs
Ischaemia involving nerve and/or neuronal cell body
MAPK activation
Neuronal apoptosis, dorsal root and sympathetic ganglia
Enhanced PKC-βII
Axonal transport deficiency
Abnormalities of axonal regeneration and synaptic plasticity
Autoimmune processes directed against axons and neuronal cell bodies

AGE, advanced glycosylation end product; BDNF, brain-derived neurotrophic factor; IGF-I, insulin-like growth factor I; MAPK, mitogen-activated protein kinase; NGF, nerve growth factor; NT-3, neurotrophin-3; PKC, protein kinase C.

normal synaptic transmission in sympathetic ganglia and normal sympathetic reflexes.[71]

Mitochondriopathy

Brownlee proposed that a diabetes-induced increase in glucose metabolism produces an exaggerated proton gradient in mitochondria, resulting in the generation of excess ubiquinone intermediates and increased superoxide production.[54] Others, however, have reported an insulin- and neurotrophin 3 (NT-3)-sensitive decrease in mitochondrial membrane potential in adult cultured dorsal root ganglion neurons.[150] Recent publications[95,96] advance the position that diabetes-induced changes in mitochondrial phenotype may represent key factors leading to altered activity of the respiratory chain and Krebs cycle components. These changes occur without a significant increase in perikaryal reactive oxygen species and are insulin sensitive.[95,96] Nutrient excess may interfere with the activity of AMP kinase, SIRT1 and PGC-1α in diabetic DRG, subsequently decreasing mitochondrial activity.[95,96]

Calcium Homeostasis

Axons of DRG neurons from diabetic rats exhibit aberrant Ca2+ homeostasis, possibly triggered by suboptimal SERCA activity, that has been proposed to contribute to distal axonopathy in diabetes.[581]

Neurotrophic Substances

Deficiencies in the amount or regulation of neurotrophic substances (e.g. NGF, NT-3, IGF, insulin) are thought to contribute to the development of both symmetrical sensorimotor neuropathy and autonomic neuropathy.[49,197] A role for NGF in somatic sensory neuropathy followed the demonstration of diminished levels of endogenous target-derived and transported NGF and reduced expression of NGF-sensitive sensory neuropeptides CGRP and substance P in somatic nerves of diabetic rats.[117] Clinical trials of exogenous recombinant human NGF (rhNGF) treatment have not demonstrated a significant beneficial effect. Nerve BDNF content is upregulated in diabetes and may exert a reparative or protective function.[149] Insulin-like growth factor I, which is decreased in diabetic serum and nerve, has antioxidant and antiapoptotic effects on glucose-treated neurons in culture, corrects hyperalgesia and deficits in axonal regeneration of diabetic rats *in vivo*,[216] and reverses experimental autonomic neuropathy.[216,387,424,451] Near-nerve or intranasal application of insulin at doses that do not affect circulating glucose levels unilaterally corrects nerve conduction velocity defects in somatic nerves of diabetic rats or mice.[155,471] C-peptide, cleaved from the pro-insulin molecule during the secretion of insulin, has also been identified as a neurotrophic factor with a pathogenetic role in the development and possible therapy of polyneuropathy in type 1 diabetes.[135,388]

Polyol Pathway

Although normally a minor pathway of glucose metabolism, the polyol pathway in diabetic nerve and ganglia converts substantial amounts of glucose to sorbitol and then to fructose using aldose reductase and sorbitol dehydrogenase, respectively, and may increase oxidative stress as the result of diminished glutathione.[354] Inhibition of the first part of the polyol pathway in experimental diabetic animals has resulted in marked improvement of various neuropathic parameters, although results in diabetic human subjects generally have been disappointing.[352]

Advanced Glycosylation End Products

Hyperglycaemia-induced glycosylation of various intracellular and extracellular proteins may be followed by chemical rearrangement into advanced glycosylation end products (AGEs), some of which may result in cross-linking of a variety of proteins and subcellular organelles.[505] Advanced glycosylation end products are thought to bind to AGE receptors (RAGEs), members of an immunoglobulin super-family, increasing oxidative stress. Inhibitors of AGE formation such as aminoguanidine have shown a positive effect on a variety of disturbed functions in diabetic somatic nerves.

Ischaemia

The relevance of ischaemia in the pathogenesis of diabetic neuropathy, particularly diffuse symmetrical sensorimotor polyneuropathy, is contentious, with groups identifying and failing to identify changes in nerve blood flow in humans and animal models.[582] However, there is evidence for tissue hypoxia in nerve and ganglia in experimental animal models and humans,[583] which may reflect endothelial damage, altered red cell deformability or defects in local oxygen release.[582] The simultaneous presence of tissue hypoxia, alterations of NO (leading to the formation of ONOO–) and other vasoactive substances such as endothelin-1, and impaired reactive hyperaemia of nerve micro-vessels may combine to place diabetic nerves at risk.[58,242,585] Nerve ischaemia is associated with nerve dysfunction but may not represent the primary or major cause; rather, it may simply accelerate the process.[281]

Mitogen-Activated Protein Kinases

Tomlinson and colleagues proposed that mitogen-activated protein kinases (MAPKs) activated by glucose and oxidative stress have an important role in the development of diabetic neuropathy, possibly by inducing excessive protein (e.g. neurofilament) phosphorylation.[399]

Neuronal Apoptosis

A role for apoptosis in the pathogenesis of diabetic neuropathy has been proposed,[88,424] largely on the basis of studies of *in vitro* glucose challenge of neurons; however, these findings conflict with the relative maintenance of neuron number in dorsal root and sympathetic ganglia and the axonal preservation in the somatic nerves of the STZ diabetic rat. Experiments with rats diabetic for 12 months showed non-lethal activated caspase 3 expression in dorsal root ganglion neurons but failed to show neuronal degeneration and loss when assessed using non-biased counting methods.[88] In contrast, mice with experimental diabetes apparently do lose sensory neurons and axons.[238]

Protein Kinase C

Enhanced activity of protein kinase C (PKC) βII isoform has been reported to contribute to structural and functional changes in the microvasculature and induction of TGF-β effects on the extracellular matrix. Inhibitors of PKC are reported to have salutary effects.[551]

Axonal Transport

Diabetes also results in diminished axonal transport of a variety of materials,[467] although the transport apparatus itself may not be the critical targeted component; instead, decreased neuronal synthesis or altered production of trophic substances by target tissues may be primary. In early experimental diabetic neuropathy, axonal atrophy may be prominent distally, perhaps because there is impaired slow axonal transport of neurofilaments.

Abnormalities of Regeneration and Synaptic Dysplasia

It has been proposed that neuroaxonal dystrophy represents a diabetes-induced abnormal outcome of ongoing cycles of synaptic turnover or remodelling, i.e. synaptic degeneration and regeneration, which may normally subserve synaptic plasticity.[446] Processes targeting synapses–particularly those related to synaptic vesicle function, membrane retrieval and turnover of subcellular organelles–are likely key targets in the pathogenesis of autonomic neuroaxonal dystrophy. Impairment of nerve regeneration following sciatic nerve crush injury has been reported in STZ[136,284] and BB/Wor[387] rats. Delayed and attenuated upregulation of IGF-I, NGF and p75 and asynchronous changes in IGF-I receptor message in distal segments of injured sciatic nerve in BB/Wor rats contrast with significantly milder changes in BBZDR/Wor rats and may account for the more efficient regenerative response in the latter model.[386]

Autoimmune Processes

An autoimmune pathogenesis has been proposed for diabetic autonomic neuropathy.[178,401] Antibodies directed against adrenal gland, sympathetic ganglia and vagus nerve may be associated with an increased incidence of autonomic neuropathy,[35] although this is controversial.

TOXIN-INDUCED NEUROPATHIES

Toxic neuropathies result from the neuropathic effect of a large collection of substances (Table 24.13), which include pharmaceutical agents, substances used in industrial processes, biological toxins and nutritional toxic states.[302] Often they produce neuropathy without a distinctive pathological signature. A few general themes have been proposed, suggesting that toxins tend to affect axons before Schwann cells, affect large myelinated axons first

TABLE 24.13 Toxic neuropathies

Toxins	Drugs
Acrylamide	Almitrine
Buckthorn	Amiodarone
Carbon disulphide	Chloroquine
Dimethylaminopropionitrile	Cisplatin
Ethylene oxide	Clioquinol
Hexacarbons and solvents	Colchicine
Organophosphorus esters	Cyanide
Trichloroethylene	Dapsone
Vacor	Disulfiram
Arsenic	Gold
Lead	Isoniazid
Mercury	Metronidazole
Thallium	Misonidazole
	Nitrofurantoin
	Nitrous oxide
	Perhexiline
	Podophyllin
	Pyridoxine (vitamin B6)
	Sodium cyanate
	Suramin
	Tacrolimus (FK506)
	Taxanes (paclitaxel, docetaxel)
	Thalidomide
	Toxic oil syndrome
	Vinca alkaloids (vincristine, vinblastine)

and most severely, and have a predilection for sensory axons, and that the severity of involvement and rate of onset parallel the dose and duration of intoxicant exposure.[324] The prompt diagnosis may permit the patient to avoid further exposure and be treated with the most appropriate regimen. In the following section we present a variety of toxins, particularly those with unusual pathological findings and distinctive clinical presentations.

Axonopathies

A large number of substances, ranging from environmental substances and industrial chemicals to drugs and cancer chemotherapeutic agents, may induce neuropathy characterized by axonal degeneration.[324,480] Some selectively target the process of axonal transport or interrupt the transport of discrete substances (Figure 24.116). Axonal transport consists of several phases, including fast and slow orthograde transport, fast retrograde transport, and turnaround transport, in which the polarity of transport is reversed, usually at the synapse but also at a site of injury. Iminodipropionitrile (IDPN), methyl-N-butyl-ketone (MnBK), 2,5-hexanedione (2,5-HD), aluminium and carbon disulphide are experimental or environmental toxins that appear to target neurofilament transport and metabolism and, as a result, cause the accumulation of neurofilaments in large swellings along the axon. Vinblastine, vincristine, podophyllin and paclitaxel (all potent cancer chemotherapeutic agents in which peripheral nerve toxicity may limit the dose and duration of clinical use) and colchicine (used in the treatment of gout) are known to interrupt microtubule function, which is critical to the process of axonal transport. Acrylamide can produce distinctive paranodal neurofilamentous accumulations or tubulovesicular aggregates involving the distal portions of axons, and also may target a phase of axonal transport or membrane dynamics at the nerve terminal. Zinc pyridinethione (ZPT; an ingredient of anti-dandruff shampoos) and bromophenylacetylurea (BPAU) preferentially target the turnaround process (by which the polarity of axonal transport is reversed), resulting in axonal swellings at nerve terminals.

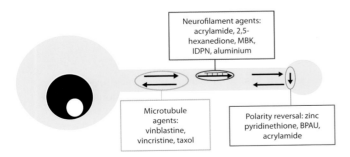

24.116 Toxic agents that interfere with axonal transport. BPAU, bromophenylacetylurea; IDPN, iminodipropionitrile; MBK, methyl-butyl-ketone.

Myelinopathy

The number of substances that produce primary myelinopathy is more limited than those resulting in axonal degeneration. Lead, diphtheria toxin, perhexilene, buckthorn toxin, lysolecithin and hexachlorophene are toxic substances directed at the Schwann cell, its myelin sheath or both, although the particular targeted elements differ between toxins.

Toxins

Acrylamide

Acrylamide (for reviews, see Gold and Schaumburg[173] and LoPachin et al.[286]), specifically its unpolymerized form, used in a variety of manufacturing processes as a grouting agent and in laboratories, can be absorbed through skin exposure to produce sensory and autonomic symptoms, frequently involving the extremities and face. Neuropathology shows loss of the most distal and longest large myelinated axons; however, severe intoxication also results in involvement of short small myelinated and unmyelinated axons, as can be demonstrated in skin biopsies.[250] The distal axonopathy is characterized by paranodal axonal neurofilamentous accumulations or tubulovesicular aggregates and may reflect interference with slow and fast axonal transport, the latter by inhibiting the interaction of kinesin, the fast axonal transport motor, with microtubules.[32,173,305] Research also suggests terminal swellings occur in response to its binding to the susceptible thiol SNARE (soluble N-ethylmaleimide sensitive factor attachment protein receptor complex) protein, which is involved in the insertion and turnover of synaptic plasmalemmal components and thus promotes the accumulation of tubulovesicular profiles.[285]

Buckthorn

Ingestion of the fruit of the *Karwinskia humboldtiana* (buckthorn shrub) causes a predominantly motor neuropathy, ultimately resulting in flaccid quadriparesis from which rapid recovery is possible. Studies have shown demyelination with superimposition of axonal degeneration.[70]

Carbon Disulphide

This industrial and experimental agent produces a central–distal axonopathy in which focal neurofilament-laden swollen axons are a pathological signature, probably resulting from cross-linking of neurofilament proteins[177,514] and culminating in nodal retraction, segmental demyelination and axonal degeneration. The pathogenetic mechanism may involve selective metal chelation, inhibition of a variety of dehydrogenases and monoamine oxidase, or generation of free radicals resulting from the cleavage of the carbon–sulphur (sulfur) bond.[32]

Dimethylaminopropionitrile

Workers involved in the manufacture of polyurethane foam may develop a constellation of distal sensory neuropathy in the lower extremities accompanied by sensory symptoms in the lower sacral dermatomes, bladder dysfunction and impotence. Neuropathological studies described both myelinated and unmyelinated axon loss and distal swollen neurofilament-containing axons, similar to experimental intoxication with β,β'-iminodipropionitrile.[380]

Ethylene Oxide

This agent, used as a gas to sterilize medical instruments, as a fumigator, and in industry in the synthesis of ethylene glycol, produces a distal, symmetrical, predominantly sensory neuropathy, characterized by organelle-laden axonal swellings and degeneration, possibly due to inhibition of axonal transport.[360]

Hexacarbons and Solvents

Exposure to n-hexane and methyl-n-butyl ketone occurs in the industrial manufacture of polyvinylchloride and shoes and by intentional inhalation ('glue-sniffing', 'huffing'), resulting in the generation of the active toxin 2,5-hexanedione and a distal sensorimotor neuropathy, in some cases accompanied by degenerative changes in the CNS. Cessation of exposure may be followed by continued worsening of the symptoms for as long as 2–4 months, a phenomenon known as 'coasting'. The neuropathy is characterized by the loss of large myelinated axons and focal axonal swellings (beginning on the proximal sides of nodes of Ranvier) containing segregated aggregates of neurofilaments, with secondary myelin thinning and distal axonal degeneration (Figure 24.117). Experimental toxicological studies show a similar distal axonopathy with preterminal axonal swellings of large myelinated axons, thought to reflect abnormal axonal transport (either increased or decreased) and cross-linking of neurofilaments due to the formation of pyrrole adducts with neurofilament amine groups and subsequent oxidation.[227,550]

Organophosphorus Esters

Most human cases have followed exposure to triorthocresylphosphate (TOCP) used as a high-temperature lubricant and as a softener in the manufacture of plastics, mostly as the result of contamination of food or beverages (such as 'ginger-jake paralysis' following contamination of Jamaican ginger extract); however, many other organophosphates with neurotoxic potential are in use. Days to weeks following TOCP exposure, the distal aspects of long large sensory and motor axons degenerate in a central–peripheral distal axonopathic pattern, which resolves, followed by a CNS deficit. Experimental studies have determined that phosphorylation of a 'neuropathy target esterase' (NTE), which is not acetylcholinesterase, plays a critical role in neurotoxicity. At one time, 'ageing' of the phosphorylated NTE complex (a non-enzymatic side-chain cleavage reaction) was thought to be critical to its neurotoxic role; however, more recent studies demonstrate that non-ageing organophosphate pesticides (e.g. chlorpyrifos) produce similar results. [230]

Toxic Oil Syndrome

An epidemic toxic neuropathy followed ingestion of adulterated rapeseed oil in Spain in the early 1980s, in which patients presented clinically with pneumonia, gastrointestinal symptoms and cutaneous lesions. Biopsies of sural

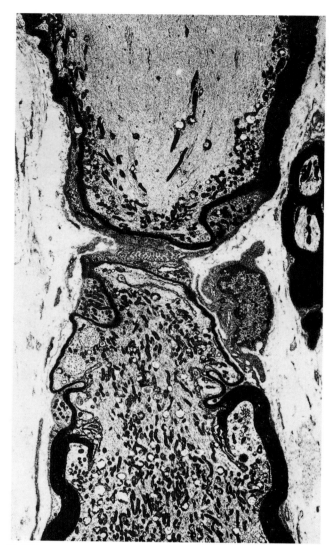

24.117 Hexacarbon neuropathy. The proximal paranode (upper) is enlarged and contains an accumulation of neurofilaments. The distal paranode (lower) contains multiple mitochondria. Electron micrograph, ×4000.

nerve[408] demonstrated an inflammatory neuropathy characterized by epineurial, perineurial and endoneurial perivascular inflammatory infiltrate in which lymphocytes and, in some cases, eosinophils were prominent, although necrotizing vasculitis was absent. The microscopic picture included perineuritis with fibrosis and axonal degeneration.

Trichloroethylene

This solvent and anaesthetic agent produces a distinctive trigeminal and facial cranial nerve functional defect resulting from degeneration of trigeminal neurons and other source nuclei.[65] The toxicity arises as trichloroethylene is converted to dichloroacetylene.

Vacor

Vacor (N-3-pyridylmethyl-N'-p-nitrophenyl urea) is a rodenticide that has structural similarities to nicotinamide, alloxan and streptozotocin, and similarly results in pancreatic islet β cell destruction and diabetes. An autonomic and sensory distal peripheral axonopathy has been reported in vacor-treated experimental animals,[549] which is thought to reflect a direct toxic effect rather than the secondary effect of diabetes.

Heavy Metals

For review, see Windebank.[560]

Arsenic

Exposure to arsenic by chronic or acute, accidental (contaminated water, foods), homicidal or intentional ingestion results in a distal, predominantly sensory neuropathy with painful dysaesthesia, accompanied by nausea, vomiting, abdominal pain and severe diarrhoea. Chronic cases feature cutaneous pigmentation and hyperkeratosis. Pathological study of the peripheral nerves of patients with arsenic poisoning demonstrated axonal degeneration involving myelinated axons of all sizes, with relative sparing of unmyelinated axons.[272] Based on the known reactivity of arsenic with sulphydryl (sulfhydryl) groups, it was proposed that arsenic interferes with pyruvate dehydrogenase activity by conversion of its cofactor lipoic acid to stable lipoic arsenate,[460] preventing the conversion of pyruvate to acetyl coenzyme A, a result similar to thiamine deficiency. However, arsenic interacts with numerous other enzymes that may also contribute to the pathogenesis of neuropathy.

Lead

Adults with lead intoxication (usually acquired from industrial exposure or contamination of drinking water) develop a predominantly motor neuropathy involving the upper, more often than the lower, extremities, producing weakness, atrophy of the wrist and finger extensor muscles and foot-drop. In experimental and clinical studies, both axonal degeneration and segmental demyelination have been described, as well as prominent endoneurial oedema.[105,559] Results vary markedly between species: in rats, an almost purely demyelinative pattern is seen but in humans axonal degeneration is primary. Intranuclear inclusions are seen in the Schwann cells and endothelial cells of humans and experimentally intoxicated animals. Although the mechanism of lead-induced neuropathy is not known, interference with calmodulin and calcium-mediated events (particularly presynaptic voltage-sensitive calcium ion channels), alterations in PKC activity, interference with mitochondrial function and changes in second messenger function have been proposed.[560]

Mercury

Methylmercury intoxication results in a variety of CNS symptoms, with a superimposed neuropathy (sensorimotor) characterized by loss of axons, comparably at thigh and ankle levels in animal studies and prominent involvement of neurons in the dorsal root ganglia, presumably from its effect on sulphydryl groups.[218,559]

Thallium

Intoxication with thallium, a sometime homicidal agent intended for use as a rodenticide and insecticide, produces a predominantly sensory, often painful, distal polyneuropathy with later motor involvement. Gastrointestinal symptoms occur acutely and, if the patient survives, characteristic alopecia develops within 2–4 weeks. Clinical cases show distal sensory and motor axonal degeneration and anterior horn motor neuron chromatolysis.[78] The early development of perinodal intra-axonal vacuoles is thought to reflect mitochondrial damage with uncoupling of oxidative phosphorylation. Thallium is known to inhibit flavin-dependent enzymes as the result of its interaction with riboflavin and interference with thiol enzymes and results in reduced antioxidant protection of cell membranes following lipid peroxidation and depletion of reduced glutathione.[304,482]

Drugs (See Also Reviews)[199,220,485]

Almitrine

Almitrine is a peripheral chemoreceptor agonist used predominantly in Europe for the treatment of chronic obstructive pulmonary disease. After 1–2 years of use, the drug may result in mild loss of predominantly large myelinated sensory axons independent of respiratory disease.[43] Experimental administration of an almitrine metabolite produces lamellated inclusions in sensory neurons, satellite cells, Schwann cells and endothelial cells of dorsal root ganglia.[567]

Amiodarone

This antiarrhythmic agent, when used over an extended period, may produce a sensorimotor neuropathy characterized by loss of myelinated and unmyelinated axons of all sizes, primary or secondary demyelination (in response to axonal atrophy), or a mixture of axonal degeneration and demyelination.[198] Experimental studies show that higher concentrations of drug result in more axonal degeneration, suggesting that different pathological changes reflect variability in blood–nerve barrier control of amiodarone concentration in nerve.[438] Electrophysiological studies may mimic CIDP. Lamellar lysosomal inclusion bodies develop in Schwann cells, perineurial cells, endoneurial fibroblasts and capillary endothelial cells. Discontinuation of the drug usually improves the neuropathy. The pathogenetic mechanism is unknown but may involve effects on ATPase activity or calcium homeostasis.

Bortezomib

Bortezomib is a proteasome inhibitor used to treat patients with multiple myeloma who are not candidates for stem cell transplantation. Severe axon degeneration and loss, endoneurial edema and inflammation with increased endoneurial macrophages have been reported.[435]

Chloroquine

Long-term use of this antimalarial and anti-inflammatory drug produces a neuropathy characterized by progressive symmetrical proximal limb weakness and distal paraesthesias. Pathological features include severe loss of myelinated axons, axonal degeneration and demyelination/remyelination in which lamellar and crystalline inclusions are found in axons (Figure 24.118), Schwann cells, perineurial and endothelial cells and presynaptic elements at the neuromuscular junction.[324,460] The pathogenetic mechanism may reflect lysosomal accumulation of the drug, which results in increased intralysosomal pH followed by the accumulation of undegraded lysosomal phospholipids and other subcellular elements.[199]

Cisplatin

This cancer chemotherapeutic agent produces a dose-related, mostly sensory neuropathy, occasionally accompanied by deafness and characterized by symmetrical

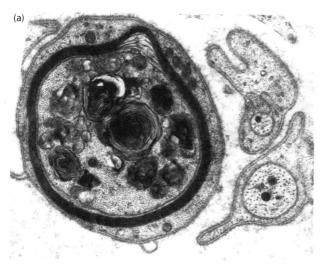

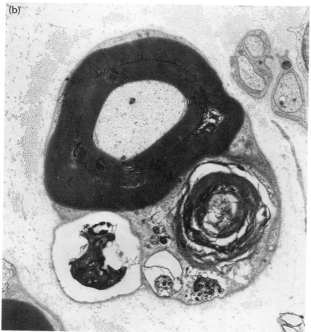

24.118 Chloroquine neuropathy. Multiple concentric membranous aggregates (arrow) are found within axons **(a)** and Schwann cells **(b)**. Electron micrographs, ×6850.

distal paraesthesias that may be potentiated by other chemotherapeutic agents such as paclitaxel. Pathological studies demonstrate loss of large myelinated axons, axonal degeneration and swollen/vacuolated dysfunctional mitochondria.[580] Other drugs, such as carboplatin, ormaplatin and oxaliplatin, produce similar toxicity. Sensory predominance may reflect access of the drug to dorsal root ganglion neurons in which there is normally a relatively permeable blood–nerve barrier. Experimental treatment results in dorsal root ganglion changes, including neuronal shrinkage, nucleolar abnormalities and changes in neurotransmitter levels.[21,507] It is thought that mitochondrial DNA damage and gradual attrition of mitochondrial function could play a role in the progressive and persistent neurotoxicity of cisplatin.[393] Treatment of experimental cisplatin neuropathy with neurotrophin-3 results in improvement of structural pathology and pathophysiology.[163]

Clioquinol

This antidiarrhoeal agent produced an epidemic of sub-acute myelo-opticoneuropathy in Japan, characterized by visual loss, paraesthesia, gait ataxia and axonal degeneration or demyelination in the posterior columns, optic nerves and peripheral nerves.[464] Animal studies showed clioquinol produced distal axonal degeneration in the ascending gracile and spinocerebellar tracts and descending corticospinal and optic tracts.[563]

Colchicine

The alkaloid of Colchicum autumnale (autumn crocus) is used in the treatment of acute gout, amyloidosis, Behçet's syndrome and familial Mediterranean fever. High doses may result in a mild to marked sensory neuropathy, with evidence of axonal degeneration, regeneration and loss that may reflect its effect on microtubular function and axonal transport.[371]

Cyanide

Often consumed accidentally in cassava-containing foods, cyanide results in an axonal and demyelinating neuropathy and is probably the cause of African tropical ataxic neuropathy.[324]

Dapsone

Dapsone (4,4′-diaminodiphenylsulphone), used as a treatment for leprosy, malaria, rheumatoid arthritis, dermatitis herpetiformis and pneumocystis pneumonia in AIDS, may produce a predominantly motor neuropathy characterized by axon loss[186] and muscle atrophy, worse in the upper limbs than the lower and worse in patients with defective liver metabolism ('slow acetylators').

Disulfiram

Disulfiram (tetraethylthiuram disulphide [disulfide]) has been used in the treatment of alcoholism. A mild sensorimotor neuropathy accompanies chronic use and is characterized by axonal degeneration in humans and experimental animals. It infrequently produces morphological giant axonal swellings (Figure 24.119) and intermolecular cross-linking produced by carbon disulphide, its apparent metabolite *in vivo*.[44,587] In experimental studies in rats, disulfiram results in Schwann cell vacuolation and segmental demyelination. Studies have suggested mitochondrial injury or inhibition of DNA topoisomerases as possible pathogenetic mechanisms.[199]

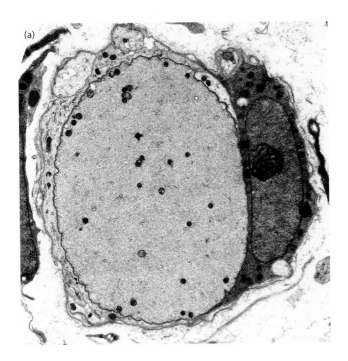

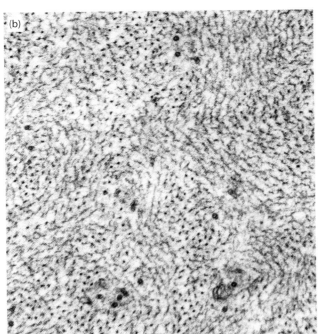

24.119 Disulfiram neuropathy. Axons may be swollen by increased numbers of neurofilaments. Electron micrographs: **(a)** ×5400; **(b)** ×19 900.

Gold

Use of gold as a treatment for rheumatoid arthritis occasionally results in the development of an acute distal polyneuropathy with sensory, motor or sensorimotor features. The neuropathy evolves over days to weeks and is characterized by both axonal degeneration and segmental demyelination[232] or, in some studies, axonal degeneration alone.

Isoniazid

Isoniazid is used as part of the therapy for tuberculosis. 'Slow acetylators' may develop increased levels of the drug, resulting in a central–distal symmetrical and predominantly sensory neuropathy. Degeneration of myelinated and unmyelinated axons occurs, often in the presence of regenerating axons. Experimental studies have shown periaxonal vacuolation and the proliferation of intra-axonal agranular reticulum and vacuoles, progressing to axonal degeneration,[219] in some cases with intraneural oedema resulting in the disruption of the blood–nerve barrier. The mechanism of isoniazid action is to inhibit pyridoxal phosphokinase, the enzyme that phosphorylates pyridoxal to form its active coenzyme and also chelates and inactivates the cofactor pyridoxal phosphate itself. The neuropathy is preventable with pyridoxine treatment.

Metronidazole and Misonidazole

Used as antiprotozoals, antibacterials and hypoxic cell radiation sensitizers in chemotherapy, both of these agents can produce a neuropathy that is a combination of axonal degeneration and demyelination,[47,513] often with large-fibre sensory predominance but extending to unmyelinated axons. Both agents can produce a CNS Wernicke-like picture in experimental animals, suggesting possible thiamine antagonism.

Nitrofurantoin

This antibiotic agent produces a subacute sensorimotor neuropathy in which axonal degeneration involving large myelinated fibres is typical.[324] One possible mechanism involves the inhibition of the synthesis of acetyl coenzyme A in the citric acid cycle by furan derivatives.[199]

Nitrous Oxide

An often abused inhalant, nitrous oxide toxicity results in a polyneuropathy (sensorimotor), occasionally accompanied by a myelopathy, which is thought to result from inactivation of cobalamin by oxidation to an inactive trivalent state and interference with vitamin B12-dependent metabolic pathways.[324]

Perhexilene

Perhexilene is used as a treatment for angina. Patients with genetically determined slow hydroxylation develop excessive blood levels of perhexilene, with a mixed sensorimotor neuropathy, occasionally with autonomic features and brain stem involvement. Nerve biopsy demonstrates both axonal degeneration and particularly extensive segmental demyelination.[426] A distinctive signature is the development of lysosomal lamellar and crystalloid inclusions in Schwann cells, smooth muscle cells, perineurial cells, pericytes and fibroblasts (as well as in liver, skin and muscle cells), as a result of perhexilene binding to polar lipids with impaired degradation and lysosomal accumulation.[292]

Podophyllin

A topical agent for the treatment of condylomata accuminatum and a constituent of some herbal preparations, podophyllin may produce a severe distal acute–subacute sensory (involving all modalities), motor and autonomic neuropathy characterized by axonal degeneration involving large myelinated and unmyelinated axons. The pathogenetic mechanism probably reflects interference with microtubule-based axonal transport.[324]

Pyridoxine (Vitamin B6)

Intake of excessive amounts of pyridoxine produces a diffuse distal sensory neuropathy in which sural nerves show non-specific axon loss,[441] which is likely to result from the degeneration of dorsal root ganglion neurons with high doses[257] or axonal atrophy with lower doses. Experimental studies demonstrate accumulated subcellular organelles in the nodal and distal paranodal axons in the dorsal root ganglia, suggesting a blockade of fast axonal transport in the proximal axon and cell body or, conversely, increased neurofilament transport. Neurotrophin-3 has been shown to be protective.

Sodium Cyanate

Used in the treatment of sickle cell anaemia, sodium cyanate produces a sensorimotor neuropathy with axonal degeneration and secondary demyelination.[324]

Suramin

Suramin is an antiparasitic and antineoplastic agent with the potential to produce a mild distal axonal sensorimotor neuropathy with axonal degeneration, and a severe subacute demyelinating neuropathy that resembles GBS.[199,324] Biopsies have shown a continuum of pathology from loss of myelinated axons to segmental demyelination with lymphocytic infiltration or macrophage infiltration,[86] in some cases resembling HIV-associated neuropathies. The mechanism is unestablished, but suramin is a known inhibitor of lysosomal enzymes and accumulates in dorsal root ganglia neurons in experimental animals; in addition, suramin blocks the receptor function of a variety of growth factors, such as IGF-I and NGF, and this may contribute to its neurotoxicity.

Tacrolimus (FK506)

This immune suppressant produces a CIDP-like picture with both axonal loss and demyelination.[324]

Taxanes (Paclitaxel, Docetaxel)

These agents were isolated from the bark of the Pacific yew (*Taxus brevifolia*) and a related species and are used as anti-tumour agents. Patients treated with these agents often develop a distal predominantly sensory neuropathy involving all modalities, which is dose-sensitive and improves on reduction or discontinuation of the drug. Pathologically, the few biopsied nerves have shown severe axon loss, atrophy and secondary demyelination, without microtubule aggregates and with inconstant evidence of regeneration.[199,425] Treatment of cultured cells with paclitaxel promotes the polymerization and inhibits the disassembly of microtubules, leading to the formation of aberrant crystalline bundles of microtubules. Local injection into rat sciatic nerve *in vivo* results in similar microtubular disorganization in Schwann cells, associated with axonal degeneration and demyelination.[273,420] Calpain inhibitors have been shown to prevent paclitaxel-induced axonal degeneration and pathophysiology in mice, without interfering with its primary antineoplastic effects.[543] A variety of neurotrophic substances, including NGF, IGF-I, ORG 2766 and LIF, are reported to protect against the neuropathy.[199]

Thalidomide

Initially released as a sedative, which resulted in a teratogenic epidemic of dysmyelia in the offspring of pregnant women, thalidomide has been reintroduced to treat Behçet's disease, graft versus host disease, various dermatological conditions, leprosy, HIV infection, plexiform neurofibromas, Crohn's disease and juvenile idiopathic arthritis, and as an antiangiogenic agent in cancer trials.[154] Thalidomide neuropathy presents as a symmetrical length-dependent axonal sensorimotor polyneuropathy, often with painful paraesthesias of the hands and feet. Sural nerve biopsies variously show axonal degeneration and loss of large myelinated axons,[87] increased numbers of regenerating axons and loss of dorsal root ganglia neurons, a pattern consistent with dying-back neuropathy and/or with sensory ganglionitis.[46,94,169]

Vinca Alkaloids (Vincristine, Vinblastine)

The frequently used chemotherapeutic agent vincristine produces a distal sensory polyneuropathy characterized by axonal degeneration and loss.[46] Studies in cats (but not typically in humans) show accumulation of focal paranodal axonal swellings, most prominent proximally, with neurofilaments and paracrystalline material in neuron cell bodies and axons.[169] The most likely pathogenetic mechanism involves the binding of vincristine to tubulin, preventing microtubular polymerization, with resultant inhibition of fast axonal transport.

METABOLIC NEUROPATHIES

Uraemia

The distal sensorimotor neuropathy accompanying chronic renal failure is characterized by both axonal degeneration[16] (larger > smaller myelinated axons) and secondary demyelination, in which analysis of teased fibres shows a concentration of demyelinated segments on some axons and complete sparing of others.[127] Loss of unmyelinated axons may be prominent, with Schwann cell processes empty of axons and often forming collagen pockets. Atrophic axons are present, even during the active phases of demyelination, suggesting that the demyelinative process is secondary. Although a number of pathogenetic mechanisms (presence of toxic circulating molecules including urea, ischaemia, etc.) have been considered; none is compelling.

Vitamin Deficiencies
Thiamine Deficiency (Beriberi)

The common aetiology of the 'dry' (neuropathic) and 'wet' (cardiac, with oedema) forms of beriberi, originally considered to be separate conditions, was recognized about 150 years ago and was established during the first decade of the twentieth century as being the result of nutritional deficiency. Although the widely held presumption is that beriberi represents a pure thiamine deficiency disease, other nutritional deficits may be superimposed. Patients have a distal symmetrical sensorimotor neuropathy in which pain, dysaesthesias and cutaneous hyperesthesia may be prominent, as may dysphonia from involvement of the recurrent laryngeal nerve. Pathological findings most consistently involve the extremities, the vagus nerve and phrenic nerves, in which axonal degeneration is most prominent in distal portions of the nerves; more proximally, segmental demyelination may reflect secondary demyelination.[520] Preservation of small myelinated and unmyelinated axons has been described in the presence of intrafascicular oedema.[361] As expected in a central–peripheral distal axonopathy, axonal degeneration is also demonstrated in the gracile columns in the spinal cord.

The biochemical mechanism appears to involve deficiency of thiamine, resulting in decreased thiamine pyrophosphate (TPP), a cofactor in the decarboxylation of α-ketoacids and the formation and degradation of α-ketols. Thiamine pyrophosphate participates in the reaction of pyruvate to acetyl coenzyme A, which is catalysed by pyruvate dehydrogenase. In experimental studies in rats, a distinctive accumulation of flattened membranous sacs and decreased numbers of neurofilaments and microtubules have been described in the distal branches of peripheral axons and central sensory projections.[397]

Niacin Deficiency (Pellagra)

Pellagra comprises a combination of cutaneous lesions, gastrointestinal disturbances, behavioural manifestations, dementia, spinal cord involvement and peripheral neuropathy. Axonal degeneration, typically mild, has been reported in peripheral nerves. An unusual outbreak of optic neuropathy and painful sensory neuropathy resembling Strachan's syndrome (amblyopia, orogenital dermatitis and painful neuropathy) developed in Cuba, also including hearing loss and myelopathy, in which large myelinated axons were lost.[40] The precise relationship of multinutritional defects to discrete syndromes has been a point of contention in patients in which a complex metabolic milieu exists.

Cobalamin (Vitamin B12) Deficiency

The symmetrical sensory polyneuropathy that develops in patients deficient in vitamin B12, which may or may not coexist with subacute combined degeneration of the spinal cord, shows axonal degeneration but not demyelination.

Experimental studies of vitamin B12 deficiency suggest that the biochemical deficit is a deficiency of methyl group addition reactions as the result of inadequate methionine and S-adenosyl methionine synthesis, a methyl folate trap and formate starvation.[501]

Vitamin E Deficiency

In conditions in which fat malabsorption develops (e.g. abetalipoproteinaemia, cystic fibrosis, congenital biliary atresia) and in patients who carry a mutation in the gene for α-tocopherol-transfer protein, vitamin E deficiency develops.[176] Vitamin E deficiency in humans, rats and monkeys results in spinocerebellar degeneration and a sensory neuropathy characterized by loss of large myelinated axons as part of a central–peripheral distal axonopathy.[176,338] Deficiency of vitamin E is presumed to produce its effects as the result of oxidative stress caused by free radical damage.

Alcoholic Neuropathy

Alcoholic neuropathy is characterized by a chronic insidious progressive distal symmetrical sensorimotor neuropathy, occasionally painful or hyperaesthetic, in which weakness of the feet, hand and thigh muscles may be prominent.[525] Initial studies of peripheral nerves in alcoholic patients reported segmental demyelination; however, more recent studies of animal models have established that distal axonal degeneration is the predominant pathology.[24] Because of the complex and abnormal nutritional status of patients with severe alcoholism who develop this neuropathy, the question of whether or not thiamine deficiency is the actual primary mechanism of alcoholic neuropathy has been debated.

MISCELLANEOUS NEUROPATHIES

Neuropathy may occur as the salient manifestation of a variety of inherited or acquired disorders, in association with involvement of the CNS, or as part of a multisystem disorder. In this section, acquired disorders, including paraneoplastic neuropathies, are discussed. Disorders associated with an inherited disease are discussed, together with other inherited diseases of peripheral nerve.

Neuropathy Related to Systemic Disease
Neuropathy Related to Liver Disease

Peripheral neuropathy has been reported in association with chronic liver disease in several studies. These may be confounded somewhat by the inclusion in the studies of patients with alcoholic liver disease and those with impaired glucose tolerance; nonetheless, patients with other liver disease aetiologies also appear to develop autonomic (44–76 per cent of patients), motor (14–52 per cent of patients) and/or sensory (20–93 per cent of patients) neuropathies on electrophysiological testing.[84,314] Histological findings in these cases have not been studied extensively, but teased fibre studies suggest that when abnormalities are present segmental demyelination and remyelination are more prominent than axonal loss.[84]

Occasional patients with primary biliary cirrhosis develop a sensory neuropathy, for which an immunological basis has been proposed.[291] An early case series reported xanthomatous deposits situated mainly in the perineurium.[502] In an autopsied case of drug-induced hepatic disease, such deposits were confined to nerves in the hilum of the liver.[291] Other reported patients with primary biliary cirrhosis and neuropathy demonstrate not xanthomatous infiltration but rather axonal loss without inflammation or demyelination.[85]

Critical Illness Polyneuropathy

Critical illness polyneuropathy (CIP) is an acute axonal neuropathy that develops in severely ill patients, typically in an intensive-care setting. Delayed weaning from the ventilator not explained by pulmonary or cardiovascular problems is the usual presentation. Critical illness polyneuropathy is common in critically ill patients, with prospective studies demonstrating the condition in 60–80 per cent of patients with severe sepsis and multiorgan failure.[31,79] However, there is some overlap with critical illness myopathy (CIM), with studies suggesting that the weakness in these critically ill patients is due to a myopathy rather than a neuropathy.[508] In fact, CIP and CIM often coexist, making their differential diagnosis difficult or even impossible. Many terms have been suggested to describe such an association, namely 'polyneuromyopathy', 'critical illness myopathy and neuropathy' (CRIMYNE) and 'critical illness polyneuropathy and myopathy'.[264]

In CIP, electrophysiological evaluation characteristically shows amplitude reduction, with preservation of conduction velocity, consistent with an axonal neuropathy.[213] This may help to distinguish it from GBS. Nerve biopsies and autopsy studies show axonal degeneration affecting motor and sensory fibres, particularly distally; neither active demyelination nor inflammation is found.[584] The pathophysiology of CIP is complex, involving metabolic, inflammatory and bioenergetic alterations. Microvascular changes in peripheral nerves due to factors mediating the systemic effects of sepsis and the systemic inflammatory response syndrome have been suggested to be responsible for the axonal degeneration of CIP.[38] Increased endothelial expression of E-selectin (considered to be a marker of endothelial cell activation) may contribute.[148] Although gross microvascular pathology is not a feature of nerve biopsies, increased microvascular permeability may allow passage of neurotoxic factors into the endoneurium.[38,121]

Neuropathy in Hypothyroidism

The most common type of peripheral nerve involvement in hypothyroidism is a focal compression neuropathy, usually carpal tunnel syndrome, which was found in 30.4 per cent of hypothyroid patients in one series.[68] In another series, 42 per cent of hypothyroid patients had electrophysiological signs of sensorimotor axonal neuropathy, and 29 per cent had carpal tunnel syndrome.[124] A more generalized sensory symptom-dominant polyneuropathy may also develop, which responds to thyroid replacement therapy. Nerve biopsy studies have concluded that segmental demyelination is the predominant abnormality.[126] Excessive

amounts of glycogen are present within the cytoplasm of Schwann, perineurial and endothelial cells and in axons. Other studies have concluded that axonal degeneration rather than demyelination is the primary abnormality.[339]

Neuropathy in Acromegaly

Carpal tunnel syndrome is the most common form of peripheral nerve involvement in acromegaly. In acromegalic patients, the metabolic syndrome may be heterogeneous and may include diabetes, which complicates the interpretation of neuropathic symptoms. A generalized neuropathy independent of the presence of diabetes is also relatively frequent.[287] The peripheral nerves show an expanded fascicular area, with an increase in subperineurial and endoneurial connective tissue and a reduction in the density of myelinated and unmyelinated axons; this is probably related both to fibre loss and to an expanded endoneurial area. Increased subperineurial and endoneurial connective tissue[287] probably reflects a growth hormone-induced increase in circulating IGF-I and the presence of IGF-I receptors on Schwann cells and fibroblasts. Teased fibre preparations demonstrate a combination of axonal degeneration and segmental demyelination. However, the basic pathological lesion described in a series of 11 sural nerve biopsies was demyelination combined with hypertrophic formations affecting the Schwann cells of the small-diameter fibres.[118] Second biopsies from two patients later in the course of their disease showed marked onion-bulb formation.

Porphyric Neuropathy

Porphyria is a term used to designate a group of rare metabolic disorders resulting from enzymatic defects in the conversion of porphyrinogens to haem, which is the oxygen carrier central to all aerobic reactions in the body.[5] Although the exact incidence of neuropathy in porphyria is unknown, estimates range from 10 per cent to 40 per cent of patients.[478] Clinically, porphyric neuropathy is a combination of autonomic and peripheral neuropathy. The autonomic neuropathy manifests as abdominal pain secondary to decreased gastric motility, constipation and pseudo-obstruction, resting tachycardia, orthostatic hypotension or labile hypertension, episodic diaphoresis and urinary or rectal incontinence.[5] The peripheral neuropathy develops after the onset of abdominal pain and CNS manifestations and generally progresses to maximum severity within 1 month. It can be life-threatening and at its peak can result in total quadriplegia and respiratory insufficiency requiring ventilatory support. It can therefore be confused with GBS and not be recognized as porphyric neuropathy until the second attack. Electrophysiological testing reveals an axonal neuropathy with low-amplitude motor responses and normal conduction velocities and distal latencies. The most consistent finding on nerve biopsy is axonal loss with wallerian degeneration.[506] Findings of demyelination are probably secondary. Pure sensory nerves are frequently spared. The mechanism of injury to the PNS is unknown but may involve a direct toxic effect of haem precursors.

Paraneoplastic Neuropathy

Paraneoplastic neuropathy occurs in about 1 per cent of all patients with malignancy.[103] Although these conditions are probably mediated by the immune system, they are frequently not associated with an identifiable onconeural antibody.[422] They may be divided into disorders associated with solid tumours and disorders associated with lymphoproliferative disorders.

Carcinomatous Neuropathy

Direct invasion of spinal roots, the limb girdle plexuses or isolated peripheral nerves by carcinoma may occur. The malignant cells penetrate the perineurium and tend to accumulate in a subperineurial position or as sheets in the endoneurial septa. However, the occurrence of peripheral neuropathy not related to direct invasion of malignant cells was first recognized clearly by Denny-Brown in 1948.[111] It is most often associated with small cell lung cancer;[103,109] in many cases, anti-Hu antibodies are found in the serum.[422] Carcinomatous neuropathies can be subdivided into a subacute sensory neuronopathy, sensorimotor neuropathy and autonomic neuropathy. The sensorimotor neuropathies are further divisible into acute and subacute or chronic forms; relapsing cases also occur.[103] These are all symmetrical polyneuropathies and are usually distal in distribution.

Classic clinical manifestations of a paraneoplastic subacute sensory neuronopathy include pain and numbness evolving over weeks, frequently with an asymmetrical onset. Facial and trunk sensation may be involved. The upper extremities may be affected first, although over time all four extremities are frequently involved. Patients develop sensory ataxia and may have pseudo-athetosis in the affected limbs.[422] Histologically, there is a loss of fibres in sensory roots and peripheral nerves.[208] This may be almost total in sensory nerves and partial in mixed nerves, because of the presence of preserved motor fibres (Figure 24.120 and 24.121). Changes in anterior horn cells and anterior roots are only mild, although degeneration of neurons may be seen (Figure 24.122). In the dorsal root ganglia (Figure 24.122) there is extensive depletion of ganglion cells and a proliferation of satellite cells, with the formation of residual nodules of Nageotte. Perivascular lymphocytic infiltrates are found in most affected ganglia. These do not usually extend into the roots. The cervical and lumbar sensory ganglia are affected more severely than those in the thoracic region, and a somewhat random involvement of the ganglia is not uncommon. Single ganglia sometimes escape from an otherwise diffuse destruction. The posterior columns show secondary axon degeneration. Concomitant inflammatory lesions elsewhere in the nervous system may be associated with carcinomatous ganglioradiculitis, including limbic encephalitis, a diffuse encephalomyelitis or a restricted myelitis.

In patients with carcinomatous sensorimotor neuropathy, the predominant change in the peripheral nerves is axonal loss, although there may be some associated segmental demyelination.[108] Sometimes there are sparse inflammatory infiltrates. Loss of dorsal root ganglion cells occurs, but not to the extent seen in carcinomatous sensory neuronopathy, together with degeneration in the posterior columns. There is some degeneration of anterior horn cells.

A chronic relapsing–remitting form of sensorimotor neuropathy also occurs but is less frequently associated with lung cancer.[103] In some cases this presents a

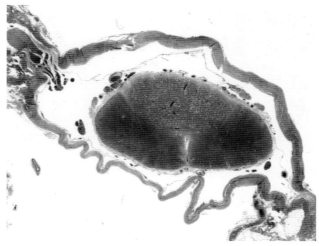

24.120 Whole mount of spinal cord, showing degeneration of dorsal columns in a patient with paraneoplastic peripheral neuropathy.

(a)

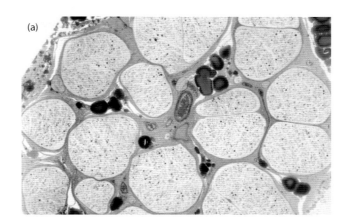

(b)

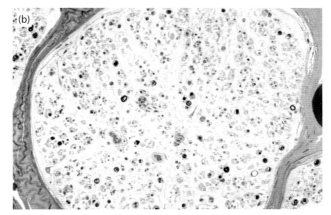

24.121 Semi-thin section of peripheral nerve from a patient with paraneoplastic peripheral neuropathy. Note the extensive fibre loss. **(a)** Low power; **(b)** high power.

CIDP-like picture and demyelination is found. In other patients a progressive asymmetrical painful neuropathy occurs, with electrophysiological study showing axonal damage; in these cases, vasculitis is found on nerve biopsy. Immunohistochemistry shows a predominance of CD8-positive T-lymphocytes.

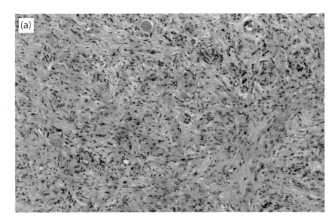

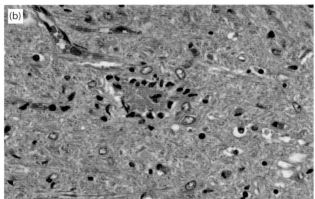

24.122 Haematoxylin and eosin (H&E)-stained paraffin section of dorsal root ganglion from a patient with paraneoplastic peripheral neuropathy. Note the extensive depletion of ganglion cells **(a)** and the histiocytic infiltrate about a degenerating ganglion cell **(b)**.

NEUROPATHIES RELATED TO LYMPHORETICULAR PROLIFERATIVE DISORDERS

Lymphoma

Cranial nerves and spinal nerve roots may be directly invaded in patients with lymphomatous involvement of the leptomeninges. Lymphomatous infiltration may also involve the limb girdle plexuses and individual peripheral nerve trunks. Spinal roots may be damaged by compression from meningeal deposits or vertebral collapse. In addition, as for carcinoma, a number of types of non-metastatic neuropathy have been recognized. These are divisible into subacute sensory neuropathy, acute or chronic relapsing demyelinating neuropathy, and subacute motor neuropathy. Widespread occlusion of the epineurial and endoneurial vasculature by intravascular lymphoma (Fig 24.123a,b) represents an unusual cause of peripheral neuropathy.

Subacute sensory neuropathy is a rare complication of both Hodgkin's[390] and non-Hodgkin's lymphoma.[515] The clinical and pathological features resemble those of carcinomatous sensory neuropathy.[208] Further, both an acute demyelinating neuropathy with clinical and pathological

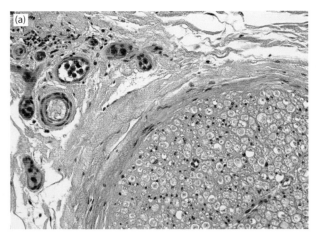

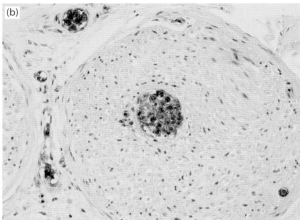

24.123 Involvement of sural nerve by intravascular lymphoma. (a) H&E, ×600 and **(b)** CD45 (leukocyte common antigen) immunostain, ×600.

features identical to those of GBS and a chronic relapsing demyelinating neuropathy may occur in patients with Hodgkin's disease, with sufficient frequency to indicate that this is not a spurious association.[279] Subacute motor neuropathy has also been described in both Hodgkin's and non-Hodgkin's lymphoma.[454,574] At autopsy, neuronal degeneration restricted to anterior horn cells, together with mild posterior column demyelination, has been described.[454]

Leukaemia

The usual explanation for peripheral nerve involvement in both acute and chronic leukaemia is direct invasion of spinal roots or peripheral nerve trunks. Occasional cases without direct involvement are encountered, sometimes with features resembling GBS.[533]

Myeloma

Peripheral nerve involvement occurs more frequently in relation to myeloma than other malignancies and may take a variety of forms. Compression of cranial nerves and spinal roots by plasmacytomas or secondary to vertebral collapse may occur, and sparse endoneurial infiltration with plasma cells has been described. Amyloidosis related to myeloma may lead to a generalized neuropathy or to compression of the median nerve in the carpal tunnel. A sensorimotor neuropathy with predominant axonal degeneration may be encountered with features resembling the sensorimotor neuropathy that is seen as a non-metastatic complication of carcinoma. The changes are more profound in distal nerves, probably representing a distal dying-back axonopathy.[526] A chronic demyelinating neuropathy, predominantly motor, is usually related to osteosclerotic myeloma (see Osteosclerotic Myeloma, POEMS Syndrome and Castleman Disease, p. 1484).

Polycythaemia Vera

A generalized sensorimotor neuropathy is a rare accompaniment of polycythaemia vera.[526]

ACKNOWLEDGEMENTS

The authors wish to record their thanks to Professor Cynthia Hawkins, co-author of the eighth edition of this chapter, for the use of the text and illustrations in the current edition. In addition, we are grateful to Professors DN Landon, RHM King and the late PK Thomas for permission to reprint some of the illustrations and for excerpts from the 'Normal Structure of the Peripheral Nerve' section in the chapter Diseases of the Peripheral Nerves, which appeared in the sixth edition of *Greenfield's Neuropathology* (1997). Normal Structure of Peripheral Nerve represents a condensed and updated version of this work. We would also like to thank Ms. Sandra Cohen for many of the electron micrographs.

REFERENCES

1. Abe T, Ogawa K, Fuziwara H, et al. Spinal ganglia and peripheral nerves from a patient with Tay–Sachs disease. Morphological and ganglioside studies. *Acta Neuropathol (Berl)* 1985;66:239–44.
2. Acheson A, Barker PA, Alderson RF, et al. Detection of brain-derived neurotrophic factor-like activity in fibroblasts and Schwann cells: inhibition by antibodies to NGF. *Neuron* 1991;7:265–75.
3. Adams D. Hereditary and acquired amyloid neuropathies. *J Neurol* 2001;248:647–57.
4. Ahmed A, Bril V, Orszag A, et al. Detection of diabetic sensorimotor polyneuropathy by corneal confocal microscopy in type 1 diabetes: a concurrent validity study. *Diabetes Care* 2012;35(4):821–8.
5. Albers JW, Fink JK. Porphyric neuropathy. *Muscle Nerve* 2004;30:410–22.
6. Ammendola A, Sampaolo S, Ambrosone L, et al. Peripheral neuropathy in hepatitis-related mixed cryoglobulinemia: electrophysiologic follow-up study. *Muscle Nerve* 2005;31:382–5.
7. Anders HJ, Goebel FD. Neurological manifestations of cytomegalovirus infection in the acquired immunodeficiency syndrome. *Int J STD AIDS* 1999;10: 151–9; quiz 160–61.
8. Ando Y, Nakamura M, Araki S. Transthyretin-related familial amyloidotic polyneuropathy. *Arch Neurol* 2005;62:1057–62.
9. Ang CW, Laman JD, Willison HJ, et al. Structure of *Campylobacter jejuni* lipopolysaccharides determines antiganglioside specificity and clinical features of Guillain–Barré and Miller Fisher patients. *Infect Immun* 2002;70:1202–8.
10. Appenzeller O, Kornfeld M. Acute pandysautonomia: clinical and morphologic study. *Arch Neurol* 1973;29:334–9.
11. Appenzeller O, Arnason BG, Adams RD. Experimental autonomic neuropathy: an immunologically induced disorder of reflex vasomotor function. *J Neurol Neurosurg Psychiatry* 1965;28:510–15.
12. Araki T, Milbrandt J. Ninjurin, a novel adhesion molecule, is induced by nerve injury and promotes axonal growth. *Neuron* 1996;17:353–61.

13. Araki T, Sasaki Y, Milbrandt J. Increased nuclear NAD biosynthesis and SIRT1 activation prevent axonal degeneration. *Science* 2004;305:1010–13.
14. Arroyo EJ, Xu YT, Zhou L, et al. Myelinating Schwann cells determine the internodal localization of Kv1.1, Kv1.2, Kvbeta2 and Caspr. *J Neurocytol* 1999;28:333–47.
15. Arthur RP, Shelley WB. The innervation of the human epidermis. *J Invest Dermatol* 1959;32:397–411.
16. Asbury AK, Victor M, Adams RD. Uremic polyneuropathy. *Arch Neurol* 1963;8: 413–28.
17. Averbuch–Heller L, Steiner I, Abramsky O. Neurologic manifestations of progressive systemic sclerosis. *Arch Neurol* 1992;49: 1292–5.
18. Axelrod F. Familial dysautonomia. *Muscle Nerve* 2004;29:352–63.
19. Ballin RH, Thomas PK. Hypertrophic changes in diabetic neuropathy. *Acta Neuropathol (Berl)* 1968;11:93–102.
20. Bandtlow CE, Heumann R, Schwab ME, Thoenen H. Cellular localization of nerve growth factor synthesis by *in situ* hybridization. *Embo J* 1987;6:891–9.
21. Barajon I, Bersani M, Quartu M, et al. Neuropeptides and morphological changes in cisplatin-induced dorsal root ganglion neuronopathy. *Exp Neurol* 1996;138: 93–104.
22. Batman PA, Miller AR, Sedgwick PM, Griffin GE. Autonomic denervation in jejunal mucosa of homosexual men infected with HIV. *AIDS* 1991;5: 1247–52.
23. Bedlack RS, Vu T, Hammans S, et al. MNGIE neuropathy: five cases mimicking chronic inflammatory demyelinating polyneuropathy. *Muscle Nerve* 2004;29: 364–8.
24. Behse F, Buchthal F. Alcoholic neuropathy: clinical, electrophysiological and biopsy findings. *Ann Neurol* 1977;2:95–110.
25. Bellavere F, Balzani I, De Masi G, et al. Power spectral analysis of heart-rate variations improves assessment of diabetic cardiac autonomic neuropathy. *Diabetes* 1992;41:633–40.
26. Ben-Othmane K, Hentati F, Lennon F, et al. Linkage of a locus (CMT4A) for autosomal recessive Charcot–Marie–Tooth

disease to chromosome 8q. *Hum Mol Genet* 1993;2:1625–8.
27. Benson MD. The hereditary amyloidoses. *Best Pract Res Clin Rheumatol* 2003;17:909–27.
28. Benz HU, Harzer K. Metachromatic reaction of pseudoisocyanine with sulfatides in metachromatic leukodystrophy: I. Technical and histochemical staining. *Acta Neuropathol* 1974;27:177–80.
29. Berciano J. Peripheral neuropathies: molecular diagnosis of Charcot–Marie–Tooth disease. *Nat Rev Neurol* 2011;7:305–6.
30. Berciano J, Combarros O, Figols J, et al. Hereditary motor and sensory neuropathy type II: clinicopathological study of a family. *Brain* 1986;109:897–914.
31. Berek K, Margreiter J, Willeit J, et al. Critical illness polyneuropathy. *Lancet* 1996;348:414.
32. Berger A, Schaumburg H. Human toxic neuropathy caused by industrial agents. In: Dyck PJ, Thomas PK eds. *Peripheral neuropathy*. Philadelphia, PA: Elsevier-Saunders, 2005:2505–25.
33. Bergstrom J, Gustavsson A, Hellman U, et al. Amyloid deposits in transthyretin-derived amyloidosis: cleaved transthyretin is associated with distinct amyloid morphology. *J Pathol* 2005;206:224–32.
34. Bilbao JM. Peripheral nerves. In: Rosai J ed. *Rosai and Ackerman's Surgical Pathology*, 9th edn. Edinburgh: Mosby, 2004:2623–62.
35. Bird SJ, Brown MJ. The clinical spectrum of diabetic neuropathy. *Semin Neurol* 1996;16: 115–22.
36. Bischoff A, Ulrich J. Peripheral neuropathy in globoid cell leukodystrophy (Krabbe's disease): ultrastructural and histochemical findings. *Brain* 1969;92:861–70.
37. Bodzioch M, Orso E, Kluchen J, et al. The gene incoding ATP-binding cassette transporter 1 is mutated in Tangier disease. *Nat Genet* 1999;22:347–51.
38. Bolton CF. Sepsis and the systemic inflammatory response syndrome: neuromuscular manifestations. *Crit Care Med* 1996;24:1408–16.
39. Bomont P, Cavalier L, Blondeau F, et al. The gene encoding gigaxonin, a new member of the cytoskeletal BTB/kelch

repeat family is mutated in giant axonal neuropathy. *Nat Genet* 2000;26:370–4.

40. Borrajero I, Perez JL, Dominguez C, *et al.* Epidemic neuropathy in Cuba: morphological characterization of peripheral nerve lesions in sural nerve biopsies. *J Neurol Sci* 1994;127:68–76.

41. Bosboom WMJ, van den Berg LH, Mollee I, *et al.* Sural nerve T-cell receptor Vbeta gene utilization in chronic inflammatory demyelinating polyneuropathy and vasculitic neuropathy. *Neurology* 2001;56:74–81.

42. Bouche P, Leger JM, Travers MA, *et al.* Peripheral neuropathy in systemic vasculitis: clinical and electrophysiologic study of 22 patients. *Neurology* 1986;36:1598–602.

43. Bouche P, Lacomblez L, Leger JM, *et al.* Peripheral neuropathies during treatment with almitrine: report of 46 cases. *J Neurol* 1989;236:29–33.

44. Bradley WG, Hewer R. Peripheral neuropathy due to disulphiram. *Br Med J* 1966;2:449–450.

45. Bradley WG, Verma A. Painful vasculitic neuropathy in HIV-1 infection: relief of pain with prednisone therapy. *Neurology* 1996;47:1446–51.

46. Bradley WG, Lassman LP, Pearce GW, Walton JN. The neuromyopathy of vincristine in man: clinical, electrophysiological and pathological studies. *J Neurol Sci* 1970;10:107–31.

47. Bradley WG, Karlsson IJ, Rassol CG. Metronidazole neuropathy. *Br Med J* 1977;2:610–11.

48. Brew BJ. The peripheral nerve complications of human immunodeficiency virus (HIV) infection. *Muscle Nerve* 2003;28:542–52.

49. Brewster WJ, Diemel LT, Leach RM, Tomlinson DR. Reduced sciatic nerve substance P and calcitonin gene-related peptide in rats with short-term diabetes or central hypoxaemia co-exist with normal messenger RNA levels in the lumbar dorsal root ganglia. *Neuroscience* 1994;58: 323–30.

50. Brimijoin S, Moser V, Hammond P, *et al.* Death of intermediolateral spinal cord neurons follows selective, complement-mediated destruction of peripheral preganglionic sympathetic terminals by acetylcholinesterase antibodies. *Neuroscience* 1993;54:201–223.

51. Brinley FJ Jr, Pardo CA, Verma A. Human immunodeficiency virus and the peripheral nervous system workshop. *Arch Neurol* 2001;58:1561–6.

52. Britland ST, Young RJ, Sharma AK, Clarke BF. Acute and remitting painful diabetic polyneuropathy: a comparison of peripheral nerve fibre pathology. *Pain* 1992;48:361–70.

53. Britton WJ, Lockwood DNJ. Leprosy. *Lancet* 2004;363:1209–19.

54. Brownlee M. Biochemistry and molecular cell biology of diabetic complications. *Nature* 2001;414:813–20.

55. Bruch L, Schmidt R. Pathology of the autonomic nervous system. In: Appenzeller O ed. *Handbook of Clinical Neurology.* Amsterdam: Elsevier, 2000:1–52.

56. Bruck W. The role of macrophages in Wallerian degeneration. *Brain Pathol* 1997;7:741–52.

57. Bruck W, Friede RL. Anti-macrophage CR3 antibody blocks myelin phagocytosis by macrophages *in vitro*. *Acta Neuropathol (Berl)* 1990;80:415–18.

58. Bucala R, Tracey KJ, Cerami A. Advanced glycosylation products quench nitric oxide and mediate defective endothelium-dependent vasodilatation in experimental diabetes. *J Clin Invest* 1991;87:432–8.

59. Buchwald B, Dudel J, Toyka KV. Neuromuscular blockade by immunoglobulin G from patients with Miller Fisher syndrome. *Ann NY Acad Sci* 1998;841:659–69.

60. Burck U, Moser HW, Goebel HH, *et al.* A case of lipogranulomatosis Farber: some clinical and ultrastructural aspects. *Eur J Pediatr* 1985;143:203–8.

61. Burnett MG, Zager EL. Pathophysiology of peripheral nerve injury: a brief review. *Neurosurg Focus* 2004;16:E1.

62. Burns TM, Mauermann ML. The evaluation of polyneuropathies. *Neurology* 2011;76 (Suppl 2):S6–13.

63. Buttmann M, Marziniak M, Toyka KV, *et al.* 'Sporadic' familial amyloidotic polyneuropathy in a German patient with B cell lymphocytic leukaemia. *J Neurol Neurosurg Psychiatry* 2002;73: 86–7.

64. Buxbaum JN. The systemic amyloidoses. *Curr Opin Rheumatol* 2004;16:67–75.

65. Buxton PH, Hayward M. Polyneuritis cranialis associated with industrial trichloroethylene poisoning. *J Neurol Neurosurg Psychiatry* 1967;30:511–18.

66. Byard RW, Lach B, Preston DN. Peripheral nerve and vasculature involvement in myophosphorylase deficiency (McArdle's disease). *Pathology* 1991;23:62–5.

67. Bywaters EG. Peripheral vascular obstruction in rheumatoid arthritis and its relationship to other vascular lesions. *Ann Rheum Dis* 1957;16:84–103.

68. Cakir M, Samanci N, Balci N, Balci MK. Musculoskeletal manifestations in patients with thyroid disease. *Clin Endocrinol (Oxf)* 2003;59:162–7.

69. Calabrese LH, Estes M, Yen-Lieberman B, *et al.* Systemic vasculitis in association with human immunodeficiency virus infection. *Arthritis Rheum* 1989;32:569–76.

70. Calderon-Gonzalez R, Rizzi-Hernandez H. Buckthorn polyneuropathy. *N Engl J Med* 1967;277:69–71.

71. Campanucci V, Krishnaswamy A, Cooper E. Diabetes depresses synaptic transmission in sympathetic ganglia by inactivating nACHRs through a conserved intracellular cysteine residue. *Neuron* 2010;66:827-34.

72. Campenot RB. Development of sympathetic neurons in compartmentalized cultures: II. Local control of neurite survival by nerve growth factor. *Dev Biol* 1982;93:13–21.

73. Carroll SL, Miller ML, Frohnert PW, *et al.* Expression of neuregulins and their putative receptors, ErbB2 and ErbB3, is induced during Wallerian degeneration. *J Neurosci* 1997;17:1642–59.

74. Carvalho AA, Vital A, Ferrer X, *et al.* Charcot–Marie–Tooth disease type 1a: clinicopathological correlation in 24 patients. *J Peripher Nerv Syst* 2005;10: 85–92.

75. Caselli RJ, Daube JR, Hunder GG, Whisnant JP. Peripheral neuropathic syndromes in giant cell (temporal) arteritis. *Neurology* 1988;38:685–9.

76. Cavanagh JB. The 'dying back' process: a common denominator in many naturally occurring and toxic neuropathies. *Arch Pathol Lab Med* 1979;103:659–64.

77. Cavanagh JB. Corpora amylacea and the family of polyglucosan diseases. *Brain Res* 1999;29:265–95.

78. Cavanagh JB, Fuller NH, Johnson HR, Rudge P. The effects of thallium salts, with particular reference to the nervous system changes: a report of three cases. *Q J Med* 1974;43:293–319.

79. Celik C, Ucan H, Alemdaroglu E, Oktay F. Critical illness polyneuropathy: a case report. *NeuroRehabilitation* 2011;29: 229–32.

80. Cellek S, Foxwell NA, Moncada S. Two phases of nitrergic neuropathy in streptozotocin-induced diabetic rats. *Diabetes* 2003;52:2353–62.

81. Chance PF. Genetic evaluation of inherited motor/sensory neuropathy. *Suppl Clin Neurophysiol* 2004;57:228–42.

82. Chance PF, Alderson MK, Leppig KA, *et al.* DNA deletion associated with hereditary neuropathy with liability to pressure palsies. *Cell* 1993;72:143–51.

83. Chaouch M, Allal T, De Sandre Giovannoli A, *et al.* The phenotypic manifestations of autosomal recessive Charcot–Marie–Tooth due to a mutation in *Lamin A/C* gene. *Neuromuscul Disord* 2003;13:60–67.

84. Chari VR, Katiyar BC, Rastogi BL, Bhattacharya SK. Neuropathy in hepatic disorders: a clinical, electrophysiological and histopathological appraisal. *J Neurol Sci* 1977;31:93–111.

85. Charron L, Peyronnard JM, Marchand L. Sensory neuropathy associated with primary biliary cirrhosis: histologic and morphometric studies. *Arch Neurol* 1980;37:84–7.

86. Chaudhry V, Eisenberger MA, Sinibaldi VJ, *et al.* A prospective study of suramin-induced peripheral neuropathy. *Brain* 1996;119 (Part 6):2039–52.

87. Chaudhry V, Cornblath DR, Corse A, *et al.* Thalidomide-induced neuropathy. *Neurology* 2002;59:1872–5.

88. Cheng C, Zochodne DW. Sensory neurons with activated caspase-3 survive long-term experimental diabetes. *Diabetes* 2003;52:2363–71.

89. Cheng HL, Randolph A, Yee D, *et al.* Characterization of insulin-like growth factor-I and its receptor and binding proteins in transected nerves and cultured Schwann cells. *J Neurochem* 1996;66: 525–36.

90. Chetty R. Vasculitides associated with HIV infection. *J Clin Pathol* 2001;54:275–8.

91. Chia L, Fernandez A, Lacroix C, *et al.* Contribution of nerve biopsy findings to the diagnosis of disabling neuropathy in the elderly: a retrospective review of 100 consecutive patients. *Brain* 1996;119:1091–8.

92. Chiba A, Kusunoki S, Obata H, *et al.* Serum anti-GQ1b IgG antibody is associated with ophthalmoplegia in Miller Fisher syndrome and Guillain–Barré syndrome: clinical and immunohistochemical studies. *Neurology* 1993;43:1911–7.

93. Chimelli L, Freitas M, Nascimento O. Value of nerve biopsy in the diagnosis and follow-up of leprosy: the role of vascular lesions and usefulness of nerve studies in the detection of persistent bacilli. *J Neurol* 1997;244:318–23.

94. Cho ES, Lowndes HE, Goldstein BD. Neurotoxicology of vincristine in the cat. Morphological study. *Arch Toxicol* 1983;52:83–90.

95. Chowdhury SKR, Dobrowsky RT, Fernyhough P. Nutrient excess and altered mitochondrial proteome and function contribute to neurodegeneration in diabetes. *Mitochondrion* 2011;11:845–54.

96. Chowdhury SKR, Zherebitskaya E, Smith DR *et al*. Mitochondrial respiratory chain dysfunction in dorsal root ganglia of streptozotocin-induced diabetic rats and its correction by insulin treatment. *Diabetes* 2010;59:1082–1091.

97. Collins MP, Mendell JR, Periquet MI, *et al*. Superficial peroneal nerve/peroneus brevis muscle biopsy in vasculitic neuropathy. *Neurology* 2000;55:636–43.

98. Collins MP, Periquet MI, Mendell JR, *et al*. Nonsystemic vasculitic neuropathy: insights from a clinical cohort. *Neurology* 2003;61:623–30.

99. Conceicao I, Sales–Luis ML, De Carvalho M, *et al*. Gelsolin-related familial amyloidosis, Finnish type, in a Portuguese family: clinical and neurophysiological studies. *Muscle Nerve* 2003;28:715–21.

100. Connors LH, Lim A, Prokaeva T, Roskens VA, Costello CE. Tabulation of human transthyretin (TTR) variants, 2003. *Amyloid* 2003;10:160–84.

101. Cooke GS, Hill AVS. Genetics of susceptibility to human infectious disease. *Nat Rev Genet* 2001;2:967–77.

102. Cooper JC, Ben-Smith A, Savage CO, Winer JB. Unusual T-cell receptor phenotype V gene usage of gamma delta T- cells in a line derived from the peripheral nerve of a patient with Guillain–Barré syndrome. *J Neurol Neurosurg Psychiatry* 2000;69:522–4.

103. Corbo M, Balmaceda C. Peripheral neuropathy in cancer patients. *Cancer Invest* 2001;19:369–82.

104. Cornblath DR, McArthur JC, Kennedy PG, *et al*. Inflammatory demyelinating peripheral neuropathies associated with human T-cell lymphotropic virus type III infection. *Ann Neurol* 1987;21:32–40.

105. Cory-Schlecta D, Schaumburg H. Lead, inorganic. In: Spencer PS, Schaumburg H eds. *Experimental and clinical neurotoxicology*. New York: Oxford University Press, 2000:708–20.

106. Court FA, Midha R, Cisterna BA, *et al*. Morphological evidence for a transport of ribosomes from Schwann cells to regenerating axons. *Glia* 2011;59:1529-39.

107. Craner MJ, Klein JP, Renganathan M, *et al*. Changes of sodium channel expression in experimental painful diabetic neuropathy. *Ann Neurol* 2002;52:786–92.

108. Croft PB, Urich H, Wilkinson M. Peripheral neuropathy of sensorimotor type associated with malignant disease. *Brain* 1967;90:31–66.

109. Dalmau J, Graus F, Rosenblum MK, Posner JB. Anti-Hu-associated paraneoplastic encephalomyelitis/ sensory neuronopathy: a clinical study of 71 patients. *Medicine (Baltimore)* 1992;71:59–72.

110. Deckwerth TL, Johnson EM Jr. Neurites can remain viable after destruction of the neuronal soma by programmed cell death (apoptosis). *Dev Biol* 1994;165:63–72.

111. Denny–Brown D. Primary sensory neuropathy with muscular changes associated with carcinoma. *J Neurol Neurosurg Psychiatry* 1948;11:73–87.

112. Dent EW, Gertler FB. Cytoskeletal dynamics and transport in growth cone motility and axon guidance. *Neuron* 2003;40:209–27.

113. Deprez M, Ceutrick-de Groote C, Gollogly L, Reznik M, Martin JJ. Clinical and neuropathological parameters affecting the diagnostic yield of nerve biopsy. *Neuromuscul Disord* 2000;10:92–8.

114. Desnick RJ, Bishop DF. Fabry disease: A-galactosidase deficiency. Schindler disease: alpha-N-acetyl galactosaminidase deficiency. In: Scriver CR, Beaudet AL, Sly WS, Valle D eds. *The metabolic basis of inherited disease*. New York: McGraw-Hill, 1989.

115. De Waegh SM, Lee VM, Brady ST. Local modulation of neurofilament phosphorylation, axonal caliber and slow axonal transport by myelinating Schwann cells. *Cell* 1992;68:451–63.

116. Diabetes Control and Complications Trial Research Group. The effect of intensive diabetes therapy on the development and progression of neuropathy. *Ann Intern Med* 1995;122:561–8.

117. Diemel LT, Brewster WJ, Fernyhough P, Tomlinson DR. Expression of neuropeptides in experimental diabetes: effects of treatment with nerve growth factor or brain-derived neurotrophic factor. *Brain Res Mol Brain Res* 1994;21:171–5.

118. Dinn JJ, Dinn EI. Natural history of acromegalic peripheral neuropathy. *Q J Med* 1985;57:833–42.

119. Dispenzieri A, Kyle RA. Neurological aspects of multiple myeloma and related disorders. *Best Pract Res Clin Haematol* 2005;18:673–88.

120. Dolman CL, MacLeod PM, Chang E. Fine structure of cutaneous nerves in ganglioside storage disease. *J Neurol Neurosurg Psychiatry* 1977;40:588–94.

121. Druschky A, Herkert M, Radespiel-Troger M, *et al*. Critical illness polyneuropathy: clinical findings and cell culture assay of neurotoxicity assessed by a prospective study. *Intensive Care Med* 2001;27:686–93.

122. Dubovy P. Wallerian degeneration and peripheral nerve conditions for both axonal regeneration and neuropathic pain induction. *Ann Anat* 2011;193:267–75.

123. Duchen LW, Anjorin A, Watkins PJ, Mackay JD. Pathology of autonomic neuropathy in diabetes mellitus. *Ann Intern Med* 1980;92(Part 2):301–3.

124. Duyff RF, Van den Bosch J, Laman DM, *et al*. Neuromuscular findings in thyroid dysfunction: a prospective clinical and electrodiagnostic study. *J Neurol Neurosurg Psychiatry* 2000;68:750–55.

125. Dyck PJ, Lambert EH. Dissociated sensation in amyloidosis: compound action potentials; quantitative histologic and teased fibers; and electron microscopic studies of sural nerve biopsies. *Trans Am Neurol Assoc* 1968;93:112–15.

126. Dyck PJ, Lambert EH. Polyneuropathy associated with hypothyroidism. *J Neuropathol Exp Neurol* 1970;29:631–58.

127. Dyck PJ, Johnson WJ, Lambert EH, O'Brien PC. Segmental demyelination secondary to axonal degeneration in uremic neuropathy. *Mayo Clin Proc* 1971;46:400–31.

128. Dyck PJ, Lais A, Karnes JL, *et al*. Fiber loss is primary and multifocal in sural nerves in diabetic polyneuropathy. *Ann Neurol* 1986;19:425–39.

129. Dyck PJ, Chance P, Lebo R, Carney JA. Neuronal atrophy and degeneration predominantly affecting peripheral sensory and autonomic neurons. In: Dyck PJ, Thomas PK eds. *Peripheral neuropathy*, Vol. 2, 3rd edn. Philadelphia, PA: W.B. Saunders, 1993:1065–93.

130. Dyck PJ, Kratz KM, Karnes JL, *et al*. The prevalence by staged severity of various types of diabetic neuropathy, retinopathy and nephropathy in a population-based cohort: the Rochester Diabetic Neuropathy Study. *Neurology* 1993;43:817–24.

131. Dyck P, Dyck J, Engelstad J. Pathologic alterations of nerves. In: Dyck P, Dyck J, Engelstad J eds. *Peripheral neuropathy*. Philadelphia, PA: Elsevier–Saunders, 2005:733–829.

132. Ebenezer GJ, O'Donnell, Hauer P *et al*. Impaired neurovascular repair in subjects with diabetes following experimental intracutaneous axotomy. *Brain* 2011;134(Part 6):1853–63.

133. Edgar JM, Garbern J. The myelinated axon is dependent on the myelinating cell for support and maintenance: molecules involved. *J Neurosci Res* 2004;76:593–8.

134. Ehlers MD. Deconstructing the axon: Wallerian degeneration and the ubiquitin–proteasome system. *Trends Neurosci* 2004;27:3–6.

135. Ekberg K, Brismar T, Johansson BL, *et al*. Amelioration of sensory nerve dysfunction by C-peptide in patients with type 1 diabetes. *Diabetes* 2003;52:536–41.

136. Ekstrom AR, Kanje M, Skottner A. Nerve regeneration and serum levels of insulin-like growth factor-I in rats with streptozotocin-induced insulin deficiency. *Brain Res* 1989;496:141–7.

137. Enzi G, Angelini C, Negrin P, *et al*. Sensory, motor, and autonomic neuropathy in patients with multiple symmetric lipomatosis. *Medicine (Baltimore)* 1985;64:388–93.

138. Esiri MM, Morris CS, Millard PR. Sensory and sympathetic ganglia in HIV-1 infection: immunocytochemical demonstration of HIV-1 viral antigens, increased MHC class II antigen expression and mild reactive inflammation. *J Neurol Sci* 1993;114:178–87.

139. Ewing DJ, Campbell IW, Clarke BF. The natural history of diabetic autonomic neuropathy. *Q J Med* 1980;49:95–108.

140. Fadic R, Russell JA, Vedanarayanan VV, *et al*. Sensory ataxic neuropathy as the presenting feature of a novel mitochondrial disease. *Neurology* 1997;49:239–45.

141. Falk RH, Comenzo RL, Skinner M. The systemic amyloidoses. *N Engl J Med* 1997;337:898–909.

142. Fathers E, Fuller GN. Vasculitic neuropathy. *Br J Hosp Med* 1996;55:643–7.

143. Fazio R, Nemni R, Quattrini A, *et al*. Acute presentation of Tangier polyneuropathy: a clinical and morphological study. *Acta Neuropathol* 1993;86:90–4.

144. Feasby TE. Axonal Guillain–Barré syndrome. *Muscle Nerve* 1994;17:678–9.

145. Feasby TE, Gilbert JJ, Brown WF, *et al*. An acute axonal form of Guillain–Barré polyneuropathy. *Brain* 1986;109(Part 6):1115–26.

146. Federico A, Palmeri S, Malandrini A, *et al*. The clinical aspects of adult hexosaminidase deficiencies. *Dev Neurosci* 1991;13:280–87.

147. Fenrich K, Gordon T. Canadian Association of Neuroscience review: axonal regeneration in the peripheral and central nervous systems. Current issues and

advances. *Can J Neurol Sci* 2004;31: 142–56.

148. Fenzi F, Latronico N, Refatti N, Rizzuto N. Enhanced expression of E-selectin on the vascular endothelium of peripheral nerve in critically ill patients with neuromuscular disorders. *Acta Neuropathol (Berl)* 2003;106:75–82.

149. Fernyhough P, Diemel LT, Brewster WJ, Tomlinson DR. Altered neurotrophin mRNA levels in peripheral nerve and skeletal muscle of experimentally diabetic rats. *J Neurochem* 1995;64:1231–7.

150. Fernyhough P, Huang TJ, Verkhratsky A. Mechanism of mitochondrial dysfunction in diabetic sensory neuropathy. *J Peripher Nerv Syst* 2003;8:227–35.

151. Ferreira-Santos R. Megacolon and megarectum in Chagas' disease. *Proc R Soc Med* 1961;54:1047–53.

152. Finn JT, Weil M, Archer F, et al. Evidence that Wallerian degeneration and localized axon degeneration induced by local neurotrophin deprivation do not involve caspases. *J Neurosci* 2000;20:1333–41.

153. Finsterer J. Mitochondrial neuropathy. *Clin Neurol Neurosurg* 2005;107:181–6.

154. Fleming FJ, Vytopil M, Chaitow J, et al. Thalidomide neuropathy in childhood. *Neuromuscul Disord* 2005;15:172–6.

155. Francis GJ, Martinez JA, Liu WQ, et al. Motor end plate innervation loss in diabetes and the role of insulin. *J Neuropathol Exp Neurol* 2011;70: 323–9.

156. Freeman R. Autonomic failure in AIDS. In: Low P ed. *Clinical autonomic disorders*. Philadelphia, PA: Lippincott Raven, 1997:727–35.

157. Fugleholm K, Schmalbruch H, Krarup C. Early peripheral nerve regeneration after crushing, sectioning, and freeze studied by implanted electrodes in the cat. *J Neurosci* 1994;14(Part 1):2659–73.

158. Fujimura H, Lacroix J, Said G. Vulnerability of nerve fibres to ischaemia. A quantitative light and electron microscope study. *Brain* 1991;114(Part 4):1929–42.

159. Gabreels-Festen A. Dejerine–Sottas syndrome grown to maturity: overview of genetic and morphological heterogeneity and follow-up of 25 patients. *J Anat* 2002;200:341–56.

160. Gabreels-Festen A, Gabreels F. Hereditary demyelinating motor and sensory neuropathy. *Brain Pathol* 1993;3:135–46.

161. Gabreels-Festen A, Hoogendijk JE, Meijerink HHS, et al. Two divergent types of nerve pathology in patients with different P0 mutations in Charcot–Marie–Tooth disease. *Neurology* 1996;47:761–5.

162. Gabreels-Festen A, Van Beersum S, Eshuis L, et al. Study on the gene and phenotypic characterisation of autosomal recessive demyelinating motor and sensory neuropathy (Charcot–Marie–Tooth disease) with a gene locus on chromosome 5q23–q33. *J Neurol Neurosurg Psychiatry* 1999;66:569–74.

163. Gao WQ, Dybdal N, Shinsky N, et al. Neurotrophin-3 reverses experimental cisplatin-induced peripheral sensory neuropathy. *Ann Neurol* 1995;38:30–37.

164. Garcia-Monco JC, Seidman RJ, Benach JL. Experimental immunization with *Borrelia burgdorferi* induces development of antibodies to gangliosides. *Infect Immun* 1995;63:4130–37.

165. Garman SC, Garboczi DN. Structural basis of Fabry disease. *Mol Genet Metab* 2002;77:3–11.

166. Gemignani F, Brindani F, Alfieri S, et al. Clinical spectrum of cryoglobulinemic neuropathy. *J Neurol Neurosurg Psychiatry* 2005;76:1410–14.

167. Gherardi RK, Chretien F, Delfau-Larue MH, et al. Neuropathy in diffuse infiltrative lymphocytosis syndrome: an HIV neuropathy, not a lymphoma. *Neurology* 1998;50:1041–4.

168. Giannini C, Dyck PJ. Basement membrane reduplication and pericyte degeneration precede development of diabetic polyneuropathy and are associated with its severity. *Ann Neurol* 1995;37:498–504.

169. Giannini F, Volpi N, Rossi S, et al. Thalidomide-induced neuropathy: A ganglionopathy? *Neurology* 2003;60:877–8.

170. Glass JD. Wallerian degeneration as a window to peripheral neuropathy. *J Neurol Sci* 2004;220:123–4.

171. Godal T, Negassi K. Subclinical infection in leprosy. *Br Med J* 1973;15:557–9.

172. Goebel HH, Wisniewski KE. Current state of clinical and morphological features in human NCL. *Brain Pathol* 2004;14:61–9.

173. Gold B, Schaumburg H. Acrylamide. In: Spencer PS, Schaumburg H eds. *Experimental and clinical neurotoxicology*. New York: Oxford University Press, 2000:124–32.

174. Goodrum JF, Brown JC, Fowler KA, Bouldin TW. Axonal regeneration, but not myelination, is partially dependent on local cholesterol reutilization in regenerating nerve. *J Neuropathol Exp Neurol* 2000;59:1002–10.

175. Goren H, Steinberg MC, Farboody GH. Familial oculoleptomeningeal amyloidosis. *Brain* 1980;103:473–95.

176. Gotoda T, Arita M, Arai H, et al. Adult onset spinocerebellar dysfunction caused by a mutation in the gene for the alpha-tocopherol transfer protein. *N Engl J Med* 1995;333:1313–8.

177. Graham D, Valentine W. Carbon disulfide. In: Spencer P, Schaumburg H eds. *Experimental and clinical neurotoxicology*. New York: Oxford University Press, 2000:315–17.

178. Granberg V, Ejskjaer N, Peakman M, Sundkvist G. Autoantibodies to autonomic nerves associated with cardiac and peripheral autonomic neuropathy. *Diabetes Care* 2005;28:1959–64.

179. Griffin JW, Sheikh K. The Guillain–Barré syndromes. In: Dyck J, Thomas PK eds. *Peripheral neuropathy*. Philadelphia, PA: Elsevier–Saunders, 2005:2197–219.

180. Griffin JW, Cornblath DR, Alexander E, et al. Ataxic sensory neuropathy and dorsal root ganglionitis associated with Sjögren's syndrome. *Ann Neurol* 1990;27:304–15.

181. Griffin JW, George R, Ho T. Macrophage systems in peripheral nerves: a review. *J Neuropathol Exp Neurol* 1993;52: 553–60.

182. Griffin JW, Li CY, Ho TW, et al. Pathology of the motor-sensory axonal Guillain–Barré syndrome. *Ann Neurol* 1996;39:17–28.

183. Griffin JW, Crawford T, McArthur JC. Peripheral neuropathies associated with HIV infection. In: Gendelman H, Lipton S, Epstein L, Swindels S eds. *The neurology of AIDS*. New York: Chapman & Hall, 1998:275–91.

184. Guazzi GC, Mandrini A, Gerli R, Federico A. Giant axonal neuropathy in two siblings: A generalized disorder of intermediate filaments. *Eur Neurol* 1991;31:50–56.

185. Guillevin L, Le Thi Huong D, Godeau P, et al. Clinical findings and prognosis of polyarteritis nodosa and Churg–Strauss angiitis: a study in 165 patients. *Br J Rheumatol* 1988;27:258–64.

186. Gutmann L, Martin JD, Welton W. Dapsone motor neuropathy: an axonal disease. *Neurology* 1976;26(Part 1): 514–16.

187. Guzik BW, Goldstein LS. Microtubule-dependent transport in neurons: steps towards an understanding of regulation, function and dysfunction. *Curr Opin Cell Biol* 2004;16:443–50.

188. Guzzetta F, Ferriere G, Lyon G. Congenital hypomyelination polyneuropathy: pathological findings compared with polyneuropathies starting later in life. *Brain* 1982;105:395–416.

189. Hahn AF. Hereditary motor and sensory neuropathy. HMSN type II (neuronal type) and X-linked HMSN. *Brain Pathol* 1993;3:147–55.

190. Hahn AF, Gilbert JJ, Kwarciak C, et al. Nerve biopsy findings in Niemann–Pick type II (NPC). *Acta Neuropathol (Berl)* 1994;87:149–54.

191. Haimanot RT, Mshana RN, McDougall AC, Andersen JO. Sural nerve biopsy in leprosy patients after varying periods of treatment: histopathological and bacteriological findings on light microscopy. *Int J Lepr* 1984;52:163–70.

192. Hammarberg H, Piehl F, Cullheim S, et al. GDNF mRNA in Schwann cells and DRG satellite cells after chronic sciatic nerve injury. *Neuroreport* 1996;7:857–60.

193. Hartung HP, Toyka KV. T-cell and macrophage activation in experimental autoimmune neuritis and Guillain–Barré syndrome. *Ann Neurol* 1990;27(Suppl):S57–63.

194. Harvey GK, Toyka KV, Zielasek J, et al. Failure of anti-GM1 IgG or IgM to induce conduction block following intraneural transfer. *Muscle Nerve* 1995;18:388–94.

195. Hawke SH, Davies L, Pamphlett R, et al. Vasculitic neuropathy: a clinical and pathological study. *Brain* 1991;114(Part 5): 2175–90.

196. Hawkins PN. Serum amyloid P component scintigraphy for diagnosis and monitoring amyloidosis. *Curr Opin Nephrol Hypertens* 2002;11:649–55.

197. Hellweg R, Hartung HD. Endogenous levels of nerve growth factor (NGF) are altered in experimental diabetes mellitus: a possible role for NGF in the pathogenesis of diabetic neuropathy. *J Neurosci Res* 1990;26:258–67.

198. Herskovitz S. Amiodarone. In: Spencer PS, Schaumburg H eds. *Experimental and clinical neurotoxicology*. New York: Oxford University Press, 2000:166–9.

199. Herskovitz S, Schaumburg HH. Neuropathy caused by drugs. In: Dyck P, Thomas PK eds. *Peripheral neuropathy*. Philadelphia, PA: Elsevier–Saunders, 2005:2553–83.

200. Hirano M, Nishigaki Y, Marti R. Mitochondrial neurogastrointestinal encephalomyopathy (MNGIE): a disease of two genomes. *Neurologist* 2004;10: 8–17.

201. Hirata K, Kawabuchi M. Myelin phagocytosis by macrophages and non-macrophages during Wallerian degeneration. *Microsc Res Tech* 2002;57:541–7.

202. Hirata K, Mitoma H, Ueno N, *et al.* Differential response of macrophage subpopulations to myelin degradation in the injured rat sciatic nerve. *J Neurocytol* 1999;28:685–95.

203. Hirschfield GM. Amyloidosis: a clinicopathophysiological synopsis. *Semin Cell Dev Biol* 2004;15:39–44.

204. Ho TW, Mishu B, Li CY, *et al.* Guillain-Barré syndrome in northern China: relationship to *Campylobacter jejuni* infection and anti-glycolipid antibodies. *Brain* 1995;118(Part 3):597–605.

205. Ho TW, Willison HJ, Nachamkin I, *et al.* Anti-GD1a antibody is associated with axonal but not demyelinating forms of Guillain–Barré syndrome. *Ann Neurol* 1999;45:168–73.

206. Holt IJ, Harding AE, Petty RK, Morgan-Hughes JA. A new mitochondrial disease associated with mitochondrial DNA heteroplasmy. *Am J Hum Genet* 1990;46:428–33.

207. Hoogendijk JE, De Visser M, Bolhuis PA, Hart AAM, Ongerboer De Visser BM. Hereditary motor and sensory neuropathy type I: clinical and neurographical features of the 17p duplication subtype. *Muscle Nerve* 1994;17:85–90.

208. Horwich MS, Cho L, Porro RS, Posner JB. Subacute sensory neuropathy: a remote effect of carcinoma. *Ann Neurol* 1977;2:7–19.

209. Houlden H, King RH, Hashemi-Nejad A, *et al.* A novel TRK A (NTRK1) mutation associated with hereditary sensory and autonomic neuropathy type V. *Ann Neurol* 2001;49:521–5.

210. Huan MC, Bromberg M. Advances in the laboratory evaluation of peripheral neuropathies. *Curr Neurol Neurosci Rep* 2012;12:84–91.

211. Hughes RA, Cornblath DR. Guillain–Barré syndrome. *Lancet* 2005;366:1653–66.

212. Hughes RA, Cameron JS, Hall SM, *et al.* Multiple mononeuropathy as the initial presentation of systemic lupus erythematosus: nerve biopsy and response to plasma exchange. *J Neurol* 1982;228:239–47.

213. Hund E. Critical illness polyneuropathy. *Curr Opin Neurol* 2001;14:649–53.

214. Hunder GG, Arend WP, Bloch DA, *et al.* The American College of Rheumatology 1990 criteria for the classification of vasculitis: introduction. *Arthritis Rheum* 1990;33:1065–7.

215. Ishibashi T, Dupree JL, Ikenaka K, *et al.* A myelin galactolipid, sulfatide, is essential for maintenance of ion channels on myelinated axon but not essential for initial cluster formation. *J Neurosci* 2002;22:6507–14.

216. Ishii DN. Insulin and related neurotrophic Factors in diabetic neuropathy. *Diabet Med* 1993;10(Suppl 2):14–15S.

217. Ito Y, Yamamoto M, Li M, *et al.* Differential temporal expression of mRNAs for ciliary neurotrophic factor (CNTF), leukemia inhibitory factor (LIF), interleukin-6 (IL-6), and their receptors (CNTFR alpha, LIFR beta,IL-6R alpha and gp130) In injured peripheral nerves. *Brain Res* 1998;793:321–7.

218. Jacobs JM, Carmichael N, Cavanagh JB. Ultrastructural changes in the dorsal root and trigeminal ganglia of rats poisoned with methyl mercury. *Neuropathol Appl Neurobiol* 1975;1–19.

219. Jacobs JM, Miller RH, Whittle A, Cavanagh JB. Studies on the early changes in acute isoniazid neuropathy in the rat. *Acta Neuropathol (Berl)* 1979;47:85–92.

220. Jaggi AS, Singh N. Mechanisms in cancer chemotherapeutic drug-induced peripheral neuropathy. *Toxicology* 2012;291:1–9.

221. Jann S, Beretta S, Bramerio MA. Different types of chronic inflammatory demyelinating polyneuropathy have a different clinical course and response to treatment. *Muscle Nerve* 2005;32:351–6.

222. Jardim MR, Antunes SL, Simons B, *et al.* Role of PGL-I antibody detection in the diagnosis of pure neural leprosy. *Lepr Rev* 2005;76:232–40.

223. Jennette JC, Falk RJ, Andrassy K, *et al.* Nomenclature of systemic vasculitides. Proposal of an international consensus conference. *Arthritis Rheum* 1994;37:187–92.

224. Job CK, Desikan KV. Pathologic changes and their distribution in peripheral nerves in lepromatous leprosy. *Int J Lepr* 1968;36:257–70.

225. Joe EH, Angelides K. Clustering of voltage-dependent sodium channels on axons depends on Schwann cell contact. *Nature* 1992;356:333–5.

226. Johnson EM Jr, Taniuchi M, DiStefano PS. Expression and possible function of nerve growth factor receptors on Schwann cells. *Trends Neurosci* 1988;11:299–304.

227. Jortner BS. Mechanisms of toxic injury in the peripheral nervous system: neuropathologic considerations. *Toxicol Pathol* 2000;28:54–69.

228. Kahn SN, Riches PG, Kohn J. Paraproteinaemia in neurological disease: incidence, associations, and classification of monoclonal immunoglobulins. *J Clin Pathol* 1980;33:617–21.

229. Kaida K, Kusunoki S, Kamakura K, *et al.* GalNAc-GD1a in human peripheral nerve: target sites of anti-ganglioside antibody. *Neurology* 2003;61:465–70.

230. Kaplan JG, Kessler J, Rosenberg N, *et al.* Sensory neuropathy associated with Dursban (chlorpyrifos) exposure. *Neurology* 1993;43:2193–6.

231. Kararizou E, Davaki P, Karandreas N, *et al.* Nonsystemic vasculitic neuropathy: a clinicopathological study of 22 cases. *J Rheumatol* 2005;32:853–8.

232. Katrak SM, Pollock M, O'Brien CP, *et al.* Clinical and morphological features of gold neuropathy. *Brain* 1980;103:671–93.

233. Kaur G, Girdhar BK, Girdhar A, *et al.* A clinical, immunological and histological study of neuritic leprosy patients. *Int J Lepr* 1991;59:385–91.

234. Kawagashira Y, Koike H, Tomita M *et al.* Morphological progression of myelin abnormalities in IgM-monoclonal gammopathy of undetermined significance anti-myelin-associated glycoprotein neuropathy. *J Neuropathol Exp Neurol* 2010;69:1143–57.

235. Kelkar P, Hammer-White S. Impaired glucose tolerance in nondiabetic lumbosacral radiculoplexus neuropathy. *Muscle Nerve* 2005;31:273–4.

236. Kelly JJ, Kyle RA, Latov N. Polyneuropathies associated with plasma cell dyscrasia. Boston, MA: Martinius Nijhoff, 1987.

237. Kelly JW, Colon W, Lai Z, *et al.* Transthyretin quaternary and tertiary structural changes facilitate misassembly into amyloid. *Adv Protein Chem* 1997;50:161–81.

238. Kennedy JM, Zochodne DW. Experimental diabetic neuropathy with spontaneous recovery: is there irreparable damage? *Diabetes* 2005;54:830–7.

239. Kennedy WR, Wendelschafer- Crabb J, Polydefkis M, McArthur JC. Pathology and quantitation of cutaneous innervation. In: Dyck PJ, Thomas PK eds. *Peripheral Neuropathy*. Philadelphia, PA: Saunders, 2005.

240. Kieseier BC, Tani M, Mahad D, *et al.* Chemokines and chemokine receptors in inflammatory demyelinating neuropathies: a central role for IP-10. *Brain* 2002;125(Part 4):823–34.

241. Kieseier BC, Kiefer R, Gold R, *et al.* Advances in understanding and treatment of immune-mediated disorders of the peripheral nervous system. *Muscle Nerve* 2004;30:131–56.

242. Kihara M, Low PA. Impaired vasoreactivity to nitric oxide in experimental diabetic neuropathy. *Exp Neurol* 1995;132:180–85.

243. Kim D, Kim HJ, Kim Y, *et al.* Kaposi's sarcoma herpesvirus-associated Castleman disease with POEMS syndrome. *Muscle Nerve* 2000;23:436–39.

244. King RH, Llewelyn JG, Thomas PK, *et al.* Diabetic neuropathy: abnormalities of Schwann cell and perineurial basal laminae. Implications for diabetic vasculopathy. *Neuropathol Appl Neurobiol* 1989;15:339–55.

245. King RH, Tournev I, Colomer J. Ultrastructural changes in peripheral nerve in hereditary motor and sensory neuropathy-LOM. *Neuropathol Appl Neurobiol* 1999;25:306–12.

246. Kioussi C, Gruss P. Making of a Schwann. *Trends Genet* 1996;12:84–6.

247. Kirchheimer WF, Storrs EE. Attempts to establish the armadillo (*Dasypus novemcinctus*) as a model for the study of leprosy: I. Report of lepromatoid leprosy in an experimentally infected armadillo. *Int J Lepr* 1971;39:693–701.

248. Kiuru-Enari S, Somer H, Seppalainen AM, *et al.* Neuromuscular pathology in hereditary gelsolin amyloidosis. *J Neuropathol Exp Neurol* 2002;61:565–71.

249. Klein CJ, Boes CJ, Chapin JE, *et al.* Adult polyglucosan body disease: core description of an expanding genetic and clinical syndrome. *Muscle Nerve* 2004;29:323–8.

250. Ko MH, Chen WP, Hsieh ST. Neuropathology of skin denervation in acrylamide-induced neuropathy. *Neurobiol Dis* 2002;11:155–65.

251. Kocen RS, King RH, Thomas PK, Haas LF. Nerve biopsy findings in two cases of Tangier disease. *Acta Neuropathol* 1973;26:317–27.

252. Koch J, Gartner S, Li CM, *et al.* Molecular cloning and characterization of a full-length complementary DNA encoding human acid ceramidase: identification of the first molecular lesion causing Farber disease. *J Biol Chem* 1996;271:33110–15.

253. Koenig M. Rare forms of autosomal recessive neurodegenerative ataxia. *Semin Pediatr Neurol* 2003;10:183–92.

254. Koga M, Yuki N, Hirata K, *et al*. Anti-GM1 antibody IgG subclass: a clinical recovery predictor in Guillain–Barré syndrome. *Neurology* 2003;60:1514–18.

255. Koller H, Kieseier BC, Jander S, Hartung HP. Chronic inflammatory demyelinating polyneuropathy. *N Engl J Med* 2005;352:1343–56.

256. Korhonen L, Lindholm D. The ubiquitin proteasome system in synaptic and axonal degeneration: a new twist to an old cycle. *J Cell Biol* 2004;165:27–30.

257. Krinke G, Naylor DC, Skorpil V. Pyridoxine megavitaminosis: an analysis of the early changes induced with massive doses of vitamin B6 in rat primary sensory neurons. *J Neuropathol Exp Neurol* 1985;44:117–29.

258. Kuhlenbaumer G, Young P, Hunermund G, Ringeslstein B, Stogbauer F. Clinical features and molecular genetics of hereditary peripheral neuropathies. *J Neurol* 2002;249:1629–50.

259. Kyle RA, Gertz MA. Primary systemic amyloidosis: clinical and laboratory features in 474 cases. *Semin Hematol* 1995;32:45–59.

260. Kyle R, Rajkumar SV. Monoclonal gammopathies of undetermined significance. *Rev Clin Exp Hematol* 2002;6:225–52.

261. Kyle R, Rajkumar SV. Monoclonal gammopathies of undetermined significance. *Best Pract Res Clin Haem* 2005;18:689–707.

262. Lachmann HJ, Booth DR, Booth SE, *et al*. Misdiagnosis of hereditary amyloidosis as AL (primary) amyloidosis. *N Engl J Med* 2002;346:1786–91.

263. Langerhans von Paul. Uber die nerven der menschlichten haut. *Virchow Arch* 1868;44:325–337.

264. Latronico N, Peli E, Botteri M. Critical illness myopathy and neuropathy. *Curr Opin Crit Care* 2005;11:126–32.

265. Lauria G, Cornblath DR, Johansson O, *et al*. EFNS guidelines on the use of skin biopsy in the diagnosis of peripheral neuropathy. *Eur J Neurol* 2005;12:747–58.

266. Lauria G, McArthur JC, Hauer PE, *et al*. Neuropathological alterations in diabetic truncal neuropathy: evaluation by skin biopsy. *J Neurol Neurosurg Psychiatry* 1998;65:762–6.

267. Lawson VH, Graham BV, Flanigan KM. Clinical and electrophysiologic features of CMT2A with mutations in the mitofusin 2 gene. *Neurology* 2005;65:197–204.

268. LeBlanc AC, Poduslo JF. Axonal modulation of myelin gene expression in the peripheral nerve. *J Neurosci Res* 1990;26:317–26.

269. Lee MK, Cleveland DW. Neuronal intermediate filaments. *Annu Rev Neurosci* 1996;19:187–217.

270. Lehmann HC, Hartung HP. Plasma exchange and intravenous immunoglobulins: mechanism of action in immune-mediated neuropathies. *J Neuroimmunol* 2001;231:61–9.

271. Leite AC, Silva MT, Alamy AH, *et al*. Peripheral neuropathy in HTLV-I infected individuals without tropical spastic paraparesis/HTLV-I-associated myelopathy. *J Neurol* 2004;251:877–81.

272. Le Quesne PM, McLeod JG. Peripheral neuropathy following a single exposure to arsenic: clinical course in four patients with electrophysiological and histological studies. *J Neurol Sci* 1977;32:437–51.

273. Letourneau PC, Ressler AH. Inhibition of neurite initiation and growth by taxol. *J Cell Biol* 1984;98:1355–62.

274. Lewis RA, Sumner AJ, Brown MJ, Asbury AK. Multifocal demyelinating neuropathy with persistent conduction block. *Neurology* 1982;32:958–64.

275. Lewis W, Dalakas MC. Mitochondrial toxicity of antiviral drugs. *Nat Med* 1995;1:417–22.

276. Lhote F, Cohen P, Guillevin L. Polyarteritis nodosa, microscopic polyangiitis and Churg–Strauss syndrome. *Lupus* 1998;7:238–58.

277. Libman BS, Quismorio FP Jr, Stimmler MM. Polyarteritis nodosa-like vasculitis in human immunodeficiency virus infection. *J Rheumatol* 1995;22:351–5.

278. Liefner M, Siebert H, Sachse T, et al. The role of TNF-alpha during Wallerian degeneration. *J Neuroimmunol* 2000;108:147–52.

279. Lisak RP, Mitchell M, Zweiman B, *et al*. Guillain–Barré syndrome and Hodgkin's disease: three cases with immunological studies. *Ann Neurol* 1977;1:72–8.

280. Liu HM, Yang LH, Yang YJ. Schwann cell properties: 3. C-fos expression, bFGF production, phagocytosis and proliferation during Wallerian degeneration. *J Neuropathol Exp Neurol* 1995;54:487–96.

281. Llewelyn J, Tomlinson D, Thomas P. Diabetic neuropathies. In: Dyck P, Thomas P eds. *Peripheral neuropathy*. Philadelphia, PA: Elsevier–Saunders, 2005:1951–91.

282. Llewelyn JG, Thomas PK, King RH. Epineurial microvasculitis in proximal diabetic neuropathy. *J Neurol* 1998;245:159–65.

283. Lombardi R, Erne B, Lauria G, *et al*. IgM deposits on skin nerves in anti-myelin-associated glycoprotein neuropathy. *Ann Neurol* 2005;57:180–7.

284. Longo FM, Powell HC, Lebeau J, *et al*. Delayed nerve regeneration in streptozotocin diabetic rats. *Muscle Nerve* 1986;9:385–93.

285. LoPachin RM, Ross JF, Lehning EJ. Nerve terminals as the primary site of acrylamide action: a hypothesis. *Neurotoxicology* 2002;23:43–59.

286. LoPachin RM, Balaban CD, Ross JF. Acrylamide axonopathy revisited. *Toxicol Appl Pharmacol* 2003;188:135–53.

287. Low PA, McLeod JG, Turtle JR, *et al*. Peripheral neuropathy in acromegaly. *Brain* 1974;97:139–52.

288. Low PA, Walsh JC, Huang CY, McLeod JG. The sympathetic nervous system in diabetic neuropathy. A clinical and pathological study. *Brain* 1975;98:341–56.

289. Lu MO, Shu J. The role of cytokines in Guillain–Barré syndrome. *J Neurol* 2011;258:533–48.

290. Luciano CA, Pardo CA, McArthur JC. Recent developments in the HIV neuropathies. *Curr Opin Neurol* 2003;16:403–9.

291. Ludwig J, Dyck PJ, LaRusso NF. Xanthomatous neuropathy of liver. *Hum Pathol* 1982;13:1049–51.

292. Lullmann H, Lullmann-Rauch R. Perhexiline induces generalized lipidosis in rats. *Klin Wochenschr* 1978;56:309–10.

293. Lunn MP, Johnson LA, Fromholt SE, *et al*. High-affinity anti-ganglioside IgG antibodies raised in complex ganglioside knockout mice: reexamination of GD1a immunolocalization. *J Neurochem* 2000;75:404–12.

294. Luo KR, Chao CC, Chen YT *et al*. Quantation of pseudomotor innervation in skin biopsies of patients with diabetic neuropathy. *J Neuropathol Exp Neurol* 2011;70:930–8.

295. Luria G. Innervation of the human epidermis: a historical review. *Ital J Neurol Sci* 1999;20:63–70.

296. Madrid R, Bradley WG. The pathology of neuropathies with focal thickening of the myelin sheath (tomaculous neuropathy). *J Neurol Sci* 1975;25:415–48.

297. Magira EE, Papaioakim M, Nachamkin I, *et al*. Differential distribution of HLA-DQ beta/DR beta epitopes in the two forms of Guillain–Barré syndrome, acute motor axonal neuropathy and acute inflammatory demyelinating polyneuropathy (AIDP): identification of DQ beta epitopes associated with susceptibility to and protection from AIDP. *J Immunol* 2003;170:3074–80.

298. Malandrini A, Guazzi GC, Alessandrini C, Federico A. Peripheral nerve involvement in ataxia telangiectasia: histological and ultrastructural studies of peroneal nerve biopsy in two cases. *Clin Neuropathol* 1990;9:109–14.

299. Malik RA, Newrick PG, Sharma AK, et al. Microangiopathy in human diabetic neuropathy: relationship between capillary abnormalities and the severity of neuropathy. *Diabetologia* 1989;32:92–102.

300. Malik RA, Tesfaye S, Thompson SD, et al. Endoneurial localisation of microvascular damage in human diabetic neuropathy. *Diabetologia* 1993;36:454–9.

301. Malik RA, Tesfaye S, Newrick PG, *et al*. Sural nerve pathology in diabetic patients with minimal but progressive neuropathy. *Diabetologia* 2005;48:578–85.

302. Manji H. Toxic neuropathy. *Curr Opin Neurol* 2011;24:484–90.

303. Manto MU. The wide spectrum of spinocerebellar ataxias (SCAs). *Cerebellum* 2005;4:2–6.

304. Manzo L. Thallium. In: Spencer PS, Schaumburg H eds. *Experimental and clinical neurotoxicology*. New York: Oxford University Press, 2000:1168–77.

305. Martenson CH, Odom A, Sheetz MP, Graham DG. The effect of acrylamide and other sulfhydryl alkylators on the ability of dynein and kinesin to translocate microtubules *in vitro*. *Toxicol Appl Pharmacol* 1995;133:73–81.

306. Martin JJ, De Barsy T, De S, *et al*. Acid maltase deficiency (type II glycogenosis): morphological and biochemical study of a childhood phenotype. *J Neurol Sci* 1976;30:155–66.

307. Martini R. Expression and functional roles of neural cell surface molecules and extracellular matrix components during development and regeneration of peripheral nerves. *J Neurocytol* 1994;23:1–28.

308. Martini R, Schachner M, Brushart TM. The L2/HNK-1 carbohydrate is preferentially expressed by previously motor axon-associated Schwann cells in reinnervated peripheral nerves. *J Neurosci* 1994;14(Part 2):7180–91.

309. Maser RE, Steenkiste AR, Dorman JS, *et al*. Epidemiological correlates of diabetic neuropathy: report from Pittsburgh Epidemiology of Diabetes Complications Study. *Diabetes* 1989;38:1456–61.

310. Maurer M, Toyka KV, Gold R. Immune mechanisms in acquired demyelinating neuropathies: lessons from animal models. *Neuromuscul Disord* 2002;12:405–14.

311. McArthur JC, Yiannoutsos C, Simpson DM, *et al.* A phase II trial of nerve growth factor for sensory neuropathy associated with HIV infection. AIDS Clinical Trials Group Team 291. *Neurology* 2000;54:1080–8.

312. McCarthy BG, Hsieh ST, Stocks A, *et al.* Cutaneous innervation in sensory neuropathies: evaluation by skin biopsy. *Neurology* 1995;45:1848–55.

313. McCombe PA, McLeod JG, Pollard JD, *et al.* Peripheral sensorimotor and autonomic neuropathy associated with systemic lupus erythematosus. Clinical, pathological and immunological features. *Brain* 1987;110(Part 2):533–49.

314. McDougall AJ, Davies L, McCaughan GW. Autonomic and peripheral neuropathy in endstage liver disease and following liver transplantation. *Muscle Nerve* 2003;28:595–600.

315. Mei FJ, Ishizu T, Murai H, *et al.* Th1 shift in CIDP versus Th2 shift in vasculitic neuropathy in CSF. *J Neurol Sci* 2005;228:75–85.

316. Mellgren SI, Conn DL, Stevens JC, Dyck PJ. Peripheral neuropathy in primary Sjögren's syndrome. *Neurology* 1989;39:390–94.

317. Mellick R, Dolan L, Kidman AD. Experimental diphtheritic neuropathy in the mouse: a study in cellular resistance. *Br J Exp Pathol* 1975;56:471–6.

318. Mendell JR, Sahenk Z, Whitaker JN, *et al.* Polyneuropathy and IgM monoclonal gammopathy: studies on the pathogenetic role of anti-myelin-associated glycoprotein antibody. *Ann Neurol* 1985;17:243–54.

319. Menicucci LA, Miranda A, Gomez Antunes SL, *et al.* Microscopic leprosy skin lesions in primary neuritic leprosy. *J Am Acad Dermatol* 2005;52:648–52.

320. Meretoja J. Familial systemic paramyloidosis with lattice dystrophy of the cornea, progressive cranial neuropathy, skin changes and various internal symptoms: a previously unrecognized heritable syndrome. *Ann Clin Res* 1969;1:314–24.

321. Merner ND, Dion PA, Rouleau GA. Recent advances in the genetics of distal hereditary motor neuropathy give insight to a disease mechanism involving copper homeostasis that may extend to other motor neuron disorders. *Clin Genet* 2011;79:23–34.

322. Meucci N, Baldini L, Capellari A, *et al.* Antimyelin- associated glycoprotein antibodies predict the development of a neuropathy in asymptomatic patients with IgM monoclonal gammopathy. *Ann Neurol* 1999;46:119–22.

323. Michailov GV, Sereda MW, Brinkmann BG, *et al.* Axonal neuregulin-1 regulates myelin sheath thickness. *Science* 2004;304:700–703.

324. Midroni G, Bilbao JM. *Biopsy diagnosis of peripheral neuropathy.* Boston, MA: Butterworth–Heinemann, 1995.

325. Midroni G, Bilbao JM. Nerve biopsy. In: Kimura J ed. *Peripheral nerve diseases: handbook of clinical neurophysiology,* Vol. 7. Edinburgh: Elsevier, 2006.

326. Miller BR, Press C, Daniels RW, *et al.* A dual leucine–kinase-dependent axon self destruction program promotes Wallerian degeneration. *Nat Neurosci* 2009;12: 387–9.

327. Misra VP, King RH, Harding AE, *et al.* Peripheral neuropathy in the Chediak–Higashi syndrome. *Acta Neuropathol (Berl)* 1991;81:354–8.

328. Mitamura T, Umata T, Nakano F, *et al.* Structure–function analysis of the diphtheria toxin receptor toxin binding site by site-directed mutagenesis. *J Biol Chem* 1997;272:27084–90.

329. Mitsumoto H, Sliman RJ, Schafer IA, *et al.* Motor neuron disease and adult hexosaminidase A deficiency in two families: evidence for multisystem degeneration. *Ann Neurol* 1985;17: 378–85.

330. Mitsuo K, Nakano T, Kobayashi T, *et al.* Juvenile Sandhoff disease: a Japanese patient carrying a mutation identical to that found earlier in a Canadian patient. *J Neurol Sci* 1990;98:277–86.

331. Monk KR, Oshima K, Heller JS, Talbot WS. Gpr126 is essential for peripheral nerve development and myelination in mammals. *Development* 2011;138: 2673–80.

332. Moore RD, Wong WM, Keruly JC, McArthur JC. Incidence of neuropathy in HIV-infected patients on monotherapy versus those on combination therapy with didanosine, stavudine and hydroxyurea. *AIDS* 2000;14:273–8.

333. Morozumi S, Koike H, Tomita M *et al.* Spatial distribution of nerve fiber pathology and vasculitis in microscopic polyangiitis-associated neuropathy. *J Neuropathol Exp Neurol* 2011;70:340–8.

334. Moser HW. Adrenoleukodystrophy: phenotype, genetics, pathogenesis and therapy. *Brain* 1997;120(Part 8):1485–508.

335. Moyle G. Clinical manifestations And management of antiretroviral nucleoside Analog-related mitochondrial toxicity. *Clin Ther* 2000;22:911–36; discussion 898.

336. Nardin RA, Johns DR. Mitochondrial dysfunction and neuromuscular disease. *Muscle Nerve* 2001;24:170–91.

337. Nardocci N, Zorzi G, Farina L, *et al.* Infantile neuroaxonal dystrophy: clinical spectrum and diagnostic criteria. *Neurology* 1999;52:1472–8.

338. Nelson JS, Fitch CD, Fischer VW, *et al.* Progressive neuropathologic lesions in vitamin E-deficient rhesus monkeys. *J Neuropathol Exp Neurol* 1981;40:166–86.

339. Nemni R, Bottacchi E, Fazio R, *et al.* Polyneuropathy in hypothyroidism: clinical, electrophysiological and morphological findings in four cases. *J Neurol Neurosurg Psychiatry* 1987;50:1454–60.

340. Nemni R, Sanvito L, Quattrini A, *et al.* Peripheral neuropathy in hepatitis C virus infection with and without cryoglobulinemia. *J Neurol Neurosurg Psychiatry* 2003;74:1267–71.

341. Nguyen QT, Sanes JR, Lichtman JW. Pre-existing pathways promote precise projection patterns. *Nat Neurosci* 2002;5:861–7.

342. Nichols WC, Gregg RE, Brewer HB Jr, Benson MD. A mutation in apolipoprotein A-I in the Iowa type of familial amyloidotic polyneuropathy. *Genomics* 1990;8:318–23.

343. Nickel FT, Seifert F, Lanz S, *et al.* Mechanisms of neuropathic pain. *Eur Neuropsychopharmacology* 2012;22: 81–91.

344. Nishimura M, Kwon KS, Shibuta K, *et al.* An improved method for DNA diagnosis of leprosy using formaldehyde-fixed, paraffin-embedded skin biopsies. *Mod Pathol* 1994;7:253–6.

345. Nishino H, Rubino FA, DeRemee RA, *et al.* Neurological involvement in Wegener's granulomatosis: an analysis of 324 consecutive patients at the Mayo Clinic. *Ann Neurol* 1993;33:4–9.

346. Nishino I, Spinazzola A, Hirano M. Thymidine phosphorylase gene mutations in MNGIE, a human mitochondrial disorder. *Science* 1999;283:689–92.

347. Nobile-Orazio E. Update on neuropathies associated with monoclonal gammopathy of undetermined significance (2008–2010). *J Peripher Nerv Syst* 2010;15:302–6.

348. Nobile-Orazio E, Cappellari A, Priori A. Multifocal motor neuropathy: current concepts and controversies. *Muscle Nerve* 2005;31:663–80.

349. Nofer JR, Ramaley AT. Tangier disease: still more questions than answers. *Cell Mol Life Sci* 2005;62:2150–60.

350. Nolano M, Provitera V, Crisci C, *et al.* Small fibers involvement in Friedreich's ataxia. *Ann Neurol* 2001;50:17–25.

351. Novella SP, Inzucchi SE, Goldstein JM. The frequency of undiagnosed diabetes and impaired glucose tolerance in patients with idiopathic sensory neuropathy. *Muscle Nerve* 2001;24:1229–31.

352. Oates P. Polyol pathway and diabetic peripheral neuropathy. In: Tomlinson DR ed. *Neurobiology of diabetic neuropathy.* Amsterdam: Academic Press, 2002:326–92.

353. Obi T, Murakami T, Takatsu M, *et al.* Clinicopathological study of an autopsy case with sensory-dominant polyradiculoneuropathy with antiganglioside antibodies. *Muscle Nerve* 1999;22: 1426–31.

354. Obrosova IG. How does glucose Generate oxidative stress in peripheral nerve? *Int Rev Neurobiol* 2002;50:3–35.

355. Obrosova IG. Diabetes and the peripheral nerve. *Biochim Biophys Acta* 2009;1792:931–40.

356. Oftebro H, Bjorkhem I, Stormer FC, Pedersen JI. Cerebrotendinous xanthomatosis: defective liver mitochondrial hydroxylation of chenodeoxycholic acid precursors. *J Lipid Res* 1981;22:632–40.

357. Oh SJ, Joy JL, Kuruoglu R. 'Chronic sensory demyelinating neuropathy': chronic inflammatory demyelinating polyneuropathy presenting as a pure sensory neuropathy. *J Neurol Neurosurg Psychiatry* 1992;55:677–80.

358. Oh SJ, Claussen GC, Odabasi Z, Palmer CP. Multifocal demyelinating motor neuropathy: pathologic evidence of inflammatory demyelinating polyradiculoneuropathy. *Neurology* 1995;45:1828–32.

359. Oh SJ, Claussen GC, Kim DS. Motor and sensory demyelinating mononeuropathy multiplex (multifocal motor and sensory demyelinating neuropathy): a separate entity or a variant of chronic inflammatory demyelinating polyneuropathy? *J Peripher Nerv Syst* 1997;2:362–9.

360. Ohnishi A. Ethylene oxide. In: Spencer PS, Schaumburg H eds. *Experimental and clinical neurotoxicology.* New York: Oxford University Press, 2000:563–6.

361. Ohnishi A, Tsuji S, Igisu H, *et al.* Beriberi neuropathy: morphometric study of sural nerve. *J Neurol Sci* 1980;45:177–90.

362. Ooi WW, Srinivasan J. Leprosy and the peripheral nervous system: basic and clinical aspects. *Muscle Nerve* 2004;30:393–409.

363. Ordog T, Takayama I, Cheung WK, et al. Remodeling of networks of interstitial cells of Cajal in a murine model of diabetic gastroparesis. *Diabetes* 2000;49:1731–9.

364. Ortiz N, Rosa R, Gallardo E, et al. IgM monoclonal antibody against terminal moiety of GM2, GalNAc-GD1a and GalNAc-GM1b from a pure motor chronic demyelinating polyneuropathy patient: effects on neurotransmitter release. *J Neuroimmunol* 2001;119:114–23.

365. Ouvrier RA, McLeod JG, Morgan GJ, Wise GA, Conchin TE. Hereditary motor and sensory neuropathy of neuronal type with onset in early childhood. *J Neurol Sci* 1981;51:181–97.

366. Oyebode OR, Hartley R, Singhota et al. Differential protection of neuromuscular sensory and motor axons and their endings in Wld(S) mutant mice. *Neuroscience* 2012;200:142–58.

367. Pagnoux C, Guillevin L. Peripheral neuropathy in systemic vasculitides. *Curr Opin Rheumatol* 2005;17:41–8.

368. Pallis CA, Scott JT. Peripheral neuropathy in rheumatoid arthritis. *Br Med J* 1965;5443:1141–7.

369. Parman Y, Battaloglu E, Baris I, et al. Clinico-pathological and genetic study of early onset demyelinating neuropathy. *Brain* 2004;127:2540–50.

370. Patterson TA, Schmued LC, Sandberg JA, Slikker W. Temporal development of 29,39-dideoxyinosine (ddI)-induced peripheral myelinopathy. *Neurotoxicol Teratol* 2000;22:429–34.

371. Paulson JC, McClure WO. Inhibition of axoplasmic transport by colchicine, podophyllotoxin, and vinblastine: an effect on microtubules. *Ann N Y Acad Sci* 1975;253:517–27.

372. Pearson J, Pytel BA. Quantitative studies of sympathetic ganglia and spinal cord intermedio-lateral gray columns in familial dysautonomia. *J Neurol Sci* 1978;39:47–59.

373. Pearson J, Pytel BA, Grover-Johnson N, Axelrod F, Dancis J. Quantitative studies of dorsal root ganglia and neuropathologic observations on spinal cords in familial dysautonomia. *J Neurol Sci* 1978;35:77–92.

374. Pedley JC, Harman DJ, Waudby H, McDougall AC. Leprosy in peripheral nerves: histopathological findings in 119 untreated patients in Nepal. *J Neurol Neurosurg Psychiatry* 1980;43:198–204.

375. Pellissier JF, Van Hoof F, Bourdet-Bonerandi D, Monier-Faugere MC, Toga M. Morphological and biochemical changes in muscle and peripheral nerve in Fabry's disease. *Muscle Nerve* 1981;4:381–7.

376. Pellissier JF, Berard-Badier M, Pinsard N. Farber's disease in two siblings: sural nerve and subcutaneous biopsies by light and electron microscopy. *Acta Neuropathol (Berl)* 1986;72:178–88.

377. Pereira JA, Lebrun-Julien F, Suter U. Molecular mechanisms regulating myelination in the peripheral nerve. *Trends Neurosci* 2012;35:123–34.

378. Periquet MI, Novak V, Collins MP, et al. Painful sensory neuropathy: prospective evaluation using skin biopsy. *Neurology* 1999;53:1641–7.

379. Pestronk A. Multifocal motor neuropathy: diagnosis and treatment. *Neurology* 1998;51(Suppl 5):S22–4.

380. Pestronk A. N,N9-dimethyl aminopropionitrile. In: Spencer PS, Schaumburg H eds. *Experimental and clinical neurotoxicology*. New York: Oxford University Press, 2000:499–502.

381. Pestronk A. Autoantibodies and immune polyneuropathies. In: Katirji B, Kaminski H, Preston D, et al. eds. *Neuromuscular disorders in clinical practice*. Boston, MA: Butterworth–Heinemann, 2002:64–73.

382. Pestronk A, Choksi R. Multifocal motor neuropathy: serum IgM anti-GM1 ganglioside antibodies in most patients detected using covalent linkage of GM1 to ELISA plates. *Neurology* 1997;49:1289–92.

383. Pestronk A, Lopate G. Polyneuropathies and antibodies to nerve components. In: Dyck P, Thomas P eds. *Peripheral neuropathy*. Philadelphia, PA: Elsevier–Saunders, 2005:2177–96.

384. Pestronk A, Choksi R, Logigian E, Al-Lozi MT. Sensory neuropathy with monoclonal IgM binding to a trisulfated heparin disaccharide. *Muscle Nerve* 2003;27:188–95.

385. Pich P, Bach D, Briones P, et al. The Charcot–Marie–Tooth type 2A gene product, Mfn2, upregulates fuel oxidation through expression of OXPHOS system. *Hum Mol Genet* 2005;14:1405–15.

386. Pierson CR, Zhang W, Murakawa Y, Sima AA. Early gene responses of trophic factors in nerve regeneration differ in experimental type 1 and type 2 diabetic polyneuropathies. *J Neuropathol Exp Neurol* 2002;61:857–71.

387. Pierson CR, Zhang W, Murakawa Y, Sima AA. Insulin deficiency rather than hyperglycemia accounts for impaired neurotrophic responses and nerve fiber regeneration in type 1 diabetic neuropathy. *J Neuropathol Exp Neurol* 2003;62:260–71.

388. Pierson CR, Zhang W, Sima AA. Proinsulin C-peptide replacement in type 1 diabetic BB/Wor-rats prevents deficits in nerve fiber regeneration. *J Neuropathol Exp Neurol* 2003;62:765–79.

389. Piette AM, Tusseau F, Vignon D, et al. Acute neuropathy coincident with seroconversion for anti-LAV/HTLV-III. *Lancet* 1986;1:852.

390. Plante-Bordeneuve V, Baudrimont M, Gorin NC, Gherardi RK. Subacute sensory neuropathy associated with Hodgkin's disease. *J Neurol Sci* 1994;121:155–8.

391. Plante-Bordeneuve V, Said G. Familial amyloid polyneuropathy. *Lancet Neurol* 2011;10:1086–97.

392. Pleasure D, Messing A. Diphtheritic polyneuropathy. In: Dyck P, Thomas P eds. *Peripheral neuropathy*. Philadelphia, PA: Elsevier–Saunders, 2005:2147–51.

393. Podratz JL, Knight AM, Ta LE, et al. Cisplatin-induced mitochondrial DNA damage in dorsal root ganglion neurons. *Neurobiol Dis* 2011;41:661–8.

394. Poncelet AN, Connolly MK. Peripheral neuropathy in scleroderma. *Muscle Nerve* 2003;28:330–35.

395. Powers JM. The pathology of peroxisomal disorders with pathogenetic considerations. *J Neuropathol Exp Neurol* 1995;54:710–19.

396. Powers JM, DeCiero DP, Ito M, et al. Adrenomyeloneuropathy: a neuropathologic review featuring its noninflammatory myelopathy. *J Neuropathol Exp Neurol* 2000;59:89–102.

397. Prineas J. Peripheral nerve changes in thiamine-deficient rats: an electron microscope study. *Arch Neurol* 1970;23:541–8.

398. Prior R, Schober R, Scharffetter K, Wechsler W. Occlusive microangiopathy by immunoglobulin (IgM-kappa) precipitation: pathogenetic relevance in paraneoplastic cryoglobulinemia neuropathy. *Acta Neuropathol* 1992;83:423–6.

399. Purves T, Middlemas A, Agthong S, et al. A role for mitogen-activated protein kinases in the etiology of diabetic neuropathy. *FASEB J* 2001;15:2508–14.

400. Quintes S, Goebbels S, Saher G et al. Neuron glia signaling and the protection of axon function by Schwann cells. *J Peripher Nerv Syst* 2010;15:10–16.

401. Rabinowe SL, Brown FM, Watts M, Smith AM. Complement-fixing antibodies to sympathetic and parasympathetic tissues in IDDM: autonomic brake index and heart-rate variation. *Diabetes Care* 1990;13:1084–8.

402. Raff MC, Whitmore AV, Finn JT. Axonal self-destruction and neurodegeneration. *Science* 2002;296:868–71.

403. Rajkumar SV, Gertz MA, Kyle RA. Prognosis of patients with primary systemic amyloidosis who present with dominant neuropathy. *Am J Med* 1998;104:232–7.

404. Rambukkana A, Selzer JL, Yurchenco PD, Tuomanen EI. Neural targeting of *Mycobacterium leprae* mediated by the G domain of the laminin-alpha 2 chain. *Cell* 1997;88:811–21.

405. Ramchandren S, Lewis RA. An update on monoclonal gammopathy and neuropathy. *Curr Neurol Neurosci Rep* 2012;12:102–10.

406. Rautenstrauss B. Targeting inherited peripheral neuropathies in the postgenomic era. *Neurology* 2011;77:540–8.

407. Reilly MM, Staunton H. Peripheral nerve amyloidosis. *Brain Pathol* 1996;6:163–77.

408. Ricoy JR, Cabello A, Rodriguez J, Tellez I. Neuropathological studies on the toxic syndrome related to adulterated rapeseed oil in Spain. *Brain* 1983;106(Part 4):817–35.

409. Ridley DS. *Pathogenesis of leprosy and related diseases*. London: Wright, 1988.

410. Ridley DS, Ridley MJ. Classification of nerves is modified by the delayed recognition of *Mycobacterium leprae*. *Int J Lepr* 1986;54:596–606.

411. Riviere JB, Ramalingam S, Lavastre V, et al. KIF1A, an axonal transporter of synaptic vesicles, is mutated in hereditary sensory and autonomic neuropathy type 2. *Am J Hum Genet* 2011;89:219–30.

412. Rizzuto N, Cavallaro T, Monaco S, et al. Role of HIV in the pathogenesis of distal symmetrical peripheral neuropathy. *Acta Neuropathol (Berl)* 1995;90:244–50.

413. Rizzuto N, Morbin M, Cavallaro T, et al. Focal lesions area feature of chronic inflammatory demyelinating polyneuropathy (CIDP). *Acta Neuropathol (Berl)* 1998;96:603–9.

414. Robert ME, Geraghty JJ 3rd, Miles SA, et al. Severe neuropathy in a patient with acquired immune deficiency syndrome (AIDS): evidence for widespread

cytomegalovirus infection of peripheral nerve and human immunodeficiency virus-like immunoreactivity of anterior horn cells. *Acta Neuropathol (Berl)* 1989;79:255–61.

415. Roberts ED, Bohm RP Jr, Lowrie RC Jr, *et al.* Pathogenesis of Lyme neuroborreliosis in the rhesus monkey: the early disseminated and chronic phases of disease in the peripheral nervous system. *J Infect Dis* 1998;178;722–32.

416. Rojas–Garcia R, Tizzano E, Cusco I, *et al.* The absence of survival motor neuron 2 gene may play a role in multifocal motor neuropathy. *Neurology* 2002;59:1112–13.

417. Ropper AH, Gorson KC. Neuropathies associated with paraproteinemia. *N Engl J Med* 1998;338:1601–7.

418. Rotthier A, Baets J, Timmerman V, Janssens K. Mechanisms of disease in hereditary sensory and autonomic neuropathies. *Nat Rev Neurol* 2012;8: 73–85.

419. Roullet E, Assuerus V, Gozlan J, *et al.* Cytomegalovirus multifocal neuropathy in AIDS: analysis of 15 consecutive cases. *Neurology* 1994;44:2174–82.

420. Roytta M, Raine CS. Taxol-induced neuropathy: chronic effects of local injection. *J Neurocytol* 1986;15:483–96.

421. Ruchoux MM, Guerouaou D, Vandenhaute B, *et al.* Systemic vascular smooth muscle cell impairment in cerebral autosomal dominant arteriopathy with subcortical infarcts and leukoencephalopathy. *Acta Neuropathol (Berl)* 1995;89:500–512.

422. Rudnicki SA, Dalmau J. Paraneoplastic syndromes of the peripheral nerves. *Curr Opin Neurol* 2005;18:598–603.

423. Rundles R. Diabetic neuropathy: general review with report of 125 cases. *Medicine* 1945;24:111–60.

424. Russell JW, Sullivan KA, Windebank AJ, *et al.* Neurons undergo apoptosis in animal and cell culture models of diabetes. *Neurobiol Dis* 1999;6:347–63.

425. Sahenk Z, Barohn R, New P, Mendell JR. Taxol neuropathy: electrodiagnostic and sural nerve biopsy findings. *Arch Neurol* 1994;51:726–9.

426. Said G. Perhexiline neuropathy: a clinicopathological study. *Ann Neurol* 1978;3:259–66.

427. Said G. Lyme disease. In: Dyck P, Thomas P eds. *Peripheral neuropathy*. Philadelphia, PA: Elsevier–Saunders, 2005:2109–16.

428. Said G, Lacroix C. Primary and secondary vasculitic neuropathy. *J Neurol* 2005;252:633–41.

429. Said G, Marion MH, Selva J, Jamet C. Hypotrophic and dying-back nerve fibers in Friedreich's ataxia. *Neurology* 1986;36:1292–9.

430. Said G, Lacroix-Ciaudo C, Fujimura H, *et al.* The peripheral neuropathy of necrotizing arteritis: a clinicopathological study. *Ann Neurol* 1988;23:461–5.

431. Said G, Lacroix C, Chemouilli P, *et al.* Cytomegalovirus neuropathy in acquired immunodeficiency syndrome: a clinical and pathological study. *Ann Neurol* 1991;29:139–46.

432. Said G, Lacroix C, Plante-Bordeneuve V, *et al.* Nerve granulomas and vasculitis in sarcoid peripheral neuropathy: a clinicopathological study of 11 patients. *Brain* 2002;125(Part 2):264–75.

433. Said G, Lacroix C, Lozeron P, *et al.* Inflammatory vasculopathy in multifocal diabetic neuropathy. *Brain* 2003;126(Part 2):376–85.

434. Said G, Lacroix C, Plante-Bordeneuve V, *et al.* Clinicopathological aspects of the neuropathy of neurogastrointestinal encephalomyopathy (MNGIE) in four patients including two with a Charcot–Marie–Tooth presentation. *J Neurol* 2005;252:655–62.

435. Saifee TA, Elliott KJ, Rabin N, *et al.* Bortezomib-induced inflammatory neuropathy. *J Peripher Nerv Syst* 2010;15:366–8.

436. Salomon B, Rhee L, Bour-Jordan H, *et al.* Development of spontaneous autoimmune peripheral polyneuropathy in B7-2-deficient NOD mice. *J Exp Med* 2001;194:677–84.

437. Sander S, Nicholson GA, Ouvrier RA, McLeod JG, Pollard JD. Charcot–Marie–Tooth disease: histopathological features of the peripheral myelin protein (PMP22) duplication (CMT1A) and Connexin32 mutations (CMTX1). *Muscle Nerve* 1998;21:217–25.

438. Santoro L, Barbieri F, Nucciotti R, *et al.* Amiodarone-induced experimental acute neuropathy in rats. *Muscle Nerve* 1992;15:788–95.

439. Saporta MA, Katona I, Zhang X *et al.* Neuropathy in a human without the PMP22 gene. *Arch Neurol* 2011;68: 814–21.

440. Scarlato M, Previtali SC, Carpo M. Polyneuropathy in POEMS syndrome: role of angiogenic factors in the pathogenesis. *Brain* 2005;128:1911–20.

441. Schaumburg H, Kaplan J, Windebank A, *et al.* Sensory neuropathy from pyridoxine abuse: a new megavitamin syndrome. *N Engl J Med* 1983;309:445–8.

442. Scherer SS. Nodes, paranodes, and incisures: from form to function. *Ann N Y Acad Sci* 1999;883:131–42.

443. Scherer SS, Wrabetz L. Molecular mechanisms of inherited demyelinating neuropathies. *Glia* 2008;56:1578–89.

444. Schmidt RE. Neuroaxonal dystrophy in aging rodent and human sympathetic autonomic ganglia: synaptic pathology as a common theme in neuropathology. *Adv Pathol Lab Med* 1993;6:505–22.

445. Schmidt RE. Neuropathology and pathogenesis of diabetic autonomic neuropathy. In: Tomlinson DR ed. *Neurobiology of diabetic neuropathy*. Amsterdam: Academic Press, 2002: 267–92.

446. Schmidt RE. Synaptic dysplasia in sympathetic autonomic ganglia. *J Neurocytol* 1996;25:777–91.

447. Schmidt RE. Non-neoplastic diseases of the peripheral nervous system. In: Nelson JS, Mena H, Parisi JE, Schochet SS eds. *Principles and practice of neuropathology*. New York: Oxford University Press, 2003;497–524.

448. Schmidt RE. Autonomic neuropathy in experimental models of diabetes mellitus. In: Zochodne D and Malik R eds. *Handbook of Clinical Neurology*, in press.

449. Schmidt RE, Plurad SB, Parvin CA, Roth KA. Effect of diabetes and aging on human sympathetic autonomic ganglia. *Am J Pathol* 1993;143:143–53.

450. Schmidt RE, Dorsey D, Parvin CA, *et al.* Dystrophic axonal swellings develop as a function of age and diabetes in human dorsal root ganglia. *J Neuropathol Exp Neurol* 1997;56:1028–43.

451. Schmidt RE, Dorsey DA, Beaudet LN, *et al.* Insulin-like growth factor I reverses experimental diabetic autonomic neuropathy. *Am J Pathol* 1999;155: 1651–60.

452. Schmitt HP, Berlet H, Volk B. Peripheral intraaxonal storage in Tay–Sachs disease (GM2-gangliosidosis type 1). *J Neurol Sci* 1979;44:115–24.

453. Schoental R, Cavanagh JB. Mechanisms involved in the dying-back process: hypothesis implicating coenzymes. *Neuropathol Appl Neurobiol* 1977;3: 145–60.

454. Schold SC, Cho ES, Somasundaram M, Posner JB. Subacute motor neuronopathy: a remote effect of lymphoma. *Ann Neurol* 1979;5:271–87.

455. Schroder J. Isoniazid. In: Spencer P, Schaumburg H eds. *Experimental and clinical neurotoxicology*. New York: Oxford University Press, 2000:690–7.

456. Schroder JM, May R, Shin YS, *et al.* Juvenile hereditary polyglucosan body disease with complete branching enzyme deficiency (type IV glycogenosis). *Acta Neuropathol (Berl)* 1993;85:419–30.

457. Scollard DM, McCormick G, Allen JL. Localization of *Mycobacterium leprae* to endothelial cell of epineurial and perineurial blood vessels and lymphatics. *Am J Pathol* 1999;154:1611–20.

458. Sendtner M, Stockli KA, Thoenen H. Synthesis and localization of ciliary neurotrophic factor in the sciatic nerve of the adult rat after lesion and during regeneration. *J Cell Biol* 1992;118:139–48.

459. Sezer O, Eucker J, Schmid P, Possinger K. New therapeutic approaches in primary systemic AL amyloidosis. *Ann Hematol* 2000;79:1–6.

460. Sghirlanzoni A, Mantegazza R, Mora M, *et al.* Chloroquine myopathy and myasthenia-like syndrome. *Muscle Nerve* 1988;11:114–9.

461. Shahrizaila N, Yuki N. Antiganglioside antibodies in Guillain–Barré syndrome and its related conditions. *Expert Rev Neurother* 2011;11:1305–13.

462. Shapshak P, Nagano I, Xin K, *et al.* HIV-1 heterogeneity and cytokines: neuropathogenesis. *Adv Exp Med Biol* 1995;373:225–38.

463. Shields ED, Russell DA, Pericak-Vance MA. Genetic epidemiology of the susceptibility to leprosy. *J Clin Invest* 1987;79:1139–43.

464. Shiraki H. The neuropathology of subacute myelo-optico-neuropathy (SMON) in humans with special reference to the quinoform intoxication. *Jpn J Med Sci Biol* 1975;28(Suppl):101–64.

465. Shy ME, Patzko A. Axonal Charcot–Marie–Tooth disease. *Curr Opin Neurol* 2011;24:475–83.

466. Sicurelli F, Dotti MT, De Stefano N, *et al.* Peripheral neuropathy in CADASIL. *J Neurol* 2005;252:1206–9.

467. Sidenius P, Jakobsen J. Axonal transport in human and experimental diabetes. In: Dyck P, Thomas PK, Asbury A, *et al.* eds. *Diabetic neuropathy*. Philadelphia, PA: WB Saunders, 1987:260–65.

468. Sigal LH, Williams S, Soltys B, Gupta R. H9724, a monoclonal antibody to *Borrelia burgdorferi* flagellin, binds to heat shock protein 60 (HSP60) within live neuroblastoma cells: a potential role for HSP60 in peptide hormone signaling and in autoimmune pathogenesis of the

neuropathy of Lyme disease. *Cell Mol Neurobiol* 2001;21:477–95.

469. Silacci P, Mazzolai L, Gauci C, *et al.* Gelsolin superfamily proteins: key regulators of cellular functions. *Cell Mol Life Sci* 2004;61:2614–23.

470. Sima AA, Zhang W, Xu G, *et al.* A comparison of diabetic polyneuropathy in type II diabetic BBZDR/Wor rats and in type I diabetic BB/Wor rats. *Diabetologia* 2000;43:786–93.

471. Singhal A, Cheng C, Sun H, Zochodne DW. Near nerve local insulin prevents conduction slowing in experimental diabetes. *Brain Res* 1997;763:209–14.

472. Siva A. Vasculitis of the nervous system. *J Neurol* 2001;248:451–68.

473. Smith AG, Ramachandran P, Tripp S, Singleton JR. Epidermal nerve innervation in impaired glucose tolerance and diabetes-associated neuropathy. *Neurology* 2001;57:1701–4.

474. Smith IS, Kahn SM, Lacey BW, *et al.* Chronic demyelinating neuropathy associated with benign IgM paraproteinemia. *Brain* 1983;106:169–95.

475. Snipes GJ, Suter U. Molecular anatomy and genetics of myelin proteins in the peripheral nervous system. *J Anat* 1995;186(Part 3):483–94.

476. Snipes GJ, McGuire CB, Norden JJ, Freeman JA. Nerve injury stimulates the secretion of apolipoprotein E by nonneuronal cells. *Proc Natl Acad Sci USA* 1986;83:1130–34.

477. Soliven B. Immune mechanisms in spontaneously occurring CIDP in NOD mice. *J Peripher Nerv Syst* 2011;16 (Suppl 1):56–59.

478. Sorensen AW, With TK. Persistent pareses after porphyric attacks. *Acta Med Scand* 1971;190:219–22.

479. Soubrier MJ, Dubost JJ, Sauvezie BJ. POEMS syndrome: a study of 25 cases and a review of the literature. French Study Group on POEMS Syndrome. *Am J Med* 1994;97:543–53.

480. Spencer PS, Schaumburg H. *Experimental and clinical neurotoxicology.* New York: Oxford University Press, 2000.

481. Spencer PS, Thomas PK. Ultrastructural studies of the dying-back process: II. The sequestration and removal by Schwann cells and oligodendrocytes of organelles from normal and diseased axons. *J Eurocytol* 1974;3:763–83.

482. Spencer PS, Peterson ER, Madrid R, Raine CS. Effects of thallium salts on neuronal mitochondria in organotypic cord–ganglia–muscle combination cultures. *J Cell Biol* 1973;58:79–95.

483. Stevens FJ. Four structural risk factors identify most fibril-forming kappa light chains. *Amyloid* 2000;7:200–211.

484. Stoll G, Muller HW. Nerve injury, axonal degeneration and neural regeneration: basic insights. *Brain Pathol* 1999;9:313–25.

485. Stubgen JP. Drug-induced dysimmune demyelinating neuropathies. *J Neurol Sci* 2011;307:1–8.

486. Sugimura K, Dyck PJ. Sural nerve myelin thickness and axis cylinder caliber in human diabetes. *Neurology* 1981;31:1087–91.

487. Sulaiman OA, Gordon T. Transforming growth factor-beta and forskolin attenuate the adverse effects of long-term Schwann cell denervation on peripheral nerve regeneration *in vivo*. *Glia* 2002;37:206–18.

488. Sumner CJ, Sheth S, Griffin JW, *et al.* The spectrum of neuropathy in diabetes and impaired glucose tolerance. *Neurology* 2003;60:108–11.

489. Susuki K, Yuki N, Hirata K. Features of sensory ataxic neuropathy associated with anti-GD1b IgM antibody. *J Neuroimmunol* 2001;112:181–7.

490. Susuki K, Yuki N, Schafer DP, *et al.* Dysfunction of nodes of Ranvier: a mechanism for anti-ganglioside antibody-mediated neuropathies. *Exp Neurol* 2012;233:534–42.

491. Suzuki K, Suzuki Y. Galactosylceramide lipidosis: globoid-cell leukodystrophy (Krabbe disease). In: Scriver CR, Beaudet al, Sly WS, Valle D eds. *The metabolic basis of inherited disease.* New York: McGraw–Hill, 1989.

492. Tafuri WL. Light and electron microscope studies of the autonomic nervous system in experimental and human American trypanosomiasis. *Virchow Arch A Pathol Anat* 1971;354:136–49.

493. Takashima H, Boerkoel CF, De Jonghe P, *et al.* Periaxin mutations cause a broad spectrum of demyelinating neuropathies. *Ann Neurol* 2002;51:709–15.

494. Tanaka K, Koyama A, Koike R, *et al.* Adrenomyeloneuropathy: report of a family and electron microscopical findings in peripheral nerves. *J Neurol* 1985;232:73–8.

495. Taniuchi M, Clark HB, Johnson EM Jr. Induction of nerve growth factor receptor in Schwann cells after axotomy. *Proc Natl Acad Sci U S A* 1986;83:4094–8.

496. Taroni F, DiDonato S. Pathways to motor incoordination: the inherited ataxias. *Nat Rev Neurosci* 2004;5:641–55.

497. Taylor P, Gerder M, Moros Z, Feldmann M. Humoral and cellular responses raised against the human HER2 oncoprotein are cross-reactive with the homologous product of the new proto-oncogene, but do not protect rats against B104 tumors expressing mutated neu. *Cancer Immunol Immunother* 1996;42:179–84.

498. Tentolouris N, Pagoni S, Tzonou A, Katsilambros N. Peripheral neuropathy does not invariably coexist with autonomic neuropathy in diabetes mellitus. *Eur J Intern Med* 2001;12:20–7.

499. Terenghi F, Allaria S, Scarlato G, Nobile-Orazio E. Multifocal motor neuropathy and *Campylobacter jejuni* reactivity. *Neurology* 2002;59:282–4.

500. Theriault M, Dort J, Sutherland G, Zochodne DW. Local human sural nerve blood flow in diabetic and other polyneuropathies. *Brain* 1997;120 (Part 7):1131–8.

501. Thomas PK, Griffin JW. Neuropathies predominantly affecting either sensory or motor function. In: Asbury AK, Thomas PK eds. *Peripheral nerve disorders.* Oxford: Butterworth–Heinemann, 1995:59–94.

502. Thomas PK, Walker JG. Xanthomatous neuropathy in primary biliary cirrhosis. *Brain* 1965;88:1079–88.

503. Thomas PK, King RH, Kocen RS, Brett EM. Comparative ultrastructural observations on peripheral nerve abnormalities in the late infantile, juvenile and late onset forms of metachromatic leukodystrophy. *Acta Neuropathol* 1977;39:237–45.

504. Thomas PK, Landon DN, King RHM. Diseases of the peripheral nerves. In: Graham DI, Lantos PL eds. *Greenfield's Neuropathology,* 6th edn. London: Arnold, 1997:367–487.

505. Thornalley P. Glycation in diabetic neuropathy: characteristics, consequences, causes and therapeutic options. In: Tomlinson DR ed. *Neurobiology of Diabetic Neuropathy.* Amsterdam: Academic Press, 2002:38–57.

506. Thorner PS, Bilbao JM, Sima AA, Briggs S. Porphyric neuropathy: an ultrastructural and quantitative case study. *Can J Neurol Sci* 1981;8:281–7.

507. Tomiwa K, Nolan C, Cavanagh JB. The effects of cisplatin on rat spinal ganglia: a study by light and electron microscopy and by morphometry. *Acta Neuropathol (Berl)* 1986;69:295–308.

508. Trojaborg W, Weimer LH, Hays AP. Electrophysiologic studies in critical illness associated weakness: myopathy or neuropathy: a reappraisal. *Clin Neurophysiol* 2001;112:1586–93.

509. Trupp M, Ryden M, Jornvall H, *et al.* Peripheral expression and biological activities of GDNF, a new neurotrophic factor for avian and mammalian peripheral neurons. *J Cell Biol* 1995;130:137–48.

510. Tzourio C, Said G, Millan J. Asymptomatic nerve hypertrophy in lepromatous leprosy: a clinical, electrophysiological and morphological study. *J Neurol* 1992;239:367–74.

511. Ugawa Y, Inoue K, Takemura T, Iwamasa T. Accumulation of glycogen in sural nerve axons in adult-onset type III glycogenosis. *Ann Neurol* 1986;19:294–7.

512. UK Prospective Diabetes Study Group. Intensive blood glucose control with sulphonylureas or insulin compared with conventional treatment and risk of complications in patients with type II diabetes. *Lancet* 1998;352:837–53.

513. Urtasun RC, Chapman JD, Feldstein ML, *et al.* Peripheral neuropathy related to misonidazole: incidence and pathology. *Br J Cancer Suppl* 1978;37:271–5.

514. Valentine WM, Amarnath V, Graham DG, *et al.* CS2-mediated cross-linking of erythrocyte spectrin and neurofilament protein: dose response and temporal relationship to the formation of axonal swellings. *Toxicol Appl Pharmacol* 1997;142:95–105.

515. Vallat JM, De Mascarel HA, Bordessoule D, *et al.* Non-Hodgkin's malignant lymphomas and peripheral neuropathies: 13 cases. *Brain* 1995;118(Part 5):1233–45.

516. Vallat JM, Funalot B, Magy L. Nerve biopsy: requirements for diagnosis and clinical value. *Acta Neuropathol* 2011;121:313–26.

517. Van Allen MW, Frohlich JA, Davis JR. Inherited predisposition to generalized amyloidosis. Clinical and pathological study of a family with neuropathy, nephropathy, and peptic ulcer. *Neurology* 1969;19:10–25.

518. Van de Warrenburg BP, Notermans NC, Schelhaas HJ, *et al.* Peripheral nerve involvement in spinocerebellar ataxias. *Arch Neurol* 2004;61:257–61.

519. Van Goethem G, Martin JJ, Dermaut B, *et al.* Recessive POLG mutations presenting with sensory and ataxic neuropathy in compound heterozygote patients with progressive external ophthalmoplegia. *Neuromuscul Disord* 2003;13:133–42.

520. Vedder E. The pathology of beriberi. *J Am Med Assoc* 1938;110:893–6.

521. Verma P, Chierzi S, Codd AM, *et al.* Axonal protein synthesis and degradation are necessary for efficient growth cone regeneration. *J Neurosci* 2005;25:331–42.

522. Vernino S, Adamski J, Kryzer TJ, *et al.* Neuronal nicotinic ACh receptor antibody in subacute autonomic neuropathy and cancer-related syndromes. *Neurology* 1998;50:1806–13.

523. Verrips A, van Engelen BG, ter Laak H, *et al.* Cerebrotendinous xanthomatosis: controversies about nerve and muscle. Observations in ten patients. *Neuromuscul Disord* 2000;10:407–14.

524. Viader A, Golden JP, Baloh RH *et al.* Schwann cell mitochondrial metabolism supports long-term axonal survival and peripheral nerve function. *J Neurosci* 2011;31:10128–40.

525. Victor M. Polyneuropathy due to nutritional deficiency and alcoholism. In: Dyck PJ, Thomas PK, Lambert H, Bunge R eds. *Peripheral neuropathy.* Philadelphia, PA: WB Saunders, 1984:1899–940.

526. Victor M, Banker BQ, Adams RD. The neuropathy of multiple myeloma. *J Neurochem* 1958;21:73–88.

527. Vincent AM, Callaghan BC, Smith AL, Feldman EL. Diabetic neuropathy: cellular mechanisms as therapeutic targets. *Nat Rev Neurol* 2011;7:573–83.

528. Vital A, Vital C. Polyarteritis nodosa and peripheral neuropathy: ultrastructural study of 13 cases. *Acta Neuropathol (Berl)* 1985;67:136–141.

529. Vital A, Vital C, Julien J, *et al.* Polyneuropathy associated with IgM monoclonal gammopathy: immunological and pathological study in 31 patients. *Acta Neuropathol* 1989;79:160–67.

530. Vital A, Vital C, Ragnaud JM, Baquey A, Aubertin J. IgM cryoglobulin deposits in the peripheral nerve. *Virchow Arch* 1991;418:83–5.

531. Vital A, Lagueny A, Julien J, *et al.* Chronic inflammatory demyelinating polyneuropathy associated with dysglobulinemia: a peripheral nerve biopsy study in 18 cases. *Acta Neuropathol* 2000;100:63–8.

532. Vital A, Ferrer X, Lagueny A, *et al.* Histopathological features of X-linked Charcot–Marie–Tooth disease in 8 patients from 6 families with different connexin 32 mutations. *J Periph Nerv System* 2001;6:79–84.

533. Vital C, Bonnaud E, Arne L, *et al.* Polyneuritis in chronic lymphoid leukaemia: ultrastructural study of the peripheral nerve (author's transl). *Acta Neuropathol (Berl)* 1975;32:169–72.

534. Vital C, Vallat JM, Deminiere C, Loubet A, Leboutet MJ. Peripheral nerve damage during multiple myeloma and Waldenström's macroglobulinemia: an ultrastructural and immunopathologic study. *Cancer* 1982;50:1491–7.

535. Vital C, Bouillot S, Vital A. Significance of uncompacted myelin lamellae in POEMS syndrome. *Muscle Nerve* 2003;27:253–4.

536. Vital C, Vital A, Bouillot S, *et al.* Uncompacted myelin lamellae in peripheral nerve biopsy. *Ultrastruct Pathol* 2003;27:1–5.

537. Vital C, Vital A, Bouillot-Eimer S, *et al.* Amyloid neuropathy: a retrospective study of 35 peripheral nerve biopsies. *J Peripher Nerv Syst* 2004;9:232–41.

538. Vlam L, van der Pol WL, Cats EA, *et al.* Multifocal motor neuropathy: diagnosis, pathogenesis and treatment strategies. *Nat Rev Neurol* 2011;8:41–58.

539. Vondracek P, Seeman P, Hermanova M, Fajkusova L. X-linked Charcot–Marie–Tooth disease: phenotypic expression of a novel mutation Ile 127 Ser in the GJB1 (connexin 32) gene. *Muscle Nerve* 2005;31:252–5.

540. Waller A. Experiments on the section of the glossopharyngeal and hypoglossal nerves of the frog, and observations on the alterations produced thereby in the structure of their primitive fibres. *Phil Trans Roy Soc Lond* (Series B) 1850;140:423–9.

541. Wang JT, Medress ZA, Barres BA. Axon degeneration: molecular mechanisms of a self-destruction pathway. *J Cell Biol* 2012;196:7–18.

542. Wang MS, Wu Y, Culver DG, Glass JD. Pathogenesis of axonal degeneration: parallels between Wallerian degeneration and vincristine neuropathy. *J Neuropathol Exp Neurol* 2000;59:599–606.

543. Wang MS, Davis AA, Culver DG, *et al.* Calpain inhibition protects against taxol-induced sensory neuropathy. *Brain* 2004;127(Part 3):671–9.

544. Wanschitz J, Maier H, Lassmann H, *et al.* Distinct time pattern of complement activation and cytotoxic T cell response in Guillain–Barré syndrome. *Brain* 2003;126(Part 9):2034–42.

545. Ward DM, Shiflett SL, Kaplan J. Chediak–Higashi syndrome: a clinical and molecular view of a rare lysosomal storage disorder. *Curr Mol Med* 2002;2:469–77.

546. Warner LE, Svaren J, Milbrandt J, Lupski JR. Functional consequences of mutations in the early growth response 2 gene (EGR2) correlate with severity of human myelinopathies. *Hum Mol Genet* 1999;8:1245–51.

547. Watkins CC, Sawa A, Jaffrey S, *et al.* Insulin restores neuronal nitric oxide synthase expression and function that is lost in diabetic gastropathy. *J Clin Invest* 2000;106:373–84.

548. Watkins PJ, Thomas PK. Diabetes mellitus and the nervous system. *J Neurol Neurosurg Psychiatry* 1998;65:620–32.

549. Watson DF, Griffin JW. Vacor neuropathy: ultrastructural and axonal transport studies. *J Neuropathol Exp Neurol* 1987;46:96–108.

550. Watson DF, Fittro KP, Hoffman PN, Griffin JW. Phosphorylation-related immunoreactivity and the rate of transport of neurofilaments in chronic 2,5-hexanedione intoxication. *Brain Res* 1991;539:103–9.

551. Way KJ, Katai N, King GL. Protein kinase C and the development of diabetic vascular complications. *Diabet Med* 2001;18:945–59.

552. Weiss MD, Luciano CA, Semino-Mora C, *et al.* Molecular mimicry in chronic inflammatory demyelinating polyneuropathy and melanoma. *Neurology* 1998;51:1738–41.

553. Westermark P, Bergstrom J, Solomon A, *et al.* Transthyretin-derived senile systemic amyloidosis: clinicopathologic and structural considerations. *Amyloid* 2003;10(Suppl 1):48–54.

554. Wetterau JR, Aggerbeck LP, Bouma MF. Absence of microsomal triglyceride transfer protein in individuals with abetalipoproteinemia. *Science* 1992;258:999–1001.

555. Wichman A, Buchthal F, Pezeshkpour GH, Gregg RE. Peripheral neuropathy in abetalipoproteinemia. *Neurology* 1985;35:1279–89.

556. Willis D, Li KW, Zheng JQ, *et al.* Differential transport and local translation of cytoskeletal, injury-response, and neurodegeneration protein mRNAs in axons. *J Neurosci* 2005;25:778–91.

557. Willison HJ, O'Hanlon GM. The immunopathogenesis of Miller Fisher syndrome. *J Neuroimmunol* 1999;100: 3–12.

558. Windebank A. Inherited focal neuropathies. In: Dyck PJ. Thomas P, Griffin J eds. *Peripheral neuropathy,* Vol. 2, 3rd edn. Philadelphia, PA: W.B. Saunders, 1993:1137–48.

559. Windebank A. Metal neuropathy. In: Dyck PJ, Thomas PK, Griffin JW eds. *Peripheral neuropathy.* Philadelphia, PA: W.B. Saunders, 1993:1549–70.

560. Windebank A. Metal neuropathy. In: Dyck P, Thomas PK eds. *Peripheral neuropathy.* Philadelphia, PA: Elsevier–Saunders, 2005:2527–51.

561. Winer J. Guillain–Barré syndrome: clinical variants and their pathogenesis. *J Neuroimmunol* 2011;231:70–2.

562. Winer J, Hughes S, Cooper J, *et al.* Gamma delta T-cells infiltrating sensory nerve biopsies from patients with inflammatory neuropathy. *J Neurol* 2002;249:616–21.

563. Worden AN, Heywood R, Prentice DE, *et al.* Clioquinol toxicity in the dog. *Toxicology* 1978;9:227–38.

564. Xie W, Strong JA, Mao J, Zhang JM. Highly localized interactions between sensory neurons and sprouting sympathetic fibers observed in a transgenic tyrosine hydrozylase reporter mouse. *Mol Pain* 2011;7:53–67.

565. Xiong X, Collins CA. A conditioning lesion protects axons from degeneration via the Wallenda/DLK MAP kinase signaling cascade. *J Neurosci* 2012;32:610–5.

566. Yamamoto M, Ito Y, Mitsuma N, *et al.* Parallel expression of neurotrophic factors and their receptors in chronic inflammatory demyelinating polyneuropathy. *Muscle Nerve* 2002;25:601–4.

567. Yamanaka Y, Sakamoto E, Sakuma Y, *et al.* Lipidosis of the dorsal root ganglia in rats treated with an almitrine metabolite. *Arch Toxicol* 1995;69:391–6.

568. Yan WX, Archelos JJ, Hartung HP, Pollard JD. P0 protein is a target antigen in chronic inflammatory demyelinating polyradiculoneuropathy. *Ann Neurol* 2001;50:286–92.

569. Yoshikawa 11, Nishimura T, Nakatsuji Y, *et al.* Elevated expression of messenger RNA for peripheral myelin protein 22 in biopsied peripheral nerves of patients with Charcot–Marie–Tooth disease type 1A. *Ann Neurol* 1994;35:445–50.

570. Yoshioka M, Shapshak P, Srivastava AK, *et al.* Expression of HIV-1 and interleukin-6 in lumbosacral dorsal root ganglia of patients with AIDS. *Neurology* 1994;44:1120–30.

571. Young P, Suter U. The causes of Charcot–Marie–Tooth disease. *Cell Mol Life Sci* 2003;60:2547–60.

572. Younger DS. Vasculitis of the nervous system. *Curr Opin Neurol* 2004;17: 317–36.

573. Younger DS. Diabetic lumbosacral radiculoplexus neuropathy: postmortem

studied patients and review of the literature. *J Neurol* 2011;258:1364–7.

574. Younger DS, Rowland LP, Latov N, *et al.* Lymphoma, motor neuron diseases and amyotrophic lateral sclerosis. *Ann Neurol* 1991;29:78–86.

575. Younger DS, Rosoklija G, Hays AP, *et al.* Diabetic peripheral neuropathy: a clinicopathologic and immunohistochemical analysis of sural nerve biopsies. *Muscle Nerve* 1996;19:722–7.

576. Yuki N. Infectious origins of, and molecular mimicry in, Guillain–Barré and Fisher syndromes. *Lancet Infect Dis* 2001;1:29–37.

577. Yuki N, Kuwabara S, Koga M, Hirata K. Acute motor axonal neuropathy and acute motor-sensory axonal neuropathy share a common immunological profile. *J Neurol Sci* 1999;168:121–6.

578. Yuki N, Yamada M, Koga M, *et al.* Animal model of axonal Guillain–Barré syndrome induced by sensitization with GM1

579. Zafeiriou DI, Triantafyllou P, Gombakis NP, *et al.* Niemann–Pick type C disease associated with peripheral neuropathy. *Pediatr Neurol* 2003;29:242–4.

580. Zheng H, Xiao WH, Bennett GJ. Functional deficits in peripheral nerve mitochondria in rats with paclitaxel- and oxaliplatin-evoked painful peripheral neuropathy. *Exp Neurol* 2011;232: 154–61.

581. Zherebitskaya E, Schapansky J, Akude E, *et al.* Sensory neurons derived from diabetic rats have diminished internal Ca2+ stores linked to impaired re-uptake by the endoplasmic reticulum. *ASN Neuro* 2012;4(1):pii:e00072.

582. Zochodne DW. Nerve and ganglion blood flow in diabetes: an appraisal. *Int Rev Neurobiol* 2002;50:161–202.

583. Zochodne DW, Ho LT. Normal blood flow but lower oxygen tension in diabetes of young rats: microenvironment and the

ganglioside. *Ann Neurol* 2001;49: 712–20.

influence of sympathectomy. *Can J Physiol Pharmacol* 1992;70:651–9.

584. Zochodne DW, Bolton CF, Wells GA, *et al.* Critical illness polyneuropathy: a complication of sepsis and multiple organ failure. *Brain* 1987;110(Part 4): 819–41.

585. Zochodne DW, Cheng C, Sun H. Diabetes increases sciatic nerve susceptibility to endothelin-induced ischemia. *Diabetes* 1996;45:627–32.

586. Zorick TS, Syroid DE, Arroyo E, *et al.* The transcription factors SCIP and Krox-20 mark distinct stages and cell fates in Schwann cell differentiation. *Mol Cell Neurosci* 1996;8:129–45.

587. Zuccarello M, Anzil AP. A localized model of experimental neuropathy by topical application of disulfiram. *Exp Neurol* 1979;64:699–703.

588. Zuchner S, Mersiyanova IV, Muglia M, *et al.* Mutations in the mitochondrial GTPase mitofusin 2 cause Charcot–Marie–Tooth neuropathy type 2A. *Nat Genet* 2004;36:449–51.

Diseases of Skeletal Muscle

Caroline A Sewry, Susan C Brown, Rahul Phadke and Francesco Muntoni

INTRODUCTION

The diagnosis of neuromuscular disorders is continuing its dramatic development of recent years. The main reasons behind this progress are related not only to improvements in protein-based assays that can directly or indirectly point towards a specific condition, but also the wider application of techniques such as magnetic resonance (MR) imaging and the molecular genetic revolution brought about by techniques such as next-generation sequencing. Indeed, following the identification of the gene responsible for Duchenne muscular dystrophy (DMD), which initiated a revolution in molecular diagnosis in the field, the defective genes of numerous neuromuscular disorders are now known, and the list is extending almost on a weekly basis (see the gene table of neuromuscular disorders at www. musclegenetable.fr). The genetic diversity of these disorders is far greater than appreciated before the 1990s, as exemplified by the number of genes responsible for the muscular dystrophies. For a few conditions, molecular analysis is now so reliable that muscle pathology often contributes little additional diagnostic information, so muscle biopsy is rarely performed. In particular, molecular analysis is now the test of choice for the diagnosis of spinal muscular atrophy (SMA), myotonic muscular dystrophies (DM1 and often DM2) and facioscapulohumeral muscular dystrophy (FSHD), and also for conditions in which there is no specific muscle pathology, such as disorders associated with mutations in the lamin A/C gene and the limb-girdle muscular dystrophy (LGMD) due to mutations in the gene encoding anoctamin 5 (ANO5). Similarly, muscle pathology may be absent, minimal or non-specific in myasthenic syndromes, where the combination of careful clinical and electrophysiological studies often provides the diagnosis.

In most other conditions, muscle pathology continues to play an important role in directing molecular analysis and in identifying morphological defects associated with specific disorders, such as in metabolic disorders and inflammatory myopathies. The need for a biopsy is sometimes questioned in disorders in which molecular defects are relatively easily identified. For example, in DMD 66 per cent of cases have a deletion or duplication that is detected by routine molecular techniques, but phenotype does not always correlate with genotype, with about 10 per cent of cases being exceptions to the reading frame rule, and therefore knowledge of protein expression and pathology is important. In cases of DMD with less common mutations (which are missed by the standard assays that readily identify the common splice site or point mutations) immunohistochemistry easily demonstrates the absence of dystrophin, which can then be followed by detailed molecular analysis.

Muscle pathology can sometimes provide a prognostic assessment of the severity of the condition, based on protein expression. The absence of dystrophin is a feature of the severe form of DMD, whereas residual expression of dystrophin is found in the milder allelic Becker muscular dystrophy (BMD) variant. In BMD there is also a broad correlation between the amount of residual protein expression and the severity of the resulting phenotype, as in many forms of recessive muscular dystrophy. Increasingly, the role for muscle pathology is to assist in directing analysis of the genes responsible for neuromuscular disorders, especially with the wider appreciation of their overlapping clinical features.

Although genetic detection techniques are rapidly changing because of the advent of next-generation sequencing, most diagnostic laboratories worldwide still rely on Sanger sequencing and/or multiple ligation-dependent probe amplification techniques. The assessment of several genes is still both expensive and slow; a final diagnosis is increasingly required for planning strategies of patient management and for accurate genetic counselling. In addition, with the increasing availability of mutation-specific experimental therapies, the need for accurate diagnosis is likely to increase further. Although it is likely that the next-generation sequencing platform will enter the diagnostic arena in the next few years, muscle pathology will still be relied on to identify the main pathological features. Indeed, it is anticipated that the immense number of sequencing studies will identify variants of unknown significance in several potential candidate genes, so the assignment of their pathogenicity will still require careful clinical and pathological skills.

The identification of defects in families of interacting proteins and the discovery that clinical boundaries between conditions caused by distinct protein products can be blurred have challenged traditional clinical classifications. In muscular dystrophies, for example, a classification based on the location of defective proteins has been proposed.[93,279] Defects in groups of proteins of the extracellular matrix, in components of the dystrophin-associated sarcolemmal protein complex and in nuclear and sarcomeric proteins are now well established. One advantage of such a classification is that the clinical phenotype is often similar among disorders of proteins with a shared location, or disorders that are part of the same functional complex. For example, the clinical features of patients whose muscles are deficient in dystrophin are difficult to distinguish from those of patients with a deficiency in one of the sarcoglycans. Similarly, defects in two nuclear proteins, emerin and lamin A/C, result in very similar forms of Emery–Dreifuss muscular dystrophy. In this chapter, we adhere to the traditional clinical classification because it is the clinical symptoms that lead to referral and to the need for a muscle biopsy. Molecular analysis and identification of the defective gene provide the ultimate diagnosis, but this is not usually the starting point. We will, however, make direct reference to both the underlying molecular defect and the best strategy for arriving at a final diagnosis.

This chapter aims to highlight the important role of muscle pathology in the diagnosis of neuromuscular disorders, while presenting relevant clinical and genetic advances. It emphasizes the importance of correlating muscle pathology with clinical, electrophysiological and biochemical data and that muscle pathology must never be assessed in isolation. The value of multidisciplinary team meetings in which the relevant aspects related to the condition affecting patients with neuromuscular disorders cannot be overemphasized.

To appreciate the spectrum of abnormal features in relation to a particular disorder, it is important to understand the structure of normal muscle and aspects of its development. The first sections of this chapter therefore summarize the anatomical features of normal muscle followed by the variety of histological, histochemical, ultrastructural and immunohistochemical changes that can occur in pathological muscle, with particular emphasis on the location of proteins assessed during the diagnostic process. This is followed by descriptions of the pathological changes associated with particular disorders and a summary of the related molecular defects.

CLINICAL ASSESSMENT OF PATIENTS WITH NEUROMUSCULAR DISEASE

The main reasons for suspecting a neuromuscular disorder are muscle weakness, muscle stiffness, muscle cramps or discomfort (especially during, or immediately following,

exercise) and muscle fatigue with activity, often associated with contractures of one or multiple joints. Occasionally, incidental elevation of serum creatine kinase (CK) can also be an indication of underlying skeletal muscle disease in the preclinical stages. A full clinical assessment of the patient is essential. Diagnosis should always be based on a detailed account of the clinical and family histories and the clinical examination. Additionally, special investigations that may be informative include the assay of serum enzymes, muscle imaging, electrophysiology in selected cases and muscle biopsy. The ultimate diagnosis in many cases relies on the identification of the causative genetic defect, which allows the patient and his/her family to receive genetic counselling.

It is important to define the onset and progression of symptoms. In general, conditions can be grouped into those with onset around the time of birth or within the first 6 months of life (e.g. severe SMAs, congenital myopathies, congenital muscular dystrophies [CMDs], congenital myotonic dystrophy), those with onset in infancy (e.g. milder SMA variants, some congenital myopathies), childhood disorders (e.g. progressive muscular dystrophies, such as DMD and various LGMDs) and muscle disorders of adolescence and adulthood (e.g. some neuropathies, some LGMDs, most of the myofibrillar myopathies, oculopharyngeal MD, myotonic dystrophy type 2 and acquired disorders). Metabolic disorders and myasthenic syndromes can present at various ages. Additional information can be gathered from the pattern of symptom progression. A static course, or a relatively static course, in a child with onset of weakness in infancy suggests a congenital myopathy or SMA rather than a more progressive form of CMD, such as merosin-deficient CMD (MDC1A). In contrast, progression of muscle weakness characterizes most of the LGMDs and DMD, but also myofibrillar myopathies. The presence or absence of associated features such as cardiac, brain or ocular involvement is also a very helpful clinical indicator. Table 25.1 summarizes key points that should be addressed during a comprehensive consultation.

Clinical Assessment

The clinical assessment of a patient with neuromuscular disease has to consider several diagnostic issues:

- differentiating weakness from hypotonia;
- presence and distribution of contractures;
- distribution of weakness (proximal versus distal/facial/ocular/bulbar);
- presence of muscle wasting or hypertrophy;
- fluctuation of muscle weakness during the course of the day or with exercise;
- involvement of other systems (e.g. heart, central nervous system, eye, skin, subcutaneous tissues).

Differentiating Weakness from Hypotonia

It is important to be aware that children with chromosomal and neurometabolic disorders can have marked central hypotonia that resembles the weakness observed in children with neuromuscular disorders. A typical example is Prader–Willi syndrome, a chromosomal disorder in which affected children are often considered weak. Similarly, in syndromes with joint hypermobility, such as Ehlers–Danlos syndrome, there can be a confusing combination of extreme hypotonia and delayed

TABLE 25.1 General clinical features for assessment of neuromuscular disorders

Age at onset of symptoms
Age developmental milestones achieved
Maximal functional ability achieved (e.g. sitting, standing, walking)
Distribution of muscle weakness
Progression of weakness
Presence of facial and/or bulbar weakness
Distribution of muscle wasting
Cramps on exercise
Presence of ptosis or ophthalmoplegia
Presence of cataracts
Presence of hypotonia associated with weakness
Ligamentous laxity
Skeletal involvement
    Contractures
    Hip dislocation
    Spinal rigidity
    Scoliosis
Central nervous system involvement
    Mental retardation
    Epilepsy
    Structural brain changes
    White matter changes on brain magnetic resonance imaging
Cardiac involvement
    Dilated cardiomyopathy
    Conduction system disease
    Restrictive cardiomyopathy
    Hypertrophic cardiomyopathy
Respiratory insufficiency
Reduced or absent reflexes

motor milestones. However, significant weakness is absent in both these conditions, and patients with Ehlers–Danlos and Prader–Willi syndromes are capable of performing unexpectedly vigorous movements against gravity and resistance that would not be expected on the basis of their extreme hypotonia. There are nevertheless conditions in which features of central nervous system involvement (i.e. central hypotonia) and skeletal muscle involvement coexists (e.g. mitochondrial diseases). There are also rare forms in which typical Ehlers–Danlos features coexist with a myopathy, such as the recently identified form due to *FKPB14* mutations (invariably associated with neurosensory hearing loss).[20] These variants often represent diagnostic challenges, which can nevertheless be helped by the study of muscle pathology.

Contractures

Limitation of joint movement is an extremely useful sign to assess. Multiple contractures at birth (arthrogryposis, if four or more joints are affected) suggest prenatal onset of immobility and weakness. A number of muscular dystrophies have a typical pattern of progressive contractures, for example Achilles tendon and elbows in Emery–Dreifuss muscular dystrophy. The presence of spinal rigidity and scoliosis is also a helpful indicator in neuromuscular disorders. Foot deformity, such as pes cavus, together with tightness of the Achilles tendons and associated distal weakness, usually, but not invariably, points towards a neurogenic disorder.

Pattern of Muscle Weakness

Different patterns of muscle weakness have traditionally helped to distinguish different types of neuromuscular disorders (Figure 25.1).[127] Muscle weakness can be generalized

(as in several congenital myopathies), or it can affect predominantly the proximal limb muscles (e.g. in DMD, some LGMDs and SMA types II and III), the distal limb muscles (e.g. in peripheral neuropathies, distal variants of SMA, distal forms of muscular dystrophies and distal myopathies), the scapulohumeral and facial muscles (e.g. in FSHD), the humeroperoneal muscles (e.g. in Emery–Dreifuss muscular dystrophy), the extraocular muscles and the levator palpebrae (e.g. in mitochondrial disorders and myasthenia), and the axial and respiratory muscles (e.g. in some forms of muscular dystrophy, the allelic conditions multi-minicore disease and rigid spine muscular dystrophy type 1 [RSMD1], and metabolic conditions such as Pompe disease and hereditary myopathy with early respiratory involvement [HMERF]).

Pattern of Muscle Wasting or Enlargement

The pattern of muscle wasting or enlargement is another useful indicator of an underlying neuromuscular disorder. Several of the childhood forms of muscular dystrophy, such as DMD, BMD and some forms of LGMD, are associated with significant calf muscle hypertrophy and, in the initial phase of the conditions, also with hypertrophy of the vastus lateralis, brachioradialis and triceps muscles. Muscle hypertrophy, especially of the leg muscles, also characterizes some of the congenital forms of muscular dystrophy, and the milder allelic LGMD variants related to abnormal expression of α-dystroglycan. In some conditions, such as LGMD2I and MDC1C, hypertrophy may also affect the tongue. Muscle enlargement is often referred to as a 'pseudo-hypertrophy' because the hypertrophy reflects an increase in fibrous and fatty tissues, rather than muscle fibres. However, a true hypertrophic component is present in the initial phases of several conditions.

In some muscular dystrophies, muscle wasting predominates. This is the case for LGMD2B (distal leg muscles), Emery–Dreifuss muscular dystrophy (generalized, but with severe involvement of humeral muscles), FSHD (scapulohumeral wasting, often asymmetrical), LGMD2A, the Ullrich form of CMD, and CMD with rigid spine (RSMD1). In most forms of muscular dystrophy, wasting and hypertrophy coexist. For example, in DMD and LGMD2I, it is common to observe striking calf hypertrophy associated with wasting of the pectoralis, whereas hypertrophy of the quadriceps and wasting of the distal leg muscles often coexist in LGMD2B. Hypertrophy (or wasting) can, in some conditions, be asymmetrical. Typical examples are asymmetrical wasting in FSHD and asymmetrical hypertrophy in female manifesting carriers of DMD, and it is a feature noted in cases of LGMD caused by defects in the *ANO5* gene. Neurogenic disorders are typically associated with muscle wasting, and in congenital myopathies there is usually generalized muscle wasting. Selective distal wasting can be feature of various myopathies of late and early onset. The complex pattern of muscle involvement in different neuromuscular conditions may in specific instances influence the selection of the site of a muscle to biopsy (see Muscle Biopsy, p. 1520).

Muscle Weakness: Static, Fluctuating or Progressive

In the majority of neuromuscular disorders, weakness is either static, or progresses slowly or more rapidly with time. However, in a few conditions, weakness fluctuates

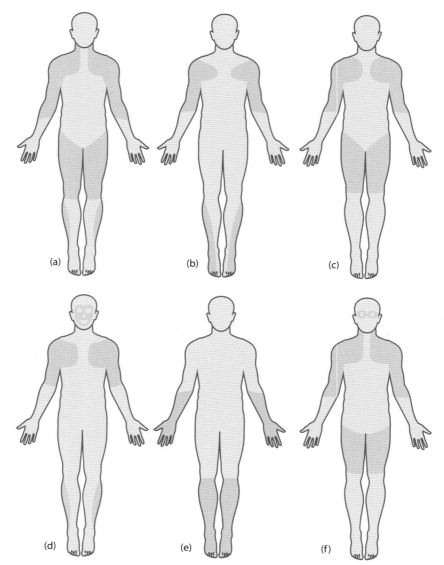

25.1 Distribution of predominant muscle weakness in various forms of muscular dystrophy. (a) Duchenne and Becker, **(b)** Emery-Dreifuss, **(c)** limb-girdle, **(d)** faci0scapulohumeral, **(e)** distal and **(f)** oculopharyngeal.

Adapted by permission from BMJ Publishing Group from Emery AE. The muscular dystrophies. BMJ 1998;317:991–5.

significantly, with relatively or completely preserved muscle strength after awakening, followed by marked fatigability within hours or shorter periods of time. Such marked fatigability is the hallmark of myasthenia but can also be found in mitochondrial disorders, whereas periodic paralysis is a feature of several channelopathies. Muscle stiffness and difficulty in relaxing muscle following exercise are features of both dystrophic and non-dystrophic myotonias, conditions in which electrophysiology plays a major role (see later).

Involvement of Other Systems

Although most myopathies and neuropathies exclusively affect their primary target organ (muscle or nerve), in a few conditions there is significant involvement of other organs. Structural brain abnormalities characterize several of the CMDs (see Congenital Muscular Dystrophies and Allied Disorders, p. 1565). Often these are associated with marked changes of signal intensity of the supratentorial white matter on MR imaging, which represents abnormal myelination and oedema, rather than loss of myelin. When present in isolation, striking white matter involvement is characteristic of merosin-deficient CMD (MDC1A). Lesions in the basal ganglia and cerebellum are common in mitochondrial disorders. Functional brain involvement (i.e. mental retardation with normal imaging) is also common in DMD and myotonic dystrophy, especially the congenital form. Structural eye involvement is found in disorders with hypoglycosylation of α-dystroglycan (Walker–Warburg syndrome, muscle–eye–brain disease, Fukuyama CMD), and retinal and auditory abnormalities can be found in a proportion of patients with FSHD. Cataracts are a feature of myotonic dystrophies, one form of dystroglycanopathy (with *GMPPB* mutations), and rare disorders such as Marinesco–Sjorgren and Vici syndromes.[99,398] Skin involvement (in the form of follicular hyperkeratosis and abnormal scar formation) is almost invariable in Ullrich CMD, whereas a characteristic rash occurs in dermatomyositis, and ichthyosis is often a feature in cases with mutations in the gene encoding choline kinase (*CHKB*).[296] Lipoatrophy affecting the limbs can be found in some patients with Emery–Dreifuss muscular dystrophy, in other conditions related to defects in proteins of the nuclear envelope and in patients with defects in the cavin-1 (*PTRF*) gene.[351] Cardiac involvement, typically in the form of a dilated cardiomyopathy, is a common secondary complication of several muscular dystrophies, in particular those associated with the dystrophin-associated glycoprotein (DAG) complex (dystrophin/sarcoglycans). Cardiac conduction defects occur in myotonic dystrophies and in Emery–Dreifuss muscular dystrophies. Hypertrophic cardiomyopathy can complicate conditions such as myosinopathies, whereas restrictive cardiomyopathies are essentially confined to myofibrillar myopathies and other rare metabolic diseases. Defects in some genes can cause predominantly a cardiomyopathy or a skeletal myopathy and occasionally both, for example the *MYH7* and the *TTN* genes encoding slow myosin and titin, respectively.

Investigations

Biochemistry

Serum enzymes are elevated in a number of muscle disorders, and CK activity is most commonly tested. The upper limit of normal varies between laboratories and must be established by each one. It can be influenced by ethnic origin, and levels may rise following exercise or intramuscular injection. There may also be extramuscular causes of CK elevation (such as bone CK in cases of fractures and bone tumours); if this situation is suspected, then bone CK can be differentiated from muscle CK by analysis of the different CK isoforms.

Elevated CK activity is considered to reflect muscle damage. The elevation can be categorized as mild if levels are two to five times normal, moderate if five to ten times normal, and markedly elevated if more than ten times normal. Very high levels (50–200 times normal) occur in some forms of muscular dystrophy, such as DMD and some forms of LGMD (Table 25.2), whereas moderate levels may occur in inflammatory myopathies (although CK can be normal in some cases of myositis and also in some LGMDs). In contrast, normal or mild to moderate elevation can be seen in patients with congenital myopathies, slowly evolving neurogenic disorders and some forms of congenital muscular dystrophy, such as Ullrich CMD and Bethlem myopathy. In metabolic disorders, CK may be normal at rest and elevated only after exercise.

In addition to CK, other enzymes and myoglobin may be elevated when there is significant muscle damage. If the levels of *myoglobin* exceed the renal threshold for reabsorption, then myoglobin becomes macroscopically visible in the

TABLE 25.2 Elevation of serum creatine kinase in the most common myopathic conditions and muscular dystrophies

Normal or mild elevation:
Nemaline myopathies
Core myopathies (central core disease/multi-minicore disease)
Centronuclear myopathies
Spinal muscular atrophy
Mitochondrial myopathies

Mild to moderate elevation:
Ullrich congenital muscular dystrophy
Bethlem myopathy
Emery–Dreifuss muscular dystrophy
Facioscapulohumeral muscular dystrophy
Myofibrillar myopathies
Limb-girdle muscular dystrophy type 2G, 2H, 1C
Oculopharyngeal muscular dystrophy
Myotonic dystrophy
Mitochondrial DNA depletion
Inflammatory myopathies

Marked elevation:
Duchenne and Becker muscular dystrophy
Limb-girdle muscular dystrophy 2A, 2B, 2C-F, 2I, 2L
Pompe disease
Congenital muscular dystrophy 1A-1D
Muscle–eye–brain disease
Fukuyama muscular dystrophy
Walker–Warburg syndrome

urine (myoglobinuria). This complication is typically associated with metabolic disorders or following general anaesthesia in malignant hyperthermia; it can, however, occur spontaneously in some patients with muscular dystrophy.[346] Table 25.2 summarizes the pattern of serum CK elevation in the most common neuromuscular conditions.

Elevation of *serum* and *cerebrospinal fluid lactate* is often seen in mitochondrial disorders and is frequently accompanied by an elevated lactate:pyruvate ratio. This is not always the case: for example, deficiency of complex I is typically associated with normal lactate levels. The study of both lactate and ammonia levels under ischaemic conditions can also provide useful information in other metabolic conditions. Elevation of serum ammonia, but not lactate, suggests a defect of glycogen metabolism (e.g. McArdle disease). In contrast, an elevation of lactate, but not ammonia, suggests a defect in purine metabolism (e.g. myoadenylate deaminase deficiency). These tests, however, are now rarely used, especially in children, and direct determination of enzymatic activity is much more precise in these conditions.

Serum autoantibodies directed against the acetylcholine receptor (AChR) and muscle-specific kinase (MuSK) can be demonstrated in the majority of patients with acquired autoimmune myasthenia, and antibodies to voltage-gated calcium channels on the presynaptic membrane cause Lambert–Eaton syndrome. Neuromyotonia results from antibodies to a presynaptic voltage-gated potassium channel. The study of autoantibodies in other neuromuscular disorders is mainly restricted to the myositic conditions, where there is an expanding list that includes anti-nuclear antibodies, anti-RNA antibodies and anti-signal recognition particle antibodies, and those associated with autoimmune neuropathies (see appropriate sections).[63]

Electrophysiology

A detailed description of electrophysiological techniques in the diagnosis of neuromuscular disease is outside the scope of this chapter, and only a summary is given here. Details can be found in appropriate textbooks.[254] Measurement of nerve conduction velocity and electromyography (EMG) are the most useful techniques. Conduction velocity is dependent on the diameter and degree of myelination of motor nerves and increases with age. In neonates, conduction velocity is only about half that of adults. in demyelinating disorders (peripheral neuropathies) and disorders associated with amyelination of axons, such as disorders linked to defects in the gene encoding laminin α2, motor nerve conduction velocity may be slower than normal.[413] In axonal neuropathies, the velocity may be normal or only slightly reduced.

Electromyography is useful in determining whether the muscle is normal or abnormal, and whether the pattern is 'myopathic' or 'neuropathic'. However, because the procedure is painful and cooperation from patients is necessary, its use should be limited to cases in which there are no other definitive clues pointing towards a primary myopathy. The muscle selected for testing should be appropriate to the clinical involvement. In myopathic conditions the potentials generated are of low amplitude, polyphasic and of short duration, whereas in neurogenic disorders spontaneous fibrillation potentials and fasciculation potentials occur. Fibrillation potentials are biphasic and of low amplitude and short duration, whereas fasciculation potentials are polyphasic and of long duration and high amplitude. In conditions associated with axonal sprouting and reinnervation, the number of muscle fibres innervated by a single motor neuron increases and 'giant' motor units are detected. Myotonic conditions produce a characteristic EMG pattern, with spontaneous bursts of potentials in rapid succession, waxing and waning, and a characteristic acoustic signal. Repetitive nerve stimulation and especially single-fibre EMG are indispensable in assessing end plate disorders.

Imaging

Imaging of muscle using ultrasound, computed tomography (CT) and MR imaging is increasingly used to diagnose muscle disorders and can help to direct molecular analysis. Muscle imaging can reveal a striking selectivity of muscle pathology, and specific patterns indicative of neuropathies, rather than myopathies, have been described.[284,431]

Imaging of the brain, in particular MR imaging, also plays a significant role in the evaluation of patients with CMDs, mitochondrial disorders, and other neurometabolic and neurodegenerative conditions, for example the variant of pontocerebellar hypoplasia associated with motor neuron degeneration or neuroaxonal dystrophy. In CMDs, abnormalities range from the abnormal signal intensity of the supratentorial white matter (in MDC1A) to the frontoparietal and, to a lesser extent, occipital pachygyria observed in Fukuyama CMD and muscle–eye–brain disease, to the severe and almost complete lissencephaly that characterizes Walker–Warburg syndrome.[87] Basal ganglia abnormalities are present in several mitochondrial disorders, but other changes, such as stroke-like areas and abnormal white matter signal intensity, can also be found in these conditions.

Muscle Biopsy

Selection of the site for muscle biopsy should take into account the distribution of weakness and any selective muscle involvement. Imaging techniques can be informative for selecting an appropriate site. It is usually advisable to select a moderately affected muscle. The vastus lateralis is often chosen in children and adults, and sometimes the deltoid or biceps, although in distal myopathies a lower limb muscle may be appropriate. One must not choose a muscle that is so severely involved that it is likely to have been replaced by fat or connective tissue and thus contains very few muscle fibres, nor choose a muscle that is so little affected that it lacks characteristic pathological changes. It is also important to remember that there are anatomical differences between muscles, particularly with regard to the proportions of fibre types,[212] and to take into account features that may relate to age, to the use of the muscle and to any previous trauma, such as sport injuries and damage that may have been caused by EMG needles. Sites near myotendinous insertions and near the fascia should also be avoided, because these often show increased numbers of internal nuclei, splitting of fibres, variation in fibre size, and inclusions.

Biopsy Technique

Muscle biopsies can be obtained by an open surgical or needle technique, provided a suitable instrument is used. Open biopsies provide a large sample, which may be required for biochemical assays, but in many situations the amount of muscle obtained with a needle technique is adequate for diagnostic purposes. The choice of technique is then dependent on local preference and expertise.

Needle muscle biopsies from adults and children can usually be taken under local anaesthesia, but many hospitals now require them to be done under general anaesthesia, and appropriate precautions are needed.[117] Local anaesthesia avoids the hazards that may occur in patients with poor respiratory function and in those at risk of malignant hyperthermia. With local anaesthetics, it is important to infiltrate only the skin and subcutaneous tissues and to avoid direct injection of the muscle because this can induce artefacts. Needle biopsies leave only a small scar a few millimetres in size, whereas the scar from an open biopsy may be considerably larger.

The biopsy needle that we favour is based on that developed by Bergström[117,123] and provides sufficient material for a variety of morphological and biochemical techniques. It is essential that needle samples are oriented under a dissecting microscope, in order to obtain good transverse alignment of as many fibres as possible. An average needle biopsy is approximately 3–4 mm³ and weighs about 20–30 mg; a typical example obtained by this method is shown in Figure 25.2. Following removal from the needle, part of the sample is mounted in a freezing compound, such as OCT (optimal cutting temperature) or Tissue-Tek, and frozen using isopentane or propane cooled in liquid nitrogen for histological, histochemical and immunohistochemical studies. A separate piece is snap frozen

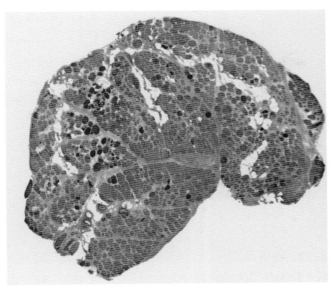

25.2 Transverse section of a whole needle biopsy from a patient with Duchenne muscular dystrophy taken with a 5 mm Bergström needle. H&E.

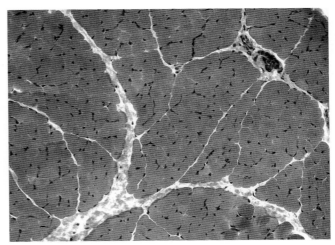

25.3 Low power view of normal muscle showing the arrangement of closely packed muscle fibres into fascicles with narrow perimysial bands of connective tissue. Note also the blood vessel in the perimysium. H&E.

directly into liquid nitrogen for immunoblotting, metabolic studies and RNA extraction, and a further small sample is fixed in glutaraldehyde for electron microscopy.[117] Samples required for studies of respiratory chain enzymes should be frozen rapidly after removal but a short delay before freezing (15 to 20 minutes) has no detrimental effect on light microscopical studies, provided the tissue is kept moist in *lightly* dampened gauze or wrapped in cling film. Delays longer than 1 or 2 hours also have a minimal effect on light microscopical studies but may affect the amount of detectable glycogen, respiratory chain enzyme activity and some ultrastructural features.

Optimal freezing of samples not only avoids the architectural distortion induced by fixation and wax embedding, but also ensures preservation of enzyme activity for histochemical and biochemical studies. An inadequately frozen sample shows holes in the muscle fibres produced by ice crystals and can influence interpretation. Some immunohistochemistry is possible on archival paraffin wax-embedded material using antigen-retrieval methods (depending on the antibody), but a full panel of studies is not possible. Samples should be frozen as soon as possible after removal, but some meaningful studies can be performed on post-mortem samples. However, enzyme activities are often altered or absent and may be difficult to interpret. Immunohistochemical studies of some proteins, such as laminins and myosins, are possible in post-mortem material but plasma membrane proteins are not always detectable, depending on the interval between death and freezing of the sample.

Use of Tissues Other Than Muscle in the Diagnosis of Neuromuscular Disorders

Although muscle is the tissue of choice for diagnosis, useful information on the immunolocalization of some proteins can be obtained from other tissues. In particular, laminin α2, collagen VI, emerin and plectin are expressed in skin. Similarly, prenatal diagnosis can be aided by studies of proteins in chorionic villi, for example laminin α2 and collagen VI (see Application of Immunohistochemistry in the Diagnosis of Neuromuscular Disorders, p. 1542; and Congenital Muscular Dystrophies and Allied Disorders, p. 1565).

Cultured fibroblasts from skin biopsies are useful for studies of mitochondrial metabolism, such as assaying cytochrome *c* oxidase (COX) and for studies of fatty acid oxidation. Research also suggests that cultured fibroblasts may be useful for assessing collagen VI and glycosylation.[225,429] Glycogen accumulation in cases with acid maltase deficiency can be demonstrated in lymphocytes with the periodic acid–Schiff (PAS) reaction, and using lymphocytes for other tests is developing, such as immunoblotting of dysferlin.[104]

NORMAL MUSCLE: STRUCTURE AND FUNCTION

Basic Organization

The word 'muscle' is derived from the Latin *mus* ('mouse') and refers to the resemblance of the muscle belly to a mouse. Muscle is a major constituent of total body mass. Individual muscles vary greatly in size, shape and architecture, and with regard to the arrangement of fibres relative to the axis of force generation.

Each muscle is composed of a variable number of muscle fibres, nerves and an associated vascular network, all enclosed within a connective tissue sheath, the epimysium, which protects the structure from the damaging effects of repeated cycles of contraction and relaxation. Collagen types I, III, IV, V and VI, and fibronectin are major components of the connective tissue in muscle, and the relative amounts of each type differ between the various connective tissue layers. These are divided into the outermost *epimysium*, surrounding the entire muscle; the *perimysium*, which is formed from extensions of the epimysium and divides the muscle fibres into bundles or fascicles; and the *endomysium*, a layer around each individual fibre (Figures 25.3 and 25.4). The epimysium, perimysium and endomysium

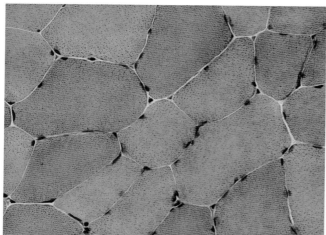

25.4 Normal muscle architecture showing the closely packed polygonal muscle fibres with multiple basophilic nuclei at their periphery. The intermyofibrillar network (including mitochondria) is seen as fine granularity. The slight difference in intensity relates to different fibre types, with type 1 fibres staining slightly darker. Note also the capillaries between the fibres, some of which lie in indentations of the sarcolemma. H&E.

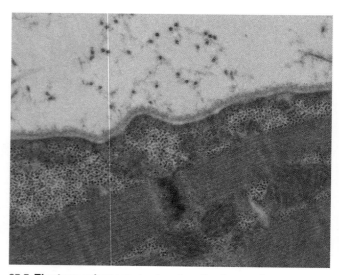

25.5 Electron micrograph showing the inner plasma membrane and outer basal lamina of the sarcolemma separated by the translucent lamina lucida. Note also the collagen in the extracellular matrix.

extend beyond the belly of the muscle into either a tendon or an aponeurosis, which connects the entire muscle to the periosteum of a bone, or to the connective tissue of other muscles. The continuity of the connective tissue network that surrounds and divides individual muscle fibres ensures that contractile force is transmitted efficiently to the bone. Genetic defects that interfere with this arrangement are the underlying cause of many forms of neuromuscular disease.

Muscle growth is associated with changes both in the connective tissue (the width of the perimysium is relatively wider in neonates than in infants and adults) and in the cross-sectional area and length of individual muscle fibres. In adult males, fibres of the quadriceps muscle are usually 40–80 μm in diameter and may reach a length of up to 10 cm.

Muscle fibres are polygonal in shape (see Figure 25.4). They are syncytial cells, and in normal mature muscle the majority of nuclei are located at the periphery of the fibre.

Muscle Fibre Basement Membrane

Individual muscle fibres are surrounded by a layer of extracellular matrix called the basement membrane, which is composed of two layers: an internal basal lamina (also referred to as the lamina densa) that directly opposes the plasma membrane and an external, fibrillar reticular lamina (Figure 25.5 and Box 25.1). The basal lamina is secreted by the muscle fibre itself and appears as an amorphous or finely granular layer. Dystroglycan and other cell surface receptors are thought to be key players in its initial deposition and organization.[505] The basal lamina is usually 20–30 nm thick, although more recent measurements of the inner limiting membrane of the human eye indicate that it may be much thicker when fully hydrated. It typically consists of non-fibrillar collagen, in particular collagen IV, a number of glycoproteins (laminins, perlecan and nidogen) and proteoglycans. Beneath the lamina densa is the lamina lucida, which appears as a 10–15 nm translucent gap between the plasma membrane and lamina lucida. The reticular layer is known to contain collagens

BOX 25.1. Basal lamina

The term 'basal lamina' is often used synonymously with 'basement membrane', and the exact structure being referred to is then unclear. The basement membrane described by early histologists refers to the lamina densa and the reticular layer. Throughout this chapter, the term 'basal lamina' is used to describe the lamina densa (the fine granular layer) and the term 'basement membrane' to indicate when the reticular layer is also included.

(including type III) and fibronectin, which are embedded in an amorphous proteoglycan-rich ground substance. Collagen VI helps to connect the basal lamina to the reticular layer.[378] In pathological muscle, the reticular layer may become thickened and prominent. Collagen IV and laminin form two distinct self-assembling networks that are linked via a number of proteins including nidogen. Both these networks have multiple binding partners in the basal lamina, reticular lamina and cell membrane, which anchor membrane-associated receptors and form a link from the cytoskeleton of the muscle fibre to the reticular lamina. This arrangement not only contributes to the tensile strength of the complete muscle fibre, but also plays an important role in development, regeneration and synaptogenesis.

The Myotendinous Junction

The myotendinous junction is the primary structure responsible for transmitting force from muscle contraction to the tendon and consequently plays a role in joint position and stabilization. The fibre membrane is highly folded in this area and interdigitates with the surrounding collagenous matrix, thus reducing the contractile stress applied per unit area of junctional membrane. Ultrastructurally, the membrane at these points shows a marked layer of electron-dense material that merges with the Z-line of the myofibrils (Figure 25.6). Internal nuclei are common at these

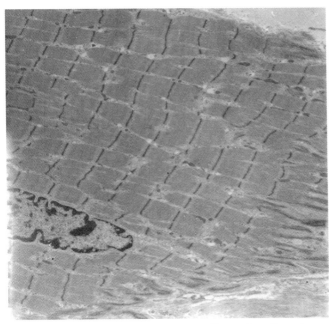

25.6 Electron micrograph of a myotendinous junction showing folds of the sarcolemma and electron-dense areas that merge with the Z-line.

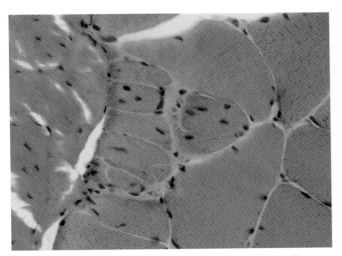

25.7 Myotendinous junctions between fibres and adjacent fascia. Note the presence of internal nuclei and how the folds give the impression of fibre size variation. H&E.

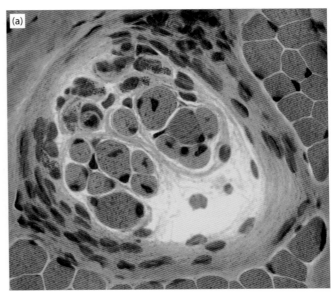

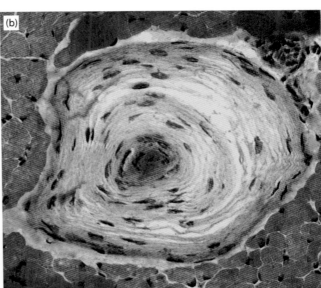

25.8 (a) A muscle spindle showing encapsulated intrafusal fibres with internal nuclei and sensory nerves. (b) A Pacinian corpuscle with concentric lamellae of fibrous connective tissue. H&E.

sites (Figure 25.7) and a number of cytoskeletal proteins appear to be increased, such as utrophin, vinculin and talin, in addition to two transmembrane receptors, DAG and integrin α7β1D.[17,201] The absence of dystrophin, utrophin or integrin α7β1D causes an alteration in the extent of membrane folding.[105] Acetylcholine receptors are also present at myotendinous junctions; the precise reason for this is unclear, but it has been suggested that they may play a role in muscle repair processes.[26]

Proprioceptors in Muscle

Limb movement and changes in position lead to deformation of tissues around the relevant joints, including skin muscles, tendons, fascia, joint capsules and ligaments. Each of these

tissues is innervated by specific types of mechanically sensitive receptors, and their density varies across muscles and regions of the body.[343] The encapsulated sensory endings of skeletal muscles are all mechanoreceptors that respond to changes in length (muscle spindle primary and secondary endings), tension (tendon organs) or pressure/vibration (lamellated corpuscles).[14] Muscle spindles are specialized structures that mediate stretch reflexes as well as limb and axial body position sensation (proprioception). Their basic structure is that of specialized, encapsulated muscle fibres (intrafusal muscle fibres) innervated by sensory (groups Ia and II) and motor (fusimotor) axons that form mechanoreceptors relaying muscle stretch sensation to the central nervous system. Spindles are usually located between the muscle fascicles in the perimysial connective tissue, often adjacent to nerves or vessels (Figure 25.8a).

They are found in all muscles except those of the face. (For details of the physiology and anatomy of the muscle spindle see Proske and Gandevia.[343]) Immature isoforms of myosin are present in some normal spindle fibres, even though the extrafusal are fully mature, and other isoforms associated with immaturity such as the brain isoform of phosphorylase and cardiac actin also occur in spindle fibres. Additional proprioceptor endings (Golgi tendon organs) are located where muscle fibres attach to tendons. These respond to tension (force) exerted by the muscle, and activity in these axons inhibits muscle contraction. Lamellated corpuscles are less numerous. Those with few lamellae are generally classified as paciniform corpuscles, whereas those with more numerous lamellae and an ovoid shape are referred to as Pacinian corpuscles, though this distinction is arbitrary. Lamellated corpuscles respond to compression, with the number of lamellae determining the sensitivity to the phasic component of the stimulus. Pacinian corpuscles are oval structures about 1 mm in length, and the lamellae are composed of layers of fibrous connective tissue derived from Schwann cells and encased in a connective tissue sheath (see Figure 25.8b).

Vasculature

Arterioles and veins of medium size run between the fascicles, whereas there is a capillary network in close relation to individual fibres within fascicles (see Figures 25.3 and 25.4). Type 1 fibres, with predominantly aerobic metabolism, have a denser capillary network than type 2 glycolytic fibres. A less extensive capillary network is apparent in muscle from neonates and in areas of regenerating muscle fibres. The vascular network is evident on routine stains and with PAS reactions, especially after diastase digestion, and with antibodies to various proteins of endothelial cells. At the ultrastructural level, muscle capillaries can often be seen as indentations of the fibre membrane. The endothelial cells contain numerous pinocytotic vesicles, but they lack tight junctions. Pericytes are applied closely to the external surface of the endothelial cells, and the capillary basal lamina covers the external surface.

Sarcoplasm

The sarcoplasm contains several organelles, including mitochondria concerned with supplying energy to the fibre and regulating intracellular calcium levels. Although the size and shape of mitochondria can be variable, they are usually small and ovoid (Figure 25.9). They have a single outer membrane and an inner membrane with deep folds known as cristae, and contain their own DNA that encodes 13 proteins involved with mitochondrial function. The central region is occupied by amorphous material that may contain small dense granules of calcium. Mitochondria are found in intermyofibrillar regions adjacent to I-bands (Figure 25.9) and also in subsarcolemmal clusters. They are often more numerous in type 1 fibres, but differences in mitochondrial volume in human muscles are not consistent enough to distinguish fibre types (see Ultrastructural Differences in Fibre Type).

The contractile apparatus is surrounded by the Golgi apparatus and a cytoskeleton of microtubules, intermediate filaments and microfilaments of actin, as well as glycogen,

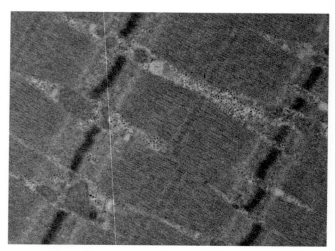

25.9 Electron micrograph showing sarcomeres and pairs of mitochondria in the intermyofibrillar space at the level of the I-band.

free ribosomes, lipid droplets and lipofuscin, an end product of lysosomal activity. Lipofuscin is usually seen in subsarcolemmal areas, often adjacent to nuclei. It is rare in children, but common in normal adults. Glycogen granules are 15–30 nm in size and, although not limited to any one part of the fibre, are more numerous at the level of the I-band than the A-band. Free ribosomes are seen in subsarcolemmal regions and are often increased in perinuclear zones, along with Golgi membranes, intermediate filaments and microtubules. Golgi elements are also observed throughout the fibre and are best seen either at the ultrastructural level or following immunolabelling of Golgi proteins in isolated fibres.[255] Microtubules are cylindrical tubes several micrometres long and 18–25 nm in diameter. They probably interact with a number of muscle proteins, including muscle-specific RING (Really Interesting New Gene) and MURF (MUscle Ring Finger) proteins, which have been implicated in linking myofibrils with other cytoskeletal elements.[170] Major proteins of microtubules are α and β isoforms of tubulin.

Contractile Apparatus

The contractile and metabolic components occupy approximately 75 per cent of the fibre volume. A single muscle fibre contains many bundles of myofibrils separated from each other by the intermyofibrillar space. Each myofibril consists of a series of sarcomeres, which are the basic unit of contraction, consisting of the thin filaments (actin, tropomyosin, troponins and nebulin) and the thick filaments (myosin). Under the light microscope the thin filaments appear bright (isotropic or I-band), whereas the thick filaments appears dark (anisotropic or A-band), thus giving rise to the characteristic striated appearance. The length of the A-band is constant at 1.5–1.6 µm, whereas I-band length varies depending on contraction, the species and muscle type. The central region of the A-band is traversed by a narrow dense line, the M-line, and is adjoined on either side by the slightly paler H-zone. The filaments of the I-band are attached to the narrow, dense Z-line (Z disc),

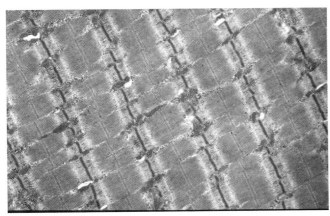

25.10 Electron micrograph showing the sarcomere pattern of a single fibre with the darker A-band and lighter I-band filaments. The A-band is traversed by the M-line and the thin filaments of the I-band are attached to dense Z-lines that mark the boundaries of each sarcomere. Note also the mitochondria and glycogen in the intermyofibrillar space.

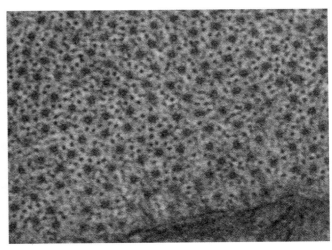

25.11 High-power electron micrograph of myofibrils sectioned transversely showing myosin surrounded by the actin lattice.

which marks the longitudinal boundary of each sarcomere (Figure 25.10). The Z-lines and the M-band are connected by transverse filaments to the sarcolemma and to neighbouring myofibrils. At rest, each sarcomere is 2.5–3.0 μm in length. Contraction of the myofibre occurs by shortening of the sarcomere and is accomplished by the I-filaments sliding towards the centre of the A-band. During this process, the I-band and H-zone shorten but the A-band remains at a constant length of 1.5–1.6 μm (Box 25.2).

BOX 25.2. Structure of the sarcomere

The A-band consists of a hexagonal lattice of thick myosin filaments 15–18 nm in diameter and 1.5–1.6 μm in length. The myosin molecules of the A-band are double-stranded helices with a rod-shaped flexible shaft of light meromyosin joined to two pear-shaped heads of heavy meromyosin. The molecules are arranged so that light meromyosin molecules oppose one another, and the heads point towards the end of the filament and lie on the surface. The region of overlap of light meromyosin tails gives rise to the central pale H-zone in the centre of the A-band. In the middle of the H-zone is the M-line, which appears as three to five lines across the thick filaments, the number being fibre type-dependent (see Figure 25.10). The M-line is believed to have a role in connecting the myosin filaments and giving stability to the A-band. Proteins localized to the M-lines include myomesin, skelemin, M protein and a fraction of creatine kinase.

The I-band filaments are mainly composed of thin actin polymers of filamentous (F) actin arranged in a double helix and are 6–7 nm in diameter. In the grooves of the actin helix is a helix of tropomyosin, to which it is attached at regular intervals. The tropomyosin spiral also has globular troponin complexes attached to it. The actin filaments are anchored at one end to the Z-line. The other end interdigitates with myosin filaments to form a lattice in which each myosin filament is surrounded by six actin filaments (Figure 25.11). The region of the A-band between two sets of I-filaments is pale, contains no myosin heads and forms the H-zone (see Figure 25.10). The length of both the I-band and the H-zone is dependent on the state of contraction of the muscle. Similarly, the prominence of the M-line that traverses the A-band varies with the state of contraction.

At the surface of the Z-line, the actin filaments are organized into a square lattice, and although this is similar to the pattern of tropomyosin crystals, this protein has only been shown in very small amounts in the Z-line. The major proteins of the Z-line are α-actinin and actin.[258] However, an increasing number of proteins are being identified as components of this structure, and the Z-line is now thought of as a nodal point for mechanosensation and mechanotransduction.[233] It also links to the T-tubular system and to the sarcoplasmic reticulum, and the presence of several E3 ubiquitin ligases suggests an association with protein turnover and possibly autophagy. Z-line width varies with fibre type, with the widest Z-line found in slow muscle.[258] Alterations in the overall protein composition of fast fibre Z-line alters their elastic properties, providing a mechanistic explanation for the loss of force generation that may explain the increased susceptibility to eccentric damage in α-actinin-3-deficient individuals.

Z-line abnormalities occur in a number of neuromuscular disorders. Some of the proteins implicated so far include desmin, αB-crystallin, filamin C, myotilin, Z-line alternatively spliced PDZ protein (ZASP) and Bcl-2-associated athanogene-3 (Bag3) (see Box 25.9). A number of additional proteins have also been studied, including telethonin (cap protein), myozenin, zeugmentin, syncoilin (see later), vinculin, obscurin and myotilin.[81,152,233,395]

Two very large proteins are also attached to the Z-line, titin (2–3 mDa) and nebulin (700–800 kDa), both of which are of pathological importance and exist in multiple isoforms that arise from splicing of the gene transcripts. Titin is the third most abundant protein in muscle (after actin and myosin), and is thought to organize the precise assembly of many of the structural, regulatory and contractile proteins of the sarcomere. It also acts as a 'molecular spring' that confers striated muscle with its distinct biomechanical properties during contraction, relaxation and stretch. A single molecule of titin stretches from the Z-line to the M-line, with its entire N terminus in the Z-line and C terminus attached to the M-line of the sarcomere.[252] Titin molecules of adjacent sarcomeres overlap

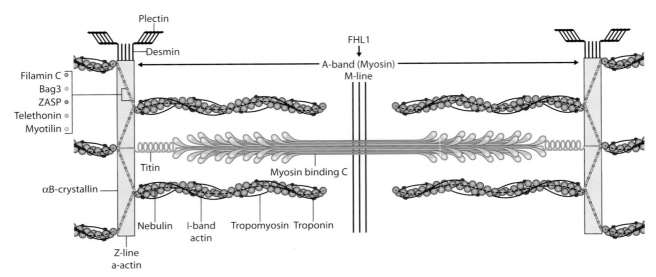

25.12 Diagram showing the major protein components of a sarcomere. The actin filaments are anchored to the Z-line and overlap with the myosin filaments. The N terminus of titin is in the Z-line and it stretches to and spans the M-line. The C terminus of nebulin inserts into the Z-line but does not fully span it. The N terminus of nebulin is located near the ends of the actin filaments. The tropomyosin–troponin complex lies in the grooves of the actin filaments. Several proteins interact with α-actinin in the Z-line; ones of known pathological significance are depicted here. Desmin is at the periphery of the Z-line and links the myofibrils to each other and to the sarcolemma. Plectin interacts with desmin.

in the Z-line and M-line. The portion of titin in the I-band is believed to be elastic and to act as a molecular ruler, having a role in passive tension during stretching of the myofibrils. Three to six titin molecules are associated with each myosin filament and there may be lateral associations with actin. Titin has binding sites for many myofibrillar proteins, including myosin, actin, α-actinin, T-cap/telethonin, myomesin, myosin-binding protein-C and obscurin. Around 10 per cent of its mass consists of non-repetitive sequences that include phosphorylation motifs, binding sites for muscle-specific calpain proteases and other proteins. These, together with a COOH-terminal serine/threonine protein kinase domain, strongly suggest an additional role in signal transduction.

Nebulin makes up 2–3 per cent of the total myofibrillar protein mass and is encoded by a 183-exon-containing gene (*NEB*). Alternative splicing of a single transcript gives rise to multiple isoforms that correspond to the various sizes of thin filaments present in developing and adult muscle fibres. A single nebulin molecule extends the length of the thin filament with its C terminus anchored at the Z-line. The extreme C terminus contains a serine-rich region with multiple phosphorylation sites and an SH3 domain that binds to myopalladin, another Z-line protein. In addition to lateral associations with actin, which are thought to play a role in determining thin filament length (a crucial role given that force production is proportional to the amount of overlap between the thick and thin filaments), the N terminus of nebulin interacts with tropomyosin, troponin I/C/T and tropomodulin.[327] More recent work implicates nebulin in mechanically linking adjacent myofibrils in addition to regulating cross-bridge cycling kinetics, potentially providing a basis for the weakness observed in patients with mutations in nebulin. There is also evidence to suggest that the C

terminus of nebulin along with titin helps to regulate Z-line width. A diagrammatic representation of the structure of a sarcomere showing proteins of pathological significance is shown in Figure 25.12.

Obscurin is another giant protein, but unlike titin and nebulin, it is not present within sarcomeres but rather around them, primarily at the level of the Z-line and M-line. It interacts with a number of other proteins, including small ankyrin 1, an integral component of the sarcoplasmic reticulum membranes, titin and sarcomeric myosin. It is thought to coordinate the assembly and organization of the sarcoplasmic reticulum with the myofibrillar elements. Titin and obscurin are thought to play important roles in signalling cascades that control homeostasis and muscle gene expression. Thus the sarcomere emerges as a structure whose function goes beyond the generation of force and motion.[236]

Plasma Membrane and Internal Membrane Systems

The plasma membrane of differentiated skeletal muscle fibres is divided into several domains: the peripheral fibre surface, the transverse (T) tubule network, the neuromuscular junction and the myotendinous junction. The plasma membrane and the T-tubule system maintain distinct protein and lipid compositions, despite being continuous with one another. The distribution of proteins spanning the lipid bilayer of the fibre surface was originally studied by freeze fracture and etching techniques, which revealed integral proteins as intramembrane particles or pits on both faces of the membrane. One notable feature using this technique is the number of caveolae that decorate the plasma membrane. Caveolae are flask-shaped

55- to 65-nm diameter invaginations of the plasma membrane. They contain a 21- to 24-kDa integral membrane protein, caveolin, of which skeletal muscle has a specific isoform, caveolin-3. Cavin-1 (also known as polymerase I and transcript release factor [PTRF]) is also localized to caveolae, and both proteins are of pathological significance (see Limb-Girdle Muscular Dystrophies, p. 1558). Immunolabelling using antibodies against membrane proteins and caveolin has shown that the entire extrajunctional plasma membrane may be seen as a mosaic of T-tubule domains, together with caveolin-associated raft and non-raft domains.[40]

The transversely oriented T-tubule system permits the rapid passage of depolarization into the interior of the fibre. Efficient excitation–contraction coupling is then achieved via specific functional associations that the T-tubule system maintains with regions of the sarcoplasmic reticulum. The sarcoplasmic reticulum is a fenestrated sheath of membranes between and around each myofibril and is responsible for the release and uptake of calcium ions during contraction and relaxation. At the level of the A/I-band interface, the sarcoplasmic reticulum forms continuous lateral sacs or terminal cisternae. Two terminal cisternae are in close contact with, but separate from, a T-system tubule and collectively these form a triad (Figure 25.13). The repetitive arrangement of triads gives a regular pattern at the A/I-band junction, along and across the length of the fibre. The lateral sacs of triads can be distinguished from the T-tubules by their amorphous or granular electron-dense material. The T-tubule of the triad is the site of the voltage-gated calcium channel, the dihydropyridine receptor (DHPR), which is activated by the action potential and induces the ryanodine receptor of the lateral sacs to release calcium. Ultrastructurally, ryanodine receptors can be seen as dense 'feet' bridging the junction of the lateral sacs and T-tubules. T-tubules of skeletal muscle differ from those in cardiac muscle in lacking laminins.

Muscle Fibre Cytoskeleton

One means by which the fibre plasma membrane is protected against the large stresses associated with contractile activity is through the regular connections it maintains with the underlying contractile apparatus. As with other cell types, the principal components of the cytoskeleton are the microfilaments, intermediate filament and microtubules. There is a distinct cytoskeletal actin filament system that interacts with dystrophin and a number of other proteins.[224] There are also a number of different intermediate filament proteins that include desmin, synemin (desmuslin), paranemin, syncoilin and members of the cytokeratin family. Many of these proteins are concentrated at the Z-line where they assist with the lateral transmission of force during contraction, emphasizing their role as integrators of structure and function, and link the myofibrils to each other, to the sarcolemma, and to other organelles.[57] Plectin belongs to a group of proteins known as cytolinkers, which also contribute to this network of proteins, as do other proteins of the costameric lattice (see Box 25.9).[497,502]

Nerves and Innervation

Each fibre is innervated by one nerve, although fibres are polyinnervated at early embryonic stages. Neuromuscular junctions are distributed in highly organized innervation zones in skeletal muscles, which in most muscles form a band across the mid-belly of the muscle. Nerves surrounded by a perineural sheath are present both between and within muscle bundles, although they may not be evident in all biopsies because of sampling variation. At the ultrastructural level, Schwann cells and both myelinated and unmyelinated axons are surrounded by layers of perineural cells and basal lamina. Within the endoneurial space, axons are surrounded by collagen. Pathological changes in peripheral nerves are usually assessed in a biopsy of the sural nerve, a sensory nerve.

Neurons innervating muscle fibres have their cell bodies in the anterior horns of the spinal cord. The axon from one cell body branches to supply a variable number of muscle fibres, but in most muscles this amounts to several hundred. The anterior horn cell, its axon and the muscle fibres it supplies constitute the motor unit. Muscle fibres of one motor unit are of uniform type; however, although confined to a limited area, they are scattered randomly and not clustered. Motor units are classified by their speed of contraction and resistance to fatigue. Physiologists have identified three main types: fast-twitch, fatigue-sensitive (FF); fast-twitch, fatigue-resistant (FR); and slow-twitch, fatigue-resistant (S). Fatigue resistance correlates with oxidative capacity and mitochondrial content, and fibres have also been classified as slow-twitch oxidative (SO), corresponding to histochemical type 1 fibres; fast-twitch glycolytic (FG), corresponding to histochemical type 2B fibres; and fast-twitch oxidative glycolytic (FOG), corresponding to type 2A fibres (Table 25.3). This classification is based on studies of non-human muscle, but evidence suggests that the situation for human muscle is similar.

Neuromuscular Junction

As the axon approaches the muscle fibre, it divides into a number of small unmyelinated terminals, each of which makes contact with the fibre. The point of contact between the nerve terminal and the muscle fibre, the neuromuscular synapse, is a specialized region designed to allow rapid transmission of the depolarizing impulse (Figure 25.14). In normal muscle, the postsynaptic

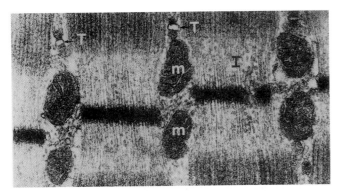

25.13 Electron micrograph showing triads at the A-band–I-band junction, with a lateral sac of sarcoplasmic reticulum containing amorphous electron-dense material on either side of a pale T-tubule (T). Note also the mitochondria (m) at the level of the I-band.

TABLE 25.3 Main characteristics of the different fibre types in human muscle

	Type 1	Type 2A	Type 2B	Type 2C
Colour	Red	White	White	
Twitch speed	Slow	Fast	Fast	Fast
Fatigability	Resistant	Resistant	Sensitive	
Twitch + oxidative and glycolytic capacity	SO	FOG	FG	
ATPase pH 9.4	+	+++	+++	+++
ATPase pH 4.6	+++	–	++	+++
ATPase pH 4.3	+++	–	–	++ or +++
NADH-TR	+++	++	+	++ or +++
Cytochrome *c* oxidase	+++	++	+	+
Succinic dehydrogenase	+++	++	+	++
Phosphorylase	+	+++	++ or +++	+++
PAS	+ or ++	+++	++	++
Lipid droplets	+++	++ or +++	+	
Antibodies to fast myosin heavy chain	–	+++	+++	++ or +++
Antibodies to slow myosin heavy chain*	+++	–	–	– or + or ++

*See text.

-, +, ++, +++ represent increasing intensity of stain.

FG, fast glycolytic; FOG, fast oxidative glycolytic; NADH-TR, nicotinamide adenine dinucleotide dehydrogenase-tetrazolium reductase; periodic acid–Schiff; SO, slow oxidative.

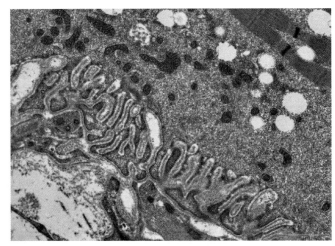

25.14 Electron micrograph of a neuromuscular junction. Basal lamina extends into the postsynaptic folds. Note the myelinated axon (bottom left).

membrane is characteristically thrown into numerous folds, the crests of which are adjacent to the nerve terminal and contain AChRs at a concentration 1000 times higher than in the extrajunctional regions of the muscle fibre. Voltage-gated sodium channels are concentrated at the base of the postsynaptic folds. This arrangement is thought to focus end plate current flow on the voltage-gated sodium channels, thereby amplifying the effect of transmitter release and ensuring effective neuromuscular transmission.[417,444]

The complexity of the postsynaptic folds differs with fibre type, and in fast-twitch fibres they are usually deeper and more branched. Under the electron microscope, regions within the postsynaptic membrane may appear darker than others because of the aggregation of AChRs (see Figure 25.14). The presynaptic nerve terminal contains numerous synaptic vesicles and organelles, in particular mitochondria. A specialized basal lamina extends into the folds and anchors neuromuscular junction-specific proteins, such as acetylcholine esterase, agrin and neuregulins, and defects in several of these proteins give rise to myasthenic syndromes (see Myasthenic Syndromes, p. 1596).[129,444] Dystrophin localizes to the troughs of the synaptic clefts along with voltage-gated sodium channels, whereas utrophin is found at the crests of the folds with AChRs. In normal mature muscle fibres, proteins such as neural cell adhesion molecule (NCAM) and utrophin are localized only to the neuromuscular junction and not to extrajunctional regions. The myonuclei around neuromuscular junctions are specialized and have a role in the transcription of the specific proteins of the neuromuscular junction.

Most of the crucial features of the neuromuscular junction are not visible with routine histological stains, but sites of innervation can be demonstrated with specific histochemical stains, antibodies and fluorescently labelled neurotoxins,

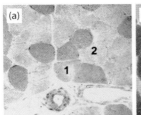
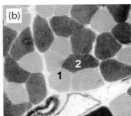

25.15 Reciprocal pattern of oxidative and phosphorylating enzymes in type 1 and 2 fibres giving a checkerboard pattern. (a) Oxidative enzymes (NADH-TR) are higher in type 1 fibres and (b) phosphorylating enzymes (ATPase pH 9.4) are higher in type 2 fibres.

such as the snake venom α-bungarotoxin, which causes paralysis by blocking AChRs. Several antibodies, including those against β-spectrin, members of the dystrophin-associated complex and laminins appear to be enhanced at neuromuscular junctions, because of the abundant folding of the sarcolemma (see Figure 25.49). With the Verhoeff–van Gieson stain, individual axons and their myelin sheaths stain black and can be readily visualized; with the Gomori trichrome stain, the myelin of individual axons stains red.

Muscle Fibre Types

Most human muscles are composed of a mosaic of two main types of fibre. The fibre type profile varies between muscles and even across different regions of the same muscle.[212] Knowledge of the site from which a biopsy has been taken is therefore essential for the assessment of fibre type proportions. The overall properties of any given muscle result largely from the proportion of its different fibre types, which are influenced by innervation/neuromuscular activity, exercise/training, mechanical loading/unloading, hormones and ageing. Alterations in fibre type profile may also be influenced by various pathological processes (see General Histological and Histochemical Abnormalities, p. 1532), making this a major aspect of any study of muscle pathology.[387]

Histochemical methods for demonstrating fibre types exploit differences in oxidative and phosphorylating enzyme activities and produce a reciprocal chequerboard pattern, which highlights the two main fibre types (Figure 25.15).[117] The considerable mitochondrial content and high oxidative enzyme activity of type 1 fibres are demonstrated well with techniques for staining reduced nicotinamide adenine dinucleotide–tetrazolium reductase (NADH-TR) and the mitochondrial-specific enzymes succinate dehydrogenase (SDH) and COX (Figure 25.16). The high oxidative metabolism of type 1 fibres is also reflected in a higher lipid content, which can be demonstrated with oil red O, Sudan black and Nile red dyes.[117] The glycolytic activity of type 2 fibres is reflected by their high phosphorylase and glycogen content and their myofibrillar adenosine triphosphatase (mATPase) activity.

The most widespread nomenclature for fibre types is based on techniques that demonstrate mATPase activity and its pH stability. Staining is performed at an alkaline pH around 9.4, with and without pre-incubation at an acid pH of 4.6 and 4.3. Three fibre types can thus be identified in normal muscle (types 1, 2A and 2B), with an additional

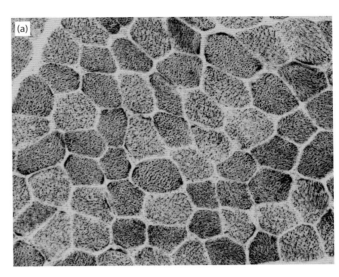

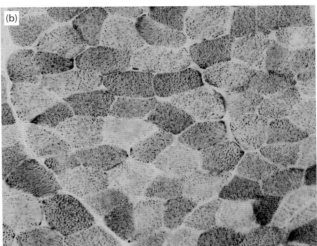

25.16 Checkerboard pattern of (a) succinate dehydrogenase and (b) cytochrome c oxidase activity with type 1 fibres staining the most intensely, 2A fibres with intermediate intensity and 2B the weakest, reflecting their different mitochondrial content.

subtype 2C, which is an immature fibre type (Figure 25.17; see also Table 25.3). Staining with acid pre-incubation at pH 4.3 gives a reciprocal pattern to that at pH 9.4, and at pH 4.6 three intensities are visible.[117] If the pH is increased up to 10, then a three-fibre pattern can also be obtained. Basophilic regenerating fibres stain as 2C fibres.

In normal muscle, this mATPase activity generally correlates with specific myosin heavy chain (MHC) isoforms and shortening velocity.[387] There are various advantages, however, to using myosin antibodies to demonstrate fibre types in pathological samples. In particular, hybrid fibres with more than one isoform can be identified; immature and regenerating fibres are more easily identified; and fibre typing in post-mortem muscle, is possible with antibodies, when ATPase activity may be lost. One disadvantage is that the equivalent of the histochemical 2B fibre (which expresses type 2X myosin) with intermediate staining for ATPase at pH 4.6, cannot easily be identified with myosin antibodies (see later). However, the identification of these fibres is now

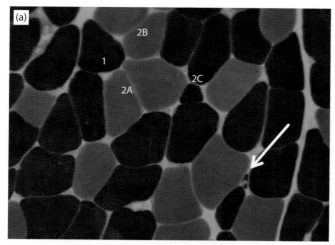

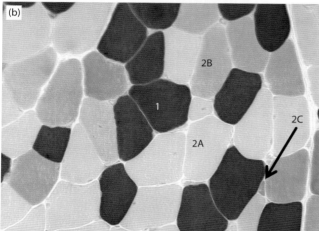

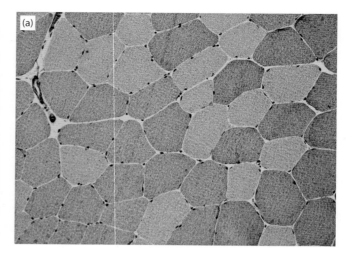

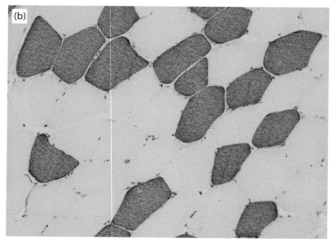

25.18 Serial sections immunolabelled with antibodies to (a) fast and (b) slow myosin heavy chains showing that most fibres in normal muscle express either fast or slow myosin.

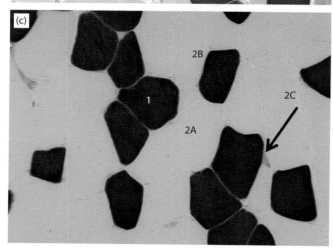

25.17 Serial sections stained for ATPase at (a) pH 9.4, with (b) pre-incubation at pH 4.6 or (c) pH 4.3 showing a checkerboard pattern and the subdivisions of the type 2 fibres into 2A and 2B. Note also the very small 2C fibre (arrow) that is stained at all pH.

of limited diagnostic value, and they can be distinguished with oxidative enzyme techniques, because these reveal three intensities of staining. In practice, the most important diagnostic distinction is between type 1 and all type 2 fibres (slow versus fast myosin). A comparison of nomenclature and fibre type properties is given in Table 25.3.

The major MHC isoforms in adult mammalian skeletal muscle associate with four main types of fibre: slow type 1 (MHC1β isoform) and three fast types, namely type IIA/2A (MHC-IIa), type IID/2D (MHCIId) and type IIB/2B (MHCIIb). Fibre type 2D (MHCIId) is considered to be equivalent to type 2X (MHCIIx). Adult human fibres, however, in common with a few other large species, do not show the fast 2B myosin protein, although the gene is present.[186,387] Thus an ATPase 2B fibre in human muscle does not have fast 2B myosin but has mainly 2X myosin. Studies with antibodies specific to fast 2X myosin are limited, and it has not been extensively studied in pathological samples. Fibres expressing only 2X myosin are usually identified by exclusion, and their histochemical equivalents in human muscle have not been elucidated fully. There are, however, a few reports using one specific antibody to myosin 2X.[30,420] In addition to these, facial and ocular muscles express unique isoforms, such as the 'super-fast' MHCII$_m$ of masticatory muscles. Although most fibres in normal mature muscle express only one heavy chain isoform (Figure 25.18), coexpression of more than one isoform (hybrid fibres) is common in pathological muscle and is a useful feature to evaluate.

In addition to MHC isoforms, fibre types also express isoforms of several other myofibrillar proteins, including myosin light chain (MLC) units, troponin subunits, tropomyosin, α-actinin and various calcium regulatory proteins. Quantitative differences in metabolic enzyme levels, especially those relating to aerobic–oxidative and anaerobic pathways of energy metabolism, may also be useful for classifying fibres types, although large overlaps in enzyme activity levels exist between fast fibre subtypes and fast and slow fibres, as defined by their MHC isoform composition.[387]

Other enzyme techniques that also distinguish fibre type and are of pathological significance include those for phosphorylase, phosphofructokinase and adenylate deaminase. In general, phosphorylase activity is higher in type 2 fibres, but the correlation with ATPase is not always direct.

Ultrastructural Differences in Fibre Type

Ultrastructural criteria can differentiate between fibre types, and this has been improved upon by the use of ultrathin frozen sections. In general, type 1 fibres have wider Z-lines and more mitochondria and lipid, but a less extensive sarcoplasmic reticulum, T-tubule system, triads and glycogen. The appearance of the M-line is also characteristic of the fibre type, muscle and species from which the section has been taken. Ultrastructural differences are less distinct in human muscle than in other species, but the Z-line and M-line, either alone or in combination, can be good indicators of fibre type in the human tibialis anterior, where type 1 fibres were shown to have broader Z-lines and five strong M-bridge lines; type 2A fibres to have intermediate Z-lines, three strong M-bridge lines and two weak M-bridge lines; and type 2B fibres to have narrow Z-lines and three strong M-bridge lines, with the two outer ones being very weak or absent.[418]

Growth and Development

Muscle fibre nuclei are usually located at the periphery of the fibre in normal muscle. Fibre nuclei align with their longitudinal axes parallel to that of the fibre, and in longitudinal section they can be seen to be elliptical and display dense peripheral heterochromatin, together with a prominent nucleolus and finely stippled nucleoplasm. A double nuclear membrane surrounds the nucleus, the outer of which is continuous with the endoplasmic reticulum. The nuclear membrane is associated with important proteins, including emerin, lamin A/C and nesprins, which can be defective in neuromuscular disorders (see Emery–Dreifuss Muscular Dystrophy, p. 1575). Emerin is a component of the inner nuclear membrane itself, whereas lamin A/C, along with other lamins and related proteins, is localized to the nuclear lamina beneath the nuclear membrane. Nesprins also interact with emerin and lamins, forming a complex known as 'linkers of the nucleoskeleton to the cytoskeleton complex' that links the nuclear membrane to the actin cytoskeleton.[275,277] The nuclear matrix contains a protein, matrin 3, which is defective in a distal myopathy with vocal cord and pharyngeal involvement.[397] Chromatin, containing the DNA and histones, is condensed in normal

muscle nuclei and is granular in appearance. It is known as heterochromatin and is anchored to the nuclear membrane. Metabolically active chromatin (euchromatin) is in the pale internal areas along with the nuclear matrix, which cannot be distinguished by electron microscopy. Each nucleus has one or two nucleoli where ribosomal transcription occurs. All nuclei are basophilic, stain blue with haematoxylin after an alkaline rinse, and usually stain red with the acid pH of the Gomori trichrome stain.

The nuclei of the syncytial adult muscle fibres are post-mitotic and unable to undergo division. Muscle fibre number in mammals is normally determined prenatally or soon after (up to 4 months in humans), and any increase in muscle size is due to increases in the size, not number, of the individual fibres. Postnatally, fibre size is regulated by both the number of nuclei incorporated into each fibre and the volume of cytoplasm that each nucleus supports, which varies between different fibre types. The main source of all new nuclei added to the fibre during growth and regeneration is the satellite cell population, where stem cell activity is thought to reside.[124] Satellite cells lie on the surface of the fibre, wedged between the fibre plasma membrane and its basal lamina. Muscle at birth contains a high proportion of satellite cells – typically 30 per cent – but this decreases to around 5 per cent in adult life.[58] Increased numbers are observed near neuromuscular junctions and in pathological situations associated with either denervation or regeneration. Satellite cell number also varies between fibre types. Ultrastructurally, satellite cells have nuclei with dense peripheral heterochromatin and a small volume of cytoplasm that contains few organelles, free ribosomes, rough endoplasmic reticulum, glycogen, microtubules and intermediate filaments. Organized contractile myofilaments are characteristically absent (Figure 25.19). Although satellite cells were originally considered to be the sole source of nuclei for postnatal growth and repair of muscle, recent work has identified a 'stem cell' population in the interstitium.

Most muscles, with the exception of some craniofacial and oesophageal muscles, are derived from the somites. Gene-targeting experiments in the mouse define a transcriptional hierarchy in which the paired-domain transcription factors

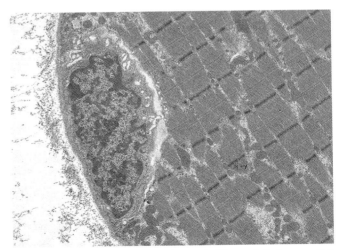

25.19 Electron micrograph of a satellite cell between the basal lamina and plasma membrane of the parent muscle fibre. Note the small volume of cytoplasm and lack of myofibrils.

Pax3 and Pax7 act upstream of the primary myogenic basic helix–loop–helix transcription factors Myf-5 and MyoD in determining the myogenic phenotype.[33] From about 7 weeks of gestation in humans, post-mitotic myoblasts fuse synchronously to form primary generation myotubes, which express a number of muscle-specific proteins such as desmin, titin and nebulin. These myotubes have large central nuclei with a prominent nucleolus, and scattered myofibrils. Early primary myotubes are initially clustered within a common basal lamina, but as differentiation continues each becomes surrounded by its own basal lamina. Secondary myotubes arise from successive waves of fusion of post-mitotic myoblasts, along the surface of the primary myotubes. These initially form within the vicinity of innervation sites on the primary myotube, and early secondary myotubes are at first encased within the same basal lamina as the parent primary myotube. With increased maturation, these secondary myotubes separate and attain their own basal lamina.

Fibre typing, particularly with antibodies to myosin isoforms, can be observed from about 10–12 weeks of gestation in human fetal quadriceps.[117] Oxidative enzyme staining, however, is often pale and more stippled than in mature muscle. Myosin heavy chain isoforms are expressed sequentially during development and are influenced by both innervation and hormones. Primary myotubes are innervated by pioneering axons at an early phase of myogenesis, and most express slow myosin and are destined to become slow, type 1 fibres. It has been proposed that these constitute the fundamental motor units of the developing neuromuscular system and are responsible for early slow movements. Secondary myotubes, however, are hybrid fibres and can express various combinations of fetal/neonatal, fast and slow myosin. These become organized into large, fast motor units later in development, eclipsing the original slow response. In human fetal quadriceps muscles, a population of very small myotubes – secondary myotubes, sometimes referred to as tertiary myotubes – appears at about 12–13 weeks of gestation.[114] These myotubes express only fast and fetal myosin, and not slow myosin. At birth, a number of fibres stain histochemically as 2C fibres and coexpress fetal myosin with fast or slow myosin. The stage at which this immature fetal/neonatal isoform is switched off in human muscle is not clear, because samples from most neonates have been taken for a medical reason and cannot unequivocally be classified as 'normal'. In our experience, many fibres from neonates express fetal/neonatal myosin; however, by 3–4 months of age very few may be seen, and a few may remain up to 1 year of age. Their pathological significance is uncertain. The embryonic isoform of myosin is not usually detected in neonatal human muscle, except in pathological situations, preterm cases or cases with delayed maturation. During the neonatal period, some fibres with a particularly large diameter stain intensely with most histological stains and have properties of type 1 fibres. These are considered to be the fibres described as 'Wohlfart B fibres' by Wohlfart in the 1930s.

Neuromuscular Transmission and Muscle Contraction

Neuromuscular transmission is the process by which an action potential generated in motor neurons passes down the axon and results in depolarization of the muscle fibre, leading to contraction of the myofibrils. A key structure in this process is the neuromuscular junction.[417,444] At this site, the action potential of the motor nerve induces the opening of presynaptic voltage-gated calcium channels. With the influx of calcium ions, synaptic vesicles containing acetylcholine (ACh) fuse with the presynaptic membrane and release ACh into the synaptic cleft. As ACh binds to the postsynaptic ligand-gated channel associated with the AChR, the channel opens and positive ions flow into the muscle fibre. This flow of ions induces a voltage change, which results in the opening of voltage-gated sodium channels in the plasma membrane of the sarcolemma, followed by depolarization. The AChR remains open for about 1 millisecond after the binding of ACh. This allows a large influx of positive ions, resulting in depolarization of the postsynaptic membrane and muscle fibre. Diffusion out of the synaptic cleft and hydrolysis by acetylcholinesterase limit the action of ACh. Cholinesterase is secreted by the muscle cell and is anchored to the basal lamina that lies between the nerve terminal and the muscle end plate.

Depolarization of the muscle cell membrane at the motor end plate triggers an action potential that spreads as a wave of excitation into the T-tubules, which penetrate transversely into the depths of the muscle fibre and form the triad of tubules with the lateral sacs of the sarcoplasmic reticulum at the level of each I-band of the sarcomere (see Figure 25.13). The action potential induces a conformational change of the DHPR, which in turn results in the release of calcium through the ryanodine receptor 1. The calcium is released from the lateral sacs of sarcoplasmic reticulum adjacent to the T-tubules, and muscle contraction is initiated within milliseconds of depolarization of the motor end plate.

Defective function of the neuromuscular junction results in muscle weakness and marked fatigability, and these conditions are collectively recognized under the term 'myasthenia'. Both genetic defects of various proteins that form the neuromuscular junction and acquired autoimmune variants are known, (see Myasthenic Syndromes, p. 1596).

According to the sliding filament model of muscle contraction, shortening of the sarcomere is achieved via the action of (thin) actin filaments sliding (or being pulled) along the (thick) myosin filaments. During this process, sarcomere length and the H-zone (the area where thin filaments do not overlap with the thick filaments) length decrease, whereas A-band length (the area containing thick filaments) remains constant at 1.5–1.6 µm. For further details on the mechanism of contraction, see Box 25.3.

GENERAL HISTOLOGICAL AND HISTOCHEMICAL ABNORMALITIES

A wide variety of abnormalities occur in diseased muscle. Few are pathognomonic of a particular disease, but a combination present in a sample, and assessed in the context of the clinical features, usually leads to identification of the type of disorder, if not an accurate diagnosis. Multidisciplinary meetings between the pathologist and clinicians play an essential part in directing further investigations. Every pathologist tends to have a favoured panel of methods to apply to a muscle biopsy,

BOX 25.3. Mechanism of contraction

Contraction of muscles occurs by the hydrolysis of adenosine triphosphate (ATP). The energy released by the splitting of ATP into adenosine diphosphate (ADP) and inorganic phosphate (P_i) is stored in the myosin molecule. The myosin–ADP–P_i complex is a high-energy state and is the predominant state at rest. Following muscle stimulation and calcium release from the sarcoplasmic reticulum, the inhibition of actin–myosin interaction, imposed by the regulatory proteins troponin and tropomyosin, is removed and the myosin (with bound ADP and P_i) attaches to actin. This interaction triggers the sequential release of P_i and ADP from the myosin head, resulting in a conformational change in the cross-bridge angle, which effectively pulls the actin filament towards the centre of the sarcomere, utilizing the energy stored in myosin. At the end of this process, myosin detaches from the actin and, with the hydrolysis of new ATP, the head returns to its original position and is thus ready to reattach to another part of the actin filament. The head of the myosin molecule therefore acts as an ATPase.

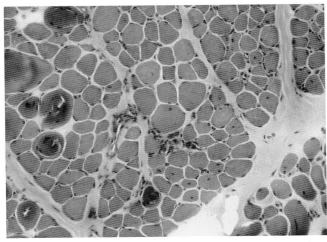

25.20 Dystrophic muscle showing fibres of varying size, split fibres, excess endomysial and perimysial connective tissue, some perimysial adipose tissue and several fibres with internal nuclei. H&E.

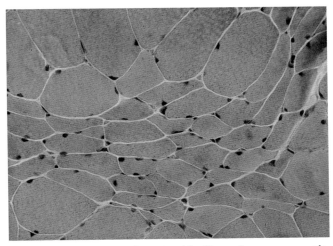

25.21 A group of angular atrophic fibres in a neurogenic disorder. Gomori trichrome.

and over the years we have adjusted ours in the light of current knowledge, the development of immunohistochemistry and the type of patient attending our clinics. In addition to a routine haematoxylin and eosin (H&E) stain, the histological techniques we find most helpful are the Gomori trichrome, PAS and oil red O stains. Routinely, we perform enzyme histochemistry for NADH-TR, COX and SDH, the combined COX/SDH method and acid phosphatase. For fibre typing, we now rely on immunohistochemical detection of different myosin isoforms in preference to ATPase reactions at varying pH. Other techniques that are applied, for example phosphorylase, phosphofructokinase and menadione NBT, are dependent on the results in the first panel and phenotype.[117,166] In this section, we summarize the main pathological features encountered in muscle and the stains most useful for demonstrating them. More details in relation to specific disorders and gene defects are described in the appropriate sections.

The abnormalities observed in pathological muscle relate to:

- changes in fibre size and shape;
- changes in fibre type proportions;
- changes in the position of nuclei;
- fibre degeneration and regeneration;
- fibrosis and adipose tissue;
- inflammatory cells;
- architectural changes in the fibres;
- structural abnormalities;
- deficiency of an enzyme;
- accumulation of intracellular material such as glycogen and lipid, or myofibrillar material.

In abnormal muscle, the normal polygonal shape of the fibres may be lost and the fibres become rounded, as often seen in muscular dystrophies (Figure 25.20). In denervation, atrophic fibres may be angular (Figure 25.21), except in SMA, where the grouped atrophic fibres are often round in shape (see Neurogenic Disorders, p. 1548). Sample handling and freezing technique, however, can influence the shape and degree of separation of the individual fibres. The assessment of changes in fibre size is fundamental to interpretation; in myopathic conditions there is a diffuse change throughout

the sample, but in neurogenic disorders there is a characteristic grouping (see Figure 25.21). Fibre sizes increase with age, and knowledge of this normal variation is important. Morphometric measurements of populations of fibres are time-consuming and do not always contribute more than the obvious. It is often sufficient to measure the smallest and largest fibres in a sample in order to obtain an approximate range of fibre sizes and to indicate whether this is appropriate for age and sex. Ideally, each pathology department should establish its own range of normal sizes, but obtaining samples from unequivocally normal individuals is ethically problematic, and many workers rely on published data.[44-47,117]

Approximate ranges are:

- birth–3 years: 15–20 µm;
- 3–10 years: 20–40 µm;
- adolescents/adults (female): 40–70 µm;
- adolescents/adults (male): 40–80 µm.

Fibre size is affected by a number of factors, including innervation, growth factors (e.g. hormones, insulin-like growth factor,

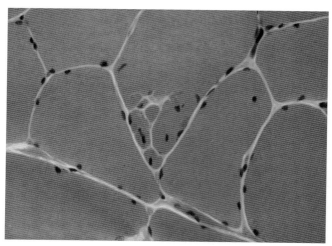

25.22 Multiple splitting of a fibre giving the impression of a cluster of fibres. Note also the internal nuclei. This appearance resembles a myotendinous junction. H&E.

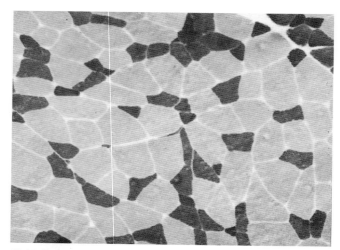

25.24 Selective atrophy of the dark type 2 fibres. ATPase pH 9.4.

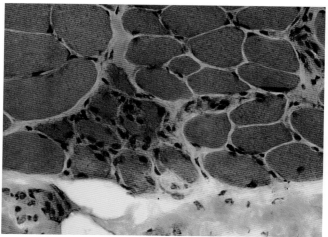

25.23 A cluster of basophilic regenerating fibres in a case of Duchenne muscular dystrophy. Note that some nuclei are internal, but several are peripheral. H&E.

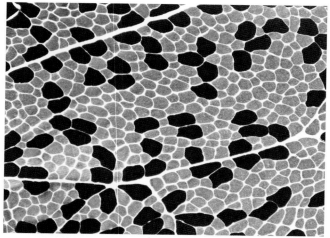

25.25 Selective atrophy/hypotrophy of type 1 fibres, which are also predominant, as seen in fibre type disproportion. ATPase 9.4.

myostatin, other members of the transforming growth factor family) and the muscle's workload. Excessive load on a muscle results in an increase in fibre size (hypertrophy), whereas disuse and denervation cause a decrease in size (atrophy). Longitudinal splitting and branching of fibres occur under certain pathological circumstances and contribute to the presence in cross-section of small fibres. Occasionally, splitting may result in the appearance in transverse sections of a small cluster of fibres (Figure 25.22). Splitting is also common near myotendinous junctions. Some small fibres in a biopsy may be regenerating and sometimes can be distinguished from atrophic fibres by their basophilia with H&E (Figure 25.23) and also by the immunohistochemical detection of particular proteins, such as embryonic and fetal/neonatal myosin, laminin α5 and utrophin (see Application of Immunohistochemistry in the Diagnosis of Neuromuscular Disorders, p. 1542).

Atrophy or hypertrophy of both fibre types occurs in most myopathic disorders, but in some instances it may specifically affect one fibre type. Atrophy of type 2 fibres, particularly 2B, is a common, non-specific myopathic finding, which can be induced by disuse and corticosteroid therapy (Figure 25.24).

Type 1 atrophy occurs in several congenital myopathies and myotonic dystrophy type 1 (Figure 25.25). Denervation results in groups of atrophic fibres of both types. In dermatomyositis, a characteristic feature is the perifascicular distribution of atrophic fibres (Figure 25.26). In chronic conditions, atrophy of a fibre may be so severe that only a clump of nuclei remains (Figure 25.27). These can be a particular early feature of myotonic dystrophy type 2 but also occur in other chronic conditions. Type-specific hypertrophy can occur, and in SMA the hypertrophic fibres are frequently type 1 (see Spinal Muscular Atrophy, p. 1551). Exercise can induce type 2 hypertrophy, and this may account for the normal difference in fibre sizes between males (in which type 2 fibres are larger than type 1) and females (in which they are approximately equal in size).

The proportion of fibre types varies in different muscles[212] and in pathological situations. As with the quantification of fibre sizes, normal baselines should be established, but published data are often consulted.[44-47,117] In myopathic disorders, an increase or predominance of type 1 fibres is common, whereas type 2 predominance occurs following spinal cord injury.[153] Collateral sprouting of surviving

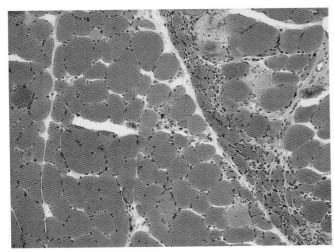

25.26 Perifascicular atrophy in a case of dermatomyositis. H&E.

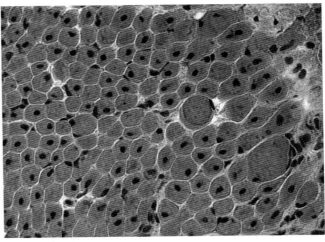

25.28 Nuclei in the centre of several fibres in a case of X-linked myotubular myopathy. H&E.

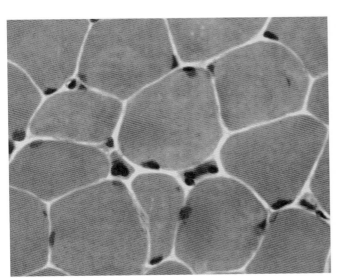

25.27 Very atrophic fibres with clumping of nuclei, sometimes called nuclear bag fibres. H&E.

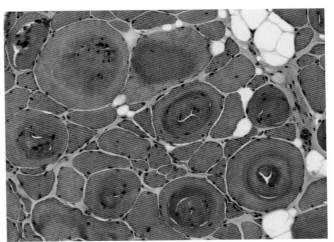

25.29 Hypertrophic, split and whorled fibres in a case of limb-girdle muscular dystrophy. Internal nuclei are often associated with the splits. Note also the increase in connective tissue and adipose tissue and the basophilic peripheral areas in the small fibres that relate to lobulation (cf Figure 25.36). H&E.

nerves following denervation results in grouping of both fibre types, and it is important to distinguish this from fibre type predominance (see Neurogenic Disorders, p. 1548).

Internal nuclei (i.e. within a fibre rather than in their normal subsarcolemmal position) are a common finding, particularly in myopathic disorders (see Figure 25.20), but they can also occur in chronic neuropathies. Sometimes more than one internal nucleus may be seen in the cross-section of a fibre. In myotonic dystrophies, and sometimes in myofibrillar myopathies, internal nuclei are particularly abundant. Occasional internal nuclei occur in normal muscle and are common near myotendinous junctions (see Figure 25.7), so care in histological interpretation in such regions is needed. It is often stated that the number of internal nuclei is not significant unless more than 3 per cent of fibres in transverse section contain one. In paediatric muscle this is probably an overestimate, and in our experience even a few internal nuclei in such cases are probably significant. In normal adults, internal nuclei are more common, particularly in individuals involved in sporting activities. In some

conditions the nuclei may be central within the fibre, and in longitudinal section they may form a chain down the centre of the fibre, for example in regenerating fibres. Central nuclei are a characteristic feature of centronuclear myopathies (Figure 25.28) and congenital myotonic dystrophy type 1, where they are regularly spaced down the fibre. Central nuclei can also occur in some fibres in cases with defects of ryanodine receptor 1, responsible for core myopathies, and titin. In other situations, internal nuclei are scattered within myofibrils. In split fibres they often occur along the internal membrane, but some of these relate to nuclei of capillary endothelial cells (Figure 25.29).

Necrosis is a feature of dystrophic muscle, in which it is associated with an increase in fibrous connective tissue. Necrotic fibres are identified by their pale staining with H&E and Gomori trichrome, and they may also contain macrophages (Figure 25.30). Round, hypercontracted fibres stain intensely with most stains and are thought to be a form of degenerating fibre, before phagocytosis. They are common in Duchenne and Becker muscular dystrophies, but

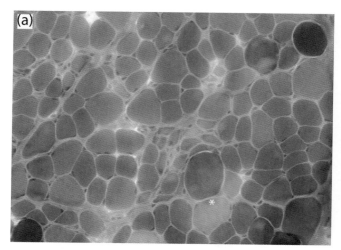

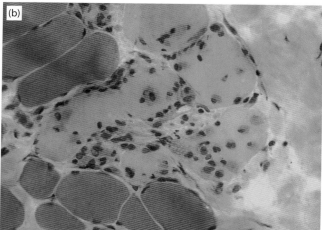

25.30 (a) Necrotic fibres (*) appear pale and (b) become invaded by macrophages. (a), Gomori trichrome; (b), H&E.

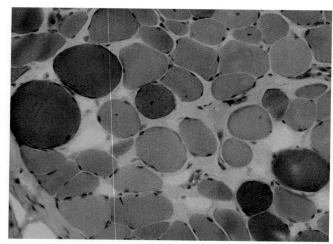

25.31 Darkly stained hypercontracted fibres in dystrophic muscle. Gomori trichrome.

they can occur in other conditions. Hypercontracted fibres are often more apparent with the Gomori trichrome stain (Figure 25.31). The Wohlfart B fibres seen in normal neonatal muscle are also stained intensely, but whether they are hypercontracted is not known. Artefactual hypercontraction of fibres can occur at the periphery of a sample and must not be overinterpreted.

Granular fibres, which are basophilic with H&E and red with the Gomori trichrome stain, are also a type of degenerating fibre and are often called 'ragged-red fibres'. They contain structurally abnormal mitochondria and may show no COX activity (Figure 25.32). They are particularly associated with some mitochondrial myopathies but occur as an incidental feature in dystrophic muscle, in inclusion body myositis and as a consequence of ageing. It is important to distinguish the normal peripheral aggregations of mitochondria that stain red with Gomori trichrome from ragged-red fibres, which often also show an abnormal basophilic granularity.

Basophilic fibres have a high RNA content and are considered to represent attempts at fibre regeneration following necrosis. They are named after their blue-purple tint in H&E sections. They also often have large nuclei with prominent nucleoli (see Figure 25.23). Basophilic fibres are common in dystrophic conditions, such as DMD, where clusters

of basophilic fibres may be seen. They can also be produced experimentally by traumatizing or producing ischaemic muscle, and may be very striking during the recovery phase after acute rhabdomyolysis. Regenerating fibres have a histochemical profile of type 2C fibres and express embryonic and fetal/neonatal myosin and other developmentally regulated proteins. At early stages of maturity, they are not innervated and therefore they also show extrajunctional NCAM. Basophilic fibres also show internal labelling with antibodies to several proteins, including utrophin, caveolin-3, dysferlin and major histocompatibility complex class I (MHC-I), but they lack neuronal nitric oxide synthase (nNOS). Split fibres sometimes appear basophilic, which may relate to myofibrillar disruption rather than to regeneration.

Damaged fibres may lose glycogen and appear as white fibres with the PAS stain (Figure 25.33), in contrast to the variable pink colour of other fibres. This is a non-specific finding. When present they suggest fibre damage, but loss of glycogen may also occur if there is a long delay before freezing. It can also occur in denervation.

Proliferation of endomysial or perimysial connective tissue is common in a number of situations and may be accompanied by varying amounts of adipose tissue (see Figure 25.20). Caution in interpreting perimysial fibrosis is needed in paediatric muscle, because wide bands of fibrous tissue separating fascicles occur in neonates and may be a normal feature, although muscle from unequivocally normal neonates is rarely studied. The endomysial connective tissue is often distinguished more easily with the Gomori trichrome technique than with an H&E preparation, but special stains such as picrosirus and Verhoff van Gieson can also be used. A variety of extracellular matrix proteins, especially various types of collagen and fibronectin, can be identified in the perimysium and endomysium. Endomysial proliferation leads to a clear separation of individual muscle fibres and is more common in myopathies than in neuropathies. It can occur, however, in chronic neurogenic disorders, but endomysial proliferation is not usually a feature of severe infantile SMA. It is a prominent feature of DMD, BMD, the LGMDs and some CMDs, and it may also be seen in FSHD. It can also occur to varying degrees in some cases of core myopathies, and this may cause diagnostic

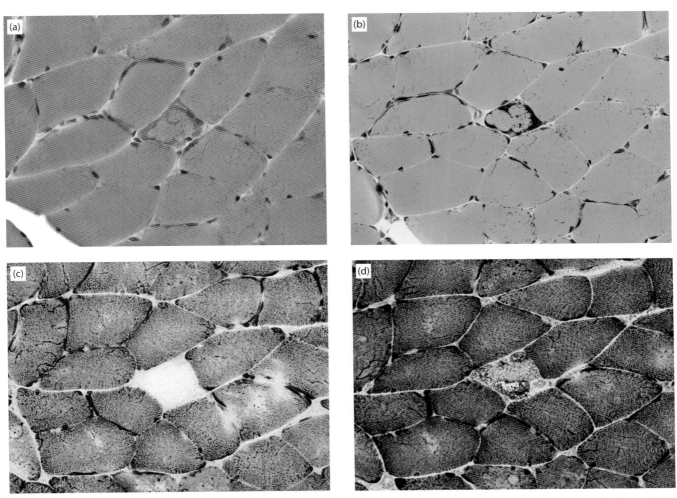

25.32 Serial sections of a ragged fibre showing (a) basophilia with haematoxylin and eosin, (b) red staining with Gomori trichrome, (c) absence of cytochrome c oxidase (COX), (d) and blue staining with the combined COX/ succinate dehydrogenase (SDH) technique due to the absence of COX but presence of SDH.

confusion with a muscular dystrophy, particularly if adipose tissue is abundant (see Congenital Myopathies and Allied Disorders, p. 1580). Necrosis and fibrosis are the two hallmarks of 'dystrophic' muscle, but necrosis may not always be apparent in the presence of fibrosis. Most disorders are characterized by muscle wasting and therefore are 'dystrophic', but the underlying cause may not always be one that involves necrosis. The term 'dystrophic' should therefore be defined, when used, in particular with regard to the presence of necrosis.

A variety of infiltrating cells may be present in a biopsy and can be visualized with routine histological stains and with specific cellular markers (see Figure 25.33). Macrophages are the most common, both classically activated M1 and alternatively activated M2 macrophages.[342] Macrophages can be seen within necrotic fibres and in the connective tissue, and stain positively for acid phosphatase. In macrophagic myofasciitis, a reaction to aluminium in vaccines, they are localized to the fascia and the muscle is otherwise relatively normal (see Figure 25.105). Inflammatory cell reactions are non-specific and can occur to varying degrees in several forms of muscular dystrophy and in inflammatory myopathies (Figure 25.34), although they are

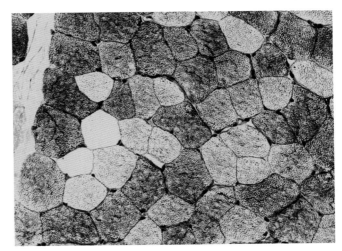

25.33 Fibres devoid of glycogen that appear white when stained with periodic acid–Schiff reagent.

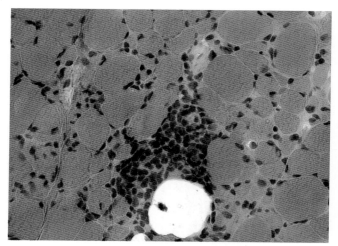

25.34 A focus of inflammatory cells in a case of muscular dystrophy. H&E.

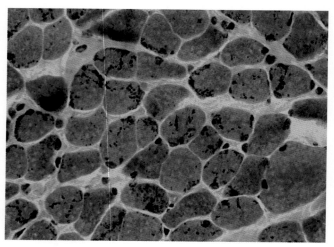

25.35 Red-stained rods in most fibres in a case of nemaline myopathy. Gomori trichrome.

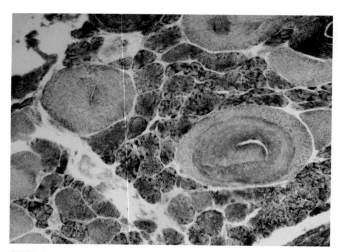

25.36 A population of small lobulated fibres with accumulations of mitochondria, particularly in peripheral triangular areas, in a case of limb-girdle muscular dystrophy with a mutation in the gene encoding calpain-3. Note also the hypertrophic fibres with whorled myofibrils. NADH-TR.

the hallmark of inflammatory myopathies. However, they are not a universal feature in inflammatory myopathies and their absence does not exclude the diagnosis. The cells may reside mainly in perivascular regions or may be endomysial, and the predominant cell type may vary with the acuteness of the condition and the timing of the biopsy. Cellular reactions are often seen in DMD and may be extensive in some cases of FSHD, the limb-girdle dystrophy with a defect in dysferlin (LGMD2B) and other forms of muscular dystrophy. Eosinophils are rarely seen in pathological muscle but have been reported to be a feature in cases with a defect in calpain (LGMD2A).[237] Cellular reactions are less common in the neurogenic atrophies, but they may occur, particularly in some of the more chronic neuropathies and inflammatory peripheral neuropathies.

Several structural changes can occur in abnormal muscle, and these are best observed with techniques such as the Gomori trichrome stain and oxidative enzyme stains. Some of these changes reflect a specific underlying pathological process, whereas others are non-specific. Electron microscopy is often helpful in defining the structural abnormalities.

Some structural defects, such as nemaline rods, abnormal mitochondria, tubular aggregates, cytoplasmic bodies and reducing bodies, are revealed by their red stain with the Gomori technique. None of these structures is specific, but an abundance of them can often suggest a diagnosis and direct further studies. Nemaline rods are the particular feature of all forms of nemaline myopathy and are associated with mutations in several genes (Figure 25.35; see Nemaline Myopathies, p. 1580). It is rarely possible to identify the affected gene from routine histological or histochemical studies.

Structurally abnormal mitochondria stain red with the Gomori trichrome technique, giving rise to fibres commonly termed 'ragged-red fibres' (see Figure 25.32). In addition to the 'ragged-red' appearance and a basophilic granular appearance with H&E, these fibres may lack COX activity and sometimes show enhanced NADH-TR and SDH reactions. Some fibres may show pronounced enhanced COX activity. The combined technique for detection of COX and SDH is useful for identifying fibres that lack COX but

retain their SDH activity and stain blue (see Figure 25.32). The absence of ragged-red fibres or fibres with enhanced oxidative enzyme activity does not exclude a mitochondrial problem (see Mitochondrial Myopathies, p. 1602).

Aggregates of mitochondria with no structural abnormality are also common. In normal muscle they often occur at the periphery of fibres or near capillaries, and they may appear as 'tram-lines' in two adjacent fibres. In lobulated fibres, aggregates of small mitochondria form triangular zones at the periphery of fibres (Figure 25.36). They can occur in a variety of conditions, but they can be a feature of some cases of the limb-girdle dystrophy caused by mutations in the gene for calpain-3 (LGMD2A). In our experience, lobulated fibres rarely occur in biopsies from children, but fibres with some resemblance to them, with pronounced peripheral aggregation of mitochondria, may occur.

Tubular aggregates also stain red with the Gomori trichrome technique, and although they can occur in a variety of disorders they are a feature of some periodic paralysis

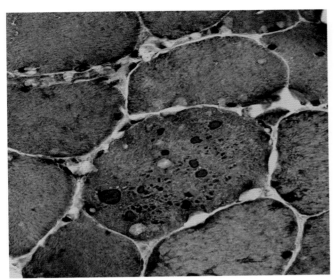

25.37 Several cytoplasmic bodies of varying size stained red with Gomori trichrome.

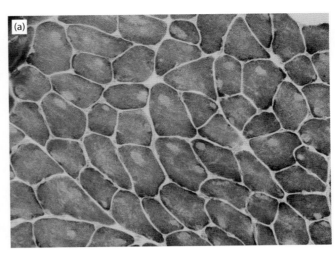

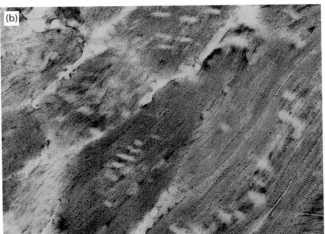

25.38 (a) Large core areas devoid of oxidative enzyme activity in a case of core myopathy caused by a mutation in the *RYR1* gene. Note also that some fibres have more than one core and the uniformity of fibre type. **(b)** Multiple minicore cores in several fibres in a molecularly unresolved myopathy; note that some fibre typing can be distinguished. NADH-TR.

and myasthenic syndromes (see Ion Channel Disorders, p. 1594; and Myasthenic Syndromes, p. 1596), and of phosphoglycerate mutase deficiency.[113] Histochemically, tubular aggregates can be identified by their lack of COX and SDH activity and by positive staining with techniques such as NADH-TR and myoadenylate deaminase. They often have a predilection for type 2 fibres and are believed to be derived from the sarcoplasmic reticulum. They can, therefore, be labelled with antibodies to the sarcoplasmic reticulum ATPase (SERCA). Dysferlin and emerin have also been shown to be associated with tubular aggregates.[202,270]

Cytoplasmic bodies are also a non-specific feature, but they are more common in disorders such as inclusion body myositis (IBM) and the myofibrillar myopathies caused by mutations in a variety of genes encoding myofibrillar proteins (Figure 25.37). They can also appear eosinophilic and in hereditary myopathy with early respiratory failure (HMERF) the eosinophilic bodies that have been described as cytoplasmic bodies bind phalloidin, indicating the presence of F-actin. Reducing bodies also stain red with the Gomori trichrome technique and may resemble cytoplasmic bodies. Reducing bodies, however, can be distinguished by their positive staining with the menadione NBT technique (without substrate). This technique, although very useful for staining reducing bodies, can also stain globular bodies in cases with acid maltase deficiency,[410] and areas of accumulated or disrupted myofibrils in some fibres in myofibrillar myopathies (see Z-line Associated Proteins and Four-and-a-Half LIM Domains Protein 1, p. 1591).

Myofibrillar disruption may occur in core-like and target lesions that are devoid of mitochondria (Figure 25.38) or in whorled or ring fibres (Figures 25.36 and 25.39). Cores can vary in size and in the degree of myofibrillar disruption (see Congenital Myopathies and Allied Disorders, p. 1580), but they are non-specific (see Figure 25.38). Large areas (central or peripheral) devoid of oxidative enzyme stains and running a considerable length down a fibre are the characteristic feature of core myopathy (also known as central core disease), caused by mutations in the ryanodine

receptor 1 gene. Multiple small areas of disruption (minicores), affecting only a few sarcomeres, occur to varying degrees in several disorders and are associated with defects in several genes, which include selenoprotein 1 (*SEPN1*), ryanodine receptor 1 (*RYR1*), collagen 6 (*COL6*), skeletal actin (*ACTA1*) and slow myosin (*MYH7*), which are responsible for various forms of congenital dystrophy, congenital myopathies and distal forms of myopathies (see relevant sections). Correlations with clinical phenotype are then particularly important when making a diagnosis. Targets are similar to cores and have a central area of disrupted myofibrils, devoid of oxidative enzymes, and surrounded by a dark staining rim (see Figure 25.56). The outer zone of the fibre usually shows a normal appearance. Cores in *RYR1*-related core disease also sometimes have a dark-stained rim around them, but target fibres are a particular feature of denervated muscle.

In ring fibres, a zone of myofibrils at the periphery of the fibre is oriented at right-angles to the long axis of the fibre, and the striations of the myofibrils in this ring can often

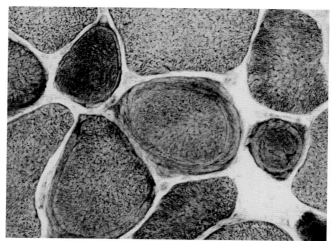

25.39 Ring fibres with a peripheral zone of myofibrils longitudinally oriented at 90° to the remaining myofibrils. NADH-TR.

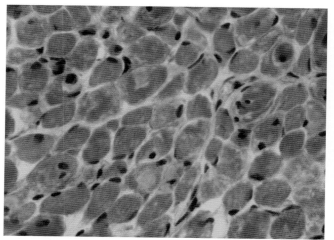

25.40 Pale-staining zones in several fibres representing an accumulation of actin filaments in a case of nemaline myopathy with a mutation in the *ACTA1* gene. H&E.

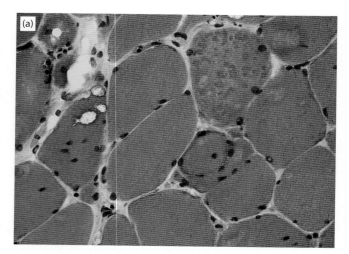

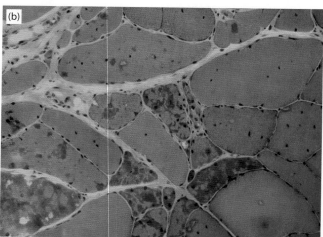

25.41 (a) Eosinophilic areas and (b) dark green areas showing accumulation of myofibrillar material in a case with a myofibrillar myopathy caused by a mutation in the gene encoding myotilin. Note also the presence of vacuoles. (a), H&E; (b), Gomori trichome.

be detected in preparations such as NADH-TR and PAS (see Figure 25.39). The myofibrillar disruption in whorled or coiled fibres is also revealed easily with NADH-TR and is more disorganized than in ring fibres (see Figure 25.36). Whorled fibres are often hypertrophic and are common in muscular dystrophies, but they can also occur in neurogenic disorders.

Pale-staining areas in routine histological stains can also reflect myofibrillar disruption, for example actin accumulation in some patients with nemaline myopathy with mutations in the *ACTA1* gene (Figure 25.40) and hyaline areas of myosin accumulation in some cases with mutations in the *MYH7* gene (see Figure 25.89).[443] Ultrastructural studies may be needed to clarify their exact nature. Other types of aggregated myofibrillar material may show enhanced eosin staining with H&E (Figure 25.41a) and appear dark green with Gomori trichrome (Figure 25.41b), which are a feature of myofibrillar myopathies. In myofibrillar myopathies and some cases of core myopathy the disrupted areas may be extensive and are devoid of oxidative enzyme stains and

ATPase activity. They may extend across the whole width of the fibre and give a 'wiped-out' or 'rubbed-out' appearance (Figure. 25.42). If the section passes through such an area, then the whole fibre may appear devoid of enzyme activity. Accumulation of myofibrillar proteins such as myotilin and desmin occurs not only in myofibrillar myopathies, but also in cores.

Vacuoles can occur in several conditions and are of different types. The disorders in which they are most common include IBM, the myofibrillar myopathies, distal myopathies, glycogenoses and periodic paralysis, although an absence of vacuoles does not exclude these diagnoses. Vacuoles rimmed by basophilia in H&E preparations and red-staining material with Gomori trichrome are the ones typically seen in IBM, some myofibrillar myopathies and some distal myopathies (Figure 25.43). The similar appearance of the vacuoles in these disorders, and the similar accumulation of proteins, particularly if no inflammatory infiltrate is present, can cause diagnostic difficulties. Some vacuoles have detectable material within them but others appear as empty spaces. It is important to distinguish

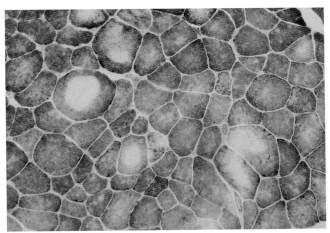

25.42 Cores and pronounced areas devoid of oxidative enzyme activity described as 'wiped-out' areas in a case with a mutation in the gene encoding ZASP. COX.

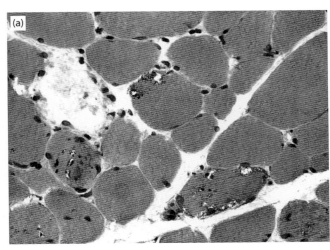

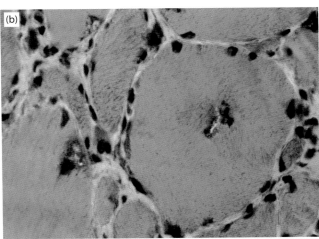

25.43 Rimmed vacuoles with associated (a) basophilia and (b) red stain in a case of inclusion body myositis. (a), H&E; (b), Gomori trichome.

freezing artefacts from this type of vacuole and not to interpret the presence of excess lipid droplets as vacuoles. Vacuoles are lined by membrane in two X-linked conditions characterized by excessive autophagic vacuoles, one caused by mutations in the *VMA21* gene encoding a V-ATPase and the other caused by a mutation in the *LAMP-2* gene.[317,352] Indentations of the sarcolemma also show sarcolemmal proteins (see Application of Immunohistochemistry in the Diagnosis of Neuromuscular Disorders, p. 1542).

A vacuolar appearance may be seen in some glycogen storage diseases with routine stains (Figure 25.44a). These areas are often where glycogen has accumulated, but it is not always detectable and may be lost during processing and staining (see Disorders of Glycogen Metabolism and Glycolysis, p. 1598). Similarly, if lipid droplets are large and prominent (Figure 25.44.b) they may appear as holes in H&E sections and have to be distinguished from freezing artefact. In type V glycogenosis (McArdle disease) the periphery of fibres may appear vacuolated, and in severe childhood cases of acid maltase deficiency (Pompe disease) vacuoles are prominent and ultrastructural studies reveal their membranes. These vacuoles do not usually label with antibodies to sarcolemmal proteins and stain intensely for acid phosphatase, indicating their lysosomal origin. In milder adult cases of acid maltase deficiency, the vacuoles are restricted mainly to type 1 fibres.

An important application of enzyme histochemistry is the detection of deficient activity, and this emphasizes the importance of freezing tissue samples and avoiding fixation. In addition to the absence of COX in scattered fibres in some mitochondrial disorders (see Figure 25.35), type V glycogenosis (McArdle disease) is characterized by a complete absence of phosphorylase from all fibres. Activity is detected in immature fibres and blood vessels, however, because of the presence of a different isoform. The only disorders where this total absence occurs are McArdle disease and the rare cases with a mutation in the *GYS1* gene that affects glycogen synthesis, because the enzyme method for detection requires endogenous glycogen l (see Figure 25.95). Damaged fibres devoid of glycogen ('white fibres') and cores show absence of phosphorylase for the same reason.

Staining for phosphofructokinase can also show an unequivocal absence of this protein, but such cases are rare. Detection of a reduction in the enzyme may be difficult to assess histochemically and requires biochemical analysis.

Myoadenylate deaminase activity may also be absent in fibres, and lack of this enzyme has been associated with myalgias and cramps during exercise. However, the clinicopathological significance of this is not entirely clear, because there is a common mutation/polymorphism of the corresponding gene in the normal population, which leads to absence of the enzyme.

Detection of excess glycogen or lipid may be useful. In glycogen storage disorders, excess glycogen may be seen throughout the fibre, peripherally, or concentrated in the vacuolated fibres. Glycogen is easily lost from fibres, and celloidin coating may be needed to demonstrate the excess glycogen.

Lipid droplets accumulate in muscle fibres in carnitine deficiency, but there is usually no detectable histochemical lipid accumulation in carnitine palmitoyl transferase deficiency. Type 1 fibres contain more mitochondria and associated lipid than type 2 fibres, and a fibre type pattern of lipid deposition is usually seen in normal muscle. Both the number and the size of the droplets may be abnormal in metabolic disorders but this is not always easy to assess, and in disorders of β-oxidation the result with oil red O or Sudan black staining may not give a clear answer.

APPLICATION OF IMMUNOHISTOCHEMISTRY TO THE DIAGNOSIS OF NEUROMUSCULAR DISORDERS

Immunohistochemical assessment of various proteins is now an essential part of the diagnostic process. Antibodies to most muscle cell components and organelles are now available. It is essential to know not only about the localization of a protein in normal muscle, but also how this varies during development because samples from fetuses and neonates and samples containing immature, regenerating fibres may have to be assessed. Several gene defects result in a change in the localization and expression of the encoded protein, particularly in recessive conditions. In dominant conditions, the normal allele produces a normal protein, and this may mask any effect of the abnormal protein. In addition, antibodies to a mutated protein may not be available or work reliably on sections and/ or immunoblots. Secondary alterations are then useful indicators of the pathological process, although they may not provide a definitive answer.

Developmental Regulation of Muscle Proteins

Several proteins in skeletal muscle are developmentally regulated. The level of detectable protein may be either higher or lower than in mature muscle, and its localization may alter (Table 25.4). In addition, different isoforms of a protein may be present at different stages of development. The following summary is not intended as a comprehensive account of the developmental regulation of muscle proteins

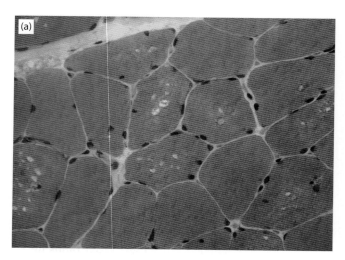

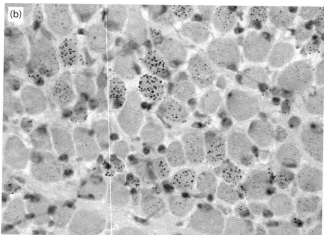

25.44 (a) Vacuoles in a population of fibres in an adult case with a deficiency of acid maltase. (H&E.) **(b)** Oil red O staining showing prominent lipid droplets in several fibres that can appear similar to vacuoles in haematoxylin and eosin-stained sections.

TABLE 25.4 Proteins relevant to pathology whose expression changes during development
Change of isoform:
Actin
Cardiac → skeletal
Myosin
Embryonic → fetal → fast or slow
Low expression on immature and regenerating fibres:
β-Spectrin (low round small regenerating fibres)
C-terminal dystrophin (sometimes)
Some dystrophin-associated proteins
Neuronal nitric oxide synthase
Integrin α7
Laminin β2
High expression on/in regenerating fibres:
Utrophin
Laminin α5
Neural cell adhesion molecule
Vimentin
Desmin
Major histocompatibility class I

but considers those relevant to the diagnostic assessment of muscle biopsies.

Studies of the developmental isoforms of myosin are useful for assessing immaturity and can sometimes help to distinguish an atrophic fibre from one that is small because it is regenerating. Antibodies to both embryonic and fetal/ neonatal myosin identify the early stages of regeneration, and immature myosins are detectable for a longer time than other developmentally regulated proteins such as utrophin, desmin and NCAM (unpublished observation).[501] Although the presence of fetal/neonatal myosin can reflect immaturity, its presence in some situations may relate to non-innervation of a fibre or possibly to a non-specific pathological response. Nuclear clumps, considered to reflect chronic atrophy, can express fetal/neonatal myosin, and experimental studies of denervated muscle suggest that embryonic myosin can be detected in this setting.[208,415] An antibody often used to detect fetal/neonatal myosin (Leica/Novocastra MHCn) is one thought to recognize the myosin encoded by the *MYH8* gene. In humans the protein is detectable in fetal muscle fibres from at least 7 weeks' gestation and is abundant during fetal development. We thus refer to this isoform as 'fetal myosin'. The number of positive fibres may be high at birth but by 4–5 months of age no, or very few, positive fibres are seen. However, the age at which MHCn is no longer detected in human muscle fibres is not clear, because muscle biopsies from neonates have all been taken for a clinical reason and may not be unequivocally normal. In animal models (e.g. rodents), muscle fibres are more immature at birth and immature myosins are abundant; however, the MHCn antibody does not cross react with myosin in all species. The antibody MHCd (Leica/Novocastra) is thought to recognize the isoform encoded by the *MYH3* gene and the terms 'embryonic' or 'developmental' myosin are often used synonymously. Thus in human muscle the MHCd antibody probably recognizes an early embryonic isoform of myosin present early in development and in regenerating fibres, whereas the MHCn antibody recognizes the fetal isoform that not only is present in immature and regenerating fibres but may also be present or re-expressed for pathological reasons. MHCd-positive fibres are not usually present at birth, except in muscle spindles, cases with delayed maturation and pathological samples.

Actin is another important myofibrillar muscle protein that changes isoform during development. Cardiac actin expression is of pathological significance in nemaline myopathies. In fetal skeletal muscle, the cardiac muscle isoform is predominant, and this is then replaced by the isoform of skeletal muscle. The two isoforms are encoded by different genes, and the proteins differ by only four amino acid residues at the N-terminal region. Several commercial antibodies therefore recognize both isoforms. Using isoform-specific antibodies, it is possible to show that the cardiac isoform is present in the small basophilic regenerating fibres of dystrophic muscle, as well as some larger fibres that are probably regenerating fibres. The switch from the cardiac to the skeletal isoform occurs at a late stage of gestation, but a few fibres with cardiac actin can be detected at birth and the number declines rapidly postnatally.[203]

In samples from neonates and those with abundant regenerating fibres, it is important to take into account immaturity, because the expression of some proteins may be greater or less in immature muscle than mature muscle, as judged by immunolabelling (see Table 25.4). Utrophin is an autosomal homologue of dystrophin and is useful for the assessment of muscular dystrophies (see Muscular Dystrophies, p. 1553). It is highly expressed on the sarcolemma of normal fetal muscle fibres and regenerating fibres, and assessment of any pathological increase in utrophin therefore requires correlation with the presence of fetal myosin (Figure 25.45).

Laminin α5 and MHC class I are also proteins that are highly expressed on regenerating fibres (see Figure 25.45), therefore any assessment of possible abnormal expression must also be related to fetal myosin. Laminin α5 is present on fetal fibres, and its presence declines during fetal development.[403] MHC-I, however, is not present on the sarcolemma of fetal muscle fibres and is found only on regenerating fibres and in pathological samples. Expression of basal lamina proteins may appear to be increased on regenerating fibres because of duplication of the basal lamina. Vimentin and desmin are also increased in fetal and regenerating fibres and downregulated during development. Vimentin is only detected on vascular tissue in mature

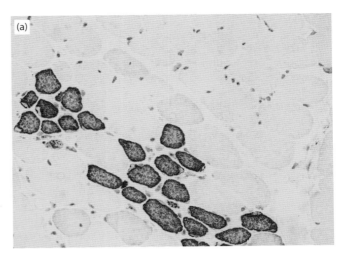

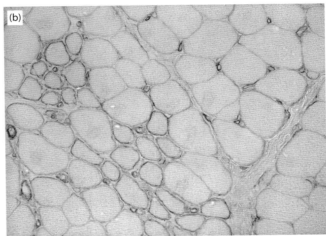

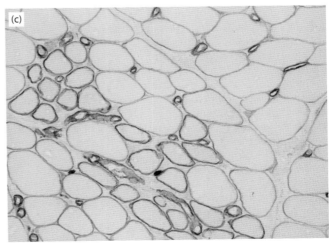

25.45 Serial sections of regenerating fibres immunolabelled for (a) fetal myosin (b) utrophin and (c) laminin α5. A higher expression of utrophin and laminin α5 is evident in fibres with fetal myosin.

muscle fibres, and desmin is found at the sarcolemma and internally in the fibres at the level of the Z-line. The neural cell adhesion molecule is present on the sarcolemma of regenerating and non-innervated fetal fibres, but following innervation NCAM, in a similar manner to utrophin, becomes localized to the neuromuscular junction; NCAM becomes extrajunctional again following denervation.[64] Extrajunctional NCAM is a common feature of DMD muscle, but the explanation for all of this, in relation to regeneration and innervation, is unclear.

Neuronal nitric oxide synthase is absent from the sarcolemma of regenerating fibres and from denervated fibres.[450] Comparing staining patterns for fetal myosin, nNOS and laminin α5, which appears unaltered by denervation, can then be helpful in distinguishing immature from denervated fibres. Fibres without both fetal myosin and nNOS and with normal levels of laminin α5 are thus likely to be denervated.

Other sarcolemmal proteins are also weakly labelled in immature neonatal muscle, and this may make pathological assessment difficult at this developmental stage. Several proteins, including β-spectrin, sarcoglycans, C-terminal dystrophin and nNOS, may appear weak on some small regenerating fibres that express fetal myosin, possibly because of immaturity and a plasma membrane that is not developed fully. Internal labelling of small basophilic fibres may also be seen with several antibodies. Sarcolemmal nNOS is labelled only weakly or is absent in neonatal muscle, and normal levels may not be reached until a few years of age.[117] Labelling of nNOS at the neuromuscular junction in immature muscle, however, is prominent.

Primary Protein Defects in Muscle Detectable with Immunohistochemistry

The growing number of defective genes and proteins responsible for a neuromuscular disorder that can be detected by immunohistochemistry are summarized in Table 25.5. These proteins are localized to diverse subcellular components, and any detectable immunohistochemical abnormalities depend upon the nature of the mutation, its effect on the protein product, and its mode of inheritance. In recessive disorders, if a mutation results in a stop codon, then an absence of protein can be demonstrated; if the mutations are missense, however, an alteration in protein may not be apparent with immunohistochemistry. In some instances, a reduction in the amount or molecular mass of protein may be visible on immunoblots. In most dominant disorders, the expression of protein from the normal allele may mask any alteration resulting from the abnormal allele. An exception to this is caveolin in LGMD1C (see Limb-Girdle Muscular Dystrophies, p. 1558). Not all antibodies recognize both native and denatured protein and may not be suitable for both immunohistochemical and immunoblot studies. For this reason, most studies of calpain-3 have been performed on immunoblots, although immunohistochemical studies have been performed and can detect an absence of the protein (see Limb-Girdle Muscular Dystrophies, p. 1558).[70] In assessing some proteins, it is important to use more than one antibody, for example dystrophin and laminin α2 (see Duchenne and Becker Muscular Dystrophy, p. 1553; and Congenital Muscular Dystrophies and Allied Disorders, p. 1565). Some proteins, such as titin and nebulin are extremely large and several alternatively spliced isoforms exist. It is then often not possible to detect a total absence of these large proteins, but specific epitopes may be absent.

In some conditions, the alteration in immunolabelling may be subtle, for example some cases of partial deficiency of laminin α2. In Ullrich CMD there may be a pronounced reduction in the expression of collagen VI in some cases, but in others the reduction may be mild and subtle and only seen at the sarcolemma, with normal reactivity in the endomysium, which is often increased in these patients (see Congenital Muscular Dystrophies and Allied Disorders, p. 1565). In these situations, immunolabelling of an additional protein, such as perlecan, to control for visualization and good preservation of the basement membrane is important. Good preservation of the sarcolemma is also important when assessing dystrophin and laminin α2, and antibodies to β-spectrin, caveolin-3 and laminin γ1 are useful for evaluating this. Slow myosin heavy chain has been localized to the hyaline bodies seen in cases with a mutation in the *MYH7* gene, but they are not seen in all cases with involvement of this gene.[162]

Accumulation of protein can occur if the corresponding gene is mutated. Actin filaments may accumulate in some neonatal cases of nemaline myopathy caused by a mutation in the *ACTA1* gene (although no mutation has been found in a few cases with actin accumulation) and they have also been observed in the reported cases of zebra body myopathy, also caused by a mutation in the *ACTA1* gene. Accumulation of actin can be suspected by the presence of pale areas in histological preparations (see Figure 25.40) and can be confirmed by electron microscopy. There are no commercial antibodies that specifically recognize skeletal muscle actin but phalloidin, which binds to F-actin, can be used to show it. Accumulation of desmin, myotillin, filamin C, Bag3 and four and a half LIM domains protein 1 (FHL1) can occur to varying degrees when the corresponding genes are mutated, and also as a secondary feature when any of them are the cause of a myofibrillar myopathy (see Myopathies Caused by Defects in Sarcomeric Proteins, p. 1589).

Secondary Protein Defects in Muscle Detectable with Immunohistochemistry

Many alterations in protein expression and/or localization that are secondary to a primary defect in another gene have been studied in pathological muscle. We list in Table 25.6 proteins that we find helpful for the assessment of pathological muscle.

Immunohistochemical studies of β-spectrin are useful for assessing the integrity of the plasmalemma, disruption of which may be induced artefactually or pathologically. Also, because it labels the periphery of fibres, β-spectrin sometimes gives a clearer indication of fibre size variability than routine histological stains. β-Spectrin is lost from the sarcolemma of necrotic fibres and labelling can appear weaker on regenerating fibres (Figure 25.46). Internal labelling is seen on the membranes of splits (Figure 25.47), some vacuoles, invaginations and branched fibres and in myofibrillar myopathies. Myotendinous and neuromuscular junctions are labelled more intensely with antibodies to several plasmalemmal and basal lamina proteins because of membrane folding (Figures 25.48 and 25.49). Invaginations of the sarcolemma, when sectioned transversely, for example at myotendinous junctions, may sometimes be confused

TABLE 25.5 Primary protein defects in neuromuscular disorder where immunochemistry can be informative

Protein defect	Neuromuscular disorder
Absence of a protein	
Sarcolemma and associated proteins	
Dystrophin	Xp21 muscular dystrophies (absent from most fibres in Duchenne, reduced in Becker muscular dystrophy)
Sarcoglycans	Limb-girdle muscular dystrophies 2C-F
Dysferlin	Limb-girdle muscular dystrophy 2B
Caveolin-3	Limb-girdle muscular dystrophy 1A, rippling muscle disease, hyperCKaemia
Laminin α2	Merosin-deficient congenital muscular dystrophy
Collagen VI	Ullrich congenital muscular dystrophy (often no detectable change in Bethlem myopathy)
Integrin α7	Mild congenital dystrophy/myopathy
Nuclear membrane	
Lamina-associated polypeptide 1B	Muscular dystrophy resembling Emery-Dreifuss but without elbow contractures
Emerin	X-linked Emery–Dreifuss muscular dystrophy
Nesprins	Autosomal Emery–Dreifuss muscular dystrophy
Sarcoplasmic reticulum	
SERCA1	Brody disease
RyR1	Some cases of core myopathy
Cytoskeleton	
Plectin	Epidermolysis bullosa with muscular dystrophy
Enzymes	
Calpain-3	Immunoblots may show an absence in limb-girdle muscular dystrophy 2A; sections may show an absence
Accumulation of the protein	
Actin	Actin- related nemaline myopathy
Myosin (slow)	Myosin storage myopathy
Desmin	Desmin-related myofibrillar myopathy
Myotilin	Myotilin-related myofibrillar myopathy
Filamin C	Filamin C-related myofibrillar myopathy
Four-and-a-half LIM domains protein 1 (FHL1)	FHL1-related myofibrillar myopathy
Vasolin-containing protein	Inclusion body myopathy with Paget's disease and frontal dementia

with vacuoles. Vacuoles of lysosomal origin, such as in acid maltase deficiency or those derived from the sarcoplasmic reticulum, do not usually label with β-spectrin or other sarcolemmal proteins, whereas the autophagic vacuoles in Danon disease (*LAMP-2* mutation) and in the X-linked myopathy with excessive autophagy (XMEA) show plasma membrane proteins on most vacuoles and basal lamina proteins on some.

Dystrophin rarely shows a secondary reduction in well-preserved muscle (but see Recessive Limb-Girdle Muscular Dystrophies, p. 1561). If dystrophin is reduced in a female patient, then careful distinction from a Duchenne carrier is needed (see Duchenne and Becker Muscular Dystrophy, p. 1553). Weak labelling with antibodies to the C terminus of dystrophin may be seen in some neonatal samples, possibly because of differential splicing at the C-terminal end of the gene.

Secondary changes in components of the DAG complex at the sarcolemma occur in DMD and LGMDs. Neuronal nitric oxide synthase is absent when dystrophin is absent and in cases of BMD with mutations in the rod domain 'hotspot' region.[279,454] This can be a quick and useful way of differentiating these mild BMDs from LGMD variants. Labelling of nNOS can also be useful in the assessment of neurogenic disorders, as discussed later (see Neurogenic Disorders, p. 1548).

Secondary modification in the O-glycosylation of a dystrophin-associated glycoprotein (DAG) is now recognized as an important pathogenic mechanism in various forms of CMD and some allelic LGMDs (see Congenital Muscular

TABLE 25.6 Secondary abnormalities in protein expression useful for assessment of pathological muscle

Protein	Disorder where useful
Utrophin	Xp21 and LGMDs
Sarcoglycans	LGMDs 2C-F
nNOS	Xp21 and disorders with denervation
Laminin α2	CMDs
Laminin β1	LGMD 2I, LGMD2L, ADEDMD, Bethlem myopathy
Laminin α5	CMDs regeneration v denervation
α-Dystroglycan	CMDs and LGMD2I
MHC class I	Pronounced in all inflammatory myopathies moderate in muscular dystrophies e.g. Xp21 & LGMD2B traces in several disorders
Myosin isoforms	Hybrid fibres in many disorders, good alternative to ATPase
Desmin accumulation	Cores, myofibrillar myopathies
Myotilin accumulation	Cores, myofibrillar myopathies
Filamin C	Myofibrillar myopathies
FHL1	Myofibrillar myopathies
Dystrophin	Myofibrillar myopathies, internal accumulation
F-actin (using phalloidin)	Eosinophilic bodies in HMERF
Cardiac actin	Regenerating fibres; nemaline myopathy null for *ACTA1*
Tau accumulation	Inclusion body myositis, myofibrillar myopathies
p62	Inclusion body myositis, autophagic vacuoles in several disorders

ADEDMD, autosomal dominant Emery–Dreifuss muscular dystrophy; CMD, congenital muscular dystrophy; FHL1, four and a half LIM domains protein 1; LGMD, limb-girdle muscular dystrophy; nNOS, neuronal nitric oxide synthase.

25.46 Immunolabelling of β-spectrin showing normal sarcolemmal labelling on most fibres, an absence on necrotic fibres and low labelling on regenerating fibres.

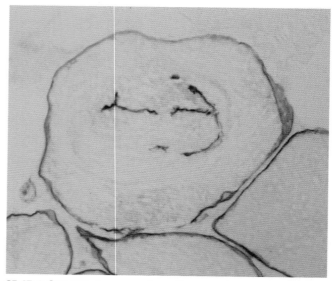

25.47 β-Spectrin is present on the sarcolemma and membranes of splits.

Dystrophies and Allied Disorders, p. 1565; and Limb-Girdle Muscular Dystrophies, p. 1558), and is therefore useful for differential diagnosis.[19,159,279] Extensive glycosylation is essential for the binding of α-dystroglycan to extracellular matrix ligands including laminins, perlecan, agrin and, in brain and the eye, neurexin, pikachurin and Slit.

Utrophin is developmentally regulated and expressed in several tissues (see Developmental Regulation of Muscle Proteins, p. 1542). Utrophin immunoreactivity is detected on blood vessels, nerves and at myotendinous and neuromuscular junctions. In addition to its expression on regenerating fibres in a variety of disorders, utrophin is prominent on the sarcolemma of mature fibres (without fetal myosin) in DMD (Figure 25.50), BMD and inflammatory myopathies,[193] although in young patients with DMD few mature fibres without fetal myosin are labelled.[447] Manifesting carriers of DMD also show overexpression on fibres with and without dystrophin. Expression of utrophin is not specific to Xp21 disorders, and low levels can be detected in neonatal muscle in a variety of disorders, and on muscle fibres adjacent to tumours.[404,408]

Two full-length forms of utrophin have been identified, regulated by alternatively spliced promoters.[52] The A isoform is present on the sarcolemma of fetal fibres and is overexpressed in dystrophic muscle. The B isoform is restricted to blood vessels. The isoform(s) recognized by commercial antibodies has not been determined.

The increase in perimysial and endomysial connective tissue that occurs in several disorders can be confirmed by demonstrating the accumulation of several extracellular matrix proteins. These include various types of collagen, such as types III, V and VI, and fibronectin. In normal muscle, several collagen types are constituents of the basement membrane and appear at the sarcolemma, and the periphery of each fibre is clearly delineated by antibodies to collagen types IV, V and VI, laminins, perlecan and nidogen. They are also seen in the extracellular matrix around blood vessels. When

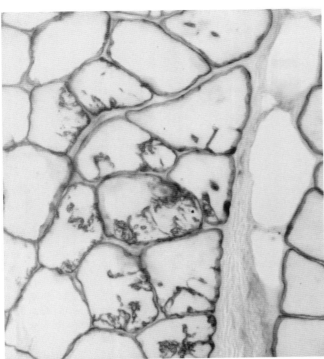

25.48 Laminin α2 immunolabelling of myotendinous junctions. The sectioning of some folds/invaginations gives the impression of vacuoles.

25.49 Enhanced immunolabelling of β-dystroglycan at a neuromuscular junction, probably due to folding of the sarcolemma.

connective tissue is increased, the sarcolemmal labelling of collagen types V and VI is usually more prominent than that of the adjacent endomysium (Figure 25.51; see Congenital Muscular Dystrophies and Allied Disorders, p. 1565).

Secondary changes in some laminin chains are seen in various muscular dystrophies, in particular various forms of CMD.[279,307] Laminin α2 is a ligand for α-dystroglycan and shows a secondary reduction in Fukuyama CMD, muscle–eye–brain disease, MDC1B and MDC1C. In LGMD2I, sarcolemmal labelling of laminin α2 usually appears normal, but may show a marked reduction on immunoblots.[54]

A reduction in laminin β1 on the sarcolemma, but not blood vessels, can be seen in some conditions, such as Bethlem

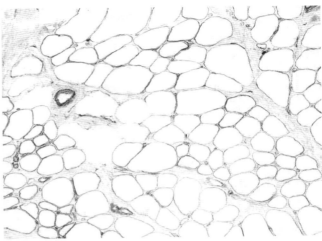

25.50 Pronounced immunolabelling of utrophin on the sarcolemma of most fibres in a case of Duchenne muscular dystrophy. Note also normal labelling of the blood vessels, including capillaries.

myopathy and autosomal dominant Emery–Dreifuss muscular dystrophy (Figure 25.52),[287,448] and has been observed in several cases with mutations in the *ANO5* gene (Barresi and Sewry, unpublished observation). However, it is not specific and has been observed in a variety of myopathies, but it is age dependent and seen in affected adults and adolescents, but rarely in biopsies from children.

Laminin α5 on the sarcolemma is increased in cases with a primary defect in laminin α2 (MDC1A), and its staining is often greater than in normal muscle in Xp21 dystrophies and inflammatory myopathies. Because expression of laminin α5 is developmentally regulated, some changes may relate to regeneration or immaturity, and careful correlation with fetal myosin is needed.

Assessment of MHC-I has been known to be useful in inflammatory myopathies for many years.[4] Normal mature muscle fibres express minimal or no detectable MHC-I, but it is detectable on the endothelial cells of blood vessels. MHC-I is expressed by regenerating fibres in all disorders, but not by fetal fibres; therefore, comparisons with fetal myosin reactivity are important for distinguishing the abnormal expression of MHC-I from that related to regeneration. In most cases of inflammatory myopathy, overexpression of MHC-I occurs on the sarcolemma, and sometimes within the fibres.[4] Overexpression of MHC-I is not specific to inflammatory myopathies and may also be seen to varying degrees in various muscular dystrophies, including DMD, BMD, LGMD2B and acid maltase deficiency.[94,131]

Studies of myosin heavy chain isoforms are informative in the assessment of fibre types in most biopsies. In diseased muscle, hybrid fibres are common and an excessive number of these can be used as an indicator of pathology. The size and number of fibres expressing fetal myosin in pathological muscle varies, and it can be useful to assess the variable patterns of their distribution in different disorders (Figure 25.53). In severe muscular dystrophies (e.g. DMD), a large diffuse population of labelled fibres of variable size and intensity is often seen. In BMD, clusters of immunopositive fibres may occur in some areas, whereas very small positive fibres are distributed diffusely elsewhere. In

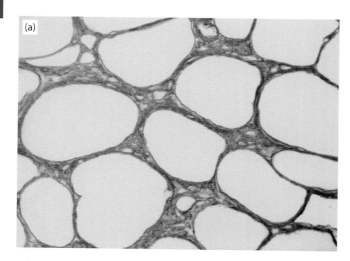

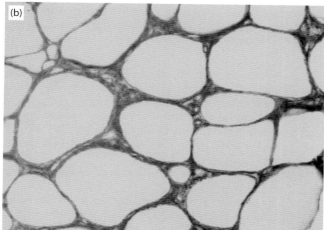

25.51 Immunolabelling of (a) collagen V and (b) collagen VI showing pronounced labelling of the excess connective tissue, but note labelling at the sarcolemmal can be distinguished.

25.52 Reduced labelling of laminin β1 at the sarcolemma, but normal intensity on all the blood vessels.

filamin C, ZASP, Bag3 and FHL1 may be seen. In IBM, several proteins accumulate in muscle, many of which are also found in the brain of patients with Alzheimer's disease (see Inflammatory Myopathies, p. 1605).[6]

NEUROGENIC DISORDERS

Inherited and acquired neurogenic disorders are caused by the defective function of, or damage to, lower motor neurons or peripheral nerves. Such disorders include motor neuron disease (amyotrophic lateral sclerosis; ALS), in which both upper and lower motor neurons are affected; the SMAs (lower motor neuron); hereditary motor and sensory neuropathies (HMSNs) or isolated hereditary motor neuropathies, which are broadly divided into demyelinating or axonal disorders;[370,500] and inflammatory peripheral neuropathies. In addition, ageing of muscle can be accompanied by a neuropathy, and involvement of lower motor neurons and peripheral nerves can also be found in some neurometabolic disorders such as peroxisomal disorders, in mitochondrial diseases, and heredodegenerative conditions such as neuroaxonal dystrophy and pontocerebellar hypoplasia type I. Peripheral neuropathy is also a component of some myofibrillar myopathies (see Myopathies Caused by Defects in Sarcomeric Proteins, p. 1589).

Several causative genes responsible for neurogenic disorders have been identified, and inheritance may be dominant or recessive (see www.musclegenetable.fr). Studies of sural nerve biopsies can be helpful in the study of peripheral neuropathies, especially in inflammatory disease, but have a limited role in the genetic variants. Because this is a specialized field it is not discussed here; further details can be found in textbooks.[102,121,227,290]

In several of the common neurogenic disorders, electrophysiology and molecular genetic analysis offers a reliable and convenient diagnostic tool. This is the case in SMA, where electrophysiology findings and deletion of exons 7 and 8 of the *SMN1* gene identifies over 95 per cent of cases, and prognosis is based on severity of clinical features, not muscle pathology. Electrophysiology and genetic analysis also play an important role in the diagnosis of demyelinating

congenital myopathies, relatively few fibres with reactivity for fetal myosin are seen; these are often only a few microns in diameter and are easily overlooked in routine histological stains. The origin of these very small fibres (sometimes described as 'pinpricks') and their properties are uncertain but they are a useful indicator of abnormality.

Actin is seen as a secondary feature of the eosinophilic bodies resembling cytoplasmic bodies in cases of HMERF caused by mutations in the A-band domain of titin (see Myopathies Caused by Defects in Sarcomeric Proteins, p. 1589). Elevated levels of desmin are seen not only in regenerating fibres, but also when genes responsible for myofibrillar myopathies are mutated (see Myopathies Caused by Defects in Sarcomeric Proteins, p. 1589). Desmin is also seen in association with structural defects, such as cores or around hyaline bodies, and in some cases with a mutation in the gene for the nuclear membrane protein lamin A/C. Cores with disruption of myofibrils may show accumulation of several additional proteins, such as filamin C, myotilin, heat-shock proteins and ubiquitin.[392,400] In myofibrillar myopathies caused by mutations in genes encoding several Z-line proteins, accumulation of desmin, myotilin (Figure 25.54),

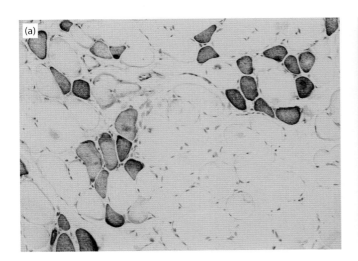

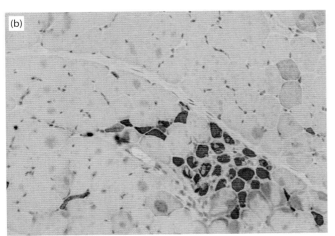

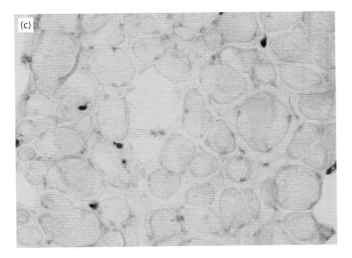

25.53 Variable number and distribution of fibres expressing fetal myosin in (a) Duchenne muscular dystrophy where a diffuse population is present, **(b)** in Becker muscular dystrophy where they are often clustered and **(c)** in a congenital myopathy where only a few very small fibres are positive.

neuropathies, where duplication of the peripheral myelin gene identifies the majority of individuals affected by this condition (HMSN1A). Genetic testing can also help in the

25.54 Pronounced accumulation of myotilin in a case of myofibrillar myopathy with a mutation in the myotilin gene.

diagnosis of other less common HMSN variants (details of the tests available can be found at www.molgen.ua.ac.be/cmtmutations/). In ALS, the yield from genetic testing is more limited, with only a minority of cases carrying a mutation in the Cu/Zn superoxide dismutase (*SOD-1*) gene. Mutations in other genes that cause forms of ALS include those that encode alsin (*ALS2*), senataxin (*SETX*), the fused in sarcoma (*FUS*), vesicle-associated membrane protein-associated protein B (*VAPB*), TAR-DNA–binding protein (TDP-43; *TARDPB*), vasolin-containing protein (*VCP*), optineurin (*OPTN)* and angiogenin (*ANG).*[414,453] In addition, mutations in the *C9ORF72* gene have been identified in cases with ALS and frontal dementia.[106,357] The majority of the defective proteins share similar biological functions, and are involved in similar pathways to those in other neurogenerative disorders, leading to the accumulation of related proteins.

Denervation of muscle in neurogenic disorders results in muscle weakness and wasting. The muscle wasting is more pronounced in cases with motor neuronal or axonal defects than in demyelinating disorders. Fasciculations may also be seen. Motor and sensory nerve conduction studies play a key role in the diagnosis of demyelinating disorders, whereas EMG readily identifies neurogenic defects caused by motor neuronal and axonal damage.

The changes seen in muscle biopsies following denervation are stereotypical, irrespective of the site of the lesion, and it is rarely possible to define the nature of the disorder from the muscle pathology, although certain patterns are suggestive. It is important to appreciate that some chronic neurogenic conditions may mimic some muscular dystrophies or myopathies. Although immunohistochemistry of the muscle may contribute to the interpretation of secondary changes in neurogenic disorders, the primary gene product is not usually studied.

The characteristic features of denervated muscle are grouping of atrophic fibres and groups of fibres of the same type, 1 and 2 (Figure 25.55). In addition, in chronic disorders, such as ALS and milder forms of SMA, dark angular fibres are seen in NADH-TR preparations and sometimes target fibres (Figure 25.56). Occasionally, split or whorled fibres are also found.

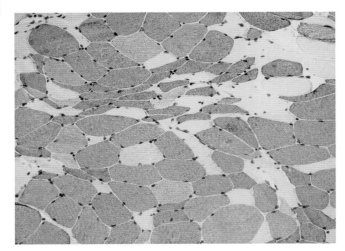

25.55 A group of angulated atrophic fibres of both types in a neurogenic disorder. Slow myosin.

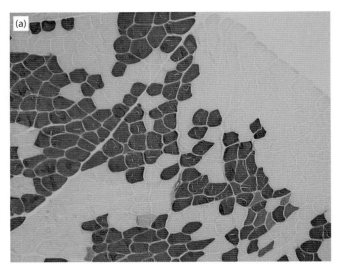

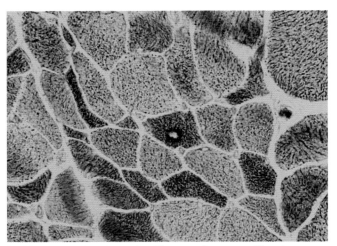

25.56 Dark-stained angular fibres and a target fibre in a neurogenic disorder. NADH-TR.

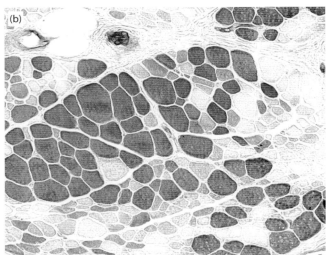

25.57 (a) Obvious and (b) less obvious fibre type grouping in two neurogenic disorders. ATPase pH 4.3.

Atrophic, denervated muscle fibres retain their internal architecture until late in the atrophic process, when all that may remain are clusters of nuclei, which may be pyknotic (see Figure 25.27). The basal lamina around individual fibres, however, is retained and may be thrown into folds. In chronic conditions such as ALS, the atrophic fibres have an angular shape, in contrast to the rounded shape of the atrophic fibres in childhood forms of SMA. ATPase and myosin immunostaining show that these fibres are of both types. These denervated fibres tend to have a positive esterase reaction but are negative for acid phosphatase activity, in contrast to regenerating or necrotic fibres, which are positive for both enzyme reactions. They may also lose their glycogen content and appear unstained and white with PAS. Some angulated fibres are immunoreactive for fetal myosin, and some may coexpress fast myosin. As discussed previously, this may reflect re-expression of fetal myosin rather than immaturity resulting from regeneration, but the possibility of regeneration stimulated by denervation cannot be excluded. Denervated fibres also show extrajunctional NCAM and lack of sarcolemmal nNOS, although reinnervated fibres express nNOS.[64,450] A number of studies of denervation and atrophy in animal species have identified quantitative alterations in several proteins that may prove in the future to be of pathological use in human conditions. In particular, the ubiquitin ligase muscle Ring finger 1 (MuRF-1), antrogen-1 and the sodium channel Nav1.5 are higher in atrophic fibres, whereas myosin-binding protein-C is reduced.[31,90,167,371]

In addition to the groups of atrophic fibres, groups of hypertrophied fibres and fibres of normal size are seen, because fibres supplied by an intact motor nerve retain their normal size or even develop compensatory hypertrophy. Surviving nerves sprout and reinnervate clusters of denervated fibres, causing them to enlarge again, and this collateral sprouting results in groups of fibres of the same type. Fibre type grouping is another pathognomonic feature of denervated muscle, but it may be difficult to assess and may not be obvious in all biopsies from neurogenic conditions (Figure 25.57). It is important to distinguish fibre type predominance from fibre type grouping, especially in a small sample, and groups of both types should be present to make a diagnosis of denervation. Coexpression of myosin isoforms may also make fibre types and grouping difficult to define in sections stained for ATPase.

Another characteristic of denervated muscle is the presence of target fibres, particularly in chronic disorders (see Figure 25.56). They are rarely seen in severe childhood forms of SMA. In some biopsies, the dark concentric rim of the target around the pale zone devoid of oxidative enzyme activity may not be prominent, and the fibres then have an appearance similar to those with central cores. Core-like areas can occur in fibres of varying size (see Spinal Muscular Atrophy) and are usually focal lesions, rarely extending down the whole length of a fibre.

Other architectural changes, such as moth-eaten and whorled fibres, may be seen occasionally with oxidative enzyme stains. Excess endomysial connective tissue and necrosis are not usually features of denervated muscle, but they can occur, particularly in chronic conditions. Similarly, internal nuclei may be seen in some hypertrophic fibres, and these features, in the absence of fibre type grouping, may make the pathology difficult to distinguish from a 'myopathic' picture.

Spinal Muscular Atrophy

Spinal muscular atrophy is one of the most common neuromuscular disorders, with an incidence of about 1 in 10 000 births. It is an autosomal recessive condition in which the degenerative process causes loss of anterior horn cells of the spinal cord. Box 25.4 gives details of the genetic defect in SMA.[66,330]

Three main SMA clinical groups, types I, II and III, are recognized on the basis of their relative severity and defined on whether the patient is able to sit or stand unaided or to walk (Table 25.7). Some clinicians also distinguish a fourth variant, in patients with adult onset (SMA IV), whereas others include these within the spectrum of SMA III. The clinical severity of SMA represents a continuum from the most severe, in type I, to milder cases with onset in adult life, and some cases fall in between the main subtypes.[116] The severest form, type I (Werdnig–Hoffmann disease), has its onset *in utero* or in very early infancy. Affected children are never able to sit or stand. In type II (intermediate) SMA, onset is usually before the first year of life; the ability to sit unsupported is achieved, but patients cannot stand or walk. The clinical spectrum of SMA III (Kugelberg–Welander disease) is broad, ranging from onset in the second year of life to adult onset. Differentiating these milder forms from a myopathic condition is important, as some patients may have a raised CK level.

The broad clinical phenotype is similar in all types of SMA, although severity is variable, with symmetrical weakness affecting the lower limbs more than the upper limbs and proximal muscles more than distal muscles. The facial and ocular muscles are typically spared. Bulbar involvement and fasciculation of the tongue are common, especially in types I and II. There is no associated sensory or upper motor neuron involvement.

The pathological changes seen in muscle biopsies in the severe infantile and intermediate forms are very similar. Although muscle biopsies are now performed less often in SMA, we summarize here the main pathological features as they highlight the characteristic features of denervated muscle.

The atrophic fibres, round in shape, often occur in large groups, which are interspersed with fascicles of

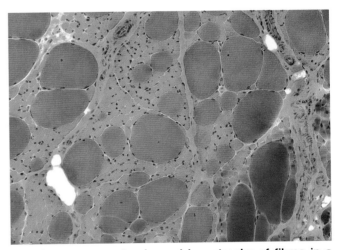

25.58 Large group atrophy and hypertrophy of fibres in a case of spinal muscular atrophy. Gomori trichrome.

hypertrophic fibres (Figure 25.58). There is usually minimal endomysial connective tissue, but the perimysium may be wide, as commonly seen in muscle from neonates. Atrophic fibres are both type 1 and 2, and large fibres are invariably type 1/slow fibres (Figure 25.59). Many of the grouped atrophic fibres may appear as type 2 with ATPase at pH 9.4, because of coexpression of more than one isoform of myosin, including fetal myosin.

The extent of atrophy may vary in different parts of the muscle. Some areas may consist entirely of atrophic fibres, whereas others may be composed entirely of normal-sized fibres. If a sample is small, it might consist entirely of small or normal fibres, or of fibres of one type. In occasional cases of severe SMA I, the sample may not show the classic features of group atrophy and fibre type grouping, and this situation has been referred to as 'pre-pathological SMA' (Figure 25.60). The

TABLE 25.7 Clinical features of spinal muscular atrophy

Type I (Werdnig–Hoffman Disease)	Type II (intermediate)	Type III (Kugelberg–Welander disease)
Onset *in utero* or within the first few months of life	Onset usually before 12 months	Onset from second year of life to childhood, adolescence or adulthood
Severe hypotonia	Hypotonia	
Severe limb and axial weakness	Symmetrical weakness of legs, predominantly proximal	Weakness static or slowly progressive
Poor head control		
Bell-shaped chest and diaphragmatic breathing		
Respiratory insufficiency that leads to early death		
Feeding difficulties		
Weak cry		
Sitting and weight bearing never achieved	Sitting unaided achieved Inability to stand unaided or walk	Difficulty running, jumping and climbing stairs Difficulty rising from floor (Gowers' manoeuvre) Ability to walk but may be limited
Fasciculation of the tongue	Fasciculation of tongue Tremor of hands common	Tongue fasciculation (variable) Hand tremor (variable)
Absent tendon jerks	Diminished or absent tendon jerks Progressive scoliosis common Intercostal muscle weakness with variable respiratory problems	
Creatine kinase normal	Creatine kinase normal or occasionally mild elevation	Creatine kinase normal or moderately elevated
EMG features of denervation with large amplitude polyphasic potential	EMG features of denervation and reinnervation with large amplitude polyphasic potentials and fasciculation	EMG features of denervation and re innervation with large amplitude polyphasic potentials
Motor nerve conduction velocity normal, although can be reduced in children at the severe end of type I spectrum	Normal nerve conduction velocity	Normal nerve conduction velocity

EMG, electromyelography.

combination of clinical features and genetic testing identifies such cases better than muscle pathology.

Degeneration, necrosis, nuclear changes (e.g. pyknotic or internal nuclei) and architectural changes within the fibres (e.g. targets, whorls) are rare in severe and intermediate SMA.

The pathological spectrum, as well as the clinical spectrum, is broad in mild cases of SMA III (Kugelberg–Welander syndrome), and the classic features of denervation may or may not be apparent. Group atrophy may occur, but the number of atrophic fibres per cluster tends to be less than in the severe forms, although it can also be extensive. Fibre type grouping also occurs, and type 2 fibre predominance may be a feature (Figure 25.61a). Architectural changes such as cores, target fibres, whorled fibres, split fibres and internal nuclei may also be seen (Figure 25.61b). Some milder cases may also have a mildly to moderately elevated serum CK level, and because focal groups of atrophic fibres are common in some forms of muscular dystrophy, such as BMD and FSHD, it is important to assess the overall pattern of abnormalities in the biopsy.

Differential Diagnosis of Neurogenic Disorders

Genes other than survival motor neuron (*SMN*) are responsible for clinical syndromes related to SMA. Some have more distal than proximal muscle involvement, and some have a dominant or X-linked inheritance. A number of genes for these variants with distal involvement, almost exclusively of the lower limbs have recently been reported, including *DYNHC1* and *TRPV4*.[10,461] An X-linked bulbospinal form with a benign course and associated facial and bulbar weakness and fasciculation, severe muscle cramps and gynaecomastia (Kennedy's disease), is caused by a CAG nucleotide expansion of the first exon of the androgen receptor on chromosome Xq11, and mutations influence the proteasomal and autophagic pathways.[141,372] A severe X-linked form with associated arthrogryposis maps to Xp13,[234] and another form is caused by mutations in the UBE1 gene that encodes for the ubiquitin-activating enzyme E1.[353] Another well-recognized autosomal recessive variant is characterized by severe diaphragmatic involvement (diaphragmatic spinal

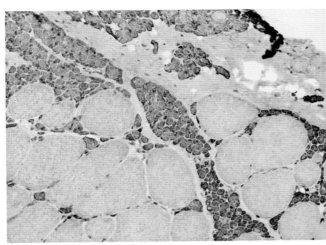

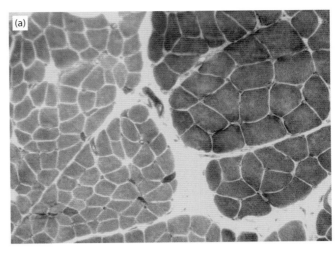

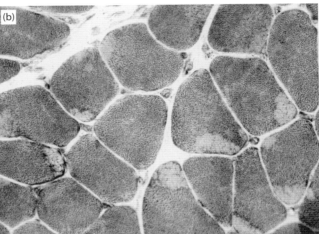

25.59 Groups of atrophic fibres in a case of spinal muscular atrophy most of which label as fast/type 2 fibres, with only an occasional slow/type 1 fibre, and hypertrophied slow/type 1 fibres. Fast myosin.

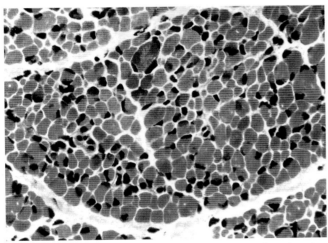

25.60 A case of severe spinal muscular atrophy showing 'pre-pathological' features with variability in fibre size but no classical group atrophy. H&E.

25.61 (a) Fibre type grouping and (b) core-like areas devoid of oxidative activity in a case of spinal muscular atrophy III. NADH-TR.

muscular atrophy with respiratory distress [SMARD1]) and is caused by mutations in the gene encoding immunoglobulin micro-binding protein 2 (IGHMBP2) on chromosome 11q13–q21.[172] The severe diaphragmatic involvement is a useful diagnostic feature when distinguishing SMARD from classic chromosome 5 SMA, in which the diaphragm is selectively spared, in spite of severe involvement of the intercostal muscles. The differential diagnosis of SMARD needs to take into consideration mutations of another gene (*MEGF10*) with several clinical similarities to SMARD1, but pathological features pointing towards a myopathy rather than a neuropathy; this gene may have a role in myogenesis.[187,253] The typical features of denervation in muscle biopsies are not always obvious in these more rare forms of SMA, and in *MEGF10* cases the features are myopathic.

Neurodegenerative disorders such as neuroaxonal dystrophy[240] and pontocerebellar hypoplasia type I may also resemble SMA pathologically[309] and to some extent clinically; however, the nature of the central nervous system

(CNS) involvement helps to differentiate them from chromosome 5-linked SMA. Mitochondrial disorders resembling severe SMA (SMA I) have also been reported and a rare variant of SMA with myoclonic epilepsy with defects in the *ASAH1* gene has been reported.[266,510]

INHERITED MUSCLE DISORDERS

Muscular Dystrophies

Duchenne and Becker Muscular Dystrophy

Duchenne muscular dystrophy is the most common form of muscular dystrophy, with an incidence usually quoted as 1 in 3500 live male births, but current data show 1 in 5000 is a more accurate estimate. The allelic Becker form (BMD) is less common, with a predicted incidence of 1 in 17 500 live male births.[126,128]

Both DMD and BMD are caused by mutations in the gene encoding the protein dystrophin on the short arm of the X chromosome.[128] Although standard genetic analysis of the gene detects many mutations, assessment of the presence of dystrophin is important.[306] Approximately 70 per cent of patients with DMD and BMD carry an intragenic deletion or duplication, and in most instances the effect of the deletion (or duplication) on the reading frame of the gene correlates with the clinical phenotype (i.e. out-of-frame deletions or duplications are associated with DMD, whereas in-frame deletions or duplications are associated with BMD; see Genotype–Phenotype Correlations, this page). However, exceptions to these rules are well documented, and in approximately 10 per cent of patients the phenotype does not correlate with the type of mutation, but correlates better with residual expression of the protein.

Clinical Features

The main clinical manifestations of DMD and BMD are summarized in Table 25.8 and are well documented elsewhere.[128] Creatine kinase levels are usually grossly elevated in both DMD and BMD (>50 × normal) at presentation and are also elevated at birth. There is no correlation between the level of CK and clinical severity. Progression of muscle weakness leads to loss of independent ambulation by the age of 12 years in boys with DMD, and is followed by scoliosis and respiratory insufficiency. Better management of these complications has improved the survival and quality of life of patients with DMD.

The clinical features of patients with BMD are milder, and age at presentation is often later than with DMD. At variance with the DMD phenotype, patients with BMD often have cramps on exercise, which can sometimes be associated with rhabdomyolysis. In the experience of the authors, a boy presenting with prominent cramps and occasional myoglobinuria following exercise is more likely to have a muscular dystrophy (such as BMD or LGMD2I) than a metabolic myopathy. Individuals with BMD are

ambulant at the age of 16 years, and in most instances these patients are still able to walk well into adulthood.

Cardiac involvement is present in most cases of DMD by late adolescence, and is common in BMD. Rare cases of X-linked cardiomyopathy, with minimal or no skeletal muscle weakness, are also caused by mutations in the dystrophin gene.[136] Immunolabelling of dystrophin in skeletal muscle of these cases appears normal but is severely reduced in their cardiac muscle. This difference in dystrophin expression is explained by differential splicing of full-length transcripts in skeletal and cardiac tissue.

Varying degrees of pathological change can be seen in DMD, even at a few months of age, and in BMD as young as 1 year, when there are no clinical manifestations of the disease other than elevated CK. The typical histopathological features of DMD and BMD are shown in Figure 25.20 and described earlier (see General Histological and Histochemical Abnormalities). It is not possible to distinguish DMD from BMD by the severity of the histopathology.

The gene encoding dystrophin that is responsible for DMD and BMD is one of the largest known, with 2.5 Mb of DNA and 79 exons. It has some very large introns and the transcribed mRNA is 14 kb. The full-length protein has a predicted molecular mass of 427 kDa and has four main domains (Figure 25.62). The N terminus is an actin-binding domain, the large rod domain has 24 spectrin-like repeats and 4 hinge regions, the cysteine-rich domain binds β-dystroglycan, and the C-terminal domain binds syntrophin, dystrobrevin and probably also F-actin and α-actinin. The dystrophin gene has at least seven promoters, with evidence from studies of lymphoblastoid cells of an eighth. The isoforms produced are of different molecular mass and are expressed differentially in skeletal, cardiac and smooth muscle, peripheral nerve, retina and brain (Figure 25.63), and there is considerable splicing at the 3' end. The various isoforms share a common C terminus (see Figure 25.63), and antibodies to C-terminal epitopes recognize all isoforms. In adult skeletal and cardiac muscles, the full-length transcripts from the muscle promoters located at the 5' end and transcribing 79 exons are the most important.[48]

Dystrophin is a cytoskeletal protein that lies on the cytoplasmic face of the plasma membrane. It interacts with the actin cytoskeleton and a complex of other proteins, the DAGs, which include α- and β-dystroglycan, sarcoglycans, dystrobrevin, syntrophin and nNOS (Figure 25.64). These interactions probably account for a number of the secondary changes in protein expression seen in DMD (see Genotype–Phenotype Correlations, below). Although the exact function of dystrophin is still unclear, it is believed to act as a link between the extracellular matrix and the cytoskeleton, stabilizing the muscle membrane during contraction, and also to have a role in signalling.

TABLE 25.8 Main clinical features of Duchenne muscular dystrophy (DMD) and Becker muscular dystrophy (BMD)

Manifests within the first 5 years of life (DMD, BMD variable)
Delayed motor milestones
Progressive proximal weakness
Contracture of Achilles tendon resulting in toe walking
Waddling gait, lumbar lordosis
Difficulty running, hopping, jumping (unable to do so in DMD)
Difficulty rising from floor (Gowers' manoeuvre, invariable in DMD)
Difficulty going up stairs
Calf hypertrophy
Cramps–Becker rather than Duchenne
Ambulation
    DMD: lost by 12 years
    BMD: ambulant beyond 16 years
Creatine kinase
    Always grossly elevated (10–50 times normal)
    Elevated at birth
Associated features
    Dilated cardiomyopathy (invariable in DMD by late teens; variable in BMD)
    Intellectual impairment (30 per cent of DMD; rare in BMD)
    Respiratory insufficiency (invariable in DMD, less common in BMD)
    Scoliosis (only DMD)

Genotype–Phenotype Correlations

About two-thirds of mutations responsible for DMD and BMD are deletions, about 20 per cent are point mutations and 10 per cent are duplications.[128] With improvements in molecular techniques, the majority of mutations can now be detected, including point mutations. There is no simple correlation

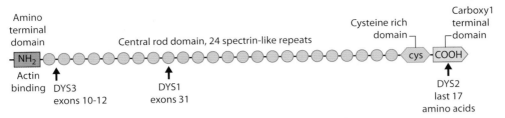

25.62 Diagram showing the four main domains of the dystrophin gene and the position of the epitopes of the dystrophin 1, 2 and 3 antibodies (Leica Biosystems, Novocastra reagents).

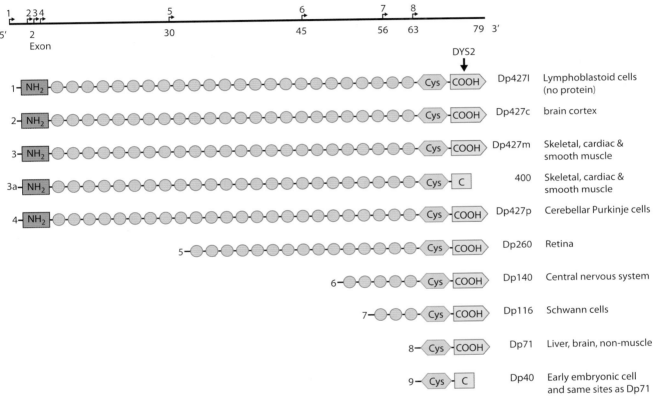

25.63 Diagram showing the main isoforms produced from the various promoters of the dystrophin gene that are expressed in different tissues. Note the presence of a common C terminus in many of them, which will be detected by antibodies recognizing a C-terminal epitope such as DYS2 (Leica Biosystems, Novocastra reagents). The most important transcripts in skeletal and cardiac muscle are transcribed from the 5′ promoters.

between the size or type of mutation and the clinical severity; some extensive deletions have been identified in patients with BMD, whereas point mutations can cause DMD. A mutation may occur in any part of the gene, but two 'hotspots' where mutations are clustered have been identified. One involves exons 45–52 and the other involves exon 3.

In DMD, dystrophin is absent, or almost absent, from the majority of muscle fibres, whereas dystrophin is retained to variable degrees in milder cases of BMD. However, a variable number of fibres with pronounced labelling of dystrophin (revertant fibres) may be present. Such fibres may be absent, diffusely distributed through a biopsy or present in clusters. The difference in labelling of dystrophin between DMD and BMD, and the presence of revertant fibres, is explained by the effect of the mutation on the reading frame of the dystrophin transcript. In the majority of DMD cases, the reading frame is disrupted, but it is maintained in BMD, allowing RNA to be transcribed and translated into protein (Figure 25.65). More than 90 per cent of cases conform to this principle, but there are

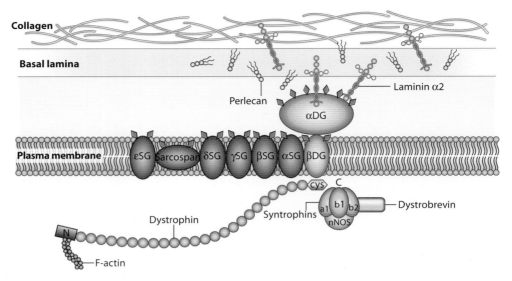

25.64 Diagram of dystrophin and its associated protein complex showing how the complex links the extracellular matrix with the actin cytoskeleton. Laminin α2 in the basal lamina binds to perlecan and to α-dystroglycan (αDG) that binds to β-dystroglycan (βDG); β-dystroglycan binds to the cysteine-rich domain of dystrophin that in turn binds to the actin cytoskeleton. The sarcoglycan complex (α, β, γ, δ) interacts with β-dystroglycan. Sarcospan also associates with the sarcoglycans, although the precise interactions are not yet clear. ε-Sarcoglycan is also present on the sarcolemma, but is thought to be part of another sarcoglycan complex. The C-terminal domain of dystrophin interacts with a complex composed of neuronal nitric oxide synthase, dystrobrevin and the syntrophins. There is also evidence of a direct interaction of β-dystroglycan with F-actin (not shown).

Redrawn from Chen YJ, Spence HJ, Cameron JM, et al. Direct interaction of beta-dystroglycan with F-actin. Biochem J 2003:15:329–37. © The Biochemical Society.

exceptions. For example, the deletion of exons 3–7 is a frameshift deletion that should result in no expression of dystrophin and a severe phenotype; however, these cases show some expression of protein, because splicing restores the reading frame. These patients often have a phenotype intermediate between DMD and BMD, emphasizing the importance of studying protein expression and not relying on molecular analysis alone.

The immunohistochemical study of dystrophin also emphasizes the importance of using antibodies to different domains of a protein, in order to avoid false negative results. If a deletion encompasses the epitope of an antibody, then labelling cannot occur and an absence of protein expression can give the impression of DMD. However, labelling with an antibody to the C-terminal domain may be present, in keeping with BMD. In practice, it is common to use three commercial antibodies, two with epitopes in the rod domain (e.g. exons 13 and 31) and one to a C-terminal domain (see Figure 25.62). Sarcolemmal damage may occur for a variety of reasons, and the plasma membrane is often lost from necrotic fibres. Therefore, an antibody to β-spectrin is commonly used as a control to assess plasmalemmal integrity. Similarly, preservation of the basal lamina, which is often retained, even on necrotic fibres, can be assessed with an antibody to laminin γ1.

Many secondary immunohistochemical changes have been identified in DMD muscle, some of which are helpful in differential diagnosis. In some BMD biopsies, dystrophin immunolabelling may appear similar to controls, and these cases must be distinguished from patients who clinically resemble BMD but who have mutations in the gene encoding fukutin-related protein (FKRP) (LGMD2I).[50] In this situation, studies of proteins in the dystrophin-associated complex (see Figure 25.64) are helpful, because they may show an absence or variable degree of reduction. Thus, both α- and β-dystroglycan are reduced in DMD and BMD, but in LGMD2I only the glycosylation of α-dystroglycan is abnormal and β-dystroglycan is usually retained. All the sarcoglycans are reduced to varying degrees in DMD, and also usually in BMD, but are retained in LGMD2I. Laminin α2, however, is usually retained in DMD and BMD, except on some necrotic fibres.

We have found that labelling of nNOS is particularly informative, especially in mild cases of BMD with a deletion in the rod domain hotspot, as these show almost complete absence of sarcolemmal nNOS, similar to DMD, whereas dystrophin immunohistochemistry can appear normal.[454]

In DMD and BMD, the A isoform of utrophin is overexpressed on the sarcolemma.[408] This increase is age dependent; muscles from young patients show very little, except on regenerating fibres.[447] Although quantifying immunohistochemical labelling is difficult, the overexpression of utrophin in DMD and BMD is usually marked, but it is not specific to Xp21 disorders and some can also occur in LGMDs, inflammatory myopathies and a variety of other disorders.[192,404] Utrophin also occurs on muscle fibres adjacent to some tumours, suggesting that cytokines may have an influence on its expression.[408]

Antibodies to the fetal isoform of myosin often reveal different patterns of labelling in DMD and BMD muscles (see Figure 25.53). In DMD, a large diffuse population of labelled fibres is usually seen, many of which are

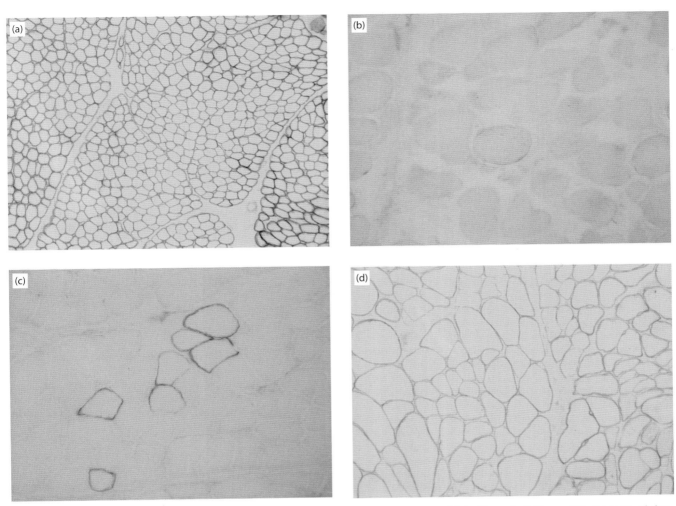

25.65 Immunolabelling of dystrophin in **(a)** a control showing normal sarcolemmal labelling of all fibres, **(b)** absence of dystrophin (except occasional slight traces) in a case of Duchenne muscular dystrophy (DMD), **(c)** a cluster of revertant fibres with dystrophin in a case of DMD and **(d)** reduced labelling of several fibres in a case of Becker muscular dystrophy. These sections have not been counterstained so that any very low levels of protein can be observed.

regenerating fibres at different stages of maturation. In BMD, the labelled fibres may be clustered, in addition to a number of scattered, very small positive fibres.

Females with X-linked Muscular Dystrophy

Rare female patients with chromosomal translocations affecting the DMD locus are affected as severely as male patients with DMD. The muscle pathology in these cases shows the typical features of DMD muscle, and dystrophin is absent, usually because the X chromosome carrying the translocation is predominantly the active chromosome. It is not certain, however, whether all cases with a translocation show a total absence of dystrophin.

Female carriers of DMD usually show no symptoms of the disease but may, on occasion, show minor features such as enlargement of a calf muscle (often unilateral) or muscle cramps. They are also susceptible to cardiomyopathy. Other carriers, in contrast, may be as severely affected as male patients with DMD. This phenotypic variability is thought to be explained by the Lyon hypothesis of random inactivation of either the normal or mutated X chromosome in every cell, and the relative proportion of these in the patient. There is also evidence of paternal transmission of mutations in the dystrophin gene.[332] Creatine kinase levels are elevated in only about 70 per cent of carriers but decrease with age; thus, a normal level does not exclude the possibility of a carrier.

Biopsies from some carriers show unequivocal histological and histochemical abnormalities, even when CK levels are normal. Often, however, only minor changes are seen, and determining their significance can be difficult. Assessment of dystrophin has a major role in distinguishing a manifesting carrier from a LGMD. Manifesting carriers show a variable number of fibres (or parts of fibres) that lack dystrophin but retain β-spectrin (Figure 25.66). These biopsies are often described as having a mosaic pattern, because of the alternating appearance of dystrophin-positive and dystrophin-negative fibres. In some asymptomatic carriers, no significant abnormality in dystrophin can be detected, or

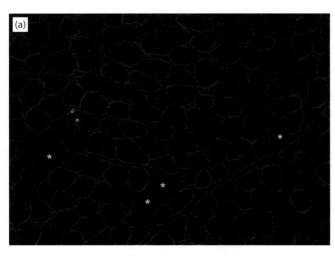

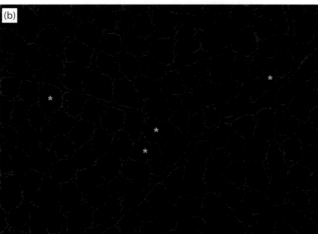

25.66 Serial sections immunolabelled for (a) dystrophin and (b) β-spectrin from a manifesting carrier of Duchenne muscular dystrophy showing fibres that lack dystrophin but have β-spectrin (*).

only occasional negative fibres are seen. These changes may be accompanied by overexpression of sarcolemmal utrophin, particularly in manifesting carriers, which is present on fibres both with and without dystrophin. Expression of the DAGs is reduced on the dystrophin-negative fibres.[117] In our experience, if the histological abnormalities in a biopsy from a female are pronounced, but dystrophin immunolabelling appears normal, then the patient is unlikely to be a DMD carrier.

Morphological changes can be detected in BMD carriers, but manifesting BMD carriers are rare, and studies of dystrophin expression in their muscles are limited.[73,157,182]

Prenatal diagnosis of DMD and BMD is reliable from chorionic villus samples if the mutation in the proband is known. If it is not known, immunolabelling of dystrophin in muscle from at-risk fetuses can be useful. Sampling of fetal muscle is usually performed after 18 weeks of gestation.[328] Dystrophin is present in fetal muscle from at least 9 weeks of gestation, and fetuses with DMD can be identified by an absence of dystrophin, provided the sarcolemma is well preserved.[88,89]

Limb-Girdle Muscular Dystrophies

The LGMDs are a heterogeneous group of disorders with either autosomal dominant or autosomal recessive inheritance (Table 25.9). Dominant forms have been classified as LGMD1 and recessive forms as LGMD2. Affected proteins are localized to various compartments of the muscle fibre, including the nuclear envelope, sarcoplasm, Golgi apparatus and endoplasmic reticulum, sarcomere and sarcolemma.[315]

The common clinical feature of all LGMDs is progressive weakness of the pelvic and shoulder muscles, although distal weakness and wasting can be observed in some (Table 25.10).[53,222,315,362]

Some LGMD variants are very rare (e.g. LGMD2G, LGMD2J), and there are geographical and ethnic differences in their incidence. For example, LGMD2C, a variant caused by mutations in the γ-sarcoglycan gene, is common in North Africans and Western European Romanies,[338] but it is rare elsewhere; on the other hand, LGMD2I (caused by mutations in the *FKRP* gene) is very common in the UK and in some other white European populations but is rare in Asian and African Caribbean populations. The recently identified LGMD2L and LGMD2A are particularly prevalent in the Caucasian population. Some forms of LGMD are caused by mutations in genes that also cause severe forms of CMD (see Congenital Muscular Dystrophy and Allied Disorders, p. 1565). Both these severe CMD and LGMD forms show hypoglycosylation of α-dystroglycan.[158,310]

Muscle pathology in LGMD shows the dystrophic changes common to all muscular dystrophies with necrosis and fibrosis (see General Histological and Histochemical Abnormalities, p. 1532). It is not possible to judge clinical severity or to identify the form of LGMD from the histological and histochemical abnormalities.

In contrast to DMD, hypercontracted fibres are less common in LGMDs, and fibre typing is often more distinct. Internal nuclei may be profuse and multiple within the cross-section of one fibre, and splitting and branching of fibres is common. Nuclear clumps may be seen in chronic cases.

Lobulated fibres (see Figure 25.36) can be a feature of adult cases of LGMD2A, which is caused by mutations in the calpain-3 gene, although they can occur in several disorders. Inflammatory cells may be present in LGMD2B, which is caused by a mutation in the dysferlin gene, and sometimes result in a misdiagnosis of myositis.[23] Eosinophils have been reported as a feature in cases with defects in the gene encoding calpain-3.[237] Vacuoles may be seen in some forms, such as LGMD1A, but are usually more abundant in other disorders such as inclusion body myositis, myofibrillar myopathies and some distal myopathies. The vacuoles are often rimmed with a basophilia that stains red with the Gomori trichrome stain (see Figure 25.43).

Immunohistochemistry and immunoblotting have a major role in directing molecular analysis, particularly in recessive forms.[18] In dominant forms, the primary defect may not lead to a detectable alteration in protein localization or its quantity, because the normal allele still produces a normal product. An exception to this is LGMD1C caused by mutations in the caveolin-3 gene (see Dominant Limb-Girdle Muscular Dystrophies, p. 1559) in which the mutant protein interferes

TABLE 25.9 Limb-girdle muscular dystrophies (LGMDs) and their gene and protein defects

LGMD	Locus	Defective protein	Subcellular localization
Dominant forms			
LGMD1A	5q31	Myotilin	Sarcomere (Z-line)
LGMD1B	1q11–q21	Lamin A/C	Nuclear envelope
LGMD1C	3p25	Caveolin- 3	Sarcolemma
LGMD1D	2q35 (previously 6q23)	Desmin	Cytoskeleton, periphery of Z-line
LGMD1E	7q36	DNAJB6	Sarcomere (Z-line)
LGMD1F	7q 32.1–q32.2	Transportin 3	Nuclear membrane
LGMD1G	4q21	HNRPDL	Ribonucleoprotein
LGMD1H	3p23–p25	?	?
Recessive forms (several rare additional forms of recessive LGMD have recently been identified [LGMD2R-2W]; see the gene table of neuromuscular disorders at www.musclegenetable.fr)			
LGMD2A	15q15.1	Calpain-3	Sarcoplasm
LGMD2B/Miyoshi	2p13	Dysferlin	Sarcolemma
LGMD2C	13q12	γ-Sarcoglycan	Sarcolemma
LGMD2D	17q 12–q21.33	α-Sarcoglycan	Sarcolemma
LGMD2E	4q12	β-Sarcoglycan	Sarcolemma
LGMD2F	5q33–q34	δ-sarcoglycan	Sarcolemma
LGMD2G	17q11–q12	Telethonin	Sarcomere (Z-line)
LGMD2H	9q31–q34	Tripartite motif containing 32 protein	Sarcoplasm
LGMD2I	19q13.3	Fukutin-related protein	Golgi
LGMD2J	2q31	Titin	Sarcomere
LGMD2K	9q3	Protein-O-mannosyl transferase 1	Endoplasmic reticulum
LGMD2L	11p13–p12	Anoctamin 5	?
LGMD2M	9q31	Fukutin	Golgi
LGMD2N	14q24	Protein-O-mannosyl transferase 2	Endoplasmic reticulum
LGMD2O	1p34.1	Protein-O-mannose β-1,2-N-acetyl- glucosaminyl-transferase	Golgi
LGMD2P	3p21	Dystroglycan	Sarcolemma
LDMD2Q	8q24	Plectin	Cytoskeleton, periphery of Z-line

with the protein from the wild-type allele, resulting in a reduction in immunolabelling. In addition, many of the mutations are missense, and the protein is still transcribed from the mutated allele. Identification of secondary changes in protein expression can be useful in the differential diagnosis of both dominant and recessive LGMDs.

Dominant Limb-Girdle Muscular Dystrophies

Limb-girdle muscular dystrophy 1A, caused by mutations in the gene for myotilin, is characterized by adult onset of proximal weakness, beginning in the pelvic girdle and progressing later to distal muscles.[188] Creatine kinase is usually mildly elevated. Several individuals exhibit a distinctive nasal dysarthric speech. In addition to the typical degenerative features of dystrophic muscle, rimmed vacuoles and striking patches of Z-line material occur. There is clinical and pathological overlap between LGMD1A and some cases of myofibrillar myopathy caused by mutations in the same gene, and some consider them allelic.[395] Cardiac involvement is present in a proportion of patients with myofibrillar myopathy, but not in LGMD1A.[188,395] Accumulation of myotilin has been reported in a cohort of cases with both LGMD1A and myofibrillar myopathy

TABLE 25.10 Main clinical features of limb-girdle muscular dystrophies (LGMDs)

Childhood or adult onset
Variable progressive weakness, may be as severe as Duchenne
Most forms associated with proximal muscle weakness of lower limb girdle and less of upper limbs
Distal weakness present in LGMD1B, Miyoshi myopathy and sometimes LGMD1C
Difficulty with gait, running, climbing steps, rising from the floor
Lumbar lordosis
Scapular winging (prominent in LGMD2A and LGMD2C–2F)
Inability to walk on tip-toes (LGMD2B/Miyoshi only)
Ambulation often retained but may be lost
Tightening of Achilles tendons: many forms, more severe in LGMD2A and LGMD1B
Muscle hypertrophy (LGMD2C–2F and LGMD2I)
Calf wasting (variable, LGMD1A, LGMD2A)
Asymmetrical muscle involvement LGMD2L
Cramps on exercise (LGMD1C, LGMD2C–2F and 2I)
Creatine kinase mildly, moderately (dominant forms), or grossly elevated (LGMD2A, 2B, 2I, 2L)
Cardiac involvement common in LGMD1A, 1B and LGMD2E, 2F and 2I

manifestations.[324] Myotilin is a Z-line protein that binds α-actinin, filamin C and F-actin, cross-linking actin and stabilizing the thin filaments.[490]

The defective gene in LGMD1B is *LMNA*, encoding lamin A/C. Mutations in this gene also give rise to other clinical variants, including autosomal dominant Emery–Dreifuss muscular dystrophy (see Emery–Dreifuss Muscular Dystrophy, p. 1575) and conditions in which skeletal muscle is not affected, such as familial partial lipodystrophy, an axonal neuropathy (Charcot–Marie–Tooth disease type 2B1), autosomal dominant dilated cardiomyopathy with conduction system disease, mandibuloacral disease and premature ageing disorders.[503]

Clinical features of LGMD1B are proximal onset of weakness in the second or third decade and relatively mild disease progression. There is no gross muscle hypertrophy, but patients tend to have a thin, wasted phenotype. The muscle wasting in these conditions can be very selective; for example, the rectus femoris is considerably less affected than the vastus lateralis and intermedius, making it essential to identify the muscle that has been biopsied. Creatine kinase is moderately elevated. The heart is invariably affected.

Although muscle pathology can help to exclude other conditions, the diagnosis is made by molecular analysis of the lamin A/C gene. Lamin A/C is localized to the nuclear membrane, but no immunohistochemical abnormalities are detected in affected patients. Mutations in several other genes encoding for nuclear membrane proteins have been identified but they appear to be very rare (see Emery–Dreifuss Muscular Dystrophy, p. 1575).

Mutations in the gene encoding caveolin-3 result in variable degrees of skeletal muscle involvement, ranging from LGMD1C to cases with little muscle weakness but with persistently high CK (hyperCKaemia). Muscle hyperexcitability following contraction and percussion is common in LGMD1C, but at times it is the predominant clinical feature (rippling muscle disease). Autoimmunity to caveolin-3

has also been identified and results in a mosaic pattern of caveolin-3 immunolabelling.[394]

The main clinical features of LGMD1C are onset in the first decade of life, with mild to moderate proximal muscle weakness and calf hypertrophy. Progression is very slow. Cramps following exercise are common, and serum CK is moderately to markedly elevated. A significant distal component with intrinsic hand wasting and pes cavus can be present in rare cases. Cardiac involvement is usually absent. The muscle pathology in cases of LGMD1C is consistent with a muscular dystrophy.

In normal muscle, caveolin-3 is situated in the caveolae of the sarcolemma, and immunolabelling clearly localizes to the sarcolemma. In all other forms of muscular dystrophy, immunolabelling is also normal, although a secondary reduction may be seen by immunoblotting in dysferlin deficiency, as caveolin-3 and dysferlin interact.[18] In contrast to most other dominant conditions, patients with a mutation in the caveolin-3 gene show a reduction in the protein with immunohistochemistry and immunoblotting,[18] and this is particularly pronounced in cases of LGMD1C. The mechanism responsible for the reduced or absent protein expression involves a toxic effect of mutant caveolin-3 and aggregates of caveolin-3 that are not targeted to the plasma membrane but are retained within the Golgi.[150] Internal localization of antibodies to caveolin-3 may be seen in several disorders, particularly in regenerating fibres.

With transmission electron microscopy, normal caveolae appear as small subsarcolemmal vesicles, but when caveolin-3 is mutated there is impairment of caveolae formation, discontinuity of the plasma membrane, subsarcolemmal vacuoles, papillary projections and disorganization of the T-system openings on the plasma membrane.[295] Mutations in the human *PTRF* gene, a caveolae component with an essential role in caveolar formation, also result in a secondary deficiency of caveolin-3 and dysferlin and a reduction in the number of caveolae, as well as being associated with lipodystrophy.[351,411]

The protein responsible for LGMD1E is desmin, which is also responsible for a typical myofibrillar myopathy. Nomenclature of LGMD1D and LGMD1E is confusing in the literature and in Online Mendelian Inheritance of Man (OMIM), as two loci on chromosomes 7q36 and 6q23 have been identified. LGMD1D/1E is often used for both. Finnish families linked to the 7q36 locus have been identified and the defective gene identified as *DNAJB6*, which encodes for a member of the heat-shock protein family (HSP40) of co-chaperones.[381] Onset of LGMD1F is in adolescence or adulthood, with proximal weakness affecting both limb girdles and involvement of axial and respiratory muscles, to produce early respiratory compromise. Serum CK in LGMD1F is only moderately elevated. The gene responsible for LGMD1F has recently been found to be transportin 3 (*TNPO3*), mapped to chromosome 7q and encoding a nuclear membrane protein.[276] Another gene at this locus, filamin C, was found to be mutated in a form of myofibrillar myopathy, but this form is phenotypically and genetically separate from LGMD1F.[484] The primary defect causing LGMD1G has recently been identified as a ribonucleoprotein, HNRPDL, but that for 1H is not known, and there are no immunohistochemical data for these conditions.

Recessive Limb-Girdle Muscular Dystrophies

The recessive forms of LGMD are more frequent than the dominant forms; in particular, LGMD2A, LGMD2B, LGMD2I and LGMD2L are relatively frequent among Caucasians. Limb-girdle muscular dystrophies 2G, 2H and 2J are rare and have been described in only a few families. The gene defects in recessive LGMDs affect a variety of proteins including enzymes (e.g. calpain-3), myofibrillar proteins (telethonin, titin), components of the DAG complex (sarcoglycans and α-dystroglycan), other sarcolemma proteins (dysferlin), a putative calcium-activated chloride channel (anoctamin 5) and a cytoskeletal protein (plectin).

Limb-girdle muscular dystrophy 2A is common and caused by defects in the gene encoding the proteolytic enzyme calpain-3, which is present in the sarcoplasm of the fibre and has a binding site on titin. Onset is in childhood or adolescence, and the phenotype is predominantly atrophic, with proximal muscle weakness affecting both the lower and the upper limb girdles, associated scapular winging and various joint contractures. Cardiac muscle is not usually affected, although there are reports,[323] and CK is usually markedly elevated.

Calpain-3 binds to the C-terminal region of titin.[421] *In vitro* studies have shown an association with filamin C, affecting its association with sarcoglycans.[484] The nature of its natural substrates suggests that it is involved in the regulation of intracellular signalling pathways, and a role in the regulation of apoptosis has been suggested.[12]

The lobulated fibres that often occur in LGMD2A, especially in adults (see Figure 25.36), are not specific for this disease; variable degrees of aggregation of tetrazolium stain may also be seen, sometimes resembling lobulation. An absence of lobulated fibres does not exclude the diagnosis of LGMD2A.

Most studies of calpain-3 have been performed on immunoblots (Figure 25.67), although the antibodies can show an absence of protein on histological sections.[70] Interpretation, however, has to take account of secondary changes that can occur when the primary defect is in genes encoding dysferlin or caveolin, and also those resulting from autolysis. This requires studies of immunoblots.[18] A normal quantity of calpain-3 on an immunoblot does not exclude a defect in the gene.

Limb-girdle muscular dystrophy 2B and Miyoshi myopathy are clinically distinct, but both are caused by defects in the dysferlin gene. The main difference between the two disorders is the site of weakness: proximal in LGMD2B and distal in Miyoshi myopathy. However, patients with LGMD2B often have noticeable distal muscle involvement, suggesting an overlap between the two entities. A characteristic feature is heel-walking, with an associated inability to stand on the toes.

Clinical presentation is usually towards the end of the second or third decade of life, with relatively rapid onset of weakness, which is preceded by a period of fully preserved strength. The clinical presentation is accompanied by gross elevation of serum CK; this, together with the rapid progression of weakness, has often led to a presumptive diagnosis of polymyositis and treatment with steroids. However, there is a poor or no response to steroids by dysferlin-deficient patients.

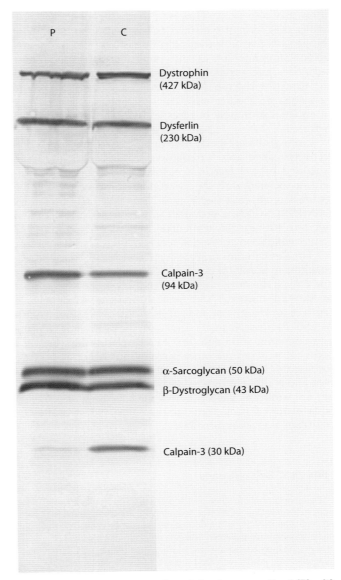

25.67 Immunoblot of several proteins from a patient (P) with a molecularly unresolved limb-girdle muscular dystrophy compared with a control (C). Note the absence of the 30 kDa calpain-3 band in the patient that was thought to be significant.

Courtesy of the late Dr Louise Anderson.

In addition to the clinical features, certain pathological features in LGMD2B and Miyoshi myopathy may lead to the suspicion of an inflammatory myopathy. As well as degenerative dystrophic changes, inflammatory infiltrates and overexpression of sarcolemmal MHC class I antigens on mature fibres are common.[94] Thus, distinction from myositis in these cases can be difficult, unless dysferlin expression is studied. The interaction of dysferlin and caveolin-3 results in similar ultrastructural abnormalities at the sarcolemma when either is defective (see Dominant Limb-Girdle Muscular Dystrophies, p. 1559).

In normal muscle, dysferlin is localized to the sarcolemma, and an absence or reduction in its immunoreactivity can be seen in both LGMD2B and Miyoshi myopathy.[18] Internal labelling of a population of fibres and regenerating fibres may also occur. However, the two commercial antibodies that recognize distinct epitopes at different ends of the protein give a clearer indication of quantity on immunoblots. Immunoblots are also important for distinguishing secondary alterations in dysferlin, which can occur when the gene for calpain-3 or caveolin-3 is defective,[18] and occasionally in other muscular dystrophies. The presence of amyloid in muscle in cases of LGMD2B has also been reported.[368,424]

Limb-girdle muscular dystrophies 2C–2F are often collectively called the 'sarcoglycanopathies', because each is caused by a defect in a member of a complex of proteins associated with the dystrophin complex and known as the sarcoglycans (see Figure 25.64). In early literature, LGMD2C, which is prevalent in North Africa, was often referred to as 'Duchenne-like muscular dystrophy' or 'severe childhood autosomal recessive muscular dystrophy'.

The sarcoglycans (α, β, γ, δ, ε, ζ) are localized to the sarcolemma in normal skeletal muscle. The sarcoglycans α, β, γ and δ form the most important complex in the sarcolemma of skeletal muscle.[329] In smooth muscle, ε-sarcoglycan replaces α-sarcoglycan and forms a different complex with β- and δ-sarcoglycan,[432] and ζ-sarcoglycan may replace γ-sarcoglycan, although the exact relationship between ζ-sarcoglycan and the other sarcoglycans is not clear.[329,496] Sarcospan (25 kDa) is also a component of the DAG complex and is thought to be associated with the sarcoglycans, but no pathogenic defects in its gene have been identified.[98] Some historical background to the nomenclature of the sarcoglycans is given in Box 25.5.[133,329]

BOX 25.5. Sarcoglycans

The sarcoglycans (α, β, γ, δ, ε and ζ) are transmembrane glycoproteins with a small intracellular domain, a single transmembrane domain and a large extracellular domain. The α, β, γ, δ units form the main complex in skeletal muscle; ε-, β-, δ- and ζ-sarcoglycans are more widely distributed. The sarcolemma labels with antibodies to ε-sarcoglycan, but this is thought to be part of another complex and to have an important role in smooth muscle. The nomenclature of the sarcoglycans has changed over the years, with the identification of additional genes. Initially, a terminology that reflected the molecular mass of these proteins and their membership of the dystrophin-associated glycoprotein (DAG) complex was introduced by Campbell and co-workers (e.g. 50-DAG, 35-DAG). Ozawa and the Japanese group, who had identified the same proteins, used a numerical terminology with 'A' as a subdivision prefix (A0–A5, e.g. A3a, A3b). The first protein of the complex to be identified was the 50-DAG-protein (now known as α-sarcoglycan), and absence of the protein was identified before the gene was cloned. The name 'adhalin' was given to it, after the Arabic name for muscle. However, the Greek lettering has now been adopted (α, β, γ, δ, ε and ζ) to refer to these proteins. The proteins ('sarcoglycans') responsible for limb-girdle dystrophies 2C–F act as a complex; these were assigned 2C–F in the order in which the loci/genes were identified. It should be noted that early papers on the dystrophin-associated proteins refer to a 43-DAG component that is now known as β-dystroglycan. Sarcospan is a 25 kDa protein associated with the sarcoglycans and is a component of the utrophin dystroglycan complex in which utrophin replaces dystrophin. No causative mutations have yet been found in the gene encoding sarcospan.

In Caucasian populations, defects in sarcoglycans are rare, but mutations in the α-sarcoglycan gene (LGMD2D) are the most frequent, with a common mutation (R77C) accounting for 50 per cent of mutated alleles. In order of frequency, LGMD2D is followed by γ-sarcoglycan (LGMD2C), β-sarcoglycan (LGMD2E) and δ-sarcoglycan (LGMD2F).[315] Mutations in the gene for ε-sarcoglycan cause myoclonus–dystonia syndrome, rather than a muscular dystrophy.[511] Severe dilated cardiomyopathy is common in LGMD2E, and the cardiomyopathic hamster is an animal model for this form.[316]

Immunohistochemistry is an important technique in the diagnosis of sarcoglycanopathies, because a reduction in protein expression can be observed. The four sarcoglycans (α, β, γ and δ) act as a complex, and a mutation in the gene for one causes a secondary reduction in the others. This reduction may be minimal or pronounced (Figure 25.68), but a total absence or a significant depletion of one of the proteins, compared with the others, is usually indicative of the primary defect. An absence of all four sarcoglycans is often associated with a defect in the β-sarcoglycan gene, whereas α- and γ-sarcoglycan mutations are typically associated with a marked reduction or absence of the mutant protein and mild or moderate reduction of the remaining sarcoglycans.[18] Careful correlation with dystrophin immunohistochemistry is required, because a secondary reduction in sarcoglycans occurs in DMD and BMD. In addition, dystrophin immunolabelling is usually normal in the sarcoglycanopathies, but a secondary reduction can occur when the β-sarcoglycan gene is the primary defect. Complementary studies of the sarcoglycans on multiplex immunoblots can be useful but also have limitations[18,231] and are rarely informative in cases with a normal CK.

Because the sarcoglycans act as a complex, it is questionable whether all four proteins need to be examined on a routine basis. It is our practice to label two of them (α- and γ-sarcoglycan) and to examine the others if results or phenotype warrant it. Secondary changes in other proteins, such as β-dystroglycan and utrophin, can help to distinguish DMD or BMD from sarcoglycanopathies. β-Dystroglycan is retained in sarcoglycan disorders but reduced in DMD and BMD. Utrophin is overexpressed in DMD and BMD but is upregulated to a lesser degree, if at all, in sarcoglycanopathies and less in other forms of LGMD.[117]

Limb-girdle muscular dystrophy 2G is rare and has been identified in only a few families.[301,314,326] The condition affects proximal muscles and is predominantly atrophic, although two families with calf hypertrophy have been described. Serum CK is moderately to markedly elevated in the initial phases of the disorder. The defective protein, telethonin, is absent with immunolabelling, and no secondary defects in the other defective proteins causing a neuromuscular defect have been reported. Rimmed vacuoles were reported in some of the cases.[470]

Limb-girdle muscular dystrophy 2H is also very rare and has been described only in the Hutterite Canadian population.[494] There are no reported studies of the expression of the defective protein, TRIM32. This is a putative E3 ubiquitin ligase. The same gene has also been shown to be responsible for cases of sarcotubular myopathy and it is considered the same disorder.[389] More recently, mutations have also been found in a Swedish family.[37]

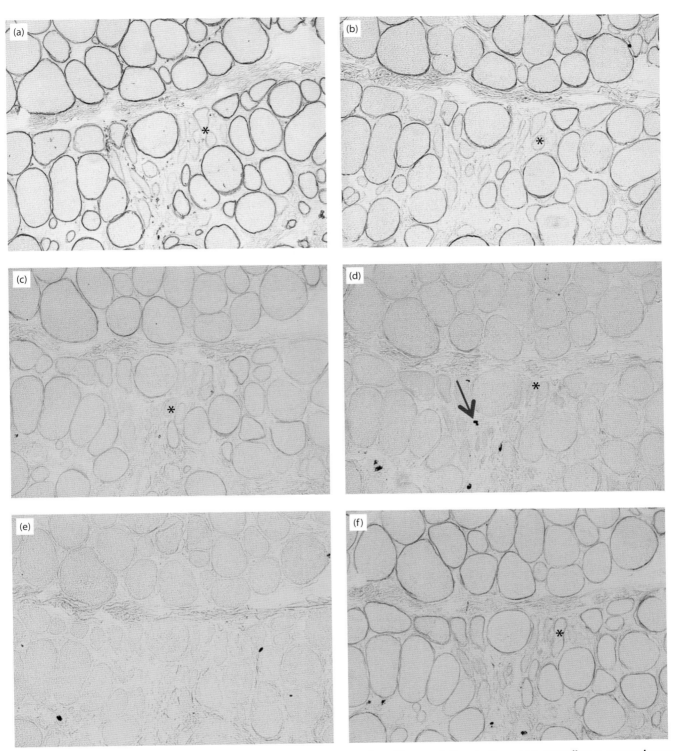

25.68 Serial sections from a case of limb-girdle muscular dystrophy with a mutation in the gene encoding γ-sarcoglycan (LGMD2C) immunolabelled with antibodies to (a) β-spectrin, **(b)** C-terminal dystrophin, **(c)** α-sarcoglycan, **(d)** β-sarcoglycan, **(e)** γ-sarcoglycan and **(f)** δ-sarcoglycan. Note the absence of γ-sarcoglycan and reduction of the other sarcoglycans but normal labelling of β-spectrin and dystrophin. Note also the reduced labelling of all these proteins in the small regenerating fibres (*) and the endogenous peroxidase in macrophages (arrow).

Limb-girdle muscular dystrophy 2I is one of the most common LGMD variants in Caucasian populations.[315] The defective gene on chromosome 19 encodes FKRP, after its sequence homology to fukutin, the defective protein in Fukuyama congenital muscular dystrophy. Allelic mutations

in the *FKRP* gene are also responsible for a severe form of congenital muscular dystrophy (MDC1C).[159]

The clinical spectrum of LGMD2I is wide, even within families. Affected individuals can present in childhood, adolescence or adulthood. Some may follow a DMD-like course, losing ambulation in the early teens; others resemble BMD.[279] Dilated cardiomyopathy, as well as respiratory impairment, develops in a significant proportion of affected individuals.

Both missense and nonsense mutations have been identified in the *FKRP* gene, but only one homozygous null mutation has been found in a patient with a severe phenotype. A homozygous *FKRP* start codon mutation is associated with Walker–Warburg syndrome, the severe end of the clinical spectrum, suggesting a complete loss of FKRP may be incompatible with life.[475] A common missense mutation, Leu276Ile, results in a milder phenotype when homozygous compared to heterozygous.[158,310] It has been suggested that the Leu276Ile mutation may be a 'founder mutation' that has dispersed among populations of European origin, although we have described the presence of different Leu276Ile haplotypes based on an intragenic single nucleotide polymorphism.[148] The protein FKRP is present in many tissues, with high levels in skeletal and cardiac muscle, and is located in the Golgi apparatus. Sequence homology suggests it is a member of the glycosyltransferase family and that it has a role in glycosylation, in particular of α-dystroglycan.

The pathological changes in muscle in LGMD2I are also variable and the histopathological distinction between BMD and LGMD2I can be difficult, especially in cases with only subtle immunohistochemical abnormalities. However, because many cases of BMD have a mutation in the rod domain hotspot, they lack sarcolemmal nNOS, in contrast to LGMD2I. Other secondary changes also have an important role in the diagnosis of LGMD2I; in particular, a common finding is reduced labelling of the glycosylated epitope of α-dystroglycan. In contrast, labelling of β-dystroglycan is normal in LGMD2I. In some cases the reduction of α-dystroglycan is unequivocal, but in patients at the mildest end of the clinical spectrum it may be subtle (Figure 25.69).[43,50] There are currently no commercial antibodies to the core protein of α-dystroglycan, but research studies have shown that it is retained in LGMD2I.

Another common secondary protein deficiency associated with mutations in the *FKRP* gene is a reduction of laminin α2, but this may only be apparent on immunoblots.[54] Laminin β1 labelling on the sarcolemma may also be reduced compared to normal labelling on capillaries, especially in adults, but this can also be seen in other conditions. Laminin γ1 labelling on these fibres is of normal intensity and makes a good control. Upregulation of utrophin can also occur on mature fibres in LGMD2I, although it is usually less pronounced than in DMD and BMD.[404]

Limb-girdle muscular dystrophy 2J is very rare and has been described in the Finnish population. The clinical hallmark of this form is distal muscle involvement, limited to the anterior compartment of the leg. Limb-girdle muscular dystrophy 2J is caused by recessive mutations in the gene for titin.[467] Dominant heterozygous mutations have also been described and give rise to a later-onset tibial muscular dystrophy,[466] which is often grouped with other distal myopathies, including Welander myopathy and the Nonaka type, allelic to hereditary inclusion body myopathy (see Distal Myopathies, p. 1593).[464,465] Dominant allelic mutations in titin also result in isolated cardiomyopathy and other phenotypes such as hereditary early

25.69 Immunolabelling of the glycosylated epitope of α-dystroglycan showing (a) normal labelling in a control but (b) absent or reduced labelling on several fibres in a case of LGMD2I.

respiratory failure (HMERF).[154,322,335] Rimmed vacuoles may be present in titin-related disorders, but not always, and accumulation of tau protein or β-amyloid, often associated with such vacuoles in other conditions, is not a feature. Rimmed vacuoles are not a feature of the recessive cases. Titin is still detectable with commercial antibodies, but an antibody raised specifically against the mutated last exon of this giant gene fails to show reactivity.[467] Titin has binding sites for calpain-3 and telethonin, and a secondary reduction in calpain-3 is associated with titin mutations.[185]

LGMD2K, LGMD2M, LGMD2N and LGMD2O (see Table 25.9) are allelic to severe congenital muscular dystrophies caused by the genes encoding the same proteins: protein-O-mannosyltransferase 1 (POMT1), Fukutin, protein-O-mannosyltransferase 2 (POMT2) and protein O-mannose beta-1,2-N-acetylglucosaminyl-transferase 1,(POMGnT1), respectively.[310] Patients with these limb-girdle phenotypes show minimal or no brain involvement, in contrast to the severe allelic cases of congenital muscular dystrophy.[159] Recently, allelic mutations in isoprenoid synthase domain-containing (ISPD) have been associated both with a severe Walker–Warburg CMD phenotype, and a milder LGMD disease course.[76,498] The degree of muscle pathology is variable and may be mild, but immunolabelling of the glycosylated epitope of α-dystroglycan is reduced. The degree of this reduction, however, does not always correlate with clinical severity, and there may be an absence or pronounced reduction of α-dystroglycan but the clinical severity relatively mild (e.g. LGMD patients with mutations in the genes encoding fukutin and ISPD).[76,159,211] As in cases with a severe CMD phenotype, immunolabelling of laminin α2 may be reduced and the number of fibres positive for fetal myosin is variable.

Limb-girdle muscular dystrophy 2L is relatively common in the Caucasian population. The condition has a relatively mild progression and onset in young adults. There is a striking predominance of affected males, the reason for which is not understood. The phenotype of affected cases resembles that associated with defects in dysferlin (LGMD2B/Myoshi myopathy) with onset of proximal weakness of the lower limbs in young adults. Weakness is frequently asymmetrical and associated with muscle atrophy, with distal weakness in cases resembling Myoshi myopathy. As in LGMD2B/Myoshi myopathy, CK levels are very high. LGMD2L is caused by mutations in the gene of a member of the anoctamin family, anoctamin 5 (*ANO5*), a putative calcium-activated chloride channel.[34] Muscle biopsies from affected patients show dystrophic changes, but there are no antibodies available to the defective protein. A secondary change that occurs in several cases is a reduction of sarcolemmal laminin β1, but this is not specific to LGMD2L (Barresi and Sewry unpublished observations). Amyloid has been observed in one case, in common with patients with a defect in dysferlin.[292]

Mutations in the *DAG1* gene encoding dystroglycan have been found in a single family with a LGMD phenotype with mental retardation but normal brain MRI, which has been designated LGMD2P.[184] This case is therefore affected by a primary dystroglycan defect in contrast to those above that have a secondary hypoglycosylation of α-dystroglycan with reduced labelling of the glycosylated epitope of α-dystroglycan and normal labelling of β-dystroglycan. Laminin α2 labelling was reported to be unaffected, although *in vitro* studies predicted the mutation affects laminin α2 binding.[184] A large heterozygous deletion of the *DAG1* gene has been found in another patient, but the contribution of this to the complex phenotype observed in this case is unclear.[149]

LGMD2Q is another rare form that has only been described in three Turkish families.[175] It is caused by homozygous mutations, probably a founder mutation, in the gene encoding plectin (*PLEC1*), which affects the 1f isoform. Allelic mutations in *PLEC1* are more typically associated with epidermolysis bullosa with muscular dystrophy and a myasthenic syndrome, but the LGMD2Q cases did not show any skin or myasthenic features. The clinical features of LGMD2Q are of a severe progressive muscular dystrophy with childhood onset that leads to loss of ambulation,

and elevated CK levels. In addition to typical pathological features of LGMDs, immunolabelling of dystrophin, sarcoglycans and dystroglycans was reported as normal. Immunolabelling of plectin, using an antibody that recognized all plectin isoforms, showed an absence of labelling at the sarcolemma but retention of the fibre typing pattern, compared with controls. This observation, however, needs to be confirmed in further cases, and possible age-related changes in the sarcolemmal labelling of plectin studied. The electron microscopy images revealed non-specific features that can be seen in several disorders.

Congenital Muscular Dystrophies and Allied Disorders

Congenital muscular dystrophies are a molecularly and clinically heterogeneous group of disorders characterized by weakness and hypotonia from birth or within the first few months of life. Major advances in clinical, molecular and biochemical aspects of CMDs have been made in recent years.[279] The most common defective proteins are components of the extracellular matrix or are involved in glycosylation, in particular of α-dystroglycan. Comprehensive epidemiological studies on CMD are lacking, and there are geographical variations in the incidence of some because of founder mutations. Various studies, however, have shown that CMDs are among the most common neuromuscular disorders, in particular Ullrich CMD.[35,86,283,288,319]

The majority of CMDs are inherited recessively, but dominant mutations in collagen VI are increasingly being recognized. Originally Ullrich CMD was thought to relate to recessively inherited defects and milder Bethlem myopathy to be dominantly inherited. Currently, however, almost 50 per cent of severely affected patients with an Ullrich CMD phenotype have *de novo* dominant mutations (see later).[35,36] There is a spectrum of phenotype associated with collagen VI defects; we discuss them all in this section, in particular Bethlem myopathy. The classification of CMDs is based on a combination of clinical and genetic data, and the biochemical defect (Table 25.11).[159,279,307] The OMIM database has recently introduced a nomenclature for the CMDs associated with hypoglycosylation of α-dystroglycan that reflects the variable involvement of the brain and clinical severity associated each gene with, but it is not yet commonly in use. Tables 25.12–25.14 summarize the major clinical features of the main molecular forms.

General Clinical Features

Congenital muscular dystrophies present at birth, or within the first 6 months of life, with hypotonia, weakness and often joint contractures. Severity of muscle involvement and progression are variable across the different disorders; in some variants, there is also involvement of the CNS. This can include white matter abnormalities and structural defects affecting the cortex, brain stem and cerebellum. Eye disease can also occur in some variants. Serum CK levels are markedly elevated in some variants but normal in others (see Tables 25.12–25.14). Rigidity of the spine, distal joint laxity, muscle hypertrophy and respiratory insufficiency are also distinctive features of some forms.

TABLE 25.11 Genetically identified forms of congenital muscular dystrophy

Protein	Protein type	Gene locus	Gene symbol	Disease phenotype	Disease abbreviations sometimes used
Laminin α2	Extracellular matrix	6q	LAMA2	'Merosin-deficient' CMD	MDC1A
Collagen VI	Extracellular matrix	21q22	COL 6A1	Ullrich CMD	UCMD
		21q22	COL 6A2		
		2q37	COL 6A3		
Integrin α7	Transmembrane (plasma membrane)	12q13	ITGA	Congenital myopathy/dystrophy	
Fukutin	Putative glycosyltransferase/phosphoryl ligand transferase	9q31–q33	FKTN	Congenital onset with brain & eye involvement	FCMD
O-mannose β-1, 2-N-acetyl-glucosaminyl-transferase	Glycosyltransferase	1p3	POMGNT1	Congenital onset with brain & eye involvement, with & without mental retardation	MEB, WWS
Protein-O-mannosyl-transferase	Glycosyltransferases	9q34	POMT1	Congenital onset with brain & eye involvement, with & without mental retardation	MEB, WWS
		14q24.3	POMT2		
Isoprenoid synthase containing domain	Cytosol	7p21	ISPD	Congenital onset with brain & eye involvement	WWS
Transmembrane protein 5	Golgi	12q14.2	TMEM5	Congenital onset with brain & eye involvement	WWS
β1,3-N-acetylgalactos-aminyltransferase 2	Endoplasmic reticulum	1q43.2	B3GALNT2	Congenital onset with brain & eye involvement	WWS
Glycosyltransferase-like domain-containing protein 2	Endoplasmic reticulum	3p22.1	GTDC2	Congenital onset with brain & eye involvement	WWS
GDP-mannose pyrophosphorylase B	Cytosol	3p21.31	GMPPB	Congenital onset with brain & eye involvement	MEB
Protein kinase-like protein SGK196	?Sarcolemma	8p11.21	SGK196	Congenital onset with brain and eye involvement	WWS
Fukutin-related protein	Putative glycosyl/phosphoryl ligand transferase	19q1	FKRP	Congenital onset with brain & eye involvement with & without mental retardation	MDC1C, WWS, MEB
LARGE	Putative bifunctional glycosyltransferase	22q12	LARGE	Congenital onset with brain & eye involvement	MDC1D
Selenoprotein N1	Glycoprotein of unknown function localized to the endoplasmic reticulum	1q36	SEPN1	Rigid spine syndrome	RSMD1

MDC1B is not included in this table as the gene has not been identified; only the locus on 1q42 is known. Muscle biopsies from the few cases identified show abnormal glycosylation of α-dystroglycan and a secondary reduction of laminin α2. The genes associated with congenital glycosylation are not included (see text). Several of the genes shown are associated with a broad clinical spectrum that includes forms of limb-girdle muscular dystrophy.

FCMD, Fukuyama CMD; MDC1A, merosin-deficient congenital muscular dystrophy; MDC1D, congenital muscular dystrophy type 1 D; MEB, muscle–eye–brain disease; RSMD1, rigid spine muscular dystrophy type 1; WWS, Walker–Warburg syndrome.

TABLE 25.12 Summary of the main clinical features of congenital muscular dystrophies (CMDs) associated with defects in extracellular matrix and sarcolemmal proteins

Features common to all forms of CMD:
Onset *in utero*, at birth or within a few months of life
Hypotonia
Muscle weakness
'Merosin-deficient' CMD (MDC1A):
Never able to walk unaided, sitting achieved
Axial weakness plus proximal > distal limb weakness
Weakness usually non-progressive
White matter changes on brain MRI in all cases by 6 months
Intelligence normal but may be reduced in cases with structural brain changes
Epilepsy common
Feeding difficulties common
Frequent spinal rigidity and scoliosis
Respiratory complications and respiratory failure common
Marked elevation of CK
Ullrich CMD:
Hyperlaxity of distal joints
Contractures of proximal joints
Dislocation of hips
Respiratory insufficiency
Delayed ambulation, achieved in some but not all
Round face with prominent ears
Hyperkeratosis; abnormal scar formation
Prominent calcanei
Scoliosis
CK normal or mildly elevated
Integrin α7 deficiency (very rare):
Delayed motor milestones
Mild muscle weakness
CK normal

CK, creatine kinase; MRI, magnetic resonance imaging.

TABLE 25.13 Main clinical features of Bethlem myopathy and variants intermediate between Bethlem and Ullrich congenital muscular dystrophies

Onset in childhood (sometimes prenatally with talipes, torticollis or hip dislocation) or within the first two decades of life
Talipes and torticollis at birth possible
Generalized joint laxity and tight Achilles tendon and mild weakness in childhood
Progressive contractures of multiple large joints in adolescence and adulthood
Characteristic contractures of long finger flexors
Moderate progression of weakness affecting proximal lower limb muscles more than upper limbs
Approximately 20 per cent of patients eventually require a wheelchair
Distal leg wasting in some cases
Abnormal skin scar formation (keloids/atrophic scars) in some cases
Absent cardiac involvement
Creatine kinase normal, or mildly elevated, occasionally moderately elevated

Note: Although described separately, Bethlem myopathy and forms intermediate between Ullrich and Bethlem congenital muscular dystrophies are essentially a continuum of clinical severity. In both these latter milder allelic variants, the general features can be similar to Ullrich congenital muscular dystrophy, but the maximum function and strength of individuals with Bethlem are significantly better (with acquisition of running abilities and forced vital capacity always above 80 per cent). Intermediate patients typically lose the ability to walk towards the late teens or early 20s, and develop respiratory insufficiency in the third decade of life.

General Pathological Features

Muscle pathology in CMDs may appear considerably more severe than expected from the clinical picture, and the degree of pathology cannot be used as an indication of disease severity or prognosis. All variants of CMD share common pathological features, although the degree of abnormality is variable. It is not possible to identify a particular form of CMD from the histological and histochemical features alone, most of which are non-specific, and immunohistochemistry is essential for making a diagnosis and directing molecular analysis. Although the name 'dystrophy' implies muscle fibre necrosis and regeneration at the pathological level, these are not striking in all variants, at least in the quadriceps muscle. Other muscles, i.e. paraspinal axial muscles, as in many disorders, show dystrophic changes. In some variants, such as RSMD1, the overall pathology may resemble a myopathy rather than a dystrophic process with necrosis.

All CMDs show the typical features of other muscular dystrophies (see General Histological and Histochemical Abnormalities). The amounts of fibrosis and adipose tissue are variable, but both may be marked (Figure 25.70). A prominent inflammatory infiltrate may be present.[331] With oxidative enzyme stains, areas of mitochondrial depletion resembling cores, or aggregation of peripheral mitochondria resembling lobulated

fibres may be present, particularly in cases of Ullrich CMD (see Figure 25.70). Some of these features also occur in some congenital myopathies, and because there is pathological and clinical overlap, these should be considered in the differential diagnosis (see Congenital Myopathies and Allied Disorders, p. 1580).

Congenital Muscular Dystrophies Associated with Sarcolemmal and Extracellular Matrix Proteins

Laminin α2-Deficient Congenital Muscular Dystrophies (Merosin-Deficient Congenital Muscular Dystrophy) This form of CMD (MDC1A) is caused by mutations in the *LAMA2* gene on chromosome 6q25. Patients invariably present at birth or in the first few weeks of life. Hypotonia and muscle weakness may be associated with failure to thrive and respiratory or feeding problems, but severe respiratory failure at birth is not a feature. Contractures may be present, but severe arthrogryposis is rare. Most mutations result in the complete absence of laminin α2 protein, or only traces of detectable protein, and are always associated with a severe phenotype. Box 25.6 gives some details of the laminin chains in skeletal muscle and their nomenclature.[11] Patients with MDC1A rarely acquire the ability to stand independently and almost invariably cannot walk unaided, but they are usually able to sit unsupported. Some *LAMA2* mutations can result in partial protein reduction and are usually associated with a milder phenotype, which can resemble a LGMD (Figure 25.71).[407] The use of two antibodies to laminin α2 is particularly useful in these cases, and a reduction in labelling is then more apparent with an antibody to the 300 kDa fragment of laminin α2. Serum CK

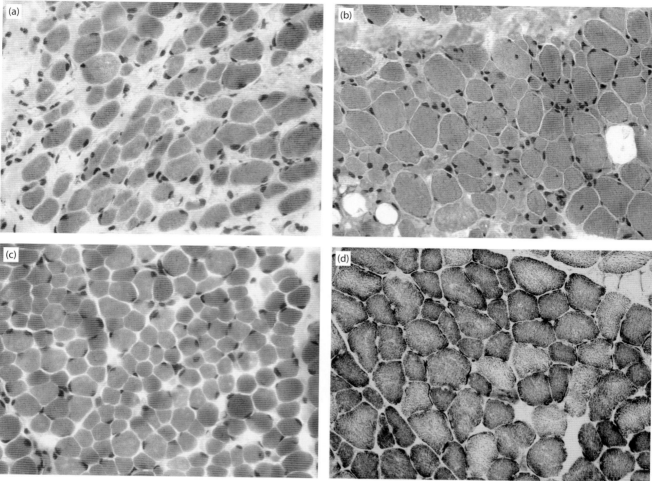

25.70 Representative views from various forms of congenital muscular dystrophy showing the variable degree of fibre size variation and fibrosis. (a) Merosin-deficient MDC1A, **(b)** Ullrich congenital muscular dystrophy, **(c)** muscle–eye–brain disease (H&E) and **(d)** the unevenness of NADH-TR staining (minicores) in a case of muscular dystrophy with rigid spine (RSMD1).

BOX 25.6. Laminins

Laminins are components of the basal lamina, and 16 variants have been identified, all of which are composed of a heterotrimer of α, β and γ chains. The previous names of merosin (M) and laminins A, B1 and B2 were replaced by a nomenclature based on the diverse α, β and γ chains. A new scheme has been proposed using three Arabic numerals, based on the α, β and γ chain numbers. For example, the laminin 211 has the chain composition α2–β1–γ1. still often referred to as merosin. The predominant trimers in muscle are 211 (laminin 2 composed of α2–β1–γ1 chains) and 221 (laminin 4, previously known as S-merosin, composed of α2–β2–γ1 chains). Thus, mutations in the gene for laminin α2 affect both variants. The laminin β2 chain has an important role at the neuromuscular junction and is also present on extrajunctional sarcolemma. Laminin α2 is important for the correct assembly and maintenance of the muscle fibre basal lamina, and ultrastructural studies reveal abnormal basal lamina surrounding the fibres in patients with 'merosin-deficient' congenital muscular dystrophy (MDC1A) and in laminin α2 *dy* mouse models. Laminin α2 undergoes spontaneous proteolytic cleavage within the C-terminal G-domain, resulting in 80-kDa and 300-kDa fragments. In cases with a partial reduction of laminin α2, the reduction may be apparent only with antibodies to the 300-kDa fragment. Western blotting can also be used to detect laminin α2 defects, but not all commercial antibodies are suitable.

levels are always elevated. Although cognitive function is usually normal, most patients with MDC1A have increased signal intensity in the white matter on T2-weighted brain MR imaging by 6 months of age, although there are a few exceptions in cases with partial reduction of laminin α2.[407] Some patients (about 5 per cent) also show structural brain changes, such as occipital agyria.[337] Mental retardation and epilepsy may be present in these cases.

Laminin α2 labelling of intramuscular nerves in cases with *LAMA2* mutations is also absent. In one rare case, absent labelling of nerves was associated with apparently normal labelling of the sarcolemma.[107] Laminin β2 is associated with laminin α2 in nerves (as a component of laminin 221), as well as being abundant at neuromuscular junctions and on the sarcolemma.[378,495] Laminin α2 immunoreactivity in the skin can be used as an alternative to muscle biopsy; it is absent from the epidermal–dermal junction, sensory nerves and glands in patients with MDC1A (Figure 25.72). Laminin α2 is absent from all blood vessels of skin and muscle but is present on blood vessels in the brain.[478]

A number of proteins are secondarily affected in MDC1A. Laminin β2 and α7 integrin are reduced on the sarcolemma, but laminin α5 and α4 chains are overexpressed.[402]

TABLE 25.14 Summary of the main clinical features of congenital muscular dystrophies associated with defects in proteins that affect the glycosylation of α-dystroglycan and may show a secondary reduction in laminin α2

Fukuyama congenital muscular dystrophy	Walker–Warburg syndrome	MDC1C ('FKRP' congenital muscular dystrophy)	Muscle–eye–brain disease	MDC1D (LARGE gene, rare, a few reported cases only)
Prevalent in Japan	Most severe form of CMD, short life expectancy	Severe muscle weakness at birth	Hypertrophy of leg muscles and tongue neonatal presentation	Severe myopia and eye involvement
Severe generalized muscle weakness at birth	Very severe muscle weakness at birth	No contractures at birth	Normal brain and intelligence in milder cases variable severity (mild to severe)	White matter changes
Standing with support achieved, rarely ambulant	Contractures at birth or soon after	Sitting delayed but usually achieved	Severe cases have structural brain changes and mental retardation	Epilepsy in about 30 per cent
Progressive contractures and scoliosis	Severe structural brain changes with type II lissencephaly	Standing with support may be temporarily achieved	Sitting and ambulation achieved in milder but not severe cases	Subtle structural brain changes
Hypertrophy of calves, quadriceps and tongue	Cerebellar hypoplasia, brain stem hypoplasia and hydrocephalus	Progressive respiratory muscle weakness	Severe cases may have eye involvement and resemble MEB or WWS muscle hypertrophy	Severe mental retardation at age 17 years
Severe brain involvement with type II lissencephaly	Severe eye abnormalities with microphthalmia, cataracts, glaucoma, cerebellar cysts, hypoplastic optic nerve		Dilated cardiomyopathy	Moderately elevated CK
Severe mental retardation	Marked elevation of CK		Joint contractures	
Epilepsy in most cases by age of 3 years	Absent psychomotor development		Pronounced elevation of CK	
Ocular involvement in about 50 per cent of cases			Severe brain involvement with type II lissencephaly	
Dilated cardiomyopathy from second decade			Cerebellar cysts, flat brain stem	
Respiratory failure in second decade			Severe mental retardation	
Marked elevation of CK				

MDC1B is not included in this table because the gene has not been identified. In common with the above disorders muscle biopsies from the few cases identified show abnormal glycosylation of α-dystroglycan and a secondary reduction of laminin α2.

Note. Each phenotype is associated with defects in more than one gene (see Table 25.11). Although the table describes the phenotype in the original group of patients in whom gene mutations were identified, there is considerable overlap in the genes responsible as well as several recently identified.

However, when assessing all these proteins, age and developmental regulation must be taken into account.

Because laminin α2 is expressed in chorionic villi on the basal lamina beneath the trophoblast, immunohistochemical studies of chorionic villi samples can be useful for prenatal diagnosis. Absence of laminin α2 from the trophoblast is highly suggestive of MDC1A, but a combined molecular genetic approach is recommended (Figure 25.73).[312] A retrospective study from five international centres confirmed the reliability of combined molecular genetic and immunohistochemical studies of chorionic villi for the prenatal diagnosis of MDC1A in cases with an absence of laminin α2.[471] Immunolabelling for laminin β2 is also reduced in

the MDC1A trophoblast. The reliability of immunohistochemical studies of chorionic villi in patients with a primary partial deficiency, and in patients with secondary deficiency, is unknown.

Integrin α7 Congenital Muscular Dystrophy This is a very rare form of CMD, and only three Japanese cases have been reported.[189] Immunohistochemical studies identified an absence of integrin α7 from the sarcolemma and mutations in the corresponding gene (*ITGA7*) were identified. The morphological changes in muscle were mild and necrosis was not a feature, although regenerating fibres were seen in one patient. Integrin β1D was slightly reduced and laminin

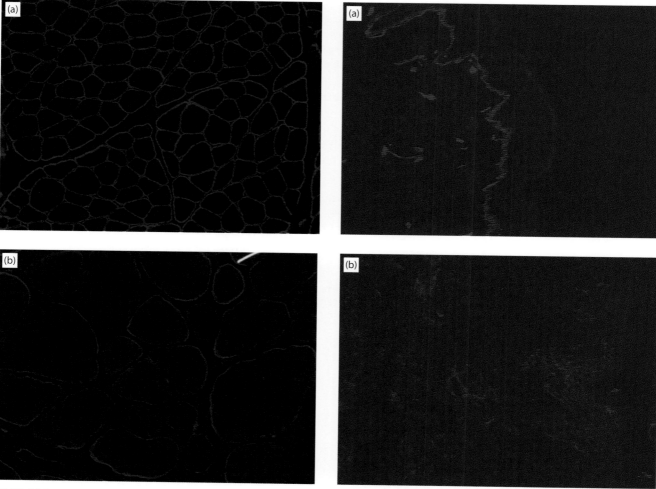

25.71 (a) Immunolabelling of laminin α2 in control muscle showing normal labelling compared with **(b)** reduced labelling on several fibres in a case with mutations in the *LAMA2* gene.

25.72 Immunolabelling of laminin α2 in skin from **(a)** a control and **(b)** a case of 'merosin-deficient' MDC1A with absence of laminin α2 at the junction of the epidermis and dermis and from the sensory nerves.

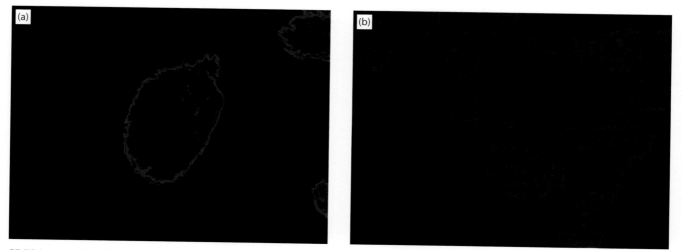

25.73 Immunolabelling of laminin α2 in a chorionic villus from **(a)** a control and **(b)** a fetus with merosin-deficient MDC1A showing an absence of laminin α2.

α2 was normal. Analysis of integrin α7 localization in CMD muscle is limited because application of commercial antibodies is limited and sarcolemmal levels are low in infants. Some details on various integrins in muscle are given in Box 25.7.[59,272]

Integrin α9 Congenital Muscular Dystrophy A locus on chromosome 3p23-21 is associated with a form of CMD with some clinical features resembling Ullrich CMD, and integrin α9 was suggested as the candidate gene.[449] Mutations in the *ITG9* gene have been reported at an international meeting but not yet published in a peer reviewed article. There are no published reports of integrin α9 expression in the cases linked to this locus, but pathological studies of a few muscle biopsies showed central nuclei in several muscle fibres and features resembling a centronuclear myopathy (see Congenital Myopathies and Allied Disorders, p. 1580).[449]

Ullrich Congenital Muscular Dystrophy and Bethlem Myopathy Ullrich CMD is one of the most common forms of CMD.[86] It is caused by defects in the genes encoding collagen VI, a major protein of the extracellular matrix with enhanced labelling seen at the sarcolemma. Collagen VI is composed of three α-chains, α1(VI), α2(VI) and α3(VI), encoded by the *COL6A1* and *COL6A2* genes on chromosome 21q25.3 and the *COL6A3* gene on chromosome 2q37. Mutations in each gene can result in Ullrich CMD. No mutations have been found in the α5 and α6 chains of collagen VI in patients with an Ullrich CMD or Bethlem phenotype.[375] In muscle, collagen VI plays a structural role and anchors the muscle fibre basement membrane to the extracellular matrix. Collagen VI may also be important for organization of components of the extracellular matrix, such as fibronectin, and for the regulation of intracellular events, including apoptosis.[205,209]

It was initially believed that recessive mutations in *COL6A* genes caused the Ullrich phenotype and that dominant mutations caused the milder Bethlem phenotype. However, dominant mutations have also been identified in severely affected patients with an Ullrich phenotype, and patients with a phenotype intermediate between Ullrich CMD and Bethlem myopathy identified.[1,35] Thus, there is a clinical spectrum, and the effect of a particular mutation on the production and function of collagen VI, rather than the mode of inheritance, determines severity.

The clinical features of patients with Ullrich CMD include contractures and hypotonia at birth, torticollis and hip dislocation, rigidity of the spine, kyphosis and follicular hyperkeratosis and keloid formation (see Table 25.12). They show marked distal laxity of the fingers and ankles, and protrusion of calcanei may also be present. There can be clinical overlap with congenital myopathies, such as those caused by mutations in the *RYR1* gene, and with connective tissue disorders such as Ehlers–Danlos syndrome.

Muscle weakness is usually milder in cases of Bethlem myopathy, particularly in adults, but weakness and progression of disease are variable. The typical features of Bethlem myopathy are summarized in Table 25.13, but as emphasized previously there is a spectrum of severity and some patients follow an intermediate course between the clinical extremes of Ullrich CMD and Bethlem myopathy. Weakness in Bethlem myopathy, as in Ullrich CMD, affects proximal more than distal muscles, and legs more than arms. A proportion of patients become wheelchair-bound during the course of adult life, although respiratory insufficiency, invariable in Ullrich CMD, is exceptional. Contractures characteristically affect the long finger flexors causing an inability to oppose the palms in a 'prayer sign'. Elbow, knee, hip and ankle contractures also occur in most patients, in association with rigidity of the spine. Abnormal scar formation (hypertrophic or atrophic) may also be seen. There is clinical overlap of some features with those that occur in the Emery–Dreifuss muscular dystrophies and LGMD2A, and sometimes they may not be easy to distinguish clinically, although the cardiac defects seen in Emery–Dreifuss muscular dystrophies are not a feature of collagen VI disorders. Muscle imaging shows a characteristic pattern in Ullrich CMD and Bethlem myopathy that is useful for differential diagnosis.[280,281] There is a characteristic pattern of muscle involvement, particularly of the vastus lateralis and rectus femoris, with the periphery more affected than the belly of the muscles. Marked, progressive replacement of muscle with fibrous and adipose tissues can also be apparent.

A variable reduction in collagen VI immunolabelling can be seen in Ullrich CMD, but normal labelling does not exclude a defect, and biopsies from patients with a mild Bethlem phenotype often show no detectable alteration. Some cases show a complete absence or an unequivocal reduction, whereas in others the reduction is subtle and may only be apparent at the sarcolemma, with normal labelling of the endomysium (Figure 25.74).[209] The absence or reduction of collagen VI may also be apparent around axons and blood vessels, but this is not a universal phenomenon. Double immunohistochemical labelling with an antibody to another protein, such as perlecan, collagen IV or collagen V, to assess the integrity of the basal lamina may be necessary to identify this subtle reduction (Figure 25.75). Laminin β1 labelling of the sarcolemma may be reduced in some cases of Bethlem myopathy compared with normal intensity of blood vessels. However, this has been observed in other

BOX 25.7. Integrins

Integrins are transmembrane heterodimers composed of α and β chains. The complex at the myotendinous junction (MTJ), neuromuscular junction (NMJ) and sarcolemma of adult muscle fibres is composed of the α7 (mainly the B-splice variant) and β1D (muscle-specific) chains. In addition, the α3 and αv subunits are also found at the NMJ and MTJ. Integrin α7β1D is a major cell surface receptor for laminin α2, and both α7 and β1D immunolabelling may be secondarily reduced in primary laminin α2 deficiency and in other forms of congenital muscular dystrophy with a secondary reduction of laminin α2.

The MTJ is severely disrupted in the muscles of integrin α7-deficient transgenic mice, with loss of the characteristic digit-like extensions and retraction of the sarcomere from the muscle membrane, suggesting that impairment of force transmission across the MTJ causes the muscle weakness.

25.74 Immunolabelling of collagen VI in (a) a control and (b) a case of Ullrich congenital muscular dystrophy (CMD) showing absence of collagen VI from the sarcolemma, perimysium and endomysium. Note also the labelling round the nerve axons and blood vessels in the control and the retained labelling around the large blood vessels in case of Ullrich CMD.

disorders and is an age-related feature usually only seen in adults and adolescents. Immunolabelling of myosins in Ullrich CMD shows a population of fibres of varying size with fetal myosin and there may be several fibres that coexpress fast and slow myosin (Figure 25.76).

Collagen VI is expressed in most connective tissues and its presence in skin can be studied immunohistochemically, and a clear reduction may be seen in some affected cases.[228,286] Normal immunolabelling of collagen VI in muscle or skin, however, does not exclude a defect in a gene for collagen VI. Studies of cultured fibroblasts suggest that changes in collagen VI may also be useful for identifying abnormalities.[210,225] Fibroblasts from cases of Ullrich CMD clearly show abnormalities, but fibroblasts from Bethlem myopathy patients show more variable results. There is also evidence from studies of cultured fibroblasts that the interaction with fibronectin may be abnormal in some cases.[373] A secondary reduction in collagen VI from fibroblasts *in vitro* is seen when tenascin-X is deficient, also reflecting the importance of the complex interactions of extracellular proteins.[294]

An absence of immunolabelling of collagen VI in chorionic villi samples can also be useful for the prenatal diagnosis of Ullrich CMD, but experience is limited to patients in whom muscle of the proband showed absent immunolabelling of collagen VI.[42]

In addition to the congenital muscular dystrophies discussed earlier, there are several other myopathies caused by defects in proteins of the extracellular network that clinically overlap with connective tissue disorders such as Ehlers–Danlos.[480] The defective proteins identified in humans include various types of collagen, tenascin-C and tenascin-X, fibrillin, perlecan, and secondary alterations of biglycan and decorin expression in human dystrophic muscle have been observed.[507] Patients with tenascin-X defects have mild muscle weakness, myalgia and fatigue, and muscle biopsies from some cases show mild myopathic features and reduced immunolabelling of tenascin-X.[479,482] In addition, mutations affecting collagen XII have recently been identified in patients with clinical similarities to UCMD and Bethlem myopathy.

Congenital Muscular Dystrophies Associated With Hypoglycosylation of α-Dystroglycan

Both α- and β-dystroglycan are central components of the DAG complex at the sarcolemma and are expressed in other tissues in addition to muscle (see Figure 25.64). They are the post-translational products of a single gene. β-Dystroglycan is the transmembrane component, the C terminus of which interacts directly with dystrophin, and the N terminus is non-covalently bound to the C terminus of α-dystroglycan. The core protein of α-dystroglycan has a predicted molecular mass of 72 kDa, but following modest N-glycosylation and extensive O-glycosylation in different tissues, its mass is increased to 156 kDa in muscle and 120 kDa in brain. O-glycosylation of several serine–threonine-rich sites on the mucin-like domain are believed to be crucial for its binding to a number of ligands, including laminin α2. The epitopes for two commercial antibodies to α-dystroglycan, IIH6 and VIA4–1, probably lie in this region. The structures of some of the O-linked mannose glycans on α-dystroglycan have been elucidated and its formation involves the action of several glycosyltransferases that add different monosaccharides in a stepwise manner.

Defects in several genes result in hypoglycosylation of α-dystroglycan. The group of muscle disorders caused by this secondary feature are collectively known as the 'dystroglycanopathies'. There is considerable overlap of phenotype with more than one gene associated with the various phenotypes. The central nervous system is frequently involved. Clinical severity associated with the genes is broad and some of the same genes are associated with limb-girdle forms of dystrophy. A new classification of this group of disorders has been proposed that takes into account the genes responsible, the involvement of the brain and eye, and the presence or absence of mental retardation.[158] This has been adopted by OMIM, but is not yet widely used and the clinical names are still relevant (see Tables 25.11 and 25.14). Several of the defective genes encode proven or putative glycosyltransferases (*POMT1, POMT2, POMGNT1, FKTN, FKRP, LARGE*). Novel methods and next-generation sequencing are identifying defects in additional genes of uncertain

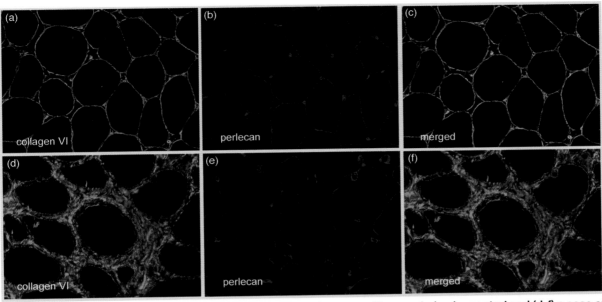

25.75 Double immunolabelling of collagen VI and perlecan and the merged images in (a-c) a control and (d-f) a case of Ullrich congenital muscular dystrophy showing the very reduced sarcolemmal collagen VI but normal labelling of perlecan.

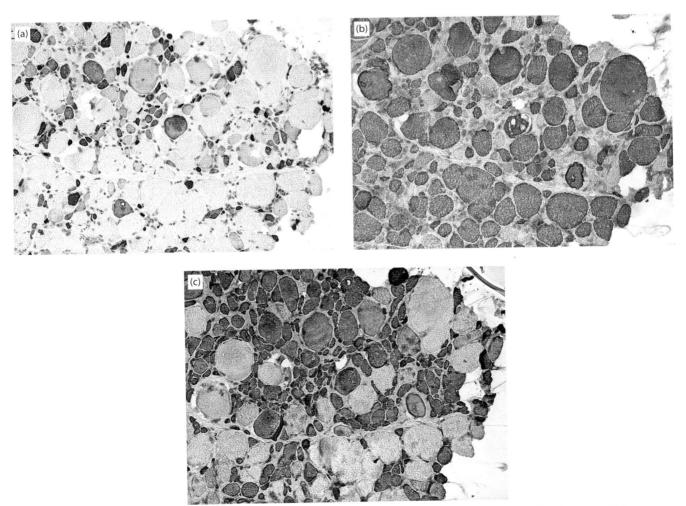

25.76 Serial sections immunolabelled for (a) fetal myosin, (b) slow and (c) fast myosin in a case of Ullrich congenital muscular dystrophy showing a population of fibres of varying size with fetal myosin and coexpression of more than one isoform in several fibres.

function that are also associated with hypoglycosylation of α-dystroglycan and its function, such as isoprenoid synthase domain-containing protein (*ISPD*), transmembrane protein 5 (*TMEM5*), β-1, 3-n-acetylglucosaminyltransferase 1 (*B3GALNT2*), guanine diphosphate mannose pyrophosphorylase B (*GMPPB*), glycosyltransferase-like containing protein (*GTDC2*) and protein kinase-like protein SgK196 (*SGK196*) (see Table 25.11).[55,61,76,159,207,271,369,428,485,498] This is an expanding area, and further causative genes will undoubtedly be identified. In addition, genes thought to only be involved with N-glycosylation also result in hypoglycosylation of α-dystroglycan. These include genes encoding members of the dolichol-phosphate-mannose synthase family of proteins (*DPM1*, *DPM2* and *DPM3*) and link disorders with glycosylation defects to the congenital muscular dystrophies.[27,204,245,289] Hypoglycosylation of α-dystroglycan has also been shown to have a role in the progression of carcinoma cells and to correlate with prognosis.[16] Mutations in the gene *DOLK*, which encodes the dolichol kinase responsible for the formation of dolichol phosphate, have so far only been associated with a dilated cardiomyopathy, although elevated serum CK was present in several patients.[244]

The hypoglycosylation of α-dystroglycan discussed earlier is a secondary phenomenon and a consequence of various gene defects. Mutations in the *DAG1* gene that encodes dystroglycan cause LGMD2P (see Recessive Limb-Girdle Muscular Dystrophies, p. 1561).

The main clinical features of each of the 'dystroglycanopathies' are listed in Table 25.14. Structural brain or eye involvement is common in patients at the severe end of the clinical spectrum of each gene defect. This suggests that the clinical features of a patient affected by a dystroglycanopathy are related to the functional effect of the mutation rather than to the gene involved. At the severe end of the spectrum, mutations in *POMT1*, *POMT2*, *FKRP*, *POMGNT1*, *FKTN*, *ISPD*, *TMEM5,*, *B3GALNT2*, *GTDC2*, *GMPPB* and *SGK196* result in type II lissencephaly, 'flat' brain stem, a hypoplastic cerebellum and absent corpus callosum.[50,207] Immunohistochemistry and immunoblotting of muscle reveal a variable reduction in glycosylation of α-dystroglycan but usually normal β-dystroglycan (in contrast to the reduction of both α- and β-dystroglycan in DMD) and is a useful control. The extent of the reduction of α-dystroglycan immunolabelling often correlates, but not always, with disease severity.[50,211] Research studies of the core protein of α-dystroglycan show that is often normal, but studies are limited by the lack of commercial antibodies that are suitable for both immunohistochemistry and immunoblotting.[211]

A secondary reduction of laminin α2 is common when α-dystroglycan is hypoglycosylated. The extent of this reduction is variable, but complete absence of laminin is never observed, in contrast to cases with a primary laminin α2 defect. Other proteins reported to show a secondary reduction in some of these CMD variants include laminin β2, perlecan, P180, and integrin α7 and β1D chains, but the maturation-related expression of some of these proteins was not always taken into account.[91,92,374,434,495]

Enzyme activity of POMGnT1 can also be assessed. It has been found to be reduced in muscle and cultured fibroblasts from patients with a mutation in the corresponding gene. Kinetic abnormalities have also been identified.[87,509]

Congenital Muscular Dystrophies due to Defects in Proteins of the Sarcoplasmic Reticulum: Rigid Spine Muscular Dystrophy

Although some degree of spinal rigidity is associated with several neuromuscular disorders, it is an invariable complication of one form of CMD (designated RSMD1). Rigid spine muscular dystrophy type 1 is caused by recessive mutations in the gene encoding selenoprotein N1 (*SEPN1*) on chromosome 1p35–36. Mutations in the *SEPN1* gene manifest pathologically as multiple cores in muscle fibres (multi-minicore disease), a myopathy with 'Mallory body'-like inclusions, and fibre type disproportion.[83,137,139] There is considerable clinical and pathological overlap between these disorders, and it is likely that they represent a clinico-pathological spectrum instead of distinct entities.

Selenoproteins constitute a family of enzymes that contain a selenium atom in the form of a seleno-cysteine in the catalytic site and are involved in oxidation–reduction reactions. Selenoprotein 1 (SEPN1) is a membrane-bound glycoprotein localizing to the rough endoplasmic reticulum. It is expressed in several tissues, including skeletal muscle, heart, brain, lung and placenta.[297] It is most highly expressed in fetal muscle. Mutations have been found in most of the 13 exons except exon 3, and most lead to a premature stop codon. The specific function of SEPN1 is not fully understood, but it is believed to be involved in oxidative stress and calcium homeostasis.[247]

Patients affected by RSMD1 usually present with axial weakness and mild proximal muscle weakness, and there is selective involvement of the diaphragm resulting in respiratory insufficiency (Table 25.15). Scoliosis typically accompanies the condition. There is clinical overlap with Emery–Dreifuss muscular dystrophy (see later), but there is no cardiac involvement in RSMD1. RSMD1 is usually stable, and most patients retain the ability to walk for life, provided that the scoliosis and respiratory problems are managed appropriately. Serum CK is usually normal.

In addition to variation in fibre size, muscle pathology may show a mild increase in endomysial connective tissue and an increase in internal nuclei, although these are not usually abundant. An uneven pattern in oxidative enzyme stains, sometimes in the form of multiple core-like lesions, is often associated with mutations in the *SEPN1* gene. Multiple cores may also be seen in cases with a mutation in the *RYR1* gene, which may cause diagnostic confusion.[214] In *SEPN1* cases, however, the core-like lesions often occur in both fibre types

TABLE 25.15 Summary of the main clinical features of the congenital muscular dystrophy with rigid spine associated with a defect in selenoprotein N1 of the endoplasmic reticulum (RSMD1)

Axial hypotonia in first few years of life
Normal motor milestones
Ambulation usually achieved and maintained into adulthood
Rigidity of spine in most cases
Progressive scoliosis
Nasal speech
Pronounced respiratory insufficiency leading to respiratory failure
Normal or mild elevation of creatine kinase
Clinical, pathological and molecular overlap with multi-minicore disease and Mallory body myopathy

and a two-fibre type pattern is usually retained, whereas in *RYR1* cases marked predominance of type 1 fibres is common and the cores are often restricted to type 1 fibres. Antibodies to SEPN1 have been used in research studies to show the absence of the 70-kDa SEPN1 band in immunoblots of fibroblasts cultured from a patient with RSMD1.[2] At present, changes in SEPN1 levels cannot be ascertained on sections by immunohistochemistry and there are no reported secondary protein abnormalities. In keeping with the absence of necrosis and low CK there are usually very few, or no, fibres with fetal myosin. Absence of the protein has been shown in fibroblasts from affected patients, but there are no studies on human sections reported. A reduced number of satellite cells has been noted in patients and in an animal model and it has been suggested that SEPN1 may function in regeneration of muscle.[65]

Congenital Muscular Dystrophies Associated with Nuclear Membrane Proteins

It is now appreciated that some early onset disorders, classified as a congenital muscular dystrophy, are caused by mutations in nuclear membrane proteins and can be lethal.[282,345,474] In early onset cases associated with mutations in the lamin A/C gene, respiratory insufficiency is rapidly progressive and spinal rigidity and scoliosis typically develop. Neck weakness resulting in a 'dropped head' may also be a feature, although not specific for lamin A/C mutations. Muscle pathology is variable and may be mild. Features include variation in fibre size, an increase in connective tissue, necrosis and regeneration and inflammation. No immunohistochemical abnormalities of sarcolemma proteins or nuclear proteins are seen.

Mutations in the *SYNE1* gene encoding nesprin-1 have been found to cause a rare congenital muscular dystrophy with adducted thumbs.[483] The two cases from the single family identified were hypotonic and had muscle weakness, ptosis, ophthalmoplegia, mild mental retardation and mild cerebellar hypoplasia. Serum CK was moderately elevated and muscle pathology showed non-specific myopathic features.

Other Congenital Muscular Dystrophies

A number of other disorders have been designated as a congenital muscular dystrophy, but not all cases have onset within the first 6 months of life or have a clear 'dystrophic' pathology with fibre necrosis, regeneration and fibrosis. For example, cases with defects in the gene encoding choline kinase B (*CHKB*) can show a spectrum of age at onset and severity.[178,296,348] The distinctive pathology of this disorder is discussed with those with mitochondrial defects (see Mitochondrial Myopathies, p. 1602).

Emery–Dreifuss Muscular Dystrophies

The clinical features of the X-linked and autosomal forms of Emery–Dreifuss muscular dystrophy are similar, but often more severe in the latter. Emery–Dreifuss muscular dystrophy is invariably associated with both cardiac and skeletal muscle involvement. Both disorders present with muscle weakness and early contractures of the elbow, the Achilles tendons and the spinal extensor muscles. The contractures

are progressive, and rigidity of the spine often becomes marked. Skeletal muscle involvement typically precedes the cardiac abnormalities, which are evident before the third decade of life and are the most deleterious aspect of both disorders, being characterized by atrioventricular conduction disturbances and heart block. Dilated cardiomyopathy can also be found in autosomal dominant Emery–Dreifuss muscular dystrophy, but less commonly in the X-linked variant.

Involvement of skeletal muscle is typically humeroperoneal, but can also feature scapular involvement. Striking wasting of the upper arms and lower legs is often apparent in both conditions, which are almost indistinguishable, although subtle differences in the pattern of muscle involvement can be demonstrated using muscle MR imaging.[280] The dominant form is more common than the X-linked form and generally more severe, with earlier onset – even congenital in a few instances.[282,285] Except in cases with onset in infancy, ambulation is usually retained for life. Serum CK levels are usually normal, or mildly or moderately elevated, but never at the levels found in DMD or BMD.

The X-linked form is caused by mutations in the *STA* gene on chromosome Xq28, which encodes for emerin.[302,504] Emerin is a 34-kDa nuclear protein with a hydrophobic C terminus anchored in the nuclear membrane and an N-terminal tail projecting into the nucleoplasm. The *STA* gene has six exons, and mutations have been found throughout the gene, with no 'hotspots'. Most are nonsense or frameshift mutations or occur at splice sites. The majority of mutations result in absence of localized protein, which can be demonstrated with antibodies.[267] Rare cases have been reported in which emerin expression is reduced rather than absent.[62,108]

Female carriers rarely manifest with muscle weakness but are at risk of cardiac involvement. The absence of emerin in a proportion of nuclei can be detected in the skin and buccal cells of carriers (Figure 25.77).[268,376] If buccal cells are investigated, it is essential that only viable cells are assessed; parallel studies of nuclear lamins are a useful control, because they appear normal.

Autosomal dominant Emery–Dreifuss muscular dystrophy is caused by dominant mutations in the *LMNA* gene on chromosome 1q11–23; *de novo* mutations are common. This gene is alternatively spliced to produce lamin A and lamin C, which are intermediate filament proteins that localize to the nuclear lamina.[503,504] The nuclear lamina has been attributed with a role in chromatin organization, gene regulation and cell signalling. A direct interaction between lamin A and emerin has been demonstrated *in vitro*, which together with the similar clinical phenotype of the two forms of Emery–Dreifuss muscular dystrophy provides evidence that these two proteins form a functional link at the nuclear envelope. Immunolabelling of emerin and lamin A/C in the autosomal dominant form of Emery–Dreifuss muscular dystrophy appears normal. Some antibodies that specifically detect lamin A but not C show labelling of very few nuclei in mature human muscle (Figure 25.78); this is thought to be due to epitope masking, because it is not seen with all antibodies. Similarly, differences in the immunolabelling of lamin B1 with different antibodies are thought to be due to epitope masking.[462] Antibodies to epitopes common to both lamin A and C show labelling of all nuclei

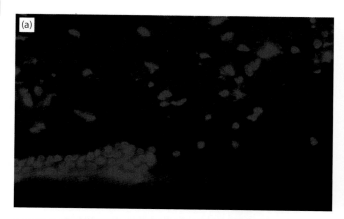

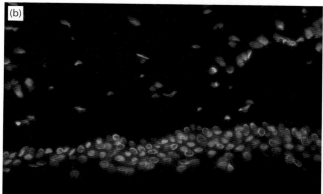

25.77 Immunolabelling of (a) emerin, (b) counterstained with DAPI in a skin biopsy from a carrier of X-linked Emery–Dreifuss muscular dystrophy showing areas of nuclei with and without emerin.

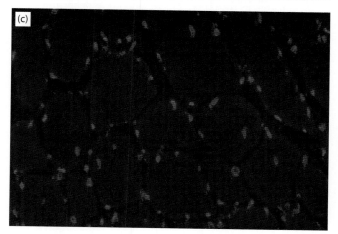

25.78 Immunolabelling of (a) lamin A (b) lamin A/C and (c) lamin B2 in a case of autosomal dominant Emery–Dreifuss muscular dystrophy that are all comparable to controls. Note the relatively few nuclei labelled with this antibody to lamin A (other antibodies can show labelling of more nuclei) and the similar labelling of internal and peripheral nuclei.

(Figure 25.78b). Some studies have suggested that there is reciprocal expression of lamin B1 and emerin, with emerin in myonuclei and lamin B1 in endothelial cell nuclei.[269] Lamin B2 appears to be present in all nuclei, and internal nuclei show similar emerin and lamin labelling as peripheral nuclei (Figure 25.78c).

In common with other intermediate filament proteins, lamins possess a highly conserved α-helical coiled-coil rod domain, which plays a crucial role in lamin–lamin interactions. Mutations occur throughout the gene, although many are found in the common α-helical rod domain of exons 1–10. These mutations result in no detectable alteration in lamin A/C immunolocalization.

Mutations in the *LMNA* gene underlie the cause of several allelic conditions, including Emery–Dreifuss muscular dystrophy, LGMD1B, dilated cardiomyopathy with conduction system disease, familial partial lipodystrophy, Charcot–Marie–Tooth disease type 2B1, mandibuloacral disostosis, premature ageing disorders and restrictive dermopathy.[504] These are now often collectively referred to as the 'laminopathies', but skeletal muscle is affected in only some of them (autosomal dominant Emery–Dreifuss muscular dystrophy, LGMD1B). Some severely affected infants with axial weakness have also been found to have *de novo* mutations in the gene encoding lamin A/C and it is often worth considering this gene in a severely affected infant or neonate in whom the muscle biopsy shows non-specific myopathic changes and/or inflammation.[345] These

cases are considered to overlap with congenital muscular dystrophies (see earlier) and some have been described as having a 'dropped head' syndrome.[71,345] The explanation for the phenotypic diversity is unclear. Research, however, suggests that tissue-specific differences in the arrangement of the lamin-associated protein complexes at the nuclear envelope may underlie some of the tissue specificity in these disorders.

Additional genes encoding proteins of the nuclear envelope are also associated with a dominant Emery–Dreifuss muscular dystrophy (EDMD) phenotype. Identification of the genes that encode nesprin 1 and 2 (*SYNE 1* and *SYNE2*), a protein known as LUMA (encoded by *TMEM43*), and identification of a mutation in the genes encoding LAP2α, LAP1B and SUN proteins (lamin A-associated protein), confirm this and emphasize the importance of the nuclear envelope and the complex of proteins that interact with emerin and lamins.[22,249,275,277,508] Defects in nesprin are also responsible for a recessive disorder that presents with arthrogryposis.[9] A protein in the nuclear matrix, matrin-3, is responsible for a dominant distal myopathy with vocal cord and pharyngeal weakness but this has a different phenotype to Emery–Dreifuss muscular dystrophy.[397]

The main histological and histochemical features of the two forms of Emery–Dreifuss muscular dystrophy are similar. In quadriceps biopsies, variation in fibre size is not markedly abnormal; occasional atrophic fibres are common, and some fibres may be hypertrophic. Internal nuclei may be few or numerous, with more than one per fibre (Figure 25.79). Necrotic fibres are generally rare, and there is usually only a mild, or little, increase in adipose or connective tissue (Figure 25.79). There are exceptions, however, such as a severely affected boy found to have a mutation in both the *STA* and the *LMNA* genes.[308] This case illustrates the importance of considering the possibility of a causative mutation in more than one gene, particularly those in which mutations are common, such as *LMNA*.

Biopsies may contain small basophilic fibres with a slightly granular appearance (Figure 25.80). These might be regenerating fibres, because they express fetal myosin and an increased amount of desmin; however, generally only a few fibres express developmental myosins, suggesting that there is little ongoing muscle fibre regeneration. It is not clear whether this reflects a lack of necrosis, which precedes regeneration, or whether there is a malfunction in the regenerative process. In support of the latter, *in vitro* studies suggest that myoblasts deficient in either lamin A/C or emerin display delayed differentiation kinetics and have a decreased differentiation potential. This may, therefore, partly explain the dystrophic phenotype observed in patients with Emery–Dreifuss muscular dystrophy.[147] A two-fibre type pattern is usually maintained with oxidative enzyme stains and ATPase. There is a tendency for the type 1 fibres to be smaller, but not usually to the degree seen in congenital myopathies. A predominance of type 1 fibres may also occur. Non-specific structural changes such as cores can also occur.

Immunolabelling of all proteins associated with the sarcolemma is normal in both forms of Emery–Dreifuss muscular dystrophy, with the exception of laminin β1. Reduced laminin β1 labelling on the sarcolemma may be apparent in some cases, but all blood vessels, including the capillary network, show normal reactivity. Labelling of laminin α2 and laminin γ1 is normal and useful as controls.[117] The reduced sarcolemmal labelling of laminin β1 is not specific for Emery–Dreifuss muscular dystrophies and may be seen in Bethlem myopathy and other

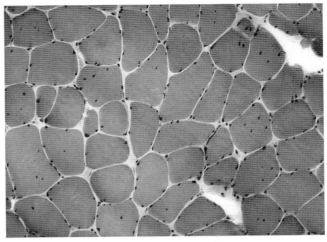

25.79 A case of autosomal dominant Emery–Dreifuss muscular dystrophy showing only mild variation in fibre size, mild fibrosis, an increase in internal nuclei and no necrosis. H&E.

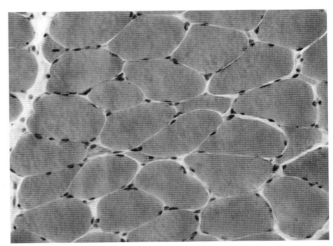

25.80 Small basophilic fibres in an 8-year-old child with autosomal dominant Emery–Dreifuss muscular dystrophy. H&E.

myopathies, including LGMD2I. It is an age-related phenomenon, observed in adult and adolescent patients, but rarely in young children.

Electron microscopy may demonstrate aggregation of chromatin and a lack of attachment of chromatin to the nuclear membrane.[49] Abnormalities of the nuclear envelope have also been reported in skeletal muscle nuclei and cultured skin fibroblasts.[140,321] The specificity of these findings to Emery–Dreifuss muscular dystrophy remains unclear.

Disorders Associated with Deletions or Expansions of Repeated Sequences

Most gene mutations responsible for a neuromuscular disorder are deletions, duplications or splice site or missense changes, which disrupt the sequence of the reading frame or, more rarely, affect their promoter regions. A few conditions, however, are caused by more unusual mechanisms, which involve deletions or expansions of a nucleotide repeat sequence. These are facioscapulohumeral muscular dystrophy (FSHD), the myotonic muscular dystrophies, and oculopharyngeal muscular dystrophy (OPMD). With the advent of reliable molecular testing for FSHD and the myotonic dystrophies, muscle biopsies are performed less often and their role has diminished.

Facioscapulohumeral muscular dystrophy (FSHD) is one of the most common muscular dystrophies, with an estimated prevalence of 1 in 20 000.[103,425,472] The clinical features of FSHD are summarized in Table 25.16.

FSHD is inherited dominantly, although cases at the severe end of the clinical spectrum are often the product of *de novo* dominant mutations. Penetrance, based on clinical presentation, is age dependent and most cases show clinical signs before the age of 20 years. Infantile cases with onset recognizable before the age of 10 years are seen in some families. Anticipation is also well recognized, although unexplained, with earlier onset in successive generations. Severity may relate to size of the deletion of the fragment associated with FSHD.

The molecular defect responsible for FSHD is a deletion of copies of a 3.3-kb DNA repeat fragment in the subtelomeric region of chromosome 4q (D4Z4) in association with a 4qA161 haplotype. In normal individuals, this fragment varies in size from 50–300 kb, with 11 or more D4Z4 repeats, but patients with FSHD have 11 or fewer repeats.[425,472] It is not clear how the reduction in the size of the 4q fragment causes disease, but recent studies indicate that a crucial step in the disease is the inefficient repression of the retrogene DUX4 in a microsatellite repeat array.[425]

Molecular diagnosis of FSHD relies on a double digest with the *Eco*RI and *Bln*I restriction enzymes, in order to distinguish the chromosome 4q fragment from the similar fragment on chromosome 10q26. The fragments from both chromosomes are detectable with the p13E–11 probe, but the chromosome 10 fragment contains a *Bln*I restriction site that is absent from the chromosome 4 fragment. Thus, these two enzymes completely digest the chromosome 10 fragment, leaving the chromosome 4-related fragments. Confusion can arise, however, because interchromosomal exchange of the repeat regions occurs in a few normal individuals, resulting in hybrids of chromosome 4 and 10 fragments. Germline mosaicism may also hamper molecular analysis, and false negative and false positive results can be obtained, requiring the use of additional probes. The double-digest analysis, however, identifies the majority of cases. About 95 per cent of cases with the typical phenotype show contraction of the 4q fragment (FSHD1) and the other 5 per cent do not show contraction, but have hypomethylation at the D4Z4 locus (FSHD2).[103]

Although muscle biopsies are now performed less often for the diagnosis of FSHD, we summarize here the pathological features that have been observed and may alert pathologists in atypical cases. The abnormalities are non-specific, and the degree of change is variable and may be influenced by the clinical involvement of the sampled muscle.

Variation in the size of both fibre types is common, but some biopsies from minimally involved muscles may show only scattered very small fibres. These fibres have been described as atrophic, but the expression of developmentally regulated proteins in them raises the possibility that they represent attempts at regeneration.[117] Fibre type grouping is not a feature, but clusters of small fibres, as in

TABLE 25.16 Main clinical features of facioscapulohumeral muscular dystrophy
Age of onset variable, congenital (rare) to adulthood. Most cases present in the first 2-3 decades of life
Autosomal dominant inheritance with variable penetrance
Facial weakness
Shoulder girdle weakness with difficulty raising arms
Peroneal muscle weakness
Scapular winging
Generalized muscle wasting, often asymmetrical
Weakness of abdominal muscles
Variable progression – minimal or slow, may lead to loss of ambulation
Hearing loss
Retinal vasculopathy
Mild to moderate elevation of CK that is age and sex dependent

Rare congenital cases with extreme repeat deletions and severe weakness, cognitive involvement and severe neurosensory hearing loss and epilepsy have been described; these cases may never acquire ambulation and need to be differentiated from congenital dystrophy.

BMD, have been put forward as evidence of denervation. These fibres, however, also show proteins associated with immaturity, and there are no electrophysiological data to support the proposal of denervation.

Fibre necrosis is not usually marked in FSHD, but it can occur. Similarly, an increase in fibrous and adipose tissues may be seen. Internal nuclei may be numerous, but they are usually not increased. An inflammatory response is frequent and may vary from mild to profuse. In contrast to inflammatory myopathies and LGMD2B, overexpression of sarcolemmal MHC class I antigens is rarely observed in FSHD.[363] There are no specific immunohistochemical abnormalities and, although reduced sarcolemmal laminin β1 has been observed, this is not a consistent feature and can be seen in other disorders.

Myotonic dystrophies are common autosomal dominant disorders. They are characterized by myotonia in association with muscle weakness and wasting. These disorders also affect several other tissues, including cardiac muscle. Two forms of myotonic dystrophy (DM1, DM2) are recognized; they are caused by defects in two different genes. Type 2 is also known as proximal myotonic myopathy (PROMM). Both DM1 and DM2 are caused by expansion of a nucleotide repeat: DM1 by expansion of a CTG repeat in the 3′ untranslated region of a gene on chromosome 19q, and DM2 by a CCTG repeat expansion in the first intron of the *ZNF9* gene on chromosome 3q. The chromosome 19 protein is a putative kinase (DM protein kinase [DMPK]) and that encoded by *ZNF9* is a zinc finger protein. Both disorders are believed to result from 'toxic RNA' produced by the expansion, which interferes with a number of RNA-binding proteins, such as muscleblind and SIX5 in the nucleus.[151,384,463]

Type 1 myotonic dystrophy is a common disorder with an estimated prevalence of about 1 in 8000 in Caucasians, whereas DM2 is rarer but is particularly common in some populations.[437] There are no reported congenital cases of DM2, but congenital presentation of DM1 is well recognized; almost invariably, a mildly affected mother transmits the mutant gene. Although clinical and electrophysiological assessments are often sufficient to make a presumptive diagnosis of DM1 or DM2, histopathological examination can help in less obvious cases and plays an important role in the diagnosis of congenital DM1 cases.

Type 1 myotonic dystrophy is caused by an increase in the number of repeats in the *DMPK* gene. In normal individuals there are between 4 and 40 CTG repeats, but in patients with DM1 this is increased to 50 or more–sometimes over 1000. In general, there is a correlation between the size of the repeat and the clinical severity and age at onset: patients with fewer than 100 repeats are affected more mildly than those with more than 1000 repeats (e.g. congenital patients). Anticipation in DM1 is common, with successive generations showing more clinical severity. There is also somatic variability and instability in the size of the repeat expansion with the number being greater and more unstable in muscle than in blood lymphocytes.

Type 2 myotonic dystrophy is caused by an increase in the number of chromosome 3 *ZNF9* gene CCTG repeats. In normal individuals, the number of repeats ranges from 10 to 30, but in patients with DM2 this is increased to many thousands. Anticipation and somatic variability also appear to occur in DM2, but the correlations are less clear than in DM1. There does not appear to be a congenital form of DM2.

Myotonia is common to both DM1 and DM2, but the pattern of muscle weakness is different. In DM2 there is early proximal muscle involvement, in contrast to the distal pattern seen in DM1, hence the name (PROMM) commonly attributed to DM2.[259,384] Facial weakness is common in DM1 but rare in DM2. Ptosis and facial/neck weakness are characteristic features of DM1. Similarly, cardiac conduction defects and CNS involvement are common in DM1 but less so in DM2. Diaphragmatic weakness leads to respiratory insufficiency and is often a cause of death in DM1. Cataracts occur in both DM1 and DM2. Other associated features of both include frontal balding and gonadal atrophy.

Molecular analysis of the myotonic dystrophies to confirm a clinical diagnosis is highly reliable and muscle biopsies are now less often performed. The diagnosis of patients with DM2, however, may not be as clinically apparent as for DM1, and a muscle biopsy from a DM2 patient is then more likely to be taken. Histopathological information on DM2 has increased, because more molecularly confirmed cases have been studied and differences between DM1 and DM2 are apparent.[117,313,391,477] Both forms show a pronounced number of multiple internal nuclei (which may be in chains) and variation in fibre size. The pathology is progressive with loss of muscle fibres and increasing amounts of fat and fibrous tissue. Sarcoplasmic masses with disorganized myofibrillar material and dilated sarcoplasmic reticulum are typical of DM1. Ring fibres are also more common in DM1 than DM2. Early changes in DM1 are atrophy of type 1 fibres and hypertrophy of type 2 fibres. In DM2, in contrast, atrophy affects type 2 fibres more than type 1 fibres. Prominent nuclear clumps are an early feature in DM2, which label with antibodies to fast and fetal myosin isoforms, but are a late feature in DM1.[391,477] Congenital forms of DM1 may show many central nuclei, and the pathology is very similar to that of myotubular myopathy. The number of fibres with slow myosin, however, is less in congenital DM1 and the two disorders can be distinguished with antibodies to muscleblind.[409,422] Molecular analysis of the DM1 locus is essential in all neonates with abundant central nuclei.

Oculopharyngeal muscular dystrophy is usually transmitted as an autosomal dominant disorder, but a few recessive cases have also been reported. The molecular defect is short GCG expansions of the first exon of the polyadenylate-binding protein nuclear 1 gene (*PABPN1*) on chromosome 14q11.1.[39] Normal individuals have six GCG repeats in the first exon of the *PABPN1* gene, but in OPMD there are an additional two to seven repeats. The disorder has a worldwide distribution, but it is particularly prevalent in French Canadian and Bukhura Jewish populations.[39]

OPMD is a late-onset disorder characterized by early ptosis and dysphagia. The disorder progresses slowly, with increasing weakness of several muscles, including those of the face, eyes and limbs; a nasal voice also develops. There is no cardiac involvement, and CK is usually normal or occasionally mildly elevated.

The pathological feature of note is the presence of rimmed vacuoles that are often more common in type 1 than type 2 fibres. The vacuoles often contain acid phosphatase. Electron microscopy shows that they are autophagic and contain osmiophilic membranous myelin-like whorls and cytoplasmic debris. Electron microscopy also reveals the other particular feature of OPMD – the presence of intranuclear tubular filaments. These can be identified in semi-thin toluidine blue-stained resin sections as pale or clear areas. These filaments are about 0.25 μm in length, with an outer diameter of 8.5 nm and an inner diameter of 3 nm. They are unbranched and their orientation is variable. They are seen only in muscle nuclei and never in the cytoplasm or nuclei of other cell types, such as satellite, endothelial and interstitial cells. Thus, the nuclear inclusions of OPMD are distinct from the 15- to 18-nm filaments seen in IBM and distal myopathies with rimmed vacuoles. The number of affected nuclei in OPMD varies between muscles (2–5 per cent) but is rarely more than 9 per cent per plane of section. Antibodies to PABPN1 localize to the nuclear inclusions, and poly(A) RNA can be detected in them with *in situ* hybridization.[21] They are also recognized by antibodies to ubiquitin and proteosomal subunits.[8]

Other pathological features of OPMD, some of which may be age-related, include variation in fibre size, nuclear clumps, occasional internal nuclei, moth-eaten fibres, core-like areas and whorled fibres. Mitochondrial aggregates, as in lobulated fibres, may be seen. A few ragged-red fibres and fibres devoid of cytochrome oxidase, reflecting the presence of abnormal mitochondria, may also occur.

Oculopharyngodistal myopathy (OPDM) is distinct from OPMD although they share some clinical and pathological similarities. It is not associated with the GCG expansion of the *PABPN1* gene and the gene responsible is not known. Both autosomal dominant and recessive inheritance of OPDM has been described.[120,293,383,473] The typical presentation is earlier than OPMD and includes ptosis, ophthalmoparesis, facial and bulbar weakness and distal limb weakness, in contrast to the proximal weakness of OPMD. Cardiomyopathy may also occur.[451] Serum CK levels are mildly elevated. Muscle biopsies show variation in fibre size, rimmed vacuoles and occasional fibres negative for cytochrome c oxidase. The 8 nm nuclear inclusions typical of OPMD are absent but nuclear and cytoplasmic tubular filaments variously reported to be 10–12 nm, 14–16 nm or 16–18 nm occur.

Congenital Myopathies and Allied Disorders

The congenital myopathies emerged as a distinct group of disorders in the 1950s and 1960s, alongside the wider application of muscle histochemistry and electron microscopy. They are clinically, genetically and pathologically a heterogeneous group of disorders defined by, and named after, characteristic morphological features on muscle biopsy, such as nemaline myopathy, central core disease, multi-minicore disease and myotubular myopathy. It is now apparent, however, that there is considerable pathological, genetic and clinical overlap with the same pathological feature being associated with more than one gene, and defects in the same gene being associated with more than one abnormal structure (Table 25.17). Onset of congenital myopathies is usually at birth or in early childhood, with hypotonia and muscle weakness ('floppy baby'), but some adult cases with similar histopathological features have been reported, and a rare case with hypertonia and a 'stiff' phenotype has been reported.[354] Muscle weakness may be predominantly proximal and of limb-girdle distribution, or it may be more generalized. In some cases, weakness may show marked involvement of the axial muscles and the face, and a few may show prominent distal involvement. A long 'myopathic' face is a common feature, particularly in nemaline myopathy and myotubular myopathies, and extraocular involvement occurs in some disorders, such as myotubular/centronuclear myopathies and in some cases with mutations in the ryanodine receptor gene (*RYR1*). The progression of the muscle weakness may be slow or minimal, but there is often disproportionately severe weakness of the respiratory muscles. Arthrogryposis may occur in some severe cases of nemaline myopathy and *RYR1*-related core disease, and in association with defects in various genes encoding myofibrillar proteins.[177,239,367,427,439,442] Lordosis, spinal rigidity, scoliosis and joint laxity are common, and hip dislocation is a particular feature of *RYR1*-related core disease. Intelligence is usually normal. Creatine kinase levels are usually normal or elevated only mildly. Differential involvement of muscles is a feature of several congenital myopathies, and muscle MR imaging reveals characteristic patterns that can help direct molecular analysis in childhood and adult cases.[284,431]

Most of the structural features that characterize these disorders are non-specific and occur to a variable extent in several disorders. As stated earlier, there is also considerable pathological overlap between the various congenital myopathies. Mutations in different genes can lead to the presence of the same histopathological feature, and mutations in the same gene can give rise to a variable clinical phenotype. Several of the genes responsible for the more common congenital myopathies have been identified (see Table 25.17) and there is now a wider appreciation of the clinical and pathological phenotypes associated with them.[217,318,489]

Inheritance of the congenital myopathies may be autosomal dominant, autosomal recessive or X-linked recessive, and there is a high incidence of *de novo* dominant mutations.

The most common congenital myopathies are nemaline myopathy, core myopathies (central core, multi-minicore) and myotubular/centronuclear myopathies. Rare disorders characterized by diverse morphological features, such as hyaline bodies, dilation of the sarcoplasmic reticulum (sarcotubular myopathy), reducing bodies, fingerprint bodies, zebra bodies, cylindrical spirals and lamellar bodies, have also been identified. Some of these have a molecular basis, but it is not clear whether they are all genetic entities.[160,400]

Most of the congenital myopathies share some histopathological features. Hypotrophy of type 1 fibres is seen in several/most of the conditions, and there is often a marked predominance or uniformity of type 1 fibres. Antibodies to myosin isoforms confirm the slow phenotype of most fibres, but there may be some hybrid fibres with more than one isoform. Necrosis and regeneration are not typical features, but they may occur. Scattered, very small fibres containing fetal myosin (sometimes referred to as 'pinpricks') are often seen, but it is not clear whether these represent attempts at regeneration, because fetal myosin can be expressed for a variety of reasons. Centrally placed nuclei characterize myotubular and centronuclear myopathies but can also occur in association with *RYR1*- related core myopathy. Fibrosis is rare in congenital myopathies, but it can occur, especially in *RYR1*-related core myopathies.

Congenital Myopathies with Structural Defects

Nemaline Myopathy

Inheritance of nemaline myopathies is autosomal dominant or autosomal recessive, with a significant number of *de novo* dominant cases. Mutations in several genes have been identified (see Table 25.17), many of which encode thin filament proteins.[405] There is further genetic heterogeneity, because some cases do not link to any of the published loci, and next-generation sequencing is identifying gene variants that are currently under investigation. Mutations in the genes encoding skeletal α-actin (*ACTA1*) and nebulin (*NEB*) are the most common. Most mutations in *ACTA1* are dominant or *de novo* dominant, with a few rare recessive cases. In contrast, all reported *NEB* mutations are recessive.[489]

Most cases of the common childhood type result from *NEB* mutations, and there is a particular deletion in the Ashkenazi Jewish population.[489] Mutations in the genes for α- and β-tropomyosin (*TPM3*, *TPM2*) are rare, and mutations in the gene for troponin T (*TNNT1*) seem to be restricted to the Amish population in North America.[489]

There is a broad clinical spectrum associated with the presence of rods.[489] The severe congenital/neonatal forms show marked hypotonia and an absence of spontaneous movements and respiration at birth. Some cases may display the fetal akinesia sequence.[239] The term nemaline myopathy is usually applied to cases with congenital hypotonia and weakness, and those of adult onset (sporadic late onset nemaline myopathy) are often of autoimmune origin, several of which have a gammopathy.[24,67,320,489] These cases are better considered as 'myopathies with rods', to distinguish them from the congenital nemaline myopathies. In addition, cases described as nemaline myopathy with onset in childhood or early adulthood, characterized by slowness of movement, have dominantly inherited mutations in the *KBTBD13* gene.[377] These cases therefore differ from

TABLE 25.17 The structural and genetic defects in congenital myopathies and allied disorders

	Gene	Gene locus	Inheritance	Protein
Nemaline rods and nemaline myopathy				
	ACTA1	1q42	AD or AR	Skeletal α-actin
	NEB	2q.2	AR	Nebulin
	TPM3	1q2	AD or AR	α-Tropomyosin
	TPM2	9p13	AD or AR	β-Tropomyosin
	TNNT1	19q13	AR	Troponin T
	CFL2	14q12	AR	Cofilin-2
	KBTBD13	15q25.31	AD	KBTBD13
	KLHL40	3p21	AR	KLHL40
	KLHL41	2q31	AR	KLHL41
Other myopathies with abundant rods				
Rods and cores	RYR1	19q13	AD	Ryanodine receptor 1
	ACTA1	1q42	AD or AR	Skeletal α-actin
	NEB	2q.2	AR	Nebulin
Rods and caps	TPM2	9q13	AD	β-Tropomyosin
Congenital myopathies with cores*				
Central core disease	RYR1	19q13	AD or AR	Ryanodine receptor 1
Multi-minicore disease	SEPN1	1p36	AR	Selenoprotein N1
Congenital myopathy +/- cardiomyopathy	TTN	2q31	AR	Titin
	MYH7	14q11	AD	Slow myosin heavy chain
Central nuclei and centronuclear myopathies				
Myotubular myopathy	MTM1	Xq28	XLR	Myotubularin
Centronuclear myopathy	DNM2	19p13	AD	Dynamin 2
	BIN1	2q14	AR	Amphiphysin 2
	RYR1	19q13	AD	Ryanodine receptor 1
	CCDC78	16p13.3	AD	Coiled-coil domain-containing protein 78
Congenital myopathy & fatal cardiomyopathy	TTN	2q31	AR	Titin
Surplus protein congenital myopathies				
Actin aggregation	ACTA1	1q42	AD	Skeletal α-actin
Zebra body myopathy	ACTA1	1q42	AD	Skeletal α-actin
Cap disease	TPM2	9q13	AD	β-Tropomyosin
	TPM3	1q2	AD	α-Tropomyosin
	ACTA1	1q42	AD	Skeletal α-actin
Congenital fibre type disproportion				
	ACTA1	1q42	AD	Skeletal α-actin
	SEPN1	1p36	AR	Selenoprotein N1
	TPM3	1q2	AD	α-Tropomyosin
	TPM2	9q13	AD	β-Tropomyosin

Continued

TABLE 25.17 The structural and genetic defects in congenital myopathies and allied disorders *(Continued)*

	Gene	Gene locus	Inheritance	Protein
	MYH7	14q11	AD	Slow myosin heavy chain
	RYR1	19q13	AD or AR	Ryanodine receptor 1
	HACD1	10p12	AR	3-hyroxyacyl-CoA dehydratase 1
Congenital myopathies characterized by distal involvement and/or distal arthrogryposis				
	NEB	2q2	AR	Nebulin
	TPM2	9q13	AD	β-Tropomyosin
	MYH3	17p13	AD	Myosin heavy chain 3
	MYH8	17p13	AD	Perinatal myosin
	TNNI2	11p15	AD	Troponin I
	TNNT3	11p15	AD	Troponin T3
	MYBPC1	12q23.2	AD	Myosin-binding protein C, slow type
	ECEL1	2q37.1	AR	Endothelin-converting enzyme-like 1

AD, autosomal dominant; AR, autosomal recessive; XLR, X-linked recessive; XLD, X-linked dominant;?, inheritance currently uncertain. +/- with or without.

Some disorders with early onset caused by mutations in myosin heavy chains, and disorders with reducing bodies and spheroid bodies are not included in this table (see section on Sarcomeric Proteins, p. 1589).

˙Core-like lesions occur in association with defects in several genes (see text).

other forms of nemaline myopathy by their lack of neonatal hypotonia and a muscle pathology that shows hypertrophy of type 1 fibres and atrophy of type 2 fibres, in addition to cores. Defects in the genes of other members of the Kelch family, however, have recently been identified as causing severe recessive forms of nemaline myopathy (*KLHL40, KLHL41*) and others are under investigation (see gene table of neuromuscular disorders at www.musclegenetable.fr).[355]

The most common form of nemaline myopathy presents with hypotonia in early infancy or childhood, and patients have delayed motor milestones and generalized weakness predominantly affecting the facial and axial muscles. There is poor muscle bulk, and feeding and respiratory problems are common. Independent ambulation is achieved, and the disorder is non-progressive or mildly progressive. Some cases show a predominant distal weakness but not all show rods.[246,488]

The characteristic feature of nemaline myopathy is the presence of rod-shaped structures staining red with Gomori trichrome (Figure 25.81). They are often in clusters at the periphery of fibres near nuclei, or they may appear throughout the fibre. If fibres are very small, rods may be difficult to identify without high-power optics. In addition to rods, varying degrees of Z-line disruption and core-like areas devoid of mitochondria and showing pronounced myofibrillar disruption may be present.[217] The areas of abundant rods do not stain for oxidative enzymes and should not be confused with cores with disrupted myofibrils. Accumulation of actin filaments can occur with or without the presence of rods in cases with *ACTA1* mutations.[163]

With electron microscopy, rods are seen as electron-dense structures, which may be rod-like or sometimes ovoid (Figure 25.82). They are frequently parallel to the longitudinal axis of the sarcomeres, and their form depends on the plane of section. Some rods may be derived from Z-lines, because they show continuity with Z-lines, have a similar lattice structure and contain similar proteins. The major constituent of both rods and Z-lines is α-actinin. They also contain tropomyosin, and proteins associated with Z-lines, such as actin and myotilin. As with Z-lines, desmin occurs at the periphery of rods, but not within them. In most cases, rods are cytoplasmic, but rare cases caused by *ACTA1* mutations also demonstrate nuclear rods.[200,220,492]

It is rarely possible to predict the defective gene from pathology, with the exception of the accumulation of actin filaments and presence of nuclear rods, which are associated with *ACTA1* mutations in most cases. Only a minority of *ACTA1* cases, however, show these features. In patients with recessive *NEB* mutations, immunohistochemistry shows nebulin is present in all muscle fibres.[400,487] In the absence of any genetic clues, molecular analysis usually begins with *ACTA1*, because it has only six exons, in contrast to the giant *NEB* gene, which has 183 exons.

Rods may also occur in normal eye muscles, at myotendinous junctions, in ageing muscle and occasionally in a variety of disorders. Nuclear rods can occur in association with mutations in the genes encoding plectin and ZASP, but the phenotype in these cases is different from the congenital nemaline myopathy cases.[15,325]

Core Myopathies

Areas devoid of oxidative enzyme stains are the characteristic pathological feature of the 'core myopathies'. However, there is considerable variability and overlap in

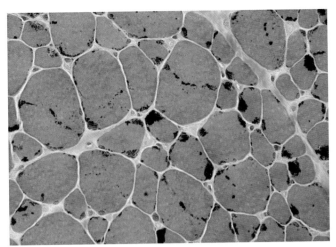

25.81 A case of nemaline myopathy showing numerous red-stained rods in peripheral clusters and throughout some fibres. Gomori trichrome.

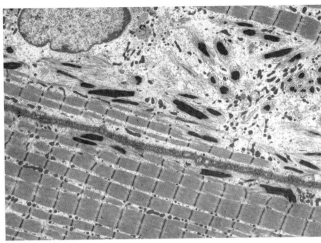

25.82 Electron micrograph of a case of nemaline myopathy showing electron-dense structures that are rod-shaped when sectioned longitudinally or ovoid in shape when sectioned transversely.

BOX 25.8. The ryanodine receptor of skeletal muscle

The *RYR1* gene consists of 106 exons with a cDNA greater than 15 kb and encodes the skeletal muscle ryanodine receptor 1 protein (RyR1). It is a large transmembrane tetrameric ligand-gated calcium-release channel in the terminal cisternae of the sarcoplasmic reticulum and has a major role in the regulation of cytosolic calcium levels and excitation–contraction coupling. The predicted structure of the ryanodine receptor suggests that the calcium-release channel is located in the C-terminal domain of the protein, whereas the remaining N-terminal domains constitute the visible foot structure that interacts with the dihydropyridine receptor (DHPR) in the T-tubule. Genotype–phenotype correlations have suggested that mutations in the cytoplasmic N-terminal domain and the cytoplasmic central domain mostly result in malignant hyperthermia susceptibility, rather than in central core disease, whereas mutations affecting the C-terminal exons are a 'hotspot' and more commonly result in central core disease. Recessive mutations associated with core-like lesions occur in all parts of the gene. The majority of mutations in the *RYR1* gene are missense mutations, although small in-frame deletions have also been detected.

the clinical phenotype and pathology that can make differential diagnosis difficult, and to refer to this group of disorders as 'core myopathies' can be helpful. We have, however, retained the two historical categories of central core disease and multi-minicore disease because these are familiar terms to pathologists, but emphasize the overlap between them.

Central Core Disease In 1956, Magee and Shy published details of muscle biopsies from a family in which fibres showed amorphous central areas.[260] The name 'central core disease' was suggested later.[169] Since then, many cases with a similar pathology have been identified, the gene responsible has been identified (the ryanodine receptor 1 gene -*RYR1* on chromosome 19q13) (Box 25.8), and a greater understanding of the phenotype appreciated.[217,229,344]

The inheritance of most *RYR1* mutations is autosomal dominant; several sporadic *de novo* dominant cases have

also been reported and there are also recessive cases.[217,405] Cases with a severe presentation, with features of the fetal akinesia sequence, have also been reported, some of which are associated with recessive inheritance.[367] These severely affected infants require ventilation at birth, and death may occur in infancy. In contrast, some of these patients may show considerable improvement, and it may be possible to wean them off ventilation; one reported child eventually became independently ambulant.[367]

The *RYR1* gene is also responsible for malignant hyperthermia susceptibility, although additional loci are also linked to this.[219] Most, if not all, patients affected by central core disease are considered to be 'at risk' of malignant hyperthermia susceptibility, and appropriate precautions need to be taken.

It is now appreciated that the range of clinical and pathological features associated with *RYR1* mutations is broad. *RYR1*-related core disease is one of the most common congenital myopathies. Patients typically have hypotonia at birth and developmental delay. Weakness is more pronounced in the pelvic girdle and axial muscles than in the upper limbs. Facial involvement is usually mild, and lack of complete eye closure may be the only finding. However, some cases show ophthalmoplegia and ptosis.[217] Orthopaedic complications such as scoliosis, talipes and dislocation of the hips are common. Contractures, other than tendon Achilles tightness, are rare, but many affected individuals have marked ligamentous laxity, occasionally associated with patellar instability. Apart from the most severe neonatal cases and some patients with congenital dislocation of the hips, most patients achieve independent walking. The course of *RYR1*-related core disease is often static or slowly progressive over prolonged periods of time.[217] Primary cardiac involvement is not a feature, and respiratory involvement is usually milder than with other congenital myopathies, except in the severe neonatal cases. Serum CK activity is usually normal or only mildly elevated. A striking feature of *RYR1*-related core disease is the differential muscle involvement, and muscle MR imaging reveals a characteristic pattern that can be helpful when selecting the site for a muscle biopsy and for directing molecular genetics.[431]

The name 'central core disease' reflects the pale central zones of muscle fibres, which are devoid of mitochondria and, therefore, oxidative enzyme staining (Figure 25.83). The core usually extends a considerable way down the fibre, and associated myofibrils are often hypercontracted (structured) or, in some cases, very disrupted (unstructured). The cores may be rimmed by PAS-positive material, and desmin may accumulate peripherally or internally within them. Additional proteins such as αB-crystallin, small heat-shock proteins, myotilin and filamin C also accumulate within cores.[117,400,405] Although cores may be central, they can also be peripheral, and more than one may be present in cross-section. Clearly demarcated cores are not always evident, and some cases may show only subtle unevenness of oxidative enzyme stains or multiple focal areas of disruption, which resemble minicores. In particular, muscles from very young patients may show only type 1 uniformity or predominance, suggesting there is an age-related development of the cores (see Figure 25.83).[406]

Fibre size variation is often mild, but fibre hypertrophy is common, particularly in adults. Some cases may show only fibre type disproportion with small type 1 fibres.[84] If fibre typing is retained, the cores have a predilection for type 1 fibres; however, fibre type uniformity is common, with most fibres staining as type 1 fibres. A few fibres may coexpress fast myosin, and there may be a few very small fibres with fetal myosin scattered through the biopsy (often referred to as 'pinpricks'; see Figure 25.53c). Some biopsies may show rods and cores, and occasionally rods may be an obvious feature.[214,299]

Cores are not specific for a *RYR1* mutation and can also occur following tenotomy or with neurogenic atrophy, where they are target-like (see Figure 25.56), and in association with several other gene defects, including mutations in the *ACTA1, MYH7, TTN, CFL2, KBTBD13* genes.[60,130,215,217,221,318,400,443,489] Cores can also coexist with rods and be associated with *RYR1, NEB, CFL2* or *KBTBD13* mutations.[300,366]

Internal nuclei had not been considered a feature of central core disease in early studies, but it is now appreciated that they can be an important indicator of *RYR1* mutations (Figure 25.84). In some cases internal nuclei

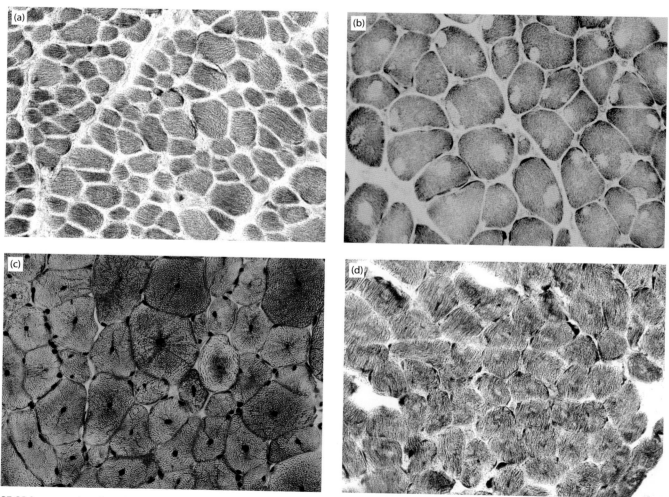

25.83 Images showing the variability of oxidative enzyme staining that can be seen in association with mutations in the RYR1 gene. In **(a)** no cores are visible but in **(b)** there are typical large cores; in **(c)** there are multiple large cores; and in **(d)** minicores and uneven staining. Note in all fibre type uniformity and absence of fibre type differentiation. (a, b, d), NADH-TR; (c), cytochrome c oxidase.

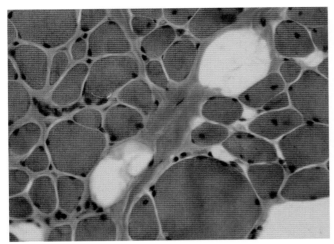

25.84 Internal nuclei and excess connective tissue and fat in a case of RYR1 core myopathy. Note also the wide variation in fibre size. H&E.

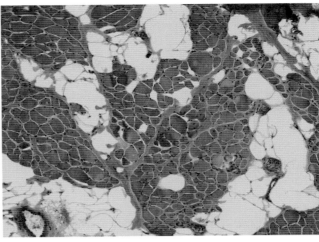

25.85 Low power view showing the pronounced adipose tissue in the same case as in Figure 25.84. H&E.

may be numerous, and several may be in a central position, resembling centronuclear myopathy.[499] Similarly, an increase in connective tissue was not considered a feature of 'classic' central core disease, but it can occur, and occasionally there may be extensive adipose tissue (Figure 25.85). In such cases, the separation of fascicles by adipose tissue and fibrous tissue has caused diagnostic confusion with a muscular dystrophy. Some of these samples may show only subtle unevenness of oxidative enzyme stains, whereas others show large classic cores or multiple small cores.

Multicore Myopathy This is a relatively non-progressive congenital myopathy characterized by multifocal areas of degeneration in muscle fibres, which prompted the name 'multicore disease'. There have been various reports of this disorder encompassing a broad range of clinical phenotypes, but with similar histopathological features. The defining histopathology consists of multiple small areas that are devoid of oxidative enzymes, lack mitochondria and show focal disruption of the sarcomeric pattern (Figure 25.86). Core-like areas, however, can be associated with defects in several genes in addition to *RYR1* and *SEPN1*, including *ACTA1, MYH7, MYH2, CFL2, TTN, CCDC78* and *KBTBD13*, as well as in some forms of muscular dystrophy, some myasthenic conditions and in association with denervation.

Four clinical categories of patients with minicores have been identified, and their molecular defects are being defined.[138] The most common phenotype shows marked axial weakness, with spinal rigidity, scoliosis, torticollis and respiratory involvement that are often disproportionate to the overall muscle weakness. This phenotype is similar to RSMD1, and the two disorders are now often considered allelic because both are caused by recessive mutations in the gene for selenoprotein N1 (*SEPN1*). The pathological spectrum associated with *SEPN1* mutations also includes cases with Mallory bodies.[137]

A second clinical group with multiple minicores and similar proximal and axial weakness also shows a variable association with external ophthalmoplegia. These cases have mutations in the *RYR1* gene.[213,298] Minicores and

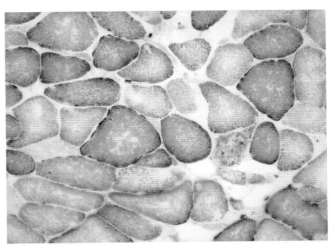

25.86 Multiple minicores in a case with 'minicore myopathy' caused by mutations in the *SEPN1* gene. Note also the two-fibre pattern and uneven staining in both fibre types. Cytochrome *c* oxidase.

opththlamoplegia are also features associated with mutations in the *MYH2* gene encoding myosin IIA (see later). *RYR1* mutations have also been found in a third phenotypic group with similarities to patients with central core disease.[298] The fourth group comprises rare patients with antenatal onset, generalized arthrogryposis, dysmorphic features and mild to moderate reduction of respiratory function. Primary cardiac dysfunction is not a feature of any of these groups. The multicore cases associated with *RYR1* mutations can be considered part of a clinicopathological spectrum of 'core myopathies', and the term 'multi-minicore' disease can then be reserved for cases with *SEPN1* mutations.

The presence of minicores or the absence of typical central cores can make it difficult to distinguish between *SEPN1* and *RYR1* cases. Pathological features that can help are the preservation of a two-fibre type pattern and the presence of minicores in both fibre types in *SEPN1* cases, versus the type 1 uniformity that is common in *RYR1* cases.

Internal nuclei may be occasional, or sometimes profuse, in *SEPN1* cases. Rods are not a feature of *SEPN1* cases, although there have been several reported cases of minicores in association with an abundance of additional structural defects, including rods and whorled fibres. Some of these cases have been shown to result from mutations in the *RYR1* gene or the *ACTA1* gene, but many of the early cases are still molecularly unresolved.[117,217,400]

Myotubular and Centronuclear Myopathies

Early descriptions of muscle biopsies with abundant central nuclei led to the introduction of the terms 'myotubular myopathy', because central nuclei are a feature of fetal myotubes, and 'centronuclear myopathy'.[412,423] The clinical and pathological features described in these early papers would probably be interpreted differently in the light of more recent advances. The term 'myotubular myopathy' is now often reserved for the X-linked disorder caused by mutations in the myotubularin gene (*MTM1*), and the term 'centronuclear myopathy' for the molecularly heterogeneous group of autosomal disorders characterized by central nuclei.[365]

X-Linked Myotubular Myopathy X-linked myotubular myopathy, caused by mutations in the *MTM1* gene on chromosome Xq28 encoding myotubularin, is a severe condition with onset *in utero*. Pregnancy is complicated by polyhydramnios, and there is often a history of miscarriages and neonatal death in the maternal line. Features include marked neonatal hypotonia, a variable degree of external ophthalmoplegia, feeding difficulties and respiratory failure at birth, which is often fatal. Some affected infants may survive if the respiratory problems in the neonatal period can be managed.[273] Female carriers may manifest with a variable degree of muscle weakness that ranges from mild to severe, usually depending on the pattern of X chromosome inactivation; hypotonia from birth and the inability to stand or to walk in a female carrier has also been reported.[216,446]

Myotubularin is expressed in most tissues. It is a dual-specificity phosphatase that dephosphorylates phosphatidylinositol 3-phosphate and phosphatidylinositol (3,5)-bisphosphate.[242] Its exact function is unclear, but evidence suggests a role in triad formation.[3,196] Preliminary studies indicated that myotubularin was localized to nuclei, but later studies showed that it is essentially cytoplasmic.[196] Antibodies to myotubularin fail to detect endogenous protein in muscle sections, but alterations in its levels have been studied by immunoprecipitation.[457] A large number of different mutations, distributed throughout the gene, have been identified, which may be missense, nonsense or splice site mutations, point mutations, small or large deletions, or insertions.

The *MTM1* gene is part of a family with several members that share sequence homology. These genes are clearly candidates for other neuromuscular disorders, and the genes for myotubularin-related protein 2 and myotubularin-related protein 13/SBF2 are mutated in forms of Charcot–Marie–Tooth neuropathy and myotubularin-related protein 14 (hJUMPY) in rare cases of autosomal centronuclear myopathy, the latter being thought to be a gene modifier.[304,456]

The characteristic pathological feature of cases with *MTM1* mutations is centrally placed nuclei that occupy a large volume of the fibre (Figure 25.87a), and are present in both fibre types. In longitudinal section, these are spaced regularly down the fibre, not in chains as in regenerating fibres (Figure 25.87b); thus, the plane of transverse section influences the number of observed central nuclei. The number of fibres with central nuclei can vary between muscles and may not be numerous at birth.[191,382] The area around the central nuclei is often devoid of myofibrils and appears as holes with ATPase staining or myosin immunolabelling. With oxidative enzyme and PAS stains, the central area is stained darkly, reflecting aggregation of mitochondria and glycogen, and there may also be pale subsarcolemmal halos around many fibres (Figure 25.88). As in many congenital myopathies, type 1 fibres may be predominant, and most fibres are small in diameter (hypotrophic and/or atrophic), particularly type 1 fibres.

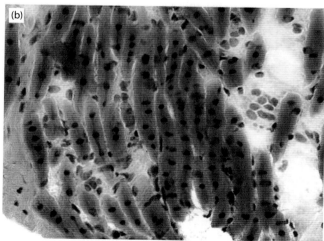

25.87 Central nuclei in a case of X-linked myotubular myopathy in (a) transverse and (b) longitudinal section. Note in transverse section not all fibres show a central nucleus that probably relates to the spacing of the nuclei down the fibre as seen in (b). The basophilic central granularity relates to accumulation of mitochondria. H&E.

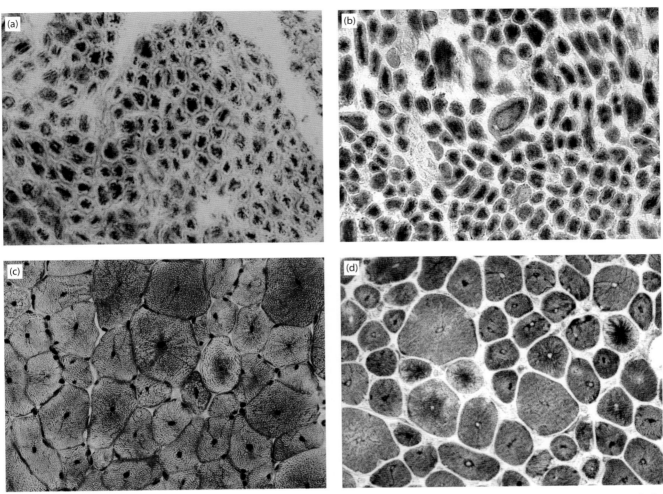

25.88 (a) NADH-TR activity concentrated in the centre of the fibres and pale peripheral halos in a case of X-linked myotubular myopathy. Note also the lack of differentiation into fibre types. **(b)** Cytochrome *c* oxidase shows similar features but one larger fibre has a loop of higher activity, as seen in necklace fibres. **(c, d)** Radial strands in an autosomal case of centronuclear myopathy with a *DNM2* mutation. (c), PAS; (d), NADH-TR.

An unusual pathological feature seen in some *MTM1* carriers and also some neonatal cases is 'necklace fibres', noted by Romero and colleagues.[28,190] A milder adult male case was also reported to show them. Necklace fibres have a basophilic loop internally within the fibre and near the sarcolemma. This loop is associated with internal nuclei, increased oxidative enzyme activity and PAS staining, and shows increased desmin, αB-crystallin and SERCA immunolabelling (Figure 25.88b). It is not yet clear if necklace fibres are specific to *MTM1* mutations, as fibres with a similar appearance but lacking the nuclei on the loop have been observed in centronuclear cases with *DNM2* mutations[250] (see later), and in one case with a *RYR1* mutation (personal observation).

The presence of abundant desmin and vimentin has been put forward as evidence of a developmental defect,[379] but it is not a feature of all fibres with central nuclei. The immunolabelling of myosin isoforms shows that fibres with central nuclei have the fast or slow isoform of mature muscle, without fetal myosin, indicating that maturation, at least with regard to myosin isoforms, does occur in myotubular myopathy.[401] Expression of NCAM, utrophin and laminin α5 has also been reported in myotubular myopathy cases.[191]

A similar pathological appearance, with abundant central nuclei, is seen in cases of congenital myotonic dystrophy, and an expansion of the *DM1* gene should always be considered in neonates with the pathological picture of myotubular myopathy (see Myotonic Dystrophies, p. 1578).

Autosomal Centronuclear Myopathies

Several cases of centronuclear myopathy not linked to Xp28 have been identified, some of which have treatable myasthenic-like symptoms.[27,361] Some are familial whereas others are sporadic. They are molecularly and clinically heterogeneous. Inheritance may be recessive or dominant and some causative genes have been identified (see Table 25.17). Mutations in the gene encoding dynamin 2 on chromosome 19q13.2 and *BIN1* encoding amphiphysin 2 are now both recognized as autosomal causes of centronuclear myopathy.[119,458] Screening of the human sequence databases has also implicated the *MTMR14* gene[456] and it is reported to have a modifying role in autophagy.[476] In addition, next-generation sequencing has identified a family with a dominant mutation in the gene encoding the coiled-coil domain-containing protein 78 (*CCDC78*), a protein enriched in the perinuclear region and triads.[261] Biopsies from this family not only showed central nuclei but also core-like lesions.

Dynamin 2 is involved in membrane remodelling, endocytosis and membrane trafficking, actin assembly and centrosome cohesion and it interacts with amphiphysin 2.[119,452] Onset in cases with mutations is usually in adolescence or adulthood, but neonatal onset has also been identified.[29,183] The condition is characterized by slowly progressive muscle weakness. Distal involvement precedes involvement of the limb girdles, trunk and neck muscles. Loss of ambulation is rare. Bilateral ptosis is almost invariable, and involvement of extraocular muscles is common. Peripheral axonal neuropathy is present in some patients, and it is notable that *DMN2* mutations are also responsible for dominant Charcot–Marie–Tooth disease type 2B.[512] The mutations responsible for centronuclear myopathy are missense changes in the central domain of the gene, whereas mutations that cause Charcot–Marie–Tooth disease type 2B are restricted to the pleckstrin homology domain.

Muscle imaging shows a pattern distinct from other neuromuscular disorders, which may help to direct molecular analysis. It is characterized predominantly by involvement of lower leg muscles, with mild involvement of the posterior thigh and gluteus maximus.[142,438]

Muscle biopsies in *DMN2* cases show central nuclei surrounded by a zone devoid of organelles, type 1 fibre hypotrophy and predominance, and oxidative enzyme and PAS stains that exhibit a spoke-like pattern radiating from the centre of the fibre (Figure 25.88c,d). It is not clear whether this is a specific feature associated with *DNM2* mutations. Radial strands were less common in the three rare cases identified with *BIN1* mutations, and electron microscopy suggests the central nuclei form chains rather than being spaced, a feature that may also be seen in *DNM2*-related cases.[458] Cases with *BIN1* mutations have shown subsarcolemmal vacuolation, and triad morphology is abnormal in *MTM1*, *DNM2* and *BIN1* related centronuclear myopathies, suggesting a common pathogenic link.[458]

The presence of cores together with central nuclei suggested a relationship with *RYR1* mutation cases and several cases with central nuclei and *RYR1* mutations have now been identified.[217,499] There are apparent founder *RYR1* mutations in the South African population.[499]

An early onset disorder, in which internal and some central nuclei are a pronounced feature, is caused by homozygous mutations in the C-terminal kinase domain in the gene encoding titin (*TTN*).[60] In addition to hypotonia and proximal and distal weakness, spinal rigidity, contractures and dilated cardiomyopathy develop. The pathological features seen in muscle biopsies include multiple internal nuclei, type 1 fibre uniformity, cores of varying size devoid of oxidative enzyme staining, and sometimes internal basophilia in occasional fibres. Immunohistochemistry shows an absence of titin only with an antibody specific to the M-line C-terminal domain and immunoblots show a secondary absence of calpain-3.

Congenital Fibre Type Disproportion

There has been a longstanding debate as to whether the presence of small type 1 fibres in the absence of other pathology (congenital fibre type disproportion [CFDP]) represents a distinct disease entity. Defects in *ACTA1*, *SEPN1*, *TPM2*, *TPM3*, *RYR1* and *MYH7* genes can all result in fibre type disproportion without any other pathological defect.[82,84,85] It is not known if the typical pathological features, such as rods or cores, associated with these genes might develop at a later age in the cases reported, because repeat muscle biopsies at a later age have not been reported. Type 1 hypotrophy has also been reported in some patients with congenital myasthenia, but these were not molecularly confirmed and myasthenic symptoms can occur in association with defects in several genes.[176] Further genetic heterogeneity associated with fibre type disproportion is likely. The *HACD1* gene is also associated with CFDP in humans and with central nuclei in dogs.

Other Early Onset Myopathies with Structural Defects

A number of other structural features are associated with early onset disorders resembling congenital myopathies, the molecular causes of which are now known. Cap-like structures of focal peripheral disorganized myofibrils are associated with defects in the *TPM2*, *TPM3* and *ACTA1* genes, all of which are also associated with other pathological features, such as nemaline rods. The caps lack, or show reduced, staining for NADH-TR and ATPase (in contrast to 'hyaline bodies' in myosin storage myopathy - see later) and reduced immunoreactivity for myosin but high reactivity for many sarcomeric proteins including actin, nebulin, tropomyosin, troponin T and desmin.

Some disorders were classified as congenital myopathies before identification of the defective gene, but they have now been reclassified as part of the clinicopathological spectrum of other disorders. For example, spheroid body myopathy is caused by defects in the gene encoding myotilin (*MYOT*) and is considered to be a variant of a myofibrillar myopathy (see later). Reducing body myopathy is a particularly severe progressive disorder with onset that is not always congenital; it is discussed later with other conditions caused by defects in the *FHL1* gene. 'Hyaline bodies' were described as a feature of a congenital myopathy and represent accumulation of slow myosin, caused by defects in the gene encoding slow myosin (*MYH7*). Disorders of *MYH7* are discussed further later (see Myopathies Caused by Defects in Sarcomeric Proteins).

A number of other cases have been reported with unusual ultrastructural features that include cylindrical spirals, fingerprint bodies, hexagonal arrays. It is not yet clear if these are all genetic entities.[160]

Congenital Myopathies Characterized by Distal Involvement and/or Distal Arthrogryposis

Distal arthrogryposis is a symptom of several disorders and several clinical forms with varying severity have been described. Distal arthrogryposis type 1, 2A and 2B have been associated with mutations in different sarcomeric proteins including β-tropomyosin (*TPM2*),[435,440] fast troponin T (*TNNT3*),[436] fast troponin I (*TNNI2*),[226] embryonic myosin heavy chain (*MYH3*),[441,460] perinatal (fetal) myosin heavy chain (*MYH8*)[459] and myosin-binding protein-C, slow type (*MYBPC1*).[177] Other forms have recently been shown to be associated with the *ECEL1* gene.[110,274]

Histopathological studies are limited, because the number of molecularly confirmed cases is small and the pathological spectra not known. The changes observed are non-specific and include small type 1 fibres in some cases with *MYH3* or *ECEL1* mutations, and small type 2 fibres cases with *TNNI2* mutations. Central basophilia has been observed in the rare cases with mutations in the slow myosin-binding protein-C.[177]

Myopathies Caused By Defects in Sarcomeric Proteins

Defects in several myofibrillar proteins of the skeletal muscle sarcomere are associated with neuromuscular disorders. Aggregation of proteins (e.g. actin, myosin, desmin) is a feature of some of these.[161,162,393] Components of the thin filaments (actin, tropomyosins, nebulin) and associated proteins are involved in nemaline myopathies (see Congenital Myopathies and Allied Disorders, p. 1580). Defects in telethonin cause a form of LGMD (see Recessive Limb-Girdle Muscular Dystrophies, p. 1561). In this section we discuss myopathies caused by defects in myosins and titin (see also Congenital Myopathies and Allied Disorders, p. 1580, and Limb-Girdle Dystrophies, p. 1561) and proteins of the Z-line that are associated with a group of disorders commonly referred to as myofibrillar myopathies. FHL1 is often also included within this group as it is a myofibrillar protein and some cases have similar pathological features to myofibrillar myopathies, although there is a broad spectrum associated with FHL1 (see Table 25.18).

Myopathies Associated with Mutations in Genes Encoding Myosin Heavy Chains

Myosins are a family of highly conserved proteins that exist is several isomeric forms encoded by different genes. The isoforms expressed in skeletal muscle currently associated with a myopathy are (i) slow myosin, expressed in type 1 fibres (and in the heart) encoded by the *MYH7* gene; (ii) myosin IIa expressed in fast 2A skeletal muscle fibres encoded by the *MYH2* gene; and (iii) embryonic and perinatal myosin expressed in developing muscle and in regenerating fibres encoded by the *MYH3* and *MYH8* genes, respectively.[439] Defects in *MYH3*, *MYH8* and *MYBPC1* are associated with syndromes characterized by distal arthrogryposis (see Congenital Myopathies and Allied Disorders, p. 1580).

The *MYH7* gene encoding slow/β-cardiac myosin is associated with either a cardiomyopathy or skeletal myopathy, or sometimes both.[162] Age of onset varies from childhood to middle age. Weakness may be predominantly distal, as in Laing early onset distal myopathy with a characteristic 'hanging big toe', or scapuloperoneal or of a limb-girdle distribution. Talipes, hip dislocation and knee flexion contractures can be present in the most severe cases. Some cases show subsarcolemmal aggregates of slow myosin in type 1 fibres. These were previously referred to as hyaline bodies ('hyaline body myopathy'), but with the identification of slow myosin within them caused by mutations in the *MYH7* gene the disorder is now referred to as 'myosin storage myopathy'. The areas of myosin aggregation

are pale pink with H&E and pale green with Gomori trichrome staining and are unstained (except at the periphery) with stains for oxidative enzymes and desmin but positive for ATPase, in contrast to caps (see Congenital Myopathies and Allied Disorders, p. 1580; Figure 25.89). With electron microscopy the accumulated material has a granular and slightly filamentous appearance.[117]

Myosin storage is not seen in other cases with *MYH7* mutations or in cases with Laing myopathy. Muscle pathology in these can include small type 1 fibres (sometimes resembling fibre type disproportion), predominance of type 1 or type 2 fibres, occasional necrotic and regenerating fibres, mild fibrosis, increased internal nuclei, core-like areas, lobulated fibres, rimmed vacuoles, tubulofilamentous inclusions and ring fibres.[117,439]

Both dominant and recessive mutations in *MYH2* can cause a myopathy. The dominant form was identified in a large Swedish family with congenital joint contractures but no hypotonia. Weakness is predominantly proximal with atrophy of the quadriceps femoris muscle, which may affect ambulation. In the recessive form, muscle weakness is mild to moderate and muscle MRI shows a distinctive pattern with predominant involvement of the medial gastrocnemius. Ophthalmoplegia is a feature of both forms. Histopathology in dominantly inherited cases shows mild changes in young cases with focal core-like areas in type 2A fibres, which are reduced in number and size. In adult cases pathological features are more pronounced and rimmed vacuoles containing p62 are present. Recessively inherited cases show an absence of 2A fibres and non-specific myopathic changes. Some cases may show fibre type uniformity and lobulated fibres. In contrast to dominant cases rimmed vacuoles or protein aggregation are absent.[439]

Disorders Associated with Defects in Titin

Titin is a giant protein that stretches from the M-line to the Z-line. Defects in only some domains have been identified, but next-generation sequencing is increasing the number of mutations detected. The phenotype of some is defined as a limb-girdle dystrophy (see Limb-Girdle Muscular

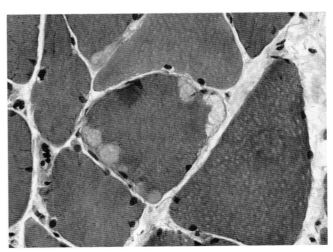

25.89 Pale-stained areas ('hyaline bodies') corresponding to accumulation of slow myosin in a case with a mutation in the *MYH7* gene. H&E.

TABLE 25.18 Features of myopathies caused by defects in sarcomeric proteins

Popular name	Locus	Gene symbol	Protein	Inheritance	Cardiac involvement	Peripheral neuropathy	Other features
Desminopathy	2q35	DES	Desmin	AD(rare AR)	Yes	Yes	
αB-crystallinopathy	11q-25.3	CRYAB	αB-crystallin	AD	Yes	Possibly	Cataracts
Myotilinopathy	5q31	MYOT (TTID)	Myotilin	AD	Yes	Yes	
Zaspopathy	10q25.3	LDB3	ZASP	AD	Yes	Yes	
Filaminopathy	7q32.1	FLNC	Filamin C	AD	Yes	Yes	
Bag3opathy	10q25	BAG3	Bag3	AD	Yes	Yes; severe axonal neuropathy	Early onset; severe progression
FHL1opathy	Xq26.3	FHL1	Fhl1	XD	Yes	Not reported	Broad phenotype; childhood onset cases with severe progression
	17p13	MYH3	Myosin heavy chain 3	AD	–	–	Arthrogryposis
	17p13	MYH8	Perinatal myosin	AD	–	–	Arthrogryposis
	12q 23.2	MYBPC1	Myosin-binding protein-C, slow type	AD	–	–	Arthrogryposis
Myosin storage myopathy and Laing distal myopathy	14q11	MHY7	Slow myosin heavy chain	AD	No	Not reported	Occasional arrthyhmias
Inclusion body myopathy	17p13	MYHC2A	Fast myosin heavy chain IIA	AD, AR	Not reported	Not reported	Ophthalmoplegia
Distal myopathy and HMERF	2q321	TTN	Titin	AD	Not reported*	Not reported	

AD, autosomal dominant; AR, autosomal recessive; Bag3, Bcl-2-associated athanogene 3; FHL1, four and a half LIM domains protein 1; HMERF, hereditary myopathy with early respiratory failure; XD, X-linked dominant; ZASP, Z-line alternatively spliced PDZ protein.

*See Limb-Girdle Muscular Dystrophies and Congenital Myopathies and Allied Disorders for recessive conditions of titin.

Dystrophies, p. 1558), whereas others have a more distal phenotype and a severe neonatal form with cardiomyopathy has been reported (see Congenital Myopathies and Allied Disorders, p. 1580).[60,466,467]

Muscle pathology in titin distal myopathy shows features of a muscular dystrophy with variation in fibre size, fibrosis, adipose tissue and internal nuclei, but necrotic fibres are rare.[181] Rimmed vacuoles are seen in the tibial muscles, which may show accumulation of ubiquitin, but the other proteins and Congo red seen in myofibrillar myopathies (see later) are not present. Immunohistochemistry using exon-specific antibodies to the C-terminal M-line M8/M9 region shows an absence of titin, but titin is detected with antibodies to other domains.[181] Titin has a binding site for calpain-3 and immunoblots show a secondary reduction of calpain.

Mutations in the A-band domain of titin are responsible for HMERF.[322,335] Presentation is from early adulthood and respiratory complications are common. Muscle MRI shows a characteristic severe involvement of the proximal parts of the thighs and the anterior and lateral compartments of the lower limbs. Muscle biopsies in HMERF show variability in muscle fibre size with atrophic and hypertrophic fibres, many fibres with numerous internal nuclei and focal areas with frequent split fibres. Eosinophilic inclusions or deposits are a typical feature but not present in all biopsies. These inclusions are reddish or dark green with Gomori trichrome staining and some of them have the appearance of cytoplasmic bodies. The cytoplasmic body-like inclusions stain positively for filamentous actin using fluorescent-labelled phalloidin. Rimmed vacuoles are usually present, and staining for oxidative enzymes shows unstained, 'rubbed-out' regions. Immunohistochemistry can show sarcolemmal NCAM and accumulation of various proteins including desmin, dystrophin, titin, myotilin and αB- crystallin.[117]

Z-Line Associated Proteins and Four-and-a-Half LIM Domain 1 (FHL1)

Disorders with various unusual inclusions have been reported, including spheroid bodies,[164] sarcoplasmic bodies,[122] cytoplasmic bodies[165] and granulofilamentous material.[132] Molecularly they are heterogeneous, but several of them share histopathological features, in particular the accumulation of proteins such as desmin. This led to the use of the terms 'desminopathies' and 'desmin-related myopathies'. Accumulation of several proteins that also occurs in IBM is seen, and the terms 'hereditary inclusion body myopathy' and 'protein surplus myopathies' have been suggested. As the molecular basis of these disorders is gradually unravelled, the term 'myofibrillar myopathies' has been adopted for those caused by or associated with defects in Z-line proteins.[403] We also include here disorders caused by abnormalities in the *FHL1* gene as some cases can have similar pathological features. Plectin is included by some authors, but these cases do not always show rimmed vacuoles, in contrast to myofibrillar myopathies. Mutations in *PLEC* cause a form of LGMD and muscular dystrophy with epidermolysis bullosa, some with a neuromuscular junction transmission defects (see Recessive Limb-Girdle Muscular Dystrophies, p. 1561; and Myasthenic Syndromes, p. 1596).

Many cases of myofibrillar myopathy are sporadic, but inheritance in most (where it can be determined) is autosomal dominant, although rare recessive mutations in the desmin and αB-crystallin genes have also been identified. Disorders associated with *FHL1* are X-linked, dominantly inherited.[146,339,393,395] Defects have been found in the genes encoding, desmin, αB-crystallin, myotilin, filamin C, ZASP, Bag3 and FHL1 (Table 25.18, Box 22.9).[395] There is further heterogeneity because no causative gene mutations have been detected in several patients with the clinicopathological phenotype of a myofibrillar myopathy. Proteins that interact with Z-line proteins or play a role in maintaining myofibrillar integrity are likely candidates.

The age at onset in myofibrillar myopathies can be in childhood, adolescence or adulthood; many occur in adulthood.[393] Although there is a spectrum of presentation many cases are of adult onset, often late (beyond the fourth decade), particularly in cases with ZASP, myotilin or filamin C defects. Cases with defects associated with the desmin gene tend to present earlier than those with ZASP, myotilin or filamin C defects. Cases with defects in FHL1, Bag3 and αB-crystallin can manifest in childhood.[393,395] Muscle weakness is slowly progressive but may be rapid in early onset cases, particularly those with FHL1 or BAG3 defects who can show a severe, rapid progression. Weakness may be proximal or, more frequently, distal or both, or scapuloperoneal, and may be asymmetrical in some cases with FHL1 defects. Muscle weakness may be accompanied by muscle wasting, stiffness or aching, cramps and sensory symptoms. Facial weakness is uncommon, but dysarthria and swallowing difficulties may occur in some older patients. Wasting of hand muscles occurs in cases with mutations in the

---

BOX 25.9. Defective proteins that cause a myofibrillar myopathy

Desmin is a highly conserved intermediate filament of skeletal, cardiac and smooth muscle. It localizes to the extramyofibrillar space around the Z-line where it forms a peripheral lattice with plectin and links the myofibrils to the nuclei, mitochondria and sarcolemma. Plectin binds to β-dystroglycan, dystrophin and utrophin, and alternative splicing of plectin transcripts gives rise to eight protein isoforms, of which four are highly expressed in muscle (1, 1b, 1d and 1f). Mutations affecting the 1f isoform have been found in a recessively inherited form of limb-girdle muscular dystrophy. Desmin filaments are 10 nm in diameter, intermediate between actin and microtubules, although originally said to be intermediate between actin and myosin. Identified mutations sometimes impair assembly of desmin filaments.

αB-Crystallin is a cytoplasmic small heat-shock protein with a chaperone role in protecting the intermediate filament network from stress-induced damage. Two α-crystallin forms (A and B), encoded by different genes, have been identified; both are abundant in the lens, where they are thought to have a role in preventing the formation of cataracts.

Myotilin is a Z-line-associated protein strongly expressed in skeletal muscle but more weakly in cardiac muscle. It binds to α-actinin and filamin C. It also binds actin and plays a role in myofibrillogenesis. Most identified mutations in the *MYOT* gene occur in the serine-rich N-terminal domain of exon 2. The antibody commonly used and marketed by Leica shows a fibre typing effect, the reason for which is not known.

ZASP is a protein of the Z-line that is predominantly expressed in skeletal and cardiac muscle. There are various splice site isoforms, three of which are expressed in skeletal muscle. All isoforms have a N-terminal PDZ domain important for protein-protein interactions, and a domain important for interaction with α-actinin.

Filamin C is part of a family of proteins and its expression is restricted to skeletal and cardiac muscle. It cross-links and stabilizes actin, and binds to several Z-line proteins, and to γ- and α-sarcoglycan at the sarcolemma. Patients with mutations in the actin-binding domain have a distal phenotype but do not show the typical muscle pathology of myofibrillar myopathies.

Bcl-2 associated athangene 3 (Bag3) is a co-chaperone protein and is also part of a family of proteins. It is highly expressed in skeletal and cardiac muscle but is also present at low levels in other tissues. It participates in the degradation of misfolded or aggregated proteins by complexing with heat-shock proteins. It has a role not only in muscle but also in neural tissues and tumour cells and various cellular activities. It also has a role in apoptosis, consistent with the finding of apoptotic nuclei in cases with a mutation.

Four and a half LIM domains protein 1 (FHL1) is another protein that is part of a family of proteins. Its function is not fully known but it is believed to participate in cell growth, differentiation, sarcomeric assembly and to be a regulator of muscle mass. It has three isoforms and mutations affecting all isoforms result in a more severe phenotype. The severity of the phenotype and presence of reducing bodies in a biopsy correlates with the domain that the mutation affects, with mutations in the LIM domain 2 being associated with the severe phenotype and the presence of reducing bodies in most cases.

---

actin-binding domain of filamin C, but the cases reported do not show the typical pathology of myofibrillar myopathies, in particular they have no vacuoles.[118] Peripheral neuropathy is present in a significant proportion of patients, particularly in cases with *BAG3* mutations, some of which show myotonic discharges. Cardiac involvement is common (arrhythmia, or dilated or hypertrophic cardiomyopathy), particularly in those cases with a mutation in the gene encoding desmin, when it may precede or coincide with skeletal muscle weakness; it is also a feature of *BAG3* cases with childhood onset. Cardiac involvement occurs in cases with mutations affecting filamin C and FHL1, but is rarer in those with defects in myotilin. Respiratory failure is present in several cases of myofibrillar myopathies, especially those that present early. Cataracts are associated with mutations in the αB-crystallin gene, but may not be present in childhood cases.[173] Scapular winging is common and other clinical features include rigid spine, scoliosis and contractures.[393] The pattern of contractures, muscle weakness and cardiac involvement in some patients with mutations in the *FHL1* gene has been assigned to a form of Emery–Dreifuss muscular dystrophy,[173,232] but the clinical and pathological features in these cases are similar to cases of myofibrillar myopathy with scapuloperoneal weakness. These cases could therefore be considered as part of the spectrum associated with mutations in *FHL1* rather than as a form of Emery–Dreifuss muscular dystrophy, which has defects in nuclear membrane proteins.[385] Serum CK is usually normal or mildly elevated, but may be more elevated in Bag3 or some myotilin-related cases. Muscle MRI can also be helpful in differential diagnosis.[143]

Mutations in the myotilin gene were first associated with a dominant form of limb-girdle muscular dystrophy, LGMD1A, but it is now appreciated that there is a spectrum of phenotypes associated with the gene defect and that this is an allelic disorder to that now known as a myofibrillar myopathy.[34] Mutations in the genes encoding myotilin and filamin C are also associated with the presence of spheroid bodies.[144,256] There are two founder mutations in ZASP, and mutations have been shown to be responsible for the late-onset distal myopathy described by Markesbery *et al.* in 1974.[171] Mutations in the actin-binding domain of filamin C cause a distal myopathy, but the pathology is not that typically observed in a myofibrillar myopathy and rimmed vacuoles are not a feature.

In addition to non-specific pathological features, such as muscle fibre atrophy and hypertrophy, fibre splitting and excess endomysial connective tissues, abundant internal nuclei and eosinophilic regions that are stained more darkly than surrounding myofibrils with the Gomori trichrome stain are characteristic (see Figure 25.41b). Some inclusions may be stained red with Gomori trichrome and are cytoplasmic bodies, spheroid bodies or reducing bodies. Reducing bodies can be distinguished from cytoplasmic bodies using the menadione NBT method without substrate, which stains reducing bodies and accompanying accumulated protein darkly (Figure 25.90). Reducing bodies are usually only seen in cases with a *FHL1* mutation in the LIM domain 2 region, most of which are the severe childhood onset cases, but some myofibrillar material may also appear darkly stained with menadione NBT or show pale staining in other cases of myofibrillar myopathy (see Figure 25.90). Female carriers with *FHL1* mutations in this domain may also show reducing bodies but are often clinically milder, possibly with X-inactivation having a role. Reducing bodies are not a feature of milder cases with mutations in other domains, although rare exceptions have been reported.[135] The pathology in *FHL1*-related cases can be focal. The dark areas with the Gomori trichrome stain represent disrupted myofibrillar material and lack staining for oxidative enzymes, contributing to a 'wiped-out' or 'rubbed-out' appearance (see Figure 25.42). Some dark areas are also congophilic, but they are not metachromatic with the crystal violet stain, in contrast to amyloid deposits in inclusion body myositis. The Congo red stain is best viewed under fluorescence, using an excitation filter in the red range, as for rhodamine or Texas red. Rimmed and unrimmed vacuoles are a feature of myofibrillar myopathies but are not apparent in all cases. A few inflammatory cells may be present, but inflammation is not usually pronounced; necrosis and regeneration may occur, but are not usually extensive.

Fibre type grouping and groups of atrophic fibres of both types may be present, consistent with a peripheral neuropathy, and nerves may show loss of myelin and increased fibrosis. Neurogenic features can be particularly apparent in *BAG3*-related cases. A predominance of type 1 fibres may occur in some cases.

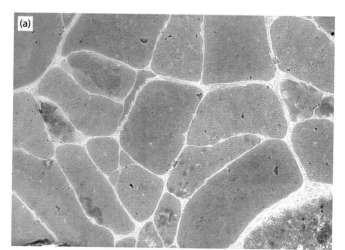 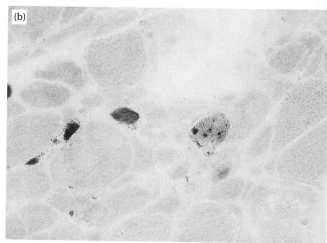

25.90 Menadione NBT staining without substrate in (a) a case of myofibrillar myopathy with a mutation in the MYOT gene and (b) a case with a mutation in the *FHL1* gene. Note the weak staining associated with the accumulated myofibrillar material in (a) and strong staining of whole fibres and focal staining corresponding to reducing bodies in (b).

Abnormal fibres demonstrate the accumulation of several proteins including desmin, αB-crystallin, syncoilin, ubiquitin, myotilin, filamin C, caveolin-3, dystrophin, β-amyloid precursor protein, Xin, filamentous actin, gelsolin, heat-shock proteins, NCAM, phosphorylated Tau, TDP43, p62 and prion protein (see Figure 25.54). Accumulation of FHL1 may also be seen. Several of these proteins are also seen in sporadic inclusion body myositis, hereditary forms of 'inclusion body myopathy' caused by defects in the *GNE* gene (UDP-N-acetylglucosamine 2-epimerase/N-acetylmannosamine kinase) and the VCP-related and other distal myopathies with rimmed vacuoles, which can cause diagnostic difficulties. For diagnosis it is rarely necessary to study a large panel of antibodies (see later).

Electron microscopy reveals various degrees of myofibrillar disruption, with Z-line streaming, accumulation of Z-line material, accumulation of granulofilamentous material (Figure 25.91) and inclusions of various types. Tubulofilamentous inclusions occur in myofibrillar as well as other myopathies with rimmed vacuoles. Cytoplasmic bodies with a halo of radiating filaments are common, as are myelin-like whorls and autophagic debris.[385,393,395]

It is rarely possible to predict the molecular defect of a myofibrillar myopathy from its histopathological features, but some features can help in the differential diagnosis from other myopathies with rimmed vacuoles (see later).

Distal Myopathies

Several disorders have predominant involvement of distal muscles and a recent paper by Udd shows a useful flow chart for diagnosis.[465] Some of these disorders have already been discussed within the spectra of conditions caused by various genes, such as nebulin (see Congenital Myopathies and Allied Disorders, p. 1580), anoctamin 5 and dysferlin (see Recessive Limb-Girdle Muscular Dystrophies, p. 1561), and titin, myosin and myofibrillar myopathies genes (see Myopathies Caused by Defects in Sarcomeric Proteins, p. 1589). In this section we discuss other disorders with distal involvement, in particular Welander myopathy, myopathy caused by mutations in the gene encoding UDP-N-acetylglucosamine-2 epimerase/N-acetylmannosamine kinase (*GNE*), myopathy caused by the gene encoding the VCP), and the rare distal myopathy with vocal cord and pharyngeal involvement (VCPDM) caused by mutations in the matrin 3 gene. Several of these are sometimes referred to as inherited inclusion body myopathies (h-IBM), because they have rimmed vacuoles and other pathological features that resembles that seen in sporadic forms of IBM (see Inflammatory Myopathies, p. 1605), but they usually lack inflammatory cells.

Welander myopathy maps to chromosome 2p13 and the defective gene has recently been shown to be the cytotoxic granule-associated RNA-binding protein, TIA1.[180] It is a late-onset disorder in which weakness initially affects the extensor muscles of the fingers and progresses to the lower legs and all muscles of the hand. Muscle biopsies show dystrophic-like features with variation in fibre size and fibrosis. Rimmed vacuoles and nuclear and cytoplasmic inclusions are a feature. Immunohistochemistry shows accumulation of several of the proteins seen in IBM, including p62 and TPD43, but inflammation is absent.

Included among 'hereditary inclusion body myopathies' is the myopathy known as 'quadriceps-sparing myopathy'. This is a slowly progressive disorder characterized by early weakness in the distal lower limb muscles that progresses to proximal weakness, but the quadriceps muscles remain relatively strong. Involvement of the upper limbs, and sometimes the distal arm and hand muscles, including the finger flexors (a feature of sporadic IBM), occurs in a few cases. Onset may be in late adolescence or more often in adulthood. It is the same disorder as Nonaka myopathy.[223] The condition is recessively inherited and a founder homozygous mutation, originally identified in the Persian Jewish population, is also present in other countries in the Middle East. This condition has also been described in other populations.[5,41]

The number of autophagic rimmed vacuoles is variable, but congophilia is reported to be absent, in contrast to myofibrillar myopathies.[41] Additional features include variation in fibre size, with fibre hypertrophy and scattered angular atrophic fibres, nuclear clumps, internal nuclei, necrosis and an increase in connective and adipose tissues. With electron microscopy, collections of cytoplasmic 15- to 21-nm tubulofilamentous structures are found, similar to those seen in sporadic IBM. The protein product of the *GNE* gene is a key enzyme involved in the synthesis of sialic acid. Reduced sialylation of NCAM has been shown on immunoblots, but it is not yet clear if this is the pathogenic mechanism in the disease. Studies of α-dystroglycan in a single study suggested a reduction in glycosylation, but this is not a consistent finding.[41]

A multisystem dominantly inherited disorder with distal involvement and rimmed vacuoles that also presents with Paget's disease and frontotemporal dementia is well recognized in some patients (e.g. inclusion body myopathy with early-onset Paget disease and frontotemporal dementia [IBMPFD]). It is caused by missense mutations of the gene encoding p97/VCP.[493] Immunolabelling of VCP and TDP-43 is useful and shows positive inclusions that can be sarcoplasmic and intranuclear in IBMPFD patients. The VCP inclusions can be present in vacuolated and non-vacuolated fibres and co-localize with ubiquitin.[493]

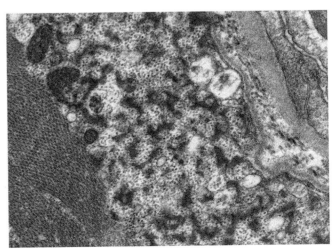

25.91 Electron micrograph of granulofilamentous material at the periphery of a fibre in a case with a mutation in the gene encoding desmin.

Rimmed vacuoles in association with distal weakness are also a feature in muscle biopsies from patients with a late-onset dominantly inherited distal myopathy with vocal cord and pharyngeal involvement (VCPDM). This was shown to be caused by defects in the gene encoding matrin 3 in the only two families described.[397] In addition, rimmed vacuoles are also seen in patients with either a dominant or recessively inherited disorder known as oculopharyngodistal myopathy that is molecularly distinct from oculopharyngeal muscular dystrophy (see section on Disorders with Deletions or Expansion of Repeat Sequence, p. 1577).[120,451]

Differential diagnosis in hereditary disorders with rimmed vacuoles and IBM is complicated by overlapping clinical and pathological features, but some pathological aspects can be useful in differential diagnosis. In myofibrillar myopathies 'rubbed-out' or 'wiped-out' fibres are reported to be a consistent feature of cases with mutations in the genes encoding desmin and αB-crystallin, whereas cases related to ZASP and myotilin are reported to show more vacuoles.[80] The large accumulations of proteins and the dark staining material seen with Gomori trichrome are features of myofibrillar myopathies not seen in IBM, and MHC-1 upregulation is less in myofibrillar myopathies compared with IBM. Inclusion body myositis and myofibrillar myopathies show congophilic amyloid deposits, but these are not a consistent feature of other myopathies with vacuoles; however, they have been observed in cases with mutations in VCP.[430] Electron microscopy studies have revealed subtle differences in relation to the genotypes of myofibrillar myopathies.[78] The granulofilamentous material is a feature of myofibrillar myopathies, but the tubulofilamentous inclusions can occur in several myopathies with vacuoles. As with all neuromuscular disorders, clinical correlations are essential and muscle MRI is having an increasing role.[143] The most useful panel of techniques for studying these disorders is H&E, Gomori trichrome, oxidative enzymes, Congo red, desmin, myotilin, αB-crystallin, dystrophin, TDP-43, VCP supplemented by menadione NBT and FHL1 (if reducing bodies are thought to be present) and electron microscopy. In HMERF, identification of F-actin with phalloidin in the cytoplasmic-like bodies can be useful.

Kelch proteins are a large family of proteins with various functions that include protein binding and transcriptional activation. A mutation in the gene encoding Kelch 9 was identified in a large family with an autosomal dominant distal myopathy. Onset was in childhood or early adulthood and muscle pathology showed atrophy and hypertrophy of fibres, increased internal nuclei, fat and connective tissue, and uniform fibre typing.[77] Mutations in Kelch 13 (*KBTBD13*) are associated with a rare form of autosomal dominant nemaline myopathy (see section on Congenital Myopathies and Allied Disorders, p. 1580). Next-generation sequencing is identifying other members of this large family that may be responsible for a neuromuscular disorder (see Nemaline Myopathies, p. 1580).

Ion Channel Disorders

Generation of action potentials and contraction of myofibrils require the movement of ions, in particular sodium, potassium, chloride and calcium ions, through channels in the sarcolemma, sarcoplasmic reticulum and T-tubules. Ion channels are complex multidomain transmembrane proteins, and numerous mutations in their genes, disrupting ion movement, have been identified (Table 25.19). These mutations result in disturbed excitability, in the form of either hyperexcitability (myotonia) or inexcitability (periodic paralysis); thus, these conditions are collectively referred to as 'ion channelopathies'. There is significant clinical overlap between the channelopathies, and defects in the same gene can give rise to different phenotypes (see Table 25.19) and fall into two main groups: those with myotonia or those with periodic paralysis.[218,350]

Defects in the calcium-release channel, the ryanodine receptor 1 of the sarcoplasmic reticulum, cause malignant hyperthermia and core myopathies, whereas Brody disease is caused by disturbances in a calcium pump of the sarcoplasmic reticulum. A number of channelopathies affecting specifically the heart or the CNS are also recognized, such as long QT syndrome and episodic ataxia, respectively.

The diagnosis of ion channelopathies is usually based on clinical assessment and detailed electrophysiological studies. Muscle biopsy does not often contribute to the process. Pathological features include variation in fibre size, increase in internal nuclei, and vacuoles or tubular aggregates (Figure 25.92). A genetic cause of tubular aggregate myopathy has recently been shown to be mutations in the calcium sensor stromal interaction molecule 1 (STIM1).[32] The vacuolation is thought to appear in a sequence that starts with focal proliferation and dilation of the sarcoplasmic reticulum and T-tubules and ends with large membrane-bound vacuoles. The dilated sarcoplasmic reticulum may contain amorphous granular material, cell debris and myelin-like whorls and stain for NADH-TR and acid phosphatase. Immunolabelling shows the presence of dystrophin and β-spectrin, but not laminin. Glycogen deposits, focal reduction of mitochondria, myofibrillar disruption and Z-line streaming have also been reported.[117]

Tubular aggregates are derived from the sarcoplasmic reticulum or endoplasmic reticulum exit sites and are often restricted to type 2 fibres.[72,386] They stain red with Gomori trichrome, are basophilic with H&E, and show reactivity for NADH-TR, myoadenylate deaminase, non-specific esterase and phosphofructokinase, but not SDH or ATPase activity (see Figure 25.92). Immunohistochemistry shows several proteins associated with them, including SERCAs, heat-shock proteins, triadin, calsequestrin, dysferlin and emerin (in one case) but not mitochondrial proteins.[72] With the electron microscope, the aggregates appear as a honeycomb of tubules, and different types have been observed.[117] Tubular aggregates are not specific for ion channel disorders and they are a feature of some inherited myasthenic disorders (see later), as well as a variety of other conditions.[156]

Malignant Hyperthermia

Malignant hyperthermia is a severe complication of general anaesthesia and is characterized by a rapid and sustained rise in temperature following the intravenous administration of anaesthetic. It is accompanied by generalized muscle rigidity, tachycardia, tachypnoea and cyanosis. Extensive

TABLE 25.19 Ion channel disorders of skeletal muscle

Clinical syndrome	Type of ion channel	Gene	Locus	Inheritance
Myotonia congenita (Becker)	Chloride channel	CLCN1	7q35	Recessive
Myotonia congenita (Thomsen)	Chloride channel	CLCN1	7q35	Dominant
Potassium-aggravated myotonia	Sodium channel	SCN4A	17q23	Dominant
Paramyotonia congenita	Sodium channel	SCN4A	17q23	Dominant
Hyperkalaemic periodic paralysis	Sodium channel	SCN4A	17q23	Dominant
Normokalaemic periodic paralysis	Sodium channel	SCN4A	17q23	Dominant
Hypokalaemic periodic paralysis	Calcium channel Sodium channel	CACNA1S SCN4A	1q32 17q23	Dominant Dominant
Hyperkalaemic or hypokalaemic periodic paralysis (Andersen's syndrome)	Potassium channel	KCNJ2	17q	Dominant
Thyrotoxic periodic paralysis	Potassium channel	KCNJ18	17p11	Unknown/ sporadic
Congenital myasthenic syndrome	Sodium channel	SCN4A	17q23	Recessive
Malignant hyperthermia	Calcium channel Calcium channel	RYR1 CACNA1S	19q13 1q32	Dominant Dominant
Tubular aggregate myopathy	Influences calcium release-activated calcium channels	STIM1	11p15	Dominant

muscle necrosis follows, with subsequent myoglobinuria and possible renal shutdown. Serum potassium is elevated and CK is grossly elevated. Many general anaesthetic agents can trigger the reaction, including those containing halogenated hydrocarbons such as halothane, and succinylcholine. Individuals 'at risk' can be diagnosed using the *in vitro* contracture test (IVCT), which measures muscle tension *in vitro* when the sample is exposed to halothane or caffeine.[13]

Malignant hyperthermia is inherited as an autosomal dominant trait. Several loci have been linked to susceptibility to malignant hyperthermia, and two genes have been identified – RYR1 and CACNA1S – that encode the calcium-release channel in terminal cisternae of the sarcoplasmic reticulum (ryanodine receptor) and the α-subunit of the voltage-gated DHPR, respectively.[13] Because mutations in RYR1 are also responsible for a core myopathy, all patients with a RYR1 defect are considered at risk for malignant hyperthermia. Linkage to chromosome 17q in several malignant hyperthermia-susceptible families suggests the sodium channel gene, SCN4A, as a possible candidate gene for malignant hyperthermia.

The muscle pathology associated with malignant hyperthermia is mild and non-specific. Rhabdomyolysis, with marked fibre necrosis and regeneration, is seen immediately after an episode of malignant hyperthermia, but samples taken at other times may show only minor changes, such as scattered smaller fibres and fibres with central nuclei. Thus, routine evaluation of muscle is not of value in diagnosing the disorder or in predicting susceptibility to malignant hyperthermia.

Brody Disease

Calcium ions are removed from the cytosol after muscle contraction by the combined action of Ca^{2+} ATPases in the sarcoplasmic reticulum (SERCA), cell membrane and mitochondrion. In mammals, type 2 fibres express the SERCA1 isoform encoded by the *ATP2A1* gene on chromosome 16p12, whereas type 1 muscle fibres express the SERCA2 isoform encoded by the *ATP2A2* gene on chromosome 12q23. Recessive mutations in the *ATP2A1* gene are responsible for Brody disease, a disorder characterized by painless cramps and impairment of muscle relaxation.[481] Muscle contraction is normal, but the relaxation phase becomes increasingly slow during exercise. An absence of SERCA1 protein from fast fibres has been detected using isoform-specific antibodies in some, but not all, patients with an *ATP2A1* mutation. This was associated with total loss of enzymatic activity. Other studies have demonstrated reduced ATPase activity and expression of a non-functional protein. Therefore, the presence of SERCA1-positive fibres does not exclude Brody disease.[481]

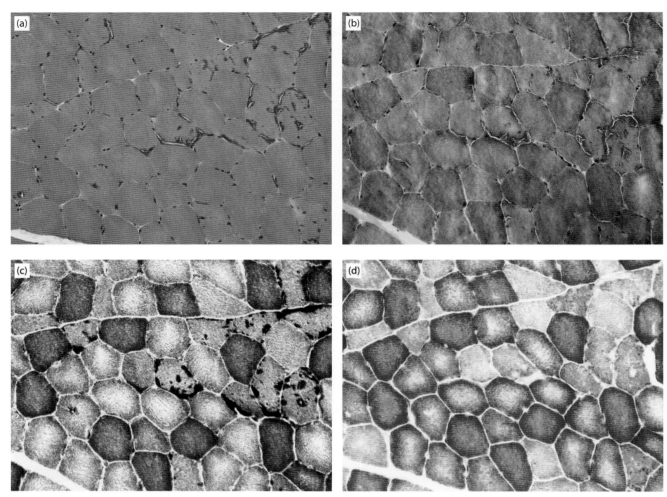

25.92 Serial sections of tubular aggregates that are (a) basophilic with H&E, (b) red with Gomori trichrome, (c) intensely stained in type 2 fibres with NADH-TR but (d) negative for cytochrome *c* oxidase activity. There is also loss of oxidative enzyme activity from the centre of several fibres in this case.

Myasthenic Syndromes

Defects of neuromuscular junction transmission are broadly categorized on the basis of their aetiology – genetic or acquired. Myasthenia gravis is an acquired autoimmune disorder in which autoantibodies against various antigens of the neuromuscular junction can be demonstrated, in particular to the AChR and to MuSK, a tyrosine kinase receptor. Both of these receptors are on the postsynaptic membrane of the neuromuscular junction.[320] Recently, autoantibodies to low density lipoprotein receptor-related protein-4 (LRPP4) have also been identified in some patients with myasthenia gravis.[334] Antibodies to voltage-gated calcium channels on the presynaptic membrane cause Lambert–Eaton syndrome, and neuromyotonia results from antibodies to a presynaptic voltage-gated potassium channel. In addition, antibodies to various muscle proteins can be detected, including to myosin, actin, α-actinin, titin, filamin, vinculin, tropomyosin and the ryanodine receptor.[134,241] Neonates of mothers with autoantibodies may show transient myasthenia (see later). There are also reports of cases with an autoimmune disorder of caveolin-3 that also have antibodies to AChR and myasthenia gravis.[390] These cases show a mosaic pattern of immunolabelling of muscle fibres with antibodies to caveolin-3. Inherited variants of myasthenia are generally congenital disorders that result from mutations in genes encoding various critical presynaptic or postsynaptic proteins (Table 25.20).[129]

Abnormal fatigability is the characteristic symptom of patients affected by most variants of myasthenia. Muscle weakness and fatigability are generalized in myasthenia gravis, with weakness of the ocular muscles and ptosis being the most common presenting symptoms. There is a high incidence of miscarriages in females with myasthenia gravis. Transient neonatal myasthenia affects about one in seven infants born to myasthenic mothers and may produce life-threatening weakness requiring urgent treatment. It results from maternal antibodies to the embryonic acetylcholine receptor.[359] The infant is usually affected at birth with general hypotonia and weakness, but symptoms may sometimes be delayed. Arthrogyposis is a severe complication in some cases. The condition is self-limiting with gradual recovery of the infant, usually within 2–4 weeks.

Confirmation of myasthenia is usually provided by pharmacological tests, such as the response to intravenous

TABLE 25.20 Congenital myasthenic syndromes and known gene defects

Location of defect	Protein	Gene	Locus	Inheritance
Presynaptic				
Defects in ACh resynthesis	ChAT	*CHAT*	10q11.2	AR
Paucity in synaptic vesicles		?		
Lambert–Eaton-like congenital myasthenia		?		
Synaptic				
End plate AChE deficiency	Collagen tail of AChE	*COLQ*	3p24.2	AR
β2 Laminin deficiency	Laminin β2 chain	*LAMB2*	3p21	AR
Postsynaptic				
Fast channel syndromes	ACh receptor α subunit	*CHRNA1*	2q24–q32	AR
	ACh receptor δ subunit	*CHRND*	2q33–q34	AR
	ACh receptor ε subunit	*CHRNE*	17p13	AR
Slow channel syndromes	ACh receptor α subunit	*CHRNA1*	2q24–q32	AD
	ACh receptor β subunit	*CHRNB1*	17p11–p12	AD
	ACh receptor δ subunit	*CHRND*	2q33–q34	AD
	ACh receptor ε subunit	*CHRNE*	17p13	AD, AR
ACh deficiency	ACh receptor β subunit	*CHRNB1*	17p11–p12	AR
	ACh receptor δ subunit	*CHRND*	2q33-q34	AR
	ACh receptor ε subunit	*CHRNE*	17p13	AR
Abnormalities in clustering of ACh receptors	Rapsyn	*RAPSYN*	1p11	AR
	MuSK	*MUSK*	9q31.3–q32	AR
Abnormalities of cytoskeleton	Plectin	*PLEC*	8q24–qter	AR
Anomaly of muscle sodium channel	Sodium channel α-subunit	*SCN4A*	17q23	AR
Defects in end plate development and maintenance				
	Docking protein 7	*DOK7*	4p16.2	AR
	Glutamine-fructose 6-phosphate transaminase 1	*GFPT1*	2p12–p15	AR
	Dolichyl-phosphate N-acetylglucosamine phosphotransferase	*DPAGT1*	11q23.3	AR
	α-1,3/1,6-mannosyltransferase homologue of yeast ALG2	*ALG2*	9q 22.33	AR
	UPD-N-acetyl glucosamine transferase subunit ALG14 homologue	*ALG14*	1p21.3	AR

ACh, acetylcholine; AChE, acetylcholinesterase; AD, autosomal dominant; AR, autosomal recessive; ChAT, choline acetyltransferase.

edrophonium (an acetylcholine esterase inhibitor), or a trial of oral pyridostigmine, or by electrophysiological studies, such as the response decrement of the motor action potential to repetitive stimulation of a nerve, or more specifically by the presence of 'jitter' on single-fibre electromyography, or by the finding of serum antibodies to acetylcholine receptors or MuSK. Electrophysiology and a response to therapy, such as pyridostigmine, have revealed an associated myasthenic syndrome in some patients with mutations in genes not known to be associated with neuromuscular junction proteins, including *TPM3*, *BIN1* and *DNM2*.[79,251,305] In addition, patients with myasthenic symptoms and muscle biopsies showing central nuclei, one of which had a mutation in the *MTM1* gene and others that have not been resolved molecularly, have been reported.[361]

Muscle biopsy has a limited role in the diagnosis of myasthenic syndromes, and pathological features, if present, are non-specific. In our experience a myasthenic or metabolic condition should be considered if a patient is clinically severely affected and the muscle pathology is minimal. The pathological features may include variation in fibre size, collections of lymphocytes, type 2 fibre predominance and core-like areas.[230] In some congenital cases (molecularly unresolved), selective atrophy of type 1 fibres resembling fibre type disproportion was reported.[176] Some cases may show pronounced fibre hypertrophy.[117] Detailed studies of nerve terminals and the neuromuscular junction in autoimmune myasthenia show abnormal binding of complement (C3, C9 and the membrane attack complex), immune complexes, and the autoantibodies derived from the serum of affected patients.

A particular and common feature of muscle biopsies from patients with congenital myasthenia caused by defects in glutamine-fructose-6-phosphate transaminase (GFPT1) and dolichyl-phosphate N-acetylglucosamine phosphotransferase (DPAGT1) and also in some cases with *ALG2* mutations is tubular aggregates.[174,199,399] These genes, together with *ALG14*, emphasize the importance of N-glycosylation at the neuromuscular junction.[96] Tubular aggregates are not usually a feature associated with defects in the other genes that cause myasthenia, for example they are absent in patients with mutations in DOK7. The involvement of the neuromuscular junction in patients with epidermolysis bullosa simplex caused by mutations in the gene encoding plectin (*PLEC*) has been noted over the years.[15,145] A detailed study of the muscle pathology in two additional rare cases showed a variety of pathological changes.[396] These included variation in fibre size, an increase in internal nuclei, large clusters of peripheral nuclei, fibrosis, necrosis and regenerating fibres, uneven distribution of oxidative enzyme stains, fibre type predominance, an increase in calcium demonstrated with alizarin red, and multiple endplates spread over a wide area. Electron microscopy revealed disruption of myofibrils, occasional nemaline rods, aggregates of mitochondria and degeneration of neuromuscular junctions. Immunolabelling of plectin with antibodies to two different domains showed a reduction in labelling from sarcoplasmic areas and a slight reduction in sarcolemmal labelling. Although both patients reported in this paper also had epidermolysis bullosa simplex with typical skin changes, not all patients with mutations in the *PLEC* gene show clinical features evocative of neuromuscular junction involvement, despite the high concentration of plectin at neuromuscular junctions.[175]

Metabolic Myopathies

There are many disorders of glycogen and lipid metabolism and of mitochondrial function, but histopathological assessment of muscle is helpful in only a few.[25] In general, defects of 'substrate utilization', whether of glycogen or fatty acids, result in two main clinical syndromes. One is associated with acute, recurrent episodes of muscle pain,

exercise intolerance, cramps and myoglobinuria, and the second with permanent muscle weakness. The diagnosis of these conditions relies on specialized biochemical techniques and confirmatory genetic testing. This section therefore concentrates on selected conditions where pathological studies are helpful in suggesting a metabolic problem. Some lysosomal diseases of muscle, such as Danon disease and the vacuolar myopathy XMEA, may have features similar to glycogenosis and are included in this section. For a description of metabolic conditions affecting muscle and their biochemical diagnosis, the reader is referred to various reviews.[112,113,248,360]

Disorders of Glycogen Metabolism and Glycolysis

Disorders due to enzymes involved in the synthesis and degradation of glycogen and in some of the steps of glycolysis are referred to as 'glycogenoses'. The numerical classification of these disorders suggested by Cori has found wide acceptance.[95] The inheritance of glycogenoses is autosomal recessive, except for type IX (phosphoglycerate mutase deficiency) and the hepatic form of type VII (phosphorylase b kinase deficiency), which are X-linked.

The following sections highlight aspects of selected glycogenoses.

Muscle Glycogen Depletion

Defects in enzymes responsible for glycogen synthesis lead to a pronounced depletion of glycogen in skeletal muscle, and the disorders described also show cardiac involvement. Defects in glycogen synthase encoded by *GSY1* have been reported in a few rare cases and designated 'muscle glycogen storage disease 0'.[235] Defects in the gene encoding glycogenin (*GYG1*) have also been identified (type XV).[303]

Type II Glycogenosis (Acid Maltase Deficiency)

Acid maltase (acid α-glucosidase) is a lysosomal enzyme that degrades glycogen by hydrolysing its 1,4-links. Absence of this enzyme results in glycogen accumulation in membrane-bound areas of lysosomal origin in several tissues, but mainly muscle. Three clinical types can be distinguished: a severe infantile form (Pompe disease), a juvenile form and a form with adult onset, although 'Pompe' is often now used for all forms.[117,278]

The severe form (Pompe disease) is usually fatal in infancy and affects both cardiac and skeletal muscles. Affected infants are usually floppy from birth or during the first few months of life, and may clinically resemble patients with infantile SMA. Pompe disease can be distinguished from SMA by diaphragmatic and cardiac involvement and a marked elevation of serum CK.

Children affected by the juvenile form have no cardiomyopathy, but have predominantly axial and proximal muscle weakness, and their symptoms may resemble those of a rigid spine syndrome. The prognosis of juvenile patients, and of adult patients presenting with limb girdle weakness, is dependent on the management of the respiratory insufficiency. These patients have often been given a clinical diagnosis of LGMD.

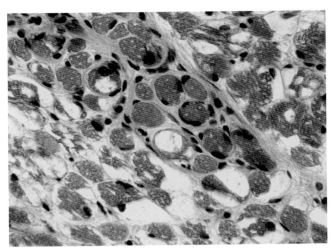

25.93 Pronounced vacuolation in a severe infantile case of Pompe disease. The spaces contain accumulation of glycogen. H&E.

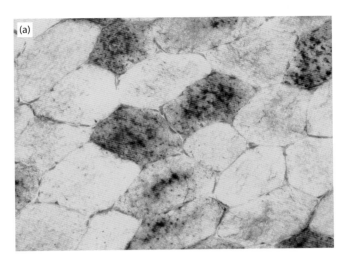

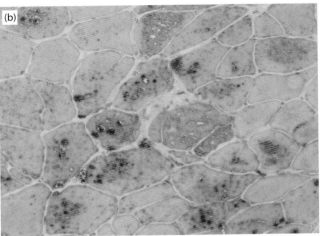

25.94 (a) Vacuoles in some fibres in an adult case of acid maltase deficiency that contain (b) acid phosphatase.

Muscle fibres in Pompe disease have a pronounced vacuolar appearance, with large PAS-positive deposits of glycogen (Figure 25.93). The glycogen is digested by diastase, but some resistant material may remain. Ultrastructurally, the glycogen is characteristically located in membrane-bound areas and in large lakes of freely dispersed granules. Glycogen is lost easily during processing, and the excess may not always be apparent. Accumulation of glycogen in vacuoles can be demonstrated easily in lymphocytes, and this is a useful diagnostic test. A dried blot spot test for testing enzyme activity is also available. Because the enzyme is lysosomal, there is also abundant acid phosphatase activity in the vacuoles. Granular bodies positive for acid phosphatase that also reduce menadione NBT (similar to reducing bodies) may also be a feature.[410]

The muscle pathology in milder cases is variable, but increased glycogen and acid phosphatase are usually apparent. The vacuolation may be extensive or minimal, or have a punctate appearance, or it may be confined mainly to type 1 fibres (Figure 25.94).

With immunohistochemistry, some vacuoles may be surrounded by dystrophin and spectrin, and sometimes also laminins, but this is not a universal feature and not as prominent as in Danon disease or XMEA, in which many vacuoles are associated with both plasmalemmal and basal lamina proteins (see later). There may also be abundant MHC-I labelling associated with the vacuoles and on the sarcolemma in acid maltase deficiency.[117] In some cases, vacuoles can be absent, and in this situation distinction from LGMD is important.

Type V Glycogenosis (McArdle Disease)

The muscle isoform of phosphorylase (myophosphorylase), which is encoded on chromosome 11, is defective in this recessive disorder.[347] The defect results in absence of enzyme activity, and in most cases this is the result of an absence of protein. There are two common hotspot mutations in northern European populations (R50X and G205s). Two other isoforms of phosphorylase, encoded by different genes on chromosomes 20 and 14, are expressed predominantly in the brain and liver, respectively. Fetal muscle, regenerating fibres and myotubes *in vitro* express the brain isoform, and this can be detected in the immature fibres in biopsies (Figure 25.95). Similarly, intrafusal fibres in muscle spindles and the smooth muscle of blood vessels express the brain isoform.

Patients with McArdle disease present with cramps on exertion. Weakness and muscle pain occur, and there may be transient myoglobinuria. There is a high incidence of chronic fatigue/pain, depression and anxiety, and a 'second wind' phenomenon (in which exercise can be endured better after a short pause) is usually present.[347]

Muscle biopsies in type V glycogenosis may show relatively few abnormalities on light microscopy. There may be some degenerating, regenerating and necrotic fibres, but the most consistent finding is the presence of subsarcolemmal 'blebs', which contain PAS-positive glycogen and resemble vacuoles but are not membrane bound (Figure 25.96). The excess glycogen may be more apparent at the ultrastructural level. Sometimes glycogen accumulates between the plasma membrane and the basal lamina.[117]

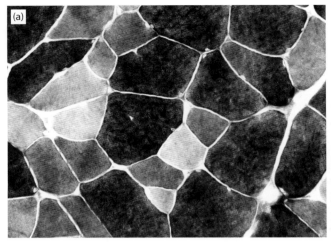

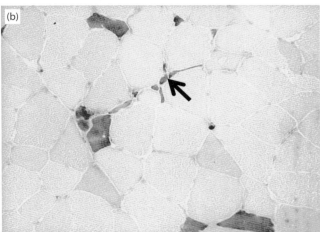

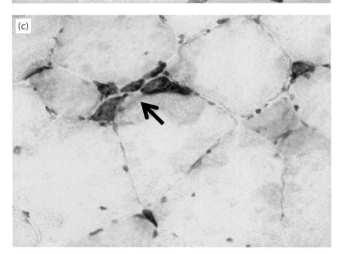

25.95 (a) Normal staining of phosphorylase in a control compared with (b) an absence from all mature fibres in a case of McArdle disease but staining of regenerating fibres that (c) express fetal myosin (arrows) because of the presence of the brain isoform encoded by a different gene.

The absence of phosphorylase can be demonstrated readily by histochemical reaction, but this must always be performed with a positive control (see Figure 25.95). The results are unequivocal, and McArdle disease is the only disorder to show a complete absence of enzyme activity,

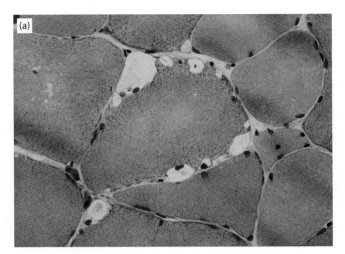

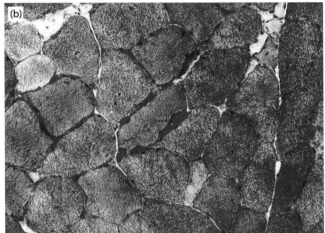

25.96 (a) Peripheral vacuolar-like 'blebs' that (b) contain glycogen in a case of McArdle disease. (a), H&E; (b), PAS.

except in cases with defects in glycogen synthase (see earlier), because endogenous glycogen is required for demonstration of the enzyme in sections. The reaction fades in aqueous mountants but is retained following dehydration and mounting in synthetic mountants, such as di-*n*-butylphthalate-polystyrene-xylene (DPX).

Type VII Glycogenosis (Tarui Disease)

This disease is caused by a deficiency of phosphofructokinase, which catalyses the conversion of fructose-6-phosphate to fructose-1,6-diphosphate.

Clinical features are similar to those of McArdle disease, but a haemolytic anaemia may also occur in phosphofructokinase deficiency.[311,455] There is a particular prevalence in Japanese and Jewish Ashkenazi populations.[349] Severe infantile and adult cases have also been described. Infants may show CNS involvement, and the distinction from CMD variants with associated brain involvement or mitochondrial diseases is important.

Muscle biopsies show non-specific changes on light microscopy and excess glycogen at the ultrastructural level, although this may not be pronounced. Diastase-resistant polyglucosan deposits positive for PAS may also be present, which accumulate with age.[262] Absence of phosphofructo-kinase activity can be detected histochemically but is better determined biochemically.

Glycogenoses with Polyglucosan Bodies

Additional disorders caused by defects of enzymes associated with glycogen metabolism have also been reported and most of them are associated with exercise intolerance, but not always with glycogen storage.[112] Mutations in the branching enzyme encoded by the *GBE1* gene cause type IV glycogenosis and result in the accumulation of abnormal glycogen, commonly referred to as polyglucosan. This is in contrast to defects in type III glycogenosis caused by defects in the debranching enzyme in which glycogen appears normal.[117] Polyglucosan bodies are often diastase-resistant PAS-positive bodies, and are the typical pathological hallmark associated with *GBE1* mutations, but some cases do not show them and not all are PAS-positive. Polyglucosan bodies are not specific for type IV glycogenosis and can also occur in phosphofructokinase deficiency, Lafora disease and an adult disease characterized by neurogenic involvement.[56,97]

Lysosomal Glycogen Storage with Normal Acid Maltase

Danon Disease

Danon disease is a vacuolar myopathy with normal acid maltase levels.[433] The gene responsible has been mapped to Xq24 and encodes the lysosomal-associated membrane 2 protein (LAMP-2). Not all cases show glycogen storage, and the disorder is sometimes referred to as 'X-linked vacuolar myopathy'.[263]

Onset is in childhood and is characterized by severe hypertrophic cardiomyopathy, a mild and relatively stable myopathy, and variable mental retardation. Creatine kinase levels are elevated, even in preclinical cases. Muscle weakness and atrophy affect the shoulder and neck muscles, but there may also be distal involvement. Female carriers may also manifest.[433]

In addition to abnormal variation in the size of both fibre types, the striking feature is the presence of numerous vacuoles containing glycogen. Invaginations of the sarcolemma are also common. The vacuoles are lined by a membrane that labels with antibodies to dystrophin, β-spectrin, laminin chains and other sarcolemmal proteins (Figure 25.97). The membrane and content of the vacuoles are labelled with some lectins, such as wheat germ agglutinin, *Ulex europaeus* I agglutinin (UEA-1) and *Limas flavus* agglutinin. This has been suggested as a possible way to distinguish the vacuoles from those seen in acid maltase deficiency, which show little or no labelling with lectins.[468] With the electron microscope, a basal lamina is seen on the inner surface of some vacuoles, which contain abundant amounts of granular, osmiophilic debris. Immunohistochemistry and immunoblots show a virtual absence of LAMP-2, indicating that this is useful in the assessment of muscle biopsies.[263,468]

X-Linked Myopathy with Excess Autophagy

The pathology in Danon disease is remarkably similar to that seen in XMEA, in which sarcolemmal proteins are also found on vacuoles but they are clinically distinct.[264] No cardiac involvement or mental retardation has been reported in XMEA. Onset is typically in adults, although a more severe and probably allelic variant with onset in childhood has been reported. Calcium deposits can be detected in subsarcolemmal areas, and complement C5b–9 (membrane attack complex) and acetylcholinesterase can be demonstrated on the sarcolemma in XMEA and may help to distinguish it from Danon disease. Duplication of the basal lamina is abundant and debris seen between the layers.[264] The genetic defect that causes XMEA is a defect in the *VMA21* gene that encodes a V-ATPase involved in lysosomal function.[352] Some similar pathological features to those described in XMEA can occur in other conditions associated with autophagy, such as Vici syndrome and in molecularly unresolved cases.[99]

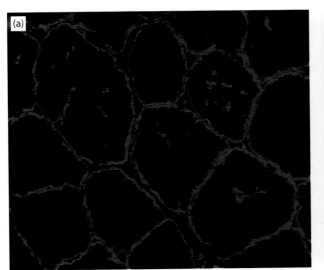 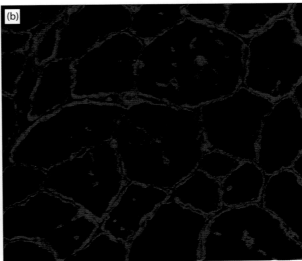

25.97 A case resembling X-linked myopathy with excessive autophagic vacuoles (XMEA) with vacuoles that are immunolabelled with antibodies to (a) β-spectrin and (b) laminin γ1. Indentations of the sarcolemma can also be seen.

Disorders of Fatty Acid Metabolism

The oxidation of fatty acids is a major energy source and occurs in mitochondria. A heterogeneous group of disorders is caused by defects in the β-oxidation metabolic pathway. These disorders fall into two broad groups: those in which muscle symptoms are the main complaint, and those in which muscle involvement is part of a systemic condition. In the former, presenting symptoms and signs may be proximal or diffuse muscle weakness, or muscle pain, particularly following prolonged exertion, which may be associated with muscle necrosis and myoglobinuria. The predominant muscle symptoms in children, in whom muscle involvement is part of a systemic illness, are hypotonia and generalized muscle weakness. There may be cardiac involvement and global delay. The two types of carnitine palmitoyltransferase M deficiency (CPTI, CPTII) are relatively common and characterized by recurrent myoglobinuria, which can be precipitated by prolonged exercise, fasting and intercurrent illnesses. Carnitine deficiency is characterized by mild weakness, hypotonia and life-threatening cardiomyopathy.

The contribution of muscle pathology to the investigation of these disorders has diminished with advances in molecular analysis and biochemical assays. In patients with carnitine deficiency, excess lipid storage gives a striking vacuolar-like appearance corresponding to the non-membrane-bound lipid droplets, and may be associated with structural abnormalities in mitochondria. In patients with CPT deficiencies, however, the amount of lipid may not be increased, and the overall pathology is minimal or absent. Similarly, in other disorders of fatty acid metabolism, including β-oxidation defects, only mild non-specific abnormalities, or no abnormalities, may be seen, and any increase in lipid is difficult to quantify. If a muscle biopsy is taken soon after an episode of myoglobinuria in CPT deficiency, necrotic or regenerating fibres may be present.[238]

Mitochondrial Myopathies

The mitochondrial myopathies are a heterogeneous group of multisystem disorders in which abnormalities in mitochondrial function may or may not be associated with structural abnormalities in the mitochondria. Overlapping clinical features are present in the various mitochondrial disorders, and further complexity arises because the same molecular abnormality may produce divergent clinical features. Particular neuromuscular features that suggest a mitochondrial disease are exercise intolerance, fatigue, rhabdomyolysis, ptosis, ophthalmoplegia and a raised serum lactate. Neonatal and infantile hypotonia are well-recognized presenting features.[336] Involvement of tissues other than skeletal muscle is common, with clinical and radiological features of CNS involvement, cardiac involvement, retinal degeneration, hearing loss, endocrine disorders, and liver, gastrointestinal and peripheral nerve involvement.

Mitochondria have a pivotal role in the final common pathway for aerobic metabolism—oxidative phosphorylation (OXPHOS), composed of five complexes. Components of these complexes are under the control of both nuclear (nDNA) and mitochondrial (mtDNA) genomes. The nuclear genome encodes most of the subunits of the enzyme complexes, assembly proteins and many of the factors necessary

for mtDNA replication, transcription and translation, and defects show Mendelian inheritance. The mitochondrial genome, however, encodes 13 subunits of the OXPHOS system, ribosomal RNA (rRNA) and transfer RNA (tRNA) involved in the mitochondrial protein synthesis, and defects are maternally inherited and influenced by heteroplasmy, threshold effect and mitotic segregation (Box 25.10).

For biochemical studies, muscle tissue must be snap frozen in liquid nitrogen within 30 minutes of performing the biopsy to avoid loss of enzyme activity. Isopentane interferes with the measurement of complexes I, II and III, but copy number can be studied in samples frozen in isopentane. Cultured skin fibroblasts are used for β-oxidation studies.

Muscle pathology is variable and can range from striking abnormalities, typical of a mitochondrial disease, to non-specific or minimal. Adults with mitochondrial disease are more likely to have an abnormal muscle biopsy than children. The absence of pathology does not exclude a mitochondrial problem. In addition to routine histological stains, enzyme histochemistry for NADH-TR (complex I),

---

BOX 25.10. Pathobiology and genetics of mitochondrial disease

Oxidative phosphorylation (OXPHOS) is carried out by the mitochondrial respiratory chain comprising five multisubunit enzyme complexes located on the inner mitochondrial membrane and the process generates adenosine triphosphate (ATP). The pathway is under dual control of both nuclear (nDNA) and mitochondrial (mtDNA) genomes. The nuclear genome encodes most of the subunits of the enzyme complexes, assembly proteins and many of the factors necessary for mtDNA replication, transcription and translation. The mitochondrial genome encodes 13 subunits of the OXPHOS system, as well as the ribosomal RNA (rRNA) and transfer RNA (tRNA) involved in the mitochondrial protein synthesis. Transmission of mitochondrial diseases is therefore governed both by Mendelian genetics and by mitochondrial genetics, the latter of which is influenced by heteroplasmy, threshold effect, mitotic segregation, and maternal inheritance. Nuclear defects are a major cause of mitochondrial disease as the majority of the mitochondrial proteins, including some respiratory chain subunits, are nuclear encoded. They can affect (i) synthesis of structural or assembly proteins of the respiratory chain; (ii) other components of the mitochondrial respiratory chain such as coenzyme Q10; (iii) intergenomic signalling impairing replication, maintenance or translation of mtDNA leading to qualitative (multiple deletions) or quantitative (depletion) alterations in mtDNA that accumulate during life; (iv) synthesis of inner mitochondrial membrane phospholipids; and (v) mitochondrial motility and fission (mitodynamics). Human mtDNA is a small 16.5 kb circular double-stranded DNA molecule of which there are many thousand copies within each nucleated cell. It contains 37 genes: 13 structural genes encoding essential mitochondrial respiratory chain subunits, 2 rRNA genes and 22 tRNA genes. With rare exceptions, all surviving mtDNA is derived from the mother's ovum at conception. mtDNA mutations are therefore inherited maternally. mtDNA mutations may affect only a proportion of mitochondria, leading to a mixture of mutant and wild-type mtDNA within a cell (heteroplasmy). The proportion of mutant mtDNA must exceed a critical threshold before a biochemical defect manifests. This threshold varies between tissues and partly explains the tissue variability in mitochondrial disease. A site-map for the mitochondrial mutation databases maintained by the Human Genome Variation Society can be accessed at www.hgvs.org/dblist/mito.html.

SDH (complex II), COX (complex IV), and the combined COX/SDH technique are the most useful techniques (see Figure 25.32). There are no reliable histochemical techniques to demonstrate complexes III and V. The role of immunohistochemistry is limited to demonstrating the presence of the enzymes and is of less diagnostic use than assay of enzyme activity.

Pathological features include fibre atrophy, but little or no hypertrophy, an increase in internal nuclei, and necrosis and fibre regeneration in cases with myoglobinuria. Fibre type differentiation is rarely abnormal, although accumulation of abnormal mitochondria may occur more often in type 1 fibres. In conditions with associated peripheral nerve involvement, there may be fibre type grouping. Mitochondrial proliferations are an important diagnostic clue, regardless of the molecular defect. Extreme mitochondrial proliferation gives rise to 'ragged-red fibres' (RRF) that show enhanced red staining with the Gomori trichrome technique and have a granular basophilic appearance with H&E (see Figure 25.32). Staining is often pronounced at the periphery of fibres and also disrupted internally. RRFs have a high proportion of mutant mitochondrial genomes that is segmental. RRFs react intensely for SDH and NADH-TR and may lack COX activity (Figure 25.98), but this is not a universal feature and fibres with enhanced COX activity may be present. Neither RRFs nor COX-negative fibres are disease specific and they can occur with ageing and as a secondary feature in several inherited and acquired disorders.[117]

Several studies have attempted to quantify the number of RRFs and/or COX-negative fibres in mitochondrial myopathies and in association with normal ageing. Various proportions of abnormal fibres have been regarded as diagnostic of mitochondrial disease including more than 2 per cent RRFs and/or more than 2 per cent COX-negative fibres if the individual is under 50 years of age, or more than 5 per cent COX-negative fibres if the individual is over the age of 50 years. It has been suggested that identification of any RRFs in an individual less than 30 years of age should raise the suspicion of mitochondrial disease. More recent work has suggested that an occurrence of more than 0.5 per cent COX-negative fibres in the absence of a primary muscle disease should raise the possibility of mitochondrial disease. In addition, the number of COX-negative fibres may vary in different muscles with more being observed in the deltoid than in the quadriceps.[419] In children, COX-negative fibres outnumber RRFs, which are rare in children below 5 years of age with mitochondrial disease.

Subsarcolemmal mitochondrial aggregates (SSMA), however, are thought to be more prevalent. The modified paediatric criteria proposed in 2002 included more than 2 per cent SSMAs as a minor diagnostic criterion and continues to be suggested for the diagnosis of mitochondrial respiratory chain disorders in children younger than 16 years of age. Recently, however, it has been proposed that muscle biopsies of paediatric patients with low a percentage of SSMA (≤4 per cent) are significantly more likely to have respiratory chain enzyme complex deficiency than patients with increased SSMA percentage (≥10 per cent). A mtDNA depletion syndrome and coenzyme Q10 deficiency should be considered in patients with a low SSMA score (≤4 per cent).[291]

Ultrastructural abnormalities of mitochondria include alteration in shape, increase in size, disruption and distortion of cristae, and paracrystalline or osmophillic inclusions (Figure 25.99). Electron microscopy may also reveal varying degrees of myofibrillar loss and disruption, and an increase in intracellular lipid, which can often be detected with oil red O or Sudan black stains. Ultrastructural changes are usually non-specific, an exception may be mitochondria with simplified cristae filled with homogenous staining material, reported to be a feature unique to mtDNA depletion.[38] In the absence of changes seen with light microscopy, mitochondria, in our experience, are usually ultrastructurally normal, except in endothelial cells (unpublished data), although some changes have been reported in endothelial cells.[364,380] Given the lack of specificity of the findings and the time and expense involved, the routine use of electron microscopy in the investigation of mitochondrial disease is questionable.

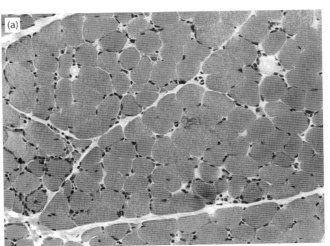 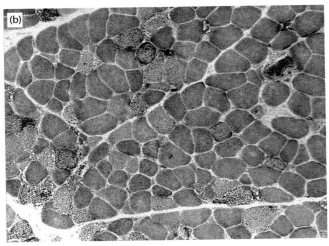

25.98 A case of a mitochondrial myopathy with mitochondrial DNA depletion caused by a TK2 mutation showing (a) granular basophilic fibres and (b) several fibres devoid of cytochrome c oxidase activity that show only blue staining for SDH that is enhanced in some fibres (ragged blue fibres). (a), H&E; (b), combined COX/SDH.

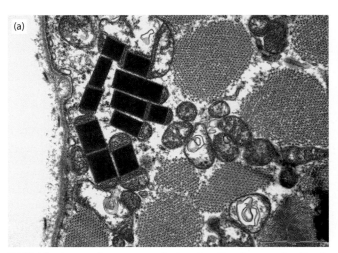 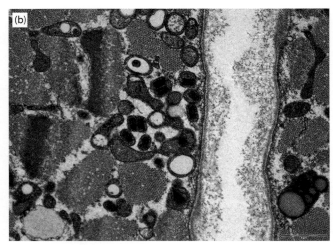

25.99 Electron microscopy of structurally abnormal mitochondria with (a) paracrystalline inclusions and abnormal cristae and (b) circular inner membranes and inclusions as well as paracrystalline inclusions.

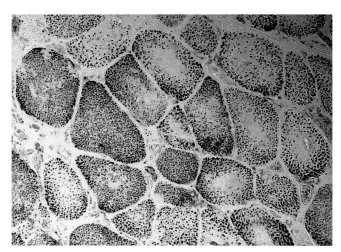

25.100 A case with mutations in the *CHKB* gene showing large mitochondria towards the periphery of the fibres and pale-stained central areas that do not show disrupted myofibrils with electron microscopy. Note also the blue staining of some fibres due to an absence of cytochrome *c* oxidase. COX/SDH.

There is no absolute correlation between genotype and the clinical, biochemical and pathological phenotype in mitochondrial disease, especially for mtDNA mutations. The presence of RRFs and COX-negative fibres in a mosaic and segmental distribution is typical of heteroplasmic mtDNA deletions seen in Kearns–Sayre syndrome (KSS) and progressive external ophthalmoplegia (PEO) or mt tRNA mutations seen in myoclonic epilepsy with ragged-red fibres (MERRF) and mitochondrial encephalomyopathy, lactic acidosis and stroke-like episodes (MELAS).[179,445] In MERRF and MELAS, mitochondrial proliferation also occurs in blood vessels that stain strongly for SDH. Both RRFs and blood vessels in MERRF are COX negative, whereas those in MELAS are typically COX positive, probably as a result of an even distribution of mutant and wild-type mtDNA in these fibres and vessels. Increased lipid in myofibres, including RRFs, is a feature seen in KSS and PEO.[388] Mutations in two genes encoding mitochondrial

tRNA cause the benign reversible infantile COX-deficient myopathy that presents as a severe myopathy at birth or in the first few weeks of life, with spontaneous recovery between 5 and 20 months of age.[198,469] An early onset myopathy with muscle wasting and mental retardation is linked to defective phosphatidylcholine biosynthesis due to mutations in the *CHKB* gene encoding choline kinase beta. The muscle pathology is distinctive, with myofibres showing central mitochondrial depletion and peripheral giant mitochondria (Figure 25.100).[296,348]

Other Metabolic Disorders

Myoadenylate Deaminase Deficiency

Myoadenylate deaminase (MAD) is the enzyme that catalyses the deamination of adenosine monophosphate (AMP) to inosine monophosphate (IMP) and there are several isoforms encoded by different genes. The muscle isoform is encoded by the myoadenylate deaminase deficiency (*AMPD1*) gene and is more abundant in type 2 fibres, giving a two-fibre type pattern on histochemistry. In addition, type 1 fibres also express the E isoform. The enzyme technique stains tubular aggregates but because they also stain without substrate present this may relate to components of the incubation medium.

The histochemical reaction for MAD is negative in affected individuals, but symptoms are mild and non-specific (exercise intolerance, aches and cramps, normal or slightly elevated CK). Because there is a common mutation in the gene in the normal population, the significance of absent enzyme activity has been questioned.

ACQUIRED DISORDERS

There are various disorders affecting muscle that are acquired rather than genetic. These include inflammatory myopathies, myopathies related to endocrine abnormalities and vitamin deficiencies, myopathies induced by drugs and toxins, critical illness myopathy, infectious myopathies and myopathies associated with neoplasia and ageing.

Inflammatory Myopathies

Idiopathic Inflammatory Myopathies

The classical idiopathic inflammatory myopathies (IIM) include polymyositis (PM), juvenile and adult dermatomyositis (JDM and DM) and IBM. However, the spectrum of inflammatory muscle diseases is much wider and includes immune-mediated and non-immune necrotizing myopathies, focal myositis, granulomatous myositis, graft-versus-host disease, fasciitis/myofasciitis, panniculitis, connective tissue diseases including overlap syndromes, brachiocervical inflammatory myopathy and the vasculitides. Overlapping clinical and pathological features between the IIMs and other inflammatory conditions can present considerable diagnostic challenges. Serology and muscle imaging have an increasing role in the diagnostic pathway for inflammatory muscle diseases.

As with other immunogenic disorders, there is evidence that implicates a role for genes, both within and outside the MHC complex, that modulate the immune response in IIM. Such associations include differing IIM phenotypes for anti-Jo-1 and anti-PM-Scl antibody cases despite a shared HLA8.1 ancestral haplotype, association of DPB1*0101 with anti-Jo-1 positivity but not anti-Scl-1, GM13 allotype being a confirmed risk factor in IIM, and potential influence of HLA8.1 ancestral haplotype on disease susceptibility and expression in IBM.[74] Specific genes at polymorphic loci such as HLA DRB1*0301, TNF-α308A and GM 3 23 5,13 are risk factors for all of the major clinical groups. Other alleles are specific to particular antibody phenotypes.[358]

Consistent and accurate classification of IIMs is more than just semantics; accurate delineation of homogenous subgroups is helpful for predicting response to treatment, clinical outcome, the development of therapeutic trials, and for epidemiological studies. The Bohan and Peter criteria formulated in 1975 have been widely used, but are limited and do not take account of pathological and clinical developments in the field. The classification excludes IBM and immune necrotizing myopathies, now well-recognized entities, and better criteria have been established.[195] Better understanding of the immunopathogenesis, histopathology, muscle imaging and specific autoantibody associations has led to refined IIM criteria through large-scale consensus efforts. (For aspects on pathogenesis see Box 25.11 and various reviews[6,100]). The European Neuromuscular Centre classification for IIMs, based on clinical, muscle pathology and other laboratory criteria, proposes five categories: (i) IBM; (ii) PM; (iii) DM; (iv) non-specific myositis; and (v) immune-mediated necrotizing myopathy.[75,111] A review encompassing historical approaches to classification as well as more recent attempts to refine knowledge of immunopathological and autoantibody associations in inflammatory myopathies has recently been published.[194]

The onset of polymyositis or dermatomyositis in adults is usually associated with muscle pain, accompanied by variable muscle weakness. The weakness may be proximal and symmetrical, as in LGMD, or asymmetrical with varying distribution, but it is rarely selective. Tenderness and swelling of muscles may accompany weakness. Progression may be rapid and severe, but most cases follow an insidious subacute or chronic course. Rapid progression is associated

---

BOX 25.11. Pathogenesis of polymyositis, dermatomyositis and inclusion body myopathy

Immunopathogenesis of polymyositis (PM) and inclusion body myositis (IBM) is based on antigen-directed cytotoxicity mediated by CD8+ T-cells invading non-necrotic, major histocompatibility class I (MHC-I) expressing muscle fibres. This CD8+/MHC-I immunological synapse is identical in PM and IBM, despite the latter being refractory to immunosuppression. The major cytotoxic effector mechanism in PM and IBM is mediated via the perforin pathway. In PM and IBM, there is evidence of variable upregulation of pro-inflammatory cytokines chemokines as well as various adhesion and extracellular matrix molecules such as VCAM, ICAM, thrombospondins and metalloproteinases on myofibres and some autoinvasive CD8+ T-cells. These molecules consolidate the immunological synapse by enhancing T-cell activation, inducing co-stimulatory molecules and facilitating cell adhesion. BB1/CD28 and ICOS/ICOS-L interactions in PM and IBM denote participation in antigen presentation, clonal expansion and T-cell co-stimulation. In IBM, in addition to the immunopathogenic changes in common with PM, there is a prominent degenerative process characterized by fibre vacuolation and accumulation of conformationally modified proteins similar to those seen in neurodegenerative diseases such as Alzheimer disease. Abnormalities in AβPP processing such as increased BACE1 and γ-secretase contribute to Aβ overproduction. Aβ has recently been demonstrated in IBM muscle and plasma. Conformationally modified Tau protein has been identified recently in IBM muscle and is implicated in IBM pathogenesis. Dermatomyositis (DM) is considered to be a humorally mediated microangiopathy; the primary antigenic target being the vascular endothelium of the endomysial capillaries and to a lesser extent of the larger blood vessels. Putative antibodies directed against the endothelial cells activate the complement cascade leading to C5b-9, the terminal lytic component of the complement pathway, being deposited early in the disease course. Demonstration of a majority of B-cells and CD4+ T-cells in the perimysial and perivascular foci and plasmacytoid dendritic cells in the perimysial foci further points to humorally mediated mechanisms in DM.

Certain immunopathogenic mechanisms are shared across the different IIM subtypes. Regenerating fibres in PM/DM express Toll-like receptors TLR3 and TLR7. Necrotic cell debris drives cytokine production *in vitro* in part through TLR3 signalling, and necrotic/regenerating fibres may amplify the immune response in PM/DM. Involvement of the type I interferon system in the pathophysiology of idiopathic inflammatory myopathies (IIMs) has emerged in recent years, as well as the role of dendritic cells (DCs). Myeloid DCs are present in substantial numbers in PM/IBM muscle, whereas in DM muscle, plasmacytoid DCs predominate. Besides innate and adaptive immune responses, non-immune mechanisms may participate in muscle damage in IIMs.

---

with gross elevation of CK. Rhabdomyolysis and myoglobinuria may also occur, but this is rare in dermatomyositis. Joint contractures affecting the ankles and other large joints are common. There is a well-established association between malignancy and dermatomyositis in adults.[506] The tumour and myopathy usually present within a short time of each other, but occasionally the myopathy may significantly precede identification of the tumour.

In dermatomyositis, involvement of skin vasculature manifests as a heliotrope or violaceous rash, particularly over the eyes and malar regions of the face, and as erythema around the nail beds and over the knees and elbows. In severe cases, the entire skin becomes tight, shiny and reddened. In chronic juvenile cases of dermatomyositis, there may be calcinosis. Calcium is deposited in the subcutaneous tissue and in the supportive connective tissues within muscle, but not in muscle fibres themselves.

Juvenile dermatomyositis differs from the adult form. It is always an idiopathic condition and is not associated with malignancy. Although muscle weakness is always present, it may be extremely variable. Children with dermatomyositis usually have systemic symptoms, such as mood swings, malaise, listlessness and lethargy, which may be the presenting feature or characterize a relapse.

Inclusion body myositis is one of the most common disorders of muscle in patients aged over 50 years. It is more common in males than females, and usually sporadic. However, some hereditary disorders sharing pathological features of inclusion body myositis, but lacking an inflammatory component, have been described and are sometimes referred to as 'hereditary inclusion body myopathies'. The underlying gene defects in some of these inherited forms have been identified, and are discussed earlier (see Z-line Associated Proteins and Four-and-a-Half LIM Domains Protein 1, p. 1591; and Distal Myopathies, p. 1593). IBM is distinguished from polymyositis and dermatomyositis by a more insidious onset, with both proximal and distal weakness, which is often asymmetrical. Dysphagia, weakness of the wrist, finger flexor muscles and of ankle dorsiflexion are common.[100] IBM patients are usually non-responsive to steroid therapy.

Serum CK activity in all forms is frequently, but not invariably, elevated, and a normal level does not exclude a diagnosis of inflammatory myopathy. Other laboratory investigations that may be helpful are a raised erythrocyte sedimentation rate (ESR), serum autoantibodies, and serum and urinary compounds such as myoglobin and neopterin. The ESR is raised in only a proportion of cases, and there is no correlation between its level and the degree of muscle weakness. Myositis-specific autoantibodies (MSAs) are detected in one-third of IIM cases. They are highly disease specific, can appear months before the onset of symptoms, correlate with disease activity and disappear on disease remission. There is increasing evidence that MSAs can allow more homogenous grouping in PM/DM, and can help in assessing prognosis and developing therapies. Antiaminoacyl-tRNA-synthetase antibodies are the most prevalent. The most common of these is anti-Jo-1; patients with these antibodies show a high frequency of moderate to severe myositis (PM or adult DM) with characteristic extramuscular manifestations, including interstitial lung disease, Raynaud's phenomenon, low grade fever, arthritis and mechanic's hands – the antisynthetase syndrome. Antisignal recognition particle (anti-SRP) and anti-3-hydroxy-3-methylglutaryl-coenzyme A reductase (HMGCR) antibodies are typically associated with immune-mediated necrotizing myopathies. It should be noted that a degree of overlap exists between MSAs and their disease associations; for instance, antisynthetase antibodies typically associated with the antisynthetase syndrome with or without myositis (PM/DM) may also occur in immune necrotizing myopathies. New autoantibodies are continually being identified and, to date, around 60–80 per cent of patients with autoimmune myositis seem to have at least one MSA.[63,74,197] The

various clinical associations with MSAs are summarized in Table 25.21.

Electromyography shows a characteristic pattern, with a combination of spontaneous fibrillation potentials, similar to those seen in denervation, and polyphasic short-duration potentials on voluntary contraction, as in myopathies. Imaging techniques are having an increasing role, and show increased signal in relation to oedema and inflammatory changes in subcutaneous fat.[486]

In muscle biopsies the presence of lymphocytes that may invade muscle fibres is a key feature of myositis, but the degree of inflammation is variable and may be absent. Some cases may show a fasciitis (see later). The presence of sarcolemmal MHC-I antigens, however, is universal in all forms and a useful diagnostic marker that can be present in the absence of other signs of inflammation or other pathology (Figure 25.101).[100,117] MHC-I immunolabelling within muscle fibres may also be seen. In DM, MHC-I upregulation may be focal or restricted to the perifascicular regions and not be as diffuse and widespread as in PM/IBM. Inflammation is not only a feature of inflammatory myopathies, but can also be prominent in various muscular

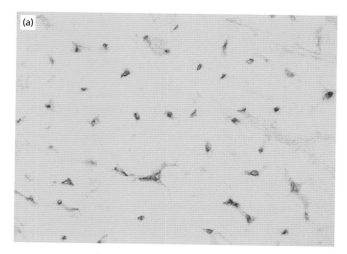

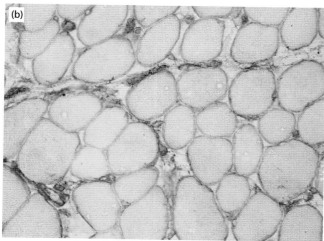

25.101 Immunolabelling of major histocompatibility class 1 antigens in (a) a control and (b) a case of juvenile dermatomyositis. Note the sarcolemmal labelling in the case of dermatomyositis and normal labelling of blood vessels in both.

TABLE 25.21 Clinical associations of myositis-specific antibodies

Antibody	Target antigen	Clinical association
Antibodies associated with antisynthetase syndrome		
Anti-amino-acyl-tRNA synthetase	Amino-acyl-tRNA synthetase	Antisynthetase syndrome (myositis, interstitial lung disease, Raynaud's phenomenon, arthritis. mechanic's hands, fever, DM skin rash)
-Jo-1 (most common)	-Histidyl	Myositis (PM/ adult DM), ILD
-PL7	-Threonyl	Hypomyopathic disease, prominent lung involvement
-PL12	-Alanyl	DM skin rash, ILD
-OJ	-Isoleucyl	DM skin rash, ILD
-EJ	-Glycyl	–
-KS	-Asparginyl	DM skin rash, ILD
-Ha	-Tyrosyl	Myositis, ILD
-Zo	-Phenylalanyl	Myositis, ILD
Antibodies associated with dermatomyositis		
Anti-Mi-2	NuRD	Classic DM, decreased risk of malignancy, more severe rash, good response to steroids, good prognosis
Anti-p155/140	TIF1 family	Children: ulceration Adults: malignancy
Anti-p140	NXP2	Children: calcinosis Adults: ILD
Anti-SAE	SAE	Skin manifestations precede myositis
Anti-CADM-140	MDA-5	CADM, ILD, cutaneous ulceration, palmar papules, rapidly progressive ILD
Anti-MJ	Nuclear matrix protein 2 (NPX2)	High frequency of calcinosis, arthritis, joint contractures and absence of truncal rash
Antibodies associated with immune-mediated necrotizing myopathies		
Anti-SRP	Signal recognition particles (cytoplasmic RNA complexes)	Aggressive disease, poor steroid response, cardiac involvement
Anti-HMGCR	3-hydroxy-3-methylglutaryl-coenzyme A reductase	Progressive myopathy in patients with statin use despite cessation of statin
Antibodies associated with inclusion body myositis		
Anti-p44	5'-nucleotidase IA	IBM

DM, dermatomyositis; HMGCR, 3-hydroxy-3-methylglutaryl-coenzyme A reductase; IBM, inclusion body myositis; ILD, interstitial lung disease; PM, polymyositis.

dystrophies, particularly in association with necrotic fibres, and MHC-I is often overexpressed on the sarcolemma (see sections on muscular dystrophies).

Abnormal variation in fibre size is often present, but hypertrophy is absent or less pronounced than in muscular dystrophies. Other pathological features include internal nuclei, basophilic fibres, an increase in connective tissue (usually less than in muscular dystrophies), moth-eaten fibres or fibres with core-like areas, and fibre splitting. There may also be loose oedematous separation of muscle fibres with interspersed fibrous tissue. Perifascicular atrophy is a particular feature of dermatomyositis, which is not seen in polymyositis or IBM, and when present should raise the suspicion of DM even in the absence of inflammation (see Figure 25.26). Histochemically, perifascicular fibres are of both types and often show intense and aggregated NADH-TR activity. Many of these small fibres express proteins associated with immaturity, such as fetal myosin, desmin and NCAM, and differentiating them from regenerating fibres is then difficult.

Necrosis and regeneration and a characteristic vacuolar degeneration may be extensive, particularly in JDM (Figure 25.102). Macrophages and T-cells invade the fibre after it becomes necrotic. Necrosis may be segmental and

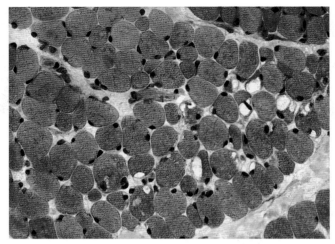

25.102 Vacuolar degeneration in a case of dermatomyositis. H&E.

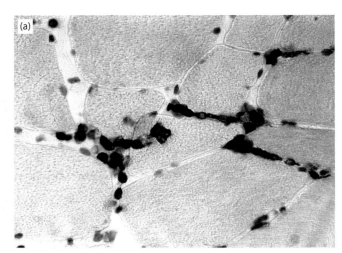

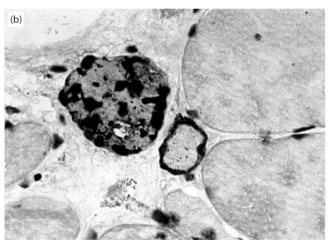

25.103 (a) Immunolabelling of CD8+ cells in the endomysium and some that appear to be invading a fibre in a case of polymyositis. (b) Immunolabelling of p62 shows cytoplasmic inclusions in a vacuolated fibre and peripheral labelling in an adjacent non-vacuolated fibre in a case of inclusion body myositis.

involve clusters of fibres, or it may involve single fibres. In dermatomyositis, areas of infarction, characterized by groups of pale-staining necrotic fibres, may be present. Necrotic fibres may show a peripheral cuff of basophilia, corresponding to regeneration, a feature rarely seen in muscular dystrophies. Acid phosphatase activity is associated with the presence of inflammatory cells and macrophages and is also increased in the fibres.[117]

T-cells, B-cells, dendritic cells and macrophages are the principal infiltrating cells. They occur in the perimysium and endomysium, are often perivascular and may partly invade blood vessel walls. However, true vasculitis is not a feature of PM/DM and if present should raise the possibility of an associated connective tissue disease. Eosinophils are not usually seen. The proportion and distribution of the various inflammatory cell types differ in polymyositis and dermatomyositis. In polymyositis, the infiltrate is predominately endomysial, with a large number of CD8+ T-lymphocytes. These surround and invade non-necrotic muscle fibres, a feature not found in dermatomyositis (Figure 25.103a). B-cells, in contrast, are predominantly perivascular and rarely located in the endomysium in polymyositis. In dermatomyositis, the cells are predominantly perivascular and perimysial, although some may be endomysial, and there is a higher proportion of B-cells and CD4+ cells than in polymyositis. A variable proportion of CD4+ cells in PM and DM are dendritic cells. Macrophages may accompany CD8+ T-cells in invading MHC-I restricted apparently non-necrotic fibres in PM. Occasionally in DM, the perimysium may harbour prominent ribbon-like configurations of macrophages with basophilic cytoplasm; this pattern has been referred to as inflammatory myopathy with abundant macrophages (IMAM), a condition that should be distinguished from macrophagic myofasciitis.[101]

Blood vessels in dermatomyositis often have thickened walls and capillaries may be enlarged. With electron microscopy, endothelial cells of capillaries and arterioles are seen to contain tubuloreticular inclusions. These are an early pathological feature. Another early feature of DM is deposition of the membrane attack complex C5b–9 on endomysial capillaries. Surface deposition of C5b–9 may be seen on a limited number of fibres and within necrotic

fibres as a non-specific feature. In both adult and juvenile dermatomyositis, there is depletion of capillaries, and this is also an early feature seen in the absence of other pathology. Because MHC-I is present on all blood vessels, it can be used to assess the number of capillaries, but this may be visualized better with the endothelial marker CD31 (PECAM-1). Basal lamina markers such as *Ulex europaeus* or laminin α5, are also useful as the capillaries are highlighted against the negative (*Ulex*) or weak (laminin α5) labelling of the sarcolemma. In DM, the perimysium contains abnormal vessel fragments, perivascular inflammation and increased CD31. Perifascicular atrophy and capillary pathology are concentrated near the avascular perimysium.[333] A scoring system has been devised for evaluating muscle biopsies in JDM assessing pathological severity in four domains (inflammatory, vascular, muscle fibre and connective tissue) and has been shown to have good interobserver reliability and correlation with clinical severity.[491]

The main pathological features of inclusion body myositis are fibre atrophy and hypertrophy, an increase in internal nuclei and endomysial connective tissue, necrosis, with invasion of fibres by phagocytes, and basophilic regenerating fibres. Cytoplasmic bodies, disruption of the myofibrillar pattern and core-like areas lacking NADH-TR activity are also seen. There is often a greater than expected number of COX-negative fibres, and electron microscopy reveals structurally abnormal mitochondria. As in PM, there is widespread MHC-I upregulation and endomysial inflammation composed predominantly of autoinvasive cytotoxic CD8+ cells and macrophages that surround and invade MHC-I restricted non-necrotic fibres. The inflammation can vary from florid to focal to sparse. Rimmed vacuoles are also a typical feature of inclusion body myositis (see Figure 25.43) but the number is variable and they may be sparse. Intranuclear inclusions may be seen. Multiple or single foci of amyloid deposits are present in vacuolated and non-vacuolated fibres, and best observed with Congo red staining viewed with fluorescence using an excitation filter suitable for rhodamine or Texas red. Some deposits are also seen with polarized light. The amyloid deposits contain Aβ42, plaque-like inclusions corresponding to 6–10 nm fibrils electron microscopically or aggregates of phosphorylated Tau, appearing with electron microscopy as 15–21 nm twisted paired helical filaments and best demonstrated as squiggly, linear or round p62/sequestrosome1 positive inclusions (Figure 25.103b).[7] Many other proteins also accumulate in IBM, including Tar-DNA–binding protein-43 (TDP-43), AβPP, ubiquitin, presenilin 1, apolipoprotein E, α-synuclein, prion protein, nuclear membrane proteins and survival motor neuron protein. Many of these proteins are found in the brains of patients with Alzheimer's disease, which has led to the hypothesis that a cascade of events leads to cell degeneration and misfolding of proteins.[6,101] TDP-43 and p62 currently seem to be the most useful to study in possible cases of IBM, but neither are specific and they can be seen in a variety of other disorders, including myofibrillar myopathies and cases with *GNE* or *VCP* mutations that show rimmed vacuoles (see Distal Myopathies, p. 1593).[115] Electron microscopy reveals cytomembranous debris, myelin-like whorls corresponding to the basophilic granules lining vacuoles. None of these changes is diagnostic for IBM, and absence of the characteristic paired helical filaments or amyloid fibrils does not exclude a diagnosis of IBM.

Immune-mediated necrotizing myopathy (IMNM), also known as necrotizing autoimmune myopathy (NAM), is a relatively newly recognized subgroup of IIM, and encompasses a heterogeneous group of diseases that share common pathological features of predominant myonecrosis, myophagocytosis and regeneration, scattered endomysial and perimysial macrophages with little or no lymphocytic inflammation in the biopsy. Some cases are associated with various autoantibodies. Clinical onset and progression are similar to PM/DM with subacute onset of symmetrical, proximal limb-girdle weakness. CK levels are usually markedly elevated (>10 times upper limit of normal) and EMG shows an irritable, myopathic pattern. Variable cardiac and lung involvement is also reported. Marked fibre size variation and hypertrophy may be seen, and this, in combination with the necrosis and regeneration and the subacute proximal weakness, may lead to the misdiagnosis of a dystrophy (Figure 25.104). IMNM can be associated with specific autoantibodies such as anti-SRP, anti-HMGCR, antisynthetase and anti-PMScl, connective tissue disease,

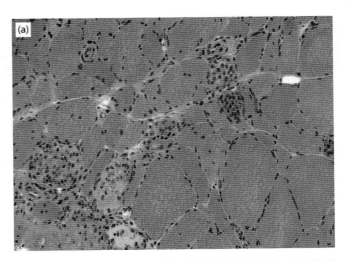

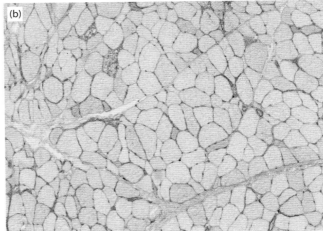

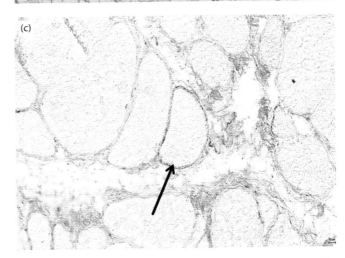

25.104 Immune-mediated anti-SRP necrotizing myopathy showing **(a)** pronounced necrosis of muscle fibres but little inflammation, **(b)** diffuse upregulation of major histocompatibility class 1 antigen on most fibres and **(c)** sarcolemmal complement C5b-9 labelling on a fibre (arrow).

paraneoplastic syndrome and viral infections such as HIV and hepatitis C. Variable, sometimes diffuse, strong MHC-I upregulation on non-necrotic fibres and prominent complement C5b-9 deposition on capillaries is reported in anti-SRP, anti-HMGCR and antisynthetase, and paraneoplastic

IMNM (see Figure 25.104). Fragmented perimysial connective tissue with alkaline phosphatase staining is seen in antisynthetase and paraneoplastic IMNM.[426] Statins (HMGCR inhibitors) can cause a toxic myopathy, which is self-limiting and may recover upon discontinuation of the drug.[265] The presentation is variable including muscle pain and weakness, raised CK, and rarely rhabdomyolysis. Muscle biopsies can reveal myonecrosis, lipid accumulation or type II atrophy.

The very rare necrotizing myopathy with pipestem capillaries shows distinct thickening of the capillary walls with complement deposition, and deposition of granular amorphous material in their basement membranes is seen electron microscopically. All reported patients had severe systemic disease such as neoplasia, vasculitis and interstitial lung disease. In contrast to non-IMNM due to exposure to drugs or toxins, IMNM cases show significantly greater MHC-I upregulation, capillary complement deposition, more inflammation and regeneration. In addition, in IMNM, a stronger Th1/classically activated macrophage M1 response was observed with elevated interferon-γ, TNF-α, interleukin-12 and STAT-1 levels in muscle. B-cells and high expression of CXCL13, a B-cell chemoattractant, were observed in a subset with defined antibodies. These findings may potentially lead to the development of new biomarkers and therapeutic targets in IMNM.[341]

Connective Tissue Disorders

Patients with IIM can present with or develop a connective tissue disease (CTD). They can have typical symptoms of CTD, such as dry mouth and eyes (Sjögren syndrome) or renal involvement (SLE), as well as IIM-related muscle symptoms – so called 'overlap myositis'. The most common secondary autoimmune diseases in overlap myositis are systemic sclerosis and mixed CTD. Myositis-associated antibodies (MSAs) are seen in both IIM as well as CTD and overlap myositis; for example, the majority of patients with myositis-scleroderma overlap syndrome are positive for anti-PM/Scl. Muscle biopsies may show fibre necrosis and inflammation, often with a vasculitis. True vasculitis is not seen in IIM and when present should prompt a search for an underlying CTD. In SLE, blood vessel walls may be thickened and may contain the tuboloreticular inclusions found in dermatomyositis. Non-specific myopathic changes, such as type 2 fibre atrophy, are also common in connective tissue disorders.

Fasciitis/Myofasciitis with Panniculitis

Fasciitis and panniculitis encompass a diverse clinicopathological spectrum of diseases where the inflammatory changes are centred on the fascia and subcutaneous fat respectively. The pathology may extend to the periphery of the fascicles. STIR MR imaging reveals hyperintense signal change in the fascial planes. A small proportion of individuals who receive vaccines containing aluminium oxyhydroxide as an adjuvant present with delayed onset of myalgia, chronic fatigue and cognitive dysfunction, and exhibit very long-term persistence of alum-loaded macrophages at the site of vaccination forming a lesion called macrophagic myofasciitis. There is focal infiltration of the epimysium, perimysium and perifascicular endomysium by circumscribed collections and sheets of CD68+ macrophages with diastase-resistant, PAS-positive basophilic cytoplasm, with a minor mainly CD8+ lymphocytic component often around blood vessels (Figure 25.105). Myofibres remote from the infiltrate are typically intact but the alum can reach the brain. Electron microscopy shows spicules of osmiophilic aluminium oxyhydroxide surrounded by discontinuous lysosomal membranes.[155]

Inflammatory myopathy with abundant macrophages is a recently defined entity. Patients present with a proximal myopathy; some are clinically diagnosed with DM based on a skin rash. The inflammation is seen typically at the periphery of the fascicles in the epimysium and perimysium comprising non-cohesive ribbons of CD68+ macrophages remote from necrotic myofibres and lacking the inclusions seen in macrophagic myofasciitis. In contrast to typical DM infiltrates, the macrophages are of the acute inflammatory MRP14+ type, CD20+ B-cells, CD3+ T-cells and CD123+ plasmacytoid dendritic cells are sparse. Capillary complement deposits are absent. Presently, it is unclear if IMAM and DM are pathogenically distinct or if they reflect different stages of the same disease.[51]

Fasciitis-panniculitis syndrome (FPS) comprises a group of disorders characterized by skin induration caused by chronic inflammation and fibrosis of the subcutaneous fascia and myosepta, as well as septal and lobular panniculitis. The prototype disorder is idiopathic eosinophilic fasciitis (Shulman syndrome) characterized by diffuse fasciitis comprising fibrosis and infiltrates of diffuse and perivascular, mainly CD8+ T-cells and/or eosinophils, eosinophilia and hypergammaglobulinaemia without visceral involvement or Raynaud's phenomenon. Eosinophils may be absent in the chronic stage or after steroid treatment. The disease can be triggered by exposure to toxins, treatment or trauma, and infections such as borreliosis and Mycoplasma arginine.[243] Histologically, FPS shows a subcutaneous septal-fascial-perimysial collagenous scaffold accompanied by an infiltrate of lymphocytes, plasma cells and histiocytes into the adjacent fat. Depending on the aetiology, eosinophils and mast cells can be identified. Secondary associations of FPS include cancer, graft-versus-host reaction, insect bites, post-traumatic or post-radiation reactions, and Sweet syndrome.

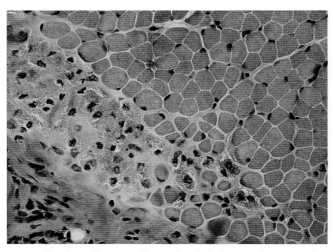

25.105 A case of macrophage fasciitis induced by vaccine showing abundant macrophages in the perimysium. H&E.

Other rare causes of fasciitis include necrotizing fasciitis due to bacterial infections, systemic non-Langerhans' histiocytosis and echovirus infection in congenital X-linked and acquired hypogammaglobulinaemia.

Granulomatous Myositis, Focal Myositis and Brachiocervical Inflammatory Myopathy

Granulomatous myositis is a rare disease characterized by discrete perimysial or endomysial epithelioid granulomas that are usually non-necrotizing, with variable interstitial inflammation and myonecrosis. Clinical presentation is usually that of proximal weakness and myalgias. Bulbar involvement may occur, and flexion contractures may be prominent in some. The association with sarcoidosis is well known and the prevalence of asymptomatic granulomatous myositis in sarcoid is reported to be as high as 50–80 per cent. Significant MHC-I upregulation may be seen in some cases mimicking IIM. Less well recognized is the association with infections (parasites, brucellosis, tuberculosis, syphilis), paraneoplastic manifestation in lymphoma, graft-versus-host disease, inflammatory bowel disease (Crohn's), CTD (rheumatoid arthritis) or as an autoimmune overlap syndrome with myasthenia gravis, myocarditis, thyroiditis and thymoma. The diagnosis of idiopathic/primary/isolated granulomatous myositis is one of exclusion.

Focal myositis is a rare entity that presents clinically as a solitary, intramuscular mass lesion and histologically corresponds to an inflammatory pseudotumour, with variable myopathic, focal neurogenic and inflammatory changes, and fibrosis. The infiltrate is macrophage and T-cell rich, with a prominent B-cell and plasmacytoid dendritic cell component present when the lesion is actively inflamed. MHC-I and IgG4 is weakly present, the latter may be linked to fibrosis. Common misdiagnoses include haematological or soft tissue malignancy, primary or proliferative myositis, myositis ossificans and inflammatory myofibroblastic tumour. Careful attention to the morphology and immunophenotype and the clinical presentation is necessary to avoid these pitfalls. Spontaneous regression is seen over time in most cases. There is no clear genetic or acquired etiological link. More recently it has been suggested that focal myositis may be a neurogenic phenomenon.[257]

Patients with brachiocervical inflammatory myopathy (BCIM) syndrome have progressive weakness in the proximal regions of the arms and neck. Histology reveals an active myopathic process with focal perimysial and perivascular inflammation with prominent B-cells, endomysial dendritic cells and complement C5b-9 staining of the endomysial connective tissue. There is a strong association with systemic autoimmune disorders and presence of antinuclear antibodies. There is a good response to steroids. It is unclear if BCIM represents a distinct form of autoimmune inflammatory myopathy.

Vasculitis of Skeletal Muscle

Vasculitis is infrequently encountered in skeletal muscle. The frequency of muscle involvement in systemic vasculitis is poorly defined. Clinicians use a two-tiered system of definite vasculitis when there is transmural inflammation with fibrinoid necrosis, mural destruction or leucocytoclasia, and probable vasculitis when there is a dense perivascular cellular cuff or transmural inflammation without the destructive features. Additional evidence of vascular damage including haemosiderin deposits, fibrous scarring or organization is used by many investigators. The presence of neurogenic atrophy, presumably due to concomitant peripheral nerve involvement (if present), points to a multisystem process. A degree of overlap occurs with IIM because perivascular inflammation can be prominent in DM an IMNM, leading to a potential misdiagnosis. However, a necrotizing component is unusual in IIM and if present points to a systemic vasculitic process such as polyarteritis nodosa, rheumatoid vasculitis, Wegener's, Churg–Strauss or drug-induced anti-neutrophil cytoplasmic antibodies (ANCA) vasculitis or sarcoidosis.[340]

Vasculitis restricted to skeletal muscle is even rarer. Granulomatous vasculitis may be seen in sarcoidosis and Wegener's disease. Eosinophils may be present in the infiltrates of Churg–Strauss vasculitis. A combined superficial peroneal nerve and peroneus brevis muscle biopsy has been shown to increase the diagnostic yield of vasculitis. However, no such advantage was noted combining sural nerve with vastus lateralis biopsy. The choice of biopsy may vary depending on the institutional preference, but the muscle and/or nerve biopsied should be clinically and/or electrophysiologically affected.

Viral and Bacterial Myositis

Several infections are known to induce an acute myositis.[125] These include influenza viruses, Coxsackie viruses, Epstein–Barr virus, cytomegalovirus, herpes simplex virus, hepatitis C virus, human immunodeficiency virus and human T-cell lymphotropic virus type 1. A variable degree of muscle fibre necrosis and inflammatory infiltration occur. Onset can be acute, with weakness and marked muscle tenderness that involves all major muscle groups. Myoglobinuria may be present. Symptoms often improve rapidly once the acute phase is over, even in the absence of specific therapy.

Drug and Toxic Myopathies

A variety of drugs and toxins can affect muscle and nerves.[117] Some of these are common, whereas others are rare. Statins are now widely prescribed and are a common cause of myalgia and raised CK. Alcohol is also a common cause of myopathy, and drugs of abuse frequently cause muscle necrosis. Several other prescribed drugs that may induce myopathy include corticosteroids, ciclosporin, D-penicillamine, chloroquine, vincristine and zidovudine. Toxic effects can be induced in muscle by various dietary supplements, such as geranium, by excess vitamin E and by snake venoms.

The pathological changes induced in muscle by drugs are non-specific, are variable in degree, and may be focal or diffuse. Necrosis, which may be acute, is common, as is type 2 fibre atrophy. A well-established side effect of steroids is type 2 fibre atrophy, particularly of type 2B fibres. Steroids can also induce selective loss of myosin from A-bands in 'critical illness myopathy'. This may affect patients receiving high doses of corticosteroids and neuromuscular blocking agents to assist mechanical ventilation and occurs when the paralysing agent is withdrawn.

A vacuolar myopathy can be induced by some anti-malarial drugs, such as chloroquine.[117] These autophagic vacuoles contain membranous myelin-like whorls, and cell debris and curvilinear bodies are a feature associated with chloroquine. Vincristine and colchicine can also induce vacuoles and the formation of spheromembranous bodies, which are thought to be derived from the sarcoplasmic reticulum (Figure 25.106). A second type of vacuolar change is associated with hypokalaemic agents, such as diuretics, laxatives and liquorice derivatives. These vacuoles are thought to originate from T-tubules.

The effects of zidovudine on mitochondria are reflected by the presence of ragged-red fibres and ultrastructurally abnormal mitochondria. Geranium-based elixirs and dietary supplements can also influence mitochondrial function, and ragged-red fibres, COX-negative fibres and ultrastructural mitochondrial damage may be seen.

Endocrine and Systemic Myopathies

Hormones have an important role in maintaining normal muscle function, and myopathies have been described in association with either an excess or a deficiency of several, in particular thyroid and parathyroid hormones, glucocorticoids, growth hormone and insulin.[117] In most cases, muscle involvement is an incidental feature of the disorder but often reversible with correction of hormone levels. Muscle symptoms may be the presenting features of endocrine imbalance and prompt the diagnosis of an underlying disorder, such as thyrotoxicosis. There is often a predominant proximal weakness with varying degrees of wasting, and in many cases the weakness is disproportional to the degree of muscle wasting. Other symptoms may include muscle pain, cramps, stiffness, periodic paralysis (hypothyroidism) and ocular involvement (hyperthyroidism). Muscle pathology may be minimal or may show non-specific changes such as type 2 fibre atrophy, type 1 fibre hypertrophy or an increase in internal nuclei. Additional pathological features may be necrosis, an increased percentage of type 1 fibres, and inflammatory infiltrates, which can make the differential diagnosis with polymyositis difficult, especially if MHC-I is not studied. Hypothyroidism during pregnancy can also affect the expression of myosin isoforms and fibre typing in the fetus.[387]

Vitamin deficiencies such as vitamin B12, C, D or E result in abnormalities, some of which affect muscle. There are both acquired and hereditary forms of vitamin E deficiency. Malabsorption of vitamin E can lead to spinocerebellar ataxia, dysmetria, areflexia and loss of vibratory sensation.[109] Muscle biopsies show typical electron-dense inclusions that are positive for acid phosphatase, non-specific esterase and are autofluorescent.[117]

Selenium deficiency, especially in association with vitamin E deficiency can result in muscle symptoms such as myalgia and weakness. Muscle biopsies can show non-specific changes such as type 2 fibre atrophy and mitochondrial changes have been reported.[69,356]

Malignancies can be associated with various neurological symptoms. Type 2 fibre atrophy is a common non-specific feature associated with malignancies. Inflammatory myopathies, in particular dermatomyositis, are associated with malignancies, especially pulmonary, gastrointestinal, ovarian and nasopharyngeal carcinomas.[506]

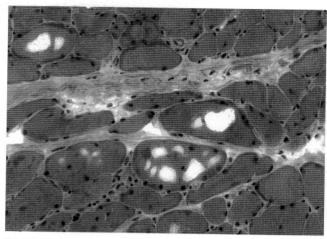

25.106 Vacuoles of varying size in a case treated with colchicine. H&E.

Amyloid is a proteinaceous material with a fibrillar structure that stains red with Congo red and is biorefringent with polarized light. It can accumulate (amyloidosis) both intracellularly and extracellularly in several tissues, and may be secondary to malignancies, chronic inflammatory conditions, genetic diseases (see Recessive Limb-Girdle Muscular Dystrophies, p. 1561) and also to ageing.[416] Amyloid myopathy in the majority of patients results from the deposition of amyloid immunoglobulin light chains, chiefly the lambda type. Clinical features include proximal muscle weakness but distal muscle weakness may occur. Dysphagia, macroglossia and/or muscle pseudo-hypertrophy are frequent but not consistent findings. Congestive heart failure and cardiomyopathy can be complications. Muscle biopsies show perivascular and endomysial/perimysial deposition of amyloid, and neurogenic atrophy of muscle fibres may be present. Electron microscopy shows blood vessels and muscle fibres coated with amyloid fibrils.[68,117]

Muscle and Ageing

Sarcopenia (loss of muscle mass) is common in ageing and there is considerable research into its pathogenesis.[206] The reduction of muscle mass is due both to muscle fibre atrophy, particularly type 2 fibres, and to loss of muscle fibres, resulting in a higher proportion of type 1 fibres. Although exercise maintains the size and strength of fibres, no way to halt the loss of type 2 fibres has been found. Mitochondrial DNA shows age-related accumulation of mutations in post-mitotic tissues, and an increase in the number of COX-negative fibres and ragged-red fibres is seen in the muscle.[168]

ACKNOWLEDGEMENTS

We are grateful to Dr Cecilia Jimenez-Mallebrera for her valuable contribution to this chapter in the previous edition. The financial support of the National Specialist Commissioning Team for Rare Neuromuscular Disorders to the Dubowitz Neuromuscular Centre for Congenital Muscular Dystrophies and Congenital Myopathies is gratefully acknowledged. Also funding from the Muscular Dystrophy Association of America to SCB is gratefully acknowledged.

REFERENCES

1. Allamand V, Brinas L, Richard P, *et al.* ColVI myopathies: where do we stand, where do we go? *Skelet Muscle* 2011;**1**:30.

2. Allamand V, Richard P, Lescure A, *et al.* A single homozygous point mutation in a 3′ untranslated region motif of selenoprotein N mRNA causes SEPN1-related myopathy. *EMBO Report* 2006;**7**:450–4.

3. Al-Qusairi L,Laporte J. T-tubule biogenesis and triad formation in skeletal muscle and implication in human diseases. *Skelet Muscle* 2011;**1**:26.

4. Appleyard ST, Dunn MJ, Dubowitz V, Rose ML. Increased expression of HLA ABC class I antigens by muscle fibres in Duchenne muscular dystrophy, inflammatory myopathy, and other neuromuscular disorders. *Lancet* 1985;**1**:361–3.

5. Argov Z,Mitrani-Rosenbaum S. Hereditary inclusion body myopathies. In: Karpati G, Hilton-Jones D, Bushby K, Griggs R eds *Disorders of voluntary muscle* 8th edn. Cambridge: Cambridge Iniversity Press, 2010.

6. Askanas V, Engel WK. Sporadic inclusion-body myositis: conformational multifactorial ageing-related degenerative muscle disease associated with proteasomal and lysosomal inhibition, endoplasmic reticulum stress, and accumulation of amyloid-beta 42 oligomers and phosphorylated tau. *Presse Med* 2011;**40**: e219–35.

7. Askanas V, Engel WK, Nogalska A. Pathogenic considerations in sporadic inclusion-body myositis, a degenerative muscle disease associated with aging and abnormalities of myoproteostasis. *J Neuropathol Exp Neurol* 2012;**71**:680–93.

8. Askanas V, Serdaroglu P, Engel WK, Alvarez RB. Immunolocalization of ubiquitin in muscle biopsies of patients with inclusion body myositis and oculopharyngeal muscular dystrophy. *Neurosci Lett* 1991;**130**:73–6.

9. Attali R, Warwar N, Israel A, *et al.* Mutation of SYNE-1, encoding an essential component of the nuclear lamina, is responsible for autosomal recessive arthrogryposis. *Hum Mol Genet* 2009;**18**:3462–9.

10. Auer-Grumbach M, Olschewski A, Papic L, *et al.* Alterations in the ankyrin domain of TRPV4 cause congenital distal SMA, scapuloperoneal SMA and HMSN2C. *Nat Genet* 2010;**42**:160–4.

11. Aumailley M, Bruckner-Tuderman L, Carter WG, *et al.* A simplified laminin nomenclature. *Matrix Biol* 2005;**24**: 326–32.

12. Baghdiguian S, Martin M, Richard I, *et al.* Calpain 3 deficiency is associated with myonuclear apoptosis and profound perturbation of the I-kappa B-alpha/NF-kappa-B pathway in limb-girdle muscular dystrophy type 2A. *Nat Med* 1999;**5**:503–11.

13. Bandschapp O, Girard T. Malignant hyperthermia. *Swiss Med Wkly* 2012;**142**:w13652.

14. Banks RW, Hulliger M, Saed HH, Stacey MJ. A comparative analysis of the encapsulated end-organs of mammalian skeletal muscles and of their sensory nerve endings. *J Anat* 2009;**214**:859–87.

15. Banwell BL, Russel J, Fukudome T, *et al.* Myopathy, myasthenic syndrome, and epidermolysis bullosa simplex due to plectin deficiency. *J Neuropathol Exp Neurol* 1999;**58**:832–46.

16. Bao X, Kobayashi M, Hatakeyama S, *et al.* Tumor suppressor function of laminin-binding alpha-dystroglycan requires a distinct beta3-N-acetylglucosaminyltransferase. *Proc Natl Acad Sci U S A* 2009;**106**:12109–14.

17. Bao ZZ, Lakonishok M, Kaufman S, Horwitz AF. Alpha 7 beta 1 integrin is a component of the myotendinous junction on skeletal muscle. *J Cell Sci* 1993;**106** (**Pt 2**):579–89.

18. Barresi R. From proteins to genes: immunoanalysis in the diagnosis of muscular dystrophies. *Skelet Muscle* 2011;**1**:24.

19. Barresi R, Campbell KP. Dystroglycan: from biosynthesis to pathogenesis of human disease. *J Cell Sci* 2006;**119**:199–207.

20. Baumann M, Giunta C, Krabichler B, *et al.* Mutations in FKBP14 cause a variant of Ehlers-Danlos syndrome with progressive kyphoscoliosis, myopathy, and hearing loss. *Am J Hum Genet* 2012;**90**:201–16.

21. Bengoechea R, Tapia O, Casafont I, *et al.* Nuclear speckles are involved in nuclear aggregation of PABPN1 and in the pathophysiology of oculopharyngeal muscular dystrophy. *Neurobiol Dis* 2012;**46**:118–29.

22. Bengtsson L, Otto H. LUMA interacts with emerin and influences its distribution at the inner nuclear membrane. *J Cell Sci* 2008;**121**:536–48.

23. Benveniste O, Romero NB. Myositis or dystrophy? Traps and pitfalls. *Presse Med* 2011;**40**: e249–55.

24. Benveniste O, Laforet P, Dubourg O, *et al.* Stem cell transplantation in a patient with late-onset nemaline myopathy and gammopathy. *Neurology* 2008;**71**:531–2.

25. Berardo A, DiMauro S, Hirano M. A diagnostic algorithm for metabolic myopathies. *Curr Neurol Neurosci Rep* 2010;**10**:118–26.

26. Bernheim L, Hamann M, Liu JH, *et al.* Role of nicotinic acetylcholine receptors at the vertebrate myotendinous junction: a hypothesis. *Neuromuscul Disord* 1996;**6**:211–4.

27. Bertini E, D'Amico A, Gualandi F, Petrini S. Congenital muscular dystrophies: a brief review. *Semin Pediatr Neurol* 2011;**18**:277–88.

28. Bevilacqua JA, Bitoun M, Biancalana V, *et al.* "Necklace" fibers, a new histological marker of late-onset MTM1-related centronuclear myopathy. *Acta Neuropathol* 2009;**117**:283–91.

29. Bitoun M, Bevilacqua JA, Prudhon B, *et al.* Dynamin 2 mutations cause sporadic centronuclear myopathy with neonatal onset. *Ann Neurol* 2007;**62**:666–70.

30. Bloemberg D, Quadrilatero J. Rapid determination of myosin heavy chain expression in rat, mouse, and human skeletal muscle using multicolor immunofluorescence analysis. *PLoS One* 2012;**7**: e35273.

31. Bodine SC, Latres E, Baumhueter S, *et al.* Identification of ubiquitin ligases required for skeletal muscle atrophy. *Science* 2001;**294**:1704–8.

32. Bohm J, Chevessier F, Maues De Paula A, *et al.* Constitutive activation of the calcium sensor STIM1 causes tubular-aggregate myopathy. *Am J Hum Genet* 2013;**92**:271–8.

33. Boldrin L, Muntoni F, Morgan JE. Are human and mouse satellite cells really the same? *J Histochem Cytochem* 2010;**58**:941–55.

34. Bolduc V, Marlow G, Boycott KM, *et al.* Recessive mutations in the putative calcium-activated chloride channel Anoctamin 5 cause proximal LGMD2L and distal MMD3 muscular dystrophies. *Am J Hum Genet* 2010;**86**:213–21.

35. Bonnemann CG. The collagen VI-related myopathies: muscle meets its matrix. *Nat Rev Neurol* 2011;**7**:379–90.

36. Bonnemann C, Bertini E. Dystrophic myopathies of early childhood onset (congenital muscular dystrophies). In: Karpati G, Hilton Jones D, Busby K, Griggs R eds. *Disorders of voluntary Muscle* 8th edn. Cambridge: Cambridge University Press, 2010:257–81.

37. Borg K, Stucka R, Locke M, *et al.* Intragenic deletion of TRIM32 in compound heterozygotes with sarcotubular myopathy/LGMD2H. *Hum Mutat* 2009;**30**:e831–44.

38. Bourgeois JM,Tarnopolsky MA. Pathology of skeletal muscle in mitochondrial disorders. *Mitochondrion* 2004;**4**:441–52.

39. Brais B. Oculopharyngeal muscular dystrophy: a polyalanine myopathy. *Curr Neurol Neurosci Rep* 2009;**9**:76–82.

40. Briand N, Dugail I, Le Lay S. Cavin proteins: New players in the caveolae field. *Biochimie* 2011;**93**:71–7.

41. Broccolini A, Gidaro T, Morosetti R, *et al.* Hereditary inclusion-body myopathy with sparing of the quadriceps: the many tiles of an incomplete puzzle. *Acta Myol* 2011;**30**:91–5.

42. Brockington M, Brown SC, Lampe A, *et al.* Prenatal diagnosis of Ullrich congenital muscular dystrophy using haplotype analysis and collagen VI immunocytochemistry. *Prenat Diagn* 2004;**24**:440–4.

43. Brockington M, Yuva Y, Prandini P, *et al.* Mutations in the fukutin-related protein gene (FKRP) identify limb girdle muscular dystrophy 2I as a milder allelic variant of congenital muscular dystrophy MDC1C. *Hum Mol Genet* 2001;**10**:2851–9.

44. Brooke MH, Engel WK. The histographic analysis of human muscle biopsies with regard to fiber types 1. Adult male and female. *Neurology* 1969;**19**:221–33.

45. Brooke MH, Engel WK. The histographic analysis of human muscle biopsies with regard to fiber types 2. Diseases of the upper and lower motor neuron. *Neurology* 1969;**19**:378–93.

46. Brooke MH, Engel WK. The histographic analysis of human muscle biopsies with regard to fiber types. 3. Myotonias, myasthenia gravis, and hypokalemic periodic paralysis. *Neurology* 1969;**19**:469–77.

47. Brooke MH, Engel WK. The histographic analysis of human muscle biopsies with regard to fiber types. 4. Children's biopsies. *Neurology* 1969;**19**:591–605.

48. Brown SC, Lucy JA eds. *Dystrophin: gene, protein and cell biology.* Cambridge: Cambridge University Press, 1997.

49. Brown SC, Muntoni F, Sewry CA. Non-sarcolemmal muscular dystrophies. *Brain Pathol* 2001;**11**:193–205.

50. Brown SC, Torelli S, Brockington M, *et al*. Abnormalities in alpha-dystroglycan expression in MDC1C and LGMD2I muscular dystrophies. *Am J Pathol* 2004;**164**:727–37.

51. Brunn A, Hans VJ, Vogelgesang S, Deckert M. Inflammatory myopathy with abundant macrophages and dermatomyositis: two stages of one disorder or two distinct entities? *Acta Neuropathol* 2009;**118**:793–801.

52. Burton EA, Tinsley JM, Holzfeind PJ, *et al*. A second promoter provides an alternative target for therapeutic up-regulation of utrophin in Duchenne muscular dystrophy. *Proc Natl Acad Sci U S A* 1999;**96**:14025–30.

53. Bushby K. Diagnosis and management of the limb girdle muscular dystrophies. *Pract Neurol* 2009;**9**:314–23.

54. Bushby K, Anderson LV, Pollitt C, *et al*. Abnormal merosin in adults. A new form of late onset muscular dystrophy not linked to chromosome 6q2. *Brain* 1998;**121**:581–8.

55. Buysse K, Riemersma M, Powell G, *et al*. Missense mutations in beta-1,3-N-acetylglucosaminyltransferase 1 (B3GNT1) cause Walker-Warburg syndrome. *Hum Mol Genet* 2013;**22**:1746–54.

56. Cafferty MS, Lovelace RE, Hays AP, *et al*. Polyglucosan body disease. *Muscle Nerve* 1991;**14**:102–7.

57. Capetanaki Y, Bloch RJ, Kouloumenta A, *et al*. Muscle intermediate filaments and their links to membranes and membranous organelles. *Exp Cell Res* 2007;**313**:2063–76.

58. Cardasis CA, Cooper GW. An analysis of nuclear numbers in individual muscle fibers during differentiation and growth: a satellite cell-muscle fiber growth unit. *J Exp Zool* 1975;**191**:347–58.

59. Carmignac V, Durbeej M. Cell-matrix interactions in muscle disease. *J Pathol* 2012;**226**:200–18.

60. Carmignac V, Salih MA, Quijano-Roy S, *et al*. C-terminal titin deletions cause a novel early-onset myopathy with fatal cardiomyopathy. *Ann Neurol* 2007;**61**:340–51.

61. Carss KJ, Stevens E, Foley AR, *et al*. Mutations in GDP-mannose pyrophosphorylase B cause congenital and limb-girdle muscular dystrophies associated with hypoglycosylation of alpha-dystroglycan. *Am J Hum Genet* 2013;**93**:29–41.

62. Cartegni L, di Barletta MR, Barresi R, *et al*. Heart-specific localization of emerin: new insights into Emery-Dreifuss muscular dystrophy. *Hum Mol Genet* 1997;**6**:2257–64.

63. Casciola-Rosen L, Mammen AL. Myositis autoantibodies. *Curr Opin Rheumatol* 2012;**24**:602–8.

64. Cashman NR, Covault J, Wollman RL, Sanes JR. Neural cell adhesion molecule in normal, denervated, and myopathic human muscle. *Ann Neurol* 1987;**21**:481–9.

65. Castets P, Bertrand AT, Beuvin M, *et al*. Satellite cell loss and impaired muscle regeneration in selenoprotein N deficiency. *Hum Mol Genet* 2011;**20**:694–704.

66. Cauchi RJ. SMN and Gemins: 'we are family' ... or are we?: insights into the partnership between Gemins and the spinal muscular atrophy disease protein SMN. *Bioessays* 2010;**32**:1077–89.

67. Chahin N, Selcen D, Engel AG. Sporadic late onset nemaline myopathy. *Neurology* 2005;**65**:1158–64.

68. Chapin JE, Kornfeld M, Harris A. Amyloid myopathy: characteristic features of a still underdiagnosed disease. *Muscle Nerve* 2005;**31**:266–72.

69. Chariot P, Bignani O. Skeletal muscle disorders associated with selenium deficiency in humans. *Muscle Nerve* 2003;**27**:662–8.

70. Charlton R, Henderson M, Richards J, *et al*. Immunohistochemical analysis of calpain 3: advantages and limitations in diagnosing LGMD2A. *Neuromuscul Disord* 2009;**19**:449–57.

71. Chemla JC, Kanter RJ, Carboni MP, Smith EC. Two children with "dropped head" syndrome due to lamin A/C mutations. *Muscle Nerve* 2010;**42**:839–41.

72. Chevessier F, Bauche-Godard S, Leroy JP, *et al*. The origin of tubular aggregates in human myopathies. *J Pathol* 2005;**207**:313–23.

73. Chevron MP, Tuffery S, Echenne B, *et al*. Becker muscular dystrophy: demonstration of the carrier status of a female by immunoblotting and immunostaining. *Neuromuscul Disord* 1992;**2**:47–50.

74. Chinoy H, Lamb JA, Ollier WE, Cooper RG. An update on the immunogenetics of idiopathic inflammatory myopathies: major histocompatibility complex and beyond. *Curr Opin Rheumatol* 2009;**21**:588–93.

75. Christopher-Stine L. Neurologists are from Mars. Rheumatologists are from Venus: differences in approach to classifying the idiopathic inflammatory myopathies. *Curr Opin Rheumatol* 2010;**22**:623–6.

76. Cirak S, Foley AR, Herrmann R, *et al*. ISPD gene mutations are a common cause of congenital and limb-girdle muscular dystrophies. *Brain* 2013;**136**:269–81.

77. Cirak S, von Deimling F, Sachdev S, *et al*. Kelch-like homologue 9 mutation is associated with an early onset autosomal dominant distal myopathy. *Brain* 2010;**133**:2123–35.

78. Claeys KG, Fardeau M, Schroder R, *et al*. Electron microscopy in myofibrillar myopathies reveals clues to the mutated gene. *Neuromuscul Disord* 2008;**18**:656–66.

79. Claeys KG, Maisonobe T, Bohm J, *et al*. Phenotype of a patient with recessive centronuclear myopathy and a novel BIN1 mutation. *Neurology* 2010;**74**:519–21.

80. Claeys KG, van der Ven PF, Behin A, *et al*. Differential involvement of sarcomeric proteins in myofibrillar myopathies: a morphological and immunohistochemical study. *Acta Neuropathol* 2009;**117**:293–307.

81. Clark KA, McElhinny AS, Beckerle MC, Gregorio CC. Striated muscle cytoarchitecture: an intricate web of form and function. *Annu Rev Cell Dev Biol* 2002;**18**:637–706.

82. Clarke NF. Congenital fibre type disproportion: a syndrome at the crossroads of the congenital myopathies. *Neuromuscul Disord* 2011;**21**:252–3.

83. Clarke NF, Kidson W, Quijano-Roy S, *et al*. SEPN1: associated with congenital fiber-type disproportion and insulin resistance. *Ann Neurol* 2006;**59**:546–52.

84. Clarke NF, Waddell LB, Cooper ST, *et al*. Recessive mutations in RYR1 are a common cause of congenital fiber type disproportion. *Hum Mutat* 2010;**31**:e1544–50.

85. Clarke NF, Waddell LB, Sie LT, *et al*. Mutations in TPM2 and congenital fibre type disproportion. *Neuromuscul Disord* 2012;**22**:955–8.

86. Clement EM, Feng L, Mein R, *et al*. Relative frequency of congenital muscular dystrophy subtypes: analysis of the UK diagnostic service 2001–2008. *Neuromuscul Disord* 2012;**22**:522–7.

87. Clement E, Mercuri E, Godfrey C, *et al*. Brain involvement in muscular dystrophies with defective dystroglycan glycosylation. *Ann Neurol* 2008;**64**:573–82.

88. Clerk A, Sewry CA, Dubowitz V, Strong PN. Characterisation of dystrophin in fetuses at risk for Duchenne muscular dystrophy. *J Neurol Sci* 1992;**111**:82–91.

89. Clerk A, Strong PN, Sewry CA. Characterisation of dystrophin during development of human skeletal muscle. *Development* 1992;**114**:395–402.

90. Cohen S, Brault JJ, Gygi SP, *et al*. During muscle atrophy, thick, but not thin, filament components are degraded by MuRF1-dependent ubiquitylation. *J Cell Biol* 2009;**185**:1083–95.

91. Cohn RD, Herrmann R, Wewer UM, Voit T. Changes of laminin beta 2 chain expression in congenital muscular dystrophy. *Neuromuscul Disord* 1997;**7**:373–8.

92. Cohn RD, Mayer U, Saher G, *et al*. Secondary reduction of alpha7B integrin in laminin alpha 2 deficient congenital muscular dystrophy supports an additional transmembrane link in skeletal muscle. *J Neurol Sci* 1999;**163**:140–52.

93. Collins J, Bonnemann CG. Congenital muscular dystrophies: toward molecular therapeutic interventions. *Curr Neurol Neurosci Rep* 2010;**10**:83–91.

94. Confalonieri P, Oliva L, Andreetta F, *et al*. Muscle inflammation and MHC class I up-regulation in muscular dystrophy with lack of dysferlin: an immunopathological study. *J Neuroimmunol* 2003;**142**:130–6.

95. Cori GT. Biochemical aspects of glycogen deposition disease. *Bibl Paediatr* 1958;**14**:344–58.

96. Cossins J, Belaya K, Hicks D, *et al*. Congenital myasthenic syndromes due to mutations in ALG2 and ALG14. *Brain* 2013;**136**:944–56.

97. Couarch P, Vernia S, Gourfinkel-An I, *et al*. Lafora progressive myoclonus epilepsy: NHLRC1 mutations affect glycogen metabolism. *J Mol Med* 2011;**89**:915–25.

98. Crosbie RH, Heighway J, Venzke DP, *et al*. Sarcospan, the 25-kDa transmembrane component of the dystrophin-glycoprotein complex. *J Biol Chem* 1997;**272**:31221–4.

99. Cullup T, Kho AL, Dionisi-Vici C, *et al*. Recessive mutations in EPG5 cause Vici syndrome, a multisystem disorder with defective autophagy. *Nat Genet* 2012;**45**:83–7.

100. Dalakas MC. Pathophysiology of inflammatory and autoimmune myopathies. *Presse Med* 2011;**40**: e237–47.

101. Dalakas MC. Review: An update on inflammatory and autoimmune myopathies. *Neuropathol Appl Neurobiol* 2011;**37**:226–42.

102. Dawson TP, Neal JW, Llewellyn L, Thomas C. *Neuropathology techniques.* London: Hodder Arnold, 2003:1–288.

103. de Greef JC, Lemmers RJ, Camano P, *et al.* Clinical features of facioscapulohumeral muscular dystrophy 2. *Neurology* 2010;**75**:1548–54.

104. De Luna N, Freixas A, Gallano P, *et al.* Dysferlin expression in monocytes: a source of mRNA for mutation analysis. *Neuromuscul Disord* 2007;**17**:69–76.

105. Deconinck AE, Rafael JA, Skinner JA, *et al.* Utrophin-dystrophin-deficient mice as a model for Duchenne muscular dystrophy. *Cell* 1997;**90**:717–27.

106. DeJesus-Hernandez M, Mackenzie IR, Boeve BF, *et al.* Expanded GGGGCC hexanucleotide repeat in noncoding region of C9ORF72 causes chromosome 9p-linked FTD and ALS. *Neuron* 2011;**72**:245–56.

107. Deodato F, Sabatelli M, Ricci E, *et al.* Hypermyelinating neuropathy, mental retardation and epilepsy in a case of merosin deficiency. *Neuromuscul Disord* 2002;**12**:392–8.

108. Di Blasi C, Morandi L, Raffaele di Barletta M, *et al.* Unusual expression of emerin in a patient with X-linked Emery-Dreifuss muscular dystrophy. *Neuromuscul Disord* 2000;**10**:567–71.

109. Di Donato I, Bianchi S, Federico A. Ataxia with vitamin E deficiency: update of molecular diagnosis. *Neurol Sci* 2010;**31**:511–5.

110. Dieterich K, Quijano-Roy S, Monnier N, *et al.* The neuronal endopeptidase ECEL1 is associated with a distinct form of recessive distal arthrogryposis. *Hum Mol Genet* 2013;**22**:1483–92.

111. Dimachkie MM. Idiopathic inflammatory myopathies. *J Neuroimmunol* 2011;**231**:32–42.

112. Dimauro S, Akman O, Hays AP. Disorders of carbohydrate metabolism. *Handb Clin Neurol* 2007;**86**:167–82.

113. DiMauro S, Spiegel R. Progress and problems in muscle glycogenoses. *Acta Myol* 2011;**30**:96–102.

114. Draeger A, Weeds AG, Fitzsimons RB. Primary, secondary and tertiary myotubes in developing skeletal muscle: a new approach to the analysis of human myogenesis. *J Neurol Sci* 1987;**81**:19–43.

115. Dubourg O, Wanschitz J, Maisonobe T, *et al.* Diagnostic value of markers of muscle degeneration in sporadic inclusion body myositis. *Acta Myol* 2011;**30**:103–8.

116. Dubowitz V. Chaos in the classification of SMA: a possible resolution. *Neuromuscul Disord* 1995;**5**:3–5.

117. Dubowitz V, Sewry CA, Oldfors A. *Muscle biopsy: a practical approach*, 4th edn. Oxford: Elsevier, 2013.

118. Duff RM, Tay V, Hackman P, *et al.* Mutations in the N-terminal actin-binding domain of filamin C cause a distal myopathy. *Am J Hum Genet* 2011;**88**:729–40.

119. Durieux AC, Prudhon B, Guicheney P, Bitoun M. Dynamin 2 and human diseases. *J Mol Med* 2010;**88**:339–50.

120. Durmus H, Laval SH, Deymeer F, *et al.* Oculopharyngodistal myopathy is a distinct entity: clinical and genetic features of 47 patients. *Neurology* 2011;**76**:227–35.

121. Dyck PJ,Thomas PK. *Peripheral neuropathies*, 4th edn. London: WB Saunders, 2005.

122. Edström L, Thornell LE, Albo J, *et al.* Myopathy with respiratory failure and typical myofibrillar lesions. *J Neurol Sci* 1990;**96**:211–28.

123. Edwards RH, Round JM, Jones DA. Needle biopsy of skeletal muscle: a review of 10 years experience. *Muscle Nerve* 1983;**6**:676–83.

124. Ehrhardt J, Morgan J. Regenerative capacity of skeletal muscle. *Curr Opin Neurol* 2005;**18**:548–53.

125. El-Beshbishi SN, Ahmed NN, Mostafa SH, El-Ganainy GA. Parasitic infections and myositis. *Parasitol Res* 2012;**110**:1–18.

126. Emery AE. Population frequencies of inherited neuromuscular diseases: a world survey. *Neuromuscul Disord* 1991;**1**:19–29.

127. Emery AE. The muscular dystrophies. *BMJ* 1998;**317**:991–5.

128. Emery AEH, Muntoni F. *Duchenne muscular dystrophy*, 3rd edn. Oxford: Oxford University Press, 2003.

129. Engel AG. Current status of the congenital myasthenic syndromes. *Neuromuscul Disord* 2012;**22**:99–111.

130. Fananapazir L, Dalakas MC, Cyran F, *et al.* Missense mutations in the beta-myosin heavy-chain gene cause central core disease in hypertrophic cardiomyopathy. *Proc Natl Acad Sci U S A* 1993;**90**:3993–7.

131. Fanin M, Angelini C. Muscle pathology in dysferlin deficiency. *Neuropathol Appl Neurobiol* 2002;**28**:461–70.

132. Fardeau M, Godet-Guillain J, Tomé FM. A new familial muscular disorder demonstrated by the intra-sarcoplasmic accumulation of a granulo-filamentous material which is dense on electron microscopy (author's translation) *Revue Neurologique (Paris)* 1978 **134**:411–25 .

133. Fardeau M, Matsumura K, Tome FM, *et al.* Deficiency of the 50 kDa dystrophin associated glycoprotein (adhalin) in severe autosomal recessive muscular dystrophies in children native from European countries. *C R Acad Sci III* 1993;**316**:799–804.

134. Farrugia ME, Vincent A. Autoimmune mediated neuromuscular junction defects. *Curr Opin Neurol* 2010;**23**:489–95.

135. Feldkirchner S, Walter MC, Muller S, *et al.* Proteomic characterization of aggregate components in an intrafamilial variable FHL1-associated myopathy. *Neuromuscul Disord* 2013;**23**:418–26.

136. Ferlini A, Sewry C, Melis MA, *et al.* X-linked dilated cardiomyopathy and the dystrophin gene. *Neuromuscul Disord* 1999;**9**:339–46.

137. Ferreiro A, Ceuterick-de Groote C, Marks JJ, *et al.* Desmin-related myopathy with Mallory body-like inclusions is caused by mutations of the selenoprotein N gene. *Ann Neurol* 2004;**55**:676–86.

138. Ferreiro A, Estournet B, Chateau D, *et al.* Multi-minicore disease: searching for boundaries: phenotype analysis of 38 cases. *Ann Neurol* 2000;**48**:745–57.

139. Ferreiro A, Quijano-Roy S, Pichereau C, *et al.* Mutations of the selenoprotein N gene, which is implicated in rigid spine muscular dystrophy, cause the classical phenotype of multiminicore disease: reassessing the nosology of early-onset myopathies. *Am J Hum Genet* 2002;**71**:739–49.

140. Fidzianska A, Toniolo D, Hausmanowa-Petrusewicz I. Ultrastructural abnormality of sarcolemmal nuclei in Emery-Dreifuss muscular dystrophy (EDMD). *J Neurol Sci* 1998;**159**:88–93.

141. Finsterer J. Perspectives of Kennedy's disease. *J Neurol Sci* 2010;**298**:1–10.

142. Fischer D, Herasse M, Bitoun M, *et al.* Characterization of the muscle involvement in dynamin 2-related centronuclear myopathy. *Brain* 2006;**129**:1463–9.

143. Fischer D, Kley RA, Strach K, *et al.* Distinct muscle imaging patterns in myofibrillar myopathies. *Neurology* 2008;**71**:758–65.

144. Foroud T, Pankratz N, Batchman AP, *et al.* A mutation in myotilin causes spheroid body myopathy. *Neurology* 2005;**65**:1936–40.

145. Forrest K, Mellerio JE, Robb S, *et al.* Congenital muscular dystrophy, myasthenic symptoms and epidermolysis bullosa simplex (EBS) associated with mutations in the PLEC1 gene encoding plectin. *Neuromuscul Disord* 2010;**20**:709–11.

146. Forrest KM, Al-Sarraj S, Sewry C, *et al.* Infantile onset myofibrillar myopathy due to recessive CRYAB mutations. *Neuromuscul Disord* 2011;**21**:37–40.

147. Frock RL, Kudlow BA, Evans AM, *et al.* Lamin A/C and emerin are critical for skeletal muscle satellite cell differentiation. *Genes Dev* 2006;**20**: 486–500.

148. Frosk P, Greenberg CR, Tennese AA, *et al.* The most common mutation in FKRP causing limb girdle muscular dystrophy type 2I (LGMD2I) may have occurred only once and is present in Hutterites and other populations. *Hum Mutat* 2005;**25**:38–44.

149. Frost AR, Bohm SV, Sewduth RN, *et al.* Heterozygous deletion of a 2-Mb region including the dystroglycan gene in a patient with mild myopathy, facial hypotonia, oral-motor dyspraxia and white matter abnormalities. *Eur J Hum Genet* 2010;**18**:852–5.

150. Galbiati F, Volonte D, Minetti C, *et al.* Phenotypic behavior of caveolin-3 mutations that cause autosomal dominant limb girdle muscular dystrophy (LGMD-1C). Retention of LGMD-1C caveolin-3 mutants within the golgi complex. *J Biol Chem* 1999;**274**:25632–41.

151. Gates DP, Coonrod LA, Berglund JA. Autoregulated splicing of muscleblind-like 1 (MBNL1) Pre-mRNA. *J Biol Chem* 2011;**286**:34224–33.

152. Gautel M. The sarcomeric cytoskeleton: who picks up the strain? *Curr Opin Cell Biol* 2011;**23**:39–46.

153. Gerrits HL, Hopman MT, Offringa C, *et al.* Variability in fibre properties in paralysed human quadriceps muscles and effects of training. *Pflugers Arch* 2003;**445**:734–40.

154. Gerull B, Gramlich M, Atherton J, *et al.* Mutations of TTN, encoding the giant muscle filament titin, cause familial dilated cardiomyopathy. *Nat Genet* 2002;**30**:201–4.

155. Gherardi RK, Authier FJ. Macrophagic myofasciitis: characterization and pathophysiology. *Lupus* 2012;**21**:184–9.

156. Ghosh A, Narayanappa G, Taly AB, *et al.* Tubular aggregate myopathy: a phenotypic spectrum and morphological study. *Neurol India* 2010;**58**:747–51.

157. Glass IA, Nicholson LV, Watkiss E, *et al.* Investigation of a female manifesting Becker muscular dystrophy. *J Med Genet* 1992;**29**:578–82.

158. Godfrey C, Clement E, Mein R, *et al.* Refining genotype phenotype correlations in muscular dystrophies with defective glycosylation of dystroglycan. *Brain* 2007;**130**:2725–35.

159. Godfrey C, Foley AR, Clement E, Muntoni F. Dystroglycanopathies: coming into focus. *Curr Opin Genet Dev* 2011;**21**:278–85.

160. Goebel HH, Bonnemann CG 169th ENMC International Workshop Rare Structural Congenital Myopathies 6–8 November 2009, Naarden, The Netherlands. *Neuromuscul Disord* 2011;**21**:363–74.

161. Goebel HH, Borchert A. Protein surplus myopathies and other rare congenital myopathies. *Semin Pediatr Neurol* 2002;**9**:160–70.

162. Goebel HH, Laing NG. Actinopathies and myosinopathies. *Brain Pathol* 2009;**19**:516–22.

163. Goebel HH, Warlo I. Nemaline myopathy with intranuclear rods--intranuclear rod myopathy. *Neuromuscul Disord* 1997;**7**:13–9.

164. Goebel HH, Muller J, Gillen HW. Autosomal dominant 'spheroid body myopathy'. *Muscle Nerve* 1978;**1**:14–26.

165. Goebel HH, Schloon H, Lenard HG. Congenital myopathy with cytoplasmic bodies. *Neuropediatrics* 1981;**12**:166–80.

166. Goebel HH, Sewry CA, Weller RO eds. *Muscle disease: pathology and genetics*, 2nd edn. Oxford: Wiley-Blackwell, 2013.

167. Gomes MD, Lecker SH, Jagoe RT, *et al.* Atrogin-1, a muscle-specific F-box protein highly expressed during muscle atrophy. *Proc Natl Acad Sci U S A* 2001;**98**:14440–5.

168. Greaves LC, Turnbull DM. Mitochondrial DNA mutations and ageing. *Biochim Biophys Acta* 2009;**1790**:1015–20.

169. Greenfield JG, Cornman T, Shy GM. The prognostic value of the muscle biopsy in the floppy infant. *Brain* 1958;**81**:461–84.

170. Gregorio CC, Perry CN, McElhinny AS. Functional properties of the titin/connectin-associated proteins, the muscle-specific RING finger proteins (MURFs), in striated muscle. *J Muscle Res Cell Motil* 2005;**26**:389–400.

171. Griggs RC, Udd BA. Markesbery disease: autosomal dominant late-onset distal myopathy: from phenotype to ZASP gene identification. *Neuromolecular Med* 2011;**13**:27–30.

172. Grohmann K, Schuelke M, Diers A, *et al.* Mutations in the gene encoding immunoglobulin mu-binding protein 2 cause spinal muscular atrophy with respiratory distress type 1. *Nat Genet* 2001;**29**:75–7.

173. Gueneau L, Bertrand AT, Jais JP, *et al.* Mutations of the FHL1 gene cause Emery-Dreifuss muscular dystrophy. *Am J Hum Genet* 2009;**85**:338–53.

174. Guergueltcheva V, Muller JS, Dusl M, *et al.* Congenital myasthenic syndrome with tubular aggregates caused by GFPT1 mutations. *J Neurol* 2011;**259**:838–50.

175. Gundesli H, Talim B, Korkusuz P, *et al.* Mutation in exon 1f of PLEC, leading to disruption of plectin isoform 1f, causes autosomal-recessive limb-girdle muscular dystrophy. *Am J Hum Genet* 2010;**87**:834–41.

176. Gurnett CA, Bodnar JA, Neil J, Connolly AM. Congenital myasthenic syndrome: presentation, electrodiagnosis, and muscle biopsy. *J Child Neurol* 2004;**19**:175–82.

177. Gurnett CA, Desruisseau DM, McCall K, *et al.* Myosin binding protein C1: a novel gene for autosomal dominant distal arthrogryposis type 1. *Hum Mol Genet* 2010;**19**:1165–73.

178. Gutierrez Rios P, Kalra AA, Wilson JD, *et al.* Congenital megaconial myopathy due to a novel defect in the choline kinase Beta gene. *Arch Neurol* 2012;**69**:657–61.

179. Haas RH, Parikh S, Falk MJ, *et al.* The in-depth evaluation of suspected mitochondrial disease. *Mol Genet Metab* 2008;**94**:16–37.

180. Hackman P, Sarparanta J, Lehtinen S, *et al.* Welander distal myopathy is caused by a mutation in the RNA-binding protein TIA1. *Ann Neurol* 2013;**73**:500–9.

181. Hackman P, Vihola A, Haravuori H, *et al.* Tibial muscular dystrophy is a titinopathy caused by mutations in TTN, the gene encoding the giant skeletal-muscle protein titin. *Am J Hum Genet* 2002;**71**:492–500.

182. Haginoya K, Yamamoto K, Iinuma K, *et al.* Dystrophin immunohistochemistry in a symptomatic carrier of Becker muscular dystrophy. *J Neurol* 1991;**238**:375–8.

183. Hanisch F, Muller T, Dietz A, *et al.* Phenotype variability and histopathological findings in centronuclear myopathy due to DNM2 mutations. *J Neurol* 2011;**258**:1085–90.

184. Hara Y, Balci-Hayta B, Yoshida-Moriguchi T, *et al.* A dystroglycan mutation associated with limb-girdle muscular dystrophy. *N Engl J Med* 2011;**364**:939–46.

185. Haravuori H, Vihola A, Straub V, *et al.* Secondary calpain3 deficiency in 2q-linked muscular dystrophy: titin is the candidate gene. *Neurology* 2001;**56**:869–77.

186. Harrison BC, Allen DL, Leinwand LA. IIb or not IIb? Regulation of myosin heavy chain gene expression in mice and men. *Skelet Muscle* 2011;**1**:5.

187. Hartley L, Kinali M, Knight R, *et al.* A congenital myopathy with diaphragmatic weakness not linked to the SMARD1 locus. *Neuromuscul Disord* 2007;**17**:174–9.

188. Hauser MA, Horrigan SK, Salmikangas P, *et al.* Myotilin is mutated in limb girdle muscular dystrophy 1A. *Hum Mol Genet* 2000;**9**:2141–7.

189. Hayashi YK, Chou FL, Engvall E, *et al.* Mutations in the integrin alpha7 gene cause congenital myopathy. *Nat Genet* 1998;**19**:94–7.

190. Hedberg C, Lindberg C, Mathe G, *et al.* Myopathy in a woman and her daughter associated with a novel splice site MTM1 mutation. *Neuromuscul Disord* 2011.

191. Helliwell TR, Ellis IH, Appleton RE. Myotubular myopathy: morphological, immunohistochemical and clinical variation. *Neuromuscul Disord* 1998;**8**:152–61.

192. Helliwell TR, Man NT, Morris GE, Davies KE. The dystrophin-related protein, utrophin, is expressed on the sarcolemma of regenerating human skeletal muscle fibres in dystrophies and inflammatory myopathies. *Neuromuscul Disord* 1992;**2**:177–84.

193. Helliwell TR, Nguyen thi Man, Morris GE. The dystrophin-related protein, utrophin, is expressed on the sarcolemma of regenerating human skeletal muscle fibres in dystrophies and inflammatory myopathies. *Neuromuscul Disord* 1992;**2**:177–84.

194. Hilton-Jones D. Observations on the classification of the inflammatory myopathies. *Presse Med* 2011;**40**: e199–208.

195. Hilton-Jones D, Miller A, Parton M, *et al.* Inclusion body myositis: MRC Centre for Neuromuscular Diseases, IBM workshop, London, 13 June 2008. *Neuromuscul Disord* 2010;**20**:142–7.

196. Hnia K, Vaccari I, Bolino A, Laporte J. Myotubularin phosphoinositide phosphatases: cellular functions and disease pathophysiology. *Trends Mol Med* 2012;**18**:317–27.

197. Holton JL, Wedderburn LR, Hanna MG. Polymyositis, dermatomyositis and inclusion body myositis. In: Goebel HH, Sewry CA, Weller RO ed. *Muscle disease: pathology and genetics*, 2nd edn. Oxford: Wiley-Blackwell, 2013.

198. Horvath R, Kemp JP, Tuppen HA, *et al.* Molecular basis of infantile reversible cytochrome c oxidase deficiency myopathy. *Brain* 2009;**132**:3165–74.

199. Huh SY, Kim HS, Jang HJ, *et al.* Limb-girdle myasthenia with tubular aggregates associated with novel GFPT1 mutations. *Muscle Nerve* 2012;**46**:600–4.

200. Hutchinson DO, Charlton A, Laing NG, *et al.* Autosomal dominant nemaline myopathy with intranuclear rods due to mutation of the skeletal muscle ACTA1 gene: clinical and pathological variability within a kindred. *Neuromuscul Disord* 2006;**16**:113–21.

201. Ibraghimov-Beskrovnaya O, Ervasti JM, Leveille CJ, *et al.* Primary structure of dystrophin-associated glycoproteins linking dystrophin to the extracellular matrix. *Nature* 1992;**355**:696–702.

202. Ikezoe K, Furuya H, Ohyagi Y. Dysferlin expression in tubular aggregates: their possible relationship to endoplasmic reticulum stress. *Acta Neuropathol* 2003;**105**:603–9.

203. Ilkovski B, Clement S, Sewry C, *et al.* Defining alpha-skeletal and alpha-cardiac actin expression in human heart and skeletal muscle explains the absence of cardiac involvement in ACTA1 nemaline myopathy. *Neuromuscul Disord* 2005;**15**:829–35.

204. Imbach T, Schenk B, Schollen E, *et al.* Deficiency of dolichol-phosphate-mannose synthase-1 causes congenital disorder of glycosylation type Ie. *J Clin Invest* 2000;**105**:233–9.

205. Irwin WA, Bergamin N, Sabatelli P, *et al.* Mitochondrial dysfunction and apoptosis in myopathic mice with collagen VI deficiency. *Nat Genet* 2003;**35**:367–71.

206. Jackson MJ, McArdle A. Age-related changes in skeletal muscle reactive oxygen species generation and adaptive responses to reactive oxygen species. *J Physiol* 2011;**589**:2139–45.

207. Jae LT, Raaben M, Riemersma M, *et al.* Deciphering the glycosylome of dystroglycanopathies using haploid screens for lassa virus entry. *Science* 2013;**340**:479–83.

208. Jakubiec-Puka A, Kordowska J, Catani C, Carraro U. Myosin heavy chain isoform composition in striated muscle after denervation and self-reinnervation. *Eur J Biochem* 1990;**193**:623–8.

209. Jimenez-Mallebrera C, Brown SC, Sewry CA, Muntoni F. Congenital muscular dystrophy: molecular and cellular aspects. *Cell Mol Life Sci* 2005;**62**:809–23.

210. Jimenez-Mallebrera C, Maioli MA, Kim J, *et al.* A comparative analysis of collagen VI production in muscle, skin and fibroblasts from 14 Ullrich congenital muscular dystrophy patients with dominant and recessive COL6A mutations. *Neuromuscul Disord* 2006;**16**:571–82.

211. Jimenez-Mallebrera C, Torelli S, Feng L, *et al.* A comparative study of alpha-dystroglycan glycosylation in dystroglycanopathies suggests that the hypoglycosylation of alpha-dystroglycan does not consistently correlate with clinical severity. *Brain Pathol* 2009;**19**:596–611.

212. Johnson MA, Polgar J, Weightman D, Appleton D. Data on the distribution of fibre types in thirty-six human muscles. An autopsy study. *J Neurol Sci* 1973;**18**:111–29.

213. Jungbluth H, Beggs A, Bonnemann C *et al.* 111th ENMC International Workshop on Multi-minicore Disease, 9–11 November 2002, Naarden, The Netherlands. *Neuromuscul Disord* 2004;**14**:754–66.

214. Jungbluth H, Muller CR, Halliger-Keller B, *et al.* Autosomal recessive inheritance of RYR1 mutations in a congenital myopathy with cores. *Neurology* 2002;**59**:284–7.

215. Jungbluth H, Sewry CA, Brown SC, *et al.* Mild phenotype of nemaline myopathy with sleep hypoventilation due to a mutation in the skeletal muscle alpha-actin (ACTA1) gene. *Neuromuscul Disord* 2001;**11**:35–40.

216. Jungbluth H, Sewry CA, Buj-Bello A, *et al.* Early and severe presentation of X-linked myotubular myopathy in a girl with skewed X-inactivation. *Neuromuscul Disord* 2003;**13**:55–9.

217. Jungbluth H, Sewry CA, Muntoni F. Core myopathies. *Semin Pediatr Neurol* 2011;**18**:239–49.

218. Jurkat-Rott K, Lehmann-Horn F. State of the art in hereditary muscle channelopathies. *Acta Myol* 2010;**29**:343–50.

219. Jurkat-Rott K, McCarthy T, Lehmann-Horn F. Genetics and pathogenesis of malignant hyperthermia. *Muscle Nerve* 2000;**23**:4–17.

220. Kaimaktchiev V, Goebel H, Laing N, *et al.* Intranuclear nemaline rod myopathy. *Muscle Nerve* 2006;**34**:369–72.

221. Kaindl AM, Ruschendorf F, Krause S, *et al.* Missense mutations of ACTA1 cause dominant congenital myopathy with cores. *J Med Genet* 2004;**41**:842–8.

222. Karpati G, Hilton-Jones D, Bushby K, Griggs RS(eds). *Disorders of voluntary muscle*, 8th edn. Cambridge: Cambridge University Press, 2010.

223. Kayashima T, Matsuo H, Satoh A, *et al.* Nonaka myopathy is caused by mutations in the UDP-N-acetylglucosamine-2-epimerase/N-acetylmannosamine kinase gene (GNE). *J Hum Genet* 2002;**47**:77–9.

224. Kee AJ, Gunning PW, Hardeman EC. Diverse roles of the actin cytoskeleton in striated muscle. *J Muscle Res Cell Motil* 2009;**30**:187–97.

225. Kim J, Jimenez-Mallebrera C, Foley AR, *et al.* Flow cytometry analysis: a quantitative method for collagen VI deficiency screening. *Neuromuscul Disord* 2012;**22**:139–48.

226. Kimber E, Tajsharghi H, Kroksmark AK, *et al.* A mutation in the fast skeletal muscle troponin I gene causes myopathy and distal arthrogryposis. *Neurology* 2006;**67**:597–601.

227. King RHM. *Atlas of peripheral nerve pathology*, London: Arnold, 1999.

228. Kirschner J, Hausser I, Zou Y, *et al.* Ullrich congenital muscular dystrophy: connective tissue abnormalities in the skin support overlap with Ehlers-Danlos syndromes. *Am J Med Genet A* 2005;**132A**:296–301.

229. Klein A, Lillis S, Munteanu I, *et al.* Clinical and genetic findings in a large cohort of patients with ryanodine receptor 1 gene-associated myopathies. *Hum Mutat* 2012;**33**:981–8.

230. Klein A, Pitt MC, McHugh JC, *et al.* DOK7 congenital myasthenic syndrome in childhood: Early diagnostic clues in 23 children. *Neuromuscul Disord* 2013.

231. Klinge L, Dekomien G, Aboumousa A, *et al.* Sarcoglycanopathies: can muscle immunoanalysis predict the genotype? *Neuromuscul Disord* 2008;**18**:934–41.

232. Knoblauch H, Geier C, Adams S, *et al.* Contractures and hypertrophic cardiomyopathy in a novel FHL1 mutation. *Ann Neurol* 2010;**67**:136–40.

233. Knoll R, Buyandelger B, Lab M. The sarcomeric Z-disc and Z-discopathies. *J Biomed Biotechnol* 2011;**2011**: 569628.

234. Kobayashi H, Baumbach L, Matise TC, *et al.* A gene for a severe lethal form of X-linked arthrogryposis (X-linked infantile spinal muscular atrophy) maps to human chromosome Xp11.3-q11.2. *Hum Mol Genet* 1995;**4**:1213–6.

235. Kollberg G, Tulinius M, Gilljam T, *et al.* Cardiomyopathy and exercise intolerance in muscle glycogen storage disease 0. *N Engl J Med* 2007;**357**:1507–14.

236. Kontrogianni-Konstantopoulos A, Ackermann MA, Bowman AL, *et al.* Muscle giants: molecular scaffolds in sarcomerogenesis. *Physiol Rev* 2009;**89**:1217–67.

237. Krahn M, Lopez de Munain A, Streichenberger N, *et al.* CAPN3 mutations in patients with idiopathic eosinophilic myositis. *Ann Neurol* 2006;**59**:905–11.

238. Laforet P, Vianey-Saban C. Disorders of muscle lipid metabolism: diagnostic and therapeutic challenges. *Neuromuscul Disord* 2010;**20**:693–700.

239. Lammens M, Moerman P, Fryns JP, *et al.* Fetal akinesia sequence caused by nemaline myopathy. *Neuropediatrics* 1997;**28**:116–9.

240. Lance JW, Evans WA. Progressive myoclonic epilepsy, nerve deafness and spinal muscular atrophy. *Clin Exp Neurol* 1984;**20**:141–51.

241. Lang B, Vincent A. Autoimmune disorders of the neuromuscular junction. *Curr Opin Pharmacol* 2009;**9**:336–40.

242. Laporte J, Biancalana V, Tanner SM, *et al.* MTM1 mutations in X-linked myotubular myopathy. *Hum Mutat* 2000;**15**:393–409.

243. Lebeaux D, Sene D. Eosinophilic fasciitis (Shulman disease). *Best Pract Res Clin Rheumatol* 2012;**26**:449–58.

244. Lefeber DJ, de Brouwer AP, Morava E, *et al.* Autosomal recessive dilated cardiomyopathy due to DOLK mutations results from abnormal dystroglycan O-mannosylation. *PLoS Genet* 2011;**7**:e1002427.

245. Lefeber DJ, Schonberger J, Morava E, *et al.* Deficiency of Dol-P-Man synthase subunit DPM3 bridges the congenital disorders of glycosylation with the dystroglycanopathies. *Am J Hum Genet* 2009;**85**:76–86.

246. Lehtokari VL, Pelin K, Herczegfalvi A, *et al.* Nemaline myopathy caused by mutations in the nebulin gene may present as a distal myopathy. *Neuromuscul Disord* 2011;**21**:556–62.

247. Lescure A, Rederstorff M, Krol A, *et al.* Selenoprotein function and muscle disease. *Biochim Biophys Acta* 2009;**1790**:1569–74.

248. Liang WC, Nishino I. Lipid storage myopathy. *Curr Neurol Neurosci Rep* 2011;**11**:97–103.

249. Liang WC, Mitsuhashi H, Keduka E, *et al.* TMEM43 mutations in Emery-Dreifuss muscular dystrophy-related myopathy. *Ann Neurol* 2011;**69**:1005–13.

250. Liewluck T, Lovell TL, Bite AV, Engel AG. Sporadic centronuclear myopathy with muscle pseudohypertrophy, neutropenia, and necklace fibers due to a DNM2 mutation. *Neuromuscul Disord* 2010;**20**:801–4.

251. Liewluck T, Shen XM, Milone M, Engel AG. Endplate structure and parameters of neuromuscular transmission in sporadic centronuclear myopathy associated with myasthenia. *Neuromuscul Disord* 2011;**21**:387–95.

252. Linke WA, Kruger M. The giant protein titin as an integrator of myocyte signaling pathways. *Physiology (Bethesda)* 2010;**25**:186–98.

253. Logan CV, Lucke B, Pottinger C, *et al.* Mutations in MEGF10, a regulator of satellite cell myogenesis, cause early onset myopathy, areflexia, respiratory distress and dysphagia (EMARDD). *Nat Genet* 2011;**43**:1189–92.

254. Logigian E, Ciafaloni E. Electrophysiological evaluation of suspected myopathy. In: Karpati G, Hilton Jones D, Bushby K, Griggs R ed. *Disorders of voluntary muscle*, 8th edn. Cambridge: Cambridge University Press, 2008: p. 81–92.

255. Lu Z, Joseph D, Bugnard E, *et al.* Golgi complex reorganization during muscle differentiation: visualization in living cells and mechanism. *Mol Biol Cell* 2001;**12**:795–808.

256. Luan X, Hong D, Zhang W, *et al.* A novel heterozygous deletion-insertion mutation (2695–2712 del/GTTTGT ins) in exon 18 of the filamin C gene causes filaminopathy in a large Chinese family. *Neuromuscul Disord* 2010;**20**:390–6.

257. Lunde HM, Skeie GO, Bertelsen AK, *et al*. Focal myositis: neurogenic phenomenon? *Neuromuscul Disord* 2012;**22**:350–4.

258. Luther PK. The vertebrate muscle Z-disc: sarcomere anchor for structure and signalling. *J Muscle Res Cell Motil* 2009;**30**:171–85.

259. Machuca-Tzili L, Brook D, Hilton-Jones D. Clinical and molecular aspects of the myotonic dystrophies: a review. *Muscle Nerve* 2005;**32**:1–18.

260. Magee KR, Shy GM. A new congenital non-progressive myopathy. *Brain* 1956;**79**:610–21.

261. Majczenko K, Davidson AE, Camelo-Piragua S, *et al*. Dominant mutation of CCDC78 in a unique congenital myopathy with prominent internal nuclei and atypical cores. *Am J Hum Genet* 2012;**91**:365–71.

262. Malfatti E, Birouk N, Romero NB, *et al*. Juvenile-onset permanent weakness in muscle phosphofructokinase deficiency. *J Neurol Sci* 2012;**316**:173–7.

263. Malicdan MC, Nishino I. Autophagy in lysosomal myopathies. *Brain Pathol* 2012;**22**:82–8.

264. Malicdan MC, Noguchi S, Nonaka I, *et al*. Lysosomal myopathies: an excessive build-up in autophagosomes is too much to handle. *Neuromuscul Disord* 2008;**18**:521–9.

265. Mammen AL. Autoimmune myopathies: autoantibodies, phenotypes and pathogenesis. *Nat Rev Neurol* 2011;**7**:343–54.

266. Mancuso M, Salviati L, Sacconi S, *et al*. Mitochondrial DNA depletion: mutations in thymidine kinase gene with myopathy and SMA. *Neurology* 2002;**59**:1197–202.

267. Manilal S, Nguyen TM, Sewry CA, Morris GE. The Emery-Dreifuss muscular dystrophy protein, emerin, is a nuclear membrane protein. *Hum Mol Genet* 1996;**5**:801–8.

268. Manilal S, Sewry CA, Man N, *et al*. Diagnosis of X-linked Emery-Dreifuss muscular dystrophy by protein analysis of leucocytes and skin with monoclonal antibodies. *Neuromuscul Disord* 1997;**7**:63–6.

269. Manilal S, Sewry CA, Pereboev A, *et al*. Distribution of emerin and lamins in the heart and implications for Emery-Dreifuss muscular dystrophy. *Hum Mol Genet* 1999;**8**:353–9.

270. Manta P, Terzis G, Papadimitriou C, *et al*. Emerin expression in tubular aggregates. *Acta Neuropathol* 2004;**107**:546–52.

271. Manzini MC, Tambunan DE, Hill RS, *et al*. Exome sequencing and functional validation in zebrafish identify GTDC2 mutations as a cause of Walker-Warburg syndrome. *Am J Hum Genet* 2012;**91**:541–7.

272. Mayer U. Integrins: redundant or important players in skeletal muscle? *J Biol Chem* 2003;**278**:14587–90.

273. McEntagart M, Parsons G, Buj-Bello A, *et al*. Genotype-phenotype correlations in X-linked myotubular myopathy. *Neuromuscul Disord* 2002;**12**:939–46.

274. McMillin MJ, Below JE, Shively KM, *et al*. Mutations in ECEL1 cause distal arthrogryposis type 5D. *Am J Hum Genet* 2013;**92**:150–6.

275. Mejat A, Misteli T. LINC complexes in health and disease. *Nucleus* 2010;**1**:40–52.

276. Melia MJ, Kubota A, Ortolano S, *et al*. Limb-girdle muscular dystrophy 1F is caused by a microdeletion in the transportin 3 gene. *Brain* 2013;**136**:1508–17.

277. Mellad JA, Warren DT, Shanahan CM. Nesprins LINC the nucleus and cytoskeleton. *Curr Opin Cell Biol* 2011;**23**:47–54.

278. Mellies U, Lofaso F. Pompe disease: a neuromuscular disease with respiratory muscle involvement. *Respir Med* 2009;**103**:477–84.

279. Mercuri E, Muntoni F. The ever-expanding spectrum of congenital muscular dystrophies. *Ann Neurol* 2012;**72**:9–17.

280. Mercuri E, Clements E, Offiah A, *et al*. Muscle magnetic resonance imaging involvement in muscular dystrophies with rigidity of the spine. *Ann Neurol* 2010;**67**:201–8.

281. Mercuri E, Lampe A, Allsop J, *et al*. Muscle MRI in Ullrich congenital muscular dystrophy and Bethlem myopathy. *Neuromuscul Disord* 2005;**15**:303–10.

282. Mercuri E, Manzur AY, Jungbluth H, *et al*. Early and severe presentation of autosomal dominant Emery-Dreifuss muscular dystrophy (EMD2). *Neurology* 2000;**54**:1704–5.

283. Mercuri E, Messina S, Bruno C, *et al*. Congenital muscular dystrophies with defective glycosylation of dystroglycan: a population study. *Neurology* 2009;**72**:1802–9.

284. Mercuri E, Pichiecchio A, Allsop J, *et al*. Muscle MRI in inherited neuromuscular disorders: past, present, and future. *J Magn Reson Imaging* 2007;**25**:433–40.

285. Mercuri E, Poppe M, Quinlivan R, *et al*. Extreme variability of phenotype in patients with an identical missense mutation in the lamin A/C gene: from congenital onset with severe phenotype to milder classic Emery-Dreifuss variant. *Arch Neurol* 2004;**61**:690–4.

286. Mercuri E, Yuva Y, Brown SC, *et al*. Collagen VI involvement in Ullrich syndrome: a clinical, genetic, and immunohistochemical study. *Neurology* 2002;**58**:1354–9.

287. Merlini L, Villanova M, Sabatelli P, *et al*. Decreased expression of laminin beta 1 in chromosome 21-linked Bethlem myopathy. *Neuromuscul Disord* 1999;**9**:326–9.

288. Messina S, Bruno C, Moroni I, *et al*. Congenital muscular dystrophies with cognitive impairment. A population study. *Neurology* 2010;**75**:898–903.

289. Messina S, Tortorella G, Concolino D, *et al*. Congenital muscular dystrophy with defective alpha-dystroglycan, cerebellar hypoplasia, and epilepsy. *Neurology* 2009;**73**:1599–601.

290. Midroni G, Bilbao JM. *Diagnosis of peripheral neuropathology*, Boston: ButterworthHeinemann, 1995 .

291. Miles L, Miles MV, Horn PS, *et al*. Importance of muscle light microscopic mitochondrial subsarcolemmal aggregates in the diagnosis of respiratory chain deficiency. *Hum Pathol* 2012;**43**:1249–57.

292. Milone M, Liewluck T, Winder TL, Pianosi PT. Amyloidosis and exercise intolerance in ANO5 muscular dystrophy. *Neuromuscul Disord* 2012;**22**:13–5.

293. Minami N, Ikezoe K, Kuroda H, *et al*. Oculopharyngodistal myopathy is genetically heterogeneous and most cases are distinct from oculopharyngeal muscular dystrophy. *Neuromuscul Disord* 2001;**11**:699–702.

294. Minamitani T, Ariga H, Matsumoto K. Deficiency of tenascin-X causes a decrease in the level of expression of type VI collagen. *Exp Cell Res* 2004;**297**:49–60.

295. Minetti C, Bado M, Broda P, *et al*. Impairment of caveolae formation and T-system disorganization in human muscular dystrophy with caveolin-3 deficiency. *Am J Pathol* 2002;**160**:265–70.

296. Mitsuhashi S, Ohkuma A, Talim B, *et al*. A congenital muscular dystrophy with mitochondrial structural abnormalities caused by defective de novo phosphatidylcholine biosynthesis. *Am J Hum Genet* 2011;**88**:845–51.

297. Moghadaszadeh B, Petit N, Jaillard C, *et al*. Mutations in SEPN1 cause congenital muscular dystrophy with spinal rigidity and restrictive respiratory syndrome. *Nat.Genet* 2001;**29**:17–8.

298. Monnier N, Ferreiro A, Marty I, *et al*. A homozygous splicing mutation causing a depletion of skeletal muscle RYR1 is associated with multi-minicore disease congenital myopathy with ophthalmoplegia. *Hum Mol Genet* 2003;**12**:1171–8.

299. Monnier N, Romero NB, Lerale J, *et al*. An autosomal dominant congenital myopathy with cores and rods is associated with a neomutation in the RYR1 gene encoding the skeletal muscle ryanodine receptor. *Hum Mol Genet* 2000;**9**:2599–608.

300. Monnier N, Romero NB, Lerale J. An autosomal dominant congenital myopathy with cores and rods is associated with a neomutation in the RYR1 gene encoding the skeletal muscle ryanodine receptor. *Hum Mol Genet* 2000 **9**:2599–608.

301. Moreira ES, Wiltshire TJ, Faulkner G, *et al*. Limb-girdle muscular dystrophy type 2G is caused by mutations in the gene encoding the sarcomeric protein telethonin. *Nat Genet* 2000;**24**:163–6.

302. Morris G, Sewry C, Wehnert M. Molecular genetics of Emery-Dreifuss muscular dystrophy. In: *Encyclopedia of life sciences*. Chichester: John Wiley & Sons Ltd, 2010.

303. Moslemi AR, Lindberg C, Nilsson J, *et al*. Glycogenin-1 deficiency and inactivated priming of glycogen synthesis. *N Engl J Med* 2010;**362**:1203–10.

304. Mruk DD, Cheng CY. The myotubularin family of lipid phosphatases in disease and in spermatogenesis. *Biochem J* 2011;**433**:253–62.

305. Munot P, Lashley D, Jungbluth H, *et al*. Congenital fibre type disproportion associated with mutations in the tropomyosin 3 (TPM3) gene mimicking congenital myasthenia. *Neuromuscul Disord* 2010;**20**:796–800.

306. Muntoni F. Is a muscle biopsy in Duchenne dystrophy really necessary? *Neurology* 2001;**57**:574–5.

307. Muntoni F, Voit T. The congenital muscular dystrophies in 2004: a century of exciting progress. *Neuromuscul Disord* 2004;**14**:635–49.

308. Muntoni F, Bonne G, Goldfarb LG, *et al*. Disease severity in dominant Emery Dreifuss is increased by mutations in

both emerin and desmin proteins. *Brain* 2006;**129**:1260–8.

309. Muntoni F, Goodwin F, Sewry C, *et al.* Clinical spectrum and diagnostic difficulties of infantile ponto-cerebellar hypoplasia type 1. *Neuropediatrics* 1999;**30**:243–8.

310. Muntoni F, Torelli S, Wells DJ, Brown SC. Muscular dystrophies due to glycosylation defects: diagnosis and therapeutic strategies. *Curr Opin Neurol* 2011;**24**:437–42.

311. Musumeci O, Bruno C, Mongini T, *et al.* Clinical features and new molecular findings in muscle phosphofructokinase deficiency (GSD type VII). *Neuromuscul Disord* 2012;**22**:325–30.

312. Naom I, D'Alessandro M, Sewry C, *et al.* The role of immunocytochemistry and linkage analysis in the prenatal diagnosis of merosin-deficient congenital muscular dystrophy. *Hum Genet* 1997;**99**:535–40.

313. Naukkarinen A. *Myotonic dystrophy type 2 (DM2): Diagnostic methods and molecular pathology.* PhD thesis. In: Department of Medical Genetics. University of Helsinki, 2011.

314. Negrao L, Matos A, Geraldo A, Rebelo O. Limb-girdle muscular dystrophy in a Portuguese patient caused by a mutation in the telethonin gene. *Acta Myol* 2010;**29**:21–4.

315. Nigro V, Aurino S, Piluso G. Limb girdle muscular dystrophies: update on genetic diagnosis and therapeutic approaches. *Curr Opin Neurol* 2011;**24**:429–36.

316. Nigro V, Okazaki Y, Belsito A, *et al.* Identification of the Syrian hamster cardiomyopathy gene. *Hum Mol Genet* 1997;**6**:601–7.

317. Nishino I, Fu J, Tanji K, *et al.* Primary LAMP-2 deficiency causes X-linked vacuolar cardiomyopathy and myopathy (Danon disease). *Nature* 2000;**406**:906–10.

318. North K. Congenital myopathies. In: Engel AG and Franzini-Armstrong CS (ed.).*Myology*, 3rd edn. New York: McGrath-Hill 2004: p 1473–533.

319. Norwood FL, Harling C, Chinnery PF, *et al.* Prevalence of genetic muscle disease in Northern England: in-depth analysis of a muscle clinic population. *Brain* 2009;**132**:3175–86.

320. Novy J, Rosselet A, Spertini O, *et al.* Chemotherapy is successful in sporadic late onset nemaline myopathy (SLONM) with monoclonal gammopathy. *Muscle Nerve* 2010;**41**:286–7.

321. Ognibene A, Sabatelli P, Petrini S, *et al.* Nuclear changes in a case of X-linked Emery-Dreifuss muscular dystrophy. *Muscle Nerve* 1999;**22**:864–9.

322. Ohlsson M, Hedberg C, Bradvik B, *et al.* Hereditary myopathy with early respiratory failure associated with a mutation in A-band titin. *Brain* 2012;**135**:1682–94.

323. Okere A, Reddy SS, Gupta S, Shinnar M. A cardiomyopathy in a patient with limb girdle muscular dystrophy type 2A. *Circ Heart Fail* 2013;**6**: e12–3.

324. Olive M, Goldfarb LG, Shatunov A, *et al.* Myotilinopathy: refining the clinical and myopathological phenotype. *Brain* 2005;**128**:2315–26.

325. Olive M, Odgerel Z, Martinez A, *et al.* Intranuclear rods in three Spanish families with Zaspopathy (abstract). *Neuromuscul Disord* 2010;**20**:623.

326. Olive M, Shatunov A, Gonzalez L, *et al.* Transcription-terminating mutation in telethonin causing autosomal recessive muscular dystrophy type 2G in a European patient. *Neuromuscul Disord* 2008;**18**:929–33.

327. Ottenheijm CA, Granzier H, Labeit S. The sarcomeric protein nebulin: another multifunctional giant in charge of muscle strength optimization. *Front Physiol* 2012;**3**:37.

328. Overton TG, Smith RP, Sewry CA, *et al.* Maternal contamination at fetal muscle biopsy. *Fetal Diagn Ther* 2000;**15**:118–21.

329. Ozawa E. Our trails and trials in the subsarcolemmal cytoskeleton network and muscular dystrophy researches in the dystrophin era. *Proc Jpn Acad Ser B Phys Biol Sci* 2010;**86**:798–821.

330. Pedrotti S,Sette C. Spinal muscular atrophy: a new player joins the battle for SMN2 exon 7 splicing. *Cell Cycle* 2010;**9**:3874–9.

331. Pegoraro E, Mancias P, Swerdlow SH, *et al.* Congenital muscular dystrophy with primary laminin alpha 2 (merosin) deficiency presenting as inflammatory myopathy. *Ann Neurol* 1996;**40**:782–91.

332. Pegoraro E, Schimke RN, Arahata K, *et al.* Detection of new paternal dystrophin gene mutations in isolated cases of dystrophinopathy in females. *Am J Hum Genet* 1994;**54**:989–1003.

333. Pestronk A, Schmidt RE, Choksi R. Vascular pathology in dermatomyositis and anatomic relations to myopathology. *Muscle Nerve* 2010;**42**:53–61.

334. Pevzner A, Schoser B, Peters K, *et al.* Anti-LRP4 autoantibodies in AChR- and MuSK-antibody-negative myasthenia gravis. *J Neurol* 2012;**259**:427–35.

335. Pfeffer G, Elliott HR, Griffin H, *et al.* Titin mutation segregates with hereditary myopathy with early respiratory failure. *Brain* 2012;**135**:1695–713.

336. Pfeffer G, Majamaa K, Turnbull DM, *et al.* Treatment for mitochondrial disorders. *Cochrane Database Syst Rev* 2012;**4**:CD004426.

337. Philpot J, Cowan F, Pennock J, *et al.* Merosin-deficient congenital muscular dystrophy: the spectrum of brain involvement on magnetic resonance imaging. *Neuromuscul Disord* 1999;**9**:81–5.

338. Piccolo F, Jeanpierre M, Leturcq F, *et al.* A founder mutation in the gamma-sarcoglycan gene of gypsies possibly predating their migration out of India. *Hum Mol Genet* 1996;**5**:2019–22.

339. Pinol-Ripoll G, Shatunov A, Cabello A, *et al.* Severe infantile-onset cardiomyopathy associated with a homozygous deletion in desmin. *Neuromuscul Disord* 2009;**19**:418–22.

340. Prayson RA. Skeletal muscle vasculitis exclusive of inflammatory myopathic conditions: a clinicopathologic study of 40 patients. *Hum Pathol* 2002;**33**:989–95.

341. Preusse C, Goebel HH, Held J, *et al.* Immune-mediated necrotizing myopathy is characterized by a specific Th1-m1 polarized immune profile. *Am J Pathol* 2012;**181**:2161–71.

342. Prokop S, Heppner FL, Goebel HH, Stenzel W. M2 polarized macrophages and giant cells contribute to myofibrosis in neuromuscular sarcoidosis. *Am J Pathol* 2011;**178**:1279–86.

343. Proske U, Gandevia SC. The proprioceptive senses: their roles in signaling body shape, body position and movement, and muscle force. *Physiol Rev* 2012;**92**:1651–97.

344. Quane KA, Healy JM, Keating KE, *et al.* Mutations in the ryanodine receptor gene in central core disease and malignant hyperthermia. *Nat.Genet* 1993;**5**:51–5.

345. Quijano-Roy S, Mbieleu B, Bonnemann CG, *et al.* De novo LMNA mutations cause a new form of congenital muscular dystrophy. *Ann Neurol* 2008;**64**:177–86.

346. Quinlivan R, Jungbluth H. Myopathic causes of exercise intolerance with rhabdomyolysis. *Dev Med Child Neurol* 2012;**54**:886–91.

347. Quinlivan R, Buckley J, James M, *et al.* McArdle disease: a clinical review. *J Neurol Neurosurg Psychiatry* 2010;**81**:1182–8.

348. Quinlivan R, Mitsuahashi S, Sewry C, *et al.* Muscular dystrophy with large mitochondria associated with mutations in the CHKB gene in three British patients: extending the clinical and pathological phenotype. *Neuromuscul Disord* 2013;**23**:549–56.

349. Raben N, Sherman JB. Mutations in muscle phosphofructokinase gene. *Hum Mutat* 1995;**6**:1–6.

350. Raja Rayan DL,Hanna MG. Skeletal muscle channelopathies: nondystrophic myotonias and periodic paralysis. *Curr Opin Neurol* 2010;**23**:466–76.

351. Rajab A, Straub V, McCann LJ, *et al.* Fatal cardiac arrhythmia and long-QT syndrome in a new form of congenital generalized lipodystrophy with muscle rippling (CGL4) due to PTRF-CAVIN mutations. *PLoS Genet* 2010;**6**:e1000874.

352. Ramachandran N, Munteanu I, Wang P, *et al.* VMA21 deficiency prevents vacuolar ATPase assembly and causes autophagic vacuolar myopathy. *Acta Neuropathol* 2013;**125**:439–57.

353. Ramser J, Ahearn ME, Lenski C, *et al.* Rare missense and synonymous variants in UBE1 are associated with X-linked infantile spinal muscular atrophy. *Am J Hum Genet* 2008;**82**:188–93.

354. Ravenscroft G, Jackaman C, Sewry CA, *et al.* Actin nemaline myopathy mouse reproduces disease, suggests other actin disease phenotypes and provides cautionary note on muscle transgene expression. *PLoS One* 2011;**3**:e28699.

355. Ravenscroft G, Miyatake S, Lehtokari VL, *et al.* Mutations in KLHL40 are a frequent cause of severe autosomal-recessive nemaline myopathy. *Am J Hum Genet* 2013;**93**:6–18.

356. Rayman MP. Selenium and human health. *Lancet* 2012;**379**:1256–68.

357. Renton AE, Majounie E, Waite A, *et al.* A hexanucleotide repeat expansion in C9ORF72 is the cause of chromosome 9p21-linked ALS-FTD. *Neuron* 2011;**72**:257–68.

358. Rider LG, Miller FW. Deciphering the clinical presentations, pathogenesis, and treatment of the idiopathic inflammatory myopathies. *JAMA* 2011;**305**:183–90.

359. Riemersma S, Vincent A, Beeson D, *et al.* Association of arthrogryposis multiplex congenita with maternal antibodies inhibiting fetal acetylcholine receptor function. *J Clin Invest* 1996;**98**:2358–63.

360. Roach PJ, Depaoli-Roach AA, Hurley TD, Tagliabracci VS. Glycogen and its metabolism: some new developments and old themes. *Biochem J* 2012;**441**:763–87.

361. Robb SA, Sewry CA, Dowling JJ, et al. Impaired neuromuscular transmission and response to acetylcholinesterase inhibitors in centronuclear myopathies. *Neuromuscul Disord* 2011;**21**:379–86.

362. Rocha CT, Hoffman EP. Limb-girdle and congenital muscular dystrophies: current diagnostics, management, and emerging technologies. *Curr Neurol Neurosci Rep* 2010;**10**:267–76.

363. Rogers M, Sewry CA, Upadhyaya M. Histological, immunocytochemical, molecular and ultrastructural characteristics of FSHD muscle In: Upadhyaya M and Cooper N (ed.). *Facioscapulohumeral muscular dystrophy (FSHD): clinical medicine and molecular cell biology.* London: BIOS Scientific Publishers, 2004: p 295–98.

364. Rollins S, Prayson RA, McMahon JT, Cohen BH. Diagnostic yield muscle biopsy in patients with clinical evidence of mitochondrial cytopathy. *Am J Clin Pathol* 2001;**116**:326–30.

365. Romero NB. Centronuclear myopathies: a widening concept. *Neuromuscul Disord* 2010;**20**:223–8.

366. Romero NB, Lehtokari VL, Quijano-Roy S, et al. Core-rod myopathy caused by mutations in the nebulin gene. *Neurology* 2009;**73**:1159–61.

367. Romero NB, Monnier N, Viollet L, et al. Dominant and recessive central core disease associated with RYR1 mutations and fetal akinesia. *Brain* 2003;**126**: 2341–9.

368. Rosales XQ, Gastier-Foster JM, Lewis S, et al. Novel diagnostic features of dysferlinopathies. *Muscle Nerve* 2010;**42**:14–21.

369. Roscioli T, Kamsteeg EJ, Buysse K, et al. Mutations in ISPD cause Walker-Warburg syndrome and defective glycosylation of alpha-dystroglycan. *Nat Genet* 2012;**44**:581–5.

370. Rossor AM, Kalmar B, Greensmith L, Reilly MM. The distal hereditary motor neuropathies. *J Neurol Neurosurg Psychiatry* 2012;**83**:6–14.

371. Rowan SL, Rygiel K, Purves-Smith FM, et al. Denervation causes fiber atrophy and myosin heavy chain co-expression in senescent skeletal muscle. *PLoS One* 2012;**7**:e29082.

372. Rusmini P, Bolzoni E, Crippa V, et al. Proteasomal and autophagic degradative activities in spinal and bulbar muscular atrophy. *Neurobiol Dis* 2010;**40**:361–9.

373. Sabatelli P, Bonaldo P, Lattanzi G, et al. Collagen VI deficiency affects the organization of fibronectin in the extracellular matrix of cultured fibroblasts. *Matrix Biol* 2001;**20**:475–86.

374. Sabatelli P, Columbaro M, Mura I, et al. Extracellular matrix and nuclear abnormalities in skeletal muscle of a patient with Walker-Warburg syndrome caused by POMT1 mutation. *Biochim Biophys Acta* 2003;**1638**:57–62.

375. Sabatelli P, Gara SK, Grumati P, et al. Expression of the collagen VI alpha 5 and alpha 6 chains in normal human skin and in skin of patients with collagen VI-related myopathies. *J Invest Dermatol* 2011;**131**:99–107.

376. Sabatelli P, Squarzoni S, Petrini S, et al. Oral exfoliative cytology for the non-invasive diagnosis in X-linked Emery-Dreifuss muscular dystrophy patients and carriers. *Neuromuscul Disord* 1998;**8**:67–71.

377. Sambuughin N, Yau KS, Olive M, et al. Dominant mutations in KBTBD13, a member of the BTB/Kelch family, cause nemaline myopathy with cores. *Am J Hum Genet* 2010;**87**:842–7.

378. Sanes JR. The basement membrane/basal lamina of skeletal muscle. *J Biol Chem* 2003;**278**:12601–4.

379. Sarnat HB. Vimentin/desmin immunoreactivity of myofibres in developmental myopathies. *Acta Paediatr Jpn* 1991;**33**:238–46.

380. Sarnat HB, Flores-Sarnat L, Casey R, et al. Endothelial ultrastructural alterations of intramuscular capillaries in infantile mitochondrial cytopathies: "Mitochondrial angiopathy." *Neuropathology* 2012;**32**:617–27.

381. Sarparanta J, Jonson PH, Golzio C, et al. Mutations affecting the cytoplasmic functions of the co-chaperone DNAJB6 cause limb-girdle muscular dystrophy. *Nat Genet* 2012;**44**:450–5.

382. Sasaki T, Shikura K, Sugai K, et al. Muscle histochemistry in myotubular (centronuclear) myopathy. *Brain Dev* 1989;**11**:26–32.

383. Satoyoshi E, Kinoshita M. Oculopharyngodistal myopathy. *Arch Neurol* 1977;**34**:89–92.

384. Schara U, Schoser BG. Myotonic dystrophies type 1 and 2: a summary on current aspects. *Semin Pediatr Neurol* 2006;**13**:71–9.

385. Schessl J, Feldkirchner S, Kubny C, Schoser B. Reducing body myopathy and other FHL1-related muscular disorders. *Semin Pediatr Neurol* 2011;**18**:257–63.

386. Schiaffino S. Tubular aggregates in skeletal muscle: just a special type of protein aggregates? *Neuromuscul Disord* 2012;**22**:199–207.

387. Schiaffino S, Reggiani C. Fiber types in mammalian skeletal muscles. *Physiol Rev* 2011;**91**:1447–531.

388. Schon EA, Dimauro S, Hirano M. Human mitochondrial DNA: roles of inherited and somatic mutations. *Nat Rev Genet* 2012;**13**:878–90.

389. Schoser BG, Frosk P, Engel AG, et al. Commonality of TRIM32 mutation in causing sarcotubular myopathy and LGMD2H. *Ann Neurol* 2005;**57**:591–5.

390. Schoser B, Jacob S, Hilton-Jones D, et al. Immune-mediated rippling muscle disease with myasthenia gravis: a report of seven patients with long-term follow-up in two. *Neuromuscul Disord* 2009;**19**:223–8.

391. Schoser BG, Schneider-Gold C, Kress W, et al. Muscle pathology in 57 patients with myotonic dystrophy type 2. *Muscle Nerve* 2004;**29**:275–81.

392. Schröder R, Reimann J, Salmikangas P, et al. Beyond LGMD1A: myotilin is a component of central core lesions and nemaline myopathy. *Neuromuscul Disord* 2003;**13**:451–5.

393. Schröder R, Schoser B. Myofibrillar myopathies: a clinical and myopathological guide. *Brain Pathol* 2009;**19**:483–92.

394. Schulte-Mattler WJ, Kley RA, Rothenfusser-Korber E, et al. Immune-mediated rippling muscle disease. *Neurology* 2005;**64**:364–7.

395. Selcen D. Myofibrillar myopathies. *Neuromuscul Disord* 2011;**21**:161–71.

396. Selcen D, Juel VC, Hobson-Webb LD, et al. Myasthenic syndrome caused by plectinopathy. *Neurology* 2011;**76**:327–36.

397. Senderek J, Garvey SM, Krieger M, et al. Autosomal-dominant distal myopathy associated with a recurrent missense mutation in the gene encoding the nuclear matrix protein, matrin 3. *Am J Hum Genet* 2009;**84**:511–8.

398. Senderek J, Krieger M, Stendel C, et al. Mutations in SIL1 cause Marinesco-Sjogren syndrome, a cerebellar ataxia with cataract and myopathy. *Nat Genet* 2005;**37**:1312–4.

399. Senderek J, Muller JS, Dusl M, et al. Hexosamine biosynthetic pathway mutations cause neuromuscular transmission defect. *Am J Hum Genet* 2011;**88**:162–72.

400. Sewry CA. Pathological defects in congenital myopathies. *J Muscle Res Cell Motil* 2008;**29**:231–8.

401. Sewry CA. The role of immunocytochemistry in congenital myopathies. *Neuromuscul Disord* 1998;**8**:394–400.

402. Sewry CA, Muntoni F. Inherited disorders of the extracellular matrix. *Curr Opin Neurol* 1999;**12**:519–26.

403. Sewry CA, Chevallay M, Tome FM. Expression of laminin subunits in human fetal skeletal muscle. *Histochem J* 1995;**27**:497–504.

404. Sewry CA, Jimenez-Mallebrera C, Feng L, et al. Overexpression of utrophin in patients with limb-girdle muscular dystrophies. *Neuromuscul Disord* 2005;**15**:717.

405. Sewry CA, Jimenez-Mallebrera C, Muntoni F. Congenital myopathies. *Curr Opin Neurol* 2008;**21**:569–75.

406. Sewry CA, Muller C, Davis M, et al. The spectrum of pathology in central core disease. *Neuromuscul Disord* 2002;**12**:930–8.

407. Sewry CA, Naom I, D'Alessandro M, et al. Variable clinical phenotype in merosin-deficient congenital muscular dystrophy associated with differential immunolabelling of two fragments of the laminin alpha 2 chain. *Neuromuscul Disord* 1997;**7**:169–75.

408. Sewry CA, Nowak KJ, Ehmsen JT, Davies KE. A and B utrophin in human muscle and sarcolemmal A-utrophin associated with tumours. *Neuromuscul Disord* 2005;**15**:779–85.

409. Sewry CA, Quinlivan RC, Squier W, et al. A rapid immunohistochemical test to distinguish congenital myotonic dystrophy from X-linked myotubular myopathy. *Neuromuscul Disord* 2012;**22**:225–30.

410. Sharma MC, Schultze C, von Moers A, et al. Delayed or late-onset type II glycogenosis with globular inclusions. *Acta Neuropathol* 2005;**110**:151–7.

411. Shastry S, Delgado MR, Dirik E, et al. Congenital generalized lipodystrophy, type 4 (CGL4) associated with myopathy due to novel PTRF mutations. *Am J Med Genet A* 2010;**152A**:2245–53.

412. Sher JH, Rimalovski AB, Athanassiades TJ, Aronson SM. Familial centronuclear myopathy: a clinical and pathological study. *Neurology* 1967;**17**:727–42.

413. Shorer Z, Philpot J, Muntoni F, *et al.* Demyelinating peripheral neuropathy in merosin-deficient congenital muscular dystrophy. *J Child Neurol* 1995;**10**:472–5.

414. Siddique T, Ajroud-Driss S. Familial amyotrophic lateral sclerosis, a historical perspective. *Acta Myol* 2011;**30**:117–20.

415. Sieck GC, Zhan WZ. Denervation alters myosin heavy chain expression and contractility of developing rat diaphragm muscle. *J Appl Physiol* 2000;**89**:1106–13.

416. Simmons Z, Specht CS. The neuromuscular manifestations of amyloidosis. *J Clin Neuromuscul Dis* 2010;**11**:145–57.

417. Sine SM. End-plate acetylcholine receptor: structure, mechanism, pharmacology, and disease. *Physiol Rev* 2012;**92**:1189–234.

418. Sjostrom M, Kidman S, Larsen KH, Angquist KA. Z- and M-band appearance in different histochemically defined types of human skeletal muscle fibers. *J Histochem Cytochem* 1982;**30**:1–11.

419. Sleigh K, Ball S, Hilton DA. Quantification of changes in muscle from individuals with and without mitochondrial disease. *Muscle Nerve* 2011;**43**:795–800.

420. Smerdu V, Soukup T. Demonstration of myosin heavy chain isoforms in rat and humans: the specificity of seven available monoclonal antibodies used in immunohistochemical and immunoblotting methods. *Eur J Histochem* 2008;**52**:179–90.

421. Sorimachi H, Kinbara K, Kimura S, *et al.* Muscle-specific calpain, p94, responsible for limb girdle muscular dystrophy type 2A, associates with connectin through IS2, a p94-specific sequence. *J Biol Chem* 1995;**270**:31158–62.

422. Soussi-Yanicostas N, Chevallay M, Laurent-Winter C, *et al.* Distinct contractile protein profile in congenital myotonic dystrophy and X-linked myotubular myopathy. *Neuromuscul Disord* 1991;**1**:103–11.

423. Spiro AJ, Shy GM, Gonatas NK. Myotubular myopathy. Persistence of fetal muscle in an adolescent boy. *Arch Neurology* 1966;**14**:1–14.

424. Spuler S, Carl M, Zabojszcza J, *et al.* Dysferlin-deficient muscular dystrophy features amyloidosis. *Ann Neurol* 2008;**63**:323–8.

425. Statland JM, Tawil R. Facioscapulohumeral muscular dystrophy: molecular pathological advances and future directions. *Curr Opin Neurol* 2011;**24**:423–8.

426. Stenzel W, Goebel HH, Aronica E. Review: immune-mediated necrotizing myopathies: a heterogeneous group of diseases with specific myopathological features. *Neuropathol Appl Neurobiol* 2012;**38**:632–46.

427. Stenzel W, Prokop S, Kress W, *et al.* Fetal akinesia caused by a novel actin filament aggregate myopathy skeletal muscle actin gene (ACTA1) mutation. *Neuromuscul Disord* 2010;**20**:531–3.

428. Stevens E, Carss KJ, Cirak S, *et al.* Mutations in B3GALNT2 cause congenital muscular dystrophy and hypoglycosylation of alpha-dystroglycan. *Am J Hum Genet* 2013;**92**:354–65.

429. Stevens E, Torelli S, Feng L, *et al.* Flow cytometry for the analysis of alpha-dystroglycan glycosylation in fibroblasts from patients with dystroglycanopathies. *PLoS One* 2013;**8**: e68958.

430. Stojkovic T, Hammouda el H, Richard P, *et al.* Clinical outcome in 19 French and Spanish patients with valosin-containing protein myopathy associated with Paget's disease of bone and frontotemporal dementia. *Neuromuscul Disord* 2009;**19**:316–23.

431. Straub V, Carlier PG, Mercuri E. TREAT-NMD workshop: pattern recognition in genetic muscle diseases using muscle MRI:25–26 February 2011, Rome, Italy. *Neuromuscul Disord* 2012;**22 Suppl 2:** S42–53.

432. Straub V, Ettinger AJ, Durbeej M, *et al.* epsilon-sarcoglycan replaces alpha-sarcoglycan in smooth muscle to form a unique dystrophin-glycoprotein complex. *J Biol Chem* 1999;**274**:27989–96.

433. Sugie K, Yamamoto A, Murayama K, *et al.* Clinicopathological features of genetically confirmed Danon disease. *Neurology* 2002;**58**:1773–8.

434. Sunada Y, Saito F, Higuchi I, *et al.* Deficiency of a 180-kDa extracellular matrix protein in Fukuyama type congenital muscular dystrophy skeletal muscle. *Neuromuscul Disord* 2002;**12**:117–20.

435. Sung SS, Brassington AM, Grannatt K, *et al.* Mutations in genes encoding fast-twitch contractile proteins cause distal arthrogryposis syndromes. *Am J Hum Genet* 2003;**72**:681–90.

436. Sung SS, Brassington AM, Krakowiak PA, *et al.* Mutations in TNNT3 cause multiple congenital contractures: a second locus for distal arthrogryposis type 2B. *Am J Hum Genet* 2003;**73**:212–4.

437. Suominen T, Bachinski LL, Auvinen S, *et al.* Population frequency of myotonic dystrophy: higher than expected frequency of myotonic dystrophy type 2 (DM2) mutation in Finland. *Eur J Hum Genet* 2011;**19**:776–82.

438. Susman RD, Quijano-Roy S, Yang N, *et al.* Expanding the clinical, pathological and MRI phenotype of DNM2-related centronuclear myopathy. *Neuromuscul Disord* 2010;**20**:229–37.

439. Tajsharghi H, Oldfors A. Myosinopathies: pathology and mechanisms. *Acta Neuropathol* 2013;**125**:3–18.

440. Tajsharghi H, Kimber E, Holmgren D, *et al.* Distal arthrogryposis and muscle weakness associated with a ß-tropomyosin mutation. *Neurology* 2007;**68**:772–5.

441. Tajsharghi H, Kimber E, Kroksmark AK, *et al.* Embryonic myosin heavy-chain mutations cause distal arthrogryposis and developmental myosin myopathy that persists postnatally. *Arch Neurol* 2008;**65**:1083–90.

442. Tajsharghi H, Ohlsson M, Palm L, Oldfors A. Myopathies associated with beta-tropomyosin mutations. *Neuromuscul Disord* 2012;**22**:923–33.

443. Tajsharghi H, Thornell LE, Lindberg C, *et al.* Myosin storage myopathy associated with a heterozygous missense mutation in MYH7. *Ann Neurol* 2003;**54**:494–500.

444. Takamori M. Structure of the neuromuscular junction: function and cooperative mechanisms in the synapse. *Ann N Y Acad Sci* 2012;**1274**:14–23.

445. Tanji K, Bonilla E. Neuropathologic aspects of cytochrome C oxidase deficiency. *Brain Pathol* 2000;**10**:422–30.

446. Tanner SM, Orstavik KH, Kristiansen M, *et al.* Skewed X-inactivation in a manifesting carrier of X-linked myotubular myopathy and in her non-manifesting carrier mother. *Hum Genet* 1999;**104**:249–53.

447. Taylor J, Muntoni F, Dubowitz V, Sewry CA. The abnormal expression of utrophin in Duchenne and Becker muscular dystrophy is age related. *Neuropathol Appl Neurobiol* 1997;**23**:399–405.

448. Taylor J, Muntoni F, Robb S, *et al.* Early onset autosomal dominant myopathy with rigidity of the spine: a possible role for laminin beta 1? *Neuromuscul Disord* 1997;**7**:211–6.

449. Tetreault M, Duquette A, Thiffault I, *et al.* A new form of congenital muscular dystrophy with joint hyperlaxity maps to 3p23–21. *Brain* 2006;**129**:2077–84.

450. Tews DS. Role of nitric oxide and nitric oxide synthases in experimental models of denervation and reinnervation. *Microsc Res Tech* 2001;**55**:181–6.

451. Thevathasan W, Squier W, MacIver DH, *et al.* Oculopharyngodistal myopathy--a possible association with cardiomyopathy. *Neuromuscul Disord* 2011;**21**:121–5.

452. Thompson HM, Cao H, Chen J, *et al.* Dynamin 2 binds gamma-tubulin and participates in centrosome cohesion. *Nat Cell Biol* 2004;**6**:335–42.

453. Ticozzi N, Tiloca C, Morelli C, *et al.* Genetics of familial Amyotrophic lateral sclerosis. *Arch Ital Biol* 2011;**149**:65–82.

454. Torelli S, Brown SC, Jimenez-Mallebrera C, *et al.* Absence of neuronal nitric oxide synthase (nNOS) as a pathological marker for the diagnosis of Becker muscular dystrophy with rod domain deletions. *Neuropathol Appl Neurobiol* 2004;**30**:540–5.

455. Toscano A, Musumeci O. Tarui disease and distal glycogenoses: clinical and genetic update. *Acta Myol* 2007;**26**:105–7.

456. Tosch V, Rohde HM, Tronchere H, *et al.* A novel PtdIns3P and PtdIns(3,5)P2 phosphatase with an inactivating variant in centronuclear myopathy. *Hum Mol Genet* 2006;**15**:3098–106.

457. Tosch V, Vasli N, Kretz C, *et al.* Novel molecular diagnostic approaches for X-linked centronuclear (myotubular) myopathy reveal intronic mutations. *Neuromuscul Disord* 2010;**20**:375–81.

458. Toussaint A, Cowling BS, Hnia K, *et al.* Defects in amphiphysin 2 (BIN1) and triads in several forms of centronuclear myopathies. *Acta Neuropathol* 2011;**121**:253–66.

459. Toydemir RM, Chen H, Proud VK, *et al.* Trismus-pseudocamptodactyly syndrome is caused by recurrent mutation of MYH8. *Am J Med Genet A* 2006;**140**:2387–93.

460. Toydemir RM, Rutherford A, Whitby FG, *et al.* Mutations in embryonic myosin heavy chain (MYH3) cause Freeman-Sheldon syndrome and Sheldon-Hall syndrome. *Nat Genet* 2006;**38**:561–5.

461. Tsurusaki Y, Saitoh S, Tomizawa K, *et al.* A DYNC1H1 mutation causes a dominant spinal muscular atrophy with lower extremity predominance. *Neurogenetics* 2012;**13**:327–32.

462. Tunnah D, Sewry CA, Vaux D, *et al.* The apparent absence of lamin B1 and emerin in many tissue nuclei is due to epitope masking. *J Mol Histol* 2005;**36**:337–44.

463. Turner C, Hilton-Jones D. The myotonic dystrophies: diagnosis and management. *J Neurol Neurosurg Psychiatry* 2010;**81**:358–67.

464. Udd B. Distal muscular dystrophies. *Handb Clin Neurol* 2011;**101**:239–62.

465. Udd B. Distal myopathies - New genetic entities expand diagnostic challenge. *Neuromuscul Disord* 2012;**22**:5–12.

466. Udd B, Partanen J, Halonen P, et al. Tibial muscular dystrophy. Late adult-onset distal myopathy in 66 Finnish patients. *Arch Neurol* 1993;**50**:604–8.

467. Udd B, Vihola A, Sarparanta J, et al. Titinopathies and extension of the M-line mutation phenotype beyond distal myopathy and LGMD2J. *Neurology* 2005;**64**:636–42.

468. Usuki F, Takenaga S, Higuchi I, et al. Morphologic findings in biopsied skeletal muscle and cultured fibroblasts from a female patient with Danon's disease (lysosomal glycogen storage disease without acid maltase deficiency). *J Neurol Sci* 1994;**127**:54–60.

469. Uusimaa J, Jungbluth H, Fratter C, et al. Reversible infantile respiratory chain deficiency is a unique, genetically heterogenous mitochondrial disease. *J Med Genet* 2011;**48**:660–8.

470. Vainzof M, Moreira ES, Suzuki OT, et al. Telethonin protein expression in neuromuscular disorders. *Biochim Biophys Acta* 2002;**1588**:33–40.

471. Vainzof M, Richard P, Herrmann R, et al. Prenatal diagnosis in laminin alpha2 chain (merosin)-deficient congenital muscular dystrophy: a collective experience of five international centers. *Neuromuscul Disord* 2005;**15**:588–94.

472. van der Maarel SM, Tawil R, Tapscott SJ. Facioscapulohumeral muscular dystrophy and DUX4: breaking the silence. *Trends Mol Med* 2011;**17**:252–8.

473. van der Sluijs BM, ter Laak HJ, Scheffer H, et al. Autosomal recessive oculopharyngodistal myopathy: a distinct phenotypical, histological, and genetic entity. *J Neurol Neurosurg Psychiatry* 2004;**75**:1499–501.

474. van Engelen BG, Muchir A, Hutchison CJ, et al. The lethal phenotype of a homozygous nonsense mutation in the lamin A/C gene. *Neurology* 2005;**64**: 374–6.

475. Van Reeuwijk J, Olderode-Berends MJ, Van den Elzen C, et al. A homozygous FKRP start codon mutation is associated with Walker-Warburg syndrome, the severe end of the clinical spectrum. *Clin Genet* 2010;**78**:275–81.

476. Vergne I, Roberts E, Elmaoued RA, et al. Control of autophagy initiation by phosphoinositide 3-phosphatase Jumpy. *EMBO J* 2009;**28**:2244–58.

477. Vihola A, Bassez G, Meola G, et al. Histopathological differences of myotonic dystrophy type 1 (DM1) and PROMM/DM2. *Neurology* 2003;**60**:1854–7.

478. Villanova M, Malandrini A, Sabatelli P, et al. Localization of laminin alpha 2 chain in normal human central nervous system: an immunofluorescence and ultrastructural study. *Acta Neuropathol* 1997;**94**:567–71.

479. Voermans NC, Altenburg TM, Hamel BC, et al. Reduced quantitative muscle function in tenascin-X deficient Ehlers-Danlos patients. *Neuromuscul Disord* 2007;**17**:597–602.

480. Voermans NC, Bonnemann CG, Huijing PA, et al. Clinical and molecular overlap between myopathies and inherited connective tissue diseases. *Neuromuscul Disord* 2008;**18**:843–56.

481. Voermans NC, Laan AE, Oosterhof A, et al. Brody syndrome: a clinically heterogeneous entity distinct from Brody disease: a review of literature and a cross-sectional clinical study in 17 patients. *Neuromuscul Disord* 2012;**22**:944–54.

482. Voermans NC, van Alfen N, Pillen S, et al. Neuromuscular involvement in various types of Ehlers-Danlos syndrome. *Ann Neurol* 2009;**65**:687–97.

483. Voit T, Parano E, Straub V, et al. Congenital muscular dystrophy with adducted thumbs, ptosis, external ophthalmoplegia, mental retardation and cerebellar hypoplasia: a novel form of CMD. *Neuromuscul Disord* 2002;**12**:623–30.

484. Vorgerd M, van der Ven PF, Bruchertseifer V, et al. A mutation in the dimerization domain of filamin c causes a novel type of autosomal dominant myofibrillar myopathy. *Am J Hum Genet* 2005;**77**:297–304.

485. Vuillaumier-Barrot S, Bouchet-Seraphin C, Chelbi M, et al. Identification of mutations in TMEM5 and ISPD as a cause of severe cobblestone lissencephaly. *Am J Hum Genet* 2012;**91**:1135–43.

486. Walker UA. Imaging tools for the clinical assessment of idiopathic inflammatory myositis. *Curr Opin Rheumatol* 2008;**20**:656–61.

487. Wallgren-Pettersson C, Donner K, Sewry C, et al. Mutations in the nebulin gene can cause severe congenital nemaline myopathy. *Neuromuscul Disord* 2002;**12**:674–9.

488. Wallgren-Pettersson C, Lehtokari VL, Kalimo H, et al. Distal myopathy caused by homozygous missense mutations in the nebulin gene. *Brain* 2007;**130**:1465–76.

489. Wallgren-Pettersson C, Sewry CA, Nowak KJ, Laing NG. Nemaline myopathies. *Semin Pediatr Neurol* 2011;**18**:230–8.

490. Wang J, Dube DK, Mittal B, et al. Myotilin dynamics in cardiac and skeletal muscle cells. *Cytoskeleton (Hoboken)* 2011;**68**:661–70.

491. Wedderburn LR, Varsani H, Li CK, et al. International consensus on a proposed score system for muscle biopsy evaluation in patients with juvenile dermatomyositis: a tool for potential use in clinical trials. *Arthritis Rheum* 2007;**57**:1192–201.

492. Weeks DA, Nixon RR, Kaimaktchiev V, Mierau GW. Intranuclear rod myopathy, a rare and morphologically striking variant of nemaline rod myopathy. *Ultrastruct. J Pathol* 2003;**27**:151–4.

493. Weihl CC, Pestronk A, Kimonis VE. Valosin-containing protein disease: inclusion body myopathy with Paget's disease of the bone and fronto-temporal dementia. *Neuromuscul Disord* 2009;**19**:308–15.

494. Weiler T, Greenberg CR, Zelinski T, et al. A gene for autosomal recessive limb-girdle muscular dystrophy in Manitoba Hutterites maps to chromosome region 9q31-q33: evidence for another limb-girdle muscular dystrophy locus. *Am J Hum Genet* 1998;**63**:140–7.

495. Wewer UM, Durkin ME, Zhang X, et al. Laminin beta 2 chain and adhalin deficiency in the skeletal muscle of Walker-Warburg syndrome (cerebro-ocular dysplasia-muscular dystrophy). *Neurology* 1995;**45**:2099–101.

496. Wheeler MT, Zarnegar S, McNally EM. Zeta-sarcoglycan, a novel component of the sarcoglycan complex, is reduced in muscular dystrophy. *Hum Mol Genet* 2002;**11**:2147–54.

497. Wiche G, Winter L. Plectin isoforms as organizers of intermediate filament cytoarchitecture. *Bioarchitecture* 2011;**1**:14–20.

498. Willer T, Lee H, Lommel M, et al. ISPD loss-of-function mutations disrupt dystroglycan O-mannosylation and cause Walker-Warburg syndrome. *Nat Genet* 2012;**44**:575–80.

499. Wilmshurst JM, Lillis S, Zhou H, et al. RYR1 mutations are a common cause of congenital myopathies with central nuclei. *Ann Neurol* 2010;**68**:717–26.

500. Wilmshurst JM, Ouvrier R. Hereditary peripheral neuropathies of childhood: an overview for clinicians. *Neuromuscul Disord* 2011;**21**:763–75.

501. Wilson LA, Dux L, Cooper BJ, et al. Experimental regeneration in canine muscular dystrophy 2. Expression of myosin heavy chain isoforms. *Neuromuscul Disord* 1994;**4**:25–37.

502. Winter L, Wiche G. The many faces of plectin and plectinopathies: pathology and mechanisms. *Acta Neuropathol* 2013;**125**:77–93.

503. Worman HJ, Bonne G. "Laminopathies": a wide spectrum of human diseases. *Exp Cell Res* 2007;**313**:2121–33.

504. Worman HJ. Nuclear lamins and laminopathies. *J Pathol* 2012;**226**: 316–25.

505. Yurchenco PD, Patton BL. Developmental and pathogenic mechanisms of basement membrane assembly. *Curr Pharm Des* 2009;**15**:1277–94.

506. Zahr ZA, Baer AN. Malignancy in myositis. *Curr Rheumatol Rep* 2011;**13**:208–15.

507. Zanotti S, Negri T, Cappelletti C, et al. Decorin and biglycan expression is differentially altered in several muscular dystrophies. *Brain* 2005;**128**:2546–55.

508. Zhang Q, Bethmann C, Worth NF, et al. Nesprin-1 and -2 are involved in the pathogenesis of Emery-Dreifuss muscular dystrophy and are critical for nuclear envelope integrity. *Hum Mol Genet* 2007;**16**:2816–33.

509. Zhang W, Vajsar J, Cao P, et al. Enzymatic diagnostic test for muscle-eye-brain type congenital muscular dystrophy using commercially available reagents. *Clin Biochem* 2003;**36**: 339–44.

510. Zhou J, Tawk M, Tiziano FD, et al. Spinal muscular atrophy associated with progressive myoclonic epilepsy is caused by mutations in ASAH1. *Am J Hum Genet* 2012;**91**:5–14.

511. Zimprich A, Grabowski M, Asmus F, et al. Mutations in the gene encoding epsilon-sarcoglycan cause myoclonus-dystonia syndrome. *Nat Genet* 2001;**29**:66–9.

512. Zuchner S, Noureddine M, Kennerson M, et al. Mutations in the pleckstrin homology domain of dynamin 2 cause dominant intermediate Charcot-Marie-Tooth disease. *Nat Genet* 2005;**37**: 289–94.

Introduction to Tumours

Arie Perry and David N Louis

EPIDEMIOLOGY AND AETIOLOGY

Intracranial and spinal tumours account for only 2 per cent of all malignant neoplasms, but in children they are the second most common tumour type and the most common cause of cancer death. Of all intracranial tumours, roughly 40 per cent originate from neuroepithelium, 35 per cent from meningothelial cells, 14.4 per cent from oral ectoderm (pituitary adenomas and craniopharyngiomas), and 7.5 per cent from peripheral nerve sheath elements. Lymphomas and germ cell tumours account for 2.3 and 0.5 per cent, respectively.[27] The 2007 classification of the World Health Organization (WHO) for central nervous system tumours lists over 120 different types and subtypes.[108] The incidence, localization, age distribution, biological behaviour and patient survival differ greatly among them. For these reasons, it is also likely that the aetiologies and biological underpinnings of many central and peripheral nervous system (CNS and PNS) tumours vary.

Incidence and Mortality

Cancer registry data are greatly influenced by whether meningeal, cranial nerve and spinal cord tumours are included in addition to neoplasms of the brain.[44] Often, incidence data include only malignant neoplasms, but the ICD-0 and efforts of the Central Brain Tumor Registry of the United States have made major strides to include all brain tumour data.

There has been some concern over a possible increase in the incidence of brain tumours since the 1980s, but most authors agree that this apparent increase is largely due to the introduction and more frequent utilization of high-resolution neuroimaging, which has greatly improved the sensitivity of detecting brain tumours.[89,121,125] Population-based studies have not shown increases in brain tumour incidence in Scandinavia since the early 1980s.[106]

Mortality in patients with brain tumours is highly dependent on the type of tumour, with some lesions (WHO grade I) acting in a relatively benign manner and others (WHO grades II–IV) representing different degrees of malignancy; patients with grade IV lesions typically have survival times of less than 2 years from diagnosis, and roughly 2–5 years for grade III, 5–10 years for grade II and >10 years for grade I. In addition, the mortality/incidence ratio for brain tumours reflects the effectiveness of diagnostic and therapeutic measures. Mortality is lower overall in women, given their lower incidence of gliomas and increased predisposition to meningiomas. Not surprisingly, mortality and morbidity are also highly associated with site of presentation, both increasing considerably when eloquent brain is involved.

Age and Sex

Preferential manifestation in specific age groups is a hallmark of CNS tumours and often yields, together with tumour site, a limited differential diagnosis. The age distribution of brain tumours is bimodal, with the first peak in children (e.g. medulloblastoma, pilocytic astrocytoma, ependymoma) and the second, larger peak in adults aged 45–70 years, mainly due to glioblastomas and meningiomas. Information for each tumour type is included under each tumour entity.

In general, gliomas and embryonal tumours occur more frequently in males, whereas meningiomas preferentially affect females. Meningiomas account for 43 per cent of primary intracranial tumours in women as compared to only 22 per cent in men.[27] In spinal meningiomas, the preferential occurrence in women is even stronger, with female/male ratios in modern surgical series ranging from 3 to 9:1.[109,122,152] Another striking preferential occurrence is germinoma of the pineal region, which occurs approximately 10 times more frequently in boys than in girls.[108]

Regional, Socioeconomic and Genetic Variation

Descriptive epidemiological studies show some geographical variation in the incidence of brain tumours, which generally tends to be highest in developed, industrial countries.[132]

In Western Europe, North America and Australia, there are between 6 and 19 new cases of primary intracranial tumours per 100 000 inhabitants each year.[27,57,132] Whereas lower frequencies were previously reported, similar incidence rates are now also seen in Japan.[121] In multiracial countries, Caucasians are affected more frequently than people of African, Hispanic, or Asian descent and this difference has also been observed in children, with some studies further suggesting genetic differences in gliomas among racial groups.[167,186] For example, glioblastomas and germ cell tumours are 3.5 times more frequent in the USA in Caucasians than in African Americans.[45] Socioeconomic associations have been found in some studies, but not in others.[8,84]

Molecular epidemiological studies over the past decade have suggested possible links between inherited genetic polymorphisms and brain tumour development. These are based on the logical premise that functional variability in genes (such as those involved in DNA repair or detoxification processes) across the population could predispose certain individuals to brain tumours and could affect the response of some people to individual therapies (the latter known as 'pharmacogenomics'). The most recent approach utilizes genome wide association studies (GWAS) with thousands of single nucleotide polymorphisms (SNPs) applied to large cohorts. For instance, one international series evaluating 75 glioma families found evidence of Mendelian inheritance and a susceptibility locus at 17q12-21.32.[161] Other GWAS have discovered and confirmed a number of risk alleles (some common and others rare), with increasing cumulative risk found with increasing numbers of risk alleles present. Of interest, several of these risk loci involve genes already known or suspected to be critical in glioma biology, including 5p15.33 (*TERT*), 7p11.2 (*EGFR*), 9p21.3 (*CDKN2A/CDKN2B*) and the *TP53* polyadenylation signal, plus several others for which the gene functions have yet to be determined with respect to gliomagenesis, including 8q24.21(*CCDC26*), 11q23.3 (*PHLDB1*) and 20q13.33 (*RTEL1*).[56,153,160,165,187] Most recently, finemapping of the 8q24.21 region revealed a variant tightly associated with risk of oligodendroglial tumours and IDH–mutant astrocytic gliomas, with odds ratios ranging from five- to six-fold risk for people carrying the risk variant in rs55705857. This result was confirmed in independent series of glioma cases and controls.[88] Approximately 40 per cent of glioma cases of the above types carry this variant compared to only about 8 per cent of controls or people with other types of glioma. Some further suggest that similar germline polymorphisms involving *SSBP2* (single-stranded DNA-binding protein 2) on 5q14.1[189] and DNA repair enzymes, such as *LIG4*, *BTBD2*, *HMGA2* and *RTEL1* genes, are associated with survival times in glioblastoma patients.[103]

Polymorphisms in DNA repair genes have similarly been implicated outside the setting of GWAS, including *ERCC1*, *ERCC2*, *XRCC1*, *XRCC3*, *MGMT*, *PARP1*, *RAD51* and *XRCC7*.[41,102,104,115,179,193] To confirm these associations, however, larger studies are required. Various individual candidate genes have also been explored, with mixed results. For example, a number of studies have evaluated glutathione S-transferase 1 (*GSTM1*), because gene deletions have been associated with increased risk for environmentally induced cancers (e.g. smoking-related lung cancer). Despite some earlier suggestions of an association, however, a recent meta-analysis of 12 published studies concluded that there is no increased risk between polymorphisms of GSTM1 or other GST variant haplotypes and glioma risk.[191]

It is also likely that there are complex interactions between race/ethnicity, genetic polymorphisms, tumour genotype, patient age and gender.[186] It has long been observed that *TP53* mutations are more common in astrocytic tumours from younger adults and, to some extent, from females.[107] In a study of *TP53* mutations from a population-based study in the San Francisco Bay area, astrocytomas were much more likely to harbour *TP53* mutations in non-white (African American and Asian) than white (Latino and non-Latino) patients with both *TP53* mutations and *EGFR* amplifications being considerably less common in carriers of the *MGMT* variant 84Phe allele.[186] Similarly, younger patients are more likely to develop low-grade gliomas and secondary glioblastomas with mutations of *IDH* mutations, *CIC*, and/or *PDGFRA*, as well as chromosome 1p/19q co-deletions, whereas older adults are more prone to primary glioblastomas with *EGFR* gene amplifications and monosomy 10.[62,70,77,116,190]

Aetiology

With the exception of inherited neoplastic syndromes (see Chapter 44, Hereditary Tumour Syndromes) and prior irradiation, the aetiology of human brain tumours is still largely unknown. Numerous epidemiological studies have been performed, but most associations with environmental, dietary and lifestyle factors either have not been statistically significant or are inconsistent.[125,129]

X-Irradiation

X-ray irradiation (both therapeutic and non-therapeutic) is the sole environmental factor clearly associated with an increased risk of brain tumours (also see Chapter 46, Reactions to Antineoplastic Therapies). In most reported cases, radiation was administered for treatment of the fungal disease tinea capitis or of a cranial tumour unrelated to the radiation-induced neoplasm, although epidemiological studies following atomic bomb detonations in Japan have similarly provided compelling evidence.[136,192]

Radiation-induced meningiomas and other tumours (schwannomas, gliomas, sarcomas and embryonal tumours) have been most frequently observed after low-dose irradiation for tinea capitis,[175] and after high-dose radiation for primary brain tumours.[6,33,151] Typically, they arise within the field of irradiation. Multiple and high-grade (II or III) lesions appear to be more frequent than among sporadic meningiomas, with latency being roughly inversely linked to radiation dose. Sarcomas (mostly fibrosarcomas and malignant peripheral nerve sheath tumours) of the dura, meninges, or nerves are less frequent but, given their extreme rarity sporadically, are highly indicative of iatrogenic origin if diagnosed in patients with prior therapeutic irradiation.[168] In a report of seven cases, the mean latency was 8 years.[28]

Children receiving prophylactic CNS irradiation for acute lymphocytic leukaemia (ALL) appear at particularly high risk for subsequent astrocytomas (low and high grade).[55,123,125] Less frequently, tumours are classified as CNS primitive neuroectodermal tumour (PNET) or other embryonal neoplasms.[33,125] In a follow-up of long-term survivors, 7 of 468 children (1.9 per cent) treated for ALL (median dose, 24 Gy) developed primary intracranial neoplasms.[177a] In a retrospective cohort study of 14 361 children treated for cancer, there was over seven-fold overall risk of subsequently developing a CNS tumour (odds ratio [OR], 7 for glioma; 10 for meningioma), the dose response for excess relative risk being linear, such that children treated with 30–44.9 Gy of cranial irradiation peaked at 21-fold increased risk of gliomas.[123] Second primary CNS tumours have similarly been observed after irradiation of pituitary adenoma,[33] craniopharyngioma,[15] pineal parenchymal tumours[74] and germinoma,[33] scalp tumours and many other lesions.

Although a causative role of radiotherapy is generally acknowledged, the possible risk of diagnostic X-rays (e.g. in dental care) has been unclear. A modern series reported a 4.9-fold increased risk (95 per cent confidence interval [CI], 1.8–13.2) of meningioma for patients getting annual panorex films before 10 years of age;[35] given that less irradiation is now given for dental series than in the past, it is unclear whether similar risks will apply going forward. Long-term low-dose radiation exposure of nuclear workers has not been definitively implicated to increase risk of brain tumours.[23] After the nuclear accident in Chernobyl, the incidence of childhood brain tumours in neighbouring Sweden did not change significantly, although further follow-up is likely needed.[172]

Occupational Exposure

Analytical epidemiological studies have revealed an increased risk of brain tumour development in association with certain occupations,[157,171] for example in physicians, farmers, dentists, firefighters, metal workers and workers in the rubber industry. Attempts to identify a specific exposure or causative environmental agent have generally been unsuccessful,[125] although a recent study suggested an association between carbon tetrachloride exposure and glioblastoma.[124] The somewhat increased incidence of CNS neoplasms in anatomists, pathologists and embalmers raised the possibility of a role for formaldehyde, but increased brain tumour risk has not been observed in workers exposed to formaldehyde in industrial settings.[125] Similarly, multicentre cohort studies have not substantiated the hypothesis that occupational exposure to vinyl chloride carries enhanced risk of developing brain tumours.[162] Polycyclic aromatic hydrocarbons have also been associated with increased brain tumour risk, including in children.[39]

Several studies have pointed to a positive association with farm work,[18,171] possibly accounted for by herbicides, pesticides and their derivatives,[10,11] but these associations remain questionable. Some studies show a slightly elevated risk for white-collar workers, including social science professionals,[18] financial workers, managers and people of higher socioeconomic status, but these trends are also inconsistent.

Parental exposure may also influence risk of paediatric gliomas. A slightly increased risk of brain tumours has been found in children of electrical or chemical workers or children of fathers involved in hobbies with toxic exposures, such as pesticides.[114,146] Once again though, such associations remain controversial as other series have shown no increased risk.[112]

Electrical and Magnetic Fields

Although a weak association of brain tumours with electromagnetic field exposure has been previously reported, over 30 years of research has failed to establish a definite link.[57,125,157] Similarly, although some studies have suggested that it is specifically residential electromagnetic field exposure (determined by the electrical wiring configuration around houses or electrical blankets) that leads to increased childhood cancer, including brain tumours,[154,182] these observations have not been subsequently confirmed.[65,127,137]

Cellular Telephones

There has been extensive media coverage addressing the question of whether cellular telephone use is associated with brain tumour risk, as well as legal cases claiming an association. Cellular phones utilize radio-frequency waves that fall between radiowaves and microwaves. Exposure is measured as the specific absorption rate (SAR), which is the amount of radio-frequency energy absorbed from the telephone into the local tissues. Radio-frequency wave exposure is related to the duration and frequency of cellular phone use, with increased use implying increased exposure.[58] Scientific studies addressing the question of whether brain tumours are related to cellular telephone use have primarily involved two approaches: (1) exposure of cells or animals to a radio-frequency field similar to that of cellular phone usage, followed by measurement of various end points, and (2) epidemiological studies. In general, the studies using experimental systems to evaluate the effects of such radio-frequency exposures have not shown biological effects that are directly relevant to the situation encountered in human brain tumours. Thus, although biological effects may be found after exposure, these may have little to do with human brain tumourigenesis. More importantly, well-conducted epidemiological studies have failed to document clear associations with increased risk of gliomas, meningiomas or vestibular schwannomas, possibly with the exception of those at the highest exposure levels, although biases in study designs have prevented definitive interpretations.[24,40,58,71,85,91] Furthermore, tumours have not occurred disproportionately on the side of head on which the telephone was used. Of note, one group from Sweden has reported an increased risk for brain tumours ipsilateral to the side of cell phone use, not for malignant tumours, but only when vestibular schwannomas are included in the analysis.[67–69] However, these data have been called into methodological question; for example, although an increased number of these tumours was noted ipsilateral to phone use, the overall number of tumours was not increased, which would problematically suggest that cell phone use may have a protective effect against tumours contralateral to the side of cell phone use. No dose–response relationships have been noted in these studies and issues of recall bias may also be operative. For these reasons, the current literature does not support a role for cellular phone use in brain tumourigenesis. Nonetheless, it has been noted that caveats remain concerning long-term cellular phone usage, i.e. that further, long-term follow-up studies are needed to exclude long-term effects. The ongoing risk may decrease with time, given the overwhelming shift from analogue to digital methodologies, because radio-frequency wave exposure appears lower with digital cellular phones.[58]

Smoking

No definite association exists between smoking and brain malignancies.[80] Despite occasional reports suggesting a weak association with passive smoking in women and during pregnancy,[38] no clear associations between parental tobacco smoking and the incidence of childhood brain tumours have been found. A prospective study of a large birth cohort in Sweden reported that children of women who smoked during pregnancy (particularly children in the 2–4-years age group) had an increased incidence of benign and malignant brain tumours (hazard ratio 1.24).[17] In addition, another study found an association between childhood astrocytomas and paternal smoking history (OR 1.4).[39] However, a meta-analysis of 12 published observational studies, representing a total of 6566 patients, showed no clear association between maternal smoking during pregnancy and risk of childhood brain tumour development.[80] Similarly, a meta-analysis of 20 previously published series found no definite link between patient smoking history and glioma development.[110] Nonetheless, limitations in study designs prevent definitive conclusions based on available data. Regardless, if an increased risk exists, then the effect appears small.

Dietary N-nitroso Compounds and Other Considerations

Because *N*-nitroso compounds are potent neurocarcinogens in rodents, numerous epidemiological studies have evaluated their possible role in brain tumourigenesis. Nitroso compounds have been detected in nitrite-preserved food and in beer, but they can also be formed in the stomach after uptake of their chemical precursors, nitrate/nitrite and secondary amines. The results of several studies suggest that the risk of developing a primary brain tumour may be slightly higher in people with a high intake of meat, in particular cooked ham, processed pork and bacon.[125] A meta-analysis of nine epidemiological studies showed that dietary cured meat intake of all types had a relative risk of 1.48, suggesting a 48 per cent increased risk of glioma in adults ingesting high levels of cured meat.[81] On the other hand, the large population-based NIH-AARP Diet and Health Study found no convincing associations.[51] Of interest, this same study found a potential protective effect of caffeine on glioma development, with a hazard ratio of roughly 0.70.[52] In some studies, an inverse association was reported for high intake of fruit and vegetables and of vitamin C, which is known to block the endogenous formation of nitrosamines;[125] in others, however, no association could be found.[51] Similarly, no associations with aspirin or non-steroidal anti-inflammatory drug (NSAID) use or with nitrite in drinking water have been found.[43,166]

Trauma

Anecdotal reports have documented the occurrence of gliomas[119,173] and meningiomas[7,156] at the site of prior head injury. A causal relationship is difficult to prove, although an association would be biologically plausible, because trauma induces a strong proliferative cellular response. Epidemiological studies have shown a weak, but inconsistent or non-significant, association with adult and perinatal traumatic head injury[73,78,94,150,158] or combined perinatal and adult head trauma.[66] A large, international case–control study revealed an elevated risk with an odds ratio of 1.5 for meningiomas in male adults.[138]

Viruses

SV40 was iatrogenically introduced on a large scale into human populations in North America and Europe between 1955 and 1962 through SV40-contaminated polio vaccines.[22] SV40 sequences have been identified in a variety of human neoplasms, raising the question of a possible aetiological role.[19] JC virus has an extensive nucleotide sequence homology with SV40, but the host range is distinctly different. Although SV40 does not infect human cells, latent JC infection is very common, with a serological prevalence of 40–60 per cent in most developed countries. In immunosuppressed patients, JC virus is reactivated and may cause progressive multifocal leukoencephalopathy (PML).

Investigations of SV40 or JC virus in brain tumourigenesis have primarily evaluated whether viral sequences can be detected in primary tumours. However, one case–control study looked at the association between antibodies to JCV and SV40 from serum collected 1–22 years before diagnosis and incidence of primary malignant brain tumours.[144] JCV and BK virus infection was high in the study population (77 and 85 per cent, respectively), whereas antibodies to SV40 were less prevalent (11 per cent). The odds ratio for subsequent brain tumour development was 1.46 for JCV, 0.66 for BKV and 1.00 for SV40. Furthermore, there were no significant differences between cases and controls in having antibodies to JCV, BKV or SV40, arguing against a major role for exposure in brain tumour risk. The literature on whether SV40 or JC virus is present in human brain tumours has reported highly variable results. In a series of papers evaluating brain tumours, SV40 sequences were detected in approximately 35 per cent of cases.[19,22,79,111] In one study, 25–56 per cent of brain tumours of Swiss patients contained SV40 sequences, but these were not detectable in a similar series from Finland, a country where SV40-contaminated polio vaccine was not used,[126] consistent with the hypothesis that SV40 in human brain tumours originates from SV40-contaminated polio vaccine. However, a selective increase in the incidence of brain tumours has not been reported in populations that received SV40-contaminated polio vaccine, and incidence rates for brain tumours are similar in countries that did or did not use SV40-contaminated vaccine.[126] Furthermore, careful study involving expert laboratories from two large centres evaluated the prevalence of SV40, JC and the related BK viral sequences in 225 brain tumours using polymerase chain reaction (PCR) followed by Southern hybridization, as well as real-time quantitative PCR. In the face of stringent controls, the laboratory using PCR followed by Southern hybridization found only three JCV-positive, three BKV-positive and three SV40-positive cases and the laboratory employing real-time quantitative PCR found only one positive tumour (for SV40). This group concluded that JCV, BKV and SV40 are rare in brain tumours.[145] When viewing the literature on this subject, one must consider that small sample sizes and differences in underlying patient populations, laboratory techniques and quality control measures could all contribute to the variability of reported results.[145] The role of these viruses in brain tumourigenesis therefore remains *sub judice*.

A somewhat more compelling case has been made for the role of human cytomegalovirus (HCMV) in gliomas, although this issue similarly remains controversial. This association was first suggested in 2002 when HCMV transcripts and proteins were detected in 22 of 22 glioblastomas, 5 of 5 lower-grade diffuse gliomas, and none of the 23 meningiomas and non-neoplastic brain samples studies.[37] Whereas some groups were unable to replicate these findings, the majority similarly found evidence of HCMV in glioblastomas using immunohistochemistry (IHC), *in situ* hybridization, PCR, electron microscopy, PCR coupled with DNA sequencing, enzyme-linked immunosorbent assay, and flow cytometry.[36,54,140] The most commonly applied method is IHC with antibodies directed against the immediate early 1 (IE1) protein. Nonetheless, methodological differences may be responsible for interlaboratory discrepancies, with ultrasensitive techniques being touted as necessary for detecting relatively low levels of infection, particularly when working with paraffin embedded tissue, which not surprisingly is less reliable than frozen tissue and generally works best if the case is relatively recent. Unlike other models of viral oncogenesis, data suggest that HCMV is not involved in neoplastic transformation, but merely facilitates malignant progression. This putative role is based on evidence that viral infection or HCMV-encoded proteins promote genomic instability, cellular proliferation, angiogenesis, evasion of growth suppressors, cellular migration, replicative immortality via telomerase activation, decreased cell death via antiapoptotic activity, and induction of tumour promoting inflammation.[36,54,140] Evidence also suggests that viral infection of glioma cells requires PDGFRA expression, a common finding in diffuse gliomas. Nonetheless, this association is still poorly understood and some have postulated that PDGFRA haplotype differences may be associated with variable levels of susceptibility to infection. Based on the lack of active viral production and the detected proteins being expressed, HCMV infection in human gliomas does not correspond to the classic definitions for either lytic or latent stages of disease, prompting the hypothesis that this is a 'persistent' form of infection. Additional evidence supporting a potential role for this virus includes: (1) a murine CMV glioma model whereby enhanced tumourigenicity and decreased survival times are reported in CMV infected versus control mice and (2) preliminary data suggesting enhanced patient survival times in two clinical trials, one from the Karolinska Institute in Stockholm utilizing the antiviral drug valgancyclovir, and the other from Duke University using autologous CMV pp65 RNA loaded dendritic cells.[36,54] One observation that is difficult to reconcile is that the viral genome only appears to involve a minority of cells within the tumour, although some data suggest a possible explanation being that the stem cell compartment is preferentially targeted.[140] Although many unresolved questions remain and there is clearly much work still to be done, the following statement was published by a group of experts: 'a consensus was reached that there is sufficient evidence to conclude that HCMV sequences and viral gene expression exist in most, if not all, malignant gliomas; that HCMV could modulate the malignant phenotype in glioblastomas by interacting with key signaling pathways; and that HCMV could serve as a novel target for a variety of therapeutic strategies'.[54]

Lastly, there are rarer tumour subsets with viral associations, including that of Epstein–Barr virus (EBV) with lymphomas (see Chapter 40, Lymphomas and Haemopoietic Neoplasms) and Smooth Muscle Tumours (see Chapter 37, Mesenchymal Non-meningothelial Tumours). EBV is a member of the herpes viral family and is one of the most common human viruses worldwide. Its potential role in lymphoproliferative disorders systemically is well known and, in the brain, it is most frequently associated with primary CNS B-cell lymphomas of immunocompromised hosts, including those with AIDS, organ transplants, or immunosuppressive regimens administered for other disorders.[14,26,97] It is similarly thought to play a role in very rare examples of intracranial leiomyomas and leiomyosarcomas in immunocompromised patients.[29,64,164]

Allergy and Autoimmune Disease

Epidemiologic studies demonstrating inverse relationships between gliomas and allergic diseases (including asthma and eczema) and/or borderline increases in serum IgE levels have been surprisingly consistent, with overall risks of roughly 0.3 to 0.7 for most associations.[20,101,113,184] Perhaps most compelling is a recent nested case–control study using archived serum specimens from Norway of 594 case subjects and 1177 controls, where IgE levels measured at least 20 years prior to diagnosis were inversely associated with subsequent risk of developing a glioma.[159] Besides asthma, the most common autoimmune disease inversely associated with gliomas is diabetes (OR, 0.63).[16] Of interest, one study found that prior exposure to chickenpox was also associated with lower risks for WHO grade II and III oligodendrogliomas (OR, 0.5–0.6).[113] Studies of meningiomas have been less constant; whereas a relatively small study of 197 meningioma patients failed to find an association,[16] a more recent investigation of 1065 patients reported a similar inverse association with allergies (OR, 0.64) as seen in gliomas.[185] Overall, the observed relationships between allergies, autoimmune disease and brain tumours suggest a role for immune regulation.

Immunosuppression

Epidemiological studies previously found an increased incidence of primary CNS lymphoma, although this may have peaked in the mid-1990s, subsequently dropping dramatically in HIV patients as a result of the efficacy of HAART therapy, but still continuing to rise slightly in immunocompetent elderly patients.[75,147,177] In non-treated or poorly treated HIV patients, the acquired immunodeficiency syndrome (AIDS) is associated with an increased risk of developing primary malignant CNS lymphomas, with the risk estimated up to 3600-fold higher for patients with AIDS than the general population.[40a] Most examples are EBV-positive diffuse large B-cell lymphomas.[14,47,83]

Primary involvement of the CNS has been found to occur in 22 per cent of patients with post-transplant non-Hodgkin's lymphoma.[135] The risk appears lower for patients with renal transplants (1–2 per cent) than for those with heart, lung or liver transplants (2–7 per cent).[155a] It has been estimated that approximately 2 per cent of all patients with prolonged immunosuppression develop primary CNS lymphomas and those with iatrogenic immunosuppression are similarly at risk.[97,133]

Familial Brain Tumour Syndromes and Clusters

A number of hereditary syndromes feature nervous system tumours; these are discussed at greater length later (see Chapter 44, Hereditary Tumour Syndromes). The syndromes and their respective nervous system tumours include neurofibromatosis 1 with diffuse astrocytomas, pilocytic astrocytomas, neurofibromas and malignant peripheral nerve sheath tumours; neurofibromatosis 2 with schwannomas, meningiomas, meningioangiomatosis and ependymomas; schwannomatosis with multiple schwannomas; tuberous sclerosis with subependymal giant cell tumours; von Hippel–Lindau disease with haemangioblastomas; Li–Fraumeni syndrome with malignant gliomas and PNETs; Turcot syndrome with malignant gliomas and PNETs; Cowden syndrome with dysplastic gangliocytoma of the cerebellum (Lhermitte–Duclos); basal cell naevus (Gorlin) syndrome with medulloblastoma; and a host of less common syndromes. For nearly all of these conditions, the respective causative genes have been identified and this knowledge has provided invaluable information concerning the molecular basis of brain tumourigenesis.

Non-syndromic clusters of brain tumours have been reported in families, but it is unclear whether such clusters arise because of genetic or environmental factors. A study of 154 patients from 72 families revealed that parents and children were affected in 33 families, siblings in 27 families, and spouses in 12 families. Notably, these tumours did not involve multiple generations or present at early age. In addition, the cases tended to cluster in time, with 47 per cent of the familial and 50 per cent of the husband–wife cases occurring within a 5-year span. These data suggested that environmental exposures may explain such clustering.[63] Another study of 25 546 relatives of 396 patients with glioma found no statistically significant increase in gliomas or other CNS tumours in these relatives.[128] Nonetheless, a report of 5088 these relatives of 639 probands with gliomas favoured a multifactorial mendelian model and rejected a model postulating a purely environmental cause.[46] Another study of the Utah Population Data Base similarly suggests an increased heritable risk in first-degree relatives of astrocytoma patients.[13] It is therefore likely that such clusters represent a combination of multigenic and environmental causes.

ANIMAL MODELS OF NERVOUS SYSTEM TUMOURS

The use of animal models has played an important role in understanding key pathways in brain tumourigenesis and in providing preclinical systems for evaluation of potential therapies. Although there are clear differences between each model and the human counterparts, knowledge of these models provides selected but important insights into human brain tumour formation and progression, and possibly response to therapy.

Spontaneously occurring nervous system tumours in animals are neither common nor stereotypical in their presentation, thus creating a substantial need for experimental tumour models. Animal models of nervous system tumours have been undertaken with a number of goals: (1) to identify environmental chemicals or viruses involved in tumour aetiology; (2) to elucidate molecular pathways operative in tumour initiation and progression; and (3) to provide preclinical models for novel therapeutic testing. Most animal modelling has shifted decidedly towards transgenic mouse models, also known as genetically engineered mouse models (GEMMs) because these can recapitulate some of the molecular and phenotypic characteristics of the human tumours. In general, such models hold greater promise for elucidating pathways and for providing as relevant preclinical models as possible. Nonetheless, xenograft models are still in common use and there is a long productive history in experimental models to evaluate chemicals and viruses that might be involved in brain tumour aetiology. The following section discusses spontaneous neoplasia, tumour xenografts, older models based on chemical or viral tumourigenesis and the transgenic approaches that are now widely used.

Spontaneous Nervous System Neoplasia in Animals

Spontaneous nervous system tumours are uncommon in animals. Some strains of mouse and rat have slightly elevated rates of primary brain tumours. This has assumed importance primarily in the determination of whether particular carcinogenic agents generate tumours above the baseline rate. Given their low incidence, such tumours are not of experimental value, although cell lines can be generated from these for subsequent use.

Glial and meningeal tumours are moderately common in dogs and cats, and are occasionally used for experimental purposes or for genetic comparisons with human counterparts.[48,72] For instance, cell lines derived from spontaneous canine gliomas can be used to generate intracerebral xenografts in dogs rendered immunotolerant after allogeneic, subcutaneous tumour growth. It has been suggested that such a model could permit evaluations of new glioma therapies for brain tumours that would not be feasible in smaller, immunocompromised or inbred animals.[9] Additionally, these tumours closely resemble the human counterpart.[21] The expense of using this model and the perceived difficulties of working with domestic dogs has, however, prevented widespread use.

Domestic dog species are highly inbred, as a result of a directed policy pursued by breeders over the past few hundred years. As a result, different breeds have different propensities to individual diseases. In dogs, brachycephalic (short-snouted) breeds have a predisposition to gliomas, whereas dolichocephalic (long-snouted) dogs more commonly get meningiomas. These canine tumours bear striking similarities to their human counterparts. Importantly, the characterization of the dog genome now creates the possibility of linking disease predisposition to the various polymorphic loci that determine breed specificity and presumably breed disease predilection.[131] It therefore remains possible that critical insights into human gliomas and meningiomas will be derived from studies linking dog brain tumours to specific genetic loci.

Xenograft Models

Xenograft models of brain tumours have been the core of experimental and preclinical brain tumour work. Most xenograft models employ well-established cell lines, either human or rodent, that are transplanted in either the brain (orthotopic) or heterotopic sites (mostly subcutaneous). Not surprisingly, the shift has been towards the former, coupled with sensitive bioluminescence techniques for monitoring tumor growth.[130] Many of these have been characterized for key genetic changes.[86] Xenograft models are highly reproducible in that tumours nearly always develop and follow stereotypical time courses, making them valuable for evaluating new therapies; indeed, most preclinical trials conducted over the past few decades have been based on xenografts. They are also relatively simple and inexpensive, not requiring complicated mouse transgenesis. However, xenograft models suffer from disadvantages as well. Nearly all glioma xenograft models are non-invasive; because glioma invasion is perhaps the cardinal feature impeding effective therapy in humans, this is a major modelling flaw and many agents that appear promising in xenografts do not fare well in human trials. In addition, some murine lines were originally induced via chemical mutagenesis (see under Chemical Models, this page), other lines appear more sarcomatous than glial and most widely used human lines have been passaged for decades. For these reasons, their direct relevance to human brain tumours remains an open question. Finally, xenografting itself raises immunological issues. For example, human cell lines transplanted into rodents will survive only in immunocompromised animals, creating a substantial complicating variable for translation to the human condition.

Major advances have recently made xenograft models more representative of the human counterparts. For instance, although most glioblastomas with gene amplifications lose amplification when grown *in vitro*, serial passaging as subcutaneous flank xenografts in nude mice yields tumours with retained *EGFR-* and *PDGFRA-* amplified status.[60] Importantly, when transplanted from the flank via short-term culture to the brain of nude mice, these lines create tumours that infiltrate into the surrounding brain. The tumours have glial characteristics, but they show necrosis only rarely and do not display microvascular proliferation.

Additionally, xenograft models have been important in formulating cell origin hypotheses and the concept of the glioma stem cell (GSC), a putative cell capable of self-renewal and recapitulation of the histopathological and molecular heterogeneity seen in the tumour of origin. Although controversial, GSCs share some properties with non-neoplastic neural stem cells (NSCs), often expressing early developmental markers, such as CD133, Nestin, SOX2, OLIG2, Bmi1, Nanog, CD44, CD15 and integrin alpha 6.[31] For instance, one study demonstrated that as few as 100 human CD133-positive GSCs injected into brains

of immunodeficient mice could generate viable xenografts, whereas as many as 100 000 CD133-negative cells could not.[163] In another example, transduction of mutant N-myc into NSCs from forebrain followed by orthotopic transplantation resulted in formation of gliomas, whereas the same approach using NSCs from cerebellum or brain stem yielded medulloblastomas and PNETs, respectively; this study suggested that both the tumour location and timing of the NSC extraction during development influenced the type of tumour that developed.[169]

Chemical and Virus-Based Models

The generation of brain tumour models in rodents through the use of chemical carcinogens or tumourigenic viruses has had a long and productive history in neuro-oncology. Such models suffer, however, from being less 'faithful' to human disease biology than more recent transgenic approaches. The following section provides a brief overview of these models and the reader is referred to earlier editions of this text,[100] as well as other reviews,[12,149] for further information.

Chemical Models

Alkylating agents are the most effective chemicals for inducing CNS neoplasms in animals. Nitrosourea derivatives, particularly methylnitrosourea (MNU) and ethylnitrosourea (ENU), cause a high incidence of CNS neoplasms in rats after systemic administration.[49] Ethyl-nitrosourea and related ethylating agents (1,2-diethylhydrazine, 1-phenyl-3,3-diethyltriazene) are particularly powerful when administered as a single dose transplacentally or shortly after birth.[87] The susceptibility of the rat CNS to these agents begins at the tenth prenatal day (E10), increases gradually and reaches its maximum at birth, when a single dose is approximately 50 times more effective than in adult rats. N-nitrosomethylurea and related methylating agents (1,2-dimethylhydrazine, 1-phenyl-3,3-dimethyltriazene) are less effective transplacentally, but induce tumours after repeated administration of small weekly doses to adult rats.[50,139,170] Of particular interest have been ENU-induced schwannomas of cranial and peripheral nerves, which invariably contain a T:A to A:T transversion at nucleotide 2012 (codon 664; Val to Glu) in the transmembrane domain of the *neu* proto-oncogene; however, no *neu* mutations have been found in human schwannomas.[155]

Oncogenic Viruses and Viral Oncogenes

Earlier studies utilized oncogenic viruses to induce brain tumours, whereas more recent approaches have expressed specific viral oncogenes in a transgenic and hence more directed fashion. The use of oncogenic viruses generates brain tumours of various sorts, depending on the virus and mode of delivery, but the relevance of such models has been questioned by the lack of direct epidemiological evidence linking such viruses to human brain tumours. Nonetheless, several oncogenic viruses induce a high incidence of tumours in rats after postnatal intracerebral injection. These are discussed briefly later, but the reader is referred to earlier editions of this text,[100] as well as other reviews,[12,149] for further information. Directed expression of viral oncogenes has found more favour in that these oncogenes affect specific pathways involved in human brain tumourigenesis, but models have shifted to direct genetic manipulation, as discussed later (see under Transgenic Mouse Models, below).

As discussed earlier (under Epidemiology and Aetiology), there have been intriguing suggestions that SV40 virus may have a role in brain tumourigenesis. This DNA virus and its transforming gene, large T antigen, exert oncogenic effects through binding and inactivation of two key cellular regulatory molecules: p53 and pRb (as well as the other pocket protein members of the pRb family). When inoculated intracerebrally in newborn hamsters, SV40 induces choroid plexus papillomas and ependymomas.[53] Transgenic expression of SV40 large T antigen can generate PNETs, retinoblastomas or choroid plexus tumours, depending on the promoter utilized.[59] Directed expression of a mutant large T antigen (T121) that specifically inactivates pRb family members, under control of the GFAP promoter, results in high-grade astrocytic tumours.[188]

JC virus has an extensive sequence homology with SV40. However, whereas SV40 does not infect human cells, latent JC infection is common, with a serological prevalence of 40–60 per cent in most developed countries. In immunosuppressed patients, JC virus is the cause of progressive multifocal leukoencephalopathy. JC virus causes brain tumours, mostly PNETs, after intracerebral injection in newborn hamsters.[178,196] Two Colombian owl monkeys inoculated with JC virus derived from human PML cases developed brain tumours after 16–25 months that closely resembled human astrocytomas.[105] Transgenic mice expressing the early region of JC virus developed medulloblastoma/PNET in the cerebellum and the surrounding brainstem at 9–13 months of age.[99]

The BK virus, which has extensive sequence homology to JC and SV40 virus, primarily affects other organs such as the urinary tract, but can induce choroid plexus papillomas and ependymomas after intracerebral injection in newborn Syrian golden hamsters.[174] Polyoma virus can be tumourigenic when inoculated at high titre into newborn mice. A variety of tumours can be induced, including gliomas in rats.[1] Intracerebral injection of various strains of Rous sarcoma virus (RSV) can produce intracranial neoplasms in a variety of animals. The resulting tumours may be malignant astrocytomas or meningeal sarcomas, depending on the site of inoculation.[12] Simian adenovirus (SA7) has induced choroid plexus papillomas and medulloblastomas in the hamster.[32,117] Transgenic mice expressing human papillomavirus (HPV16) E6 and E7 open reading frames under control of the human beta-actin promoter developed brain tumours at a penetrance of 71 per cent between 2.5 and 10 months of age.[2a] Most frequent were anaplastic neuroepithelial tumours associated with the ependyma of the third ventricle; other tumours were choroid plexus neoplasms and pituitary carcinomas.

Transgenic Mouse Models

Transgenic mouse models have revolutionized experimental neurooncology. These models all employ genetic manipulation to generate mice that are highly susceptible to specific brain tumour types. There are numerous approaches to generating such mice. Some of the key issues relating to

> **BOX 26.1. Considerations in evaluating mouse brain tumour models**
>
> Is the genetic manipulation that results in the mouse brain tumour also found in human brain tumours?
>
> Is there a reasonable genotype–phenotype correlation between mouse and human disease?
>
> Does the model overexpress a tumour-promoting oncogene or inactivate a tumour suppressor gene? Furthermore, is overexpression to physiological or supraphysiological levels, and is inactivation complete or partial downregulation?
>
> Is the nature of the genetic manipulation homozygous or hemizygous? This applies not only for the original genetic manipulation, but also for subsequent experiments in which one line is crossed into a second transgenic line. Additionally, somatic events must be evaluated to determine if, for example, the second copy of a hemizygously inactivated tumour suppressor has been lost during the process of tumourigenesis.
>
> Is the genetic manipulation in all cells or is it confined to a particular cell type or set of cell types? In this regard, the use of cell-specific promoters can direct an oncogenic effect to one organ and cell type.
>
> Is the genetic deregulation constant or inducible? Use of a particular promoter will direct expression or inactivation to cells when that promoter is 'turned on'. However, use of an inducible promoter, which involves addition or removal of a compound from the animal's drinking water, can turn on and/or turn off gene expression according to an experimental protocol. Another method to induce genetic deregulation at a specific time involves introduction of viruses bearing oncogenes or other genes that induce subsequent genetic consequences (e.g. Cre recombinase). Because the deregulation of some genes during development can be lethal or can produce a phenotype altered in many undesirable ways, inducible systems may allow distinctions to be made between developmental and non-developmental effects.
>
> Are there strain-specific effects on the expression of the phenotype? Some genetic manipulations produce gliomas in one genetic strain, but nerve sheath tumours in another.[141]
>
> How penetrant is the model? If the model is not highly penetrant, can the phenotype be clearly separated from age-dependent tumour development in inbred strains?

evaluating the models are listed in Box 26.1. The optimal preclinical model would: (1) accurately reproduce the human phenotype histopathologically and molecularly, (2) deliver short latency and high penetrance, (3) be easy to generate and utilize, and (4) incorporate a built-in molecular mechanism to assess therapeutic efficacy, such as a bioluminescent reporter.[82] Achieving all of these in one model has not been possible to date and one must consider that even in primary human tumours, genomic studies have revealed multiple molecular subsets for each diagnostic category, such that there are now attempts at modelling individual genetic subtypes. Therefore, each model offers its own distinct advantages and disadvantages, although testing prospective therapeutic agents on multiple genetically distinct GEMMs would likely provide the highest yield and reduce potential false negatives. Additionally, there has been an increasing recognition that not only the neoplastic cells themselves, but also their microenvironment is critical in determining tumour development and phenotype.[82,120,148] For instance, data suggest that *Nf1* heterozygous (one mutant and one wild-type allele) inflammatory cells, such as mast cells and microglia, are necessary for the formation of neurofibromas and optic gliomas in GEMMs.[5,194]

To date, GEMMs have been generated using many approaches. Modelling has focused most heavily on malignant gliomas, although GEMMs have been generated for a wide variety of tumour types. Some of these models have been more 'true' to the human condition, either in their genetic makeup or in their histological characteristics, than others. Some of the more relevant models of gliomas, medulloblastomas, nerve sheath tumours and meningiomas are covered elsewhere and the reader is referred to a number of reviews for additional information.[25,31,82,90,118,120,180] Models of other nervous system tumours are discussed in subsequent chapters.

Malignant Gliomas

The suggested approach to classification of GEM gliomas follows the nomenclature of the WHO systems.[180] GEM high-grade astrocytomas have been generated using a wide variety of approaches,[82] many employing GFAP promoters to encourage oncogenic events in astrocytic cells. Whereas most strategies targeting only a single tumour suppressor or oncogene have failed, highly efficient tumourigenesis has generally been achieved by combining activation of receptor tyrosine kinase (RTK) pathways with dysregulation of the cell cycle,[31] with some models appearing more discrete and others more infiltrative as in the human counterpart. Further incorporation of progression associated alterations, such as *Pten* loss, generally results in high-grade gliomas exclusively. Most recently, GEM glioblastomas have begun to be used to understand the role of cancer stem cells and the relationship of such cells to chemotherapeutic resistance in glioblastomas.[2,30]

More focal malignant gliomas have been generated via combined inactivation of the *Nf1* and *Tp53* genes. One approach generated mice with heterozygous inactivation of *Nf1* and *Trp53* in a *cis* configuration (residing on the same chromosome). These animals developed a range of histologically typical low-grade astrocytomas to glioblastomas with a penetrance of 100 per cent at 6 months.[141] Strikingly, this was strain-specific, because the same transgenic manipulation in a different strain resulted in malignant peripheral nerve sheath tumours.[34] A more directed approach was achieved via inactivation of both *Nf1* and *Trp53*, specifically in astrocytic cells or their precursors, with GFAP driving Cre expression.[195] Low-grade astrocytomas developed in 100 per cent of these mice, eventually progressing to high-grade tumours with all of the classic histological findings of glioblastoma. For these reasons, such mice may prove to be a highly useful model of astrocytoma formation and progression.

The most directed approach to yield high-grade astrocytomas that closely recapitulate the histological features of human glioblastoma involves the avian retrovirus RCAS system.[76] In this approach, transgenic expression of an avian retroviral receptor is driven by either the nestin or GFAP promoter; viruses expressing specific oncogenes are then introduced via intracerebral injection. Only those cells expressing the retroviral receptor can be infected by the virus and express the oncogene. Mimicking activation of the EGFR pathway by introducing activated Ras and mimicking inactivation of the PTEN pathway by introducing Akt expression, both in nestin-expressing progenitor cells, produces histologically classic glioblastomas in about one-quarter of mice by approximately 2 months of age.[76]

Other methods have been utilized to generate astrocytoma models, including introduction of activated EGFR into cultured cortical astrocytes from *Ink4a*-deficient mice, recapitulating two cardinal events in glioblastoma formation (EGFR overexpression and p16 deletion).[3] Overexpression of EGFR drives these astrocytes to a less differentiated state. Remarkably, these cells will then generate tumours of divergent (astrocytic, oligodendroglial and neuronal) differentiation when introduced into nude mouse brains.

Oligodendrogliomas have resulted from a variety of genetic manipulations. Driving v-erbB expression (homologous to EGFR) under control of the *S-100B* promoter generates diffuse tumours that are histologically identical to oligodendrogliomas. Crossing these mice into an *Ink4a*-deficient or *Tp53*-deficient background then produces high-grade oligodendrogliomas.[181] Using the RCAS system, oligodendrogliomas have been produced by overexpressing PDGF-B in nestin-expressing neural progenitors, inducing oligodendrogliomas in about 60 per cent of mice by 3 months of age; on the other hand, PDGF transfer to GFAP-expressing astrocytes more often produced oligoastrocytomas, in about 40 per cent of mice by 3 months. Additional loss of Ink4a, as in other models, created high-grade tumours.[42]

Medulloblastomas and Embryonal Neoplasms

Medulloblastomas and other embryonal neoplasms have been generated using a variety of genetic manipulations.[118] One of the most relevant to human medulloblastoma has been heterozygous inactivation of the *Ptc* gene, which results in medulloblastoma in fewer than 20 per cent of mice.[61] Penetrance jumps to over 95 per cent and is accelerated to under 12 weeks of age in mice that lack *p53*.[183] Other groups have targeted a variety of other molecules in various combinations, including *Tp53*, *Rb1*, *Shh*, *SmoA1*, *Inc4c*, *N-Myc* and *c-Myc* producing models of medulloblastoma and/or CNS PNET,[118] with overexpression of the latter often associated with large cell or anaplastic features.[134] For atypical teratoid/rhabdoid tumour, a *Smarcb1+/−* GEMM has been reported, although the majority of tumours develop in the soft tissue rather than the CNS.[142]

Nerve Sheath Tumours

Genetically engineered murine nerve sheath tumours have primarily involved genetic inactivation of *Nf1*, *Nf2*, *Smarcb1* and *Prkar1a*, mimicking human neurofibromatosis 1 (NF1), neurofibromatosis 2 (NF2), schwannomatosis and Carney complex, respectively; a full description of these models is beyond the scope of this text and the reader is referred to an excellent review.[25] As mentioned, the microenvironment appears to be key in some of these models and Schwann cell conditional knockouts are needed in others. Similar to GEM gliomas, strain background similarly has an influence in GEM nerve sheath tumours.

CLASSIFICATION AND GRADING

Classification and Grading Systems

Tumours of the nervous system present a bewildering variety of histological appearances. Therefore, it is not surprising that many attempts have been made to produce classifications that accurately reflect prognosis and response to particular therapies. The aim to produce such a classification has been frustrated not only by lack of knowledge concerning histogenesis and tumourigenesis at a biological level, but also by the variably subjective nature of histological parameters. The classification of neoplasms can be based on morphological features, biological behaviour, cells of origin, histological resemblances, expression of particular molecules and genetic abnormalities.

The introduction of modern investigative methods into neuro-oncology has been instrumental in devising classifications that take more than one aspect of each tumour into consideration. Electron microscopy, tissue culture, immunohistochemistry, biology and molecular genetics have all substantially contributed to the understanding of the neoplastic process and, in doing so, have greatly improved the definitional criteria on which tumour classifications are based. It must be emphasized that tumour classification is a dynamic process that is nestled between pathological approaches to diagnosis, radiological techniques, biological advances and improvements in therapy. Classification can, and must, change in response to improved understanding and abilities in each of these areas. For example, the advent of a new effective therapy raises the possibility that particular histological or molecular features correlate with response to the new therapy. On the other hand, molecular advances now commonly outpace clinical neuro-oncology. For instance, recent high throughput genomics data suggest that there are at least four molecular subtypes each of glioblastoma and medulloblastoma.[98,143,176] Nevertheless, there are not targeted therapies available for each of these subtypes. Furthermore, although classification systems must be dynamic, they must refrain from excessive flux, in order to retain stability in the treatment of individual patients. In this regard, changes in classification must be based on high-quality validated data.

Many classification systems have been put forth for brain tumours over the past 100 years.[4,92,95,96,149,197,198] In 1979, the WHO published histological typing of tumours of the CNS.[197] It was subsequently revised multiple times by teams of experts with subsequent publications in 1993, 2000 and 2007.[95,96,108]

The WHO classification adopted the basic principle of histological typing: tumour entities are defined primarily by morphological appearances, including constituent cell types and tissue patterns. However, the results of modern investigative techniques, particularly those of genetics and immunohistochemistry, were taken into consideration when available. The overall aim was to classify, whenever possible, neoplasms according to their biological properties. That being said, there are numerous, mostly rare entities for which no significant biological information exists, and these tumours are classified solely on the basis of their light-microscopic characteristics. In this regard, it must be recognized that histological appearances may not reflect cells of origin, i.e. that a tumour having cells resembling astrocytes does not necessarily result from transformation of astrocytes.

Grading attempts to assign numerical values to expected 'natural' biological behaviours. This immensely complex problem is unlikely to be sufficiently addressed by simply assigning histological grades to intracranial neoplasms ranging from I (benign) to IV (most malignant). This numerical system, based on the similar grading of carcinomas, was first developed by Kernohan and colleagues.[93] The revised classification has adapted these criteria within the framework of the internationally accepted coding system.[108] However, the grading of rare or newly defined tumour entities requires continuous reassessment, because their biological behaviour becomes clearer with longer follow-up studies of larger cohorts. Two general points should also be emphasized. First, histological variations within the same tumour may render grading of small biopsies a treacherous exercise, a difficulty that may be overcome by multiple, image-guided stereotactic biopsies and close communication between the neuropathologist and the neurosurgeon. Second, the importance of factors independent of histology should not be overlooked in prognosis: patient age, extent of surgical removal and clinical performance status are the most important prognostic factors for high-grade malignant gliomas.

Clinical Approach to Brain Tumour Diagnosis

Brain tumour diagnosis by the pathologist is based on amalgamation of a wide variety of data derived from clinical information and specialized assays. In general, knowledge of clinical history, radiological features, neurosurgical findings and histopathological evaluation is required for accurate diagnosis. In many cases, immunohistochemistry and special stains provide valuable ancillary information. Less commonly, electron microscopy is used. Increasingly, molecular diagnostic assays also provide valuable diagnostic, prognostic, or even predictive information. The basic features of each of these parameters are discussed later.

From a clinical point of view, the following information must be found before evaluating a brain tumour sample: patient age and gender; the location of the tumour; neuroradiological findings; and pertinent past medical history. For example, with knowledge of patient age and tumour location, the differential diagnostic possibilities can be narrowed and prioritized to a remarkable degree. Neuroradiological features, including the exact location, nature of the margins and imaging characteristics (e.g. enhancing versus non-enhancing, pattern of enhancement, perfusion and diffusion weighted imaging data, etc.), also allow prioritization of the diagnostic possibilities. Moreover, imaging features may provide information not available from the tissue sample; for instance, the finding of a ring-enhancing parenchymal tumour on neuroimaging in the presence of a WHO grade II or III astrocytoma on biopsy argues strongly that a glioblastoma has been sampled inadequately.

Histochemical stains do not play a major role in the classification of brain tumours, but may be of help to demonstrate reticulin or mucin or other structures of diagnostic importance. Immunohistochemistry, on the other hand, is of great importance in tumour classification and, to a lesser extent, tumour grading by use of proliferation markers. Most immunohistochemical assays evaluate lines of differentiation, for example GFAP in glial tumours and cytokeratins in epithelial malignancies. This application is covered in the following chapters, when each of the entities is discussed. It should be borne in mind that 'differentiation' in malignant tumours may be biologically distinct from normal development and that tumours may undergo divergent differentiation. In this regard, one should not conclude tumour cell of origin from studies of tumour differentiation.

The need for electron microscopy has diminished in diagnostic neuropathology with the advent of improved immunohistochemical approaches and the emerging role of molecular genetic analysis, but may still be of great utility in rare settings, such as histologically atypical ependymal neoplasms or poorly differentiated tumours in general. Molecular analysis has made considerable inroads into diagnostic tumour neuropathology. The application of molecular genetics to neuro-oncology is well established in the field of lymphoma diagnosis, where monoclonality of immunoglobulin and T-cell receptor gene rearrangements may be diagnostically useful. Other molecular alterations characterize particular tumours and can be used for diagnosis, such as specific translocations in sarcomas or chromosome 22 loss and *INI1* mutations in atypical teratoid/rhabdoid tumours (ATRT). In addition to diagnostic aid, some markers are associated with enhanced prognosis, such as the presence of *MGMT* promotor methylation in glioblastomas or *IDH* gene mutations in diffuse gliomas in general. Most widespread are assays for parameters that potentially affect treatment decisions such as the type of chemotherapy or radiation therapy; 1p and 19q testing in oligodendroglial tumours conforms to this scenario, as may *EGFR* analysis in non–small cell lung carcinoma or ER, PR and *HER2* studies in metastatic breast cancer. Of interest, some assays initially assessable only through molecular techniques may now be interrogated with standard immunohistochemistry. Examples include the loss of INI1 protein expression in ATRT and the detection of the R132H mutant IDH1 protein in diffuse gliomas.

The following two sections closely follow the 2007 WHO classification. It should be stressed, however, that not all tumours fit well within the standard WHO entities. Not uncommonly, individual brain tumours defy exact classification. In such a situation, it makes little sense to attempt to force a lesion into one of the existing entities, because the behaviour of the tumour may not correspond with that of the existing entity. For tumours that do not conform to the WHO definitions, descriptive diagnoses suffice, as long as they convey the critical prognostic and predictive information needed by the clinician. Caveats must also be issued regarding WHO grades because these primarily reflect 'natural history'. Grade I tumours are benign in the sense that, if they can be resected, they can be cured, but not all grade I brain tumours can be resected, particularly those lying deep within the brain. Grade IV tumours, at the other end of the spectrum, are highly malignant tumours with a generally poor prognosis, but the natural behaviour can be altered radically using available therapies (e.g. medulloblastoma). Furthermore, although all tumours can be assigned a WHO grade, most clinicians only utilize grades in the management of gliomas, particularly for the astrocytic group of neoplasms.

ACKNOWLEDGEMENTS

The authors are grateful to Dr Margaret Wrensch, Neurological Surgery and Institute of Human Genetics, University of California San Francisco, for providing valuable input regarding the latest GWAS and allergy study data.

REFERENCES

1. Aguzzi A, Kleihues P, Heckl K, Wiestler OD. Cell type-specific tumour induction in neural transplants by retrovirus-mediated oncogene transfer. *Oncogene* 1991;6:113–18.
2. Alcantara Llaguno S, Chen J, Kwon CH, et al. Malignant astrocytomas originate from neural stem/progenitor cells in a somatic tumor suppressor mouse model. *Cancer Cell* 2009;15:45–56.
2a. Arbeit JM, Munger K, Howley PM, Hanahan D. Neuroepithelial carcinomas in mice transgenic with human papillomavirus type 16 E6/E7 ORFs. *Am J Pathology* 1993;142:1187–97.
3. Bachoo RM, Maher EA, Ligon K, et al. Epidermal growth factor receptor and Ink4a/Arf: convergent mechanisms governing terminal differentiation and transformation along the neural stem cell to astrocyte axis. *Cancer Cell* 2002;1:269–77.
4. Bailey P, Cushing H. *A classification of tumors of the glioma group on a histogenetic basis with a correlation study of prognosis.* Philadelphia, PA: Lippincott, 1926.
5. Bajenaru ML, Hernandez MR, Perry A, et al. Optic nerve glioma in mice requires astrocyte Nf1 gene inactivation and Nf1 brain heterozygosity. *Cancer Res* 2003;63:8573–7.
6. Banerjee J, Paakko E, Harila M, et al. Radiation-induced meningiomas: a shadow in the success story of childhood leukemia. *Neuro Oncol* 2009;11:543–9.
7. Barnett GH, Chou SM, Bay JW. Posttraumatic intracranial meningiomas: a case report and review of the literature. *Neurosurgery* 1986;18:75–8.
8. Benson VS, Pirie K, Green J, Casabonne D, Beral V. Lifestyle factors and primary glioma and meningioma tumours in the Million Women Study cohort. *Br J Cancer* 2008;99:185–90.
9. Berens ME, Giese A, Shapiro JR, Coons SW. Allogeneic astrocytoma in immune competent dogs. *Neoplasia* 1999;1:107–12.
10. Berleur MP, Cordier S. The role of chemical, physical, or viral exposures and health factors in neurocarcinogenesis: implications for epidemiological studies of brain tumours. *Cancer Causes Control* 1995;6:240–56.
11. Bhat AR, Wani MA, Kirmani AR. Brain cancer and pesticide relationship in orchard farmers of Kashmir. *Indian J Occup Environ Med* 2010;14:78–86.
12. Bigner D, Swenberg J. *Experimental tumors of the central nervous system.* Kalamazoo, MI: Upjohn Company, 1977.
13. Blumenthal DT, Cannon-Albright LA. Familiality in brain tumors. *Neurology* 2008;71:1015–20.
14. Bossolasco S, Cinque P, Ponzoni M, et al. Epstein-Barr virus DNA load in cerebrospinal fluid and plasma of patients with AIDS-related lymphoma. *J Neurovirol* 2002;8:432–8.
15. Brat DJ, James CD, Jedlicka AE, et al. Molecular genetic alterations in radiation-induced astrocytomas. *Am J Pathol* 1999;154:1431–8.
16. Brenner AV, Linet MS, Fine HA, et al. History of allergies and autoimmune

diseases and risk of brain tumors in adults. *Int J Cancer* 2002;**99**:252–9.

17. Brooks DR, Mucci LA, Hatch EE, Cnattingius S. Maternal smoking during pregnancy and risk of brain tumors in the offspring. A prospective study of 1.4 million Swedish births. *Cancer Causes Control* 2004;**15**:997–1005.

18. Brownson RC, Reif JS, Chang JC, Davis JR. An analysis of occupational risks for brain cancer. *Am J Publ Health* 1990;**80**:169–72.

19. Butel JS, Lednicky JA. Cell and molecular biology of simian virus 40: implications for human infections and disease. *J Natl Cancer Inst* 1999;**91**:119–34.

20. Calboli FC, Cox DG, Buring JE, et al. Prediagnostic plasma IgE levels and risk of adult glioma in four prospective cohort studies. *J Natl Cancer Inst* 2011;**103**:1588–95.

21. Candolfi M, Curtin JF, Nichols WS, et al. Intracranial glioblastoma models in preclinical neuro-oncology: neuropathological characterization and tumor progression. *J Neurooncol* 2007;**85**:133–48.

22. Carbone M, Rizzo P, Pass HI. Simian virus 40, poliovaccines and human tumors: a review of recent developments. *Oncogene* 1997;**15**:1877–88.

23. Cardis E, Gilbert ES, Carpenter L, et al. Effects of low doses and low dose rates of external ionizing radiation: cancer mortality among nuclear industry workers in three countries. *Radiat Res* 1995;**142**:117–32.

24. Cardis E, Richardson L, Deltour I, et al. The INTERPHONE study: design, epidemiological methods, and description of the study population. *Eur J Epidemiol* 2007;**22**:647–64.

25. Carroll SL. Molecular mechanisms promoting the pathogenesis of Schwann cell neoplasms. *Acta Neuropathol* 2012;**123**:321–48.

26. Castellano-Sanchez AA, Li S, Qian J, et al. Primary central nervous system posttransplant lymphoproliferative disorders. *Am J Clin Pathol* 2004;**121**:246–53.

27. CBTRUS. CBTRUS Statistical Report: Primary brain tumors in the United States, 2004-2008. Hinsdale, IL: Central Brain Tumor Registry of the United States, 2012.

28. Chang SM, Barker FG, Larson DA, et al. Sarcomas subsequent to cranial irradiation. *Neurosurgery* 1995;**36**:685–90.

29. Chaves NJ, Kotsimbos TC, Warren MA, et al. Cranial leiomyosarcoma in an Epstein-Barr virus (EBV)-mismatched lung transplant recipient. *J Heart Lung Transplant* 2007;**26**:753–5.

30. Chen J, Li Y, Yu TS, et al. A restricted cell population propagates glioblastoma growth after chemotherapy. *Nature* 2012;**488**:522–6.

31. Chen J, McKay RM, Parada LF. Malignant glioma: lessons from genomics, mouse models, and stem cells. *Cell* 2012;**149**:36–47.

32. Chen T, Mora E, Mealey JJ. Cultivation of medulloblastoma cells derived from simian adenovirus SA7-induced hamster brain tumour. *Cancer Res* 1975;**35**:3566–70.

33. Chowdhary A, Spence AM, Sales L, et al. Radiation associated tumors following therapeutic cranial radiation. *Surg Neurol Int* 2012;**3**:48–58.

34. Cichowski K, Shih TS, Schmitt E, et al. Mouse models of tumor development in neurofibromatosis type 1. *Science* 1999;**286**:2172–6.

35. Claus EB, Calvocoressi L, Bondy ML, et al. Dental x-rays and risk of meningioma. *Cancer* 2012;**118**:4530–7.

36. Cobbs CS. Evolving evidence implicates cytomegalovirus as a promoter of malignant glioma pathogenesis. *Herpesviridae* 2011;**2**:10.

37. Cobbs CS, Harkins L, Samanta M, et al. Human cytomegalovirus infection and expression in human malignant glioma. *Cancer Res* 2002;**62**:3347–50.

38. Cordier S, Iglesias MJ, Le Goaster C, et al. Incidence and risk factors for childhood brain tumors in the Ile de France. *Int J Cancer* 1994;**59**:776–82.

39. Cordier S, Monfort C, Filippini G, et al. Parental exposure to polycyclic aromatic hydrocarbons and the risk of childhood brain tumors: The SEARCH International Childhood Brain Tumor Study. *Am J Epidemiol* 2004;**159**:1109–16.

40. Corle C, Makale M, Kesari S. Cell phones and glioma risk: a review of the evidence. *J Neurooncol* 2012;**106**:1–13.

40a. Cote TR, Manns A, Hardy CR, et al. Epidemiology of brain lymphoma among people with or without acquired immunodeficiency syndrome. AIDS/Cancer Study Group. *J Natl Cancer Inst* 1996;**15**;88:675–9.

41. Custodio AC, Almeida LO, Pinto GR, et al. Analysis of the polymorphisms XRCC1Arg194Trp and XRCC1Arg399Gln in gliomas. *Genet Mol Res* 2011;**10**:1120–9.

42. Dai C, Celestino JC, Okada Y, et al. PDGF autocrine stimulation dedifferentiates cultured astrocytes and induces oligodendrogliomas and oligoastrocytomas from neural progenitors and astrocytes in vivo. *Genes Dev* 2001;**15**:1913–25.

43. Daugherty SE, Moore SC, Pfeiffer RM, et al. Nonsteroidal anti-inflammatory drugs and glioma in the NIH-AARP Diet and Health Study cohort. *Cancer Prev Res (Phila)* 2011;**4**:2027–34.

44. Davis FG, Bruner JM, Surawicz TS. The rationale for standardized registration and reporting of brain and central nervous system tumors in population-based cancer registries. *Neuroepidemiology* 1997;**16**:308–16.

45. Davis FG, McCarthy B, Jukich P. The descriptive epidemiology of brain tumors. *Neuroimag Clin N Am* 1999;**9**:581–94.

46. De Andrade M, Barnholtz JS, Amos CI, et al. Segregation analysis of cancer in families of glioma patients. *Genet Epidemiol* 2001;**20**:258–70.

47. DeAngelis LM, Wong E, Rosenblum M, Ferneaux H. Epstein–Barr virus in acquired immune deficiency syndrome (AIDS) and non-AIDS primary central nervous system lymphoma. *Cancer* 1992;**70**:1607–11.

48. Dickinson PJ, LeCouteur RA, Higgins RJ, et al. Canine spontaneous glioma: a translational model system for convection-enhanced delivery. *Neuro Oncol* 2010;**12**:928–40.

49. Druckrey H, Preussmann R, Ivankovic S, Schmahl D. Organotrope cancerogene Wirkungen bei 65 verschiedenen N-Nitroso-Verbindungen an BD-Ratten. *Z Krebsforsch* 1967;**69**:103–201.

50. Druckrey H, Ivankovic S, Preussmann R, et al. Transplacental induction of neurogenic malignancies by 1,2-diethylhydrazine, azo-, and azoxyethane in rats. *Experientia* 1968;**24**:561–2.

51. Dubrow R, Darefsky AS, Park Y, et al. Dietary components related to N-nitroso compound formation: a prospective study of adult glioma. *Cancer Epidemiol Biomarkers Prev* 2010;**19**:1709–22.

52. Dubrow R, Darefsky AS, Freedman ND, Hollenbeck AR, Sinha R. Coffee, tea, soda, and caffeine intake in relation to risk of adult glioma in the NIH-AARP Diet and Health Study. *Cancer Causes Control* 2012;**23**:757–68.

53. Duffell D, Hinz R, Nelson E. Neoplasms in hamsters induced by simian virus 40. Light and electron microscopic observations. *Am J Pathol* 1964;**45**:59–73.

54. Dziurzynski K, Chang SM, Heimberger AB, et al. Consensus on the role of human cytomegalovirus in glioblastoma. *Neuro Oncol* 2012;**14**:246–55.

55. Edwards MK, Terry JG, Montebello JF, et al. Gliomas in children following radiation therapy for lymphoblastic leukemia. *Acta Radiol [Suppl] (Stockh)* 1986;**369**:651–3.

56. Egan KM, Thompson RC, Nabors LB, et al. Cancer susceptibility variants and the risk of adult glioma in a US case-control study. *J Neurooncol* 2011;**104**:535–42.

57. Filippini G. Epidemiology of primary central nervous system tumors. *Handb Clin Neurol* 2012;**104**:3–22.

58. Frumkin H, Jacobson A, Gansler T, Thun MJ. Cellular phones and risk of brain tumors. *CA Cancer J Clin* 2001;**51**:137–41.

59. Fung K, Trojanowski J. Animal models of medulloblastomas and related primitive neuroectodermal tumors. A review. *J Neuropathol Exp Neurol* 1995;**54**:285–96.

60. Giannini C, Sarkaria JN, Saito A, et al. Patient tumor EGFR and PDGFRA gene amplifications retained in an invasive intracranial xenograft model of glioblastoma multiforme. *J Neurooncol* 2005;**7**:164–76.

61. Goodrich LV, Milenkovic L, Higgins KM, Scott MP. Altered neural cell fates and medulloblastoma in mouse patched mutants. *Science* 1997;**277**:1109–13.

62. Gorovets D, Kannan K, Shen R, et al. IDH mutation and neuroglial developmental features define clinically distinct subclasses of lower-grade diffuse astrocytic glioma. *Clin Cancer Res* 2012;**18**:2490–501.

63. Grossman SA, Osman M, Hruban R, Piantadosi S. Central nervous system cancers in first-degree relatives and spouses. *Cancer Invest* 1999;**17**:299–308.

64. Gupta SY, Havens PL, Southern JF, Firat SY, Jogal SS. Epstein-Barr virus-associated intracranial leiomyosarcoma in an HIV-positive adolescent. *J Pediatr Hematol Oncol* 2010;**32**:e144–7.

65. Gurney JG, Mueller BA, Davis S, et al. Childhood brain tumour occurrence in relation to residential power line configurations, electric heating sources, and electric appliance use. *Am J Epidemiol* 1996;**143**:120–8.

66. Gurney JG, Preston-Martin S, McDaniel AM, et al. Head injury

as a risk factor for brain tumors in children: results from a multicenter case–control study. *Epidemiology* 1996;**7**:485–9.

67. Hardell L, Nasman A, Pahlson A, et al. Use of cellular telephones and the risk for brain tumours: a case–control study. *Int J Oncol* 1999;**15**:113–16.

68. Hardell L, Mild KH, Pahlson A, Hallquist A. Ionizing radiation, cellular telephones and the risk for brain tumours. *Eur J Cancer Prev* 2001;**10**:523–9.

69. Hardell L, Hallquist A, Mild KH, et al. Cellular and cordless telephones and the risk for brain tumours. *Eur J Cancer Prev* 2002;**11**:377–86.

70. Hartmann C, Meyer J, Balss J, et al. Type and frequency of IDH1 and IDH2 mutations are related to astrocytic and oligodendroglial differentiation and age: a study of 1,010 diffuse gliomas. *Acta Neuropathol* 2009;**118**:469–74.

71. Hepworth SJ, Schoemaker MJ, Muir KR, et al. Mobile phone use and risk of glioma in adults: case-control study. *BMJ* 2006;**332**:883–7.

72. Higgins RJ, Dickinson PJ, LeCouteur RA, et al. Spontaneous canine gliomas: overexpression of EGFR, PDGFRalpha and IGFBP2 demonstrated by tissue microarray immunophenotyping. *J Neurooncol* 2010;**98**:49–55.

73. Hochberg F, Toniolo P, Cole P. Head trauma and seizures as risk factors of glioblastoma. *Neurology* 1984;**34**:1511–14.

74. Hodges LC, Smith JL, Garrett A, Tate S. Prevalence of glioblastoma multiforme in subjects with prior therapeutic radiation. *J Neurosci Nurs* 1992;**24**:79–83.

75. Hoffman S, Propp JM, McCarthy BJ. Temporal trends in incidence of primary brain tumours in the United States, 1985–1999. *J Neurooncol* 2006;**8**:27–37.

76. Holland EC, Celestino J, Dai C, et al. Combined activation of Ras and Akt in neural progenitors induces glioblastoma formation in mice. *Nat Genet* 2000;**25**:55–7.

77. Homma T, Fukushima T, Vaccarella S, et al. Correlation among pathology, genotype, and patient outcomes in glioblastoma. *J Neuropathol Exp Neurol* 2006;**65**:846–54.

78. Howe GR, Burch JD, Chiarelli AM, et al. An exploratory case–control study of brain tumors in children. *Cancer Res* 1989;**49**:4349–52.

79. Huang H, Reis R, Yonekawa Y, et al. Identification in human brain tumors of DNA sequences specific for SV40 large T antigen. *Brain Pathol* 1999;**9**:33–42.

80. Huncharek M, Kupelnick B, Klassen H. Maternal smoking during pregnancy and the risk of childhood brain tumors: a meta-analysis of 6566 subjects from twelve epidemiological studies. *J Neurooncol* 2002;**57**:51–7.

81. Huncharek M, Kupelnick B, Wheeler L. Dietary cured meat and the risk for adult glioma: a meta-analysis of nine observational studies. *J Environ Pathol Toxicol Oncol* 2003;**22**:129–37.

82. Huse JT, Holland EC. Genetically engineered mouse models of brain cancer and the promise of preclinical testing. *Brain Pathol* 2009;**19**:132–43.

83. Iglesias-Rozas JR, Bantz B, Adler T, et al. Cerebral lymphoma in AIDS. Clinical, radiological, neuropathological and immunopathological study. *Clin Neuropathol* 1991;**10**:65–72.

84. Inskip PD, Tarone RE, Hatch EE, et al. Sociodemographic indicators and risk of brain tumours. *Int J Epidemiol* 2003;**32**:225–33.

85. INTERPHONE Study Group. Brain tumour risk in relation to mobile telephone use: results of the INTERPHONE international case-control study. *Int J Epidemiol* 2010;**39**:675–94.

86. Ishii N, Maier D, Merlo A, et al. Frequent co-alterations of TP53, p16/CDKN2A, p14ARF, PTEN tumor suppressor genes in human glioma cell lines. *Brain Pathol* 1999;**9**:469–79.

87. Ivankovic S, Druckrey H. Transplacentare Erzeugung maligner Tumoren des Nervensystems. I. Athyl-nitroso-harnstoff (ANH) an BD IX-Ratten. *Z Krebsforsch* 1968;**71**:320–60.

88. Jenkins R, Xiao Y, Sicotte H, et al. A low frequency variant at 8q24.21 is strongly associated with risk of oligodendroglial tumors and IDH mutated astrocytomas. *Nat Genet* 2012;**44**:1122–5.

89. Kaderali Z, Lamberti-Pasculli M, Rutka JT. The changing epidemiology of paediatric brain tumours: a review from the Hospital for Sick Children. *Childs Nerv Syst* 2009;**25**:787–93.

90. Kalamarides M, Stemmer-Rachamimov AO, Takahashi M, et al. Natural history of meningioma development in mice reveals a synergy between Nf2 and p16(Ink4a) mutations. *Brain Pathol* 2008;**18**:62–70.

91. Kan P, Simonsen SE, Lyon JL, Kestle JR. Cellular phone use and brain tumor: a meta-analysis. *J Neurooncol* 2008;**86**:71–8.

92. Kernohan J, Sayre G. Tumors of the central nervous system. In: Kernohan J, Sayre G eds. *Atlas of tumour pathology.* Washington DC: Armed Forces Institute of Pathology, 1952.

93. Kernohan JW, Mabon RF, Svien HJ, Adson AW. A simplified classification of gliomas. *Proc Staff Meet Mayo Clin* 1949;**24**:71–5.

94. Khan S, Evans AA, Rorke-Adams L, et al. Head injury, diagnostic X-rays, and risk of medulloblastoma and primitive neuroectodermal tumor: a Children's Oncology Group study. *Cancer Causes Control* 2010;**21**:1017–23.

95. Kleihues P, Cavenee WK eds. *World Health Organization classification of tumours. Pathology and genetics: tumours of the nervous system.* Lyon: IARC Press, 2000.

96. Kleihues P, Burger P, Scheithauer B. Histological typing of tumours of the central nervous system. In: Sobin L ed. *World Health Organization. International histological classification of tumours.* Berlin: Springer, 1993.

97. Kleinschmidt-Demasters BK, Damek DM, Lillehei KO, Dogan A, Giannini C. Epstein Barr virus-associated primary CNS lymphomas in elderly patients on immunosuppressive medications. *J Neuropathol Exp Neurol* 2008;**67**:1103–11.

98. Kool M, Korshunov A, Remke M, et al. Molecular subgroups of medulloblastoma: an international meta-analysis of transcriptome, genetic aberrations, and clinical data of WNT, SHH, Group 3, and Group 4 medulloblastomas. *Acta Neuropathol* 2012;**123**:473–84.

99. Krynska B, Otte J, Franks R, et al. Human ubiquitous JCV.CV T-antigen gene induces brain tumors in experimental animals. *Oncogene* 1998;**18**:39–46.

100. Lantos P, Louis D, Rosenblum M, Kleihues P. Tumours of the nervous system. In: Graham D, Lantos P eds. *Greenfield's neuropathology.* London: Arnold, 2001:767–1052.

101. Linos E, Raine T, Alonso A, Michaud D. Atopy and risk of brain tumors: a meta-analysis. *J Natl Cancer Inst* 2007;**99**:1544–50.

102. Liu Y, Scheurer ME, El-Zein R, et al. Association and interactions between DNA repair gene polymorphisms and adult glioma. *Cancer Epidemiol Biomarkers Prev* 2009;**18**:204–14.

103. Liu Y, Shete S, Etzel CJ, et al. Polymorphisms of LIG4, BTBD2, HMGA2, and RTEL1 genes involved in the double-strand break repair pathway predict glioblastoma survival. *J Clin Oncol* 2010;**28**:2467–74.

104. Liu Y, Shete S, Wang LE, et al. Gamma-radiation sensitivity and polymorphisms in RAD51L1 modulate glioma risk. *Carcinogenesis* 2010;**31**:1762–9.

105. London WT, Houff SA, Madden DL, et al. Brain tumors in owl monkeys inoculated with human polyomavirus. *Science* 1978;**201**:1246–9.

106. Lonn S, Klaeboe L, Hall P, et al. Incidence trends of adult primary intracerebral tumors in four Nordic countries. *Int J Cancer* 2004;**108**:450–5.

107. Louis DN, von Deimling A, Chung RY, et al. Comparative study of p53 gene and protein alterations in human astrocytic tumors. *J Neuropathol Exp Neurol* 1993;**52**:31–8.

108. Louis DN, Ohgaki H, Wiestler OD, Cavenee WK eds. *World Health Organization classification of tumours of the central nervous system.* Lyon: IARC Press, 2007.

109. Maiuri F, De Caro ML, de Divitiis O, Vergara P, Mariniello G. Spinal meningiomas: age-related features. *Clin Neurol Neurosurg* 2011;**113**:34–8.

110. Mandelzweig L, Novikov I, Sadetzki S. Smoking and risk of glioma: a meta-analysis. *Cancer Causes Control* 2009;**20**:1927–38.

111. Martini F, Iaccheri L, Lazzarin L, et al. SV40 early region and large T antigen in human brain tumors, peripheral blood cells, and sperm fluids from healthy individuals. *Cancer Res* 1996;**56**:4820–5.

112. Mazumdar M, Liu CY, Wang SF, et al. No association between parental or subject occupation and brain tumor risk. *Cancer Epidemiol Biomarkers Prev* 2008;**17**:1835–7.

113. McCarthy BJ, Rankin KM, Aldape K, et al. Risk factors for oligodendroglial tumors: a pooled international study. *Neuro Oncol* 2011;**13**:242–50.

114. McKean-Cowdin R, Preston-Martin S, Pogoda JM, et al. Parental occupation and childhood brain tumors: astroglial and primitive neuroectodermal tumors. *J Occup Environ Med* 1998;**40**:332–40.

115. McKean-Cowdin R, Barnholtz-Sloan J, Inskip PD, et al. Associations between polymorphisms in DNA repair genes and glioblastoma. *Cancer Epidemiol Biomarkers Prev* 2009;**18**:1118–26.

116. Mellai M, Piazzi A, Caldera V, et al. IDH1 and IDH2 mutations, immunohistochemistry and associations in a series of brain tumors. *J Neurooncol* 2011;**105**:345–57.

117. Merkow LP, Slifkin M, Pardo M, Rapoza NP. Pathogenesis of oncogenic simian adenoviruses: VIII. The histopathology and ultrastructure of simian adenovirus 7-induced intracranial neoplasms. *Exp Mol Pathol* 1970;**12**:264–74.

118. Momota H, Holland EC. Mouse models of CNS embryonal tumors. *Brain Tumor Pathol* 2009;**26**:43–50.

119. Mrowka R, Bogunska C, Kulesza J, et al. Grave cranio-cerebral trauma 30 years ago as cause of the brain glioma at the locus of the trauma: particulars of the case. *Zentralbl Neurochir* 1978;**39**:57–64.

120. Munoz DM, Guha A. Mouse models to interrogate the implications of the differentiation status in the ontogeny of gliomas. *Oncotarget* 2011;**2**:590–8.

121. Nakamura H, Makino K, Yano S, Kuratsu J. Epidemiological study of primary intracranial tumors: a regional survey in Kumamoto prefecture in southern Japan--20-year study. *Int J Clin Oncol* 2011;**16**:314–21.

122. Nakamura M, Tsuji O, Fujiyoshi K, et al. Long-term surgical outcomes of spinal meningiomas. *Spine* 2012;**37**:E617–23.

123. Neglia JP, Robison LL, Stovall M, et al. New primary neoplasms of the central nervous system in survivors of childhood cancer: a report from the Childhood Cancer Survivor Study. *J Natl Cancer Inst* 2006;**98**:1528–37.

124. Nelson JS, Burchfiel CM, Fekedulegn D, Andrew ME. Potential risk factors for incident glioblastoma multiforme: the Honolulu Heart Program and Honolulu-Asia Aging Study. *J Neurooncol* 2012;**109**:315–21.

125. Ohgaki H. Epidemiology of brain tumors. *Methods Mol Biol* 2009;**472**:323–42.

126. Ohgaki H, Huang H, Haltia M, et al. More about: cell and molecular biology of simian virus 40: implications for human infections and disease. *J Natl Cancer Inst* 2000;**92**:495–7.

127. Olsen JH, Nielsen A, Schulgen G. Residence near high voltage facilities and risk of cancer in children. *BMJ* 1993;**307**:891–5.

128. O'Neill BP, Blondal H, Yang P, et al. Risk of cancer among relatives of patients with glioma. *Cancer Epidemiol Biomarkers Prev* 2002;**11**:921–4.

129. Ostrom QT, Barnholtz-Sloan JS. Current state of our knowledge on brain tumor epidemiology. *Curr Neurol Neurosci Rep* 2011;**11**:329–35.

130. Ozawa T, James CD. Establishing intracranial brain tumor xenografts with subsequent analysis of tumor growth and response to therapy using bioluminescence imaging. *J Vis Exp* 2010;**41**:1988–96.

131. Parker HG, Kim LV, Sutter NB, et al. Genetic structure of the purebred domestic dog. *Science* 2004;**304**:1160–4.

132. Parkin D, Muir C, Whelan S, et al. *Cancer incidence in five continents*. Lyon: IARC Press, 1992.

133. Patchell RA. Primary central nervous system lymphoma in the transplant patient. *Neurol Clin* 1988;**6**:297–303.

134. Pei Y, Moore CE, Wang J, et al. An animal model of MYC-driven medulloblastoma. *Cancer Cell* 2012;**21**:155–67.

135. Penn I, Porat G. Central nervous system lymphomas in organ allograft recipients. *Transplantation* 1995;**59**:240–4.

136. Preston DL, Ron E, Yonehara S, et al. Tumors of the nervous system and pituitary gland associated with atomic bomb radiation exposure. *J Natl Cancer Inst* 2002;**94**:1555–63.

137. Preston-Martin S, Navidi W, Thomas D, et al. Los Angeles study of residential magnetic fields and childhood brain tumors. *Am J Epidemiol* 1996;**143**:105–19.

138. Preston-Martin S, Pogoda JM, Schlehofer B, et al. An international case–control study of adult glioma and meningioma: the role of head trauma. *Int J Epidemiol* 1998;**27**:579–86.

139. Preussmann R, Ivankovic S, Landschutz C, et al. Carcinogene Wirkungen von 13 Aryldialky-triazenen an Ratten. *Z Krebsforsch* 1974;**81**:285–310.

140. Ranganathan P, Clark PA, Kuo JS, Salamat MS, Kalejta RF. Significant association of multiple human cytomegalovirus genomic loci with glioblastoma multiforme samples. *J Virol* 2012;**86**:854–64.

141. Reilly KM, Loisel DA, Bronson RT, et al. Nf1;Trp53 mutant mice develop glioblastoma with evidence of strain-specific effects. *Nat Genet* 2000;**26**:109–13.

142. Roberts CW, Galusha SA, McMenamin ME, Fletcher CD, Orkin SH. Haploinsufficiency of Snf5 (integrase interactor 1) predisposes to malignant rhabdoid tumors in mice. *Proc Natl Acad Sci U S A* 2000;**97**:13796–800.

143. Robinson G, Parker M, Kranenburg TA, et al. Novel mutations target distinct subgroups of medulloblastoma. *Nature* 2012;**488**:43–8.

144. Rollison DE, Helzlsouer KJ, Alberg AJ, et al. Serum antibodies to JC virus, BK virus, simian virus 40, and the risk of incident adult astrocytic brain tumors. *Cancer Epidemiol Biomarkers Prev* 2003;**12**:460–3.

145. Rollison DE, Utaipat U, Ryschkewitsch C, et al. Investigation of human brain tumors for the presence of polyomavirus genome sequences by two independent laboratories. *Int J Cancer* 2005;**113**:769–74.

146. Rosso AL, Hovinga ME, Rorke-Adams LB, Spector LG, Bunin GR. A case-control study of childhood brain tumors and fathers' hobbies: a Children's Oncology Group study. *Cancer Causes Control* 2008;**19**:1201–7.

147. Rubenstein J, Ferreri AJ, Pittaluga S. Primary lymphoma of the central nervous system: epidemiology, pathology and current approaches to diagnosis, prognosis and treatment. *Leuk Lymphoma* 2008;**49**(Suppl 1):43–51.

148. Rubin JB. Only in congenial soil: the microenvironment in brain tumorigenesis. *Brain Pathol* 2009;**19**:144–9.

149. Russell D, Rubinstein L. *Pathology of tumours of the nervous system*, 5th edn. London: Edward Arnold, 1989.

150. Rutherford GW, Wlodarczyk RC. Distant sequelae of traumatic brain injury: premature mortality and intracranial neoplasms. *J Head Trauma Rehabil* 2009;**24**:468–74.

151. Sadetzki S, Flint-Richter P, Ben-Tal T, Nass D. Radiation-induced meningioma: a descriptive study of 253 cases. *J Neurosurg* 2002;**97**:1078–82.

152. Sandalcioglu IE, Hunold A, Muller O, et al. Spinal meningiomas: critical review of 131 surgically treated patients. *Eur Spine J* 2008;**17**:1035–41.

153. Sanson M, Hosking FJ, Shete S, et al. Chromosome 7p11.2 (EGFR) variation influences glioma risk. *Hum Mol Genet* 2011;**20**:2897–904.

154. Savitz DA, Kaune WT. Childhood cancer in relation to a modified residential wire code. *Environ Health Perspect* 1993;**101**:76–80.

155. Saya H, Ara S, Lee PS, et al. Direct sequencing analysis of transmembrane region of human Neu gene by polymerase chain reaction. *Mol Carcinog* 1990;**3**:198–201.

155a. Schabet M. Epidemiology of primary CNS lymphoma. *J Neuro-oncol* 1999;**43**:199–201.

156. Schiffer J, Avidan D, Rapp A. Posttraumatic meningioma. *Neurosurgery* 1985;**17**:84–7.

157. Schlehofer B, Kunze S, Sachsenheimer W, et al. Occupational risk factors for brain tumors: results from a population-based case–control study in Germany. *Cancer Causes Control* 1990;**1**:209–15.

158. Schlehofer B, Blettner M, Becker N, et al. Medical risk factors and the development of brain tumors. *Cancer* 1992;**69**:2541–7.

159. Schwartzbaum J, Ding B, Johannesen TB, et al. Association between prediagnostic IgE levels and risk of glioma. *J Natl Cancer Inst* 2012;**104**:1251–9.

160. Shete S, Hosking FJ, Robertson LB, et al. Genome-wide association study identifies five susceptibility loci for glioma. *Nat Genet* 2009;**41**:899–904.

161. Shete S, Lau CC, Houlston RS, et al. Genome-wide high-density SNP linkage search for glioma susceptibility loci: results from the Gliogene Consortium. *Cancer Res* 2011;**71**:7568–75.

162. Simonato L, L'Abbe KA, Andersen A, et al. A collaborative study of cancer incidence and mortality among vinyl chloride workers. *Scand J Work Environ Health* 1991;**17**:159–69.

163. Singh SK, Hawkins C, Clarke ID, et al. Identification of human brain tumour initiating cells. *Nature* 2004;**432**:396–401.

164. Sivendran S, Vidal CI, Barginear MF. Primary intracranial leiomyosarcoma in an HIV-infected patient. *Int J Clin Oncol* 2011;**16**:63–6.

165. Stacey SN, Sulem P, Jonasdottir A, et al. A germline variant in the TP53 polyadenylation signal confers cancer susceptibility. *Nat Genet* 2011;**43**:1098–103.

166. Steindorf K, Schlehofer B, Becher H, et al. Nitrate in drinking water: a case–contol study on primary brain tumours with an embedded drinking water survey in Germany. *Int J Epidemiol* 1994;**23**:451–7.

167. Stiller CA, Nectoux J. International incidence of childhood brain and spinal tumours. *Int J Epidemiol* 1994;**23**:458–64.

168. Stucky CC, Johnson KN, Gray RJ, et al. Malignant peripheral nerve sheath tumors (MPNST): the Mayo Clinic experience. *Ann Surg Oncol* 2011;**19**:878–85.

169. Swartling FJ, Savov V, Persson AI, et al. Distinct neural stem cell populations give rise to disparate brain tumors in response to N-MYC. *Cancer Cell* 2012;**21**:601–13.

170. Swenberg J, Cooper H, Bucheler J, Kleihues P. 1,2-Dimethylhydrazine-induced methylation of DNA bases in various rat organs and the effect of

pretreatment with disulfiram. *Cancer Res* 1979;**39**:465–7.

171. Thomas TL, Waxweiler RJ. Brain tumors and occupational risk factors. *Scand J Work Environ Health* 1986;**12**:1–15.

172. Tondel M, Carlsson G, Hardell L, *et al.* Incidence of neoplasms in ages 0–19 y in parts of Sweden with high 137Cs fallout after the Chernobyl accident. *Health Phys* 1996;**71**:947–50.

173. Troost D, Tulleken CAF. Malignant glioma after bombshell injury. *Clin Neuropathol* 1984;**3**:139–42.

174. Uchida S, Watanabe S, Aizawa T, *et al.* Polyoncogenicity and insulinoma-inducing ability of BK virus, a human papovavirus, in Syrian golden hamsters. *J Natl Cancer Inst* 1979;**63**:119–26.

175. Umansky F, Shoshan Y, Rosenthal G, Fraifeld S, Spektor S. Radiation-induced meningioma. *Neurosurg Focus* 2008;**24**:E7.

176. Verhaak RG, Hoadley KA, Purdom E, *et al.* Integrated genomic analysis identifies clinically relevant subtypes of glioblastoma characterized by abnormalities in PDGFRA, IDH1, EGFR, and NF1. *Cancer Cell* 2010;**17**:98–110.

177. Villano JL, Koshy M, Shaikh H, Dolecek TA, McCarthy BJ. Age, gender, and racial differences in incidence and survival in primary CNS lymphoma. *Br J Cancer* 2011;**105**:1414–18.

177a. Vowels MR, Tobias V, Mameghan H. Second intracranial neoplasms following treatment of childhood acute lymphoblastic leukaemia. *J Paediatr Child Health* 1991;**27**:43–6.

178. Walker D, Padgett B, ZuRhein G, *et al.* Human papovavirus (JC): induction of brain tumors in hamsters. *Science* 1973;**181**:674–6.

179. Wang LE, Bondy ML, Shen H, *et al.* Polymorphisms of DNA repair genes and risk of glioma. *Cancer Res* 2004;**64**:5560–3.

180. Weiss WA, Israel M, Cobbs C, *et al.* Neuropathology of genetically engineered mice: consensus report and recommendations from an international forum. *Oncogene* 2002;**21**:7453–63.

181. Weiss WA, Burns MJ, Hackett C, *et al.* Genetic determinants of malignancy in a mouse model for oligodendroglioma. *Cancer Res* 2003;**63**:1589–95.

182. Wertheimer N, Leeper E. Electrical wiring configurations and childhood cancer. *Am J Epidemiol* 1979;**109**:273–84.

183. Wetmore C, Eberhart DE, Curran T. Loss of p53 but not ARF accelerates medulloblastoma in mice heterozygous for patched. *Cancer Res* 2001;**61**:513–16.

184. Wiemels JL, Wilson D, Patil C, *et al.* IgE, allergy, and risk of glioma: update from the San Francisco Bay Area Adult Glioma Study in the temozolomide era. *Int J Cancer* 2009;**125**:680–7.

185. Wiemels JL, Wrensch M, Sison JD, *et al.* Reduced allergy and immunoglobulin E among adults with intracranial meningioma compared to controls. *Int J Cancer* 2011;**129**:1932–9.

186. Wiencke JK, Aldape K, McMillan A, *et al.* Molecular features of adult glioma associated with patient race/ethnicity, age, and a polymorphism in O6-methylguanine-DNA-methyltransferase. *Cancer Epidemiol Biomarkers Prev* 2005;**14**:1774–83.

187. Wrensch M, Jenkins RB, Chang JS, *et al.* Variants in the CDKN2B and RTEL1 regions are associated with high-grade glioma susceptibility. *Nat Genet* 2009;**41**:905–8.

188. Xiao A, Wu H, Pandolfi PP, *et al.* Astrocyte inactivation of the pRb pathway predisposes mice to malignant astrocytoma development that is accelerated by PTEN mutation. *Cancer Cell* 2002;**1**:157–68.

189. Xiao Y, Decker PA, Rice T, *et al.* SSBP2 variants are associated with survival in glioblastoma patients. *Clin Cancer Res* 2012;**18**:3154–62.

190. Yan H, Parsons DW, Jin G, *et al.* IDH1 and IDH2 mutations in gliomas. *N Engl J Med* 2009;**360**:765–73.

191. Yao L, Ji G, Gu A, Zhao P, Liu N. An updated pooled analysis of glutathione S-transferase genotype polymorphisms and risk of adult gliomas. *Asian Pacific J Cancer Prev* 2012;**13**:157–63.

192. Yonehara S, Brenner AV, Kishikawa M, *et al.* Clinical and epidemiologic characteristics of first primary tumors of the central nervous system and related organs among atomic bomb survivors in Hiroshima and Nagasaki, 1958-1995. *Cancer* 2004;**101**:1644–54.

193. Yosunkaya E, Kucukyuruk B, Onaran I, *et al.* Glioma risk associates with polymorphisms of DNA repair genes, XRCC1 and PARP1. *Br J Neurosurg* 2010;**24**:561–5.

194. Zhu Y, Ghosh P, Charnay P, Burns DK, Parada LF. Neurofibromas in NF1: Schwann cell origin and role of tumor environment. *Science* 2002;**296**:920–2.

195. Zhu Y, Guignard F, Zhao D, *et al.* Early inactivation of p53 tumor suppressor gene cooperating with NF1 loss induces malignant astrocytoma. *Cancer Cell* 2005;**8**:119–30.

196. Zu Rhein GM, Varakis JN. Perinatal induction of medulloblastomas in Syrian golden hamsters by a human polyoma virus (JC). *Natl Cancer Inst Monogr* 1979;**51**:205–8.

197. Zülch K. *Histological typing of tumours of the central nervous system. International histological classification of tumours.* Geneva: World Health Organization, 1979.

198. Zülch K. *Brain tumours. Their biology and pathology.* Berlin: Springer, 1986.

Astrocytic Tumours

Daniel J Brat

INTRODUCTION

Astrocytomas are central nervous system (CNS) tumours formed by neoplastic cells displaying astrocytic differentiation. They include the common diffusely infiltrative astrocytomas, as well as the less common, low-grade circumscribed variants. Although there is occasional histological overlap, these two groups should be considered clinically and biologically distinct. The diffusely infiltrative astrocytomas are subdivided by degree of malignancy into diffuse astrocytoma, WHO grade II, anaplastic astrocytoma (AA), WHO grade III and glioblastoma, WHO grade IV.[143] The circumscribed astrocytic tumours are distinctive clinicopathologic entities, yet share a more indolent clinical course; they include pilocytic astrocytoma, pleomorphic xanthoastrocytoma (PXA) and subependymal giant cell astrocytoma (SEGA).

OVERVIEW AND BIOLOGY OF DIFFUSE ASTROCYTIC TUMOURS

The astrocytic neoplasms, collectively referred to as 'diffuse astrocytic tumours, (WHO grade II diffuse astrocytoma, WHO grade III anaplastic astrocytoma and WHO grade IV glioblastoma), are the most common primary tumours of the cerebral hemispheres in adults.[52,143] They are related both clinically and biologically and share two cardinal characteristics: (1) diffuse infiltration of involved CNS structures and (2) an inherent tendency to progress to a more malignant phenotype. Also characteristic are preferential location in the cerebral hemispheres, more frequent presentation in adults than children, and a wide range of histopathological features, genetic alterations and biological behaviour.[143]

Incidence

Diffusely infiltrating astrocytic tumours are the most frequent CNS neoplasms and account for more than 60 per cent of all intra-axial brain tumours.[52] Although there may be slight regional variation, estimates suggest an annual incidence of 0.58, 0.36 and 3.19 per 100 000 for grade II (diffuse astrocytoma), grade III (anaplastic astrocytoma) and grade IV (glioblastoma), respectively.[52]

Age and Gender

Histological grade correlates directly with age of presentation. Entities within the grade I category, such as pilocytic astrocytoma and SEGA, tend to arise in childhood and adolescence. Diffusely infiltrative astrocytomas, WHO grade II, typically affect young adults, whereas glioblastoma shows a peak incidence in the sixth decade. Anaplastic astrocytoma occupies an intermediate position. Population-based studies show a mean age at diagnosis of 39 years for diffuse astrocytoma, WHO grade II and 61 years for glioblastoma.[174,176] Children may also develop the entire range of diffuse astrocytomas, although less frequently than adults. Males are affected more frequently, with a male-female ratio ranging from 1.4 to 1.5:1.

Sites

Diffuse astrocytomas preferentially arise in the cerebral hemispheres, particularly the frontotemporal region, often occupying the subcortical or deep white matter. However, they can occur throughout the neuraxis, including the spinal cord. Interestingly, diffuse astrocytomas rarely involve the cerebellum as a primary site. In children, the brain stem and thalamus are characteristic locations for diffuse astrocytomas. Circumscribed forms of astrocytomas tend to occur in stereotypic locations. Pilocytic astrocytomas arise most frequently in the cerebellum, brain stem, optic pathways and hypothalamus. SEGAs are almost always localized to the lateral ventricle near the foramen of Monro. PXAs arise most frequently in the temporal lobes, but also in other cerebral hemispheric locations.

Clinical Features

Focal neurological deficits are related to tumour location and may include weakness, sensory abnormalities or visual disturbance. Non-localizing signs and symptoms are also common, particularly headaches, seizures and altered consciousness. In the setting of lower-grade lesions, seizures may be present for years before the onset of other clinical signs and symptoms. Ultimately, patients develop increased intracranial pressure owing to mass effect.

Grading of Diffuse Astrocytomas and Survival

Diffuse astrocytic tumours range from slowly growing, relatively localized lesions to high-grade malignancies that involve large expanses of brain. Significant indicators of increasing grade in gliomas include cytological atypia, cellular density, mitotic activity, microvascular proliferation and necrosis. The grading system that is most widely utilized is the WHO classification.[143]

As with other forms of neoplasia, grading of astrocytomas is based on the most malignant areas, assuming that this population drives the course of disease. Importantly, both astrocytic differentiation and tumour grading are determined morphologically and subject to interpretation.[70] The diagnosis of an infiltrative astrocytoma (WHO grade II) is applied when individual tumour cells showing astrocytic differentiation infiltrate CNS parenchyma.[47,143] Classification of infiltrating tumours as astrocytic versus oligodendroglial depends on cell shape, appearance and the character of the nuclei.[70] In astrocytomas, nuclei are elongate, hyperchromatic and irregular, generally lacking prominent nucleoli and perinuclear halos. The histopathologic distinction of grade II from grade III depends on the identification of mitotic activity, with the finding of even a few mitotic figures sufficient to establish the diagnosis of anaplastic astrocytoma, WHO grade III. As compared to grade II astrocytoma, AA also has increased cellular density, as well as greater nuclear pleomorphism and atypia. For the diagnosis of glioblastoma (GBM; WHO grade IV), either microvascular hyperplasia or necrosis, often with pseudopalisading (or both), is required.[26,143] In the past, necrosis within a malignant glioma was often viewed as the sole criterion for the diagnosis of GBM. However, studies have emphasized that vascular proliferation and necrosis are biologically linked, so that either feature can be used for the diagnosis of GBM.[20,47]

In addition to histological grade, patient survival depends on a variety of clinical features, including patient age[29,228] and neurological status, as reflected in the Karnofsky performance score,[228] tumour location and treatment, e.g. extent of surgical resection,[2,15,165] radiotherapy[2,128] and chemotherapy.[231,232] Data from clinical trials and institutional

series reveal patient survivals of 6–8 years for diffuse astrocytomas, 2–4 years for anaplastic astrocytomas and 12–16 months for patients with glioblastoma.[143,231] Population-based studies that include all patients with disease rather than only those who qualify for clinical trials indicate survival times of 5.6 years for diffuse astrocytoma, 1.6 years for AA, and less than 6 months for GBM patients.[170]

Cells of Origin

The cells of origin for astrocytomas and other malignant gliomas remain enigmatic. Most glioma classifications have postulated that astrocytomas arise from astrocytes, and oligodendrogliomas from oligodendrocytes.[142] However, the number of actively dividing glial cells in the normal brain is low, making this possibility unlikely. Work in both animal models and primary gliomas has suggested that malignant gliomas arise from progenitor cells (Figure 27.1).[75,76] Neuroectodermal stem cells that reside in adult mammalian brains have a proliferative potential, are migratory and can pursue diverse paths of differentiation – all features intrinsic to glioma cells and likely characteristics for neoplastic cells of origin. Differential targeting of oncogenic alterations to either progenitor

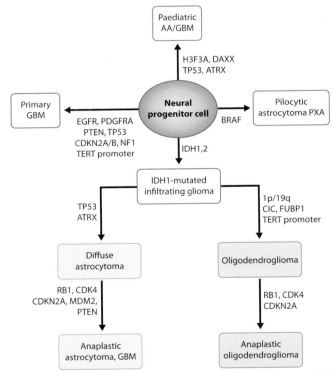

27.1 Progenitor cells, genetic alterations and tumour differentiation. A glioma progenitor cell could arise either from a stem cell population or from a differentiating progenitor cell population. Astrocytomas can develop through numerous pathways of acquired gene mutations, amplifications and deletions. Those that are *IDH* mutant are clinically and biologically distinct from those that are *IDH* wild type. Among *IDH* mutant gliomas, the resultant phenotype of astrocytoma or oligodendroglioma depends on specific sets of genetic changes. *TP53* and *ATRX* mutations are typical of astrocytomas, whereas co-deletion of 1p and 19q and mutations of *CIC* and *FUBP1* are typical of oligodendroglioma.

cells or maturing astrocytes has demonstrated that glial progenitors are more permissive to oncogenic transformation than mature astrocytes. For instance, overexpressing oncogenic Ras and Akt in progenitors results in mouse brain tumours that are histologically similar to glioblastomas, yet targeting more mature astrocytic progenitors is less oncogenic.[92] Furthermore, malignant gliomas themselves likely contain tumour stem cells, a relatively primitive population responsible for repopulating tumours as they develop and progress; such cells may represent transformed variants of normal neural progenitors.[50,134,223] The existence of tumour stem cells may have major therapeutic implications as well, because therapies that do not ablate them will ultimately prove ineffective.

Neoplastic Transformation

In many epithelial malignancies, genetic changes occurring in the progression from normal to hyperplastic to dysplastic to malignant have been identified. For diffuse astrocytic tumours, the first identifiable step is already a low-grade malignancy (WHO grade II astrocytoma) and knowledge of the earliest oncogenic events is limited.

Mutations in isocitrate dehydrogenase 1 (*IDH1*) gene are frequent (70–80 per cent) in grade II and III astrocytomas, oligodendrogliomas, and oligoastrocytomas, as well as the GBMs resulting from progression of lower grade gliomas (secondary GBMs).[177,264] Mutations in *IDH2* have also been described, but are much less frequent. *IDH* mutations are infrequent in primary (*de novo*) GBMs. Because mutations are common to both grade II astrocytomas and oligodendrogliomas, it has been suggested that this oncogenic step is one of the first to occur in the development of diffuse gliomas, with later genetic alterations determining astrocytoma or oligodendroglioma lineages, such as *TP53* mutations and 1p/19q losses, respectively (Figure 27.1). *IDH* mutations lead to the production of the oncometabolite 2-hydroxyglutarate, which inhibits the function of numerous α-ketoglutarate–dependent enzymes.[243] Inhibition of the family of histone demethylases and the TET family of 5-methylcytosine hydroxylases has profound epigenetic effects and leads directly to a hypermethylator phenotype that has been referred to as the CpG Island Methylator Phenotype (G-CIMP).[167]

Importantly, over 90 per cent of *IDH1* mutations in the diffuse gliomas occur at a specific site and are characterized by a base exchange of guanine to adenine within codon 132, resulting in an amino acid change from arginine to histidine (R132H). Because of this consistent protein alteration, a monoclonal antibody has been developed to the mutant protein, allowing its detection in paraffin-embedded specimens (mIDH1R132H).[37] The reported sensitivity and specificity for identifying IDH1 mutant gliomas using this antibody was 94 and 100 per cent, respectively. Furthermore, the ability of this antibody to detect only minor mIDH1R132H populations makes this method more sensitive than sequencing in specimens with minimal tumour.

The p53 tumour suppressor protein encoded by the *TP53* gene on chromosome 17p plays a central role in numerous cellular processes, including cell cycle arrest, response to DNA damage, apoptosis, angiogenesis and differentiation. In grade II astrocytomas that are *IDH* mutant, inactivating mutations are present in the vast majority.[176] In glioblastoma, the p53 pathway may be deregulated by alterations of other components in the signalling pathway, including amplifications of *MDM2* or *MDM4* or losses of *CDKN2A-ARF*.[95,96] Indeed, The Cancer Genome Atlas (TCGA) project has catalogued these related gene alterations, finding that this family is dysregulated in nearly 90 per cent of GBM.[27,36]

A small number of genes related to histone modification, chromatin remodelling and telomere maintenance are mutated in diffuse astrocytomas as an early event and are tightly coupled to *TP53* mutation. *ATRX* (α-thalassaemia/mental-retardation-syndrome-X-linked) mutations are present in 33 per cent of grade II and 46 per cent of grade III gliomas and are highly correlated with astrocytic differentiation, both by morphologic and molecular assessment.[139] They are also present in 80 per cent of secondary, but only 7 per cent of primary GBMs. *ATRX* alterations are closely coupled with mutations in *IDH1/2* and *TP53* across all astrocytoma grades. Mutations of *ATRX* lead to alternative lengthening of telomeres (ALT), a telomerase independent mechanism of maintaining telomeres in cancer.[83,219] Interestingly, ATRX mutations are uncommon in lower-grade paediatric astrocytomas and in gliomas from adults appear to be mutually exclusive with 1p/19q co-deletions and gene mutations associated with oligodendrogliomas (*CIC, FUBP1*).

Another gene related to chromatin remodeling, *H3F3A*, is mutated in astrocytomas and appears to be an early event, mostly in paediatric high-grade astrocytomas.[219] In one series, *H3F3A* mutations were noted in over 40 per cent of such cases. *ATRX* and *TP53* mutations were also present in these samples and showed a considerable degree of overlap with *H3F3A* mutations. There are two types of recurrent somatic mutations that occur in *H3F3A*, with one resulting in amino acid substitution at K27 and the other at G34. Each of these has an impact on the ability of H3.3 to regulate gene expression and leads to alterations in transcriptional profile.[233] The K27 mutated tumours occur in the youngest children in midline sites (thalamus and pons), whereas the G34 mutated tumours preferentially involve teenagers and young adults with cerebral hemispheric gliomas. *H3F3A* mutations are mutually exclusive with *IDH* mutations.

Mutations in *DAXX* (death-domain associated protein), encoding yet another chromatin remodelling subunit, have also been described in paediatric high-grade astrocytomas, but at a much lower frequency.[219] The presence of mutations in these chromatin remodelling genes is also tightly coupled to the finding of ALT. ALT occurred most frequently in those astrocytomas with combined *ATRX/H3F3A/TP53* mutations.

Many growth factors and their receptors are overexpressed in grade II astrocytomas, including platelet-derived growth factor (PDGF), fibroblast growth factors (FGFs), vascular endothelial growth factor (VEGF) and EGFR. PDGF ligands and receptors are expressed approximately equally in all astrocytoma grades, suggesting that overexpression is an initial event.[35] Introduction of PDGF into the rodent white matter is sufficient to induce neoplasia and malignant transformation, highlighting the role of this signal transduction network in gliomagenesis.[5,6]

Differentiation and Tumour Phenotype

A wide variety of cellular patterns have been described in astrocytomas, including fibrillary, gemistocytic, small cell, protoplasmic, sarcomatous, epithelioid, granular cell, giant cell and mixed with oligodendroglioma (oligoastrocytoma). Factors that determine tumour phenotypes are unclear. Mouse modelling studies have shown variations in tumour morphology depending on the type of cell transformed, as well as the oncogenic combination.[92] For example, overexpression of Ras and Akt in progenitors yields tumours with astrocytic differentiation, whereas overexpression of PDGF-B in the same cells produces tumours resembling oligodendroglioma.[7,46]

The occurrence of oligoastrocytomas in both humans and animal models provides insight to the origins and pathways of glial differentiation. Morphologically distinct regions in oligoastrocytomas have similar genetic alterations, indicating that these are clonal lesions, albeit with striking phenotypic diversity.[120]

Most human astrocytomas do not display overt neuronal differentiation. Nonetheless, as more sensitive neuronal markers are utilized, many glial neoplasms seemingly coexpress neuronal and glial antigens, either uniformly or focally. This includes rare but distinct variants, such as malignant gliomas with PNET foci and rosetted glioneuronal tumours.[186,238] It is likely that most 'gliomas' will prove to be more heterogeneous, particularly when developing from pluripotent progenitors.

Understanding glioma phenotype must also take into account that astrocytic tumours are associated with specific genetic alterations, including *TP53* and *ATRX* mutations, whereas oligodendrogliomas are strongly associated with 1p/19q losses, CIC mutations and FUBP1 mutations. In this regard, it may be possible that astrocytomas and oligodendrogliomas arise from the same cells of origin, yet genetic events drive differentiation along one or another pathway (Figure 27.1). It is interesting to note, however, that those oligodendroglial tumours with 1p and 19q loss preferentially affect particular areas of the brain, raising the possibility that specific precursor populations in different brain regions transform along distinct genetic pathways to reach common phenotypic end points, such as oligodendroglioma.[268]

Invasion

Diffuse gliomas of all grades and morphologies display a remarkable tendency to infiltrate the brain, confounding therapeutic attempts at local control (Figure 27.2). Patterns of brain invasion by gliomas are stereotypic.[266] For instance, there is preferential invasion along white matter tracts: many gliomas cross the corpus callosum to form 'butterfly' lesions; other gliomas remain confined to the white matter, stopping abruptly at the grey–white matter junction. Still other migratory patterns give rise to the so-called 'secondary structures of Scherer', including preferential growth

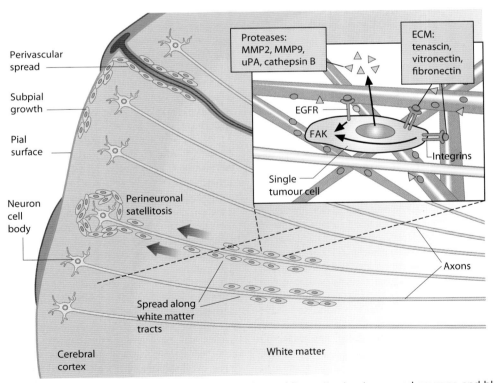

27.2 Invasion. Malignant glioma cells show preferential invasion along white matter tracts, around neurons and blood vessels, and in the subpial region. Molecular events relating to invasion of single cells include elaboration of proteases such as MMP2, MMP9, uPA and cathepsin B; expression of integrins that interact with extracellular matrix (ECM) components, such as tenascin, vitronectin and fibronectin, that are themselves expressed by tumour cells; and activation of FAK-mediated cellular signalling pathways either via EGFR or integrin signalling.

Adapted with permission from DN Louis.[141]

around neurons ('perineuronal satellitosis'), perivascular aggregation and subpial spread.

These infiltrative tendencies suggest that glioma cells have either a tropism for particular sites or a restricted ability to invade other regions. Moreover, glioma invasion is best viewed as the combined ability to migrate and to modulate the extracellular space. Unfortunately, investigations of glioma invasion have been hampered by a paucity of representative experimental models that mimic the human disease.

Invasion by glioma cells reflects a dynamic interplay between cell–cell adhesion, remodelling of the extracellular matrix and cell motility.[14,143] Glioma invasion of brain is biologically distinct from carcinoma invasion because of the single cell nature of the former and the distinctive extracellular matrix of the brain. In general, the extracellular matrix of the brain is ill defined and scant, consisting primarily of hyaluronic acid, except in two areas: around blood vessels and at the pial surface (glia limitans). At these sites, there is a well-defined and more traditional basal lamina that includes collagens. Notably, glioma cells preferentially involve the perivascular and subpial spaces – places where basal lamina is well defined – but they also involve perineuronal and white matter locations – places where it is not. It has been suggested that the expression of the chemokine SDF-1α by neurons, blood vessels, subpial regions and white matter tracts may guide the infiltration of glioma cells towards these structures, because tumour cells express the receptor for SDF-1α, CXCR4, with highest expression by those invading glioma cells organized around neurons and blood vessels, in subpial regions, and along white matter tracts.[266] Moreover, neuronal and endothelial cells exposed to VEGF upregulate the expression of SDF-1α, thereby enhancing the chemoattraction in hypoxia.

Investigations into astrocytoma invasion have highlighted the complex nature of cell–cell and cell–extracellular matrix interactions.[14,196] Proteases are elaborated by glioma cells, which appear to play a significant role, including cysteine, serine and metalloproteinases. These degrade the extracellular environment to facilitate migration, but also remodel the environment in a manner that facilitates tumour cell growth. Most studies have focused on matrix metalloproteinases MMP2 and MMP9, the serine protease urokinase-type plasminogen activator (uPA) and its receptor (uPAR), and the cysteine protease cathepsin B.[196] Their expression increases with glioma grade, and their interference *in vitro* results in decreased invasive and/or migratory properties.

Studies of interactions between glioma cell surface molecules and extracellular matrix molecules have shown that gliomas express a variety of integrin receptors that mediate interactions with molecules in the extracellular space. The integrin heterodimers most clearly implicated have been α2β1 (interacting with tenascin), α5β1 (interacting with fibronectin), α6β1 (interacting with laminin) and αvβ3 (interacting with vitronectin).[246] Activation of integrins through interactions with extracellular ligands results in alterations of the cellular cytoskeleton, promoting locomotion. Focal adhesion kinase (FAK), an intermediate signalling molecule in glioma migration, is a cytoplasmic tyrosine kinase expressed in high-grade gliomas and activated by EGFR and integrins such as αvβ3 and αvβ5.[202] FAK subsequently signals through pathways that affect proliferation, survival and migration.[164]

Many of the growth factors expressed in astrocytomas, such as FGF, EGF and VEGF, also stimulate migration. Significantly, those glioblastomas with *EGFR* gene amplification do not demonstrate uniform distribution of the amplified cells within the tumour.[175] Rather, *EGFR*-amplified cells are preferentially located at the infiltrating edges.[229] Given that *EGFR* gene amplicons are found on double minute chromosomes, which must be maintained by positive selection during cell division, this suggests that *EGFR* amplification provides selective advantage at the infiltrating edge. Further support that EGFR signalling contributes to invasion is provided by gene expression profiling data. Overexpression of the vIII EGFR mutant, a constitutively active EGFR variant, results in upregulated expression of multiple genes associated with invasion, including metalloproteinases (MMP1 and MMP13) and collagens.[125] Furthermore, inhibition of EGFR appears to reduce invasion.[180]

Tumour Progression

Diffuse astrocytomas nearly always recur, typically showing histopathological evidence of tumour progression, including increased nuclear atypia, mitotic activity and, eventually, microvascular proliferation and/or necrosis. Glioblastomas developing along this pathway have been termed secondary glioblastomas,[215] in contrast to primary glioblastomas, which develop clinically *de novo*, i.e. without an identifiable, less malignant precursor lesion.[171] Nearly all *de novo* GBMs are *IDH* wild type, whereas the vast majority of secondary GBMs are *IDH1* or *IDH2* mutant.[264] Although the acquisition of anaplastic features is an inherent property of diffuse astrocytomas, there is temporal variability in progression. Occasional WHO grade II astrocytomas do not change histological grade for over ten years.[173] Others, especially those that are *IDH* wild type, rapidly progress to malignancy within one or two years.

Molecular changes underlying malignant progression of astrocytomas parallel histological changes and clinical course.[171] Deregulation of cell cycle control as well as activation of receptor tyrosine kinase (RTK) and PI3K-AKT-mediated signalling pathways is strongly related to progression of grade II gliomas to higher-grade counterparts, including glioblastoma. At a simplified level, many alterations can be divided into two large groups: those related to deregulated RTK-AKT signalling and those related to deregulated p53-Rb cell cycle control/apoptosis cascade (Figure 27.3). At a histological level, WHO grade III tumours have increased cellular density, mitotic activity and proliferative indices compared to grade II tumours. At a molecular level, many genetic alterations target cell cycle regulatory genes. Most of these converge on critical cell-cycle regulatory complexes that include the CDKN2A/p16, cyclin-dependent kinase 4 (CDK4), CDK6 and retinoblastoma (Rb) proteins. Individual components in this pathway are altered in up to 50 per cent of anaplastic astrocytomas, higher in those that are *IDH* wild type, and in nearly all glioblastomas. In the TCGA analysis of Rb pathway genetic alterations, the most frequent alterations included *CDKN2A/p16* deletions (52 per cent), *CDKN2B* deletions (47 per cent), *CDK4* amplification (18 per cent),

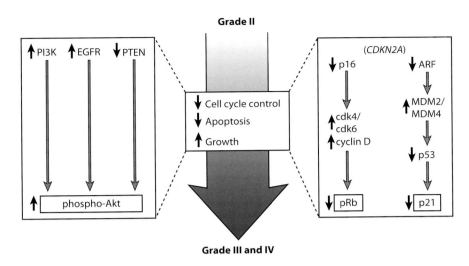

27.3 Progression from grade II to grade III and IV malignant gliomas is associated in nearly all cases with genetic changes that activate the growth receptor tyrosine kinase signalling pathways that include EGFR, PDGFR, PTEN, Akt and NF1 and that inactivate the cell cycle control pathways that feature p53 and pRb. ↑, upregulation; ↓, downregulation.

Adapted with permission from DN Louis.[141]

RB1 mutation (11 per cent), *CCND2* amplification (2 per cent) and *CDK6* amplification (1 per cent).[27,36]

Chromosome 9p loss occurs in approximately 50 per cent of anaplastic astrocytomas and glioblastomas, with 9p deletions primarily affecting the region of the *CDKN2A* gene, which encodes the p16 and the ARF proteins. The *CDKN2A* gene is inactivated either by homozygous deletion or, less commonly, by point mutations or hypermethylation. The role of p16 in progression has been confirmed in mouse models overexpressing either PDGF or EGFR, in which a p16 null background is sufficient to change the phenotype from low-grade to anaplastic.[46,260] Loss of chromosome 13q occurs in one-third to one-half of high-grade astrocytomas, with the *RB1* gene preferentially targeted by losses and inactivating mutations. *RB1* and *CDKN2A* alterations rarely occur together in the same tumour, suggesting that their losses are functionally similar. Amplification of the *CDK4* gene, located on chromosome 12q13-14, provides an alternative to subvert cell-cycle control and facilitate progression to glioblastoma. *CDK4* amplification, *CDK6* amplification and cyclin D1 or D2 overexpression appear to represent alternative events to *CDKN2A* deletions and *RB* alterations, because these genetic changes only rarely occur in the same tumours.[95,245]

Chromosome 10 loss occurs in 60–95 per cent of glioblastomas, but less commonly in grade II or III diffuse astrocytomas.[172] The *PTEN* gene at 10q23.3 has been strongly implicated as a glioma-related tumour suppressor on chromosome 10q, with mutations identified in about 25–30 per cent of glioblastomas. PTEN functions as a protein tyrosine phosphatase and has 3′ phosphoinositol phosphatase activity; in addition, PTEN has an amino-terminal domain with homologies to tensin and auxilin. Thus, PTEN may regulate cell migration via affecting focal adhesion kinase (FAK) and may regulate cell proliferation via control of the Akt serine/threonine kinase. Introduction of wild-type *PTEN* into glioma cells with mutant *PTEN* leads to growth suppression.[263] Allelic losses have been found at other loci in high-grade astrocytomas, particularly on 19q (up to 40 per cent of anaplastic astrocytomas and glioblastomas), suggesting a progression-associated glial tumour suppressor gene.

EGFR is a transmembrane receptor tyrosine kinase, whose ligands include EGF and TGF-α. The *EGFR* gene is the most frequently amplified oncogene in astrocytic tumours, being amplified in approximately 40 per cent of all glioblastomas, but rarely in lower grade astrocytomas.[171,172] Glioblastomas with *EGFR* gene amplification display overexpression of EGFR at both the mRNA and protein levels, suggesting that activation of this growth signal pathway is integral to malignant progression. Downstream targets include the Shc-Grb2-ras pathway and the PI3K-AKT pathway. Approximately one-third of glioblastomas with *EGFR* gene amplification also have specific *EGFR* deletions (the vIII mutant), which produce truncated cell surface receptors with constitutive tyrosine kinase activity. Such truncated EGFR receptors are capable of conferring dramatically enhanced tumorigenicity to glioblastoma cells.

Although *EGFR* amplification is the most frequent and best studied oncogenic event involving a receptor tyrosine kinase with downstream signalling of PI3K-ATK and Ras pathways, other family members have also been implicated. Amplification of *PDGFRA* is noted in approximately 13 per cent of glioblastomas, based on high density SNP analysis of copy number alterations.[36,248] Fluorescence *in situ* hybridization (FISH) – based assays of *PDGFRA*, which can identify lower level copy number alterations than genomic averaging techniques, suggest that *PDGFRA* amplifications occur in a higher frequency, one study finding *PDGFRA* amplifications in 21 per cent of adult GBMs and 29 per cent of paediatric GBMs.[189] This study also concluded that the *PDGFRA* amplification was a poor prognostic feature in *IDH1* mutated adult GBM, removing the prognostic advantage normally associated with *IDH1* mutations.

In addition to *EGFR* and *PDGFRA* amplification, less frequent alterations that enhance intracellular signalling of the RTK, PI3K and Ras pathways include *c-Met* amplification, activating mutations in *PI3K*, mutations and deletions of *PTEN* and mutations and deletions of *NF1*.[27,36]

Necrosis and Hypoxia

Necrosis is one of the diagnostic features of glioblastoma and a key driving force behind its behaviour.[197,208] Indeed, no histological feature is more powerful in predicting prognosis among the diffuse gliomas.[143] The accelerated tumour growth that accompanies necrosis could be due to a highly malignant state achieved by the neoplasm, a selection pressure due to necrosis that encourages outgrowth of highly malignant cells, or the effects of hypoxia and other factors that are associated with necrosis (Figure 27.4).

Necrosis could potentially arise from a number of mechanisms. In the setting of rapidly dividing cells with high metabolic demands, regions of tumour distant from blood vessels may develop necrosis when metabolic demands exceed supply (diffusion-limited hypoxia and necrosis).[208] Necrosis may also arise following vaso-occlusion associated with intravascular thrombosis, which is frequently seen in GBM, but not lower-grade gliomas (perfusion-limited hypoxia and necrosis).[236] One possible molecular culprit that could promote intravascular thrombosis is tissue factor,

which is highly overexpressed by neoplastic cells and could act as a local pro-coagulant.[22,209]

One theory suggests hypoxia follows vaso-occlusion and thrombosis within a high-grade astrocytoma and leads to the active migration of tumour cells outward towards a more functional vascular supply, thus 'clearing' a central region that undergoes necrosis. The latter hypothesis is based on work showing that those glioblastoma tumour cells surrounding necrotic centres (so-called 'pseudo-palisades') are less proliferative and more apoptotic than adjacent cells, suggesting that they accumulate from their migration.[22,23] These perinecrotic cells also express hypoxia-inducible genes, such as HIF1α and VEGF;[23] and *in vitro* studies have demonstrated that hypoxia induces an increase in cellular migration and in gelatinase activity. Morphometric analysis of the central necrotic zones of pseudo-palisades in glioblastomas

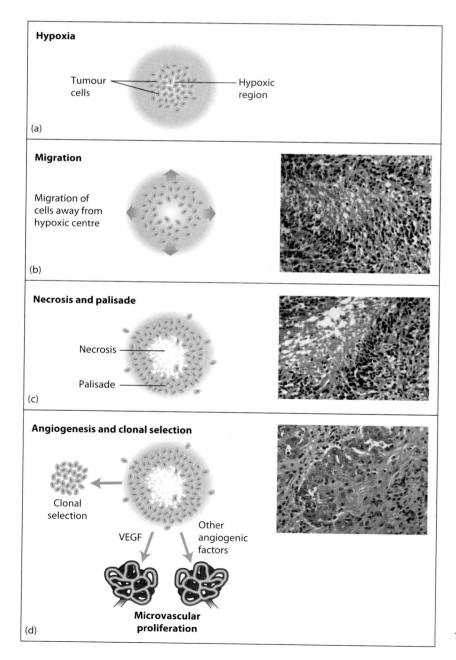

27.4 Hypoxia, necrosis and angiogenesis. The development of hypoxia, necrosis and angiogenesis is biologically linked. **(a)** Localized hypoxia appears to upregulate migration-associated genes, leading to migration of tumour cells away from a central hypoxic centre **(b)**. **(c)** Necrosis then ensues in the central region, sometimes in association with vascular thrombosis and a 'palisade' of densely packed tumour cells develops. **(d)** Palisading cells express angiogenic factors such as VEGF, leading to adjacent angiogenesis that includes so-called 'glomeruloid' microvascular proliferation. Another consequence of hypoxia may be clonal selection of malignant cells that are able to survive selection pressure.

Adapted with permission from DN Louis.[141]

have demonstrated abnormal and sometimes thrombosed vessels in over half, suggesting an initial vaso-occlusive event may have initiated the hypoxia/necrosis cycle. Factors that initiate vaso-occlusion are not clear, yet endothelial cells of small vessels may be driven toward apoptosis and regression as a result of angiopoietin 2 expression.[91,265]

The development of hypoxia may have other downstream effects as well. For example, hypoxia may act as a selective force that leads to the emergence of highly malignant and apoptosis-resistant tumour cells bearing inactivated p53.[69] Hypoxia also facilitates angiogenesis by the release of growth factors such as VEGF and IL-8.[25] Expression profiling of pseudo-palisading cells of glioblastomas also supports the notion that perinecrotic regions contain highly malignant clones.[53] These, in turn, imply increased metabolic demand, likely causing greater hypoxia or necrosis and feeding a vicious cycle. Lastly, the development of hypoxia occurs centrally in the neoplasm, with many of its influences leading to the radial expansion of GBM in a rapid fashion.

Angiogenesis

Markedly increased vascular density is a hallmark of glioblastoma and occurs in two pathologically discernible forms: (1) increase in vessel number because of enhanced small vessel formation and (2) an abnormal form of angiogenesis most commonly known as 'microvascular proliferation' (Figure 27.4). The diffuse increase in vascular density is not always an obvious feature on haematoxylin and eosin (H&E)-stained sections, but can be appreciated using immunohistochemistry for endothelial cells.

Microvascular proliferation is a complex accumulation of proliferating endothelial and perivascular cells that lead to tufting and budding of the vasculature within neoplastic tissue. The multilayering of these often hyperplastic-appearing cells is a feature that correlates with aggressive behaviour in GBM.[47] The most characteristic form is the so-called 'glomeruloid' body (because of their resemblance to renal glomeruli), which are large and complex three-dimensional structures composed of both proliferating endothelial and smooth muscle cells, representing the most exuberant form of angiogenesis.[21,74,143]

Microvascular proliferation is irregularly distributed in glioblastomas. Most notably, complex glomeruloid bodies form semicircular garlands that hug regions of necrosis, highlighting the interrelationship between hypoxia/necrosis and angiogenesis. Less commonly, microvascular proliferation can be found at the invading edges, far from necrosis, and presumably as a result of angiogenic factors expressed by invading glioma cells.

The biological underpinnings of microvascular proliferation are complex, with many angiogenic growth factors and their receptors found in glioblastomas. VEGF and PDGF are expressed by tumour cells whereas their tyrosine kinase receptors, VEGF receptors 1 and 2 for VEGF and the PDGF-β-receptor for PDGF, are expressed on endothelial cells.[21] VEGF and its receptors may also be responsible for breakdown of the blood–brain barrier and tumoural oedema in glioblastoma, by causing vascular permeability. VEGF is a downstream target of a number of the activated signalling pathways, e.g. via EGFR and Akt, and is upregulated by numerous oncogenic events. Interleukin-8 (IL-8)

is another hypoxia-inducible cytokine that is expressed in gliomas and has potent angiogenic activity.[25]

Numerous lines of investigation support the notion that angiogenesis within gliomas is supported and enhanced by bone marrow progenitor cells. Studies in animal models indicate that these progenitors localize to angiogenic vessels in high-grade gliomas and are incorporated into their walls. Whether these cells are capable of transdifferentiating into endothelial cells or pericytes or have additional roles continues to be investigated.[55]

DIFFUSE ASTROCYTOMA (WHO GRADE II)

Diffuse astrocytoma, WHO grade II, is characterized by advanced cellular differentiation and widespread brain invasion by individual neoplastic cells. It manifests most frequently in young adults, with a peak incidence in the fourth and fifth decades. It may be located in any region of the CNS, including the spinal cord, but preferentially involves the cerebral hemispheres. Symptoms depend on location, but seizures are common.[143]

Neuroimaging

By computed tomography (CT), diffuse astrocytomas present as ill-defined, homogeneous masses of low density without contrast enhancement. Magnetic resonance (MR) imaging demonstrates low signal intensity on T1-weighted and higher signal intensity with better defined borders on T2-weighted sequences (Figure 27.5a). Diffusion weighted imaging (DWI), perfusion weighted imaging (PWI) and MR spectroscopy (MRS) are helpful in estimating tumour grade pre-operatively, with diffuse astrocytomas typically having low relative cerebral blood volume (rCBV), high apparent diffusion coefficients and low Cho/Cr and Cho/NAA ratios as compared to higher grade astrocytomas.[4,9]

Macroscopic Appearances

Astrocytomas expand the involved brain, have ill-defined borders and are slightly firm, yellow-white and homogeneous, with occasional cysts. Infiltration often leads to enlargement and distortion, but not destruction, of involved grey or white matter. Extensive micro-cyst formation may cause a gelatinous appearance.

Microscopy

Diffuse astrocytomas infiltrate the involved brain as single cells of variable density and cytologic atypia (Figure 27.5b–h). Normal nervous system cells and structures, including neurons, their axons, glial cells and blood vessels, are all typically entrapped within the lesion. Mitotic activity is generally absent, although isolated mitoses found after long searches of large resection specimens may not connote increased malignancy in the same way as finding a single mitosis in a needle biopsy.[63] Three major variants have been distinguished: fibrillary, gemistocytic and protoplasmic, with granular cell morphology representing a rare, yet intriguing variation (Figure 27.6a–c).

27.5 Diffuse astrocytoma, WHO grade II. **(a)** On MRI, diffuse astrocytomas, such as that in the right frontal lobe in this axial FLAIR image, are hyperintense on T2-weighted or FLAIR imaging, typically centred in the white matter and expand the involved brain. **(b)** In tissue sections, individual astrocytoma cells with enlarged, atypical nuclei are noted infiltrating the CNS parenchyma. **(c)** Cytologic preparations demonstrate the oblong nuclei of astrocytoma cells and thin, elongate fibrillary processes. **(d)** Diffuse astrocytomas will occasionally show prominent microcystic architecture. **(e)** Invasion of the cortex by diffuse astrocytomas is often accompanied by peri-neuronal satellitosis. **(f)** Infiltrating astrocytoma cells occasionally accumulate in the subpial zone of the cortex. **(g)** Astrocytoma cells infiltrating along white matter tracts. **(h)** Immunohistochemistry for neurofilament highlights the entrapped axons adjacent to infiltrating neoplastic cells..

Fibrillary astrocytomas are most common, being characterized by scant to indiscernible cytoplasm, creating the appearance of 'naked nuclei' (Figure 27.5b). Cytologic preparations are better for demonstrating the elongate, delicate eosinophilic glial process that emerge from individual tumour cells (Figure 27.5c). Nuclear atypia, i.e. enlarged, irregular hyperchromatic nuclei, often resembling 'Idaho potatoes' is a histological hallmark distinguishing tumour cells from normal and reactive astrocytes. Neoplastic cell processes form a loose fibrillary matrix that is most often indiscernibly intertwined with the neuropil meshwork of the normal brain parenchyma. A gradient of increasing cell density from normal brain to hypercellular tumour can often be appreciated in fibrillary astrocytomas and is helpful in establishing a diagnosis of an infiltrative form of glioma (Figure 27.6a). Micro-cysts containing mucinous fluid dominate the histological picture in a subset (Figure 27.5d). The diffusely infiltrative pattern sometimes forms so-called 'secondary structures of Scherer': perivascular satellitosis, subpial growth and perivascular spread (Figure 27.5e–h). Immunohistochemistry for neurofilament can be used to highlight the infiltration of white matter tracts by neoplastic astrocytes (Figure 27.5h). GFAP is usually expressed by neoplastic cells, although the GFAP-positive fibrillary matrix of the brain parenchyma may render interpretation difficult. Nuclear staining with OLIG2 may be helpful in establishing glial lineage.[104,136] Tumour cells also usually show S-100 protein immunoreactivity in the nucleus and cell processes. Proliferative activity, as determined by the Ki-67/MIB-1 labelling index, is usually less than 4 per cent.

Gemistocytic astrocytomas are characterized by a conspicuous fraction of cells with abundant glassy eosinophilic cytoplasm and eccentric nuclei (Figure 27.6b). Stout, randomly oriented processes extend from cells and intermix with the normal neuropil. The cells consistently express GFAP. Perivascular lymphocyte cuffing is frequent. MIB-1 labelling is usually less than 4 per cent, with the gemistocytic cells having a lower rate of proliferation than intermixed fibrillary or small astrocytoma cells.

Granular cell astrocytomas are characterized by sheets or interspersed large, round tumour cells packed with eosinophilic, PAS-positive granules (Figure 27.6c).[38] They may be confused with macrophage-rich lesions in some instances, given the abundance of large, lysosome-filled cells. Transition to typical infiltrating astrocytoma is noted in the majority of cases, yet others consist almost entirely of atypical granular cells. Lymphocytic infiltrates are common. Given their highly unusual morphology, determining their glial differentiation often requires immunohistochemistry for GFAP, S-100 protein or OLIG2.

Protoplasmic astrocytoma, a less common variant, has been described as containing neoplastic astrocytes with small cell bodies with few, thin processes and a low content of glial filaments. Nuclei are mostly round to oval and the cellularity is low. Mucoid degeneration and micro-cyst formation are common and the MIB-1 labelling index, is often less than 1 per cent. This lesion is not well defined and is considered by some to be a non-specific pattern, rather than a true variant.

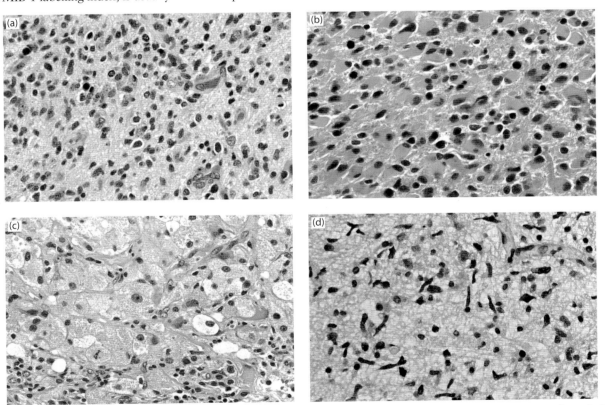

27.6 Astrocytoma variants. (a) Fibrillary astrocytomas are the most frequent morphology and typically appear as elongate hyperchromatic nuclei haphazardly arranged in a densely fibrillar matrix. Note the gradient of increasing cellular density, which is helpful in establishing an infiltrative pattern of neoplasia. **(b)** Gemistocytic astrocytoma with copious eosinophilic cytoplasm. **(c)** Granular cell astrocytomas contain neoplastic cells with abundant cytoplasm packed with lysosomes. **(d)** Diffuse astrocytomas sometimes contain long, thin 'microglia-like' neoplastic cells, and this finding is particularly characteristic of gliomatosis cerebri.

Gliomatosis cerebri is a clinicopathologic diagnosis that implies extensive concurrent involvement of multiple lobes (at least three) or brain compartments by an infiltrating glioma.[114] Most examples appear astrocytic, yet oligodendroglial forms have also been described. Microscopically they usually resemble fibrillary astrocytomas of grade II or III. Long, thin mildly hyperchromatic 'microglia-like' astrocytoma nuclei are typical (Figure 27.6d). As with other infiltrating gliomas, there are often secondary structures, including subpial or subependymal condensation, perivascular aggregates, and perineuronal satellitosis. Although gliomatosis is characterized by widespread involvement by diffusely infiltrating astrocytoma, foci of dedifferentiation to GBM may also develop, either at the time of clinical presentation or later in the disease progression.

Grading

Diffuse astrocytomas correspond to WHO grade II.[143]

Molecular Genetics

Mutations in isocitrate dehydrogenase 1 (*IDH1*) are frequent (60–80 per cent) in grade II astrocytomas,[177,264] with mutations in IDH2 much less common. In all forms of diffuse gliomas, the mutant forms of *IDH1* and IDH2 cause the accumulation of the oncometabolite 2-hydroxyglutarate, which leads to the hypermethylator (G-CIMP) phenotype. Immunohistochemistry for mutant IDH1 (mIDH1R132H) is highly valuable in distinguishing grade II astrocytomas from diagnostically challenging reactive astrocytic proliferations.[37] The sensitivity for identifying IDH1 mutant gliomas of any kind using this monoclonal antibody was 94 per cent and the specificity was 100 per cent.

TP53 mutations are present in over 60 per cent of grade II astrocytomas,[255] even higher in those that are *IDH* mutant, and in up to 80 per cent of gemistocytic variants.[257] Nuclear p53 protein accumulation is similarly frequent but does not always reflect a mutation.[255] During malignant progression of astrocytomas, the frequency of *TP53* mutations does not increase significantly, indicating that this is an early genetic event and already present in the first biopsy in the vast majority of cases.[222,254,255] The association of germline *TP53* mutations and predilection to astrocytomas also argues for a role for p53 deregulation early in tumorigenesis.[116]

Genomic and gene expression studies on the diffusely infiltrative astrocytomas of grades II and III have shown three clearly distinguishable classes.[68,106] One group is characterized by both *IDH* and *TP53* mutations; the second group is characterized by *IDH* mutations, with wild-type *TP53*; and the third group is *IDH* wild type. The last group behaves very aggressively and is associated with much shorter survival times.

ATRX (α-thalassaemia/mental-retardation-syndrome-X-linked) mutations are also common in grade II astrocytomas, but are uncommon in oligodendrogliomas.[139] *ATRX* alterations occur nearly exclusively in astrocytomas harbouring mutations in *IDH* and *TP53*; they are associated with alternative lengthening of telomeres (ALT), a telomerase independent mechanism for maintaining long telomeres in neoplasms.

Comparative genomic hybridization (CGH) analyses have repeatedly demonstrated that the most frequent genomic imbalances are the gain of chromosome 7q and amplification of 8q.[166,218] Less common alterations include chromosome 22q loss[100] and chromosome 6 deletions.[153]

Methylation of the gene encoding O6-methylguanine-DNA methyltransferase (MGMT), a DNA repair protein that directly and specifically repairs promutagenic DNA lesions by removing alkyl groups from the O6 position of guanine, is present in about half of grade II diffuse astrocytomas and may also be related to p53 alterations. Loss of MGMT expression could be an early change that facilitates *TP53* mutations in astrocytomas.[163]

Prognosis

The mean survival time after diagnosis is approximately 6–8 years, with marked individual variation.[143,231] Five- and 10-year survival rates for diffuse fibrillary astrocytomas are 65 and 31 per cent, respectively.[176] In addition to the extent of resection, the prognosis depends on whether or not the glioma progresses to a higher grade. Several reports indicate that the gemistocytic variant appears particularly prone to malignant progression,[121,176,256] whereas protoplasmic forms and tumours with extensive microcystic change may follow a slower course, often with a history of chronic seizures.[194]

Proliferative potential correlates inversely with time to recurrence and survival in grade II astrocytomas, but does not allow a prediction of clinical outcome in individual cases. Higher Ki-67/MIB-1 labelling indices (>5 per cent) correlate with more rapid progression and shorter survival,[101,155] but precise cut-off values are difficult to establish. Grade II astrocytomas with *IDH* mutations have a better prognosis than wild-type counterparts. Those with evidence of genetic changes more typical of high-grade astrocytomas, such as *PTEN* mutation, *CDKN2A* deletion or *RB1* loss/mutation, may follow more aggressive courses.[88]

ANAPLASTIC ASTROCYTOMA

Anaplastic astrocytomas are diffuse astrocytomas with mitotic activity, and are designated as grade III by the World Health Organization (WHO).[143] They may arise following progression from a grade II diffuse astrocytoma, but are also frequently diagnosed at first biopsy, without indication of a lower grade precursor. The terms 'malignant astrocytoma' and 'high-grade astrocytoma' are also sometimes applied to this lesion, but should be avoided, because all diffuse astrocytomas (grades II–IV) are malignant and glioblastomas are also high grade.

Neuroimaging

Anaplastic astrocytomas present as ill-defined intrinsic masses of low signal intensity on T1-weighted MRI and high signal intensity on T2-weighted and FLAIR MRI (Figure 27.7a). In contrast to grade II counterparts, partial contrast enhancement can be observed. However, the rim-like enhancement pattern typical of glioblastoma is not a feature. Grade III astrocytomas have higher rCBV than

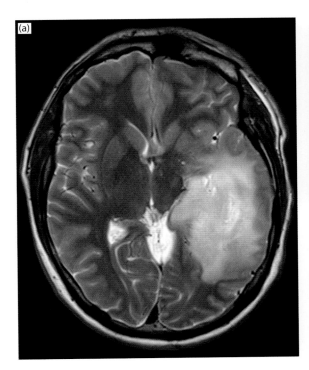

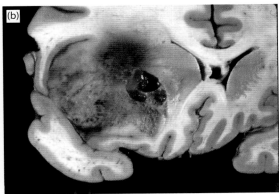

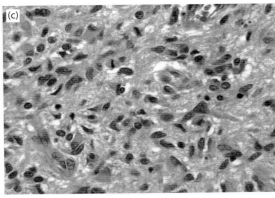

27.7 Anaplastic astrocytoma. (a) MRI demonstrates a large, T2-hyperintense lesion involving the left temporal and parietal lobes. **(b)** Large, partially cystic left temporal lobe mass. **(c)** Hypercellular invasive astrocytoma with mitotic activity.

grade II lesions and also show lower apparent diffusion coefficients and higher Cho/Cr and Cho/NAA ratios.[4,9]

Macroscopic Appearances

The higher cell density of anaplastic astrocytomas produces a more discernible tumour mass that may appear more solid than grade II counterparts (Figure 27.7b). Nonetheless, there is infiltration without tissue destruction, often leading to enlargement of invaded structures. Macroscopic cysts are uncommon. Rapid tumour growth and peritumoral oedema may lead to mass shifts and increased intracranial pressure.

Microscopy

Compared with grade II diffuse astrocytomas, there is increased cellular density, and individual cells contain enlarged, irregular, hyperchromatic nuclei (Figure 27.7c). Anaplastic astrocytomas often contain cells with scant cytoplasm ('naked nuclei'), with glial processes merging with the surrounding neuropil. On cytologic preparations, the glial differentiation is usually more appreciable, with elongate cellular processes extending from individual neoplastic cells. Gemistocytic tumour cells may be present and are more common in anaplastic astrocytomas than in grade II lesions. Capillaries are lined by a single endothelial layer with frank microvascular proliferation, and necrosis is absent by definition. Immunoreactivity for GFAP and S-100 protein is typical. Mitotic activity is the defining feature (Figure 27.7c). The growth fraction, as determined by

the antibodies Ki-67/MIB-1, is usually in the range of 4–10 per cent, but overlaps with grade II diffuse astrocytomas on one side and glioblastoma on the other.

Grading

Anaplastic astrocytomas correspond to WHO grade III.[143]

Molecular Genetics

IDH1 mutations are frequent (60–80 per cent) in grade III astrocytomas, with *IDH2* less commonly implicated.[177,264] These mutations are associated with prolonged survival in comparison to *IDH* wild-type anaplastic astrocytomas. *ATRX* mutations are present in 46 per cent and typically occur in combination with *IDH* and *TP53* mutations.[139]

Anaplastic astrocytomas have *TP53* mutation rates as grade II astrocytomas. Alterations of the RB pathway (CDKN2A/p16, CDK4, Rb1) and of the long arm of chromosome 19, however, are found more often in anaplastic astrocytomas, implicating these events in tumour progression. Allelic losses of chromosome 19q occur in 40–55 per cent.[162,225] Typically, when the genetic events associated strongly with glioblastoma are found in cases of anaplastic astrocytoma, there is shortened survival, presumably because such cases represent incipient transformation to glioblastoma, sampling error or both. For instance, loss of *CDKN2A*, *CDKN2B* and *RB1*, or *CDK4* gene amplification, are associated with worse prognosis in anaplastic astrocytomas.[8] Chromosome

10 losses and *EGFR* amplifications are less common in anaplastic astrocytoma, yet the former may be accompanied by *PTEN* mutation and both are associated with shorter survival.[226] In a series of 80 anaplastic astrocytomas, even simple gains of chromosome 7 were associated with shorter survival, independent of patient age.[123]

Prognosis

The prognosis for patients with anaplastic astrocytoma, WHO grade III, lies between that of grade II and grade IV counterparts, with considerable survival ranges. Traditional estimates have been approximately 2–4 years. In a population-based study, the median survival time was only 1.6 years, with only 11 per cent of patients alive at 5 years after diagnosis.[170] *IDH* mutant anaplastic astrocytomas are associated with improved survival.[264] In one study, the median survival was 65 months for such cases, compared with 20 months for *IDH* wild-type anaplastic astrocytomas.[264] This same study also demonstrated that *IDH* wild-type anaplastic astrocytomas had worse prognosis than *IDH* mutant GBMs.

GLIOBLASTOMA

Glioblastoma is the most malignant neoplasm among the diffuse astrocytic tumours and is designated as WHO grade IV. They typically affect adults and are preferentially localized to cerebral hemispheres. In less than 10 per cent of cases,[174] they develop from low-grade or anaplastic astrocytomas ('secondary glioblastoma'). The rest arise *de novo* after a short clinical history, without evidence of a less malignant precursor lesion ('primary glioblastoma').

Incidence

Glioblastoma accounts for approximately 12–15 per cent of all intracranial neoplasms,[269] and 50–60 per cent of all astrocytic tumours. The incidence in the general population is two to four new cases per 100 000 for most European and North American countries.

Age and Gender

Glioblastomas manifest at all ages, but preferentially affect adults, with a peak incidence between 40 and 70 years. In a review of 715 glioblastomas, approximately two-thirds fell into this age group.[174] Primary glioblastomas typically develop in older patients (mean age 62 years), whereas secondary glioblastomas manifest in younger patients (mean age approximately 45 years).[174] The overall male:female ratio is roughly 1.3:1, but primary glioblastomas are more frequent in males, whereas secondary glioblastomas are more common in females.[174] In a series of 488 glioblastomas, 8.8 per cent were diagnosed in children.[51]

Site, Spread and Metastasis

Glioblastomas preferentially affect the cerebral hemispheres (Figure 27.8a,b). Tumour infiltration is typically widespread, often extending deep into the basal ganglia and thalamus, and frequently to the opposite hemisphere (Figure 27.8c). Glioblastomas of the brain stem are less frequent and often affect children (Figure 27.8d), whereas the cerebellum and the spinal cord are rarer sites.

Although occasional glioblastomas may appear deceptively circumscribed by neuroimaging and seem to be 'shelled out' surgically, these tumours are notorious for their extensive parenchymal invasion.[30] The poor clinical prognosis is largely a result of this extensive spread, particularly along myelinated tracts, making complete resection impossible. Extension through the corpus callosum (Figure 27.8b,c) into the contralateral hemisphere is common, occasionally creating the image of a bilateral, symmetrical lesion ('butterfly glioma'). Similarly, spread is observed in the internal capsule, fornix, anterior commissure and optic radiation, with these structures becoming enlarged and distorted. New masses may then arise at distant sites, thereby leading to the neuroradiological image of a multifocal glioblastoma. Most cases of multifocality on neuroimaging likely represent spread from an original lesion, followed by distant expansion at a second or third location.[11,13,109]

Despite their highly infiltrative growth pattern, glioblastomas do not routinely invade the subarachnoid space and only rarely disseminate through the cerebrospinal fluid (CSF). Extension within and along perivascular spaces is another mode of infiltration, yet invasion through the vascular wall resulting in haematogenous spread to extraneural tissues is very rare in patients without previous surgical intervention; similarly, dural, venous sinus and bone penetration are exceptional.

Clinical Features

Clinical history is usually less than 3 months, unless the neoplasm has developed from a lower-grade astrocytoma. Patients typically present with non-specific neurological symptoms, headache, personality changes and epilepsy, and sometimes focal signs.

Neuroimaging

On CT scans, glioblastomas usually present as irregularly shaped lesions that are hypodense or isodense to brain and typically have a peripheral rim-like zone of contrast enhancement around a dark area of central necrosis. On contrast-enhanced MR images, the contrast-enhancing rim corresponds to the cellular and highly vascularized region that surrounds the central, hypointense area of necrosis (Figure 27.8a). The rim of intense contrast enhancement does not represent the outer tumour border, because infiltrating glioma cells are noted well outside this region and beyond a 2-cm margin.[30] In T2-weighted images, this zone is broader and less well defined, and overlaps with surrounding vasogenic oedema. Advanced MR imaging including DWI, PWI and MRS are being increasingly used for the characterization of diffuse gliomas. Compared to lower-grade gliomas, glioblastomas have high rCBV, low apparent diffusion coefficients and high Cho/Cr and Cho/NAA ratios.[4,9]

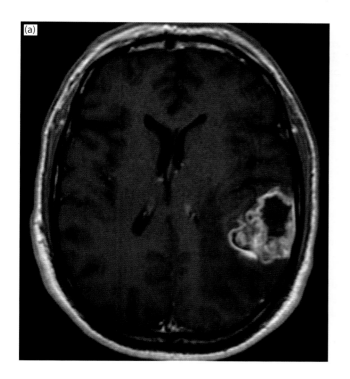

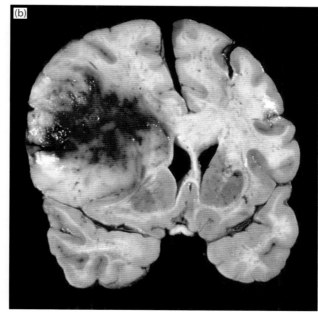

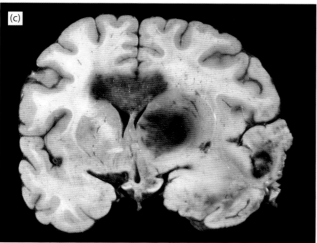

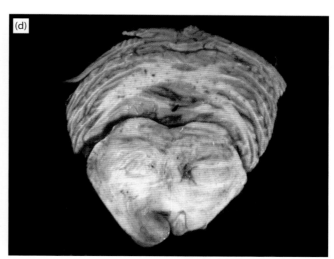

27.8 Glioblastoma. (a) Contrast-enhanced, T1-weighted MR image of rim-enhancing left parietal lobe mass. **(b)** Large, haemorrhagic glioblastoma of the left frontal lobe with expansion of the corpus callosum. **(c)** Apparently multifocal glioblastoma involving the right temporal lobe, deep right hemispheric grey matter and corpus callosum. **(d)** Glioblastoma of the pons in a child ('brain stem glioma'), with ventral extension wrapping around the basilar artery.

Macroscopic Appearances

Glioblastomas are poorly delineated with respect to adjacent brain. The cut surface shows heterogeneity with peripheral greyish tumour masses, yellowish necrosis and single or multiple haemorrhages (Figure 27.8b–d). The central necrosis may occupy as much as 90 per cent of the total tumour mass. Macroscopic cysts, if present, contain a turbid fluid and represent liquefied necrotic tumour tissue. Haemorrhages are usually small and dispersed throughout the neoplasm. However, extensive haemorrhages may occur and evoke stroke-like symptoms, which are sometimes the first clinical sign of tumour manifestation.

Microscopy

The histopathology of glioblastoma is highly variable and regional heterogeneity is found in nearly all cases. Although some lesions show a high degree of cellular density, nuclear pleomorphism and multiple patterns of differentiation, others have a high cell density, but are rather monotonous. The astrocytic nature of neoplastic cells can be appreciated morphologically, at least focally, in the majority of tumours, but can be difficult to recognize in others, owing to poor or metaplastic differentiation. Cytologic preparations are often helpful, because the astrocytic processes can be best appreciated using this technique. There are multiple variants, including gliosarcoma, giant cell glioblastoma, small cell glioblastoma and glioblastoma with an oligodendroglioma component (Figure 27.9a–d).

The combination of diffusely infiltrative astrocytoma cells, mitotic activity and microvascular proliferation and/or necrosis is diagnostic (Figure 27.10a–d). The distribution of these key elements within the tumour is variable, but usually, large necrotic areas occupy the tumour centre, whereas viable tumour cells tend to accumulate in the periphery and infiltrate at the leading edge. The gradient from hypercellular neoplasm centrally to a low-density, infiltrative periphery is nearly pathognomonic, because non-glial neoplasms do not infiltrate as readily or with the same pattern (Figure 27.6a). Microvascular proliferation can be seen throughout the lesion, yet preferentially localizes around necrotic foci and at the peripheral infiltration zone. The infiltrating edges display the same propensity to create 'secondary structures of Scherer' as do lower-grade counterparts; subpial growth, perineuronal satellitosis and perivascular accumulation are all common findings.

Few human neoplasms are as cytologically heterogeneous as glioblastomas. Although poorly differentiated,

fusiform, round or pleomorphic cells may prevail, more differentiated neoplastic astrocytes are usually discernible, at least focally and particularly in secondary glioblastomas. The transition between areas with still recognizable astrocytic differentiation and highly anaplastic cells may be either gradual or abrupt. Some tumours are dominated by giant cells (Figure 27.9b), small monotonous anaplastic cells (Figure 27.9c), spindle-shaped cells (Figure 27.9a), large epithelioid cells, PNET-like foci, granular cells (Figure 27.6c) or lipidized cells, and therefore a host of other neoplasms may come into the differential diagnosis; immunohistochemistry may be helpful in ruling in a diagnosis of glioblastoma and in excluding other possibilities. Many of these differentiation patterns may be secondary in nature and do not necessarily designate a specific biological form of glioblastoma, especially when focal.

Glioblastomas occasionally contain foci with glandular and ribbon-like epithelial ('adenoid') structures or even squamous epithelial-like cells, which may be well delineated from the remaining tumour areas. Others may

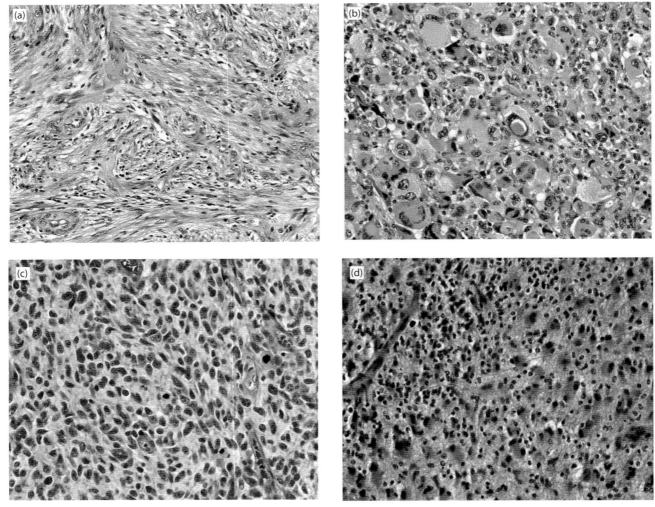

27.9 Glioblastoma variants. (a) Gliosarcoma with spindled sarcomatous regions growing in fascicles and interspersed with collagen. **(b)** Giant cell GBM with markedly pleomorphic enlarged cells. **(c)** Small cell glioblastoma with monomorphic cells growing in sheets with high mitotic rate. **(d)** GBM with oligodendroglioma component contains regions of astrocytic differentiation and oligodendroglial differentiation.

show mesenchymal changes, including cartilage and bone formation. Both epithelial and mesenchymal metaplastic changes are more common in the gliosarcoma variant. Significantly, genetic studies of histologically biphasic tumours have generally shown clonal genetic changes between the histologically distinct regions, including in oligoastrocytomas, gliosarcomas and glioblastomas with metaplastic changes. For instance, glial and sarcomatous,[118] as well as glial and epithelial areas[56,156] have the same *TP53* mutations. In a recently described variant, glioblastoma with PNET-like foci, both components may share common features such as 10q loss, but the PNET foci may additionally show unique alterations, such *MYCC* or *MYCN* amplification.[186]

Proliferative activity is usually prominent, with numerous typical and atypical mitoses. The Ki-67/MIB-1 proliferation index varies considerably, but is generally greater than 5 per cent and may be very high (>50 per cent). Whereas the Ki-67/MIB-1 proliferative index is prognostic in grades II and III astrocytomas, its value as a prognostic marker in glioblastoma has not been adequately demonstrated.[26] It is likely that biologic forces other than proliferation, such as hypoxia and angiogenesis, become more relevant to tumour behaviour at this level.

The cardinal diagnostic features of glioblastoma are microvascular proliferation and necrosis (Figure 27.10a–d). The biological underpinnings of these phenomena were previously discussed. Microvascular changes take on many morphologies including hypertrophy, hyperplasia of endothelial and pericytic cells, and endothelial layering within the lumen (Figure 27.10c). The most complex arrangements are glomeruloid bodies (Figure 27.10d), which are often arranged in a festoon-like pattern, typically immediately adjacent to regions of necrosis. The latter may extend over considerable distances, suggesting that they form a three-dimensional network, around the central necrotic core. Microvascular proliferation is a signpost for the presence of necrosis and either feature justifies classifying a high-grade astrocytoma as glioblastoma. The glomeruloid appearance is based on multilayered hyperplastic endothelial cells, which typically show mitotic activity and high MIB-1 labelling. In nearly all glioblastomas, intravascular thrombosis can be appreciated, both within larger calibre vessels extending into the neoplasm and within vessels near or within necrotic foci (Figure 27.10b). Neurosurgeons are well acquainted with the association of thrombosed blood vessels seen at surgery and the diagnosis of glioblastoma. It has been speculated that intravascular thrombosis either

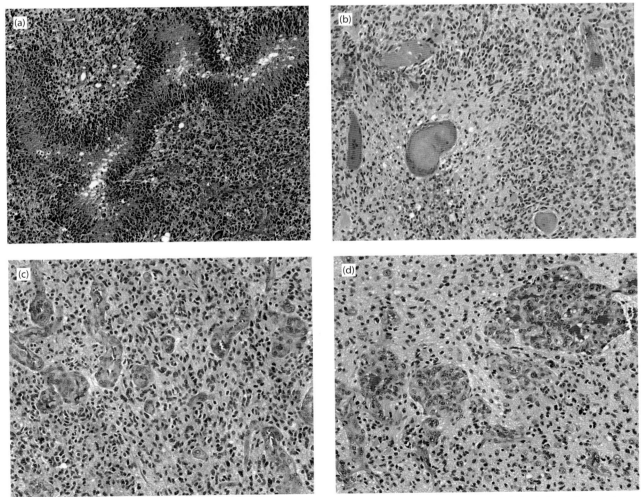

27.10 Glioblastoma. (a) Pseudo-palisading necrosis. **(b)** Foci of necrosis often show thrombosed vessels in their centres and around edges. **(c)** Vessels in GBM show endothelial hypertrophy, hyperplasia and multilayering. **(d)** Glomeruloid microvascular proliferation.

initiates or propagates hypoxia and necrosis and may be a fundamental property of this tumour type.[208,236]

Necrosis (Figure 27.10a,b) is found in nearly all glioblastomas, depending on the diagnostic criteria employed. Using the WHO criteria, in which glioblastoma can be diagnosed on the basis of either microvascular proliferation or necrosis, one study found necrosis in 88 per cent of glioblastomas.[10] In some, necrosis comprises the vast majority of the tumour, creating diagnostic challenges for the pathologist. The most characteristic form, however, consists of multiple small, irregularly shaped necrotic foci, surrounded by radially oriented, small fusiform glioma cells–'pseudo-palisading' pattern (Figure 27.10a). The central area of such geographical necrosis sometimes consists of a fine fibrillar network in which neither viable nor necrotic glioma cells are identified. It has been suggested that these small foci of necrosis are growing outwardly and enlarging, eventually coalescing into larger zones that merge to form the central necrotic core of glioblastoma.[208,236]

Grading

Glioblastomas are WHO grade IV.[143]

Immunohistochemistry and Differential Diagnosis

Glioblastomas show variable staining for GFAP. In general, astrocyte-like tumour cells, in particular gemistocytes, are strongly positive, whereas small, undifferentiated cells may stain weakly or not at all. Giant cells stain variably, with marked differences in GFAP expression even among neighbouring cells. Although large portions may lack GFAP expression, wider sampling usually reveals at least occasional immunoreactive tumour cells. GFAP expression tends to decrease during glioma progression, but there is no indication that its extent is prognostic. Vimentin, S-100 protein and OLIG2 are usually expressed widely.

The primary utility of GFAP immunohistochemistry is in the differential diagnosis of glioblastoma from other poorly differentiated malignancies. As mentioned earlier, the marked cytological heterogeneity of glioblastoma may bring metastatic carcinoma, sarcoma, melanoma, lymphoma or even anaplastic meningioma into the histological differential diagnosis. GFAP positivity is rare in other tumours and its presence therefore strongly supports a glioma diagnosis in the appropriate clinicopathological setting. Moreover, an immunohistochemical panel for epithelial, mesenchymal, melanocytic and lymphoid markers will typically exclude other diagnostic possibilities.

Molecular Genetics: Subtypes of Glioblastoma

Two clinically distinctive subtypes of glioblastoma are now well established: *primary glioblastoma* arises *de novo* as a grade IV neoplasm, whereas the *secondary glioblastoma* arises following the progression of a lower-grade glioma. By definition, these clinically defined primary and secondary glioblastomas do not overlap.

There is good correlation between these two clinical pathways and genetic alterations, because the majority of secondary glioblastomas have *IDH* mutations, also with frequent *TP53* and *ATRX* mutations, whereas these mutations are much less frequent in *de novo* glioblastomas. *EGFR* gene amplification is rare in secondary glioblastoma and is relatively frequent in primary glioblastomas.[174] However, true secondary glioblastomas are much less common than primary glioblastomas, accounting for only 5 per cent in a population-based study.[174] A considerable number of primary, *de novo* glioblastomas have *TP53* mutations.[174,217] Thus, although *TP53* mutations are more frequent (as a percentage) in secondary glioblastomas, the absolute number of *TP53* mutations is greater in primary glioblastomas.

Molecular Genetics: Key Genetic Events

As discussed earlier, glioblastoma may arise through alterations in multiple genetic pathways, yet there is strong convergence on particular sets of pathways that govern cell growth, cell death, invasion and angiogenesis. Genetic pathways clearly implicated in glioblastoma include those involving (1) p53 (*TP53*, *MDM2/MDM4*, *ARF*), (2) retinoblastoma (*Rb1*, *cdk4*, *CDKN2A/p16*) and (3) receptor tyrosine kinases (*EGFR*, *PDGFR*, *MET*, *PI3-kinase*, *PTEN*, *Neurofibromatosis 1*). These pathways are deregulated by particular genetic events, such as gene mutations, deletion and amplifications, but may also be influenced by other growth promoting and growth suppressing molecules.

The *EGFR* gene is involved in the control of cell proliferation. It is amplified in about 40 per cent of glioblastomas, of which roughly 40 per cent include a truncated variant known as the vIII mutant,[61] rarely with other mutations,[61] and often together with neighbouring genes at 7p12.[138] Only 8 per cent of secondary glioblastomas show *EGFR* amplification.[174] EGFR protein is also overexpressed in primary glioblastomas: more than 60 per cent of cases versus 10 per cent in secondary glioblastomas.[254] There is a close but imperfect correlation between gene amplification and overexpression. In particular, expression of the vIII mutant correlates closely with underlying *EGFR* amplification.[1] Glioblastomas with *EGFR* amplification typically show simultaneous chromosome 10 loss.[249]

PDGFRA amplification is the second most frequent RTK amplification in glioblastoma. Most investigations using genome averaging techniques, such as array-based CGH, have found high level amplification in 10–15 per cent of cases.[36] However, increased PDGF pathway activity has been documented in higher fractions, suggesting other mechanisms. A recent FISH-based analysis documented *PDGFRA* amplification in 23 per cent of adult and 39 per cent of paediatric GBM. In this study, both low- and high-level amplification events could be detected, because FISH allows detection at the individual tumour cell level.[189]

Recent studies have noted that *EGFR* and *PDGFRA* amplifications occasionally occur within the same tumour.[229,234] In most, *EGFR* and *PDGFRA* are not amplified within the same cells and the amplifications seem to be spatially distinct, with most *EGFR* amplification noted peripherally and most *PDGFRA* amplification present centrally.[175,229] Signalling networks and drug-sensitive targets downstream of these RTKs would also be expected to vary with these amplification events, because EGFR and PDGFRA are powerful oncogenic stimuli in GBM.[36,234]

A key pathway that regulates cell cycle control and apoptosis, among other functions, involves p53, mdm2 and ARF.[96] *TP53* mutations were among the first genetic alterations identified in astrocytic brain tumours.[42] In glioblastoma series, the reported frequencies vary considerably, with a mean of 25–30 per cent.[174] *TP53* mutations are uncommon in primary or *de novo* glioblastomas, whereas secondary glioblastomas have a high incidence (approximately 65 per cent), of which over 90 per cent are already present in the first biopsy.[173,254,255] The incidence of p53 protein accumulation is observed more frequently than *TP53* mutations,[255] but is also significantly higher in secondary (>90 per cent) than in primary glioblastomas (<35 per cent).[254] The percentage of glioma cells with p53 accumulation appears to increase from the first biopsy to recurrent tumours,[255] and one study suggests that this reflects the clonal expansion of glioma cells carrying a *TP53* mutation.[222]

The MDM2 protein forms a complex with p53, thereby abolishing its transcriptional activity and constituting an alternative mechanism to escape from p53-regulated control of cell growth. Amplification of *MDM2* on 12q is present in about 8 per cent of glioblastomas,[198] all of which appear to be primary glioblastomas that lack *TP53* mutation.[16,198] The related *MDM4* gene on 1q is likely the primary gene underlying the occasional glioblastomas with amplifications at 1q32.[201] A detailed analysis of the p53 pathway by the TCGA project, including *TP53*, *MDM2/4* and *CDKN2A-ARF*, found that this family is altered in nearly 90 per cent of GBMs.[36]

A second key regulatory pathway, primarily affecting cell cycle control, involves p16, cdk4 and pRb, which is deregulated in the vast majority of glioblastomas.[95] The *CDKN2A* locus on chromosome 9p21[94,244] encodes two distinct proteins: the product of exons 1α, 2 and 3 (CDKN2A/INK4A transcript) is the p16 tumour suppressor that induces a G1 cell-cycle arrest by inhibiting phosphorylation of the RB1 protein through binding of CDK4; the product of exons 1β, 2 and 3 (ARF transcript) is most commonly termed ARF, which binds MDM2, resulting in the stabilization of both p53 and MDM2. In glioblastomas, *CDKN2A* deletion and *RB1* alterations appear mutually exclusive,[17,33,245] and these changes occur in both primary and secondary glioblastomas.[17,163] *CDKN2A* deletion occurs frequently together with *EGFR* amplification.[84] ARF alterations (either promoter hypermethylation or homozygous deletion) occur in 50 per cent of primary and 75 per cent of secondary glioblastomas,[163] but the 9p deletions are large and often also affect other genes in addition to *CDKN2B*,[102] and therefore the significance of these changes is not clear.

Mutations of the *RB1* gene, as well as corresponding loss of the remaining 13q allele, are found in about one-quarter of high-grade astrocytic tumours.[86] Promoter hypermethylation of the *RB1* gene also occurs, more often in secondary (43 per cent) than in primary (14 per cent) glioblastomas, and hypermethylation correlates closely with gene silencing as shown by a lack of RB1 immunoreactivity.[163] In addition to pRb and p16 inactivation, this pathway is also

deregulated by amplification and overexpression of *CDK4*, which occurs in up to 15 per cent of glioblastomas.[95,96]

Losses of large regions at 10p, 10q23 and 10q25-26 loci or an entire chromosome 10 are the most frequent genetic alterations in glioblastomas.[251] Loss of the long arm, which occurs more frequently than the short arm, occurs equally in primary (70 per cent) and secondary (63 per cent) glioblastomas.[174] Of the various candidate genes on 10q, only *PTEN* has been strongly implicated.

The *PTEN* gene on chromosome 10q23.3[131,230] is mutated in approximately 25–30 per cent of unselected glioblastomas.[19] In one study, *PTEN* mutations were found almost exclusively in primary glioblastomas (32 per cent) and rarely (4 per cent) in secondary glioblastomas,[240] whereas another study suggests that *PTEN* inactivation is involved in both pathways.[267] Importantly, PTEN is central to regulating growth and apoptosis, and possibly cell migration and angiogenesis. This pathway involves PI3 (phosphatidylinositol 3) kinase, PTEN, pAKT, tuberin/hamartin and mTOR as important regulatory molecules. PTEN itself plays a key role in inhibiting the activation state of signalling lipids, such as phosphoinositols, through removal of phosphates, whereas PI3 kinase has an opposing role through phosphorylation and hence activation. In general, alterations of the *PI3K* genes occur in glioblastomas with wild-type *PTEN*,[154] demonstrating that PTEN inactivation and PI3 kinase activation are alternative means to activate the Akt pathway.

It has long been known that germline mutations of the Neurofibromatosis 1 (*NF1*) gene lead to the NF1 syndrome, which predisposes to the development of neurofibromas systemically and to the development of pilocytic astrocytomas of the optic pathways.[252] Patients with NF1 are also at risk for the development of high-grade gliomas, but not to the same extent as pilocytic astrocytomas.[103] The description of *NF1* as a tumour suppressor in sporadic glioblastoma has been more recent,[36,177] mutations being noted in approximately 15 per cent and hemizygous deletions in another 15–20 per cent. *NF1* encodes a Ras-GTPase activating protein (RasGAP), referred to as neurofibromin, and its loss of function activates the Ras pathway. *NF1* mutations and deletions are strongly associated with the mesenchymal transcriptional class of glioblastoma and are uncommon in the proneural, neural and classical classes.[248]

Paediatric glioblastomas appear to have a set of genetic alterations that is distinct and may indicate a differing molecular pathogenesis than in adults. For example, mutations in the chromatin remodeling gene *H3F3A* are much more specific to paediatric high-grade astrocytomas,[219] where they are found in 40 per cent, many of these neoplasms also showing *ATRX* and *TP53* mutations. *H3F3A* mutations can lead to an amino acid substitution either at K27 or at G34.[233] K27-mutated tumours occur in the youngest children and in the midline (thalamus and pons), whereas the G34-mutated tumours occur in the cerebral hemispheres of teenagers and young adults. Mutations in *DAXX* (death-domain associated protein) are also relatively specific to high-grade paediatric astrocytomas, but occur at much lower frequency.[219]

A number of groups have investigated large series of glioblastoma to determine if there are distinct subsets based on gene expression profile.[36,188,248] TCGA found that there were four distinct transcriptional classes following unsupervised hierarchical clustering and, based on the signature genes within each class, referred to them as proneural, neural, classical and mesenchymal. The prognostic significance of these four classes was not substantial, yet enthusiasm remains high that subsets such as these will serve as a platform for targeted therapies. There is relatively good correlation between genomic alterations, including mutation and copy number changes, and gene expression class, but this association is not exact. The proneural class contains nearly all of the tumours with *IDH* mutations and is also enriched with *PDGFRA* amplified and *TP53* mutant tumours. The classical subtype is represented by *EGFR* amplifications and *CDKN2A* deletions, whereas the mesenchymal class contains tumours with *NF1* mutations and deletions, as well as a subset of *TP53* mutant tumours. The neural class includes a variety of genomic alterations that do not seem cohesive.

Other large-scale molecular studies based on DNA methylation patterns have uncovered an important subset of glioblastomas with a hypermethylator phenotype referred to as the CpG island methylator phenotype (G-CIMP).[167] This subset, which also harbours *IDH1* or *IDH2* mutations, is a part of the proneural transcriptional class and has an improved survival compared to non-G-CIMP glioblastomas. The presence of *IDH* mutations leads to the accumulation of the oncometabolite 2-hydroxyglutarate, which inhibits a large number of α-ketoglutarate-dependent enzymes. Inhibition of the family of histone demethylases and the TET family of 5-methylcytosine hydroxylases has profound epigenetic effects in mutated cells leading directly to the G-CIMP phenotype.[243]

Prognosis

Clinical trials from the past three decades have revealed consistent prognostic factors for glioblastoma patients. One of the most solid is the correlation of patient age with prognosis. Young patients (under 45 years of age) have substantially improved clinical outcomes compared to older counterparts.[29] The clinically assessed performance status at the time of diagnosis is also associated, such that among glioblastoma patients over 50 years of age, those with Karnofsky performance status (KPS) >70 have substantially improved outcomes.[44,132] KPS is also an important prognostic factor for younger patients and other histologies, but the threshold KPS score varies. In general, patients with higher performance status show improved clinical outcomes. Numerous investigations have also indicated that the extent of surgical resection can have an impact on survival. In one large retrospective series, neurosurgical resection greater than 78 per cent based on neuroimaging assessment was associated with prolonged survival, with additional survival advantages noted with increasing extents of resection.[211]

Because the WHO allows the diagnosis of glioblastoma based on the histologic presence of either microvascular proliferation or necrosis, one study evaluated the prognostic effect of necrosis. In a series of 275 glioblastomas, the absence of necrosis (in 12 per cent of cases) was associated with younger age, less extensive surgical resection and a median survival of 12.5 months, compared to 10.9 months in those with tumour necrosis.[10] Although it has been repeatedly demonstrated that the Ki-67/MIB-1 labelling index correlates with tumour grade, proliferative potential does not provide additional independent prognostic information once the glioblastoma histology is achieved.

Many studies have attempted to correlate molecular alterations with prognosis in glioblastoma. Mutations in *IDH1/2* are strongly associated with survival. One study demonstrated that glioblastomas with *IDH* mutations had a median survival of 31 months as compared to 15 months for *IDH* wild-type glioblastomas.[264] This relationship is more complex, however, because most patients with *IDH*-mutated GBM are younger and have secondary GBM, which are both associated with improved survival as well.

Another approach compares long- versus short-term GBM survivors for key molecular differences. A CGH study of 39 glioblastomas from patients who survived longer than three years and from 24 short-term survivors showed that 6q loss, 10q loss and 19q gain were associated with short survival times and loss of 19q with long survival times.[34] Most investigations of prognostic molecular markers have not shown simple associations, but have suggested complex interplays between patient age, genetic parameters and possibly treatment response. Associations between older age and *EGFR* gene amplification,[251] as well as younger age and *TP53* mutation are strong; as mentioned earlier, age itself is a powerful prognostic factor.[29] For example, in one report, *EGFR* amplification was an independent predictor of prolonged survival only in patients with glioblastoma who were older than 60 years of age.[226] Furthermore, in addition to *TP53* and *EGFR* alterations, the prognostic effects of *CDKN2A* deletions,[12,105] also appear dependent on the age of the patient, being more pronounced in patients older than 70 years of age.[12]

Predictive molecular parameters, i.e. those that address response to therapy rather than prognosis, have drawn less attention in glioblastomas than in oligodendrogliomas, largely because measurable therapeutic responses are less common in glioblastomas. Most studies of astrocytic tumours have not found prognostic importance for 1p/19q loss,[224] arguing against a role for 1p/19q testing in glioblastoma management.[24] The demonstration that concomitant temozolomide treatment provided a 2-month survival advantage in patients with glioblastoma[231] prompted correlative studies related to *MGMT* promoter methylation status.[258] Glioblastomas with *MGMT* promoter methylation would be predicted to have better prognosis because the ability to repair DNA damage from alkylating agents is impaired in MGMT-deficient tumours. Indeed, such tumours were found to have improved overall survival and enhanced responses to temozolomide.[85] Studies of glioblastoma patients who were treated in the era before the use of temozolomide indicate that GBMs with *MGMT* methylation also have improved survival following radiation alone, suggesting that this alteration may identify GBMs with a more general survival advantage.[203] Thus, *MGMT* methylation is an important prognostic marker in GBM and appears to predict sensitivity to therapy.

The advent of targeted molecular therapies provides potential for molecular markers as predictors of treatment response. Given the role of EGFR in tumorigenesis, a number of clinical trials have investigated small molecule inhibitors of EGFR for efficacy against glioblastoma.

Unfortunately, only a small subset of patients have benefited.[200] Others have investigated molecular determinants of response to EGFR inhibitors among this small group of responders. In a series of 41 patients with malignant glioma treated with erlotinib, eight responded to treatment and response was associated with EGFR expression and EGFR amplification (but not vIII mutant expression), particularly in the 29 patients with glioblastoma. Interestingly, none of the 22 tumours with high levels of phosphorylated PKB/Akt responded to erlotinib treatment, suggesting further that PI3 kinase–PTEN pathway disruption predicted poor response.[73] Similarly, another study found that only those tumours that had coexpression of both EGFRvIII and PTEN showed substantial response to EGFR inhibitors.[150] In both studies, the suggestion is that downstream activation of Akt, due to PTEN loss or other mechanisms, renders EGFR antagonism ineffective.

Gene expression profiling is a powerful manner to estimate prognosis of malignant gliomas. In one study, a set of approximately 70 genes separated glioblastomas into two groups that differed over four-fold in median duration of survival.[135] Another study explored diagnostically difficult cases, in which glioblastoma was not easily distinguished from anaplastic oligodendroglioma pathologically and demonstrated that a model of about 19 differentially expressed genes was superior in estimating prognosis than standard histopathological classification.[168]

Large-scale gene expression profiles have been developed that identify a more aggressive form of glioblastoma, which has been referred to as the mesenchymal class, dominated by genes related to angiogenesis and mesenchymal cell differentiation.[188] Upon recurrence of high-grade gliomas, many show conversion to the mesenchymal expression class, suggesting that it may represent an end-stage, highly malignant form. There have been additional efforts to develop a smaller panel of genes that could predict prognosis and be more clinically useful than large-scale gene expression platforms. One such study took the gene expression and clinical outcomes data from four large, independent GBM data sets and identified a group of nine genes that could be used on formalin-fixed material and reliably predict prognosis on multivariate analysis.[43]

GLIOBLASTOMA VARIANTS

Gliosarcoma

Gliosarcoma, defined as a glioblastoma admixed with a 'sarcomatous' component, accounts for approximately 2 per cent of all glioblastomas.[119,149] A preferential location in the temporal lobe has been observed.[149] Gliosarcomas can arise as primary, recurrent or radiation-induced neoplasms.[80,81] Clinical features are generally similar to those of classic glioblastoma with regard to age, gender, race, tumour size or use of adjuvant radiation therapy.[119] The prognosis is dismal, with survivals similar to or slightly shorter than that of glioblastoma.[119] In cases with a predominant sarcomatous component, the tumour appears as a well-demarcated hyperdense mass with homogeneous contrast enhancement. Those that are peripherally located and abut the dura may mimic a meningioma. A recent study indicates that this subset of gliosarcomas that mimic meningioma may have a better prognosis.[79]

Essential for the diagnosis of the gliosarcoma is a biphasic tissue pattern with areas displaying gliomatous or mesenchymal differentiation (Figure 27.9a). The glial portion usually resembles glioblastoma. Although the large majority have astrocytic differentiation, gliosarcomas have also been described as arising with oligodendroglial, PNET and ependymal differentiation.[89,107,205] The mesenchymal areas may show the typical herringbone pattern of fibrosarcomas, with densely packed long bundles of spindle cells. Occasionally, they resemble features of a pleomorphic sarcoma. The sarcomatous component also often shows signs of malignant transformation, such as nuclear atypia, mitotic activity and necrosis. It forms a rich reticulin network, in which the sarcomatous areas are well demarcated from the glial elements. Some show additional lines of mesenchymal differentiation, such as cartilage, bone and muscle. Furthermore, epithelial metaplasia with clusters of keratinizing stratified epithelia and adenoid formations have been noted. The occasional occurrence of spindle cells within a glioblastoma does not justify the diagnosis of gliosarcoma. Moreover, the infiltration of otherwise typical glioblastoma into the overlying leptomeninges and dura may lead to the erroneous impression of gliosarcoma because of the incorporation of reactive and collagen-rich elements.

Gliosarcomas show variable genetic aberrations similar to those occurring in glioblastomas, i.e. gain of chromosome 7, loss of chromosomes 10 and 17, deletions of the short arm of chromosome 9 and alterations of chromosome 3. TP53 mutations are common, as are PTEN mutations and CDKN2A deletions.[18,178,199] In one series, however, no gliosarcomas showed EGFR amplification or overexpression.[199] Only a small percentage of primary gliosarcomas (7.7 per cent) showed IDH1/2 mutations, similar to primary glioblastomas. More distinctive was the low percentage of MGMT promoter methylation in gliosarcoma (11.5 per cent) as compared to typical glioblastomas (35–45 per cent).[127]

Genetic analyses of gliosarcomas[18,178] and comparison of the mutational pattern in the gliomatous and sarcomatous components have demonstrated that each have identical TP53 and PTEN mutations, suggesting a monoclonal origin.[18,199] More recent investigations using high density genomic array techniques have demonstrated focal amplification of a chromosomal region, 13q13.3-q14.1, containing the genes STOML3, FREM2 and LHFP, exclusively within the sarcomatous component.[159] The overexpression of these genes and proteins was confirmed predominantly in the sarcomatous elements, suggesting that additional genomic alterations in the sarcomatous component lead to its distinctive phenotype. The finding that transcription factors known to drive the epithelial-mesenchymal transition (EMT) in other forms of cancer, such as Twist and Slug, are expressed exclusively in the sarcomatous elements of gliosarcoma indicate that these factors drive the mesenchymal transition.[160]

Giant Cell Glioblastoma

This histological variant has a marked predominance of bizarre, multinucleated giant cells and, on occasion, an abundant stromal reticulin network (Figure 27.9b). The consistent expression of GFAP has firmly established its astrocytic nature and this is confirmed by the genetic profile.[182]

It accounts for approximately 1 per cent of all glioblastomas. The race and gender profiles are similar to conventional glioblastomas. However, giant cell glioblastomas tend to occur at a younger age (mean 51 years).[118]

Giant cell glioblastomas are more circumscribed than other glioblastomas and often located subcortically in the temporal and parietal lobe. As a result, they may mimic a metastasis on neuroimaging. If they abut the dura, they can be confused with meningioma by neuroimaging and intra-operatively. Giant cell glioblastomas are completely resected with greater frequency than other glioblastomas, most likely because of their peripheral location and their circumscription. There is also evidence indicating that the survival of patients with giant cell glioblastoma is longer than those with typical glioblastoma, perhaps because of in part the younger patient age and the improved likelihood of complete resection. However, even after correcting for other features associated with survival, the giant cell histology was independently prognostic.[118] Importantly, the improved survival of giant cell glioblastoma has not been noted in the paediatric population.[108]

On microscopic examination, tumour cells may be extremely bizarre and up to 400 µm in diameter. The number of nuclei per cell varies from one to more than 20. They are often angulated, may contain prominent nucleoli and, on occasion, cytoplasmic inclusions. Atypical mitoses can be observed, but the overall proliferation rate is similar to that of ordinary glioblastomas. Expression of GFAP is highly variable, and perivascular lymphocyte cuffing may be present.

Giant cell glioblastomas are characterized by frequent *TP53* (75–90 per cent of cases) and *PTEN* mutations (33 per cent of cases), but typically lack homozygous *CDKN2A* deletion and *EGFR* amplification/overexpression.[151,181,182]

The primary diagnostic concern is pleomorphic xanthoastrocytoma (PXA), which is also a peripherally located, circumscribed neoplasm that contains large, bizarre tumour cells. However, PXA also usually contains more abundant xanthomatous cells, eosinophilic granular bodies, as well as a substantially lower proliferative rate.

Small Cell Glioblastoma

Small cell glioblastoma is less clearly defined than gliosarcoma and giant cell glioblastoma, but is recognized as a pattern with distinctive genetic and clinical associations in the WHO classification.[143] The tumour is characterized by monotonous, generally bland appearing cells with round-to-ovoid nuclei that are mildly hyperchromatic and resemble oligodendroglioma at lower magnifications (Figure 27.9c). The cell density is variable, but the nuclear:cytoplasmic ratio and mitotic index are high. The amount of small cell phenotype necessary for the diagnosis has not been established and foci of small cells can be noted in otherwise standard glioblastoma. Immunohistochemistry is helpful in the differential diagnosis, because these tumours are generally positive for GFAP, although the elongate processes may appear wispy or the stain may be mostly negative because of the presence of minimal cytoplasm. The small cell phenotype appears to correlate strongly with *EGFR* gene amplification. In a study of 79 glioblastomas, *EGFR* amplification was found in 14 of 21 (67 per cent) glioblastomas that were composed exclusively of small cells, in 8 of 25 (32 per cent) glioblastomas with both small cell and non – small cell areas, and in 3 of 33 (9 per cent) glioblastomas without small cells.[31] The nosological position of so-called small cell astrocytomas lacking microvascular proliferation and necrosis is less clear, because they often behave like glioblastomas even when otherwise qualifying only for a WHO grade III designation.[185] Small cell glioblastoma shares histological features with oligodendroglioma, including chicken-wire vasculature, haloes, perineuronal satellitosis and micro-calcifications, although typically lacking microcystic spaces and minigemistocytes. In contrast to oligodendrogliomas, *EGFR* amplification was present in 69 per cent, with 10q deletions in 97 per cent, but 1p and 19q losses were not present in one series.[185] In another study of glioblastoma variants, none of the 45 small cell glioblastomas showed immunohistochemical evidence of *IDH1* mutation.[104]

Glioblastoma with Oligodendroglioma Component

Glioblastoma with oligodendroglioma component (GBM-O), WHO grade IV ('grade IV oligoastrocytoma'), is essentially a high-grade oligoastrocytoma with necrosis.[253] These tumours contain either admixed tumour cells with oligodendroglioma and astrocytoma differentiation or distinct regions containing these cell types (Figure 27.9d). GBM-O was only recently accepted following extensive clinicopathologic investigations of anaplastic oligoastrocytomas.[152,227,247] Miller et al. studied the overall survival of 215 patients with anaplastic oligoastrocytoma as it related to age, gender, type of surgical procedure, necrosis and endothelial hyperplasia.[152] A significantly shorter median survival was found for patients with anaplastic oligoastrocytomas with necrosis than for those without it. In contrast, the presence of endothelial proliferation was not found to be prognostically important in this subset. Thus, these data indicated that patients with anaplastic oligoastrocytomas with necrosis had shorter survival and that such tumours should be considered grade IV. In the fourth edition, the WHO classified GBM-O as grade IV.[143]

One recent investigation found that GBM-O accounts for 12 per cent of all glioblastomas.[3] They were found to arise in younger patients than other forms of GBMs (50.7 versus 58.7 years, respectively) and were also more frequently secondary. Compared to other GBMs, they had a higher frequency of *IDH1* mutations and a lower frequency of *PTEN* deletions. Survival was longer in GBM-O patients compared to conventional GBM, with median survivals of 16.2 and 8.1 months, respectively.

Most of the survival advantage appeared to be associated with younger age at presentation. Among patients with GBM-O, younger age at presentation and 1p deletion were most significant in conferring prolonged survival.

PILOCYTIC ASTROCYTOMA

The pilocytic astrocytoma is a slowly growing, circumscribed astrocytic neoplasm, predominantly of childhood, composed of a compact arrangement, well-differentiated tumour cells with highly elongate ('hair-like') glial processes. These tumours arise in stereotypic locations within the CNS and are associated with favourable prognosis.

Incidence

The pilocytic astrocytoma accounts for approximately 1.5 per cent of all intracranial tumours and has an incidence of 0.33 per 100 000.[52] It is the most common low-grade brain tumour of childhood, accounting for 23.5 per cent in this age group. In adults, it comprises less than 1 per cent of brain tumours.

Age and Sex

More than 75 per cent of pilocytic astrocytomas occur in children and adolescents, with a peak incidence between 8 and 13 years. Tumours of the cerebral hemispheres and spinal cord tend to manifest at an older age than those of the optic nerve and chiasm, brain stem and cerebellum. Males and females are affected equally, independent of site.

Sites

The cerebellum is most frequently affected (Figure 27.11a), with cerebellar hemispheres (>80 per cent) more frequently affected than the vermis (20 per cent). Optic nerve (Figure 27.11b) and chiasmatic gliomas are second most common. Of the latter, a significant fraction involves the adjacent hypothalamus and third ventricle. Those of the cerebral hemispheres are less frequent, except for temporal lobe, in particular its medial portion. Tumours of the brain stem are next in frequency, followed by rarer locations, such as the infundibulum, hypothalamus (without optic chiasm) and spinal cord. In the brain stem, they tend to occupy the dorsal regions and pontomedullary junction, often with exophytic growth, in contrast to diffusely infiltrating fibrillary astrocytomas, which typically develop in the ventral pons.[59] Some hypothalamic-chiasmatic lesions of infancy appear to be associated with leptomeningeal seeding and a poor outcome,[183] but it is unclear whether such tumours constitute a distinct entity because this region predisposes to the more aggressive pilomyxoid variants.[239] Pilocytic astrocytomas may occur simultaneously or subsequently at different CNS sites, usually in the setting of NF1.

Clinical Features

In cerebellar astrocytomas, symptoms and signs of increased intracranial pressure (headache and papilloedema) prevail, together with ataxia, nausea and cranial nerve deficit. In optic gliomas, reduced visual acuity and visual field defects are most common. Hypothalamic involvement is typically associated with endocrine syndromes (e.g. diabetes insipidus, precocious puberty), electrolyte imbalance and autonomic dysregulation (e.g. hyperthermia). Astrocytomas of the brain stem typically cause cranial nerve deficits, whereas supratentorial tumours usually manifest with seizures or raised intracranial pressure.

Neuroimaging

CT scans usually reveal cystic, round to oval lesions with isodense to slightly hypodense signal, which enhance with contrast media. On MR imaging, tumours appear hypointense or isointense on T1- and hyperintense on T2-weighted images. The presence of a mural tumour nodule within a macroscopic cyst (Figure 27.11a) is particularly characteristic for cerebellar and supratentorial hemispheric tumours. Optic nerve tumours appear as fusiform enlargements (Figure 27.11b), whereas a more globular contour is often encountered in chiasmatic examples. Brain stem astrocytomas are usually dorsal and exophytic. Spinal lesions appear as fusiform intramedullary thickenings as a result of a longitudinal extension over several segments ('pencil-shaped glioma'). Positron-emission tomography scans show a high rate of glucose utilization. MRS shows elevated choline and lactate peaks, with low NAA levels. These findings can be misleading because they are more typical of a high-grade neoplasms overall.

Macroscopic Appearances

In the cerebellum, pilocytic astrocytoma is well delineated and appears to expand rather than infiltrate adjacent brain structures. At other sites, the border with adjacent structures is less defined. The cut surface is greyish-pink and often shows mucoid degeneration, leading to the formation of cysts, a hallmark present in more than 80 per cent of cerebellar astrocytomas.[97] In large cysts, the main tumour mass typically forms a mural nodule. The consistency is firm, unless there is extensive mucoid degeneration.

Microscopy

The histopathology of pilocytic astrocytomas varies considerably and the diagnosis is occasionally challenging. Typical, particularly of cerebellar lesions, is a biphasic pattern with compact highly fibrillated areas intermingled with loosely structured, micro-cystic tumour that displays a mucinous background (Figure 27.11c,d). In many instances, cells within the microcystic regions will be composed of cells that resemble oligodendroglioma, with round regular nuclei and perinuclear haloes. Although a biphasic pattern is classic, in some pilocytic astrocytomas one pattern will predominate. Those in the optic nerve typically have an exclusively more compact pattern, with abundant Rosenthal fibres. Furthermore, in the optic nerve, the connective tissue septa remain largely intact, but the fascicles are enlarged with nerve fibres being progressively replaced by tumour cells. Extension into the

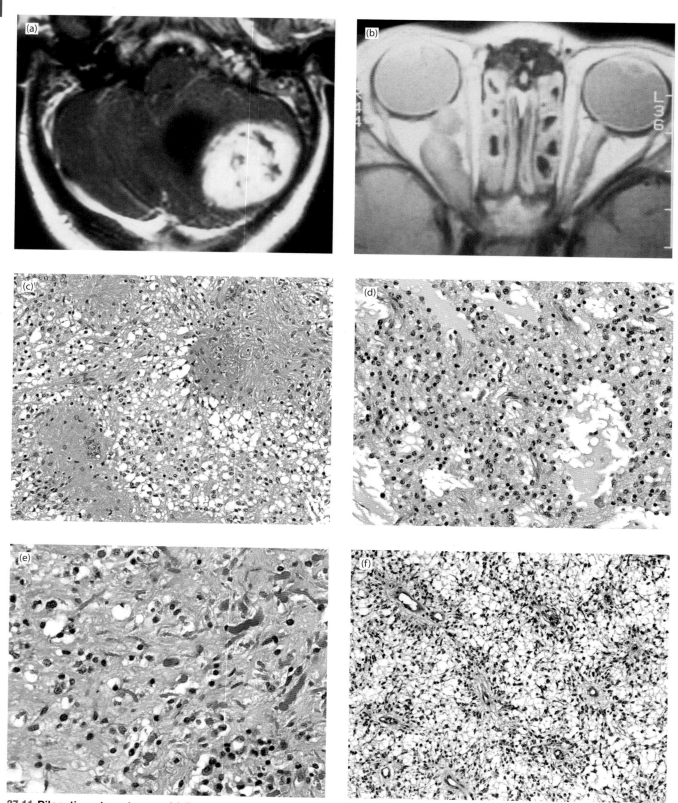

27.11 Pilocytic astrocytomas. (a) Post-contrast T1-weighted magnetic resonance (MR) image showing characteristic enhancing mass associated with a cyst. **(b)** T2-weighted MR image of a pilocytic astrocytoma ('optic glioma') diffusely expanding the optic nerve. **(c)** Biphasic pattern with compact fibrillar and looser, microcystic areas. **(d)** Oligodendroglioma-like cells and microcysts are often seen in pilocytic astrocytoma. **(e)** Rosenthal fibres mainly involve compact regions. **(f)** Pilomyxoid astrocytoma contains cells with an angiocentric orientation and a myxoid background.

meninges further contributes to the marked, fusiform enlargement of the optic nerve.

As its name suggests, the prevailing cell type in the pilocytic astrocytoma is elongated, unipolar or bipolar, with thin hair-like (Greek *pilos*, hair) processes packed with intermediate filaments, which often form parallel or interdigitating bundles. Although the pilocytic astrocytoma does not have a high cell density, the tumour cell processes produce a coarsely fibrillated, dense matrix. Piloid cells are strongly immunoreactive for GFAP. Focal mucoid degeneration is typical and associated with marked changes in morphology; cells become round or stellate, with or without discernible processes and lack GFAP gene expression, thus mimicking protoplasmic astrocytes or oligodendrocytes. This change is usually accompanied by micro-cyst formation.

Highly characteristic of pilocytic astrocytomas are Rosenthal fibres and eosinophilic granular bodies. Rosenthal fibres are bright eosinophilic bodies, with a shape resembling a sausage, corkscrew or carrot (Figure 27.11e). Their presence is mostly restricted to compact areas and are generally rare in cases with extensive mucoid change. The number of Rosenthal fibres varies considerably, but in their absence a lesion should be diagnosed as pilocytic astrocytoma with caution. The expression of GFAP in Rosenthal fibres may be strong, intermediate or absent, and often confined to the periphery. More specific is the presence of αB-crystallin.[242]

Eosinophilic granular bodies are cytoplasmic inclusions that are also highly characteristic, although not specific for pilocytic astrocytoma. They appear as multiple 'granular' bright eosinophilic deposits that may share with Rosenthal fibres, immunoreactivity for GFAP and αB-crystallin.[158] Their presence is most frequent in loose, micro-cystic areas.

Pilocytic astrocytomas may display histological features that raise the spectre of malignancy, although they almost never assume a malignant character clinically. There may be a remarkable degree of nuclear pleomorphism and multinucleated giant cells may occur. Although mitoses are absent or rare and MIB-1 indices are generally less than 1 per cent, occasional pilocytic astrocytomas show increased proliferative activity, some of which often reflects inflammatory infiltrates.[63] Microvascular proliferation may be extensive and often resembles glomerular tufts, although the more commonly found blood vessels are small and have thick, hyalinized walls. They are particularly prominent along the wall of tumour cysts and may occasionally resemble vascular malformations. As in malignant gliomas, their growth is due to secretion by neoplastic astrocytes of VEGF.[129] Finally, necrosis may occur, but usually has an infarcted appearance and does not feature pseudo-palisading.

Pilocytic astrocytomas have a tendency to invade the leptomeninges, particularly in optic gliomas and in patients with NF1. Neoplastic invasion of the meninges results from the extension of delicate cellular bridges from the cerebellar cortex through the pia mater into the subarachnoid space. Focal desmoplasia may form broad fibrocollagenous septa, but has also been observed in sulci adjacent to the tumour border.[97] Meningeal invasion is not considered an aggressive feature and has been associated with improved survival in some studies. Seeding via CSF is uncommon.

Grading

Pilocytic astrocytomas correspond to WHO grade I.[36] The rare malignant (anaplastic) pilocytic astrocytoma accounts for less than 2 per cent of all cases and has a biological behaviour similar to that of grade II or grade III astrocytomas.[206]

Differential Diagnosis

The histological diagnosis of pilocytic astrocytoma can be challenging on occasion. The differential diagnosis with diffuse astrocytomas is most important, particularly in the brain stem and other sites affected by both astrocytoma types.[59] Helpful in this distinction, particularly in small biopsies, is the use of neurofilament immunohistochemistry to highlight the axons of infiltrated neuropil. Axons are usually conspicuous in the background of diffuse astrocytic tumours, but absent or scant in pilocytic astrocytomas, except at the edges of some pilocytic lesions. Any slow-growing lesion in the CNS, particularly in the brain stem and spinal cord, may produce Rosenthal fibres and thus mimic a pilocytic astrocytoma. This can be most misleading around a cystic cerebellar haemangioblastoma or around a suprasellar/third ventricular tumour, such as a craniopharyngioma; further searching for diagnostic features is therefore critical. Gangliogliomas may also include a pilocytic component; identification of neoplastic ganglion cells ensures a correct diagnosis. The dysembryoplastic neuroepithelial tumour (DNT) may be difficult to delineate from the pilocytic astrocytoma of the temporal lobe. The multinodularity of the DNT, its preferred cortical location and the presence of a specific glioneuronal elements make it a distinct lesion, even if some areas resemble pilocytic differentiation. Immunoreactivity for mutant IDH1 is helpful in distinguishing diffuse astrocytomas, because pilocytic astrocytomas will be negative, although lack of staining does not exclude the former, particularly in children where the majority are negative. In the appropriate clinical and radiological setting, alterations in *BRAF*, particularly *BRAF* gene fusion/duplication, favours the diagnosis of pilocytic astrocytoma.

Histogenesis

The cellular origin of pilocytic astrocytoma has remained enigmatic. It seems likely that they arise from a progenitor-like cell, via acquisition of specific genetic changes, particularly involving the *BRAF* and *NF1* genes. In addition, the developmental transcription factor OLIG2, which is restricted to oligodendrocyte and spinal motor neuron formation during embryogenesis, is widely expressed in non-ependymal gliomas, including pilocytic astrocytomas.[136]

Molecular Genetics

Cytogenetic analyses of pilocytic astrocytomas have revealed either a normal karyotype or a variety of aberrations without a distinct pattern suggesting the loss of a particular tumour suppressor gene.[146] Gains of chromosomes 5, 7 and 8 are the most frequent finding.[262] Conventional CGH has shown a variety of changes, although none are either frequent or consistent.[212,235]

In contrast, more recent array CGH studies have identified a low-level copy number gain of the *BRAF* gene on 7q34 in a large proportion of cerebellar pilocytic astrocytomas.[146,187] *BRAF* is a proto-oncogene within the MAPK/ERK signalling pathway and is a regulator of cellular differentiation, proliferation and migration. The *BRAF* copy gain is due to a tandem duplication producing a KIAA1549:BRAF fusion protein with loss of its Ras-binding domain and constitutive BRAF activity.

BRAF fusions are present in 70 per cent of all pilocytic astrocytomas, but are rare in high-grade paediatric gliomas. These fusions are found in approximately 75 per cent of cerebellar, but only 55 per cent of non-cerebellar pilocytic astrocytomas.[93] The frequency of BRAF-KIAA1549 fusions also appears to vary with patient age, decreasing in frequency with increasing age. Approximately 50 per cent of pilomyxoid astrocytomas contain *BRAF* fusions.

The constitutively active V600E point mutation of *BRAF* is present in about 10 per cent of pilocytic astrocytomas, but is much less frequent in cerebellar tumours.[216] The V600E is more common in other low-grade tumours in the differential, including 25 per cent of gangliogliomas and 80 per cent of pleomorphic xanthoastrocytomas. Thus, over 75 per cent of sporadic PAs have some sort of *BRAF* alteration. Less than 10 per cent of *NF1*-associated PAs contain a *BRAF* fusion or mutation, because *NF1* loss similarly leads to activation of the MAPK/ERK signalling pathway.

Those gliomas of childhood that have *BRAF* fusion events usually behave as a typical grade I pilocytic astrocytomas, whereas those without *BRAF* fusion are more likely to behave in a more aggressive fashion. Detection of *BRAF* fusion is feasible via several strategies, including reverse transcriptase polymerase chain reaction (PCR) analysis and FISH.

Approximately 15 per cent of patients with NF1 develop pilocytic astrocytomas,[130] particularly of the optic nerve, and up to one-third of patients with a pilocytic astrocytoma in this location fulfil the diagnostic criteria of NF1. Occasionally, sporadic pilocytic astrocytomas show a loss of chromosome 17q, including the region encoding the *NF1* gene.[250] Because the *NF1* gene has tumour suppressor functions, loss of neurofibromin expression likely plays a tumorigenic role. However, screening of *NF1* coding sequences, including the critical GRD region, has failed to detect mutations in sporadic cases.[191] Immunohistochemically, neurofibromin is overexpressed,[191] but a study of eight pilocytic astrocytomas from six patients with NF1 showed loss of neurofibromin expression, with *NF1* loss in two of four studied tumours.[71] These results raise the possibility that the role of the *NF1* gene may be different in NF1 associated versus sporadic pilocytic astrocytomas.

Inactivation of the *TP53* gene does not seem to play a role in pilocytic astrocytoma.[126] Increased levels of the p53 protein may be found in pilocytic astrocytomas without *TP53* mutations.[126] Other alterations commonly involved in diffuse astrocytomas are also not frequently found in pilocytic astrocytomas. For example, a study of the *CDNK2A*, *TP53*, *CDK4* and *PTEN* genes in 29 pilocytic astrocytomas showed only one *TP53* mutation and one *PTEN* mutation.[40] However, activation of the PI3-kinase/

Akt pathway has been associated with aggressive clinical behaviour in pilocytic astrocytomas.[207]

Prognosis and Treatment

In contrast to diffusely infiltrating astrocytomas, pilocytic astrocytomas do not have an intrinsic tendency to undergo malignant progression. Even after many years, recurrences usually display histopathological features similar to those of the primary lesion, without aggressive behaviour. Observed survival rates have been 100 per cent at 5 years and 95.8 per cent at 10 years after diagnosis.[32] Nevertheless, exceptional cases of malignant recurrence from benign pilocytic astrocytoma have been reported.[98]

Occasionally, neuroradiological examination reveals multiple lesions (multicentric pilocytic astrocytoma). If association with NF1 is ruled out, metastatic spread via the CSF is the most likely cause. In the majority of cases reported, primary tumours were located in the hypothalamus and patients had undergone neurosurgical intervention followed by radiotherapy, chemotherapy or both.[145,148] Meningeal spread may be associated with malignant progression, but it has also been observed in tumours with benign morphology.[145,169,192]

Pilocytic astrocytomas are considered most benign of the gliomas, with recurrence-free intervals of up to more than 20 years.[60] Complete surgical resection is most effective but often impossible to achieve, particularly in midline structures, e.g. the optic chiasm, the hypothalamus and the brain stem. Radiotherapy may be carried out, particularly in the setting of subtotally resected but symptomatic tumours. Given adverse sequelae from radiation to the developing brain, however, chemotherapy has been advocated, particularly for progressing, surgically unresectable lesions.

The recurrence-free survival of patients with pilocytic astrocytoma largely depends on whether or not complete surgical resection is possible. Histopathological criteria that allow a prediction of the clinical outcome have not been identified.[63] Even in the rare cases of late malignant recurrence, the initial biopsy did not contain features indicative of incipient malignant transformation.[241]

Variants of Pilocytic Astrocytoma

The pilomyxoid astrocytoma (PMA), WHO grade II is typically a tumour of infancy[239] and is considered a variant of pilocytic astrocytoma, with characteristic clinical, neuroimaging and pathologic features. PMAs most often arise in hypothalamic region, with symptoms referable to that site, including failure to thrive, developmental delay, vomiting and feeding difficulties. In older children, headaches, nausea and visual symptoms are more common.[117] By MR imaging, they are well circumscribed, generally solid and homogeneously contrast-enhancing midline masses, mostly in the suprasellar and hypothalamic region.

The histologic appearance of PMA is dominated by a hypercellular, monomorphous population of piloid cells that are typically embedded within a rich myxoid matrix and often display an angiocentric arrangement (Figure 27.11f). It has a compact architecture, with only a slight tendency for peripheral infiltration of adjacent brain. Individual tumour cells have elongate fibrillar processes, are moderate in size, and contain hyperchromatic nuclei with only modest nuclear pleomorphism. The mitotic index is typically low. The diagnosis of PMA is made only when this tissue pattern is predominant, because focal myxoid or angiocentric cell arrangement may be noted in typical pilocytic or infiltrating astrocytomas. Unlike ordinary pilocytic astrocytomas, PMA typically lack a biphasic appearance, do not contain Rosenthal fibres, and only exceptionally contain eosinophilic granular bodies.

Immunohistochemically, PMAs label strongly and diffusely for GFAP and vimentin but are typically negative for the neuronal markers neurofilament and chromogranin. Synaptophysin immunoreactivity has been reported in a subset of PMAs, especially in a perivascular distribution.[62] The MIB-1 labelling index is often around 5 per cent. The relation of PMA to pilocytic astrocytoma is still debated. Reports of hybrid tumours that contain components of both conventional pilocytic astrocytoma and PMA, as well as 'maturation' of the latter into the former on recurrence, suggest that the two tumours are related and form a spectrum. This concept is reflected in the new WHO classification, with PMA categorized as a variant of pilocytic astrocytoma. Nevertheless, PMAs are associated with a more aggressive clinical course, resulting in a WHO grade II designation.[41,58,117]

Anaplastic pilocytic astrocytoma refers to the rare examples that have undergone malignant transformation. In one systematic review of over 2000 pilocytic astrocytomas, 1.7 per cent were found to have anaplastic features, which included mitotic figures >4 per 10 HPF, moderate to severe nuclear atypia, hypercellularity or necrosis.[206] Nearly a quarter of these arose in the setting of NF1 and 12 per cent arose following radiation therapy. Median overall and progression-free survivals after diagnosis for the entire study group were 24 and 14 months.

Importantly, several histopathological features indicative of progression to anaplasia in diffuse astrocytomas are not associated with malignancy in the pilocytic astrocytoma, e.g. nuclear polymorphism, vascular proliferation and invasion of the meninges. The diagnosis of anaplastic (pilocytic) astrocytoma requires overt anaplasia with significant proliferative activity. Foci of necrosis are often present but not diagnostic in the absence of mitoses.[241]

PLEOMORPHIC XANTHOASTROCYTOMAS

Pleomorphic xanthoastrocytoma (PXA) is a rare, superficially located neuroepithelial neoplasm characterized by pleomorphic and lipidized cells, typically with a rich reticulin network.

Incidence, Age and Sex

The PXA accounts for less than 1 per cent of astrocytic tumours.[64,112] Without obvious predilection for either sex, these tumours typically manifest in children and young adults with a longstanding history of seizures. Two-thirds of patients are under the age of 20 years. Cases have been noted in the setting of NF1, including those with malignant features.[161,210]

Sites

The vast majority of tumours arise in superficial supratentorial locations, with extensive involvement of overlying subarachnoid space and a proclivity for the temporal lobe. Dural involvement is, however, exceptional.[111,112] Neoplasms with the typical histopathological features of PXAs occasionally develop in other locations, including cerebellum[137] and spinal cord;[87] their biological behaviour potentially differing from supratentorial tumours.

Neuroimaging

Neuroimaging typically demonstrates a cerebral cortical neoplasm with deep extension to the grey-white junction and superficial extension to the leptomeningeal surface. Both CT and MR images usually show clearly demarcated borders, cyst formation with proteinaceous contents and a mural nodule with strong contrast enhancement (Figure 27.12a). The tumour mass is often isointense to grey matter on T1-weighted and mildly hyperintense on T2-weighted MR imaging. Leptomeningeal contrast enhancement is seen occasionally.

Macroscopic Appearances

PXA commonly have solid and cystic components. The cysts may be conspicuous, containing large amounts of dark golden, somewhat xanthochromic, serous fluid. The mural nodule has variable appearance, with a predominant yellow-orange hue that may be punctuated by focal haemorrhage. The tumours are usually firmer than the adjacent brain.

Microscopy

The striking histopathological features are multinucleated, occasionally lipidized giant cells with bizarre, often hyperchromatic nuclei. In addition, there are small, round, polygonal and fusiform cells, often arranged in fascicular patterns (Figure 27.12b). As the name of the lesion suggests, cytological diversity is the rule. The astroglial nature is shown by GFAP immunoreactivity in plump polygonal cells without processes, and in the more fusiform cells arranged in interlacing bundles (Figure 27.12c). Cytoplasmic lipidization, especially in the large cells, may be prominent but is usually a minor feature and may be absent in some. Of particular importance is the presence of eosinophilic granular bodies, which are often numerous and an important clue to the diagnosis. Mitoses are infrequent. Perivascular lymphocytic infiltration is common. A reticulin-positive stroma is a hallmark of PXA, but is not universal. When present, it is most prominent in tumour involving the subarachnoid space. Reticulin deposition may delineate fascicles of cells or may envelop single tumour cells. Ultrastructural studies have demonstrated a basal lamina separating cells.[113,261]

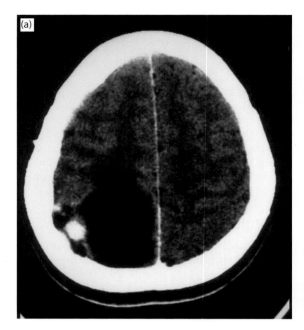

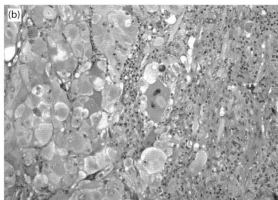

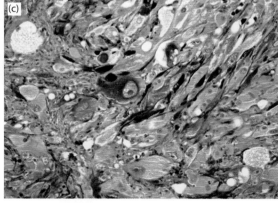

27.12 Pleomorphic xanthoastrocytoma. (a) Contrast-enhanced computed tomography (CT) scan showing superficial large cyst with an enhancing mural nodule. **(b)** Large, markedly pleomorphic cells with some lipidization; note also smaller cells and scattered lymphocytes. **(c)** Variable immunoreactivity for GFAP.

Although PXA appear well demarcated macroscopically, portions of the tumour invade the adjacent brain and perivascular spaces. The involvement of the superficial Virchow–Robin spaces may be striking in otherwise usual tumours. Several cases without a prominent reticulin stroma, but otherwise typical features, have also been described.[111]

Evidence of neuronal differentiation may be found in otherwise typical PXA, although as opposed to ganglioglioma, synaptophysin or neurofilament positive cells often do not resemble ganglion cells. A study of 40 cases found immunopositivity for GFAP and S-100 protein in 100 per cent of cases, class III beta-tubulin in 73 per cent, synaptophysin in 38 per cent, and neurofilaments and MAP2 in 8 per cent, but no staining for chromogranin A.[66] Another report documented staining for neuronal markers (class III beta-tubulin, neuronal nuclear antigen, neurofilament protein, synaptophysin) at least focally in all nine tumours studied.[147] Ultrastructural analyses have also demonstrated neuronal features in 20 per cent of tumours, including dense-core granules, microtubules and clear vesicles.[90] Cases have also been reported in which PXA constitutes the glial component of a ganglioglioma or forms a combined collision-type tumour[66,137] and tumours, particularly of the temporal lobe, have been observed in association with cortical dysplasia[99,124] or arising in the setting of a prior cortical malformation.[195] Thus, although the tumour is designated as an 'astrocytoma', neuronal differentiation is common.

Grading

Pleomorphic xanthoastrocytomas are designated WHO grade II. For lesions with significant mitotic activity (>5 mitoses per 10 high-power fields), areas of necrosis, or both, the designation 'pleomorphic xanthoastrocytoma with anaplastic features' has been proposed,[64] but this variant has not yet been designated a particular grade.[143]

Differential Diagnosis

The main differential diagnosis for PXA is that of malignant astrocytic tumours, such as giant cell glioblastoma. Most helpful in this setting is the presence of eosinophilic granular bodies, because these are rare in glioblastomas. Features such as reticulin deposition, xanthomatous change, relatively sharp borders and inflammation are not definitive, because other gliomas may occasionally show these findings. Documentation of neuronal differentiation may favour a diagnosis of PXA, but this is similarly not definitive, because more malignant gliomas are also showing positivity for neuronal markers on immunohistochemistry.

Histogenesis

PXAs were originally suggested to arise from subpial astrocytes, because such cells elaborate basal lamina and would explain the superficial localization. The demonstration of neuronal differentiation in some PXA suggests a more complex histogenesis.[66,147,193] Moreover, the reported association with cortical dysplasia[99,124,195] suggests a link to developmental dysregulation. It seems likely that PXA are derived from a cell of origin that is cortical and that has bipotential differentiation capability.

Cytogenetics and Molecular Genetics

Complex karyotypes have been documented, with gains on chromosomes 3 and 7,[213] as well as alterations of chromosome 1q.[133,214]

The activating *BRAF* mutation V600E has been documented in 60–70 per cent of PXA.[48,216] However, the *BRAF* fusion that is typical of pilocytic astrocytomas is not seen in PXA.[54] *IDH1* and *IDH2* mutations are also not typical.[54,264]

In two studies of a total of 14 PXAs, three tumours contained a *TP53* missense mutation.[157,179] In a larger series of 55 PXAs studied, two thirds of tumours were p53 immunonegative, and only a single *TP53* mutation was detected.[65] Another large series of 62 PXAs had only three tumours with *TP53* mutation, and no tumours with homozygous *CDKN2A* deletion or amplifications of *CDK4*, *MDM2* or *EGFR*.[110] Although there are no definite tumorigenic associations with the *NF1* gene, cases of PXA have been reported in NF1 patients.[161,210]

Prognosis

A recent analysis of the Surveillance, Epidemiology, and End Results (SEER) database demonstrated 5- and 10-year overall survival rates of 75 and 67 per cent, respectively.[184] On multivariate analysis, male gender and increasing age were associated with worse overall survival.

The average interval to recurrence appears to be longer in cases lacking histological evidence of anaplasia.[112,113,144261] However, malignant recurrence after an interval of 15 years has been documented.[113] Increased mitotic rates may be predictive of tumour recurrence,[144] but not necessarily of malignant progression. A study of 71 cases confirmed that mitotic index and extent of surgical resection appear to be the main predictors of recurrence-free survival.[82]

SUBEPENDYMAL GIANT-CELL ASTROCYTOMAS

Subependymal giant-cell astrocytomas (SEGAs) are WHO grade I neuroepithelial tumours that primarily develop within the setting of the tuberous sclerosis complex (TSC).[143] Located in the wall of the lateral ventricles, they are of uncertain histogenesis and composed of large cells having both astrocytic and neuronal features.

Incidence, Age and Sex

SEGAs typically present clinically within the first two decades of life (median age about 13 years, range 1–31 years) without any gender predilection. The incidence of TSC is approximately 1/5000, and SEGAs occur in 5 to 15 per cent of TSC patients.[259] In a large series of 345 well-documented cases of TSC,[221] histopathological examination confirmed that SEGAs were present in about 6 per cent of cases. Their true incidence is likely higher, because not all SEGAs warrant surgical intervention.

Clinical Features

Patients with SEGA typically present with symptoms of hydrocephalus or acute haemorrhage. In some cases, it may be the first manifestation, but more frequently, patients have longstanding, antecedent seizures due to disease-related cortical tubers and have other evidence of TSC.

Tumour Sites, Neuroimaging and Macroscopic Appearances

The most common location of SEGA is in the wall of the lateral ventricles near the foramen of Monro. In the more anterior portion of the ventricle, smaller nodules of discrete subependymal hamartomas situated in the caudothalamic groove often coexist with a larger tumour. Neuroimaging shows a well-delineated, heterogeneous neoplasm with mixed hypodense and isodense regions on CT and mixed signal intensities on both T1- and T2-weighted MR imaging. The heterogeneity is due partly to the nodular and multicystic architecture of the tumours, which are variably calcified and have a marked but heterogeneous vascular component. Macroscopic examination of unfixed tissue reveals firm, tan-white nodules with multiple microcysts and occasional small or massive haemorrhages (Figure 27.13a).

Microscopy, Immunohistochemistry and Electron Microscopy

SEGAs are characterized by an admixture of heterogeneous cell populations. Three major cell types are present, to varying degrees in different tumours, in a fibrillar background: small spindle-shaped or elongated cells often arranged in sweeping fascicles; intermediate-sized polygonal or 'gemistocyte-like' cells; and globoid or ganglion-like cells (Figure 27.13b). Nuclei are usually pleomorphic, round to oval, and contain finely granular chromatin with distinct, sometimes prominent, nucleoli. The spindle and polygonal cells are often randomly oriented, whereas in some areas the elongated cells appear to stream from the blood vessel walls in a manner reminiscent of ependymal pseudo-rosettes. Elongated cells commonly have broader, fibrillated cytoplasmic processes than is typical of ependymomas (Figure 27.13c). The polygonal cells may be conspicuous with eccentric nuclei and enlarged globoid cells often have eosinophilic, homogeneous cytoplasm. Giant cells, with a 'ganglion cell-like' appearance, are not uncommon and multinucleated cells can usually be found. The tumour microvasculature is often prominent, not uncommonly forming dilated channels with either thin or hyalinized walls that may bleed, either spontaneously or after surgical manipulation. Calcification may be dense (Figure 27.13d). Some SEGAs have occasional mitoses, moderate atypia, focal necrosis or vascular hyperplasia, but such features do not connote more aggressive behaviour.

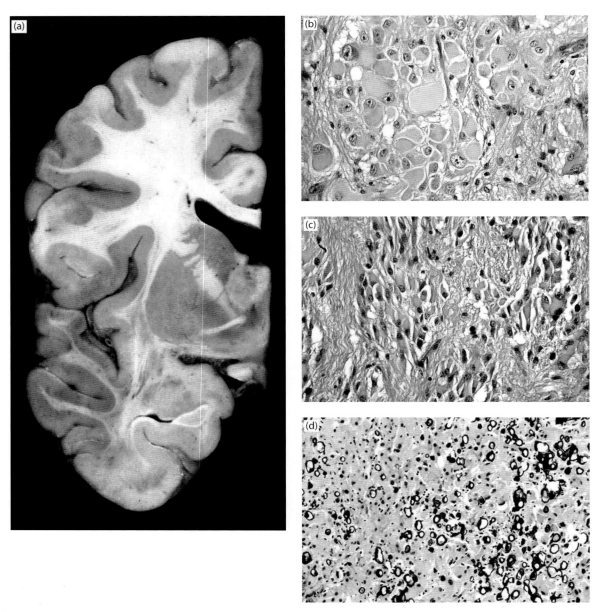

27.13 Subependymal giant-cell astrocytoma. (a) SEGA in the anterior lateral ventricle in a TSC patient; also note the cortical tubers. **(b)** Ganglioid and epithelioid cells within a fibrillar matrix. **(c)** Areas with more elongate and spindled cells intermingled among spans of dense fibrillarity. **(d)** Marked calcification.

GFAP expression is variably demonstrated in cellular processes and the cytoplasm of spindle, polygonal and ganglioid cells. S-100 protein is also typically present. A study of 20 cases showed immunoreactivity for class III β-tubulin (TUJ-1), a neuron-associated β-tubulin, in about 85 per cent of cases.[140] Staining for TUJ-1 was found in the cytoplasm of most cell types; however, it was most apparent in the polygonal and ganglion-like cells. Epitopes for the medium and high molecular weight neurofilament proteins (NF-M/H) were less readily demonstrable; nevertheless, the patterns of the various phosphorylation-dependent epitopes in the cell bodies and processes were consistent with neuronal differentiation. Other studies have documented synaptophysin and neuron-specific enolase immunoreactivity.[28] Some neoplastic cells express both glial- and neuron-associated antigens, suggesting a capacity for differentiation along glioneuronal, as well as neuroendocrine lineages.[140] Although some TSC-associated lesions react with HMB-45, a melanoma marker, SEGA do not.[72,115]

Ultrastructural features of SEGA include cytoplasmic intermediate filaments within cellular processes, multiple mitochondria, ribosomes, microtubules, Golgi and endoplasmic reticulum profiles.[28] Cells with secretory granules and rare synapse-like structures reflect neuronal differentiation.

Grading

SEGA are designated WHO grade I.[143]

Treatment and Prognosis

Symptomatic tumours are treated with resection. SEGAs are generally detected in patients with TSC who are imaged for other reasons. In this setting, depending on the size of the lesion, careful monitoring of tumour growth may be indicated rather than immediate surgery. These tumours have an almost uniformly favourable prognosis.[220] Despite the potential for late recurrence, reported as late as 22 or 47 years after initial therapy,[77,220] cases with malignant transformation have not been described, although rare cases may have drop metastases.[237]

Because the genetic alterations that lead to the development of SEGAs—mutations in either TSC1 or TSC2—are known to lead to upregulation of the mTOR pathway by neoplastic cells, clinical trials have evaluated the potential efficacy of an mTOR inhibitor, everolimus, for SEGA patients.[122] Initial experience with everolimus has been positive, with patients showing marked reduction of SEGA volume and seizure frequency, suggesting that pharmacologic therapy may be a viable alternative when complete resection is not possible.

Histogenesis

The histogenesis of SEGA is poorly understood. That these tumours are histologically identical to the subependymal nodules ('candle gutterings') that stud the ventricles in TSC patients strongly suggests that they are derived from these hamartomatous lesions.[49] In this regard, their histogenesis is most likely related to other hamartomatous lesions in TSC. SEGA demonstrate variable glial (astrocytic/ependymal), neuronal or mixed glial-neuronal differentiation on the basis of ultrastructural and immunohistochemical features.[28] Therefore, SEGA may eventually be more properly classified as a glioneuronal, rather than purely astrocytic tumour.

Molecular Genetics

SEGA is a major diagnostic criteria for TSC (see Chapter 44), an autosomal dominant disorder characterized by hamartomas and benign neoplasms of multiple organ systems.[49,67,204] There are two related genes linked to TSC:[45,190,204] TSC1 on chromosome 9q34 encodes hamartin, whereas TSC2 on chromosome 16p encodes tuberin.[45,143,190] Tuberin and hamartin interact physically within the cell cytoplasm to form a tumour suppressor complex that inhibits the function of mTOR (mammalian target of rapamycin). Loss of function of either results in upregulation of mTOR and increased proliferative activity.

Immunohistochemical and genetic analyses of SEGAs from seven patients with TSC (four with TSC1 mutations and three with TSC2 mutations) showed that tumour cells had high levels of phospho-S6K, phospho-S6 and phospho-Stat3, indicating activation of the PTEN-mTOR pathway. In addition, five of six tumours also had biallelic mutations of TSC1 or TSC2.[39] Inactivation of tuberin may also occur via phosphorylation, suggesting another possible mechanism for altering the pathway.[78] Furthermore, expression of hamartin and tuberin tend to be mutually exclusive, suggesting a need to inactivate both copies of one or other of these molecules.[57]

REFERENCES

1. Aldape KD, Ballman K, Furth A, *et al.* Immunohistochemical detection of EGFRvIII in high malignancy grade astrocytomas and evaluation of prognostic significance. *J Neuropathol Exp Neurol* 2004;63:700–707.
2. Ammirati M, Vick N, Liao YL, *et al.* Effect of the extent of surgical resection on survival and quality of life in patients with supratentorial glioblastomas and anaplastic astrocytomas. *Neurosurgery* 1987;21:201–6.
3. Appin CL, Gao J, Chisolm C, *et al.* Glioblastoma with oligodendroglioma component (GBM-O): molecular genetic and clinical characteristics. *Brain Pathol* 2013;23:454–61.
4. Arvinda HR, Kesavadas C, Sarma PS, *et al.* Glioma grading: sensitivity, specificity, positive and negative predictive values of diffusion and perfusion imaging. *J Neurooncol* 2009;94:87–96.
5. Assanah M, Lochhead R, Ogden A, *et al.* Glial progenitors in adult white matter are driven to form malignant gliomas by platelet-derived growth factor-expressing retroviruses. *J Neurosci* 2006;26:6781–90.
6. Assanah MC, Bruce JN, Suzuki SO, *et al.* PDGF stimulates the massive expansion of glial progenitors in the neonatal forebrain. *Glia* 2009;57:1835–47.

7. Bachoo RM, Maher EA, Ligon K, *et al.* Epidermal growth factor receptor and Ink4a/Arf: covergent mechanisms governing terminal differentiation and transformation along the neural stem cell to astrocyte axis. *Cancer Cell* 2002;1:269–77.
8. Backlund LM, Nilsson BR, Liu L, *et al.* Mutations in Rb1 pathway-related genes are associated with poor prognosis in anaplastic astrocytomas. *Br J Cancer* 2005;93:124–30.
9. Bai X, Zhang Y, Liu Y, *et al.* Grading of supratentorial astrocytic tumors by using the difference of ADC value. *Neuroradiology* 2011;53:533–9.
10. Barker FG 2nd, Davis RL, Chang SM, Prados MD. Necrosis as a prognostic factor in glioblastoma multiforme. *Cancer* 1996;77:1161–6.
11. Barnard RO, Geddes JF. The incidence of multifocal cerebral gliomas. A histologic study of large hemisphere sections. *Cancer* 1987;60:1519–31.
12. Batchelor TT, Betensky RA, Esposito JM, *et al.* Age-dependent prognostic effects of genetic alterations in glioblastoma. *Clin Cancer Res* 2004;10:228–33.
13. Batzdorf U, Malamud U. The problem of multicentric gliomas. *J Neurosurg* 1963;20:122–36.

14. Bellail AC, Hunter SB, Brat DJ, *et al.* Microregional extracellular matrix heterogeneity in brain modulates glioma cell invasion. *Int J Biochem Cell Biol* 2004;36:1046–69.
15. Berger MS, Deliganis AV, Dobbins J, Keles GE. The effect of extent of resection on recurrence in patients with low grade cerebral hemisphere gliomas. *Cancer* 1994;74:1784–91.
16. Biernat W, Kleihues P, Yonekawa Y, Ohgaki H. Amplification and overexpression of MDM2 in primary (de novo) glioblastomas. *J Neuropathol Exp Neurol* 1997;56:180–85.
17. Biernat W, Tohma Y, Yonekawa Y, *et al.* Alterations of cell cycle regulatory genes in primary (de novo) and secondary glioblastomas. *Acta Neuropathol (Berl)* 1997;94:303–9.
18. Boerman RH, Anderl K, Herath J, *et al.* The glial and mesenchymal elements of gliosarcomas share similar genetic alterations. *J Neuropathol Exp Neurol* 1996;55:973–81.
19. Bostrom J, Cobbers JM, Wolter M, *et al.* Mutation of the PTEN (MMAC1) tumour suppressor gene in a subset of glioblastomas but not in meningiomas with loss of chromosome arm 10q. *Cancer Res* 1998;58:29–33.

20. Brat DJ, Mapstone TB. Malignant glioma physiology: cellular response to hypoxia and its role in tumor progression. *Ann Intern Med* 2003;**138**:659–68.

21. Brat DJ, Van Meir EG. Glomeruloid microvascular proliferation orchestrated by VPF/VEGF: a new world of angiogenesis research. *Am J Pathol* 2001;**158**:789–96.

22. Brat DJ, Van Meir EG. Vaso-occlusive and prothrombotic mechanisms associated with tumor hypoxia, necrosis, and accelerated growth in glioblastoma. *Lab Invest* 2004;**84**:397–405.

23. Brat DJ, Castellano-Sanchez AA, Hunter SB, et al. Pseudopalisades in glioblastoma are hypoxic, express extracellular matrix proteases, and are formed by an actively migrating cell population. *Cancer Res* 2004;**64**:920–27.

24. Brat DJ, Seiferheld WF, Perry A, et al. Analysis of 1p, 19q, 9p, and 10q as prognostic markers for high-grade astrocytomas using fluorescence in situ hybridization on tissue microarrays from Radiation Therapy Oncology Group trials. *Neuro Oncol* 2004;**6**:96–103.

25. Brat DJ, Bellail AC, Van Meir EG. The role of interleukin-8 and its receptors in gliomagenesis and tumoral angiogenesis. *Neuro Oncol* 2005;**7**:122–33.

26. Brat DJ, Prayson RA, Ryken TC, Olson JJ. Diagnosis of malignant glioma: role of neuropathology. *J Neurooncol* 2008;**89**:287–311.

27. Brennan CW, Verhaak RG, McKenna A, et al. The somatic genomic landscape of glioblastoma. *Cell* 2013;**155**:462–77.

28. Buccoliero AM, Franchi A, Castiglione F, et al. Subependymal giant cell astrocytoma (SEGA): is it an astrocytoma? Morphological, immunohistochemical and ultrastructural study. *Neuropathology* 2009;**29**:25–30.

29. Burger PC, Green SB. Patient age, histologic features, and length of survival in patients with glioblastoma multiforme. *Cancer* 1987;**59**:1617–25.

30. Burger PC, Heinz ER, Shibata T, Kleihues P. Topographic anatomy and CT correlations in the untreated glioblastoma multiforme. *J Neurosurg* 1988;**68**:698–704.

31. Burger PC, Pearl DK, Aldape K, et al. Small cell architecture– a histological equivalent of EGFR amplification in glioblastoma multiforme? *J Neuropathol Exp Neurol* 2001;**60**:1099–104.

32. Burkhard C, Di Patre PL, Schuler D, et al. A population-based study of the incidence and survival rates in patients with pilocytic astrocytoma. *J Neurosurg* 2003;**98**:1170–74.

33. Burns KL, Ueki K, Jhung SL, et al. Molecular genetic correlates of p16, cdk4, and pRb immunohistochemistry in glioblastomas. *J Neuropathol Exp Neurol* 1998;**57**:122–30.

34. Burton EC, Lamborn KR, Feuerstein BG, et al. Genetic aberrations defined by comparative genomic hybridization distinguish long-term from typical survivors of glioblastoma. *Cancer Res* 2002;**62**:6205–10.

35. Calzolari F, Malatesta P. Recent insights into PDGF-induced gliomagenesis. *Brain Pathol* 2010;**20**:527–38.

36. Cancer Genome Atlas Research Network. Comprehensive genomic characterization defines human glioblastoma genes and core pathways. *Nature* 2008;**455**:1061–8.

37. Capper D, Weissert S, Balss J, et al. Characterization of R132H mutation-specific IDH1 antibody binding in brain tumors. *Brain Pathol* 2010;**20**:245–54.

38. Castellano-Sanchez AA, Ohgaki H, Yokoo H, et al. Granular cell astrocytomas show a high frequency of allelic loss but are not a genetically defined subset. *Brain Pathol* 2003;**13**:185–94.

39. Chan JA, Zhang H, Roberts PS, et al. Pathogenesis of tuberous sclerosis subependymal giant cell astrocytomas: biallelic inactivation of TSC1 or TSC2 leads to mTOR activation. *J Neuropathol Exp Neurol* 2004;**63**:1236–42.

40. Cheng Y, Pang JC, Ng HK, et al. Pilocytic astrocytomas do not show most of the genetic changes commonly seen in diffuse astrocytomas. *Histopathology* 2000;**37**:437–44.

41. Chikai K, Ohnishi A, Kato T, et al. Clinico-pathological features of pilomyxoid astrocytoma of the optic pathway. *Acta Neuropathol (Berl)* 2004;**108**:109–14.

42. Chung R, Whaley J, Kley N, et al. TP53 gene mutations and 17p deletions in human astrocytomas. *Genes Chromosomes Cancer* 1991;**3**:323–31.

43. Colman H, Zhang L, Sulman EP, et al. A multigene predictor of outcome in glioblastoma. *Neuro Oncol* 2010;**12**:49–57.

44. Curran WJ Jr, Scott CB, Horton J, et al. Recursive partitioning analysis of prognostic factors in three Radiation Therapy Oncology Group malignant glioma trials. *J Natl Cancer Inst* 1993;**85**:704–10.

45. Dabora SL, Jozwiak S, Franz DN, et al. Mutational analysis in a cohort of 224 tuberous sclerosis patients indicates increased severity of TSC2, compared with TSC1, disease in multiple organs. *Am J Hum Genet* 2001;**68**:64–80.

46. Dai C, Celestino JC, Okada Y, et al. PDGF autocrine stimulation dedifferentiates cultured astrocytes and induces oligodendrogliomas and oligoastrocytomas from neural progenitors and astrocytes in vivo. *Genes Dev* 2001;**15**:1913–25.

47. Daumas-Duport C, Scheithauer B, O'Fallon J, Kelly P. Grading of astrocytomas. A simple and reproducible method. *Cancer* 1988;**62**:2152–65.

48. Dias-Santagata D, Lam Q, Vernovsky K, et al. BRAF V600E mutations are common in pleomorphic xanthoastrocytoma: diagnostic and therapeutic implications. *PLoS One* 2011;**6**:e17948.

49. DiMario FJ, Jr. Brain abnormalities in tuberous sclerosis complex. *J Child Neurol* 2004;**19**:650–57.

50. Dirks PB. Brain tumor stem cells: bringing order to the chaos of brain cancer. *J Clin Oncol* 2008;**26**:2916–24.

51. Dohrmann GJ, Farwell JR, Flannery JT. Glioblastoma multiforme in children. *J Neurosurg* 1976;**44**:442–8.

52. Dolecek TA, Propp JM, Stroup NE, Kruchko C. CBTRUS statistical report: primary brain and central nervous system tumors diagnosed in the United States in 2005–2009. *Neuro Oncol* 2012;**14**(Suppl 5):v1–49.

53. Dong S, Nutt CL, Betensky RA, et al. Histology-based expression profiling yields novel prognostic markers in human glioblastoma. *J Neuropathol Exp Neurol* 2005;**64**:948–55.

54. Dougherty MJ, Santi M, Brose MS, et al. Activating mutations in BRAF characterize a spectrum of pediatric low-grade gliomas. *Neuro Oncol* 2010;**12**:621–30.

55. Du R, Lu KV, Petritsch C, et al. HIF1alpha induces the recruitment of bone marrow-derived vascular modulatory cells to regulate tumor angiogenesis and invasion. *Cancer Cell* 2008;**13**:206–20.

56. Du Plessis DG, Rutherfoord GS, Joyce KA, Walker C. Phenotypic and genotypic characterization of glioblastoma multiforme with epithelial differentiation and adenoid formations. *Clin Neuropathol* 2004;**23**:141–8.

57. Ess KC, Kamp CA, Tu BP, Gutmann DH. Developmental origin of subependymal giant cell astrocytoma in tuberous sclerosis complex. *Neurology* 2005;**64**:1446–9.

58. Fernandez C, Figarella-Branger D, Girard N, et al. Pilocytic astrocytomas in children: prognostic factors--a retrospective study of 80 cases. *Neurosurgery* 2003;**53**:544–53; discussion 554–5.

59. Fisher PG, Breiter SN, Carson BS, et al. A clinicopathologic reappraisal of brain stem tumour classification. Identification of pilocytic astrocytoma and fibrillary astrocytoma as distinct entities. *Cancer* 2000;**89**:1569–76.

60. Forsyth PA, Shaw EG, Scheithauer BW, et al. Supratentorial pilocytic astrocytomas. A clinicopathologic, prognostic, and flow cytometric study of 51 patients. *Cancer* 1993;**72**:1335–42.

61. Frederick L, Wang XY, Eley G, James CD. Diversity and frequency of epidermal growth factor receptor mutations in human glioblastomas. *Cancer Res* 2000;**60**:1383–7.

62. Fuller CE, Frankel B, Smith M, et al. Suprasellar monomorphous pilomyxoid neoplasm: an ultrastructural analysis. *Clin Neuropathol* 2001;**20**:256–62.

63. Giannini C, Scheithauer BW, Burger PC, et al. Cellular proliferation in pilocytic and diffuse astrocytomas. *J Neuropathol Exp Neurol* 1999;**58**:46–53.

64. Giannini C, Scheithauer B, Burger P, et al. Pleomorphic xanthoastrocytoma: what do we really know about it? *Cancer* 1999;**85**:2033–45.

65. Giannini C, Hebrink D, Scheithauer BW, et al. Analysis of p53 mutation and expression in pleomorphic xanthoastrocytoma. *Neurogenetics* 2001;**3**:159–62.

66. Giannini C, Scheithauer BW, Lopes MB, et al. Immunophenotype of pleomorphic xanthoastrocytoma. *Am J Surg Pathol* 2002;**26**:479–85.

67. Gomez MR. Phenotypes of the tuberous sclerosis complex with a revision of diagnostic criteria. *Ann N Y Acad Sci* 1991;**615**:1–7.

68. Gorovets D, Kannan K, Shen R, et al. IDH mutation and neuroglial developmental features define clinically distinct subclasses of lower grade diffuse astrocytic glioma. *Clin Cancer Res* 2012;**18**:2490–501.

69. Graeber TG, Osmanian C, Jacks T, et al. Hypoxia-mediated selection of cells with diminished apoptotic potential in solid tumors. *Nature* 1996;**379**:88–91.

70. Gupta M, Djalilvand A, Brat DJ. Clarifying the diffuse gliomas: an update on the morphologic features and markers that discriminate oligodendroglioma from astrocytoma. *Am J Clin Pathol* 2005;**124**:755–68.

71. Gutmann DH, Donahoe J, Brown T, *et al.* Loss of neurofibromatosis 1 (NF1) gene expression in NF1-associated pilocytic astrocytomas. *Neuropathol Appl Neurobiol* 2000;**26**:361–7.

72. Gyure KA, Prayson RA. Subependymal giant cell astrocytoma: a clinicopathologic study with HMB-45 and MIB1 immunohistochemistry. *Mod Pathol* 1997;**10**:313–17.

73. Haas-Kogan DA, Prados MD, Tihan T, *et al.* Epidermal growth factor receptor, protein kinase B/Akt, and glioma response to erlotinib. *J Natl Cancer Inst* 2005;**97**:880–87.

74. Haddad SF, Moore SA, Schelper RL, Goeken JA. Vascular smooth muscle hyperplasia underlies the formation of glomeruloid vascular structures of glioblastoma multiforme. *J Neuropathol Exp Neurol* 1992;**51**:488–92.

75. Hadjipanayis CG, Van Meir EG. Brain cancer propagating cells: biology, genetics and targeted therapies. *Trends Mol Med* 2009;**15**:519–30.

76. Hadjipanayis CG, Van Meir EG. Tumor initiating cells in malignant gliomas: biology and implications for therapy. *J Mol Med (Berl)* 2009;**87**:363–74.

77. Halmagyi GM, Bignold LP, Allsop JL. Recurrent subependymal giant-cell astrocytoma in the absence of tuberous sclerosis. *J Neurosurg* 1979;**50**:106–9.

78. Han S, Santos TM, Puga A, *et al.* Phosphorylation of tuberin as a novel mechanism for somatic inactivation of the tuberous sclerosis complex proteins in brain lesions. *Cancer Res* 2004;**64**:812–6.

79. Han SJ, Yang I, Ahn BJ, *et al.* Clinical characteristics and outcomes for a modern series of primary gliosarcoma patients. *Cancer* 2010;**116**:1358–66.

80. Han SJ, Yang I, Tihan T, *et al.* Primary gliosarcoma: key clinical and pathologic distinctions from glioblastoma with implications as a unique oncologic entity. *J Neurooncol* 2010;**96**:313–20.

81. Han SJ, Yang I, Tihan T, *et al.* Secondary gliosarcoma: a review of clinical features and pathological diagnosis. *J Neurosurg* 2010;**112**:26–32.

82. Hasselblatt M, Bohm C, Tatenhorst L, *et al.* Identification of novel diagnostic markers for choroid plexus tumors: a microarray-based approach. *Am J Surg Pathol* 2006;**30**:66–74.

83. Heaphy CM, Subhawong AP, Hong SM, *et al.* Prevalence of the alternative lengthening of telomeres telomere maintenance mechanism in human cancer subtypes. *Am J Pathol* 2011;**179**:1608–15.

84. Hegi ME, Zur HA, Ruedi D, *et al.* Hemizygous or homozygous deletion of the chromosomal region containing the p16INK4a gene is associated with amplification of the EGF receptor gene in glioblastomas. *Int J Cancer* 1997;**73**:57–63.

85. Hegi ME, Diserens AC, Gorlia T, *et al.* MGMT gene silencing and benefit from temozolomide in glioblastoma. *N Engl J Med* 2005;**352**:997–1003.

86. Henson JW, Schnitker BL, Correa KM, *et al.* The retinoblastoma gene is involved in malignant progression of astrocytomas. *Ann Neurol* 1994;**36**:714–21.

87. Herpers MJHM, Freling G, Beuls EAM. Pleomorphic xanthoastrocytoma in the spinal cord. Case report. *J Neurosurg* 1994;**80**:564–9.

88. Hilton DA, Penney M, Evans B, *et al.* Evaluation of molecular markers in low-grade diffuse astrocytomas: loss of p16 and retinoblastoma protein expression is associated with short survival. *Am J Surg Pathol* 2002;**26**:472–8.

89. Hiniker A, Hagenkord JM, Powers MP, *et al.* Gliosarcoma arising from an oligodendroglioma (oligosarcoma). *Clin Neuropathol* 2013;**32**:165–70.

90. Hirose T, Giannini C, Scheithauer BW. Ultrastructural features of pleomorphic xanthoastrocytoma: a comparative study with glioblastoma multiforme. *Ultrastruct Pathol* 2001;**25**:469–78.

91. Holash J, Maisonpierre PC, Compton D, *et al.* Vessel cooption, regression, and growth in tumors mediated by angiopoietins and VEGF. *Science* 1999;**284**:1994–8.

92. Holland EC, Celestino J, Dai C, *et al.* Combined activation of Ras and Akt in neural progenitors induces glioblastoma formation in mice. *Nat Genet* 2000;**25**:55–7.

93. Horbinski C. To BRAF or not to BRAF: is that even a question anymore? *J Neuropathol Exp Neurol* 2013;**72**:2–7.

94. Ichimura K, Schmidt EE, Yamaguchi N, *et al.* A common region of homozygous deletion in malignant human gliomas lies between the IFN alpha/omega gene cluster and the D9S171 locus. *Cancer Res* 1994;**54**:3127–30.

95. Ichimura K, Schmidt EE, Goike HM, Collins VP. Human glioblastomas with no alterations of the CDKN2 (p16INK4A, MTS1) and CDK4 genes have frequent mutations of the retinoblastoma gene. *Oncogene* 1996;**13**:1065–1072.

96. Ichimura K, Bolin MB, Goike HM, *et al.* Deregulation of the p14ARF/MDM2/p53 pathway is a prerequisite for human astrocytic gliomas with G1-S transition control gene abnormalities. *Cancer Res* 2000;**60**:417–24.

97. Ilgren EB, Stiller CA. Cerebellar astrocytomas. Part I. Macroscopic and microscopic features. *Clin Neuropathol* 1987;**6**:185–200.

98. Ilgren EB, Stiller CA. Cerebellar astrocytomas. Part II. Pathologic features indicative of malignancy. *Clin Neuropathol* 1987;**6**:201–14.

99. Im SH, Chung CK, Kim SK, *et al.* Pleomorphic xanthoastrocytoma: a developmental glioneuronal tumor with prominent glioproliferative changes. *J Neurooncol* 2004;**66**:17–27.

100. Ino Y, Silver JS, Blazejewski L, *et al.* Common regions of deletion on chromosome 22q12.3–13.1 and 22q13.2 in human astrocytomas appear related to malignancy grade. *J Neuropathol Exp Neurol* 1999;**58**:881–5.

101. Jaros E, Perry RH, Adam L, *et al.* Prognostic implications of p53 protein, epidermal growth factor receptor, and Ki-67 labelling in brain tumours. *Br J Cancer* 1992;**66**:373–85.

102. Jen J, Harper JW, Bigner SH, *et al.* Deletion of p16 and p15 genes in brain tumors. *Cancer Res* 1994;**54**:6353–8.

103. Jett K, Friedman JM. Clinical and genetic aspects of neurofibromatosis 1. *Genet Med* 2010;**12**:1–11.

104. Joseph NM, Phillips J, Dahiya S, *et al.* Diagnostic implications of IDH1-R132H and OLIG2 expression patterns in rare and challenging glioblastoma variants. *Mod Pathol* 2013;**26**:315–26.

105. Kamiryo T, Tada K, Shiraishi S, *et al.* Analysis of homozygous deletion of the p16 gene and correlation with survival in patients with glioblastoma multiforme. *J Neurosurg* 2002;**96**:815–22.

106. Kannan K, Inagaki A, Silber J, *et al.* Whole-exome sequencing identifies ATRX mutation as a key molecular determinant in lower-grade glioma. *Oncotarget* 2012;**3**:1194–203.

107. Kaplan KJ, Perry A. Gliosarcoma with primitive neuroectodermal differentiation: case report and review of the literature. *J Neurooncol* 2007;**83**:313–18.

108. Karremann M, Butenhoff S, Rausche U, *et al.* Pediatric giant cell glioblastoma: new insights into a rare tumor entity. *Neuro Oncol* 2009;**11**:323–9.

109. Kase CS, Louis DN. Case records of the Massachusetts General Hospital: 'Astrocytoma with multiple foci of glioblastoma and hemorrhage'. *N Engl J Med* 1990;**322**:1866–78.

110. Kaulich K, Blaschke B, Numann A, *et al.* Genetic alterations commonly found in diffusely infiltrating cerebral gliomas are rare or absent in pleomorphic xanthoastrocytomas. *J Neuropathol Exp Neurol* 2002;**61**:1092–9.

111. Kawano N. Pleomorphic xanthoastrocytoma (PXA) in Japan: its clinico-pathologic features and diagnostic clues. *Brain Tumour Pathol* 1991;**8**:5–10.

112. Kepes JJ, Rubinstein LJ, Eng LF. Pleomorphic xanthoastrocytoma: a distinctive meningocerebral glioma of young subjects with relatively favorable prognosis; a study of 12 cases. *Cancer* 1979;**44**:1839–52.

113. Kepes JJ, Rubinstein LJ, Ansbacher L, Schreiber DJ. Histopathological features of recurrent pleomorphic xanthoastrocytomas: further corroboration of the glial nature of this neoplasm. A study of three cases. *Acta Neuropathol (Berl)* 1989;**78**:585–93.

114. Kim DG, Yang HJ, Park IA, *et al.* Gliomatosis cerebri: clinical features, treatment, and prognosis. *Acta Neurochir (Wien)* 1998;**140**:755–62.

115. Kimura N, Watanabe M, Date F, *et al.* HMB-45 and tuberin in hamartomas associated with tuberous sclerosis. *Mod Pathol* 1997;**10**:952–9.

116. Kleihues P, zur Hausen A, Schauble B, Ohgaki H. Tumours associated with p53 germline mutations. A synopsis of 91 families. *Am J Pathol* 1997;**150**:1–13.

117. Komotar RJ, Mocco J, Carson BS, *et al.* Pilomyxoid astrocytoma: a review. *MedGenMed* 2004;**6**:42.

118. Kozak KR, Moody JS. Giant cell glioblastoma: a glioblastoma subtype with distinct epidemiology and superior prognosis. *Neuro Oncol* 2009;**11**:833–41.

119. Kozak KR, Mahadevan A, Moody JS. Adult gliosarcoma: epidemiology, natural history, and factors associated with outcome. *Neuro Oncol* 2009;**11**:183–91.

120. Kraus JA, Koopmann J, Kaskel P, *et al.* Shared allelic losses on chromosomes 1p and 19q suggest a common origin of oligodendroglioma and oligoastrocytoma. *J Neuropathol Exp Neurol* 1995;**54**:91–5.

121. Krouwer HG, Davis RL, Silver P, Prados M. Gemistocytic astrocytomas: a reappraisal. *J Neurosurg* 1991;**74**:399–406.

122. Krueger DA, Care MM, Holland K, et al. Everolimus for subependymal giant-cell astrocytomas in tuberous sclerosis. N Engl J Med 2010;363:1801–11.
123. Kunwar S, Mohapatra G, Bollen A, et al. Genetic subgroups of anaplastic astrocytomas correlate with patient age and survival. Cancer Res 2001;61:7683–8.
124. Lach B, Duggal N, DaSilva VF, et al. Association of pleomorphic xanthoastrocytoma with cortical dysplasia and neuronal tumors. A report of three cases. Cancer 1996;78:2551–63.
125. Lal A, Glazer CA, Martinson HM, et al. Mutant epidermal growth factor receptor up-regulates molecular effectors of tumor invasion. Cancer Res 2002;62:3335–9.
126. Lang FF, Miller DC, Pisharody S, et al. High frequency of p53 protein accumulation without p53 gene mutation in human juvenile pilocytic, low grade and anaplastic astrocytomas. Oncogene 1994;9:949–54.
127. Lee D, Kang SY, Suh YL, et al. Clinicopathologic and genomic features of gliosarcomas. J Neurooncol 2012;107:643–50.
128. Leibel SA, Scott CB, Loeffler JS. Contemporary approaches to the treatment of malignant gliomas with radiation therapy. Semin Oncol 1994;21:198–219.
129. Leung SY, Chan AS, Wong MP, et al. Expression of vascular endothelial growth factor and its receptors in pilocytic astrocytoma. Am J Surg Pathol 1997;21:941–50.
130. Lewis RA, Gerson LP, Axelson KA, et al. von Recklinghausen neurofibromatosis. II. Incidence of optic gliomata. Ophthalmology 1984;91:929–35.
131. Li J, Yen C, Liaw D, et al. PTEN, a putative protein tyrosine phosphatase gene mutated in human brain, breast, and prostate cancer. Science 1997;275:1943–7.
132. Li J, Wang M, Won M, et al. Validation and simplification of the Radiation Therapy Oncology Group recursive partitioning analysis classification for glioblastoma. Int J Radiat Oncol Biol Phys 2011;81:623–30.
133. Li YS, Ramsay DA, Fan YS, et al. Cytogenetic evidence that a tumour suppressor gene in the long arm of chromosome 1 contributes to glioma growth. Cancer Genet Cytogenet 1995;84:46–50.
134. Li Z, Bao S, Wu Q, et al. Hypoxia-inducible factors regulate tumorigenic capacity of glioma stem cells. Cancer Cell 2009;15:501–13.
135. Liang Y, Diehn M, Watson N, et al. Gene expression profiling reveals molecularly and clinically distinct subtypes of glioblastoma multiforme. Proc Natl Acad Sci U S A 2005;102:5814–19.
136. Ligon KL, Alberta JA, Kho AT, et al. The oligodendroglial lineage marker OLIG2 is universally expressed in diffuse gliomas. J Neuropathol Exp Neurol 2004;63:499–509.
137. Lindboe C, Cappelen J, Kepes J. Pleomorphic xanthoastrocytoma as a component of a cerebellar ganglioglioma: case report. Neurosurgery 1992;31:353–5.
138. Liu L, Ichimura K, Pettersson EH, Collins VP. Chromosome 7 rearrangements in glioblastomas; loci adjacent to EGFR are independently amplified. J Neuropathol Exp Neurol 1998;57:1138–45.

139. Liu XY, Gerges N, Korshunov A, et al. Frequent ATRX mutations and loss of expression in adult diffuse astrocytic tumors carrying IDH1/IDH2 and TP53 mutations. Acta Neuropathol 2012;124:615–25.
140. Lopes MBS, Altermatt HJ, Scheithauer BW, VandenBerg SR. Immunohistochemical characterization of subependymal giant cell astrocytomas. Acta Neuropathol (Berl) 1996;91:368–75.
141. Louis DN. Molecular pathology of malignant gliomas. Ann Rev Pathol Mech Dis 2006;1:97–117.
142. Louis DN, Holland EC, Cairncross JG. Glioma classification: a molecular reappraisal. Am J Pathol 2001;159:779–786.
143. Louis DN, Ohgaki H, Wiestler OD, Cavenee WK. WHO Classification of tumours of the central nervous system, 4th ed. Lyon: International Agency for Research, 2007.
144. Macaulay R, Jay V, Hoffman H, Becker L. Increased mitotic activity as a negative prognostic indicator in pleomorphic xanthoastrocytoma. J Neurosurg 1993;79:761–8.
145. Mamelak AN, Prados MD, Obana WG, et al. Treatment options and prognosis for multicentric juvenile pilocytic astrocytoma. J Neurosurg 1994;81:24–30.
146. Marko NF, Weil RJ. The molecular biology of WHO grade I astrocytomas. Neuro Oncol 2012;14:1424–31.
147. Martinez-Diaz H, Kleinschmidt-DeMasters BK, Powell SZ, Yachnis AT. Giant cell glioblastoma and pleomorphic xanthoastrocytoma show different immunohistochemical profiles for neuronal antigens and p53 but share reactivity for class III beta-tubulin. Arch Pathol Lab Med 2003;127:1187–91.
148. Matsumoto T, Uekusa T, Abe H, et al. Multicentric astrocytomas of the optic chiasm, brain stem and spinal cord. Acta Pathol Jpn 1989;39:664–9.
149. Meis JM, Martz KL, Nelson JS. Mixed glioblastoma multiforme and sarcoma. A clinicopathologic study of 26 radiation therapy oncology group cases. Cancer 1991;67:2342–9.
150. Mellinghoff IK, Wang MY, Vivanco I, et al. Molecular determinants of the response of glioblastomas to EGFR kinase inhibitors. N Engl J Med 2005;353:2012–24.
151. Meyer-Puttlitz B, Hayashi Y, Waha A, et al. Molecular genetic analysis of giant cell glioblastoma. Am J Pathol 1997;151:853–7.
152. Miller CR, Dunham CP, Scheithauer BW, Perry A. Significance of necrosis in grading of oligodendroglial neoplasms: a clinicopathologic and genetic study of newly diagnosed high-grade gliomas. J Clin Oncol 2006;24:5419–26.
153. Miyakawa A, Ichimura K, Schmidt EE, et al. Multiple deleted regions on the long arm of chromosome 6 in astrocytic tumours. Br J Cancer 1999;82:543–9.
154. Mizoguchi M, Nutt CL, Mohapatra G, Louis DN. Genetic alterations of phosphoinositide 3-kinase subunit genes in human glioblastomas. Brain Pathol 2004;14:372–7.
155. Montine TJ, Vandersteenhoven JJ, Aguzzi A, et al. Prognostic significance of Ki-67 proliferation index in supratentorial fibrillary astrocytic neoplasms. Neurosurgery 1994;34:674–8.
156. Mueller W, Lass U, Herms J, et al. Clonal analysis in glioblastoma with

epithelial differentiation. Brain Pathol 2001;11:39–43.
157. Munoz EL, Eberhard DA, Lopes MBS, et al. Proliferative activity and p53 mutation as prognostic indicators in pleomorphic xanthoastrocytoma. J Neuropathol Exp Neurol 1996;55:606.
158. Murayama S, Bouldin TW, Suzuki K. Immunocytochemical and ultrastructural studies of eosinophilic granular bodies in astrocytic tumors. Acta Neuropathol (Berl) 1992;83:408–14.
159. Nagaishi M, Kim YH, Mittelbronn M, et al. Amplification of the STOML3, FREM2, and LHFP genes is associated with mesenchymal differentiation in gliosarcoma. Am J Pathol 2012;180:1816–23.
160. Nagaishi M, Paulus W, Brokinkel B, et al. Transcriptional factors for epithelial-mesenchymal transition are associated with mesenchymal differentiation in gliosarcoma. Brain Pathol 2012;22:670–76.
161. Naidich MJ, Walker MT, Gottardi-Littell NR, et al. Cerebellar pleomorphic xanthoastrocytoma in a patient with neurofibromatosis type 1. Neuroradiology 2004;46:825–9.
162. Nakamura M, Yang F, Fujisawa H, et al. Loss of heterozygosity on chromosome 19 in secondary glioblastomas. J Neuropathol Exp Neurol 2000;59:539–43.
163. Nakamura M, Watanabe T, Klangby U, et al. P14ARF deletion and methylation in genetic pathways to glioblastomas. Brain Pathol 2001;11:159–68.
164. Natarajan M, Hecker TP, Gladson CL. FAK signaling in anaplastic astrocytoma and glioblastoma tumors. Cancer J 2003;9:126–33.
165. Nazzaro JM, Neuwelt EA. The role of surgery in the management of supratentorial intermediate and high-grade astrocytomas in adults. J Neurosurg 1990;73:331–44.
166. Nishizaki T, Ozaki S, Harada K, et al. Investigation of genetic alterations associated with the grade of astrocytic tumour by comparative genomic hybridization. Genes Chromosomes Cancer 1998;21:340–46.
167. Noushmehr H, Weisenberger DJ, Diefes K, et al. Identification of a CpG island methylator phenotype that defines a distinct subgroup of glioma. Cancer Cell 2010;17:510–22.
168. Nutt CL, Mani DR, Betensky RA, et al. Gene expression-based classification of malignant gliomas correlates better with survival than histological classification. Cancer Res 2003;63:1602–7.
169. Obana WG, Cogen PH, Davis RL, Edwards MS. Metastatic juvenile pilocytic astrocytoma: case report. J Neurosurg 1991;75:972–5.
170. Ohgaki H, Kleihues P. Population-based studies on incidence, survival rates, and genetic alterations in astrocytic and oligodendroglial gliomas. J Neuropathol Exp Neurol 2005;64:479–89.
171. Ohgaki H, Kleihues P. Genetic pathways to primary and secondary glioblastoma. Am J Pathol 2007;170:1445–53.
172. Ohgaki H, Kleihues P. Genetic alterations and signaling pathways in the evolution of gliomas. Cancer Sci 2009;100:2235–41.
173. Ohgaki H, Vogeley KT, Kleihues P, Wechsler W. Neu mutations and loss of

normal allele in schwannomas induced by N-ethyl-N-nitrosourea in rats. *Cancer Lett* 1993;**70**:45–50.

174. Ohgaki H, Dessen P, Jourde B, *et al.* Genetic pathways to glioblastoma: a population-based study. *Cancer Res* 2004;**64**:6892–9.

175. Okada Y, Hurwitz EE, Esposito JM, *et al.* Selection pressures of TP53 mutation and microenvironmental location influence EGFR gene amplification in human glioblastomas. *Cancer Res* 2003;**63**: 413–16.

176. Okamoto Y, Di Patre PL, Burkhard C, *et al.* Population-based study on incidence, survival rates, and genetic alterations of low-grade diffuse astrocytomas and oligodendrogliomas. *Acta Neuropathol (Berl)* 2004;**108**:49–56.

177. Parsons DW, Jones S, Zhang X, *et al.* An integrated genomic analysis of human glioblastoma multiforme. *Science* 2008;**321**:1807–12.

178. Paulus W, Bayas A, Ott G, Roggendorf W. Interphase cytogenetics of glioblastoma and gliosarcoma. *Acta Neuropathol (Berl)* 1994;**88**:420–25.

179. Paulus W, Lisle DK, Tonn JC, *et al.* Molecular genetic alterations in pleomorphic xanthoastrocytoma. *Acta Neuropathol (Berl)* 1996;**91**:293–7.

180. Penar PL, Khoshyomn S, Bhushan A, Tritton TR. Inhibition of epidermal growth factor receptor-associated tyrosine kinase blocks glioblastoma invasion of the brain. *Neurosurgery* 1997;**41**:141–51.

181. Peraud A, Watanabe K, Plate KH, *et al.* p53 Mutations versus EGF receptor expression in giant cell glioblastomas. *J Neuropathol Exp Neurol* 1997;**56**:1235–41.

182. Peraud A, Watanabe K, Schwechheimer K, *et al.* Genetic profile of the giant cell glioblastoma. *Lab Invest* 1999;**79**:123–9.

183. Perilongo G, Carollo C, Salviati L, *et al.* Diencephalic syndrome and disseminated juvenile pilocytic astrocytomas of the hypothalamic–optic chiasm region. *Cancer* 1997;**80**:142–6.

184. Perkins SM, Mitra N, Fei W, Shinohara ET. Patterns of care and outcomes of patients with pleomorphic xanthoastrocytoma: a SEER analysis. *J Neurooncol* 2012;**110**:99–104.

185. Perry A, Aldape KD, George DH, Burger PC. Small cell astrocytoma: an aggressive variant that is clinicopathologically and genetically distinct from anaplastic oligodendroglioma. *Cancer* 2004;**101**:2318–26.

186. Perry A, Miller CR, Gujrati M, *et al.* Malignant gliomas with primitive neuroectodermal tumor-like components: a clinicopathologic and genetic study of 53 cases. *Brain Pathol* 2009;**19**:81–90.

187. Pfister S, Janzarik WG, Remke M, *et al.* BRAF gene duplication constitutes a mechanism of MAPK pathway activation in low-grade astrocytomas. *J Clin Invest* 2008;**118**:1739–49.

188. Phillips HS, Kharbanda S, Chen R, *et al.* Molecular subclasses of high-grade glioma predict prognosis, delineate a pattern of disease progression, and resemble stages in neurogenesis. *Cancer Cell* 2006;**9**:157–73.

189. Phillips JJ, Aranda D, Ellison DW, *et al.* PDGFRA amplification is common in pediatric and adult high-grade astrocytomas and identifies a poor prognostic group in IDH1 mutant glioblastoma. *Brain Pathol* 2013;**23**:565–73.

190. Plank TL, Yeung RS, Henske EP. Hamartin, the product of the tuberous sclerosis 1 (TSC1) gene, interacts with tuberin and appears to be localized to cytoplasmic vesicles. *Cancer Res* 1998;**58**:4766–70.

191. Platten M, Giordano MJ, Dirven CM, *et al.* Up-regulation of specific NF 1 gene transcripts in sporadic pilocytic astrocytomas. *Am J Pathol* 1996;**149**:621–7.

192. Pollack IF, Hurtt M, Pang D, Albright AL. Dissemination of low grade intracranial astrocytomas in children. *Cancer* 1993;**73**:2869–78.

193. Powell SZ, Yachnis AT, Rorke LB, *et al.* Divergent differentiation in pleomorphic xanthoastrocytoma: evidence for a neuronal element and possible relationship to ganglion cell tumors. *Am J Surg Pathol* 1996;**20**:80–85.

194. Prayson RA, Estes ML. Protoplasmic astrocytoma. A clinicopathologic study of 16 tumors. *Am J Clin Pathol* 1995;**103**:705–9.

195. Ramelli GP, von der Weid N, Remonda L, *et al.* Pleomorphic xanthoastrocytoma derived from glioneuronal malformation in a child with intractable epilepsy. *J Child Neurol* 2000;**15**:270–72.

196. Rao JS. Molecular mechanisms of glioma invasiveness: the role of proteases. *Nat Rev Cancer* 2003;**3**:489–501.

197. Raza SM, Lang FF, Aggarwal BB, *et al.* Necrosis and glioblastoma: a friend or a foe? A review and a hypothesis. *Neurosurgery* 2002;**51**:2–12; discussion 13.

198. Reifenberger G, Liu L, Ichimura K, *et al.* Amplification and overexpression of the MDM2 gene in a subset of human malignant gliomas without p53 mutations. *Cancer Res* 1993;**53**:2736–9.

199. Reis RM, Konu-Leblebicioglu D, Lopes JM, *et al.* Genetic profile of gliosarcomas. *Am J Pathol* 2000;**156**:425–32.

200. Rich JN, Reardon DA, Peery T, *et al.* Phase II trial of gefitinib in recurrent glioblastoma. *J Clin Oncol* 2004;**22**:133–42.

201. Riemenschneider MJ, Knobbe CB, Reifenberger G. Refined mapping of 1q32 amplicons in malignant gliomas confirms MDM4 as the main amplification target. *Int J Cancer* 2003;**104**:752–7.

202. Riemenschneider MJ, Mueller W, Betensky RA, *et al.* In situ analysis of integrin and growth factor receptor signaling pathways in human glioblastomas suggests overlapping relationships with FAK activation. *Am J Pathol* 2005;**167**:1379–87.

203. Rivera AL, Pelloski CE, Gilbert MR, *et al.* MGMT promoter methylation is predictive of response to radiotherapy and prognostic in the absence of adjuvant alkylating chemotherapy for glioblastoma. *Neuro Oncol* 2010;**12**:116–21.

204. Roach ES, DiMario FJ, Kandt RS, Northrup H. Tuberous Sclerosis Consensus Conference: recommendations for diagnostic evaluation. National Tuberous Sclerosis Association. *J Child Neurol* 1999;**14**:401–7.

205. Rodriguez FJ, Scheithauer BW, Perry A, *et al.* Ependymal tumors with sarcomatous change ("ependymosarcoma"): a clinicopathologic and molecular cytogenetic study. *Am J Surg Pathol* 2008;**32**:699–709.

206. Rodriguez FJ, Scheithauer BW, Burger PC, *et al.* Anaplasia in pilocytic astrocytoma predicts aggressive behavior. *Am J Surg Pathol* 2010;**34**:147–60.

207. Rodriguez EF, Scheithauer BW, Giannini C, *et al.* PI3K/AKT pathway alterations are associated with clinically aggressive and histologically anaplastic subsets of pilocytic astrocytoma. *Acta Neuropathol* 2011;**121**:407–20.

208. Rong Y, Durden DL, Van Meir EG, Brat DJ. 'Pseudopalisading' necrosis in glioblastoma: a familiar morphologic feature that links vascular pathology, hypoxia, and angiogenesis. *J Neuropathol Exp Neurol* 2006;**65**:529–39.

209. Rong Y, Belozerov VE, Tucker-Burden C, *et al.* Epidermal growth factor receptor and PTEN modulate tissue factor expression in glioblastoma through JunD/activator protein-1 transcriptional activity. *Cancer Res* 2009;**69**:2540–49.

210. Saikali S, Le Strat A, Heckly A, *et al.* Multicentric pleomorphic xanthoastrocytoma in a patient with neurofibromatosis type 1: case report and review of the literature. *J Neurosurg* 2005;**102**:376–81.

211. Sanai N, Polley MY, McDermott MW, *et al.* An extent of resection threshold for newly diagnosed glioblastomas. *J Neurosurg* 2011;**115**:3–8.

212. Sanoudou D, Tingby O, Ferguson-Smith MA, *et al.* Analysis of pilocytic astrocytoma by comparative genomic hybridization. *Br J Cancer* 2000;**82**:1218–22.

213. Sawyer JR, Roloson GJ, Chadduck WM, *et al.* Cytogenetic findings in a pleomorphic xanthoastrocytoma. *Cancer Genet Cytogenet* 1991;**55**: 225–30.

214. Sawyer JR, Thomas EL, Roloson GJ, *et al.* Telomeric associations evolving to ring chromosomes in a recurrent pleomorphic xanthoastrocytoma. *Cancer Genet Cytogenet* 1992;**60**:152–7.

215. Scherer HJ. Cerebral astrocytomas and their derivatives. *Am J Cancer* 1940;**40**:159–98.

216. Schindler G, Capper D, Meyer J, *et al.* Analysis of BRAF V600E mutation in 1,320 nervous system tumors reveals high mutation frequencies in pleomorphic xanthoastrocytoma, ganglioglioma and extra-cerebellar pilocytic astrocytoma. *Acta Neuropathol* 2011;**121**:397–405.

217. Schmidt MD, Antweller S, Urban N, *et al.* Impact of genotype and morphology on the prognosis of glioblastoma. *J Neuropathol Exp Neurol* 2002;**61**:321–8.

218. Schrock E, Blume C, Meffert MC, *et al.* Recurrent gain of chromosome arm 7q in low-grade astrocytic tumors studied by comparative genomic hybridization. *Genes Chromosomes Cancer* 1996;**15**:199–205.

219. Schwartzentruber J, Korshunov A, Liu XY, *et al.* Driver mutations in histone H3.3 and chromatin remodelling genes in paediatric glioblastoma. *Nature* 2012;**482**:226–31.

220. Sharma MC, Ralte AM, Gaekwad S, *et al.* Subependymal giant cell astrocytoma: a clinicopathological study of 23 cases with special emphasis on histogenesis. *Pathol Oncol Res* 2004;**10**:219–24.

221. Shepherd CW, Scheithauer BW, Gomez MR, *et al.* Subependymal giant cell astrocytoma: a clinical, pathological,

and flow cytometric study. *Neurosurgery* 1991;**28**:864–8.

222. Sidransky D, Mikkelsen T, Schwechheimer K, et al. Clonal expansion of p53 mutant cells is associated with brain tumour progression. *Nature* 1992;**355**:846–7.

223. Singh SK, Hawkins C, Clarke ID, et al. Identification of human brain tumour initiating cells. *Nature* 2004;**432**:396–401.

224. Smith JS, Perry A, Borell TJ, et al. Alterations of chromosome arms 1p and 19q as predictors of survival in oligodendrogliomas, astrocytomas, and mixed oligoastrocytomas. *J Clin Oncol* 2000;**18**:636–45.

225. Smith JS, Tachibana I, Pohl U, et al. A transcript map of the chromosome 19 q-arm tumour suppressor region. *Genomics* 2000;**64**:44–50.

226. Smith JS, Tachibana I, Passe SM, et al. PTEN mutation, EGFR amplification, and outcome in patients with anaplastic astrocytoma and glioblastoma multiforme. *J Natl Cancer Inst* 2001;**93**:1246–56.

227. Smith SF, Simpson JM, Brewer JA, et al. The presence of necrosis and/or microvascular proliferation does not influence survival of patients with anaplastic oligodendroglial tumours: review of 98 patients. *J Neurooncol* 2006;**80**:75–82.

228. Sneed PK, Prados MD, McDermott MW, et al. Large effect of age on the survival of patients with glioblastoma treated with radiotherapy and brachytherapy boost. *Neurosurgery* 1995;**36**:898–904.

229. Snuderl M, Fazlollahi L, Le LP, et al. Mosaic amplification of multiple receptor tyrosine kinase genes in glioblastoma. *Cancer Cell* 2011;**20**:810–17.

230. Steck PA, Pershouse MA, Jasser SA, et al. Identification of a candidate tumour suppressor gene, MMAC1, at chromosome 10q23.3 that is mutated in multiple advanced cancers. *Nat Genet* 1997;**15**:356–62.

231. Stupp R, Mason WP, van den Bent MJ, et al. Radiotherapy plus concomitant and adjuvant temozolomide for glioblastoma. *N Engl J Med* 2005;**352**:987–96.

232. Stupp R, Hegi ME, Mason WP, et al. Effects of radiotherapy with concomitant and adjuvant temozolomide versus radiotherapy alone on survival in glioblastoma in a randomised phase III study: 5-year analysis of the EORTC-NCIC trial. *Lancet Oncol* 2009;**10**:459–66.

233. Sturm D, Witt H, Hovestadt V, et al. Hotspot mutations in H3F3A and IDH1 define distinct epigenetic and biological subgroups of glioblastoma. *Cancer Cell* 2012;**22**:425–37.

234. Szerlip NJ, Pedraza A, Chakravarty D, et al. Intratumoral heterogeneity of receptor tyrosine kinases EGFR and PDGFRA amplification in glioblastoma defines subpopulations with distinct growth factor response. *Proc Natl Acad Sci U S A* 2012;**109**:3041–6.

235. Szymas J, Wolf G, Petersen S, et al. Comparative genomic hybridization indicates two distinct subgroups of pilocytic astrocytomas. *Neurosurg Focus* 2000;**8**:1–6.

236. Tehrani M, Friedman TM, Olson JJ, Brat DJ. Intravascular thrombosis in central nervous system malignancies: a potential role in astrocytoma progression to glioblastoma. *Brain Pathol* 2008;**18**:164–71.

237. Telfeian AE, Judkins A, Younkin D, et al. Subependymal giant cell astrocytoma with cranial and spinal metastases in a patient with tuberous sclerosis: case report. *J Neurosurg* 2004;**100**(5 Suppl):498–500.

238. Teo JG, Gultekin SH, Bilsky M, et al. A distinctive glioneuronal tumor of the adult cerebrum with neuropil-like (including "rosetted") islands: report of 4 cases. *Am J Surg Pathol* 1999;**23**:502–10.

239. Tihan T, Fisher PG, Kepner JL, et al. Pediatric astrocytomas with monomorphous pilomyxoid features and a less favorable outcome. *J Neuropathol Exp Neurol* 1999;**58**:1061–8.

240. Tohma Y, Gratas C, Biernat W, et al. PTEN (MMAC1) mutations are frequent in primary glioblastomas (de novo) but not in secondary glioblastomas. *J Neuropathol Exp Neurol* 1998;**57**:684–9.

241. Tomlinson FH, Scheithauer BW, Hayostek CJ, et al. The significance of atypia and histologic malignancy in pilocytic astrocytoma of the cerebellum: a clinicopathologic and flow cytometric study. *J Child Neurol* 1994;**9**:301–10.

242. Tomokane N, Iwaki T, Tateishi J, et al. Rosenthal fibers share epitopes with alpha B-crystallin, glial fibrillary acidic protein, and ubiquitin, but not with vimentin: immunoelectron microscopy with colloidal gold. *Am J Pathol* 1991;**138**:875–85.

243. Turcan S, Rohle D, Goenka A, et al. IDH1 mutation is sufficient to establish the glioma hypermethylator phenotype. *Nature* 2012;**483**:479–83.

244. Ueki K, Rubio MP, Ramesh V, et al. MTS1/CDKN2 gene mutations are rare in primary human astrocytomas with allelic loss of chromosome 9p. *Hum Mol Genet* 1994;**3**:1841–5.

245. Ueki K, Ono Y, Henson JW, et al. CDKN2/p16 or RB alterations occur in the majority of glioblastomas and are inversely correlated. *Cancer Res* 1996;**56**:150–53.

246. Uhm JH, Gladson CL, Rao JS. The role of integrins in the malignant phenotype of gliomas. *Front Biosci* 1999;**4**:D188–99.

247. van den Bent MJ, Carpentier AF, Brandes AA, et al. Adjuvant procarbazine, lomustine, and vincristine improves progression-free survival but not overall survival in newly diagnosed anaplastic oligodendrogliomas and oligoastrocytomas: a randomized European Organisation for Research and Treatment of Cancer phase III trial. *J Clin Oncol* 2006;**24**:2715–22.

248. Verhaak RG, Hoadley KA, Purdom E, et al. Integrated genomic analysis identifies clinically relevant subtypes of glioblastoma characterized by abnormalities in PDGFRA, IDH1, EGFR, and NF1. *Cancer Cell* 2010;**17**:98–110.

249. Von Deimling A, Louis DN, von Ammon K, et al. Association of epidermal growth factor receptor gene amplification with loss of chromosome 10 in human glioblastoma multiforme. *J Neurosurg* 1992;**77**:295–301.

250. Von Deimling A, Louis DN, Menon AG, et al. Deletions on the long arm of chromosome 17 in pilocytic astrocytoma. *Acta Neuropathol (Berl)* 1993;**86**:81–5.

251. Von Deimling A, von Ammon K, Schoenfeld D, et al. Subsets of glioblastoma multiforme defined by molecular genetic analysis. *Brain Pathol* 1993;**3**:19–26.

252. Von Deimling A, Krone W, Menon AG. Neurofibromatosis type 1: pathology, clinical features and molecular genetics. *Brain Pathol* 1995;**5**:153–62.

253. Wang Y, Li S, Chen L, et al. Glioblastoma with an oligodendroglioma component: distinct clinical behavior, genetic alterations, and outcome. *Neuro Oncol* 2012;**14**:518–25.

254. Watanabe K, Tachibana O, Sato K, et al. Overexpression of the EGF receptor and p53 mutations are mutually exclusive in the evolution of primary and secondary glioblastomas. *Brain Pathol* 1996;**6**:217–24.

255. Watanabe K, Sato K, Biernat W, et al. Incidence and timing of p53 mutations during astrocytoma progression in patients with multiple biopsies. *Clin Cancer Res* 1997;**3**:523–50.

256. Watanabe K, Tachibana O, Yonekawa Y, et al. Role of gemistocytes in astrocytoma progression. *Lab Invest* 1997;**76**:277–84.

257. Watanabe K, Peraud A, Gratas C, et al. p53 and PTEN gene mutations in gemistocytic astrocytomas. *Acta Neuropathol (Berl)* 1998;**95**:559–64.

258. Watanabe T, Katayama Y, Komine C, et al. O6-methylguanine-DNA methyltransferase methylation and TP53 mutation in malignant astrocytomas and their relationships with clinical course. *Int J Cancer* 2005;**113**:581–7.

259. Webb DW, Osborne JP. Tuberous sclerosis. *Arch Dis Child* 1995;**72**:471–4.

260. Weiss WA, Israel M, Cobbs C, et al. Neuropathology of genetically engineered mice: consensus report and recommendations from an international forum. *Oncogene* 2002;**21**:7453–63.

261. Weldon-Linne GM, Victor TA, Groothuis DR, Vick NA. Pleomorphic xanthoastrocytoma: ultrastructural and immunohistochemical study of a case with a rapidly fatal outcome following surgery. *Cancer* 1983;**52**:2055–63.

262. White FV, Anthony DC, Yunis EJ, et al. Non random chromosomal gains in pilocytic astrocytomas of childhood. *Hum Pathol* 1995;**26**:979–86.

263. Xiao A, Wu H, Pandolfi PP, et al. Astrocyte inactivation of the pRb pathway predisposes mice to malignant astrocytoma development that is accelerated by PTEN mutation. *Cancer Cell* 2002;**1**:157–68.

264. Yan H, Parsons DW, Jin G, et al. IDH1 and IDH2 mutations in gliomas. *N Engl J Med* 2009;**360**:765–73.

265. Zagzag D, Hooper A, Friedlander DR, et al. In situ expression of angiopoietins in astrocytomas identifies angiopoietin-2 as an early marker of tumor angiogenesis. *Exp Neurol* 1999;**159**:391–400.

266. Zagzag D, Esencay M, Mendez O, et al. Hypoxia- and vascular endothelial growth factor-induced stromal cell-derived factor-1alpha/CXCR4 expression in glioblastomas: one plausible explanation of Scherer's structures. *Am J Pathol* 2008;**173**:545–60.

267. Zhou XP, Li YJ, Hoang-Xuan K, et al. Mutational analysis of the PTEN gene in gliomas: molecular and pathological correlations. *Int J Cancer* 1999;**84**:150–54.

268. Zlatescu MC, TehraniYazdi AR, Sasaki H, et al. Tumor location and growth pattern correlate with genetic signature in oligodendroglial neoplasms. *Cancer Res* 2001;**61**:6713–15.

269. Zülch K. *Brain tumours. Their biology and pathology.* Berlin: Springer, 1986.

Oligodendroglial Tumours

Guido Reifenberger

OLIGODENDROGLIOMA

Oligodendroglioma is defined as a diffusely infiltrating low-grade glioma composed of neoplastic cells morphologically resembling oligodendroglia. Most oligodendrogliomas carry an *IDH1* or *IDH2* mutation combined with deletion of chromosomal arms 1p and 19q.

Incidence, Age and Sex Distribution

Oligodendroglioma accounts for approximately 2 per cent of all primary brain tumours and 6 per cent of all gliomas. For the United States of America, the overall annual incidence rate during the years 2004 to 2008 has been estimated as 0.28 per 100 000 persons.[16] The incidence rate increased over time, in particular during the late 1990s and early 2000s, which has been attributed to a less stringent use of diagnostic criteria at that time; more recently, the incidence has stabilized at the rate given earlier.[67]

Oligodendrogliomas develop at any age, but the majority arise in adults with an incidence peak in the fourth and fifth decades of life.[77] In children younger than 14 years of age, oligodendroglial tumours account for only 1.1 per cent of brain tumours.[16] Oligodendrogliomas are more common in white than in black people, with a corresponding ratio of 2.43. Males are more often affected than females (male to female ratio: 1.26).[16]

Clinical and Radiological Features

Seizures are the most common presenting symptom that is seen in approximately two thirds of the patients.[63,78] Additional clinical symptoms include headache and other signs of increased intracranial pressure, focal neurological deficits and cognitive or mental changes. In older studies, patient histories were often long-standing with intervals greater than 5 years between the first symptom and the final diagnosis being common.[75,104] Today, patient histories are usually shorter because computed tomography (CT) and magnetic resonance imaging (MRI) are widely available for diagnosis of patients with suspicious neurological signs and symptoms. On CT, oligodendrogliomas appear as hypo- or isodense, well-demarcated, frequently calcified masses most commonly located in the subcortical white matter with extension into the adjacent cortex. MRI typically reveals a T1-hypointense and T2-hyperintense lesion, which appears well-demarcated and shows little perifocal oedema (Figure 28.1). Some tumours demonstrate heterogeneity as a result of intratumoural haemorrhages and/or cystic degeneration. Gadolinium enhancement is commonly seen in anaplastic oligodendrogliomas. Contrast enhancement in low-grade tumours has been linked to less favourable prognosis.[120] Perfusion and diffusion imaging may help to distinguish low-grade oligodendrogliomas from diffuse astrocytomas of WHO grade II, because regional cerebral blood volume (rCBV) and apparent diffusion coefficient (ADC) values are frequently higher in oligodendrogliomas.[6] Positron emission tomography (PET) imaging with amino acid tracers often shows increased tumour/brain ratios in oligodendrogliomas as compared to diffuse astrocytomas.[106] Tumour/brain ratios are higher in anaplastic as compared to low-grade oligodendroglial tumours.[34]

Paediatric oligodendrogliomas less frequently show calcification, contrast enhancement and oedema, when compared to adult counterparts.[111] Oligodendrogliomas without 1p/19q deletions more often demonstrate mixed T1- and T2-weighted signal intensities.[47,68] In addition, 1p/19q deletion appears to be associated with indistinct tumour borders on T1-weighted images, paramagnetic susceptibility and calcification.[68] However, these findings were not confirmed by others.[47] Recent studies indicate that elevated levels of 2-hydroxyglutarate, the oncometabolite aberrantly produced by mutant *IDH1* and IDH2 proteins, can be readily detected by magnetic resonance spectroscopy,[18] thereby allowing for the non-invasive identification

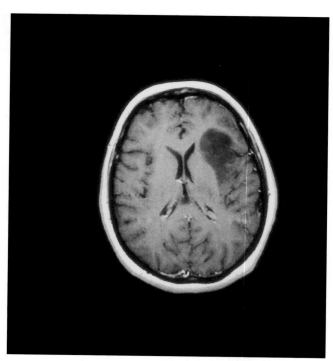

28.1 Oligodendroglioma. Low-signal, non-enhancing, well-defined lesion on axial, T1-weighted, post-gadolinium MRI.

Courtesy of Dr CC Penney, King's Healthcare NHS Trust, London, UK.

of *IDH1/2*-mutant gliomas, including the vast majority of oligodendrogliomas.

Macroscopy

Oligodendrogliomas may arise anywhere in the central nervous system but most develop in the cerebral hemispheres. The frontal lobe is involved in approximately 50–65 per cent of patients. With decreasing frequencies, oligodendrogliomas manifest in the temporal, parietal and occipital lobes. Infiltrative growth involving more than one cerebral lobe or both hemispheres is not uncommon. Oligodendrogliomas are far less frequent in the basal ganglia, thalamus, brain stem or cerebellum. Primary oligodendrogliomas of the spinal cord are rare, accounting for only 1.5 per cent of all oligodendrogliomas and 2 per cent of all spinal cord tumours.[32] Occasional patients present with primary leptomeningeal oligodendroglioma or diffuse leptomeningeal oligodendrogliomatosis, respectively. Patients with oligodendroglial gliomatosis cerebri have also been reported.[109] Moreover, rare oligodendrogliomas arising in ovarian teratomas are on record.[114]

Macroscopically, the typical oligodendroglioma appears variably well-defined, grayish-pink and soft, growing in cerebral cortex and subcortical white matter. The affected gyrus is expanded and the gray-white matter junction is blurred. Oligodendrogliomas may focally infiltrate adjacent leptomeninges, sometimes with an accompanying desmoplastic reaction leading to a more firm, rubbery consistency of the superficial component. Calcifications are frequently present and may impart a gritty texture to the tumour, with occasional densely calcified lesions demonstrating intratumoural 'stones'. Rare cases appear as very soft, gelatinous masses due to

extensive mucoid degeneration. Areas of macrocystic degeneration are not unusual. Non-therapy associated necrosis suggests anaplasia. Oligodendrogliomas are densely vascularized tumours and intratumoural haemorrhages are frequent.

Microscopy

Oligodendrogliomas are monomorphous, moderately cellular, diffusely infiltrating gliomas composed of cells with uniform, round to slightly oval nuclei and perinuclear halos on routinely formalin-fixed paraffin sections (Figure 28.2a). The nuclei are slightly larger than those of normal oligodendrocytes, with a chromatin pattern that is less coarse with small nucleoli evident in well preserved specimens. Occasional mitotic figures are still compatible with a low-grade oligodendroglioma. The typical nuclear features are best demonstrated in tissue smears and in well-fixed, paraffin-embedded specimens. On smear preparations, oligodendroglioma cells have a small rim of cytoplasm and processes are sparse. In fixed tissue sections, cellular swelling and retraction of the delicate cytoplasmic processes produces the variable, but hallmark, perinuclear halos resulting in the characteristic 'honeycomb' or 'fried egg' appearance. However, in optimally preserved specimens, smear preparations, frozen sections and paraffin sections made from frozen tumour tissue this artefact is not present and the tumour cells have scant but distinct cytoplasm. There is a notable paucity of fibrillarity in solid regions of oligodendrogliomas, whereas the infiltrative edge incorporates background neuropil. This entrapped neuropil should not be confused with the inherent fibrillarity of astrocytic gliomas, or on immunohistochemistry, with its inherent synaptophysin positivity.

On low-power examination of tissue sections, a striking feature of most oligodendrogliomas is their cellular uniformity. In this regard, the diagnosis of oligodendroglioma should be considered in the setting of any moderately hypercellular glioma with uniform nuclei. This may be particularly useful in frozen sections, where the presence of a hypercellular glioma without much nuclear pleomorphism, spindled cells or mitoses should prompt consideration of oligodendroglioma. However, pathologists should be reluctant to make a definite diagnosis of oligodendroglioma based on intraoperative frozen sections alone.

The tumour cells are usually arranged in diffuse sheets, often conspicuously grouped by a branching capillary network. Some tumours contain rather distinct nodules that must be distinguished from those seen in dysembryoplastic neuroepithelial tumours. Nodular areas may show increased cellularity, which is not indicative of anaplasia as long as mitotic activity is low. Occasional tumours contain a spongioblastic pattern with parallel, palisaded rows of somewhat fusiform cells (Figure 28.2b), although this pattern is not specific as it may be encountered in several other tumor types. Extracellular mucin deposition and microcyst formation are prominent in some cases.

Oligodendrogliomas can show varying 'astrocytoma-like' features. For instance, tumour cells with a rim of glial fibrillary acidic protein (GFAP) positivity have been called 'gliofibrillary oligodendrocytes'.[41] Other neoplastic cells with eccentric, rounded, eosinophilic bellies of GFAP positive cytoplasm are referred to as 'minigemistocytes' or 'microgemistocytes'. Neither of these cell types necessarily

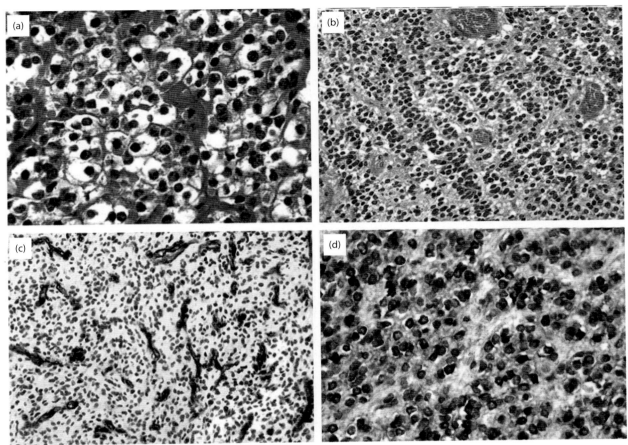

28.2 Oligodendroglioma. (a) The typical 'honeycomb' appearance: groups of cells, with regular, round nuclei and artificially swollen, empty-looking cytoplasm, bounded by distinct cell membrane. Haematoxylin and eosin (H&E). **(b)** Parallel rows of cells forming spongioblastoma-like palisades. H&E. **(c)** The delicate vascular pattern demonstrated by lectin histochemistry. *Ulex europaeus* antigen I. **(d)** Immunoreactivity for the *R132H* mutant form of *IDH1* is common.

implies a transition to oligoastrocytoma. Similarly, hypertrophic reactive astrocytes are typically scattered throughout oligodendrogliomas and should not be confused with the neoplastic astrocytes in oligoastrocytomas. Individual cases of oligodendroglioma composed predominantly of GFAP-negative signet-ring cells have been reported.[62] Rarely, eosinophilic granular cells are prominent.[19] Individual tumours, including cases with 1p/19q-deletion, demonstrate evidence of neuronal or neurocytic differentiation, i.e. contain neoplastic cells with expression of neuronal markers and formation of neurocytic rosettes.[81] Moreover, ganglioglioma-like foci have been reported in rare instances.[80]

Oligodendrogliomas have a characteristic delicate, branching, arcuate 'chicken wire' like vasculature (Figure 28.2c); when present, this pattern should prompt consideration of an oligodendroglioma, although this feature alone is not sufficiently specific. In some tumours, the capillary network subdivides the tumour tissue into smaller and larger lobules. Probably because of their dense vascularization, oligodendrogliomas have a tendency for intratumoural haemorrhages. Microvascular proliferation and necrosis are absent in low-grade oligodendroglioma.

The infiltration patterns of oligodendroglioma parallel those of other diffuse gliomas, although 'secondary structures of Scherer' tend to be more pronounced. These 'secondary

structures' include perineuronal satellitosis, perivascular aggregations and subpial spread. Oligodendrogliomas may also spread into the leptomeninges and, occasionally, grow primarily as leptomeningeal masses. Calcification is typical of oligodendroglioma, albeit not invariable. Calcification varies from minute particles to large, grossly visible 'stones', with intermediate-sized calcospherites being the most frequent. Calcospherites are irregular or spherical, sometimes lamellated calcifications. When large deposits are present, they are usually centrally localized. Minute calcifications are most common alongside or within the delicate vasculature.

Grading

Oligodendrogliomas are slowly growing neoplasms that histologically correspond to World Health Organization (WHO) grade II.[87] Various morphological features have been associated with higher malignancy and poor prognosis. These include nuclear atypia and pleomorphism, high cellularity, brisk mitotic activity, endothelial hypertrophy and microvascular proliferation, as well as necrosis. Collectively, these morphological features are similar to those commonly used for the grading of diffuse astrocytic gliomas. However, their individual impact on grading and their integration into an objective and reproducible grading system of oligodendrogliomas is less established. A study by seven independent neuropathologists identified older patient age, high cellularity, presence of mitoses, endothelial hypertrophy and proliferation, and necrosis significantly associated with shorter survival on univariate analysis in a cohort of 124 patients.[35] On multivariate analysis, however, only patient age and endothelial proliferation were independently associated with survival.

The WHO classification separates oligodendroglial tumours into well-differentiated tumours of WHO grade II and anaplastic (malignant) tumours of WHO grade III.[87,88] The value of the WHO grade as a significant predictor of survival has been confirmed in various studies.[35,63,77,100] The WHO criteria for anaplasia in oligodendroglial tumours leave some room for subjectivity because neither the impact of the various parameters, i.e. 'increased cellularity, marked cytological atypia, high mitotic activity, microvascular proliferation and necrosis', nor the number of required parameters are precisely defined. As a rule, the histological diagnosis of an anaplastic oligodendroglioma should require either the presence of conspicuous endothelial proliferation and/or high mitotic activity. In borderline cases, immunostaining for MIB–1 and attention to clinical and neuroradiological features, such as rapid symptomatic growth and contrast enhancement, may provide helpful additional information.

In addition to patient age, clinical performance score, contrast enhancement on neuroimaging and histological grading, there is increasing evidence that the expression of proliferation markers and, in particular, genetic alterations, such as *IDH1/2* mutation and 1p/19q deletion, are important prognostic factors for patients with oligodendroglial tumours, in particular when patients are treated with radio- and/or chemotherapy. Thus, modern assessment of oligodendroglioma behaviour should consider clinical and neuroimaging findings, histological grading, proliferation indices and molecular genetic characteristics.

Immunohistochemistry

Immunohistochemical studies may provide useful information for the classification and grading of oligodendroglial tumours. However, a specific and sensitive immunohistochemical marker of oligodendroglial tumours is still lacking. Nevertheless, certain immunohistochemical staining patterns may be helpful to distinguish oligodendrogliomas from most other brain tumour entities.

Differential Diagnostic Markers

Most oligodendrogliomas stain strongly and uniformly with the monoclonal antibody against the *IDH1* R132H mutant protein (Figure 28.2d), thereby distinguishing these tumours from non-neoplastic lesions and a variety of other 'clear cell neoplasms' of the central nervous system.[15] However, absence of *IDH1* R132H immunostaining does not exclude an oligodendroglioma because other, less common *IDH1* mutations as well as *IDH2* mutations are not detected by this antibody. In contrast to the majority of diffuse astrocytomas, oligodendrogliomas usually lack widespread nuclear p53 staining, a finding corresponding to the rarity of *TP53* mutations in these tumours. In fact, *TP53*

mutation and widespread nuclear p53 immunopositivity are mutually exclusive to 1p/19q deletion in gliomas.[93]

Oligodendrogliomas commonly show immunoreactivity for S–100 protein, CD57 (anti-Leu-7, HNK–1) and the microtubule-associated protein 2 (MAP2), the latter often in a characteristic perinuclear cytoplasmic immunostaining without significant process labelling.[8] Unfortunately, immunoreactivity is not restricted to oligodendrogliomas but is also found in various other neuroectodermal tumours. Similarly, expression of the oligodendrocyte lineage-associated transcription factors OLIG1 and OLIG2 is found not only in oligodendrogliomas but also in astrocytomas.[93] The transcription factor Sox10, another key determinant of oligodendroglial differentiation, is expressed in both oligodendrogliomas and astrocytic tumours.[4]

Immunohistochemical analyses for several proteins related either to myelin or to particular oligodendrocytic developmental stages have been performed on tissue sections of oligodendroglial tumours, but are generally not useful in diagnostic practice. The investigated markers include major protein components of central nervous system (CNS) myelin, such as myelin basic protein (MBP) and proteolipid protein (PLP), which were shown by some to be highly expressed in oligodendrogliomas.[36] However, others did not identify MBP immunoreactivity in neoplastic oligodendrocytes.[74] Immunoreactivity for myelin-associated glycoprotein (MAG) has been demonstrated in only occasional oligodendrogliomas.[74] Membrane proteoglycans, neutral glycolipids, gangliosides and other proteins that are regulated during oligodendrocyte development are inconstantly or inconsistently expressed by neoplastic oligodendrocytes in routinely processed tissues.

GFAP positive cytoplasmic processes are typical of astrocytomas but not oligodendrogliomas. However, as discussed earlier, both 'gliofibrillary oligodendrocytes' and 'minigemistocytes' are strongly GFAP positive and may predominate in some oligodendrogliomas.[41,74] Vimentin is infrequently expressed in low-grade oligodendrogliomas but is more often found in anaplastic oligodendrogliomas.[57] Dot-like immunoreactivity for epithelial membrane antigens (EMA) has been reported in a small fraction of oligodendrogliomas.[57]

Synaptophysin immunoreactivity due to residual neuropil is frequently observed in oligodendrogliomas, in particular at the infiltrating tumour borders. Such staining of tumour-infiltrated neuropil should not be mistaken as neuronal or neurocytic tumour differentiation. However, some oligodendrogliomas, including cases with combined losses of 1p and 19q, contain tumour cells with morphological features indicative of neuronal/neurocytic differentiation and immunohistochemical positivity for synaptophysin and other neuronal markers.[81] Moreover, immunoreactivity for α–internexin, a proneural gene encoding a neurofilament interacting protein, is frequent in oligodendroglioma and has been proposed as a marker for 1p/19q-deleted tumours.[26] Other authors confirmed frequent α–internexin positivity in oligodendrogliomas, but reported that immunoreactivity was regionally heterogeneous and not reliably linked to 1p/19q deletion.[28]

Proliferation Markers

Ki–67 (MIB–1) has been widely studied in oligodendroglial tumours for tumour grading and prognostic assessment. In general, the mean fraction of positive tumour cells is significantly higher in anaplastic oligodendrogliomas as compared to low-grade oligodendrogliomas. Although independent review of the same set of MIB–1-stained slides from 30 oligodendrogliomas by six different pathologists revealed good interobserver agreement (concordance rate of 0.832),[83] interlaboratory staining and scoring variability for MIB–1 constitutes a major obstacle in defining reproducible diagnostic cut-off values. Published data suggest that oligodendrogliomas with MIB–1 labelling indices above 5 per cent are more likely to behave aggressively with less favourable outcomes. For example, a study of 89 patients reported a 5-year survival rate of 83 per cent for patients whose tumours had labelling indices below 5 per cent compared with 24 per cent for patients with tumours with >5 per cent MIB–1 positive cells.[22] Other authors also found statistically significant median survival differences based on a 5 per cent cut-off.[20] Within the group of WHO grade II oligodendrogliomas, one report found no significant correlation between MIB–1 staining and survival[124] whereas other authors reported that a MIB–1 index above 5 per cent was indicative of significantly shorter disease-free survival.[89] In a series of 20 paediatric low-grade oligodendrogliomas, the MIB–1 labelling index was generally low and not associated with survival.[9] In contrast, the MIB–1 index had a strong prognostic impact in anaplastic oligodendroglioma patients on univariate, but not multivariate, analyses, casting doubt that it represents an independent prognostic factor.[84]

Studies on the expression of other proliferation-associated antigens, such as the proliferating cell nuclear antigen (PCNA),[89] topoisomerase II α (Ki–S1)[58] and minichromosome maintenance 2 (MCM2) protein,[124] also revealed associations with tumour grade and survival. However, none of these markers provide a significant advantage over MIB–1 in the routine diagnostic setting.

Electron Microscopy

Oligodendroglioma cannot reliably be distinguished from other gliomas by means of electron microscopy because none of its ultrastructural features are entirely specific. Tumours are typically composed of small, round tumour cells showing a paucity of cytoplasmic intermediate glial filaments, which are otherwise common in normal and neoplastic astrocytes. Gliofibrillary oligodendrocytes and minigemistocytes contain cytoplasmic skeins or whorls of intermediate filaments, in contrast to the notably random distribution of short intermediate filaments in the gemistocytic astrocytoma tumour cells.[60] The nucleus of oligodendroglioma cells is usually round to oval and contains abundant euchromatin. In comparison with other gliomas, cytoplasm is sparse and processes tend to be short and tapered. Variable numbers of randomly arranged microtubules may be observed, and there may be moderate amounts of endoplasmic reticulum, moderately to well-developed Golgi complex, and variable numbers of mitochondria. Signet-ring cells in oligodendroglioma have their cytoplasm filled with degenerating mitochondria and irregularly and widely dilated cisternae of rough endoplasmic reticulum containing granular material.[62] In contrast, eosinophilic granular cells in oligodendrogliomas exhibit abundant autophagic type vacuoles and lysosomes containing electron-dense pleomorphic material.[19]

Differential Diagnosis

Several macrophage-rich lesions, including demyelinating disease, infarct and progressive multifocal leukoencephalopathy may mimic oligodendroglioma, in particular in small specimens with freezing artefacts. Cytological preparations from tissue smears most readily permit the identification of macrophages with their vacuolated cytoplasm and accompanying reactive astrocytes. Stains for myelin, e.g. Luxol fast blue, coupled with the periodic acid Schiff (PAS) reaction, allow the identification of myelin loss and infiltrating macrophages. Immunostains for macrophage markers such as CD68, CD163, or HAM–56 also facilitate the identification of macrophages. These cells often lie clustered around blood vessels in association with lymphocytes, but perivascular macrophages may also be present in otherwise typical oligodendrogliomas.

Partial lobectomy specimens performed for intractable seizures not infrequently have seemingly increased numbers of oligodendrocytes. In such instances, however, the white matter is condensed with resultant crowding of oligodendroglial nuclei, whereas the accompanying astrogliosis further contributes to the increased cellularity. Similar histological features may be seen adjacent to arteriovenous malformations. However, in these situations, oligodendroglial atypia is usually lacking. Smear preparations also help to distinguish well-differentiated oligodendroglioma from gliosis, in that normal oligodendrocytes possess little discernible cytoplasm and no nuclear lobation, and reactive astrocytes typically have more open chromatin, ample cytoplasm, and symmetrically radiating tapered processes. Moreover, *IDH1/2* mutations are generally absent in these non-neoplastic lesions, making the demonstration of such mutations by immunohistochemistry or DNA sequencing a powerful tool for the identification of oligodendroglial neoplasms.

With respect to the differential diagnosis of neoplasms, the distinction of oligodendroglioma from astrocytomas, in particular diffuse and pilocytic subtypes, bears important clinical implications (Box 28.1). This differential diagnosis can be quite challenging. For example, a central pathology review of of low-grade oligodendrogliomas submitted for 1p deletion testing could confirm this diagnosis in only half of the cases.[98] Differential diagnosis is particularly difficult in specimens lacking the characteristic honeycomb appearance, such as frozen sections or small, rapidly fixed paraffin specimens like stereotactic biopsy samples. In the absence of the typical perinuclear clearing, the distinction of oligodendroglioma from diffuse astrocytoma is largely based on the roundness and uniformity of nuclei. In addition, infiltration into the cortex and formation of secondary structures is more typical of oligodendrogliomas, but not specific. Overall GFAP and vimentin expression is usually less prominent in oligodendrogliomas than in fibrillary or gemistocytic astrocytomas. However, neither stain is specific. Strong nuclear immunoreactivity for p53 and loss of *ATRX* staining argue in favour of a diffuse astrocytoma, but lack of p53 and retained *ATRX* expression does not exclude this diagnosis.[65]

Some pilocytic astrocytomas mimic oligodendroglioma. In most instances, however, at least focally classic pilocytic features are present. In addition, typical clinical and neuroradiological features, such as paediatric presentation,

BOX 28.1. Diagnostic overview

The histopathological differential diagnosis of oligodendroglioma involves the recognition of both reactive and neoplastic
lesions. Concerning reactive lesions, oligodendrogliomas
need to be distinguished from macrophage-rich processes
such as demyelinating diseases or cerebral infarcts. The differential diagnosis towards neoplastic lesions includes a
variety of different tumour types, in particular those that may
present with clear cells, such as clear cell ependymoma,
neurocytoma, dysembryoplastic neuroepithelial tumour (DNT),
clear cell meningioma and metastatic clear cell carcinoma.
Immunohistochemical analysis usually helps distinguish these
entities. In particular, positivity for mutant *IDH1* rules out non-
neoplastic lesions and other clear cell tumours. It is also important to know if a biopsy comes from the temporal lobe because
normal perineuronal oligodendrocytes may be numerous there
and may mimic neoplastic perineuronal satellitosis. Freezing
artefacts that cause loss of detail in chromatin structure, chromatin hyperchromasia and nuclear irregularity are problematic
in low-grade oligodendrogliomas by eliminating salient nuclear
features. Molecular genetics is also playing a growing role in
differential diagnosis, particularly *IDH1/2* mutation and 1p/19q
deletion analyses (see text following).

location in the cerebellum, brain stem or spinal cord, and mural nodule/cyst formation argue in favour of pilocytic astrocytoma. In children, molecular analysis is of limited help because paediatric oligodendrogliomas usually lack *IDH1/2* mutations and 1p/19q deletions.[108] Moreover, *BRAF* gain/duplication or *KIAA1549–BRAF* fusion, i.e., characteristic aberrations in pilocytic astrocytomas, have also been detected in subsets of *IDH1*-mutant and 1p/19q-deleted oligodendroglial tumours.[3,56]

In paediatric patients, disseminated oligodendroglial-like leptomeningeal tumours have been suggested as a distinctive clinicopathologic entity.[94] These tumours show widespread leptomeningeal spread, sometimes with an associated intra-spinal mass. Histologically, they contain oligodendroglial-like tumour cells with frequent immunopositivity for OLIG2 and S–100 and variable GFAP and synaptophysin expres-sion. In contrast to the vast majority of oligodendrogliomas, these tumours generally lack staining for the mutant *IDH1* R132H protein and only rarely demonstrate 1p/19q dele-tions, although solitary 1p deletion is common.

Ependymomas, particularly those of the clear cell type, may also be mistaken for oligodendroglioma. The scattered presence of perivascular pseudorosettes with elongated, often tapering processes, vimentin, as well as dot- or ring-like EMA immunoreactivity and the typical ultrastructural features of ependymomas are helpful. Sharp demarcation from adjacent brain is also typical. In addition, genetic analysis may be helpful because clear cell ependymomas lack *IDH1/2* mutation[15] and 1p/19q deletions.[90]

Dysembryoplastic neuroepithelial tumour (DNT) consti-tutes another important differential diagnosis of low-grade oligodendroglioma. DNT consists of patterned mucin-rich nodules with oligodendrocyte-like cells that often line capil-laries or axonal bundles; they are largely limited to the cere-bral cortex and may be associated with cortical dysplasia. Prominent intercellular mucin surrounds mature or occa-sionally dysmorphic neurons, which appear to 'float'. The highly characteristic, complex nodules vary considerably in morphology, a minority being composed of astrocytic cells

with pilocytic or other gliomatous features. The perineu-ronal satellitosis and subpial spread is not as prominent in DNT as in oligodendroglioma. Furthermore, these tumours neither show *IDH1/2* mutations nor 1p/19q deletions.[15,33]

The distinction of oligodendroglioma from neurocytic tumours can pose considerable problems. The finding of perinuclear halos, arborizing vasculature and not infrequent calcification in both tumours contributes to the possible confusion. However, unlike oligodendroglioma, the clas-sic central neurocytoma is an intraventricular tumour that is typically attached to the septum pellucidum. This unique loca-tion combined with neurocytic rosettes, immunohistochemical reactivity for synaptophysin, lack of diffuse immunoreactivity for S–100 protein, and the characteristic neuronal ultrastruc-tural features provide the definitive diagnosis. Nevertheless, neurocytic tumours also arise outside the ventricular system, including the cerebral hemispheres.[10] Such extraventricu-lar neurocytomas may be very difficult to distinguish from oligodendroglioma, particularly as rare cases of diffusely infiltrating 'oligodendrogliomas' with deletion of 1p/19q and clear evidence of neurocytic differentiation have been reported.[81] Combined deletion of 1p and 19q, the genetic hallmark of oligodendroglioma, is rare in neurocytoma,[33] as is *IDH1/2* mutation.[15] Thus, mutant *IDH1* immunostaining and, if necessary, molecular testing for *IDH1/2* mutations and 1p/19q deletions may distinguish these entities.

Nuclear regularity, similar to oligodendrogliomas, may be noted in rare cases of cerebral neuroblastomas and other primitive neuroectodermal tumours of the central nervous system (CNS PNET). The differences in cellular-ity and mitotic activity, and the immunohistochemistry for neurofilaments and synaptophysin are features that dis-tinguish them from oligodendrogliomas. Cerebellar lipo-neurocytoma also comes into the differential diagnosis. Distinguishing points are similar to those of neurocytoma, with the additional feature of lipidized cells that resemble adipocytes, and the preferential cerebellar location.

Clear cell meningiomas rarely enter the differential diag-nosis, but should be considered in the setting of a primarily leptomeningeal oligodendroglioma. The immunopositiv-ity for epithelial membrane antigen, lack of mutant *IDH1* expression, PAS–positive cytoplasm and presence of more classical meningothelial areas usually ensure an accurate diagnosis of clear cell meningioma.

Histogenesis

The precise histogenesis of human oligodendrogliomas is still unknown. The immunocytochemical profile of oligoden-droglioma cells is more reminiscent of immature glial cells than mature oligodendroglia. Furthermore, the finding that oligo-dendroglioma cells may occasionally express markers of other lineages, including astrocytic and neuronal antigens, might favour the hypothesis of an origin from neural stem or progen-itor cells rather than mature oligodendrocytes. Nonetheless, it is important to stress that neoplastic development is not nec-essarily analogous to the highly regulated and co-ordinated normal glial development, and caution should be exercised in the histogenetic interpretation of immunohistochemical data using 'differentiation' markers on primary tumours. In transgenic mice, oligodendrogliomas could be induced by expression of platelet-derived growth factor (PDGF) under the control of promoters for the nestin, GFAP or 2′,3′–cyclic nucleotide 3′–phosphodiesterase (CNP) genes, suggesting that these neoplasms can arise from different stem/precursor cell types, including oligodendrocyte precursors.[129] Oligodendrogliomas and oligoastrocytomas could also be induced in mice by combined expression of H–ras and epidermal growth factor receptor (*EGFR*) from the GFAP promoter, as well as *EGFR* from the S–100 beta promoter. More recent data on murine and human oligodendrogliomas suggest an origin from NG2–positive and asymmetric division-defective oligodendroglial progenitor cells in the cerebral white matter rather than from neural stem cells.[82,107]

Molecular Genetics

Deletions of Chromosomal Arms 1p and 19q

Combined deletion of chromosomal arms 1p (Figure 28.3) and 19q constitutes the hallmark alteration in oligodendrogliomas and is found in up to 80 per cent of cases, typically on the background of *IDH1* or *IDH2* mutation and frequently associated with *MGMT* promoter methylation[91] (Figure 28.4). Diagnostically, the demonstration of 1p/19q deletion may serve to confirm the diagnosis of oligodendroglioma versus other clear cell tumours. However, absence of detectable 1p and 19q deletion does not exclude an oligodendroglioma. In particular, paediatric oligodendrogliomas often lack these deletions but may represent a distinct entity.[86]

Combined 1p and 19q deletion is typically caused by an unbalanced t(1;19)(q10;p10) translocation, with the chromosomal breakpoints located close to the centromeres of both chromosomes, thus resulting in complete losses of one copy of 1p and 19q, respectively.[45] Concerning oligodendroglioma-associated tumour suppressor genes on these chromosome arms, recent large-scale sequencing studies have identified frequent mutations in the far-upstream element binding protein 1 (*FUBP1*) gene on 1p31.1 and the *CIC* (homologue of the *Drosophila* gene capicua) gene on 19q13.2.[5,127] In fact, most oligodendrogliomas are genetically characterized by concurrent mutations in *IDH1/2* and *CIC* as well as 1p/19q deletion,[97,127] whereas most diffuse astrocytomas show concurrent mutations in *IDH1/2*, *TP53* and *ATRX* (Jiao *et al.* 2012).[65] *FUBP1* mutations are restricted to a smaller subset of *IDH1/2*-mutant and 1p/19q-deleted oligodendroglial tumours.[97,127] Several other genes located on 1p or 19q have been suggested as oligodendroglioma-associated tumour suppressor gene candidates.[92] For example, mutations or homozygous deletions of the cyclin-dependent kinase inhibitor 2C gene (*CDKN2C*) at 1p32 have been detected in a minor fraction of mostly anaplastic oligodendrogliomas. Other candidate genes on 1p include the calmodulin-binding transcription activator 1 gene (*CAMTA1*, 1p36), the chromodomain helicase DNA binding domain 5 gene (*CHD5*, 1p36), the DNA fragmentation factor subunit β gene (*DFFB*, 1p36), the adherens junction–associated protein 1 gene (*AJAP1*, 1p36.32), the transcriptional coactivator 4 gene (*CITED4*, 1p34), the peroxiredoxin 1 gene (*PRDX1*, 1p34), and the RAS homolog gene family gene *DIRAS3* (1p31). Candidate tumour suppressor genes on 19q other than *CIC* include the *p190RhoGAP* gene (19q13.3), the myelin-related epithelial membrane

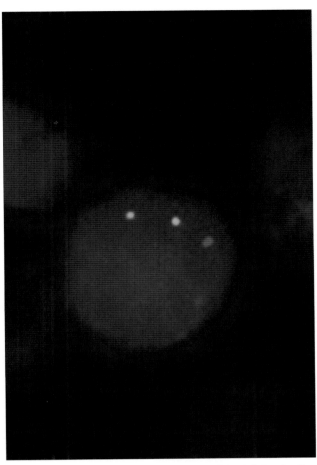

28.3 Oligodendroglioma. Demonstration of 1p deletion by fluorescent *in situ* hybridisation (FISH) on interphase nuclei. Note two green signals from probes to the long arm of chromosome 1 (1q), but only a single red signal from the probe to the short arm of chromosome 1(1p).

Courtesy of Dr Gayatry Mohapatra, Massachusetts General Hospital, Boston, MA, USA.

protein gene 3 (*EMP3*) at 19q13.3, *ZNF342*, a zinc-finger transcription factor gene at 19q13, and the maternally imprinted *PEG3* gene at 19q13.4. However, in contrast to *CIC*, *FUBP1* and *CDKN2C*, the other reported 1p or 19q genes are generally not inactivated by structural DNA alterations, such as point mutations or homozygous deletions, but show frequent epigenetic silencing due to aberrant promoter methylation. Hypermethylation of these and further genes located on other chromosomes is likely related to global changes in DNA methylation referred to as the Glioma CpG Island Methylator Phenotype (G–CIMP).[76] This widespread aberration is particularly common in oligodendroglial tumours but also present in *IDH1/2*-mutant diffuse astrocytomas. G–CIMP has been mechanistically linked to reduced activity of certain α–ketoglutarate-dependent DNA and histone demethylases as a consequence of *IDH1* or *IDH2* mutation.[113] In line with these findings, the *MGMT* gene promoter is hypermethylated in the vast majority of oligodendroglial tumours.[71] At the transcriptional level, 1p/19q-deleted oligodendrogliomas typically display a proneural gene

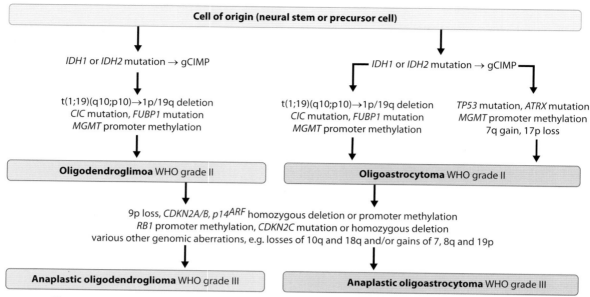

28.4 Summary of important molecular aberrations associated with the initiation and progression of oligodendrogliomas and oligoastrocytomas (modified according to Riemenschneider and Reifenberger,[93] with kind permission from Springer Science and Business Media).

expression signature,[27] which again is linked to *IDH1/2* mutation and G–CIMP.[76,113]

Chromosomal aberrations that are less frequent than 1p/19q deletion but still occur at more than random frequency include gains on chromosome 7 as well as losses on chromosomes 4, 6, 11p, 14, and 22q.[92] In contrast to diffuse astrocytomas, losses on 17p and *TP53* gene mutations are rare in oligodendrogliomas and mutually exclusive to 1p/19q losses. Nonetheless, the p53 pathway is frequently deregulated in oligodendrogliomas, e.g. by epigenetic silencing of the *p14^ARF* gene, which encodes a negative regulator of p53 activity that binds to Mdm2 and inhibits the Mdm2-mediated degradation of p53.[92]

Growth Factors and Receptors

Both low-grade and anaplastic oligodendrogliomas frequently demonstrate increased expression of epidermal growth factor receptor (*EGFR*) mRNA and protein.[92] The mechanisms causing upregulation of *EGFR* expression in these tumours are as yet unknown, because *EGFR* gene amplification is sufficiently rare that its presence strongly favours small cell glioblastoma over anaplastic oligodendroglioma.[79] The PDGF/PDGFR growth factor/receptor system also is of paramount importance in oligodendrogliomas as indicated by the finding that gene transfer of PDGF to neural stem or progenitor cells can induce oligodendrogliomas in mice.[2] Furthermore, both PDGF and PDGF receptors are frequently co-expressed in oligodendroglial tumours, suggesting auto- and/or paracrine growth stimulatory activities of this signalling pathway.[24] Expression of vascular endothelial growth factor (VEGF) and its receptors has been documented in oligodendroglial tumours, with increased expression levels in anaplastic tumours.[92]

Prognostic Significance of Genetic Alterations

The prognostic significance of genetic alterations in WHO grade II oligodendrogliomas is still unclear, largely because studies are usually based on small cohorts. In fact, low-grade gliomas are difficult to study because they rarely show dramatic radiological responses to therapy and require long follow-up times. In addition, *IDH1* mutation, 1p/19q losses and *MGMT* promoter methylation are so common in WHO grade II oligodendrogliomas that it is difficult to identify larger numbers of tumours without such aberrations. Recent data suggest that none of these genetic alterations are prognostic in WHO grade II glioma patients who are not treated with radio- or chemotherapy.[38] Other authors reported that 1p/19q deletion is associated with significantly longer survival for patients with WHO grade II gliomas.[55] Data on the prognostic role of *IDH1* or *IDH2* mutation in low-grade glioma patients are similarly controversial.[38,55] A clinical trial on low-grade oligodendroglioma patients treated with temozolomide revealed that 1p/19q loss, *MGMT* promoter methylation and *IDH1* mutation were associated with better therapeutic response and longer survival.[53] Taken together, the favourable prognostic role of *IDH1* mutation, 1p/19q losses and *MGMT* promoter methylation in low-grade oligodendroglioma patients is most evident when patients receive cytotoxic adjuvant treatment.

Aetiology and Genetic Susceptibility

The aetiology of human oligodendrogliomas is still unclear. In rodents, oligodendroglioma can be induced by various carcinogens; in particular administration of ethylnitrosourea and methylnitrosourea in rats frequently causes glial tumours with the morphology of oligodendrolioma. However, a role of these carcinogens in human gliomas is unclear. Cranial irradiation clearly is a risk factor, as indicated by individual patients who developed oligodendrogliomas after radiation therapy for other tumours. Several studies proposed a role for viral infections, in particular the SV40, JC and BK papoviruses, which can cause gliomas in experimental animals. In addition, viral DNA sequences and proteins have been detected in human oligodendrogliomas.[23] However, other authors failed to detect any JC, BK or SV40 viral sequences in oligodendrogliomas.[96] Therefore, it seems unlikely that these viruses play a causal role in human oligodendroglioma formation.

The vast majority of oligodendrogliomas arise sporadically, i.e. in patients without an apparent cancer predisposition. Recent single nucleotide polymorphism (SNP) genotyping data indicate an association between a low-frequency SNP variant at 8q24.21[21] and the risk of oligodendroglioma, irrespective of *IDH1/2* and 1p/19q status.[46] Rare cases of oligodendroglioma in patients with a hereditary tumour syndrome have been documented, including one patient with hereditary breast and ovarian cancer,[56] one child with retinoblastoma syndrome,[1] a child with cafe-au-lait spots, oligodendroglioma and rectal cancer on the basis of hereditary nonpolyposis colorectal cancer (HNPCC) syndrome,[69] and oligodendroglioma in identical twins with Ollier's disease.[17] Taylor *et al.*[110] reported a patient with Turcot syndrome who developed two metachronous glioblastomas showing histological features of oligodendroglial differentiation. The patient's sister also had a glioblastoma with oligodendroglial features.[110] Familial clustering of oligodendroglial tumours has been documented in a few instances, including individual case reports on oligodendrogliomas in two brothers, in a mother and a daughter, in twin sisters, and in a father and a son, as well as polymorphous oligodendrogliomas in a brother and a sister.[31] Additional studies identified familial oligoastrocytomas, including one study in identical twins, another study on two siblings with glioblastoma and oligoastrocytoma and an example of anaplastic oligoastrocytomas in two brothers with an oligodendroglioma in their maternal grandmother.[31]

Biological Behaviour and Prognosis

WHO grade II oligodendrogliomas are slowly growing tumours usually associated with long postoperative survival. However, the vast majority of tumours recur locally and malignant progression on recurrence is not uncommon. A population-based study from Switzerland revealed a median overall survival (OS) of 11.6 years and a 10-year survival rate of 51 per cent for patients with WHO grade II oligodendroglioma.[77] This was significantly longer than oligoastrocytoma patients (median OS: 6.6 years, 10-year survival: 49 per cent) or diffuse astrocytoma patients (median OS: 5.9 years, 10-year survival: 31 per cent). Data from the Central Brain Tumour Registry of the United States (CBTRUS) show 5- and 10-year survival rates of 79.25 per cent and 62.62 per cent, respectively, which again are longer than those of diffuse astrocytoma (47.58 per cent and 35.36 per cent) and mixed glioma (58.35 per cent and 45.42 per cent).[16] Clinical parameters that have been associated with longer survival include younger age at diagnosis, frontal tumour location, presentation with seizures, high Karnofsky performance status, lack of contrast enhancement on neuroimaging and complete tumour resection.[120] The optimal postoperative treatment of patients with WHO grade II oligodendroglioma is a matter of ongoing clinical investigations. Because late toxicity is a major concern for such patients with expected longterm survival, radio- and/or chemotherapy is often deferred until tumour progression, in particular in young patients presenting with seizures

only.[120] On the other hand, patients with symptomatic residual and/or progressive tumours after surgery, anaplastic tumours or enhancing lesions should be treated. A randomized trial on 314 patients with low-grade astrocytomas and oligodendrogliomas revealed that early radiotherapy after surgery lengthens the period without progression but does not affect overall survival.[115] Radiotherapy could therefore be deferred for patients who are in good condition, provided they are carefully monitored. Another phase III trial compared radiotherapy versus radiotherapy plus procarbazine, CCNU, and vincristine (PCV) chemotherapy in 251 adult patients with low-grade gliomas.[105] Progression-free survival, but not overall survival, was longer for patients receiving combined treatment. In addition, combined treatment provided a survival benefit in patients alive beyond two years, suggesting a delayed benefit for chemotherapy. A phase II study also suggested a role of upfront chemotherapy with temozolomide for patients with progressive low-grade oligodendroglioma.[53] Radiotherapy or chemotherapy with either PCV or temozolomide is usually administered to patients with recurrent tumours showing histological and/or clinical progression.[120]

ANAPLASTIC OLIGODENDROGLIOMA

Anaplastic oligodendroglioma is defined by the WHO classification of tumours of the central nervous system as an oligodendroglioma with either focal or diffuse histological features of anaplasia and less favourable prognosis.[88]

Incidence, Age and Gender Distribution

Anaplastic oligodendroglioma accounts for approximately 0.6 per cent of all primary brain tumours and 30 per cent of the oligodendroglial tumours; the adjusted annual incidence rate has been estimated as 0.12 per 100 000 population.[16] The vast majority develop in adults, peaking between 45 and 50 years of age, i.e. approximately 7–8 years later on average than low-grade oligodendroglioma.[77] In children, anaplastic oligodendrogliomas are very rare. Caucasians are more commonly affected than black people, as indicated by incidence rates of 0.13 versus 0.05 per 100 000 persons, with rates slightly higher for males (0.14 per 100 000) than for females (0.11 per 100 000).[16]

Clinical and Radiological Features

Anaplastic oligodendroglioma either may develop *de novo* or secondarily via progression from a low-grade oligodendroglioma. Patients with secondary tumours are younger than their *de novo* counterparts.[63] The preoperative history of patients with *de novo* tumours is usually short, but clinical symptoms and signs do not significantly differ from those of other primary anaplastic gliomas. Epilepsy is the most common presenting symptom.[63] In patients with secondary forms, the mean time to progression from low-grade oligodendroglioma has been estimated at 6.6 ± 4.2 years.[77] Other authors reported a slightly shorter interval of 72 months, but a similar survival time from WHO grade III diagnosis in primary and secondary anaplastic oligodendrogliomas.[63] However, previous resection for lower grade tumour has also been reported as a prognostically favourable factor.[120]

On neuroimaging, anaplastic oligodendrogliomas may show heterogeneous patterns owing to the variable presence of necrosis, cystic degeneration, intratumoural haemorrhages and calcification. The majority of tumours demonstrate contrast enhancement on CT and MRI, which can be either patchy or homogeneous.[47,63] However, lack of contrast enhancement does not exclude an anaplastic oligo-dendroglioma. Ring enhancement is uncommon and associated with less favourable prognosis.[13]

Macroscopy

The vast majority of anaplastic oligodendrogliomas are located in the cerebral hemispheres with a preference for the frontal lobe, followed by the temporal lobe. The macroscopic appearance does not allow for a reliable distinction from low-grade oligodendrogliomas, although anaplastic oligodendrogliomas often show a more heterogeneous cut surface due to haemorrhages, cyst formations and areas of necrosis (Figure 28.5a).

Microscopy

According to the WHO classification, the histological features that separate anaplastic oligodendroglioma from low-grade oligodendroglioma include high cellularity, nuclear pleomorphism and hyperchromasia, moderate to high mitotic activity, microvascular proliferation and necrosis.[88] Anaplastic oligodendrogliomas usually show a number of these features. Unfortunately, it is not possible to equate anaplastic oligodendroglioma with the presence of any one of the above histological characteristics, although it has been argued that endothelial proliferation and brisk mitotic activity (at least 6 mitoses/10 HPF) are of particular importance.[35]

In general, anaplastic oligodendrogliomas are cellular, mitotically active, diffusely infiltrating gliomas composed of neoplastic cells showing morphological features indicative of oligodendroglial cells, i.e. rounded nuclei, perinuclear halos in routinely processed tissue samples and few cellular processes. In comparison to low-grade oligodendroglioma, there is often increased cytoplasm, more open chromatin and increased nucleolar prominence. The characteristic vascular pattern of branching capillaries is often still recognizable, although additional microvascular proliferation is usually obvious. Focal microcalcifications are frequent. Rare cases demonstrate marked desmoplasia.[48] Gliofibrillary oligo-dendrocytes and minigemistocytes (Figure 28.5b) are more common in anaplastic oligodendrogliomas but are not of prognostic relevance. Occasional tumours show marked cellular pleomorphism including multinucleated giant cells. In addition, rare anaplastic oligodendrogliomas may present with a sarcomatous component.[95] Infiltration of the cerebral cortex is often associated with the formation of secondary structures, in particular perineuronal satellitosis.

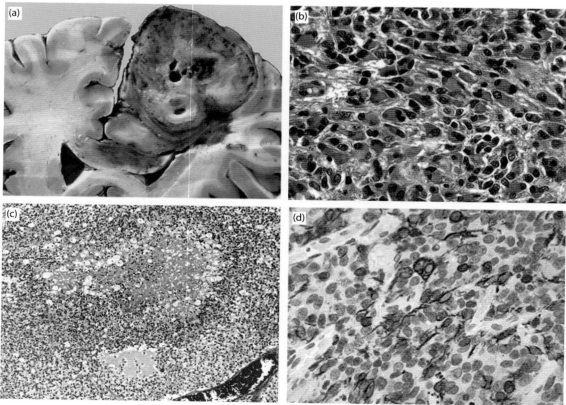

28.5 Anaplastic oligodendroglioma. (a) Large tumour with haemorrhage, necrosis and cysts, involving the frontal lobe and spreading to the corpus callosum. **(b)** Minigemistocytes with eccentric nuclei and eosinophilic cytoplasm. **(c)** Pseudopalisading necrosis. **(d)** Immunohistochemistry for GFAP demonstrating positivity in a subset of tumour cells.

Courtesy of Dr Arie Perry, UCSF, San Francisco, CA, USA.

Some anaplastic oligodendrogliomas feature necrosis, including rare cases with pseudopalisades resembling those of glioblastoma (Figure 28.5c). As long as the tumour shows the typical cytological and histological hallmarks of oligodendroglioma, the WHO classification recommends classifying these tumours as anaplastic oligodendroglioma of WHO grade III.[88] In contrast to patients with malignant oligoastrocytomas, the presence of necrosis did not have an adverse prognostic effect in anaplastic oligodendroglioma patients.[70]

Grading

Anaplastic oligodendrogliomas correspond to WHO grade III.

Immunohistochemistry

The immunohistochemical profile of anaplastic oligodendrogliomas is similar to that of low-grade oligodendrogliomas, including frequent positivity for *IDH1* R132H and MAP2. GFAP-immunoreactive cells such as gliofibrillary oligodendrocytes and microgemistocytes are occasionally numerous (Figure 28.5d). Vimentin immunopositivity is also more common in anaplastic than in low-grade oligodendrogliomas. The MIB–1 labelling index is significantly higher in anaplastic oligodendrogliomas as compared to their low-grade counterparts, reflecting the more rapid tumour growth. Several studies suggested a MIB–1 index of 5 per cent as a cut-off value to distinguish two groups of oligodendroglial tumours with significantly different outcome.[20,89] A study based on a prospective phase III trial revealed a strong prognostic impact of the MIB–1 index on univariate analysis, but no independent influence on multivariate analysis.[84]

Differential Diagnosis

Similar to low-grade oligodendrogliomas, the differential diagnosis includes a variety of other clear cell tumour entities. Occasional anaplastic oligodendrogliomas may superficially resemble metastatic clear cell carcinomas. Unlike the latter, which are solid and sharply demarcated, oligodendrogliomas are infiltrative. Although immunohistochemistry readily permits their distinction, caution is recommended because there is a misleading cross-reactivity with certain broad-spectrum cytokeratin antibodies and GFAP. By contrast, stains for low molecular weight cytokeratin are negative in oligodendrogliomas and therefore reliably exclude metastatic carcinoma. In a fraction of anaplastic oligodendrogliomas, the differential diagnosis with anaplastic oligoastrocytoma may be problematic and associated with considerable interobserver variability. Moreover, it is important to separate anaplastic oligodendrogliomas from malignant small cell astrocytic neoplasms, i.e. 'small cell astrocytoma/glioblastoma', which behave much more aggressively, akin to conventional glioblastomas.[11,79] Molecular genetic analyses can be helpful to solve this differential diagnosis because small cell astrocytic tumours lack 1p/19q deletion but often demonstrate *EGFR* amplification and chromosome 10 losses. Conversely, *IDH1* (R132H) immunoreactivity and *IDH1/2* mutations are found in most anaplastic oligodendrogliomas, but not in small cell glioblastomas.[52]

Molecular Genetics

Anaplastic oligodendrogliomas share with low-grade oligodendrogliomas the frequent mutations in *IDH1* or IDH2, detectable in up to 80 per cent of cases (Box 28.2).[39] 1p and 19q codeletions are found in 50–70 per cent, with frequent *CIC* mutation in 1p/19q-deleted tumours and additional *FUBP1* mutations in a subset of cases.[97] Anaplastic oligodendrogliomas display a higher degree of genomic instability as indicated by aberrations involving genes or chromosomal segments from several other chromosomes. These include homozygous deletions on 9p21 involving the tumour suppressor genes *CDKN2A*, *p14^{ARF}* and *CDKN2B* in up to one third of anaplastic oligodendrogliomas. Such deletions are particularly common in anaplastic oligodendrogliomas without 1p and 19q losses, but may also be present in 1p/19q-deleted cases. Other chromosomal imbalances detected at more than random frequency include deletions on 4q, 10q and 18q as well as gains on 7, 8q and 19p.[112] *PTEN* mutations are rare in anaplastic oligodendrogliomas.[99] Large-scale sequencing efforts revealed individual mutations in a large variety of genes, with recurrent changes affecting the *PIK3CA*, *NOTCH1*, *NOTCH2* and *HDAC2* genes in a study of seven tumours.[5] Whole exome sequencing of ten 1p/19q-deleted oligodendroglial tumours, including three anaplastic oligodendrogliomas, also revealed mutations across the genome, with the *IDH1/2*, CIC and *NOTCH1* genes most commonly affected.[127] Gene amplifications targeting the *EGFR*, *PDGFRA*, *CDK4*, *MDM4*, *MYC* or *MYCN* are uncommon (generally <10 per cent).[92]

BOX 28.2. Assessment of prognostic and predictive molecular markers in anaplastic glioma patients

There are currently three clinically relevant molecular markers that provide strong prognostic and/or predictive information beyond the histological classification of anaplastic oligodendroglial tumours. These are *IDH1* or *IDH2* mutation, *MGMT* promoter methylation and 1p/19q deletion.[91,126] *IDH1/2* mutation is a strong prognostic marker for longer survival in anaplastic glioma patients treated with radiotherapy, chemotherapy or combined radiochemotherapy. Similarly, in *IDH1/2* mutant tumours, which constitute the majority of anaplastic oligodendrogliomas and oligoastrocytomas, *MGMT* promoter methylation is linked to a more favourable prognosis independent of the type of adjuvant therapy. Patients whose tumours carry codeletion of 1p and 19q also show significantly longer overall survival, both when treated with radiotherapy or radiotherapy plus PCV chemotherapy. However, this molecular marker is additionally useful to predict a benefit from the addition of alkylating chemotherapy to radiotherapy, i.e. patients with 1p/19q-deleted anaplastic gliomas survive significantly longer following combined modality treatment as compared to radiotherapy alone. Thus, testing for 1p/19q deletion may guide treatment decisions in patients with anaplastic oligodendroglial tumours in addition to serving as a prognostic marker. Various methods are available for the testing of these clinically relevant molecular markers in the routine diagnostic setting, each associated with distinct advantages and disadvantages.[91] Diagnostic application of these methods requires experience in the interpretation of their results and knowledge of potential pitfalls. Moreover, appropriate methods of quality control need to be established to avoid unacceptable intra- and interlaboratory variability in molecular testing results.

Correlation of Genetic Aberrations with Tumour Location

Oligodendrogliomas located in the frontal, parietal and occipital lobes have more frequent 1p and 19q allelic losses than anaplastic oligodendrogliomas in the temporal lobe, insula and diencephalon.[72,128] In addition, tumours with 1p and 19q losses more often show bilateral tumour growth.[128]

Clinical Significance of Genetic Alterations

The first report on an important prognostic role of 1p (or 1p and 19q) deletions dates back to 1998 when Cairncross and colleagues provided the first evidence that anaplastic oligodendroglioma patients treated with procarbazine, vincristine and CCNU (PCV) chemotherapy demonstrated significantly longer survival if their tumours had lost 1p.[13] Since then, numerous retrospective as well as three large prospective phase III trials have corroborated that anaplastic glioma patients with 1p/19q-deleted tumours show longer survival when treated with radiotherapy, alkylating chemotherapy or both.[12,117,125] Although these studies originally suggested that the favourable prognostic effect of 1p/19q deletion is independent of the type of adjuvant therapy, i.e. radiotherapy or chemotherapy, recent long-term follow-up data of two of these trials (RTOG 9402 and EORTC 26951) support a survival benefit of initial combined modality treatment using PCV plus radiotherapy over radiotherapy alone in patients with 1p/19q-deleted tumours.[14,116] Thus, 1p/19q deletion not only is a prognostic marker but may also guide therapeutic decisions in anaplastic glioma patients.[126]

The molecular mechanisms underlying the predictive significance of 1p and 19q losses in patients with anaplastic oligodendroglial tumours are still unknown. In particular, it is unclear whether mutations of genes located on either chromosomal arm, e.g. CIC and FUBP1, may be responsible for the clinically less aggressive behaviour and better sensitivity to cytotoxic therapy. Alternatively, the 1p/19q status may just represent a molecular signpost for genetic/epigenetic alterations on other chromosomes that influence treatment response and survival. The observation that MGMT promoter methylation is common in oligodendrogliomas with IDH1/2 mutation and losses on 1p and 19q may point to a possible mechanism contributing to the chemosensitivity of these tumours.[71,73] Furthermore, 1p/19q-deleted and IDH1/2-mutant anaplastic oligodendroglial tumours commonly demonstrate global changes in DNA methylation, which lead to hypermethylation of numerous genes, possibly including genes linked to therapy resistance and/or poor prognosis. Moreover, anaplastic gliomas without 1p/19q deletion may carry more prognostically unfavourable genetic aberrations, such as homozygous deletion of CDKN2A, loss of chromosome 10, mutation of PTEN, gain on 8q, EGFR amplification and others.[92]

With respect to diagnostic testing for 1p and 19q deletion, only whole arm deletions of both chromosomes, usually as a consequence of the unbalanced t(1;19)(q10;p10) translocation,[45] are clearly indicative of favourable prognosis. In fact, malignant gliomas carrying deletions of just one chromosomal arm or deletions of only parts of these arms often demonstrate more aggressive behavior, even when compared to 1p/19q-undeleted cases.[91]

IDH1 or IDH2 mutation is a strong prognostic factor for patients with anaplastic oligodendroglial tumours, irrespective of whether they were treated with radiotherapy, chemotherapy or both.[118,125] In contrast to its predictive role in primary glioblastomas, MGMT promoter methylation has been linked to longer survival of anaplastic glioma patients not only when treated with chemotherapy but also when treated with radiotherapy alone.[125] The different roles of MGMT promoter methylation (predictive versus prognostic) in glioblastoma versus anaplastic glioma patients likely depend on the distinct IDH1/2 mutation status in these entities, with anaplastic oligodendrogliomas frequently showing IDH1/2 mutation and the associated glioma CpG island methylator phenotype (CIMP). In fact, data from the EORTC 26951 trial suggest that the presence of CIMP is a better predictor of survival than MGMT promoter methylation in patients with anaplastic oligodendroglial tumours.[119] The individual genes whose inactivation contributes to this favourable prognostic effect are still unknown. One candidate gene that is commonly inactivated in oligodendroglial tumours by 1p loss and promoter methylation is the pH-regulatory gene NHE1, silencing of which leads to lower intracellular pH and inhibition of tumour growth due to impaired neutralization of the lactic acidosis generated in tumour cells.[7]

Biological Behaviour and Prognosis

Anaplastic oligodendrogliomas are malignant tumours that grow rapidly and tend to recur after treatment. The prognosis is less favourable when compared to low-grade oligodendroglioma but significantly better when compared to malignant astrocytic tumours.[77,125] Nonetheless, reported survival data vary considerably depending on the patient populations and treatment. A population-based analysis from Switzerland reported a median survival of 3.5 years.[77] A retrospective study on 106 anaplastic oligodendroglioma patients revealed a considerably longer median OS of 7.3 years, and a 5-year survival rate of 62 per cent.[85] Data from long-term follow-up of patients enrolled in the RTOG 9402 and EORTC 26951 prospective trials indicate that the type of adjuvant treatment strongly influences survival of patients with anaplastic oligodendroglial tumours when stratified according to 1p/19q deletion. In both trials, patients were either treated by operation and radiotherapy or by operation, radiotherapy and PCV chemotherapy. In the RTOG 9402 trial, median overall survival times were 2.6 years (radiotherapy) versus 2.7 years (radiotherapy plus PCV) in the patient group with 1p/19q intact tumours.[14] In contrast, patients having 1p/19q-deleted tumours had median overall survival times of 14.7 years (radiotherapy plus PCV) versus 7.3 years (radiotherapy), respectively. Similarly, longterm follow up of the EORTC 26951 patients revealed median overall survival times of only 25 months (combined treatment) and 21 months (radiotherapy only) in patients whose tumours lacked 1p/19q deletions, whereas median overall survival was not reached after more than 10 years' follow-up in the patients with 1p/19q-deleted anaplastic gliomas treated by radiotherapy plus PCV, and was 9.3 years in the patients treated with radiotherapy alone.[116] These data not only indicate a marked survival benefit for patients having

1p/19q-deleted anaplastic oligodendroglial tumours but also argue that chemotherapy should be part of their initial treatment.[126]

In addition to *IDH1* mutation, *MGMT* promoter methylation and 1p/19q deletion, several clinical factors have been associated with longer survival, including young age at diagnosis, high Karnofsky performance score and extent of resection.[12,117,125] The majority of patients with anaplastic oligodendroglioma die from local tumour recurrence. Occasional patients develop cerebrospinal fluid (CSF) spread or even systemic metastases outside the nervous system.

OLIGOASTROCYTOMA

Oligoastrocytoma is defined by the WHO classification of tumours of the central nervous system as a diffusely infiltrating glioma composed of a conspicuous mixture of two distinct neoplastic cell types morphologically resembling the tumour cells in oligodendroglioma or diffuse astrocytoma of WHO grade II.[121] The oligodendroglial and astroglial components may either be diffusely intermingled or separated into distinct, biphasic areas. Most oligoastrocytomas carry *IDH1* or *IDH2* mutations, with distinct subsets either showing additional 1p/19q deletions or additional *TP53* and *ATRX* mutations.

Incidence, Age and Sex Distribution

Definitive diagnostic criteria remain controversial. Accordingly, the estimated incidence of these tumours varies from study to study. In a population-based study of 987 glioma patients from Switzerland, WHO grade II oligoastrocytomas accounted for only 2 per cent of the cases and showed an annual incidence rate of 0.1 per 100 000 population.[77] The CBTRUS estimates the annual incidence rate of mixed gliomas (without grading) at 0.20 per 100 000 population.[16] It has been reported that the incidence of oligoastrocytomas increased annually by approximately 4 per cent.[43] However, it cannot be excluded that this increase simply reflects changes in the histological classification of diffuse gliomas over time. The fraction of oligoastrocytomas among all low-grade diffuse gliomas also varies considerably among studies, with values ranging from 16 per cent up to 33 per cent in larger series.[16,77] Oligoastrocytomas usually develop in middle-aged individuals, with a peak incidence between 40 and 45 years of age.[77] There is a slight male preponderance.[16]

Clinical and Radiological Features

Most patients initially present with seizures. Other common presenting signs and symptoms include focal neurological deficits, personality changes, headaches, and other signs of increased intracranial pressure. Areas with contrast enhancement on CT or MRI may be seen but are more common in anaplastic tumours.[47] Similarly, undefined margins and inhomogeneity on T1 and T2 signals are more common in high-grade oligoastrocytomas. Approximately 25 per cent of oligoastrocytomas demonstrate calcifications on neuroimaging.

Macroscopy

The vast majority of oligoastrocytomas arise in the cerebral hemispheres, with the frontal lobe being the most common localization, followed by temporal and parietal locations. The macroscopic appearance is indistinguishable from other diffusely infiltrative gliomas, i.e. diffuse astrocytomas and oligodendrogliomas.

Microscopy

Oligoastrocytomas are diffusely infiltrating gliomas of moderate cellularity and low mitotic activity. Microcalcifications and microcystic degeneration are commonly seen. Necrosis and vascular endothelial proliferation are absent. The tumour consists of two distinct neoplastic cell populations showing either astrocytic or oligodendroglial phenotypes. However, neoplastic cells with ambiguous (transitional) phenotypes that are difficult to assign to either the astrocytic or the oligodendroglial lineage are often present. Only a minority of tumours clearly demonstrate regionally distinct areas of classic oligodendroglial and classic fibrillary or gemistocytic astrocytic differentiation. This pattern has been described as the 'compact' or 'biphasic' variant of oligoastrocytoma (Figure 28.6). In most cases, however, both populations are intimately admixed. Of these two patterns, the 'biphasic' type is easier to recognize whereas distinction of oligoastrocytomas with 'admixed' growth pattern from either oligodendrogliomas or diffuse astrocytomas is problematic. The absence of objective diagnostic criteria for these lesions and the desire not to miss any tumour that potentially responds to adjuvant chemotherapy may have increased the tendency for neuropathologists to identify an 'oligodendroglial component' in diffuse gliomas.[67] Indiscriminate placement of morphologically ambiguous and poorly preserved gliomas into the 'wastebasket' of the mixed gliomas may further increase the problem. Because the intermingled type of oligoastrocytoma is relatively loosely defined, these developments have essentially led to an increase in the diagnosis of the admixed type of oligoastrocytoma at some institutions, whereas others prefer to classify such tumours either as oligodendroglioma or diffuse astrocytoma, depending on the prevailing differentiation. Unfortunately, this diagnostic

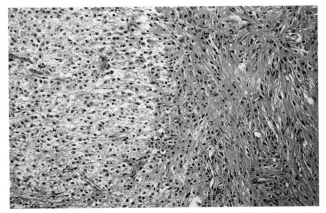

28.6 Oligoastrocytoma. There are clearly two different neoplastic cell populations: oligodendroglial on the left and astrocytic on the right.

variability causes considerable interobserver variability, which is particularly pronounced in the classification of anaplastic oligoastrocytomas.[61]

Given the characteristic moderate pleomorphism in diffuse astrocytomas, it is not surprising to find rounded nuclei in these tumours that raise the possibility of oligodendroglioma cells; however, it remains unclear how many rounded, oligodendroglioma-like nuclei are required for a diagnosis of oligoastrocytoma or whether such cells even constitute evidence for an oligodendroglial component. In addition, oligodendrogliomas may include cells with astrocytic features and/or GFAP-positivity, such as gliofibrillary oligodendrocytes and minigemistocytes, and reactive astrocytes are commonly trapped in oligodendrogliomas. Thus, at present, the diagnosis of oligoastrocytoma remains controversial and more objective genetic or epigenetic parameters are needed to improve the classification of such neoplasms (Box 28.3).

The role of quantitative assessments of each cytological component in oligoastrocytomas is disputed because precise percentages are difficult to determine given limited tumour sampling and the presence of tumour cells with ambiguous phenotypes. Therefore, a definite diagnostic threshold that is minimally required for the minor tumour component is not provided by the WHO.[121] Nevertheless, further histological subdivision into oligodendroglioma-predominant or astrocytoma-predominant oligoastrocytomas has long been suggested.[37] Again, such histological subdivision is fraught with marked interobserver variability. Moreover, its clinical role in terms of prognostic significance is unclear. An older study reported that patient survival was similar irrespective of whether oligodendrocytes or astrocytes predominated or whether the proportion of these two cell types was approximately equal.[103] A prospective study by the same group evaluated oligodendroglioma-predominant mixed gliomas together with 'pure' oligodendrogliomas versus astrocytoma-predominant mixed gliomas together with 'pure' astrocytomas, and found significantly shorter 2-year and 5-year survival rates in the latter group.[102] In the NOA–04 phase III trial on anaplastic gliomas, patients whose tumours were centrally classified as anaplastic oligoastrocytomas showed similar survival as anaplastic oligodendroglioma patients, whereas survival of anaplastic astrocytoma patients was significantly shorter.[125]

Grading

Oligoastrocytomas correspond to WHO grade II.

Immunohistochemistry

There is no immunohistochemical marker that can reliably distinguish the astrocytic and oligodendroglial components in oligoastrocytomas. GFAP immunoreactivity is usually strong in fibrillary and gemistocytic astroglial cells and more variable in the oligodendroglial fractions. Most oligoastrocytomas express the *IDH1* R132H mutant protein, which may help to distinguish these tumours from non-neoplastic lesions but does not aid the differential diagnosis towards diffuse astrocytoma or oligodendroglioma, respectively. Approximately one third of the oligoastrocytomas demonstrate strong nuclear

> ### BOX 28.3. Mixed gliomas
>
> Mixed gliomas are defined by the coexistence of at least two distinct glioma phenotypes, with oligoastrocytomas representing by far the most common type of mixed glioma. The hypothesis that mixed gliomas are 'collision' tumours, in which two separate glial neoplasms arose side by side in a patient unfortunate enough to have a local propensity towards glioma formation, appears unlikely. Molecular analysis of phenotypically different components in mixed oligoastrocytomas has revealed uniform genetic changes.[59] Thus, mixed gliomas are indeed monoclonal tumours that display phenotypic heterogeneity at the histological level. This might occur because of variable epigenetic changes and/or regional variations in growth factors or other signals that promote differentiation along different glial lineages. The nosological position of oligoastrocytomas is controversial and their very existence can be questioned in light of genetic studies showing that they lack a distinctive pattern of genetic alterations but rather carry mutations typical for either oligodendroglial or astrocytic tumours. Therefore, it is possible that oligoastrocytomas may no longer be considered as a distinct entity when genetic alterations are being used for subclassification of diffuse gliomas. Along this line, the observation that 1p/19q-deleted oligoastrocytomas behave clinically like oligodendrogliomas whereas oligoastrocytomas without these deletions show a clinical course similar to diffuse astrocytomas suggests that the combination of morphological and molecular parameters could indeed reshape the definition of oligoastrocytomas. However, unless a general consensus concerning the implementation of molecular parameters into the routine classification of these neoplasms is achieved, classification should still primarily rely on histological features, bearing in mind that morphological criteria leave considerable space for subjectivity and interobserver variability.

p53 positivity, which is in line with the presence of *TP53* mutations in a similar fraction of cases (see Molecular Genetics, later). MIB–1 proliferation index is usually low (<5 per cent) in WHO grade II oligoastrocytomas. One study reported that patients with histologically low-grade oligoastrocytoma but a Ki–67 labelling index of ≥10 per cent showed a reduced time to progression that was similar to that of anaplastic oligoastrocytoma patients.[101]

Differential Diagnosis

The differential diagnosis of oligoastrocytoma includes both oligodendroglioma and diffuse astrocytoma. An admixture of GFAP positive minigemistocytes and gliofibrillary oligodendrocytes with typical oligodendroglial cells is not sufficient to shift a diagnosis from oligodendroglioma to oligoastrocytoma. Only tumours with an additional classic astroglial component should be diagnosed as oligoastrocytoma. It remains to be determined whether immunohistochemical testing for loss of *ATRX* expression, which is frequent in *IDH1* and *TP53* mutant astrocytic gliomas but rare in 1p/19q-deleted oligodendrogliomas,[44] provides helpful information in the routine diagnostic setting. Molecular analyses, in particular testing for 1p and 19q, is often performed to supplement the diagnostic and prognostic assessment of oligoastrocytomas or diffuse gliomas with ambiguous histology, and may indeed assist therapeutic decision making in progressive and anaplastic oligoastrocytomas concerning the best type of adjuvant treatment.[126]

Histogenesis

The histogenesis of human oligoastrocytomas is unclear. The observation of common genetic alterations in the different histological components of individual tumours are consistent with oligoastrocytomas arising from a glial precursor cell able to undergo bipotential differentiation. An oligodendrocyte/type 2 astrocyte (O–2A) progenitor-like cell might be a good candidate for the cell of origin in both oligodendrogliomas and oligoastrocytomas, but this remains speculative. In addition, epigenetic events and regional changes in the tumour microenvironment, e.g. regional heterogeneity in PDGF or Akt/Ras signalling activity,[21] are likely to contribute to the phenotypic variability in oligoastrocytomas.

Molecular Genetics

The molecular genetic changes observed in oligoastrocytomas either correspond to those commonly present in oligodendrogliomas, i.e. *IDH1/2* mutation and 1p/19q loss, often accompanied by *CIC* mutation, or resemble the genetic aberration pattern typically seen in diffuse astrocytomas, i.e. mutation of *IDH1/2* and *TP53*. Similar to diffuse astrocytomas, the latter type of oligoastrocytoma may show additional *ATRX* mutation and/or loss of expression.[65] However, a specific pattern of genetic abnormalities that would reliably distinguish oligoastrocytomas from oligodendrogliomas and diffuse astrocytomas has not yet emerged. Molecular analyses of microdissected oligodendroglial and astrocytic regions revealed common genetic alterations in most instances, indicating a monoclonal origin of both components.[59] Approximately 30–50 per cent of the oligoastrocytomas show allelic losses on 1p and 19q.[93] *TP53* mutations, often combined with loss of heterozygosity on 17p, have been detected in approximately 30–40 per cent of the cases, with *TP53* mutation being mutually exclusive to 1p/19q deletion.[93] Mutations in *IDH1* or *IDH2* are present in approximately 80 per cent of oligoastrocytomas, including tumours with either 1p/19q deletion or *TP53* mutations.[39,55] Concerning outcome, patients with low-grade gliomas carrying 1p/19q deletion and *IDH1/2* mutation appear to survive longer than patients with *TP53* and *IDH1/2* mutant tumours.[55] One study suggested that the rare low-grade gliomas without any of these alterations, i.e. 'triple-negative' tumours, frequently demonstrate genetic aberrations in genes encoding members of the retinoblastoma (RB1) pathway and show a less favourable clinical outcome.[54]

Histologically, oligoastrocytomas with 1p/19q loss are more frequently oligodendroglioma-predominant, whereas oligoastrocytomas with *TP53* mutations are more often astrocytoma-predominant.[66] In addition, 1p/19q deletions have been detected less commonly than *TP53* mutation in oligoastrocytomas of the temporal lobe, whereas the opposite pattern predominates in other locations.[29,72] Comparative genomic hybridisation analysis of oligoastrocytomas suggested 4 distinct genetic subtypes: a '–1p/–19q' subtype, a '+7/–10' subtype, an 'intermediate' (–1p/–19q plus other chromosomal imbalances) subtype, and a subtype characterized by imbalances of other chromosomes.[49] Taken together, the available molecular data suggest that genetic analysis could prove useful in distinguishing those oligoastrocytomas that behave clinically like oligodendrogliomas from those that behave like astrocytomas.

Biological Behaviour and Prognosis

Oligoastrocytomas are slowly growing tumours that tend to recur locally and may progress to anaplastic gliomas and eventually, secondary glioblastoma. Several studies suggest that oligoastrocytoma follows a clinical course intermediate between that of oligodendroglioma or diffuse astrocytoma.[77,103] Based on a study of 60 patients with low-grade oligoastrocytomas, Shaw *et al.*[103] determined a median survival time of 6.3 years and 5- and 10-year survival rates of 58 per cent and 32 per cent, respectively. A population-based survey calculated a median survival time of 6.6 years and a 10-year survival rate of 49 per cent for patients with WHO grade II oligoastrocytomas.[77] Data from the Central Brain Tumor Registry of the United States show 5- and 10-year survival rates of 58.35 per cent and 45.42 per cent for mixed gliomas.[16] Progressive oligoastrocytomas with 1p/19q deletion are more likely to respond favourably to adjuvant therapy including chemotherapy when compared to 1p/19q-intact tumours.[42,64] Other prognostic factors that have been associated with longer survival of oligoastrocytoma patients are similar to those in oligodendroglioma.

ANAPLASTIC OLIGOASTROCYTOMA

Anaplastic oligoastrocytoma is defined by the WHO classification of tumours of the central nervous system as an oligoastrocytoma with focal or diffuse histologic features of anaplasia, such as increased cellularity, nuclear atypia, pleomorphism and increased mitotic activity.[122] Necrosis is absent. Oligoastrocytomas with necrosis are classified as 'glioblastoma with oligodendroglial component'.

Incidence, Age and Sex Distribution

Data on the incidence of anaplastic oligoastrocytomas are sparse and confounded by the variability in the histological classification of these tumours. Ohgaki and Kleihues[77] reported an adjusted annual incidence rate of 0.07 per 100 000 population. In their series of 987 patients with oligodendroglial, mixed or astrocytic tumours, only 11 (1.1 per cent) were diagnosed as anaplastic oligoastrocytomas of WHO grade III, but this may reflect relative underdiagnosis of this entity in the contributing institutions. In the CBTRUS database, anaplastic oligoastrocytomas are not listed as a separate histological entity.[16] Anaplastic oligoastrocytomas are most common in the fifth and sixth decades, with a mean age at diagnosis of 45–50 years.[77] Males are slightly more commonly affected than females.

Clinical and Radiological Features

The clinical signs and symptoms of anaplastic oligoastrocytomas do not differ from those of patients with other anaplastic gliomas. Most anaplastic oligoastrocytomas are primary tumours that present with a short clinical history. However, tumours may also develop by progression from pre-existing low-grade tumours. In such patients, clinical histories of several years may be encountered. CT and MRI readily detect the space-occupying lesion, which usually demonstrates at least focal contrast enhancement. However, some tumours may lack detectable enhancement. Undefined margins and inhomogeneous T1/T2 signals were found more commonly in anaplastic than low-grade oligoastrocytomas.[29]

Macroscopy, Microscopy and Immunohistochemistry

Anaplastic oligoastrocytomas are predominantly hemispheric tumours with a preference for the frontal lobes, followed by the temporal lobes. The macroscopic appearance is similar to other anaplastic gliomas. Microscopy shows a diffusely infiltrating oligoastrocytoma with focal or diffuse histologic signs of anaplasia. These include high cellularity, nuclear atypia, cellular pleomorphism and obvious mitotic activity. Microvascular proliferation may also be present. However, the identification of necrotic areas indicates progression towards glioblastoma with oligodendroglial component. Most commonly, the astrocytic and oligodendroglial components both demonstrate anaplastic features. In some cases, however, anaplasia may be focal and restricted to either component.

Immunohistochemically, anaplastic oligoastrocytomas share with other diffuse gliomas the frequent positivity for IDH1 R132H, which is detectable in approximately 65 per cent of the cases.[39] A recent study similarly found immunoreactivity in 55 per cent of glioblastomas with oligodendroglial component.[52] A subset of anaplastic oligoastrocytomas demonstrates strong nuclear p53 immunoreactivity. MIB–1 labelling indices are higher than in WHO grade II oligoastrocytomas, i.e., generally more than 5 per cent of tumour cells are positive for MIB–1.

Grading

Anaplastic oligoastrocytomas correspond to WHO grade III, whereas 'glioblastoma with oligodendroglial component' corresponds to WHO grade IV.

Differential Diagnosis

The most important differential diagnoses are anaplastic oligodendroglioma, anaplastic astrocytoma and glioblastoma. Among these, the distinction from anaplastic astrocytoma poses no problem when a definite oligodendroglioma component is identified. The identification of an oligodendroglial component is prognostically important, as indicated by the study of Donahue et al.[25] who reported a median overall survival of 3.0 years for patients with anaplastic astrocytomas, compared with 7.3 years for patients with an oligodendroglial component (anaplastic oligoastrocytoma). Similarly, data from the NOA–04 trial showed longer survival for patients with anaplastic oligodendroglioma or anaplastic oligoastrocytoma than with anaplastic astrocytoma.[125] The histological separation of anaplastic oligoastrocytoma

from anaplastic oligodendroglioma may be more challenging because some anaplastic oligodendrogliomas show considerable cellular pleomorphism, including tumour cells with transitional phenotypes such as gliofibrillary oligodendrocytes and minigemistocytes. The differential diagnosis between anaplastic oligoastrocytoma and 'glioblastoma with oligodendroglial component' is based on the presence of necrosis in the latter. This distinction was originally based on a retrospective analysis of a large series of malignant glioma patients that revealed significantly shorter survival of patients with anaplastic oligoastrocytomas containing areas of necrosis.[70] Although some studies suggested that 'glioblastoma with oligodendroglial component' is associated with longer survival as compared to classic glioblastoma,[70,123] other authors observed no clear survival benefit.[40] Again, this discrepancy likely reflects differences in the histological criteria that suffice to constitute an 'oligodendroglial component' within highly heterogeneous malignant gliomas, including common misdiagnosis of small cell glioblastomas as having oligodendroglial features.

Molecular Genetics

Mutations in IDH1 or IDH2 are detectable in approximately 65–70 per cent of anaplastic oligoastrocytomas.[39] Combined deletions of 1p and 19q are present in up to 50 per cent of the cases, whereas allelic losses on 17p and/or TP53 mutations are found in one third of cases, predominantly those that lack 1p/19q losses and are located in the temporal lobe.[29,91] MGMT promoter methylation is frequent in anaplastic oligoastrocytomas, in particular those carrying 1p/19q deletions and/or IDH1/2 mutations.[71,73] Progression-associated changes include allelic losses on 9p and homozygous deletion of CDKN2A, as well as losses on chromosomes 10, 11p and 13q. Amplification of proto-oncogenes, e.g. EGFR or PDGFRA, may be present but are much less common than in primary glioblastomas.[50,92]

Biological Behaviour and Prognosis

Anaplastic oligoastrocytomas are rapidly growing malignant tumours that tend to recur after treatment, which usually consists of a multimodal regimen involving resection, radiotherapy and/or chemotherapy. In patients not stratified according to the 1p/19q genotype, median overall survival of 2.8 years and 5- and 10-year survival rates of 36 per cent and 9 per cent have been reported.[103] However, similar to anaplastic oligodendroglioma, survival of anaplastic oligoastrocytoma patients is significantly longer in patients with 1p/19q-deleted tumours.[12,117] Moreover, IDH1 mutation and MGMT promoter methylation are favourable prognostic factors.[118,125] On the other hand, loss of chromosome 10 seems to be an unfavourable prognostic factor with significantly shorter progression free (13 vs 60 months) and overall survival times (24 vs 108 months).[29] Concerning the prognostic role of necrosis, a study on 866 adult patients with high-grade diffuse gliomas, including 180 anaplastic oligoastrocytoma patients, indicated that the presence of necrosis in an anaplastic oligoastrocytoma indicates a significantly worse prognosis, i.e. median overall survival of 20.7 months versus >96 months in patients whose tumours lacked necrosis.[70] As stated earlier, based on these data and others, the WHO classification recommended stratifying high-grade oligoastrocytomas into either anaplastic oligoastrocytomas (WHO grade III) or glioblastoma with oligodendroglial component (WHO grade IV) based on absence or presence of necrosis.[122]

OTHER MIXED GLIOMAS

In the older literature, rare cases of mixed gliomas other than oligoastrocytomas have been reported, including a few tumours reportedly composed of oligodendroglioma and ependymoma,[37] as well as individual cases of mixed ependymoma–astrocytomas located in the cerebral cortex or cerebello–pontine angle. However, the existence of truly mixed 'oligoependymomas' is questionable, in particular because it is known that clear cell ependymoma may closely mimic the morphological appearance of oligodendroglioma. Similarly, it remains open whether mixed 'ependymoma–astrocytoma' truly exists. The differential diagnosis would include other entities that may demonstrate both a fibrillar matrix and variably angiocentric features, such as subependymoma, tanycytic ependymoma, astroblastoma, pilomyxoid astrocytoma and angiocentric glioma.

REFERENCES

1. Aerts I, Pacquement H, Doz F, et al. Outcome of second malignancies after retinoblastoma: a retrospective analysis of 25 patients treated at the Institut Curie. *Eur J Cancer* 2004;**40**:1522–9.
2. Appolloni I, Calzolari F, Tutucci E, et al. PDGF–B induces a homogeneous class of oligodendrogliomas from embryonic neural progenitors. *Int J Cancer* 2009;**124**:2251–9.
3. Badiali M, Gleize V, Paris S, et al. KIAA1549–BRAF fusions and IDH mutations can coexist in diffuse gliomas of adults. *Brain Pathol* 2012;**22**(6):841–7.
4. Bannykh SI, Stolt CC, Kim J, Perry A, Wegner M. Oligodendroglial-specific transcriptional factor SOX10 is ubiquitously expressed in human gliomas. *J Neurooncol* 2006;**76**:115–27.
5. Bettegowda C, Agrawal N, Jiao Y, et al. Mutations in CIC and FUBP1 contribute to human oligodendroglioma. *Science* 2011;**333**:1453–5.
6. Bian W, Khayal IS, Lupo JM, et al. Multiparametric characterization of grade 2 glioma subtypes using magnetic resonance spectroscopic, perfusion and diffusion imaging. *Transl Oncol* 2009;**2**:271–80.
7. Blough MD, Al-Najjar M, Chesnelong C, et al. DNA hypermethylation and 1p Loss silence NHE–1 in oligodendroglioma. *Ann Neurol* 2012;**71**:845–9.
8. Blümcke I, Becker AJ, Normann S, et al. Distinct expression pattern of microtubule-associated protein–2 in human oligodendrogliomas and glial precursor cells. *J Neuropathol Exp Neurol* 2001;**60**:984–93.
9. Bowers DC, Mulne AF, Weprin B, et al. Prognostic factors in children and adolescents with low-grade oligodendrogliomas. *Pediatr Neurosurg* 2002;**37**:57–63.
10. Brat DJ, Scheithauer BW, Eberhart CG, Burger PC. Extraventricular neurocytomas: pathologic features and clinical outcome. *Am J Surg Pathol* 2001;**25**:1252–60.
11. Burger PC, Pearl DK, Aldape K, et al. Small cell architecture – a histological equivalent of EGFR amplification in glioblastoma multiforme? *J Neuropathol Exp Neurol* 2001;**60**:1099–104.
12. Cairncross G, Berkey B, Shaw E, et al. Phase III trial of chemotherapy plus radiotherapy compared with radiotherapy alone for pure and mixed anaplastic oligodendroglioma: Intergroup Radiation Therapy Oncology Group Trial 9402. *J Clin Oncol* 2006;**24**:2707–14.
13. Cairncross JG, Ueki K, Zlatescu MC, et al. Specific genetic predictors of chemotherapeutic response and survival in patients with anaplastic oligodendrogliomas. *J Natl Cancer Inst* 1998;**90**:1473–9.
14. Cairncross JG, Wang M, Shaw EG, et al. Phase III trial of chemoradiotherapy for anaplastic oligodendroglioma: long-term results of RTOG 9402. *J Clin Oncol* 2013;**31**:337–43.
15. Capper D, Reuss D, Schittenhelm J, et al. Mutation-specific IDH1 antibody differentiates oligodendrogliomas and oligoastrocytomas from other brain tumors with oligodendroglioma-like morphology. *Acta Neuropathol* 2011;**121**:241–52.
16. CBTRUS (2012). *CBTRUS statistical report: primary brain and central nervous system tumors diagnosed in the United States in 2004–2008* (March 23, 2012 Revision). Source: Central Brain Tumor Registry of the United States, Hinsdale, IL. website:www.cbtrus.org
17. Chang S, Prados MD. Identical twins with Ollier's disease and intracranial gliomas: case report. *Neurosurgery* 1994;**34**:903–6.
18. Choi C, Ganji SK, DeBerardinis RJ, et al. 2–hydroxyglutarate detection by magnetic resonance spectroscopy in IDH-mutated patients with gliomas. *Nat Med* 2012;**18**:624–9.
19. Chorneyko K, Maguire J, Simon GT. Oligodendroglioma with granular cells: a case report. *Ultrastruct Pathol* 1998;**22**:79–82.
20. Coons SW, Johnson PC, Pearl DK. The prognostic significance of Ki–67 labelling indices for oligodendrogliomas. *Neurosurgery* 1997;**41**:878–84.
21. Dai C, Lyustikman Y, Shih A, et al. The characteristics of astrocytomas and oligodendrogliomas are caused by two distinct and interchangeable signaling formats. *Neoplasia* 2005;**7**:397–406.
22. Dehghani F, Schachenmayr W, Laun A, Korf HW. Prognostic implication of histopathological, immunohistochemical and clinical features of oligodendrogliomas: a study of 89 cases. *Acta Neuropathol* (Berl) 1998;**95**:493–504.
23. Del Valle L, Enam S, Lara C, et al. Detection of JC polyomavirus DNA sequences and cellular localization of T-antigen and agnoprotein in oligodendrogliomas. *Clin Cancer Res* 2002;**8**:3332–40.
24. Di Rocco F, Carroll RS, Zhang J, Black PM. Platelet-derived growth factor and its receptor expression in human oligodendrogliomas. *Neurosurgery* 1998;**42**:341–6.
25. Donahue B, Scott CB, Nelson JS, et al. Influence of an oligodendroglial component on the survival of patients with anaplastic astrocytomas: a report of Radiation Therapy Oncology Group 83–02. *Int J Radiat Oncol Biol Phys* 1997;**38**:911–4.
26. Ducray F, Crinière E, Idbaih A, et al. alpha–Internexin expression identifies 1p19q codeleted gliomas. *Neurology* 2009;**72**:156–61.
27. Ducray F, Idbaih A, de Reyniès A, et al. Anaplastic oligodendrogliomas with 1p19q codeletion have a proneural gene expression profile. *Mol Cancer* 2008;**7**:41.
28. Eigenbrod S, Roeber S, Thon N, et al. Internexin in the diagnosis of oligodendroglial tumors and association with 1p/19q status. *J Neuropathol Exp Neurol* 2011;**70**:970–8.
29. Eoli M, Bissola L, Bruzzone MG, et al. Reclassification of oligoastrocytomas by loss of heterozygosity studies. *Int J Cancer* 2006;**119**:84–90.
30. Feigin I, Epstein F, Mangiardi J. Extensive advanced maturation of medulloblastoma to astrocytoma and ependymoma. *J Neurooncol* 1983;**1**:95–108.
31. Flannery T, Cawley D, Zulfiger A, et al. Familial occurrence of oligodendroglial tumours. *Br J Neurosurg* 2008;**22**:436–8.
32. Fountas KN, Karampelas I, Nikolakakos LG, Troup EC, Robinson JS. Primary spinal cord oligodendroglioma: case report and review of the literature. *Childs Nerv Syst* 2005;**21**:171–5.
33. Fujisawa H, Marukawa K, Hasegawa M, et al. Genetic differences between neurocytoma and dysembryoplastic neuroepithelial tumour and oligodendroglial tumours. *J Neurosurg* 2002;**97**:1350–5.
34. Giammarile F, Cinotti LE, Jouvet A, et al. High and low grade oligodendrogliomas

(ODG): correlation of amino-acid and glucose uptakes using PET and histological classifications. *J Neurooncol* 2004;68:263–74.

35. Giannini C, Scheithauer BW, Weaver AL, et al. Oligodendrogliomas: reproducibility and prognostic value of histologic diagnosis and grading. *J Neuropathol Exp Neurol* 2001;60:248–62.

36. Golfinos JG, Norman SA, Coons SW, et al. Expression of the genes encoding myelin basic protein and proteolipid protein in human malignant gliomas. *Clin Cancer Res* 1997;3:799–804.

37. Hart MN, Petito CK, Earle KM. Mixed gliomas. *Cancer* 1974;33:134–140.

38. Hartmann C, Hentschel B, Tatagiba M, et al. Molecular markers in low-grade gliomas: predictive or prognostic? *Clin Cancer Res* 2011;17:4588–99.

39. Hartmann C, Meyer J, Balss J, et al. Type and frequency of *IDH1* and IDH2 mutations are related to astrocytic and oligodendroglial differentiation and age: a study of 1010 diffuse gliomas. *Acta Neuropathol* 2009;118:469–74.

40. Hegi ME, Janzer RC, Lambiv WL, et al. Presence of an oligodendroglioma-like component in newly diagnosed glioblastoma identifies a pathogenetically heterogeneous subgroup and lacks prognostic value: central pathology review of the EORTC_26981/NCIC_CE.3 trial. *Acta Neuropathol* 2012;123:841–52.

41. Herpers MJ, Budka H. Glial fibrillary acidic protein (GFAP) in oligodendroglial tumours: gliofibrillary oligodendroglioma and transitional oligoastrocytoma as subtypes of oligodendroglioma. *Acta Neuropathol* (Berl) 1984;64:265–72.

42. Hoang–Xuan K, Capelle L, Kujas M, et al. Temozolomide as initial treatment for adults with low-grade oligodendrogliomas or oligoastrocytomas and correlation with chromosome 1p deletions. *J Clin Oncol* 2004;22:3133–8.

43. Hoffman S, Propp JM, McCarthy BJ. Temporal trends in incidence of primary brain tumours in the United States, 1985–1999. *Neuro Oncol* 2006;8:27–37.

44. Jiao Y, Killela PJ, Reitman ZJ, et al. Frequent *ATRX*, *CIC* , and *FUBP1* mutations refine the classification of malignant gliomas. *Oncotarget* 2012;3:709–22.

45. Jenkins RB, Blair H, Ballman KV, et al. A t(1;19)(q10;p10) mediates the combined deletions of 1p and 19q and predicts a better prognosis of patients with oligodendroglioma. *Cancer Res* 2006;66:9852–61.

46. Jenkins RB, Xiao Y, Sicotte H, et al. A low-frequency variant at 8q24.21 is strongly associated with risk of oligodendroglial tumors and astrocytomas with *IDH1* or IDH2 mutation. *Nat Genet* 2012;44(10):1122–5.

47. Jenkinson MD, du Plessis DG, Smith TS, et al. Histological growth patterns and genotype in oligodendroglial tumours: correlation with MRI features. *Brain* 2006;129:1884–91.

48. Jentoft M, Giannini C, Rossi S, et al. Oligodendroglial tumors with marked desmoplasia: clinicopathologic and molecular features of 7 cases. *Am J Surg Pathol* 2011;35:845–52.

49. Jeuken JW, Sprenger SH, Boerman RH, et al. Subtyping of oligo-astrocytic tumours by comparative genomic hybridization. *J Pathol* 2001;194:81–7.

50. Jeuken JW, von Deimling A, Wesseling P. Molecular pathogenesis of oligodendroglial tumours. *J Neurooncol* 2004;70:161–81.

51. Johannsson O, Ostermeyer EA, Hakansson S, et al. Founding BRCA1 mutations in hereditary breast and ovarian cancer in southern Sweden. *Am J Hum Genet* 1996;58:441–50.

52. Joseph NM, Phillips J, Dahiya S, et al. Diagnostic implications of *IDH1*–R132H and OLIG2 expression patterns in rare and challenging glioblastoma variants. *Modern Pathology* 2013;26(3):315–26.

53. Kesari S, Schiff D, Drappatz J, et al. Phase II study of protracted daily temozolomide for low-grade gliomas in adults. *Clin Cancer Res* 2009;15:330–7.

54. Kim YH, Lachuer J, Mittelbronn M, et al. Alterations in the RB1 pathway in low-grade diffuse gliomas lacking common genetic alterations. *Brain Pathol* 2011;21:645–51.

55. Kim YH, Nobusawa S, Mittelbronn M, et al. Molecular classification of low-grade diffuse gliomas. *Am J Pathol* 2010;177:2708–14.

56. Kim YH, Nonoguchi N, Paulus W, et al. Frequent *BRAF* gain in low-grade diffuse gliomas with 1p/19q loss. *Brain Pathol* 2012;22(6):834–40.

57. Koperek O, Gelpi E, Birner P, et al. Value and limits of immunohistochemistry in differential diagnosis of clear cell primary brain tumours. *Acta Neuropathol* (Berl) 2004;108:24–30.

58. Korshunov A, Golanov A, Sycheva R. Immunohistochemical markers for prognosis of oligodendroglial neoplasms. *J Neurooncol* 2002;58:237–53.

59. Kraus JA, Koopmann J, Kaskel P, et al. Shared allelic losses on chromosomes 1p and 19q suggest a common origin of oligodendroglioma and oligoastrocytoma. *J Neuropathol Exp Neurol* 1995;54:91–5.

60. Kros JM, de Jong AA, van der Kwast TH. Ultrastructural characterization of transitional cells in oligodendrogliomas. *J Neuropathol Exp Neurol* 1992;51:186–93.

61. Kros JM, Gorlia T, Kouwenhoven MC, et al. Panel review of anaplastic oligodendroglioma from European Organization for Research and Treatment of Cancer Trial 26951: assessment of consensus in diagnosis, influence of 1p/19q loss, and correlations with outcome. *J Neuropathol Exp Neurol* 2007;66:545–51.

62. Kros JM, van den Brink WA, van Loon–van Luyt JJ, Stefanko SZ. Signet-ring cell oligodendroglioma – report of two cases and discussion of the differential diagnosis. *Acta Neuropathol* (Berl) 1997;93:638–43.

63. Lebrun C, Fontaine D, Ramaioli A, et al. Longterm outcome of oligodendrogliomas. *Neurology* 2004;62:1783–7.

64. Levin N, Lavon I, Zelikovitsh B, et al. Progressive low-grade oligodendrogliomas: response to temozolomide and correlation between genetic profile and O6–methylguanine DNA methyltransferase protein expression. *Cancer* 2006;106:1759–65.

65. Liu XY, Gerges N, Korshunov A, et al. Frequent *ATRX* mutations and loss of

expression in adult diffuse astrocytic tumors carrying *IDH1*/IDH2 and *TP53* mutations. *Acta Neuropathol* 2012;124(5):615–25.

66. Maintz D, Fiedler K, Koopmann J, et al. Molecular genetic evidence for subtypes of oligoastrocytomas. *J Neuropathol Exp Neurol* 1997;56:1098–104.

67. McCarthy BJ, Propp JM, Davis FG, Burger PC. Time trends in oligodendroglial and astrocytic tumor incidence. *Neuroepidemiology* 2008;30:34–44.

68. Megyesi JF, Kachur E, Lee DH, et al. Imaging correlates of molecular signatures in oligodendrogliomas. *Clin Cancer Res* 2004;10:4303–6.

69. Menko FH, Kaspers GL, Meijer GA, et al. A homozygous MSH6 mutation in a child with cafe-au-lait spots, oligodendroglioma and rectal cancer. *Fam Cancer* 2004;3:123–7.

70. Miller CR, Dunham CP, Scheithauer BW, Perry A. Significance of necrosis in grading of oligodendroglial neoplasms: a clinicopathologic and genetic study of newly diagnosed high-grade gliomas. *J Clin Oncol* 2006;24:5419–26.

71. Möllemann M, Wolter M, Felsberg J, Collins VP, Reifenberger G. Frequent promoter hypermethylation and low expression of the *MGMT* gene in oligodendroglial tumours. *Int J Cancer* 2005;113:379–85.

72. Mueller W, Hartmann C, Hoffmann A, et al. Genetic signature of oligoastrocytomas correlates with tumour location and denotes distinct molecular subsets. *Am J Pathol* 2002;161:313–9.

73. Mulholland S, Pearson DM, Hamoudi RA, et al. MGMT CpG island is invariably methylated in adult astrocytic and oligodendroglial tumors with *IDH1* or IDH2 mutations. Int *J Cancer* 2012;131:1104–13.

74. Nakagawa Y, Perentes E, Rubinstein LJ. Immunohistochemical characterization of oligodendrogliomas: an analysis of multiple markers. *Acta Neuropathol* (Berl) 1986;72:15–22.

75. Nijjar TS, Simpson WJ, Gadalla T, McCartney M. Oligodendroglioma. The Princess Margaret Hospital experience (1958–1984). *Cancer* 1993;71:4002–6.

76. Noushmehr H, Weisenberger DJ, Diefes K, et al. Identification of a CpG island methylator phenotype that defines a distinct subgroup of glioma. *Cancer Cell* 2010;17:510–22.

77. Ohgaki H, Kleihues P. Population-based studies on incidence, survival rates and genetic alterations in astrocytic and oligodendroglial gliomas. *J Neuropathol Exp Neurol* 2005;64:479–89.

78. Olson JD, Riedel E, DeAngelis LM. Longterm outcome of low-grade oligodendroglioma and mixed glioma. *Neurology* 2000;54:1442–8.

79. Perry A, Aldape KD, George DH, Burger PC. Small cell astrocytoma: an aggressive variant that is clinicopathologically and genetically distinct from anaplastic oligodendroglioma. *Cancer* 2004;101:2318–26.

80. Perry A, Burton SS, Fuller GN, et al. Oligodendroglial neoplasms with ganglioglioma-like maturation: a diagnostic pitfall. *Acta Neuropathol* 2010;120:237–52.

81. Perry A, Scheithauer BW, Macaulay RJ, et al. Oligodendrogliomas with neurocytic differentiation. A report of 4 cases with diagnostic and histogenetic implications. *J Neuropathol Exp Neurol* 2002;61:947–55.

82. Persson AI, Petritsch C, Swartling FJ, et al. Non-stem cell origin for oligodendroglioma. *Cancer Cell* 2010;18:669–82.

83. Prayson RA, Castilla EA, Hembury TA, et al. Interobserver variability in determining MIB–1 labelling indices in oligodendrogliomas. *Ann Diagn Pathol* 2003;7:9–13.

84. Preusser M, Hoeftberger R, Woehrer A, et al. Prognostic value of Ki67 index in anaplastic oligodendroglial tumours – a translational study of the European Organization for Research and Treatment of Cancer Brain Tumor Group. *Histopathology* 2012;60:885–94.

85. Puduvalli VK, Hashmi M, McAllister LD, et al. Anaplastic oligodendrogliomas: prognostic factors for tumour recurrence and survival. *Oncology* 2003;65:259–66.

86. Raghavan R, Balani J, Perry A, et al. Pediatric oligodendrogliomas: a study of molecular alterations on 1p and 19q using fluorescence *in situ* hybridization. *J Neuropathol Exp Neurol* 2003;62:530–7.

87. Reifenberger G, Kros JM, Louis DN, Collins VP. Oligodendroglioma. In: Louis DN, Ohgaki H, Wiestler OD, Cavenee WK eds. *World Health Organization classification of tumours of the central nervous system.* Lyon: IARC, 2007:54–59.

88. Reifenberger G, Kros JM, Louis DN, Collins VP. Anaplastic Oligodendroglioma. In: Louis DN, Ohgaki H, Wiestler OD, Cavenee WK eds. *World Health Organization classification of tumours of the central nervous system.* Lyon: IARC, 2007:60–62.

89. Reis–Filho JS, Faoro LN, Carrilho C, Bleggi–Torres LF, Schmitt FC. Evaluation of cell proliferation, epidermal growth factor receptor and bcl–2 immunoexpression as prognostic factors for patients with World Health Organization grade 2 oligodendroglioma. *Cancer* 2000;88:862–9.

90. Rickert CH, Korshunov A, Paulus W. Chromosomal imbalances in clear cell ependymomas. *Mod Pathol* 2006;19:958–62.

91. Riemenschneider MJ, Jeuken JW, Wesseling P, Reifenberger G. Molecular diagnostics of gliomas: state of the art. *Acta Neuropathol* 2010 Nov;120(5):567–84.

92. Riemenschneider MJ, Reifenberger G. Molecular neuropathology of gliomas. *Int J Mol Sci* 2009;10:184–212.

93. Riemenschneider MJ, Reifenberger G. Molecular neuropathology of low-grade gliomas and its clinical impact. *Adv Tech Stand Neurosurg* 2010;35:35–64.

94. Rodriguez FJ, Perry A, Rosenblum MK, et al. Disseminated oligodendroglial-like leptomeningeal tumor of childhood: a distinctive clinicopathologic entity. *Acta Neuropathol* 2012;124(5):627–41.

95. Rodriguez FJ, Scheithauer BW, Jenkins R, et al. Gliosarcoma arising in oligodendroglial tumors ('oligosarcoma'): a clinicopathologic study. *Am J Surg Pathol* 2007;31:351–62.

96. Rollison DE, Utaipat U, Ryschkewitsch C, et al. Investigation of human brain tumours for the presence of polyomavirus genome sequences by two independent laboratories. *Int J Cancer* 2005;113:769–74.

97. Sahm F, Koelsche C, Meyer J, et al. *CIC* and *FUBP1* mutations in oligodendrogliomas, oligoastrocytomas and astrocytomas. *Acta Neuropathol* 2012;123:853–60.

98. Sasaki H, Zlatescu MC, Betensky RA, et al. Histopathological-molecular genetic correlations in referral pathologist-diagnosed low-grade 'oligodendroglioma'. *J Neuropathol Exp Neurol* 2002;61:58–63.

99. Sasaki H, Zlatescu MC, Betensky RA, et al. *PTEN* is a target of chromosome 10q loss in anaplastic oligodendrogliomas and *PTEN* alterations are associated with poor prognosis. *Am J Pathol* 2001;159:359–67.

100. Scheie D, Meling TR, Cvancarova M, et al. Prognostic variables in oligodendroglial tumors: a single-institution study of 95 cases. *Neuro Oncol* 2011;13:1225–33.

101. Shaffrey ME, Farace E, Schiff D, et al. The Ki–67 labelling index as a prognostic factor in grade II oligoastrocytomas. *J Neurosurg* 2005;102:1033–9.

102. Shaw E, Arusell R, Scheithauer B, et al. Prospective randomized trial of low- versus high-dose radiation therapy in adults with supratentorial low-grade glioma: initial report of a North Central Cancer Treatment Group/Radiation Therapy Oncology Group/Eastern Cooperative Oncology Group study. *J Clin Oncol* 2002;20:2267–76.

103. Shaw EG, Scheithauer BW, O'Fallon JR, Davis DH. Mixed oligoastrocytomas: a survival and prognostic factor analysis. *Neurosurgery* 1994;34:577–82.

104. Shaw EG, Scheithauer BW, O'Fallon JR, Tazelaar HD, Davis DH. Oligodendrogliomas: the Mayo Clinic experience. *J Neurosurg* 1992;76:428–34.

105. Shaw EG, Wang M, Coons SW, et al. Randomized trial of radiation therapy plus procarbazine, lomustine, and vincristine chemotherapy for supratentorial adult low-grade glioma: initial results of RTOG 9802. *J Clin Oncol* 2012;30:3065–70.

106. Shinozaki N, Uchino Y, Yoshikawa K, et al. Discrimination between low-grade oligodendroglioma and diffuse astrocytoma with the aid of 11C–methionine positron emission tomography. *J Neurosurg* 2011;114:1640–7.

107. Sugiarto S, Persson AI, Munoz EG, et al. Asymmetry-defective oligodendrocyte progenitors are glioma precursors. *Cancer Cell* 2011;20:328–40.

108. Suri V, Jha P, Agarwal S, et al. Molecular profile of oligodendrogliomas in young patients. *Neuro Oncol* 2011;13:1099–106.

109. Taillibert S, Chodkiewicz C, Laigle–Donadey F, et al. Gliomatosis cerebri: a review of 296 cases from the ANOCEF database and the literature. *J Neurooncol* 2006;76:201–5.

110. Taylor MD, Perry J, Zlatescu MC, et al. The hPMS2 exon 5 mutation and malignant glioma. Case report. *J Neurosurg* 1999;90:946–50.

111. Tice H, Barnes PD, Goumnerova L, Scott RM, Tarbell NJ. Pediatric and adolescent oligodendrogliomas. *AJNR Am J Neuroradiol* 1993;14:1293–300.

112. Trost D, Ehrler M, Fimmers R, et al. Identification of genomic aberrations associated with shorter overall survival in patients with oligodendroglial tumors. *Int J Cancer* 2007;120:2368–76.

113. Turcan S, Rohle D, Goenka A, et al. IDH1 mutation is sufficient to establish the glioma hypermethylator phenotype. *Nature* 2012;483:479–83.

114. Ud Din N, Memon A, Aftab K, et al. Oligodendroglioma arising in the glial component of ovarian teratomas: a series of six cases and review of literature. *J Clin Pathol* 2012;65:631–4.

115. van den Bent MJ, Afra D, de Witte O, et al. Longterm efficacy of early versus delayed radiotherapy for low-grade astrocytoma and oligodendroglioma in adults: the EORTC 22845 randomized trial. *Lancet* 2005;366:985–90.

116. van den Bent MJ, Brandes AA, Taphoorn MJ, et al. Adjuvant procarbazine, lomustine, and vincristine chemotherapy in newly diagnosed anaplastic oligodendroglioma: longterm follow-up of EORTC Brain Tumor Group Study 26951. *J Clin Oncol* 2013;49(16):3477–85.

117. van den Bent MJ, Carpentier AF, Brandes AA, et al. Adjuvant procarbazine, lomustine, and vincristine improves progression-free survival but not overall survival in newly diagnosed anaplastic oligodendrogliomas and oligoastrocytomas: a randomized European Organisation for Research and Treatment of Cancer phase III trial. *J Clin Oncol* 2006;24:2715–22.

118. van den Bent MJ, Dubbink HJ, Marie Y, et al. IDH1 and IDH2 mutations are prognostic but not predictive for outcome in anaplastic oligodendroglial tumors: a report of the European Organization for Research and Treatment of Cancer Brain Tumor Group. *Clin Cancer Res* 2010;16:1597–604.

119. van den Bent MJ, Gravendeel LA, Gorlia T, et al. A hypermethylated phenotype is a better predictor of survival than MGMT methylation in anaplastic oligodendroglial brain tumors: a report from EORTC study 26951. *Clin Cancer Res* 2011;17:7148–55.

120. van den Bent MJ, Reni M, Gatta G, Vecht C. Oligodendroglioma. *Crit Rev Oncol Hematol* 2008;66:262–72.

121. von Deimling A, Reifenberger G, Kros JM, Louis DN, Collins VP. Oligoastrocytoma. In: Louis DN, Ohgaki H, Wiestler OD, Cavenee WK eds. *World Health Organization classification of tumours of the central nervous system.* Lyon: IARC, 2007:63–65.

122. von Deimling A, Reifenberger G, Kros JM, Louis DN, Collins VP. Anaplastic oligoastrocytoma. In: Louis DN, Ohgaki H, Wiestler OD, Cavenee WK eds. World Health Organization Classification of Tumours of the Central Nervous System. Lyon: IARC, 2007:66–67.

123. Wang Y, Li S, Chen L, et al. Glioblastoma with an oligodendroglioma component: distinct clinical behavior, genetic alterations, and outcome. *Neuro Oncol* 2012;14:518–25.

124. Wharton SB, Chan KK, Anderson JR, Stoeber K, Williams GH. Replicative Mcm2 protein as a novel proliferation marker in oligodendrogliomas and its relationship to Ki67 labelling index, histological grade and prognosis. *Neuropathol Appl Neurobiol* 2001;27:305–13.

125. Wick W, Hartmann C, Engel C, *et al.* NOA–04 randomised phase III trial of sequential radiochemotherapy of anaplastic glioma with procarbazine, lomustine, and vincristine or temozolomide. *J Clin Oncol* 2009;**27**:5874–80.

126. Weller M, Stupp R, Hegi ME, *et al.* Personalized care in neuro-oncology coming of age: why we need *MGMT* and 1p/19q testing for malignant glioma patients in clinical practice. *Neuro Oncol* 2012;**14**(4):iv100–8.

127. Yip S, Butterfield YS, Morozova O, *et al.* Concurrent *CIC* mutations, IDH mutations, and 1p/19q loss distinguish oligodendrogliomas from other cancers. *J Pathol* 2012;**226**:7–16.

128. Zlatescu MC, Tehrani-Yazdi A, Sasaki H, *et al.* Tumour location and growth pattern correlate with genetic signature in oligodendroglial neoplasms. *Cancer Res* 2001;**61**:6713–5.

129. Zong H, Verhaak RG, Canolk P. The cellular origin for malignant glioma and prospects for clinical advancements. *Expert Rev Mol Diagn* 2012;**12**:383–94.

Ependymal Tumours

Guido Reifenberger

INTRODUCTION

This group of gliomas comprises neoplasms of ependymal differentiation, including ependymomas and its variants, anaplastic (malignant) ependymomas, myxopapillary ependymomas and subependymomas. The rare ependymoblastoma is discussed in Chapter 34, Embryonal Tumours.

EPENDYMOMA

Ependymoma is defined as a slowly growing glioma composed of neoplastic cells with ependymal differentiation, commonly originating from the walls of the cerebral ventricles or spinal canal. Ependymomas mostly manifest in children and young adults. Key histological features include perivascular pseudorosettes and true ependymal rosettes.

Incidence, Age and Sex Distribution

According to the Central Brain Tumor Registry of the United States (CBTRUS), ependymoma, anaplastic ependymoma and ependymoma variants account for approximately 1.8 per cent of all primary brain tumours and 5.8 per cent of all gliomas.[8] The adjusted overall annual incidence rate is estimated at 0.36 per 100 000 population.[8] In children below 14 and between 15 and 19 years of age, ependymal tumours are estimated to account for 5.7 per cent and 4.5 per cent of all primary central nervous system (CNS) tumours, respectively.[8] A population-based study on paediatric brain tumours in England and Wales reported that 6.7 per cent of all gliomas in children below 15 years were ependymomas.[79] Data from the European Automated Childhood Cancer Information System (ACCIS) database indicate an annual incidence rate of 0.34 per 100 000 in children aged 0–14 years,[53] whereas CBTRUS[8] estimates incidence rates of 0.26 per 100 000 in children below 14 years and 0.39 per 100 000 in infants below 4 years of age. Ependymoma is the most common glioma in the spinal cord.

Ependymomas can develop at any age. However, there are two distinct incidence peaks: the first one in children below 14 years of age and the second one in adults between 35 and 45 years of age. Supratentorial ependymomas affect both children and adults, infratentorial tumours predominate in children and spinal cord ependymomas usually present in adults. Ependymal tumours are more common in white than in black people.[8] There is a slight male predominance.[8,42]

Clinical and Radiological Features

Clinical manifestations depend on tumour location. Posterior fossa ependymomas often present with nausea, vomiting and headache related to hydrocephalus and raised intracranial pressure caused by obstruction of the fourth ventricle. Other symptoms include ataxia, nystagmus, gaze palsy, dizziness, hemiparesis and neck pain. Infants under 2 years of age may show increased head circumference because their cranial sutures are still open. The clinical symptomatology of supratentorial ependymomas results from a combination of mass effect and focal neurological deficit to produce headache, nausea, vomiting, seizure, papilloedema, hemiparesis, apraxia, visual field loss, intellectual impairment and/or behavioural changes. Under 3 years of age, intracranial ependymomas present, in order of decreasing frequency, with vomiting, ataxia, headache, lethargy, increased head circumference and irritability.[9] Spinal tumours manifest with motor and sensory disturbances caused by compression of the relevant tracts.

On computed tomography (CT) imaging, intracranial ependymomas are isodense or of mixed density and show contrast enhancement. Cystic changes, calcifications and intratumoural haemorrhages may be present. On T1-weighted MRI, ependymomas typically present as hypointense or isointense

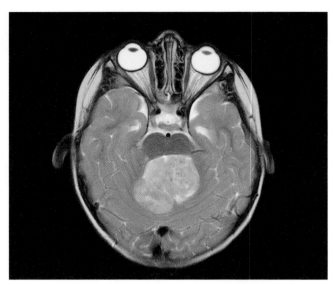

29.1 Ependymoma. Magnetic resonance imaging of a well-demarcated tumour in the fourth ventricle of a 3-year-old girl.

Courtesy of Dr B Turowski, Department of Neuroradiology, Heinrich Heine University, Düsseldorf, Germany.

lesions with varying contrast enhancement. On T2-weighted, proton density and FLAIR images, ependymomas are hyperintense to grey matter (Figure 29.1). The tumours generally appear as well circumscribed lesions, usually with no or only little perifocal oedema. Obstructive hydrocephalus is a common feature. Supratentorial parenchymal ependymomas are often large, cystic mass lesions in children and young adults, sometimes with no clear ventricular involvement. Their neuroradiological distinction from other primary brain tumours is difficult. Spinal cord ependymomas typically present as well circumscribed intramedullary tumours, most commonly in the cervical and cervicothoracic cord. They are often associated with rostral or caudal syrinx formation. On MRI, spinal intramedullary ependymomas are usually iso- to hypointense on T1-weighted images and hyperintense on T2-weighted images. Gadolinium enhancement is invariable.

Localization and Macroscopy

Ependymomas can occur anywhere along the craniospinal axis. Intracranial ependymomas are solid, well circumscribed, soft and greyish-red tumours. Some show cystic degeneration, necrosis or haemorrhage. Approximately 60 per cent of all intracranial ependymomas present in the fourth ventricle. Depending on tumour location and growth pattern, midfloor, lateral and roof types have been distinguished, with survival being shorter in patients with lateral, as compared to medial, tumours.[23] Interestingly, molecular analyses have linked these regional differences to distinct gene expression profiles that define prognostically distinct molecular subtypes of posterior fossa ependymoma.[87] Macroscopically, ependymomas of the fourth ventricle usually form an exophytic growth filling the cavity, encroaching surrounding structures and causing obstructive hydrocephalus (Figure 29.2a). Some tumours grow extraventricularly, extending through the foramina into the cerebellopontine angle, or protruding into the cisterna magna, sometimes

extending through the foramen magnum to the cervical cord. These extracerebral extensions may undergo degenerative changes, cyst formation and calcification.

Approximately 40 per cent of all intracranial ependymomas are supratentorial, with the majority being located near the lateral ventricles. These tumours often involve the adjacent cerebral parenchyma. They are well demarcated and do not diffusely infiltrate the brain. Ependymomas of the third ventricle are rare. Occasionally, ependymomas arise as primary intraparenchymal brain lesions without any contact to the ventricular system, including rare cases of primary cortical ependymoma.[64] In the spinal cord, ependymomas appear as intramedullary, well demarcated but unencapsulated lesions involving several spinal segments. An accompanying syrinx is seen in approximately 65 per cent of cases. Two thirds arise from or extend into the cervical cord.

Rare ependymomas have been reported in the sellar region[72] or the trigeminal nerve.[38] Other uncommon sites of primary extraneural ependymomas include the ovaries, liver, soft tissues and mediastinum.

Microscopy

Ependymomas are moderately cellular tumours with neoplastic cells maintaining many features of normal ependymal cells (Figure 29.2b,c). The tumour cells usually have monomorphic round or oval nuclei with abundant, clumped chromatin. Mitotic activity is absent or low. Thin cytoplasmic processes often impart a gliofibrillary background, which is variable from area to area. The most important diagnostic hallmark of ependymoma is the formation of two characteristic rosette-like structures, namely the perivascular pseudorosette and the true ependymal rosette (Figure 29.2b,c). The former consists of neoplastic cells arranged circumferentially with processes projecting towards a centrally located blood vessel. Perivascular pseudorosettes are seen in the vast majority of ependymomas. In contrast, ependymal rosettes occur only in a minor fraction of tumours. These diagnostic structures are composed of columnar cells that mimic the normal ventricular lining and the central canal by forming rounded ependymal rosettes (Figure 29.2c) or sometimes slit-like or tubular structures known as ependymal canals. In contrast to the diffuse gliomas, ependymomas feature a sharp interface with surrounding CNS parenchyma. Some ependymomas demonstrate regressive changes such as mucoid or cystic degeneration as well as focal calcifications. Hyalinisation and thickening of blood vessel walls is common. In the absence of other features of anaplasia, areas of non-palisading necrosis are still compatible with a WHO grade II ependymoma.

Histological Variants

The WHO classification distinguishes four variants: cellular, papillary, clear cell and tanycytic ependymoma.[44]

Cellular ependymoma is the most common, characterized by solid growth of densely packed tumour cells with fewer tendencies to form rosettes and perivascular pseudorosettes. In contrast to anaplastic ependymoma and medulloblastoma, mitotic activity is low and primitive features are absent.

Papillary ependymomas are rare and are characterized by gliovascular papillary structures with tumour cells forming perivascular pseudorosettes (Figure 29.2d). On haematoxylin and eosin (H&E)-stained sections, papillary ependymoma may mimic other papillary tumours, such as choroid plexus papilloma, papillary meningioma or metastatic papillary carcinoma. However, immunocytochemical studies readily distinguish these entities.

Clear cell ependymoma constitutes a rare variant preferentially developing supratentorially in children and young adults, with spinal examples being less common. The tumours are composed of oligodendroglia-like cells

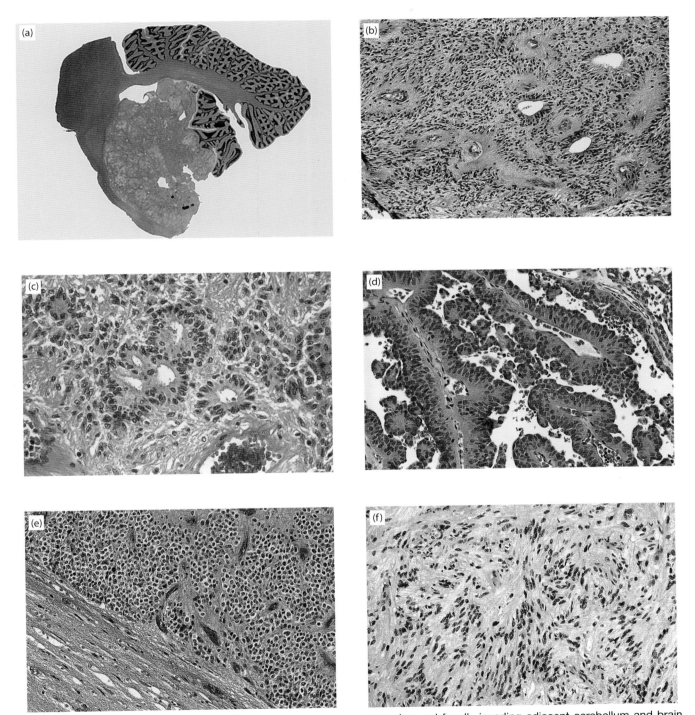

29.2 Ependymoma. (a) The neoplasms fill the fourth ventricle, compressing and focally invading adjacent cerebellum and brain stem. Haematoxylin and eosin (H&E). **(b)** The neoplastic cells form perivascular pseudorosettes, ependymal canals or solid islands with a fibrillary stroma. H&E. **(c)** Ependymal rosette formation. H&E. **(d)** Papillary ependymoma resembling a choroid plexus papilloma. H&E. **(e)** Clear cell ependymoma showing a well-defined border with adjacent brain. The cells with clear cytoplasm mimic oligodendroglioma. H&E. **(f)** Tanycytic ependymoma composed of elongated fibrillary cells. H&E.

Continued

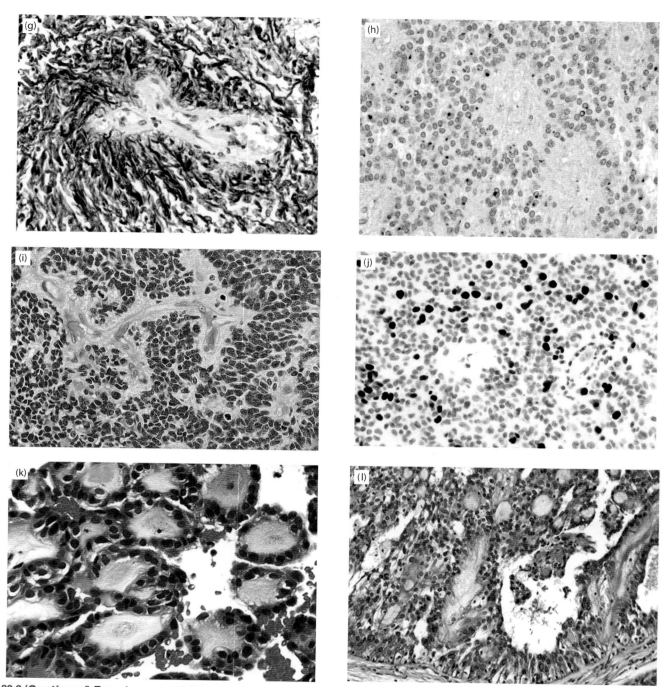

29.2 (Continued) Ependymoma. (g) Ependymoma with pronounced GFAP immunoreactivity in perivascular tumour cell processes. **(h)** Ependymoma with characteristic dot- and ring-like intracytoplasmic EMA-positivity. **(i)** Increased cell density in an anaplastic ependymoma with mitotic activity. H&E. **(j)** High Ki–67 (MIB–1) staining index in an anaplastic ependymoma. **(k)** Myxopapillary ependymoma. Columnar and cuboidal cells line the acellular stroma. H&E. **(l)** Myxopapillary ependymoma showing the typical architecture. Glial fibrillary acidic protein (GFAP) immunostaining and periodic acid Schiff (PAS).

(a) Courtesy of Dr HC Grant, formerly of the Middlesex Hospital, London, UK.

with clear cytoplasm and conspicuous cell membranes (Figure 29.2e). Calcifications may be present. The presence of sharp demarcation and occasional perivascular pseudorosettes helps distinguish clear cell ependymoma from oligodendroglioma. In many cases, signs of anaplasia are evident, including cytological atypia, increased mitotic activity and microvascular proliferation.[14] Thus, the clinical course of being clear cell ependymoma often corresponds to anaplastic ependymoma and combined treatment by surgical resection and local radiotherapy is recommended.[14]

The microscopic picture of tanycytic ependymomas may imitate pilocytic astrocytoma or schwannoma

(Figure 29.2f). The tumours are of low to moderate cellularity and composed of elongated, bipolar cells with fibrillar processes and a fascicular architecture. The term 'tanycytic' refers to morphologic similarities of the tumour cells with so-called tanycytes, a specialised form of paraventricular cells with long processes extending to the ependymal surface. Perivascular pseudorosettes are less prominent and true ependymal rosettes are usually absent.

Other rare variants have been reported, including individual cases of melanotic ependymoma, signet ring cell ependymoma and ependymoma with extensive tumour cell vacuolation.[44] Formation of bizarre multinucleated giant cells occasionally becomes a striking feature ('giant cell ependymoma'). Such tumours appear to be more common in extraventricular locations, with spinal and infratentorial cases showing more frequent low-grade histologies, whereas supratentorial giant cell ependymomas often show anaplastic features.[36] Rare cases demonstrate cartilaginous or osseous metaplasia. Individual ependymomas contain areas of lipidization with neoplastic cells that are indistinguishable from adipocytes by traditional stains but show rim-like immunostaining for glial fibrillary acidic protein (GFAP).[67] The term 'desmoplastic ependymoma' has been proposed for a supratentorial neoplasm composed of large, true ependymal rosettes and thick fibrous septa.[88] Ependymal tumours with sarcomatous changes have been referred to as 'ependymosarcomas'.[62] Another study reported on three patients with 'epithelioid ependymomas' showing a diffuse myxoid background, often containing tightly clustered cells that mimicked multinucleated giant cells, but lacked perivascular pseudorosettes or central lumen rosettes. A dot-like cytoplasmic immunoreactivity for epithelial membrane antigen (EMA) was detected in two of the tumours and electron microscopy revealed cells with extensive surface microvilli.[26] An ependymal tumour composed of mitochondrion-rich epithelioid cells has also been reported and referred to as 'oncocytic ependymoma'.[81] Synaptophysin-positive neuropil-like islands have been observed in a paediatric ependymoma.[15]

Grading

Classic ependymoma corresponds histologically to WHO grade II. The WHO classification also considers the cellular, papillary, clear cell and tanycytic ependymoma variants as WHO grade II neoplasms.[44] However, the clear cell variant frequently shows histological signs of anaplasia and rapid disease progression, as indicated by local recurrence within the first year after diagnosis in 5 of 10 patients and extraneural metastases in 2 of 10 patients.[14] Thus, depending on the absence or presence of anaplastic features, this particular variant may correspond either to WHO grade II or, more often, to WHO grade III.[14,61]

General Aspects Concerning Grading of Ependymal Tumours

The WHO classification separates the ependymal tumours into three grades, with subependymoma and myxopapillary ependymoma corresponding to WHO grade I, ependymoma

and its variants to WHO grade II, and anaplastic ependymoma to WHO grade III.[44] However, the prognostic value of grading in ependymomas, in particular concerning the distinction between WHO grade II and III, has been questioned based on several clinical study cohorts.[13] In contrast, histological grade has been confirmed as a significant predictor of survival in several other studies and brain tumour registries.[1,32] In part, this discrepancy may be due to the fact that the criteria for grading, in particular concerning the distinction between WHO grade II and WHO grade III (anaplastic) ependymoma, are disputed and less well established than for astrocytomas. Histological features associated with higher tumour grade and shorter survival have included mitotic activity, nuclear atypia, hypercellularity, loss of differentiation, microvascular proliferation and pseudopalisading necrosis. Unfortunately, neither the individual impact of these features nor the number or combination of parameters required for an anaplastic ependymoma are precisely defined in the WHO classification. Several studies implicated high mitotic activity as the histological finding most consistently associated with poor prognosis. In addition, anaplastic ependymomas are usually hypercellular, nearly always demonstrate microvascular proliferation, and may contain areas with glioblastoma-like pseudopalisading necrosis. Nuclear atypia, cellular pleomorphism, nodules of increased cellularity, and necrosis without pseudopalisading are also common in anaplastic ependymoma but may additionally be observed in some WHO grade II ependymomas. In borderline cases, immunostaining for MIB–1 is helpful because a high labelling index has been repeatedly reported as an independent predictor of shorter survival. Additional attention should be paid to clinical and neuroradiological features, such as patient age and tumour location, because anaplastic changes are more common in intracranial tumours in children and adolescents, whereas spinal ependymomas in adults are usually low-grade lesions. Moreover, new molecular and immunohistochemical markers have been proposed that may help distinguish prognostically distinct subgroups of ependymoma (see Molecular Genetics).

Immunohistochemistry

Ependymomas are positive for GFAP; however, expression is variable. Ependymal cells forming perivascular pseudorosettes give the strongest and most consistent GFAP immunostaining: cell processes radiating towards blood vessels are strongly positive (Figure 29.2g). Other cells stain variably, including those forming tubules, rosettes, papillae or solid aggregates. Reactive astrocytes, present in the tumour or at the periphery, stand out with uniformly strong reaction.

Other intermediate filament proteins, in particular vimentin, are often expressed in ependymomas. In fact, vimentin expression may be more widespread than GFAP immunoreactivity. Expression of nestin has also been noted and implicated as an independent marker for poor outcome.[49] Ependymomas typically express S-100 protein and are usually, but not invariably, negative for neuronal markers, such as neurofilaments, synaptophysin and NeuN.[63] Data on the expression of cytokeratins are controversial. Certain cytokeratin antibodies, in particular the monoclonal antibodies AE1/AE3, showed frequent positivity in ependymomas, likely representing cross reactivity to GFAP.[83] However, immunoreactivity with various other cytokeratin antibodies was either absent or limited to occasional cells and processes.[83] Thus, strong cytokeratin expression is not typical. On the other hand, the majority of ependymal tumours exhibit a characteristic dot-like positivity for EMA, whereas a ring-like staining pattern and linear labelling of luminal surfaces are other characteristic but less common findings (Figure 29.2h).[19] The presence of 5 EMA-positive dots per microscopic high-power field was found to be associated with a sensitivity of 72 per cent and a specificity of 81 per cent in the differential diagnosis of ependymoma versus other glioma subtypes. The presence of ring-like EMA positive structures was less sensitive (32 per cent), but highly specific (100 per cent). Thus, distinct punctate and ring-like EMA staining may serve as sensitive and specific markers for ependymomas.[19] In contrast to the majority of diffuse gliomas, ependymal tumours generally lack *IDH1* or *IDH2* mutations and thus do not stain with antibodies detecting mutant IDH1 protein.[7] Strong nuclear positivity for p53, as seen in the majority of diffuse astrocytomas, is rare in ependymomas.

Immunohistochemical Markers Linked to Tumour Grade and Prognostic Subgroups

Expression of the Ki–67 (MIB–1) antigen has been extensively studied in ependymal tumours, indicating that the labelling index is higher in anaplastic than low-grade ependymomas and that a high MIB–1 index appears to be associated with shorter patient survival.[58] However, a commonly accepted diagnostic cut-off for the percentage of MIB–1 positive cells has not been established, with various studies reporting on prognostically relevant cut-off values ranging from 5 per cent[35] to 20.7 per cent.[58] In addition, interlaboratory differences yield considerable variability in MIB–1 indices.[58] Thus, although commonly used in the routine setting, the MIB–1 index needs to be interpreted with caution.

In addition to MIB–1, several other proliferation-associated antigens, such as topoisomerase II α[29] and proliferating cell nuclear antigen (PCNA),[84] have been linked to higher tumour grade and poor prognosis in ependymal tumours. Other immunohistochemical markers reported as being associated with less favourable outcome include nuclear p53 positivity,[84] loss of p14[ARF] expression and positivity for tenascin C,[29] as well as upregulated expression of the human telomerase reverse transcriptase (hTERT),[45,50] the anti-apoptotic protein survivin,[59] epidermal growth factor receptors,[45] nucleolin and nestin.[49,50] In addition, high-level coexpression of ERBB2 and ERBB4 has been linked to increased proliferative activity and poor outcome.[17] However, the prognostic impact of these immunohistochemical parameters in the routine diagnostic assessment is still limited and needs further evaluation. Similarly, it remains to be confirmed in independent studies whether the distinction of two prognostically relevant molecular subgroups of posterior fossa ependymomas based on immunohistochemical stains for LAMA2 and NELL2[87] can be successfully translated into routine diagnostics.

Electron Microscopy

Ultrastructurally, ependymomas have three salient features reminiscent of normal ependymal cells. First, neoplastic ependymal cells have intermediate filaments of 10 nm in diameter; thus, they maintain glial fibrillogenesis. This explains the variable, but positive immunoreactivities to GFAP and vimentin. Secondly, neoplastic cells also preserve some of the polarity of normal ependyma and feature surface specializations, including microvilli and cilia. These structures are of various dimensions and project from the cell surface. Two cells may form a microrosette, the lumen of which is filled with these surface protrusions. The basal bodies of cilia are easy to discern as the normal 9 + 2 triplets, which give rise to the axial fibrils of cilia. Abnormal configuration of the basal bodies is also seen. The third feature is the presence of complex intercellular junctions similar to those of normal ependyma. These junctions are zonulae adherentes rather than zonulae occludentes; the extracellular space is not sealed completely by the fusion of the cell membrane, leaving a gap in between. They may be of considerable length ('zipper-like') and their intracellular surface may be lined by dense material, similar to that seen in desmosomes.

Although the presence of these ultrastructural features is helpful in the diagnosis, the vast majority of ependymomas can be diagnosed without electron microscopy. However, in individual cases lacking decisive morphological and immunohistochemical features, electron microscopy may be helpful. Nevertheless, rare tumours may also lack typical ultrastructural features and present problems even ultrastructurally.

Differential Diagnosis

Histological classification is straightforward in the presence of perivascular pseudorosettes, ependymal rosettes, and ependymal tubules and clefts, sometimes complete with cilia and microvilli. However, small biopsy specimens or the presence of extensive secondary changes, but particularly the histological variants of cellular, clear cell, tanycytic and papillary ependymomas, may pose differential diagnostic problems. Cellular ependymoma shows a conspicuous cellularity but, in contrast to anaplastic ependymoma, lacks additional features of anaplasia. In particular, mitotic count and proliferative activity are not significantly elevated. Clear cell ependymomas may be difficult to distinguish from oligodendrogliomas, central neurocytomas and metastatic renal cell carcinomas. However, in most instances GFAP-positive perivascular pseudorosettes are detected at least focally. Immunohistochemistry for EMA is helpful by demonstrating a characteristic dot- or ring-like immunoreactivity. Furthermore, clear cell ependymomas differ from oligodendrogliomas by their non-infiltrative growth. Thus, staining for neurofilaments usually shows no or only few residual axons in the tumour. Moreover, clear cell ependymomas lack immunostaining with the IDH1 R132H mutation-specific antibody.[7] Nuclear positivity for OLIG2 is more widespread and stronger in oligodendrogliomas as compared to clear cell ependymomas.[57] If neither morphology nor immunohistochemistry allows for a definite classification, electron microscopy shows typical ultrastructural features of ependymal cells, including intercellular junctions, microvilli and cilia. These features are absent in the three other tumour types. In contrast to clear cell ependymoma, central neurocytomas are diffusely positive for synaptophysin, often express NeuN focally, and ultrastructurally show evidence of neuronal differentiation, including dense secretory granules, growth cones and synaptic structures. Metastatic renal carcinomas usually are more vascular, lack pseudorosettes, stain with antibodies to cytokeratins, and lack GFAP expression.

Tanycytic ependymoma may be difficult to distinguish from an astrocytoma, in particular because perivascular pseudorosettes are sparse. Similar to pilocytic astrocytoma, tanycytic ependymoma grows non-invasively. However, other features of pilocytic differentiation are absent and ultrastructural investigation reveals ependymal characteristics. Some resemble schwannoma, but differ in their intramedullary localization and lack of dense intercellular reticulin or basement membrane deposition.

Papillary ependymomas should be distinguished from other papillary tumours, including metastatic carcinomas, choroid plexus tumours, papillary pituitary adenomas, astroblastomas, papillary tumours of the pineal region and papillary meningiomas. The use of immunohistochemistry, including GFAP, vimentin, EMA, S–100 protein, cytokeratins, transthyretin (prealbumin), neuronal markers and antibodies to pituitary hormones, enables the distinction of these tumours. Both ependymomas and astroblastomas express GFAP and vimentin. Furthermore, the perivascular pseudorosettes of ependymomas resemble those of astroblastomas, albeit with a more distinctly fibrillar quality. Additionally, in ependymomas the cells have no footplates on the vascular wall, the perikaryon is less intimately related to the blood vessels, and the intervascular spaces are compact and filled with cells. Choroid plexus tumours are positive for cytokeratins, which are usually negative in ependymomas and astroblastomas. Immunoreactivity for prealbumin (transthyretin) and several novel choroid plexus markers, such as Kir7.1 and stanniocalcin–1, is commonly seen in choroid plexus papillomas.[20] Papillary meningiomas coexpress vimentin and EMA but usually lack GFAP immunoreactivity and do not show dot- or ring-like EMA staining. The presence of at least focal whorl formation further aids their distinction. Papillary pituitary adenomas also lack GFAP but express neuroendocrine markers and often, specific pituitary hormones. Finally, metastatic papillary carcinomas stain strongly positive for cytokeratins and lack GFAP immunoreactivity.

In tumours of the third ventricular/suprasellar region, a rare location of ependymomas, pilomyxoid astrocytoma (PMA) needs to be considered in the differential diagnosis because its perivascular pseudorosette-like formations may suggest ependymoma. The strongly myxoid background and the loose tissue texture, together with the typical location and age group, argue in favour of PMA.

In paediatric ependymomas of the posterior fossa, medulloblastoma represents an important differential diagnosis. Medulloblastomas are more cellular and primitive appearing. Furthermore, the neuropil-rich Homer Wright rosettes in medulloblastoma are distinct from ependymal rosettes or pseudorosettes, although the latter may be seen in medulloblastomas as well.

Histogenesis

The proximity to ventricular walls or the central canal and their shared morphological and ultrastructural features, suggest that ependymomas likely develop from ependymal cells. However, it is unclear whether these tumours originate from mature (post-mitotic) ependymal cells, which dedifferentiate into a more immature form capable of self-renewal, or arise from glial progenitor cells. Data obtained by genomic and expression profiling of ependymal tumours from different locations showed that histologically similar ependymomas from different parts of the CNS (supratentorial, posterior fossa, spinal) represent molecularly and clinically distinct disease subgroups.[31,76] Interestingly, ependymomas from different locations exhibited gene expression signatures that closely recapitulated those of radial glia in the corresponding CNS region. Furthermore, stem-like cancer cells isolated from ependymomas displayed a radial glia phenotype and were able to generate ependymomas when transplanted into nude mice. Thus, radial glia represent attractive candidate stem cells of ependymoma.[76] An origin of ependymomas from regionally distinct types of neural stem cells was supported by comparison of transcriptomes obtained in human tumours with those of murine neural stem cells isolated from distinct brain regions at different developmental stages.[25] Thereby, it was found that a genetically defined subgroup of supratentorial ependymomas with amplification of *EPHB2* and loss of *INK4A/ARF* shared a similar transcriptional profile as embryonic neural stem cells obtained from *INK4A/ARF*-deficient mice. Moreover, activation of ephrinB2 signalling in these specific neural stem cells resulted in the first transgenic mouse model for ependymoma.[25] Taken together, current data favour an origin from neural stem or progenitor cells, in particular radial glia, rather than from differentiated ependymal cells. It remains to be shown whether this hypothesis holds true for all ependymoma subtypes or whether other cell types, e.g. tanycytes, may also give rise to certain tumours such as the tanycytic variant.

Molecular Genetics

A review of conventional cytogenetic findings in 125 ependymal tumours revealed abnormal karyotypes in 83 (66 per cent), of which 24 had a sole autosomal abnormality.[41] About one-third had monosomy 22 or chromosomal loss at breakpoint 22q11–13, with a higher incidence in adults (56 per cent) than in children (28 per cent). Structural abnormalities of chromosomes 1, 6 and 17, and numerical abnormalities of chromosomes 7, 9, 12 and 20 were also noted.[41] Studies employing genome- and transcriptome-wide molecular profiling approaches characterized different molecular subgroups of ependymal tumours that appear to be associated with distinct biological and clinical features.[25,32,86,87] Overall, the most common gene copy number changes in ependymal tumours are losses of chromosomes 6q, 10, 13, 14 and 22q, as well as gains of chromosomes 1q, 7, 9, 12q, 15q and 18. Spinal intramedullary ependymomas preferentially demonstrate losses of chromosomes 22q and 14q and gains on chromosomes 7q, 9p and 16. In contrast, intracranial ependymomas frequently carry gains of 1q and losses on 6q. Among the various genomic imbalances, gains on 1q have been correlated with the presence of structural chromosomal aberrations, paediatric age, high-grade histology and aggressive clinical behaviour.[32,45] Based on distinct patterns of DNA copy number aberrations, three prognostically relevant molecular subgroups of intracranial ependymomas have been proposed:[32] Group 1 tumours (favourable prognosis) carry gains on chromosomes 9, 15q and 18 or loss of chromosome 6; Group 2 tumours (intermediate prognosis) have largely balanced genomic profiles; Group 3 tumours (poor prognosis) are characterized by 1q gains and/or homozygous CDKN2A deletions. Another study identified three genetic subgroups among posterior fossa ependymomas that were characterized either by (i) multiple concurrent DNA amplifications, (ii) gain of 1q, or (iii) a balanced karyotype.[76] In this study, ependymomas from different regions (spinal, infratentorial, supratentorial) also showed distinct mRNA expression signatures, with supratentorial ependymomas expressing elevated levels of members of the EPHB–EPHRIN and NOTCH families, whereas spinal ependymomas show up-regulated expression of multiple HOX gene family members.[76] Another mRNA profiling study identified two molecularly and clinically distinct subgroups of posterior fossa ependymomas that are characterized by distinct expression signatures:[87] Group A tumours (poor prognosis with frequent relapse and metastatic seeding) occur in younger patients, are located laterally in the 4th ventricle and are more frequent in males. They have mostly balanced genomes with frequent gain of 1q and loss of 22. Group B tumours (favourable prognosis) are genetically more unstable with frequent gains and losses on various chromosomes. These tumours are more prevalent in adults and located in the midline. Interestingly, both ependymoma subgroups could be distinguished based on immunohistochemical surrogate markers, with group A tumours being positive for LAMA2 but negative for NELL2, and group B tumours demonstrating the inverse immunostaining pattern.[86,87]

Comparative genomic hybridization (CGH) analysis of clear cell ependymomas showed loss of chromosome 9 as the most common genomic change, which separates these tumours from the other ependymomas as well as oligodendrogliomas and neurocytomas.[61] Other recurrent aberrations, which were more common in anaplastic clear cell variants, included losses of chromosomes 3 and 22q as well as gains on 1q.

Molecular genetic studies on selected candidate genes revealed frequent NF2 gene mutations in intramedullary spinal ependymomas but not in intracranial ependymomas, myxopapillary ependymomas or subependymomas.[12] Mutations in the TP53, IDH1/2, PTEN and INI1 tumour suppressor genes are rare or absent in ependymomas. Deletions of the CDKN2A gene are frequent in supratentorial ependymomas, in particular anaplastic variants, but rare in ependymomas from other locations.[25,76] Large-scale genomic profiling of ependymomas identified numerous focal gene amplifications and gene deletions targeting various known proto-oncogenes and tumour suppressor genes.[25] One of the focal amplifications often found together with CDKN2A deletions in a subset of supratentorial ependymomas, i.e. amplification of EPHB2, was shown to drive ependymoma development in INK4A/ARF-deficient mice.[25]

In addition to chromosomal and genetic aberrations, epigenetic changes contribute to ependymoma pathogenesis, with several genes being reported as epigenetically silenced by aberrant promoter methylation in these tumours, including the known tumour suppressor genes RASSF1, CDKN2A, CDKN2B, p14ARF and TP73, as well as several other genes.[18,66] Of clinical importance concerning the response to adjuvant alkylating chemotherapy is the finding that MGMT promoter methylation is less frequent in ependymomas as compared to malignant astrocytic gliomas.[28]

Aetiology and Genetic Susceptibility

The aetiology of ependymomas is essentially unknown. Only a few cases linked to ionizing irradiation are documented. The aetiological role of oncogenic viruses, such as SV40, JC and BK, is unclear. The vast majority of ependymomas arise sporadically. However, it is well established that patients with neurofibromatosis type 2 (NF2) carry a significantly increased risk for ependymomas, in particular intramedullary spinal tumours, which account for the vast majority of NF2-associated gliomas. NF2 patients represent approximately 2.5 per cent of all patients with intramedullary spinal cord tumours. Most of these tumours are located in the cervical cord, with multifocality being common. Histologically, NF2-associated ependymomas are mostly WHO grade II and classic, albeit individual tanycytic variants have also been documented.[27] NF2-associated spinal ependymomas typically follow an indolent clinical course.[54]

Only rare cases of ependymoma have been reported in other hereditary cancer syndromes, including a single patient with an intracranial ependymoma and a TP53 germline mutation,[48] one patient with ependymoma and familial cutaneous melanoma syndrome[4] and one patient with cervical ependymoma in familial leukonychia with sebaceous cysts (Bauer syndrome).[51] In addition, familial ependymomas outside any known syndrome have been published, including intracranial ependymomas in three members of one family, a family with two members diagnosed with spinal anaplastic ependymoma, a family with four affected members having anaplastic ependymomas and fourth ventricular ependymomas in a father and son.[39]

Biological Behaviour and Prognosis

Ependymomas are well-differentiated tumours with relatively slow growth and modest potential to invade. In general, spinal intramedullary ependymomas in adults are associated with long-term, recurrence-free and overall survival after complete resection.[16] The prognosis of spinal ependymomas in children is also favourable following gross total resection.[6] The value of adjuvant therapy is disputed. Radiotherapy is often administered in those lesions that cannot be resected completely, show disseminated tumour growth or histological features of anaplasia. Incompletely resected tumours have a higher risk for local recurrence.[16]

The prognosis of intracranial ependymomas is more variable and less favourable as compared to spinal ependymomas.[1,42] Local recurrence rates ranging between 44 per cent[30] up to 89 per cent[22] have been reported. In addition, a small subset of intracranial ependymomas may give rise to cerebrospinal fluid (CSF) metastases,[30] which are best demonstrated by MR imaging; CSF cytology is of limited value.[55] Survival data vary considerably depending on the type of study and patient cohorts. A European population-based analysis estimated a 5-year overall survival rate of 83.5 per cent for patients with ependymomas and choroid plexus tumours.[70] The CBTRUS database reports 5- and 10-year survival rates for patients with ependymomas/anaplastic ependymomas of 82 per cent and 77 per cent, respectively.[8] Even better prognosis, with 5-year progression-free and overall survival rates of 90 per cent and 93 per cent, was determined in a retrospective study of 131 patients with low-grade ependymomas.[30] In contrast, an analysis of paediatric supratentorial ependymoma patients treated in an Italian trial revealed a 10-year overall survival rate of only 55 per cent for patients with WHO grade II ependymoma.[50]

Survival is influenced by several parameters, including, most notably, treatment-related factors and, in particular, extent of surgical resection and administration of adjuvant radiotherapy. This is in addition to biological factors, such as patient age, tumour location, disease dissemination, histological grade and certain immunohistochemical and molecular parameters (see earlier). Surgery is the most important variable, with complete resection being the best predictor of favourable prognosis in patients with localized disease.[16] Advances in microsurgical techniques have increased the rate of gross total resections up to 85 per cent in some series, and modern radiation techniques have further improved outcome along with reductions in treatment-related side effects.[46]

Age at diagnosis has been reported as a prognostically important parameter, with younger patients showing less favourable likelihood of survival.[30] A multi-institutional, retrospective study of 83 paediatric patients with intracranial ependymomas also revealed that children younger than 3 years of age had significantly worse outcome.[22] Moreover, a population-based analysis involving 635 patients registered in the Surveillance Epidemiology End Results (SEER) database confirmed an independent prognostic role of age in paediatric ependymomas.[42]

Only rarely do ependymomas give rise to extraneural metastases. In a series of 81 patients, 5 instances were encountered (6.2 per cent), including 2 patients with ventriculoperitoneal shunts and peritoneal metastases.[52] Among 258 patients studied by Korshunov et al.,[30] 5 patients with primary anaplastic ependymomas (2 per cent) developed extraneural metastases. Another evaluation of 1011 children with primary intracranial tumours identified extraneural metastases in only 10 (0.98 per cent), with metastatic ependymoma being restricted to a single case.[82]

ANAPLASTIC EPENDYMOMA

Anaplastic ependymoma constitutes a malignant variant associated with rapid growth and less favourable prognosis. Anaplastic ependymomas are particularly prevalent in children and are far more common among intracranial lesions, in particular infratentorial lesions, as compared to spinal lesions. Histologically, the tumours are characterized by features of anaplasia, particularly high mitotic activity and increased cellularity, often in conjunction with microvascular proliferation and areas of pseudo-palisading necrosis.

Incidence, Age and Sex Distribution

The incidence of anaplastic ependymomas is difficult to assess as different histological criteria have been used in various studies and data on ependymal tumours in CBTRUS are not stratified according to WHO grade.[8] In a population-based study of 2802 ependymoma patients in the SEER programme, 328 patients (11.7 per cent) were registered with anaplastic ependymoma.[1] In several retrospective single- or multi-institutional studies, the fractions of anaplastic ependymomas were considerably higher.[30,73] The gender distribution and associations with race do not differ from those of ependymal tumours in general[8] or low-grade ependymomas.[1]

Clinical Features and Neuroimaging

The clinical signs and symptoms of patients with anaplastic ependymomas are similar to those of lower-grade ependymomas. However, the clinical symptomatology may develop and progress more rapidly. They usually demonstrate contrast enhancement on CT and MR imaging. In contrast to malignant astrocytic and oligodendroglial tumours, most anaplastic ependymomas are still well-demarcated with only limited invasion into adjacent parenchyma. However, more extensive brain invasion is seen in rare instances, in particular in children and young adults with intracerebral masses that are neuroradiologically indistinguishable from other malignant gliomas.

Location and Macroscopy

The frequency of anaplastic ependymomas varies according to site. In contrast to intracranial tumours, intraspinal ependymomas rarely show anaplastic features. The population-based SEER series lists only 26 examples among 1108 spinal ependymomas.[1] The macroscopic appearance is similar to other ependymomas, except that anaplastic ependymomas may show large areas of necrosis, as well as focal invasion and destruction of brain parenchyma.

Microscopy

Anaplastic ependymomas are highly cellular tumours composed of closely packed polygonal, rounded or epithelial-like tumour cells (Figure 29.2i). Mitotic activity is prominent. Cellular pleomorphism may be striking, including the presence of large atypical or even multinucleated giant cells. On the other hand, poorly differentiated, small anaplastic cells may predominate in some tumours, eliciting a differential diagnosis with embryonal tumours, e.g. medulloblastoma, often requiring immunohistochemical or ultrastructural studies to resolve. Perivascular pseudorosettes are usually recognizable in anaplastic ependymoma whereas other features of well-differentiated ependymoma, such as ependymal rosettes, ependymal tubules and clefts lined by ependymal cells are often absent. Areas of tumour necrosis can be extensive, and glioblastoma-like features, such as pseudopalisading necrosis and/or microvascular proliferation are often present. In contrast to WHO grade II ependymomas, some anaplastic tumours invade and destroy surrounding structures.

Grading

Anaplastic ependymoma corresponds histologically to WHO grade III.

Immunohistochemistry

The expression patterns of GFAP, S–100 protein, vimentin and EMA are similar to those in WHO grade II ependymomas, but may be less pronounced. Proliferative activity as determined by MIB–1 immunostaining is generally high (Figure 29.2j). However, a definitive MIB–1 cut-off value that separates anaplastic ependymoma from WHO grade II ependymoma has not been established.

Differential Diagnosis

Anaplastic ependymoma should be distinguished from ependymoblastoma, a very rare embryonal tumour containing multi-layered, ependymoblastic rosettes of mitotically active tumour cells around small round lumina (see Chapter 34, Embryonal Tumours). In anaplastic ependymomas with marked microvascular proliferation and pseudopalisading necrosis, the differential diagnosis of glioblastoma can arise. However, glioblastomas are usually more invasive, do not show unequivocal ependymal features, and usually lack dots and rings upon immunohistochemistry for EMA. Nevertheless, a subset of anaplastic ependymomas is frankly invasive and occasional glioblastomas show perivascular pseudorosette-like architectures reminiscent of ependymal differentiation. In such cases, consideration of clinical features, such as patient age and tumour location, may provide helpful clues. In rare cases, ultrastructural features of ependymoma or a molecular signature of glioblastoma resolves this differential.

Biological Behaviour and Prognosis

Anaplastic ependymomas are associated with unfavourable outcome in most patients. Complete surgical resection is the treatment of choice. In addition, patients are usually treated with adjuvant radiotherapy and/or chemotherapy. Despite aggressive treatment, tumours tend to recur locally. CSF dissemination is seen in a subset whereas metastatic seeding outside the CNS may occur, albeit rarely. Data from the German prospective trials HIT 88/89 and HIT 91, which included 55 children with newly diagnosed anaplastic ependymoma treated by operation, radio- and multiagent chemotherapy revealed an overall survival rate of 75.6 per cent at 3 years after surgery.[77] In children below 3 years of age treated in the

HIT–SKK 87 and HIT–SKK 92 trials, 3-year overall survival was lower, i.e. 55.9 per cent.[78] A more recent Italian study reported a 10-year survival rate of 19 per cent for children with anaplastic ependymoma.[50]

The prognostic relevance of anaplastic histological features is controversial. For example, survival analysis in a series of 298 patients failed to demonstrate a worse outcome for patients with anaplastic as compared to classic ependymoma.[73] Similarly, a study of several prospective clinical trials did not identify a prognostic role for tumour grading.[13] However, other studies, including prospective cohorts and population-based registries, suggested that anaplastic ependymomas were associated with shorter survival than low-grade ependymomas.[1,30,47,50] Concerning other prognostic factors, a review of 127 patients with high-grade ependymomas identified the following parameters on univariate analyses: age (<16 years vs ≥16 years), tumour location (infratentorial vs supratentorial), extent of resection (gross total vs subtotal), and radiotherapy (yes vs no).[30] Significant prognostic factors in the HIT 88/89 and HIT 91 trials were extent of resection (estimated 3-year progression-free survival of 83.3 per cent after complete resection and 38.5 per cent after incomplete resection) and metastatic disease at diagnosis (0 per cent vs 65.8 per cent estimated 3-year progression-free survival in localized tumours).[77]

MYXOPAPILLARY EPENDYMOMA

Myxopapillary ependymoma constitutes a distinct low-grade ependymal neoplasm that typically arises in the conus/cauda equina/filum terminale region of the spinal cord. Histologically, myxopapillary ependymoma is characterized by tumour cells forming papillary structures around vascular mucoid stromal cores.

Incidence, Age and Sex Distribution

Precise incidence data are not available. Among 298 ependymomas collected from different institutions, 13 per cent corresponded to the myxopapillary type.[73] A multicentre retrospective review of 231 adult patients with cauda equina tumours revealed myxopapillary ependymoma in 79 patients, thus constituting the second most common tumour type in this region after schwannomas.[85] Myxopapillary ependymomas commonly arise in young adults, with an average age of 36.4 years (range from 6 to 82 years); the male/female ratio is 1.7–1.0.[74]

Clinical and Radiological Features

In a clinicopathological study of 14 cases, the preoperative symptoms lasted from 2 months to 18 years with a median of 12 months, most commonly including lower back pain.[56] Disturbances of sphincter function, sexual dysfunction and neurological deficits caused by compression of the conus medullaris or sacral nerve roots may also be seen. MRI shows a well-demarcated contrast-enhancing lesion that is hyperintense on T1-weighted sequences. Areas of cystic degeneration or haemorrhage may be seen.

Localization and Macroscopy

Myxopapillary ependymomas are almost exclusively located in the region of the conus medullaris, cauda equina and filum terminale. Rare cases have been reported in other locations, including the cerebral hemispheres,[80] cerebral ventricles,[37] cerebellopontine angle,[75] medulla oblongata,[11] thoracic–cervical spinal cord, and spinal nerve roots.[74] Rare instances of multifocality are also on record.[2] Extraneural tumours also occur, most commonly in the subcutaneous sacrococcygeal and presacral regions. Macroscopically, the tumours are solitary, lobulated and often encapsulated, soft, greyish and translucent lesions. Large growths may compress or even envelop the cauda equina, but invasion of the nerve roots is rare: these cases present surgical difficulties. Exceptionally large tumours may erode adjacent bones. Occasionally, myxopapillary ependymoma may arise in conjunction with malformative lesions such as tethered cord, dermal sinus and dermoid cyst.

Microscopy

Histologically, the tumours are composed of cuboidal or columnar cells mounted on well-vascularised, acellular cores of connective tissue (Figure 29.2k,l). The cells covering the papillary fronds are regular, well-defined and usually single layered. The connective tissue stroma frequently undergoes hyaline and mucoid degeneration. The distinctive histology of myxopapillary ependymomas may result from this mucinous stromal change. In addition to the variable papillary arrangement, more solid, epithelial-like areas, tubules and clefts lined by cuboidal or low columnar cells are often present. Fibrillar areas may also be seen. Mitotic activity is either absent or low. Some tumours feature so-called balloons, i.e. small, spherical eosinophilic structures consisting of stromal collagen fibrils highlighted on Masson's trichrome and PAS stains. Rare cases showing marked cellular pleomorphism and nuclear atypia with or without myxopapillary features have been referred to as 'giant cell ependymoma of the filum terminale'.[89] Very exceptionally, myxopapillary ependymomas may present with histological features of anaplasia.[2,3]

Grading

Myxopapillary ependymomas are slowly growing tumours that histologically correspond to WHO grade I.

Immunohistochemistry

The glial derivation of the neoplastic cells can be demonstrated by immunostaining for GFAP (Figure 29.2l) and S–100 protein. Vimentin may be positive in tumour cells, in addition to the connective tissue stroma and blood vessels. The tumours are usually negative for cytokeratins and often lack the dot- or ring-like EMA staining pattern typically seen in other ependymomas.[19] Immunostaining for p53 shows only rare labelled nuclei. Immunoreactivity for three marker proteins, namely HOXB13, NEFL and PDGFR alpha, was reported to be particularly strong in myxopapillary ependymoma as compared to absent, weak or focal staining in other ependymoma types.[5] The MIB1

index is low, with a median of 0.9 per cent reported in one series.[56] Higher values are not necessarily related to recurrence or distant metastases.

Electron Microscopy

Ultrastructurally, these tumours show similarities with other ependymal tumours, including the presence of few cilia and complex cellular interdigitations. However, they additionally demonstrate abundant basement membrane material. The latter feature, together with the presence of collagen fibres, reflects the normal architecture of the filum terminale in which ependymal cells rest on connective tissue derived from the leptomeninges and not on the neuropil of the CNS. Abundant microtubular aggregates within rough endoplasmic reticulum have been detected in some cases and may represent a unique feature.[21]

Differential Diagnosis

The differential diagnosis with schwannoma and paraganglioma, two other common intradural tumours in the conus–cauda–filum terminale region, is usually straightforward. Other tumours that need to be considered include chordoma, myxoid (chordoid) chondrosarcoma, mesothelioma and metastases from adenoid cystic carcinoma or mucinous adenocarcinoma. Chordoma, mesothelioma and secondary carcinomas all stain with cytokeratin antibodies but are GFAP-negative. Soft-tissue myxoid (chordoid) chondrosarcoma can also be eliminated by its lack of GFAP expression. Sometimes the question arises whether the myxoid and pseudopapillary features of an ependymal tumour in the lumbosacral region are pronounced enough to justify the diagnosis of myxopapillary ependymoma. At present, there is no evidence that the extent of myxopapillary features (widespread vs focal) is associated with different biological behaviours.

Molecular Genetics

Despite their benign clinical behaviour, myxopapillary ependymomas are often aneuploid or tetraploid tumours that carry numerous chromosomal imbalances as determined by CGH analysis. In fact, the average number of chromosomal aberrations per tumour is higher than in ependymomas and anaplastic ependymomas.[71] Characteristic genomic changes detected by high-resolution array-CGH are concurrent gains of chromosomes 5, 7, 9, 16 and 18.[65] Molecular genetic analyses of a small number of cases revealed no PTEN, NF2 or INI1 mutations.[12,33] Thus, current data indicate that the genetic alterations in myxopapillary ependymoma are distinct from those of other ependymal tumours. The different pathogenesis is further corroborated by microarray-based expression profiles demonstrating specific gene expression signatures in myxopapillary ependymomas.[5,31]

Aetiology and Genetic Susceptibility

The aetiology of myxopapillary ependymoma is unclear. The tumours develop sporadically. Familial cases have not been reported.

Biological Behaviour and Prognosis

Myxopapillary ependymomas usually demonstrate a favourable prognosis after gross total resection; the vast majority of patients enjoy long-term, recurrence-free survivals over 10 years.[74] However, late recurrences may develop and CSF dissemination and distant metastases are occasionally observed. Thus, regular clinical follow-up is recommended. Adjuvant radiotherapy has been reported as being beneficial for patients with incompletely resected tumours.[74] The prognosis of lumbosacral ependymomas appears to be unrelated to myxopapillary versus classical ependymoma subtype.[24]

Primary Extraspinal Myxopapillary Ependymoma

Primary extraspinal myxopapillary ependymomas of the subcutaneous sacrococcygeal and presacral regions form a rare, but clinically important subgroup.[40] Subcutaneous sacrococcygeal tumours are thought to arise either from the coccygeal medullary vestige, an ependymal lined cavity forming the remnant of the caudal portion of the neural tube, or from heterotopic ependymal cell nests, whereas presacral tumours probably originate from extradural remnants of the filum terminale or an extension of the intradural filum. Most patients are children and young adults, with a reported age range from 2 months to 67 years. Both sexes are affected equally. Clinically, sacrococcygeal myxopapillary ependymoma typically presents as an asymptomatic, slowly growing subcutaneous mass, which is often misinterpreted as a pilonidal cyst or sinus. Presacral tumours more often produce symptoms, such as bowel and bladder dysfunction, paraesthesia or lower limb weakness. Most extraspinal myxopapillary ependymomas are well-demarcated lesions that can be completely resected. Some cases show invasion into adjacent soft tissue or the sacral bone. Histology, ultrastructure and immunocytochemistry are essentially the same as in the intraspinal myxopapillary ependymomas (Figure 29.3a). However, despite benign morphology, these tumours may recur locally and up to 20 per cent metastasize, most often to regional lymph nodes, lungs, liver or bone. Rare cases show anaplastic progression on recurrence (Figure 29.3a,b). Late metastases may develop 10–20 years after initial presentation. Unfortunately, there are no clinical or histological features that would allow for reliable prediction of metastatic potential. Complete surgical resection is the treatment of choice, whereas radiotherapy is reserved for cases with incomplete resection or metastasis. Because of the risk of late development of recurrences and distant metastases, regular follow-up over many years is recommended.

SUBEPENDYMOMA

Subependymoma is defined as a slowly growing, benign intraventricular or spinal neoplasm composed of clusters of glial tumour cells with small rounded nuclei embedded in a densely fibrillar, often microcystic matrix.

Incidence, Age and Sex Distribution

Subependymomas, in particular those located in the ventricles, often remain asymptomatic. Therefore, precise

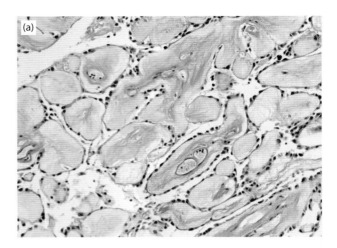

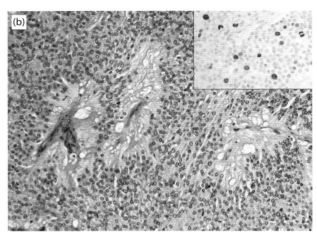

29.3 Presacral myxopapillary ependymoma with anaplastic progression. (a) Primary presacral myxopapillary ependymoma with standard myxopapillary phenotype. Haematoxylin and eosin (H&E). **(b)** Local recurrence of the tumour with increased cell density, mitotic activity and microvascular proliferation, now corresponding histologically to an anaplastic ependymoma (WHO grade III). Note residual foci of myxoid degeneration around blood vessels. H&E. Inset shows high proliferative activity in the recurrent tumour. Ki–67 immunohistochemistry.

estimation of the incidence is difficult. In a retrospective series of 298 ependymal tumours, subependymoma accounted for 8.3 per cent of the cases.[73] The tumours occur in all age groups and both genders. Middle-aged and elderly men are most commonly affected.

Clinical and Radiological Features

The clinical presentation depends on the tumour location and size. Small intraventricular lesions often remain clinically silent and are detected only incidentally by neuroimaging for other reasons or at autopsy. Larger tumours may become symptomatic, with tumours in the lateral ventricles showing symptoms more often than lesions in the fourth ventricle. Typically, the tumours cause obstructive hydrocephalus and signs of increased intracranial pressure, such as headache, nausea and vomiting. Other presenting symptoms include seizures, ataxia and dizziness/vertigo.[60] Large tumours of the fourth ventricle can cause symptoms by brainstem compression. Individual patients may present with intratumoural and subarachnoid haemorrhage. Spinal subependymomas become symptomatic with motor and/or sensory deficits attributable to the affected spinal cord segment.

On neuroimaging, intracranial subependymomas present as well demarcated, nodular masses attached to the ventricular walls. The tumours are isodense on CT and show minimal enhancement. Dystrophic calcifications are often seen, in particular in fourth ventricular lesions. On MRI, subependymomas appear as hypo- to isointense lesions on T1-weighted and hyperintense lesions on T2-weighted sequences. Contrast enhancement is usually absent or only scarce, but may be more prominent in fourth ventricular tumours. Intramedullary subependymomas are often located eccentrically, which contrasts with the typically central location of intraspinal ependymomas. However, neuroimaging does not provide a definite pre-operative diagnosis.

Localization and Macroscopy

Most subependymomas arise in the fourth ventricle, followed by the lateral ventricles. Other locations include the third ventricle, septum pellucidum, cerebral aqueduct and spinal cord. Rare cases have been reported in the cerebral parenchyma[60] or cerebellopontine angle.[10] Spinal subependymomas are well-demarcated, somewhat eccentrically located intramedullary lesions that favour the cervical and the cervicothoracic segments. Rare examples present as extramedullary tumours. Macroscopically, subependymomas are well-demarcated, soft, often lobulated, white-tan masses that are firmly attached to the ventricular wall (Figure 29.4a). Fourth ventricular tumours are often calcified whereas cystic degeneration is more common in tumours of the lateral ventricles.

Microscopy

Subependymomas are paucicellular tumours composed of clusters of uniform, cytologically bland cells embedded in a densely fibrillar glial matrix (Figure 29.4b). Microcystic degeneration is often prominent, particularly in supratentorial tumours (Figure 29.4c). Other frequently encountered secondary changes are haemosiderin deposition, hyalinised blood vessels and dystrophic calcifications, the latter most common in fourth ventricular tumours. In long-standing cases, scattered nuclear atypia may be seen but are not indicative of malignancy. Mitoses are usually inconspicuous. Necrosis and microvascular proliferation are absent. Formation of perivascular pseudorosettes is indistinct and true ependymal rosettes are not found. However, some tumours display combined features of typical ependymoma and subependymoma. These appear to be more common among the fourth ventricular lesions and have been referred to as 'mixed ependymoma/subependymoma WHO grade II'.[43] Rare cases of subependymoma have presented with rhabdomyosarcomatous transformation, osseous metaplasia or melanin pigmentation.

Grading

Subependymomas are benign tumours corresponding to WHO grade I.

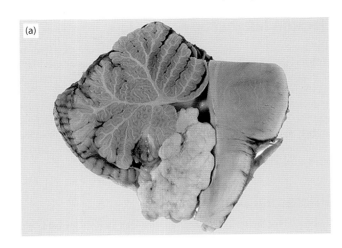

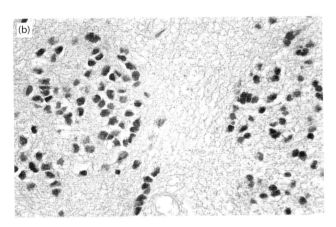

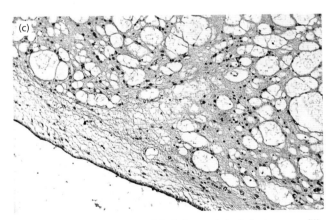

29.4 Subependymoma. (a) A large lobulated mass filling the fourth ventricle and extending caudally to compress the brain stem. **(b)** Typical histology with clusters of isomorphic cells in a densely fibrillar matrix. H&E. **(c)** Microcystic degeneration in a subependymoma of the lateral ventricle. H&E.

Immunohistochemistry

Subependymomas are immunohistochemically positive for GFAP, S–100 protein and vimentin. Focal dot-like EMA staining may be seen. The MIB–1 labelling index is generally low.

Electron Microscopy

Ultrastructural examination reveals small groups of tumour cell perikarya widely separated by a meshwork of abundant cell processes densely filled with intermediate filaments. In addition to large cells showing ultrastructural similarities with ependymal precursor cells, other cells demonstrate astrocytic or poorly developed ependymal features, such as microvilli, cilia formation and cell junctions, or transitional features between astrocytes and ependymal cells.

Differential Diagnosis

Subependymomas are histologically distinctive lesions that usually do not pose differential diagnostic problems, except that their distinction from ependymoma can occasionally be difficult. Focal areas resembling subependymoma are often encountered in otherwise typical ependymomas, in particular in tumours of the fourth ventricle. However, cellularity is usually higher and perivascular pseudorosettes are more prominent. Furthermore, whereas fourth ventricular ependymomas are most common in children, subependymomas usually present in adults. Nevertheless, some are difficult to assign to either category and the WHO suggests the term 'mixed ependymoma/subependymoma' for these tumours.[43] Subependymomas of the spinal cord need to be separated from other intramedullary gliomas, in particular classic and tanycytic ependymomas, as well as astrocytomas.

Histogenesis

The histogenesis of subependymomas is unclear. Various cells of origin have been suggested, including subependymal glia, astrocytes of the subependymal plate, ependymal cells and both ependymal cells and astrocytes.[43] Experimental data point to the radial glia as a possible cell of origin.[76] However, it remains to be seen whether this hypothesis holds true. It has also been speculated that small, asymptomatic subependymomas may represent hamartomas rather than true neoplasms. Moreover, multiple small lesions have been considered to result from reactive ependymal and subependymal glial proliferation as a response to long-term hydrocephalus or chronic ependymitis, or in association with longstanding tumours, such as choroid plexus papilloma and craniopharyngioma.[68]

Molecular Genetics

Genome-wide profiling of 12 subependymomas using high-resolution array-CGH analysis revealed genomic copy number changes in 5 tumours, including losses on chromosomes 6 and 8 in two cases each, as well as losses on chromosome 14 and trisomy 7 in one case each.[34] Allelic losses on chromosome arms 10q and 22q and mutations in the *hSNF5/INI1*, *NF2* and *PTEN* genes were not detected.[12,33]

Aetiology and Genetic Susceptibility

The aetiology of subependymomas is unknown. The vast majority arise sporadically. However, rare familial cases have been reported, including the simultaneous occurrence of fourth ventricular tumours in monozygotic twins, familial clustering of three subependymomas in a family of 11 siblings, and subependymomas in a father and son.[69]

Biological Behaviour and Prognosis

Subependymomas are slowly growing benign tumours associated with a favourable prognosis.[60] The treatment of choice in both symptomatic intracranial and spinal subependymoma consists of surgical resection, which usually results in long-term, recurrence-free survival. Radiation therapy or radiosurgery may be used for the treatment of symptomatic residual or recurrent subependymomas. Mixed ependymoma/subependymoma tumours are assumed to follow a clinical course similar to WHO grade II ependymomas.

REFERENCES

1. Amirian ES, Armstrong TS, Aldape KD, Gilbert MR, Scheurer ME. Predictors of survival among paediatric and adult ependymoma cases: a study using Surveillance, Epidemiology, and End Results data from 1973 to 2007. *Neuroepidemiology* 2012;39:116–24.
2. Andoh H, Kawaguchi Y, Seki S, *et al.* Multifocal myxopapillary ependymoma in the lumbar and sacral regions requiring cranio–spinal radiation therapy: a case report. *Asian Spine J* 2011;5:68–72.
3. Awaya H, Kaneko M, Amatya VJ, *et al.* Myxopapillary ependymoma with anaplastic features. *Pathol Int* 2003;53:700–3.
4. Azizi E, Friedman J, Pavlotsky F, *et al.* Familial cutaneous malignant melanoma and tumours of the nervous system. A hereditary cancer syndrome. *Cancer* 1995;76:1571–8.

5. Barton VN, Donson AM, Kleinschmidt–DeMasters BK, *et al.* Unique molecular characteristics of pediatric myxopapillary ependymoma. *Brain Pathol* 2010;20:560–70.
6. Benesch M, Weber–Mzell D, Gerber NU, *et al.* Ependymoma of the spinal cord in children and adolescents: a retrospective series from the HIT database. *J Neurosurg Pediatr* 2010;6:137–44.
7. Capper D, Reuss D, Schittenhelm J, *et al.* Mutation-specific IDH1 antibody differentiates oligodendrogliomas and oligoastrocytomas from other brain tumours with oligodendroglioma-like morphology. *Acta Neuropathol* 2011;121:241–52.
8. CBTRUS (2012). *CBTRUS statistical report: primary brain and central nervous system tumours diagnosed in the United States in 2004–2008* (March 23, 2012 Revision). Source: Central Brain Tumour

Registry of the United States, Hinsdale, IL. website:www.cbtrus.org.
9. Comi AM, Backstrom JW, Burger PC, Duffner PK. Clinical and neuroradiologic findings in infants with intracranial ependymomas. Pediatric Oncology Group. *Pediatr Neurol* 1998;18:23–9.
10. Cunha AM, Brito AC, de Almeida Lima G, *et al.* Cerebellopontine angle subependymoma without fourth ventricle extension: an uncommon tumour in a rare location. *Neuropathology* 2012;32:164–70.
11. DiLuna ML, Levy GH, Sood S, Duncan CC. Primary myxopapillary ependymoma of the medulla: case report. *Neurosurgery* 2010;66:E1208–9.
12. Ebert C, von Haken M, Meyer–Puttlitz B, *et al.* Molecular genetic analysis of ependymal tumours. NF2 mutations and chromosome 22q loss occur preferentially

in intramedullary spinal ependymomas. *Am J Pathol* 1999;**155**:627–32.

13. Ellison DW, Kocak M, Figarella–Branger D, *et al*. Histopathological grading of pediatric ependymoma: reproducibility and clinical relevance in European trial cohorts. *J Negat Results Biomed* 2011;**10**:7.

14. Fouladi M, Helton K, Dalton J, *et al*. Clear cell ependymoma: a clinicopathologic and radiographic analysis of 10 patients. *Cancer* 2003;**98**:2232–44.

15. Gessi M, Marani C, Geddes J, *et al*. Ependymoma with neuropil-like islands: a case report with diagnostic and histogenetic implications. *Acta Neuropathol* (Berl) 2005;**109**:231–4.

16. Gilbert MR, Ruda R, Soffietti R. Ependymomas in adults. *Curr Neurol Neurosci Rep* 2010;**10**:240–7.

17. Gilbertson RJ, Bentley L, Hernan R, *et al*. ERBB receptor signaling promotes ependymoma cell proliferation and represents a potential novel therapeutic target for this disease. *Clin Cancer Res* 2002;**8**:3054–64.

18. Hamilton DW, Lusher ME, Lindsey JC, Ellison DW, Clifford SC. Epigenetic inactivation of the RASSF1A tumour suppressor gene in ependymoma. *Cancer Lett* 2005;**227**:75–81.

19. Hasselblatt M, Paulus W. Sensitivity and specificity of epithelial membrane antigen staining patterns in ependymomas. *Acta Neuropathol* (Berl) 2003;**106**:385–8.

20. Hasselblatt M, Bohm C, Tatenhorst L, *et al*. Identification of novel diagnostic markers for choroid plexus tumours: a microarray-based approach. *Am J Surg Pathol* 2006;**30**:66–74.

21. Ho KL. Microtubular aggregates within rough endoplasmic reticulum in myxopapillary ependymoma of the filum terminale. *Arch Pathol Lab Med* 1990;**114**:956–60.

22. Horn B, Heideman R, Geyer R, *et al*. A multi-institutional retrospective study of intracranial ependymoma in children: identification of risk factors. *J Pediatr Hematol Oncol* 1999;**21**:203–11.

23. Ikezaki K, Matsushima T, Inoue T, *et al*. Correlation of microanatomical localization with postoperative survival in posterior fossa ependymomas. *Neurosurgery* 1993;**32**:38–44.

24. Jeibmann A, Egensperger R, Kuchelmeister K, *et al*. Extent of surgical resection but not myxopapillary versus classical histopathological subtype affects prognosis in lumbo–sacral ependymomas. *Histopathology* 2009;**54**:260–2.

25. Johnson RA, Wright KD, Poppleton H, *et al*. Cross-species genomics matches driver mutations and cell compartments to model ependymoma. *Nature* 2010;**466**:632–6.

26. Kleinman GM, Zagzag D, Miller DC. Epithelioid ependymoma: a new variant of ependymoma: report of three cases. *Neurosurgery* 2003;**53**:743–7.

27. Kobata H, Kuroiwa T, Isono N, *et al*. Tanycytic ependymoma in association with neurofibromatosis type 2. *Clin Neuropathol* 2001;**20**:93–100.

28. Koos B, Peetz–Dienhart S, Riesmeier B, Frühwald MC, Hasselblatt M. O(6)–methylguanine–DNA methyltransferase (MGMT) promoter methylation is significantly less frequent in ependymal tumours as compared to malignant astrocytic gliomas. *Neuropathol Appl Neurobiol* 2010;**36**:356–8.

29. Korshunov A, Golanov A, Timirgaz V. Immunohistochemical markers for prognosis of ependymal neoplasms. *J Neurooncol* 2002;**58**:255–70.

30. Korshunov A, Golanov A, Sycheva R, Timirgaz V. The histologic grade is a main prognostic factor for patients with intracranial ependymomas treated in the microneurosurgical era: an analysis of 258 patients. *Cancer* 2004;**100**:1230–7.

31. Korshunov A, Neben K, Wrobel G, *et al*. Gene expression patterns in ependymomas correlate with tumour location, grade, and patient age. *Am J Pathol* 2003;**163**:1721–7.

32. Korshunov A, Witt H, Hielscher T, *et al*. Molecular staging of intracranial ependymoma in children and adults. *J Clin Oncol* 2010;**28**:3182–90.

33. Kraus JA, de Millas W, Sorensen N, *et al*. Indications for a tumour suppressor gene at 22q11 involved in the pathogenesis of ependymal tumours and distinct from hSNF5/INI1. *Acta Neuropathol* (Berl) 2001;**102**:69–74.

34. Kurian KM, Jones DT, Marsden F, *et al*. Genome-wide analysis of subependymomas shows underlying chromosomal copy number changes involving chromosomes 6, 7, 8 and 14 in a proportion of cases. *Brain Pathol* 2008;**18**:469–73.

35. Kurt E, Zheng PP, Hop WC, *et al*. Identification of relevant prognostic histopathologic features in 69 intracranial ependymomas, excluding myxopapillary ependymomas and subependymomas. *Cancer* 2006;**106**:388–95.

36. Li JY, Lopez JI, Powell SZ, Coons SW, Fuller GN. Giant cell ependymoma-report of three cases and review of the literature. *Int J Clin Exp Pathol* 2012;**5**:458–62.

37. Lim SC, Jang SJ. Myxopapillary ependymoma of the fourth ventricle. *Clin Neurol Neurosurg* 2006;**108**:211–4.

38. Little NS, Morgan MK, Eckstein RP. Primary ependymoma of a cranial nerve. Case report. *J Neurosurg* 1994;**81**:792–4.

39. Lord H, Ironside J, Summers D, *et al*. Fourth ventricle ependymoma in father and son. *Br J Neurosurg* 2008;**22**:423–5.

40. Ma YT, Ramachandra P, Spooner D. Case report: primary subcutaneous sacrococcygeal ependymoma: a case report and review of the literature. *Br J Radiol* 2006;**79**:445–7.

41. Mazewski C, Soukup S, Ballard E, Gotwals B, Lampkin B. Karyotype studies in 18 ependymomas with literature review of 107 cases. *Cancer Genet Cytogenet* 1999;**113**:1–8.

42. McGuire CS, Sainani KL, Fisher PG. Incidence patterns for ependymoma: a surveillance, epidemiology, and end results study. *J Neurosurg* 2009;**110**:725–9.

43. McLendon RE, Schiffer D, Rosenblum MK, Wiestler OD. Subependymoma. In Louis DN, Ohgaki H, Wiestler OD, Cavenee WK (Eds.). *WHO classification of tumours of the central nervous system*. IARC, Lyon, 2007:70–71.

44. McLendon RE, Wiestler OD, Kros JM, Korshunov A, Ng HK. Ependymoma. In Louis DN, Ohgaki H, Wiestler OD, Cavenee WK (Eds.). *WHO classification of tumours of the central nervous system*. IARC, Lyon, 2007:74–78.

45. Mendrzyk F, Korshunov A, Benner A, *et al*. Identification of gains on 1q and epidermal growth factor receptor overexpression as independent prognostic markers in intracranial ependymoma. *Clin Cancer Res* 2006;**12**:2070–9.

46. Merchant TE, Fouladi M. Ependymoma: new therapeutic approaches including radiation and chemotherapy. *J Neurooncol* 2005;**75**:287–99.

47. Merchant TE, Mulhern RK, Krasin MJ, *et al*. Preliminary results from a phase II trial of conformal radiation therapy and evaluation of radiation-related CNS effects for pediatric patients with localized ependymoma. *J Clin Oncol* 2004;**22**:3156–62.

48. Metzger AK, Sheffield VC, Duyk G, *et al*. Identification of a germ-line mutation in the p53 gene in a patient with an intracranial ependymoma. *Proc Natl Acad Sci USA* 1991;**88**:7825–9.

49. Milde T, Hielscher T, Witt H, et al. Nestin expression identifies ependymoma patients with poor outcome. *Brain Pathol* 2012;**22**:848–860.

50. Modena P, Buttarelli FR, Miceli R, et al. Predictors of outcome in an AIEOP series of childhood ependymomas: a multifactorial analysis. *Neuro Onco* 2012;**14**:1346–56.

51. Morin G, Desenclos C, Jeanpetit C, et al. Additional familial case of subtotal leukonychia and sebaceous cysts (Bauer syndrome): belong the nervous tumours to the phenotype? *Eur J Med Genet* 2008;**51**:436–43.

52. Newton HB, Henson J, Walker RW. Extraneural metastases in ependymoma. *J Neurooncol* 1992;**14**:135–42.

53. Peris–Bonet R, Martinez–Garcia C, et al. Childhood central nervous system tumours –incidence and survival in Europe (1978–1997): Report from Automated Childhood Cancer Information System project. *Eur J Cancer* 2006;**42**:2064–80.

54. Plotkin SR, O'Donnell CC, Curry WT, et al. Spinal ependymomas in neurofibromatosis type 2: a retrospective analysis of 55 patients. *J Neurosurg Spine* 2011;**14**:543–7.

55. Poltinnikov IM, Merchant TE. CSF cytology has limited value in the evaluation of patients with ependymoma who have MRI evidence of metastasis. *Pediatr Blood Cancer* 2006;**47**:169–73.

56. Prayson RA. Myxopapillary ependymomas: a clinicopathologic study of 14 cases including MIB–1 and p53 immunoreactivity. *Mod Pathol* 1997;**10**:304–10.

57. Preusser M, Budka H, Rössler K, Hainfellner JA. OLIG2 is a useful immunohistochemical marker in differential diagnosis of clear cell primary CNS neoplasms. *Histopathology* 2007;**50**:365–70.

58. Preusser M, Heinzl H, Gelpi E, et al. Ki67 index in intracranial ependymoma: a promising histopathological candidate biomarker. *Histopathology* 2008;**53**:39–47.

59. Preusser M, Wolfsberger S, Czech T, et al. Survivin expression in intracranial

ependymomas and its correlation with tumour cell proliferation and patient outcome. *Am J Clin Pathol* 2005;**124**:543–9.

60. Ragel BT, Osborn AG, Whang K, et al. Subependymomas: an analysis of clinical and imaging features. *Neurosurgery* 2006;**58**:881–90.

61. Rickert CH, Korshunov A, Paulus W. Chromosomal imbalances in clear cell ependymomas. *Mod Pathol* 2006;**19**:958–62.

62. Rodriguez FJ, Scheithauer BW, Perry A, et al. Ependymal tumours with sarcomatous change ('ependymosarcoma'): a clinicopathologic and molecular cytogenetic study. *Am J Surg Pathol* 2008;**32**:699–709.

63. Rodriguez FJ, Scheithauer BW, Robbins PD, et al. Ependymomas with neuronal differentiation: a morphologic and immunohistochemical spectrum. *Acta Neuropathol* 2007;**113**:313–24.

64. Roncaroli F, Consales A, Fioravanti A, Cenacchi G. Supratentorial cortical ependymoma: report of three cases. *Neurosurgery* 2005;**57**: E192.

65. Rousseau A, Idbaih A, Ducray F, et al. Specific chromosomal imbalances as detected by array CGH in ependymomas in association with tumour location, histological subtype and grade. *J Neurooncol* 2010;**97**:353–64.

66. Rousseau E, Ruchoux MM, Scaravilli F, et al. CDKN2A, CDKN2B and p14ARF are frequently and differentially methylated in ependymal tumours. *Neuropathol Appl Neurobiol* 2003;**29**:574–83.

67. Ruchoux MM, Kepes JJ, Dhellemmes P, et al. Lipomatous differentiation in ependymomas: a report of three cases and comparison with similar changes reported in other central nervous system neoplasms of neuroectodermal origin. *Am J Surg Pathol* 1998;**22**:338–46.

68. Russell DS, Rubinstein LJ. *Pathology of tumours of the nervous system*, 5th edn. London: Edward Arnold, 1989:206–212

69. Ryken TC, Robinson RA, VanGilder JC. Familial occurrence of subependymoma.

Report of two cases. *J Neurosurg* 1994;**80**:1108–11.

70. Sant M, Minicozzi P, Lagorio S, et al. Survival of European patients with central nervous system tumors. *Int J Cancer* 2012;**131**:173–85.

71. Scheil S, Bruderlein S, Eicker M, et al. Low frequency of chromosomal imbalances in anaplastic ependymomas as detected by comparative genomic hybridization. *Brain Pathol* 2001;**11**:133–43.

72. Scheithauer BW, Swearingen B, Whyte ET, Auluck PK, Stemmer–Rachamimov AO. Ependymoma of the sella turcica: a variant of pituicytoma. *Hum Pathol* 2009;**40**:435–40.

73. Schiffer D, Chio A, Giordana MT, et al. Histologic prognostic factors in ependymoma. *Childs Nerv Syst* 1991;**7**:177–82.

74. Sonneland PR, Scheithauer BW, Onofrio BM. Myxopapillary ependymoma. A clinicopathologic and immunocytochemical study of 77 cases. *Cancer* 1985;**56**:883–93.

75. Sparaco M, Morelli L, Piscioli I, et al. Primary myxopapillary ependymoma of the cerebellopontine angle: report of a case. *Neurosurg Rev* 2009;**32**:241–4.

76. Taylor MD, Poppleton H, Fuller C, et al. Radial glia cells are candidate stem cells of ependymoma. *Cancer Cell* 2005;**8**:323–35.

77. Timmermann B, Kortmann RD, Kühl J, et al. Combined postoperative irradiation and chemotherapy for anaplastic ependymomas in childhood: results of the German prospective trials HIT 88/89 and HIT 91. *Int J Radiat Oncol Biol Phys* 2000;**46**:287–95.

78. Timmermann B, Kortmann RD, Kühl J, et al. Role of radiotherapy in anaplastic ependymoma in children under age of 3 years: results of the prospective German brain tumour trials HIT–SKK 87 and 92. *Radiother Oncol* 2005;**77**:278–85.

79. Tseng JH, Tseng MY. Survival analysis of children with primary malignant brain tumours in England and Wales: a population-based study. *Pediatr Neurosurg* 2006;**42**:67–73.

80. Tzerakis N, Georgakoulias N, Kontogeorgos G, et al. Intraparenchymal myxopapillary ependymoma: case report. *Neurosurgery* 2004;**55**:981.

81. Vajtai I, von Gunten M, Fung C, et al. Oncocytic ependymoma: a new morphological variant of high-grade ependymal neoplasm composed of mitochondrion-rich epithelioid cells. *Pathol Res Pract* 2011;**207**:49–54.

82. Varan A, Sari N, Akalan N, et al. Extraneural metastasis in intracranial tumours in children: the experience of a single center. *J Neurooncol* 2006;**79**:187–90.

83. Vege KD, Giannini C, Scheithauer BW. The immunophenotype of ependymomas. *Appl Immunohistochem Mol Morphol* 2000;**8**:25–31.

84. Verstegen MJ, Leenstra DT, Ijlst–Keizers H, Bosch DA. Proliferation- and apoptosis-related proteins in intracranial ependymomas: an immunohistochemical analysis. *J Neurooncol* 2002;**56**:21–8.

85. Wager M, Lapierre F, Blanc JL, Listrat A, Bataille B. Cauda equina tumours: a French multicenter retrospective review of 231 adult cases and review of the literature. *Neurosurg Rev* 2000;**23**:119–29

86. Wani K, Armstrong TS, Vera–Bolanos E, et al. A prognostic gene expression signature in infratentorial ependymoma. *Acta Neuropathol* 2012;**123**:727–38.

87. Witt H, Mack SC, Ryzhova M, et al. Delineation of two clinically and molecularly distinct subgroups of posterior fossa ependymoma. *Cancer Cell* 2011;**20**:143–57.

88. Yoshida K, Sato K, Kubota T, et al. Supratentorial desmoplastic ependymoma with giant ependymal rosettes. *Clin Neuropathol* 2000;**19**:186–91.

89. Zec N, De Girolami U, Schofield DE, Scott RM, Anthony DC. Giant cell ependymoma of the filum terminale. A report of two cases. *Am J Surg Pathol* 1996;**20**:1091–101.

Choroid Plexus Tumours

Hope T Richard, Jason F Harrison and Christine E Fuller

INTRODUCTION

Tumours of the choroid plexus include the World Health Organization's (WHO's) classification of nervous system tumours designated choroid plexus papilloma (WHO grade I), atypical choroid plexus papilloma (WHO grade II) and choroid plexus carcinoma (WHO grade III).[15] These lesions are nearly always located within the ventricles and are derived from specialized neuroepithelial cells that recapitulate the histologic and physiologic characteristics of normal choroid plexus. In fact, excessive production of cerebrospinal fluid by these tumours has been shown in some cases to be a direct cause or complicating factor in the development of hydrocephalus.[64] Surgical resection and histological assessment are essential in the treatment of these lesions. Although tumour location and grade are key factors in patient outcome, good long-term survival is achievable even in higher grade lesions. This chapter presents the classic neuroimaging and clinicopathologic characteristics of choroid plexus neoplasms and a guide to differentiating these lesions from diagnostic mimics.

EPIDEMIOLOGY

Choroid plexus tumours are rare, with an average annual incidence of about 0.3 per million.[11,64] Accounting for approximately 0.3 per cent of central nervous system (CNS) tumours, most occur in childhood particularly in the first decade of life. They constitute 10–20 per cent of brain tumours in infancy and 2.3 per cent of primary intracranial neoplasms in childhood.[34,54] In one study of over 265 cases, 74 per cent developed during the first decade of life and 45 per cent during the first year of life.[34] Fetal choroid plexus papillomas are relatively more common constituting 5–20 per cent of all perinatal brain tumours.[3,51]

Choroid plexus carcinomas are rarer than papillomas by a ratio of 1:5.[15,38] Unlike carcinomas that arise elsewhere in the body, choroid plexus carcinoma is primarily a tumour of childhood with 70 per cent occurring before 2 years of age; the median age of occurrence is 26–32 months.[6] Adult examples are exceedingly rare. Most choroid plexus carcinomas arise in the lateral ventricles with rare exceptions.[10,53]

In terms of tumour location, 40–50 per cent of choroid plexus tumours arise in the lateral ventricle, 5–10 per cent in the third ventricle and 40 per cent in the fourth ventricle.[38,42,47] Rare extraventricular locations have been described, including the cerebellopontine angle, cerebellomedullary cistern, suprasellar cistern and even the sacral canal.[31,33,43,52,57] The age distribution of patients with choroid plexus tumours varies by site.[23] Whereas approximately 80 per cent of tumours in the lateral ventricles occur in children, tumours in the fourth ventricle are more evenly distributed across all age groups. Meta-analysis has shown a significant correlation between age and tumour location with a median age at diagnosis of 1.5 years for lateral and third ventricular tumours compared to 23.5 years for fourth ventricular tumours.[64]

There is a slight male predominance,[32] with male:female ratios of 3:2 for fourth ventricular versus 1:1 for lateral ventricular tumours.

CLINICAL FEATURES

As with most intracranial lesions, the signs and symptoms at presentation for patients with choroid plexus tumours may include focal neurological deficits depending upon tumour location. However, the most common findings are associated with increased intracranial pressure resulting directly from tumoural mass effects and/or indirectly from hydrocephalus.[23] Often there is generalized hydrocephalus with ventricular enlargement caused by obstruction of cerebrospinal fluid (CSF) flow and possibly complicated by overproduction of CSF.[19] Although increased production of CSF has only been shown in a few patients, these findings are supported by ultrastructural analysis consistent with CSF production, resolution of non-obstructive hydrocephalus following tumour resection and the development of ascites following ventriculoperitoneal shunt placement in patients with choroid plexus tumours.[22,46,62]

Headache, nausea and vomiting are common symptoms of increased intracranial pressure; however, findings vary with age at presentation.[23] Cranial sutures have yet to fuse in children younger than 2 years of age; thus patients with hydrocephalus may first present with macrocephaly in association with signs that include strabismus, ataxia and delayed development. Shunt-resistant hydrocephalus in infants can occasionally be caused by bilateral choroid plexus papillomas of the lateral ventricles.[14]

The majority of choroid plexus tumours are sporadic in nature; however, a number of cases have been linked to familial tumour syndromes and other inherited developmental disorders. Choroid plexus papillomas are associated with Aicardi syndrome, an X-linked dominant condition defined by agenesis of the corpus callosum, chorioretinal lacunae and infantile spasms.[51,56] A high incidence of choroid plexus tumours has been identified in females with this syndrome; thus females diagnosed with choroid plexus papillomas should be carefully evaluated for Aicardi syndrome. Scattered case reports have also described a link between choroid plexus papillomas and von Hippel–Lindau disease.[9] The association between choroid plexus carcinoma and Li–Fraumeni syndrome is well established.[20,36,51,55] These patients harbour germline mutations of the *TP53* tumour suppressor gene, leading to increased risk and early onset of soft-tissue sarcomas, osteosarcomas, premenopausal breast cancer, adrenocortical tumours and brain tumours. Choroid plexus carcinomas have also been reported in the context of rhabdoid predisposition syndrome with germline mutations of the *hSNF5/INI1/SMARCB1* gene, although it is also possible that some of these represent misdiagnosed atypical teratoid/rhabdoid tumour given considerable overlap in the histological features of these two entities.[50,65]

RADIOLOGY

From a neuroimaging standpoint, choroid plexus tumours typically present as isodense to hyperdense intraventricular masses on computed tomography (CT) imaging. They are usually well demarcated and may display foci of calcifications and haemorrhage. On magnetic resonance imaging (MRI) they appear as isointense to grey matter on T1, hyperintense on T2 and enhance intensely following contrast administration (Figure 30.1a); thus, rare extraventricular examples may be difficult to distinguish from meningiomas. Multiple flow voids on T2 MRI reflect a robust vascular support system. Radiographically, the distinction between choroid plexus papilloma and choroid plexus carcinoma can be elusive.[58] In comparison to choroid plexus papillomas, choroid plexus carcinomas are often larger with increased parenchymal invasion and associated vasogenic oedema

(Figure 30.1g).[66] CSF dissemination correlates with leptomeningeal enhancement.

MACROSCOPIC APPEARANCES

Upon gross inspection, choroid plexus papilloma has features often likened to that of a cauliflower floret. Its bosselated, cobbled surface may have a gritty consistency as a result of calcification (Figure 30.1b). *In situ*, these villiform lesions are pink and friable; however, the tissue loses its characteristic hyperaemic appearance when robbed of its rich blood supply following resection. These tumours tend to expand within the ventricular cavity, often causing compression of surrounding structures, most often without evidence of invasion. Because they obstruct CSF pathways, hydrocephalus is invariably present. Choroid plexus papillomas are prone to haemorrhage, and this may be macroscopically evident. Degenerative changes, such as cyst formation or calcification, are infrequently found in some large tumours.[39]

Choroid plexus carcinomas tend to be more solid, filling the ventricle and often invading adjacent brain. Intratumoural haemorrhage and necrosis may be evident. Metastatic spread through the CSF pathways can be a feature.

MICROSCOPIC APPEARANCES

Choroid plexus tumours are epithelial neoplasms, resembling normal choroid plexus tissue with varying degrees of differentiation. Choroid plexus papillomas (WHO grade I) are the most well differentiated, composed of delicate papillary cores of fibrovascular tissue draped by a single layer of cuboidal to columnar epithelium (Figure 30.1c, d). The branching and papillary architecture of these tumours is striking. Similar to normal choroid plexus epithelium, the epithelial cells of papillomas exhibit monotonously round-to-oval nuclei usually basally oriented within either clear or eosinophilic cytoplasm. In contrast to its non-neoplastic counterpart, epithelial cells in papillomas tend to be more crowded with evidence of stratification and loss of the normal cobblestone-like surface, mildly increased nuclear to cytoplasmic ratio, nuclear hyperchromasia and rare mitotic figures.[44,64] Cytoplasmic vacuolation may be prominent, and unusual phenotypes include oncocytic change, osseous and adipose metaplasia, production of melanin and mucinous material with gland-like or tubular arrangements.[12,17] The latter example has been referred to as choroid plexus (tubular) adenoma.[4] Foci of calcification with psammoma body formation, hyalinization of connective tissue and stromal oedema may also be seen. The borders of papillomas are generally well demarcated from surrounding parenchyma, without evidence of invasion. The presence of necrosis, increased cellularity, loss of papillary structure or foci of superficial parenchymal invasion should prompt a search for higher grade features as described later.

A subset of choroid plexus papillomas exhibit modestly increased mitotic activity (more than two mitoses per high-powered field) and more complex architecture with

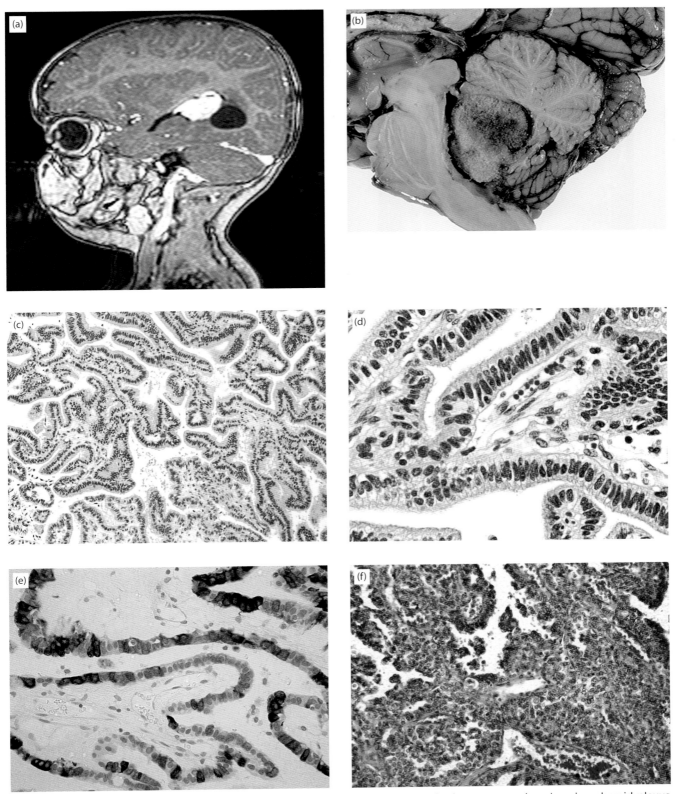

30.1 Choroid plexus tumours. (a) Sagittal T1-weighted MR scan post-contrast of a homogeneously enhancing choroid plexus papilloma of the lateral ventricle. **(b)** Midline sagittal section showing a choroid plexus papilloma in the fourth ventricle, which compresses but does not invade the brain stem and cerebellum. **(c)** Choroid plexus papilloma mimics the architecture of the normal choroid plexus. **(d)** Choroid plexus papilloma. A simple epithelium in which surface cilia are often visualized overlies fibrovascular tissue. **(e)** Choroid plexus papilloma. The epithelium is immunoreactive for cytokeratin. **(f)** Atypical choroid plexus papilloma. A focal syncytial pattern replaces the papillary architecture and may be associated with increased cytological pleomorphism and proliferative activity.

Continued

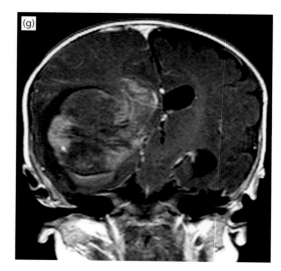

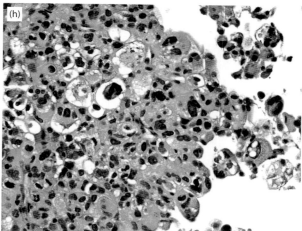

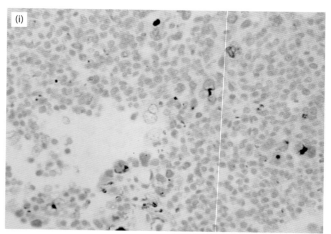

30.1 (*Continued*) **Choroid plexus tumours. (g)** Coronal T1-weighted MR scan, post-contrast, of a large choroid plexus carcinoma within the right lateral ventricle showing heterogeneous enhancement and focal parenchymal invasion. **(h)** Choroid plexus carcinoma. Loss of papillary architecture, cytological pleomorphism and abundant mitotic figures characterize this tumour. **(i)** Choroid plexus carcinomas may show only focal immunoreactivity for cytokeratins.

Courtesy of P Kleihues.

cribriforming and anastomosing. Falling short of established diagnostic criteria for malignancy, they are designated atypical choroid plexus papillomas and assigned a WHO grade II (Figure 30.1f). Increased cellularity, nuclear pleomorphism and focal necrosis with penetration of juxtatumoural brain tissue may also be evident focally.[27] Although the atypical papilloma designation as a distinct variant remains somewhat controversial, an increased likelihood of recurrence and progression to anaplasia has been observed.[27,41]

Choroid plexus carcinomas are at the most poorly differentiated end of the spectrum; they bear frankly malignant histologic features and are designated WHO grade III. Unlike choroid plexus papillomas, which are generally similar to one another, carcinomas are highly variable, often generating significant diagnostic confusion with other primary CNS and metastatic lesions. A syncytial or solid architecture is generally present, although papillary structures may be focally evident (Figure 30.1h). Areas of necrosis and haemorrhage are common, and extensive parenchymal invasion can be identified. Marked cytologic atypia with nuclear pleomorphism and hyperchromasia as well as high mitotic activity are characteristic. Uncommonly, features of rhabdoid or small (primitive) cell morphology and melanin pigment production are identified, raising differential diagnoses with atypical teratoid/rhabdoid tumour, medulloblastoma/primitive neuroectodermal tumour (PNET), or even melanoma.[5,59]

Ultrastructural analysis of choroid plexus papillomas recapitulates the cytoarchitecture of normal choroid plexus.[37] The epithelial layer is shown to rest on an uninterrupted basement membrane outlining the basal contour of the cells. They are joined with elaborate junctional complexes and topped by microvilli and occasional cilia on their apical surface.[37] The cytoplasm includes pinocytotic and coated vesicles in addition to rough endoplasmic reticulum and Golgi complexes. As with normal choroid plexus, the papillary fibrous stroma may be conspicuously infiltrated by foamy macrophages. Aggregates of glycogen can be seen in infantile and childhood examples. Ultrastructural examination of choroid plexus carcinomas confirms the histological features of anaplasia often with an abnormal arrangement of cilia abnormal cilia, but at least some features resembling normal choroid plexus.[37]

GRADING

As noted earlier, the WHO classification of nervous system tumours assigns choroid plexus tumours to the following grades: papillomas (grade I), atypical papillomas (grade II) and carcinomas (grade III).[15] Although pathologically similar to its grade I counterpart, there is evidence that atypical choroid plexus papillomas exhibit a more aggressive biological behaviour with higher rates of recurrence and progression to histological anaplasia.[28] Cytological pleomorphism may increase focally and may be associated with an increased mitotic index.[41] However, it is a widespread loss of papillary architecture and cytological anaplasia that are considered characteristic of choroid plexus carcinoma.

IMMUNOHISTOCHEMISTRY

Choroid plexus tumours are typically immunoreactive for epithelial markers (Figure 30.1e). Papillomas are consistently positive for pancytokeratin and vimentin, with pancytokeratin often producing a diffuse or dot-like cytoplasmic pattern of reactivity.[44] Variable immunoreactivity can be seen with cytokeratin (CK) 7 and CK20, with the most common pattern being CK7+/CK20 .[24] Although nonspecific, epithelial membrane antigen (EMA) and carcinoembryonic antigen (CEA) are usually negative whereas up to 90 per cent of papillomas are at least focally positive for S-100, thus distinguishing choroid plexus tumours from metastatic carcinoma.[37] Focal glial fibrillary acidic protein (GFAP) reactivity is also seen in 50 per cent of cases, whereas synaptophysin is positive in a minority of cases.[30,41] Transthyretin is positive in most choroid plexus papillomas though not entirely specific, as papillary carcinomas from alternate body sites may be similarly positive. Collagen IV or laminin staining is helpful in highlighting the subepithelial basement membrane.[1]

Choroid plexus carcinomas also show immunoreactivity for pancytokeratin (Figure 30.1i) and vimentin; however, transthyretin and S-100 staining are not as consistently positive. Synaptophysin, GFAP and carbohydrate antigen 19-9 may be focally expressed. EMA and CEA reactivity is uncommon. Some evidence suggests choroid plexus carcinomas and atypical choroid plexus papillomas express the standard isoform of an adhesion molecule (CD44H), which is not detected in normal choroid plexus or WHO grade I papillomas.[61] Choroid plexus carcinomas have also been shown to contain globular hyaline deposits of α1-antitrypsin and nuclear p53 staining.[26] Nuclear staining for *INI1* is retained in choroid plexus carcinomas, including those with rhabdoid morphology; in contradistinction, true rhabdoid tumours, including atypical teratoid/rhabdoid tumour (AT/RT), lose nuclear expression of *INI1*.[29]

Immunoprofiles may vary with anatomical site and patient age. S-100 immunoreactivity is greater in fourth ventricular tumours compared to those of the lateral ventricle. Additionally, tumours in older patients (older than 20 years) exhibit higher GFAP and transthyretin staining than those of younger patients.[41]

As previously discussed, the mitotic rate is a helpful tool in distinguishing between choroid plexus papillomas of varying grade (I versus II) and carcinomas. To that end, MIB-1/Ki-67 immunostaining can be used as a diagnostic adjunct by providing the proliferation index. Although MIB-1 staining is variable in choroid plexus carcinomas, the labelling index is typically high, with an average of 14 per cent staining compared to 3.7 per cent in papillomas.[60]

Microarray based studies have identified several other potential diagnostic markers for choroid plexus tumours.[25] Positive staining for an inward rectifier potassium channel (Kir7.1), stanniocalcin-1, E-cadherin[18] and excitatory amino acid transporter-1 (EAAT-1)[8] have all been reported. Further studies have shown that expression of EAAT-1 may be helpful in distinguishing reactive choroid plexus epithelium from its neoplastic counterparts.[7]

DIFFERENTIAL DIAGNOSIS

First and foremost, choroid plexus tumours must always be included within the differential diagnosis for patients presenting with an intraventricular mass. In adults, other intraventricular tumours include subependymomas, subependymal giant cell astrocytomas, meningiomas, ependymomas or metastases. In children the differential includes ependymomas, medulloblastomas/PNETs, teratomas, AT/RTs and astrocytomas. The majority of these can be easily differentiated from choroid plexus tumours based on simple histologic findings, with a few exceptions as detailed later.

Differential diagnostic considerations encompass several histopathologically similar primary and secondary tumours with papillary architecture, as well as normal choroid plexus. The distinction between papilloma and normal/hyperplastic choroid plexus can be difficult, particularly in the setting of a tiny biopsy. However, papillomas typically lose the characteristic cobblestone-like surface of normal choroid plexus with the latter showing partial spaces between surface epithelial cells. Evaluation of mitotic activity, epithelial architecture and cellular atypia, along with careful consideration of the clinical context, can also help distinguish papillomas from reactive proliferations.[14] Choroid plexus tumours may share similar microscopic features with several primary CNS tumours, including AT/RT, ependymoma, medulloepithelioma, astroblastoma and embryonal carcinoma. These neoplasms are most often considered in the differential diagnosis in children, whereas metastatic papillary carcinoma must be excluded in adults with suspected choroid plexus carcinoma.

Similar to choroid plexus papillomas, papillary ependymoma and astroblastoma all feature papillary architecture, but differ in their immunoprofiles. A laminin-positive basement membrane underlying a cytokeratin-positive epithelium is characteristic of papillomas, whereas papillary ependymoma and astroblastoma exhibit GFAP-positive perivascular pseudorosettes; astroblastomas differ from ependymoma in their lack of fibrillary processes.[2]

Choroid plexus carcinomas, in contrast to anaplastic ependymomas, exhibit strong cytokeratin staining in the presence of a sometimes fragmented basement membrane without GFAP staining of pseudorosettes. Additionally, E-cadherin positivity and absence of nerve cell adhesion molecule staining supports a diagnosis of choroid plexus carcinoma.[18] Medulloepithelioma and embryonal carcinoma can also mimic choroid plexus carcinoma, although the primitive epithelioid cells of medulloepithelioma are cytokeratin negative and embryonal carcinoma is typically positive for placental alkaline phosphatase, OCT-3/4 and CD30. Another important differential in the diagnosis of choroid plexus carcinoma especially in cases with significant rhabdoid morphology is AT/RT. As noted elsewhere, choroid plexus carcinomas retain nuclear *INI1* expression, whereas this is lost in AT/RT.[29,48]

When an intracerebral papillary carcinoma arises in an adult patient, metastatic carcinoma is considerably more likely than choroid plexus carcinoma, with the immunoprofiles generally reflecting their primaries of origin. Although lacking absolute specificity, transthyretin and S-100 positivity supports choroid plexus carcinoma.[1] Additionally,

GFAP positivity is often focally present in choroid plexus tumours and lacking in metastatic neoplasms. As a general rule, few metastatic papillary carcinomas appear as well differentiated as choroid plexus papillomas, and choroid plexus carcinomas are so rare in adults that metastatic papillary carcinoma must be the presumptive diagnosis until proven otherwise.

HISTOGENESIS

There is speculation and some limited scientific support for a viral role in choroid plexus tumorigenesis. For instance, DNA sequences of the simian papova virus SV40 have been detected in choroid plexus tumours, and this virus has been further implicated in animal models.[40] Additionally, expression of a segment of the SV40 T-antigen has been reported in paediatric choroid plexus tumours.[40,63] It is hypothesized that these and other similar polyomaviruses may induce neoplastic transformation by interfering with key cell cycle regulatory proteins. Interactions of viral proteins with p53 and pRb have been identified; however, the biological significance of these interactions has not been fully elucidated.[16] Importantly, the presence of these sequences does not definitively prove a causal link and may merely indicate that these neoplasms provide a microenvironment that favours viral replication.

MOLECULAR GENETICS

Classic and molecular cytogenetic assessments of choroid plexus tumours show that chromosomal imbalance is common in both papillomas and carcinomas. Choroid plexus papillomas are typically hyperdiploid, with gains identified on chromosomes 5, 7, 9, 12, 15, 17, 18, 20 and 21, and losses on chromosomes 10 and 22q.[21,45] Losses on chromosomes 5, 10q, 18q, and 22q and gains on 1, 4, 8q, 9p, 12, 14q, 20q and 21 have been encountered in choroid plexus carcinoma. These differences in genetic abnormalities support the theory that choroid plexus tumours of different grade develop *de novo*, with malignant transformation from papilloma to carcinoma seldom occurring.

The significance of reported *hSNF5/INI1* (at 22q11.2) mutations in choroid plexus tumours is controversial.[65] Despite the frequent (40–70 per cent) loss of chromosome 22q in choroid plexus papillomas and carcinomas, very few mutations of the *INI1* gene have been detected. Further complicating this issue is the histopathological resemblance of choroid plexus carcinoma to AT/RT, the latter characterized by *hSNF5/INI1* gene mutations. Although loss of chromosome 22q and alterations of *INI1* (mainly in the form of deletions) have been reported

in some well-documented choroid plexus carcinomas (including those with rhabdoid phenotypes), immunohistochemistry confirms that INI1 protein expression remains intact, thus maintaining the distinction between these two neoplasms described earlier.[29]

Choroid plexus tumours have been associated with several familial tumour syndromes, including Li–Fraumeni syndrome (see Chapter 44). Germline *TP53* mutations are the hallmark of this syndrome, and recent studies suggest a strong association between a specific *TP53* mutation (R337H) and choroid plexus carcinomas. In multiple studies of populations with a high prevalence of Li–Fraumeni syndrome, an increased ratio of carcinomas to papillomas (1:0.6) was identified when compared to the normal population (1:5).[13,49,55]

BIOLOGICAL BEHAVIOUR AND THERAPEUTIC CONSIDERATIONS

The most important factors determining outcomes in patients with choroid plexus tumours are the extent of surgical resection and histologic grade.[15,64] Five-year survival rates for patients diagnosed with choroid plexus papillomas approach 100 per cent, where surgery alone is often curative. Although recurrences are unusual, papillomas may recur many years after initial presentation, particularly in the context of subtotal removal. Additionally, there have been rare cases of CSF seeding described in patients with this otherwise indolent neoplasm.[35] In contrast to papillomas, choroid plexus carcinomas are aggressive tumours with poor prognosis. Five-year survival rates for carcinomas are roughly 40–50 per cent. Complete surgical resection in these cases is often difficult because of the tumour's propensity to invade adjacent brain and metastasize through CSF pathways.[38] Atypical choroid plexus papillomas exhibit intermediate behaviour, which manifests predominantly as recurrence risks.[27] Of note, all choroid plexus neoplasms regardless of grade are highly vascular tumours with a propensity to bleed profusely upon manipulation, thereby making surgical resection challenging.

Chemotherapy is usually employed as adjuvant treatment for carcinomas, and radiation may be appropriate for adults and older children. Craniospinal irradiation may be helpful in those cases with subtotal resection and/ or leptomeningeal dissemination. A recent study showed a significantly lower survival rate in patients diagnosed with choroid plexus carcinoma exhibiting *TP53* alterations.[55] Such mutations confer resistance to chemotherapy and radiation in other cancers suggesting that further investigation may be similarly warranted in choroid plexus tumours.

REFERENCES

1. Albrecht S, Rouah E, Becker LE, Bruner J. Transthyretin immunoreactivity in choroid plexus neoplasms and brain metastases. *Mod Pathol* 1991;4:610–4.
2. Ang LC, Taylor AR, Bergin D, Kaufmann JC. An immunohistochemical study

of papillary tumors in the central nervous system. *Cancer* 1990;65: 2712–9.
3. Anselem O, Mezzetta L, Grange G, et al. Fetal tumors of the choroid plexus: is differential diagnosis between papilloma

and carcinoma possible? *Ultrasound Obstet Gynecol* 2011;38:229–32.
4. Aquilina K, Nanra JS, Allcutt DA, Farrell M. Choroid plexus adenoma: case report and review of the literature. *Childs Nerv Syst* 2005;21:410–5.

5. Barreto AS, Vassallo J, Queiroz Lde S. Papillomas and carcinomas of the choroid plexus: histological and immunohistochemical studies and comparison with normal fetal choroid plexus. *Arq Neuropsiquiatr* 2004;**62** (Part 3A):600–7.

6. Berger C, Thiesse P, Lellouch-Tubiana A, Kalifa C, Pierre-Kahn A, Bouffet E. Choroid plexus carcinomas in childhood: clinical features and prognostic factors. *Neurosurgery* 1998;**42**:470–5.

7. Beschorner R, Pantazis G, Jeibmann A, et al. Expression of EAAT-1 distinguishes choroid plexus tumors from normal and reactive choroid plexus epithelium. *Acta Neuropathol* 2009;**117**:667–75.

8. Beschorner R, Schittenhelm J, Schimmel H, et al. Choroid plexus tumors differ from metastatic carcinomas by expression of the excitatory amino acid transporter-1. *Hum Pathol* 2006;**37**:854–60.

9. Blamires TL, Maher ER. Choroid plexus papilloma. A new presentation of von Hippel-Lindau (VHL) disease. *Eye (Lond)* 1992;**6**:90–2.

10. Carter AB, Price DL, Jr., Tucci KA, Lewis GK, Mewborne J, Singh HK. Choroid plexus carcinoma presenting as an intraparenchymal mass. *J Neurosurg* 2001;**95**:1040–4.

11. CBTRUS. *CBTRUS statistical report: primary brain and central nervous system tumors diagnosed in the United States in 2004–2007*. www.cbtrus.org [accessed July 2012].

12. Corcoran GM, Frazier SR, Prayson RA. Choroid plexus papilloma with osseous and adipose metaplasia. *Ann Diagn Pathol* 2001;**5**:43–7.

13. Custodio G, Taques GR, Figueiredo BC, et al. Increased incidence of choroid plexus carcinoma due to the germline TP53 R337H mutation in southern Brazil. *PLoS One* 2011;**6**: e18015.

14. D'Ambrosio AL, O'Toole JE, Connolly ES, Jr., Feldstein NA. Villous hypertrophy versus choroid plexus papilloma: a case report demonstrating a diagnostic role for the proliferation index. *Pediatr Neurosurg* 2003;**39**:91–6.

15. Louis DN, Ohgaki H, Wiestler OD, et al eds. *WHO classification of tumours of the central nervous system*. 4th ed. Lyon, France: International Agency for Research on Cancer, 2007.

16. DeCaprio JA, Ludlow JW, Figge J, et al. SV40 large tumor antigen forms a specific complex with the product of the retinoblastoma susceptibility gene. *Cell* 1988;**54**:275–83.

17. Diengdoh JV, Shaw MD. Oncocytic variant of choroid plexus papilloma. Evolution from benign to malignant "oncocytoma". *Cancer* 1993;**71**:855–8.

18. Figarella-Branger D, Lepidi H, Poncet C, et al. Differential expression of cell adhesion molecules (CAM), neural CAM and epithelial cadherin in ependymomas and choroid plexus tumors. *Acta Neuropathol* 1995;**89**:248–57.

19. Fujimura M, Onuma T, Kameyama M, et al. Hydrocephalus due to cerebrospinal fluid overproduction by bilateral choroid plexus papillomas. *Childs Nerv Syst* 2004;**20**:485–8.

20. Gozali AE, Britt B, Shane L, et al. Choroid plexus tumors; management, outcome, and association with the Li–Fraumeni syndrome: the Children's Hospital Los Angeles (CHLA) experience, 1991–2010. *Pediatr Blood Cancer* 2012;**58**:905–9.

21. Grill J, Avet-Loiseau H, Lellouch-Tubiana A, et al. Comparative genomic hybridization detects specific cytogenetic abnormalities in pediatric ependymomas and choroid plexus papillomas. *Cancer Genet Cytogenet* 2002;**136**:121–5.

22. Gudeman SK, Sullivan HG, Rosner MJ, Becker DP. Surgical removal of bilateral papillomas of the choroid plexus of the lateral ventricles with resolution of hydrocephalus. Case report. *J Neurosurg* 1979;**50**:677–81.

23. Gupta N. Choroid plexus tumors in children. *Neurosurg Clin N Am* 2003;**14**:621–31.

24. Gyure KA, Morrison AL. Cytokeratin 7 and 20 expression in choroid plexus tumors: utility in differentiating these neoplasms from metastatic carcinomas. *Mod Pathol* 2000;**13**:638–43.

25. Hasselblatt M, Bohm C, Tatenhorst L, et al. Identification of novel diagnostic markers for choroid plexus tumors: a microarray-based approach. *Am J Surg Pathol* 2006;**30**:66–74.

26. Jay V, Ho M, Chan F, Malkin D. P53 expression in choroid plexus neoplasms: an immunohistochemical study. *Arch Pathol Lab Med* 1996;**120**:1061–5.

27. Jeibmann A, Hasselblatt M, Gerss J, et al. Prognostic implications of atypical histologic features in choroid plexus papilloma. *J Neuropathol Exp Neurol* 2006;**65**:1069–73.

28. Jeibmann A, Wrede B, Peters O, Wolff JE, Paulus W, Hasselblatt M. Malignant progression in choroid plexus papillomas. *J Neurosurg* 2007;**107** (Suppl 3):199–202.

29. Judkins AR, Burger PC, Hamilton RL, et al. INI1 protein expression distinguishes atypical teratoid/rhabdoid tumor from choroid plexus carcinoma. *J Neuropathol Exp Neurol* 2005;**64**:391–7.

30. *J Neuropathol Exp Neurol* 1999;**58**:398–401.

31. Kimura M, Takayasu M, Suzuki Y, et al. Primary choroid plexus papilloma located in the suprasellar region: case report. *Neurosurgery* 1992;**31**:563–6.

32. Knierim DS. Choroid plexus tumors in infants. *Pediatr Neurosurg* 1990;**16**:276–80.

33. Kurtkaya-Yapicier O, Scheithauer BW, Van Peteghem KP, Sawicki JE. Unusual case of extradural choroid plexus papilloma of the sacral canal. Case report. *J Neurosurg* 2002;**97** (Suppl 1):102–5.

34. Laurence KM. The biology of choroid plexus papilloma in infancy and childhood. *Acta Neurochir (Wien)* 1979;**50**:79–90.

35. Leblanc R, Bekhor S, Melanson D, Carpenter S. Diffuse craniospinal seeding from a benign fourth ventricle choroid plexus papilloma. Case report. *J Neurosurg* 1998;**88**:757–60.

36. Magnusson S, Gisselsson D, Wiebe T, Kristoffersson U, Borg A, Olsson H. Prevalence of germline TP53 mutations and history of Li–Fraumeni syndrome in families with childhood adrenocortical tumors, choroid plexus tumors, and rhabdomyosarcoma: A population-based survey. *Pediatr Blood Cancer* 2012;**59**:846–53.

37. Matsushima T. Choroid plexus papillomas and human choroid plexus. A light and electron microscopic study. *J Neurosurg* 1983;**59**:1054–62.

38. Meyers SP, Khademian ZP, Chuang SH, Pollack IF, Korones DN, Zimmerman RA. Choroid plexus carcinomas in children: MRI features and patient outcomes. *Neuroradiology* 2004;**46**:770–80.

39. Miyagi Y, Natori Y, Suzuki SO, et al. Purely cystic form of choroid plexus papilloma with acute hydrocephalus in an infant. Case report. *J Neurosurg* 2006;**105** (Suppl 6):480–4.

40. Okamoto H, Mineta T, Ueda S, et al. Detection of JC virus DNA sequences in brain tumors in pediatric patients. *J Neurosurg* 2005;**102** (Suppl 3):294–8.

41. Paulus W, Janisch W. Clinicopathologic correlations in epithelial choroid plexus neoplasms: a study of 52 cases. *Acta Neuropathol* 1990;**80**:635–41.

42. Pencalet P, Sainte-Rose C, Lellouch-Tubiana A, et al. Papillomas and carcinomas of the choroid plexus in children. *J Neurosurg* 1998;**88**:52128.

43. Peyre M, Bah A, Kalamarides M. Multifocal choroid plexus papillomas: case report. *Acta Neurochir (Wien)* 2012;**154**:295–9.

44. Rickert CH, Paulus W. Tumors of the choroid plexus. *Microsc Res Tech* 2001;**52**:104–11.

45. Rickert CH, Wiestler OD, Paulus W. Chromosomal imbalances in choroid plexus tumors. *Am J Pathol* 2002;**160**:1105–1113.

46. Sahar A, Feinsod M, Beller AJ. Choroid plexus papilloma: hydrocephalus and cerebrospinal fluid dynamics. *Surg Neurol* 1980;**13**:476–8.

47. Schijman E, Monges J, Raimondi AJ, Tomita T. Choroid plexus papillomas of the III ventricle in childhood. Their diagnosis and surgical management. *Childs Nerv Syst* 1990;**6**:331–4.

48. Schittenhelm J, Nagel C, Meyermann R, Beschorner R. Atypical teratoid/rhabdoid tumors may show morphological and immunohistochemical features seen in choroid plexus tumors. *Neuropathology* 2011;**31**:461–7.

49. Seidinger AL, Mastellaro MJ, Paschoal Fortes F, et al. Association of the highly prevalent TP53 R337H mutation with pediatric choroid plexus carcinoma and osteosarcoma in southeast Brazil. *Cancer* 2011;**117**:2228–35.

50. Sevenet N, Lellouch-Tubiana A, Schofield D, et al. Spectrum of hSNF5/INI1 somatic mutations in human cancer and genotype-phenotype correlations. *Hum Mol Genet* 1999;**8**:2359–68.

51. Severino M, Schwartz ES, Thurnher MM, Rydland J, Nikas I, Rossi A. Congenital tumors of the central nervous system. *Neuroradiology* 2010;**52**:531–48.

52. Stafrace S, Molloy J. Extraventricular choroid plexus papilloma in a neonate. *Pediatr Radiol* 2008;**38**:593.

53. Stevens EA, Stanton CA, Nichols K, Ellis TL. Rare intraparenchymal choroid plexus carcinoma resembling atypical teratoid/rhabdoid tumor diagnosed by immunostaining for INI1 protein. *J Neurosurg Pediatr* 2009;**4**:368–71.

54. Strojan P, Popovic M, Surlan K, Jereb B. Choroid plexus tumors: a review of 28-year experience. *Neoplasma* 2004;**51**:306–12.

55. Tabori U, Shlien A, Baskin B, et al. TP53 alterations determine clinical subgroups and survival of patients with choroid plexus tumors. *J Clin Oncol* 2010;**28**:1995–2001.

56. Taggard DA, Menezes AH. Three choroid plexus papillomas in a patient with Aicardi syndrome. A case report. *Pediatr Neurosurg* 2000;**33**:219–23.

57. Talacchi A, De Micheli E, Lombardo C, Turazzi S, Bricolo A. Choroid plexus papilloma of the cerebellopontine angle: a twelve patient series. *Surg Neurol* 1999;**51**:621–9.

58. Taylor MB, Jackson RW, Hughes DG, Wright NB. Magnetic resonance imaging in the diagnosis and management of choroid plexus carcinoma in children. *Pediatr Radiol* 2001;**31**:624–30.

59. Tena-Suck ML, Gomez-Amador JL, Ortiz-Plata A, Salina-Lara C, Rembao-Bojorquez D, Vega-Orozco R. Rhabdoid choroid plexus carcinoma: a rare histological type. *Arq Neuropsiquiatr* 2007;**65** (Part 3A):705–9.

60. Vajtai I, Varga Z, Aguzzi A. MIB-1 immunoreactivity reveals different labelling in low-grade and in malignant epithelial neoplasms of the choroid plexus. *Histopathology* 1996;**29**:147–51.

61. Varga Z, Vajtai I, Aguzzi A. The standard isoform of CD44 is preferentially expressed in atypical papillomas and carcinomas of the choroid plexus. *Pathol Res Pract* 1996;**192**:1225–31.

62. Welch K, Strand R, Bresnan M, Cavazzuti V. Congenital hydrocephalus due to villous hypertrophy of the telencephalic choroid plexuses. Case report. *J Neurosurg* 1983;**59**:172–5.

63. White MK, Gordon J, Reiss K, et al. Human polyomaviruses and brain tumors. *Brain Res Brain Res Rev* 2005;**50**:69–85.

64. Wolff JE, Sajedi M, Brant R, Coppes MJ, Egeler RM. Choroid plexus tumours. *Br J Cancer* 2002;**87**:1086–91.

65. Zakrzewska M, Wojcik I, Zakrzewski K, et al. Mutational analysis of hSNF5/INI1 and TP53 genes in choroid plexus carcinomas. *Cancer Genet Cytogenet* 2005;**156**:179–82.

66. Zhang TJ, Yue Q, Lui S, Wu QZ, Gong QY. MRI findings of choroid plexus tumors in the cerebellum. *Clin Imaging* 2011;**35**:64–7.

Other Glial Neoplasms

Daniel J Brat

INTRODUCTION

Three rare glial tumour types are grouped together in this category: astroblastoma, chordoid glioma of the third ventricle and angiocentric glioma. These entities are separated from the more common astrocytic, oligodendroglial and ependymal tumour categories because their undefined histogenesis precludes a definite assignment to any other group.

ASTROBLASTOMA

The term 'astroblastoma' was first mentioned in the classification scheme of Bailey and Cushing in 1926,[3] with a more detailed description by Bailey and Bucy[2] following in 1930. Because of its rarity in pure form and the fact that focal astroblastic features may be encountered in otherwise typical astrocytic and ependymal tumours, it is not entirely clear whether astroblastoma should be regarded as a distinct tumour entity. However, based on several well-defined patient series and a greater emphasis on definitive diagnostic elements, astroblastoma is now generally regarded as a unique type of glial neoplasm with distinctive clinical, radiological, pathological and genetic features.[1,4,5,22,33,39]

Incidence, Age and Sex Distribution

Astroblastomas are rare and epidemiological data are imprecise. The tumours commonly affect adolescents and young adults, with most cases presenting in the first three decades.[37] However, congenital astroblastomas and examples in patients over 50 years of age have also been reported. Recent reviews indicate a female predilection.[37]

Clinical and Radiological Features

Patients most commonly present with seizures, focal neurologic deficits and/or signs of increased intracranial pressure, including headache, nausea and vomiting.[4,5,22,37] Rarely,

they present with intracranial haemorrhage.[15,39] The typical radiological appearance is a large, superficial, lobulated and well-defined lesion.[27] Tumours can arise throughout the CNS, with cerebral hemispheres being the most common location by far. Rare examples have been reported in the cerebellum, brain stem, optic nerves and cauda equina. On magnetic resonance imaging (MRI), astroblastomas usually consist of heterogeneously contrast enhancing, solid and cystic components (Figure 31.1a), with a characteristic 'bubbly' appearance of the solid parts on T2-weighted images.[27] Well differentiated examples show relatively little peritumoural T2 hyperintensity (vasogenic oedema) and/or infiltration of adjacent brain tissue. Anaplastic forms may demonstrate greater peritumoural oedema as a result of their rapid growth. On computed tomography (CT) scans, there may be punctate calcifications. Taken together, the radiological features may help distinguish astroblastomas from ependymomas and diffusely infiltrating gliomas.

Macroscopy

Most tumours are superficially located and macroscopically appear as well circumscribed, often large solid and cystic masses. Areas of necrosis may be discernible, particularly in large lesions and anaplastic variants.

Microscopy

Astroblastomas are solid, non-infiltrative cellular and well-vascularized tumours. In contrast to diffusely infiltrating gliomas, entrapped brain is usually absent within the tumour and so-called 'pushing borders' are observed at the tumour/brain interface. Anaplastic variants may show focal, but not diffuse, brain invasion. The histological hallmark of astroblastomas is a distinctive type of perivascular orientation by elongate to cuboidal tumour cells, the 'astroblastic pseudorosette' (Figure 31.1b,c).[4,5] This structure is formed by a single layer of tumour cells with eosinophilic, epithelioid cytoplasm and broad, non-tapering processes

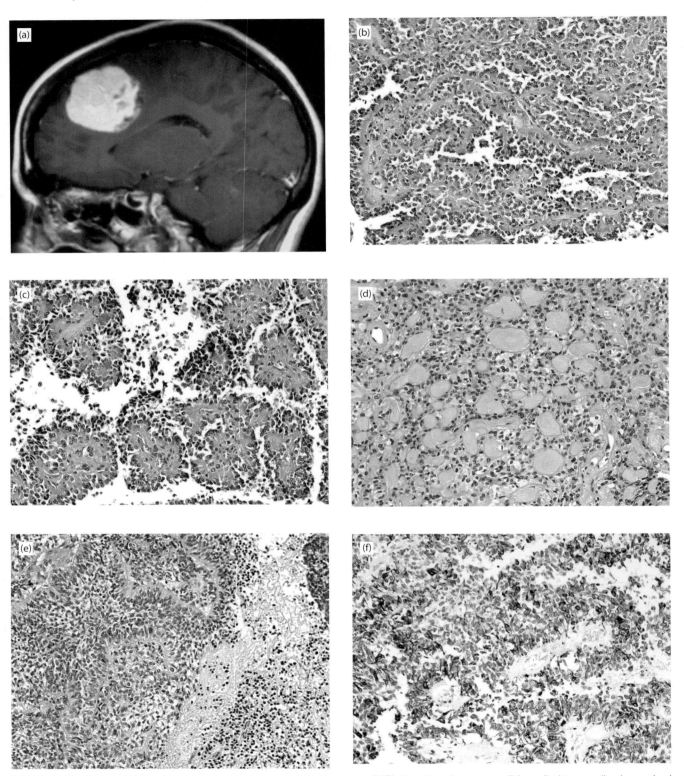

31.1 Astroblastoma. (a) Sagittal, post-contrast magnetic resonance (MR) imaging shows a solid, well-circumscribed, cerebral hemispheric mass with contrast enhancement and a bubbly internal appearance. In this instance, in which the tumour was well differentiated, there is only slight peritumoural oedema with partial compression of the adjacent ventricle. **(b)** The histologic hallmark of astroblastomas is the astroblastic pseudorosette, composed of cuboidal or elongate cells with columnar or slightly tapering processes oriented around a central vessel. Unlike ependymoma, glial fibrillarity is lacking. **(c)** Astroblastomas occasionally appear papillary as a result of perivascular stromal thickening or hyalinization of astroblastic pseudorosettes and a lack of fibrillar stroma. **(d)** Perivascular hyalinization ranges from mild to extensive and is present to a variable degree in nearly all astroblastomas. **(e)** Anaplastic variants of astroblastoma show high cellular density, solid growth patterns, nuclear atypia, mitotic activity and coagulative necrosis. **(f)** Astroblastomas are immunoreactive for GFAP and these stains also highlight the elongate 'stout' processes of astroblastoma.

that radiate towards a central vessel. In tissue sections and on smear preparations, there is a paucity of glial fibrillarity. Artificial tissue shrinkage often causes the formation of pseudo-papillae. Other areas often lack astroblastic pseudorosettes, consisting of solid sheets of moderately pleomorphic epithelioid cells with eccentric round to oval nuclei. Another characteristic feature is the presence of prominent perivascular hyalinization, which may coalesce into large stromal areas (Figure 31.1d). Dystrophic calcifications are not uncommon in these areas.

Grading

The World Health Organization (WHO) classification does not recommend a definite grade for astroblastomas.[22] However, histological subdivision into low-grade (well-differentiated) and high-grade (anaplastic) lesions has been suggested and appears to be prognostic.[5,38] Low-grade tumours are non-invasive lesions with orderly astroblastic pseudorosettes, minimal atypia, sparse mitotic activity and no microvascular proliferation. High-grade astroblastomas show foci of increased cellularity and atypia, obvious mitotic activity (usually >5 mitoses/10 HPF), microvascular proliferation, and often, pseudopalisading necrosis. Non-palisading necrosis can be observed in both low- and high-grade examples (Figure 31.1e).

Immunohistochemistry

Astroblastomas show immunoreactivity for GFAP (Figure 31.1f), S-100 protein and vimentin.[5,18,33] Expression of GFAP, however, may be variable and restricted to small areas in some cases. At least partial immunoreactivity for epithelial membrane antigen (EMA), sometimes noted with a dot-like pattern, is also common. Neuronal markers, such as synaptophysin and neurofilaments, are negative. Astroblastomas typically lack cytokeratin expression, although there has been one report of positivity for low molecular weight cytokeratins. The MIB1 proliferation index varies greatly and is generally greater in high-grade examples. One report showed a mean labeling index of 15.5 per cent in high grade versus 3.2 per cent in low-grade astroblastomas.[5]

Electron Microscopy

Several ultrastructural studies have been published.[12,14] Tumour cells are typically oriented towards blood vessels and often contain abundant intermediate filaments. Coated vesicles have also been reported.[17] Blood vessels frequently exhibit fenestrated endothelial cells and are surrounded by abundant lamellated basal laminae and collagen fibres. Two tumours displayed intermediate ultrastructural features between those of astrocytes and ependymal cells.[32]

Differential Diagnosis

Astroblastomas must be distinguished from diffuse astrocytomas, ependymomas and papillary meningiomas. Focal perivascular orientation resembling astroblastic pseudorosettes may be seen in otherwise typical diffuse astrocytomas, including glioblastomas. However, in contrast to diffuse gliomas, astroblastomas usually feature a well-demarcated solid growth pattern. In contrast to ependymomas, astroblastomas typically arise superficially in the cerebral hemispheres. The presence of classic ependymal pseudorosettes, as well as true ependymal canals and rosettes, helps to distinguish ependymoma. Cytologically, astroblastomas appear more epithelioid and lack the thin fibrillar processes of ependymoma. In addition, perivascular hyalinisation is usually more prominent in astroblastomas than in ependymomas. Papillary meningiomas usually contain areas of classic meningothelial histology, and show stronger and more widespread EMA expression. As a rule, papillary meningiomas lack GFAP immunoreactivity. The angiocentric glioma combines the histopathological features of a diffuse astrocytoma and ependymoma, and may focally resemble an astroblastoma. However, the predominant wrapping around small blood vessels is distinct from the astroblastic pseudorosette, whereas the infiltrative growth is more readily apparent.

Histogenesis

The cellular origin of astroblastoma is disputed. Bailey and Bucy[1] suggested an origin from the 'astroblast', which they considered an astroglial precursor cell. On the other hand, Rubinstein and Herman found ultrastructural characteristics suggesting an origin from tanycytes.[32]

Molecular Genetics

Comparative genomic hybridization (CGH) analysis revealed gains of chromosome arm 20q and chromosome 19 as the most frequent genomic alterations in 7 astroblastomas.[3] Recurrent losses were found on chromosomes 9q, 10 and X. Taken together, these data suggest that astroblastomas have a cytogenetic profile that differs from more common astrocytic, oligodendroglial and ependymal tumours. However, further studies are needed to substantiate this hypothesis and to identify astroblastoma-specific gene alterations.

Biological Behaviour and Prognosis

Prediction of biological behaviour in individual cases is difficult. Studies with well-described histologic criteria revealed a better prognosis for low-grade than high-grade (anaplastic) variants, with higher recurrence rates in the latter.[4,5,38] Most astroblastomas are resectable, with one recent review indicating that gross total resection was achievable in 84 per cent of patients.[37] Those with completely resected tumours often attain long-term survival. However, recurrences may develop at the original tumour site and/or at distant sites within the central nervous system (CNS).

CHORDOID GLIOMA OF THE THIRD VENTRICLE

Chordoid glioma of the third ventricle was first described in 1998.[7,22] Since then, small series and case reports have been published, with over 50 tumours documented.[10]

Incidence, Age and Sex Distribution

Chordoid gliomas are rare and preferentially manifest in adults, peaking in the fourth and fifth decades. However, age ranges from 5 to 75 years. Rare cases of paediatric chordoid glioma have been reported.[8] Females outnumber males by a ratio of 2:1.

Clinical and Radiological Features

Most patients present with signs and symptoms of obstructive hydrocephalus and raised intracranial pressure, in particular headache, nausea and vomiting.[10] Other clinical features are endocrine abnormalities reflecting hypothalamic compression, e.g. hypothyroidism, amenorrhea and diabetes insipidus, visual field disturbances due to compression/displacement of the optic chiasm, as well as personality changes, including psychiatric symptoms and memory abnormalities. Neuroradiologically, chordoid gliomas present with strikingly similar imaging features.[26] The anterior third ventricle tumours appear well circumscribed, ovoid and hyperdense to grey matter on CT scans, but isointense on T1-weighted MR images. Administration of contrast agents results in strong, homogeneous enhancement (Figure 31.2a). Mass effect is generally distributed symmetrically and causes vasogenic oedema (T2-weighted hyperintensity) in compressed adjacent CNS structures including the optic tracts, basal ganglia and internal capsules. Most tumours abut the hypothalamus and some appear to have an intrinsic anterior hypothalamic component, suggesting a potential site of origin.[19]

Macroscopy

Chordoid gliomas are well-circumscribed, usually solid tumours located in the anterior portion of the third ventricle. They typically adhere to the ventricular walls, expand the third ventricle and cause obstructive hydrocephalus. Occasionally, they include a cystic component.

Microscopy

Chordoid gliomas are solid tumours of moderate cell density, characterized by clusters, ribbons and cords of epithelioid tumour cells with prominent eosinophilic cytoplasm, relatively uniform nuclei and inconspicuous nucleoli (see Figure 31.2b–e). Tumour cells may form coarsely fibrillar processes, embedded in an Alcian blue positive, mucinous and sometimes vacuolated matrix. Other minor architectural patterns include papillary, alveolar and pseudoglandular forms. A stromal reticulin network frequently surrounds small groups of tumour cells. Lymphoplasmacytic infiltrates are a regular feature (Figure 31.2d) and Russell bodies may be prominent. Mitotic activity is low and high-grade histological features are absent. The tumours are sharply demarcated from the surrounding brain tissue, which typically shows marked reactive astrogliosis, often with Rosenthal fibres (Figure 31.2e).

Grading

Chordoid gliomas are designated as WHO grade II.[22]

Immunohistochemistry

The immunoprofile of chordoid gliomas greatly aids in the diagnosis. They generally show strong immunopositivity for GFAP, vimentin and CD34 (Figure 31.2f).[7,13,34] Immunoreactivity for S-100, EMA and cytokeratins is more variable and often restricted to minor tumour fractions. Epidermal growth factor receptors and merlin/schwannomin are expressed, whereas nuclear p53 staining is weak or absent. Neuronal and neuroendocrine markers (synaptophysin, neurofilaments, chromogranin A) are consistently negative. The MIB1 index is generally low (<5 per cent).

Electron Microscopy

Brat and colleagues[7] studied four cases and reported abundant intermediate filaments, focal projections resembling microvilli, scattered intermediate junctions and focal basal lamina formation, but no desmosomes or cilia. Other studies observed ultrastructural features suggestive of ependymal lineage, including the formation of microvilli and cilia.[9,24,35] Whereas some authors have noted ultrastructural similarities to the specialized secretory ependymal cells of the so-called subcommissural organ,[9] others have suggested tanycytic differentiation.[35]

Differential Diagnosis

The specific localization of chordoid glioma to the anterior third ventricle is extremely helpful in narrowing the differential diagnosis to regional neoplasms including meningioma, pituitary adenoma, craniopharyngioma, ependymoma, other low-grade gliomas, central neurocytoma and germ cell neoplasms. The most important alternative histological diagnoses to consider are chordoid meningioma and chordoma. Chordoid meningiomas usually contain small foci of classic meningioma with whorl formation and psammoma bodies; they are also immunopositive for EMA, but negative for GFAP and CD34. In contrast to chordoid glioma, chordomas involve bone (e.g. clivus), strongly express cytokeratins and brachyury, but lack immunoreactivity for GFAP and CD34. In addition, chordomas contain physalipherous cells, which are not seen in chordoid gliomas. Other radiological differential diagnoses are readily distinguished by histopathological evaluation.

Histogenesis

One of the most striking features of chordoid gliomas is their predilection for the anterior third ventricle and hypothalamus. Based on ultrastructural features, Cenacchi et al.[9] hypothesized a 'cell of origin'. In keeping with other studies, they found evidence of ependymal differentiation (microvilli and hemidesmosome-like structures).[7,24,30] In addition, they described a zonation of organelles, filaments and secretory vessels that was suggestive of the specialized ependymal cells of subventricular organs. Further evidence of specialized ependymal differentiation has come from a report that demonstrated abnormal cilia in a juxtanuclear location.[24] Based on ultrastructural findings and the localization of these tumours to the anterior third ventricular, it has been proposed that chordoid gliomas might arise from a circumventricular organ located in the anterior third ventricle, the organum vasculosum of the lamina terminalis (OVLT).[19,24]

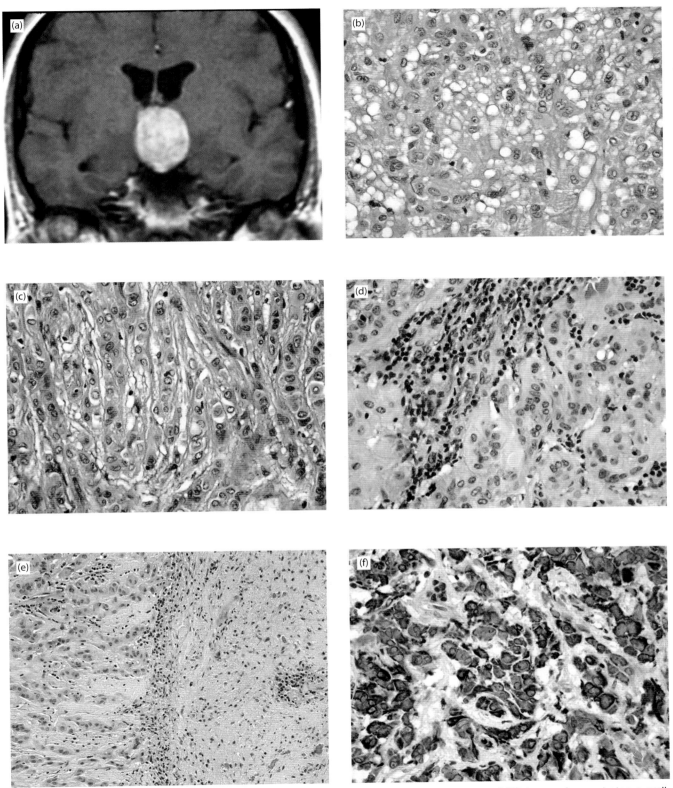

31.2 Chordoid glioma of the third ventricle. (a) Post-contrast coronal magnetic resonance (MR) image demonstrates a well-circumscribed, contrast-enhancing mass within the third ventricle. **(b)** Histologically, tumours are characterized by cohesive clusters of epithelioid cells with abundant pink cytoplasm and a bubbly, bluish, mucin-rich stroma. **(c)** In almost every instance, tumour cells also form solid arrangements comprised of either nests or linear arrays. **(d)** A lymphoplasmacytic infiltrate is present in nearly all chordoid gliomas and Russell bodies can often be identified. **(e)** The border between chordoid glioma and adjacent brain is well defined with little evidence of tumour infiltration. Borders typically show chronic inflammation and Rosenthal fibres within the neighbouring brain. **(f)** Immunohistochemistry typically demonstrates strong GFAP expression.

Molecular Genetics

To date, only a few cases of chordoid glioma have been subjected to molecular analysis. A recent array CGH and *fluorescence in situ hybridization* (FISH) study documented that loss at 11q13 was a frequent finding. Loss at 9p21 was another consistent finding. No EGFR amplifications, chromosome 7 gain or TP53 mutations were noted.[13] In another study using PCR-based techniques, DNA sequencing, and CGH, no consistent chromosomal imbalances were detected, nor were alterations of *TP53, p16(CDKN2A), EGFR, CDK4* and *MDM2*.[31]

Biological Behaviour and Prognosis

Chordoid gliomas are slowly growing lesions. Gross total resection is the treatment of choice and may result in long-term recurrence-free survival.[7,10] However, complete resection can be difficult and hazardous in patients with tumours attached to the hypothalamus and suprasellar structures. Consequently, several patients have been reported with disabling post-operative neurological complications and/or early postoperative death. Indeed, the majority of deaths recorded for patients with chordoid glioma occur in the first four weeks post-operatively.[10] Specific post-operative complications include diabetes insipidus, amnesia and pulmonary emboli.[10] Patients with residual tumour have been treated with radiation therapy or radiosurgery, whereas the use of chemotherapy has not been reported in this setting.

ANGIOCENTRIC GLIOMA

In 2005, two groups simultaneously described series of low-grade brain tumours in children and young adults that were associated with seizures and a distinctive histology.[20,40] Although only recently described, the unique clinical, radiologic and pathologic features led to the acceptance of angiocentric glioma as a new entity by the WHO in 2007.[6,22]

Incidence, Age and Sex Distribution

This tumour is rare, with less than 50 cases reported to date. It occurs mostly in children and young adults. There does not appear to be a gender predilection.[20,28,40]

Clinical and Radiological Features

Angiocentric glioma presents as a slowly growing, cerebral hemispheric mass, most often involving the frontal, parietal and temporal lobes. Nearly all patients have long-standing epilepsy that is refractory to medical treatment. Tumours are typically centred in the cortex, but often extend into subcortical regions. On magnetic resonance (MR) imaging, these lesions expand the involved cortex and are T2- or fluid-attenuated inversion recovery (FLAIR) hyperintense but generally lack contrast enhancement (Figure 31.3a).[16] There is often only minimal mass effect.[36] A stalk-like extension towards the ventricular system has been reported.[20]

Macroscopy

Angiocentric gliomas are supratentorial tumours that are centred in the cortex and extend focally into the white matter. Mass effects of the lesion can be apparent, yet subtle.

Microscopy

The defining histologic feature of angiocentric glioma is the presence of monomorphous, bipolar tumour cells intimately associated with blood vessels of the involved cortex and white matter (Figure 31.3b–e). Tumour cells are uniform, spindled with oval or elongated nuclei and speckled chromatin as well as pink, tapering cytoplasm. These slender cells are most frequently oriented parallel to vessels, sometimes expanding perivascular spaces with streaming arrays of either single or multilayered cells. In some examples, tumour cells are radially oriented to vessels in a pattern, highly reminiscent of ependymal pseudorosettes. In a small subset, a similar tendency to orient perpendicularly to the pia mater is seen, giving a palisading appearance at the brain surface. In addition to the perivascular and subpial distribution, scattered single cells or cell clusters are present at low density within the cortical and subcortical parenchyma. Non-neoplastic elements, including cortical neurons and neuropil, are entrapped within the tumour, consistent with an infiltrative growth pattern. In lesions resected from adults with long-standing histories of seizures, neurofibrillary tangles may be seen in native neurons.[28] In one recent study, evidence of adjacent malformation of cortical development/focal cortical dysplasia was observed in all four cases.[23] Mitoses are generally absent and the MIB1 proliferation index ranges from 1 to 5 per cent. Cases with higher indices have been described, yet it is unclear if this has an impact on clinical behaviour.[21,25]

Grading

Angiocentric glioma is histologically low grade and has been designated WHO grade I.[22]

Immunohistochemistry

Immunoreactivity is consistently strong for GFAP (Figure 31.3e), S-100 and vimentin often showing 'dot-like' cytoplasmic staining for EMA – a pattern typical of ependymoma (Figure 31.3f).[23,28,36] Staining for CD99 is variable. The infiltrative growth pattern is also highlighted with stains for neurofilament protein, which show entrapped intratumoural axons. Ependymal differentiation is also seen on electron microscopy, which demonstrates microlumen formation, microvilli, cilia, and complex, zipper-like intermediate junctions.

Differential Diagnosis

The angiocentric pattern of these tumours, especially when cells are oriented radially, resembles classic ependymoma. The distinction can be more problematic when ependymomas occur within the brain parenchyma, such as is seen with cortical ependymoma.[11] Immunohistochemical and ultrastructural data have supported the ependymal differentiation of angiocentric glioma. However, unlike classic

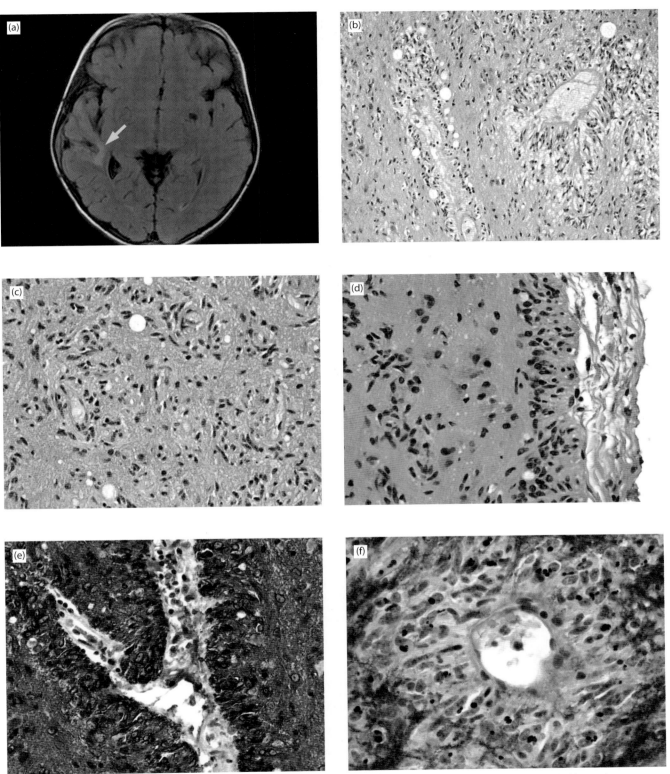

31.3 Angiocentric glioma. (a) On magnetic resonance (MR) imaging, tumours (arrow) are T2- or fluid-attenuated inversion recovery (FLAIR) hyperintense but generally lack contrast enhancement. **(b)** The defining histologic feature is the presence of monomorphous, bipolar tumour cells intimately associated with blood vessels of the involved cortex and white matter. **(c)** In addition to their perivascular location, elongate, slender cells are noted to be embedded within the neuropil of cortex and white matter, either singly or in small clusters. **(d)** There is a tendency for angiocentric glioma cells to accumulate perpendicular or parallel to the pia mater, giving them a palisading appearance at the brain surface. **(e)** Immunoreactivity is consistently strong for GFAP, highlighting thin processes that are often arranged either parallel to blood vessels or radially surrounding them. **(f)** Immunoreactivity for epithelial membrane antigen (EMA) is typical, sometimes with a cytoplasmic dot-like pattern, similar to ependymoma.

ependymoma, angiocentric glioma does not form a discrete mass, but rather infiltrates the brain in a combined diffuse and angiocentric fashion. As such, the magnetic resonance image (MRI) shows a T2-bright region of invaded brain, rather than a solid contrast-enhancing mass. Pilocytic astrocytoma is composed of cytologically bland, often spindled GFAP-positive cells, much like angiocentric glioma. Although pilocytic astrocytomas can have a perivascular growth pattern and orient toward vessels, the degree is usually less dramatic than that of angiocentric glioma. Moreover, unlike angiocentric glioma, pilocytic astrocytomas tend to form solid components that push aside, rather than invade adjacent brain. Diffuse astrocytoma shares the infiltrative growth pattern and elongate nuclei seen in angiocentric glioma, but it lacks the angiocentricity, typically involves larger portions of the brain, and shows greater nuclear hyperchromasia and pleomorphism.

Histogenesis

The histogenesis of angiocentric glioma remains unsettled. Ependymal differentiation is seen on electron microscopy.[40]

Despite these ependymal features, however, tumours show an infiltrative growth pattern.

Molecular Genetics

A CGH investigation of eight cases uncovered a single a loss of chromosomal band 6q24-q25 in one tumour.[28] A gain at chromosome 11p11.2, the site of protein tyrosine phosphatase receptor J, was found on high resolution array-CGH in a second tumour. In a small series of three cases, immunohistochemistry for mutant IDH1 (R132H) failed to reveal any mutations.[29]

Biological Behaviour and Prognosis

The behaviour of those tumours documented thus far suggests a stable clinical course and probable cure by surgical resection alone. The majority of patients undergoing subtotal resections have shown stable, residual tumour on MR imaging.[20,40] Therefore, angiocentric glioma has been given a WHO grade I designation.

REFERENCES

1. Alaraj A, Chan M, Oh S, *et al*. Astroblastoma presenting with intracerebral hemorrhage misdiagnosed as dural arteriovenous fistula: review of a rare entity. *Surg Neurol* 2007;**67**:308–13.
2. Bailey P, Bucy PC. Astroblastomas of the brain. *Acta Psychiatr Neurol* 1930;**5**:439–61.
3. Bailey P, Cushing H. *A classification of tumors of the glioma group on a histogenetic basis with a correlated study of prognosis*. Philadelphia, PA: JB Lippincott, 1926.
4. Bonnin JM, Rubinstein LJ. Astroblastomas: a pathological study of 23 tumors, with a postoperative follow-up in 13 patients. *Neurosurgery* 1989;**25**:6–13.
5. Brat DJ, Hirose Y, Cohen KJ, *et al*. Astroblastoma: clinicopathologic features and chromosomal abnormalities defined by comparative genomic hybridization. *Brain Pathol* 2000;**10**:342–52.
6. Brat DJ, Scheithauer BW, Fuller GN, Tihan T. Newly codified glial neoplasms of the 2007 WHO Classification of Tumours of the Central Nervous System: angiocentric glioma, pilomyxoid astrocytoma and pituicytoma. *Brain Pathol* 2007;**17**:319–24.
7. Brat DJ, Scheithauer BW, Staugaitis SM, *et al*. Third ventricular chordoid glioma: a distinct clinicopathologic entity. *J Neuropathol Exp Neurol* 1998;**57**:283 90.
8. Castellano-Sanchez AA, Schemankewitz E, Mazewski C, Brat DJ. Pediatric chordoid glioma with chondroid metaplasia. *Pediatr Dev Pathol* 2001;**4**:564–7.
9. Cenacchi G, Roncaroli F, Cerasoli S, *et al*. Chordoid glioma of the third ventricle: an ultrastructural study of three cases with a histogenetic hypothesis. *Am J Surg Pathol* 2001;**25**:401–5.
10. Desouza RM, Bodi I, Thomas N, *et al*. Chordoid glioma: ten years of a low-grade tumor with high morbidity. *Skull Base* 2010;**20**:125–38.

11. Hiniker A, Lee HS, Chang S, *et al*. Cortical ependymoma with unusual histologic features. *Clin Neuropathol* 2013;**32**:318–23.
12. Hoag G, Sima AA, Rozdilsky B. Astroblastoma revisited: a report of three cases. *Acta Neuropathol* 1986;**70**:10–16.
13. Horbinski C, Dacic S, McLendon RE, *et al*. Chordoid glioma:a case report and molecular characterization of five cases. *Brain Pathol* 2009;**19**:439–48.
14. Jay V, Edwards V, Squire J, Rutka J. Astroblastoma: report of a case with ultrastructural, cell kinetic, and cytogenetic analysis. *Paediatr Pathol* 1993;**13**:323–32.
15. Johnson KA, Bonnin JM, Boaz JC, *et al*. Anaplastic astroblastoma presenting as massive, sudden-onset, intraparenchymal hemorrhage. *Pediatr Neurosurg* 2010;**46**:457–61.
16. Koral K, Koral KM, Sklar F. Angiocentric glioma in a 4-year-old boy: imaging characteristics and review of the literature. *Clin Imaging* 2012;**36**:61–4.
17. Kubota T, Hirano A, Sato K, Yamamoto S. The fine structure of astroblastoma. *Cancer*. 1985;**55**:745–50.
18. Kubota T, Sato K, Arishima H, *et al*. Astroblastoma: immunohistochemical and ultrastructural study of distinctive epithelial and probable tanycytic differentiation. *Neuropathology* 2006;**26**:72–81.
19. Leeds NE, Lang FF, Ribalta T, *et al*. Origin of chordoid glioma of the third ventricle. *Arch Pathol Lab Med* 2006;**130**:460–4.
20. Lellouch-Tubiana A, Boddaert N, Bourgeois M, *et al*. Angiocentric neuroepithelial tumor (ANET): a new epilepsy-related clinicopathological entity with distinctive MRI. *Brain Pathol*. 2005;**15**:281–6.
21. Li JY, Langford LA, Adesina A, *et al*. The high mitotic count detected by phospho-histone H3 immunostain does not alter the benign behavior of angiocentric glioma. *Brain Tumor Pathol* 2012;**29**:68–72.

22. Louis DN, Ohgaki H, Wiestler OD, Cavenee WK. *WHO classification of tumours of the central nervous system*, 4th edn. Lyon: Internationl Agency for Research, 2007.
23. Marburger T, Prayson R. Angiocentric glioma: a clinicopathologic review of 5 tumors with identification of associated cortical dysplasia. *Arch Pathol Lab Med* 2011;**135**:1037–41.
24. Pasquier B, Peoc'h M, Morrison AL, *et al*. Chordoid glioma of the third ventricle: a report of two new cases, with further evidence supporting an ependymal differentiation, and review of the literature. *Am J Surg Pathol* 2002;**26**:1330–42.
25. Pokharel S, Parker JR, Parker JC Jr, *et al*. Angiocentric glioma with high proliferative index: case report and review of the literature. *Ann Clin Lab Sci* 2011;**41**:257–61.
26. Pomper MG, Passe TJ, Burger PC, *et al*. Chordoid glioma: a neoplasm unique to the hypothalamus and anterior third ventricle. *AJNR Am J Neuroradiol* 2001;**22**:464–9.
27. Port JD, Brat DJ, Burger PC, Pomper MG. Astroblastoma: radiologic-pathologic correlation and distinction from ependymoma. *AJNR Am J Neuroradiol* 2002;**23**:243–7.
28. Preusser M, Hoischen A, Novak K, *et al*. Angiocentric glioma: report of clinico-pathologic and genetic findings in 8 cases. *Am J Surg Pathol* 2007;**31**:1709–18.
29. Raghunathan A, Olar A, Vogel H, *et al*. Isocitrate dehydrogenase 1 R132H mutation is not detected in angiocentric glioma. *Ann Diagn Pathol* 2012;**16**:255–9.
30. Raizer JJ, Shetty T, Gutin PH, *et al*. Chordoid glioma: report of a case with unusual histologic features, ultrastructural study and review of the literature. *J Neurooncol* 2003;**63**:39–47.
31. Reifenberger G, Weber T, Weber RG, *et al*. Chordoid glioma of the third ventricle: immunohistochemical and molecular

genetic characterization of a novel tumour entity. *Brain Pathol* 1999;**9**:617–26.

32. Rubinstein LJ, Herman MM. The astroblastoma and its possible cytogenetic relationship to the tanycyte. An electron microscopic, immunohistochemical, tissue- and organ-culture study. *Acta Neuropathol (Berl)* 1989;**78**:472–83.

33. Salvati M, D'Elia A, Brogna C, *et al.* Cerebral astroblastoma: analysis of six cases and critical review of treatment options. *J Neurooncol* 2009;**93**:369–78.

34. Sangoi AR, Dulai MS, Beck AH, *et al.* Distinguishing chordoid meningiomas from their histologic mimics: an immunohistochemical evaluation. *Am J Surg Pathol* 2009;**33**:669–81.

35. Sato K, Kubota T, Ishida M, *et al.* Immunohistochemical and ultrastructural study of chordoid glioma of the third ventricle: its tanycytic differentiation. *Acta Neuropathol* 2003;**106**:176–80.

36. Shakur SF, McGirt MJ, Johnson MW, *et al.* Angiocentric glioma: a case series. *J Neurosurg Pediatr* 2009;**3**:197–202.

37. Sughrue ME, Choi J, Rutkowski MJ, *et al.* Clinical features and post-surgical outcome of patients with astroblastoma. *J Clin Neurosci* 2011;**18**:750–4.

38. Thiessen B, Finlay J, Kulkarni R, Rosenblum MK. Astroblastoma: does histology predict biologic behavior? *J Neurooncol* 1998;**40**:59–65.

39. Tumialan LM, Brat DJ, Fountain AJ, Barrow DL. An astroblastoma mimicking a cavernous malformation: case report. *Neurosurgery* 2007;**60**:E569–70; discussion E70.

40. Wang M, Tihan T, Rojiani AM, *et al.* Monomorphous angiocentric glioma: a distinctive epileptogenic neoplasm with features of infiltrating astrocytoma and ependymoma. *J Neuropathol Exp Neurol* 2005;**64**:875–81.

Neuronal and Mixed Neuronal–Glial Tumours

Daniel J Brat

GANGLIOCYTOMAS

Gangliocytomas are World Health Organization (WHO) grade I neoplasms composed almost entirely of well-differentiated but dysmorphic ganglion cells.[150] This mature neuronal population lacks a substantial neoplastic glial, schwannian or neuroblastic component and is therefore distinct from ganglioglioma, ganglioneuroma and embryonal neoplasms, respectively. However, gangliocytomas can be regarded as part of the 'ganglion cell tumour' spectrum that includes ganglioglioma. The latter are described separately later, but there is substantial overlap in the clinical, neuroimaging and histopathologic features of these variants. Another form of 'gangliocytoma' – the dysplastic gangliocytoma of the cerebellum or Lhermitte–Duclos disease – is a unique clinicopathologic entity that is also treated separately. See Chapter 41, Pituitary and Suprasellar Tumours, regarding gangliocytomas of the pituitary gland, a heterogeneous collection of lesions mostly arising within growth hormone-producing adenomas.

Epidemiology and Clinical Features

Pure gangliocytomas are rare. Together with gangliogliomas, which are much more frequent, they account for just over 1 per cent of all central nervous system (CNS) tumours.[150] Most arise in younger patients, presenting within the first three decades of life.[65] The majority occur in children and there are even examples of prenatal detection.[43] They are occasionally discovered in older adults and, like other WHO grade I tumours, may have been present for decades before becoming symptomatic.[65] Frequent locations include the cerebral hemispheres, particularly the temporal lobes and cervicothoracic spinal cord, although gangliocytomas may also arise in the suprasellar region, cerebellum, brainstem and pineal region.[43,59,65,110] A protracted clinical course is typical. Seizures and headaches are the most frequent manifestations of cerebral lesions, whereas spinal tumours produce slowly progressive long tract signs and may be associated with scoliosis.[217] Symptomatic hydrocephalus results from pineal and third ventricular/hypothalamic examples. Gangliocytomas are surgically curable tumours that only rarely recur and even less commonly disseminate through the subarachnoid space.[15,65]

Radiology

Gangliocytomas cannot be definitively diagnosed on the basis of their neuroradiological features, yet there are a few stereotypical findings on computed tomography (CT) and magnetic resonance imaging (MRI).[4] These lesions are most often discrete, sometimes cystic and have variable signal intensities. They are typically hypointense on T1-weighted and hyperintense on T2-weighted MRI.[230] Solid components nearly always show contrast enhancement. Calcifications are best appreciated on CT. Peritumoural oedema is not present and mass effect is modest or absent. Intramedullary examples may extend over multiple segments. A distinct tissue plane at the interface of tumour and adjacent parenchyma has been noted.[217]

Microscopy

Gangliocytomas consist of a moderate to high density of well-differentiated ganglion cells that display architectural disarray and cytological dysmorphism (Figure 32.1). The cell density is generally greater than that noted in normal grey matter, which is an important, yet inconstant, diagnostic feature. More importantly, these neuronal cells are spatially disordered, with no evidence of shared polarity, layering or respect for territory.[150] Indeed, close clustering of multiple disoriented, well-differentiated neurons is a

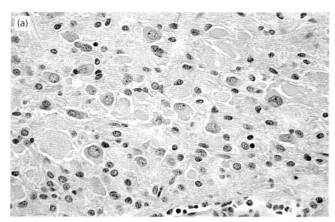 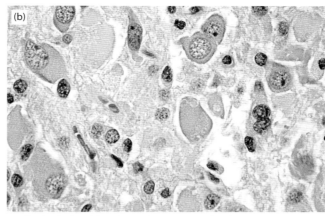

32.1 Gangliocytoma. (a,b) Clusters of atypical, pleomorphic ganglion cells, including binucleate forms are embedded in a haphazard manner within a delicate neuropil matrix. No neoplastic glial cells are present in a gangliocytoma.

diagnostic feature that can help distinguish gangliocytomas (or cortical dysplasias) from normal brain. Individual neurons possess large, vesicular nuclei, prominent and centrally positioned nucleoli, abundant cytoplasm with Nissl substance, and multipolar processes that are better visualized using silver stains or neurofilament immunohistochemistry. Cellular gigantism, coarse cytoplasmic vacuolisation and multinucleation are common. Gangliocytomas occasionally show evidence of neurofibrillary cytoskeletal changes, including well-defined tangles, as well as granulovacuolar degeneration and other neurodegenerative alterations.[29,138] The pleomorphic and disoriented neurons of gangliocytoma are usually embedded within a hypocellular and rarefied meshwork comprised mostly of cell processes. This 'stroma' may also contain delicate reticulin fibres and a minor glial population of hyperplastic astrocytes. By definition, a neoplastic glial population is absent. Some investigators suggest that nearly all ganglion cell tumours contain at least a minor neoplastic glial component and that true gangliocytomas are rare or nonexistent.[23]

Immunohistochemistry and Electron Microscopy

Neurons of gangliocytoma express synaptophysin and neurofilament protein, some also labelling with antibodies to chromogranin A.[65] Synaptophysin labelling of perikaryal membranes may be observed, a phenomenon also characteristic of gangliogliomas. Immunoreactivity for NeuN, an antigen present in nuclei of well-differentiated cortical neurons, is surprisingly negative to weakly positive in most ganglion cell tumours.[185] Immunostaining for a variety of neuropeptides and biogenic amines has been noted, including somatostatin, met– and leu–enkephalins, corticotrophin-releasing hormone, VIP, beta–endorphin, calcitonin and serotonin. The few ultrastructural investigations have emphasized neuronal dysmorphism and neurodegenerative features, depicting a variety of abnormal cytoplasmic inclusions (e.g. curvilinear bodies, concentric laminated bodies and branched tubular structures), whereas documenting evidence of ganglion cell-like maturation includes well-developed rough endoplasmic reticulum, abundant free ribosomes, neuritic processes with parallel microtubular arrays, clear and dense-core vesicles and, in some cases, synaptic contacts.[109,120]

Histogenesis

The origins of gangliocytomas are obscure and their neoplastic, as opposed to hamartomatous, nature remains unsettled. The cytological anomalies present in the neuronal population are shared to some extent, although usually in a less pronounced form, by the abnormal neuronal elements in malformations of cortical development (e.g. cortical dysplasias and hemi-megalencephaly; see Chapter 4, Malformations, and Chapter 11, Epilepsy). However, this does not necessarily imply a unifying histogenesis.

GANGLIOGLIOMAS

Epidemiology

Although uncommon, gangliogliomas are the most frequent mixed glioneuronal tumours,[150] constituting approximately 1.3 per cent of all CNS tumours. Although gangliogliomas may be encountered at any age, 80 per cent present within the first three decades. Depending on the study, a mean age of 8.5 to 25 years at diagnosis has been documented, with male to female ratios ranging from 1.1:1 to 1.9:1.[23,102,141] One study of 99 childhood examples found a mean age at diagnosis of 9.5 years without a significant sex bias, whereas a series of 326 gangliogliomas from an epilepsy surgery centre reported a mean age of 22.1 years and a male to female ratio of 1.3:1.[23,115] Gangliogliomas arise throughout the central neuraxis. They are most common in the cerebral hemispheres, with a strong predilection for the temporal lobes. Indeed, this location accounts for 60–70 per cent of cases.[23] Other cerebral hemispheric locations, in decreasing order of frequency, are the frontal, parietal and occipital lobes. Also recognized are gangliogliomas of the brainstem, cerebellum and spinal cord. Some observers report a relatively high incidence of bulbar and intramedullary examples in paediatric patients.[45,157] Overall, gangliogliomas account for 1.1 per cent of spinal cord tumours and most often involve the cervical region.[111]

Clinical Features

Manifestations of these slowly growing tumours generally reflect their location. Cerebral examples are mostly associated with protracted, often medically refractory epilepsy. Gangliogliomas may account for over 20 per cent of all lesions involved in temporal lobe epilepsy resections, representing the most common neoplasm encountered in this clinical setting.[281,282] Gangliogliomas may similarly account for up to 20 per cent of chronic convulsive disorders localizing to extratemporal sites.[75] The mean preoperative duration of symptoms exceeds 5 years.[141] By contrast, pre-detection symptomatic intervals are usually shorter for bulbar and intramedullary variants. Spinal cord tumours most often present with paraparesis and segmental pain.[111] In addition, a spinal location is occasionally associated with scoliosis, which may be the presenting manifestation in some children without neurological complaints.[45]

Gangliogliomas generally arise sporadically, but there are isolated examples associated with neurofibromatosis 1, neurofibromatosis 2, Down syndrome, type 1 Turcot syndrome and Martin–Bell [fra(x)–XLMR] syndrome.[178,212,219,248] In one large series, approximately 5 per cent of cases occurred in association with congenital anomalies that included partial agenesis of the corpus callosum, orofaciodigital synostosis, leptomeningeal glioneuronal ectopias, cortical glioneuronal malformations, cerebellar polymicrogyria and Down syndrome.[216] Gangliogliomas are often associated with microscopic glioneuronal cortical malformations.[22] Isolated accounts describe gangliogliomas arising in association with vascular malformations and Rasmussen's encephalitis.[42,72]

Gangliogliomas are WHO grade I tumours that are treated surgically with gross total resection being the goal.[150,181] Rates of recurrence following complete resection are low and CSF dissemination is rare. Eighty-eight per cent of chronic epilepsy patients treated surgically and diagnosed with ganglioglioma were seizure free after 7 years' follow-up.[23] Among patients with low grade gangliogliomas, tumour recurrence was noted in less than 2 per cent of cases within this same interval, although this series may be biased toward temporal lobe lesions where complete surgical resection is more common. In a more general population of patients with ganglioglioma, local recurrence has been reported in 17–33 per cent.[102,141] Local recurrence of spinal gangliogliomas occurs in approximately 30 per cent of cases.[111] Patients do not generally succumb to disease, with an overall survival of 84 per cent at 10 years.[141]

Radiology

Intracranial gangliogliomas exhibit a constellation of CT and MR features. They are generally circumscribed and either solid, or solid and cystic.[230,283] The solid component, which may be a mural nodule within the cyst wall, almost always shows contrast enhancement (Figure 32.2a). Mass effect and surrounding oedema are generally minimal. Foci of calcification are frequently seen, especially on CT. Occasional solid gangliogliomas are less discrete and some fail to enhance or do so in a patchy or ring-like fashion. The solid components of gangliogliomas are usually hypodense to isodense in precontrast CT studies, tending to

be T1 hypointense and T2 hyperintense on MRI. Scalloping of the calvarium attests to the slow expansion of cerebral gangliogliomas, most of which are superficial (involving the cortical mantle).

A study of 27 gangliogliomas of the spinal cord described a characteristic, but not pathognomonic, MR profile as compared with intramedullary fibrillary astrocytomas and ependymomas.[182] Features that correlated with ganglioglioma included tumour length (eight vertebral segments for gangliogliomas vs four for astrocytomas and ependymomas), the presence of intratumoural cysts, bone changes (scoliosis or erosion), mixed signal intensity on T1-weighted images, absence of associated oedema, patchy contrast enhancement and extension to the cord surface.

Macroscopic Appearances

A mural nodule is often noted bulging into a serous fluid-filled cyst. In other instances, these tumours may exhibit more limited cystic changes or may be entirely solid with tan or grey-white tissue. Most tumours are relatively demarcated, especially the cystic variants, and can acquire a firm texture owing to desmoplasia or a palpable grittiness due to calcification. Haemorrhage is rare and necrosis is mostly limited to previously treated or high-grade examples.

Microscopy

Gangliogliomas, by definition, contain a neoplastic glial population admixed with an atypical, mature neuronal component.[23,150] The relative representation of these cellular constituents varies considerably. Neuronal elements may be easily seen, occasionally dominating the histological picture, or are evident only after extensive searching, in some cases being sparsely distributed or regionally segregated. Well-differentiated ganglion cell constituents possess round, vesicular, centrally placed nuclei, variably prominent nucleoli, amphophilic or eosinophilic cytoplasm and peripherally distributed Nissl substance (Figure 32.2b). Whereas native ganglion cells are evenly distributed with orderly polarity and relatively unaltered cytology, neuronal cells in gangliogliomas usually lie in obvious architectural disarray, often clustering, and may exhibit pronounced dysmorphism. Chief among the latter are conspicuous variation in size and shape, multinucleation, cytoplasmic vacuolation, clumped Nissl substance and thickened, tortuous neuritic processes that sprout irregularly from cell bodies. Giant and bizarre forms that prove to be neuronal only on immunohistochemical assessment may be encountered, while some neurons bear neurofibrillary tangles and other abnormal cytoplasmic inclusions associated with neurodegenerative changes.[29,235]

A delicate, neurite-rich matrix that is prone to spongy rarefaction is typical in regions of high ganglion cell density. These gangliocytic regions also often display a characteristic perivascular and interstitial infiltrate of lymphocytes and plasma cells (Figure 32.2c). Stromal fibrosis of gangliogliomas consists of a reticulin or collagenous network that can be minor and form wispy bridges between blood vessels or a more substantial spindle cell proliferation with fascicular or storiform patterns. Particularly prevalent in neuron-rich zones are stromal calcifications, mural calcification and

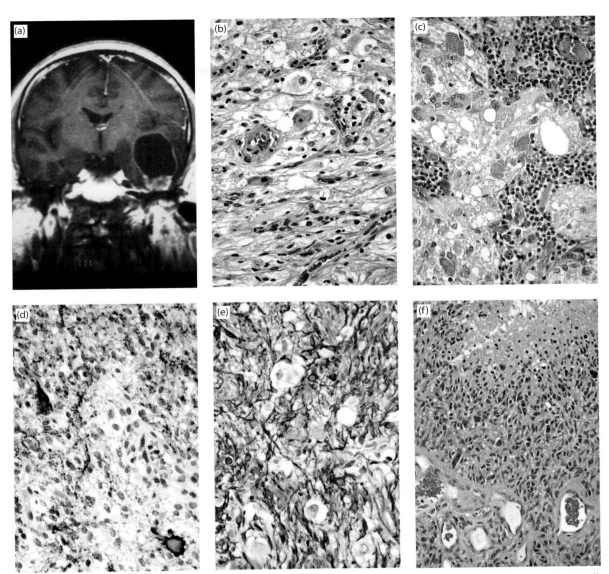

32.2 Ganglioglioma and anaplastic ganglioglioma. (a) Post-contrast coronal magnetic resonance (MR) image of a ganglioglioma in the left temporal lobe demonstrating the characteristic cyst and mural nodule pattern, with intense contrast enhancement of the solid component. **(b)** Large, atypical and unoriented ganglion cells are seen admixed with neoplastic, mildly pleomorphic astroglia. **(c)** Typical features noted in gangliogliomas are lymphocytic infiltrates and eosinophilic granular bodies (EGBs). **(d)** Synaptophysin immunoreactivity highlights the ganglion cells of ganglioglioma, especially the cell surfaces, and also demonstrates the extensive network of neuronal processes in the tumour stroma. **(e)** The astroglial component of ganglioglioma stains strongly for glial fibrillary acidic protein (GFAP). **(f)** Anaplastic ganglioglioma contains a high-grade glial component, including hypercellularity, nuclear atypia, mitotic activity, necrosis and vascular proliferation.

sclerosis of blood vessels and 'eosinophilic granular bodies' (EGBs) (Figure 32.2c). The latter are lysosomally derived, spherical proteinaceous deposits dispersed in the supporting matrix and cell processes of gangliogliomas and other low-grade CNS tumours, including pilocytic astrocytoma and pleomorphic xanthoastrocytoma (PXA). Both EGBs and lymphocytic infiltrates serve as signposts of low-grade biology in CNS tumours and are generally absent in higher-grade neuroepithelial lesions. Some gangliogliomas feature extensive large vascular channels, resembling an arteriovenous malformation.

In the great majority of cases, the glial component is astrocytic (Figure 32.2) and assumes the appearance of a low-grade fibrillary or pilocytic astrocytoma.[102,283] Rarely, gemistocytic elements are present and some contain patterns similar to PXA.[197] Oligodendrocyte-like populations are occasionally identified, with immunohistochemistry required to distinguish these from neurocytes.[102,157] Ependymal differentiation is a curiosity, as is melanin production.[107,234]

Conventional WHO grade I gangliogliomas exhibit little, if any, mitotic activity, usually limited to the glial elements. Isolated mitoses, glial atypia (which may be pronounced, particularly in piloid regions), microvascular proliferation, leptomeningeal invasion (a common feature) and microscopic infiltration of adjoining brain tissue do not predictably affect outcome. Extension into the sub-arachnoid space and contact with the pia–arachnoid may provoke a florid fibroblastic response, with occasional gangliogliomas developing dural attachments. These phenomena may prompt differential diagnostic consideration of desmoplastic infantile ganglioglioma or meningioma. The current WHO includes grade I (benign) and grade III (anaplastic) designations for ganglioglioma.[150] The designation of 'atypical ganglioglioma' has been used by some for those tumours that display increased cellularity and proliferative activity of the glial component, but do not fulfil criteria for anaplasia.[23]

Cerebral gangliogliomas are not infrequently associated with nearby malformative lesions, including focal cortical dysplasia (mostly type I) and mild malformations of cortical development.[197,274] Some tumours combine features of ganglioglioma and dysembryoplastic neuroepithelial tumour, the latter being also associated with cortical maldevelopment.[102,194]

Immunohistochemistry

The neuronal components of gangliogliomas may be labelled by antibodies against neuron-associated cytoskeletal proteins, biogenic amines and related enzymes, neuropeptides, calcium-binding proteins, or neurosecretory/synaptic vesicle components.[102] Especially common is cytoplasmic immunoreactivity for neurofilament, synaptophysin (Figure 32.2d) and occasionally chromogranin A. In addition to highlighting neuronal cell bodies, antibodies to neurofilament proteins may delineate abnormal neuritic processes. Particularly striking in synaptophysin immunostains is the reaction pattern along perikaryal surfaces in a coarsely granular or linear fashion, a phenomenon that may reflect synapse formation and one that has been reproduced with antibodies to another synaptic vesicle-associated protein, synapsin I.[157,233] This pattern of perikaryal synaptophysin labelling is not typical of native cerebrocortical neurons, but is a normal property of certain neuronal populations in the striatum, thalamus, brain stem and spinal cord.[202,284] The dense and diffuse perikaryal immunoreactivity for chromogranin A is also helpful in the diagnosis of ganglioglioma, because CNS neurons outside the hypothalamus and brain stem react only weakly, if at all, for this protein.[102] A large variety of other neuronal antigens have been demonstrated within the neuronal component of gangliogliomas, including class III β–tubulin and MAP–2, PGP–9.5, calcineurin and calbindin D28k, the neuronal nuclear proteins Hu and NeuN, α–synuclein, tyrosine hydroxylase, dopamine β–hydroxylase, VIP, neuropeptide Y, met–enkephalin, β–endorphin, substance P and somatostatin.[102,150] Gangliogliomas containing paired helical filaments typical of neurofibrillary tangles were found to label for tau protein, ubiquitin and phosphorylated neurofilaments.[29,235]

GFAP immunoreactivity is restricted to the cytoplasm of glial cells within gangliogliomas (Figure 32.2e) and may unmask some ganglion cell-like forms as astrocytic. Glial cells also label for OLIG2, S–100 protein and vimentin, but the latter two stain some tumoural neurons as well. Oligodendrocyte-like cells may be reactive for S–100 protein and negative for GFAP, vimentin and all neuronal

markers or lie in a synaptophysin-rich matrix and exhibit nuclear NeuN immunolabelling indicative of a neurocytic character. Laminin and type IV collagen deposition are more common in gangliogliomas than in conventional gliomas, especially in those with inflammatory infiltrates and long preoperative symptom intervals.

Greater than 80 per cent of gangliogliomas display some immunoreactivity for CD34. This epitope is normally expressed exclusively by endothelial cells in the adult brain, but is also transiently expressed by early developmental precursors in the CNS.[21,23] Cells that stain with CD34 in gangliogliomas co-stain with NeuN but not GFAP, suggesting they are neuronal in nature, although their precise identity has not been determined. Because normal brain and spinal cord does not express CD34, this marker may be helpful in establishing a diagnosis in some histologically ambiguous cases by identifying a dysplastic neuronal population. Those neurons that express CD34 also express MAP–2.[23]

The proliferative activity of gangliogliomas is generally low as determined by MIB–1 immunohistochemistry.[102] With rare exception, reactivity has been restricted to glial elements. MIB–1 labelling indices recorded in the larger series varied from less than 1.0 to over 10 per cent, with mean values in the 1.1–2.7 per cent range. Although the WHO classification does not include MIB–1 expression as a grading criterion, some investigators suggest that a labelling index over 5 per cent is a feature of 'atypical' ganglioglioma.[23] Others have demonstrated that elevated MIB–1 indices correlate with high-grade (anaplastic) histology or recurrence.[102] Immunoreactivity for p53 has been reported in a subset of gangliogliomas, most notably in the glial component, with a variable labelling index that correlated with tumour recurrence.[102]

Electron Microscopy

Ultrastructurally, tumoural neurons vary from small neurocytic forms to much larger ganglionic profiles showing expansive cytoplasm, well-developed Golgi complexes, polyribosomes, lamellar mitochondria and stacked rough endoplasmic reticulum.[102] Dense-core granules are usually abundant (explaining the aberrant labelling for chromogranin A) and located in cell bodies, as well as in neuritic processes containing parallel microtubular arrays. These granules measure 100–230 nm in diameter, similar to those of autonomic ganglion cells. Because such granules are not generally present in normal cortical neurons, they may be of diagnostic utility. Clear vesicles and synapses, including axosomatic contacts, may also be identified.[157] Neuronal elements may contain densely osmiophilic and laminated bodies, as well as paired helical filaments and other abnormal cytoplasmic inclusions. Glial elements typically exhibit astrocytic features; their cell processes contain intermediate filaments and, in some cases, are covered by basal lamina where they abut the extracellular matrix. Oligodendrocyte-like cells with well-formed Golgi bodies, centrioles, mitochondria and microtubules may be identified. A rare instance of ependymal differentiation has been confirmed by ultrastructural demonstration of elaborate zonulae adherentes, microvilli and cilia.[98]

ANAPLASTIC GANGLIOGLIOMAS

A small subset of gangliogliomas show frankly malignant histology on initial assessment or upon recurrence and aggressive transformation sometimes occurs many years (even decades) into the clinical course.[8,51,92,150,158,163] Interestingly, anaplastic variants of ganglioglioma do not show the strong temporal lobe predilection seen in grade I lesions, but are more evenly distributed throughout the cerebral hemispheres and spinal cord.[23] High-grade elements are almost invariably astrocytic, rarely assuming oligodendroglial appearances, and are characterized by dense cellularity, conspicuous mitotic activity and, in some cases, necrosis (Figure 32.2f). The histological picture may be indistinguishable, save for the presence of tumoural neurons, from that of glioblastoma. The MIB–1 proliferation index is high in the glial component of anaplastic ganglioglioma, generally exceeding 10 per cent.[23,197] In contrast to conventional cases, anaplastic (grade III) gangliogliomas show a lower frequency of CD34 reactivity. Interestingly, a recent study showed that these neoplasms were clonal throughout both benign and malignant components; however, the malignant component was characterized by addition chromosomal gains that may be relevant to progression, in addition to *TP53* mutation.[176]

Tumours containing glial components equivalent to WHO grade III or IV are appropriately designated as anaplastic ganglioglioma, WHO grade III, which can behave in a locally aggressive fashion, seed the leptomeninges and lead to death. However, there are documented cases of anaplastic tumours faring well following complete excision, likely reflecting that some of these neoplasms retain compact, relatively non-infiltrative growth patterns amenable to surgical excision.[114,141] A predictably poor outlook is associated with partial resection or biopsy, but the optimal management of these rare tumours remains to be defined.[224] A recent study using Surveillance, Epidemiology, and End Results (SEER) cancer registry data determined that the median overall survival for anaplastic ganglioglioma was 28.5 months and that unifocal disease and surgical treatment were the most important predictors of survival.[225]

Histogenesis of Gangliocytomas and Gangliogliomas

Much speculation has centered on whether gangliogliomas represent neoplasms, hamartomatous malformations or both. Their frequent association with developmental anomalies and typically indolent behaviour have prompted speculation that gangliogliomas represent tumoural forms of cortical dysplasia or benign neoplasms arising on a background of dysembryogenesis.[22,23,197] An extension of this hypothesis suggests that neoplastic transformation selectively targets the glial elements in neuronal or glioneuronal hamartomas. Clonality studies have suggested a monoclonal origin for the glial and neuronal populations, but have not been conclusive.[287] Further evidence of such an origin comes from the shared immunolabelling of gangliogliomas and glioneuronal hamartias/hamartomas for CD34, an oncofoetal antigen that may be involved in dysregulated neuronal migration in such lesions.[22,23] Gangliogliomas

could represent embryonal neoplasms programmed to advanced differentiation or could be derived from bipotential neuroepithelial progenitors. In this regard, the reelin signalling pathway has been investigated for its potential involvement in the development of ganglioglioma. Reelin signalling regulates neuronal development and cortical architecture mainly through its downstream effectors, doublecortin (DXC) and cyclin dependent kinase 5 (CDK5).[86] Preliminary studies of the reelin pathway in gangliogliomas have not shown any mutations in DXC or CDK5, as they are seen in neuronal migration disorders; however, levels of DXC and CDK5 mRNA are reduced in gangliogliomas in comparison to normal brain.[46] These findings could implicate dysregulated reelin signalling in the abnormal neuronal migration and maturation that leads to ganglioglioma.

Molecular Genetics

One the most complete studies of cytogenetic alterations screened 61 grade I gangliogliomas and found aberrations in 66 per cent.[103] Frequent gains were noted on chromosomes 7 (21 per cent), 5 (16 per cent), 8 (13 per cent), and 12 (12 per cent), with frequent losses on 22q (16 per cent), 9 (10 per cent), and 10 (8 per cent). Recurrent partial imbalances comprised the minimal overlapping regions dim(10)(q25) and enh(12)(q13.3–q14.1). Unsupervised cluster analysis of genomic profiles detected two major subgroups: 1) complete gain of 7 and additional gains of 5, 8 or 12; and 2) no major recurring imbalances or mainly losses. Interestingly, interphase fluorescence *in situ* hybridization (FISH) demonstrated that cytogenetic aberrations were localized to the glial rather than neuronal cells.

Molecular genetic analysis of gangliogliomas has been fragmentary. The recent recognition of the role of activating *BRAF* mutations and subsequent activation of the MEK/ERK pathway in low grade gliomas has led to their study in gangliogliomas as well.[97] The activating V600E mutation in *BRAF* was found in a substantial subset of gangliogliomas (14/77; 18 per cent) and anaplastic gangliogliomas (3/6; 50 per cent).[222] Other studies, although smaller in scope, have demonstrated *BRAF* mutations in approximately 50 per cent of gangliogliomas.[57] Further study of prognostic or therapeutic implications and additional mechanisms of signalling pathway activation are in order.

Unlike the diffusely infiltrating gliomas, only a small percentage of gangliogliomas are characterized by mutations in isocitrate dehydrogenase 1 or 2 (*IDH1*, *IDH2*).[57,105] Horbinski *et al.* found that approximately 8 per cent of gangliogliomas had mutations in *IDH1*; however, this subset was shown to have a greater risk of recurrence and a higher risk of malignant transformation.[105] Thus, *IDH1* mutations identify a subset of gangliogliomas that behave more like diffuse gliomas and the question remains whether these simply represent diffuse gliomas with entrapped dysmorphic cortical neurons rather than true gangliogliomas.

Because of the histological similarity of gangliogliomas to some malformative lesions such as focal cortical dysplasia and cortical tubers, in which the *TSC1* and *TSC2* genes have been implicated, these genes have also been investigated for their possible role in ganglioglioma development. One study uncovered polymorphisms of the *TSC2* locus involving intron 4 at a significantly higher incidence than in control patients or in patients with other brain tumours.[190] A more detailed analysis of 20 epilepsy patients with gangliogliomas identified 7 polymorphisms of the *TSC1* gene and 28 polymorphisms, as well as a single mutation, in the *TSC2* gene.[17] The frequency of *TSC2* polymorphisms in intron 4 and exon 41 in gangliogliomas was much higher than in the control population. The clustering of these *TSC2* polymorphisms near the GAP-related domain and the hamartin-interacting domain of the gene suggest that these alterations could have functional significance, but further evidence is needed.

DESMOPLASTIC INFANTILE ASTROCYTOMA/DESMOPLASTIC INFANTILE GANGLIOGLIOMA

The desmoplastic infantile ganglioglioma is a low-grade neuroepithelial tumour that affects the very young and is typically classified together with the desmoplastic infantile astrocytoma, which only differs by its lack of a neuronal component. Accordingly, they are linked under the designation of 'desmoplastic infantile astrocytoma and ganglioglioma' in the WHO classification of nervous system tumours.[150] These lesions have previously been described by a variety of terms, including 'superficial cerebral astrocytomas attached to dura' and 'desmoplastic supratentorial neuroepithelial tumours of infancy with divergent differentiation'.[249,260]

Epidemiology

Desmoplastic infantile astrocytomas and gangliogliomas occur in the supratentorial compartment with the vast majority presenting in the first 2 years of life (mean age 6 months).[150] Overall, they account for approximately 1 per cent of all paediatric CNS neoplasms, but may constitute 15 per cent of those encountered in infants. Several reports have now described such tumours arising in older children, adolescents and young adults.[179,191,272] A survey of 84 published cases revealed a male to female ratio of 1.5:1.[150]

Clinical Features

Clinical manifestations most commonly include rapidly increasing head circumference, bulging fontanelles, hypertonus and forced downward deviation of the eyes (the 'sunset sign'). Seizures and paresis may also be observed, as may VIth and VIIth cranial nerve palsies.

Desmoplastic infantile astrocytomas and gangliogliomas are classified as WHO grade I tumours and long-term follow-up studies have consistently reported a favourable outcome following gross total resection.[150,252,259,260] In those with subtotal resection or biopsy, most tumours are stable or regrow slowly.[58] Two tumours showed radiological evidence of tumour regression following subtotal resection.[247] On the other hand, some cases have been reported to behave more aggressively.[149,189] One desmoplastic infantile ganglioglioma that could not be surgically resected due to an unusually deep location progressed and caused death.[132,177] CSF dissemination has been reported, but is rare.[50,56] Adjuvant therapy is generally reserved for patients who are not candidates for resection.[58]

Radiology

Desmoplastic infantile astrocytomas and gangliogliomas share a sufficiently distinctive neuroradiological presentation to suggest the diagnosis in patients of appropriate age.[241,253,258] Supratentorial lesions most often arise in the frontoparietal regions, are typically quite large and often span multiple cerebral lobes.[150] Particularly characteristic is the finding on CT or MRI study of a superficially positioned, multinodular and brightly contrast-enhancing mass with plaque-like attachment to the dura and a subjacent, uni- or multiloculated cyst (Figure 32.3a). In fact, it is the large cystic component that is frequently responsible for the mass effect. Solid components may appear isodense or slightly hyperdense in non-enhanced CT studies, isointense relative to cortex in precontrast T1-weighted MR images and heterogeneous on T2-weighted assessment. Cystic elements are typically T1 hypointense and T2 bright. Despite the large size, there is only mild oedema and communication with the ventricular system is rare.[258] Other common features include erosion of the neighbouring inner table and sutural diastases, both evident on plain skull films.

Macroscopic Appearances

At operation, desmoplastic infantile astrocytomas and gangliogliomas are often large, not infrequently measuring 10 cm in greatest dimension. Their solid components lie largely outside the cerebrum proper, commonly being anchored to adjacent dura; they are grey-white and rubbery or firm owing to the large amounts of collagen.[150] A clear or xanthochromic fluid fills the cystic components. The tumour adheres to adjacent brain and these seemingly discrete neoplasms can demonstrate variable infiltration of neighbouring cerebral cortex.

Microscopy

Histological examination confirms their largely extracerebral localization, while also revealing invasion of adjoining cerebral cortex (often via Virchow–Robin spaces and only superficial in extent). A distinctly biphasic morphology is characteristic. Collagen- and reticulin-rich regions populated principally by elongate or plump spindled cells in loose fascicular or storiform array dominate most, leading to a decidedly mesenchymal appearance, which abruptly gives way to tissue of neuroepithelial character (Figure 32.3). The latter typically contain small cells of embryonal or astroglial appearance densely aggregated within a reticulin-free fibrillar matrix. Polygonal and gemistocytic cells may be seen in both fibrillar and desmoplastic regions. The presence of neuronal elements leads to the designation of desmoplastic infantile ganglioglioma rather than astrocytoma. Neuronal cells are most prevalent in the non-collagenous portions, range considerably in size and include ganglion cells that are fully differentiated, yet show dysmorphic features. Mitotic activity and necrosis are not conspicuous and are typically restricted to primitive small cell components.

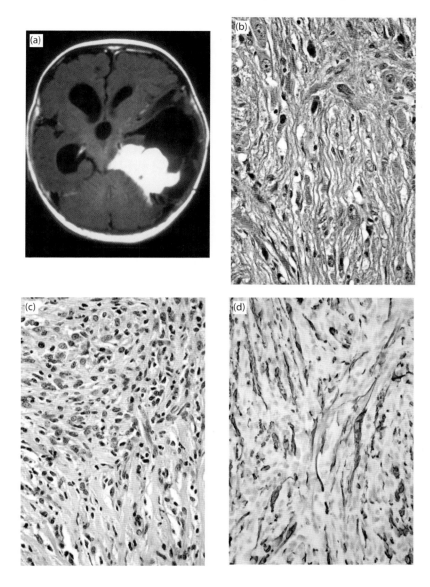

32.3 Desmoplastic infantile ganglioglioma. (a) MR image of a desmoplastic infantile ganglioglioma demonstrates large size, super-ficial localization, broad attachment to the dura, intense contrast enhancement of solid components and a large associated cyst. **(b)** Collagen-rich spindled region with arrays of elongate stromal cells and occasional interspersed ganglion-like cells. **(c)** Other regions show higher cellularity with atypical cells that can be either embryonal or astroglial in morphology. **(d)** Desmoplastic regions are rich in elongate glial fibrillary acidic protein (GFAP)-positive glial cells.

Examples with high mitotic rate, microvascular prolifera-tion and necrosis have been documented, yet a more aggres-sive biology has not been demonstrated.[56,136]

Immunohistochemistry

GFAP labels the astrocytic elements (Figure 32.3d), which constitute a surprisingly large percentage of the spindle cells in desmoplastic regions.[259] Individual tumour cells are out-lined by antibodies to type IV collagen, mirroring the pattern of reticulin stains and suggesting basal lamina deposition.[151] The visualization of neuronal constituents is greatly facilitated by immunoreactivity for synaptophysin, class III β–tubulin and neurofilament epitopes.[259] These neuronal markers may also be expressed by less differentiated, small cell popula-tions common to these tumour types as may MAP–2, the

neuron-associated Hu antigen and, in demonstration of their plasticity, GFAP and desmin.[166,183,215] MIB–1 labelling indices range from less than 0.5 per cent to 7 per cent.[150]

Electron Microscopy

Ultrastructural studies have confirmed the deposition of basal lamina material around individual tumour cells in regions of desmoplasia.[10,48] These cells are astrocytic and possess extended cytoplasmic processes rich in intermediate filaments. There is also a modest population of fibroblasts with characteristically well-developed Golgi complexes and abundant rough endoplasmic reticulum that may be distended by granular material. Neuronal elements elabo-rate neuritic processes replete with microtubules, dense core granules and neurofilaments.[260] Synapses are generally lacking.

Molecular Genetics

Classic cytogenetic analysis has been carried out on only a limited number of cases. In each case, either a normal karyotype or non-clonal abnormalities were described.[34] Molecular studies of DIA revealed no loss of heterozygosity on chromosomes 10 and 17 and no *TP53* mutations.[151,249] A comparative genomic hybridization study of 3 cases of DIA and DIG did not reveal any consistent chromosomal gains or losses.[134] One DIG showed a loss on 8p22–pter, whereas one DIA showed gain on 13q21.[34] Hypermethylation of the *P14ARF* gene was reported in one tumour.

Because DIGs are rare, large studies of *BRAF* gene fusions and activating mutations have not fully characterized their frequency. One study of activating V600E mutations did not find any mutations.[222] Another found it in 1 of 2 DIGs.[57]

Differential Diagnosis

Neuroepithelial neoplasms that exhibit fibrosis and harbour spindle-shaped, astrocytic tumour cells invested by basal lamina include pleomorphic xanthoastrocytoma (PXA) and tumours that have been referred to as 'gliofibromas'.[32,193] 'Gliofibromas' are a heterogeneous group of neoplasms that have no stereotypical age of onset, localization within the CNS or neuroradiological features and include aggressive, as well as relatively indolent variants. PXAs usually arise in older children or young adults, exhibiting bizarre cytological alterations and cellular lipidization not found in desmoplastic infantile tumours. Neither PXAs nor gliofibromas contain the primitive-appearing components of desmoplastic infantile ganglioglioma. Cellular aggregates of undifferentiated and embryonal appearance are lacking in conventional ganglion cell tumours, although these may demonstrate considerable reticulin and collagen deposition. Fibroblastic meningiomas and other mesenchymal tumours do not contain neuroepithelial constituents that are immunoreactive for GFAP or neuronal antigens.

Histogenesis

The cellular origins of desmoplastic infantile astrocytomas and gangliogliomas remain to be clarified. The presentation of these tumours in early life and their content of seemingly primitive small cell populations that can express both glial and neuronal proteins suggest that these are embryonal neoplasms programmed to undergo progressive maturation and, as judged by their generally benign clinical behaviour, eventual senescence. It has been suggested that basal lamina-associated constituents of these neoplasms, which are generally abundant, may inhibit tumour cell proliferation, and induce their terminal differentiation.[151,218,259] An origin from the specialized subpial astrocytes that form a continuous, limiting basal lamina investing their terminal processes could account for a comparable phenomenon occurring in desmoplastic infantile astrocytomas and for the superficial localization of these tumours, but is difficult to reconcile with the complex immunophenotypic potential of their small cell components.[10,151] Whatever their histogenesis, it would appear that the molecular events common to diffuse fibrillary astrocytomas do not play a similar tumourigenic

role. Specifically, the desmoplastic infantile astrocytomas assessed to date have not demonstrated either *TP53* mutations or LOH involving chromosomes 10 or 17.[151,252] Isolated examples of desmoplastic infantile astrocytoma and ganglioglioma have been described as having normal karyotypes or as exhibiting a variety of non-clonal structural cytogenetic anomalies.[48,179]

CENTRAL NEUROCYTOMAS AND OTHER NEUROCYTIC NEOPLASMS

The central neurocytoma is a well-defined clinicopathological entity that primarily affects young adults.[150] It is typically located in the lateral ventricles in the region of the foramen of Monro, shows a consistent pattern of neuronal differentiation and usually carries a favourable clinical prognosis. Its neuronal nature was first described by electron microscopy.[95] The name 'central neurocytoma' was proposed to distinguish these well-differentiated tumours from the more malignant neuroblastoma. The clinical, neuroimaging and histopathological features of central neurocytoma have been extensively reviewed.[41,96,223]

Epidemiology

Central neurocytomas are uncommon, likely comprising 0.25 to 0.5 per cent of all intracranial neoplasms.[96,124] In an evaluation of 300 published cases, there was no significant sex preference.[40] The mean age at clinical manifestation was 29 years; 46 per cent were diagnosed in the third decade and approximately two-thirds between the ages of 20 and 40 years.

Clinical Features

The majority of patients present with signs and symptoms of increased intracranial pressure, such as papilloedema, headache, nausea and vomiting, rather than a distinct neurological deficit. Other patients experience mental disturbances, visual changes, paraesthesias, lethargy, loss of balance or tinnitus.[221] The clinical history is usually short (mean 3.2 months).[96] Symptoms related to hormonal dysfunction have been reported in cases involving the septum, the third ventricle and the hypothalamus. In a series of 45 cases, the 10-year overall survival and local control rates were 83 per cent and 60 per cent, respectively.[142] Central neurocytoma has been designated as a WHO grade II neoplasm.[150]

Central neurocytomas are typically located supratentorially in the lateral ventricles and/or the third ventricle. The anterior portion of one lateral ventricle is the most frequent site (50 per cent), followed by the combined involvement of the lateral and third ventricles (15 per cent) and the involvement of both lateral ventricles (13 per cent) (Figure 32.4a).[96,223] Tumour growth limited to the third ventricle is observed in less than 3 per cent of cases.[71] In one case, the tumour extended over the entire ventricular system, including the fourth ventricle.[279] Small neurocytomas have been documented with precise sites of origin at the foramen of Monro, septum pellucidum, corpus callosum, hypothalamus and thalamus.

Occasionally, tumours with histopathological features similar to those of the central neurocytoma are found outside the ventricles, within the cerebral hemispheric parenchyma or other sites throughout the neuroaxis.[28,83,84,170] Infratentorial neurocytomas have been reported in the fourth ventricle, cerebellum, brain stem, spinal cord and cauda equina.[228,244,265] Given their locations, these neuronal neoplasms outside the lateral ventricles do not fit into the classic definition of central neurocytoma, yet appear to have similar histological, immunohistological and biological properties. In addition, extraventricular neoplasms have been described that, at least partially, contain neurocytic elements, yet are thought to represent distinct pathologic entities.[40,84,240] The term 'central neurocytoma' is typically used for those tumours within the lateral and third ventricles, whereas those outside have been referred to as 'extraventricular neurocytoma'.[28]

The cerebellar liponeurocytoma in particular appears to represent a unique clinicopathologic entity that is defined both by its peculiar predilection for the posterior fossa and for its lipomatous differentiation.[40,84,240]

Radiology

On CT scans, central neurocytomas appear as isodense or slightly hyperdense, well-demarcated, lobulated, intraventricular masses.[269,279] In about half of the cases, the lesion is calcified, hyperdense and irregularly enhancing. Low-density areas suggestive of cystic degeneration are less frequent. T1- and T2-weighted MR imaging reveal predominantly solid masses that are isointense or slightly hyperintense relative to the cortex (see Figure 32.4a)[37,269,279] They usually have moderate contrast enhancement, which is irregular in cases with calcification or cysts. Hydrocephalus due to obstruction of the foramen of Monro may be present. Intratumoural haemorrhage with or without extension into the ventricular lumen is exceptional.[37,174] Proton MR spectroscopy has demonstrated elevated choline and decreased creatine and N-acetylaspartate.[125]

Macroscopic Appearances

On cut section, these tumours are greyish and finely granular. Calcification can be extensive, with the lesion presenting occasionally as a 'stone'.[95] The neoplasm is attached to the ventricular wall only regionally. Invasion of neighbouring structures occurs but is rarely extensive.

Microscopy

Central neurocytoma can be tentatively identified on the basis of its histopathological appearance, but verification of the diagnosis usually requires immunohistochemical or electron microscopic evidence of neuronal differentiation. Central neurocytoma is a tumour of small to medium sized mature neurons arranged in a sheet-like, monotonous architecture with round, regular tumour cells densely packed close to one another and separated only by a delicate neuropil background (Figure 32.4b). Tumour cells grow either in a solid pattern or in linear arrays and often cluster around small blood vessels. In most instances, a pattern of neurocytic rosettes can be noted and these range

from being poorly formed and loose to tight Homer Wright or Flexner–Wintersteiner-type rosettes.[71] Within the centre of rosettes and also within larger expanses between tumour cell clusters are zones of finely fibrillar neuropil (Figure 32.4c). Such neuropil arises from the delicate extensions from tumour cells and is distinctive from the coarser fibrillarity of astrocytic neoplasms. Tumour cell nuclei are round or oval, with finely granular chromatin and small nucleoli. The cytoplasm is generally sparse and either finely pink or clear. In some lesions, abundant clear cells mimic oligodendroglioma (Figure 32.4c). Similar to oligodendroglioma, calcifications and 'chicken wire'-like capillaries are common.

Central neurocytoma includes neuronal differentiation by definition, which can often be appreciated on haematoxylin and eosin (H&E)-stained sections, but is more definitively established using immunohistochemistry or electron microscopy. Ganglionic cell differentiation is rare in central neurocytomas,[155,169] but is relatively common (about 50 per cent) in extraventricular neurocytomas.[28]

Calcification is common and reported in approximately one-third of cases.[96] It is distributed throughout the tumour, in contrast to oligodendrogliomas in which calcification predominates at the tumour margins. Necrosis occurs in rare cases that otherwise lack malignant features, but an association with aggressive growth has also been reported.[262,263] Occasionally, intratumoural haemorrhage is observed.[252]

Immunohistochemistry

Immunohistochemical studies have shown a consistent pattern of immunoreactivity for a variety of neuronal proteins. The most commonly used method for demonstrating neuronal differentiation is immunohistochemistry for synaptophysin, a structural component of the synaptic vesicle membrane.[262,263] Synaptophysin staining is typically strong and diffuse in both neuropil islands and cell bodies (Figure 32.4d).

A variety of other neuronal marker proteins have been identified in central neurocytomas, including synapsin, neuron-associated class III β–tubulin, MAP–2, tau, calcineurin, the neuron-specific antigen L1, the isoform 180 of the neural cell adhesion molecule (NCAM) and NeuN.[71,88,96,99] Neurocytoma cells with advanced neuronal differentiation defined by their nuclear NeuN immunoreactivity have been shown to be the least proliferative.[64] Immunoreactivity to neurofilament proteins is less consistent.[71,262] OLIG2 has been reported to be positive in only a small percentage of neurocytomas, a finding of potential aid in distinguishing neurocytic tumours from oligodendrogliomas.[198] Another neuronal marker, the anti-Hu antibody, selectively labels the nuclei of neurocytes and has been proposed as a reliable tool for the diagnosis of neurocytoma.[89] Photoreceptor differentiation, as indicated by the retinal S–antigen expression, has been observed in the majority of cases.[155] Although α–synuclein, a presynaptic nerve terminal protein, is expressed in a variety of neuronal and mixed neuronal/glial tumours, central neurocytomas lack alpha-synuclein immunoreactivity.[207] Similarly, neurocytomas seem to lack immunoreactivity to the neurotrophin receptors TrkA and TrkB.[171] Neuroendocrine features may be reflected by chromogranin and vasopressin immunoreactivities.[71,153]

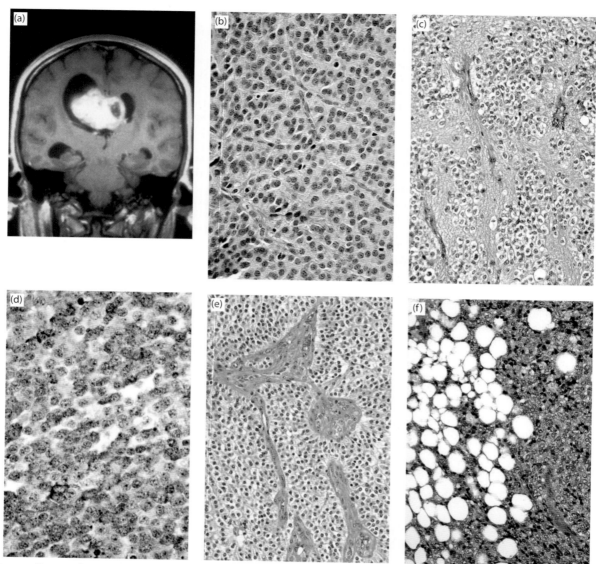

32.4 Neurocytic neoplasms. (a) Coronal, post-contrast magnetic resonance (MR) imaging of a central neurocytoma demonstrating its typical location in the midline, between the lateral ventricles near the foramen of Monro. **(b)** Typical appearance of densely packed small, round bland tumour cells and small, delicate blood vessels in central neurocytoma. **(c)** Tumour cells with clear cytoplasm have features similar to oligodendroglioma, but the presence of neurocytic rosettes and neuropil islands is characteristic of neurocytoma. **(d)** Neurocytomas are strongly and diffusely positive for synaptophysin by immunohistochemistry. **(e)** Atypical neurocytomas are highly cellular and show increased mitotic activity. The example here shows extensive microvascular proliferation. **(f)** Liponeurocytoma. A rare subtype of neurocytic neoplasm, most often arising in the cerebellum, shows well-defined lipomatous differentiation by neoplastic cells.

Expression of GFAP has been reported in up to 17 per cent of central neurocytomas and in nearly half of all extraventricular neurocytomas.[28,239,262,263] Some GFAP-positive central neurocytomas show marked mitotic activity, vascular proliferation or necrosis, suggesting that these may be more aggressive or represent a more primitive form.[60,71,160] It remains unclear whether GFAP and synaptophysin are expressed by the same cells within these neoplasms.[108,263] The GFAP-positive cells usually have either non-specific or astrocytic morphology, but in rare instances, ependymal differentiation has been described.[3,117]

Lipomatous differentiation is noted in occasional neurocytomas, especially those that arise in the fourth ventricle (see Cerebellar Liponeurocytoma, p. 1738). An unusual rhabdomyomatous differentiation (myoneurocytoma) has also been reported.[175] Other neurocytomas demonstrate dark cellular pigment representing lipofuscin, neuromelanin or haemosiderin (pigmented central neurocytoma).[123,167]

Electron Microscopy

The identification of central neurocytoma as a neuronal neoplasm by Hassoun and colleagues was based on ultrastructural identification of neuronal features.[95] This and subsequent reports described features that can be summarized as follows: (i) abundance of 60–160 nm dense-core vesicles, 40–60 nm clear vesicles of the presynaptic type and specialized synaptic junctions; and (ii) numerous thin cell processes with morphological characteristics of non-myelinated neurites, including 20-nm microtubules.[96] Intermediate filaments have infrequently been detected.[85] A single case has been reported with the ultrastructural presence of concentric lamellar structures, suggesting dual differentiation into neurocytes and oligodendrocytes.[180]

Proliferative Activity

Mitoses are infrequent or absent in the majority of central neurocytomas and the growth fraction as defined by the antibody Ki–67/MIB–1 is usually less than 2 per cent.[13,239] However, cases with brisk mitotic activity and higher MIB–1 values have been observed.[239,262,263] The proliferation potential of neurocytoma is a useful predictor of clinical outcome. Early investigations suggested that a labelling index greater than 2 per cent was associated with a significantly shorter recurrence-free interval.[239] Meta-analysis of reported studies indicates that a MIB–1 proliferation index greater than 3 per cent is associated with worse prognosis, both in terms of local control and for survival.[205]

Atypical Neurocytoma

A subset of neurocytomas are encountered that either have histopathologic features suggestive of aggressive behaviour or demonstrate an unusually elevated MIB–1 proliferation index (>2–3 per cent), warranting the diagnosis of 'atypical central neurocytoma' or 'atypical extraventricular neurocytoma'. Microvascular proliferation, focal necrosis and/or marked mitotic activity are the histological features of atypical central or extraventricular neurocytomas (Figure 32.4e).[28,126,152,239]

It remains unclear whether there are 'anaplastic' or 'malignant' neurocytomas. These terms have been used for cases that histopathologically showed even more exuberant microvascular proliferation, necrosis and mitotic activity.[262,263,279] However, follow-up revealed recurrence-free survival of several years in some cases. The overall experience with neurocytic tumours, including the atypical variants, suggests that their prognosis is still much better than that of malignant gliomas and therefore the modifiers 'atypical' and 'proliferating' have been more widely used than 'anaplastic' or 'malignant'.[152,279]

Histogenesis

The histogenesis of the central neurocytoma has remained enigmatic. The stereotypic location in the anterior part of the lateral ventricles and its consistent neuronal differentiation have led to the suggestion that it originates from small grey nuclei of the septum pellucidum.[95,168] Although this is a frequent site of attachment, subsequent studies show that central neurocytomas may arise from any part of the ventricular wall, including the third ventricle. Another hypothesis is that central neurocytomas originate postnatally from remnants of the subependymal plate of the lateral ventricles, which during development gives rise to neurons, glial and ependymal cells.[262,263] Remnants of the germinal zone persist and maintain a proliferative potential. An origin of central neurocytomas from the subependymal plate could explain their intraventricular location and the capacity for neuronal and occasional glial differentiation, but attachment would be expected at the lateral wall of the ventricles rather than at the septum pellucidum. Those who are sceptical of the capacity for GFAP expression maintain that neurocytomas are formed from cells committed to a neuronal phenotype and not from multipotent cells.[71]

Other investigations have suggested a shared histogenesis between neurocytomas and oligodendrogliomas. Support comes from the finding that tumours histologically identical to oligodendrogliomas can also show variable degrees of neuronal differentiation by immunohistochemical and ultrastructural studies; that there is substantial morphologic overlap between neurocytomas and oligodendroglioma; and that tumours have been reported that have both oligodendroglial and neurocytic differentiation, including the presence of neurocytic rosettes with synaptophysin staining.[180,188] A subset of neurocytomas show expression of OLIG2, a marker that is more commonly expressed by developing and mature oligodendrocytes and other glial cells.[146,198] Combined, these findings could indicate that neurocytic neoplasms and oligodendroglioma form a biological and diagnostic spectrum.

Genetics

Cytogenetic data on central neurocytoma are scarce, probably because of their low proliferation rates. In two cases, an isochromosome 17 and complex karyotype were reported.[33,112] Gains on chromosomes 7, 2p, 10q and 18q were observed by FISH and comparative genomic hybridization (CGH), respectively.[251,280] *TP53* mutations and *MYCN* amplification have not been found in neurocytomas.[112,173]

Numerous investigations have attempted to provide genetic markers that can distinguish neurocytomas from oligodendrogliomas, because these two tumours have significant morphologic overlap.[186,257] Investigation of 1p and 19q allelic loss by FISH analysis or by micro-satellite markers has demonstrated these losses in 70–85 per cent of oligodendrogliomas, whereas these losses are rare in central neurocytomas.[78] In contrast, losses of 1p and 19q have been identified in a few extraventricular neurocytomas.[161,186] More recently, a FISH analysis identified 1p/19q codeletion in 5 of 24 (24 per cent) extraventricular neurocytomas, with isolated 1p deletion in another 2 (10 per cent). Most of the co-deleted cases were associated with the translocation t(1:19)(q10:p10). Interestingly, those tumours with this translocation showed atypical histologic features, increased mitotic figures and a greater frequency of recurrence.[213] It is increasingly recognized that there is histologic, immunohistochemical and molecular genetic overlap of extraventricular neurocytomas and oligodendrogliomas. The finding of 1p and 19q codeletions in extraventricular neurocytomas likely identifies a subset with biologic similarity to oligodendroglioma.

Biological Behaviour

In accordance with its low grade histopathological features and the generally low proliferative activity, the clinical course of patients with central neurocytoma is usually favourable.[96] The goal of therapy is to control the tumour locally, because most cases of recurrence and progression occur at the original tumour site. Therefore, most therapeutic consideration is given to the extent of surgical resection and postoperative radiation therapy. Only in rare instances has craniospinal dissemination of central neurocytoma been documented.[246]

Most studies have indicated that gross total resection of central neurocytoma is associated with better local tumour control and longer patient survival than subtotal resection.[203] Local control following gross total resection ranges from 85 to 100 per cent at 5 years with overall survival at 80 to 95 per cent.[203,221] Other investigations have indicated slightly higher rates of tumour recurrence after both total and subtotal resection.[19,279] For those neurocytomas with mitoses <3 per 10 high power fields (i.e. those that are not 'atypical'), the survival and local control rates at 10 years were 89 per cent and 74 per cent, respectively.[142] A review of the literature has indicated that radiation therapy does not necessarily improve local control or survival for patients following the complete surgical resection of central neurocytoma. Following incomplete resection, however, radiation appears to improve local tumour control, but may not alter overall survival after 5 or 10 years.[203] In the setting of radiotherapy following subtotal resection, partial and complete tumour regression have been reported, yet long disease-free intervals have also been observed in patients treated by surgery alone.[279] Atypical central neurocytomas are associated with worse prognosis, both in terms of local tumour control and long-term survival.[204] Survival and local control rates at 10 years for atypical neurocytomas (≥3 mitoses per 10 hpf) are reported as 63 per cent and 46 per cent, respectively.[142] The addition of radiation therapy improves local tumour control for atypical neurocytomas, especially in the setting of incompletely resected tumour. Chemotherapy has not been investigated as thoroughly, but may be associated with tumour stabilization in progressive disease in some instances.[223]

CEREBELLAR LIPONEUROCYTOMA

Cerebellar liponeurocytoma is a rare, yet distinct, clinicopathological entity.[240] It occurs in adults and exhibits the unusual combination of advanced neurocytic and focal lipomatous differentiation. The tumour has low proliferative activity and a favourable prognosis as compared to medulloblastoma, yet recurrence occurs in over 50 per cent of patients, leading to its designation as WHO grade II.[106,150]

The first case of 'lipomatous medulloblastoma' was reported in 1978.[16] Subsequently, a number of case reports and small series of these unusual neoplasms appeared.[40,54,62,83] Various terms have been proposed for this neoplasm, including lipomatous medulloblastoma, neurocytoma/lipoma (neurolipocytoma), medullocytoma, lipomatous glioneurocytoma and lipidized mature neuroectodermal tumour of the cerebellum. The WHO classification adopted the term 'cerebellar liponeurocytoma' to emphasize its neurocytic character and its distinction from medulloblastoma.[150]

Epidemiology and Clinical Features

Cerebellar liponeurocytoma occurs almost exclusively in adults. Patients present with symptoms of a posterior fossa

tumour in their fifth to sixth decades, ranging in age from 24 to 77 (mean: 50) years. This age distribution contrasts with that of classic medulloblastomas, which manifests in children in 70 per cent and is rare over the age of 40 years. The retrospective screening of 354 paediatric medulloblastomas failed to identify any with significant lipomatous differentiation.[239] No sex predilection is noted.

The vast majority arise from the cerebellum, either in the vermis or hemispheres, occasionally presenting as an exophytic mass in the cerebellopontine angle. Headache and symptoms related to increased intracranial pressure are the most common clinical presentations. There have been scattered reports of neurocytomas with lipomatous differentiation in non-cerebellar locations, including the supratentorial compartment, the third ventricle and the lateral ventricle.[80,90,135] In contrast, neurocytic neoplasms of the cerebellum are nearly always lipidized.

Microscopy and Immunohistochemistry

The neurocytic component is similar to central neurocytoma and exhibits a monotonous pattern of round to oval cells with clear cytoplasm and ill-defined cell membranes. Necrosis and microvascular proliferation are usually absent. The histological hallmark of the liponeurocytoma is the focal accumulations of lipid-laden cells (Figure 32.4f). Immunohistochemical studies indicate that these cells are not adipocytes but rather neuroepithelial tumour cells displaying lipomatous differentiation. The possibility of fatty degeneration (lipidization) of tumour cells is less likely but cannot be ruled out.

Another consistent characteristic of liponeurocytoma is advanced neuronal/neurocytic differentiation, indicated histologically by the presence of oligodendroglia-like cells with perinuclear halos, small fibrillary anuclear zones and immunoreactivity for neuron-specific enolase (NSE), synaptophysin and MAP–2. Well developed neurocytic rosettes are occasionally encountered, sometimes resembling Homer Wright (neuroblastic) rosettes, but generally lacking the primitive, mitotically active cells that characterize the latter. Ultrastructural features of neuronal differentiation include dense core and clear vesicles, microtubule-containing neurites and rare synapse-like structures. The presence of Homer Wright-like and neurocytic rosettes led initially to variably proposed designations of neuroblastoma and cerebellar neurocytoma.[62,240]

Astrocytic differentiation, as identified by GFAP expression, is present in the majority.[189,240] In contrast to neuronal differentiation, it is more focal and easily missed without immunohistochemistry. Individual cases with myoid and ependymal differentiation have been described.[87,117]

Mitotic activity is absent or low, with MIB–1 labelling indices of 2–3 per cent (range, 1–6 per cent), significantly lower than those typical of paediatric and adult medulloblastomas.[62,240]

Histogenesis and Molecular Genetics

Immunoreactivity to neuronal antigens and GFAP is not restricted to small non-lipidized cells, but is also present in cells containing fat globules.[240] Together with ultrastructural studies, this further suggests that the fat-laden cells result from lipomatous differentiation of tumour cells rather than from non-neoplastic mesenchymal elements. The histogenesis of this lesion remains enigmatic. It remains possible that these fourth ventricular tumours arise along the same route as medulloblastomas, but represent a better differentiated form, with lower proliferative potential and lipomatous differentiation. In a large international consortium effort to characterize these rare tumours, *TP53* mutations were found in 4 of 20 cases, which is a higher rate than in medulloblastoma and not a common property of central neurocytoma.[106] None of the cerebellar liponeurocytomas had isochromosome 17 or mutations of *PTCH*, *APC* or the β–catenin (*CTNNB1*) genes, each of which are seen in subsets of medulloblastoma. Gene expression profiling and cluster analysis of cerebellar liponeurocytomas showed that they have profiles more similar to central neurocytomas than medulloblastomas. Thus, although the location of liponeurocytoma is similar to medulloblastoma, genetic alterations and gene expression studies suggest that it is biologically distinct and has more features in common with central neurocytoma.

Biological Behaviour

Previously, it was thought that cerebellar liponeurocytomas had uniformly favourable clinical courses. However, longer follow-up revealed higher rates of recurrence and fatality. Over half of the patients have developed recurrences, ranging from 1 to 12 years.[106,113,150] Among those patients with adequate follow-up (n=21), 29 per cent died within 2 years, 24 per cent died at 2–4 years and 48 per cent survived from 5–16 years. Because of these rates of tumour progression, the cerebellar liponeurocytoma is designated WHO grade II.

DYSEMBRYOPLASTIC NEUROEPITHELIAL TUMOUR (DNT)

Epidemiology and Clinical Features

Originally described as a clinicopathological entity by Daumas–Duport and colleagues, the dysembryoplastic neuroepithelial tumour (DNT) is currently classified as a WHO grade I glioneuronal neoplasm.[53,150] They are uncommon, comprising only 1.2 per cent of brain tumours encountered in patients under 20 years of age and 0.2 per cent of those identified in older subjects.[250] However, DNTs rank highly among space-occupying lesions resected for control of chronic, medically refractory epilepsy.[274] Particularly characteristic is a protracted history of partial seizures with onset before 20 years of age and without focal neurological deficits. Dysembryoplastic neuroepithelial tumours are typically discovered in the second or third decade, but have also been documented in older patients. Occasional examples have been found in the setting of neurofibromatosis 1, but there is not a clear association with any familial condition.[143] Some observers have noted a male predisposition. Although DNTs have been described involving striatal, septal, cerebellar and bulbar regions, the overwhelming majority are localized to cerebral cortex.[12,35,77,137,144] There is a clear predilection for the temporal lobe, particularly its medial structures.[172,201] Multifocal examples have been described.[144,268] Intratumoural haemorrhage

has been described as a presenting manifestation, but is exceptional.[254]

Radiology

Neuroradiological features are critical for distinguishing DNTs from conventional glial neoplasms (particularly oligodendrogliomas and oligoastrocytomas) that figure prominently in their differential diagnosis.[52,129] On MR studies, most DNTs are largely restricted, if not entirely confined, to an expanded cerebral cortex. They tend to be well demarcated, T1-hypointense and often display internal nodularity. They are best appreciated on T2-weighted or FLAIR images, which show a tumour with bright signal compared with adjacent brain (Figure 32.5a). High resolution MR images demonstrate thin septations within the tumour that have the same signal intensity as cortex.[67] A pseudo-cystic appearance may result from the intralesional accumulation of mucoid matrix, but true cystic change is not common. Non-enhanced CT studies, in which DNTs are hypodense or isodense, may disclose calcifications and rarely intratumoural haemorrhage.[254] Most DNTs are not contrast enhancing, but about one third contain discrete foci of nodular, homogeneous or ring-like enhancement. Oedema and mass effect (other than that related to associated cysts) are not typical, but deformation and/or thinning of the adjacent calvarium supports the chronicity of this superficially situated, indolent lesion.

Macroscopic Appearances

The study of lobectomy and *en bloc* resection specimens has revealed the essentially cortical topography of the DNT.[52,53] Typical is a thickened cortical mantle in which multiple, often gelatinous or mucoid nodules are apparent. The underlying white matter is usually minimally involved, although temporal lobe examples more often extend into subcortical tissues than do extratemporal variants.

Microscopy

Dysembryoplastic neuroepithelial tumours can be divided into 'simple' and 'complex' histological variants, although there does not appear to be a clinically compelling reason to do so. Common to both is the presence of mucin-rich intracortical nodules with patterned, microcystic or alveolar substructures (Figure 32.5b, c). Additionally, a 'specific glioneuronal element' is defined by the presence of small, oligodendrocyte-like cells aligned in columnar fashion along bundled axons and capillaries that are arrayed perpendicular to the pial surface and variably separated by a myxoid matrix in which mature neurons seem to float (Figure 32.5c, d).[52,53] Stellate astrocytes may be admixed. Whereas simple DNTs consist solely of these elements, complex variants additionally harbour spacially distinct glial nodules with histologic similarity to pilocytic (or less frequently, fibrillary) astrocytoma, oligodendroglioma or oligoastrocytoma. These glial components may be associated with a malformative-appearing and calcified vasculature. Dysembryoplastic neuroepithelial tumours of either type often display cytoarchitectural abnormalities (dysplasia) of the internodular or adjoining cerebral cortex that include neuronal

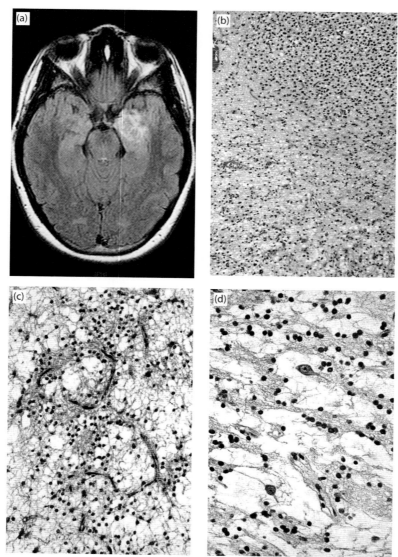

32.5 Dysembryoplastic neuroepithelial tumour (DNT). (a) Axial magnetic resonance (MR) imaging (fluid-attenuated inversion recovery [FLAIR]), showing a well-circumscribed, lobulated, hyperintense lesion involving the left anterior temporal lobe. **(b)** Tumours are often macroscopically and microscopically multinodular, with individual nodules demonstrating well-defined borders with adjacent brain. **(c)** The cytoarchitecture of DNTs varies, but a nearly constant feature is the presence of glioneuronal units (columns) with small, bland oligodendrocyte-like cells lining vascular elements and neuronal processes. **(d)** Mucin-filled microcysts are frequent in DNTs and 'floating neurons' are often appreciated within them.

disorganization and effacement of cortical lamination. Other histological features that may be encountered include micro-calcifications, oligodendrocyte-like cells arrayed around fibrillar cores in rosetted or cribriform fashion and 'knotted' tumour cell nuclei lying within a microcystic matrix. A melanotic example has been described, as have lesions combining elements of DNT and ganglioglioma.[61,100,196,229] In a recent series of eight cases of composite DNT/ganglioglioma, most were found to involve the temporal lobes and to contain multiple nodules with distinctive histologies.

Immunohistochemistry and Electron Microscopy

DNTs are complex neoplasms composed of glial and neuronal cells. The stellate and piloid astroglial forms encountered within DNTs are GFAP immunoreactive, whereas floating (likely entrapped) neurons have been reported to label variably for class III β–tubulin, NSE, neurofilament protein, NeuN, N–methyl–D–aspartate receptor subunit (NR–1), glutamate decarboxylase, γ–aminobutyric acid–A (GABA$_A$) receptor and synaptophysin.[52,104,250] Synaptophysin decoration of neuropil-like matrix components is also common, although this may reflect the fact that DNTs characteristically colonise synaptophysin-rich cortex. Oligodendrocyte-like cells of the specific glioneuronal element are generally immunoreactive for S–100 protein and GFAP negative, although some observers have noted occasional GFAP labelling of this population.[101] Small subsets of oligodendrocyte-like forms have been reported to show immunolabelling for synaptophysin, class III β–tubulin, NR1 and NeuN, findings taken as evidence of neuronal differentiation, albeit not dissimilar to findings also reported in oligodendroglioma cells.[101,273] Other workers, however, have described the immunoreactivity of such cells for myelin oligodendrocyte glycoprotein, a marker of mature oligodendroglia, and have provided *in situ* hybridization evidence that they transcribe the myelin-associated *PLP* gene.[275] Expression of OLIG2 has been noted to be strongly and diffusely expressed in DNTs.[146,198] MIB–1 labelling indices do not usually exceed 1–2 per cent, and are often well below 1 per cent, but values of up to 8 per cent have been noted.

Ultrastructural studies have yielded conflicting findings regarding the differentiation potential of the oligodendrocyte-like cells in DNTs.[101,133] These have been variously described as uncommitted in appearance, showing neuronal features (neurite-like processes, clear and dense core vesicles, and axosomatic synaptic complexes) and manifesting characteristics of early oligodendroglial differentiation (such as rudimentary lamellar membrane formations and perineuritic infoldings). Such cells may, therefore, constitute a population of heterogeneous lineage or cells capable of divergent glioneuronal differentiation.

Differential Diagnosis

The diagnosis of DNT rests on recognition of its principally intracortical localization and demonstration of its characteristically patterned specific glioneuronal element. These are readily appreciated in *en bloc* resection or lobectomy specimens; they may be difficult or impossible to discern, however, in fragmented neurosurgical specimens. Favouring DNT are associations with seizures in a young subject, a cortical-based abnormality without mass effect or oedema, adjacent calvarial thinning, and adjacent cortical dysplasia. In contrast, the presence of *IDH* mutations or chromosome 1p/19q codeletion essentially excludes DNT, although care must be exercised in paediatric cases where even classic oligodendrogliomas lack these alterations. Lesions combining DNT and ganglioglioma have also been described, yet in its pure form, DNT does not show the pronounced neuronal dysmorphism or inflammatory infiltrates characteristic of the latter.[100]

Genetics

DNTs have been investigated for potential genetic similarity to other more frequently encountered CNS neoplasms. Most studies have concluded that these lesions do not display 1p or 19q deletions or *TP53* mutations[113,186] yet other more recent studies have reported rare examples of 1p and 19q codeletion and other alterations more typical of diffuse gliomas;[78,116,255] whether such cases could represent misdiagnosed oligodendrogliomas remains uncertain. A recent investigation of *IDH1* mutations in DNTs found that none of the 21 cases examined showed immunoreactivity for the mutant protein,[31] although as indicated earlier, rare positive cases have been reported by others, with the same caveat about rare misdiagnoses potentially applying. Two studies of activating *BRAF* mutations in low grade paediatric gliomas, each including 4 DNTs, did not identify any mutations,[57,222] although more recent studies found it in roughly 30 per cent.[38,192]

Biological Behaviour and Histogenesis

Dysembryoplastic neuroepithelial tumours are classified as WHO grade I lesions.[150] Follow-up studies indicate that histologically conventional variants have limited growth potential and gross total resection usually controls seizures and achieves cures.[52,53] In one study, 85 per cent of children with DNTs were seizure free at 1 year and 62 per cent were seizure free at longer intervals (mean 4.3 years' follow-up).[172] Patients who are older at presentation and those with longer duration of seizures are at greatest risk for seizure recurrence. Extent of resection has also been found to be associated with the control of seizures.[36] Although most DNTs remain radiologically stable following subtotal surgical resection, the presence of residual tumour is associated with recurrence of seizures.[172] Additionally, true tumoural recurrences have been reported, occasionally with only the glial nodule component (e.g. resembling pilocytic astrocytoma) evident on repeat surgery.[208] Cases with malignant transformation are rare and may relate to radiation therapy. Also, although DNTs are generally associated with a favourable prognosis and seizure control, neuropsychological testing of patients who undergo resection has revealed that the majority of patients do not achieve a level of neurocognitive function similar to age-matched peers.[201]

The presence of features typically associated with aggressive behaviour, such as conspicuous mitotic activity, complex microvascular proliferation and necrosis have not been shown to impact postoperative outcome. However, because only a few complex DNTs showing these atypical characteristics have been studied, their biological potential remains at issue. Aggressive behaviour has been documented for a small subset, yet features predicting this outcome have not been elucidated.

The regular association of DNTs with cortical dysplasia has been taken as evidence of their dysembryogenetic origins, and their clinical stability raises further questions regarding whether such lesions are more akin to hamartomas than neoplasms.[52,53] On the other hand, occasional recurrences and demonstrable growth on serial imaging studies are more like the behaviour of benign neoplasms. DNTs may be congenital neoplasms that are regulated in their growth and induced to mature by elements of the cortical micro-environment. The histogenesis of these unusual lesions is uncertain, but an origin from secondary germinal layers (e.g. the subpial and subependymal layers, or the foetal external granular layer of the cerebellum) has been suggested to account for the superficial cortical or periventricular topography of most recorded examples.

DYSPLASTIC GANGLIOCYTOMA OF THE CEREBELLUM (LHERMITTE–DUCLOS DISEASE)

Epidemiology and Clinical Features

The dysplastic gangliocytoma of the cerebellum, eponymously known as Lhermitte–Duclos disease, is a rare and enigmatic lesion that usually comes to attention in the third to fourth decade, although congenital presentation and patients up to 74 years of age have been reported.[5,1175] There does not appear to be a significant sex predilection. The clinical behaviour is that of a posterior fossa mass and the associated neurological manifestations evolve chronically, with a mean predetection symptomatic interval of 40 months. In the majority of cases, symptoms include ataxia and seizures or are related to obstructive hydrocephalus, increased intracranial pressure or cerebellar injury. Cranial nerve deficits may be observed, with atypical presentations including severe orthostatic hypotension and acute subarachnoid haemorrhage.[214,227,242] Both the vermis and hemispheric cerebellar cortex may be involved.

Patients with dysplastic gangliocytomas of the cerebellum may show evidence of extracerebellar brain dysfunction, which generally takes the form of mild intellectual disability, seizure disorders or a variety of less common CNS and systemic anomalies. These include neuronal heterotopias in the white matter, olivary nuclear hypertrophy, hydromyelia, cervical syrinx, vascular malformations, polydactyly and partial gigantism. Dysplastic gangliocytomas of the cerebellum is recognized as a component of Cowden syndrome (CS; see Chapter 44, Hereditary Tumour Syndromes), an autosomal dominant phakomatosis that has been linked to germline *PTEN/MMAC–1* mutations.[63] Among patients with CS, there is cumulative lifetime risk of 32 per cent for the development of dysplastic gangliocytoma.[211] Germline intragenic *PTEN* mutations have been demonstrated in 81 per cent of CS patients and at least some of the non-mutated cases may be accounted for by alterations of the *PTEN* promoter.[286] The precise relationship between *PTEN* mutations, CS and dysplastic gangliocytoma remains to be defined, however, because not all patients with dysplastic gangliocytoma develop other manifestations of CS and some patients with dysplastic gangliocytoma do not have germline *PTEN* mutations, especially in paediatric examples.[1,211,285] Patients with such cerebellar lesions should be evaluated and followed carefully, because female patients with CS have a high incidence of breast carcinoma and therefore warrant careful surveillance.

Although there is debate whether this lesion should be considered neoplastic or hamartomatous, it is considered benign and is designated WHO grade I.[150] Surgical resection is curative in the majority, but local recurrence also occurs in a substantial fraction with long-term follow-up. Many have suggested that recurrence of these dysplastic gangliocytomas favours a neoplastic rather than hamartomatous designation for these lesions.[242,271] Others have speculated that clinical recurrence may be caused by hypertrophy of residual, genetically affected tissue rather than a recurrence related to proliferation.[1]

Radiology

Dysplastic gangliocytoma is typically a non-enhancing, unilateral hemispheric expansion of the cerebellum (Figure 32.6a). They are hypointense on T1-weighted MR images and hyperintense on T2-weighted images. In both instances, parallel linear striations (tiger stripes) are present on the surface that are nearly pathognomonic and represent affected, abnormally thickened cerebellar folia.[128,237] Calcifications are best seen on CT. Advanced MR imaging has shown that these lesions have mildly increased diffusivity and perfusion imaging demonstrates increased relative cerebral blood volume, blood flow and mean transit time.[256]

Macroscopic Appearances, Microscopy and Immunochemistry

Dysplastic gangliocytoma is evident on macroscopic examination as a region of folial thickening that blends into adjacent, unaltered cerebellar cortex. The enlarged folia often exhibit surface pallor or yellow-white discoloration (reflecting aberrant myelination), may be unusually firm and frequently have some white matter cavitation.

The most obvious histological change is the variable replacement of the internal granule layer of the cerebellar folia by moderate to large hypertrophic ganglion cells (Figure 32.6b–d). The degree of granular cell layer changes ranges from modest replacement of only superficial cells by a ganglion cell population to complete granular cell layer replacement. In the most severe cases, the molecular layer also shows increased numbers of granular or atypical ganglion cells. Occasionally, a collection of granular cell and abnormal ganglion cells are seen in the subpial zone of the molecular layer, hinting at disrupted neuronal migration of the external granular cell layer during cerebellar development. Another consistent finding is the abnormal myelination of the molecular layer. The abnormal neurons that populate the granule cell layer extend axons into the molecular zone that run, relative to the pial surface, in parallel stacks within its deeper layers and in perpendicular array more superficially. These axons become myelinated (unlike the neuronal processes that normally populate the molecular layer) and electron microscopic studies demonstrate that myelin sheaths in this condition are disproportionately thin given the 3–7 μm axonal diameters.[200,210] Other histological findings include a reduction in the number of Purkinje cells, microcalcification, large bizarre neurons, dense capillary networks and vacuolation of cerebellar white matter.[1]

Morphological, immunohistochemical and electron microscopic studies suggest that the neuronal populations in dysplastic gangliocytomas of the cerebellum are heterogeneous.[69,200,210,277] Large, polygonal neurons with prominent nucleoli contain numerous mitochondria, moderately developed Golgi complexes but inconspicuous Nissl substance and cytoplasmic processes filled with densely packed intermediate filaments and microtubules. A second, generally predominant class of smaller neurons with hyperchromatic nuclei, possess fewer mitochondria and more abundant free ribosomes and are often multipolar with tangled cell processes. Both neuronal variants contain clear and dense-core vesicles, with synapse formation being apparent in some cases. The fine structure of most dysplastic cells, along with the orientation of their axonal processes support the hypothesis that the neuronal constituents of the dysplastic gangliocytoma are principally of granule cell type, albeit substantially enlarged. Elongated and branching neurites with claw-shaped terminals, which are not found in conventional cerebral or cerebellar gangliogliomas, have also been demonstrated.[68,70] Patterns of neurofilament expression further suggest a granule cell histogenesis, yet a minor subset of the large neuronal forms share antigenic features with Purkinje cells.[231,277] These include immunoreactivity to

32

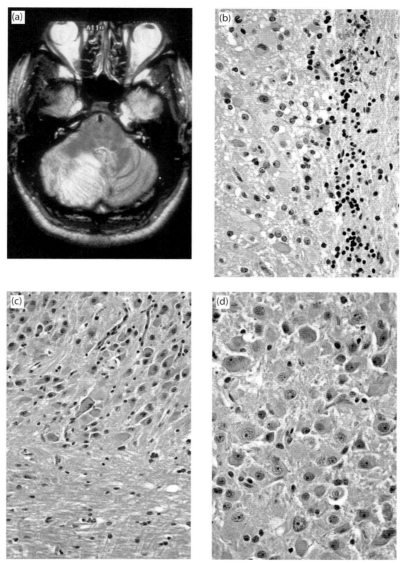

32.6 Dysplastic gangliocytoma of the cerebellum (Lhermitte–Duclos disease). (a) Axial magnetic resonance (MR) imaging (fluid-associated inversion recovery (FLAIR)) demonstrating a ribbon-like pattern of alternating high and low signal intensities in the right cerebellar hemisphere that cause expansion of the affected region. **(b)** Atypical pyramidal-type neurons seen in the top half of the picture replace the remnant internal granule cell noted on the left. **(c)** The high density of atypical ganglion cells ends abruptly at the interface with adjacent white matter. **(d)** The dysplastic ganglion cells present in these lesions have morphologic similarity to other forms of gangliocytomas.

the Leu–4 epitope, as well as to L7, PEP–19 and calbindin, and the observation that some of these demonstrate circumferential, membranous immunolabelling for the synaptic vesicle glycoprotein SV2, a phenomenon that presumably reflects the formation of Purkinje cell-like axosomatic synapses.[69,91,231] A similar labelling pattern may be appreciated for synaptophysin.

Histogenesis

The varied names attached over the years to the dysplastic gangliocytoma of the cerebellum – Purkinjeoma, gangliomatosis of the cerebellum, granule cell hypertrophy of the cerebellum and diffuse hypertrophy of the cerebellar cortex – attest to the diversity of opinions regarding its histogenesis and malformative vs neoplastic nature. One theory suggests that this lesion represents an incomplete development of the foetal external granular layer that results in a reduced population of the internal granule cell layer, forcing the remaining internal granular neurons to undergo compensatory hypertrophy. The presence of neuronal subpopulations with Purkinje cell features has been taken as evidence that the basic process is hamartomatous and not a simple reaction of internal granule cells to malformative events. Dysplastic gangliocytomas exhibit little, if any, proliferative activity and only rarely contain mitotic figures, also consistent with a hamartomatous origin.[1,91]

More recent investigations have emphasized the *PTEN* signalling cascade as a central node that is disrupted in the development of dysplastic gangliocytoma and leads to both abnormal cell migration and aberrant ganglionic maturation of neurons.[1,285] Mice that have the *PTEN* gene conditionally knocked out in the CNS develop cerebellar lesions similar to dysplastic ganglioglioma in humans.[11,139] In these animals and in the human disease, there are often abnormal collections of cerebellar granular cells and hyperplastic ganglion cells in the subpial zone, strongly suggesting that the inward cell migration of the external granular cell layer is disrupted during cerebellar development following *PTEN* loss. *PTEN* loss leads to downstream activation of AKT, mTor and S6 kinase, all of which have been clearly demonstrated in the large ganglionic cells of dysplastic gangliocytoma.[1] *PTEN* loss is also apparently responsible for the abnormal ganglionic differentiation of granular cells. Because the proliferation of these ganglionic cells is low, it has been speculated that the mass-like growth of these lesions is due to hypertrophy of individual ganglionic cells rather than to increased proliferation.

OTHER GLIONEURONAL NEOPLASMS

A number of less common glioneuronal tumours with unique histopathological features have been described. The most distinctive of this group is the papillary glioneuronal tumour (PGNT) (Figure 32.7a).[102,115,195,567] This tumour was first reported in 1998 and recognized as a variant of ganglioglioma in the 3rd WHO edition in 2000.[27,30,131] Increased recognition of its unique morphologic and clinical features has led to its classification as a new entity in the 4th edition of the WHO.[150] PGNTs arise predominantly in the cerebral hemispheres of adults where they are seen by MRI as well-circumscribed, contrast-enhancing lesions with little mass effect or surrounding oedema. Common clinical presentations include seizures, headaches and other focal neurologic manifestations related to tumour location. The histopathologic and immunohistochemical features of these circumscribed, non-invasive tumours are distinctive. The papillary or pseudopapillary architecture at low magnification is readily identified and closer inspection at high magnification reveals that the central fibrovascular core is surrounded by two distinct cell types. The innermost layer is composed of small, cuboidal cells with eosinophilic cytoplasm and round nuclei, whereas the outer layer in between the papillae contains larger clear cells with neurocytic or ganglioid appearance.

Immunohistochemistry highlights the biphasic nature of these papillary structures by demonstrating strong GFAP labelling of the inner layer and strong reactivity for neuronal markers (synaptophysin or NeuN) in the outer layers. Molecular characterization of these tumours is incomplete. Of 4 tested in one series, none were 1p/19q co-deleted, but 3 showed methylation of the *MGMT* promoter.[162] Both the inner glial cells and the outer neuronal cells are cytologically low grade and mitoses are generally difficult to find or absent. The MIB–1 proliferation index is low (1–2 per cent). Two cases of PGNT have been described that displayed atypical features, including elevated mitotic counts, microvascular hyperplasia and necrosis.[162] Although clinical follow-up is limited, the current data on outcome for classical cases are favourable and these tumours have been designated as WHO grade I.

The 'rosette-forming glioneuronal tumour of the fourth ventricle' is a recently described entity.[130,199] This rare tumour is found most commonly in the posterior fossa, where it arises in the midline, usually occupying a substantial fraction of the fourth ventricle, and is noted by MR imaging as a circumscribed, solid mass with heterogeneous contrast enhancement. Other locations have also been described, including the septum pellucidum, the lateral ventricular walls, pineal gland, the cerebellar vermis and the spinal cord.[7,121,226,276] It mostly afflicts adults (mean age: 30 yrs)[236] who present with headache, ataxia or hydrocephalus due to obstructed cerebrospinal fluid (CSF) flow. Although no firm association with predisposing genetic syndrome has been established, these tumours have occurred in patients with neurofibromatosis 1 and Noonan syndrome.[119,120] On microscopic examination, tumours are biphasic, with clearly defined and spatially separate neurocytic and glial components. The neurocytic component contains a homogeneous population of small clear cells that are arranged in either a rosetted pattern with central neuropil or papillae around central vessels (Figure 32.7b). A microcystic component with blue mucinous extracellular

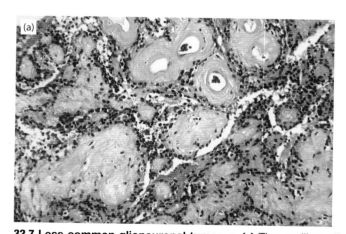 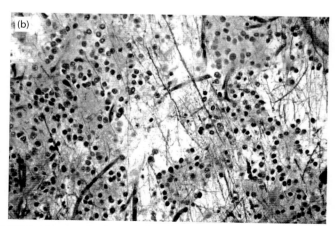

32.7 Less common glioneuronal tumours. (a) The papillary glioneuronal tumour is characterized by pseudo-papillary structures composed of hyalinised blood vessels surrounded by glial fibrillary acidic protein (GFAP)-positive glial tumour cells. Admixed are neuronal cells that range in differentiation from neurocyte-like to mature ganglion cells. **(b)** The rosette-forming glioneuronal tumour of the fourth ventricle consists of a monotonous population of well-differentiated neurocytic cells, generally with clear cytoplasm, that form rosettes and pseudorosettes in the setting of a finely fibrillar neuropil-rich background.

matrix may be present as well. Delicate processes form a neuropil matrix adjacent to tumour cells and extending to central vessels. The glial component of this tumour is solid and composed of cells resembling pilocytic astrocytoma. Also like pilocytic astrocytoma, this glial component may have an oligodendroglioma-like tissue pattern, microcysts, Rosenthal fibres and eosinophilic granular bodies. Both the neuronal and glial elements are histologically low grade and these tumours do not generally display overtly invasive properties. Mitoses are only rarely encountered and the MIB–1 proliferation index ranges from 1 to 3 per cent. The limited testing of these tumours has shown that they do not have *BRAF* alterations, 1p/19q co-deletion or *IDH1* or *IDH2* mutations.[119,276] The current experience suggests they are clinically benign, with low rates of recurrence and little propensity for malignant transformation. They have been suggested to behave as WHO grade I neoplasms.

Another morphologically distinctive lesion is the mixed glioneuronal tumour with neuropil-like islands or, more simply, 'rosetted' glioneuronal tumour.[1128] The cases described thus far have affected adults (ages 25–40 years), involved the cerebral hemispheres as infiltrative growths and were non-enhancing, T1 hypointense and T2 hyperintense on presentation. All were dominated by astrocytomas of fibrillary, gemistocytic or protoplasmic cytology (WHO grades II or III, with MIB–1 labelling indices ranging from 2.0 to 8.2 per cent) containing intensely synaptophysin-immunoreactive, neuropil-like islands rimmed in a rosetted fashion or occupied by neurocytes and atypical neuronal forms. Well-differentiated, medium to large ganglion cell-sized neurons were also identified. An intramedullary case and an example composed mainly of proliferating neuronal nodules have been reported.[93,122] A guarded prognosis is reported, because their infiltrative nature appears to predispose to recurrence and progression after surgery. There is likely overlap of these glioneuronal tumours with those described in a small series of oligodendrogliomas that contain advanced neurocytic differentiation, including synaptophysin-staining rosettes.[188] Potentially distinguishing these from the rosetted glioneuronal tumour are the oligodendroglial nature of the infiltrating glioma and chromosomal losses of 1p and 19q.

PARAGANGLIOMA

Classification

Paragangliomas represent a diverse group of neuroendocrine tumours that arise from either the adrenal medulla (phaeochromocytomas) or from the extra-adrenal paraganglion cells. The WHO and molecular classifications have converged on a unitary view of this category: tumours of the adrenal and extra-adrenal chromaffin tissues, the chemodectomas and histologically similar neoplasms have all been included in the paraganglioma/phaeochromocytoma family.[49,55,270] Consequently, three main groups are distinguished: (i) phaeochromocytomas originating from the adrenal medulla, (ii) sympathetic paragangliomas arising from neuroendocrine cells associated with the sympathetic chain and (iii) parasympathetic paragangliomas derived from cells that have chemoreceptor function and parasympathetic innervation. Collectively, these belong to the larger group of neuroendocrine neoplasms capable of synthesizing biogenic amines and peptide hormones, which together have been classified as tumours of the amine precursor uptake and decarboxylation (APUD) system.[184] Tumours arising from the carotid body and the glomus jugulare account for over 90 per cent of the extra-adrenal paragangliomas, the latter often encountered by neuropathologists. In regions of the central nervous system, most paragangliomas additionally arise in the region of the cauda equina.[264] Only intracranial and intraspinal paragangliomas are considered in this section.

Epidemiology

Paragangliomas within the neural axis are rare. Even in the region of the cauda equina, where these tumours are most common, they account for only 3.5 per cent of neoplasms.[4,156,238] There is a male predominance (male to female ratio of 1.5:1) and a peak in middle decades of life (ranging from 12 to 71 years, mean of 48 years).

Most neuraxial paragangliomas are located in the region of the cauda equina and over 80 per cent show a physical association with the filum terminale, either directly or through attachment to a vascular pedicle.[156,238] Other primary spinal paragangliomas have been described in the lumbar, thoracic and cervical cord.[159,232] Only one case has been documented within the conus medullaris.[238] Paragangliomas can also involve the CNS by direct extension of glomus jugulare tumours into the intracranial compartment.[140] Rare paragangliomas appear primary to the cerebral hemispheres, the sella turcica, cavernous sinus, pineal gland, cerebellopontine angle or the petrous ridge.[209,243,278]

Clinical Features

Paragangliomas of the cauda equina manifest clinically with low back pain (90 per cent) that is usually associated with sciatica.[4,156,238] Less common are motor and sensory deficits of the lower limbs (35 per cent), rarely including paraplegia.[238] Other regional symptoms include urinary or faecal incontinence and impotence. Unlike phaeochromocytomas and other extra-adrenal paragangliomas, systemic manifestations associated with bioamine and neuropeptide production are rare. One unusual case presented with a flushing-like syndrome and another showed symptoms of a more severe vasomotor syndrome.[25,267]

Radiology

Twenty-five per cent of cases show bony erosion of the surrounding vertebral structures. Specific findings include flattening or destruction of the pedicles, an increase in interpedicular distance, or scalloping of vertebra. MR imaging features of cauda equina paragangliomas are characteristic, but not diagnostic.[9,26,145] A mass lesion that is isointense or slightly hypointense as compared with spinal cord on T1-weighted images and hyperintense to CSF on T2-weighted images is typical. There is usually substantial contrast enhancement, which is either heterogeneous or homogeneous. Cystic change has been described, but is uncommon. More specific is a serpiginous pattern of flow void surrounding the mass that is due to congested and distorted vasculature. Paragangliomas are nearly always encapsulated and this component appears as a rim of T2 hypointensity, presumably because of the paramagnetic properties of haemosiderin deposition.

Macroscopic Appearances

Paragangliomas of the cauda equina range from small nodules of a few centimetres in diameter to large masses, reaching 10–15 cm.[238] They are encapsulated, rubbery, firm, nodular or lobulated masses, and the pinkish-grey cut surface may be speckled with haemorrhages. Calcification is rare. Although tumours do not invade neural tissues, their expansive growth, often in a limited space, may compress and eventually erode adjacent bony structures. Most tumours in this region are physically associated with the filum, and only occasional examples originate from the caudal nerve roots, or involve both filum and conus.

Microscopy, Electron Microscopy and Immunohistochemistry

Paragangliomas characteristically feature tight nests of cells, known as zellballen (Figure 32.8). Individual cells are small, round or polygonal and nuclei are round to oval with finely stippled chromatin and inconspicuous nucleoli. The cytoplasm is eosinophilic and finely granular. Based on cytoarchitecture, three histological types can be distinguished. The first and most typical is organoid: a lobulated pattern results from the groups of cells being surrounded by vascular or sinusoidal channels. The second, adenomatous type is characterized by a more diffuse epithelial-like pattern, sometimes with sinusoidal papillary arrangements. In the third, angiomatous type, vascular channels predominate. In any of these, there may be cellular pleomorphism, including multinucleated giant cells, but mitoses are rare or absent. Because the tumour is highly vascular, recent and old haemorrhages are common. Variable populations of thinly elongate or stellate satellite or sustentacular cells are typically admixed.

In the cauda equina region, paragangliomas often show adenomatous and angiomatous patterns (see Figure 32.8).[159,238] In some areas, there are also more elongate cells, their processes often oriented towards blood vessels, thus giving rise to pseudorosette formation reminiscent of ependymomas. A substantial subset show ganglionic differentiation. These cells are often arranged in clusters. Intermediate forms between the main neoplastic cell type and the ganglionic cells suggest a potential for transition or maturation. Haemorrhagic necrosis and scattered mitoses occur, but have not been associated with more aggressive behaviour.

Histochemical stains further characterize these tumours. Reticulin is found in the fibrovascular stroma, outlining the overall pattern of the lesion. Grimelius preparations show the argyrophilic cytoplasmic granules and argentaffin stains show scattered reactive cells.

By electron microscopy, paragangliomas are composed of 'light' and 'dark' cells, with a predominance of the former.[238] The main cytoplasmic features include well-developed organelles associated with intense protein production and storage, typical of neuroendocrine cells: rough endoplasmic reticulum and Golgi complexes, dense core neurosecretory vesicles with diameters between 100 and 200 nm and small numbers of intermediate filaments forming paranuclear whorls or 'fibrous bodies'. Close clusters of neoplastic cells are often joined together by desmosomes and are surrounded by a basal lamina, which separates them from the fibrovascular stroma. Dark, sustentacular cells found at the periphery of cell clusters may send stout processes among the neoplastic cells.[118] An important ultrastructural feature is the heterogeneity of secretory granules:

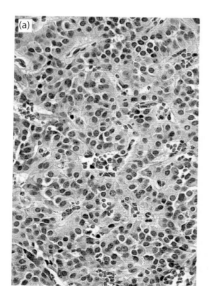
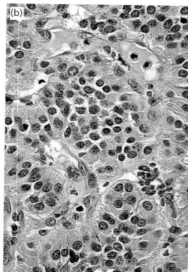
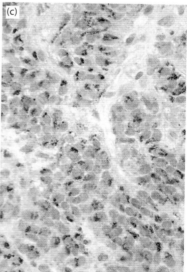

32.8 Paraganglioma of the cauda equina. (a) Many paragangliomas that arise in this region are highly vascular or show a dominant angiomatous pattern. **(b)** The histological signature of paraganglioma is the zellballen arrangement of tumour cells in moderate sized aggregates surrounded by a delicate fibrovascular stroma. **(c)** Individual chief cells of paraganglioma are positive by immunohistochemistry for neuronal markers, such as chromogranin.

they vary in size, shape and electron density, indicating that paragangliomas are capable of producing a range of neuropeptides and bioamines.[245]

The combination of ultrastructural studies and immunohistochemistry has identified two distinct cell populations in paraganglioma: chief cells (type I) and sustentacular cells (type II).[74,127,266] Chief cells are immunoreactive for chromogranin, synaptophysin and NSE (see Figure 32.8c).[159] Variable staining has been reported for neurofilament proteins. Both chief cells and ganglion cells show expression of somatostatin and serotonin (5–hydroxytryptamine), but other neuropeptides and gut hormones are not expressed. A subset of tumours arising in the cauda equina exhibit strong cytokeratin immunoreactivity, suggesting a dual paraganglionic and epithelial phenotype.[39] The sustentacular (satellite) cells of paraganglioma are immunoreactive for S–100 protein as are the chief cells in some examples.[156,159,238] GFAP may also be identified in sustentacular cells in a minority of cases.

Histogenesis

The histogenesis of paragangliomas within the central nervous system has not been fully elucidated. In particular, it is not clear if precursor paraganglia cells are a normal constituent in these regions or whether disrupted or incomplete migration of neuroblasts during development results in rests of precursor paraganglia.[20,206,243] Paraganglia may be neural crest-derived and of sufficient number in the foetus to account for the sporadic occurrence of paragangliomas in specific sites in the CNS because of altered neuroblast migration. However, there has been no evidence of mature paraganglia in the filum terminale.[243] It also remains possible that paragangliomas in the neural axis may arise from paraganglion cells associated with blood vessels or autonomic nerves.[148]

Molecular Biology and Genetics

Specific germline mutations and genetic syndromes are associated with the development of phaeochromocytoma and paragangliomas: multiple endocrine neoplasia type 2 (MEN2) characterized by germline *RET* mutations; von Hippel–Lindau syndrome characterized by germline *VHL* mutation; neurofibromatosis type 1 characterized by mutations in the *NF1* gene; and the four clinical entities of paraganglioma syndrome – PGL1, PGL2, PGL3 and PGL4 (see Chapter 44, Hereditary Tumour Syndromes).[14,24,73,164,165,220] PGL1, PGL2, PGL3 and PGL4 are associated with mutations of genes that encode separate subunits or co-factors of succinate dehydrogenase (SDH), a key enzyme complex in the Krebs cycle and respiratory chain. Germline mutations of *SDHB*, *SDHC* and *SDHD* are associated with PGL4, PGL3 and PGL1, respectively. Germline mutations of the fourth subunit of SDH, *SDHA*, have been demonstrated in phaeochromocytoma and paragangliomas, yet they appear to be extremely rare. The gene associated with PGL2 is *SDHAF2* (also known as SDH5), which is a co-factor of SDH that is required for its proper enzymatic activity. In population-based studies of patients with head and neck paragangliomas, germline *SDHB* mutations were noted in 7 per cent, *SDHC* mutations

in 4 per cent and *SDHD* mutations in 17 per cent.[165,200] Two other susceptibility genes have more recently been described included *MAX*, which is also known as Myc-associated factor, and *TMEM127*.

In combination, approximately one-third of patients with phaeochromocytoma or paraganglioma have germline mutations in a known susceptibility gene. Twenty-five per cent of patients carry germline mutations that involve the SDH complex, including *SDHA*, *SDHB*, *SDHC*, *SDHD*, or *SDHAF2*, with the clinical presentations differing among the genotypes. Immunohistochemistry for the SDHB protein subunit has been shown to be relatively sensitive and specific for mutations in the SDH subunits.[261] SDHB protein was absent in all 102 cases of phaeochromocytoma and paraganglioma with mutations in *SDHB*, *SDHC* or *SDHD* mutation, but was present in nearly all of those tumours that were sporadic or associated with MEN2, NF1 or VHL. Thus far, only one paraganglioma of the cauda equina has been associated with a germline mutation of an *SDH* subunit gene.[154] This tumour occurred in a 39-year-old man with a germline mutation of *SDHD*, but no family history of paraganglioma. This tumour was the only one of 22 cauda equina paragangliomas screened for *SDHD* mutations. Interestingly, this tumour recurred 22 years after its initial resection, and at the time of recurrence, the patient was found to have multiple cerebellar metastases. Further study is needed in order to determine whether cauda equina paragangliomas are associated with *SDHB* or *SDHC* mutations or other genetic alterations.

Biological Behaviour and Prognosis

Nearly all paragangliomas of the neural axis are histologically benign. Histological features associated with a more aggressive clinical course have not been identified.[4,147,156,238] It has been suggested that more aggressive paragangliomas outside the CNS have either lower numbers or absent sustentacular cells, but this observation has not been extended to cauda equina tumours.[127] The treatment of choice is surgical removal and, in 90 per cent of cases, total excision is possible. In other cases, the tumour vascularity, local adherence or rare infiltrative behaviour cause surgical difficulties. There are only scattered reports of tumour recurrence following gross total resection. Approximately 10 per cent of tumours regrow within one year following subtotal resection, and this percentage may be higher with longer follow-up, because cauda equina paragangliomas have recurred after extended periods.[154,238] Radiation therapy is an option for recurrent tumours.[156] Although uncommon, CSF dissemination of cauda equina paraganglioma has been reported.[44] Only one case of cauda equina paraganglioma has been reported to metastasize outside the CNS.[159]

Differential Diagnosis

The location, imaging appearance and histological pattern of paragangliomas usually enable a correct diagnosis, but other tumours can arise in this region and metastatic carcinoma, meningioma and ependymoma should be considered in the differential diagnosis. Metastatic carcinomas are more destructive of bone and tend to be more histologically anaplastic. Meningiomas most often show meningothelial whorls and psammoma bodies and can otherwise be distinguished by their immunoreactivity for epithelial membrane antigen (EMA) and lack of staining for neuronal markers. The occasional pseudorosettes of paragangliomas may mimic ependymomas, but other ependymal structures are not seen, and ependymal tumours in the cauda equina region tend to be myxopapillary variants. Furthermore, the immunohistochemical profile of paragangliomas, particularly the negative staining for glial antigens and positive staining for chromogranin, should secure the diagnosis.

HYPOTHALAMIC HAMARTOMA

Epidemiology and Clinical Features

Hypothalamic hamartomas (HH) are developmental/malformative masses that arise from the hypothalamus and tuber cinereum.[6,46,66] They are relatively uncommon, affecting 1 in 200 000 children and adolescents. No gender or racial predilection has been noted. HH may be asymptomatic and noted only as an incidental finding or may present with gelastic (laughing) seizures and precocious puberty in childhood. Hypothalamic hamartomas arise in two distinct locations within the region of the hypothalamus.[6,46] The intrahypothalamic subset accounts for the large majority (90 per cent) and these are centered within the walls of the third ventricle. The parahypothalamic subset accounts for less than 10 per cent and is centred inferior to the hypothalamus, with only minimal attachment to it. Intrahypothalamic HHs are associated with gelastic epilepsy, cognitive impairment and psychiatric disturbance. Gelastic seizures are highly associated with HH, but not entirely pathognomonic, because they can occasionally occur in other seizure syndromes.

The gelastic form of epilepsy associated with HH seems to be specific to childhood presentation; adults who become symptomatic are more likely to present with other, non-gelastic seizures. It is relatively common for the seizure syndrome of HH to progress in type and severity. Within the course of 4–10 years, the initial seizure syndrome may evolve to complex partial, tonic clonic, tonic or 'falling' types of seizures. Both the primary gelastic seizure and the secondary, generalized seizures that progress from them arise primarily from the intrinsic epileptogenic potential of the HH.[66] Those less common HHs that are localized inferiorly to the hypothalamus, the parahypothalamic subset, are not as likely to be associated with gelastic seizures. Because of their location near the infundibulum and pituitary gland, these are more likely to present with precocious puberty. The majority of HHs are sporadic. However, approximately 5 per cent occur in the setting of Pallister–Hall syndrome, an autosomal dominant disease that also includes skeletal dysmorphism, especially polydactyly, and other developmental anomalies such as imperforate anus.

Radiology

By MR imaging, HHs are hypothalamic mass lesions that vary from 8–40 mm (average: 19 mm) (Figure 32.9a).[76] The smallest are located typically within the hypothalamus

and third ventricle, whereas the larger lesions also extend inferiorly to occupy the space between cerebral peduncles. MR imaging studies indicate a nearly constant involvement of the mammillary bodies, fornix and mammillothalamic tracts, which may be responsible for the generation of seizure activity. HHs are modestly T2-bright, T1-isointense or slightly hypointense and non-enhancing. There is typically no enlargement of HHs on repeat imaging. MR spectroscopy performed on HHs has demonstrated increased peak intensity of myoinositol and decreased intensity of the N–acetylaspartate peak.

Macroscopic Appearances, Microscopy and Immunochemistry

Grossly, HHs are sessile or pedunculated, often resembling the consistency and colour of cerebral gray matter. Microscopically, the vast majority feature mildly disordered collections of mature neurons and glia, which may appear only subtly abnormal on a biopsy specimen (Figure 32.9b,c).[46] In most, the neuronal component is dominant, with small to intermediate sized neurons typically arranged in a multinodular pattern. Nodules vary in size, ranging from 10 to >100 neurons, and are separated by hypocellular neuropil populated by scattered neurons and glia. The large ganglionic cells that normally occupy hypothalamic nuclei are not prominent in HH. Less commonly, well-differentiated glial elements are the main cellular constituent. Fibrillary astrocytes are most frequent, and are noted together with scattered oligodendrocytes and microglia. The background stroma of HH is composed of a fine, slightly vacuolated collection of neuronal and glial processes that resembles normal CNS neuropil, a finding that accounts for similarity of HH to normal brain on MR imaging. There is no histologic difference between sporadic HH and those associated with Pallister–Hall.

The diagnosis of HH is usually established upon evaluation of H&E-stained slides with no further ancillary studies being necessary. Nonetheless, neurons of HH are immunoreactive for non-phosphorylated neurofilament protein (NF) and synaptophysin,[46] with small neurocytic cells being variably NeuN positive (Figure 32.9d). Immunohistochemistry for phosphorylated NF shows only minimal staining within cellular processes. Only rare, scattered MIB–1 reactive cells are noted in HH.

Molecular Genetics

The Pallister–Hall syndrome, which includes HH as one of its manifestations, is associated with a germ-line defect in the GLI3 gene. Genetic analysis of HH from sporadic cases has not identified specific mutations in GLI3; however, chromosomal abnormalities on chromosome 7p within and surrounding the GLI3 locus were detected in 15 per cent of cases.[47]

Differential Diagnosis

The regional differential diagnosis of a hypothalamic or third ventricular mass includes ganglioglioma, pilocytic astrocytoma, chordoid glioma, Rathke's cleft cyst, craniopharyngioma and germinoma. Among these, the main histologic concern would be ganglioglioma, which is composed

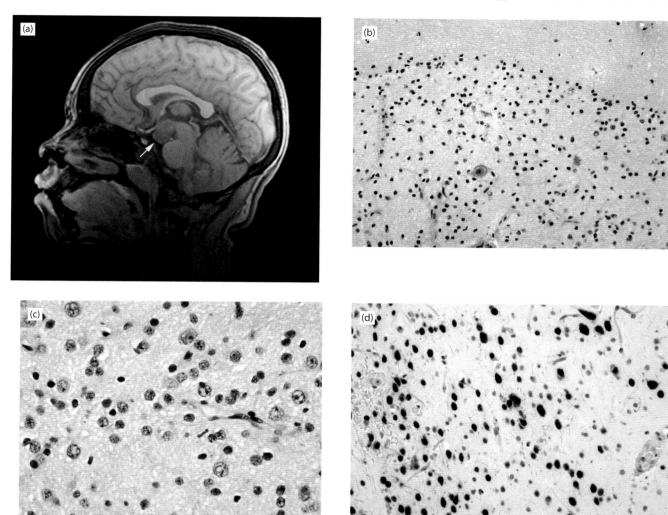

32.9 Hypothalamic hamartoma. (a) Sagittal T1-weighted magnetic resonance (MR) image showing a pedunculated hypothalamic mass (arrow), consistent with a hypothalamic hamartoma. **(b)** The lesion is peripherally well demarcated from adjacent normal myelinated fibres (top portion). **(c)** There is a predominance of cytologically normal small to medium sized neurons that differ from normal hypothalamus, the latter of which features dense collections of large ganglion cells. **(d)** Small neurocytic neurons are variably NeuN positive, with this example showing intense immunoreactivity.

Images provided by Dr Arie Perry, UCSF, San Francisco, CA, USA.

of well-differentiated neurons and a low grade glial component. However, HHs are composed of cytologically normal-appearing neurons, which are typically much smaller than the pyramidal-type cells of ganglioglioma. The glial population of HH also appears normal rather than neoplastic.

Perhaps of greater diagnostic concern, especially in the setting of a small biopsy, is the distinction from normal brain, which requires familiarity with the normal regional histology. The nuclei of the hypothalamus contain large pyramidal neurons with abundant cytoplasm, large nuclei with dispersed chromatin and prominent cellular processes. These types of neurons are not typical of HH. Between nuclei of the hypothalamus are regions of lower cellular density that contain bundles of myelinated fibres that are best recognized by Luxol fast blue (LFB) staining. These fibre tracts are not a component of HH and are only noted on the periphery (Figure 32.9b).

Biological Behaviour

The primary treatment for symptomatic HH is neurosurgery,[94] with the primary goal being to alleviate symptoms, including gelastic seizures, secondary seizures or precocious puberty. In many instances, these goals can be achieved by disconnective rather than resective surgical procedures. For example, it has been suggested that the improvement of seizure symptoms following surgery was independent from the extent of resection, indicating that the disconnective aspect of surgery may be most critical to its success. The majority of patients who undergo surgery for HH are seizure free or experience reduced symptoms following resection or disconnective surgery. The postoperative control of secondary generalized seizures in patients with HH remains a challenge in many instances.

REFERENCES

1. Abel TW, Baker SJ, Fraser MM, *et al.* Lhermitte–Duclos disease: a report of 31 cases with immunohistochemical analysis of the PTEN/AKT/mTOR pathway. *J Neuropathol Exp Neurol* 2005;64:341–9.

2. Aghakhani N, George B, Parker F. Paraganglioma of the cauda equina region – report of two cases and review of the literature. *Acta Neurochir* (Wien) 1999;141:81–7.

3. Alleyne CH Jr, Hunter S, Olson JJ, *et al.* Lipomatous glioneurocytoma of the posterior fossa with divergent differentiation: case report. *Neurosurgery* 1998;42:639–43.

4. Altman NR. MR and CT characteristics of gangliocytoma: a rare cause of epilepsy in children. *AJNR Am J Neuroradiol* 1988;9:917–21.

5. Ambler M, Pogacar S, Sidman R. Lhermitte–Duclos disease (granule cell hypertrophy of the cerebellum) pathological analysis of the first familial cases. *J Neuropathol Exp Neurol* 1969;28:622–47.

6. Amstutz DR, Coons SW, Kerrigan JF, Rekate HL, Heiserman JE. Hypothalamic hamartomas: Correlation of MR imaging and spectroscopic findings with tumor glial content. *AJNR Am J Neuroradiol* 2006;27(4):794–8.

7. Anan M, Inoue R, Ishii K, *et al.* A rosette-forming glioneuronal tumor of the spinal cord: the first case of a rosette-forming glioneuronal tumor originating from the spinal cord. *Hum Pathol* 2009;40(6):898–901.

8. Araki M, Fan J, Haraoka S, *et al.* Extracranial metastasis of anaplastic ganglioglioma through a ventriculoperitoneal shunt: a case report. *Pathol Int* 1999;49:258–63.

9. Araki Y, Ishida T, Ootani M, *et al.* MRI of paraganglioma of the cauda equina. *Neuroradiology* 1993;35:232–3.

10. Aydin F, Ghatak NR, Salvant J, Muizelaar P. Desmoplastic cerebral astrocytoma of infancy. A case report with immunohistochemical, ultrastructural and proliferation studies. Acta *Neuropathol* (Berl) 1993;86:666–70.

11. Backman SA, Stambolic V, Suzuki A, *et al.* Deletion of Pten in mouse brain causes seizures, ataxia and defects in soma size resembling Lhermitte–Duclos disease. *Nat Genet* 2001;29:396–403.

12. Baisden BL, Brat DJ, Melham ER, *et al.* Dysembryoplastic neuroepithelial tumour (DNT) – like neoplasm of the septum pellucidum: a lesion often misdiagnosed as glioma. Report of ten cases. *Am J Surg Pathol* 2001;25:494–9.

13. Barbosa MD, Balsitis M, Jaspan T, Lowe J. Intraventricular neurocytoma: a clinical and pathological study of three cases and review of the literature. *Neurosurgery* 1990;26:1045–54.

14. Bardella C, Pollard PJ, Tomlinson I. SDH mutations in cancer. *Biochim Biophys Acta* 2011;1807(11):1432–43.

15. Beal MF, Kleinman GM, Ojemann RG, Hochberg FH. Gangliocytoma of third ventricle: hyperphagia, somnolence and dementia. *Neurology* 1981;31:1224–8.

16. Bechtel JT, Patton JM, Takei Y. Mixed mesenchymal and neuroectodermal tumour of the cerebellum. *Acta Neuropathol* (Berl) 1978;41:261–3.

17. Becker AJ, Lobach M, Klein H, *et al.* Mutational analysis of TSC1 and TSC2 genes in gangliogliomas. *Neuropathol Appl Neurobiol* 2001;27:105–14.

18. Becker AJ, Klein H, Baden T, *et al.* Mutational and expression analysis of the reelin pathway components CDK5 and double cortin in gangliogliomas. *Acta Neuropathol* (Berl) 2002;104:403–8.

19. Bertalanffy A, Roessler K, Koperek O, *et al.* Recurrent central neurocytomas. *Cancer* 2005;104:135–42.

20. Binkley W, Vakili ST, Worth R. Paraganglioma of the cauda equina. Case report. *J Neurosurg* 1982;56:275–9.

21. Blümcke I, Giencke K, Wardelmann E, *et al.* The CD34 epitope is expressed in neoplastic and malformative lesions associated with chronic, focal epilepsies. *Acta Neuropathol* (Berl) 1999;97:481–90.

22. Blümcke I, Lobach M, Wolf HK, Wiestler OD. Evidence for developmental precursor lesions in epilepsy-associated glioneuronal tumors. *Microsc Res Tech* 1999;46:53–8.

23. Blümcke I, Wiestler OD. Gangliogliomas: an intriguing tumor entity associated with focal epilepsies. *J Neuropathol Exp Neurol* 2002;61:575–84.

24. Boedeker CC, Neumann HP, Ridder GJ, *et al.* Paragangliomas in patients with mutations of the SDHD gene. *Otolaryngol Head Neck Surg* 2005;132:467–70.

25. Boker DK, Wassmann H, Solymosi L. Paragangliomas of the spinal canal. *Surg Neurol* 1983;19:461–8.

26. Boukobza M, Foncin JF, Dowling–Carter D. Paraganglioma of the cauda equina: magnetic resonance imaging. *Neuroradiology* 1993;35:459–60.

27. Bouvier–Labit, C, Daniel L, Dufour H, Grisoli F, Figarella–Branger D. Papillary glioneuronal tumour: clinicopathological and biochemical study of one case with 7-year follow up. *Acta Neuropathol* (Berl), 2000;99:321–6.

28. Brat DJ, Scheithauer BW, Eberhart CG, Burger PC. Extraventricular neurocytomas: pathologic features and clinical outcome. *Am J Surg Pathol* 2001;25:1252–60.

29. Brat DJ, Gearing M, Goldthwaite PT, *et al.* Tau-associated neuropathology in ganglion cell tumours increases with patient age but appears unrelated to ApoE genotype. *Neuropathol Appl Neurobiol* 2001;27:197–205.

30. Broholm H, Madsen FF, Wagner AA, Laursen H. Papillary glioneuronal tumour – a new tumor entity. *Clin Neuropathol* 2002;21(1):1–4.

31. Capper D, Reuss D, Schittenhelm J, *et al.* Mutation-specific IDH1 antibody differentiates oligodendrogliomas and oligoastrocytomas from other brain tumors with oligodendroglioma-like morphology. *Acta Neuropathol* 2011;121(2):241–52.

32. Cerda–Nicolas M, Kepes JJ. Gliofibromas (including malignant forms), and gliosarcomas: a comparative study and review of the literature. *Acta Neuropathol* (Berl) 1993;85:349–61.

33. Cerda–Nicolas M, Lopez–Gines C, Peydro–Olaya A, *et al.* Central neurocytoma: a cytogenetic case study. *Cancer Genet Cytogenet* 1993;65:173–4.

34. Cerda–Nicolas M, Lopez–Gines C, Gil–Benso R, *et al.* Desmoplastic infantile ganglioglioma. Morphological,

35. Cervera–Pierot P, Varlet P, Chodkiewicz J, Daumas–Duport C. Dysembryoplastic neuroepithelial tumors located in the caudate nucleus area: report of four cases. *Neurosurgery* 1997;40:1065–9.

36. Chang EF, Christie C, Sullivan JE, *et al.*, Seizure control outcomes after resection of dysembryoplastic neuroepithelial tumor in 50 patients. *J Neurosurg Pediatr* 2010;5(1):123–30.

37. Chang KH, Han MH, Kim DG, *et al.* MR appearance of central neurocytoma. *Acta Radiol* 1993;34:520–26.

38. Chappe C, Padovani L, Scavarda D, *et al.* Dysembryoplastic Neuroepithelial tumors share with pleomorphic xanthoastrocytomas and gangliogliomas BRAF(V600E) mutation and expression. *Brain Pathol* 2013;23(5):574–83.

39. Chetty R, Pillay P, Jaichand V. Cytokeratin expression in adrenal phaeochromocytomas and extra-adrenal paragangliomas. *J Clin Pathol* 1998;51:477–8.

40. Chimelli L, Hahn MD, Budka H. Lipomatous differentiation in a medulloblastoma. *Acta Neuropathol* (Berl) 1991;81:471–3.

41. Choudhari KA, Kaliaperumal C, Jain A, *et al.* Central neurocytoma: a multi-disciplinary review. *Br J Neurosurg* 2009;23(6):585–95.

42. Chovanes GI, Truex RC Jr. Association of a ganglioneuroma with an arteriovenous malformation: case report. *Neurosurgery* 1987;21:241–3.

43. Chung SN, Rosemond RL, Graham D. Prenatal diagnosis of a foetal intracranial tumour. *J Ultrasound Med* 1998;17:521–3.

44. Constantini S, Soffer D, Siegel T, Shalit MN. Paraganglioma of the thoracic spinal cord with cerebrospinal fluid metastasis. *Spine* 1989;14:643–5.

45. Constantini S, Houten J, Miller DC, *et al.* Intramedullary spinal cord tumors in children under the age of 3 years. *J Neurosurg* 1996;85:1036–43.

46. Coons SW, Rekate HL, Prenger EC, *et al.* The histopathology of hypothalamic hamartomas: study of 57 cases. *J Neuropathol Exp Neurol* 2007;66(2):131–41.

47. Craig DW, Itty A, Panganiban C, *et al.*, Identification of somatic chromosomal abnormalities in hypothalamic hamartoma tissue at the GLI3 locus. *Am J Hum Genet* 2008;82(2):366–74.

48. Craver RD, Nadell J, Nelson JS. Desmoplastic infantile ganglioglioma. *Pediatr Dev Pathol* 1999;2:582–7.

49. Dahia PL. Evolving concepts in pheochromocytoma and paraganglioma. *Curr Opin Oncol* 2006;18:1–8.

50. Darwish B, Arbuckle S, Kellie S, Besser M, Chaseling R, Desmoplastic infantile ganglioglioma/astrocytoma with cerebrospinal metastasis. *J Clin Neurosci* 2007;14(5):498–501.

51. Dash RC, Provenzale JM, McComb RD, *et al.* Malignant supratentorial ganglioglioma (ganglion cell-giant cell glioblastoma): a case report and review of the literature. *Arch Pathol Lab Med* 1999;123:342–5.

52. Daumas–Duport C. Dysembryoplastic neuroepithelial tumors. *Brain Pathol* 1993;3:283–95.

53. Daumas–Duport C, Scheithauer BW, Chodkiewicz JP, et al. Dysembryoplastic neuroepithelial tumour: a surgically curable tumour of young patients with intractable partial seizures. Report of thirty-nine cases. *Neurosurgery* 1988;23:545–56.

54. Davis DG, Wilson D, Schmitz M, Markesbery WR. Lipidized medulloblastoma in adults. *Hum Pathol* 1993;24:990–95.

55. DeLellis RA. Pathology and genetics of tumours of endocrine organs. In: *World Health Organization classification of tumours.* Lyon: International Agency for Research on Cancer, 2004:320 .

56. De Munnynck K, Van Gool S, Van Calenbergh F, et al. Desmoplastic infantile ganglioglioma: a potentially malignant tumor? *Am J Surg Pathol* 2002;26: 1515–22.

57. Dougherty MJ, Santi M, Brose MS, et al. Activating mutations in BRAF characterize a spectrum of pediatric low-grade gliomas. *Neuro Oncol* 2010;12(7):621–30.

58. Duffner PK, Burger PC, Cohen ME, et al. Desmoplastic infantile gangliogliomas: an approach to therapy. *Neurosurgery* 1994;34:583–9.

59. Ebina K, Suzuki S, Takahashi T, et al. Gangliocytoma of the pineal body. A case report and review of the literature. *Acta Neurochir* (Wien) 1985;74:134–40.

60. Elek G, Slowik F, Eross L, et al. Central neurocytoma with malignant course. Neuronal and glial differentiation and craniospinal dissemination. *Pathol Oncol Res* 1999;5:155–9.

61. Elizabeth J, Bhaskara RM, Radhakrishnan VV, et al. Melanotic differentiation in dysembryoplastic neuroepithelial tumour. *Clin Neuropathol* 2000;19:38–40.

62. Ellison DW, Zygmunt SC, Weller RO. Neurocytoma/lipoma (neurolipocytoma) of the cerebellum. *Neuropathol Appl Neurobiol* 1993;19:95–8.

63. Eng C. PTEN: one gene, many syndromes. *Hum Mutat* 2003;22:183–98.

64. Englund C, Alvord EC Jr, Folkerth RD, et al. NeuN expression correlates with reduced mitotic index of neoplastic cells in central neurocytomas. *Neuropathol Appl Neurobiol* 2005;31:429–38.

65. Felix I, Bilbao JM, Asa SL, et al. Cerebral and cerebellar gangliocytomas: a morphological study of nine cases. *Acta Neuropathol* (Berl) 1994;88:246–51.

66. Fenoglio KA, Wu J, Kim do Y, et al. Hypothalamic hamartoma: basic mechanisms of intrinsic epileptogenesis. *Semin Pediatr Neurol* 2007;14(2):51–9.

67. Fernandez C, Girard N, Paz Paredes A, et al. The usefulness of MR imaging in the diagnosis of dysembryoplastic neuroepithelial tumor in children: a study of 14 cases. *AJNR Am J Neuroradiol* 2003;24:829–34.

68. Ferrer I, Isamat F, Acebes J. A Golgi and electron microscopic study of a dysplastic gangliocytoma of the cerebellum. *Acta Neuropathol* (Berl) 1979;47:163–5.

69. Ferrer I, Isamat F, López–Obarrio L, et al. Parvalbumin and calbindin D-28K immunoreactivity in central ganglioglioma and dysplastic gangliocytoma of the cerebellum. Report of two cases. *J Neurosurg* 1993;78:133–7.

70. Ferrer I, Marti E, Guionnet N, et al. Studies with the Golgi method in central gangliogliomas and dysplastic gangliocytoma of the cerebellum. *Histol Histopathol* 1990;5:329–36.

71. Figarella–Branger D, Pellissier JF, Daumas–Duport C, et al. Central neurocytomas. Critical evaluation of a small-cell neuronal tumour. *Am J Surg Pathol* 1992;16:97–109.

72. Firlik KS, Adelson PD, Hamilton RL. Coexistence of a ganglioglioma and Rasmussen's encephalitis. *Pediatr Neurosurg* 1999;30:278–82.

73. Fishbein L, Nathanson KL, Pheochromocytoma and paraganglioma: understanding the complexities of the genetic background. *Cancer Genet* 2012;205(1–2):1–11.

74. Fraga M, Garcia–Caballero T, Antúnez J, et al. Gastric paraganglioma: an immunohistological and ultrastructural case study. *J Submicroscop Cytol Pathol* 1990;22:401–8.

75. Frater JL, Prayson RA, Morris HH III, Bingaman WE. Surgical pathologic findings of extratemporal-based intractable epilepsy. A study of 133 consecutive resections. *Arch Pathol Lab Med* 2000;124:545–9.

76. Freeman JL, Coleman LT, Wellard RM, et al. MR imaging and spectroscopic study of epileptogenic hypothalamic hamartomas: analysis of 72 cases. *AJNR Am J Neuroradiol* 2004;25(3):450–62.

77. Fujimoto K, Ohnishi H, Tsujimoto M, et al. Dysembryoplastic neuroepithelial tumour of the cerebellum and brainstem. Case report. *J Neurosurg* 2000;93:487–9.

78. Fujisawa H, Marukawa K, Hasegawa M, et al. Genetic differences between neurocytoma and dysembryoplastic neuroepithelial tumor and oligodendroglial tumors. *J Neurosurg* 2002;97:1350–55.

79. Geddes JF, Jansen GH, Robinson SFD, et al. 'Gangliocytomas' of the pituitary. A heterogeneous group of lesions with differing histogenesis. *Am J Surg Pathol* 2000;24:607–13.

80. George DH, Scheithauer BW. Central liponeurocytoma. *Am J Surg Pathol* 2001;25:1551–5.

81. Gessi M, Giangaspero F, Pietsch T. Atypical teratoid/rhabdoid tumors and choroid plexus tumors: when genetics 'surprise' pathology. *Brain Pathol* 2003;13:409–14.

82. Gessi M, Marani C, Geddes J, et al. Ependymoma with neuropil-like islands: a case report with diagnostic and histogenetic implications. *Acta Neuropathol* (Berl) 2005;109(2): 231–4.

83. Giangaspero F, Cenacchi G, Losi L, et al. Extraventricular neoplasms with neurocytoma features. A clinicopathological study of 11 cases. *Am J Surg Pathol* 1997;21:206–12.

84. Giangaspero F, Cenacchi G, Roncaroli F, et al. Medullocytoma. A cerebellar neoplasm of adults with favorable prognosis. *Am J Surg Pathol* 1996;20:656–64.

85. Giroux M, Farmer JP, Meagher Villemure KM, et al. Intraventricular central neurocytoma. *Can J Neurol Sci* 1992;19:392–6..

86. Gleeson JG, Walsh CA. Neuronal migration disorders: from genetic diseases to developmental mechanisms. *Trends Neurosci* 2000;23:352–9.

87. Gonzalez–Campora R, Weller RO. Lipidized mature neuroectodermal tumour of the cerebellum with myoid differentiation. *Neuropathol Appl Neurobiol* 1998;24:397–402.

88. Goto S, Nagahiro S, Ushio Y, et al. Immunocytochemical detection of calcineurin and microtubule-associated protein 2 in central neurocytoma. *J Neurooncol* 1993;16:19–24.

89. Gultekin SH, Dalmau J, Graus Y, et al. Anti-Hu immuno labelling as an index of neuronal differentiation in human brain tumors: a study of 112 central neuroepithelial neoplasms. *Am J Surg Pathol* 1998;22:195–200.

90. Gupta K, Salunke P, Kalra I, Vasishta RK. Central liponeurocytoma: case report and review of literature. *Clin Neuropathol* 2011;30(2):80–5.

91. Hair LS, Symmans F, Powers JM, Carmel P. Immunohistochemistry and proliferative activity in Lhermitte–Duclos disease. *Acta Neuropathol* (Berl) 1992;84:570–73.

92. Hakim R, Loeffler JS, Anthony DC, Black PM. Gangliogliomas in adults. *Cancer* 1997;79:127–31.

93. Harris BT, Horoupian DS. Spinal cord glioneuronal tumor with 'rosetted' neuropil islands and meningeal dissemination: a case report. *Acta Neuropathol* (Berl) 2000;100:575–9.

94. Harvey AS, Freeman JL, Berkovic SF, Rosenfeld JV. Transcallosal resection of hypothalamic hamartomas in patients with intractable epilepsy. *Epileptic Disord* 2003;5(4):257–65.

95. Hassoun J, Gambarelli D, Grisoli F, et al. Central neurocytoma. An electron-microscopic study of two cases. *Acta Neuropathol* (Berl) 1982;56:151–6.

96. Hassoun J, Soylemezoglu F, Gambarelli D, et al. Central neurocytoma: a synopsis of clinical and histological features. *Brain Pathol* 1993;3:297–306.

97. Hawkins C, Walker E, Mohamed N, et al., BRAF–KIAA1549 fusion predicts better clinical outcome in pediatric low-grade astrocytoma. *Clin Cancer Res* 2011;17(14):4790–8.

98. Hayashi S, Kameyama S, Fukuda M, Takahashi H. Ganglioglioma with a tanycytic ependymoma as the glial component. *Acta Neuropathol* (Berl) 2000;99:310–16.

99. Hessler RB, Lopes MB, Frankfurter A, et al. Cytoskeletal immunohistochemistry of central neurocytomas. *Am J Surg Pathol* 1992;16:1031–8.

100. Hirose T, Scheithauer BW. Mixed dysembryoplastic neuroepithelial tumour and ganglioglioma. *Acta Neuropathol* (Berl) 1998;95:649–54.

101. Hirose T, Scheithauer BW, Lopes MBS, VandenBerg S. Dysembryoplastic neuroepithelial tumour (DNT): an immunohistochemical and ultrastructural study. *J Neuropathol Exp Neurol* 1994;53:184–95.

102. Hirose T, Scheithauer BW, Lopes MB, et al. Ganglioglioma: an ultrastructural and immunohistochemical study. *Cancer* 1997;79:989–1003.

103. Hoischen A, Ehrler M, Fassunke J, et al. Comprehensive characterization of genomic aberrations in gangliogliomas by CGH, array-based CGH and interphase FISH. *Brain Pathol* 2008;18(3): 326–37.

104. Honavar M, Janota I, Polkey CE. Histological heterogeneity of dysembryoplastic neuroepithelial tumour: identification and differential diagnosis in a series of 74 cases. *Histopathology* 1999;34:342–56.

105. Horbinski C, Kofler J, Yeaney G, et al., Isocitrate dehydrogenase 1 analysis differentiates gangliogliomas from infiltrative gliomas. *Brain Pathol* 2011;21(5):564–74.

106. Horstmann S, Perry A, Reifenberger G, et al. Genetic and expression profiles of cerebellar liponeurocytomas. *Brain Pathol* 2004;**14**:281–9.

107. Hunt SJ, Johnson PC. Melanotic ganglioglioma of the pineal region. *Acta Neuropathol* (Berl) 1989;*79*:222–5.

108. Ishiuchi S, Nakazato Y, Iino M, et al. *In vitro* neuronal and glial production and differentiation of human central neurocytoma cells. *J Neurosci Res* 1998;51:526–35.

109. Itoh Y, Yagishita S, Chiba Y. Cerebral gangliocytoma. An ultrastructural study. *Acta Neuropathol* (Berl) 1987;74:169–78.

110. Jacob JT, Cohen–Gadol AA, Scheithauer BW, Krauss WE. Intramedullary spinal cord gangliocytoma: case report and a review of the literature. *Neurosurg Rev* 2005;28:326–9.

111. Jallo GI, Freed D, Epstein FJ. Spinal cord gangliogliomas: a review of 56 patients. *J Neurooncol* 2004;68:71–7.

112. Jay V, Edwards V, Hoving E, et al. Central neurocytoma: morphological, flow cytometric, polymerase chain reaction, fluorescence in situ hybridization, and karyotypic analyses. Case report. *J Neurosurg* 1999;90:348–54.

113. Jenkinson MD, Bosma JJ, Du Plessis D, et al. Cerebellar liponeurocytoma with an unusually aggressive clinical course: case report. *Neurosurgery* 2003;53(6):1425–7;discussion 1428.

114. Johannsson JH, Rekate HL, Roessmann U. Gangliogliomas: pathological and clinical correlation. *J Neurosurg* 1981;54: 58–63.

115. Johnson JH Jr, Hariharan S, Berman J, et al. Clinical outcome of pediatric gangliogliomas: ninety-nine cases over 20 years. *Pediatr Neurosurg* 1997;27: 203–7.

116. Johnson MD, Vnencak–Jones CL, Toms SA, Moots PM, Weil R. Allelic losses in oligodendroglial and oligodendroglioma-like neoplasms: analysis using microsatellite repeats and polymerase chain reaction. *Arch Pathol Lab Med* 2003;127(12): 1573–9.

117. Jouvet A, Lellouch–Tubiana A, Boddaert N, et al. Fourth ventricle neurocytoma with lipomatous and ependymal differentiation. *Acta Neuropathol* (Berl) 2005;109:346–51.

118. Kamalian N, Abbassioun K, Amirjamshidi A, Shams–Shahrabadi M. Paraganglioma of the filum terminale. Report of a case and review of the literature. *J Neurol* 1987;235:56–9.

119. Karafin M, Jallo GI, Ayars M, Eberhart CG, Rodriguez FJ. Rosette forming glioneuronal tumor in association with Noonan syndrome: pathobiological implications. *Clin Neuropathol* 2011;30(6):297–300.

120. Kawamoto K, Yamanouchi Y, Suwa J, et al. Ultrastructural study of a cerebral gangliocytoma. *Surg Neurol* 1985;24:541–9.

121. Kemp S, Achan A, Ng T, Dexter MA. Rosette-forming glioneuronal tumour of the lateral ventricle in a patient with neurofibromatosis 1. J Clin Neurosci 2012;19(8):1180–1.

122. Keyvani K, Rickert C, von Wild K, et al. Rosetted glioneuronal tumour: a case with proliferating neuronal nodules. *Acta Neuropathol* 2001;101:525–8.

123. Kiehl TR, Kalkanis SN, Louis DN. Pigmented central neurocytoma. *Acta Neuropathol* (Berl) 2004;1076:571–4.

124. Kim DG, Chi JG, Park SH, et al. Intraventricular neurocytoma: clinicopathological analysis of seven cases. *J Neurosurg* 1992;76:759–65.

125. Kim DG, Choe WJ, Chang KH, et al. *In vivo* proton magnetic resonance spectroscopy of central neurocytomas. *Neurosurgery* 2000;46:329–33.

126. Kim DG, Kim JS, Chi JG, et al. Central neurocytoma:proliferative potential and biological behavior. *J Neurosurg* 1996;84:742–7.

127. Kliewer KE, Cochran AJ. A review of the histology, ultrastructure, immunohistology, and molecular biology of extra-adrenal paragangliomas. *Arch Pathol Lab Med* 1989;113:1209–18.

128. Klisch J, Juengling F, Spreer J, et al. Lhermitte–Duclos disease: assessment with MR imaging, positron emission tomography, single-photon emission CT and MR spectroscopy. *AJNR Am J Neuroradiol* 2001;22:824–30.

129. Koeller KK, Dillon WP. Dysembryoplastic neuroepithelial tumors: MR appearance. *AJNR Am J Neuroradiol* 1992;13: 1319–25.

130. Komori T, Scheithauer BW, Hirose T. A rosette-forming glioneuronal tumor of the fourth ventricle: infratentorial form of dysembryoplastic neuroepithelial tumor? *Am J Surg Pathol* 2002;26(5):582–91.

131. Komori T, Scheithauer BW, Anthony DC, et al., Papillary glioneuronal tumour: a new variant of mixed neuronal–glial neoplasm. *Am J Surg Pathol* 1998;22:1171–83.

132. Komori T, Scheithauer BW, Parisi JE, et al. Mixed conventional and desmoplastic infantile ganglioglioma: an autopsied case with 6-year follow-up. *Mod Pathol* 2001;14:720–26.

133. Kordek R, Biernat W, Zakrzewski K, et al. Dysembryoplastic neuroepithelial tumour (DNT): an ultrastructural study of six cases. *Folia Neuropathol* 1999;37:167–70.

134. Kros JM, Delwel EJ, de Jong TH, et al. Desmoplastic infantile astrocytoma and ganglioglioma: a search for genomic characteristics. *Acta Neuropathol* 2002;104(2):144–8.

135. Kuchelmeister, K., Nestler U, Siekmann R, Schachenmayr W. Liponeurocytoma of the left lateral ventricle – case report and review of the literature. *Clin Neuropathol* 2006;25(2): 86–94.

136. Kuchelmeister K, Schonmeyr R, Albani M, Schachenmayr W. Anaplastic desmoplastic infantile ganglioglioma. *Clin Neuropathol* 1998;17:269.

137. Kuchelmeister K, Demirel T, Schlorer E, et al. Dysembryoplastic neuroepithelial tumour of the cerebellum. *Acta Neuropathol* (Berl) 1995;89:385–90.

138. Kudo M. Hypothalamic gangliocytoma. Selective appearance of neurofibrillary changes, granulovacuolar degeneration, and argentophilic bodies. *Acta Pathol Jpn* 1986;36:1225–9.

139. Kwon CH, Zhu X, Zhang J, et al. Pten regulates neuronal soma size: a mouse model of Lhermitte–Duclos disease. *Nat Genet* 2001;29:404–11.

140. Lack EE, Cubilla AL, Woodruff JM. Paragangliomas of the head and neck region. A pathologic study of tumors from 71 patients. *Hum Pathol* 1979;10:191–218.

141. Lang FF, Epstein FJ, Ransohoff J, et al. Central nervous system gangliogliomas. Part 2: Clinical outcome. *J Neurosurg* 1993;79:867–73.

142. Leenstra JL, Rodriguez FJ, Frechette CM, et al. Central neurocytoma: management recommendations based on a 35-year experience. *Int J Radiat Oncol Biol Phys* 2007;67(4):1145–54.

143. Lellouch–Tubiana A, Bourgeois M, Vekemans M, Robain O. Dysembryoplastic neuroepithelial tumors in two children with neurofibromatosis type 1. *Acta Neuropathol* (Berl) 1995;90:319–22.

144. Leung SY, Gwi E, Ng HK, et al. Dysembryoplastic neuroepithelial tumour. A tumour with small neuronal cells resembling oligodendroglioma. *Am J Surg Pathol* 1994;18:604–14.

145. Levy RA. Paraganglioma of the filum terminale: MR findings. *Am J Roentgenol* 1993;160:851–2.

146. Ligon KL, Alberta JA, Kho AT, et al. The oligodendroglial lineage marker OLIG2 is universally expressed in diffuse gliomas. *J Neuropathol Exp Neurol* 2004;63: 499–509.

147. Linnoila RI, Lack EE, Steinberg SM, Keiser HR. Decreased expression of neuropeptides in malignant paragangliomas: an immunohistochemical study. *Hum Pathol* 1988;19:41–50.

148. Lipper S, Decker RE. Paraganglioma of the cauda equina. A histologic, immunohistochemical, and ultrastructural study and review of the literature. *Surg Neurol* 1984;22:415–20.

149. Loh JK, Lieu AS, Chai CY, Howng SL. Malignant transformation of a desmoplastic infantile ganglioglioma. *Pediatr Neurol* 2011;45(2):135–7.

150. Louis DN, Ohgaki H, Wiestler OD, Cavenee WK. *WHO Classification of Tumours of the Central Nervous System.* 4th edn. Lyon: International Agency for Research on Cancer, 2007:309.

151. Louis DN, von Deimling A, Dickersin GR, et al. Desmoplastic cerebral astrocytomas of infancy: a histopathologic, immunohistochemical, ultrastructural, and molecular genetic study. *Hum Pathol* 1992;23:1402–9.

152. Mackenzie IR. Central neurocytoma: histologic atypia, proliferation potential and clinical outcome. *Cancer* 1999;85:1606–10.

153. Maguire JA, Bilbao JM, Kovacs K, Resch L. Hypothalamic neurocytoma with vasopressin immunoreactivity: immunohistochemical and ultrastructural observations. *Endocr Pathol* 1992;3:99–104.

154. Masuoka J, Brandner S, Paulus W, et al. Germline SDHD mutation in paraganglioma of the spinal cord. *Oncogene* 2001;20:5084–6.

155. Mena H, Morrison AL, Jones RV, Gyure KA. Central neurocytomas express photoreceptor differentiation. *Cancer* 2001;91:136–43.

156. Miliaras GC, Kyritsis AP, Polyzoidis KS. Cauda equina paraganglioma: a review. *J Neurooncol* 2003;65:177–90.

157. Miller DC, Lang FF, Epstein FJ. Central nervous system gangliogliomas: part 1: pathology. *J Neurosurg* 1993;79: 859–66.

158. Mittler M, Walters B, Fried A, *et al.* Malignant glial tumour arising from the site of a previous hamartoma/ganglioglioma: coincidence or malignant transformation? *Pediatr Neurosurg* 1999;30:132–4.

159. Moran CA, Rush W, Mena H. Primary spinal paragangliomas: a clinicopathological and immunohistochemical study of 30 cases. *Histopathology* 1997;31:167–73.

160. Mrak RE. Malignant neurocytic tumour. *Hum Pathol* 1994;25:747–52.

161. Mrak RE, Yasargil MG, Mohapatra G, *et al.* Atypical extraventricular neurocytoma with oligodendroglioma-like spread and an unusual pattern of chromosome 1p and 19q loss. *Hum Pathol* 2004;35:1156–9.

162. Myung JK, Byeon SJ, Kim B, *et al.* Papillary glioneuronal tumors: a review of clinicopathologic and molecular genetic studies. *Am J Surg Pathol* 2011;35(12):1794–805.

163. Nakajima M, Kidooka M, Nakasu S. Anaplastic ganglioglioma with dissemination to the spinal cord: a case report. *Surg Neurol* 1998;49:445–8.

164. Neumann HP, Bausch B, McWhinney SR, *et al.* Germ-line mutations in nonsyndromic pheochromocytoma. *N Engl J Med* 2002;346:1459–66.

165. Neumann HP, Pawlu C, Peczkowska M, *et al.* Distinct clinical features of paraganglioma syndromes associated with SDHB and SDHD gene mutations. *JAMA* 2004;292:943–51.

166. Ng TH, Fung CF, Ma LT. The pathological spectrum of desmoplastic infantile gangliogliomas. *Histopathology* 1990;16:235–41.

167. Ng TH, Wong AY, Boadle R, *et al.* Pigmented central neurocytoma: case report and literature review. *Am J Surg Pathol* 1999;23:1136–40.

168. Nishio S, Fujiwara S, Tashima T. Tumours of the lateral ventricular wall, especially the septum pellucidum: clinical presentation and variations in pathological features. *Neurosurgery* 1990;27:224–30.

169. Nishio S, Takeshita I, Fukui M. Primary cerebral ganglioneurocytoma in an adult. *Cancer* 1990;66:358–62.

170. Nishio S, Takeshita I, Kaneko Y, Fukui M. Cerebral neurocytoma: a new subset of benign neuronal tumors of the cerebrum. *Cancer* 1992;70:529–37.

171. Nishio S, Morioka T, Hamada Y, *et al.* Immunohistochemical expression of tyrosine kinase (Trk) receptor proteins in mature neuronal cell tumors of the central nervous system. *Clin Neuropathol* 1998;17:123–30.

172. Nolan MA, Sakuta R, Chuang N, *et al.* Dysembryoplastic neuroepithelial tumors in childhood: long-term outcome and prognostic features. *Neurology* 2004;62:2270–76.

173. Ohgaki H, Eibl RH, Schwab M, *et al.* Mutations of the p53 tumour suppressor gene in neoplasms of the human nervous system. *Mol Carcinog* 1993;8:74–80.

174. Okamura A, Goto S, Sato K, Ushio Y. Central neurocytoma with hemorrhagic onset. *Surg Neurol* 1995;43:252–5.

175. Pal L, Santosh V, Gayathri N, *et al.* Neurocytoma/rhabdomyoma (myoneurocytoma) of the cerebellum. *Acta Neuropathol* (Berl) 1998;95:318–23.

176. Pandita A, Balasubramaniam A, Perrin R, Shannon P, Guha A. Malignant and benign gangliogliomas: a pathological and molecular study. *Neuro Oncol* 2007;9(2):124–34.

177. Parisi J, Scheithauer B, Priest J, *et al.* Desmoplastic infantile ganglioglioma (DIG): a form of ganglioglio\matosis? *J Neuropathol Exp Neurol* 1992;51:365.

178. Parizel PM, Martin JJ, van Vyve M, *et al.* Cerebral ganglioglioma and neurofibromatosis type I: case report and review of the literature. *Neuroradiology* 1991;33:357–9.

179. Park JP, Dossu JR, Rhodes CH. Telomere associations in desmoplastic infantile ganglioglioma. *Cancer Genet Cytogenet* 1996;92:4–7.

180. Park SH, Ostrzega N, Akers MA, *et al.* Intraventricular neurocytoma with prominent myelin figures. *Ultrastruct Pathol* 1999;23:311–17.

181. Park YS, Kim DS, Shim KW, Kim JH, Choi JU. Factors contributing to resectability and seizure outcomes in 44 patients with ganglioglioma. *Clin Neurol Neurosurg* 2008;110(7):667–73.

182. Patel U, Pinto RS, Miller DC, *et al.* MR of spinal cord ganglioglioma. *AJNR Am J Neuroradiol* 1998;19:879–87.

183. Paulus W, Schlote W, Perentes E, *et al.* Desmoplastic supratentorial neuroepithelial tumours of infancy. *Histopathology* 1992;21:43–9.

184. Pearse AGE. The cytochemistry and ultrastructure of polypeptide hormone-producing cells of the APUD series and the embryologic, physiological and pathologic implications of the concept. *J Histochem Cytochem* 1969;17:303–13.

185. Perry A, Brat DJ. *Practical Surgical Pathology: A Diagnostic Approach.* Philadelphia: Elsevier, 2010.

186. Perry A, Fuller CE, Banerjee R, *et al.* Ancillary FISH analysis for 1p and 19q status: preliminary observations in 287 gliomas and oligodendroglioma mimics. *Front Biosci* 2003;8:1–9.

187. Perry A, Giannini C, Scheithauer BW, *et al.* Composite pleomorphic xanthoastrocytoma and ganglioglioma: report of four cases and review of the literature. *Am J Surg Pathol* 1997;21:763–71.

188. Perry A, Scheithauer BW, Macaulay RJ, *et al.* Oligodendrogliomas with neurocytic differentiation: a report of 4 cases with diagnostic and histogenetic implications. *J Neuropathol Exp Neurol* 2002;61:947–55.

189. Phi JH, Koh EJ, Kim SK, *et al.* Desmoplastic infantile astrocytoma: recurrence with malignant transformation into glioblastoma: a case report. *Childs Nerv Syst* 2011;27(12):2177–81.

190. Platten M, Meyer–Puttlitz B, Blumcke I, *et al.* A novel splice site-associated polymorphism in the *tuberous sclerosis 2 (TSC2)* gene may predispose to the development of sporadic gangliogliomas. *J Neuropathol Exp Neurol* 1997;56:806–10.

191. Pommepuy I, Delage–Corre M, Moreau JJ, Labrousse F. A report of a desmoplastic ganglioglioma in a 12-year-old girl with review of the literature. *J Neurooncol* 2006;76:271–5.

192. Prabowo AS, Iyer AM, Veersema TJ, *et al.* BRAF V600E mutation is associated with mTOR signalling activation in glioneuronal tumours. *Brain Pathol* 2013;24(1):52–66.

193. Prayson RA. Gliofibroma: a distinct entity or a subtype of desmoplastic astrocytoma? *Hum Pathol* 1996;27:610–13.

194. Prayson RA. Composite ganglioglioma and dysembryoplastic neuroepithelial tumour. *Arch Pathol Lab Med* 1999;123:247–50.

195. Prayson RA. Papillary glioneuronal tumor. *Arch Pathol Lab Med* 2000;124:1820–23.

196. Prayson RA, Napekoski KM. Composite ganglioglioma/dysembryoplastic neuroepithelial tumor: a clinicopathologic study of 8 cases. *Hum Pathol* 2012;43(7):1113–8.

197. Prayson RA, Khajavi K, Comair YG. Cortical architectural abnormalities and MIB1 immunoreactivity in gangliogliomas: a study of 60 patients with intracranial tumors. *J Neuropathol Exp Neurol* 1995;54:513–20.

198. Preusser M, Budka H, Rössler K, Hainfellner JA. OLIG2 is a useful immunohistochemical marker in differential diagnosis of clear cell primary CNS neoplasms. *Histopathology* 2007;50(3):365–70.

199. Preusser M, Dietrich W, Czech T, *et al.* Rosette-forming glioneuronal tumor of the fourth ventricle. *Acta Neuropathol* (Berl), 2003;106(5):506–8.

200. Pritchett PS, King TI. Dysplastic gangliocytoma of the cerebellum: an ultrastructural study. *Acta Neuropathol* (Berl) 1978;42:1–5.

201. Qaddoumi I, Ellison DW, Morris EB, *et al.*, Dysembryoplastic neuroepithelial tumours and cognitive outcome: cure at a price? *Cancer* 2010;116(23): 5461–9.

202. Quinn B. Synaptophysin staining in normal brain: importance for diagnosis of ganglioglioma. *Am J Surg Pathol* 1998;22:550–56.

203. Rades D, Fehlauer F. Treatment options for central neurocytoma. *Neurology* 2002;59:1268–70.

204. Rades D, Fehlauer F, Schild SE. Treatment of atypical neurocytomas. *Cancer* 2004;100:814–17.

205. Rades D, Schild SE, Fehlauer F. Prognostic value of the MIB–1 labelling index for central neurocytomas. *Neurology* 2004;62:987–9.

206. Raftopoulos C, Flament–Durand J, Brucher JM, *et al.* Paraganglioma of the cauda equina: report of 2 cases and review of 59 cases from the literature. *Clin Neurol Neurosurg* 1990;92:263–70.

207. Raghavan R, White CL III, Rogers B, *et al.* Alpha–synuclein expression in central nervous system tumors showing neuronal or mixed neuronal/glial differentiation. *J Neuropathol Exp Neurol* 2000;59:490–94.

208. Ray WZ, Blackburn SL, Casavilca–Zambrano S, *et al.*, Clinicopathologic features of recurrent dysembryoplastic neuroepithelial tumor and rare malignant transformation: a report of 5 cases and review of the literature. *J Neurooncol* 2009;94(2):283–92.

209. Reithmeier T, Gumprecht H, Stolzle A, Lumenta CB. Intracerebral paraganglioma. *Acta Neurochir* (Wien) 2000;142:1063–6.

210. Reznik M, Schoenen J. Lhermitte–Duclos disease. *Acta Neuropathol* (Berl) 1983;59:88–94.

211. Riegert–Johnson DL, Gleeson FC, Roberts M, *et al.* Cancer and Lhermitte–Duclos disease are common in Cowden syndrome

patients. *Hered Cancer Clin Pract* 2010;**8**(1):6.

212. Rodewald L, Miller DC, Sciorra L, *et al.* Central nervous system neoplasm in a young man with Martin–Bell syndrome–fra(X)–XLMR. *Am J Med Genet* 1987;**26**:7–12.

213. Rodriguez FJ, Mota RA, Scheithauer BW, *et al.* Interphase cytogenetics for 1p19q and t(1;19)(q10;p10) may distinguish prognostically relevant subgroups in extraventricular neurocytoma. *Brain Pathol* 2009;**19**(4):623–9.

214. Ruchoux MM, Gray F, Gherardi R, *et al.* Orthostatic hypotension from a cerebellar gangliocytoma: case report. *J Neurosurg* 1986;**65**:245–8.

215. Rushing EJ, Rorke LB, Sutton L. Problems in the nosology of desmoplastic tumors of childhood. *Pediatr Neurosurg* 1993;**19**: 57–62.

216. Russell D, Rubinstein L. *Pathology of Tumours of the Nervous System*. 5th edn. London: Edward Arnold, 1989.

217. Russo CP, Katz DS, Corona RJ Jr, Winfield JA. Gangliocytoma of the cervicothoracic spinal cord. *AJNR Am J Neuroradiol* 1995;**16**:889–91.

218. Rutka JT, Giblin JR, Apodaca G, *et al.* Inhibition of growth and induction of differentiation in a malignant human glioma cell line by normal leptomeningeal extracellular matrix proteins. *Cancer Res* 1987;**47**:3515–22.

219. Sawin PD, Theodore N, Rekate HL. Spinal cord ganglioglioma in a child with neurofibromatosis type 2: case report and literature review. *J Neurosurg* 1999;**90**:231–3.

220. Schiavi F, Boedeker CC, Bausch B, *et al.* Predictors and prevalence of paraganglioma syndrome associated with mutations of the SDHC gene. *JAMA* 2005;**294**:2057–63.

221. Schild SE, Scheithauer BW, Haddock MG, *et al.* Central neurocytomas. Cancer 1997;**79**:790–95.

222. Schindler G, Capper D, Meyer J, *et al.*, Analysis of *BRAF* V600E mutation in 1320 nervous system tumors reveals high mutation frequencies in pleomorphic xanthoastrocytoma, ganglioglioma and extra-cerebellar pilocytic astrocytoma. *Acta Neuropathol* 2011;**121**(3):397–405.

223. Schmidt MH, Gottfried ON, von Koch CS, *et al.* Central neurocytoma: a review. *J Neurooncol* 2004;**66**:377–84.

224. Selch MT, Goy BW, Lee SP, *et al.* Gangliogliomas: experience with 34 patients and review of the literature. *Am J Clin Oncol* 1998;**21**:557–64.

225. Selvanathan SK, Hammouche S, Salminen HJ, Jenkinson MD. Outcome and prognostic features in anaplastic ganglioglioma: analysis of cases from the SEER database. *J Neurooncol* 2011;**105**(3):539–45.

226. Shah MN, Leonard JR, Perry A. Rosette-forming glioneuronal tumors of the posterior fossa. *J Neurosurg Pediatr* 2010;**5**(1):98–103.

227. Shanley DJ, Vassallo CJ. Atypical presentation of Lhermitte–Duclos disease: preoperative diagnosis with MRI. *Neuroradiology* 1992;**34**:103–4.

228. Sharma S, Sarkar C, Gaikwad S, *et al.* Primary neurocytoma of the spinal cord: a case report and review of literature. *J Neurooncol* 2005;**74**:47–52.

229. Shimbo Y, Takahashi H, Hayano M, *et al.* Temporal lobe lesion demonstrating features of dysembryoplastic neuroepithelial tumour and ganglioglioma: a transitional form? *Clin Neuropathol* 1997;**16**:65–8.

230. Shin JH, Lee HK, Khang SK, *et al.* Neuronal tumors of the central nervous system: radiologic findings and pathologic correlation. *Radiographics* 2002;**22**:1177–89.

231. Shiurba RA, Gessaga EC, Eng LF, *et al.* Lhermitte–Duclos disease: an immunohistochemical study of the cerebellar cortex. *Acta Neuropathol* (Berl) 1988;**75**:474–80.

232. Silverstein AM, Quint DJ, McKeever PE. Intradural paraganglioma of the thoracic spine. *AJNR Am J Neuroradiol* 1990;**11**:614–16.

233. Smith TW, Nikulasson S, de Girolami U, de Gennaro LJ. Immunohistochemistry of synapsin I and synaptophysin in human nervous system and neuroendocrine tumors: applications in diagnostic neuro-oncology. *Clin Neuropathol* 1993;**12**:335–42.

234. Soffer D, Lach B, Constantini S. Melanotic cerebral ganglioglioma: evidence for melanogenesis in neoplastic astrocytes. *Acta Neuropathol* (Berl) 1992;**83**:315–23.

235. Soffer D, Umansky F, Goldman JE. Ganglioglioma with neurofibrillary tangles (NFTs): neoplastic NFTs share antigenic determinants with NFTs of Alzheimer's disease. *Acta Neuropathol (Berl)* 1995;**89**:451–3.

236. Solis OE, Mehta RI, Lai A, *et al.* Rosette-forming glioneuronal tumor: a pineal region case with IDH1 and IDH2 mutation analyses and literature review of 43 cases. *J Neurooncol* 2011;**102**(3):477–84.

237. Sonier CB, Feve JR, de Kersaint–Gilly A, *et al.* Lhermitte–Duclos disease: a rare cause of intracranial hypertension in adults. *J Neuroradiol* 1992;**19**:133–8.

238. Sonneland PRL, Scheithauer BW, LeChago J, *et al.* Paraganglioma of the cauda equina region: clinicopathologic study of 31 cases with special reference to immunocytology and ultrastructure. *Cancer* 1986;**58**:1720–35.

239. Soylemezoglu F, Scheithauer BW, Esteve J, Kleihues P. Atypical central neurocytoma. *J Neuropathol Exp Neurol* 1997;**56**:551–6.

240. Soylemezoglu F, Soffer D, Onol B, *et al.* Lipomatous medulloblastoma in adults: a distinct clinicopathological entity. *Am J Surg Pathol* 1996;**20**:413–18.

241. Sperner J, Gottschalk J, Neumann K, *et al.* Clinical, radiological and histological findings in desmoplastic infantile ganglioglioma. *Childs Nerv Syst* 1994;**10**:458–63.

242. Stapleton SR, Wilkins PR, Bell BA. Recurrent dysplastic cerebellar gangliocytoma (Lhermitte–Duclos disease) presenting with subarachnoid haemorrhage. *Br J Neurosurg* 1992;**6**:153–6.

243. Steel TR, Dailey AT, Born D, *et al.* Paragangliomas of the sellar region: report of two cases. *Neurosurgery* 1993;**32**:844–7.

244. Stephan CL, Kepes JJ, Arnold P, *et al.* Neurocytoma of the cauda equina: case report. *J Neurosurg* 1999;**90**:247–51.

245. Takahashi H, Nakashima S, Kumanishi T, Ikuta F. Paragangliomas of the craniocervical region; an immunohistochemical study on tyrosine hydroxylase. *Acta Neuropathol* (Berl) 1987;**73**:227–32.

246. Takao H, Nakagawa K, Ohtomo K. Central neurocytoma with craniospinal dissemination. *J Neurooncol* 2003;**61**: 255–9.

247. Takeshima H, Kawahara Y, Hirano H, *et al.* Postoperative regression of desmoplastic infantile gangliogliomas: report of two cases. *Neurosurgery* 2003;**53**:979–83;discussion 983–4.

248. Tamiya T, Hamazaki S, Ono Y, *et al.* Ganglioglioma in a patient with Turcot syndrome: case report. *J Neurosurg* 2000;**92**:170–75.

249. Taratuto AL, Monges J, Lylyk P, Leiguarda R. Superficial cerebral astrocytoma attached to dura. Report of six cases in infants. *Cancer* 1984;**54**:2505–12.

250. Taratuto AL, Pomata H, Sevlever G, *et al.* Dysembryoplastic neuroepithelial tumour: morphological, immunocytochemical, and deoxyribonucleic acid analyses in a pediatric series. *Neurosurgery* 1995;**36**:474–81.

251. Taruscio D, Danesi R, Montaldi A, *et al.* Nonrandom gain of chromosome 7 in central neurocytoma: a chromosomal analysis and fluorescence in situ hybridization study. *Virchows Arch* 1997;**430**:47–51.

252. Taylor CL, Cohen ML, Cohen AR. Neurocytoma presenting with intraparenchymal cerebral hemorrhage. *Pediatr Neurosurg* 1998;**29**:92–5.

253. Tenreiro–Picon OR, Kamath SV, Knorr JR, *et al.* Desmoplastic infantile ganglioglioma: CT and MRI features. *Pediatr Radiol* 1995;**25**:540–43.

254. Thom M, Gomez–Anson B, Revesz T, *et al.* Spontaneous intralesional haemorrhage in dysembryoplastic neuroepithelial tumours: a series of five cases. *J Neurol Neurosurg Psychiatry* 1999;**67**:97–101.

255. Thom M, Toma A, An S, *et al.* One hundred and one dysembryoplastic neuroepithelial tumors: an adult epilepsy series with immunohistochemical, molecular genetic, and clinical correlations and a review of the literature. *J Neuropathol Exp Neurol* 2011;**70**(10):859–78.

256. Thomas B, Krishnamoorthy T, Radhakrishnan VV, Kesavadas C. Advanced MR imaging in Lhermitte–Duclos disease: moving closer to pathology and pathophysiology. *Neuroradiology* 2007; 49(9):733–8.

257. Tong CY, Ng HK, Pang JC, *et al.* Central neurocytomas are genetically distinct from oligodendrogliomas and neuroblastomas. *Histopathology* 2000;**37**:160–65.

258. Trehan G, Bruge H, Vinchon M, *et al.* MR imaging in the diagnosis of desmoplastic infantile tumor: retrospective study of six cases. *AJNR Am J Neuroradiol* 2004;**25**:1028–33.

259. Deleted in proof.

260. VandenBerg SR, May EE, Rubinstein LJ, *et al.* Desmoplastic supratentorial neuroepithelial tumors of infancy with divergent differentiation potential: report on 11 cases of a distinctive embryonal tumour with favorable prognosis. *J Neurosurg* 1987;**66**:58–71.

261. van Nederveen FH, Gaal J, Favier J, *et al.* An immunohistochemical procedure to detect patients with paraganglioma and phaeochromocytoma with germline *SDHB*, *SDHC*, or *SDHD* gene mutations: a retrospective and prospective analysis. *Lancet Oncol* 2009;**10**(8): 764–71.

262. Von Deimling A, Janzer R, Kleihues P, Wiestler OD. Patterns of differentiation

in central neurocytoma: an immunohistochemical study of eleven biopsies. *Acta Neuropathol* (Berl) 1990;**79**:473–9.

263. Von Deimling A, Kleihues P, Saremaslani P, *et al.* Histogenesis and differentiation potential of central neurocytomas. *Lab Invest* 1991;**64**:585–91.

264. Wager M, Lapierre F, Blanc JL, Listrat A, Bataille B. Cauda equina tumours: a French multicenter retrospective review of 231 adult cases and review of the literature. *Neurosurg Rev* 2000;**23**:119–29.

265. Warmuth–Metz M, Klein R, Sorensen N, *et al.* Central neurocytoma of the fourth ventricle: case report. *J Neurosurg* 1999;**91**:506–9.

266. Warren WH, Lee I, Gould VE, *et al.* Paragangliomas of the head and neck: ultrastructural and immunohistochemical analysis. *Ultrastruct Pathol* 1985;**8**:333–43.

267. Wester DJ, Falcone S, Green BA, *et al.* Paraganglioma of the filum: MR appearance. *J Comput Assist Tomogr* 1993;**17**:967–9.

268. Whittle IR, Dow GR, Lammie GA, Wardlaw J. Dysembryoplastic neuroepithelial tumour with discrete bilateral multifocality: further evidence for a germinal origin. *Br J Neurosurg* 1999;**13**:508–11.

269. Wichmann W, Schubiger O, von Deimling A, *et al.* Neuroradiology of central neurocytoma. *Neuroradiology* 1991;**33**:143–8.

270. Wick MR. Neuroendocrine neoplasia. Current concepts. *Am J Clin Pathol* 2000;**113**(3):331–5.

271. Williams DW III, Elster AD, Ginsberg LE, Stanton C. Recurrent Lhermitte–Duclos disease: report of two cases and association with Cowden's disease. *ANJR Am J Neuroradiol* 1992;**13**:287–90.

272. Woesler B, Kuwert T, Kurlemann G, *et al.* High amino acid uptake in a low-grade desmoplastic infantile ganglioglioma in a 14-year-old patient. *Neurosurg Rev* 1998;**21**:31–5.

273. Wolf HK, Buslei R, Blümcke I, *et al.* Neural antigens in oligodendrogliomas and dysembryoplastic neuroepithelial tumors. *Acta Neuropathol* (Berl) 1997;**94**:436–43.

274. Wolf HK, Wellmer J, Müller MB, *et al.* Glioneuronal malformative lesions and dysembryoplastic neuroepithelial tumors in patients with chronic pharmacoresistant epilepsies. *J Neuropathol Exp Neurol* 1995;**54**:245–54.

275. Wong K, Gyure KA, Prayson RA, *et al.* Dysembryoplastic neuroepithelial tumour: *in situ* hybridization of proteolipid protein. *J Neuropathol Exp Neurol* 1999;**58**:542 .

276. Xiong J, Liu Y, Chu SG, *et al.* Rosette-forming glioneuronal tumor of the septum pellucidum with extension to the supratentorial ventricles: rare case with genetic analysis. *Neuropathology* 2012;**32**(3):301–5.

277. Yachnis AT, Trojanowski JQ, Memmo M, Schlaepfer WW. Expression of neurofilament proteins in the hypertrophic granule cells of Lhermitte–Duclos disease:an explanation for the mass effect and the myelination of parallel fibers in the disease state. *J Neuropathol Exp Neurol* 1988;**47**:206–16.

278. Yamauchi T, Kubota M, Saeki N, *et al.* Paraganglioma in the frontal skull base: case report. *Neurol Med Chir* (Tokyo) 1999;**39**:308–12.

279. Yasargill MG, von Ammon K, von Deimling A, *et al.* Central neurocytoma: histopathological variants and therapeutic approaches. *J Neurosurg* 1992;**76**:32–7.

280. Yin XL, Pang JC, Hui AB, *et al.* Detection of chromosomal imbalances in central neurocytomas by using comparative genomic hybridization. *J Neurosurg* 2000;**93**: 77–81.

281. Zentner J, Hufnagel A, Wolf HK, *et al.* Surgical treatment of temporal lobe epilepsy: clinical, radiological, and histopathological findings in 178 patients. *J Neurol Neurosurg Psychiatry* 1995;**58**:666–73.

282. Zentner J, Hufnagel A, Wolf HK, *et al.* Surgical treatment of neoplasms associated with medically intractable epilepsy. *Neurosurgery* 1997;**41**:378–86.

283. Zentner J, Wolf HK, Ostertun B, *et al.* Gangliogliomas: clinical, radiological, and histopathological findings in 51 patients. *J Neurol Neurosurg Psychiatry* 1994;**57**:1497–502.

284. Zhang PJ, Rosenblum MK. Synaptophysin expression in the human spinal cord: diagnostic implications of an immunohistochemical study. *Am J Surg Pathol* 1996;**20**:273–6.

285. Zhou XP, Marsh DJ, Morrison CD, *et al.* Germline inactivation of PTEN and dysregulation of the phosphoinositol–3–kinase/Akt pathway cause human Lhermitte–Duclos disease in adults. *Am J Hum Genet* 2003;**73**:1191–8.

286. Zhou XP, Waite KA, Pilarski R, *et al.* Germline PTEN promoter mutations and deletions in Cowden/Bannayan–Riley–Ruvalcaba syndrome result in aberrant PTEN protein and dysregulation of the phosphoinositol–3–kinase/Akt pathway. *Am J Hum Genet* 2003;**73**:404–11.

287. Zhu JJ, Leon SP, Folkerth RD, *et al.* Evidence for clonal origin of neoplastic neuronal and glial cells in gangliogliomas. *Am J Pathol* 1997;**151**:565–71.

Neuroepithelial Tumours of the Pineal Region

Alexandre Vasiljevic, Anne Jouvet and Michelle Fevre Montange

INTRODUCTION

Neuroepithelial tumours of the pineal region are rare, accounting for less than 1 per cent of primary central nervous system (CNS) tumours. They include pineal parenchymal tumours (PPTs), glial tumours and papillary tumour of the pineal region (PTPR), the latter described as a novel neoplasm in this region.[40] The neuroglial cyst (pineal cyst) is a frequent non-neoplastic lesion of the pineal gland that needs to be distinguished from pineal tumours, particularly pineocytomas.

PINEAL PARENCHYMAL TUMOURS

PPTs account for approximately 30 per cent of tumours in the pineal region.[21] Histopathologically, they constitute a morphologic continuum from slowly growing well-differentiated lesions to highly proliferative tumours. The 2007 WHO classification includes three distinct categories: pineocytoma (PC), pineal parenchymal tumour of intermediate differentiation (PPTID) and pineoblastoma (PB).[63] A four-tiered subclassification of PPTs, based on mitotic count and immunohistochemical staining for neurofilament proteins (NFP), has also been proposed.[39]

Pineocytoma

PCs are circumscribed, slowly growing neoplasms composed of uniform cells resembling pineocytes. A characteristic architectural feature is the formation of pineocytomatous rosettes.

Incidence, Age and Sex Distribution

In a literature review of 16 papers covering 326 PPTs, 145 (44 per cent) were found to be PC.[21] This percentage might be an overestimate, as some PPTIDs were classified as PC before the 2007 WHO classification. Others have estimated that PCs account for 14 to 30 per cent of all PPTs[15] and

may present at any age, but mostly occur in adults, with a peak incidence between the third and sixth decades of life.[63] There is no gender preference.

Clinical and Radiological Features

PCs, like other pineal region tumours, often cause obstructive hydrocephalus and thus increased intracranial pressure. Headache is the most common presenting symptom. Ocular movement disturbances due to midbrain compression, e.g. up-gaze palsy and nystagmus (Parinaud syndrome), are seen in a subset of patients. Compression of cerebellar structures can cause ataxia and dysmetria.[30]

On computed tomography (CT) scans, PCs are well demarcated, usually less than 3 cm and iso- to hyperdense. Central or peripheral areas of calcification may be visible on the CT scan, whereas macrocystic lesions more likely represent a non-neoplastic pineal cyst.[30] On magnetic resonance imaging (MRI), they appear as well-circumscribed lesions that are hypo- to iso-intense on T1-weighted images and hyperintense on T2-weighted images. On post-contrast images, they show homogeneous enhancement (Figure 33.1a).[83] Tumoural haemorrhage (pineal apoplexy) rarely occurs.

Macroscopic Examination

PCs are circumscribed, grey or grey-brown tumours (Figure 33.1b), with a cut surface that is homogeneous and finely granular. Some show degenerative changes, such as small cysts. Necrosis is rare.

Microscopy

Typical PCs are composed of well-differentiated tumour cells that resemble pineocytes and grow in a sheet-like pattern. The tumour cells are uniform, with sparse, eosinophilic cytoplasm, short processes and round-to-oval nuclei with finely dispersed chromatin and inconspicuous nucleoli. Silver impregnation techniques highlight short cytoplasmic processes, often with bulbous or club-shaped terminations. Micro-calcifications may be seen. Mitotic

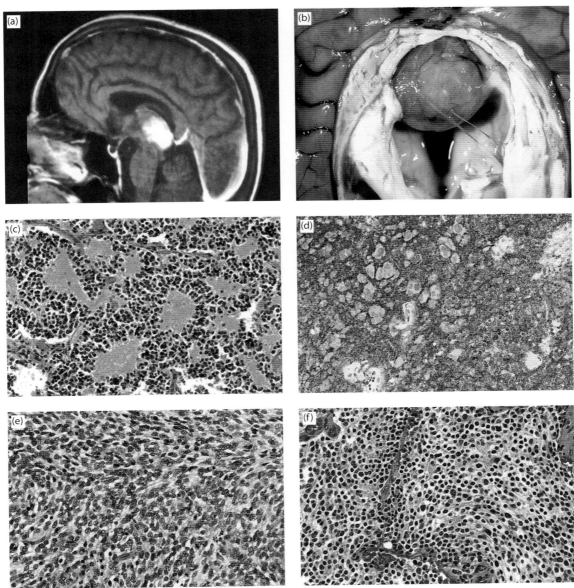

33.1 Pineal tumours. (a) Sagittal, post-contrast T1-weighted magnetic resonance imaging, showing an enhancing pineal tumour, with obstructive hydrocephalus due to compression of the cerebral aqueduct. **(b)** Pineocytoma with well-delineated macroscopic borders protruding into the third ventricle. **(c)** Typical pineocytomatous rosettes in a pineocytoma. **(d)** Diffuse synaptophysin immuno-labelling is characteristic of pineocytomas. **(e)** Pineoblastoma showing dense cellularity, primitive cells and mitotic activity. **(f)** Pineal parenchymal tumour of intermediate differentiation. This tumour lacks typical pineocytomatous rosettes. However, it does not display the primitive 'small blue cell' histology of a pineoblastoma. Note the isomorphic cells with round nuclei and a clear cytoplasm mimicking neurocytoma or oligodendroglioma.

(a) Courtesy of Dr TCS Cox, formerly of The Bethlem and Maudsley NHS Trust, London, UK. (f) Courtesy of Professor W Paulus, University of Münster, Germany.

figures are absent or rare. Necrosis is very rare. The most characteristic feature is the formation of large, sometimes confluent 'pineocytomatous' rosettes (Figure 33.1c). These structures appear as ovoid eosinophilic areas composed of a meshwork of tumour cell processes without a central blood vessel. Pineocytomatous rosettes are similar to neuroblastic rosettes of the Homer Wright type, but considerably larger and not surrounded by primitive tumour cells.

A subset of PC is characterized by the presence of large ganglionic cells and/or pleomorphic multinucleated giant cells.[24,39,48] They show low proliferative activity and are biologically indolent.

Immunohistochemistry

PCs are diffusely immunopositive for neuron-specific enolase (NSE), synaptophysin (SYN) (Figure 33.1d) and NFP, with strong reactivity in pineocytomatous rosettes. Immunoreactivity for several other neuronal or neuroendocrine antigens, including class III beta-tubulin, microtubule-associated protein 2 (MAP2), tau protein and chromogranin A, is also common.[11,39,66] In pleomorphic PC, the pleomorphic cells show strong expression of SYN, NFP and sometimes chromogranin A.[24,48] PCs can demonstrate a photoreceptor-like immunophenotype, with patchy positivity for retinal S-antigen and/or rhodopsin.[46,69] They also express hydroxy-indole-O-methyltransferase (HIOMT), the enzyme that catalyses the final reaction in melatonin biosynthesis.[28] S-100 protein (PS100) immunoreactivity is seen in the interstitial astrocytic cells and sometimes in the neoplastic cells, to varying degrees. Glial fibrillary acidic protein (GFAP) expression is seen in reactive astrocytes.[11,39] Proliferative activity, as assessed by the Ki-67 labelling index (LI), is low.[3,26,66]

Electron Microscopy

PCs are composed of clear cells with a varying number of dark cells, sometimes joined by zonula adherentes.[38] Their cytoplasm is relatively abundant and contains well-developed organelles, including smooth and rough endoplasmic reticulum, Golgi complex, mitochondria, multivesicular bodies and lysosomes. The cells share many ultrastructural features with normal pineocytes, such as dense-core (neurosecretory) vesicles, clear (synaptic-type) vesicles, vesicle-crowned rodlets (synaptic ribbons), paired twisted filaments and 'fibrous filaments'.[16,22,34,35,38] Tumour cell processes are filled with microtubules and terminate in vesicle-rich club-like expansions, which may show synapse-like junctions. Some tumours show signs of photoreceptor differentiation, including the presence of cytoplasmic annulate lamellae, as well as cilia with a 9+0 configuration.[38]

Differential Diagnosis

The distinction between PC and normal pineal gland can be difficult with a small biopsy. However, in normal gland, lobulation is more prominent, whereas proliferative activity and pineocytomatous rosettes are absent. Immunostaining for neuronal markers further highlights the lobularity. The presence of prominent pineocytomatous rosettes and lower proliferation indices favours PCs over PPTID.

Molecular Genetics

Cytogenetic studies on PC are rare and have not shown any non-randomly distributed abnormalities, although both numerical and structural aberrations are common. In three studies, the karyotype of PC was mostly pseudodiploid with losses of chromosomes 4, 5, 14 and 15 being common; in two, loss of all, or part of chromosomes 22, 11 and 1 was observed.[4,16,72] On comparative genomic hybridization (CGH), these tumours similarly lack signature alterations.[76] TP53 mutation and p53 protein accumulation were not detected in five PCs.[91]

Biological Behaviour and Prognosis

PCs grow slowly, are associated with favourable prognosis after surgery (5-year overall survival ranging from 86 to 91 per cent) and do not metastasize.[21,56,80] The literature is primarily composed of case reports and small case series, in which low-grade PPTIDs were sometimes included as PCs. A recent review indicates that surgical resection is the appropriate treatment.

Adjuvant fractionated radiotherapy does not improve tumour control or survival when used to treat a subtotally resected tumour, but close radiological follow-up is recommended.[9,10] However, others suggest that radiosurgery has a role as an alternative primary therapy for small lesions, as well as in the treatment of residual and recurrent tumours.[19,74]

Pineoblastoma

This is a highly malignant, dense, 'small blue cell' tumour arising in the pineal gland and is indistinguishable from medulloblastomas or other CNS primitive neuroectodermal tumours (PNET).

Age and Sex Distribution

They typically occur in children, with a mean age of 12.6 years, but adults may also be affected,[21,56] with rare reports involving patients older than 60 years.[53,55] There is no gender predilection.

Clinical and Radiological Features

PB share with other pineal region tumours a clinical presentation dominated by signs and symptoms of obstructive hydrocephalus and raised intracranial pressure. However, compared to PC, the history is usually shorter and more rapidly progressive. On neuroimaging, PB usually present as large (typically >3 cm), poorly demarcated masses, with invasion into adjacent brain parenchyma and meninges.[47,62] Tumoural calcification is peripheral, giving rise to the 'exploded' calcification appearance.[30] On MRI, PB are heterogeneous, with the solid portion appearing hypo- to iso-intense on T1-weighted images and iso- to mildly hyper-intense relative to the cortex on T2-weighted images. They demonstrate heterogeneous enhancement on post-contrast images.[83] Craniospinal dissemination is frequent, but metastases outside the CNS are exceptional.[13,21]

Macroscopic Examination

PB are poorly demarcated, soft or gelatinous, grey-pink tumours. Haemorrhagic and necrotic areas may be present. The tumours often destroy the pineal gland, bulge into the posterior third ventricle and compress the colliculi and the aqueduct.

Microscopy

PB are composed of densely packed small cells with scant cytoplasm, hyperchromatic, round to oval nuclei (Figure 33.1e) and high nuclear/cytoplasmic ratios. The tumour lacks any obvious lobular architecture or pineocytomatous rosettes. However, PB often contain Homer Wright (neuroblastic) and/or Flexner–Wintersteiner (retinoblastic) rosettes. Large cell/anaplastic features, as seen in medulloblastomas, can be present. PB occasionally show evidence of advanced photoreceptor differentiation, with the formation of 'fleurettes'. Rare tumours contain cells with melanin pigment. Mitotic figures are frequent. Apoptotic bodies and areas of necrosis may be prominent, the latter sometimes being associated with microcalcifications. Vessels are usually thin walled, but focal endothelial proliferation may be seen.

Immunohistochemistry

A dot-like or diffuse immunoreactivity for SYN is common in PB.[39,56] NSE is also expressed, whereas immunoreactivity for NFPs and/or chromogranin A is inconsistent and tends to be restricted to individual tumour cells.[39,56] PB can contain cells with immunoreactivity for photoreceptor markers, such as retinal S-antigen.[69] GFAP and PS100 immunoreactivity is rare.[39] The Ki-67 LI is high (>20 per cent).[26]

Electron Microscopy

In line with ultrastructural findings for other CNS PNETs, PB contain poorly differentiated cells with a few short processes lacking the bulbous terminations typical of PC.[38,66] Scant microtubules and occasional dense-core vesicles may be observed. However, specialized structures, such as paired twisted filaments, vesicle-crowned rodlets or synaptic junctions are absent.

Differential Diagnosis

The differential diagnosis includes embryonal tumours that can seed or infiltrate the pineal region, in particular, medulloblastoma, CNS PNET and primitive appearing gliomas. PB must also be distinguished from higher-grade PPTID. The distinction hinges upon degrees of cellularity, atypia, mitotic activity and necrosis. In adults, metastatic small-cell carcinoma can be distinguished by their immunoreactivity for epithelial markers, such as cytokeratins. Malignant germ cell tumours can resemble PB on imaging, but the two can usually be easily distinguished histologically.

Molecular Genetics

Conventional and CGH cytogenetic studies have shown frequent numerical and structural abnormalities.[6,54,76,87,88] The karyotypes are mostly near-diploid, but hypertetraploidy has been reported. Recurrent aberrations include gains of 1q, 5p, 5q, 6p and 14q and losses of chromosomes 20 and 22, as well as isochromosome 17q (i[17q]), or unbalanced gain of 17q. In cytogenetic reports of 13 PB, i[17q] or unbalanced 17q gain was described in four cases, including two tumours and two cell lines.[6,54] In contrast, CGH studies have shown that most PB do not exhibit 17q gain.[76,77] Thus, whether PB are genetically related to medulloblastomas remains unclear.

In vitro, PB cell lines showed enhanced N-myc expression in the absence of *MYCN* gene amplification, in contrast to the situation in medulloblastomas.[42,43] No *TP53* mutations were demonstrated in four PB.[91]

The *RB1* gene has not been studied for genetic alterations in sporadic PB.[54,88] However, studies on knock-out mice indicate that the simultaneous inactivation of p53 and Rb results in an increased rate of PB.[94] Interestingly, patients with familial retinoblastoma syndrome have an increased risk of developing PB, a condition known as 'trilateral retinoblastoma'.[18,44] PB that arise in this setting have a more aggressive course than sporadic cases.[70] However, no specific abnormalities of chromosome 13q in the region of the *Rb* gene have been found in the latter.[6,76] One case of PB associated with familial adenomatous polyposis has been reported as a potential variant of Turcot's syndrome type 2 (see Chapter 44).[29] This case remains isolated, and no association has been made between *APC* gene mutation and PB, in contrast to the firm association between mutation of this gene and medulloblastomas.

Biological Behaviour and Prognosis

PB are locally invasive and tend to disseminate via the cerebrospinal fluid (CSF), requiring aggressive treatment. In adults, stereotactic biopsy or open surgery is usually followed by adjuvant radiotherapy and chemotherapy.[53,55,85,86] Nevertheless, the prognosis is poor, as indicated by the median survival time of 16 months and 10 per cent 5-year survival rate.[21] A slightly better median overall survival has been reported for adult patients, ranging from 25.7 to 77 months.[53,55] The extent of disease at diagnosis, the histology (PB versus PPTID) and the degree of residual disease after initial treatment are independent prognostic factors in adult patients.[55] The prognosis in infants younger than 18 months is even more dismal.[37] In children treated with radiotherapy and chemotherapy, a 3-year progression-free survival rate of 61 per cent has been reported, albeit commonly with severe developmental side effects in children younger than 9 years of age.[37] In children pineoblastomas appear to do slightly better than CNS PNETs.[12,89]

Pineal Parenchymal Tumour of Intermediate Differentiation

Synonyms and Historical Overview

PPTIDs are cellular tumours with variable architectural features. First proposed in 1993,[79] they were subsequently recognized by the World Health Organization (WHO).

Incidence, Age and Sex Distribution

The relative frequency of PPTID varies greatly in the literature, reflecting the difficulties in establishing reproducible definitional criteria. In carefully defined series, PPTIDs represent 20 to 62 per cent of PPTs.[3,21,79] They occur mostly in adults, with a peak incidence in young adults (20–40 years of age). Most present as localized disease, with CSF dissemination less common than for PB.[21,80]

Clinical and Radiological Features

The clinical signs are similar to those of other pineal region tumours.[21] Imaging findings are similarly non-specific. PPTIDs are heterogeneously hypointense on T1-weighted and hyperintense on T2-weighted images; they are contrast enhancing. Cystic areas may be seen.[45,83]

Macroscopic Examination

The gross appearance of PPTIDs is similar to that of PC, with no gross evidence of necrosis.

Microscopy

Histologically, PPTIDs are variable.[39] One pattern shows endocrine-like lobular/diffuse architecture with isomorphic tumour cells containing round nuclei and clear cytoplasm (Figure 33.1f). Another phenotype, the 'transitional variant', has mixed lobular/diffuse areas, in addition to regions with

PC-like morphology. Finally, some rare tumours may present with a biphasic pattern combining the typical features of PC and PB. Neoplastic cells have less cytoplasm than in PC, but it is still visible on standard staining. Nuclear atypia is moderate. Mitotic activity is usually present, but may vary considerably. Foci of necrosis or vascular proliferation have been reported in subsets of PPTID tumours, although they lack the primitive 'small blue cell' appearance of PB.[39] A pleomorphic variant may be encountered in low-grade PPTIDs.[24]

Immunohistochemistry

In PPTID, expression of neuronal markers is variable. Cytoplasmic SYN labelling is usually diffuse, but of variable intensity. NFP can be expressed in a variable number of cells, and this variability has been used together with morphology and proliferation to discriminate low-grade from high-grade PPTID. Chromogranin A may be seen in PPTID, especially those with a lobulated architecture.[39]

Electron Microscopy

PPTIDs display short cytoplasmic processes and rare bulbous endings. In lobulated PPTID, the organelles characteristic of neurosensory/photoreceptor differentiation are usually absent, but the cell processes contain oriented microtubules, clear and dense-cored vesicles.

Differential Diagnosis

PPTID should not be mistaken for neurocytoma or oligodendroglioma. The clear cells and sheet-like growth patterns of some oligodendrogliomas and neurocytomas, as well as the presence of fibrillary areas or perivascular neuritic processes in the latter, may lead to misdiagnosis, but PPTIDs do not express OLIG2 or NeuN. PPTIDs are distinguished from PC and PB on the basis of histopathological criteria, mitotic activity and NFP expression. More particularly, high-grade PPTIDs need to be distinguished from PB, which, in contrast, presents a higher cellular density and small cells with scant cytoplasm and hyperchromatic nuclei.

Molecular Genetics

One CGH study of PPTID showed overlap with PB in terms of chromosome 22 loss and similar proportions of chromosomal imbalances per case (5.3 for PPTID and 5.6 for PB).[76]

Biological Behaviour and Prognosis

The clinical outcome for patients with PPTID is highly variable, so the WHO classification does not assign a definite grade to these neoplasms. Other studies have proposed that intermediate tumours can be subdivided histologically into two grades associated with significantly different outcomes: grade II for tumours with <6 mitoses per 10 high-power fields (HPF) and strong NFP expression and grade III for tumours with either 6 or more mitoses per 10 HPF or low mitotic index, but with negligible NFP immunoreactivity.[21,39] The 5-year survival rates are 74 per cent for grade II and 42 per cent for grade III tumours.[21] In a series of 37 adult patients with PPTID who were not grade stratified, the median overall survival was 165 months, whereas the 5- and 10-year survival rates were 80 and 72 per cent, respectively.[55]

Grading of PPT

Classification of PPT is difficult, especially when using small biopsy samples. PC and pleomorphic PC are well-differentiated tumours and correspond to WHO grade I.[63] PB correspond to WHO grade IV. PPTID may correspond to WHO grade II or III, but the grading criteria described in the prior section have yet to be validated. The Ki-67 LI may also be a useful tool.[3,26]

Histogenesis of PPT

PPTs are thought to originate from cells of pineocytic lineage. Pineocytes have photosensory and neuroendocrine functions and constitute the major cell population within the normal pineal gland.[60] They develop from neuroepithelial precursors in the roof of the diencephalon and are ontogenetically related to retinal photoreceptor cells. Pineocyte development depends crucially on the homeobox transcription factor Otx2, because Otx2 knock-out mice lack these cells.[64] Otx2 expression is maintained in adult pineocytes and may control the expression of genes associated with phototransduction and melatonin synthesis.[73] Although a study has demonstrated amplification and frequent overexpression of the *OTX2* gene in medulloblastomas,[5] a role for aberrant Otx2 expression in PPT remains to be established. PB probably originate from these same neuroepithelial precursors, a hypothesis based on ultrastructural and immunohistochemical similarities between PB cells and cells of the developing pineal gland,[38,59,60] as well as similarities with retinoblastomas, and the common occurrence of both tumour types in patients with trilateral retinoblastoma.[44]

Gene Expression in PPT

Gene expression studies of pineal region tumours have shown that PPTs cluster together.[23] Classic PC and pleomorphic variants have similar profiles, perhaps implying that pleomorphism is not related to anaplasia. A few genes coding for enzymes of melatonin biosynthesis, such as *TPH1* (tryptophan hydroxylase) and *HIOMT*, are expressed in PPT, with higher levels in PC than in PB.[23] Some genes involved in phototransduction, such as *OPN4*, coding for the photoreceptor pigment melanopsin, are also expressed in PPT. Transcript profiles of four genes (*PRAME*, *CD24*, *HOXD13* and *POU4F2*) can divide PPTID into high- and low-grade tumours, the former showing higher expression of all four.[23]

OTHER NEUROEPITHELIAL TUMOURS OF THE PINEAL REGION AND PINEAL CYST

Papillary Tumour of the Pineal Region

Historical Overview

PTPR was described as a new entity in 2003[40] and was included in the 2007 WHO classification scheme.[41] It is a neuroepithelial tumour arising in the pineal region, characterized by papillary architecture and epithelial cytology.

Incidence, Age and Sex Distribution

PTPRs are rare with only 123 cases reported to date. They affect both children and adults, with a peak age between 20 and 30 years.[25,71,75] There is no sex predilection.

Clinical and Radiological Features

The most common symptom at presentation is increased intracranial pressure. Other frequent symptoms are Parinaud syndrome, ataxia and isolated diplopia.[52,95] On neuroimaging, PTPRs are usually well circumscribed, mildly lobulated, partially cystic, heterogeneously enhancing masses, usually associated with obstructive hydrocephalus.[2,71,82] They are difficult to distinguish from other clinical entities, especially PCs.[2,71]

Macroscopic Examination

PTPRs are usually large (2–4 cm),[41] well-circumscribed masses. The tumours may be reddish, pink or yellowish, with a soft to friable consistency, with occasional cystic components.[81]

Microscopy

Histological examination reveals papillary formations with epithelial cytology (Figure 33.2a). PTPRs present two morphological variants: a papillary growth pattern or a mixture of solid and papillary regions.[25] True rosettes, as well as occasional perivascular pseudorosettes are observed. The tumour cells usually appear columnar or cuboidal, with a defined cytoplasmic membrane. Vacuolated cells, partially positive with the periodic acid-Schiff reaction, have been described.[40,49] Mitotic activity is generally moderate and areas of necrosis may be present. Blood vessel walls are frequently hyalinized.

Grading

Histological grading criteria for PTPRs remain to be defined. The biological behaviour may correspond to WHO grade II or III.

Immunohistochemistry

Immunohistochemistry reveals strong reactivity for cytokeratins (CKs), particularly CK18 (Figure 33.2b).[25,33,41] whereas CK7, CK20 and CK5/6 expression is absent or weak. Weak epithelial membrane antigen (EMA) immunoreactivity may be present, but dot-like or ring-like EMA positivity is rare. Although E-cadherin is negative, claudins 1 and 3 are expressed.[25] Immunoreactivity for PS100 and vimentin is invariable, whereas GFAP positivity is rare. Neuroendocrine markers (NSE, chromogranin A and SYN) may be immunoreactive, whereas NCAM and nestin are always expressed. NFP is rarely positive,[14,61] whereas MAP2 staining is found in the majority. In contrast to their high expression in choroid plexus tumours, stanniocalcin and Kir-7 are only weakly expressed in PTPRs.[33] Transthyretin is expressed, whereas germ cell tumour markers are negative, except for c-Kit.[14]

Electron Microscopy

PTPRs display ultrastructural evidence of ependymal differentiation, including abundant microvilli at the apical pole and numerous interdigitated ependyma-like processes[14,25,40] surrounded by basement membrane at the basal pole.[25,40]

Differential Diagnosis

The differential diagnosis includes a variety of other papillary tumours, most notably papillary ependymoma, choroid plexus papilloma, papillary meningioma, astroblastoma and metastatic papillary carcinoma. However, these can usually be excluded on the basis of their distinct morphological features and immunophenotypes. Rare cases of PPT with papillary features have been reported, including a papillary pineocytoma[92] and a malignant pineocytoma with prominent papillary features.[90] In contrast to PPT, PTPRs usually do not express retinal S-antigen or NFP and show prominent epithelial features, as well as cytokeratin, PS100 and vimentin immunoreactivity.

Histogenesis

On the basis of their ultrastructural and immunohistochemical features, it has been suggested that PTPRs arise from specialized cytokeratin-positive and nestin-positive ependymal cells that are derived from the subcommissural organ (SCO).[40,41] Supporting this hypothesis, a micro-array study

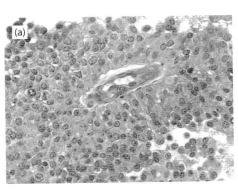

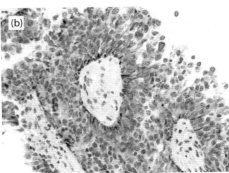

33.2 Papillary tumour of the pineal gland. (a) This cellular tumour consists of neuroectodermal cells showing an epithelial-like growth pattern with formation of papillary features. **(b)** Strong expression of cytokeratin 18 in tumoural cells comprising papillary structures.

has shown high expression of genes that are also expressed in the rodent SCO.[23]

Molecular Genetics

CGH analysis of five cases of PTPR showed frequent losses on chromosomes 10 and 22 and gains on chromosomes 4, 8, 9 and 12.[33] A micro-array study shows high expression of *SPDEF*, *KRT18* and genes coding for proteins reported to be expressed in the animal SCO, namely *ZFH4*, *RFX3*, *TTR* and *CGRP*.[23]

Biological Behaviour and Prognosis

The biological behaviour of PTPR is unclear, although local tumour recurrence appears to be common. Long survival times are reported.[52]

Pineal Cyst

Incidence, Age and Sex Distribution

Glial cysts of the pineal gland are common incidental findings on MRI, with reported frequencies of cysts larger than 5 mm ranging from 1.4 to 4.3 per cent in healthy subjects.[58,68] Autopsy data suggest a prevalence of up to 40 per cent in the elderly, when cysts larger than 2 mm across are considered.[32] Rare studies have suggested a higher incidence in females.[1,51,78]

Clinical and Radiological Features

Almost all pineal cysts remain asymptomatic, but rare examples become large enough to produce clinical symptoms, usually between the third and fifth decades of life.[57] A symptomatic presentation in childhood is also possible.[51] Symptoms and signs usually relate to obstructive hydrocephalus, but others associated with compression of adjacent structures may occur.[57] Prevalence and cyst appearance are comparable in children with or without central precocious puberty.[51] Haemorrhage may rarely cause an abrupt onset of symptoms, a condition referred to as 'pineal cyst apoplexy'.[68]

On MRI, pineal cysts appear as round midline lesions with a smooth margin and a homogeneous liquid content that is either iso-intense or slightly hyperintense relative to the CSF on T1-weighted images.[27,47,57] The lesion appears bright on T2-weighted images. Enhancement with gadolinium is seen in the majority of cases.[27] Calcification of the cyst wall has been observed in a subset of patients.[27] On high resolution MRI, fine internal septations or small internal cysts are common.[51] On FLAIR, pineal cysts have relaxation times that differ from those of CSF.[67]

Macroscopic Examination

Macroscopically, pineal cysts are filled with a clear or pale yellow proteinaceous fluid and have a smooth lining that sometimes shows siderotic discolouration due to old haemorrhage.

Microscopy

Histological examination demonstrates a characteristic pattern in the cyst wall. This consists of a paucicellular and finely fibrillary gliotic inner layer, with Rosenthal fibres, eosinophilic granular bodies and some deposits of haemosiderin. This gliotic layer is bordered by pineal parenchyma and an outer fibrovascular capsule. The pineal tissue is sharply demarcated from the inner gliotic layer and often appears somewhat disorganized as a result of chronic compression. However, its lobular architecture is usually still recognizable and the small calcifications of the normal pineal gland ('acervulus' or 'brain sand') are still present.

Immunohistochemistry

Immunohistochemistry shows strong expression of GFAP and PS100 in the gliotic layer of the cyst wall. The adjacent pineal parenchyma stains strongly for SYN. The strong NFP immunopositivity makes the lobularity of the pineal parenchyma more obvious.[38] Proliferative activity, as determined by Ki-67, is absent.

Electron Microscopy

The normal and cystic pineal gland is characterized by the juxtaposition of clear and dark cells. The dark cells contain numerous organelles, specifically clusters of mitochondria, dense-core vesicles, 'synaptic ribbons' and paired twisted filaments.[38,50]

Differential Diagnoses

The two principal differential diagnoses to pineal cyst are PC and pilocytic astrocytoma. On MRI, PCs are not truly cystic[20] and pineal cysts are stable lesions.[7] Microscopically, PCs are recognized by their pineocytomatous rosettes and lack the normal lobularity of the pineal gland. In addition, PCs are rarely cystic and do not form a gliotic zone with Rosenthal fibres and haemosiderin deposits. In contrast to pilocytic astrocytomas, which are rare in the pineal gland, the gliotic layer of a pineal cyst is less cellular and lacks a biphasic architecture including microcystic areas. However, the diagnosis is particularly challenging on small biopsy specimens when tectal glioma coexists with fragments of a pineal cyst.

Histogenesis

The origin of pineal cysts is unknown. Various hypotheses have been raised, including an embryologic origin, development from a diverticulum of the third ventricle or a degenerative or post-haemorrhagic origin.[1,68]

Treatment

Symptomatic pineal cysts are benign lesions with a favourable prognosis after surgical resection or endoscopic treatment,[57,58] but incidentally discovered pineal cysts almost never require surgery.[1]

Other Neuroepithelial Tumors of the Pineal Region

In addition to PPT, a variety of other neuroepithelial tumours can originate in the pineal region. These include astrocytic tumours, such as pilocytic, diffuse and anaplastic astrocytomas,[36] glioblastomas,[93] pleomorphic xanthoas-trocytomas and granular astrocytoma-like lesions.[65,84] The histogenesis of these gliomas is unclear; however, they could arise from stromal astrocytes within the pineal parenchyma. A case of pineal subependymal giant cell astrocytoma has also been reported.[17] In addition, individual cases of pineal ganglioglioma and melanotic neuroectodermal tumour (melanotic progonoma) of the pineal gland have been reported.[8,31]

REFERENCES

1. Al-Holou WN, Garton HJ, Muraszko KM, et al. Prevalence of pineal cysts in children and young adults. Clinical article. *J Neurosurg Pediatr* 2009;4:230–6.
2. Amemiya S, Shibahara J, Aoki S, et al. Recently established entities of central nervous system tumors: review of radiological findings. *J Comput Assist Tomogr* 2008;32:279–85.
3. Arivazhagan A, Anandh B, Santosh V, et al. Pineal parenchymal tumors – utility of immunohistochemical markers in prognostication. *Clin Neuropathol* 2008;27:325–33.
4. Bello MJ, Rey JA, de Campos JM, et al. Chromosomal abnormalities in a pineocytoma. *Cancer Genet Cytogenet* 1993;71:185–6.
5. Boon K, Eberhart CG, Riggins GJ. Genomic amplification of orthodenticle homologue 2 in medulloblastomas. *Cancer Res* 2005;65:703–7.
6. Brown AE, Leibundgut K, Niggli FK, et al. Cytogenetics of pineoblastoma: four new cases and a literature review. *Cancer Genet Cytogenet* 2006;170:175–9.
7. Cauley KA, Linnell GJ, Braff SP, et al. Serial follow-up MRI of indeterminate cystic lesions of the pineal region: experience at a rural tertiary care referral center. *AJR Am J Roentgenol* 2009;193:533–7.
8. Chang YL, Lin SZ, Chiang YH, et al. Pineal ganglioglioma with premature thelarche. Report of a case and review of the literature. *Childs Nerv Syst* 1996;12:103–6.
9. Clark AJ, Ivan ME, Sughrue ME, et al. Tumor control after surgery and radiotherapy for pineocytoma. *J Neurosurg* 2010;113:319–24.
10. Clark AJ, Sughrue ME, Aranda D, et al. Contemporary management of pineocytoma. *Neurosurg Clin N Am* 2011;22:403–7.
11. Coca S, Vaquero J, Escandon J, et al. Immunohistochemical characterization of pineocytomas. *Clin Neuropathol* 1992;11:298–303.
12. Cohen BH, Zeltzer PM, Boyett JM, et al. Prognostic factors and treatment results for supratentorial primitive neuroectodermal tumors in children using radiation and chemotherapy: a Childrens Cancer Group randomized trial. *J Clin Oncol* 1995;13:1687–96.
13. Constantine C, Miller DC, Gardner S, et al. Osseous metastasis of pineoblastoma: a case report and review of the literature. *J Neurooncol* 2005;74:53–7.
14. Cykowski MD, Wartchow EP, Mierau GW, et al. Papillary tumor of the pineal region: ultrastructural study of a case. *Ultrastruct Pathol* 2012;36:68–77.
15. Dahiya S, Perry A. Pineal tumors. *Adv Anat Pathol* 2010;17:419–27.
16. Dario A, Cerati M, Taborelli M, et al. Cytogenetic and ultrastructural study of a pineocytoma case report. *J Neurooncol* 2000;48:131–4.
17. Dashti SR, Robinson S, Rodgers M, et al. Pineal region giant cell astrocytoma associated with tuberous sclerosis: case report. *J Neurosurg* 2005;102:322–5.
18. De Potter P, Shields CL, Shields JA. Clinical variations of trilateral retinoblastoma: a report of 13 cases. *J Pediatr Ophthalmol Strabismus* 1994;31:26–31.
19. Deshmukh VR, Smith KA, Rekate HL, et al. Diagnosis and management of pineocytomas. *Neurosurgery* 2004;55:349–55; discussion 55–7.
20. Fakhran S, Escott EJ. Pineocytoma mimicking a pineal cyst on imaging: true diagnostic dilemma or a case of incomplete imaging? *AJNR Am J Neuroradiol* 2008;29:159–63.
21. Fauchon F, Jouvet A, Paquis P, et al. Parenchymal pineal tumors: a clinicopathological study of 76 cases. *Int J Radiat Oncol Biol Phys* 2000;46:959–68.
22. Fevre-Montange M, Jouvet A, Privat K, et al. Immunohistochemical, ultrastructural, biochemical and in vitro studies of a pineocytoma. *Acta Neuropathol* 1998;95:532–9.
23. Fevre-Montange M, Champier J, Szathmari A, et al. Microarray analysis reveals differential gene expression patterns in tumors of the pineal region. *J Neuropathol Exp Neurol* 2006;65:675–84.
24. Fevre-Montange M, Szathmari A, Champier J, et al. Pineocytoma and parenchymal tumors of intermediate differentiation presenting cytologic pleomorphism: a multicenter study. *Brain Pathol* 2008;18:354–9.
25. Fevre-Montange M, Vasiljevic A, Bergemer Fouquet AM, et al. Histopathological and ultrastructural features and claudin expression in papillary tumors of the pineal region: a multicenter analysis. *Am J Surg Pathol* 2012; 36: 916–28.
26. Fevre-Montange M, Vasiljevic A, Frappaz D, et al. Utility of Ki67 immunostaining in the grading of pineal parenchymal tumours: a multicentre study. *Neuropathol Appl Neurobiol* 2012;38:87–94.
27. Fleege MA, Miller GM, Fletcher GP, et al. Benign glial cysts of the pineal gland: unusual imaging characteristics with histologic correlation. *AJNR Am J Neuroradiol* 1994;15:161–6.
28. Fukuda T, Akiyama N, Ikegami M, et al. Expression of hydroxyindole-O-methyltransferase enzyme in the human central nervous system and in pineal parenchymal cell tumors. *J Neuropathol Exp Neurol* 2010;69:498–510.
29. Gadish T, Tulchinsky H, Deutsch AA, et al. Pinealoblastoma in a patient with familial adenomatous polyposis: variant of Turcot syndrome type 2? Report of a case and review of the literature. *Dis Colon Rectum* 2005;48:2343–6.
30. Gaillard F, Jones J. Masses of the pineal region: clinical presentation and radiographic features. *Postgrad Med J* 2010;86:597–607.
31. Gorhan C, Soto-Ares G, Ruchoux MM, et al. Melanotic neuroectodermal tumour of the pineal region. *Neuroradiology* 2001;43:944–7.
32. Hasegawa A, Ohtsubo K, Mori W. Pineal gland in old age; quantitative and qualitative morphological study of 168 human autopsy cases. *Brain Res* 1987;409:343–9.
33. Hasselblatt M, Blumcke I, Jeibmann A, et al. Immunohistochemical profile and chromosomal imbalances in papillary tumours of the pineal region. *Neuropathol Appl Neurobiol* 2006;32:278–83.
34. Hassoun J, Gambarelli D, Peragut JC, et al. Specific ultrastructural markers of human pinealomas. A study of four cases. *Acta Neuropathol* 1983;62:31–40.
35. Hassoun J, Devictor B, Gambarelli D, et al. Paired twisted filaments: a new ultrastructural marker of human pinealomas? *Acta Neuropathol* 1984;65:163–5.
36. Hirato J, Nakazato Y. Pathology of pineal region tumors. *J Neurooncol* 2001;54:239–49.
37. Jakacki RI, Zeltzer PM, Boyett JM, et al. Survival and prognostic factors following radiation and/or chemotherapy for primitive neuroectodermal tumors of the pineal region in infants and children: a report of the Childrens Cancer Group. *J Clin Oncol* 1995;13:1377–83.
38. Jouvet A, Fevre-Montange M, Besancon R, et al. Structural and ultrastructural characteristics of human pineal gland, and pineal parenchymal tumors. *Acta Neuropathol* 1994;88:334–48.
39. Jouvet A, Saint-Pierre G, Fauchon F, et al. Pineal parenchymal tumors: a correlation of histological features with prognosis in 66 cases. *Brain Pathol* 2000;10:49–60.
40. Jouvet A, Fauchon F, Liberski P, et al. Papillary tumor of the pineal region. *Am J Surg Pathol* 2003;27:505–12.
41. Jouvet A, Nakazato Y, Scheithauer BW, Paulus W. Papillary tumour of the pineal region. In: Louis DN, Ohgaki H, Wiestler OD, Cavenee WK eds. *WHO classification of tumours of the central nervous system*. Lyon: International Agency for Research on Cancer, 2007;128–129.
42. Kees UR, Biegel JA, Ford J, et al. Enhanced MYCN expression and isochromosome 17q in pineoblastoma cell lines. *Genes Chromosomes Cancer* 1994;9:129–35.
43. Kees UR, Spagnolo D, Hallam LA, et al. A new pineoblastoma cell line, PER-480, with der(10)t(10;17), der(16)t(1;16), and enhanced MYC expression in the absence

of gene amplification. *Cancer Genet Cytogenet* 1998;**100**:159–64.

44. Kivela T. Trilateral retinoblastoma: a meta-analysis of hereditary retinoblastoma associated with primary ectopic intracranial retinoblastoma. *J Clin Oncol* 1999;**17**:1829–37.

45. Komakula S, Warmuth-Metz M, Hildenbrand P, et al. Pineal parenchymal tumor of intermediate differentiation: imaging spectrum of an unusual tumor in 11 cases. *Neuroradiology* 2011;**53**:577–84.

46. Korf HW, Klein DC, Zigler JS, et al. S-antigen-like immunoreactivity in a human pineocytoma. *Acta Neuropathol* 1986;**69**:165–7.

47. Korogi Y, Takahashi M, Ushio Y. MRI of pineal region tumors. *J Neurooncol* 2001;**54**:251–61.

48. Kuchelmeister K, von Borcke IM, Klein H, et al. Pleomorphic pineocytoma with extensive neuronal differentiation: report of two cases. *Acta Neuropathol* 1994;**88**:448–53.

49. Kuchelmeister K, Hugens-Penzel M, Jodicke A, et al. Papillary tumour of the pineal region: histodiagnostic considerations. *Neuropathol Appl Neurobiol* 2006;**32**:203–8.

50. Kurumado K, Mori W. Synaptic ribbon in the human pinealocyte. *Acta Pathol Jpn* 1976;**26**:381–4.

51. Lacroix-Boudhrioua V, Linglart A, Ancel PY, et al. Pineal cysts in children. *Insights Imaging* 2011;**2**:671–8.

52. Lechapt-Zalcman E, Chapon F, Guillamo JS, et al. Long-term clinicopathological observations on a papillary tumour of the pineal region. *Neuropathol Appl Neurobiol* 2011;**37**:431–5.

53. Lee JY, Wakabayashi T, Yoshida J. Management and survival of pineoblastoma: an analysis of 34 adults from the brain tumor registry of Japan. *Neurol Med Chir (Tokyo)* 2005;**45**: 132–41; discussion 41–2.

54. Li MH, Bouffet E, Hawkins CE, et al. Molecular genetics of supratentorial primitive neuroectodermal tumors and pineoblastoma. *Neurosurg Focus* 2005;**19**:E3.

55. Lutterbach J, Fauchon F, Schild SE, et al. Malignant pineal parenchymal tumors in adult patients: patterns of care and prognostic factors. *Neurosurgery* 2002;**51**:44–55; discussion 56.

56. Mena H, Rushing EJ, Ribas JL, et al. Tumors of pineal parenchymal cells: a correlation of histological features, including nucleolar organizer regions, with survival in 35 cases. *Hum Pathol* 1995;**26**:20–30.

57. Mena H, Armonda RA, Ribas JL, et al. Nonneoplastic pineal cysts: a clinicopathological study of twenty-one cases. *Ann Diagn Pathol* 1997;**1**:11–18.

58. Michielsen G, Benoit Y, Baert E, et al. Symptomatic pineal cysts: clinical manifestations and management. *Acta Neurochir (Wien)* 2002;**144**:233–42; discussion 42.

59. Min KW, Seo IS, Song J. Postnatal evolution of the human pineal gland. An immunohistochemical study. *Lab Invest* 1987;**57**:724–8.

60. Min KW, Scheithauer BW, Bauserman SC. Pineal parenchymal tumors: an ultrastructural study with prognostic implications. *Ultrastruct Pathol* 1994;**18**:69–85.

61. Nakamura H, Makino K, Kochi M, et al. Successful treatment of neoadjuvant therapy for papillary tumor of the pineal region. *Brain Tumor Pathol* 2009;**26**:73–7.

62. Nakamura M, Saeki N, Iwadate Y, et al. Neuroradiological characteristics of pineocytoma and pineoblastoma. *Neuroradiology* 2000;**42**:509–14.

63. Nakazato Y, Jouvet A, Scheithauer BW. Tumours of the pineal region. In: Louis DN, Ohgaki H, Wiestler OD, Cavenee WK, eds. *WHO classification of tumours of the central nervous system*. Lyon: International Agency for Research on Cancer, 2007;122–7.

64. Nishida A, Furukawa A, Koike C, et al. Otx2 homeobox gene controls retinal photoreceptor cell fate and pineal gland development. *Nat Neurosci* 2003;**6**:1255–63.

65. Nitta J, Tada T, Kyoshima K, et al. Atypical pleomorphic astrocytoma in the pineal gland: case report. *Neurosurgery* 2001;**49**:1458–60; discussion 60–1.

66. Numoto RT. Pineal parenchymal tumors: cell differentiation and prognosis. *J Cancer Res Clin Oncol* 1994;**120**:683–90.

67. Pastel DA, Mamourian AC, Duhaime AC. Internal structure in pineal cysts on high-resolution magnetic resonance imaging: not a sign of malignancy. *J Neurosurg Pediatr* 2009;**4**:81–4.

68. Patel AJ, Fuller GN, Wildrick DM, et al. Pineal cyst apoplexy: case report and review of the literature. *Neurosurgery* 2005;**57**:E1066.

69. Perentes E, Rubinstein LJ, Herman MM, et al. S-antigen immunoreactivity in human pineal glands and pineal parenchymal tumors. A monoclonal antibody study. *Acta Neuropathol* 1986;**71**:224–7.

70. Plowman PN, Pizer B, Kingston JE. Pineal parenchymal tumours: II. On the aggressive behaviour of pineoblastoma in patients with an inherited mutation of the RB1 gene. *Clin Oncol (R Coll Radiol)* 2004;**16**:244–7.

71. Poulgrain K, Gurgo R, Winter C, et al. Papillary tumour of the pineal region. *J Clin Neurosci* 2011;**18**:1007–17.

72. Rainho CA, Rogatto SR, de Moraes LC, et al. Cytogenetic study of a pineocytoma. *Cancer Genet Cytogenet* 1992;**64**:127–32.

73. Rath MF, Munoz E, Ganguly S, et al. Expression of the Otx2 homeobox gene in the developing mammalian brain: embryonic and adult expression in the pineal gland. *J Neurochem* 2006;**97**:556–66.

74. Reyns N, Hayashi M, Chinot O, et al. The role of gamma knife radiosurgery in the treatment of pineal parenchymal tumours. *Acta Neurochir (Wien)* 2006;**148**:5–11; discussion.

75. Rickard KA, Parker JR, Vitaz TW, et al. Papillary tumor of the pineal region: two case studies and a review of the literature. *Ann Clin Lab Sci* 2011;**41**:174–81.

76. Rickert CH, Simon R, Bergmann M, et al. Comparative genomic hybridization in pineal parenchymal tumors. *Genes Chromosomes Cancer* 2001;**30**:99–104.

77. Russo C, Pellarin M, Tingby O, et al. Comparative genomic hybridization in patients with supratentorial and infratentorial primitive neuroectodermal tumors. *Cancer* 1999;**86**:331–9.

78. Sawamura Y, Ikeda J, Ozawa M, et al. Magnetic resonance images reveal a high incidence of asymptomatic pineal cysts in young women. *Neurosurgery* 1995;**37**: 11–15; discussion 5–6.

79. Schild SE, Scheithauer BW, Schomberg PJ, et al. Pineal parenchymal tumors. Clinical, pathologic, and therapeutic aspects. *Cancer* 1993;**72**:870–80.

80. Schild SE, Scheithauer BW, Haddock MG, et al. Histologically confirmed pineal tumors and other germ cell tumors of the brain. *Cancer* 1996;**78**:2564–71.

81. Sharma MC, Jain D, Sarkar C, et al. Papillary tumor of the pineal region – a recently described entity: a report of three cases and review of the literature. *Clin Neuropathol* 2009;**28**:295–302.

82. Shibahara J, Todo T, Morita A, et al. Papillary neuroepithelial tumor of the pineal region. A case report. *Acta Neuropathol* 2004;**108**:337–40.

83. Smith AB, Rushing EJ, Smirniotopoulos JG. From the archives of the AFIP: lesions of the pineal region: radiologic–pathologic correlation. *Radiographics* 2010;**30**:2001–20.

84. Snipes GJ, Horoupian DS, Shuer LM, et al. Pleomorphic granular cell astrocytoma of the pineal gland. *Cancer* 1992;**70**:2159–65.

85. Stoiber EM, Schaible B, Herfarth K, et al. Long term outcome of adolescent and adult patients with pineal parenchymal tumors treated with fractionated radiotherapy between 1982 and 2003 – a single institution's experience. *Radiat Oncol* 2010;**5**:122.

86. Tate MC, Rutkowski MJ, Parsa AT. Contemporary management of pineoblastoma. *Neurosurg Clin N Am* 2011;**22**:409–12.

87. Taylor M, Mainprize TG, Squire JA, et al. Molecular genetics of pineal region neoplasms. *J Neurooncol* 2001;**54**:219–38.

88. Taylor MD, Mainprize TG, Rutka JT. Molecular insight into medulloblastoma and central nervous system primitive neuroectodermal tumor biology from hereditary syndromes: a review. *Neurosurgery* 2000;**47**:888–901.

89. Timmermann B, Kortmann RD, Kuhl J, et al. Role of radiotherapy in the treatment of supratentorial primitive neuroectodermal tumors in childhood: results of the prospective German brain tumor trials HIT 88/89 and 91. *J Clin Oncol* 2002;**20**:842–9.

90. Trojanowski JQ, Tascos NA, Rorke LB. Malignant pineocytoma with prominent papillary features. *Cancer* 1982;**50**:1789–93.

91. Tsumanuma I, Sato M, Okazaki H, et al. The analysis of p53 tumor suppressor gene in pineal parenchymal tumors. *Noshuyo Byori* 1995;**12**:39–43.

92. Vaquero J, Coca S, Martinez R, et al. Papillary pineocytoma. Case report. *J Neurosurg* 1990;**73**:135–7.

93. Vaquero J, Ramiro J, Martinez R. Glioblastoma multiforme of the pineal region. *J Neurosurg Sci* 1990;**34**:149–50.

94. Williams BO, Remington L, Albert DM, et al. Cooperative tumorigenic effects of germline mutations in Rb and p53. *Nat Genet* 1994;**7**:480–4.

95. Yano H, Ohe N, Nakayama N, et al. Clinicopathological features from long-term observation of a papillary tumor of the pineal region (PTPR): a case report. *Brain Tumor Pathol* 2009;**26**:83–8.

CHAPTER

34

Embryonal Tumours

Charles Eberhart

INTRODUCTION

Of the central nervous system (CNS) embryonal tumours, the medulloblastoma is by far the most common, accounting for approximately 90 per cent of cases. Other embryonal neoplasms listed in the World Health Organization (WHO) classification of nervous system tumours are the medulloepithelioma, ependymoblastoma, atypical teratoid/rhabdoid tumour (ATRT) and CNS primitive neuroectodermal tumour (PNET).[116] Medulloblastoma includes several variants, such as desmoplastic/nodular medulloblastoma and large cell/anaplastic medulloblastoma, and these are increasingly being linked to molecular classification schemes. Although undifferentiated neuroepithelial cells characterize all CNS embryonal tumours, ATRT, medulloepithelioma and ependymoblastoma each exhibit idiosyncratic histopathological features that have historically set these three tumours apart from the medulloblastoma and most CNS PNET.

The term 'primitive neuroectodermal tumour' was introduced for all embryonal neuroepithelial tumours composed of undifferentiated small cells with a high nuclear:cytoplasmic (N/C) ratio, but without distinctive architectural or cytological features.[82] Thus, it was a diagnosis of exclusion, once medulloepithelioma, ependymoblastoma, central neuroblastoma and medulloblastoma had been eliminated. Later, a proposal was advanced to draw together all of these embryonal tumours under the PNET umbrella, with some separation based on the degree of differentiation along neuronal, glial and ependymal lines.[164]

The conceptual basis for classifying various embryonal tumours together as PNETs was that they all have the capacity for neuronal and glial differentiation and might share a common cell of origin from the subependymal germinal matrix. This principle also has the potential advantage that these tumours can be assimilated for therapeutic purposes. However, it has become clear that the various embryonal tumours harbour distinct genetic abnormalities and may show different responses to the same treatment regimens; thus medulloblastoma and CNS PNET are now regarded as distinct entities. Indeed, multiple discrete subtypes showing specific clinical, pathological and molecular features are being described within the broader medulloblastoma and CNS PNET groups.[132,193]

In this section on embryonal tumours, medulloblastoma and CNS PNET not otherwise specified are discussed first because of their histopathological similarities and the tendency for most epidemiological, clinical and molecular studies to amalgamate these two entities, whereas rarer and histopathologically distinct CNS embryonal tumours are considered later.

MEDULLOBLASTOMA AND PRIMITIVE NEUROECTODERMAL TUMOURS

Epidemiology

Embryonal neoplasms represent 1.1 per cent of all benign and malignant brain tumours according to the 2012 report of the Central Brain Tumor Registry of the United States (www.cbtrus.org). They occur predominantly in childhood, and a significant proportion present in the first few years of life. The medulloblastoma is by far the most common, with a peak age of about 7 years.[116] Several congenital cases have been reported, indicating the potential for neoplastic transformation during prenatal development. In the first year of life, medulloblastomas account for 13–25 per cent of all intracranial tumours.[187] An analysis of Surveillance, Epidemiology and End Results (SEER) data from 1973 to 2007 identified an overall medulloblastoma incidence of 6.0 per million in children 1 to 9 years of age, compared to an incidence of 0.6 per million in adults over 19 years of age.[184] Although some reports have suggested these tumours are being more commonly encountered, this recent SEER analysis found that the incidence of medulloblastoma has not increased over time. Medulloblastoma is a tumour that preferentially affects males. In two International Society of Paediatric Oncology (SIOP) trials, a male:female ratio of about 1.6:1 has been reported.[10,194] However, this difference in incidence between males and females is not observed in medulloblastoma arising in adults.[184] Both age and gender have been shown to associate in specific ways with emerging molecular subgroups.[193]

The precise incidence of CNS PNET is difficult to determine because of differing viewpoints on classification, but collectively they likely account for 1 per cent or less of primary brain tumours. Many supratentorial PNETs show some signs of morphological differentiation along neuronal lines, being designated as cerebral neuroblastomas or ganglioneuroblastomas, but others are indistinguishable from the medulloblastoma.[15,116] Over 80 per cent of cases registered in the largest cerebral neuroblastoma series reported to date occurred in the first decade of life, over half in children 5 years old or younger and about 25 per cent in infants, with no evident sex predilection.[15] In a more recently reported cohort of 142 molecularly analysed hemispheric CNS PNET, more than 50% arose in children over 4 years of age.[149] Cerebral PNETs have been reported in the elderly.[136] However, it is not clear if embryonal-appearing tumours showing only glial differentiation are a glioblastoma variant or CNS PNET. Unusual sites for PNET include the bulbar region, cerebellopontine angle, spinal cord and cauda equina.[101,116]

Clinical Features

Patients with embryonal tumours tend to present acutely with raised intracranial pressure. Some with epilepsy or focal neurological signs reflect tumour location. In the case of childhood medulloblastoma, which is located in the cerebellar vermis in at least 75 per cent of children, raised intracranial pressure is frequently a consequence of acute obstructive hydrocephalus. In infants with embryonal tumours, lethargy and increased head circumference are common presenting features. When metastatic disease within the neuraxis exists at presentation, spinal cord disease may manifest as subtle, non-specific symptoms and signs, such as backache and difficulty with micturition. In this clinical context, neuroimaging usually identifies the tumour, but is not sufficiently specific to indicate a diagnosis of embryonal tumour.

Radiology

Despite a propensity to invade adjacent brain, many embryonal tumours appear demarcated on neuroimaging. They can be hypodense, isodense or hyperdense on precontrast computed tomography (CT) scans, and generally show patchy enhancement with contrast. The detection of metastatic disease, which occurs at presentation in up to a third of patients, is important for therapeutic stratification and prognosis. Gadolinium-enhanced magnetic resonance (MR) images are a good way to detect the spread of small metastatic deposits of tumour to the spinal cord and nerves.

Medulloblastomas appear as solid, contrast-enhancing masses (Figure 34.1). Those in the vermis are usually circumscribed, and descend into the fourth ventricle from its roof; this is in contrast to ependymomas, which usually grow out from its floor. Calcifications are usually absent. The T2-weighted MR images are usually isodense or hypodense compared with normal grey matter. Medulloblastomas involving the lateral cerebellar hemispheres occasionally

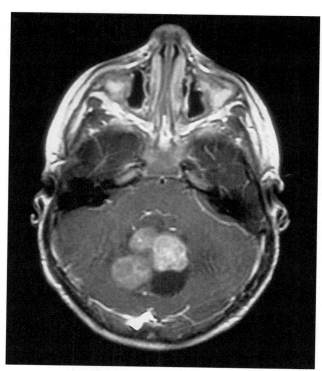

34.1 Medulloblastoma. Axial T1-weighted, post-gadolinium magnetic resonance imaging, showing an enhancing mass posterior to the fourth ventricle.

Courtesy of Dr CC Penney, King' Healthcare NHS Trust, London, UK.

appear as extra-axial lesions simulating meningiomas or vestibular schwannomas.[13] The medulloblastoma with extensive nodularity (MBEN), a variant of desmoplastic medulloblastoma, often looks like a bunch of grapes on MR imaging because of its distinctive and extensive nodular architecture.[71] Similarly, medullomyoblastomas containing large islands of rhabdomyoblastic and neuroectodermal cells can demonstrate a nodular pattern.[85] Diffusion-weighted imaging can have utility in distinguishing medulloblastoma from other paediatric cerebellar tumours such as ependymoma and pilocytic astrocytoma, but some overlap exists.[75,92] A neuroradiological scheme for grading the extent of metastatic spread shown by medulloblastomas (Chang stage) is used widely in therapeutic stratification.[34]

CNS PNETs can be extensive, often combining large mass with evidence of cerebrospinal fluid (CSF) spread. They often present a striking picture, which includes marked midline shift, cyst formation associated with necrosis, haemorrhage and focal calcification.[151] Signal heterogeneity in non-enhanced CT and T1- or T2-weighted MR images is common.

Macroscopic Appearances

Many medulloblastomas are located in the midline, appearing as pink or grey masses that arise in the region of the vermis to occupy the fourth ventricle (Figure 34.2). Lateral placement is more frequent in adulthood and with the desmoplastic

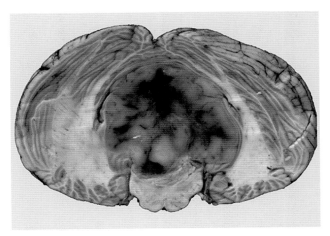

34.2 Medulloblastoma. Large medulloblastoma occupying the fourth ventricle and compressing the cerebellar hemispheres and the medulla oblongata.

variant.[73] The desmoplastic medulloblastoma tends to be more firm and circumscribed than the classic variant. Neoplastic cells may spread over the surface of the cerebellar hemisphere or the floor of the fourth ventricle and usually invade the cerebellar cortex. Involvement of the subarachnoid space is common. Metastatic spread may occur within the neuraxis producing distinct nodules of tumour or, less often, a coating of the pial or ventricular surfaces. Evidence of spread outside the CNS is rare and usually late in the evolution of disease.[33] Medulloblastoma most often spreads to lymph nodes or bone marrow, but there are also examples of peritoneal seeding through a ventriculoperitoneal shunt.[48]

Not surprisingly, cerebral PNETs and medulloblastomas have similar macroscopic appearances. Some cerebral PNETs appear quite circumscribed, but invasion of the brain can produce a multifocal appearance. When tumour cells invade the ventricular system, multiple deposits are evident throughout the neuraxis. Large areas of necrosis can produce a cystic appearance.

In surgical biopsy specimens, embryonal tumours are soft, but not mucoid, and sometimes appear to have a slightly granular surface. The fresh specimen usually appears deep pink. In contrast to high-grade gliomas, macroscopic necrosis or a filigree of angiogenesis is uncommon. During craniotomy for resection of a medulloblastoma, the first neoplastic tissue encountered by the surgeon is often that submitted to the pathologist, and it is not uncommon to receive leptomeningeal deposits of tumour in this situation. This tissue is firm because of the leptomeningeal desmoplasia provoked by neoplastic infiltration. If the leptomeningeal location of the sample is confirmed during intraoperative histopathological assessment, it is important to request further sampling of the tumour in order to gauge the full range of the tumour's architectural and cytological features.

Microscopic Appearances

Classic Medulloblastoma

The most common variant of medulloblastoma consists of sheets of primitive appearing cells with round or oval hyperchromatic nuclei surrounded by scant cytoplasm

(Figure 34.3a). The resultant high N/C ratio is characteristic. In addition, groups of monomorphic neurocyte-like cells with round nuclei, in which the chromatin is less condensed, are occasionally found.

Neuroblastic (Homer Wright) rosettes consisting of tumour nuclei arranged in a circular fashion around fine cytoplasmic processes may be observed (Figure 34.3b). However, prominent perivascular anuclear zones and true rosettes with central lumens are not typical, and when present raise the diagnostic possibility of ependymoma. Ribbons of medulloblastoma nuclei may be arranged with their long axes in parallel, resembling a picket fence, a pattern seen when columns of tumour cells invade along radial glia through the molecular layer of the cerebellum (Figure 34.3c). Other patterns of invasion observed in biopsy material include diffuse permeation of cerebellar tissue and subpial accumulation of neoplastic cells resembling a persistent fetal external granular layer. When medulloblastoma cells spread within the subarachnoid space, they may take the path of least resistance when invading back into cerebellar cortex, spreading along the perivascular (Virchow–Robin) spaces of penetrating vessels. Tumour cells in the subarachnoid space may elicit a considerable desmoplastic reaction with ribbons or small clusters of neoplastic cells entrapped among collagenous fibres. Surrounded by desmoplasia in this location, tumour cells often appear more pleomorphic than within parenchymal masses.

Other architectural features include angiogenesis and foci of necrosis. A supporting network of small blood vessels is usually present, but only rarely do the new vessels exhibit mural hyperplasia as exemplified by the glomeruloid vessels of high-grade gliomas. Areas of necrosis are less common than expected for a primitive neoplasm, but in rare cases, may show circumferential pseudopalisading similar to that observed in glioblastomas.

Morphological differentiation in medulloblastomas may take various forms, but is principally along neuroepithelial lines; other types of differentiation, such as rhabdomyoblastic (medullomyoblastoma) are rare. Neuronal differentiation is most common, but is often only apparent upon immunohistochemical analysis.[29] Small irregularly outlined groups of mature neurocytic or ganglion cells are found in a small number of medulloblastomas (Figure 34.3d). Glial differentiation is uncommon and usually takes the form of scattered small groups of cells with an astrocytic phenotype.[29,54] If the glial features predominate, however, one should consider a cellular glioblastoma in the differential diagnosis. Mitotic figures are readily detected but can be surprisingly difficult to find in some medulloblastomas. Apoptotic bodies are usually frequent and often outnumber mitoses.

Large Cell/Anaplastic Medulloblastoma

The rare large cell medulloblastoma contains cells at least twice the size of those in classic medulloblastomas.[123] It has an idiosyncratic phenotype characterized by often discohesive cells with uniform round vesicular nuclei and a single prominent nucleolus (Figure 34.4a).[46,54,72,123] The tumour cells are arranged in sheets and have the high N/C ratio expected of a medulloblastoma, though some exhibit more cytoplasm than most cells in a classic medulloblastoma.

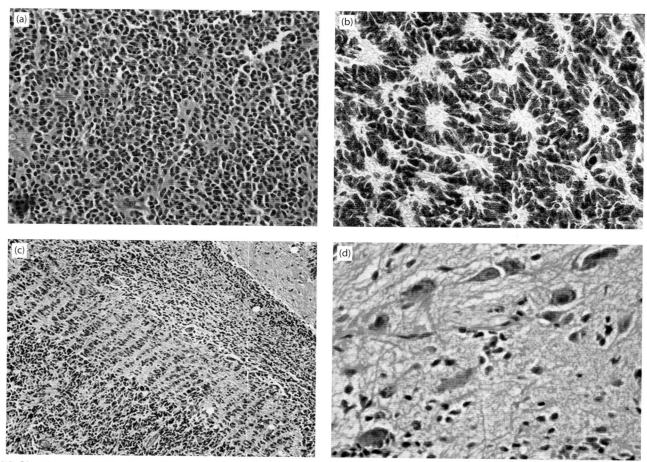

34.3 Classic medulloblastoma. (a) A sheet of uniform cells with a high cell density. **(b)** Numerous neuroblastic (Homer Wright) rosettes. **(c)** Formation of parallel bands of tumour cells at right angles to the pial surface. **(d)** Some ganglion cells are admixed with a lower density of small hyperchromatic tumour cells against a neuropil-like background.

Mitotic figures are readily found and large cell medulloblastomas have a higher average mitotic index than classic medulloblastomas.[123] Although large cell medulloblastoma sometimes appears pure, many tumours are heterogeneous, consisting of mixtures of enlarged and either classic or anaplastic elements (Figure 34.4b).

Anaplastic medulloblastoma cells are characterized by enlarged, pleomorphic polyhedral nuclei and a distinctive nuclear moulding, which produces a paving-like or mosaic pattern (Figure 34.4c).[46,72] Cannibalistic wrapping of one cell around another, with the engulfed cell often undergoing cell death, is an additional feature of diagnostic utility (Figure 34.4d). As in large cell medulloblastoma, mitotic and apoptotic rates are typically high.[46] Because large cell and anaplastic elements often coexist, this group of tumours is often combined into a single large cell/anaplastic category, accounting for roughly 10-15 per cent of all medulloblastomas. Individual large or anaplastic cells can be found focally in many medulloblastoma, but should comprise a significant fraction (ideally the majority) of a lesion before it is designated large cell/anaplastic.

Desmoplastic/Nodular Medulloblastoma

Desmoplasia may occur focally in many medulloblastomas.[50,54,144] It invariably occurs as a reactive phenomenon where tumour cells invade the leptomeninges. However, it manifests as a specific phenomenon in the desmoplastic/nodular medulloblastoma, in which collagen deposition is not secondary to meningeal invasion. Instead, it surrounds round to oval reticulin-free zones or 'pale islands'. These nodules, which represent zones of neuronal maturation, exhibit a reduced N/C ratio, a fibrillary neuropil-like matrix and uniform cells with neurocytic appearance (Figure 34.5a). This intranodular maturation is accompanied by decreased proliferative activity and increased apoptosis.[49] Internodular zones are characterized by densely packed mitotically active cells with hyperchromatic and moderately pleomorphic nuclei. Coursing through the internodular zones is a network of reticulin-positive fibres (Figure 34.5b).

In the typical desmoplastic/nodular medulloblastoma, neurocytic nodules and desmoplastic internodular regions are readily identified, but nodules may be more obvious in some areas than others. In a few 'paucinodular' cases, nodules can be hard to find and may only evince marginally decreased cellularity compared with internodular zones. In this situation, a reticulin preparation and immunohistochemistry for neuronal markers helps to delineate the subtle pattern of nodule formation and differentiation.

In contrast, nodules are large and patently obvious in the MBEN, a variant previously designated 'cerebellar neuroblastoma'. It occurs in infants and is associated with a good

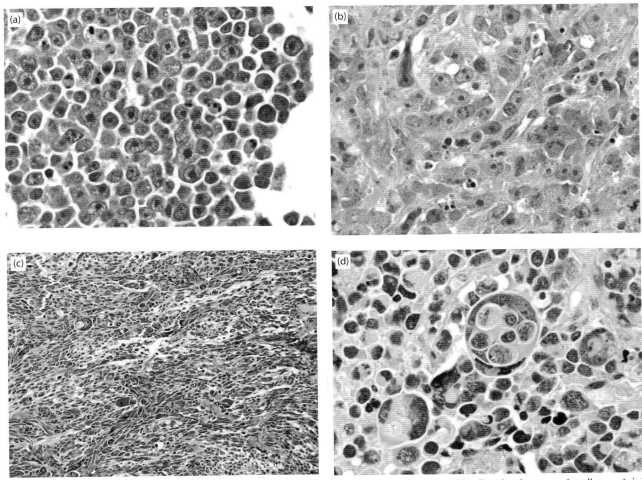

34.4 Large cell and anaplastic medulloblastomas. (a) Large cell medulloblastoma with discohesive round cells containing prominent single central nucleoli. **(b)** In another region, this tumour had a more anaplastic phenotype. **(c)** Anaplasia combines large polyhedral cells with a paving-like pattern and high mitotic and apoptotic counts. **(d)** Marked anaplasia is sometimes associated with cellular cannibalism with some tumour cells phagocytosing others.

Images (c) and (d) courtesy of Arie Perry, UCSF, San Francisco, CA, USA.

prognosis.[71] It differs from the typical nodular/desmoplastic variant by having an expanded lobular architecture, in which the neurocytic nodules become elongated, or sometimes reniform, and unusually neuropil rich (Figure 34.5c). Within the nodules, neurocytic cells exhibit a remarkable uniformity and are essentially devoid of mitotic activity. Streaming patterns and circumferential anuclear zones are characteristic. The internodular component is markedly reduced in some areas, but retains the architectural and cytological features of this component in others. Following radiotherapy and/or chemotherapy, MBENs occasionally undergo further maturation to tumours dominated by ganglion cells.[37]

Medulloblastoma with Myogenic or Melanotic Differentiation

Given the multipotent nature of embryonal tumours, it is not surprising that both myogenic and melanotic differentiation are occasionally present in medulloblastoma, leading to tumours once referred to as medullomyoblastoma

and melanocytic medulloblastoma. These were previously regarded as distinct but rare medulloblastoma variants; however, because the genetic changes and clinical outcomes are not clearly distinct from other embryonal tumours, they are now considered intriguing differentiation patterns rather than true tumour variants.[116]

In medullomyoblastoma the myoblastic elements may form either distinct groups or scattered cells (Figure 34.5d). Early reported examples were identified by the presence of elongated rhabdomyoblasts with cross-striations. However, globular myoblastic cells that dwarf the neuroectodermal cells can also be present. Although in the majority of reported cases, the neuroectodermal component has features of classic medulloblastoma, nodular/desmoplastic and large cell/anaplastic phenotypes have also been reported.[85,111]

Melanotic medulloblastomas are extremely rare (Figure 34.5e), and are characterized by neuroectodermal cells displaying intracytoplasmic melanin pigment.[42] The melanotic cells may have an epithelioid phenotype and occasionally form small acinar structures, reminiscent of pigmented retinal epithelium. Case reports

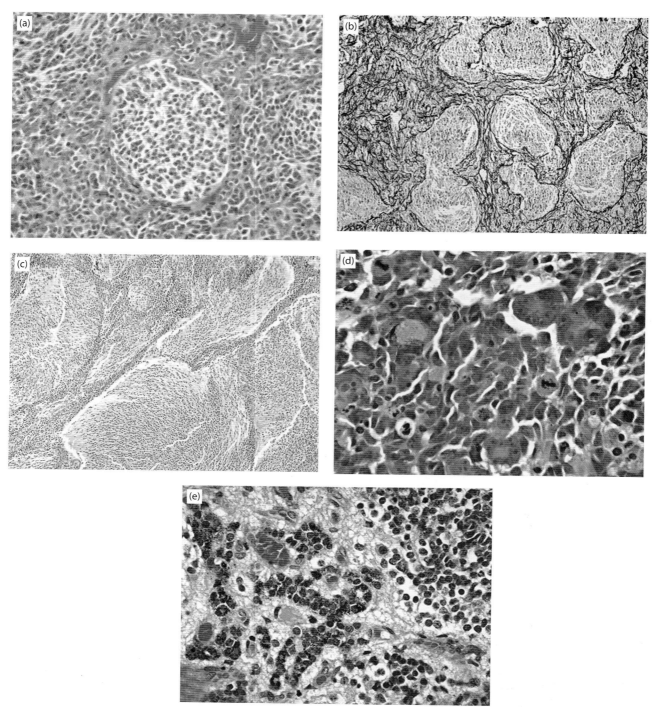

34.5 Desmoplastic/nodular medulloblastoma. (a) Round to oval islands with low cellularity are typical of desmoplastic medulloblastoma. **(b)** Reticulin-free islands, surrounded by highly cellular reticulin-forming tumour cells. Gomori's reticulin stain. **(c)** Extensive nodularity with typical cell streaming in the fibrillary background. **(d)** Medullomyoblastoma. These large pleomorphic cells with eosinophilic cytoplasm were immunoreactive for desmin. **(e)** Melanotic medulloblastoma. Note the pseudo-glandular architecture of melanin-containing tumour cells.

describing a melanotic desmoplastic medulloblastoma and a cerebellar neoplasm that contains both pigmented and rhabdomyoblastic cells support a link between melanotic medulloblastoma, medullomyoblastoma and the more common medulloblastoma variants.[98,152,182] The melanotic medulloblastoma shares some histopathological features with melanotic neuroectodermal tumours of infancy, which develop outside the CNS, typically in the bones of the jaw and skull base, and have a biphasic phenotype consisting of neuroblastic and epithelioid elements.[99,125] However, the two tumours are biologically distinct and most melanotic neuroectodermal tumours of infancy have a much better prognosis than melanotic medulloblastomas.

Extracerebellar Primitive Neuroectodermal Tumours (CNS PNET)

Embryonal tumours located outside the cerebellum, including those with features of neuroblastoma, ganglioneuroblastoma, medulloepithelioma or ependymoblastoma fall under the general designation CNS PNET in the 2007 WHO classification.[116] Those lacking specific morphological features of the above mentioned entities can be classified as CNS PNET not otherwise specified (NOS). Because many occur in the cerebral hemispheres, the term 'supratentorial PNET' is sometimes used, but they can also be encountered at other sites such as the brain stem and spinal cord. It has also recently been suggested that ependymoblastoma is not a distinct diagnostic entity[94] and that many of these lesions represent a CNS PNET variant often referred to as embryonal tumour with abundant neuropil and true rosettes (ETANTR).

Typical CNS neuroblastomas are densely populated by small cells of undifferentiated appearance, which are arranged in patternless sheets or occasionally in regimented palisades.[88,136] Neuroblastic rosettes can be a feature of these tumours, but probably not more frequently than in medulloblastomas (Figure 34.6a). The tumour cells have hyperchromatic nuclei of round, oval or angular contour. Mitotic figures and apoptotic bodies are readily found. Areas of necrosis are present, occasionally with a 'pseudopalisading' pattern reminiscent of glioblastomas, or with dense calcifications as seen in neuroblastomas of the adrenal gland. Desmoplasia is encountered in regions of leptomeningeal invasion, but is not accompanied by the formation of neurocytic nodules. The ganglioneuroblastoma is characterized by a combination of ganglion cells and the neuroblastic phenotype described earlier, either scattered among the small cells or in groups (Figure 34.6b). The ganglion cells can show a range of dysmorphic morphologies but appear terminally differentiated.

Other CNS PNETs look like medulloblastomas and potentially include astrocytic, as well as a neuronal differentiation. Several cases have been described in which mesenchymal elements, including rhabdomyoblastic, smooth muscle, melanotic and lipomatous elements, are present. CNS PNET can show a degree of nuclear pleomorphism and moulding that would approximate the anaplastic variant of medulloblastoma. In one analysis of 33 CNS PNET cases, significant anaplasia was present in 18 (55%) and was associated with decreased survival.[14]

ETANTRs were first described as distinctive paediatric neuroblastic brain tumours containing abundant neuropil and true rosettes.[45] An expanded series of 29 cases found that the tumours were most common in the cerebral cortex of infants, although the cerebellum and brain stem could also be affected.[68] Unlike other embryonal tumours of the CNS, girls were more commonly affected than boys. The microscopic features of ETANTR include prominent mature neuropil and scattered true rosettes formed by pseudo-stratified embryonal cells circumferentially arranged around a central lumen (Figure 34.7). In some cases that otherwise fit the molecular and clinical profile of ETANTR, either the neuropil or true rosettes are absent. This issue usually arises when only small biopsies are obtained. In others, the neuropil-rich zones may be associated with extensive neurocytic differentiation.[43]

Immunohistochemistry

Most commonly, and particularly in cerebral cases, the neuroepithelial lineage of embryonal tumours manifests immunophenotypically as expression of neuronal antigens. Synaptophysin is demonstrated, at least focally, in many PNETs (Figure 34.8a), with Homer Wright rosettes and the 'pale islands' of the nodular/desmoplastic medulloblastoma also strongly expressing this marker (Figure 34.8b). Antibodies to class III β-tubulin and microtubule-associated protein 2 also label these architectural features. Neurofilament protein (NFP) expression occurs less commonly than synaptophysin immunoreactivity among medulloblastomas (Figure 34.8c). However, anti-NFP antibodies pick out ganglion cells in medulloblastomas and ganglioneuroblastomas. Expression of retinal proteins such as retinal S-antigen has also been demonstrated.[190]

Only a minority of medulloblastomas and PNETs contain glial fibrillary acidic protein (GFAP)-positive cells, and these often have the typical spider-like appearance of entrapped reactive astrocytes that are sparsely distributed among the poorly differentiated tumour cells. However,

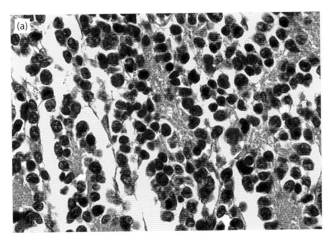
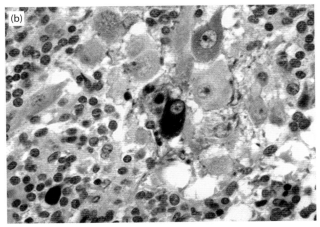

34.6 Central nervous system neuroblastoma and ganglioneuroblastoma. (a) Neuroblastomas are composed of small hyperchromatic cells with delicate fibrillary processes that typically form Homer Wright rosettes. **(b)** Focal ganglion cell maturation is accompanied by the expression of neurofilament proteins. Immunohistochemistry for neurofilament protein.

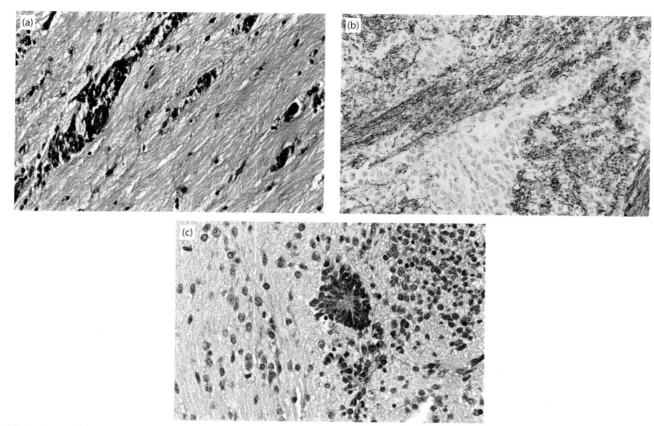

34.7 Embryonal tumour with abundant neuropil and true rosettes. (a) Fine neuropil with only scattered primitive-appearing neoplastic cells is a distinctive element. **(b)** Neurofilament immunostains highlight the neuronal differentiation. **(c)** Both neuroblastic and true rosettes can be found, sometimes standing alone in a neuropil-rich region.

Courtesy of Peter Burger, Johns Hopkins University, Baltimore, MD, USA.

antibodies to this glial intermediate filament also label scattered undifferentiated cells in approximately 10 per cent of tumours (Figure 34.8d). GFAP-positive tumour cells tend to be most abundant in nodular/desmoplastic medulloblastomas where they are concentrated within and rimming the 'pale islands'.

Although they have the capacity to express various markers of neuroepithelial lineage, PNETs may be immunonegative with a standard panel of antibodies to NFP, synaptophysin and GFAP. The immunophenotype of the CNS PNET can also include reactivities for vimentin, neuronal cell adhesion molecules, nerve growth factors and even photoreceptor-associated proteins such as rhodopsin and retinal S-antigen.[23,62,104,190] Neural stem/progenitor markers, including CD133, LIN28, OLIG2, nestin, BMI1, and CD15, have also been detected in medulloblastoma and CNS PNET using immunohistochemistry.[149]

Immunohistochemistry with antibodies to cell cycle antigens reveals a high proportion of proliferating tumour cells in medulloblastoma and PNETs. Labelling indices with Ki-67 antibodies are usually above 30 per cent and are among the highest shown by CNS tumours. However, Ki-67 nuclear labelling may vary greatly and is notably low in regions of neuronal differentiation, such as 'pale islands' of desmoplastic/nodular tumours. Though large cell/ anaplastic variants typically have mitotic counts that are greater than those of classic medulloblastomas, the Ki-67 labelling indices were no different in one study.[123]

Differential Diagnosis

Age is clearly a critical factor to consider when encountering embryonal-appearing tumours. In a child, the presentation of a systemic tumour as metastatic disease in the CNS is an exceptional clinicopathological scenario, though metastatic neuroblastoma, retinoblastoma or lymphoma could enter the differential diagnosis of CNS PNET in the appropriate setting. Alternatively, other considerations include primary poorly differentiated CNS tumours such as high-grade glioma, ependymoma, choroid plexus carcinoma, pineoblastoma, ATRT and germ cell tumour (mainly immature teratoma). This list also applies to an adult patient with a suspected PNET, but choroid plexus carcinoma and ATRT are less likely, whereas the possibility of a metastatic tumour, particularly secondary small cell lung carcinoma, should be considered.

Small cell glioblastomas and anaplastic oligodendrogliomas can occasionally resemble medulloblastoma and PNET because of their hypercellularity and high N/C ratios. Artefactual perinuclear clearing may be histopathological features in either of these gliomas, yet would not be expected in PNET. A predominantly neuronal immunophenotype supports a diagnosis of PNET, but otherwise, distinguishing

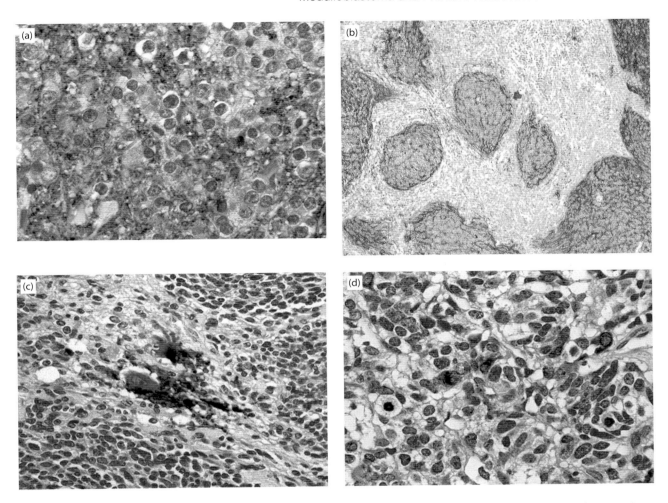

34.8 Medulloblastoma. (a) Synaptophysin expression with predominant immunoreactivity at the cell membrane and between tumour cells. **(b)** Synaptophysin expression in nodular islands of low cellularity. Immunohistochemistry for synaptophysin. **(c)** Focal expression of neurofilament protein (NFP) in neurons. Immunohistochemistry for NFP. **(d)** Astrocytic differentiation indicated by contain glial fibrillary acidic protein immunoreactivity.

these entities is occasionally difficult. Molecular studies can be of use, because loss of chromosomal arms 1p and 19q or mutations in *IDH1* would support a diagnosis of anaplastic oligodendroglioma, whereas amplification of *EGFR* is more frequent in small cell glioblastoma. In both children and adults, it is increasingly recognized that PNET-like regions can arise in the setting of malignant glioma,[185] with *N-myc* and *c-myc* gene amplification associated with the embryonal phenotype in a significant number of cases.[145] Such cases share the increased propensity to metastasize through the CSF as primary embryonal tumours, although the optimal therapy for such patients has yet to be determined.

From a therapeutic perspective, ependymoma is an important tumour to distinguish from embryonal tumours, especially from childhood medulloblastoma in the region of the fourth ventricle. Ependymomas lack the propensity of PNETs to invade adjacent brain and often display idiosyncratic architectural features, such as nodules of increased cell density and ependymal rosettes or canals. Ependymomas usually lack a neuronal immunophenotype and display immunoreactivity for epithelial membrane antigen (EMA), often as dot-like intracytoplasmic deposits.

In infants, choroid plexus carcinomas may present as large intracerebral masses that resemble PNETs at both macroscopic and microscopic levels. Choroid plexus carcinomas may retain a papillary architecture and an epithelioid phenotype in some regions, which set them apart from PNETs. Additionally, the diagnosis of choroid plexus carcinoma is supported by immunoreactivity for cytokeratins, Kir7.1 and stanniocalcin.[83]

In the 1993 WHO classification of nervous system tumours, pineoblastomas were included among the embryonal tumours because of their close histopathological resemblance to PNETs. Only site reliably sets these two entities apart. Though among the differential diagnosis of PNET, teratoma only poses a problem when immature neuroepithelium dominates a small biopsy; the presence of more mature elements from the three tissue lineages reveals the true nature of the neoplasm.

Finally, clusters of rhabdoid cells in an embryonal tumour can alert the pathologist to the diagnosis of ATRT. However, these may not be present, and *SMARCB1/INI1* immunohistochemistry is now routinely used to rule out ATRT in embryonal neoplasms, particularly those from infants.[14,93] Additional markers highlighting the polyphenotypic profile of ATRT and distinguishing it from medulloblastoma and CNS PNET are EMA and actin, with the former often showing strong but very focal immunoreactivity in small clusters of cells.

Histogenesis of Embryonal Brain Tumours

Increasingly detailed profiling of genetic alterations and mRNA expression, complemented by transgenic mouse models, has begun to unravel the complex histogenesis of medulloblastoma and other embryonal brain tumours. In general, these studies suggest that various embryonal tumour subgroups arise from cells that are distinct in terms of their location and differentiation status. They also support the notion that oncogenic molecular 'drivers' do not efficiently promote tumour formation in all cells; rather, the inciting genetic event must occur in specific cells of origin in order for tumours to arise. It also seems that despite the multipotent, stem-like phenotype displayed by embryonal tumours, in some animal models genetically altered cells must commit to a specific lineage before exuberant neoplastic growth can occur.

Histogenesis of Medulloblastoma

Theories of histogenesis have long revolved around ventricular zone stem cells[164] and progenitors in the cerebellar external granule cell layer (EGL).[4,97,166] The EGL is formed when undifferentiated neuroepithelial cells migrate from the roof of the fourth ventricle to the rhombic lip and then onto the surface of the nascent cerebellar cortex. These cells proliferate in the EGL before migrating inward through the molecular layer to form internal granule cell layer neurons. Because the EGL is unique to the cerebellum, it provides an intriguing substrate in which medulloblastomas localized to this portion of the brain could form.

Over the last decade it has become clear that the medulloblastoma subgroup associated with Sonic Hedgehog (Shh) signalling indeed arise from EGL progenitors. Proliferation of these superficial cells during normal cerebellar development is strongly promoted by Shh activity, and genetic alterations activating the pathway are sufficient to induce medulloblastoma formation in EGL progenitors in transgenic mouse models.[77,137] Interestingly, when the pathway is activated in periventricular stem cells, medulloblastomas only form after cells commit to the rhombic lip lineage, which forms the EGL.[178,210]

Other molecular subgroups seem to have distinct cellular origins. Although Shh-associated tumours usually arise in the lateral cerebellar hemispheres where the bulk of EGL progenitors reside, medulloblastomas with high levels of WNT signalling more often localize to the midline of the posterior fossa.[73] Consistent with this distribution in humans, WNT activation in transgenic mice generates medulloblastoma from midline neural progenitors in the dorsal brain stem, but not from EGL precursors.[73] Clinically aggressive tumours associated with high c-myc (MYC) levels have a more stem-like phenotype, and can be generated most efficiently in mice from stem cells located in postnatal animals in the cerebellar white matter and other sites.[100,142] EGL precursors can also be transformed by increased MYC activity and loss of p53 function, but lose their lineage markers and take on a stem-like phenotype, suggesting that de-differentiation can play a role in the final cellular phenotypes of medulloblastoma.

Molecular Abnormalities in Medulloblastoma and Primitive Neuroectodermal Tumours

Medulloblastoma: Molecular Genetics Overview

The application of array-based comparative genomic hybridization, advanced expression profiling and next-generation sequencing to increasingly larger medulloblastoma cohorts has resulted in an explosion of molecular knowledge. It has become clear that four main molecular medulloblastoma subgroups exist, each with significant clinical and pathological associations. These are outlined in Figure 34.9, and specific genetic and epigenic changes are probably best considered within the framework of this molecular subgroup structure. Important early discoveries as well as more recent analyses of medulloblastoma genetics are summarized later.

Medulloblastoma: Cytogenetics and General Features

Abnormalities affecting chromosome 17 are most common and are concentrated in medulloblastoma subgroups 3 and 4. Isochromosome or isodicentric 17q (i[17q]), which is characterized by common breakpoints at 17p11.2 or in the pericentromeric region of chromosome 17, is present in about one-third of cases (Figure 34.10a).[18,130,175] Although i[17q] is the most common mechanism for loss of 17p in medulloblastomas, partial or complete loss of 17p occurs through interstitial deletion, unbalanced translocation or in monosomy 17, and up to 50 per cent of tumours show this abnormality. Loss of chromosome 6 is associated with the WNT subgroup, whereas loss of chromosomal arm 9q is found predominantly in tumours with high levels of Shh activity.[36,133,193] Cytogenetic methods have also suggested the presence of gene amplifications (see next section).

Medulloblastoma: Molecular Genetics, General Features

Gene amplification is featured in a subset of medulloblastomas. Double minute chromosomes are observed in some tumours, frequently involving amplification of the myc family of oncogenic transcription factors.[20] Amplification of MYC is evident in a significantly higher proportion of medulloblastoma cell lines than tumour samples, suggesting that the oncogene may confer a growth advantage *in vitro* (Figure 34.10b). Amplifications of the MYCN (at 2p24) and MYC (at 8q24) genes have each been reported in 5–15 per cent of medulloblastomas, and have been linked with both poor prognosis and the large cell and anaplastic variants.[3,51,108] Amplifications of both MYCN and MYC are rarely found together in a medulloblastoma.

Another oncogene strongly implicated in the pathogenesis of medulloblastoma is orthodenticle homologue 2 (*OTX2*). Two studies independently revealed a novel amplicon at 14q22, which included the *OTX2* gene, in about 20 per cent of medulloblastoma cell lines and many primary tumours with anaplastic features.[24,39] RNA and protein analyses of OTX2 in a larger cohort of medulloblastoma demonstrated expression in over 70 per cent of tumours.[38] It was subsequently shown that OTX2 is altered predominantly in group

	WNT	SHH	Group 3	Group 4
Subgroup Prevalence	7–8%	28–32%	26–27%	34–38%
Common Histology	Classic	Desmoplastic/ Nodular	Classic LC/A	Classic
Clinical Outcome	Very Good	Good to Intermediate	Poor	Intermediate
Chromosomal Changes	–6	–9q, GLI2 Amp MYCN Amp	i(17q), –17p MYCC Amp	i(17q), –17p, –X CDK6 Amp MYCN Amp
Mutations	CTNNB1	PTCH, SMO SUFU		
Gene Expression	WNT	SHH	MYC,GABAergic Photoreceptor OTX2	Neuronal, OTX2 Glutamatergic
Cellular Origin/ Phenotype	Dorsal Brainstem Progenitor	Cerebellar EGL	Cerebellar Stem Cell	?

34.9 Molecular subtypes of medulloblastoma. EGL, external granule cell layer; LC/A, large cell/anaplastic; Shh, Sonic hedgehog; SMO, smoothened; SUFU, Suppressor of Fused.

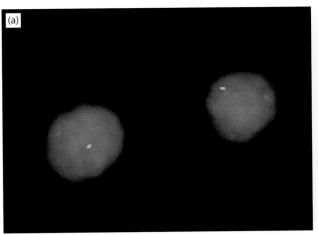
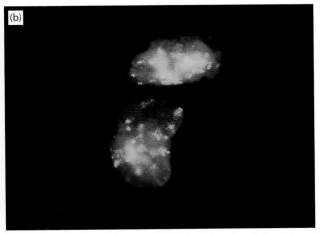

34.10 Medulloblastoma. (a) Loss of chromosome 17p. One green signal from the 17p13.3 probe is detected and focal loss is inferred from the presence of two red signals from a centromeric probe. **(b)** MYC amplification. On a background of four red centromeric signals, there are multiple speckled green MYC signals from scattered double minute chromosomes.

3 and 4 tumours lacking WNT and Shh expression signatures, and that it is required for growth of tumour xenografts.[1] Increased OTX2 expression in the murine hindbrain caused aberrant proliferation of precursor cells but did not generate tumours.[208] Chromatin binding studies have also suggested functional interactions between OTX2 and MYC proteins in regulating gene expression in medulloblastoma.[27]

Epigenetic events are increasingly recognized as important processes in the development of tumours, and transcriptional silencing by hypermethylation of CpG islands in the promoter regions of tumour suppressor genes is a frequent finding in medulloblastomas.[12,40] Genes that are silenced by this mechanism in a significant proportion of medulloblastomas include *RASSF1A* (93 per cent of tumours), *CASP8* (36 per cent of tumours) and *HIC1* (38 per cent of tumours).[114,163,215] *RASSF1A* is mainly inactivated by hypermethylation of both alleles, whereas

hypermethylation of one allele of *HIC1* (at 17p13.3) is associated with the chromosome 17p loss that is a feature of up to 50 per cent of medulloblastomas. HIC1 is a direct repressor of Atonal Homolog 1 (Atoh1), a proneural transcription factor important in cerebellar development, and loss of HIC1 is thought to promote medulloblastoma growth by modulating differentiation of neoplastic cells.[25] Epigenome-wide screens using pharmacological demethylating agents have identified a number of genes, including the HGF/MET regulator *SPINT2* and the collagen *COL1A2*, as being altered in many medulloblastomas.[5,102] Overall, methylation profiles correlate well with gene expression subgroups in medulloblastoma, and may prove to be a more robust way to classify tumours molecularly when only formalin-fixed tissue is available.[179]

Genes that regulate epigenetic changes are being identified as potential drivers of medulloblastoma growth, because high throughput analyses have revealed that they are commonly altered in medulloblastoma. High-resolution single nucleotide polymorphism genotyping of 212 medulloblastomas identified previously unknown amplifications and homozygous deletions in genes targeting histone lysine methylation, particularly that of histone 3, lysine 9 (H3K9).[134] Sequencing of all known protein-coding and miRNA genes in 22 medulloblastomas identified only a small number of alterations in each tumour (11 on average), but among the most common were mutations in the histone-lysine N-methyltransferase genes *MLL2* and *MLL3*.[141]

MicroRNAs are also emerging as important players in pathogenesis, and their expression can help define molecular tumour subgroups.[12,36] A microRNA-regulated circuit involving miR199b, Hes factors and stem cell markers including CD133 and CD15 has been shown to affect stem cell properties in medulloblastoma cell lines and primary cultures.[6,67] Increased expression of the miR-183~96~182 cluster has been noted in the more aggressive medulloblastoma group 3 and regulates proliferation and migration of tumour cells.[201] miR-512-2 is also thought to regulate MYC and aggressive medulloblastoma behaviour,[120] whereas the miR-17~92 cluster collaborates with the Shh pathway.[197] These represent only a fraction of the growing list of miRNA shown to be dysregulated in medulloblastoma.

Medulloblastoma: Molecular Genetics, Specific Cell Signalling Pathways

Several pathways involved in the development of sporadic medulloblastoma were first suggested by their involvement in hereditary tumour syndromes (reviewed in Chapter 44). Mutations in *APC*, a member of the WNT pathway, are associated with medulloblastoma arising in the context of type 2 Turcot syndrome.[81] Similarly, inactivating genetic alterations in *PTCH*, a gene located at 9q22 that encodes for an inhibitory receptor in the Shh pathway, were identified in both medulloblastoma associated with naevoid basal cell carcinoma syndrome (NBCCS, also known as Gorlin syndrome) and sporadic lesions.[150,155] The tumour suppressor gene *TP53* and other members of the p53 pathway are altered in some medulloblastomas,[64] and Li–Fraumeni syndrome patients occasionally have embryonal brain tumours. Medulloblastoma has in rare cases been associated with germline *BRCA2* mutations in Fanconi anaemia subtype D1,[87] Rubenstein–Taybi syndrome and Coffin–Siris syndrome, but it is not clear if the same genetic elements are altered in sporadic cases.[161,192]

The Shh pathway represents the best understood driver of medulloblastoma initiation and growth. Germline mutations of *PTCH* cause NBCCS/Gorlin syndrome, and approximately 4 per cent of patients with NBCCS, mostly infants, develop a medulloblastoma. Of patients developing medulloblastoma, 1–2 per cent have NBCCS.[54,189] The *PTCH* gene product and the Shh pathway play a key role in normal CNS development.[200] As a cell surface receptor, PTCH is activated by a family of ligands, of which Shh is the best described. In the developing cerebellum, Shh is secreted by Purkinje cells and promotes the replication of cells in the EGL. It binds to PTCH receptors, causing derepression of another transmembrane protein, Smoothened (SMO),

which PTCH inhibits. SMO can then activate downstream mediators in Gli transcription factors. Mutational inactivation of *PTCH* and activating mutations of *SMO* lead to constitutive activation of the Shh/PTCH pathway. In addition, Suppressor of Fused (SUFU) acts to inhibit Shh signalling. It has been shown that localization of Shh components to the primary cilia in cells is critical for pathway activity.[118]

Shh pathway activation occurs in over 25 per cent of medulloblastomas. Nonsense, missense or frameshift *PTCH* mutations (at 9q22) have been reported in 8–12 per cent, and comparative genomic hybridization and loss of heterozygosity data show losses of chromosome 9q22 in 8–18 per cent of cases.[199,205] Activating mutations of *SMO* occur in approximately 5 per cent, whereas *SUFU* mutations have been variously reported in 0–10 per cent of tumours.[159,191] Mutations of *PTCH* and *SUFU* are typically accompanied by genetic loss of their second allele, consistent with a tumour suppressor gene role. Mutations in other elements of the pathway, such as *SHH* and *BTRCP*, have not been found.

NBCCS medulloblastomas are generally of the nodular/desmoplastic variant.[177] In addition, several molecular genetic studies have found a close association between the nodular/desmoplastic variant and either loss of chromosome 9q22 or *PTCH* mutations.[150] However, this does not appear to be an absolute association.[54,205] *SUFU* mutations have also been reported to segregate preferentially with nodular/desmoplastic tumours.[191] As noted previously, Shh tumours are generally found in the lateral hemispheres.

The role of the Shh pathway in the development of medulloblastoma is further supported by the generation of murine medulloblastomas following loss of *PTCH* or mutational activation of *SMO*.[80,202] Such models have been very useful in testing novel therapies that target Shh.[16,162] Unfortunately, although such targeted therapies show initial efficacy in patients and in mice, resistance mediated by mutations in *SMO* or amplification of Gli factors can rapidly emerge.[28,167,211] However, other inhibitors are effective even in the setting of resistance-promoting alterations to SMO and Gli.[110]

Activation of the WNT pathway defines another major medulloblastoma subgroup. A major downstream effector of the WNT pathway is β-catenin, which accumulates and translocates to the nucleus when the pathway is activated (a diagnostically useful pattern on immunohistochemistry). In the nucleus, β-catenin associates with Tcf/Lef transcriptional complexes, regulating the function of multiple genes, including cyclin D1 and *MYC*. WNT ligand binding to the Frizzled receptor produces inhibition of glycogen synthase kinase-3β (GSK-3β), which is part of a multimeric protein complex that binds β-catenin along with APC and AXIN1, resulting in the accumulation and nuclear translocation of β-catenin.

Abnormalities of the Wnt/Wg pathway have been demonstrated in a subset of sporadic medulloblastomas. Mutations of *CTNNB1* (encoding β-catenin) have been reported in 5–15 per cent of tumours.[53,214] Missense mutations of *APC* or *AXIN1* affect approximately 2 per cent of cases, whereas mutation of the *GSKβ* gene does not appear to play a significant role in pathogenesis.[9,89] A strong relationship is observed between *CTNNB1* mutations and nuclear accumulation of β-catenin in medulloblastomas.[58] Nuclear accumulation of β-catenin has been associated with excellent clinical outcomes.[57,58]

The p53 pathway also plays an important role in medulloblastoma. Loss of chromosome 17p occurs in up to 50 per cent of medulloblastomas, and *TP53* (at 17p13.1) has been investigated as a possible tumour suppressor gene in medulloblastoma on this basis, although the presence of tumour suppressor genes other than *TP53* (at 17p13.1) on chromosome 17p are also suggested by mapping of a consensus region of loss to 17p13.3. Approximately 10 per cent of sporadic tumours have a *TP53* mutation.[64] In addition, *TP53* deletion accelerates tumour development in murine genetic models of medulloblastoma, and widespread accumulation of p53 protein has been reported to be associated with poor prognosis.[203] Most recently, it has been shown that early *TP53* mutations in human tumours are associated with massive chromosomal rearrangements known as chromothripsis.[158]

The *TP53* pathway includes p14*ARF*, a cell cycle inhibitor encoded by the *INK4A/ARF* gene complex. p14*ARF* liberates p53 by sequestering Mdm2, a negative regulator of *TP53*, promoting either cell cycle arrest or apoptosis.[183] Aside from *TP53* mutation, the pathway can be disrupted by various genetic events, including loss of p14*ARF* function following mutation or promoter hypermethylation and amplification of the *MDM2* oncogene. Approximately 10 per cent of medulloblastomas contain mutually exclusive homozygous deletion or promoter hypermethylation of *ARF*, but *MDM2* amplification is rare.[2,64] Thus, genetic abnormalities of the *TP53* pathway occur in up to 20 per cent of medulloblastomas. An association between *TP53* pathway abnormalities and cytological anaplasia has been reported for medulloblastomas, but the biological significance of this has yet to be established.

A wide range of other genes and pathways have been implicated in medulloblastoma pathogenesis. Notch signalling is important in neural stem cells, and agents inhibiting this pathway have shown promise in some preclinical studies.[60,61,80] The c-met pathway can also modulate the growth of human medulloblastoma cells and murine tumours,[21,113] and may be regulated by epigenetic mechansisms.[102] Insulin-like growth factors promote medulloblastoma formation and growth, particularly in association with Shh activity,[26,121,157] and are being targeted in preclinical studies. Like Shh and WNT, all of these pathways play an important

role in the fetal cerebellum, further emphasizing the links be developmental biology and medulloblastoma.

CNS Primitive Neuroectodermal Tumours: Cytogenetics and Molecular Genetics

Because of their rarity, relatively few molecular studies of extracerebellar PNETs have been undertaken. Some molecular changes are found in both medulloblastoma and CNS PNET, including *MYC* and *MYCN* amplification, elevated WNT activity and mutations in *CTNNB1*.[14,160] However, many molecular abnormalities in medulloblastomas and CNS PNETs appear to differ.[90,168] Early chromosomal analysis studies revealed that abnormalities of chromosome 17, including i[17q], are rare in cerebral PNETs, which tend to have aberrations, such as losses on chromosomes 14q and 19q, that are infrequent or undetected in medulloblastomas. Both array-based and more focused profiling of mRNA expression also support the notion that these are distinct neoplasms.[148,153] CNS PNET are also distinct from those arising outside the nervous system. The *EWS-FLI1* chimeric gene and expression of MIC2 glycoprotein associated with a t(11;22) in peripheral PNETs/Ewing's sarcomas is not a feature of CNS PNETs, but has been recorded in dural PNETs.[14,91]

As in medulloblastoma, molecular analysis has suggested that CNS PNETs contain distinct subgroups, and these correlate at least in part with clinical and morphological features (Figure 34.11). Array comparative genomic hybridization analysis of 45 patients with CNS PNET identified amplification of the microRNA cluster C19MC at chromosome 19q13 in 11 cases (24 per cent) that had distinct gene expression profiles, very poor survival and histological features of ETANTR in many tumours.[112] Fluorescence *in situ* hybridization analysis of the 19q13 locus by another group in 20 histologically defined ETANTRs and 20 ependymoblastomas identified amplicons in 37 tumours (93 per cent) and confirmed the dismal outcomes in these patients.[105] Because of the partially overlapping clinical and morphological features of ETANTR and ependymoblastoma, and their common genetic changes, the authors suggested that they represent a single biological entity best regarded as

	Group 1	Group 2	Group 3
Demographics	Age < 4 years F>M	Age > 4 years M>F	All Children M>F
Histology/IHC	ETANTR/ LIN28+, OLIG2–	LIN28–, OLIG2+	LIN28–, OLIG2–
Clinical Outcome	Very Poor	Poor	Poor, Metastases Common
Chromosomal Changes	19q13 Amp +2, +3	CDKN2 loss +8p, +13, +20	CDKN2 loss –14
Gene Expression	C19MC, Lin28, WNT, Stem Cell	OLIG1/2 SOX8/10	TGFβ, PTEN Mesenchymal

34.11 Genetics of central nervous system primitive neuroectodermal tumours. PNET, primitive neuroectodermal tumour; TGFβ, transforming growth factor β.

ETANTR. Others have also argued that the term 'ependymoblastoma' is confusing and imprecise, and suggested that it does not represent a true diagnostic entity.[94] Although some CNS PNETs with 19q13 gains lack neuropil and true rosettes, the recent report of an ETANTR that lost these morphological features on recurrence but retained the key genetic signature provides a possible explanation.[204]

An expanded analysis of 142 hemispheric CNS PNET genetic profiles suggested that tumours could be separated into three groups.[149] The first was characterized by DNA amplifications at 19q13, high expression of LIN28 mRNA and protein, younger age, increased proportion of females, and worse prognosis than other CNS PNETs. Other studies have also suggested that immunohistochemical detection of LIN28 protein is relatively specific in identifying PNETs with ETANTR morphology.[106] Immunohistochemical detection of OLIG2 has been suggested as a marker of group 2 CNS PNET, whereas group 3 PNETs are negative for both proteins.[149]

Biological Behaviour of Medulloblastomas and CNS PNETs

All embryonal tumours are classified as WHO grade IV and have an aggressive natural history, being prone to recurrence and dissemination throughout the neuraxis. Despite this, approximately 80 per cent of children with standard-risk medulloblastoma are now cured with a combination of surgery and intensive radiochemotherapy regimens.[55,65,66] Outcomes for high-risk medulloblastoma and other embryonal tumours are less favourable, and the intensive nature of the therapies produces significant long-term adverse effects in surviving children, such as cognitive decline and neuroendocrine problems. Adults have somewhat poorer outcomes, with a recent population-based study of adult Europeans reporting a 45 per cent overall 5-year survival rate.[171]

The important clinical variables that determine outcome are age and metastatic status, and these are used in therapeutic stratification.[66] Children less than 3 years old and those with evidence of metastatic disease, either by cytological analysis of CSF or on neuroimaging, have a poor prognosis. The pairing of innovative murine models and advanced molecular analysis has recently revealed that only a limited number of genetic clones within medulloblastoma appear responsible for metastatic spread, emphasizing the need to account for intratumoural heterogeneity in profiling tumours.[209] The role played by cancer stem cell subpopulations in mediating treatment resistance in long-term growth is also linked to the issue of intratumoural heterogeneity and, as in malignant gliomas, has been controversial.[59]

For medulloblastoma, an aggressive biology has been established for the large cell/anaplastic variant, which often presents with metastatic disease.[50,72,123] At the other end of the biological scale, the MBEN is associated with good prognosis.[71] It is unclear whether this association is related to the extensive differentiation demonstrated by this variant or an idiosyncratic therapeutic response. Desmoplastic medulloblastomas have been variously described to have a prognosis that is the same as, better than, or worse than classic medulloblastomas.[35,76,108,122] These conflicting data have generally been based on small cohorts of patients

treated in various different ways. However, when the prognostic significance of the nodular/desmoplastic variant has been sought in infants treated on a therapeutic trial, there is a strong association of nodules with a good outcome.[50,169]

The relationship between measures of tumour cell proliferation and outcome has been the subject of various studies, without firm conclusions. In a few studies, high mitotic counts or indices have a negative correlation with survival, as have some, but not all, estimates of increased growth fraction (e.g. with Ki-67 antibodies).[74,124,206]

Many studies have attempted to relate the presence of molecular abnormalities to biological behaviour. Mutation of the *TP53* gene or accumulation of p53 protein has been identified as a predictor of poor outcome in some studies,[47,70,188] but can also be compatible with long survival, particularly in the WNT subgroup.[146] An association between poor outcome and amplification or overexpression of the *MYC* oncogene has been reported in a number of studies,[3,8,51,52,78,170,174] and *MYC* plays a key role in promoting anaplastic transformation in murine and human models.[100,142,186] *MYC* expression is also a defining feature of the aggressive medulloblastoma group 3 (see Figure 34.9), and most *MYC*-amplified tumours are found in this subgroup.

In contrast, the group of tumours with WNT pathway activity generally have the best outcomes. This group can be defined by expression profiling, but immunohistochemical demonstration of nuclear β-catenin is also often used to identify these tumours.[58] Loss of chromosome 6 is also tightly associated with this low-risk WNT group.[57] Indeed, a combination of MYC and chromosome 6 copy number assessment by fluorescence *in situ* hybridization, and nuclear accumulation of β-catenin determined by immunohistochemistry is planned for an upcoming Children's Oncology Group medulloblastoma trial.

The future, however, most likely lies in more comprehensive categorization of medulloblastoma into molecular subgroups as shown in Figure 34.9. The method by which this will be accomplished is not yet clear. Immunohistochemical marker panels have been proposed, but may prove difficult to standardize across institutions in a robust and reproducible way.[56,133] Recent attempts to measure expression of a small number of genes using mRNA extracted from paraffin by NanoString technology appear to generate robust and reproducible results in several test sets and centres,[135] and this approach seems promising, as does categorization using global methylation changes.[179]

ATYPICAL TERATOID/RHABDOID TUMOURS

Clinical Aspects

Improved diagnostic criteria and a growing recognition among pathologists of the existence of the ATRT have prompted re-evaluation of its rarity, and in early series many were likely misdiagnosed as PNET variants.[17,30,165] In a review of cases from two European trials for infants with brain tumours and children aged 3–16 years with PNETs, ATRTs represented 2.9 and 0.7 per cent of tumours, respectively.[194]

Over 90 per cent of ATRTs are encountered in children under 5 years of age, but several examples have now been described in adults as well.[119,156] Males are affected more frequently than females, at a ratio of 1.4:1.[116] The posterior fossa is affected more frequently than supratentorial sites (52 per cent versus 44 per cent in one series).

ATRTs are aggressive tumours with a dismal prognosis; many have seeded the CSF pathways by presentation. Outcomes have been significantly worse than in other embryonal tumours, but studies describe survival of over 2 years in children treated with radiation and high-dose alkylator-based chemotherapy or other multiagent approaches.[63,195,213] Radiation therapy was significantly associated with improved survival in some retrospective reviews,[31] but not in others.[107] Tandem high-dose chemotherapy and autologous stem cell transplantation was has also been used, with an overall 3-year survival of 53 per cent.[139]

Histopathology

Atypical teratoid/rhabdoid tumours are soft pink neoplasms containing foci of necrosis. Microscopically, the ATRT is a polymorphous tumour, often with a striking repertoire of cell types and a somewhat 'jumbled' appearance. Rhabdoid cells are often present in small groups or scattered among undifferentiated embryonal cells (Figure 34.12a), but may be absent. Resembling a typical PNET, masses of cells with a high N/C ratio and negligible differentiation are characteristically found. A fine fibrovascular network divides the tumour, but glomeruloid hyperplasia of endothelial cells is unusual. The undifferentiated cells often show less nuclear hyperchromasia than those in most PNETs (Figure 34.12b)

and may contain single nucleoli. Other regions may contain more pleomorphic cells with vague neuronal or glial features or even mesenchymal or epithelial features. Multinucleated or pleomorphic giant cells are occasionally present. Mitoses are frequent and necrosis or apoptotic lakes are common. Wrapping and moulding of cells similar to that seen in anaplastic medulloblastoma can be present.

ATRTs show a diverse polyphenotypic immunoprofile. Groups of cells typically express GFAP, EMA (Figure 34.12c) and smooth muscle α-actin, but immunoreactivities for NFP, synaptophysin, cytokeratins, desmin and HMB-45 among scattered cells are not uncommon.[30] The rhabdoid cells and many others in an ATRT are vimentin-positive, often highlighting the paranuclear inclusions composed of whorled bundles of intermediate filaments as visualized by electron microscopy.

Antibodies to the protein product of the *SMARCB1/INI1* gene are diagnostically useful (Figure 34.12d), demonstrating loss of the normal nuclear immunoreactivity in ATRTs,[96] but not in PNETs, gliomas or composite rhabdoid tumours, such as the rhabdoid meningioma.[143] Because rhabdoid cells can sometimes be absent, particularly in small specimens, routine immunohistochemical testing for SMARCB1/INI1 protein in embryonal tumours has been advocated.[79,96] Although there was initially some controversy over *SMARCB1* gene involvement in choroid plexus carcinoma, most now believe that previously published choroid plexus carcinomas with INI1 loss are in fact ATRT.[69,95,128,181,212] However, SMARCB1/INI1 protein loss is not completely specific for ATRT in the brain, as distinctive periventricular cribriform

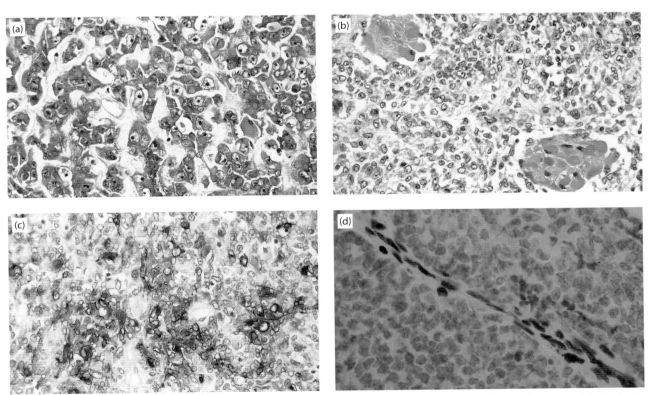

34.12 Atypical teratoid/rhabdoid tumour. (a) The cells forming trabeculae have abundant cytoplasm with eosinophilic inclusions. **(b)** An area composed of primitive cells with neuroepithelial differentiation: the clumps of large eosinophilic cells were strongly positive for GFAP. **(c)** Evidence of epithelial differentiation. Immunohistochemistry for EMA. **(d)** In contrast to immunopositive vascular cells, surrounding tumour cells do not show expression of the SMARCB1/INI1 protein.

neuroepithelial tumours with SMARCB1/INI1 protein loss, relatively good outcomes and no rhabdoid features have been reported.[84,140] Claudin 6 has recently been proposed as a novel immunohistochemical marker expressed in ATRT but not in other embryonal brain tumours.[22]

Molecular Genetics

A nosological relationship between the ATRT and malignant rhabdoid tumour (MRT) of the kidney and soft tissue has been established through cytogenetic and molecular genetic analyses, which have demonstrated a characteristic profile for these tumours. This involves monosomy 22 in association with mutation of the tumour suppressor gene *SMARCB1 (SNF5/INI1)* at 22q11.2, or a homozygous deletion of this locus.[19,180,198] This can involve a germline mutation which predisposes to MRTs at various sites, a condition known as rhabdoid tumour predisposition syndrome (see Chapter 44).[181] In one rhabdoid tumour registry, 10 out of 41 patients with CNS disease had germline *SMARCB1* mutations.[103] *SMARCB1* functions in an ATP-dependent chromatin remodelling complex, and cells derived from rhabdoid tumours show polyploidy and chromosomal instability. In rare cases, *SMARCB1* is intact in ATRT, although genetic alterations in other members of the protein complex such as *SMARCA4* have been identified.[176]

EPENDYMOBLASTOMA

Clinical and Molecular Aspects

The ependymoblastoma is conceptually aligned to other embryonal tumours by the formation of sheets of undifferentiated neuroepithelial cells, but also elaborates distinctive rosettes with ependymal features.[127] Recorded ependymoblastomas have nearly all occurred in the first decade of life[41] and some appear to have been congenital.[115] There is no clear predilection for either sex. Ependymoblastomas have mainly been located in the cerebrum, particularly deep paraventricular structures, but other sites have been described, including the leptomeninges. Most ependymoblastomas prove fatal within 2 years of diagnosis.

However, it has now been suggested that ependymoblastoma are not a distinct entity, as 'ependymoblastic' rosettes can be seen in a variety of contexts.[94] Molecular studies showing the same 19q13 amplifications in ependymoblastoma and ETANTR, as well as their overlapping morphological appearance, has led a number of neuropathologists and other investigators to suggest that these represent a single entity.[44,94,105,147] What to call this potential entity is not yet fully established. However, because of the neuronal differentiation, ependymoblastoma does not seem appropriate.

Histopathology

The ependymoblastoma shows no distinctive macroscopic features. Microscopic evaluation centres on finding ependymoblastomatous rosettes, which consist of multiple layers of monomorphic undifferentiated cells with a high N/C ratio (Figure 34.13). The fine processes of these cells are arranged radially and terminate abruptly on a central

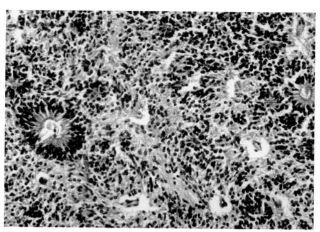

34.13 Ependymoblastoma. The hallmark of the restricted differentiation is a tubular pseudo-stratified structure; these ependymoblastomatous rosettes are randomly admixed with small to medium primitive cells with variably developed fibrillary processes.

slit-like lumen. The ependymal ultrastructural characteristics of the periluminal cells include polarization, junctional complexes of variable length (including zonulae adherentes), blepharoplasts, basal bodies, microvilli and cilia, and the apical granular stippling and epithelial qualities of the periluminal cells at the light microscopic level might be a manifestation of these features.[109] Mitotic figures are found among the cells of ependymoblastomatous rosettes. Elsewhere, the tumour is characterized by focally necrotic sheets of densely packed undifferentiated cells with minimal cytoplasm. Immunohistochemical studies of ependymoblastomas have reported focal reactivity for GFAP, but there may be none, whereas synaptophysin and neurofilament stains are generally positive.[94]

The differential diagnosis of ependymoblastoma includes anaplastic ependymoma, medulloepithelioma and immature teratoma. Occasionally, examples of anaplastic ependymoma achieve a cell density that rivals that of embryonal tumours. However, if sampled sufficiently, they will show typical perivascular rosettes and may show the true rosettes or canals of classic ependymoma, which consist of a monolayer of differentiated ependymal cells. Glomeruloid vascular proliferation, which is usually present in the anaplastic ependymoma, is usually absent from ependymoblastoma. Ependymoblastoma-like elements are found within some examples of medulloepithelioma and immature teratoma, but the ependymoblastoma does not contain tubulopapillary or canalicular structures delimited by an external basement membrane, and it does not exhibit divergent neuronal or glial differentiation. The presence of non-neuroepithelial elements reflecting somatic differentiation readily removes the immature teratoma from further consideration.

MEDULLOEPITHELIOMA

Clinical Aspects

In replicating the architectural and cytological features of the embryonic neural tube, the medulloepithelioma is sometimes considered the most primitive of CNS embryonal neoplasms. However, although this suggests that it is derived from an early neuroepithelial stem cell, its histogenesis is obscure. Indeed, it is possible that these tumours are also part of the ETANTR spectrum, because they show some morphological overlap, and the molecular ETANTR subgroup is now thought to be the most stem-like of CNS PNETs.[149]

This exceedingly rare neoplasm is generally encountered in children aged less than 5 years, but examples do present in older patients.[126] Males and females appear equally affected, and clinical outcomes have traditionally been extremely poor, although some long-term survivors have been reported following combined radiation and chemotherapy.[129] Tumours are often hypodense or isodense, rather than hyperdense, on precontrast CT images, and frequently evince no contrast enhancement on CT/MR imaging. The medulloepithelioma is an aggressive neoplasm, recurring readily at the site of surgical resection and spreading through CSF pathways.[126] Tumours also known as medulloepithelioma can arise in the ciliary body of the eye, but have a somewhat different microscopic appearance and are associated with generally good outcomes; they therefore are thought to represent a distinct type of neoplasm.[172] Medulloepithelioma can arise in the retrobulbar optic nerve or optic nerve head, but these have some morphological features not commonly seen in other CNS medulloepithelioma, and they may represent part of the intraocular medulloepithelioma spectrum.[154]

Histopathology

Like other embryonal tumours, the medulloepithelioma usually appears circumscribed upon macroscopic examination, but then demonstrates invasion of adjacent tissues at microscopy. Recalling the primitive medullary epithelium, medulloepitheliomas exhibit complex architectural arrangements of tubular or papillary structures, which are formed by undifferentiated columnar or cuboidal cells in a single layer or a pseudo-stratified pattern (Figure 34.14a). The cells are delimited by a periodic

acid–Schiff (PAS)-positive basement membrane and a fine fibrovascular stroma. An ill-defined layer of PAS-positive material often covers their apical surfaces, but cilia are not present. Mitotic figures are readily found, especially in the basal layer of multilayered structures. Aside from areas exhibiting the distinctive architectural phenotype described earlier, medulloepitheliomas usually contain sheets of undifferentiated neuroepithelial cells, like other embryonal tumours. Some examples contain foci of neuronal differentiation, which can amount to ganglion cell formation, or areas of astrocytic, oligodendroglial or ependymal differentiation.[173] Medulloepitheliomas can even harbour mesenchymal tissues.

Ultrastructural examination has shown that features of the primitive medullary epithelium, few organelles and apical zonulae adherentes, are recapitulated by the undifferentiated cells of the medulloepithelioma. Similarly, immunohistochemistry demonstrates a shared antigenic profile between the medullary epithelium and medulloepitheliomas, including reactivities for vimentin (Figure 34.14b), nestin and microtubule-associated protein type 5. Apical cell immunoreactivities for EMA and cytokeratins have also been described. The undifferentiated cells are usually immunonegative for GFAP or markers of mature neuronal differentiation, such as NFP, but foci of morphological differentiation show the expected immunophenotypes.[32,196]

The differential diagnosis of medulloepithelioma includes choroid plexus carcinoma, ependymoblastoma and immature teratoma. Choroid plexus carcinomas may show a focal papillary architecture and do not contain differentiating glioneuronal elements. Generally, they are focally immunopositive for cytokeratins. Ependymoblastic rosettes are not delimited by a basement membrane, and ependymoblastomas do not show mature neuronal differentiation. Immature teratomas should contain tissues of somatic ectodermal and endodermal origins, and may be part of a mixed germ cell tumour with elements of embryonal carcinoma or yolk sac tumour. A medulloepithelioma with ETANTR components and a 19q13.42 amplicon has been reported.[131]

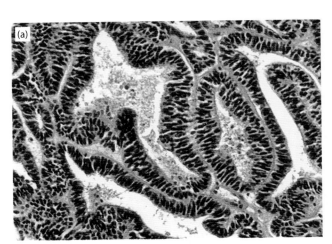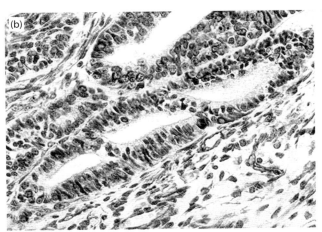

34.14 Medulloepithelioma. (a) Tubules and rosettes, composed of multiple-layered and pseudo-stratified arrangements of slightly elongated, primitive cells, usually delineated by an external basal lamina, recall the primitive ventricular matrix zone of the embryonal CNS. **(b)** The primitive cells that constitute these neuroepithelial tubules are typically immunoreactive for vimentin.

OLFACTORY NEUROBLASTOMA (AESTHESIONEUROBLASTOMA)

Clinical Aspects

In the WHO classification, this tumour is grouped with neuroblastic tumours, rather than embryonal tumours, but is included in this chapter because it may spread to the cranial cavity.[117] Other neuroblastic tumours (of the peripheral nervous system) are beyond the scope of this book.

Olfactory neuroblastomas are rare. Unlike many CNS embryonal tumours and peripheral neuroblastomas, they are not limited to childhood and most present in the second and fifth decades.[11,138] There is no gender bias. Most tumours appear to arise in the nasal vault in association with the cribriform plate, but an intracranial presentation is possible, albeit rare, and initial symptoms are sometimes referable to involvement of the anterior cranial fossa. Therapy involves open or endoscopic surgical excision, radiotherapy and sometimes chemotherapy.[11,138]

In addition to standard CT and MR imaging, in which olfactory neuroblastomas are visualized as masses of variable signal intensity and relatively uniform contrast enhancement, PET imaging has been used to help stage metastatic tumours.[11]

Histopathology

Macroscopically, olfactory neuroblastomas are soft polypoid tumours. Microscopically, the classic olfactory neuroblastoma presents a sheet-like arrangement of small cells with round hyperchromatic nuclei and a high N/C ratio (Figure 34.15a). This pattern may be interrupted by a vascular network that produces a vague nodular pattern, but a prominent nodularity is characteristic of the variant resembling paraganglioma, which typically contains larger, more epithelioid cells. Other architectural features include rosette formation, of both Homer Wright (neuroblastic) and Flexner–Wintersteiner (with central lumen) varieties (Figure 34.15b), although these are often absent. Neuronal differentiation in the form of ganglion cells and the presence of rhabdomyoblasts are rare events. Mitotic activity and extent of necrosis are variable.

The immunophenotype of olfactory neuroblastomas typically includes reactivities for neurone specific enolase and synaptophysin, with variable labelling of tumour cells for neurofilament proteins, microtubule-associated protein 2 and chromogranin A. In examples with a nodular phenotype, circumferential cells immunopositive for S-100 mimic the sustentacular cells of paraganglioma. This variant is particularly prone to express chromogranin A. In contrast, immunoreactivity for neurofilament proteins is characteristic of the neuroblastic phenotype. Isolated examples have also demonstrated focal immunolabelling for ACTH, vasopressin, tyrosine or dopamine hydroxylase, and neuropeptides such as met-enkephalin, VIP and substance P.[86] It has been suggested that diffuse calretinin expression can help to differentiate olfactory neuroblastomas from other small round blue cell tumours of the sinonasal tract.[207]

The olfactory neuroblastoma probably derives from the olfactory neuroepithelium. This view accounts best for the neurosensory/neurosecretory ultrastructural features and immunophenotype of the tumour.[86] It does not show the expression of CD99 or the t(11;22) translocation characteristic of peripheral PNET/Ewing's sarcoma.[7]

Paraganglioma-like features, particularly the presence of sustentacular-like cells, can help to distinguish olfactory neuroblastoma from cerebral PNETs. Immunohistochemistry to demonstrate an epithelial phenotype, with extensive reactivities for cytokeratins and EMA, can help to delineate sinonasal neuroendocrine carcinomas that can mimic olfactory neuroblastoma.

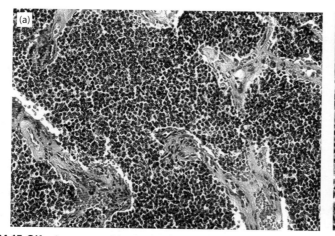
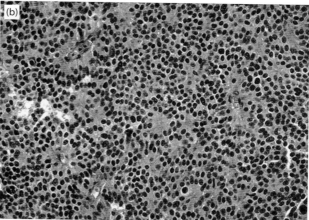

34.15 Olfactory neuroblastoma. (a) Amorphous, densely cellular sheets of small, primitive cells that are irregularly interrupted by hypocellular zones of fibrovascular stroma. **(b)** A field of typical neuroblastic (Homer Wright) rosettes.

REFERENCES

1. Adamson DC, Shi Q, Wortham M, Northcott PA, Di C, Duncan CG, et al. OTX2 is critical for the maintenance and progression of Shh-independent medulloblastomas. *Cancer Res* 2010;**70**:181–91.

2. Adesina AM, Nalbantoglu J, Cavenee WK. p53 gene mutation and mdm2 gene amplification are uncommon in medulloblastoma. *Cancer Res* 1994;**54**:5649–51.

3. Aldosari N, Bigner SH, Burger PC, et al. MYCC and MYCN oncogene amplification in medulloblastoma. A fluorescence in situ hybridization study on paraffin sections from the Children' Oncology Group. *Arch Pathol Lab Med* 2002;**126**:540–4.

4. Amacher AL, Torres QU, Rittenhouse S. Congenital medulloblastoma: an inquiry into origins. *Childs Nerv Syst* 1986;**2**: 262–5.

5. Anderton JA, Lindsey JC, Lusher ME, Gilbertson RJ, Bailey S, Ellison DW, et al. Global analysis of the medulloblastoma epigenome identifies disease-subgroup-specific inactivation of COL1A2. *Neuro Oncol* 2008;**10**:981–94.

6. Andolfo I, Liguori L, De Antonellis P, Cusanelli E, Marinaro F, Pistollato F, et al. The micro-RNA 199b-5p regulatory circuit involves Hes1, CD15, and epigenetic modifications in medulloblastoma. *Neuro Oncol* 2012;**14**:596–612.

7. Argani P, Perez-Ordonez B, Xiao H, et al. Olfactory neuroblastoma is not related to the Ewing family of tumors: absence of EWS/FLI1 gene fusion and MIC2 expression. *Am J Surg Pathol* 1998;**22**:391–8.

8. Badiali M, Pession A, Basso G, Andreini L, Rigobello L, Galassi E, et al. N-myc and c-myc oncogenes amplification in medulloblastomas. Evidence of particularly aggressive behavior of a tumor with c-myc amplification. *Tumori* 1991;**77**:118–21.

9. Baeza N, Masuoka J, Kleihues P, Ohgaki H. AXIN1 mutations but not deletions in cerebellar medulloblastomas. *Oncogene* 2003;**22**:632–6.

10. Bailey CC, Gnekow A, Wellek S, et al. Prospective randomised trial of chemotherapy given before radiotherapy in childhood medulloblastoma. International Society of Paediatric Oncology (SIOP) and the (German) Society of Paediatric Oncology (GPO): SIOP II. *Med Pediatr Oncol* 1995;**25**:166–78.

11. Bak M, Wein RO. Esthesioneuroblastoma: a contemporary review of diagnosis and management. *Hematol Oncol Clin North Am* 2012;**26**:1185–207.

12. Batora NV, Sturm D, Jones DT, Kool M, Pfister SM, Northcott PA. Transitioning from genotypes to epigenotypes: Why the time has come for medulloblastoma epigenomics. *Neuroscience* 2014;**264**(Part C):171–85.

13. Becker RL, Becker AD, Sobel DF. Adult medulloblastoma: review of 13 cases with emphasis on MRI. *Neuroradiology* 1995; **37**:104–8.

14. Behdad A, Perry A. Central nervous system primitive neuroectodermal tumors: a clinicopathologic and genetic study of 33 cases. *Brain Pathol* 2010;**20**:441–50.

15. Bennett JP Jr, Rubinstein LJ. The biological behavior of primary cerebral neuroblastoma: a reappraisal of the clinical course in a series of 70 cases. *Ann Neurol* 1984;**16**:21–7.

16. Berman DM, Karhadkar SS, Hallahan AR, Pritchard JI, Eberhart CG, Watkins DN, et al. Medulloblastoma growth inhibition by hedgehog pathway blockade. *Science* 2002;**297**:1559–61.

17. Biegel JA, Rorke LB, Emanuel BS. Monosomy 22 in rhabdoid or atypical teratoid tumors of the brain. *N Engl J Med* 1989;**321**:906.

18. Biegel JA, Rorke LB, Packer RJ, et al. Isochromosome 17q in primitive neuroectodermal tumors of the central nervous system. *Genes Chromosomes Cancer* 1989;**1**:139–47.

19. Biegel JA, Tan L, Zhang F, et al. Alterations of the hSNF5/INI1 gene in central nervous system atypical teratoid/rhabdoid tumors and renal and extrarenal rhabdoid tumors. *Clin Cancer Res* 2002;**8**:3461–7.

20. Bigner SH, Mark J, Friedman HS, et al. Structural chromosomal abnormalities in human medulloblastoma. *Cancer Genet Cytogenet* 1988;**30**:91–101.

21. Binning MJ, Niazi T, Pedone CA, Lal B, Eberhart CG, Kim KJ, et al. Hepatocyte growth factor and Sonic Hedgehog expression in cerebellar neural progenitor cells costimulate medulloblastoma initiation and growth. *Cancer Res* 2008;**68**:7838–45.

22. Birks DK, Kleinschmidt-DeMasters BK, Donson AM, Barton VN, McNatt SA, Foreman NK, et al. Claudin 6 is a positive marker for atypical teratoid/rhabdoid tumors. *Brain Pathol* 2010;**20**:140–50.

23. Bonnin JM, Perentes E. Retinal S-antigen immunoreactivity in medulloblastomas. *Acta Neuropathol* 1988;**76**:204–7.

24. Boon K, Eberhart CG, Riggins GJ. Genomic amplification of orthodenticle homologue 2 in medulloblastomas. *Cancer Res* 2005;**65**:703–7.

25. Briggs KJ, Corcoran-Schwartz IM, Zhang W, Harcke T, Devereux WL, Baylin SB, et al. Cooperation between the Hic1 and Ptch1 tumor suppressors in medulloblastoma. *Genes Dev* 2008;**22**:770–85.

26. Browd SR, Kenney AM, Gottfried ON, Yoon JW, Walterhouse D, Pedone CA, et al. N-myc can substitute for insulin-like growth factor signaling in a mouse model of sonic hedgehog-induced medulloblastoma. *Cancer Res* 2006;**66**:2666–72.

27. Bunt J, Hasselt NE, Zwijnenburg DA, Koster J, Versteeg R, Kool M. Joint binding of OTX2 and MYC in promotor regions is associated with high gene expression in medulloblastoma. *PLoS One* 2011;**6**:e26058.

28. Buonamici S, Williams J, Morrissey M, Wang A, Guo R, Vattay A, et al. Interfering with resistance to smoothened antagonists by inhibition of the PI3K pathway in medulloblastoma. *Sci Transl Med* 2010;**2**:51ra70.

29. Burger PC, Grahmann FC, Bliestle A, Kleihues P. Differentiation in the medulloblastoma. A histological and immunohistochemical study. *Acta Neuropathol* 1987;**73**:115–23.

30. Burger PC, Yu IT, Tihan T, et al. Atypical teratoid/rhabdoid tumor of the central nervous system: a highly malignant tumor of infancy and childhood frequently mistaken for medulloblastoma: a Pediatric Oncology Group study. *Am J Surg Pathol* 1998;**22**:1083–92.

31. Buscariollo DL, Park HS, Roberts KB, Yu JB. Survival outcomes in atypical teratoid rhabdoid tumor for patients undergoing radiotherapy in a Surveillance, Epidemiology, and End Results analysis. *Cancer* 2012;**118**:4212–9.

32. Caccamo DV, Herman MM, Rubinstein LJ. An immunohistochemical study of the primitive and maturing elements of human cerebral medulloepitheliomas. *Acta Neuropathol* 1989;**79**:248–254.

33. Campbell AN, Chan HS, Becker LE, et al. Extracranial metastases in childhood primary intracranial tumors. A report of 21 cases and review of the literature. *Cancer* 1984;**53**:974–81.

34. Chang CH, Housepian EM, Herbert C Jr. An operative staging system and a megavoltage radiotherapeutic technic for cerebellar medulloblastomas. *Radiology* 1969;**93**:1351–9.

35. Chatty EM, Earle KM. Medulloblastoma. A report of 201 cases with emphasis on the relationship of histological variants to survival. *Cancer* 1971;**28**:977–83.

36. Cho YJ, Tsherniak A, Tamayo P, Santagata S, Ligon A, Greulich H, et al. Integrative genomic analysis of medulloblastoma identifies a molecular subgroup that drives poor clinical outcome. *J Clin Oncol* 2011;**29**:1424–30.

37. De Chadarévian JP, Montes JL, O'Gorman AM, Freeman CR. Maturation of cerebellar neuroblastoma into ganglioneuroma with melanosis. A histological, immunocytochemical, and ultrastructural study. *Cancer* 1987;**59**:69–76.

38. De Haas T, Oussoren E, Grajkowska W, et al. OTX1 and OTX2 expression correlates with the clinicopathologic classification of medulloblastomas. *J Neuropathol Exp Neurol* 2006;**65**:176–86.

39. Di C, Liao S, Adamson DC, et al. Identification of OTX2 as a medulloblastoma oncogene whose product can be targeted by all-trans retinoic acid. *Cancer Res* 2005;**65**:919–24.

40. DNA methylation of developmental genes in pediatric medulloblastomas identified by denaturation analysis of methylation differences. *Proc Natl Acad Sci U S A* 2010;**107**:234–9.

41. Dohrmann GJ, Farwell JR, Flannery JT. Ependymomas and ependymoblastomas in children. *J Neurosurg* 1976;**45**:273–83.

42. Dolman CL. Melanotic medulloblastoma. A case report with immunohistochemical and ultrastructural examination. *Acta Neuropathol* 1988;**76**:528–31.

43. Dunham C, Sugo E, Tobias V, Wills E, Perry A. Embryonal tumor with abundant neuropil and true rosettes (ETANTR):

report of a case with prominent neurocytic differentiation. *J Neurooncol* 2007;**84**:91–8.

44. Eberhart CG. Molecular diagnostics in embryonal brain tumors. *Brain Pathol* 2011;**21**:96–104.

45. Eberhart CG, Brat DJ, Cohen KJ, Burger PC. Pediatric neuroblastic brain tumors containing abundant neuropil and true rosettes. *Pediatr Dev Pathol* 2000;**3**:346–52.

46. Eberhart CG, Burger PC. Anaplasia and grading in medulloblastomas. *Brain Pathol* 2003;**13**:376–85.

47. Eberhart CG, Chaudhry A, Daniel RW, Khaki L, Shah KV, Gravitt PE. Increased p53 immunopositivity in anaplastic medulloblastoma and supratentorial PNET is not caused by JC virus. *BMC Cancer* 2005;**5**:19.

48. Eberhart CG, Cohen KJ, Tihan T, Goldthwaite PT, Burger PC. Medulloblastomas with systemic metastases: evaluation of tumor histopathology and clinical behavior in 23 patients. *J Pediatr Hematol Oncol* 2003;**25**:198–203.

49. Eberhart CG, Kaufman WE, Tihan T, Burger PC. Apoptosis, neuronal maturation, and neurotrophin expression within medulloblastoma nodules. *J Neuropathol Exp Neurol* 2001;**60**:462–9.

50. Eberhart CG, Kepner JL, Goldthwaite PT, *et al.* Histopathologic grading of medulloblastoma: a Pediatric Oncology Group study. *Cancer* 2002;**94**:552–60.

51. Eberhart CG, Kratz JE, Schuster A, *et al.* Comparative genomic hybridization detects an increased number of chromosomal alterations in large cell/anaplastic medulloblastomas. *Brain Pathol* 2002;**12**:36–44.

52. Eberhart CG, Kratz J, Wang Y, Summers K, Stearns D, Cohen K, *et al.* Histopathological and molecular prognostic markers in medulloblastoma: c-myc, N-myc, TrkC, and anaplasia. *J Neuropathol Exp Neurol* 2004;**63**:441–9.

53. Eberhart CG, Tihan T, Burger PC. Nuclear localization and mutation of beta-catenin in medulloblastomas. *J Neuropathol Exp Neurol* 2000;**59**:333–7.

54. Ellison D. Classifying the medulloblastoma: insights from morphology and molecular genetics. *Neuropathol Appl Neurobiol* 2002;**28**:257–82.

55. Ellison DW, Clifford SC, Gajjar A, Gilbertson RJ. What' new in neuro-oncology? Recent advances in medulloblastoma. *Eur J Paediatr Neurol* 2003;**7**:53–66.

56. Ellison DW, Dalton J, Kocak M, Nicholson SL, Fraga C, Neale G, *et al.* Medulloblastoma: clinicopathological correlates of SHH, WNT, and non-SHH/WNT molecular subgroups. *Acta Neuropathol* 2011;**121**:381–96.

57. Ellison DW, Kocak M, Dalton J, Megahed H, Lusher ME, Ryan SL, *et al.* Definition of disease-risk stratification groups in childhood medulloblastoma using combined clinical, pathologic, and molecular variables. *J Clin Oncol* 2011;**29**:1400–7.

58. Ellison DW, Onilude OE, Lindsey JC, *et al.* Beta-catenin status predicts a favorable outcome in childhood medulloblastoma. *J Clin Oncol* 2005;**23**:7951–7.

59. Fan X, Eberhart CG. Medulloblastoma stem cells. *J Clin Oncol* 2008;**26**:2821–7.

60. Fan X, Matsui W, Khaki L, Stearns D, Chun J, Li YM, *et al.* Notch pathway inhibition depletes stem-like cells and blocks engraftment in embryonal brain tumors. *Cancer Res* 2006;**66**:7445–52.

61. Fan X, Mikolaenko I, Elhassan I, Ni X, Wang Y, Ball D, *et al.* Notch1 and notch2 have opposite effects on embryonal brain tumor growth. *Cancer Res* 2004;**64**:7787–93.

62. Figarella-Branger DF, Durbec PL, Rougon GN. Differential spectrum of expression of neural cell adhesion molecule isoforms and L1 adhesion molecules on human neuroectodermal tumors. *Cancer Res* 1990;**50**:6364–70.

63. Finkelstein-Shechter T, Gassas A, Mabbott D, Huang A, Bartels U, Tabori U, *et al.* Atypical teratoid or rhabdoid tumors: improved outcome with high-dose chemotherapy. *J Pediatr Hematol Oncol* 2010;**32**:e182–6.

64. Frank AJ, Hernan R, Hollander A, *et al.* The TP53-ARF tumor suppressor pathway is frequently disrupted in large/cell anaplastic medulloblastoma. *Brain Res Mol Brain Res* 2004;**121**:137–40.

65. Gajjar A, Hernan R, Kocak M, *et al.* Clinical, histopathologic, and molecular markers of prognosis: toward a new disease risk stratification system for medulloblastoma. *J Clin Oncol* 2004;**22**:984–93.

66. Gajjar A, Packer RJ, Foreman NK, Cohen K, Haas-Kogan D, Merchant TE. Children's Oncology Group 2013 blueprint for research: central nervous system tumors. *Pediatr Blood Cancer* 2013;**60**:1022–6.

67. Garzia L, Andolfo I, Cusanelli E, Marino N, Petrosino G, De Martino D, *et al.* MicroRNA-199b-5p impairs cancer stem cells through negative regulation of HES1 in medulloblastoma. *PLoS One* 2009;**4**:e4998.

68. Gessi M, Giangaspero F, Lauriola L, Gardiman M, Scheithauer BW, Halliday W, *et al.* Embryonal tumors with abundant neuropil and true rosettes: a distinctive CNS primitive neuroectodermal tumor. *Am J Surg Pathol* 2009;**33**:211–7.

69. Gessi M, Giangaspero F, Pietsch T. Atypical teratoid/rhabdoid tumors and choroid plexus tumors: when genetics 'surprise' pathology. *Brain Pathol* 2003;**13**:409–14.

70. Gessi M, von Bueren AO, Rutkowski S, Pietsch T. p53 expression predicts dismal outcome for medulloblastoma patients with metastatic disease. *J Neurooncol* 2012;**106**:135–41.

71. Giangaspero F, Perilongo G, Fondelli MP, *et al.* Medulloblastoma with extensive nodularity: a variant with favorable prognosis. *J Neurosurg* 1999;**91**:971–7.

72. Giangaspero F, Rigobello L, Badiali M, *et al.* Large-cell medulloblastomas. A distinct variant with highly aggressive behavior. *Am J Surg Pathol* 1992;**16**:687–93.

73. Gibson P, Tong Y, Robinson G, Thompson MC, Currle DS, Eden C, *et al.* Subtypes of medulloblastoma have distinct developmental origins. *Nature* 2010;**468**:1095–9.

74. Gilbertson RJ, Jaros E, Perry RH, *et al.* Mitotic percentage index: a new prognostic factor for childhood medulloblastoma. *Eur J Cancer* 1997;**33**:609–15.

75. Gimi B, Cederberg K, Derinkuyu B, Gargan L, Koral KM, Bowers DC, *et al.* Utility of apparent diffusion coefficient ratios in distinguishing common pediatric cerebellar tumors. *Academic Radiol* 2012;**19**:794–800.

76. Giordana MT, Cavalla P, Chio A, *et al.* Prognostic factors in adult medulloblastoma. A clinico-pathologic study. *Tumori* 1995;**81**:338–46.

77. Goodrich LV, Milenkovic L, Higgins KM, Scott MP. Altered neural cell fates and medulloblastoma in mouse patched mutants. *Science* 1997;**277**:1109–13.

78. Grotzer MA, Hogarty MD, Janss AJ, Liu X, Zhao H, Eggert A, *et al.* MYC messenger RNA expression predicts survival outcome in childhood primitive neuroectodermal tumor/medulloblastoma. *Clin Cancer Res* 2001;**7**:2425–33.

79. Haberler C, Laggner U, Slavc I, Czech T, Ambros IM, Ambros PF, *et al.* Immunohistochemical analysis of ini1 protein in malignant pediatric CNS tumors: lack of ini1 in atypical teratoid/rhabdoid tumors and in a fraction of primitive neuroectodermal tumors without rhabdoid phenotype. *Am J Surg Pathol* 2006;**30**:1462–8.

80. Hallahan AR, Pritchard JI, Hansen S, Benson M, Stoeck J, Hatton BA, *et al.* The SmoA1 mouse model reveals that notch signaling is critical for the growth and survival of Sonic Hedgehog-induced medulloblastomas. *Cancer Res* 2004;**64**:7794–800.

81. Hamilton SR, Liu B, Parsons RE, Papadopoulos N, Jen J, Powell SM, *et al.* The molecular basis of Turcot' syndrome. *N Engl J Med* 1995;**332**:839–47.

82. Hart MN, Earle KM. Primitive neuroectodermal tumors of the brain in children. *Cancer* 1973;**32**:890–7.

83. Hasselblatt M, Bohm C, Tatenhorst L, *et al.* Identification of novel diagnostic markers for choroid plexus tumors: a microarray-based approach. *Am J Surg Pathol* 2006;**30**:66–74.

84. Hasselblatt M, Oyen F, Gesk S, Kordes U, Wrede B, Bergmann M, *et al.* Cribriform neuroepithelial tumor (CRINET): a nonrhabdoid ventricular tumor with INI1 loss and relatively favorable prognosis. *J Neuropathol Exp Neurol* 2009;**68**:1249–55.

85. Helton KJ, Fouladi M, Boop FA, *et al.* Medullomyoblastoma: a radiographic and clinicopathologic analysis of six cases and review of the literature. *Cancer* 2004;**101**:1445–54.

86. Hirose T, Scheithauer BW, Lopes MBS, *et al.* Olfactory neuroblastoma: an immunohistochemical, ultrastructural, and flow cytometric study. *Cancer* 1995;**76**:4–19.

87. Hirsch B, Shimamura A, Moreau L, *et al.* Association of biallelic BRCA2/FANCD1 mutations with spontaneous chromosomal instability and solid tumors of childhood. *Blood* 2004;**103**:2554–9.

88. Horten BC, Rubinstein LJ. Primary cerebral neuroblastoma. A clinicopathological study of 35 cases. *Brain* 1976;**99**:735–56.

89. Huang H, Mahler-Araujo BM, Sankila A, *et al.* APC mutations in sporadic medulloblastomas. *Am J Pathol* 2000;**156**:433–7.

90. Inda MM, Perot C, Guillaud-Bataille M, et al. Genetic heterogeneity in supratentorial and infratentorial primitive neuroectodermal tumours of the central nervous system. *Histopathology* 2005;47:631–7.

91. Ishii N, Hiraga H, Sawamura Y, et al. Alternative EWS-FLI1 fusion gene and MIC2 expression in peripheral and central primitive neuroectodermal tumors. *Neuropathology* 2001;21:40–4.

92. Jaremko JL, Jans LB, Coleman LT, Ditchfield MR. Value and limitations of diffusion-weighted imaging in grading and diagnosis of pediatric posterior fossa tumors. *AJNR Am J Neuroradiol* 2010;31: 1613–6.

93. Judkins AR. Immunohistochemistry of INI1 expression: a new tool for old challenges in CNS and soft tissue pathology. *Adv Anat Pathol* 2007;14:335–9.

94. Judkins AR, Ellison DW. Ependymoblastoma: dear, damned, distracting diagnosis, farewell! *Brain Pathol* 2010;20:133–9.

95. Judkins AR, Burger PC, Hamilton RL, et al. INI1 protein expression distinguishes atypical teratoid/rhabdoid tumor from choroid plexus carcinoma. *J Neuropathol Exp Neurol* 2005;64:391–7.

96. Judkins AR, Mauger J, Ht A, et al. Immunohistochemical analysis of hSNF5/INI1 in pediatric CNS neoplasms. *Am J Surg Pathol* 2004;28:644–50.

97. Kadin ME, Rubinstein LJ, Nelson JS. Neonatal cerebellar medulloblastoma originating from the fetal external granular layer. *J Neuropathol Exp Neurol* 1970;29:583–600.

98. Kalimo H, Paljarvi L, Ekfors T, Pelliniemi LJ. Pigmented primitive neuroectodermal tumour with multipotential differentiation in cerebellum (pigmented medullomyoblastoma). A case with light- and electron-microscopic, and immunohistochemical analysis. *Pediatr Neurosci* 1987;13:188–95.

99. Kapadia SB, Frisman DM, Hitchcock CL, et al. Melanotic neuroectodermal tumour of infancy. Clinicopathological, immunohistochemical, and flow cytometric study. *Am J Surg Pathol* 1993;17:566–73.

100. Kawauchi D, Robinson G, Uziel T, Gibson P, Rehg J, Gao C, et al. A mouse model of the most aggressive subgroup of human medulloblastoma. *Cancer Cell* 2012;21:168–80.

101. Kepes JJ, Belton K, Roessmann U, Ketcherside WJ. Primitive neuroectodermal tumors of the cauda equina in adults with no detectable primary intracranial neoplasm – three case studies. *Clin Neuropathol* 1985;4:1–11.

102. Kongkham PN, Northcott PA, Ra YS, Nakahara Y, Mainprize TG, Croul SE, et al. An epigenetic genome-wide screen identifies SPINT2 as a novel tumor suppressor gene in pediatric medulloblastoma. *Cancer Res* 2008;68:9945–53.

103. Kordes U, Gesk S, Fruhwald MC, Graf N, Leuschner I, Hasselblatt M, et al. Clinical and molecular features in patients with atypical teratoid rhabdoid tumor or malignant rhabdoid tumor. *Genes Chromosomes Cancer* 2010;49:176–81.

104. Korf HW, Czerwionka M, Reiner J, et al. Immunocytochemical evidence of molecular photoreceptor markers in cerebellar medulloblastomas. *Cancer* 1987;60:1763–6.

105. Korshunov A, Remke M, Gessi M, Ryzhova M, Hielscher T, Witt H, et al. Focal genomic amplification at 19q13.42 comprises a powerful diagnostic marker for embryonal tumors with ependymoblastic rosettes. *Acta Neuropathol* 2010;120:253–60.

106. Korshunov A, Ryzhova M, Jones DT, Northcott PA, van Sluis P, Volckmann R, et al. LIN28A immunoreactivity is a potent diagnostic marker of embryonal tumor with multilayered rosettes (ETMR). *Acta Neuropathol* 2012;124:875–81.

107. Lafay-Cousin L, Hawkins C, Carret AS, Johnston D, Zelcer S, Wilson B, et al. Central nervous system atypical teratoid rhabdoid tumours: the Canadian Paediatric Brain Tumour Consortium experience. *Eur J Cancer* 2012;48:353–9.

108. Lamont JM, McManamy CS, Pearson AD, et al. Combined histopathological and molecular cytogenetic stratification of medulloblastoma patients. *Clin Cancer Res* 2004;10:5482–93.

109. Langford LA. The ultrastructure of the ependymoblastoma. *Acta Neuropathol* 1986;71:136–41.

110. Lee MJ, Hatton BA, Villavicencio EH, Khanna PC, Friedman SD, Ditzler S, et al. Hedgehog pathway inhibitor saridegib (IPI-926) increases lifespan in a mouse medulloblastoma model. *Proc Natl Acad Sci U S A* 2012;109:7859–64.

111. Leonard JR, Cai DX, Rivet DJ, et al. Large cell/anaplastic medulloblastomas and medullomyoblastomas: clinicopathological and genetic features. *J Neurosurg* 2001;95:82–8.

112. Li M, Lee KF, Lu Y, Clarke I, Shih D, Eberhart C, et al. Frequent amplification of a chr19q13.41 microRNA polycistron in aggressive primitive neuroectodermal brain tumors. *Cancer Cell* 2009;16: 533–46.

113. Li Y, Lal B, Kwon S, Fan X, Saldanha U, Reznik TE, et al. The scatter factor/hepatocyte growth factor: c-met pathway in human embryonal central nervous system tumor malignancy. *Cancer Res* 2005;65:9355–62.

114. Lindsey JC, Lusher ME, Anderton JA, et al. Identification of tumour-specific epigenetic events in medulloblastoma development by hypermethylation profiling. *Carcinogenesis* 2004;25:661–8.

115. Lorentzen M, Hagerstrand I. Congenital ependymoblastoma. *Acta Neuropathol* 1980;49:71–4.

116. Louis DN, Ohgaki H, Wiestler OD, Cavenee WK eds. *World Health Organization classification of tumours of the central nervous system.* Lyon: IARC Press, 2007.

117. Louis DN, Ohgaki, H, Wiestler OD, Cavenee WK, Burger PC, Jouvet A, Scheithauer BW, Kleihues P. The 2007 WHO classification of tumours of the central nervous system. *Acta Neuropathol* 2007;114:97–109.

118. Louvi A, Grove EA. Cilia in the CNS: the quiet organelle claims center stage. *Neuron* 2011;69:1046–60.

119. Lutterbach J, Liegibel J, Koch D, et al. Atypical teratoid/rhabdoid tumors in adult patients: case report and review of the literature. *J Neurooncol* 2001;52:49–56.

120. Lv SQ, Kim YH, Giulio F, Shalaby T, Nobusawa S, Yang H, et al. Genetic alterations in microRNAs in medulloblastomas. *Brain Pathol* 2012;22:230–9.

121. Mainwaring LA, Kenney AM. Divergent functions for eIF4E and S6 kinase by Sonic Hedgehog mitogenic signaling in the developing cerebellum. *Oncogene* 2011;30:1784–97.

122. McLendon RE, Friedman HS, Fuchs HE, et al. Diagnostic markers in paediatric medulloblastoma: a Paediatric Oncology Group Study. *Histopathology* 1999;34:154–62.

123. McManamy CS, Lamont JM, Taylor RE, et al. Morphophenotypic variation predicts clinical behavior in childhood non-desmoplastic medulloblastomas. *J Neuropathol Exp Neurol* 2003;62:627–32.

124. Miralbell R, Tolnay M, Bieri S, et al. Pediatric medulloblastoma: prognostic value of p53, bcl-2, Mib-1, and microvessel density. *J Neurooncol* 1999;45:103–10.

125. Mirich DR, Blaser SI, Harwood-Nash DC, et al. Melanotic neuroectodermal tumour of infancy: clinical, radiologic, and pathologic findings in five cases. *AJNR Am J Neuroradiol* 1991;12:689–97.

126. Molloy PT, Yachnis AT, Rorke LB, et al. Central nervous system medulloepithelioma: a series of eight cases including two arising in the pons. *J Neurosurg* 1996;84:430–6.

127. Mork SJ, Rubinstein LJ. Ependymoblastoma: a reappraisal of a rare embryonal tumor. *Cancer* 1985;55:1536–42.

128. Mueller W, Eum JH, Lass U, et al. No evidence of hSNF5/INI1 point mutations in choroid plexus papilloma. *Neuropathol Appl Neurobiol* 2004;30:304–7.

129. Müller K, Zwiener I, Welker H, Maass E, Bongartz R, Berthold F, et al. Curative treatment for central nervous system medulloepithelioma despite residual disease after resection. Report of two cases treated according to the GPHO Protocol HIT 2000 and review of the literature. *Strahlenther Onkol* 2011;187:757–62.

130. Nicholson JC, Ross FM, Kohler JA, Ellison DW. Comparative genomic hybridization and histological variation in primitive neuroectodermal tumours. *Br J Cancer* 1999;80:1322–31.

131. Nobusawa S, Yokoo H, Hirato J, Kakita A, Takahashi H, Sugino T, et al. Analysis of chromosome 19q13.42 amplification in embryonal brain tumors with ependymoblastic multilayered rosettes. *Brain Pathol* 2012;22:689–97.

132. Northcott PA, Jones DT, Kool M, Robinson GW, Gilbertson RJ, Cho YJ, et al. Medulloblastomics: the end of the beginning. *Nat Rev Cancer* 2012;12:818–34.

133. Northcott PA, Korshunov A, Witt H, Hielscher T, Eberhart CG, Mack S, et al. Medulloblastoma comprises four distinct molecular variants. *J Clin Oncol* 2011;29:1408–14.

134. Northcott PA, Nakahara Y, Wu X, Feuk L, Ellison DW, Croul S, et al. Multiple recurrent genetic events converge on control of histone lysine methylation in medulloblastoma. *Nat Genet* 2009;41:465–72.

135. Northcott PA, Shih DJ, Remke M, Cho YJ, Kool M, Hawkins C, et al. Rapid, reliable, and reproducible molecular sub-grouping of clinical medulloblastoma samples. *Acta Neuropathol* 2012;**123**:615–26.

136. Ojeda VJ, Stokes BA, Lee MA, et al. Primary cerebral neuroblastomas: a clinicopathological study of one adolescent and five adult patients. *Pathology* 1986;**18**:41–9.

137. Oliver TG, Read TA, Kessler JD, Mehmeti A, Wells JF, Huynh TT, et al. Loss of patched and disruption of granule cell development in a pre-neoplastic stage of medulloblastoma. *Development* 2005;**132**:2425–39.

138. Ow TJ, Bell D, Kupferman ME, Demonte F, Hanna EY. Esthesioneuroblastoma. *Neurosurg Clin N Am* 2013;**24**:51–65.

139. Park ES, Sung KW, Baek HJ, Park KD, Park HJ, Won SC, et al. Tandem high-dose chemotherapy and autologous stem cell transplantation in young children with atypical teratoid/rhabdoid tumor of the central nervous system. Journal of Korean medical science 2012;**27**:135–40.

140. Park JY, Kim E, Kim DW, Chang HW, Kim SP. Cribriform neuroepithelial tumor in the third ventricle: A case report and literature review. *Neuropathology* 2012;**32**:570–6.

141. Parsons DW, Li M, Zhang X, Jones S, Leary RJ, Lin JC, et al. The genetic landscape of the childhood cancer medulloblastoma. *Science* 2011;**331**:435–9.

142. Pei Y, Moore CE, Wang J, Tewari AK, Eroshkin A, Cho YJ, et al. An animal model of MYC-driven medulloblastoma. *Cancer Cell* 2012;**21**:155–67.

143. Perry A, Fuller CE, Judkins AR, et al. INI1 expression is retained in composite rhabdoid tumors, including rhabdoid meningiomas. *Mod Pathol* 2005;**18**:951–8.

144. Perry A. Medulloblastomas with favorable versus unfavorable histology: how many small blue cell tumor types are there in the brain? *Adv Anat Pathol* 2002;**9**:345–50.

145. Perry A, Miller CR, Gujrati M, Scheithauer BW, Zambrano SC, Jost SC, et al. Malignant gliomas with primitive neuroectodermal tumor-like components: a clinicopathologic and genetic study of 53 cases. *Brain Pathol* 2009;**19**:81–90.

146. Pfaff E, Remke M, Sturm D, Benner A, Witt H, Milde T, et al. TP53 mutation is frequently associated with CTNNB1 mutation or MYCN amplification and is compatible with long-term survival in medulloblastoma. *J Clin Oncol* 2010;**28**:5188–96.

147. Pfister SM, Korshunov A, Kool M, Hasselblatt M, Eberhart C, Taylor MD. Molecular diagnostics of CNS embryonal tumors. *Acta Neuropathol* 2010;**120**:553–66.

148. Phi JH, Kim JH, Eun KM, Wang KC, Park KH, Choi SA, et al. Upregulation of SOX2, NOTCH1, and ID1 in supratentorial primitive neuroectodermal tumors: a distinct differentiation pattern from that of medulloblastomas. *J Neurosurg Pediatr* 2010;**5**:608–14.

149. Picard D, Miller S, Hawkins CE, Bouffet E, Rogers HA, Chan TS, et al. Markers of survival and metastatic potential in childhood CNS primitive neuro-ectodermal

brain tumours: an integrative genomic analysis. *Lancet Oncol* 2012;**13**:838–48.

150. Pietsch T, Waha A, Koch A, et al. Medulloblastomas of the desmoplastic variant carry mutations of the human homologue of Drosophila patched. *Cancer Res* 1997;**57**:2085–8.

151. Pigott TJ, Punt JA, Lowe JS, et al. The clinical, radiological and histopathological features of cerebral primitive neuroectodermal tumours. *Br J Neurosurg* 1990;**4**:287–97.

152. Polydorides AD, Perry A, Edgar MA. Large cell medulloblastoma with myogenic and melanotic differentiation: a case report with molecular analysis. *J Neurooncol* 2008;**88**:193–7.

153. Pomeroy SL, Tamayo P, Gaasenbeek M, Sturla LM, Angelo M, McLaughlin ME, et al. Prediction of central nervous system embryonal tumour outcome based on gene expression. *Nature* 2002;**415**: 436–42.

154. Pushker N, Shrey D, Bajaj MS, Kashyap S, Yadav P, Mehta M, et al. Malignant non-teratoid medulloepithelioma of the optic nerve with intraocular extension. *Clin Exp Ophthalmol* 2010;**38**:731–3.

155. Raffel C, Jenkins RB, Frederick L, Hebrink D, Alderete B, Fults DW, et al. Sporadic medulloblastomas contain PTCH mutations. *Cancer Res* 1997;**57**:842–5.

156. Raisanen J, Biegel JA, Hatanpaa KJ, et al. Chromosome 22q deletions in atypical teratoid/rhabdoid tumors in adults. *Brain Pathol* 2005;**15**:23–8.

157. Rao G, Pedone CA, Valle LD, Reiss K, Holland EC, Fults DW. Sonic hedgehog and insulin-like growth factor signaling synergize to induce medulloblastoma formation from nestin-expressing neural progenitors in mice. *Oncogene* 2004;**23**:6156–62.

158. Rausch T, Jones DT, Zapatka M, Stutz AM, Zichner T, Weischenfeldt J, et al. Genome sequencing of pediatric medulloblastoma links catastrophic DNA rearrangements with TP53 mutations. *Cell* 2012;**148**:59–71.

159. Reifenberger J, Wolter M, Weber RG, et al. Missense mutations in SMOH in sporadic basal cell carcinomas of the skin and primitive neuroectodermal tumors of the central nervous system. *Cancer Res* 1998;**58**:1798–803.

160. Rogers HA, Miller S, Lowe J, Brundler MA, Coyle B, Grundy RG. An investigation of WNT pathway activation and association with survival in central nervous system primitive neuroectodermal tumours (CNS PNET). *Br J Cancer* 2009;**100**:1292–302.

161. Rogers L, Pattisapu J, Smith RR, Parker P. Medulloblastoma in association with the Coffin–Siris syndrome. *Childs Nerv Syst* 1988;**4**:41–4.

162. Romer JT, Kimura H, Magdaleno S, Sasai K, Fuller C, Baines H, et al. Suppression of the Shh pathway using a small molecule inhibitor eliminates medulloblastoma in Ptc1(+/-)p53(-/-) mice. *Cancer Cell* 2004;**6**:229–40.

163. Rood BR, Zhang H, Weitman DM, Cogen PH. Hypermethylation of HIC-1 and 17p allelic loss in medulloblastoma. *Cancer Res* 2002;**62**:3794–7.

164. Rorke LB. The cerebellar medulloblastoma and its relationship

to primitive neuroectodermal tumors. *J Neuropathol Exp Neurol* 1983;**42**:1–15.

165. Rorke LB, Packer RJ, Biegel JA. Central nervous system atypical teratoid/rhabdoid tumors of infancy and childhood: definition of an entity. *J Neurosurg* 1996;**85**:56–65.

166. Rubinstein LJ. Embryonal central neuroepithelial tumors and their differentiating potential: a cytogenetic view of a complex neuro-oncological problem. *J Neurosurg* 1985;**62**:795–805.

167. Rudin CM, Hann CL, Laterra J, Yauch RL, Callahan CA, Fu L, et al. Treatment of medulloblastoma with hedgehog pathway inhibitor GDC-0449. *N Engl J Med* 2009;**361**:1173–8.

168. Russo C, Pellarin M, Tingby O, et al. Comparative genomic hybridization in patients with supratentorial and infratentorial primitive neuroectodermal tumors. *Cancer* 1999;**86**: 331–9.

169. Rutkowski S, Bode U, Deinlein F, et al. Treatment of early childhood medulloblastoma by postoperative chemotherapy alone. *N Engl J Med* 2005;**352**:978–86.

170. Ryan SL, Schwalbe EC, Cole M, Lu Y, Lusher ME, Megahed H, et al. MYC family amplification and clinical risk-factors interact to predict an extremely poor prognosis in childhood medulloblastoma. *Acta Neuropathol* 2012;**123**:501–13.

171. Sant M, Minicozzi P, Lagorio S, Borge Johannesen T, Marcos-Gragera R, Francisci S. Survival of European patients with central nervous system tumors. *Int J Cancer* 2012;**131**:173–85.

172. Saunders T, Margo CE. Intraocular medulloepithelioma. *Arch Pathol Lab Med* 2012;**136**:212–6.

173. Scheithauer BW, Rubinstein LJ. Cerebral medulloepithelioma: report of a case with multiple divergent neuroepithelial differentiation. *Childs Brain* 1979;**5**:62–71.

174. Scheurlen WG, Schwabe GC, Joos S, Mollenhauer J, Sorensen N, Kuhl J. Molecular analysis of childhood primitive neuroectodermal tumors defines markers associated with poor outcome. *J Clin Oncol* 1998;**16**:2478–85.

175. Scheurlen WG, Schwabe GC, Seranski P, et al. Mapping of the breakpoints on the short arm of chromosome 17 in neoplasms with an i(17q). *Genes Chromosomes Cancer* 1999;**25**:230–40.

176. *Am J Hum Genet* 2010;**86**:279–84.

177. Schofield D, West DC, Anthony DC, et al. Correlation of loss of heterozygosity at chromosome 9q with histological subtype in medulloblastomas. *Am J Pathol* 1995;**146**:472–80.

178. Schuller U, Heine VM, Mao J, Kho AT, Dillon AK, Han YG, et al. Acquisition of granule neuron precursor identity is a critical determinant of progenitor cell competence to form Shh-induced medulloblastoma. *Cancer Cell* 2008;**14**:123–34.

179. *Acta Neuropathol* 2013;**125**:359–71.

180. Sevenet N, Lellouch-Tubiana A, Schofield D, et al. Spectrum of hSNF5/INI1 somatic mutations in human cancer and genotype–phenotype correlations. *Hum Mol Genet* 1999;**8**:2359–68.

181. Sevenet N, Sheridan E, Amram D, *et al.* Constitutional mutations of the hSNF5/INI1 gene predispose to a variety of cancers. *Am J Hum Genet* 1999;65:1342–8.

182. Sharma MC, Agarwal M, Suri A, *et al.* A melanotic desmoplastic medulloblastoma: report of a rare case and review of the literature. *Brain Tumor Pathol* 2002;19:93–6.

183. Sherr CJ, McCormick F. The RB and p53 pathways in cancer. *Cancer Cell* 2002;2:103–12.

184. Smoll NR, Drummond KJ. The incidence of medulloblastomas and primitive neurectodermal tumours in adults and children. *J Clin Neurosci* 2012;19:1541–4.

185. Song X, Andrew Allen R, Terence Dunn S, Fung KM, Farmer P, Gandhi S, *et al.* Glioblastoma with PNET-like components has a higher frequency of isocitrate dehydrogenase 1 (IDH1) mutation and likely a better prognosis than primary glioblastoma. *Int J Clin Exp Pathol* 2011;4:651–60.

186. Stearns D, Chaudhry A, Abel TW, Burger PC, Dang CV, Eberhart CG. c-myc overexpression causes anaplasia in medulloblastoma. *Cancer Res* 2006;66:673–81.

187. Stiller CA, Bunch KJ. Brain and spinal tumours in children aged under two years: incidence and survival in Britain, 1971–85. *Br J Cancer* 1992;66:S50–3.

188. Tabori U, Baskin B, Shago M, Alon N, Taylor MD, Ray PN, *et al.* Universal poor survival in children with medulloblastoma harboring somatic TP53 mutations. *J Clin Oncol* 2010;28:1345–50.

189. Taipale J, Beachy PA. The Hedgehog and Wnt signalling pathways in cancer. *Nature* 2001;411:349–54.

190. Tajima Y, Molina RP Jr, Rorke LB, *et al.* Neurotrophins and neuronal versus glial differentiation in medulloblastomas and other pediatric brain tumors. *Acta Neuropathol* 1998;95:325–32.

191. Taylor MD, Liu L, Raffel C, *et al.* Mutations in SUFU predispose to medulloblastoma. *Nat Genet* 2002;31:306–10.

192. Taylor MD, Mainprize TG, Rutka JT, *et al.* Medulloblastoma in a child with Rubenstein–Taybi syndrome: case report and review of the literature. *Pediatr Neurosurg* 2001;35:235–8.

193. Taylor MD, Northcott PA, Korshunov A, Remke M, Cho YJ, Clifford SC, *et al.* Molecular subgroups of medulloblastoma: the current consensus. *Acta Neuropathol* 2012;123:465–72.

194. Taylor RE, Bailey CC, Robinson K, *et al.* Results of a randomized study of preradiation chemotherapy versus radiotherapy alone for nonmetastatic medulloblastoma: The International Society of Paediatric Oncology/United Kingdom Children' Cancer Study Group PNET-3 Study. *J Clin Oncol* 2003;21:1581–91.

195. Tekautz TM, Fuller CE, Blaney S, *et al.* Atypical teratoid/rhabdoid tumors (ATRT): improved survival in children 3 years of age and older with radiation therapy and high-dose alkylator-based chemotherapy. *J Clin Oncol* 2005;23:1491–9.

196. Troost D, Jansen GH, Dingemans KP. Cerebral medulloepithelioma: electron microscopy and immuno-histochemistry. *Acta Neuropathol* 1990;80:103–7.

197. *Proc Natl Acad Sci U S A* 2009;106:2812–7.

198. Versteege I, Sevenet N, Lange J, *et al.* Truncating mutations of hSNF5/INI1 in aggressive paediatric cancer. *Nature* 1998;394:203–6.

199. Vorechovsky I, Tingby O, Hartman M, *et al.* Somatic mutations in the human homologue of Drosophila patched in primitive neuroectodermal tumours. *Oncogene* 1997;15:361–6.

200. Wechsler-Reya R, Scott MP. The developmental biology of brain tumors. *Annu Rev Neurosci* 2001;24:385–428.

201. Weeraratne SD, Amani V, Teider N, Pierre-Francois J, Winter D, Kye MJ, *et al.* Pleiotropic effects of miR-183~96~182 converge to regulate cell survival, proliferation and migration in medulloblastoma. *Acta Neuropathol* 2012;123:539–52.

202. Wetmore C, Eberhart DE, Curran T. The normal patched allele is expressed in medulloblastomas from mice with heterozygous germline mutation of patched. *Cancer Res* 2000;60:2239–46.

203. Wetmore C, Eberhart DE, Curran T. Loss of p53 but not ARF accelerates medulloblastoma in mice heterozygous for patched. *Cancer Res* 2001;61:513–16.

204. Woehrer A, Slavc I, Peyrl A, Czech T, Dorfer C, Prayer D, *et al.* Embryonal tumor with abundant neuropil and true rosettes (ETANTR) with loss of morphological but retained genetic key features during progression. *Acta Neuropathol* 2011;122:787–90.

205. Wolter M, Reifenberger J, Sommer C, *et al.* Mutations in the human homologue of the Drosophila segment polarity gene patched (PTCH) in sporadic basal cell carcinomas of the skin and primitive neuroectodermal tumors of the central nervous system. *Cancer Res* 1997;57:2581–5.

206. Woodburn RT, Azzarelli B, Montebello JF, Goss IE. Intense p53 staining is a valuable prognostic indicator for poor prognosis in medulloblastoma/central nervous system primitive neuroectodermal tumors. *J Neurooncol* 2001;52:57–62.

207. Wooff JC, Weinreb I, Perez-Ordonez B, Magee JF, Bullock MJ. Calretinin staining facilitates differentiation of olfactory neuroblastoma from other small round blue cell tumors in the sinonasal tract. *Am J Surg Pathol* 2011;35:1786–93.

208. Wortham M, Jin G, Sun JL, Bigner DD, He Y, Yan H. Aberrant otx2 expression enhances migration and induces ectopic proliferation of hindbrain neuronal progenitor cells. *PLoS One* 2012;7:e36211.

209. Wu X, Northcott PA, Dubuc A, Dupuy AJ, Shih DJ, Witt H, *et al.* Clonal selection drives genetic divergence of metastatic medulloblastoma. *Nature* 2012;482:529–33.

210. Yang ZJ, Ellis T, Markant SL, Read TA, Kessler JD, Bourboulas M, *et al.* Medulloblastoma can be initiated by deletion of Patched in lineage-restricted progenitors or stem cells. *Cancer Cell* 2008;14:135–45.

211. Yauch RL, Dijkgraaf GJ, Alicke B, Januario T, Ahn CP, Holcomb T, *et al.* Smoothened mutation confers resistance to a Hedgehog pathway inhibitor in medulloblastoma. *Science* 2009;326: 572–4.

212. Zakrzewska M, Wojcik I, Zakrzewski K, *et al.* Mutational analysis of hSNF5/INI1 and TP53 genes in choroid plexus carcinomas. *Cancer Genet Cytogenet* 2005;156:179–82.

213. Zimmerman MA, Goumnerova LC, Proctor M, *et al.* Continuous remission of newly diagnosed and relapsed central nervous system atypical teratoid/rhabdoid tumor. *J Neurooncol* 2005;72:77–84.

214. Zurawel RH, Chiappa SA, Allen C, Raffel C. Sporadic medulloblastomas contain oncogenic beta-catenin mutations. *Cancer Res* 1998;58:896–9.

215. Zuzak TJ, Steinhoff DF, Sutton LN, *et al.* Loss of caspase-8 mRNA expression is common in childhood primitive neuroectodermal brain tumour/medulloblastoma. *Eur J Cancer* 2002;38:83–91.

Tumours of the Peripheral Nerves

Arie Perry and Robin Reid

INTRODUCTION

Most tumours that develop in association with the peripheral nervous system (PNS) arise from the neural crest-derived and mesenchymal cells that form the nerve sheath.[5,113] Cellular lineages for neoplastic transformation include: (i) Schwann cells, (ii) perineurial cells and (iii) fibroblasts.

The vast majority of nerve sheath tumours are sporadic, without clear aetiologies. There are, however, some well-defined predisposing factors for the development of particular nerve sheath tumours, notably schwannomas, neurofibromas and malignant peripheral nerve sheath tumours (MPNSTs). The most common underlying syndromes are neurofibromatosis type 1 (NF1) or type 2 (NF2), schwannomatosis and Carney complex (see Chapter 44, Hereditary Tumour Syndromes). Patients with NF1 develop multiple neurofibromas and, to a lesser but significant degree, MPNSTs.[66,114] Indeed, plexiform neurofibromas and certain variants of MPNST (malignant Triton tumour, glandular MPNST and MPNST with angiosarcoma) are highly characteristic of NF1. In contrast, patients with NF2 develop multiple schwannomas, among other tumours, and bilateral vestibular schwannomas are diagnostic for NF2. Schwannomatosis patients are predisposed to multiple non-vestibular schwannomas, whereas patients with Carney complex may develop psammomatous melanotic schwannomas.[18,114,116] Prior irradiation predisposes to occasional schwannomas and up to 10 per cent of all MPNSTs.[108,118,127,154]

SCHWANNOMAS

Incidence, Age and Sites

Schwannomas (also known as neurilemmomas or neurinomas) account for roughly 8.5–10 per cent of all primary intracranial tumours,[22,96,125] of which 80–90 per cent are vestibular schwannomas, often referred to clinically as 'acoustic neuromas', which is a misnomer because they arise from the vestibular (rather than acoustic) branch of the eighth cranial nerve and represent true neoplasms rather than reactive proliferations. The incidence of vestibular schwannomas has been steadily increasing over the past two decades, likely because of increased use and resolution of neuroimaging studies, improved and more readily available audiology testing and longer life spans.[125] These factors similarly account for the fact that these tumours are now more commonly identified at an earlier (smaller sized) stage.

Patients typically present with a gradual and progressive asymmetrical or unilateral sensorineural hearing loss, preferentially targeting high frequencies. Sudden hearing loss can occur in 10 per cent of cases, secondary to vascular compromise of the auditory nerve or cochlea.

Overall incidence ranges from about 1.4 to 2 per 100 000,[22,96,125] and the age-related incidence increases between the fourth and sixth decades, with a mean age of clinical presentation of 58 years.[125] Most series show a female to male ratio of 1.5–2:1.[22,96,125] Most tumours (95 per cent) are solitary, whereas 3 per cent are multiple, occurring as part of NF2, 2 per cent are multiple in the setting of schwannomatosis and 13 per cent of all spinal schwannomas are associated with NF2.[55] Paediatric vestibular schwannomas are exceptional and, as such, should provoke suspicion of NF2.

Schwannomas generally arise in sensory, rather than motor cranial and spinal nerves, including posterior spinal nerve roots. After the vestibular branch of the eighth nerve, the next most frequent extramedullary intracranial sites are the trigeminal nerve root, the gasserian ganglion and the three major trigeminal divisions, accounting for about 0.2 per cent of all intracranial tumours.[71] Tumours may also develop within motor nerves, especially in association with NF2.[69] Involvement of other cranial nerves has been reported.[25,68,105,151] Schwannomas of the spinal nerve roots account for 16–30 per cent of all spinal tumours. Any region may be affected, with the lower segments, the lumbosacral region and the cauda equina being most frequent, although patients with NF2 may more often develop cervicothoracic root lesions.[54] About 20–25 per cent of all spinal root schwannomas are located in the cauda equina,[23] where the tumours grow either as exophytic lesions or as intraneural masses intermingled with nerve fibres. Patients complain of lower back pain and sciatica, often for several years. In contrast to the intracranial sites, there is a male sex preference (male to female ratio of 3:1).[23]

Schwannomas may arise in association with any peripheral nerve, especially cutaneous and autonomic nerves in the head and neck, and on the flexor surfaces of the extremities. In the gastrointestinal (GI) tract, they may involve the stomach and other sites, but must be distinguished from more common tumours, such as GI stromal tumours (GIST).[58,113,139] Other less common locations include the mediastinum, retroperitoneum and orbit.[10,128,142]

Intraparenchymal schwannomas arise exceptionally, with a slight male predilection (1.6:1), within both intracranial[21,47,80,132] and spinal locations.[62,83,115] Most affect cerebral hemispheres (75 per cent) or cerebellum (20 per cent), with 20 per cent of the former located close to the lateral ventricles. Less common sites include the brain stem, the sella and the fourth ventricle. Intraparenchymal schwannomas may arise from perivascular Schwann cells derived from the innervation of intracerebral arteries or dural cranial nerve (trigeminal) fibres (for convexity schwannomas) or from ectopic developmental Schwann cell rests.

Schwannomas can be cured if surgically resectable, their demarcation from the adjacent nerve often allowing removal with preservation of nerve function. The exceedingly rare documented cases of malignant transformation to MPNST affect mainly sporadic schwannomas.[2,18,77,85,149] The malignant component is often epithelioid in pattern and it has been suggested that transformation may arise within foci of single or grouped large rounded atypical cells, a phenomenon described as epithelioid malignant change.[85]

Neuroimaging

Most tumours are isointense or hypodense by computed tomography (CT), and visualization without contrast is inconsistent, but usually possible with contrast administration, owing to avid tumour enhancement. Calcification is either absent or minimally detectable in rare cases. The overall shape with magnetic resonance imaging (MRI) is that of a relatively round, globular and partially cystic, non-calcified cerebellopontine angle mass involving the internal auditory canal, which is often penetrated or eroded by the lesion, which is a useful distinction from other considerations such as meningioma.[76] On T1-weighted images, the signal intensity is higher than cerebrospinal fluid (CSF) and usually lower than surrounding brain. Significant heterogeneity may result from cystic degeneration and focal haemorrhage.[111] MRI most effectively detects involvement of the internal auditory canal owing to the relatively homogeneous tumoural enhancement after gadolinium administration (Figure 35.1). On T2-weighted images, the intensity

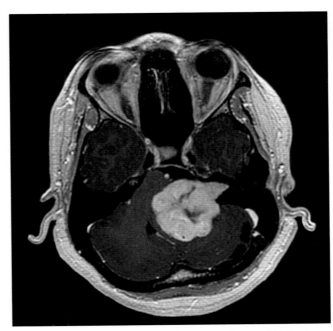

35.1 Post-contrast magnetic resonance image (MRI) showing an avidly enhancing mass in the left cerebellopontine angle. The nipple-like extension into the internal auditory canal is typical of vestibular schwannoma.

is variable: heterogeneously increased signal intensity is associated with cystic degeneration. Peritumoural oedema is usually insignificant. Outside the cranial compartment, schwannomas are typically well-delineated T1 isodense, marked T2 hyperintense masses compared with adjacent muscle.

Macroscopic Appearances

Schwannomas are typically well-encapsulated globoid lesions with a soft, rubbery texture. Unlike neurofibromas, they tend to leave the parent nerve as splayed fibres or an intact bundle at the edge of the tumour. Vestibular schwannomas most probably arise at the transition zone of central nervous system (CNS) and peripheral nervous system (PNS) tissue within the internal auditory meatus and typically expand medially into the cerebellopontine angle. Spinal examples tend to grow through the intervertebral foramina to produce a dumbbell configuration seen on neuroimaging. The cut surface is predominantly tan in colour, with variable cystic and haemorrhagic degeneration accompanied by yellow, lipid-laden areas, particularly in large tumours (Figure 35.2) and those of the lower spinal regions. Fewer than 5 per cent of cutaneous schwannomas are plexiform, mostly as sporadic examples, but occasionally in association with NF2 or schwannomatosis.

Microscopy and Immunohistochemistry

Schwannoma cells are usually spindle-shaped with tapered nuclei, these being two to three times the size of neurofibroma nuclei. The two classic architectural patterns termed Antoni A and Antoni B may be randomly admixed or

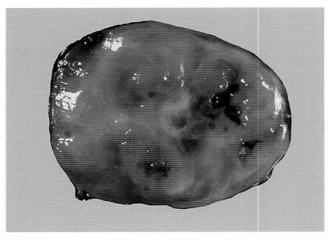

35.2 Schwannoma. Gelatinous, slightly opalescent appearance of a schwannoma with typical foci of haemorrhage.

partitioned as distinctive zones (Figure 35.3a). Antoni A tissue demonstrates compact fascicles of spindle cells with long nuclei and indistinct cytoplasmic borders. Verocay bodies, well-defined palisaded structures (Figure 35.3b), may assume an exaggerated radial orientation so as to resemble a rosette. Verocay bodies are typical of spinal schwannomas and are less common in vestibular tumours. Antoni B tissue contains more stellate cells dispersed in a loose matrix with regions of microcystic and myxoid changes resembling those of neurofibroma. Hyalinized blood vessels are prominent, some dilated with fibrinous degeneration and thrombosis. Spontaneous haemorrhage and necrosis may be accompanied by chronic inflammation and haemosiderin deposition and tumours often have numerous lipid-laden macrophages. Considerable pleomorphism and atypia, a finding that in the absence of excess mitotic activity has no sinister significance, has been dubbed 'ancient change' (Figure 35.3c).

Schwannomas are diffusely immunoreactive for S–100 protein and basement membrane components, the latter highlighted by either a reticulin stain or immunohistochemical stains for collagen IV and laminin.[70,98,119] Immunoreactivity for glial fibrillary acidic protein (GFAP) has been demonstrated in schwannomas, neurofibromas and MPNSTs.[49,51] CD34 highlights a specialized fibroblastic or dendritic cell, which may be selectively detected in Antoni B zones, especially in areas with marked myxoid stroma.[113,143] Antibodies to the Schwann cell and melanocytic specific transcription factor, SOX10, may also be useful.[70,97] Another marker reportedly expressed more commonly in schwannoma than in neurofibroma is calretinin.[41] A significant proportion of retroperitoneal schwannomas expresses cytokeratins.[36] Scattered, presumably entrapped, perineurial cells in the capsule express epithelial membrane antigen (EMA).

Electron Microscopy

The ultrastructural features of neoplastic Schwann cells include elongate nuclei and relatively attenuated cytoplasm from which flattened elongate cytoplasmic processes emanate and intertwine, often encircling collagen. The cells are

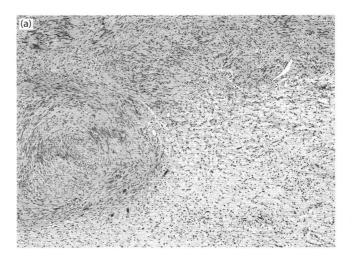

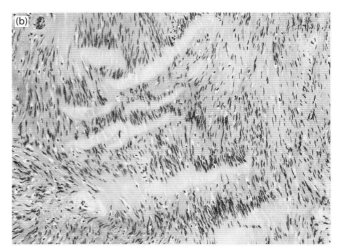

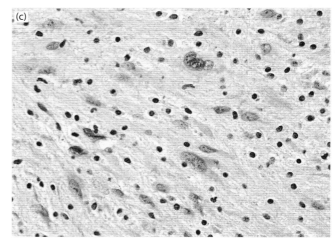

35.3 Schwannoma. **(a)** The tumour features a mixture of compact Antoni A (upper left) and loose Antoni B (lower right) patterns. **(b)** Rhythmic nuclear palisading represents Verocay bodies. **(c)** The presence of scattered bizarre nuclei in the absence of mitotic activity characterizes 'ancient change'.

surrounded by continuous, multi-layered, pericellular and intercellular basal laminae.[34] The Antoni B tissue is less cellular and is characterized by multipolar cells with rounded nuclei.

Molecular Genetics

Whether familial or sporadic, the majority of schwannomas show biallelic loss of the *NF2* gene on chromosome 22, resulting in loss of schwannomin (also known as merlin) protein expression.[1,19] Tumours associated with either sporadic or familial forms of schwannomatosis are more complex and follow a 'four-hit model' wherein both pairs of *NF2* and *INI1 (SMARCB1/hSNF5/BAF47)* genes on chromosome 22 are inactivated during tumorigenesis (see Chapter 44, Hereditary Tumour Syndromes).[11,53,121] Furthermore, it was recently found that in contrast to sporadic schwannomas where INI1 protein expression is retained, the majority of familial counterparts (schwannomatosis or NF2) demonstrate a peculiar mosaic pattern of expression,[100] wherein some nuclei are positive and others negative (Figure 35.4).

Variants of Schwannoma

Cellular Schwannoma

This variant represents about 10 per cent of schwannomas and is important because of the ease with which it can be overdiagnosed as MPNST. Typically these tumours are large and deeply located, e.g. the mediastinum or retroperitoneum, with a quarter or so arising in the extremities.[42,86,144,148] Rare intracranial examples are reported.[101] Most patients are young or middle-aged adults, with a peak incidence in the fifth decade. These lesions may behave in a locally aggressive manner with erosion of bone but, unlike MPNST, they have no metastatic potential.

Like conventional schwannomas, they are grossly encapsulated, lobular tan tumours with focal haemorrhages and cystic degeneration; however, they are somewhat firmer. Microscopically, Antoni A regions dominate (Figure 35.5), Verocay bodies are almost never seen and Antoni B tissue is sparse by definition. The nuclear to cytoplasmic ratio is high. There is often xanthomatous change, subcapsular chronic inflammation and hyalinized vessels.

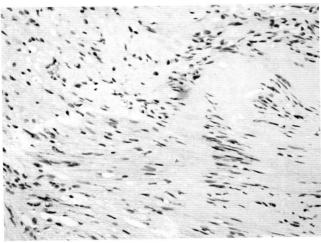

35.4 INI1 immunostain. A mosaic pattern of INI1 expression, with mixtures of immunopositive and immunonegative tumour cells, is typical of hereditary forms of schwannoma.

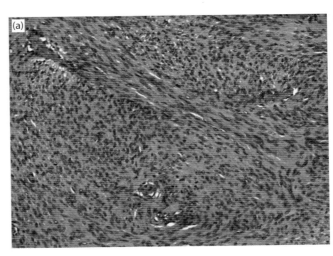

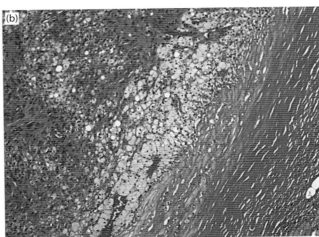

35.5 Cellular schwannoma. (a) This lesion consists largely of cellular spindle cell tissue, without Verocay body formation or palisading. **(b)** The periphery shows a fibrous capsule and there are prominent foam cells. With immunohistochemistry, the tumour strongly expressed S–100 protein.

Nuclear hyperchromasia and pleomorphism is typically mild, but there may be increased mitotic activity of up to 10/10 high-power fields and even foci of necrosis. Unlike MPNST, there is strong generalized S–100 protein and collagen IV or laminin immunoreactivity.

Cellular schwannomas have an excellent prognosis, but it is notable that tumours in paravertebral, sacral or intracranial locations are more likely to recur than peripherally situated tumours.

Epithelioid Schwannoma

This term is used to describe rare schwannomas and other similar but more difficult to classify tumours ('benign epithelioid nerve sheath tumours of soft tissue'), usually affecting peripheral nerves and skin, in which there are foci of epithelioid S–100 and collagen IV-rich cells arranged in cords and nests, often surrounded by EMA positive perineurium.[78,117] These cells may line variably sized cystic spaces and simulate glandular spaces or form rosette-like structures.[72] Fortunately, there are usually regions of typical schwannoma present. Although this variant, with its cellularity, epithelioid features and cord-like growth pattern, may simulate a high-grade lesion, it has an indolent behaviour. The epithelioid cells do not express cytokeratins distinguishing them from the rare benign schwannoma with true glandular structures.[15,146] These cases probably represent a combination of true neoplastic epithelial formations and entrapped adnexal structures.

Melanotic and Psammomatous Melanotic Schwannomas

Melanotic schwannoma is an uncommon variant, characterized by pigmented neoplastic Schwann cells.[18,62,75,123] The psammomatous melanotic schwannoma additionally contains PAS-positive, laminated calcified bodies resembling psammoma bodies. These, in particular, are strongly associated with the autosomal dominant Carney complex (see Chapter 44, Hereditary Tumour Syndromes).[1,113,123,138] These patients tend to present a decade earlier than those with the sporadic form, for which the mean age at presentation is 35 years. Approximately 20 per cent present with multiple tumours, 80 per cent of which occur in Carney complex patients. Tumours have been described in numerous sites, including the gastrointestinal tract, retroperitoneum, liver, spinal nerve roots, soft tissue of the trunk and extremities, bone, chest wall, heart, bronchus and trigeminal ganglion.

Grossly, they are circumscribed, lobulated tumours ranging from grey to black or blue, with uneven pigmentation and variable cystic change. In lightly pigmented tumours, fatty change may produce intense yellow foci.

On microscopy, the tumour cells may be spindle-shaped, dendritic and epithelioid forming ill-defined palisading or whorled structures. These cells are immunoreactive for S–100, HMB–45, and Melan–A and may contain large amounts of melanin. Psammoma bodies are present in varying numbers and small amounts of mature adipose tissue are often present. Areas of degenerative change with cyst formation, haemorrhage and necrosis are not uncommon. In the absence of psammoma bodies, these tumours may be extremely difficult to distinguish from melanocytic neoplasms, such as melanocytoma, although the majority of the latter are now known to harbour *GNAQ* and *GNA11* gene mutations similar to those encountered in blue nevi.[75]

Ultrastructural studies demonstrate cells with elongated and interdigitating processes enclosed by a continuous basal lamina. Cytoplasmic premelanosomes and melanosomes are usually conspicuous.

Although most tumours are indolent, malignant transformation occurs in a subset.[18,123] Approximately 10 per cent follow an aggressive course, including systemic metastases. Usually, but not always, such tumours have large nuclei with prominent nucleoli, frequent mitoses and large areas of necrosis.

Plexiform Schwannoma

These tumours most commonly arise in the skin and subcutis, consisting of multiple expanded nerve fascicles forming a rope-like, or plexiform, mass (Figure 35.6), but deeply situated examples are also recognized.[10,57,113,118]

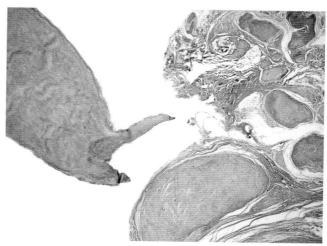

35.6 Plexiform schwannoma, characterized by a multinodular growth pattern. Note the Verocay bodies in the upper left nodule.

They show a histological spectrum across cellular, classic and mixed schwannoma and are typically dominated by dense Antoni A tissue. They occur mostly sporadically, occasionally in patients with NF2 or schwannomatosis, and rarely in patients with NF1.

Most tumours diagnosed as 'plexiform neurofibroma' in NF2 patients turn out to be plexiform schwannomas on review, thus supporting the association of plexiform schwannoma with NF2,[67] which is an important distinction because plexiform schwannomas are typically not deep-seated and do not progress to MPNST. The deeply located examples, in particular, should not be overdiagnosed as MPNST, despite increased cellularity and mild atypia.[3] The entity originally described as plexiform MPNST of infancy and childhood[88] is now regarded by many pathologists as a cellular variant of plexiform schwannoma because of its good prognosis.[150]

NEUROFIBROMAS

Incidence, Age and Sites

Solitary neurofibroma, the most common tumour of peripheral nerves, usually arises during early adulthood without sex predilection. Cutaneous, deep and visceral autonomic nerves are most commonly affected (Figure 35.7), followed by spinal nerve roots. Unlike schwannomas, intracranial neurofibromas are extremely rare. Neurofibromas may be classified as intraneural or diffusely infiltrative. Intraneural lesions may be solitary, fusiform or multinodular with involvement of multiple fascicles. Whereas this latter 'plexiform' growth pattern is seen almost exclusively in NF1 (see Chapter 44, Hereditary Tumour Syndromes), the presence of a single plexiform neurofibroma is not sufficient by itself for a diagnosis of NF1.[114] Intraneural neurofibromas frequently involve cervical, brachial and lumbosacral nerves.[119] Intraspinal neurofibromas are frequently associated with NF1.[54] Multiple neurofibromas are the hallmark of NF1 (Figure 35.8).

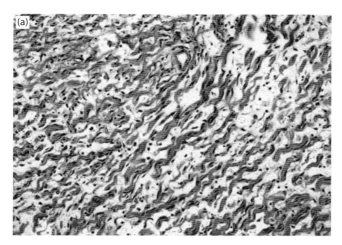

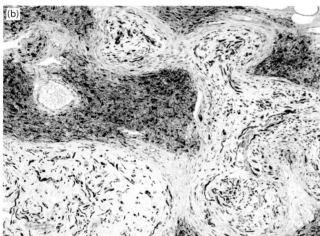

35.7 Neurofibroma. (a) Neurofibroma showing the typical wavy arrays of tumour cells within a loose matrix. **(b)** S–100 protein immunoreactivity is typically variable given the presence of intermixed non-Schwann cell elements.

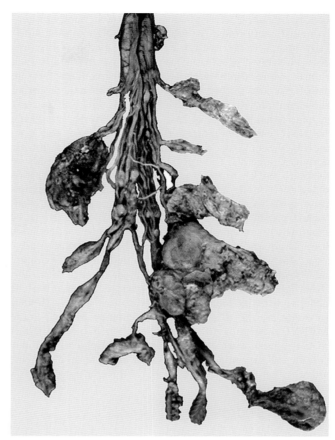

35.8 Neurofibromatosis type 1. Multiple neurofibromas of the lumbosacral plexus and the cauda equina in a patient with neurofibromatosis type 1.

Neurofibromas can be cured by resection, but the intimate mixture of tumour cells and axons renders dissection from the parent nerve impossible, so that complete resection of neurofibromas is associated with greater morbidity than that of schwannomas.

Neuroimaging and Macroscopic Appearances

Neurofibromas, like peripheral schwannomas, but in contrast to many malignant soft-tissue tumours, have irregular T2-weighted and gadolinium-enhanced T1-weighted signals. The tumours are not encapsulated, unless confined within the original epineurium. Most cutaneous growths are not obviously associated with a parent nerve. Solitary tumours grow by diffusely expanding the central endoneurial spaces producing a fusiform enlargement of the affected nerve. Plexiform tumours involve multiple fascicles with either thickening of nerve branches within a plexus ('bag of worms' appearance) or a ropy thickening of large complex nerves.[119] Neurofibromas tend to be soft, almost gelatinous, in consistency and somewhat translucent to homogeneously grey–tan.

Microscopy and Immunohistochemistry

Solitary and plexiform neurofibromas are similar histologically, being composed of spindle-shaped, wavy cells arranged in loose bundles within a matrix rich in collagen and mucopolysaccharide (Figure 35.7a). Varying proportions of Schwann cells, perineurial-like cells, fibroblasts and various inflammatory components, including mast cells, are present. The nuclei are typically much smaller than those in schwannomas. Blood vessels are delicate and relatively inconspicuous. Centrally placed myelinated and non-myelinated neurofilament immunopositive axons may be found within neurofibromas, facilitating their distinction from schwannomas. Diffuse cutaneous neurofibromas, often affecting the head and neck of patients with NF1, may contain distinctive Meissner-like corpuscles (see Figure 44.1b, p. 1929), stacked membranous structures, which are strongly S–100 immunopositive.

Neurofibromas show more variable, less pronounced S–100 staining (Figure 35.7b) than schwannomas and CD34 immunoreactivity is variably present in thin spindled cells.[95,113,143]

Unlike schwannomas, a subset of mostly non-cutaneous neurofibromas are predisposed to malignant transformation, most notably in 5–10 per cent of plexiform neurofibromas and less often in intraneural neurofibromas.[35,119] Malignancy is suggested clinically by rapid enlargement of a pre-existing neurofibroma, pain or a change in neurological symptoms, particularly in NF1 patients.[30,73] Histological diagnosis can be difficult because this process probably represents a continuum. Many classify such tumours into three categories based on nuclear atypia, cellularity and mitotic activity. 'Neurofibroma' describes those of typical appearance or those showing only nuclear atypia, either focal or diffuse. A diagnosis of 'low-grade MPNST' can be made if there is increased cell size, increased cellularity, nuclear hyperchromasia and mitotic activity; indeed, if the cellularity is such that the cells lie 'back to back', mitotic activity is not essential for this diagnosis.[119] The term 'atypical neurofibroma' describes those with occasional mitoses, but lacking sufficient cytological pleomorphism or cellularity to allow a definitive diagnosis of malignancy. Of interest, recent studies have found frequent losses of the *CDKN2A* gene in such cases, suggesting that they are either premalignant or already malignant.[8] The process may be focal or extensive, and thorough examination of the specimen is required in order to identify focal progression to low-grade MPNST. In contrast, the diagnosis of malignancy in high-grade MPNST is seldom difficult, although it is often difficult to distinguish such tumours from histologically similar spindle cell sarcomas in the absence of nerve involvement, a history of NF1 or clear-cut neural differentiation.

Electron Microscopy

Ultrastructural studies confirm the variability of cellular types. Schwann cells predominate and may invest the residual small axons engulfed during tumour growth. Perineurial-like and fibroblastic cells are also present in varying proportions and stages of differentiation. The former typically have entangled elongated processes with an incomplete pericellular basal lamina, a well-developed Golgi apparatus, abundant endoplasmic reticulum and surface-orientated pinocytotic vesicles, whereas the latter lack basal lamina and commonly have a very prominent, well-developed endoplasmic reticulum.

Molecular Genetics

Most plexiform neurofibromas, including the rare sporadic examples, harbour demonstrable losses of the *NF1* gene on chromosome 17, with other subtypes showing deletions slightly less often.[9,28,79,81,103] The resulting loss of the neurofibromin protein expression is felt to be critical to tumorigenesis. However, studies have shown that within these neurofibromas, only the Schwann cells are neoplastic, whereas the many other non-neoplastic cell types are presumably entrapped and/or recruited into the tumour.[81,103] Cutaneous neurofibromas are now thought to arise from a more primitive dermal progenitor cell.[79] Of interest, murine models that selectively target the *NF1* gene for inactivation in Schwann cells only develop neurofibromas in the presence of heterozygous *NF1* mutant/wild type stromal cells, with mast cells, in particular, being critical to tumorigenesis.[156] During malignant transformation to MPNST, additional genetic alterations occur.

PERINEURIOMAS

Perineuriomas are rare sporadic tumours composed of cells with the immunohistochemical and ultrastructural properties of perineurial cells. Two major variants exist: intraneural perineuriomas and soft-tissue perineuriomas.[63,113,119]

Intraneural perineurioma mainly elicits a differential diagnosis with localized hypertrophic neuropathy, a non-neoplastic mononeuropathy characterized by focal nerve hypertrophy and a fusiform mass. The histological features of the latter are dominated by classical onion bulbs, concentrically laminated proliferations of S–100 immunoreactive Schwann cells around central axons. In contrast, intraneural perineuriomas feature pseudo-onion bulbs composed of neoplastic EMA positive perineurial-like cells (Figure 35.9) that have incomplete basal lamina and numerous pinocytotic vesicles at the ultrastructural level.[32] Immunostains for neurofilament and S–100 highlight residual, often centrally placed axons and Schwann cells, respectively. These lesions vary considerably in length, but may extend up to 30 cm in rare examples.[32] Children and young adults are especially affected.

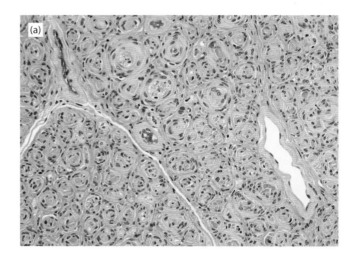

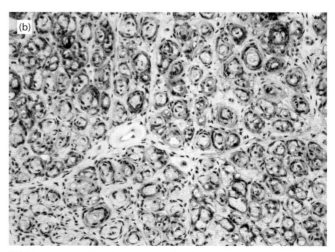

35.9 Intraneural perineurioma. (a) Cross section of the tumour reveals numerous pseudo-onion bulbs composed of concentric rings of perineurial cell cytoplasm, which is highlighted on the EMA stain **(b)**.

In these lesions, Ki–67 labelling indices may be elevated (4–17 per cent),[32] but the lesions behave in a benign manner. Although the fusiform nature of the lesion suggests a discrete border, a variable ingrowth of EMA-positive cells into apparently normal fascicles at the margins of the lesion may occur.[126] Proliferation of perineurial cells within the lesion may be multifocal[126] and molecular cytogenetic studies reveal that such lesions can be associated with clonal chromosome 22 losses.[32]

Soft-tissue perineuriomas usually develop between the third and fifth decades, with no sex predilection and no clear association with peripheral nerve;[63] they are most common in superficial soft tissues, especially in the hand. The tumours are circumscribed nodular masses ranging from 0.3 to 7 cm in maximum dimension with a firm texture and a pale cut surface. Tumour cells are typically arranged in short bundles with whorling, or a fascicular to laminar pattern, but the tight pseudo-onion bulb formations of intraneural perineuriomas are generally not seen. A storiform pattern can be conspicuous. The tumour cells of soft-tissue perineuriomas are thin and fusiform, with bipolar cellular processes and spindled nuclei with light-staining chromatin and inconspicuous nucleoli. Cellularity may be uniformly high or variable with lower density foci in association with a myxohyaline stroma. Small clusters of xanthomatous cells may also be detected within the lesion. The intercellular matrix usually contains copious collagen, but extensive hyalinization is uncommon. The vasculature is relatively delicate and inconspicuous.

Immunohistochemistry for EMA, claudin–1, glucose transporter 1, and vimentin shows consistent reactivity in the tumour cells, which are otherwise negative for S–100 protein, neurofilament epitopes, desmin, CD117 and smooth-muscle actin.

A variant, 'sclerosing perineurioma',[39,42] occurs in the hands of young men and consists of round cells arranged in often concentric cords, in a densely collagenous background. This subtype may strongly express CD34, a potential pitfall with other diagnostic considerations.[45] The term 'reticular perineurioma' has been applied to a variant with a net-like pattern of cells in a myxoid background. This entity was reported in a very small series of tumours tending to affect the upper limbs of young women.[50]

Follow-up suggests that perineuriomas have an indolent growth potential without recurrence after local excision.

Rare MPNSTs showing perineurial differentiation characterized by EMA expression and a whorled architecture have also been reported.[59]

Molecular Genetics

In contrast to schwannomas and neurofibromas, familial associations with perineuriomas are exceptionally rare.[7] Chromosome 10 aberrations, including translocation t(2;10)(p23;q24) and monosomy 10 have been reported in sclerosing perineuriomas.[14] All subtypes have also been associated with chromosome 22q losses.[14,32,48] Whether these deletions target the *NF2* gene or other chromosome 22q genes is yet to be determined.

HYBRID NERVE SHEATH TUMOURS

Although the vast majority of benign nerve sheath tumours conform to a single category, rare cases combining features of neurofibroma, schwannoma and perineurioma have now been reported.[113] One controversial pairing is the hybrid neurofibroma-schwannoma,[38,56] wherein distinct regions of each classical morphology present together as a single collision tumour–like mass. However, the definitions remain vague and the findings are potentially subject to varying interpretations, such as 'schwannoma-like nodules' within pure neurofibromas and the fact that Antoni B areas may resemble neurofibroma within otherwise pure schwannomas. The plexiform architecture of some cases further complicates interpretations and, because these hybrid tumours have now been described in NF1, NF2, and schwannomatosis, a diagnosis of hybrid neurofibroma-schwannoma may also engender diagnostic confusion for geneticists and neurologists attempting to diagnose a specific syndrome. As such, more objective clinicopathological and genetic definitions are still needed. Perhaps a more clearly defined and widely accepted pairing is the hybrid schwannoma–perineurioma.[64,91,99] These neoplasms often resemble the soft tissue perineurioma on routine histology, but include intermixed populations of S–100 positive Schwann cells with EMA, claudin–1 and CD34 positive perineurial cells on immunohistochemical and ultrastructural studies. To date, no hereditary associations have been identified, although a single example of progression to MPNST has been reported.[111] Otherwise, these hybrid tumours are considered benign.

NERVE SHEATH MYXOMA AND NEUROTHEKEOMA

Nerve sheath myxoma and neurothekeoma were formerly thought to form a single group of benign, primarily cutaneous tumours[109] characterized by lobular aggregates of cells; however, they are now considered separate entities.[119]

Nerve sheath myxoma (previously termed 'classic neurothekeoma') is mainly a tumour of adults, typically presenting as a slow-growing, painless, solitary, multinodular mass in the extremities, especially the hand, pretibial region and foot, whereas less common sites include oral mucosa.[40,137] The tumours involve the dermis or subcutis and consist of multinodular myxoid lobules containing spindled to stellate cells separated by collagenous bands. These cells are immunoreactive for S–100 and GFAP (neoplastic Schwann cells), and sometimes show mild nuclear atypia. CD34-immunopositive intraneural cells are present in small numbers. Mitotic figures are uncommon. However, these tumours often recur following local excision.

Neurothekeomas and cellular neurothekeomas usually affect children and young adults, are more common in females and mostly occur on the face.[46,106] On microscopy, they consist of variably cellular lobules, with a myxoid background in conventional neurothekeoma, but only scant mucin in the cellular variant. The cells are typically epithelioid, with abundant eosinophilic cytoplasm. The cells are immunonegative for S–100 and GFAP, but variably positive for MiTF, S–100A6, smooth muscle actin and PGP9.5.[46,106,140] Overall, the constituent cell is probably not of nerve sheath origin, but fibroblastic or fibrohistiocytic in nature.

GRANULAR CELL TUMOURS

The granular cell tumour (also known as granular cell schwannoma; previously termed granular cell myoblastoma) is a relatively common neoplasm. It is currently regarded as a poorly circumscribed nerve sheath tumour with extensive lysosomal accumulation.[4,119] Granular cell tumours develop at any age, but are most common between the fourth and sixth decades, more often afflicting women. They occur anywhere, but most commonly in the tongue and the breast; other sites in the head and neck, chest wall and upper extremities are frequently affected, and rarely granular tumours occur in the respiratory or gastrointestinal systems. Occasional patients develop multiple granular cell tumours. Macroscopically, granular cell tumours are yellow and usually 1–2 cm in diameter, but may be up to 5 cm.

Microscopic examination reveals a collection of polyhedral cells with abundant eosinophilic, granular, periodic acid Schiff (PAS)-positive cytoplasm and small hyperchromatic nuclei (Figure 35.10). Occasional examples appear plexiform.[4] The tumour cells are immunoreactive for S–100 protein, NSE and CD68. On occasion, there is such dense collagenisation that the granular cells are obscured. Ultrastructurally, the cytoplasmic granules are large secondary lysosomes containing debris that resembles myelin breakdown products. As in other schwannian neoplasms, the cells produce extensive basal lamina and long-spacing collagen may be present.

The vast majority are benign, but occasionally, typical examples develop systemic metastases.[119] The rare, histologically malignant granular cell tumours show marked hypercellularity, pleomorphism, spindle cell morphology,

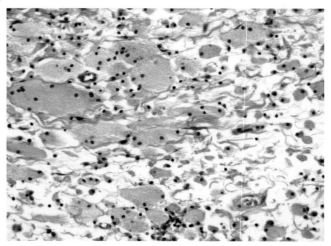

35.10 Granular cell tumour. This example is characterized by clusters of cells with abundant lysosome-rich cytoplasm and small, rounded nuclei.

high nuclear to cytoplasmic ratio, prominent nucleoli, frequent mitoses and conspicuous necrosis.[37] Granular cell tumours must be distinguished from a wide variety of tumours with granular cytoplasm, including the dermal non-neural granular cell tumour.[24]

MALIGNANT PERIPHERAL NERVE SHEATH TUMOURS

Incidence, Age and Sex

The diagnosis of malignant peripheral nerve sheath tumour (MPNST) should be considered for malignant spindle cell tumours that (i) arise in a peripheral nerve; (ii) develop in the setting of a benign nerve sheath tumour, especially plexiform neurofibroma; (iii) occur in a patient with NF1; and/or (iv) show immunohistochemical and/or ultrastructural evidence of nerve sheath differentiation.[113,127] Previously utilized synonyms that should now be avoided include malignant schwannoma, neurogenic sarcoma and neurofibrosarcoma. Roughly half occur sporadically and half in patients with NF1.

The incidence of MPNST in the general population is estimated at 1:100 000 according to a large Mayo Clinic series,[30] whereas in patients with NF1 the lifetime risk is estimated at 8–13 per cent.[35] Tumours most frequently involve adults, with NF1 patients tending to be younger (mean age: 26–29 years) than sporadic counterparts (mean age: 40–53 years).[30,107] MPNSTs involving children and adolescents are rare[29,87] with a lower proportion suffering from NF1.[17] In sporadic cases, the sex incidence is equal, whereas in NF1, there is a male predominance.

About 10 per cent of all soft-tissue sarcomas are MPNSTs.[142] They may occur *de novo* within a normal nerve, but often arise as a result of malignant transformation of a solitary intraneural or a plexiform neurofibroma. The concurrence of a neurofibromatous component has been demonstrated in about 60 per cent, with 81 per cent of those arising in NF1 patients.[30] Also, MPNSTs may arise from a peripheral nerve exposed to radiation,[1] with post-radiation examples documented both in patients with and without NF1.[31,43,118,127] Exceptionally, MPNSTs may arise secondary to malignant transformation of schwannomas, phaeochromocytomas and ganglioneuromas.[20,52,85,112,118,149]

The anatomical distribution of MPNSTs is similar to that of solitary and plexiform neurofibromas. They tend to be deep tumours associated with a major nerve trunk, most frequently located in the proximal limbs and in the trunk, and less commonly in the head and neck region.[1,30,142] Tumours in NF1 patients are more often centrally located, a factor that may underlie their poorer prognosis. Rare MPNSTs involving cranial nerves have been reported, more commonly arising from schwannomas in this location. Reported cases have involved trigeminal, vestibular and other nerves.[118]

The main presenting complaint is an expanding mass accompanied by pain and neurological symptoms related to the involved nerve.[30,136] Many factors contribute to the clinical outcome of MPNST patients.[30,87,107,127,157] Centrally located tumours, including paraspinal lesions, fare worse than those arising in extremities. Large tumours (e.g. >5 cm) similarly fare worse, though this is defined variably by different groups.[127,157] Tumours of higher histological grade and those with higher proliferation indices may also follow a more aggressive course, but such associations have not been found in all studies, possibly reflecting the highly variable grading schemes applied. Other prognostic factors include extent of surgery, positive surgical margins, presence of metastatic disease, p53 expression and lack of S–100 positivity. The presence or absence of NF1 significantly impacts survival rates, with 5-year survival rates of 16–50 per cent for patients with NF1 vs 44–82 per cent in patients without the disorder. However, this difference could represent the predominance of large, more centrally located tumours in NF1 patients.

Macroscopic Appearances

Most MPNSTs present as large deep-seated masses. In cases arising superficially in the extremities, the tumours present as fusiform or eccentric masses within a major nerve. On cut surface, MPNSTs vary from white-tan, yellow or red-brown with patchy discolouration from necrosis and haemorrhage. The consistency is usually firm, with softer foci representing myxoid degeneration or necrosis. Although tumours may appear deceptively well-circumscribed, infiltration of adjacent soft tissues is common.

Microscopy and Immunohistochemistry

Considerable histological variation is encountered in MPNSTs. Most tumours are composed of densely cellular fascicles of spindle cells (Figure 35.11a), sometimes exhibiting a herring-bone or storiform pattern. Patterns resembling the nuclear palisading and meissnerian differentiation of schwannomas and neurofibromas are rare, but hypocellular myxoid areas similar to Antoni B tissue are common and often impart a two-toned dark blue/light blue appearance at low magnification. Perivascular accumulation of tumour cells and proliferation of cells into subendothelial regions are typical of MPNSTs, as is high mitotic activity. Necrosis is often prominent and may exhibit pseudopalisading. Some tumours are markedly pleomorphic. Between 10 and 20 per cent of tumours demonstrate heterologous differentiation, particularly in NF1 patients.[110,118]

In about 50–80 per cent, S–100 protein is expressed; however, the staining tends to be focal and limited to small subpopulations (Figure 35.11b).[145] Indeed, a strongly and diffusely S–100-immunopositive tumour is unlikely to be an MPNST, but rather a desmoplastic/spindle cell melanoma or a cellular schwannoma. However, the epithelioid MPNST is the exception to this rule. Additional, albeit poorly specific markers of Schwann cell differentiation include Leu–7 and collagen IV.[87,145] A more recent marker with increased specificity and similar sensitivity is SOX10, a transcription factor expressed in both Schwann cell and melanocytic neoplasms.[70,92,97] SOX9 is often highly expressed, although its diagnostic utility in this setting has yet to be explored.[92,93,134] In the rare perineurial MPNSTs, EMA is at least focally positive. However, another important consideration in this situation is synovial sarcoma, particularly the

monophasic variant, which commonly expresses EMA (and cytokeratin) and may also express S–100 protein.[120] Demonstration of the characteristic X:18 (SYT–SSX) translocation of synovial sarcoma enables the distinction in most cases, whereas immunoreactivity for TLE1 can similarly be helpful.[44,74] This potential diagnostic pitfall is particularly relevant because not only may synovial sarcoma arise within a peripheral nerve[26,120] but also intraneural metastasis from a primary synovial sarcoma elsewhere is also possible.[84]

Electron Microscopy

Ultrastructural studies may assist in the differential diagnosis when tumours are poorly differentiated, although it is not uncommon, unfortunately, for electron microscopy to similarly show non-specific features. MPNSTs are characterized by many of the features seen in benign nerve sheath tumours, but with less differentiation. Helpful features include branching cytoplasmic processes with interdigitating cell membranes and cytoplasm containing microtubules and microfilaments.[34,133] In the more differentiated tumours, a basal lamina is present and Luse bodies (long-spacing collagen) may be found. In less differentiated tumours, the cell

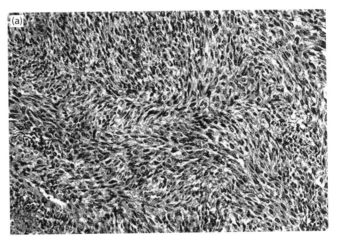

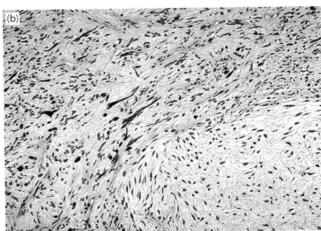

35.11 Malignant peripheral nerve sheath tumour (MPNST). **(a)** MPNST showing hypercellularity and the typical dense, fascicular arrangement of spindle cells. **(b)** S–100 protein positivity, although present, is not abundant.

processes are broader and the basal lamina is incomplete or only focally present.

Molecular Genetics

Molecular studies have generally shown highly complex karyotypes and genomic profiles in MPNSTs, with great overlap in sporadic versus NF1 associated MPNSTs, often featuring allelic losses of 17q loci, including the *NF1* gene.[12,13,19,82,89,135,141,153,155] Current models posit that inactivation of the *NF1* gene occurs at the stage of neurofibroma development, whereas additional events account for malignant progression. The *TP53* gene on chromosome 17p and the *CDKN2A/p16* gene on chromosome 9p are two tumour suppressor genes that are most commonly inactivated during progression to MPNST.[19,33,89,104] In addition, expression of the p27[Kip-1] cell cycle regulator and miR–34a appear to be downregulated in the progression from neurofibroma to MPNST, whereas PDGFRs, EGFR, insulin receptor substrate (IRS) and focal adhesion kinase (FAK) are upregulated.[61,102,122,129,131] A genomic study of MPNSTs suggests that *CDK4* gene amplification and FOXM1 overexpression are associated with decreased patient survival times.[155]

MPNSTS with Divergent Mesenchymal Differentiation

Approximately 15 per cent of MPNSTs display mesenchymal differentiation, most commonly rhabdomyoblastic, warranting the designation 'malignant Triton tumour'.[110,118] Other heterologous elements include malignant cartilage and bone. Malignant Triton tumours and other heterologous MPNST tumours are rare and around two-thirds of the cases reported in the literature arise in patients with NF1,[16] with additional cases reported in patients without NF1 after radiation.[152] The tumours usually arise in relatively young patients, with an average age of 35 years. The great majority involve peripheral nerves in a wide distribution including head, neck and trunk. A few have arisen in cranial nerves, particularly in the vestibular nerve.[118]

The characteristic histopathological feature of malignant Triton tumour is the presence of variable numbers of rhabdomyoblasts distributed singly or in groups within an otherwise typical MPNST (Figure 35.12a). The rhabdomyoblasts have abundant eosinophilic cytoplasm and hyperchromatic nuclei. Less frequently, spindled or strap-like cells displaying cytoplasmic cross-striations can be identified. Mitotic figures tend to be abundant and foci of necrosis are present. Immunohistochemistry reveals reactivities for desmin (Figure 35.12b), myogenin and myoD1 within rhabdomyoblasts, along with patchy S–100 protein reactivity within typical MPNST cells. Because the differential diagnosis includes rhabdomyosarcoma, the identification of a focal MPNST phenotype is critical, especially in small biopsies.

Epithelioid MPNSTs

The epithelioid variant accounts for less than 5 per cent of MPNSTs, with less association with NF1.[77] Unlike classic MPNSTs, the majority localize to the deep dermis or subcutis, although some may be deep-seated and involve nerve trunks.[20,77,130] They consist of groups of plump epithelioid

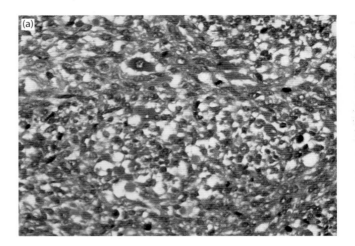

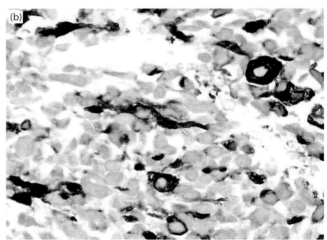

35.12 Malignant Triton tumour. (a) This is a malignant spindle cell tumour and its cytological features would fit well with a diagnosis of malignant peripheral nerve sheath tumour (MPNST). The presence of large rhabdomyoblasts with copious eosinophilic cytoplasm indicates heterologous skeletal muscle differentiation, which is further substantiated on a desmin immunostain **(b)**.

cells with abundant eosinophilic granular cytoplasm, round vesicular nuclei and prominent nucleoli, which are arranged in nests or cords (Figure 35.13a). Immunoreactivity for S–100 protein is strong and diffuse (Figure 35.13b).[145] Some are purely epithelioid, whereas in others, a spindle cell element is admixed. The epithelioid cells are usually immunonegative for cytokeratins, a feature differentiating these tumours from carcinomas. Given an often superficial location, epithelioid features and S–100 immunopositivity, these tumours may be difficult to distinguish from some melanomas, particularly neurotropic melanomas.[130] Very rarely, epithelioid MPNSTs may even demonstrate focal immunoreactivity for melanoma antigens, e.g. HMB–45.[124] Electron microscopy may thus be helpful because epithelioid MPNSTs show schwannian differentiation with the presence of pericellular basal lamina, variable cell junctions and epithelioid differentiation with microvilli and lumen formation, but no premelanosomes.[94,130] Additionally, these tumours not infrequently show loss of INI–1 (BAF47) expression, a finding that should not prompt reclassification as either malignant rhabdoid tumour or epithelioid sarcoma.[20,60,65]

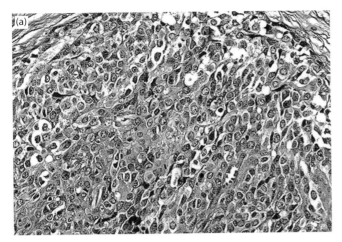

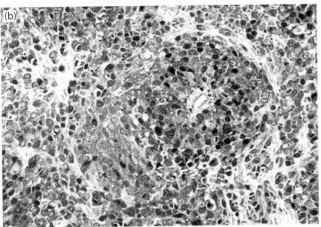

35.13 Epithelioid malignant peripheral nerve sheath tumour (MPNST). **(a)** Large, epithelioid tumour cells with relatively well-delineated borders in an epithelioid MPNST. **(b)** The characteristic tumour cells in the epithelioid MPNST display prominent S–100 immunoreactivity.

Glandular MPNSTs

Glandular MPNSTs are rare tumours in which neoplastic epithelial glands are scattered throughout an otherwise typical MPNST. These glands appear cytologically benign and immunostain strongly for epithelial markers, such as cytokeratins and EMA. They are usually of intestinal type; columnar, goblet and neuroendocrine cells may be present. There is a strong association between glandular MPNST and NF1, with nearly 75 per cent occurring in NF1 patients.[147] The mean age of onset is low: 29 years. The prognosis is poor, most patients dying within 2 years. The major differential diagnosis is biphasic synovial sarcoma, although gland-like elements appear malignant in this tumour.

MPNST with Angiosarcoma

This rare tumour nearly always occurs in association with NF1, with most occurring in young adults (mean age: 23 years).[85,90] It follows an aggressive course, with average survival typically under 2 years. Histologically, angiosarcomatous components are densely cellular regions consisting of small vascular spaces lined by neoplastic cells that stain immunohistochemically for endothelial markers, such as factor VIII-related antigen and *Ulex europaeus* lectin. These elements may also arise rarely in benign nerve sheath tumours.[90]

MPNST Arising from Ganglioneuroma and Phaeochromocytoma

In exceptional circumstances, MPNSTs arise in the setting of other nerve sheath or neural crest tumours, such as schwannoma (mostly epithelioid MPNSTs), ganglioneuroma, ganglioneuroblastoma, or phaeochromocytoma.[20,52,85,112,118,149] Most are aggressive tumours, mainly affecting young adults.

REFERENCES

1. Adamson DC, Cummings TJ, Friedman AH. Malignant peripheral nerve sheath tumour of the spine after radiation therapy for Hodgkin's lymphoma. Clin Neuropathol 2004;23:245–5.
2. Agaimy A, Stachel KD, Jungert J, et al. Malignant epithelioid peripheral nerve sheath tumour with prominent reticular/microcystic pattern in a child: a low-grade neoplasm with 18-years follow-up. Appl Immunohistochem Mol Morphol 2011 Jul 15 [Epub ahead of print].
3. Agaram NP, Prakash S, Antonescu CR. Deep-seated plexiform schwannoma: a pathological study of 16 cases and comparative analysis with the superficial variety. Am J Surg Pathol 2005;29: 1042–8.
4. Aldabagh B, Azmi F, Vadmal M, Neider S, Usmani AS. Plexiform pattern in cutaneous granular cell tumours. J Cutan Pathol 2009;36(11):1174–6.
5. Antonescu CR, Woodruff JM, Scheithauer BW. Tumours of the peripheral nervous system, 4th edn. Washington DC: American Registry of Pathology, 2012.
6. Deleted in proof.

7. Ausmus GG, Piliang MP, Bergfeld WF, Goldblum JR. Soft-tissue perineurioma in a 20-year-old patient with neurofibromatosis type 1 (NF1): report of a case and review of the literature. J Cutan Pathol 2007;34(9):726–30.
8. Beert E, Brems H, Daniels B, et al. Atypical neurofibromas in neurofibromatosis type 1 are premalignant tumours. Genes Chromosomes Cancer 2011;50(12):1021–32.
9. Beert E, Brems H, Renard M, et al. Biallelic inactivation of NF1 in a sporadic plexiform neurofibroma. Genes Chromosomes Cancer 2012;51(9):852–7.
10. Berg JC, Scheithauer BW, Spinner RJ, Allen CM, Koutlas IG. Plexiform schwannoma: a clinicopathologic overview with emphasis on the head and neck region. Hum Pathol 2008;39(5):633–40.
11. Boyd C, Smith MJ, Kluwe L, et al. Alterations in the SMARCB1 (INI1) tumour suppressor gene in familial schwannomatosis. Clin Genet 2008;74(4):358–66.
12. Brekke HR, Ribeiro FR, Kolberg M, et al. Genomic changes in chromosomes 10,

16 and X in malignant peripheral nerve sheath tumours identify a high-risk patient group. J Clin Oncol 2010;28(9): 1573–82.
13. Bridge RS Jr, Bridge JA, Neff JR, et al. Recurrent chromosomal imbalances and structurally abnormal breakpoints within complex karyotypes of malignant peripheral nerve sheath tumour and malignant triton tumour: a cytogenetic and molecular cytogenetic study. J Clin Pathol 2004;57(11):1172–8.
14. Brock JE, Perez–Atayde AR, Kozakewich HP, et al. Cytogenetic aberrations in perineurioma: variation with subtype. Am J Surg Pathol 2005;29:1164–9.
15. Brooks J, Draffen R. Benign glandular schwannoma. Arch Pathol Lab Med 1992;116:192–5.
16. Brooks JSJ, Freeman M, Enterline HT. Malignant 'triton' tumours. Natural history and immunohistochemistry of nine new cases with literature review. Cancer 1985;55:2543–9.
17. Carli M, Ferrari A, Mattke A. Paediatric malignant peripheral nerve sheath tumour: the Italian and German soft tissue

sarcoma cooperative group. J Clin Oncol 2005;23:8422–30.

18. Carney JA. Psammomatous melanotic schwannoma: a distinctive, heritable tumour with special associations, including cardiac myxoma and the Cushing syndrome. Am J Surg Pathol 1990;14:206–22.

19. Carroll SL. Molecular mechanisms promoting the pathogenesis of Schwann cell neoplasms. Acta Neuropathol 2012;123(3):321–48.

20. Carter JM, O'Hara C, Dundas G, et al. Epithelioid malignant peripheral nerve sheath tumour arising in a schwannoma, in a patient with 'neuroblastoma-like' schwannomatosis and a novel germline SMARCB1 mutation. Am J Surg Pathol 2012;36(1):154–60.

21. Casadei GP, Komori T, Scheithauer BW, et al. Intracranial parenchymal schwannoma. A clinicopathological and neuroimaging study of nine cases. J Neurosurg 1993;79(2):217–22.

22. CBTRUS. CBTRUS Statistical Report: Primary brain tumours in the United States, 2004–2008. Hinsdale, IL: Central Brain Tumour Registry of the United States, 2012.

23. Cervoni L, Celli P, Scarpinati M, Cantore G. Neurinomas of the cauda equina clinical analysis of 40 surgical cases. Acta Chir 1994;127:199–202.

24. Chaudhry IH, Calonje E. Dermal non-neural granular cell tumour (so-called primitive polypoid granular cell tumour a distinctive entity further delineated in a clinicopathological study of 11 cases. Histopathology 2005;47:179–85.

25. Chewning RH, Sasson AD, Jordan LC, Tamargo RJ, Gailloud P. Acute third cranial nerve palsy from a third cranial nerve schwannoma presenting as a saccular aneurysm on three-dimensional computed tomography angiography: case illustration. J Neurosurg 2008;108(5):1037.

26. Chu PG, Benhattar J, Weiss LM, Meagher–Villemure K. Intraneural synovial sarcoma: two cases. Mod Pathol 2004;17:258–63.

27. Deleted in proof.

28. De Raedt T, Maertens O, Chmara M, et al. Somatic loss of wild type NF1 allele in neurofibromas: Comparison of NF1 microdeletion and non-microdeletion patients. Genes Chromosomes Cancer 2006;45(10):893–904.

29. Demir HA, Varan A, Yalcn B, et al. Malignant peripheral nerve sheath tumours in childhood: 13 cases from a single centre. J Pediatr Hematol Oncol 2012;34(3):204–7.

30. Ducatman BS, Scheithauer BW, Piepgras DG, et al. Malignant peripheral nerve sheath tumours: a clinicopathological study of 120 cases. Cancer 1986;57:2006–21.

31. Ducatman BS, Scheithauer BW. Postirradiation neurofibrosarcoma. Cancer 1983;51(6):1028–33.

32. Emory TS, Scheithauer BW, Hirose T, et al. Intraneural perineurioma: a clonal neoplasm associated with abnormalities of chromosome 22. Am J Clin Pathol 1995;103:696–704.

33. Endo M, Kobayashi C, Setsu N, et al. Prognostic significance of p14ARF, p15INK4b, and p16INK4a inactivation in malignant peripheral nerve sheath tumours. Clin Cancer Res 2011;17(11):3771–82.

34. Erlandson RA, Woodruff JM. Peripheral nerve sheath tumours: an electron microscopic study of 43 cases. Cancer 1982;49:273–87.

35. Evans DG, Baser ME, McGaughran J, et al. Malignant peripheral nerve sheath tumours in neurofibromatosis 1. J Med Genet 2002;39:311–14.

36. Fanburg–Smith JC, Majidi M, Miettinen M. Keratin expression in schwannoma: a study of 115 retroperitoneal and 22 peripheral schwannomas. Mod Pathol 2006;19:115–21.

37. Fanburg–Smith JC, Meis–Kindblom JM, Fante R, Kindblom LG. Malignant granular cell tumour of soft tissue: diagnostic criteria and clinicopathological correlation. Am J Surg Pathol 1998;22:779–94.

38. Feany MB, Anthony DC, Fletcher CD. Nerve sheath tumours with hybrid features of neurofibroma and schwannoma: a conceptual challenge. Histopathology 1998;32(5):405–10.

39. Fetsch JF, Miettinen M. Sclerosing perineurioma: a clinicopathological study of 19 cases of a distinctive soft tissue lesion with a predilection for the fingers and palms of young adults. Am J Surg Pathol 1997;21:1433–42.

40. Fetsch JF, Laskin WB, Miettinen M. Nerve sheath myxoma: a clinicopathological and immunohistochemical analysis of 57 morphologically distinctive, S–100 protein- and GFAP-positive, myxoid peripheral nerve sheath tumours with a predilection for the extremities and a high local recurrence rate. Am J Surg Pathol 2005;29:1615–24.

41. Fine SW, McClain SA, Li M. Immunohistochemical staining for calretinin is useful for differentiating schwannomas from neurofibromas. Am J Clin Pathol 2004;122(4):552–9.

42. Fletcher CDM, Davies SE, McKee PH. Cellular schwannoma: a distinct pseudosarcomatous entity. Histopathology 1987;11:21–35.

43. Foley KM, Woodruff JM, Ellis FT, Posner JB. Radiation-induced malignant and atypical peripheral nerve sheath tumours. Ann Neurol 1980;7:311–18.

44. Foo WC, Cruise MW, Wick MR, Hornick JL. Immunohistochemical staining for TLE1 distinguishes synovial sarcoma from histologic mimics. Am J Clin Pathol 2011;135(6):839–44.

45. Fox MD, Gleason BC, Thomas AB, Victor TA, Cibull TL. Extra-acral cutaneous/soft tissue sclerosing perineurioma: an under-recognized entity in the differential of CD34-positive cutaneous neoplasms. J Cutan Pathol 2010;37(10):1053–6.

46. Fox MD, Billings SD, Gleason BC, et al. Expression of MiTF may be helpful in differentiating cellular neurothekeoma from plexiform fibrohistiocytic tumour (histiocytoid predominant) in a partial biopsy specimen. Am J Dermatopathol 2012;34(2):157–60.

47. Frim DM, Ogilvy CS, Vonsattal J–P, Chapman PH. Is intracerebral schwannoma a developmental tumour of children and young adults? Pediatr Neurosurg 1992;1:190–4.

48. Giannini C, Scheithauer BW, Jenkins RB, et al. Soft-tissue perineurioma. Evidence for an abnormality of chromosome 22, criteria for diagnosis, and review

of the literature. Am J Surg Pathol 1997;21:164–73.

49. Gould VE, Moll I, Lee I, et al. The intermediate filament complement of the spectrum of nerve sheath neoplasms. Lab Invest 1986;55:463–4.

50. Graadt van Roggen JF, McMenamin ME, Belchis DA, et al. Reticular perineurioma: a distinctive variant of soft tissue perineurioma. Am J Surg Pathol 2001;25:485–93.

51. Gray MH, Rosenberg AE, Dickersin GR, Bhan AK. Glial fibrillary acidic protein and keratin expression by benign and malignant nerve sheath tumours. Hum Pathol 1989;20:1089–96.

52. Gupta R, Sharma A, Arora R, Vijayaraghavan M. Composite phaeochromocytoma with malignant peripheral nerve sheath tumour and rhabdomyosarcomatous differentiation in a patient without von Recklinghausen disease. J Clin Pathol 2009;62(7):659–61.

53. Hadfield KD, Newman WG, Bowers NL, et al. Molecular characterization of SMARCB1 and NF2 in familial and sporadic schwannomatosis. J Med Genet 2008;45(6):332–9.

54. Halliday AL, Sobel RA, Martuza RL. Benign spinal nerve sheath tumours: their occurrence sporadically and in neurofibromatosis types 1 and 2. J Neurosurg 1991;74:248–53.

55. Hanemann CO, Evans DG. News on the genetics, epidemiology, medical care and translational research of Schwannomas. J Neurol 2006;253(12):1533–41.

56. Harder A, Wesemann M, Hagel C, et al. Hybrid neurofibroma/schwannoma is overrepresented among schwannomatosis and neurofibromatosis patients. Am J Surg Pathol 2012;36(5):702–9.

57. Hebert–Blouin MN, Amrami KK, Scheithauer BW, Spinner RJ. Multinodular/plexiform (multifascicular) schwannomas of major peripheral nerves: an underrecognized part of the spectrum of schwannomas. J Neurosurg 2010;112(2):372–82.

58. Hemminger J, Iwenofu OH. Discovered on gastrointestinal stromal tumours 1 (DOG1) expression in non-gastrointestinal stromal tumour (GIST) neoplasms. Histopathology 2012;61(2):170–7.

59. Hirose T, Scheithauer BW, Sano, T. Perineurial malignant peripheral nerve sheath tumour (MPNST): a clinicopathologic, immunohistochemical, and ultrastructural study of seven cases. Am J Surg Pathol 1998;22:1368–78.

60. Hollmann TJ, Hornick JL. INI1-deficient tumours: diagnostic features and molecular genetics. Am J Surg Pathol 2011;35(10):e47–63.

61. Holtkamp N, Malzer E, Zietsch J, et al. EGFR and erbB2 in malignant peripheral nerve sheath tumours and implications for targeted therapy. Neuro Oncol 2008;10(6):946–57.

62. Hoover JM, Bledsoe JM, Giannini C, Krauss WE. Intramedullary melanotic schwannoma. Rare Tumors 2012;4(1):e3.

63. Hornick JL, Fletcher CD. Soft tissue perineurioma: clinicopathologic analysis of 81 cases including those with atypical histologic features. Am J Surg Pathol 2005;29(7):845–58.

64. Hornick JL, Bundock EA, Fletcher CD. Hybrid schwannoma/perineurioma:

clinicopathologic analysis of 42 distinctive benign nerve sheath tumours. Am J Surg Pathol 2009;33(10):1554–61.

65. Hornick JL, Dal Cin P, Fletcher CD. Loss of INI1 expression is characteristic of both conventional and proximal-type epithelioid sarcoma. Am J Surg Pathol 2009;33(4):542–50.

66. Ingham S, Huson SM, Moran A, et al. Malignant peripheral nerve sheath tumours in NF1: Improved survival in women and in recent years. Eur J Cancer 2011;47(18):2723–8.

67. Ishida T, Kuroda M, Motoi T, et al. Phenotypic diversity of neurofibromatosis 2: association with plexiform schwannomas. Histopathology 1998;32:264–70.

68. Jackowski A, Weiner G, O'Reilly G. Trochlear nerve schwannomas: a case report and literature review. Br J Neurosurg 1994;8:219–23.

69. Josty IC, Sykes PJ. An unusual schwannoma of the median nerve: effects on the motor branch. Br J Plast Surg 2001;54(1):71–3.

70. Karamchandani JR, Nielsen TO, van de Rijn M, West RB. Sox10 and S100 in the diagnosis of soft-tissue neoplasms. Appl Immunohistochem Mol Morphol 2012;20(5):445–50.

71. Kepes JJ, Chen WY, Pang LC, Kepes M. Tumours of the central nervous system in Taiwan, Republic of China. Surg Neurol 1984;22:149–56.

72. Kindblom LG, Meis-Kindblom JM, Havel G, Busch C. Benign epithelioid schwannoma. Am J Surg Pathol 1998;22:762–70.

73. King AA, Debaun MR, Riccardi VM, Gutmann DH. Malignant peripheral nerve sheath tumours in neurofibromatosis 1. Am J Med Genet 2000;93(5):388–92.

74. Knosel T, Heretsch S, Altendorf-Hofmann A, et al. TLE1 is a robust diagnostic biomarker for synovial sarcomas and correlates with t(X;18): analysis of 319 cases. Eur J Cancer 2010;46(6):1170–6.

75. Kusters–Vandevelde HV, van Engen–van Grunsven IA, Kusters B, et al. Improved discrimination of melanotic schwannoma from melanocytic lesions by combined morphological and GNAQ mutational analysis. Acta Neuropathol 2010;120(6):755–64.

76. Lalwani AK. Meningiomas, epidermoids and other nonacoustic tumours of the cerebellopontine angle. Otolaryngol Clin North Am 1992;25:707–28.

77. Laskin WB, Weiss SW, Bratthauer GL. Epithelioid variant of malignant peripheral nerve sheath (malignant epithelioid schwannoma). Am J Surg Pathol 1991;15:1136–45.

78. Laskin WB, Fetsch JF, Lasota J, Miettinen M. Benign epithelioid peripheral nerve sheath tumours of the soft tissues: clinicopathologic spectrum of 33 cases. Am J Surg Pathol 2005;29(1):39–51.

79. Le LQ, Shipman T, Burns DK, Parada LF. Cell of origin and microenvironment contribution for NF1-associated dermal neurofibromas. Cell Stem Cell 2009;4(5):453–63.

80. Louis E, Cret C, Poirier J, et al. Intra-cerebral schwannoma simulating glioma. J Neurooncol 2003;64:279–82.

81. Maertens O, Brems H, Vandesompele J, et al. Comprehensive NF1 screening on cultured Schwann cells from neurofibromas. Hum Mutat 2006;27(10):1030–40.

82. Mantripragada KK, Spurlock G, Kluwe L, et al. High-resolution DNA copy number profiling of malignant peripheral nerve sheath tumours using targeted microarray-based comparative genomic hybridization. Clin Cancer Res 2008;14(4):1015–24.

83. Marchese MJ, McDonald JV. Intramedullary melanotic schwannoma of the cervical spinal cord: report of a case. Surg Neurol 1990;33:353–5.

84. Matsumine A, Kusuzaki K, Hirata H, et al. Intraneural metastasis of a synovial sarcoma to a peripheral nerve. J Bone Joint Surg Br 2005;87:1553–5.

85. McMenamin ME, Fletcher CD. Expanding the spectrum of malignant change in schwannomas: epithelioid malignant change, epithelioid malignant peripheral nerve sheath tumour, and epithelioid angiosarcoma:a study of 17 cases. Am J Surg Pathol 2001;25:13–25.

86. Megahed M, Ruzicka T. Cellular schwannoma. Am J Dermatopathol 1994;16:418–21.

87. Meis JM, Enzinger FM, Martz KL, Neal JA. Malignant peripheral nerve sheath tumours (malignant schwannomas) in children. Am J Surg Pathol 1992;16:694–707.

88. Meis–Kindblom JM, Enzinger FM. Plexiform malignant peripheral nerve sheath tumour of infancy and childhood. Am J Surg Pathol 1994;18:479–85.

89. Menon AG, Anderson KM, Riccardi VM, et al. Chromosome 17p deletions and p53 gene mutations associated with the formation of malignant neurofibrosarcomas in von Recklinghausen neurofibromatosis. Proc Natl Acad Sci USA 1990;87:5435–9.

90. Mentzel T, Katenkamp D. Intraneural angiosarcoma and angiosarcoma arising in benign and malignant peripheral nerve sheath tumours: clinicopathological and immunohistochemical analysis of four cases. Histopathology 1999;35:114–20.

91. Michal M, Kazakov DV, Belousova I, et al. A benign neoplasm with histopathological features of both schwannoma and retiform perineurioma (benign schwannoma-perineurioma): a report of six cases of a distinctive soft tissue tumour with a predilection for the fingers. Virchows Arch 2004;445(4):347–53.

92. Miller SJ, Rangwala F, Williams J, et al. Large-scale molecular comparison of human Schwann cells to malignant peripheral nerve sheath tumour cell lines and tissues. Cancer Res 2006;66(5):2584–91.

93. Miller SJ, Jessen WJ, Mehta T, et al. Integrative genomic analyses of neurofibromatosis tumours identify SOX9 as a biomarker and survival gene. EMBO Mol Med 2009;1(4):236–48.

94. Morgan KG, Gray C. Malignant epithelioid schwannoma of superficial soft tissue: a case report with immunohistology and electron microscopy. Histopathology 1985;9:765–75.

95. Naber U, Friedrich RE, Glatzel M, Mautner VF, Hagel C. Podoplanin and CD34 in peripheral nerve sheath tumours: focus on neurofibromatosis 1-associated atypical neurofibroma. J Neurooncol 2011;103(2):239–45.

96. Nakamura H, Makino K, Yano S, Kuratsu J. Epidemiological study of primary intracranial tumours: a regional survey in Kumamoto prefecture in southern Japan – 20-year study. Int J Clin Oncol 2011;16(4):314–21.

97. Nonaka D, Chiriboga L, Rubin BP. Sox10: a pan-schwannian and melanocytic marker. Am J Surg Pathol 2008;32(9):1291–8.

98. Ogawa K, Oguchi M, Yamabe H, Nakashima Y, Hamashima Y. Distribution of collagen type IV in soft tissue tumours. An immunohistochemical study. Cancer 1986;58(2):269–77.

99. Ohata C, Imai N, Hinogami H, Akamatsu K, Sumimura Y. Hybrid schwannoma/perineurioma: a report of two cases including a possible radiation-induced case. J Cutan Pathol 2012;39(1):56–62.

100. Patil S, Perry A, Maccollin M, et al. Immunohistochemical analysis supports a role for INI1/SMARCB1 in hereditary forms of schwannomas, but not in solitary, sporadic schwannomas. Brain Pathol 2008;18(4):517–9.

101. Perez MT, Farkas J, Padron S, et al. Intrasellar and parasellar cellular schwannoma. Ann Diagn Pathol 2004;8:142–50.

102. Perrone F, Da Riva L, Orsenigo M, et al. PDGFRA, PDGFRB, EGFR and downstream signaling activation in malignant peripheral nerve sheath tumour. Neuro Oncol 2009;11(6):725–36.

103. Perry A, Roth KA, Banerjee R, Fuller CE, Gutmann DH. NF1 deletions in S–100 protein-positive and negative cells of sporadic and neurofibromatosis 1 (NF1)-associated plexiform neurofibromas and malignant peripheral nerve sheath tumours. Am J Pathol 2001;159(1):57–61.

104. Perry A, Kunz SN, Fuller CE, et al. Differential NF1, p16, and EGFR patterns by interphase cytogenetics (FISH) in malignant peripheral nerve sheath tumour (MPNST) and morphologically similar spindle cell neoplasms. J Neuropathol Exp Neurol 2002;61(8):702–9.

105. Petrela E, Hodge CJ, Hahn SS, Chung CT, Mejico LJ. Stereotactic radiosurgery in two cases of presumed fourth cranial nerve schwannoma. J Neuroophthalmol 2009;29(1):54–7.

106. Plaza JA, Torres–Cabala C, Evans H, Diwan AH, Prieto VG. Immunohistochemical expression of S100A6 in cellular neurothekeoma: clinicopathologic and immunohistochemical analysis of 31 cases. Am J Dermatopathol 2009;31(5):419–22.

107. Porter DE, Prasad V, Foster L, et al. Survival in malignant peripheral nerve sheath tumours: a comparison between sporadic and neurofibromatosis type 1-associated tumours. Sarcoma 2009;2009:756395.

108. Preston DL, Ron E, Yonehara S, et al. Tumours of the nervous system and pituitary gland associated with atomic bomb radiation exposure. J Natl Cancer Inst 2002;94(20):1555–63.

109. Pultizer DR, Reed RJ. Nerve sheath myxoma (perineurial myxoma). Am J Dermatopathol 1985;7:409–21.

110. Ramanathan RC, Thomas JM. Malignant peripheral nerve sheath tumours

associated with von Recklinghausen's neurofibromatosis. Eur J Surg Oncol 1999;25(2):190–3.

111. Rekhi B, Jambhekar NA. Malignant transformation in a hybrid schwannoma/perineurioma: addition to the spectrum of a malignant peripheral nerve sheath tumour. Indian J Pathol Microbiol 2011;54(4):825–8.

112. Ricci A, Parham DM, Woodruff JM, et al. Malignant peripheral nerve sheath tumours arising from ganglioneuromas. Am J Surg Pathol 1984;8:19–29.

113. Rodriguez FJ, Folpe AL, Giannini C, Perry A. Pathology of peripheral nerve sheath tumours: diagnostic overview and update on selected diagnostic problems. Acta Neuropathol 2012;123(3):295–319.

114. Rodriguez FJ, Stratakis CA, Evans DG. Genetic predisposition to peripheral nerve neoplasia: diagnostic criteria and pathogenesis of neurofibromatoses, Carney complex and related syndromes. Acta Neuropathol 2012;123(3):349–67.

115. Ross DA, Edwards MS, Wilson CB. Intramedullary neurilemomas of the spinal cord: report of two cases and review of the literature. Neurosurgery 1986;19:458–64.

116. Rothenbuhler A, Stratakis CA. Clinical and molecular genetics of Carney complex. Best Pract Res Clin Endocrinol Metab [Review] 2010;24(3):389–99.

117. Saad AG, Mutema GK, Mutasim DF. Benign cutaneous epithelioid schwannoma: case report and review of the literature. Am J Dermatopathol 2005;27(1):45–7.

118. Scheithauer BW, Erdogan S, Rodriguez FJ, et al. Malignant peripheral nerve sheath tumours of cranial nerves and intracranial contents: a clinicopathologic study of 17 cases. Am J Surg Pathol 2009;33:325–38.

119. Scheithauer BW, Woodruff JM, Spinner RJ. Peripheral nerve sheath tumours. In: Perry A, Brat DJ eds. Practical surgical neuropathology. Philadelphia: Churchill Livingstone, 2010:235–85.

120. Scheithauer BW, Amrami KK, Folpe AL, et al. Synovial sarcoma of nerve. Hum Pathol 2011 Apr;42(4):568–77.

121. Sestini R, Bacci C, Provenzano A, Genuardi M, Papi L. Evidence of a four-hit mechanism involving SMARCB1 and NF2 in schwannomatosis-associated schwannomas. Hum Mutat 2008;29(2):227–31.

122. Shaw CM, Grobmyer SR, Ucar DA, et al. Elevated expression of IRS2 in the progression from neurofibroma to malignant peripheral nerve sheath tumour. Anticancer Res 2012;32(2):439–43.

123. Shields LB, Glassman SD, Raque GH, Shields CB. Malignant psammomatous melanotic schwannoma of the spine: A component of Carney complex. Surg Neurol Int 2011;2:136.

124. Shimizu S, Teraki Y, Ishiko A, et al. Malignant epithelioid schwannoma of the skin showing partial HMB–45 positivity. Am J Dermatopathol 1993;15(4):378–84.

125. Stangerup SE, Caye–Thomasen P. Epidemiology and natural history of vestibular schwannomas. Otolaryngol Clin North Am 2012;45(2):257–68.

126. Stanton C, Perentes E, Phillips L, VandenBerg SR. The immunohistochemical demonstration of early perineurial change in the development of localized hypertrophic neuropathy. Hum Pathol 1988;19:1455–7.

127. Stucky CC, Johnson KN, Gray RJ, et al. Malignant peripheral nerve sheath tumours (MPNST): the Mayo Clinic experience. Ann Surg Oncol 2011;19(3):878–85.

128. Subramanian N, Rambhatia S, Mahesh L, et al. Cystic schwannoma of the orbit – a case series. Orbit 2005;24(2):125–9.

129. Subramanian S, Thayanithy V, West RB, et al. Genome-wide transcriptome analyses reveal p53 inactivation mediated loss of miR–34a expression in malignant peripheral nerve sheath tumours. J Pathol 2009;220(1):58–70.

130. Suster S, Amazon K, Rosen LB, Ollague JM. Malignant epithelioid schwannoma of the skin: a low-grade neurotropic malignant melanoma? Am J Dermatopathol 1989;11:338–44.

131. Tabone–Eglinger S, Bahleda R, Cote JF, et al. Frequent EGFR positivity and overexpression in high-grade areas of human MPNSTs. Sarcoma 2008;2008:849156.

132. Takei H, Schmiege L, Buckleair L, Goodman JC, Powell SZ. Intracerebral schwannoma clinically and radiologically mimicking meningioma. Pathol Int 2005;55(8):514–9.

133. Taxy JB, Battifora H, Trujillo Y, Dorfman HD. Electron microscopy in the diagnosis of malignant schwannoma. Cancer 1981;48:1381–91.

134. Upadhyaya M. Genetic basis of tumorigenesis in NF1 malignant peripheral nerve sheath tumours. Front Biosci (Landmark Ed) 2011;16:937–51.

135. Upadhyaya M, Spurlock G, Thomas L, et al. Microarray-based copy number analysis of neurofibromatosis type-1 (NF1)-associated malignant peripheral nerve sheath tumours (MPNSTs) reveals a role for Rho–GTPase pathway genes in NF1 tumorigenesis. Hum Mutat 2012;33(4):763–76.

136. Valeyrie–Allanore L, Ismaili N, Bastuji–Garin S, et al. Symptoms associated with malignancy of peripheral nerve sheath tumours: a retrospective study of 69 patients with neurofibromatosis 1. Br J Dermatol 2005;153(1):79–82.

137. Vered M, Fridman E, Carpenter WM, Buchner A. Classic neurothekeoma (nerve sheath myxoma) and cellular neurothekeoma of the oral mucosa: immunohistochemical profiles. J Oral Pathol Med;40(2):174–80.

138. Vezzosi D, Vignaux O, Dupin N, Bertherat J. Carney complex: Clinical and genetic 2010 update. Ann Endocrinol (Paris) 2010;71(6):486–93.

139. Voltaggio L, Murray R, Lasota J, Miettinen M. Gastric schwannoma: a clinicopathologic study of 51 cases and critical review of the literature. Hum Pathol 2012;43(5):650–9.

140. Wang AR, May D, Bourne P, Scott G. PGP9.5: a marker for cellular neurothekeoma. Am J Surg Pathol 1999;23:1401–7.

141. Watson MA, Perry A, Tihan T, et al. Gene expression profiling reveals unique molecular subtypes of neurofibromatosis type I-associated and sporadic malignant peripheral nerve sheath tumours. Brain Pathol 2004;14(3):297–303.

142. Weiss SW, Goldblum JR eds. Enzinger and Weiss's soft tissue tumours, 4th edn. St Louis: Mosby, 2001.

143. Weiss SW, Nickoloff BJ. CD–34 is expressed by a distinctive cell population in peripheral nerve, nerve sheath tumours and related lesions. Am J Surg Pathol 1993;17:1039–45.

144. White W, Shiu MH, Rosenblum MK, et al. Cellular schwannoma: a clinicopathological study of 57 patients and 58 tumours. Cancer 1990;66:1266–75.

145. Wick MR, Swanson PE, Scheithauer BW, Manivel JC. Malignant peripheral nerve sheath tumour: an immunohistochemical study of 62 cases. Am J Clin Pathol 1987;87:425–33.

146. Woodruff JM. Peripheral nerve tumours showing glandular differentiation (glandular schwannoma). Cancer 1976;37:2399–413.

147. Woodruff JM. Pathology of tumours of the peripheral nerve sheath in type 1 neurofibromatosis. Am J Med Genet 1999;89:23–30.

148. Woodruff JM, Goodwin TA, Erlandson RA, et al. Cellular schwannoma: a variety of schwannoma sometimes mistaken for a malignant tumour. Am J Surg Pathol 1981;5:733–44.

149. Woodruff JM, Selig AM, Crowley K, Allen PW. Schwannoma (neurilemoma) with malignant transformation. Am J Surg Pathol 1994;18:882–95.

150. Woodruff JM, Scheithauer BW, Kurtkaya–Yapicier O, et al. Congenital and childhood plexiform (multinodular) cellular schwannoma: a troublesome mimic of malignant peripheral nerve sheath tumour. Am J Surg Pathol 2003;27:1321–9.

151. Xu X, Tong Y, Jin J, Zhan R, Zhou Y. A giant facial nerve schwannoma extending from the middle cranial fossa to the mastoid region: case report. J Int Med Res 2009;37(1):247–52.

152. Yakulis R, Manack L, Murphy AI. Postradiation malignant Triton tumour: case report and review of the literature. Arch Pathol Lab Med 1996;120:541–8.

153. Yang J, Ylipaa A, Sun Y, Zheng H, Chen K, Nykter M, et al. Genomic and molecular characterization of malignant peripheral nerve sheath tumour identifies the IGF1R pathway as a primary target for treatment. Clin Cancer Res 2011;17(24):7563–73.

154. Yonehara S, Brenner AV, Kishikawa M, et al. Clinical and epidemiologic characteristics of first primary tumours of the central nervous system and related organs among atomic bomb survivors in Hiroshima and Nagasaki, 1958–1995. Cancer 2004;101(7):1644–54.

155. Yu J, Deshmukh H, Payton JE, et al. Array-based comparative genomic hybridization identifies CDK4 and FOXM1 alterations as independent predictors of survival in malignant peripheral nerve sheath tumour. Clin Cancer Res 2011;17(7):1924–34.

156. Zhu Y, Ghosh P, Charnay P, Burns DK, Parada LF. Neurofibromas in NF1: Schwann cell origin and role of tumour environment. Science 2002;296(5569):920–2.

157. Zou C, Smith KD, Liu J, et al. Clinical, pathological, and molecular variables predictive of malignant peripheral nerve sheath tumour outcome. Ann Surg 2009;249(6):1014–22.

Tumours of the Meninges

Arie Perry

This group covers a wide range of neoplasms originating from either meningothelial (arachnoidal cap cell) or other meningeal cell types. The 2007 World Health Organization (WHO) classification divides these into meningiomas, mesenchymal non-meningothelial tumours, haemangiopericytomas, melanocytic lesions and haemangioblastomas.[103]

TUMOURS OF MENINGOTHELIAL/ARACHNOIDAL CELLS

Meningiomas are by far the single largest and most important group of meningeal tumours. This group comprises benign and more aggressive subsets, the latter including clear cell, chordoid, papillary, rhabdoid, atypical, brain invasive and anaplastic (malignant) meningiomas. Much progress has been made in terms of of meningioma classification, grading and molecular subtyping.[109]

Meningiomas

Incidence

Meningioma is now considered the most common central nervous system (CNS) neoplasm, accounting for 35.5 per cent of over 310 000 primary tumours reported to the Central Brain Tumor Registry of the United States in the 2005–2009 census.[55] Spinal cord meningiomas are less common than their intracranial counterparts and have a particular predilection for the thoracic regions, particularly in older women.[163]

The estimated incidence of meningiomas is 7.22 per 100 000 person years, with a mean age of 65 years at diagnosis.[55] Over time, this incidence has steadily increased, likely reflecting enhanced detection of incidental meningiomas. Similarly, when considering frequency, a distinction should be made between biopsy and post-mortem series, because incidental meningiomas may be seen in as many as 2.3 per cent of autopsies and 0.9 per cent of magnetic resonance (MR) images, particularly in the elderly.[116,188] Meningiomas have been found to be the most common incidentally detected intracranial tumour, accounting for 56 per cent of such cases in one series.[188] The majority of these incidental meningiomas appear to be indolent.

Meningiomas may develop in families, in association with neurofibromatosis type 2 (NF2) and rarely in Gorlin's syndrome, Cowden's syndrome, Li–Fraumeni syndrome, Turcot's/Gardener's syndrome and von Hippel-Lindau disease[109] (see Chapter 44). They may also occur uncommonly in families without an established tumour syndrome or with rare germline mutations involving *SMARCB1*, *SMARCE1* or *SUFU* genes.[1,16,44,175] Meningiomas are rarely found in combination with glial neoplasms, and meningiomas are among the most common neoplastic hosts of systemic metastases, especially breast carcinoma.[5,149,182]

Age and Sex

Meningiomas are mostly neoplasms of middle-aged to elderly adults, with a peak incidence in the sixth to seventh decades of life; there are no obvious race predilections.[197] The age-adjusted incidence rates per 100 000 steadily increase throughout life from 0.09 below 14 years of age to 44.90 in those over 85 years old.[55] Meningiomas are comparatively rare in infants and children.[134,185] Unique aspects within this age group include higher risks of large tumour size, cyst formation, lack of dural attachment, high-grade histology, aggressive behaviour and aggressive variant histology, particularly the clear cell and papillary subtypes. They are also more likely to present in unusual locations, such as lateral ventricles, posterior fossa and spinal epidural regions. NF2 and prior irradiation are common predisposing factors and they lack the female predilection of their adult counterparts. The behaviour of paediatric meningiomas is less predictable and more often aggressive. Meningiomas are significantly more common in women than in men, with a female/male ratio of 2:1.[197] The female/male ratio is even higher for thoracic spinal meningiomas, where it approaches 7:1.[197]

Aetiology

Various aetiological factors, both environmental and genetic, have been implicated in the development of meningiomas. The genetic aspects of meningiomas have been considered briefly earlier, and tumours associated with NF2 are also discussed in the section on hereditary tumour syndromes (see later). The environmental factors include irradiation and trauma. Trauma has been suggested as a causative agent, which occasionally raises medicolegal issues. In Cushing and Eisenhardt's ground-breaking monograph, a surprising 32 per cent of intracranial meningiomas had a prior history of head injury.[53] An epidemiologic study estimated an odds ratio of 4.33 (4.33; 95% CI = 2.06, 9.10) for meningiomas occurring 10 to19 years after head trauma,[144] and the association appears to be stronger for men, likely reflecting the fact that head trauma is more common in men than in women. Nonetheless, the role of head injury remains controversial and unproven.[197] No convincing evidence to date of increased risk with the use of mobile phones has been found, although longer follow-up may still be needed to prove this notion.[70]

Meningiomas caused by irradiation are well documented. A causal association is supported by their presentation within the field of irradiation, long latency (usually several years), differing histology from the original disease being treated, and higher frequency in irradiated cohorts than in control patients. Radiation-induced meningiomas have been divided into those associated with low-dose (<10 Gy), medium-dose and miscellaneous (10–20 Gy) and high-dose (>20 Gy) radiation. Most reported cases followed low-dose irradiation (less than 2 Gy) to the scalp for tinea capitis, whereas about 10 per cent resulted from high-dose irradiation of primary brain tumours. The miscellaneous group refers to modalities such as direct application of radium, thorotrast ventriculography and myelography. Radiation-induced meningiomas present at a younger age than sporadic counterparts, average ages being 45, 32.3 and 34.2 years for high-, medium- and low-dose groups, respectively. Although any grade may be encountered, higher grade or more aggressive variants are encountered more commonly than with sporadic examples. Average latency is 35.2 years for the low-dose category, with 26.1 and 19.5 years for the moderate- and high-dose groups, respectively. As a general rule, the greater the dose, the shorter the latency and the younger the patient at presentation.[186] The latency is also influenced by patient age, being particularly short in children, the mean being about 10 years. Meningiomas among atomic bomb survivors in Japan have continued to increase over time, the incidence associated with distance from the epicentre of the explosion.[205]

Sites

Meningiomas can occur anywhere along the neuraxis, including intracranial, spinal, intraventricular and extracranial sites (Figure 36.1). In the cranial cavity, they most frequently

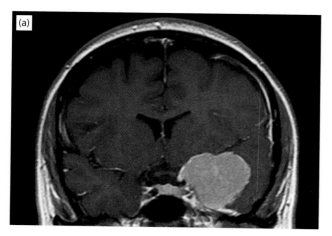
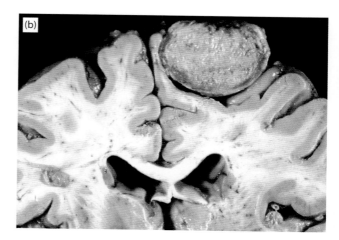
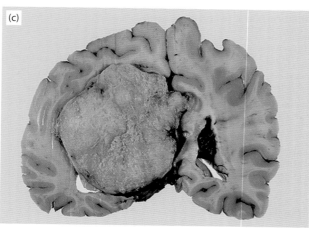
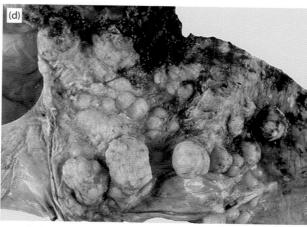

36.1 Meningioma. (a) T1-weighted, post-contrast, parasagittal MRI of a skull base (sphenoid ridge) meningioma. **(b)** Parasagittal meningioma. **(c)** Large intraventricular tumour compressing the surrounding brain. **(d)** Multiple growths on the dura.

develop over the convexity, approximately half adjoining the sagittal sinus (Figure 36.1b). These parasagittal tumours usually develop over the middle third of the convexity, with frontal regions favoured over occipital. Other convexity lesions are more lateral, including over the Sylvian fissures and parietal regions. Falcine tumours differ from parasagittal meningiomas in that they are not associated with the sagittal sinus, but adhere firmly to the falx itself. At the base of the brain, the olfactory grooves, parasellar areas, sphenoidal ridges (Figure 36.1a) and tuberculum sellae are common. Optic nerve meningiomas account for roughly 2 per cent of cases and are often clinically aggressive, despite a benign histologic appearance; nonetheless, radiotherapy improves the outcome for subtotally resected cases.[56,176] In the posterior fossa, they may develop in the area of the petrous bone, tentorium cerebelli and foramen magnum. Meningiomas arising from the tentorium may be supratentorial, infratentorial or both. The pineal region is rarely affected.

Spinal meningiomas most often develop in the thoracic region, although this site predilection is mainly seen in women. Cervical tumours occur most commonly anterior to the cord, whereas thoracic cases usually localize posteriorly. They are firmly attached to the dura, usually dorsolaterally, and cover several segments. In the cervical and lumbar regions they may be more extensive and are occasionally leptomeningeal-based or epidural.

Intraventricular meningiomas represent 0.5–3 per cent of intracranial meningiomas and are thought to arise from the tela choroidea in the choroid plexus (Figure 36.1c).[102] They most often develop in the trigone of the lateral ventricles, with a curious preference for the left side. They are often large and may be difficult to resect. Of 675 reported cases, 15.6 per cent and 6.6 per cent occurred in the third and fourth ventricles respectively.[102]

Extracranial or extradural meningiomas may occur in the orbit, skin and subcutis of the scalp, paranasal sinuses, nasal cavities and bone, including the calvaria. Although some of the latter are purely intraosseous, bone invasion from an adjacent thin, *en plaque* or carpet-like dural meningioma must first be ruled out.[52,97] Of 504 primary extraneuraxial meningiomas, 58 per cent occurred in the orbit, 16 per cent in the skin and subcutis, 14 per cent in the bone including the middle ear, and 11 per cent in the nasal cavity, nasopharynx and paranasal sinus.[172] The origin of these tumours is controversial. They may occasionally represent extensions of intracranial tumours, but in many cases such a connection cannot be established. In these cases an origin from ectopic meningothelial remnants appears most likely. Even rarer sites include peripheral nerve, lung, salivary gland and the soft tissue of the little finger. In the lung, rare arachnoid-like clusters known as minute meningothelial pulmonary nodules represent one potential histogenetic explanation. It also remains possible that some cases diagnosed as extracranial meningioma represent misdiagnoses (e.g. perineurioma).[31,38]

Multiple Meningiomas

Multiple meningiomas occur commonly in NF2 patients, but can be found in approximately 3 per cent of patients with sporadic disease in surgical series and 8 per cent in autopsy series (Figure 36.1d). However, the true incidence of multiple lesions remains difficult to establish. In a review of 427 cases of multiple meningiomas, 86 were definitely associated with NF2 and only in 239 cases was it stated that there was no evidence of any nerve sheath tumours. Multicentricity was initially diagnosed in only half of cases.[128] It is not unusual to find a large tumour and then smaller ones either in the vicinity of the main lesion or at some distance and, histologically, they generally tend to be of the same type. Histologically, a higher frequency of transitional and psammomatous types has been noted, and evidence of an increased rate for recurrence is lacking.[170] The number of multiple meningiomas varies, with as many as 47 separate tumours of the same histology reported in a patient without any sign of NF2 or evidence of a molecular genetic abnormality.[43] Interestingly, studies have shown identical point mutations of the *NF2* gene as well as inactivation of the same X-chromosome in over half of multiple meningioma cases, indicating their monoclonal origin.[178] Some have speculated that subarachnoid spread is the mechanism for such cases. However, they do not conform to the typical pattern of cerebrospinal fluid (CSF) dissemination with drop metastases and leptomeningeal carcinomatosis. When combined with the frequent finding of microscopic meningothelial nests in random dural strip samplings from meningioma patients[27] and the frequent finding of dural invasion and peripheral migration by meningiomas in general, intradural spread seems a more reasonable explanation.[109] The presence of multiple meningiomas in children is even more often due to NF2 than in adults.[60,134,185]

Clinical Features and Neuroimaging

Because meningiomas can occur anywhere along the neural axis, clinical features are extremely variable and mostly reflect mass effects. Intracranial examples most commonly present with headache, seizures and increasing neurological deficits such as hemiparesis, cortical sensory deficits, ataxia and personality changes. Parasagittal meningiomas, when compressing the motor cortex, may cause leg weakness together with urinary incontinence. Parasellar and optic nerve tumours often produce visual symptoms, whereas those in the cerebellopontine angle lead to hearing loss. Spinal lesions, compressing the cord, may interfere with motor and sensory tracts. Meningiomas in certain locations, particularly in the ventricles and, to a lesser extent, sphenoidal and subfrontal examples, may remain symptomless for many years, reaching large sizes before coming to clinical attention.

Modern neuroimaging plays a critical role in the diagnosis and management planning of meningiomas. On nonenhanced computed tomography (CT) and T1-weighted MR images, meningiomas are often isodense to grey matter, making them difficult to visualize. However, they enhance avidly on post-contrast images (Figure 36.1a), with tumours less than 3 mm detectable with 1.5T and more powerful scanners. The contrast enhancement often trails beyond the tumour in a tail-like fashion, although this 'dural tail' sign is non-specific, because it is encountered in nearly all dural-based processes, neoplastic or otherwise. Interestingly, this dural tail often consists of reactive hypervascular tissue alone, although microscopic nests of tumour can be seen in a subset, either within the dural tail itself or in randomly sampled strips of peritumoural dura.[27] T2-weighted images vary greatly, depending mostly on tumoural consistency. Hypointense tumours are more likely to be firm and fibroblastic, whereas T2 bright examples are more often soft, vascular and/or meningothelial in appearance.[59] Calcifications are common, being dark on T1 MR images and bright on CT scans. Foci of necrosis are hypointense on T1 and hyperintense on T2 scans.

Patient morbidity and mortality may also be related to accompanying peritumoural cerebral oedema. Moreover, psychiatric symptoms have been specifically associated with oedema, particularly in frontal lobe examples.[94] Peritumoural oedema is highly variable and, as expected, is much more common in symptomatic than incidental meningiomas. Greater degrees of oedema have also been associated with large tumour size, parasitization of pial vasculature, convexity/middle fossa localization, irregular tumour–brain interface, hyperintensity on T2-weighted images, brain invasion, malignancy, and the secretory, microcystic, angiomatous and lymphoplasmacyte-rich variants.[125] Data further suggest that elevated tumoural vascular endothelial growth factor (VEGF) expression is associated with cerebral oedema.[207]

Whereas most meningiomas have a smooth, rounded contour, those with an irregular tumour–brain interface are more likely to show brain invasion and high-grade histology. In one study, the combination of an irregular interface and heterogeneous contrast enhancement was associated with higher grade in 98 per cent of cases.[79]

Macroscopic Appearances

The gross pathology of meningiomas varies greatly based on location, size, growth pattern and histologic subtype. Most are well-circumscribed, spherical growths firmly attached to the dura (Figure 36.1b). The surface is smooth or bosselated with variable collagenization making most meningiomas firm. These slow-growing tumours often compress and mold the adjacent brain, and most can be easily dissected away from the adjacent parenchyma (Figure 36.1b,c). Lack of a clear cleavage or resection plane suggests the possibility of brain invasion, although the gross impression is relatively unreliable, because many are merely adherent to the adjacent pia without true parenchymal invasion.[140] Meningiomas arising from dural reflections that separate intracranial compartments may assume more irregular, dumb-bell shapes. For example, falcine meningiomas may involve both frontal lobes and those of the tentorium may spread towards both superiorly and inferiorly. Intraventricular meningiomas may reach considerable size, often filling and distorting the ventricle (Figure 36.1c).

Unlike the more typical tumours, *en plaque* meningiomas grow within and expand the dura in a more diffuse carpet-like fashion, without forming discrete masses. They frequently permeate adjacent bony structures, causing hyperostosis. These occur most frequently in the skull base region, particularly the sphenoid wing.

Whereas brain invasion is relatively rare, infiltration of the dura, venous sinuses, bones and surrounding soft tissue is fairly common, even with histologically benign examples.

Bone invasion is particularly common, especially in skull base tumours. Although osteolytic lesions may also be seen, hyperostosis is fairly typical and nearly always signifies bone invasion.[146] This suggests that meningiomas secrete osteoblast-stimulating factors. Alkaline phosphatase may be one such substance, because it is often increased in tumours with hyperostosis and/or numerous psammoma bodies; other possibilities include platelet-derived growth factor (PDGF), insulin-related growth factor 1 (IGF1), IGF2, fibroblast growth factors (FGF) and transforming growth factor beta (TGF-β).[164]

Most often, the cut surface is firm and lobulated; the colour is dependent on vascularity, ranging from pinkish-white through red to tan (Figure 36.1b,c). Large, spherical tumours tend to be softer, rubbery or even friable. At their dural attachment, they are tougher with radiating fibrous bands attesting to their intimate association with dura. Extensive psammoma bodies impart a gritty quality to the cut surface, whereas xanthomatous change results in yellowish areas. Haemorrhages are rare and metaplastic bone, cartilage or fat is occasionally found.

Grossly evident cysts are seen in 2–4 per cent of meningiomas, mostly in benign tumours.[193] Any meningioma subtype may become cystic, although the microcystic variant is most common, with macrocysts presumably resulting from the coalescence of smaller ones. The dural attachment is often subtle and there may be ring enhancement. Cysts may be either intratumoural or peritumoural and are thought to develop from secretory, reactive or degenerative changes, or possibly as a result of meningioma arising within a pre-existing developmental abnormality such as an arachnoid cyst. The cyst fluid is protein-rich and may appear xanthochromic.

Histological Variants

Meningiomas present a bewildering array of histological patterns, with mixtures being common. In the classical study by Cushing and Eisenhardt, 9 main types and 20 subtypes were distinguished.[53] Although some of these have now been reclassified as other entities (e.g. meningeal hemangiopericytoma), the 2007 WHO classification nevertheless still includes nine benign (grade I: meningothelial, fibrous, transitional, psammomatous, angiomatous, microcystic, secretory, lymphoplasmacyte-rich and metaplastic), three intermediate category (grade II: atypical, clear cell and chordoid) and three malignant (grade III: anaplastic/malignant, papillary, and rhabdoid) subtypes.[136] For many of these variants, the minimum quantity needed for its designation is unclear. Because four have significant grade implications, it is proposed that the majority of the tumour (>50 per cent) should show the defining morphology before the tumour is reflexively 'upgraded'.[109]

Grading and Prognosis

Based on histological criteria discussed later, the 2007 WHO classification provides a grading system for estimating meningioma prognosis.[136] The high-grade variants are associated with significantly increased risks of recurrence and death (see Table 36.1 and later). However, because the majority of meningiomas are considered benign, the risk of recurrence is often influenced more by the site and

TABLE 36.1 Meningiomas with a greater likelihood of recurrence and/or aggressive behaviour

Type of meningioma	WHO grade
Atypical	II
Clear cell	II
Choroid	II
Brain invasive (but not anaplastic)	II
Anaplastic (malignant)	III
Papillary	III
Rhabdoid	III
Any histological subtype or grade with high proliferative index	

WHO, World Health Organization.

the surgeon than histological subtype, because extent of surgical removal is highly correlated with recurrence rates. When operative mortality is excluded, meningioma patients treated with complete resection do not seem to suffer any excess mortality when compared with age- and sex-matched controls.[77,177] On the other hand, there is a small but statistically significant increased risk with subtotal resection. Additionally, estimated 5- and 10-year recurrence rates increase from 5 and 25 per cent with gross total to 40 and 61 per cent with subtotal resections, respectively.[177] On multivariate analyses from large series, negative prognostic variables besides extent of resection include higher histologic grade, male gender, young patient age (<40 years), involvement of the anterior visual pathway, and elevated mitotic/proliferative indices.[14,88,141,177]

Surgery is the treatment of choice, but radiation therapy is also important in reducing recurrence rates, particularly when surgery is contraindicated or if the tumour is subtotally resected and/or higher grade.[2,4,26] Nonetheless, the risks of radiation-induced secondary neoplasms and other complications of radiation (see Chapter 46) must be weighed against these potential benefits, particularly

in young patients with a presumably long life expectancy ahead of them. Additionally, a wide range of newer radiotherapeutic modalities are gaining popularity, including stereotactic radiosurgery, such as gamma knife, as well as fractionated stereotactic, intensity modulated and proton beam forms of radiotherapy.

WHO Grade I Meningiomas

Meningothelial Meningioma

These consist of lobulated to whorled masses of polygonal or epithelioid meningothelial cells (Figure 36.2a,b). The nuclei are round to oval, with delicate chromatin and often either clear intranuclear inclusions or eosinophilic pseudoinclusions formed by intranuclear invaginations of cytoplasm. The cell membranes appear indistinct, imparting a syncytium-like appearance and justifying the synonym, syncytial meningioma. Nuclear atypia may occur and occasionally, even bizarre mononucleate or multinucleated giant cells may be seen. This pleomorphism, however, does not indicate higher grade because it is usually degenerative in nature. Large nests or islands of cells are surrounded by variable fibrous tissue.

Fibrous (Fibroblastic) Meningioma

These tumours are composed of fibroblast-like spindled cells arranged in intersecting fascicles or a storiform growth pattern (Figure 36.2c,d). The nuclei, although elongated, retain the overall features of meningothelial cells. They are rich in collagen and reticulin. The typical whorl formation and psammoma bodies are only present focally.

Transitional Meningioma

As the name implies, this variant includes features of both the meningothelial and fibrous types, with syncytial islands of epithelioid cells alternating with bundles of spindled cells. These meningiomas have a striking tendency for whorl formation and nearly always form psammoma bodies (Figure 36.2e).

Psammomatous Meningioma

These essentially represent transitional meningiomas with psammoma bodies obscuring or replacing most of

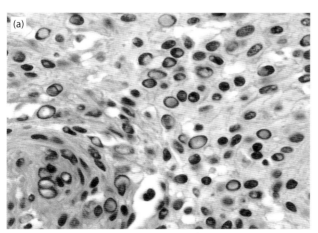
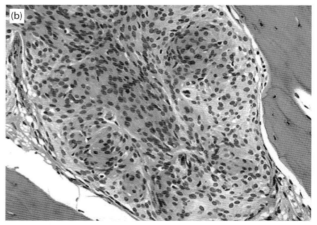

36.2 Meningioma, WHO grade I. (a) Meningothelial meningioma with epithelioid cells, ill-defined cell membranes imparting a syncytial-like appearance, and numerous intranuclear clearings and pseudoinclusions. **(b)** Meningothelial meningioma. Infiltration of bone is not a sign of malignancy.

Continued

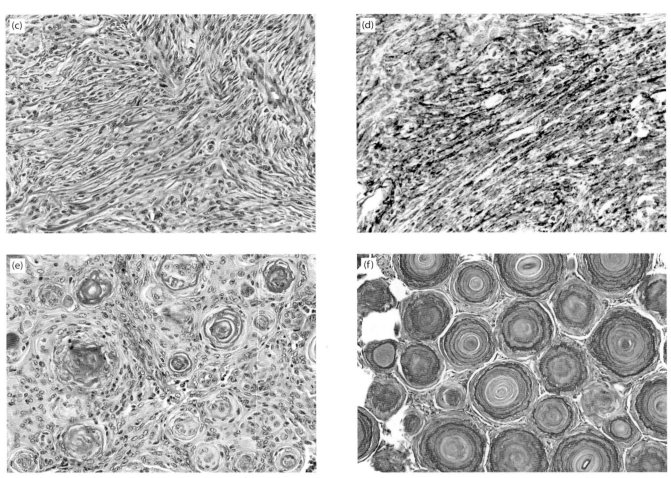

36.2 (*Continued*) Meningioma, WHO grade I. (c) Fibrous meningioma composed of spindled cells arranged in intersecting fascicles. **(d)** Epithelial membrane antigen immunoreactivity in a fibrous meningioma. **(e)** Transitional meningioma. Whorl formation is the predominant histological feature. **(f)** Psammomatous meningioma: a sparsely cellular tumour with abundant, calcified psammoma bodies.

the viable tumour (Figure 36.2f). They are encountered most often as thoracic spinal tumours in elderly women. The mRNA of bone-related proteins is expressed in these meningiomas, with osteopontin, a major phosphory-lated glycoprotein of bone, produced by CD68-positive macrophages.[68] Psammomatous meningiomas are also more likely to contain stromal amyloid than are other variants.[61]

Angiomatous (Vascular) Meningioma

This subtype has been defined as having a vascular com-ponent that exceeds 50 per cent of the tumour volume[65] (Figure 36.3a,b). The larger blood vessels are often mark-edly hyalinized, although smaller, capillary-type blood vessels often predominate; a vacuolated appearance may lead to confusion with haemangioblastomas. Among the vascular channels, islands of meningothelial cells can still be recognized, often with pleomorphic nuclei representing degenerative atypia. This variant often coexists with the microcystic subtype and is often associated with cerebral oedema.[65,125]

Microcystic Meningioma

This subtype is usually soft with a glistening cut sur-face, justifying its original name of *humid meningioma*. Cyst formation may be noted even macroscopically in some cases. High levels of VEGF, the flt-1 receptor and various tissue matrix proteins may account for the cyst formation, high vascularity and associated peritumoura-loedema commonly encountered.[45,125,127] Histologically, the tumour cells are stellate with long processes sur-rounding clear spaces (Figure 36.3c,d) that sometimes contain pale eosinophilic mucin. The precise mechanism of microcyst formation is controversial; secretory activ-ity by the tumour cells, degenerative process, penetra-tion of the CSF into the tumour and vascular changes have all been implicated. This is the one subtype that at light microscopic and ultrastructural levels bears a greater resemblance to arachnoidal trabecular, rather than cap cells.[121] The cytoplasm, when preserved, is faintly eosinophilic or finely vacuolated. Whorls and psammoma bodies are rare. Pleomorphism may be prominent and a concomitant angiomatous component is common.

Secretory Meningioma

This variant is typically seen on a background of meningothelial or transitional meningioma displaying advanced epithelial differentiation in the form of intracellular 'gland-like' spaces (Figure 36.3e,f). There is an even more striking female predominance than normally seen, with a predilection for frontal convexity or sphenoid ridge sites and for peritumoural oedema.[125,153] Lumens contain periodic acid–Schiff (PAS)-positive secretions termed *pseudopsammoma bodies*, both within intracellular lumina and between flattened neoplastic cells. They may be single or multiple, and vary in size and staining intensity. The inclusions may be evenly distributed throughout the meningioma or concentrated in a small area. The tumour cells associated with the gland-like spaces are usually strongly immunoreactive for cytokeratin and carcinoembryonic antigen (CEA). Occasionally, there is sufficient production to elevate serum levels of CEA and there are enhanced pericytic, mast cell and histiocytic elements in comparison to other variants.[34] Driver mutations of the *KLF4* and *TRAF7* genes are nearly universal.[155]

Lymphoplasmacyte-Rich Meningioma

Of all meningiomas, this is perhaps the most poorly defined subtype. It is defined by dense infiltrates of lymphocytes and plasma cells that often obscure the intermingled meningothelial nests.[32,101] Clinically, patients may have an associated monoclonal gammopathy and anaemia. Other common features that are more akin to an inflammatory process than a true meningioma include young age of onset, *en plaque* growth pattern, multifocality, spontaneous regressions and recurrences over multiple sites. Therefore, it is possible that the meningothelial proliferation in some cases is hyperplastic rather than neoplastic in nature. Diagnostically, therefore, one needs to exclude other lymphoplasmacyte-rich meningeal disorders, such as infection, Rosai–Dorfman disease, plasma cell granuloma/inflammatory myofibroblastic tumour, Castleman's disease, collagen vascular disorders and either primary or secondary low-grade lymphomas. One group found that half of their 10 previously diagnosed cases qualified for the alternate diagnosis of IgG4-related meningeal disease on further workup.[100]

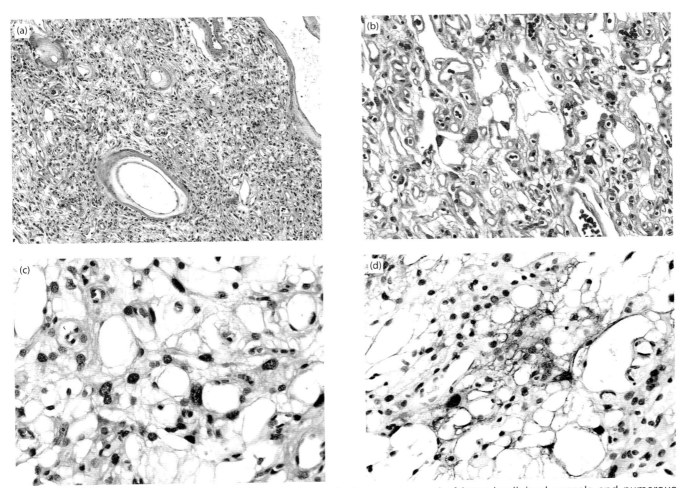

36.3 Meningioma, WHO grade I. (a,b) Angiomatous meningioma composed of large hyalinized vessels and numerous capillaries. The scattered meningothelial cells may be hard to recognize as such and often display degenerative nuclear atypia. **(c)** Microcystic meningioma. The histology is dominated by cysts of various size and a cobweb-like appearance. **(d)** Patchy epithelial membrane antigen positivity in a microcystic meningioma.

Continued

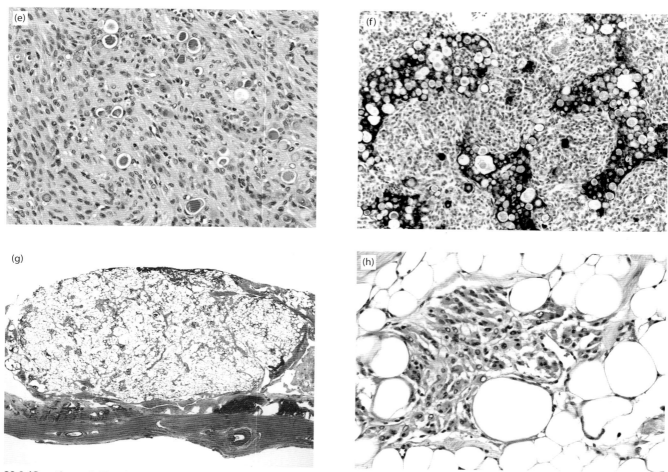

36.3 (*Continued*) Meningioma, WHO grade I. (e) Secretory meningioma with numerous gland-like spaces filled with eosinophilic pseudopsammoma bodies. **(f)** Epithelial features are demonstrated by strong immunostaining for cytokeratin in the meningioma cells surrounding pseudopsammoma bodies. **(g,h)** Metaplastic meningioma with extensive lipidization ('lipomatous meningioma').

Metaplastic Meningiomas

Various meningioma subtypes may be associated with mesenchymal 'metaplasia', including cartilaginous, osseous, lipomatous (Figure 36.3g,h), xanthomatous and myxoid foci that alternate with more classic patterns. Careful scrutiny suggests that, in most, it is probably not true metaplasia, but merely cytoplasmic fat accumulation, vacuolation or other changes within otherwise epithelial membrane antigen (EMA)-immunoreactive meningothelial cells that retain their characteristic ultrastructural features.[21,50,90] For example, Roncaroli *et al.* proposed the term *lipidized*, rather than lipomatous meningioma.[160] As in other subtypes, the degree of these changes needed to diagnose these rare subvariants is not defined; indeed, the not infrequent presence of scattered collections of foamy cells in otherwise typical meningiomas does not occasion a diagnosis of xanthomatous meningioma in everyday practice.

WHO Grade II Meningiomas

Tumours assigned a WHO grade II, which include atypical meningiomas as well as specific histological variants, have a considerably greater chance of recurrence, even after seemingly complete resection. They also have a modest but statistically significant increase in mortality.[109] Their accurate identification is therefore of clinical importance.

Atypical Meningioma

Atypical meningioma is a histological diagnosis; notably, gross invasion of adjacent dura, bones and soft tissue does not warrant a higher grade, although it makes complete resection more difficult. Similarly, features such as cytologic atypia and embolization-induced necrosis should not be overinterpreted as high-grade features (Figure 36.4). Atypical meningiomas may arise from any of the more commonly benign histological patterns noted earlier. Whereas prior grading schemes were often vague and poorly reproducible, the 2000 and 2007 WHO schemes incorporated stricter guidelines based primarily on data from two large Mayo Clinic series.[136,139,140] Atypical meningiomas are currently defined by the presence (even focally) of at least four mitoses per 10 high-power field (HPF) or at least three of the following five features: high cellularity, clusters of small cells (high nuclear/cytoplasmic ratio), prominent nucleoli, loss of architectural pattern ('sheeting') and spontaneous necrosis, i.e. not due to pre-operative embolization or radiation

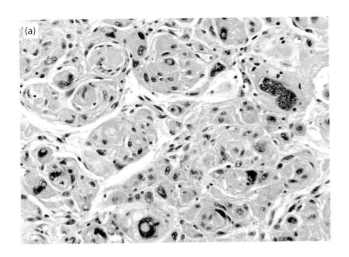

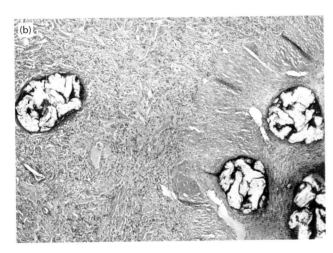

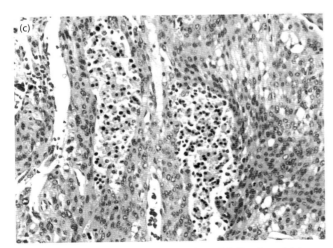

36.4 Pitfalls in meningioma grading. (a) Scattered bizarre or markedly 'atypical' nuclei likely represent degenerative atypia in this meningioma, analogous to that seen in ancient schwannomas. **(b)** Embolized meningioma with large vessels containing polyvinyl alcohol (translucent blue) and fibrin. **(c)** Embolization-induced necrosis often appears acute in nature containing numerous pyknotic nuclei; this iatrogenically induced necrosis should not be utilized as a criterion for meningioma grading.

(Figure 36.5). Additionally, brain invasive meningiomas are now also considered WHO grade II.[136] Whereas these features are often found at first diagnosis, they may also present first at recurrence as evidence of tumour progression.

Based on current criteria, atypical meningiomas are more common than previously believed. Whereas older studies quote frequencies of 5–7 per cent, in contemporary series, they comprise 20-35 per cent of cases.[17,130,140,158,198] In an audit of 314 consecutive meningiomas, the most common reason for upgrade was the formal mitotic count, emphasizing the need for a careful search even when other worrisome features are lacking.[198] As currently defined, they have an enhanced risk of recurrence compared with benign meningiomas and are therefore assigned a WHO grade of II. For example, Perry and colleagues reported a 5-year recurrence rate of 40 per cent after gross total resection, as compared to a figure of 5 per cent in similarly treated benign meningiomas.[140] After subtotal resection, the vast majority of atypical meningiomas recur. These tumours require careful radiological follow-up; whether they should be treated with ancillary radiation therapy remains debated.

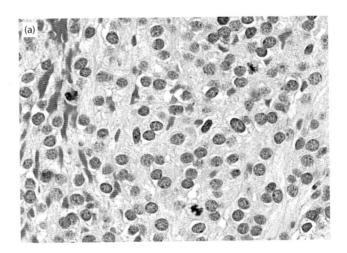

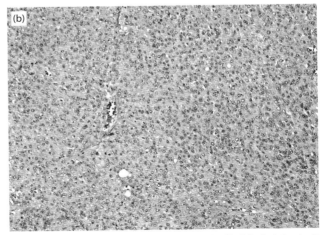

36.5 Atypical meningioma, WHO grade II. (a) Cytologically bland meningioma with increased mitotic activity. **(b)** Hypercellular meningioma with sheeting architecture.

Continued

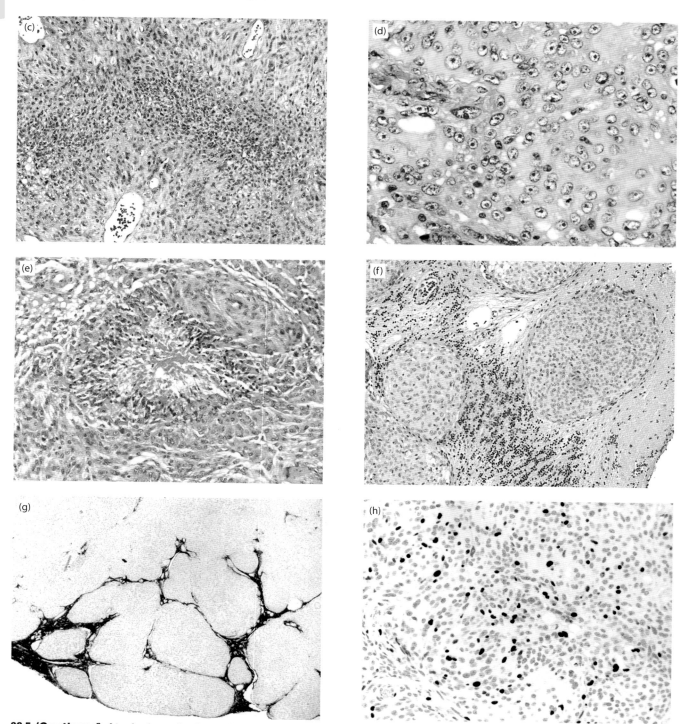

36.5 (Continued) Atypical meningioma, WHO grade II. (c) Small cell formation. **(d)** Macronucleoli. **(e)** Focus of spontaneous micronecrosis. **(f)** Brain invasion with finger-like tumour nodules protruding into the cerebellum. **(g)** Entrapped glial fibrillary acidic protein-positive central nervous system parenchyma at the periphery of a brain invasive meningioma. **(h)** Elevated MIB-1 (Ki-67) labelling index.

Clear Cell Meningioma

These tumours are composed of sheets of polygonal cells with clear cytoplasm, resulting from increased diastase-digestible PAS positivite glycogen (Figure 36.6a–c). Whorl formation and psammoma bodies are absent or poorly developed. Extensive interstitial and perivascular hyalinization is characteristic, occasionally forming thick amianthoid collagen fibres.[148,212] There is a predilection for the spinal cord and posterior fossa, often afflicting children and young adults. Despite a typically bland histology, the behaviour is aggressive, warranting its WHO grade II designation. Zorludemir and colleagues originally reported 14 cases with 61 per cent recurrence and 23 per cent mortality rates,

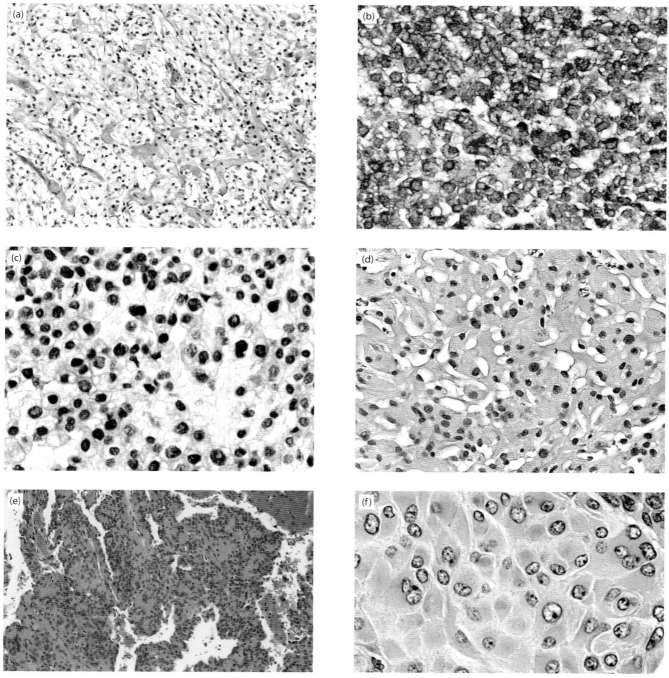

36.6 Aggressive meningioma variants. Clear cell meningioma, WHO grade II with **(a)** blocky perivascular collagen and glycogen-rich clear cytoplasm, highlighted by histochemical stains for PAS without **(b)** and with **(c)** diastase. **(d)** Chordoid meningioma, WHO grade II with a mucin-rich extracellular matrix and bubbly cytoplasm mimicking physaliferous cells. **(e)** Papillary meningioma, WHO grade III with uniform population of cells arranged in a perivascular pattern typical of these tumours. **(f)** Rhabdoid meningoma, WHO grade III with a sheet of rhabdoid cells containing paranuclear eosinophilic inclusions.

one also showing CSF dissemination.[212] Recurrences may be local or distant.[69]

Chordoid Meningioma

As the name implies, these meningiomas bear a striking resemblance to chordoma. They usually present as large, difficult to resect supratentorial masses.[51,82,184] The tumour is predominantly composed of eosinophilic epithelioid to spindled and clear vacuolated cells forming trabeculae (Figure 36.6d). The overall pattern is lobulated and the stroma may contain a lymphoplasmacytic infiltrate. This chordoid pattern is often intermingled with foci of conventional meningioma, but may also be purely chordoid. Psammoma bodies are not common. Although initially described in children with Castleman's disease and other haematological abnormalities,[82] larger series have found such associations rare.[51] However, chordoid meningiomas display a greater likelihood of recurrence after subtotal resection and have therefore been classified as WHO grade II;[136] nevertheless, the behaviour of completely resected chordoid meningiomas may parallel that of typical meningioma.

Oncocytic Meningioma

A small series of six meningiomas with marked oncocytic change was initially reported in 1997.[159] Histologically, these were characterized by granular eosinophilic cytoplasm that corresponded ultrastructurally to mitochondrial accumulations. Clinically, these tumours demonstrated a greater likelihood for recurrence. However, because of the paucity of additional experience with this subtype, it has yet to be officially recognized by the WHO.

WHO Grade III (Malignant) Meningiomas

Tumours assigned a WHO grade of III have a greater chance not only of recurrence, but also of widespread dissemination and tumour-related patient death. WHO grade III meningiomas include anaplastic (malignant) meningiomas, as well as papillary and rhabdoid histological variants.

Anaplastic (Malignant) Meningioma

These are highly malignant tumours exhibiting cellular anaplasia and/or excessive proliferative activity. Earlier definitions of malignancy presented considerable problems, because the association with poor prognosis was inconsistent.[109] However, the 2000 and 2007 WHO schemes have attempted to rectify this problem by adopting stricter criteria: at least 20 mitoses per 10 HPF and/or frank anaplasia (i.e. resembling sarcoma, carcinoma or melanoma)[136,139] (Figure 36.7). In contrast to prior definitions, brain invasion no longer constitutes an absolute criterion for malignancy. As such, whereas the diagnosis of atypical meningioma has increased, the more stringent definition of malignancy has led to a decrease in anaplastic meningiomas, with current estimates at 1–3 per cent of cases.[64,139,198] Furthermore, anaplastic forms should not be confused with meningeal sarcomas, and thus the term 'sarcomatous meningioma' referring to anaplastic spindle-celled or collagen-rich lesions should not be used.

The usual female predominance of meningiomas is not observed in malignant meningiomas. They present either as anaplastic from the outset (*de novo*) or via progression from atypical or benign meningiomas (secondary).[89] Either way, using the strict WHO definitions, the prognosis is poor with median survival times of 18 to 40 months.[139,204] Roughly one-quarter of patients live longer and most of their tumours lack 9p21 deletions (see Molecular Genetics).[132]

Papillary Meningioma

Papillary meningiomas are rare cellular tumours characterized by pseudorosette-like structures and a pseudopapillary pattern resulting from decreased cohesion and perivascular preservation (Figure 36.6e). This pattern was originally described by Cushing and Eisenhardt in a patient who underwent 17 operations, ultimately succumbing to pulmonary metastases.[53] Histologically, these tumours are composed of a rather uniform population of cells with meningothelial cytological features. Cell processes radiate towards blood vessels, mimicking ependymal pseudorosettes. The vascular walls may occasionally show hyaline thickening. This papillary pattern usually develops from more common meningioma subtypes; indeed, the papillary pattern predominates in only 25 per cent of cases, but may increase in prominence with each recurrence. Mitotic activity is variable, although additional high-grade features are typically found. The immunocytochemical profile is similar to that of other meningiomas. Papillary meningiomas histologically correspond to WHO grade III. They are unusually aggressive and have a propensity to invade, recur and metastasize.[105,190] In one series, 75 per cent invaded the brain or other adjacent structures, 55 per cent recurred and 20 per cent metastasized.[129] Half of the patients die from the tumour, and the patients are often younger with roughly half presenting in children.[105] Some combine papillary architecture with rhabdoid cytology.[201]

Rhabdoid Meningioma

Rhabdoid meningiomas contain collections of discohesive rhabdoid cells (Figure 36.6f).[83,138] As with rhabdoid tumours elsewhere, cells contain large eccentric nuclei, prominent nucleoli and eosinophilic cytoplasm that often has a whorled filamentous appearance. Most rhabdoid meningiomas have other features of malignancy, including high mitotic counts, cytological atypia and necrosis. As a result, most follow a course similar to malignant meningiomas, justifying the assigned WHO grade of III.[136,138,211] Rhabdoid cells may first present at recurrence, often heralding a more aggressive course. However, the behaviour of focally rhabdoid meningiomas that otherwise lack malignant features remains to be determined. Such tumours should probably be graded as usual, perhaps with the patient being followed more carefully. As mentioned earlier, rhabdoid cytology is occasionally combined with a papillary architecture, occasional cases also showing an unexpected glial fibrillary acidic protein (GFAP) immunoreactivity.[8,138]

Brain Invasion and Metastasis

The significance of brain invasion and metastasis in meningioma are complex issues, possibly relating more to tumour staging rather than grading. Brain invasion is defined as extension of meningothelial cells beyond the pial surface into the brain parenchyma (see Figure 36.5f,g), which must be distinguished from extension along superficial Virchow–Robin spaces. It is typically found at the periphery of larger meningiomas as irregular tongue-like protrusions that incite a brisk reactive astrocytosis in adjacent brain. The previously held opinion that brain invasion is synonymous with malignancy in meningiomas is no longer tenable.[139] Clearly, brain invasion connotes a greater likelihood of recurrence (see Table 36.1). The distinction between brain invasive and otherwise malignant meningiomas is further supported by molecular genetic investigations, because brain invasive meningiomas without malignant cytological features rarely harbour the genetic changes characteristic of malignant meningiomas.[35,95,194] Nevertheless, in

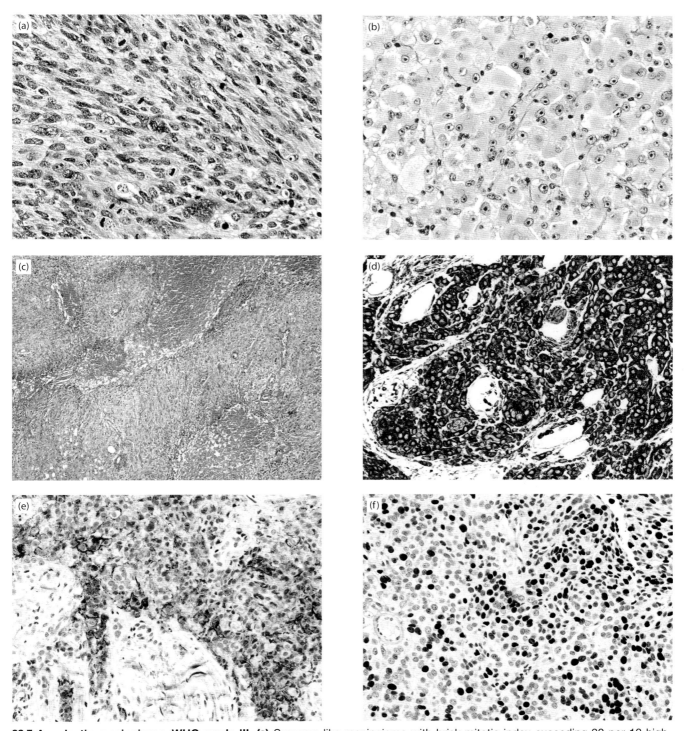

36.7 Anaplastic meningioma, WHO grade III. (a) Sarcoma-like meningioma with brisk mitotic index exceeding 20 per 10 high-power fields. **(b)** Melanoma-like cytology. **(c)** Extensive geographic necrosis. **(d)** Diffuse vimentin immunoreactivity. **(e)** Patchy membrane pattern staining for epithelial membrane antigen. **(f)** Markedly elevated MIB-1 (Ki-67) labelling index.

the absence of frank anaplasia, recurrence and mortality rates of brain invasive meningiomas are similar to atypical meningiomas.[139] As such, the 2007 WHO scheme considers them as grade II prognostically.[136]

Metastasis is a rare complication, involving only 0.1 per cent of meningiomas. It is generally a feature of malignant meningioma, although clinically indolent WHO grade I meningiomas ('benign metastasizing meningioma') may rarely seed distant organs.[3,118] The lungs and the pleura are the most frequent sites of metastasis, followed by the musculoskeletal system, liver, reticuloendothelial system and kidneys, in decreasing order of involvement. Increased risk of metastasis is associated with prior craniotomy, venous sinus invasion, local recurrence, histological malignancy and papillary and/or rhabdoid morphology.[3]

Immunohistochemistry

Immunohistochemistry supports the dual mesenchymal and epithelial-like nature of meningeal cells. The vast majority of meningiomas coexpress vimentin and EMA, the latter representing the most commonly utilized antibody for support of meningothelial derivation (Figures 36.2d, 36.3d and 36.7d,e). Unlike most carcinomas, cytokeratin is usually negative or only focally positive. Secretory meningiomas represent an exception, however, strongly expressing keratin in the cells surrounding pseudopsammoma bodies (Figure 36.3f). The latter is also true of CEA, which is correlated with degree of surrounding oedema and is typically negative in other types of meningioma.[153] S-100 protein expression is variable, but is most commonly encountered in the fibrous subtype. Immunoreactivity may create diagnostic confusion with schwannoma, but differs by its focal or patchy expression, rather than the diffuse pattern of schwannoma. Staining for GFAP is essentially negative, except in rare examples, but can be useful for confirming the presence of brain invasion in equivocal cases (Figure 36.5g). Antibodies to the desmosomal plaque proteins (desmoplakins I and II) and ultrastructural immunolocalization show that vimentin filaments are anchored to the desmosomal plaques. The exclusive combination of vimentin intermediate filaments and desmoplakin, found only in arachnoid cells, may therefore be a useful diagnostic feature of meningiomas.[6] Additional potentially useful markers include progesterone receptor, cathepsin D, E-cadherin, claudin-1, platelet-derived growth factor receptor beta and somatostatin receptor 2A,[15,106] although most of these lack specificity.

Other particularly useful ancillary markers for grading and prognosis include progesterone receptor and MIB-1/Ki-67 (see Figures 36.5h and 36.7f). Whether elevated proliferative labelling indices represent an independent prognostic variable has been debated, because they generally increase proportionally to mitotic indices and histologic grade in general.[141,162] Additionally, interlaboratory variability in staining and counting methods make it difficult to extrapolate results from one study to another. Nonetheless, MIB-1 and progesterone receptor (PR) immunostains may both be useful in borderline grade I–II or II–III meningiomas, potentially providing information that helps the clinician direct follow-up care. However, it is possible that focal elevations in proliferative index may not be as biologically significant as more diffuse ones.[117] PR expression is inversely associated with tumour grade, but as with Ki-67, the association with clinical behaviour remains imperfect.[161]

Electron Microscopy

Characteristic features common to most meningiomas, regardless of subtype, include complex intercellular junctions, interdigitating cell processes and intracellular filaments. The light microscopic impression of fuzzy cell borders and a syncitial quality in meningothelial and transitional meningiomas is due to interdigitating cell processes. Similar to normal arachnoidal cap cells, neoplastic cells maintain desmosomes, hemidesmosomes and gap junctions. Another feature is the abundance of intermediate (10 nm) filaments, corresponding to vimentin, which tend to converge on the cytoplasmic surface of desmosomes or may also show a pronounced whorling pattern. The common nuclear pseudoinclusions represent cytoplasmic invaginations, whereas the clear vacuoles may contain glycogen, but more often appear as empty non-membranebound spaces.[206]

Psammoma bodies are formed by dystrophic calcification associated with arachnoid cells and hyalinized whorls.[7,202] Extracellular matrix vesicles with or without hydroxyapatite crystals are occasionally present at the periphery. Moreover, many small aggregates of crystals are seen adjacent and parallel to the collagen and reticulin fibres. These observations indicate that the matrix vesicles, presumably produced by meningothelial cells, serve as nidi of calcification, whereas the collagen and reticulin fibres may guide the deposition of apatite crystals. Scanning electron microscopy further reveals that the dense amorphous calcified core of each psammoma body is surrounded by an outer coating of entwined collagen fibres.

Various histological types may show unique ultrastructural characteristics. In microcystic meningiomas, spider-like delicate processes line the microcystic spaces and interdigitate with scattered desmosomes, reminiscent of normal arachnoid trabecular cells.[121] The presence of pinocytotic vesicles and prominent Golgi complexes indicates active cytoplasmic vesicular transport. The widened extracellular space is filled with finely granular material. Despite the xanthoma-like appearance of some cells by light microscopy, they do not contain lipid droplets. Secretory meningiomas contain inclusions, originally described as pseudopsammoma bodies,[80] that are contained in gland-like spaces lined by microvilli. The inclusions may be amorphous or more complex, displaying particulate, vesicular or lamellar structures. The cells surrounding the inclusions have dense cytoplasm, abundant filaments and desmosomes. The endothelial lining of small blood vessels may be surrounded by multiple layers of pericytes, which themselves are invested by basal lamina.[120] Ultrastructural examination of clear cell meningiomas confirms their rich glycogen content and occasional amianthoid type collagen fibres.[147] Rhabdoid meningiomas feature whorled bundles of intermediate filaments as encountered in rhabdoid cells generally,[138] whereas the rare oncocytic variant is defined by mitochondrial accumulations.[159] The finding of typical meningothelial features ultrastructurally can be extremely helpful in establishing the diagnosis of poorly differentiatied variants, such as anaplastic and papillary meningioma, each of which may engender an extensive differential diagnosis.[10,139] Lastly, as stated earlier, metaplastic meningiomas typically retain meningothelial ultrastructural features, suggesting that most are probably not truly metaplastic, but instead, simply accumulate cytoplasmic lipid, lysosomes, etc.[160]

Cytogenetics

Consistent cytogenetic abnormalities are found in most meningiomas and involve both chromosomal losses and structural rearrangements.[84,208] The most frequent chromosomal abnormality is monosomy 22 in about 50–60 per cent of cases. Less often, a 22q deletion occurs. Following monosomy 22, numerical losses of chromosomes 14, 18 and 19 are most frequent, with losses of 6 and 10 slightly less common. In terms of structural alterations, 1p loss is by far the most common. It is possible that chordoid meningiomas are associated with a characteristic translocation of chromosome arms 1p and 3p:t(1;3)(p12–13;q11),[179] a site that is also implicated in radiation-induced meningiomas.[151,171,209]

Benign meningiomas are likely to have a normal karyotype or monosomy 22 alone.[84,208] As the neoplasm progresses, the karyotype becomes increasingly hypodiploid and later structural rearrangements may occur, including translocations and telomeric associations resulting in ring and dicentric chromosomes.[9,135] Increasingly abnormal karyotypes may be associated with malignant progression. In a study of 198 gross totally resected meningiomas, the tumours were stratified into four cytogenetic groups: 0, normal diploid karyotype; 1, monosomy 22 only; 2, hypodiploid with loss of additional autosomes; and 3, 1p deletion and, often, other alterations. Recurrence rates were highly associated with these groupings, being 4.3 per cent in groups 0 and 1, 10.5 per cent in group 2 and 30 per cent in group 3.[84] Furthermore, these patterns were highly associated with WHO grade and tumour location, such that the more aggressive group 2 and 3 meningiomas tended to be atypical or anaplastic meningiomas of the convexity. In contrast, the majority of spinal and skull base meningiomas were benign tumours with group 0 or 1 patterns.

Molecular Genetics

Molecular genetic and molecular cytogenetic approaches have also demonstrated frequent losses of chromosome 22q in benign meningiomas, and losses of other chromosomal regions as meningiomas progress to atypical and malignant forms.[136] In particular, losses of 1p, 10 and 14q are frequent in atypical and malignant meningiomas. Of interest, such alterations encountered in recurrent high-grade meningiomas may already be present in the primary tumour at a time when it appears otherwise benign.[9] In fact, comparisons of benign meningiomas with and without subsequent recurrences revealed statistically increased likelihoods of 1p and 14q deletions in the former.[20,35] Providing further support, a comparative genomic hybridization (CGH) study found average chromosomal alteration numbers of 2.9, 9.2 and 13.3 in grade I, II and III meningiomas, respectively. The most common changes were losses of 22q in 58 per cent of benign tumours; losses of 1p (76 per cent), 22q (71 per cent), 14q (43 per cent), 18q (43 per cent), 10 (38 per cent) and 6q (33 per cent) as well as gains of 20q (48 per cent), 12q (43 per cent), 15q (43 per cent), 1q (33 per cent), 9q (33 per cent) and 17q (33 per cent) in atypical meningiomas; and, in malignant meningiomas, these alterations with increased frequencies for losses of 6q (53 per cent), 10 (68 per cent), 14q (63 per cent) and 9p (32 per cent).[194]

Similar findings have been reported in numerous studies using loss of heterozygosity (LOH) and fluorescence *in situ* hybridization (FISH).[109] (Figure 36.8).

The consistent losses of 22q, followed by 1p, 10 and 14q, strongly suggest the presence of meningioma tumour suppressor genes on these chromosomal arms. Of these, the most studied has been chromosome 22q. Detailed analyses of the NF2 gene in meningiomas have now confirmed that this gene is altered in both sporadic and NF2-associated meningiomas, including the vast majority of meningiomas that display chromosome 22q loss.[136] Genetic studies suggest that other chromosome 22q loci besides NF2, including AP1B1/BAM22, MN1 and SMARCB1 (INI1/hSNF5) may play a role in rare examples. The latter is particularly interesting because it is the tumour suppressor implicated in malignant rhabdoid tumours and atypical teratoid/rhabdoid tumours (see Chapter 34). Nevertheless, expression of the protein is typically retained in rhabdoid meningiomas, suggesting that it does not play a significant role in these morphologically similar tumours.[133] Nonetheless, this gene has now been implicated in rare meningiomas, particularly in families with schwannomatosis[12,16,44,187] (see Chapter 44). In atypical and anaplastic meningiomas, NF2 gene mutations occur in approximately 70 per cent of cases, matching the frequency of NF2 mutations in benign fibroblastic and transitional meningiomas; this is consistent with a role for NF2 inactivation in the formation, rather than progression, of meningiomas. Most mutations are small insertions or deletions, or nonsense mutations that affect splice sites, create stop codons or result in frameshifts and that occur predominantly in the most 5′ two-thirds of the gene.[104] Therefore, these mutations would be predicted to result in a truncated, and presumably non-functional, merlin (schwannomin) protein. Interestingly, the frequency of NF2 gene mutations varies among the three most common variants of meningioma: fibroblastic and transitional meningiomas carry NF2 gene mutations in approximately 70–80 per cent of cases; meningothelial meningiomas, particularly those encountered at the skull base, have NF2 gene mutations in only 25 per cent of cases,[91,195] suggesting that many meningothelial meningiomas have a genetic origin distinct from NF2 gene mutation.

Genomic studies have now identified additional driver mutations in the roughly half of meningiomas that are NF2 intact, many of which correspond to midline skull base, meningothelial and/or secretory examples.[30,47,155] Most frequent among these are TRAF7 gene mutations, often in association with either K409Q mutations of KLF4 or E17K mutations of the AKT1 genes.[47,155] Such cases account for roughly 25 per cent of all meningiomas, whereas driver mutations of SMO that activate the sonic hedgehog pathway roughly represent another 5 per cent.[30,47] Along with NF2 then, driver mutations can now be identified in up to 80 per cent of all meningiomas. Multiple different point mutations of the tumour necrosis factor receptor-associated factor 7 (TRAF7) gene on chromosome 16p have been reported, nearly all involving the seven WD40 repeat regions at the C terminus. This proapoptotic transcription factor is thought to inhibit NF-κB activation and promote the JNKAP1 pathway. The KLF4 gene on chromosome 9q, encodes a zinc finger-containing protein that is thought to

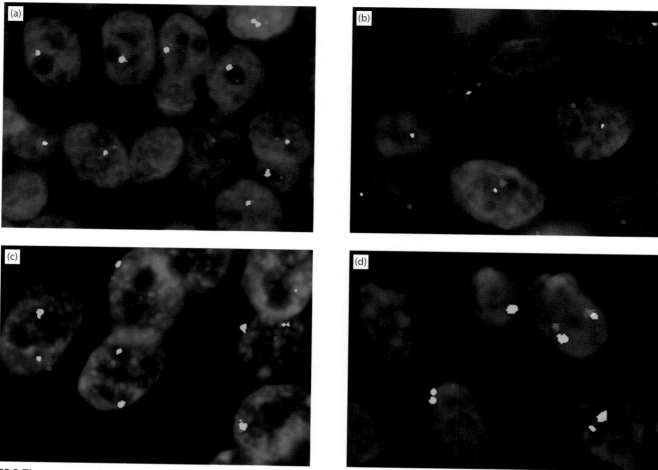

36.8 Fluorescence *in situ* hybridization studies with common genetic alterations in meningiomas. (a) 22q loss or monosomy 22; most nuclei have only one red NF2 (22q12) and one green BCR (22q11.2) signal. **(b)** Deletions of 1p (green) and 14q (red), consistent with a higher grade or more aggressive meningiomas. **(c)** Loss of the p16 (9p21) region in an anaplastic meningioma, with most cells showing one red (9p21) and two green (centromere 9) signals. **(d)** Another case displays homozygous p16 (9p21) deletions with only green centromere 9 signals seen in most tumour nuclei.

have context-dependent roles in transcriptional activation and repression, including oncogenic activation and tumour suppression. It is expressed in several cell types, including meningothelial, and is thought to promote the conversion of differentiated cells into pluripotent stem cells.[47] The *AKT1* mutation is well known for its activating role in PI3K signalling. Of additional interest, germline mutations of *SMARCE1*, another member of the chromatin remodeling pathway similar to *SMARCB1*, have been implicated in familial examples of clear cell meningioma.[175] Whether this might similarly serve as the driver mutation in sporadic cases of this rare but aggressive variant requires further study.

Analysis of predicted amino acid sequences have demonstrated homologies between the *NF2* gene product, merlin and other members of the protein 4.1 family, including ezrin, radixin and moesin (ERM proteins). Although the functions of most of these proteins remain unclear, data support a role for merlin via its stromal interactions in the regulation of proliferation, apoptosis, survival, motility, adhesion, and invasion.[113] Merlin has also been shown to interact with several potentially important interacting proteins, including a sodium-hydrogen exchange regulatory factor (NHE-RF), βII-spectrin (fodrin), hepatocyte growth factor-regulated tyrosine kinase substrate (HRS), schwannomin interacting protein-1 (SCHIP-1), paxillin and other ERM proteins. One downstream oncogene that appears to be activated by merlin is yes-associated protein 1 (YAP1).[18] Merlin also binds several transmembrane signalling proteins, including β1-integrin and CD44. CD44 is a hyaluronic acid receptor that binds ERM proteins through amino acid residues in its carboxyl-terminal cytoplasmic tail domain. Hyaluronic acid has been shown to promote proliferation and motility in some cells, suggesting that the association between merlin and CD44 might influence growth regulation and motility. This may partially explain the peculiar ability of meningiomas to invade dura, bone and soft tissue, even when histologically benign.

Although cytogenetic and CGH studies have not shown consistent losses of other chromosomal arms in benign meningiomas, it is likely that other suppressor loci exist as well. For example, a few cases of meningiomas have been reported that lack 22q loss, but have losses of 1p and 3p.[39]

This is of further interest given reports of a characteristic translocation of 1p and 3p in chordoid meningiomas[179] and the importance of 1p losses in radiation-induced meningiomas.[57] Moreover, the loss of both *VHL* alleles on 3p26–p25 in a case is intriguing, given some suggestions of increased meningioma risks in patients with von Hippel–Lindau syndrome (see Chapter 44).[78] Nonetheless, additional studies are needed to prove a causal relationship. Finally, it is clear that non-*NF2*-associated familial meningiomas exist.[67] Rare examples have been linked to *SMARCB1*, *SMARCE1* and *SUFU*, although other genes likely contribute as well.[1,44,175,187]

Among the other genomic regions frequently lost in atypical and malignant meningiomas, studies have focused primarily on 1p, 6q, 10, 14q and 18q.[109] Investigations of chromosome 1p and 14q have shown losses of one or both in the vast majority of atypical and malignant meningiomas.[35] The localization of putative tumour suppressors has been hindered by the fact that the entire 1p arm and chromosome 14 are lost in most cases. On chromosome 1, at least two regions on 1p32 and 1p36 have been suggested, with the *4.1R* (also known as *EPB4.1*) gene on 1p36 as one interesting candidate.[157] However, losses of *4.1R* mRNA expression in meningiomas have not correlated with 1p LOH, nor have data supported a role for *GADD45A* on 1p31.[145] A number of other putative tumour suppressors have been considered, but lack compelling evidence of a causal role.[180] One exception may be the *NDRG2* gene on 14q11.2;[108] by expression profiling, *NDRG2* was expressed in all five benign and lost in all five anaplastic meningiomas. Validation studies showed diminished or absent *NDRG2* expression in the majority of anaplastic and clinically aggressive atypical meningiomas, with promoter methylation raised as an explanation for loss of expression of the second allele. Similarly, the maternally expressed gene 3 (*MEG3*) has been proposed as another 14q candidate.[19,210] An imprinted gene on 14q32 encoding a non-coding RNA with antiproliferative effects, its loss of expression, genomic deletion and degree of promoter methylation have been associated with aggressive biology.

Investigations of known tumour suppressor genes have revealed only rare alterations in meningiomas. For instance, mutations of *TP53* are extremely rare in meningiomas, although hypermethylation of the *p14^{ARF}* gene is occasionally seen.[11] Nevertheless, wild-type p53 protein accumulates in occasional meningiomas.[58] Deletions of the *CDKN2A/p16* gene on 9p and the *PTCH* gene on 9q are also rare in benign meningiomas, but losses of the *CDKN2A/p16* region on 9p21 are seen in the majority of anaplastic (malignant) meningiomas, where they are associated with poor survival.[28,132] The importance of this gene is further supported by the finding that adding its inactivation to that of *NF2* promotes faster development and higher grade histology in mouse models of meningioma.[142]

Consistent oncogene abnormalities have not been demonstrated in benign, atypical or malignant meningiomas, although amplifications involving 17q23 are common and the *S6K* gene may be involved in a minority of such cases.[33,36,181] Nonetheless, this signalling pathway may be activated in larger subsets of tumours as evidenced by decreased growth in mouse models using an mTORC1

inhibitor.[126] Rare amplifications have also been noted involving the *CDK4* and *MDM2* genes on 12q13–15 and the *HER2* (*ERBB2*) gene on 17q12, the latter often co-associated with 1p14q deletions.[63,194]

Molecular and Cell Biology

Molecular insights are progressively emerging as specific gene functions are elucidated. As stated earlier, *NF2* gene inactivation with loss of merlin expression accounts for roughly half of benign meningiomas, with *TRAF7*, *KLF4*, *AKT1* and/or *SMO* mutations found in many of the rest. However, downstream changes in cell biology are less understood. Oncogene and growth factor expression studies are often difficult to interpret because alterations in a single protein may affect multiple signalling pathways with extensive 'cross talk' among pathways, often frustrating single-agent targeted therapy strategies.[24,74,76,98,99,143,165] Altered signalling pathways include the smoothened/sonic hedgehog, WNT/beta-catenin, ERBB1 (EGFR), ERBB2 (HER2), VEGF and many others. The PDGF and its receptors have been particularly well studied.[75] PDGF-A, PDGF-B and PDGF-β receptor are all expressed in meningiomas and the β-receptor, when activated, increases c-fos levels. PDGF is also found in CSF. PDGF-BB and PDGF-β receptors appear to be involved in the growth control of meningiomas through autocrine and/or paracrine mechanisms. This signalling pathway appears to be activated in the majority of meningiomas, regardless of grade,[75,115] although high-grade meningiomas activate additional mitogenic pathways.[115] Other alterations, such as *CDKN2A/p16* losses, alter cell cycle regulation, potentially accounting for their high proliferative rates encountered.

The epidermal growth factor receptor (EGFR) is expressed in over half of meningiomas and can be detected even in subsets of normal and hyperplastic meningothelial cells.[137,196] The phosphorylation of downstream signalling proteins suggests that EGFR is activated in meningiomas.[41] However, no consistent associations with tumour grade, patient age, clinical outcome or responses to pharmacological inhibitors have been found.[37,122,196] Increased TGF-α and TGF-β expression levels have also been variably encountered in fibroblastic and aggressive meningiomas.[62,191] TGF-α is also found in the CSF, suggesting the possibilities of both autocrine and paracrine stimulation.[76] Both the PDGF and EGF receptors activate the p21RAS-Raf1-MEK1-MAPK/ERK signalling pathway that ultimately upregulates many cellular growth-associated transcription factors.

Somatostatin (sst) receptors have been found in the majority of meningiomas, the sst2A subtype being most common and potentially providing both diagnostic and therapeutic utilities.[13,15,168] Whereas somatostatin analogues have not led to measurable responses in most, stable disease has been achieved in a subset of meningiomas that were otherwise challenging to control.[71,167] Meningiomas also overexpress growth hormone receptors, as well as related insulin-like growth factors and their binding proteins, particularly IGF-1 and IGF-2.[112] In this regard, growth inhibition may be achieved with growth hormone receptor antagonists, such as pegvisomant. Expression levels of several *IGF-2* transcripts are particularly upregulated in high-grade examples.[99,192,200]

Significant levels of basic fibroblast growth factor (bFGF) and its receptors, FGFR1 and FGFR2 have been detected in both leptomeninges and meningiomas.[73,96] FGFs, being mitogens as well as differentiation and angiogenic agents, may affect tumour progression as autocrine growth factors. Prolactin and dopamine receptors are also commonly expressed in meningiomas,[42,46] as is the apoptosis inhibitor, survivin.[66,106] CSF itself has been shown to stimulte meningioma growth, possibly via STAT3 activation.[72] Other forms of oncogene activation in meningiomas of various grades includes the PI3K-AKT-S6K and c-myc signalling pathways.[75,110,115]

Vascular endothelial growth factor/vascular permeability factor (VEGF/VPF) is a potent angiogenic and vascular permeability molecule. In a study of 60 meningiomas, VEGF/VPF immunoreactivity was found in the endothelium of over half of the tumours, along with expression of one of the VEGF receptors, flt-1.[45] Expression of VEGF/VPF was particularly common in microcystic meningiomas (75 per cent), suggesting that the vascular permeability effects could mediate microcyst formation in this subtype of meningioma. Other investigators, however, have found little correlation with vascular pattern in meningiomas and VEGF, VEGFR1 and VEGFR2 expression patterns, possibly explaining the only modest responses to bevacizumab observed to date.[24,119,123]

Another important area of meningioma cell biology involves extracellular matrix (ECM) maintenance, degradation and remodeling, especially in reference to disordered growth, invasion, cellular migration, ECM-mediated cell signalling, angiogenesis and cerebral oedema. Potentially relevant regulators include plasminogens, matrix metalloproteinases (MMP) and their tissue inhibitors (TIMP), as well as adhesion factors and integrins, such as galectin-3, laminin, vitronectin, osteonectin (SPARC) and fibronectin, some of which are themselves regulated by growth factors already discussed.[25,54,85,154] For instance, most meningiomas express urokinase plasminogen activator (uPA), MMP-2, MMP-9, TIMP-1, galectin-3 and fibronectin.[54,173] Additionally, high-grade and aggressive meningiomas often have increased MMP-9, SPARC, uPA, stromelysin-3 and oncofetal ECM proteins, such as tenascin and fibronectin, as well as decreased CD13/aminopeptidase N (APN), integrin alpha-3 and alpha-6 expression levels in comparison to conventional benign counterparts.[23,25,29,85,86,111,131,154] Differential expression of ECMs is also seen in rare variants such as secretory, clear cell and rhabdoid meningiomas.[93]

Role of Hormones

Sex hormones and their receptors have been studied extensively in meningiomas. Support for a biological association comes from the female predominance, reports of rapidly worsening visual symptoms during pregnancy, and modest epidemiologic links with exogenous hormones and with breast carcinoma, another hormone-related tumour of women.[48,152] In terms of rapid pregnancy-associated growth, such cases are relatively rare and lack a convincing epidemiologic link; nonetheless, they can be clinically dramatic with symptoms most often due to optic nerve compression, presenting typically in the third trimester, resolving postpartum, and then recurring in subsequent

pregnancies.[107,174] Because of this reversible nature and a general lack of increased mitotic figures on histology, the 'growth' is thought to primarily result from vascular congestion and cytotoxic oedema, rather than a true hormone-induced tumour proliferation; extensive intercellular and intracellular oedema can occasionally cause diagnostic challenges.[107] Additionally, reports of PR expression in 50–80 per cent of meningiomas have generated great interest. Initially, oestrogen receptors were also detected, although the vast majority of studies since have found measurable expression levels to be relatively rare.[109]

The range of PR expression is highly variable, but is roughly inversely proportional to grade, such that the majority of benign meningiomas are strongly immunoreactive, especially in young patients with the meningothelial variant; in contrast, most atypical, anaplastic and clinically aggressive meningiomas are negative or show only focal staining.[106,161,199] Unfortunately, in most large series, there is substantial overlap in expression levels among meningiomas of varying grade and clinical behaviour and as such, an independent prognostic role remains uncertain. Therefore, its routine use is not warranted. Nonetheless, immunostaining for PR may be helpful for gauging recurrence risks in borderline atypical cases, especially when utilized in combination with MIB-1 (Ki-67) labelling indices.

The precise biological role of PR also remains unclear. Arguing in favour of a tumourigenic or growth stimulatory function is the female predominance and a modest increased risk of meningioma formation for women using oral contraceptives or hormone replacement therapy.[48] Against a critical role, however, is the presence of PR in tumours from men and children nearly as often as from women, a lack of compelling growth stimulation by progesterone *in vitro* and a peak incidence in women at roughly 60 years of age, beyond child-bearing years or periods when circulating progesterone levels are normally high. Despite these observations, it had been hoped that therapy with anti-progestational agents such as mifepristone (RU-486) might be useful as an ancillary therapy for unresectable meningiomas; unfortunately, a recent large clinical trial did not show significant efficacy.

Additional hormone receptors detected in meningiomas include the androgen, prolactin, growth hormone, thyroid hormone, erythropoietin and cholecystokinin receptors.[46,87,92,112,114,124,183,189] The potential biological roles of these receptors have yet to be fully elucidated, although data suggest that high-grade meningiomas more often express androgen receptor.

Histogenesis

The histogenesis of meningiomas has been controversial.[81] The uncertainty of derivation was reflected in the abundance of misleading terminology and it was only in 1922 that Cushing's proposed term of meningioma rendered the many prior names obsolete. For the cell of origin, various cell types were suggested, including dural, endothelial, fibroblastic and epithelial. Some features are entirely consistent with mesenchymal origin in that spindled meningothelial resemble fibroblasts, they produce collagen and other extracellular matrix proteins, various forms of mesenchymal metaplasia are seen in meningiomas, and some anaplastic examples resemble sarcomas. Epithelial characteristics include desmosomal intercellular attachments, EMA expression, the capacity for a papillary pattern, the formation of cytokeratin and CEA-positive cells with gland-like spaces in the secretory variant, and a carcinoma-like appearance in some anaplastic forms.

The original observation by Cleland,[49] confirmed later by Schmidt,[166] indicated that these tumours were morphologically similar to cell clusters capping the arachnoidal villi. Since then, arachnoidal cap cells have been regarded as the most likely cell of origin based on the striking light- and electron-microscopic similarities, including intranuclear inclusions, plasmalemmal interdigitations, desmosomes, hemidesmosome-like junctions and cytoplasmic filaments.[203] Arachnoidal cap cells are encountered not only in arachnoid granulations, but also throughout external portions of the leptomeninges and in the tela choroidea at the stromal base of the choroid plexus. They are unique in the body and are endowed with multiple functions: (1) similar to meningiomas, they ensheath or wrap around multiple structures, notably the surface of the CNS and proximal portions of nerve roots where they form part of the CNS–CSF and blood–CSF barriers; (2) they participate in CSF homeostasis, both in terms of protein secretion and the regulation of intracranial pressure; (3) they provide trophic support for neuroglial cells during development; and (4) they take part in the mononuclear phagocytic system.[109]

Differential Diagnosis

In most cases meningiomas can be diagnosed without any difficulty, from haematoxylin and eosin (H&E)-stained sections alone. However, these tumours display a remarkably varied histological spectrum that may cause considerable diagnostic difficulties in selected cases (Table 36.2), particularly the rarer variants. However, the typical immunocytochemical profile of meningiomas, with EMA immunopositivity, often aids in the diagnosis. Only rare cases, usually highly anaplastic examples, require ultrastructural or genetic studies for diagnosis.[109]

Schwannomas may be occasionally difficult to distinguish from fibrous meningiomas, particularly in NF2 patients who have a susceptibility to both lesions and in whom both tumour types can be found in a single resection specimen. Generally, fibrous meningiomas will have at least focal whorls and psammoma bodies, but one is occasionally surprised to find schwannomas with well-developed whorls and meningiomas with Verocay body-like structures. Similarly, it is important to note that up to 70 per cent of fibrous meningiomas are S-100 positive, although they usually lack the more diffuse staining pattern of schwannomas. Also, reticulin histochemical stains and type IV collagen immunohistochemistry highlight the diffuse delicate peritumoural basement membrane network of schwannomas in contrast to the coarser, patchy reticulin pattern of meningiomas, the latter often showing minimal collagen IV deposition beyond perivascular spaces. Lastly, schwannomas are consistently negative for EMA. Electron microscopy also confirms the basal lamina closely apposed to neoplastic Schwann cells versus the complex imbricating processes and intercellular junctions

of meningioma. The occasional difficulty with the differential diagnosis with astrocytomas can usually be resolved by GFAP immunostaining, which is positive in astrocytomas and nearly always negative in meningiomas (see earlier). Meningiomas, particularly the meningothelial type, may superficially mimic carcinomas, especially in higher grade examples. Whereas both tumours are positive for EMA, only meningiomas give consistently positive immunostaining for vimentin, whereas carcinomas generally display far more extensive cytokeratin immunoreactivity. In this differential diagnosis, it is also important to remember that carcinomas may metastasize to meningiomas, particularly breast carcinomas.

TABLE 36.2 Common differential diagnoses for meningioma variants

Variant	Differential diagnosis
Meningothelial or transitional	Metastatic carcinoma Meningothelial hyperplasia
Fibroblastic	Schwannoma Solitary fibrous tumour/haemangiopericytoma Fibrosis or fibromatosis Fibrosarcoma
Psammomatous	Meningothelial hyperplasia Calcifying pseudotumour of the neural axis
Angiomatous (vascular)	Haemangioblastoma
Microcystic	Diffuse or pilocytic astrocytoma Clear cell meningioma
Secretory	Metastatic adenocarcinoma
Lymphoplasmacyte-rich	Inflammatory process Rosai–Dorfman disease
Metaplastic (bone, cartilage, xanthomatous, myxoid, fat, etc.)	Soft tissue tumours
Clear cell (WHO grade II)	Metastatic renal cell carcinoma Microcystic meningioma Hemangioblastoma
Chordoid (WHO grade II)	Chordoma Chordoid glioma of the third ventricle Epithelioid hemangioendothelioma
Papillary (WHO grade III)	Papillary ependymoma Astroblastoma Haemangiopericytoma Metastatic malignancy Meningeal melanocytoma
Rhabdoid (WHO grade III)	Metastatic malignancy Atypical teratoid/rhabdoid tumour Glioblastoma/gliosarcoma

WHO, World Health Organization.

Of the rarer histological subtypes of meningiomas, the secretory, microcystic, lymphoplasmacytoid and chordoid variants require special consideration. Secretory meningiomas may be confused with adenocarcinomas, because the acini contain PAS-positive pseudopsammoma bodies expressing both keratin and CEA. However, regions of typical meningioma are usually present and should confirm the meningothelial nature of the neoplasm. Microcystic meningiomas may superficially resemble low-grade protoplasmic and pilocytic astrocytomas, especially at the time of frozen section. However, the dural attachment is an important clue and GFAP is consistently negative. Lymphoplasmacytoid meningiomas should be distinguished from a variety of meningeal processes rich in chronic inflammation, including infections, sarcoidosis, plasma cell granuloma/inflammatory myofibroblastic tumour, meningeal rheumatoid nodules, Wegener's granulomatosis, Rosai–Dorfman disease (extranodal sinus histiocytosis), Castleman's disease, and low-grade lymphomas, such as marginal zone lymphoma.

Chordoid meningiomas present particular problems when they are situated near the midline at the base of the skull, although this is a rare occurrence because most present as large, obviously dura-based supratentorial masses. Nevertheless, neuroimaging and immunocytochemistry are helpful in distinguishing these lesions. Whereas chordomas infiltrate the bone and are strongly cytokeratin and S-100 positive, chordoid meningiomas involve the dura, often causing hyperostosis in the surrounding bones and are only inconsistently and focally immunoreactive for S-100 and cytokeratin. Clear cell meningiomas may superficially resemble metastatic renal cell carcinoma, although they have a relatively unique dense perivascular and intercellular collagen pattern.[212] Both entities may show PAS-positive diastase-digestible glycogen-rich cytoplasm, although this is not true of microcystic meningioma, which may also enter the differential. Renal cell carcinomas are more likely to be PR negative and immunoreactive for cytokeratin, CD10, RCC and PAX8 than clear cell meningiomas.[40,148,212]

Papillary meningiomas should be distinguished from other papillary neoplasms, including ependymomas, choroid plexus tumours, astroblastomas, adenocarcinomas, melanocytomas and melanomas. Strong GFAP positivity should aid in establishing a diagnosis of ependymoma or astroblastoma. Melanocytomas and melanomas are vimentin and S-100 positive, but immunonegative for EMA and additionally stain with more specific melanocytic markers, such as HMB-45 and Melan-A. Haemangiopericytomas and solitary fibrous tumours are mostly EMA negative, strongly express BCL2 and CD99, and display nuclear rather than cytoplasmic STAT6 expression.[150,169] Haemangioblastomas are also EMA negative, with stromal cells typically expressing alpha inhibin, podoplanin (D2-40) and brachyury.[22,156] Rhabdoid meningiomas may look similar to other rhabdoid neoplasms; however, atypical teratoid/rhabdoid tumours are mostly tumours of infancy, whereas rhabdoid meningiomas afflict adult patients. The latter also do not inactivate the *INI1/hSNF5* (*SMARCB1*) gene and therefore, the protein product is readily identified by immunohistochemistry.[133]

REFERENCES

1. Aavikko M, Li SP, Saarinen S, Alhopuro P, Kaasinen E, Morgunova E, *et al.* Loss of SUFU function in familial multiple meningioma. *Am J Hum Genet* 2012;**91**:520–6.
2. Adeberg S, Hartmann C, Welzel T, Rieken S, Habermehl D, von Deimling A, *et al.* Long-term outcome after radiotherapy in patients with atypical and malignant meningiomas—clinical results in 85 patients treated in a single institution leading to optimized guidelines for early radiation therapy. *Int J Radiat Oncol Biol Phys* 2012;**83**:859–64.
3. Adlakha A, Rao K, Adlakha H, Perry A, Crotty TB, Scheithauer BW, *et al.* Meningioma metastatic to the lung. *Mayo Clin Proc* 1999;**74**:1129–33.
4. Aghi MK, Carter BS, Cosgrove GR, Ojemann RG, Amin-Hanjani S, Martuza RL, *et al.* Long-term recurrence rates of atypical meningiomas after gross total resection with or without postoperative adjuvant radiation. *Neurosurgery* 2009;**64**:56–60.
5. Aghi M, Kiehl TR, Brisman JL. Breast adenocarcinoma metastatic to epidural cervical spine meningioma: case report and review of the literature. *J Neurooncol* 2005;**75**:149–55.
6. Akat K, Mennel HD, Kremer P, Gassler N, Bleck CK, Kartenbeck J. Molecular characterization of desmosomes in meningiomas and arachnoidal tissue. *Acta Neuropathol* 2003;**106**:337–47.
7. Alcolado JC, Moore IE, Weller RO. Calcification in the human choroid plexus, meningiomas and pineal gland. *Neuropathol Appl Neurobiol* 1986;**12**:235–50.
8. Al-Habib A, Lach B, Al Khani A. Intracerebral rhabdoid and papillary meningioma with leptomeningeal spread and rapid clinical progression. *Clin Neuropathol* 2005;**24**:1–7.
9. Al-Mefty O, Kadri PA, Pravdenkova S, Sawyer JR, Stangeby C, Husain M. Malignant progression in meningioma: documentation of a series and analysis of cytogenetic findings. *J Neurosurg* 2004;**101**:210–8.
10. Al-Sarraj S, King A, Martin AJ, Jarosz J, Lantos PL. Ultrastructural examination is essential for diagnosis of papillary meningioma. *Histopathology* 2001;**38**:318–24.
11. Amatya VJ, Takeshima Y, Inai K. Methylation of p14(ARF) gene in meningiomas and its correlation to the p53 expression and mutation. *Mod Pathol* 2004;**17**:705–10.
12. Ammerlaan AC, Houben MP, Tijssen CC, Wesseling P, Hulsebos TJ. Secondary meningioma in a long-term survivor of atypical teratoid/rhabdoid tumour with a germline INI1 mutation. *Childs Nerv Syst* 2008;**24**:855–7.
13. Arena S, Barbieri F, Thellung S, Pirani P, Corsaro A, Villa V, *et al.* Expression of somatostatin receptor mRNA in human meningiomas and their implication in in vitro antiproliferative activity. *J Neurooncol* 2004;**66**:155–66.
14. Ayerbe J, Lobato RD, de la Cruz J, Alday R, Rivas JJ, Gomez PA, *et al.* Risk factors predicting recurrence in patients operated on for intracranial meningioma. A multivariate analysis. *Acta Neurochir (Wien)* 1999;**141**:921–32.
15. Bacchi CE, Kandalaft PL, Hwang HC, Goldstein LC, Lopes LL, Bacchi LM, *et al.* Somatostatin receptor 2A: A novel immunohistochemical marker of meningioma (abstract 1725). *Mod Pathol* 2013;**26**:414A.
16. Bacci C, Sestini R, Provenzano A, Paganini I, Mancini I, Porfirio B, *et al.* Schwannomatosis associated with multiple meningiomas due to a familial SMARCB1 mutation. *Neurogenetics* 2010;**11**:73–80.
17. Backer-Grondahl T, Moen BH, Torp SH. The histopathological spectrum of human meningiomas. *Int J Clin Exp Pathol* 2012;**5**:231–42.
18. Baia GS, Caballero OL, Orr BA, Lal A, Ho JS, Cowdrey C, *et al.* Yes-Associated Protein 1 is activated and functions as an oncogene in meningiomas. *Mol Cancer Res* 2012;**10**:904–13 .
19. Balik V, Srovnal J, Sulla I, Kalita O, Foltanova T, Vaverka M, *et al.* MEG3: a novel long noncoding potentially tumour-suppressing RNA in meningiomas. *J Neurooncol* 2013;**112**:1–8.

20. Barbera S, San Miguel T, Gil-Benso R, Munoz-Hidalgo L, Roldan P, Gonzalez-Darder J, et al. Genetic changes with prognostic value in histologically benign meningiomas. *Clin Neuropathol* 2013;32:311–7.

21. Barresi V, Caffo M, Ieni A, Alafaci C, Tuccari G. Osteoblastic meningiomas: clinico-pathological and immunohistochemical features of an uncommon variant. *J Neurooncol* 201;105:225–32.

22. Barresi V, Vitarelli E, Branca G, Antonelli M, Giangaspero F, Barresi G. Expression of brachyury in hemangioblastoma: potential use in differential diagnosis. *Am J Surg Pathol* 2012;36:1052–7.

23. Barresi V, Vitarelli E, Tuccari G, Barresi G. MMP-9 expression in meningiomas: a prognostic marker for recurrence risk? *J Neurooncol* 2011;102:189–96.

24. Baumgarten P, Brokinkel B, Zinke J, Zachskorn C, Ebel H, Albert FK, et al. Expression of vascular endothelial growth factor (VEGF) and its receptors VEGFR1 and VEGFR2 in primary and recurrent WHO grade III meningiomas. *Histol Histopathol* 2013;28:1157–66.

25. Beschet I, Brunon J, Scoazec JY, Mosnier JF. Expression of beta1 and beta4 integrins in normal arachnoid membrane and meningiomas. *Cancer* 1999;86:2649–58.

26. Bloch O, Kaur G, Jian BJ, Parsa AT, Barani IJ. Stereotactic radiosurgery for benign meningiomas. *J Neurooncol* 2012;107:13–20.

27. Borovich B, Doron Y. Recurrence of intracranial meningiomas: the role played by regional multicentricity. *J Neurosurg* 1986;64:58–63.

28. Bostrom J, Meyer-Puttlitz B, Wolter M, Blaschke B, Weber RG, Lichter P, et al. Alterations of the tumor suppressor genes CDKN2A (p16(INK4a)), p14(ARF), CDKN2B (p15(INK4b)), and CDKN2C (p18(INK4c)) in atypical and anaplastic meningiomas. *Am J Pathol* 2001;159:661–9.

29. Bozkurt SU, Ayan E, Bolukbasi F, Elmaci I, Pamir N, Sav A. Immunohistochemical expression of SPARC is correlated with recurrence, survival and malignant potential in meningiomas. *APMIS* 2009;117:651–9.

30. Brastianos PK, Horowitz PM, Santagata S, Jones RT, McKenna A, Getz G, et al. Genomic sequencing of meningiomas identifies oncogenic SMO and AKT1 mutations. *Nat Genet* 2013;45:285–9.

31. Brock JE, Perez-Atayde AR, Kozakewich HP, Richkind KE, Fletcher JA, Vargas SO. Cytogenetic aberrations in perineurioma: variation with subtype. *Am J Surg Pathol* 2005;29:1164–9.

32. Bruno MC, Ginguene C, Santangelo M, Panagiotopoulos K, Piscopo GA, Tortora F, et al. Lymphoplasmacyte rich meningioma. A case report and review of the literature. *J Neurosurg Sci* 2004;48:117–24.

33. Buschges R, Ichimura K, Weber RG, Reifenberger G, Collins VP. Allelic gain and amplification on the long arm of chromosome 17 in anaplastic meningiomas. *Brain Pathol* 2002;12:145–53.

34. Caffo M, Caruso G, Germano A, Galatioto S, Meli F, Tomasello F. CD68 and CR3/43 immunohistochemical expression in secretory meningiomas. *Neurosurgery* 2005;57:551–7.

35. Cai DX, Banerjee R, Scheithauer BW, Lohse CM, Kleinschmidt-DeMasters BK, Perry A. Chromosome 1p and 14q FISH analysis in clinicopathologic subsets of meningioma: diagnostic and prognostic implications. *J Neuropathol Exp Neurol* 2001;60:628–36.

36. Cai DX, James CD, Scheithauer BW, Couch FJ, Perry A. PS6K amplification characterizes a small subset of anaplastic meningiomas. *Am J Clin Pathol* 2001;115:213–8.

37. Caltabiano R, Barbagallo GM, Castaing M, Cassenti A, Senetta R, Cassoni P, et al. Prognostic value of EGFR expression in de novo and progressed atypical and anaplastic meningiomas: an immunohistochemical and fluorescence in situ hybridization pilot study. *J Neurosurg Sci* 2013;57:139–51.

38. Canales-Ibarra C, Magarinos G, Olsoff-Pagovich P, Ortiz-Hidalgo C. Cutaneous sclerosing perineurioma of the digits: an uncommon soft-tissue neoplasm. Report of two cases with immunohistochemical analysis. *J Cutan Pathol* 2003;30:577–81.

39. Carlson KM, Bruder C, Nordenskjold M, Dumanski JP. 1p and 3p deletions in meningiomas without detectable aberrations of chromosome 22 identified by comparative genomic hybridization. *Genes Chromosomes Cancer* 1997;20:419–24.

40. Carney EM, Banerjee P, Ellis CL, Albadine R, Sharma R, Chaux AM, et al. PAX2(-)/PAX8(-)/inhibin A(+) immunoprofile in hemangioblastoma: a helpful combination in the differential diagnosis with metastatic clear cell renal cell carcinoma to the central nervous system. *Am J Surg Pathol* 2011;35:262–7.

41. Carroll RS, Black PM, Zhang J, Kirsch M, Percec I, Lau N, et al. Expression and activation of epidermal growth factor receptors in meningiomas. *J Neurosurg* 1997;87:315–23.

42. Carroll RS, Schrell UM, Zhang J, Dashner K, Nomikos P, Fahlbusch R, et al. Dopamine D1, dopamine D2, and prolactin receptor messenger ribonucleic acid expression by the polymerase chain reaction in human meningiomas. *Neurosurgery* 1996;38:367–75.

43. Chaparro MJ, Young RF, Smith M, Shen V, Choi BH. Multiple spinal meningiomas: a case of 47 distinct lesions in the absence of neurofibromatosis or identified chromosomal abnormality. *Neurosurgery* 1993;32:298–301.

44. Christiaans I, Kenter SB, Brink HC, van Os TA, Baas F, van den Munckhof P, et al. Germline SMARCB1 mutation and somatic NF2 mutations in familial multiple meningiomas. *J Med Genet* 2011;48:93–7.

45. Christov C, Lechapt-Zalcman E, Adle-Biassette H, Nachev S, Gherardi RK. Vascular permeability factor/vascular endothelial growth factor (VPF/VEGF) and its receptor flt-1 in microcystic meningiomas. *Acta Neuropathol* 1999;98:414–20.

46. Ciccarelli E, Razzore P, Gaia D, Todaro C, Longo A, Forni M, et al. Hyperprolactinaemia and prolactine binding in benign intracranial tumours. *J Neurosurg Sci* 2001;45:70–4.

47. Clark VE, Erson-Omay EZ, Serin A, Yin J, Cotney J, Ozduman K, et al. Genomic analysis of non-NF2 meningiomas reveals mutations in TRAF7, KLF4, AKT1, and SMO. *Science* 2013;339:1077–80.

48. Claus EB, Calvocoressi L, Bondy ML, Wrensch M, Wiemels JL, Schildkraut JM. Exogenous hormone use, reproductive factors, and risk of intracranial meningioma in females. *J Neurosurg* 2013;118:649–56.

49. Cleland J. Description of two tumours adherent to the deep surface of the dura mater. *Glasgow Med J* 1864;11:148–59.

50. Colnat-Coulbois S, Kremer S, Weinbreck N, Pinelli C, Auque J. Lipomatous meningioma: report of 2 cases and review of the literature. *Surg Neurol* 2008;69:398–402.

51. Couce ME, Aker FV, Scheithauer BW. Chordoid meningioma: a clinicopathologic study of 42 cases. *Am J Surg Pathol* 2000;24:899–905.

52. Crawford TS, Kleinschmidt-DeMasters BK, Lillehei KO. Primary intraosseous meningioma. Case report. *J Neurosurg* 1995;83:912–5.

53. Cushing H, Eisenhardt L. *Meningiomas: their classification, regional behaviour, life history, and surgical end results.* Springfield, IL: CC Thomas; 1938.

54. Das A, Tan WL, Smith DR. Expression of extracellular matrix markers in benign meningiomas. *Neuropathology* 2003;23:275–81.

55. Dolecek TA, Propp JM, Stroup NE, Kruchko C. CBTRUS statistical report: primary brain and central nervous system tumors diagnosed in the United States in 2005–2009. *Neuro Oncol* 2012;14(Suppl 5):1–49.

56. Eddleman CS, Liu JK. Optic nerve sheath meningioma: current diagnosis and treatment. *Neurosurg Focus* 2007;23:E4.

57. Elbabaa SK, Gokden M, Crawford JR, Kesari S, Saad AG. Radiation-associated meningiomas in children: clinical, pathological, and cytogenetic characteristics with a critical review of the literature. *J Neurosurg Pediatr* 2012;10:281–90.

58. Ellison DW, Lunec J, Gallagher PJ, et al. Accumulation of wild-type p53 in meningiomas. *Neuropathol Appl Neurobiol* 1995;21:136–42.

59. Engelhard HH. Progress in the diagnosis and treatment of patients with meningiomas. Part I: diagnostic imaging, preoperative embolization. *Surg Neurol* 2001;55:89–101.

60. Evans DG, Watson C, King A, Wallace AJ, Baser ME. Multiple meningiomas: differential involvement of the NF2 gene in children and adults. *J Med Genet* 2005;42:45–8.

61. Foschini MP, D'Adda T, Bordi C, Eusebi V. Amyloid stroma in meningiomas. *Virchows Arch A Pathol Anat Histopathol* 1993;422:53–9.

62. Halper J, Jung C, Perry A, Suliman H, Hill MP, Scheithauer B. Expression of TGF-alpha in meningiomas. *J Neurooncol* 1999;45:127–34.

63. Hamilton BO, Sy JS, Megyesi JF, Ang LC. Her2neu amplification associates with co-deletion 1p/14q in recurrent meningiomas. *Can J Neurol Sci* 2013;40:361–5.

64. Hanft S, Canoll P, Bruce JN. A review of malignant meningiomas: diagnosis, characteristics, and treatment. *J Neurooncol* 2010;99:433–43.

65. Hasselblatt M, Nolte KW, Paulus W. Angiomatous meningioma: a

clinicopathologic study of 38 cases. *Am J Surg Pathol* 2004;**28**:390–3.

66. Hassounah M, Lach B, Allam A, Al-Khalaf H, Siddiqui Y, Pangue-Cruz N, et al. Benign tumors from the human nervous system express high levels of survivin and are resistant to spontaneous and radiation-induced apoptosis. *J Neurooncol* 2005;**72**:203–8.

67. Heinrich B, Hartmann C, Stemmer-Rachamimov AO, Louis DN, MacCollin M. Multiple meningiomas: investigating the molecular basis of sporadic and familial forms. *Int J Cancer* 2003;**103**:483–8.

68. Hirota S, Nakajima Y, Yoshimine T, Kohri K, Nomura S, Taneda M, et al. Expression of bone-related protein messenger RNA in human meningiomas: possible involvement of osteopontin in development of psammoma bodies. *J Neuropathol Exp Neurol* 1995;**54**:698–703.

69. Hori S, Hayashi N, Ishizawa S, Hayashi S, Sato H, Nagao S, et al. Clear cell meningioma with histologically aggressive appearance and clinically aggressive behavior: a case report. *Neuropathology* 2012;**32**:415–9.

70. INTERPHONE Study Group. Brain tumour risk in relation to mobile telephone use: results of the INTERPHONE international case-control study. *Int J Epidemiol* 2010;**39**:675–94.

71. Johnson DR, Kimmel DW, Burch PA, Cascino TL, Giannini C, Wu W, et al. Phase II study of subcutaneous octreotide in adults with recurrent or progressive meningioma and meningeal hemangiopericytoma. *Neuro Oncol* 2011;**13**:530–5.

72. Johnson MD, O'Connell M, Facik M, Maurer P, Jahromi B, Pilcher W. Cerebrospinal fluid stimulates leptomeningeal and meningioma cell proliferation and activation of STAT3. *J Neurooncol* 2012;**107**:121–31.

73. Johnson MD, O'Connell MJ, Pilcher W, Reeder JE. Fibroblast growth factor receptor-3 expression in meningiomas with stimulation of proliferation by the phosphoinositide 3 kinase-Akt pathway. *J Neurosurg* 2010;**112**:934–9.

74. Johnson MD, O'Connell MJ, Vito F, Pilcher W. Bone morphogenetic protein 4 and its receptors are expressed in the leptomeninges and meningiomas and signal via the Smad pathway. *J Neuropathol Exp Neurol* 2009;**68**:1177–83.

75. Johnson MD, Okedli E, Woodard A, Toms SA, Allen GS. Evidence for phosphatidylinositol 3-kinase-Akt-p7S6K pathway activation and transduction of mitogenic signals by platelet-derived growth factor in meningioma cells. *J Neurosurg* 2002;**97**:668–75.

76. Johnson MD, Sade B, Milano MT, Lee JH, Toms SA. New prospects for management and treatment of inoperable and recurrent skull base meningiomas. *J Neurooncol* 2008;**86**:109–22.

77. Kallio M, Sankila R, Hakulinen T, Jaaskelainen J. Factors affecting operative and excess long-term mortality in 935 patients with intracranial meningioma. *Neurosurgery* 1992;**31**:2–12.

78. Kanno H, Yamamoto I, Yoshida M, Kitamura H. Meningioma showing VHL gene inactivation in a patient with von Hippel-Lindau disease. *Neurology* 20038;**60**:1197–9.

79. Kawahara Y, Nakada M, Hayashi Y, Kai Y, Uchiyama N, Nakamura H, et al. Prediction of high-grade meningioma by preoperative MRI assessment. *J Neurooncol* 2012;**108**:147–52.

80. Kepes JJ. The fine structure of hyaline inclusions (pseudopsammoma bodies) in meningiomas. *J Neuropathol Exp Neurol* 1975;**34**:282–94.

81. Kepes J. *Meningiomas: biology, pathology, and differential diagnosis.* New York: Masson; 1982.

82. Kepes JJ, Chen WY, Connors MH, Vogel FS. "Chordoid" meningeal tumors in young individuals with peritumoral lymphoplasmacellular infiltrates causing systemic manifestations of the Castleman syndrome. A report of seven cases. *Cancer* 1988;**62**:391–406.

83. Kepes JJ, Moral LA, Wilkinson SB, Abdullah A, Llena JF. Rhabdoid transformation of tumor cells in meningiomas: a histologic indication of increased proliferative activity: report of four cases. *Am J Surg Pathol* 1998;**22**:231–8.

84. Ketter R, Henn W, Niedermayer I, Steilen-Gimbel H, Konig J, Zang KD, et al. Predictive value of progression-associated chromosomal aberrations for the prognosis of meningiomas: a retrospective study of 198 cases. *J Neurosurg* 2001;**95**:601–7.

85. Kilic T, Bayri Y, Ozduman K, Acar M, Diren S, Kurtkaya O, et al. Tenascin in meningioma: expression is correlated with anaplasia, vascular endothelial growth factor expression, and peritumoral edema but not with tumor border shape. *Neurosurgery* 2002;**51**:183–92.

86. Kitange G, Tsunoda K, Anda T, Nakamura S, Yasunaga A, Naito S, et al. Immunohistochemical expression of Ets-1 transcription factor and the urokinase-type plasminogen activator is correlated with the malignant and invasive potential in meningiomas. *Cancer* 2000;**89**:2292–300.

87. Konstantinidou AE, Korkolopoulou P, Mahera H, Kotsiakis X, Hranioti S, Eftychiadis C, et al. Hormone receptors in non-malignant meningiomas correlate with apoptosis, cell proliferation and recurrence-free survival. *Histopathology* 2003;**43**:280–90.

88. Korshunov A, Shishkina L, Golanov A. DNA topoisomerase II-alpha and cyclin A immunoexpression in meningiomas and its prognostic significance: an analysis of 263 cases. *Arch Pathol Lab Med* 2002;**126**:1079–86.

89. Krayenbuhl N, Pravdenkova S, Al-Mefty O. De novo versus transformed atypical and anaplastic meningiomas: comparisons of clinical course, cytogenetics, cytokinetics, and outcome. *Neurosurgery* 2007;**61**:495–503.

90. Krisht KM, Altay T, Couldwell WT. Myxoid meningioma: a rare metaplastic meningioma variant in a patient presenting with intratumoral hemorrhage. *J Neurosurg* 2012;**116**:861–5.

91. Kros J, de Greve K, van Tilborg A, Hop W, Pieterman H, Avezaat C, et al. NF2 status of meningiomas is associated with tumour localization and histology. *J Pathol* 2001;**194**:367–72.

92. Kuster O, Simon P, Mittelbronn M, Tabatabai G, Hermann C, Strik H, et al. Erythropoietin receptor is expressed in meningiomas and lower levels are associated with tumour recurrence. *Neuropathol Appl Neurobiol* 2009;**35**:555–65.

93. Kwon MJ, Sung CO, Kang SY, Do IG, Suh YL. Differential expression of extracellular matrix-related genes in rare variants of meningioma. *Hum Pathol* 2013;**44**:260–8.

94. Lampl Y, Barak Y, Achiron A, Sarova-Pinchas I. Intracranial meningiomas: correlation of peritumoral edema and psychiatric disturbances. *Psychiatry Res* 1995;**58**:177–80.

95. Lamszus K. Meningioma pathology, genetics, and biology. *J Neuropathol Exp Neurol* 2004;**63**:275–86.

96. Lamszus K, Lengler U, Schmidt NO, Stavrou D, Ergun S, Westphal M. Vascular endothelial growth factor, hepatocyte growth factor/scatter factor, basic fibroblast growth factor, and placenta growth factor in human meningiomas and their relation to angiogenesis and malignancy. *Neurosurgery* 2000;**46**:938–47.

97. Lang FF, Macdonald OK, Fuller GN, DeMonte F. Primary extradural meningiomas: a report on nine cases and review of the literature from the era of computerized tomography scanning. *J Neurosurg* 2000;**93**:940–50.

98. Laurendeau I, Ferrer M, Garrido D, D'Haene N, Ciavarelli P, Basso A, et al. Gene expression profiling of ErbB receptors and ligands in human meningiomas. *Cancer Invest* 2009;**27**:691–8.

99. Laurendeau I, Ferrer M, Garrido D, D'Haene N, Ciavarelli P, Basso A, et al. Gene expression profiling of the Hedgehog signaling pathway in human meningiomas. *Mol Med* 2010;**16**:262–70.

100. Lindstrom KM, Cousar JB, Lopes MB. IgG4-related meningeal disease: clinicopathological features and proposal for diagnostic criteria. *Acta Neuropathol* 2010;**120**:765–76.

101. Liu JL, Zhou JL, Ma YH, Dong C. An analysis of the magnetic resonance imaging and pathology of intracal lymphoplasmacyte-rich meningioma. *Eur J Radiol* 2012;**81**:968–73.

102. Liu M, Wei Y, Liu Y, Zhu S, Li X. Intraventricular meninigiomas: a report of 25 cases. *Neurosurg Rev* 2006;**29**:36–40.

103. Louis DN, Ohgaki H, Wiestler OD, Cavenee WK. *WHO classification of tumours of the central nervous system* 4th edn. Lyon: IARC; 2007.

104. Louis DN, Ramesh V, Gusella JF. Neuropathology and molecular genetics of neurofibromatosis 2 and related tumors. *Brain Pathol* 1995;**5**:163–72.

105. Ludwin SK, Rubinstein LJ, Russell DS. Papillary meningioma: a malignant variant of meningioma. *Cancer* 1975;**36**:1363–73.

106. Lusis EA, Chicoine MR, Perry A. High throughput screening of meningioma biomarkers using a tissue microarray. *J Neurooncol* 2005;**73**:219–23.

107. Lusis EA, Scheithauer BW, Yachnis AT, Fischer BR, Chicoine MR, Paulus W, et al. Meningiomas in pregnancy: a clinicopathologic study of 17 cases. *Neurosurgery* 2012;**71**:951–61.

108. Lusis EA, Watson MA, Chicoine MR, Lyman M, Roerig P, Reifenberger G, et al. Integrative genomic analysis identifies NDRG2 as a candidate tumor suppressor gene frequently inactivated in clinically aggressive meningioma. *Cancer Res* 2005;**65**:7121–6.

109. Mawrin C, Perry A. Pathological classification and molecular genetics of meningiomas. *J Neurooncol* 2010;99:379–91.

110. Mawrin C, Sasse T, Kirches E, Kropf S, Schneider T, Grimm C, et al. Different activation of mitogen-activated protein kinase and Akt signaling is associated with aggressive phenotype of human meningiomas. *Clin Cancer Res* 2005;11:4074–82.

111. Mawrin C, Wolke C, Haase D, Kruger S, Firsching R, Keilhoff G, et al. Reduced activity of CD13/aminopeptidase N (APN) in aggressive meningiomas is associated with increased levels of SPARC. *Brain Pathol* 2010;20:200–10.

112. McCutcheon IE, Flyvbjerg A, Hill H, Li J, Bennett WF, Scarlett JA, et al. Antitumor activity of the growth hormone receptor antagonist pegvisomant against human meningiomas in nude mice. *J Neurosurg* 2001;94:487–92.

113. Morrow KA, Shevde LA. Merlin: the wizard requires protein stability to function as a tumor suppressor. *Biochim Biophys Acta* 2012;1826:400–6.

114. Muccioli G, Ghe C, Faccani G, Lanotte M, Forni M, Ciccarelli E. Prolactin receptors in human meningiomas: characterization and biological role. *J Endocrinol* 1997;153:365–71.

115. Nagashima G, Aoyagi M, Yamamoto S, Wakimoto H, Tamaki M, Yamamoto K, et al. Involvement of disregulated c-myc but not c-sis/PDGF in atypical and anaplastic meningiomas. *Clin Neurol Neurosurg* 2001;103:13–8.

116. Nakasu S, Hirano A, Shimura T, Llena JF. Incidental meningiomas in autopsy study. *Surg Neurol* 1987;27:319–22.

117. Nakasu S, Li DH, Okabe H, Nakajima M, Matsuda M. Significance of MIB-1 staining indices in meningiomas: comparison of two counting methods. *Am J Surg Pathol* 2001;25:472–8.

118. Nakayama Y, Horio H, Horiguchi S, Hato T. Pulmonary and pleural metastases from benign meningeal meningioma: a case report. *Ann Thorac Cardiovasc Surg* 2013 Jan 31 [Epub ahead of print].

119. Nayak L, Iwamoto FM, Rudnick JD, Norden AD, Lee EQ, Drappatz J, et al. Atypical and anaplastic meningiomas treated with bevacizumab. *J Neurooncol* 2012;109:187–93.

120. Nishio S, Morioka T, Suzuki S, Hirano K, Fukui M. Secretory meningioma: clinicopathologic features of eight cases. *J Clin Neurosci* 2001;8:335–9.

121. Nishio S, Takeshita I, Fukui M. Microcystic meningioma: tumors of arachnoid cap vs trabecular cells. *Clin Neuropathol* 1994;13:197–203.

122. Norden AD, Raizer JJ, Abrey LE, Lamborn KR, Lassman AB, Chang SM, et al. Phase II trials of erlotinib or gefitinib in patients with recurrent meningioma. *J Neurooncol* 2010;96:211–7.

123. Nunes FP, Merker VL, Jennings D, Caruso PA, di Tomaso E, Muzikansky A, et al. Bevacizumab Treatment for Meningiomas in NF2: A Retrospective Analysis of 15 Patients. *PLoS One* 2013;8:e59941.

124. Oikonomou E, Machado AL, Buchfelder M, Adams EF. Meningiomas expressing and responding to cholecystokinin (CCK). *J Neurooncol* 2005;73:199–204.

125. Osawa T, Tosaka M, Nagaishi M, Yoshimoto Y. Factors affecting peritumoral brain edema in meningioma: special histological subtypes with prominently extensive edema. J Neurooncol 2013;111:49–57.

126. Pachow D, Andrae N, Kliese N, Angenstein F, Stork O, Wilisch-Neumann A, et al. mTORC1 inhibitors suppress meningioma growth in mouse models. *Clin Cancer Res* 2013;19:1180–9.

127. Paek SH, Kim DG, Park CK, Phi JH, Kim YY, Im SY, et al. The role of matrix metalloproteinases and tissue inhibitors of matrix metalloproteinase in microcystic meningiomas. *Oncol Rep* 2006;16:49–56.

128. Parent A. Multiple meningiomas. In: Al Mefty O ed. *Meningiomas*. New York: Raven Press; 1991:75–85.

129. Pasquier B, Gasnier F, Pasquier D, Keddari E, Morens A, Couderc P. Papillary meningioma. Clinicopathologic study of seven cases and review of the literature. *Cancer* 1986;58:299–305.

130. Pearson BE, Markert JM, Fisher WS, Guthrie BL, Fiveash JB, Palmer CA, et al. Hitting a moving target: evolution of a treatment paradigm for atypical meningiomas amid changing diagnostic criteria. *Neurosurg Focus* 2008;24:E3.

131. Perret AG, Duthel R, Fotso MJ, Brunon J, Mosnier JF. Stromelysin-3 is expressed by aggressive meningiomas. *Cancer* 2002;94:765–72.

132. Perry A, Banerjee R, Lohse CM, Kleinschmidt-DeMasters BK, Scheithauer BW. A role for chromosome 9p21 deletions in the malignant progression of meningiomas and the prognosis of anaplastic meningiomas. *Brain Pathol* 2002;12:183–90.

133. Perry A, Fuller CE, Judkins AR, Dehner LP, Biegel JA. INI1 expression is retained in composite rhabdoid tumors, including rhabdoid meningiomas. *Mod Pathol* 2005;18:951–8.

134. Perry A, Giannini C, Raghavan R, Scheithauer BW, Banerjee R, Margraf L, et al. Aggressive phenotypic and genotypic features in pediatric and NF2-associated meningiomas: a clinicopathologic study of 53 cases. *J Neuropathol Exp Neurol* 2001;60:994–1003.

135. Perry A, Jenkins RB, Dahl RJ, Moertel CA, Scheithauer BW. Cytogenetic analysis of aggressive meningiomas: possible diagnostic and prognostic implications. *Cancer* 1996;77:2567–73.

136. Perry A, Louis DN, Scheithauer BW, Budka H, Von Deimling A. Meningiomas. In: Louis DN, Ohgaki H, Wiestler OD, Cavenee WK eds. *WHO classification of tumours of the central nervous system* 4th edn. Lyon: IARC; 2007:164–72.

137. Perry A, Lusis EA, Gutmann DH. Meningothelial hyperplasia: a detailed clinicopathologic, immunohistochemical and genetic study of 11 cases. *Brain Pathol* 2005;15:109–15.

138. Perry A, Scheithauer BW, Stafford SL, Abell-Aleff PC, Meyer FB. "Rhabdoid" meningioma: an aggressive variant. *Am J Surg Pathol* 1998;22:1482–90.

139. Perry A, Scheithauer BW, Stafford SL, Lohse CM, Wollan PC. "Malignancy" in meningiomas: a clinicopathologic study of 116 patients, with grading implications. *Cancer* 1999;85:2046–56.

140. Perry A, Stafford SL, Scheithauer BW, Suman VJ, Lohse CM. Meningioma grading: an analysis of histologic parameters. *Am J Surg Pathol* 1997;21:1455–65.

141. Perry A, Stafford SL, Scheithauer BW, Suman VJ, Lohse CM. The prognostic significance of MIB-1, p53, and DNA flow cytometry in completely resected primary meningiomas. *Cancer* 1998;82:2262–9.

142. Peyre M, Stemmer-Rachamimov A, Clermont-Taranchon E, Quentin S, El-Taraya N, Walczak C, et al. Meningioma progression in mice triggered by Nf2 and Cdkn2ab inactivation. *Oncogene* 2013;32:4264–72.

143. Pham MH, Zada G, Mosich GM, Chen TC, Giannotta SL, Wang K, et al. Molecular genetics of meningiomas: a systematic review of the current literature and potential basis for future treatment paradigms. *Neurosurg Focus* 2011;30:E7.

144. Phillips LE, Koepsell TD, van Belle G, Kukull WA, Gehrels JA, Longstreth WT, Jr. History of head trauma and risk of intracranial meningioma: population-based case-control study. *Neurology* 2002;58:1849–52.

145. Piaskowski S, Rieske P, Szybka M, Wozniak K, Bednarek A, Pluciennik E, et al. GADD45A and EPB41 as tumor suppressor genes in meningioma pathogenesis. *Cancer Genet Cytogenet* 2005;162:63–7.

146. Pieper DR, Al-Mefty O, Hanada Y, Buechner D. Hyperostosis associated with meningioma of the cranial base: secondary changes or tumor invasion. *Neurosurgery* 1999;44:742–6.

147. Pimentel J, Fernandes A, Pinto AE, Fonseca I, Moura Nunes JF, Lobo Antunes J. Clear cell meningioma variant and clinical aggressiveness. *Clin Neuropathol* 1998;17:141–6.

148. Prayson RA, Chamberlain WA, Angelov L. Clear cell meningioma: a clinicopathologic study of 18 tumors and examination of the use of CD10, CA9, and RCC antibodies to distinguish between clear cell meningioma and metastatic clear cell renal cell carcinoma. *Appl Immunohistochem Mol Morphol* 2010;18:422–8.

149. Prayson RA, Chowdhary S, Woodhouse S, Hanson M, Nair S. Collision of a syncytial meningioma and malignant astrocytoma. *Ann Diagn Pathol* 2002;6:44–8.

150. Rajaram V, Brat DJ, Perry A. Anaplastic meningioma versus meningeal hemangiopericytoma: immunohistochemical and genetic markers. *Hum Pathol* 2004;35:1413–8.

151. Rajcan-Separovic E, Maguire J, Loukianova T, Nisha M, Kalousek D. Loss of 1p and 7p in radiation-induced meningiomas identified by comparative genomic hybridization. *Cancer Genet Cytogenet* 2003;144:6–11.

152. Rao G, Giordano SH, Liu J, McCutcheon IE. The association of breast cancer and meningioma in men and women. *Neurosurgery* 2009;65:483–9.

153. Regelsberger J, Hagel C, Emami P, Ries T, Heese O, Westphal M. Secretory meningiomas: a benign subgroup causing life-threatening complications. *Neuro Oncol* 2009;11:819–24.

154. Rempel SA, Ge S, Gutierrez JA. SPARC: a potential diagnostic marker of invasive meningiomas. *Clin Cancer Res* 1999;5:237–41.

155. Reuss DE, Piro RM, Jones DT, Simon M, Ketter R, Kool M, et al. Secretory meningiomas are defined by combined KLF4 K409Q and TRAF7 mutations. *Acta Neuropathol* 2013;**125**:351–8.

156. Rivera AL, Takei H, Zhai J, Shen SS, Ro JY, Powell SZ. Useful immunohistochemical markers in differentiating hemangioblastoma versus metastatic renal cell carcinoma. *Neuropathology* 2010;**30**:580–5.

157. Robb VA, Li W, Gascard P, Perry A, Mohandas N, Gutmann DH. Identification of a third Protein 4.1 tumor suppressor, Protein 4.1R, in meningioma pathogenesis. *Neurobiol Dis* 2003;**13**:191–202.

158. Rogers L, Gilbert M, Vogelbaum MA. Intracranial meningiomas of atypical (WHO grade II) histology. *J Neurooncol* 2010;**99**:393–405.

159. Roncaroli F, Riccioni L, Cerati M, Capella C, Calbucci F, Trevisan C, et al. Oncocytic meningioma. *Am J Surg Pathol* 1997;**21**:375–82.

160. Roncaroli F, Scheithauer BW, Laeng RH, Cenacchi G, Abell-Aleff P, Moschopulos M. Lipomatous meningioma: a clinicopathologic study of 18 cases with special reference to the issue of metaplasia. *Am J Surg Pathol* 2001;**25**:769–75.

161. Roser F, Nakamura M, Bellinzona M, Rosahl SK, Ostertag H, Samii M. The prognostic value of progesterone receptor status in meningiomas. *J Clin Pathol* 2004;**57**:1033–7.

162. Roser F, Samii M, Ostertag H, Bellinzona M. The Ki-67 proliferation antigen in meningiomas. Experience in 600 cases. *Acta Neurochir (Wien)* 2004;**146**:37–44.

163. Sandalcioglu IE, Hunold A, Muller O, Bassiouni H, Stolke D, Asgari S. Spinal meningiomas: critical review of 131 surgically treated patients. *Eur Spine J* 2008;**17**:1035–41.

164. Sanson M, Cornu P. Biology of meningiomas. *Acta Neurochir (Wien)* 2000;**142**:493–505.

165. Saydam O, Shen Y, Wurdinger T, Senol O, Boke E, James MF, et al. Downregulated microRNA-200a in meningiomas promotes tumor growth by reducing E-cadherin and activating the Wntβ catenin signaling pathway. *Mol Cell Biol* 2009;**29**:593–23–40.

166. Schmidt MB. Ueber die Pacchioni'schen Granulationen und ihr Verhältniss zu den Sarcomen und Psammomen der Dura mater. *Virchows Arch Pathol Anat Physiol Klin Med* 1902;**170**:429–64.

167. Schulz C, Mathieu R, Kunz U, Mauer UM. Treatment of unresectable skull base meningiomas with somatostatin analogs. *Neurosurg Focus* 2011;**30**:E11.

168. Schulz S, Pauli SU, Schulz S, Handel M, Dietzmann K, Firsching R, et al. Immunohistochemical determination of five somatostatin receptors in meningioma reveals frequent overexpression of somatostatin receptor subtype sst2A. *Clin Cancer Res* 2000;**6**:1865–74.

169. Schweizer L, Koelsche C, Sahm F, Piro RM, Capper D, Reuss DE, et al. Meningeal hemangiopericytoma and solitary fibrous tumors carry the NAB2-STAT6 fusion and can be diagnosed by nuclear expression of STAT6 protein. *Acta Neuropathol* 2013;**125**:651–8.

170. Sheehy JP, Crockard HA. Multiple meningiomas: a long-term review. *J Neurosurg* 1983;**59**:1–5.

171. Shoshan Y, Chernova O, Juen SS, Somerville RP, Israel Z, Barnett GH, et al. Radiation-induced meningioma: a distinct molecular genetic pattern? *J Neuropathol Exp Neurol* 2000;**59**:614–20.

172. Shuangshoti S. Primary meningiomas outside the central nervous system. In: Al Mefty O, ed. *Meningiomas*. New York: Raven; 1991:107–28.

173. Siddique K, Yanamandra N, Gujrati M, Dinh D, Rao JS, Olivero W. Expression of matrix metalloproteinases, their inhibitors, and urokinase plasminogen activator in human meningiomas. *Int J Oncol* 2003;**22**:289–94.

174. Smith JS, Quinones-Hinojosa A, Harmon-Smith M, Bollen AW, McDermott MW. Sex steroid and growth factor profile of a meningioma associated with pregnancy. *Can J Neurol Sci* 2005;**32**:122–7.

175. Smith MJ, O'Sullivan J, Bhaskar SS, Hadfield KD, Poke G, Caird J, et al. Loss-of-function mutations in SMARCE1 cause an inherited disorder of multiple spinal meningiomas. *Nat Genet* 2013;**45**:295–8.

176. Stafford SL, Perry A, Leavitt JA, Garrity JA, Suman VJ, Scheithauer BW, et al. Anterior visual pathway meningiomas primarily resected between 1978 and 1988: the Mayo Clinic Rochester experience. *J Neuroophthalmol* 1998;**18**:206–10.

177. Stafford SL, Perry A, Suman VJ, Meyer FB, Scheithauer BW, Lohse CM, et al. Primarily resected meningiomas: outcome and prognostic factors in 581 Mayo Clinic patients, 1978 through 1988. *Mayo Clin Proc* 1998;**73**:936–42.

178. Stangl AP, Wellenreuther R, Lenartz D, Kraus JA, Menon AG, Schramm J, et al. Clonality of multiple meningiomas. *J Neurosurg* 1997;**86**:853–8.

179. Steilen-Gimbel H, Niedermayer I, Feiden W, Freiler A, Steudel WI, Zang KD, et al. Unbalanced translocation t(1;3)(p12–13;q11) in meningiomas as the unique feature of chordoid differentiation. *Genes Chromosomes Cancer* 1999;**26**:270–2.

180. Sulman EP, White PS, Brodeur GM. Genomic annotation of the meningioma tumor suppressor locus on chromosome 1p34. *Oncogene* 2004;**23**:1014–20.

181. Surace EI, Lusis E, Haipek CA, Gutmann DH. Functional significance of S6K overexpression in meningioma progression. *Ann Neurol* 2004;**56**:295–8.

182. Takei H, Powell SZ. Tumor-to-tumor metastasis to the central nervous system. *Neuropathology* 2009;**29**:303–8.

183. Tao Y, Liang G, Li Z, Wang Y, Wu A, Wang H, et al. Clinical features and immunohistochemical expression levels of androgen, estrogen, progesterone and Ki-67 receptors in relationship with gross-total resected meningiomas relapse. *Br J Neurosurg* 2012;**26**:700–4.

184. Tena-Suck ML, Collado-Ortiz MA, Salinas-Lara C, Garcia-Lopez R, Gelista N, Rembao-Bojorquez D. Chordoid meningioma: a report of ten cases. *J Neurooncol* 2010;**99**:41–8.

185. Thuijs NB, Uitdehaag BM, Van Ouwerkerk WJ, van der Valk P, Vandertop WP, Peerdeman SM. Pediatric meningiomas in The Netherlands 1974–2010: a descriptive epidemiological case study. *Childs Nerv Syst* 2012;**28**:1009–15.

186. Umansky F, Shoshan Y, Rosenthal G, Fraifeld S, Spektor S. Radiation-induced meningioma. *Neurosurg Focus* 2008;**24**:E7.

187. van den Munckhof P, Christiaans I, Kenter SB, Baas F, Hulsebos TJ. Germline SMARCB1 mutation predisposes to multiple meningiomas and schwannomas with preferential location of cranial meningiomas at the falx cerebri. *Neurogenetics* 2012;**13**:1–7.

188. Vernooij MW, Ikram MA, Tanghe HL, Vincent AJ, Hofman A, Krestin GP, et al. Incidental findings on brain MRI in the general population. *N Engl J Med* 2007;**357**:1821–8.

189. Wang CJ, Lin PC, Howng SL. Expression of thyroid hormone receptors in intracranial meningiomas. *Kaohsiung J Med Sci* 2003;**19**:334–8.

190. Wang DJ, Zheng MZ, Gong Y, Xie Q, Wang Y, Cheng HX, et al. Papillary meningioma: clinical and histopathological observations. *Int J Clin Exp Pathol* 2013;**6**:878–88.

191. Wang X, Gong Y, Wang D, Xie Q, Zheng M, Zhou Y, et al. Analysis of gene expression profiling in meningioma: deregulated signaling pathways associated with meningioma and EGFL6 overexpression in benign meningioma tissue and serum. *PLoS One* 2012;**7**:e52707.

192. Watson MA, Gutmann DH, Peterson K, Chicoine MR, Kleinschmidt-DeMasters BK, Brown HG, et al. Molecular characterization of human meningiomas by gene expression profiling using high-density oligonucleotide microarrays. *Am J Pathol* 2002;**161**:665–72.

193. Weber J, Gassel AM, Hoch A, Kilisek L, Spring A. Intraoperative management of cystic meningiomas. *Neurosurg Rev* 2003;**26**:62–6.

194. Weber RG, Bostrom J, Wolter M, Baudis M, Collins VP, Reifenberger G, et al. Analysis of genomic alterations in benign, atypical, and anaplastic meningiomas: toward a genetic model of meningioma progression. *Proc Natl Acad Sci U S A* 1997;**94**:14719–24.

195. Wellenreuther R, Waha A, Vogel Y, Lenartz D, Schramm J, Wiestler OD, et al. Quantitative analysis of neurofibromatosis type 2 gene transcripts in meningiomas supports the concept of distinct molecular variants. *Lab Invest* 1997;**77**:601–6.

196. Wernicke AG, Dicker AP, Whiton M, Ivanidze J, Hyslop T, Hammond EH, et al. Assessment of epidermal growth factor receptor (EGFR) expression in human meningioma. *Radiat Oncol* 2010;**5**:46.

197. Wiemels J, Wrensch M, Claus EB. Epidemiology and etiology of meningioma. *J Neurooncol* 2010;**99**:307–14.

198. Willis J, Smith C, Ironside JW, Erridge S, Whittle IR, Everington D. The accuracy of meningioma grading: a 10-year retrospective audit. *Neuropathol Appl Neurobiol* 2005;**31**:141–9.

199. Wolfsberger S, Doostkam S, Boecher-Schwarz HG, Roessler K, van Trotsenburg M, Hainfellner JA, et al. Progesterone-receptor index in meningiomas: correlation with clinico-pathological parameters and review of the literature. *Neurosurg Rev* 2004;**27**:238–45.

200. Wrobel G, Roerig P, Kokocinski F, Neben K, Hahn M, Reifenberger G, et al. Microarray-based gene expression profiling of benign, atypical and anaplastic meningiomas identifies novel genes

References **1827**

36

associated with meningioma progression. *Int J Cancer* 2005;**114**:249–56.

201. Wu YT, Ho JT, Lin YJ, Lin JW. Rhabdoid papillary meningioma: A clinicopathologic case series study. *Neuropathology* 2011;**31**:599–605.

202. Yamashima T, Kida S, Kubota T, Yamamoto S. The origin of psammoma bodies in the human arachnoid villi. *Acta Neuropathol* 1986;**71**:19–25.

203. Yamashima T, Kida S, Yamamoto S. Ultrastructural comparison of arachnoid villi and meningiomas in man. *Mod Pathol* 1988;**1**:224–34.

204. Yang SY, Park CK, Park SH, Kim DG, Chung YS, Jung HW. Atypical and anaplastic meningiomas: prognostic implications of clinicopathological features. *J Neurol Neurosurg Psychiatry* 2008;**79**:574–80.

205. Yonehara S, Brenner AV, Kishikawa M, Inskip PD, Preston DL, Ron E, et al.
Clinical and epidemiologic characteristics of first primary tumors of the central nervous system and related organs among atomic bomb survivors in Hiroshima and Nagasaki, 1958–1995. *Cancer* 2004;**101**:1644–54.

206. Yoshida T, Hirato J, Sasaki A, Yokoo H, Nakazato Y, Kurachi H. Intranuclear inclusions of meningioma associated with abnormal cytoskeletal protein expression. *Brain Tumor Pathol* 1999;**16**:86–91.

207. Yoshioka H, Hama S, Taniguchi E, Sugiyama K, Arita K, Kurisu K. Peritumoral brain edema associated with meningioma: influence of vascular endothelial growth factor expression and vascular blood supply. *Cancer* 1999;**85**:936–44.

208. Zang KD. Meningioma: a cytogenetic model of a complex benign human tumor, including data on 394 karyotyped cases. *Cytogenet Cell Genet* 2001;**93**:207–20.

209. Zattara-Cannoni H, Roll P, Figarella-Branger D, Lena G, Dufour H, Grisoli F, et al. Cytogenetic study of six cases of radiation-induced meningiomas. *Cancer Genet Cytogenet* 2001;**126**:81–4.

210. Zhang X, Gejman R, Mahta A, Zhong Y, Rice KA, Zhou Y, et al. Maternally expressed gene 3, an imprinted noncoding RNA gene, is associated with meningioma pathogenesis and progression. *Cancer Res* 2010;**70**:2350–8.

211. Zhou Y, Xie Q, Gong Y, Mao Y, Zhong P, Che X, et al. Clinicopathological analysis of rhabdoid meningiomas: report of 12 cases and a systematic review of the literature. *World Neurosurg* 2013;**79**:724–32.

212. Zorludemir S, Scheithauer BW, Hirose T, Van Houten C, Miller G, Meyer FB. Clear cell meningioma. A clinicopathologic study of a potentially aggressive variant of meningioma. *Am J Surg Pathol* 1995;**19**:493–505.

Mesenchymal Non-meningothelial Tumours

Christine E Fuller and Knarik Arkun

A wide variety of benign and malignant mesenchymal non-meningothelial tumours are encountered within the central nervous system (CNS). As a general rule, they share histologic, immunohistochemical and molecular alterations with their soft tissue and bone counterparts. Haemangiopericytoma (HPC) and the histologically similar solitary fibrous tumour (SFT) are by far the most commonly encountered subtypes and generate the most diagnostic confusion with meningiomas. Because of this, HPC and SFT will be discussed first, with the remainder of less common, histologically distinct benign and malignant mesenchymal lesions to follow.

MENINGEAL HAEMANGIOPERICYTOMA AND SOLITARY FIBROUS TUMOURS

Haemangiopericytoma

Formerly regarded as an angioblastic variant of meningiomas, CNS haemangiopericytoma (HPC) is a relatively common meningeal tumour, felt by some to represent the most common primary CNS sarcoma. Showing neither true meningothelial nor pericytic differentiation, its histogenesis remains a mystery. Despite this, the 2007 World Health Organization (WHO) classification scheme considers HPC as a distinct biologically aggressive entity, correspondingly designated WHO grade II or III depending on criteria noted later.[39] It is, however, recognized that this tumour overlaps significantly with the extrapleural SFT and that the two entities may form part of a single spectrum,[8,18] although this view is not universally held.[59]

Meningeal haemangiopericytomas are tumours of young to middle-aged adults, peaking in the fourth decade and with a male predominance.[44] They typically arise as solitary dural masses, compressing or invading the underlying brain. Rare intraparenchymal, intraventricular and spinal cases have been reported.[17,44,47,52] On neuroimaging studies, HPCs are well demarcated, dural based and intensely contrast enhancing (Figure 37.1a) with surrounding oedema,

not unlike meningiomas. Unlike the latter, however, intratumoural calcifications are lacking and HPCs may erode adjacent bony structures rather than inducing hyperostosis as is typical of meningiomas.[56]

Haemangiopericytomas are cellular tumours composed of monotonous oval to spindle-shaped cells with inconspicuous borders, dense chromatin and no intranuclear pseudoinclusions (Figure 37.1b). The characteristic vascular pattern features numerous branched thin-walled blood vessels lined by a single layer of flat endothelium, likened to a deer antler or 'staghorn' appearance (Figure 37.1c). A reticulin-rich network surrounding individual tumour cells is usually present, though with significant intertumoural and intratumoural variability.[44] Focal hyalinization and myxoid change may be present, but is more characteristic of SFT. Mitotic activity is variable. The diagnosis of anaplastic HPC (WHO grade III) requires a mitotic rate in excess of 5 per 10 high-power fields and/or necrosis plus at least two of the following: haemorrhage, at least moderate nuclear atypia, and hypercellularity (Figure 37.1d).[39]

The differentiation of haemangiopericytoma from meningioma and other entities is aided by immunocytochemistry and molecular pathology.[52] Haemangiopericytoma and SFT both show extensive vimentin, CD99 and BCL-2 expression whereas, occasionally, focal epithelial membrane antigen positivity causes confusion with meningioma. Claudin-1 appears to be a more specific, though not especially sensitive, marker for meningiomas.[24] In contrast to SFT where CD34 immunoreactivity is characteristically strong and diffuse, CD34 staining in haemangiopericytoma is patchy, weak or absent.[51] Individual cell positivity for factor XIIIa, CAM 5.2, cytokeratin and desmin may also be seen.[51,52] In one series, p53 immunoreactivity was demonstrated in over 50 per cent of HPCs, whereas it was infrequent in both SFTs and meningiomas.[51] From a molecular standpoint, meningeal haemangiopericytomas were recently found to harbour *NAB2-STAT6* fusions, a signature that they share with both meningeal and peripheral SFTs. This fusion results in nuclear accumulation of STAT6 protein; immunohistochemical detection of nuclear STAT6 positivity is useful because it

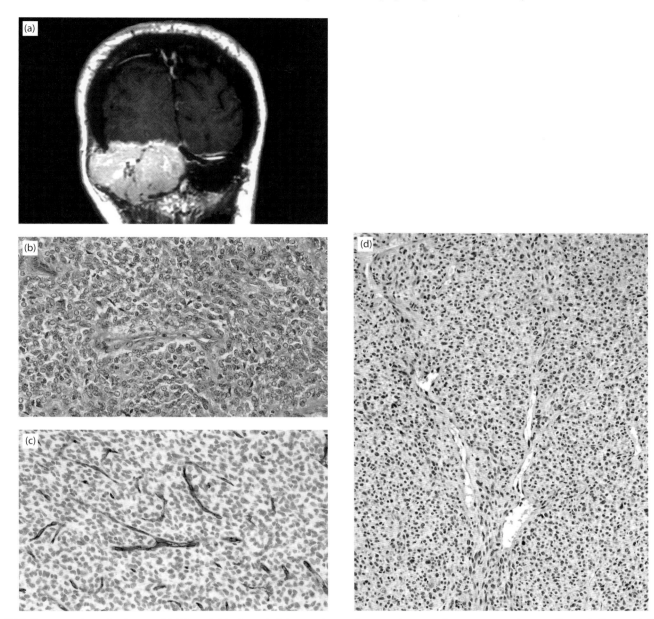

37.1 Haemangiopericytoma. (a) T1-weighted, gadolinium-enhanced coronal magnetic resonance image, through the occipital lobe, showing a large mass eroding the skull. The tumour contains multiple signal voids, indicating the highly vascular nature of the lesion. **(b)** Well-vascularized, cellular neoplasm composed of elongated and polygonal, tightly packed, mitotically active cells. **(c)** The neoplasm is endowed with slit-like, branching vascular channels. Immunohistochemistry for CD34. **(d)** Anaplastic haemangiopericytoma showing hypercellularity, nuclear atypia and numerous mitoses.

(a) Courtesy of Dr TCS Cox, formerly of the Bethlem and Maudsley NHS Trust, London, UK.

is a consistent finding in meningeal HPCs and SFTs, but not found in meningiomas.[55] Unlike meningiomas, HPCs also do not contain losses or mutations of the *NF2* gene.[31,52]

As a rule, HPC is more biologically aggressive then both meningioma and SFT. The vast majority eventually recur despite complete excision and often metastasize within and to sites external to the CNS.[61] Time to recurrence ranges from 47 to 104 months in separate series.[23,34] Within the CNS, most recurrences occur at the primary site, although diffuse leptomeningeal seeding has been documented.[34] Common sites of extraneural metastasis include bone, liver, lung and the abdominal cavity.[23,34,44] Completeness

of surgical excision[23,34] and tumour grade[16,44] are both significantly associated with recurrence-free survival. One series cited 144 months overall survival time for grade II versus only 62 months for grade III HPCs.[44] Chemotherapy has thus far proven to be ineffective.[16]

Solitary Fibrous Tumour

Solitary fibrous tumour (SFT) of the CNS, as noted earlier, shares many histopathologic and immunohistochemical features with HPC, but exhibits a significantly more benign biologic behaviour. Most SFTs are dural based, more frequently supratentorial and display a female predominance.[10,59] Occasional examples arise in subpial, intraparenchymal, intraventricular or radicular sites,[5] with brain invasion being rarely encountered.[10,11] The majority present between the third and fifth decades, with rare paediatric case reports.[41] Although there is no single neuroradiologic finding to reliably differentiate SFT from meningioma and other dural lesions, a 'black-and-white mixed' pattern of signal intensity on T2-weighted images, heterogeneous enhancement and absence of dural tail are all features that may favour SFT.[62]

Solitary fibrous tumours are characteristically heterogeneous on microscopic examination with alternating hypocellular and hypercellular areas. The spindle cells are described as being arranged in a 'patternless pattern', with irregular fascicular arrangements interrupted by prominent bands of collagen (Figure 37.2a).[10,59] Foci of hyalinization are consistent, albeit varying markedly in extent from tumour to tumour; thick hyalinized vessels are also commonly seen. Whorls and storiform arrangements are rarely present.[10] Staghorn-like vasculature is present at least focally in most cases, and in hypercellular regions, raises the differential with HPC.[59] The individual tumour cells tend to be uniform with elongate profiles, indistinct cell boarders, bland oval nuclei and finely dispersed chromatin. Reticulin fibres may be detected, mostly surrounding groups of tumour cells.

Strong diffuse positivity for antibodies against CD34 (Figure 37.2b) is a consistent finding in SFT and is particularly helpful in differentiating this tumour from meningioma and HPC, both of which typically show patchy to no staining. Consistently strong staining is also seen for vimentin, CD99 and BCL2, whereas stains for S100 and epithelial membrane antigen are usually negative.[5] Approximately one half will show positivity for oestrogen receptor, whereas nearly all will be positive for progesterone receptor.[10] Focal factor XIIIa staining is common and may represent infiltrating dendritic cells, whereas CD31 is consistently negative in tumour cells (but highlights intratumoural vasculature).[59] As noted earlier, *NAB2-STAT6* fusion is a consistent feature of SFTs as well as HPCs; this shared genetic signature provides strong evidence in support of the concept that meningeal HPC and SFT represent variants of a single entity.[55] Gene expression profiling studies also indicate that SFTs, regardless of site, have distinct expression profiles from all other sarcomas, and that IGF2 is consistently overexpressed.[25]

The behaviour of meningeal SFT is generally indolent following gross total resection.[5,58] Recurrences are most frequently associated with incomplete resection or atypical histology, particularly elevated mitotic rate/Ki-67 proliferation index. Up to 10–15 per cent show malignant behaviour with local recurrence, cerebrospinal fluid dissemination or metastatic disease.[5] Brain invasion may also be an adverse prognostic factor.[11]

OTHER MENINGEAL MESENCHYMAL NEOPLASMS

In addition to HPC and SFT, a wide spectrum of mesenchymal neoplasms form primary tumours within the craniospinal vault, the majority involving the meninges. Although benign examples are known, the vast majority represent

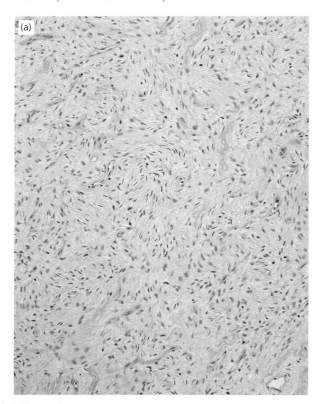
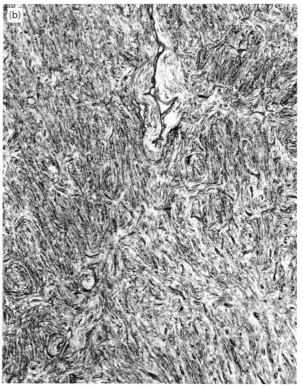

37.2 Solitary fibrous tumour. (a) Moderately cellular tumour composed of spindle cells embedded in abundant collagenous matrix. **(b)** Immunohistochemistry for CD34 is diffusely positive.

primary meningeal sarcomas. All are rare, constituting <1 per cent of intracranial tumours.[54] True primary meningeal sarcomas must be distinguished from both metastatic sarcomas and gliosarcomas. Cranial irradiation is a well-known risk factor for the development of meningeal sarcoma in general, and Epstein–Barr virus (EBV) has been implicated in smooth muscle tumours in immunocompromised patients (see later).

Meningeal sarcomas occur preferentially in younger patients, including children, and without obvious sex predilections. Most are clearly associated with the dura or leptomeninges, and the base of the skull is a common sight. Rarely, they may arise from the spinal meninges. Meningeal sarcomas are usually massive and, although they may appear well demarcated in places, they are not encapsulated and tend to invade the brain. In this context, they are often mistaken for meningiomas on radioimaging studies. Alternately, some do not form a definable mass, instead arising from and diffusely invading the meninges; this has been termed 'meningeal sarcomatosis', which not surprisingly could mimic a host of diffuse meningeal processes on imaging studies.

Historically, only a few variants of meningeal sarcoma were recognized, with the descriptive names of fibrosarcomas, spindle cell sarcomas and polymorphic cell sarcomas.[13] This descriptive terminology has been abandoned, and intracranial mesenchymal tumours are currently classified similar to soft tissue and bone tumours occurring elsewhere in the body, with corresponding histologic and immunohistochemical features.[50] The following is a brief survey of the types encountered in neuropathological practice.

Fibrosarcoma and Other Fibrohistiocytic/Myofibroblastic Lesions

Primary fibrosarcoma of the craniospinal vault, though rare, represents one of the more common subtypes. The majority arise in adults and are dural based, although occasional intraparenchymal examples have been encountered.[9,21,50] Most are high-grade lesions composed of generally uniform spindle cells arranged in bundles, often with a herringbone-like architecture. Occasional pleomorphic cells, including multinucleate forms, or focal necrosis are seen. The review by Gaspar and colleagues demonstrated the propensity of primary intracranial fibrosarcoma to show local and distant recurrence, meningeal seeding and systemic metastases. Intracerebral tumours tended towards shorter survival times.[21] Immunohistochemistry is more helpful in ruling out similar-appearing spindle cell lesions (e.g. meningioma, SFT, HPC) than in directly diagnosing fibrosarcoma, with vimentin being the only consistently positive stain in the latter.

Pleomorphic sarcomas, not otherwise specified, are identical to their counterparts in soft tissues, containing a storiform pattern of spindle-shaped cells interspersed with large pleomorphic, often lipidized cells. Mitoses are frequent and necrosis may be seen. Osteoclast-like giant cells may be prominent.[42] The immunohistochemical profile shows non-specific positivity with antibodies to α_1-antichymotrypsin, CD68 and vimentin, but lack of desmin and S-100 protein expression.[27] Benign fibrous histiocytoma may also arise in dura or brain parenchyma, containing a similar mix of spindle and pale/foamy cells arranged in a cartwheel architecture; these lesions lack obvious malignant features and have a correspondingly benign behaviour following excision.[46] Both pleomorphic sarcomas and benign fibrous histiocytomas are mainly tumours of adults, with only rare paediatric examples appearing as case reports.[14]

Inflammatory myofibroblastic tumours (IMT) may occur over a wide age range, with a tendency for male predominance.[30] They may present as either a localized dural-based mass or diffuse dural thickening. Extension into adjacent structures is not uncommon and may include leptomeningeal involvement, invasion of extradural structures or venous sinus thrombosis.[33] Neuroimaging studies show a dural-based lesion with diffuse contrast enhancement, mimicking meningioma.[33] Microscopically, IMT is composed of a mixture of myofibroblastic and chronic inflammatory cells, the former being immunopositive for smooth muscle actin.[30] Variable patterns resembling nodular fasciitis, fibromatosis or scar have been described.[18] Although anaplastic lymphoma kinase (ALK) protein overexpression is a common feature of peripheral IMTs, this is less common in the CNS.[30] Most IMTs have a favourable outcome following gross total excision, though some recurrences have been reported.[30]

Vascular Tumours

Though characteristically presenting as intraparenchymal/intra-axial lesions, some vascular neoplasms arise from the meninges. At the low grade end of the spectrum are cavernous haemangiomas, comprised of thin-walled gaping vascular channels lined by a single layer of bland endothelium. Most frequently presenting with seizures as a supratentorial intraparenchymal lesion with a surrounding rim of microhaemorrhage and hemosiderin deposition, cavernous haemangioma has on rare occasions been encountered arising from the dura at the floor of the middle cranial fossa.[36,53] Angiosarcoma and Kaposi's sarcoma represent malignant vascular tumours that on rare occasions involve the dura;[43,50] of interest, one AIDS patient with dural-based Kaposi's sarcoma came to clinical attention because of subdural hematoma.[2] Epithelioid haemangioendothelioma, with histologic and clinical features of a low-grade malignancy, may also present as a meningeal or parenchymal lesion; invasion into surrounding tissues, recurrence and metastasis may, however, be encountered in a subset of cases. Similar to its extracranial counterpart, complete resection affords a favourable outcome.[66]

Chondroid and Osteogenic Tumours

Intracranial chondrosarcomas mostly arise from the skull base or infrequently from cartilaginous rests in dura mater.[6,12,22,50] Rare intraparenchymal and spinal examples have also been encountered.[22,37] Intralesional calcifications are frequently present on neuroimaging studies.[12,22] Mesenchymal, myxoid and conventional subtypes have all been reported.[6,12,22,37] Likewise, the majority of intracranial chondromas involve the skull base, although cases arising from the falx/dura have also been described.[4,19] Dural-based and parenchymal osteosarcomas are exceedingly rare.[3] Surgical excision is the primary therapy for all of these lesions.

Ewing Sarcoma Family of Tumours (Ewing Sarcoma/Peripheral Primitive Neuroectodermal Tumour)

Representing the small round blue cell tumours, the Ewing sarcoma family of tumours arise either in bone (Ewing sarcoma) or in soft tissues (peripheral primitive neuroectodermal tumour [pPNET]). They share common expression of the MIC2 antigen (CD99), as well as translocations mostly involving the *EWS* gene on chromosome 22q12, with the t(11;22)(q24;q12) resulting in fusion of *EWS* and *FLI1* accounting for roughly 90% of cases. Though more frequently arising in the surrounding bony structures, cases inside the craniospinal vault have been encountered. Spinal examples are generally intradural and extramedullary, often arising in association with nerve roots,[26,45,60] whereas intracranial Ewing's sarcoma/pPNET is most often dural based, mimicking meningioma.[1,15,20,32,45,49,50] Ewing's sarcoma/pPNET must be distinguished from central embryonal neoplasms, particularly CNS PNET, medulloblastoma, and atypical teratoid/rhabdoid tumours, all of which lack EWS-related translocations typical of Ewing's sarcoma/pPNET.

Smooth Muscle Tumours

Leiomyosarcoma and its benign counterpart leiomyoma are rare intracranial lesions, and have been reported involving the dura/meninges, brain parenchyma and the ventricular system.[29,35,40,57,64] Similar to corresponding smooth muscle tumours from elsewhere in the body, these intracranial lesions feature fascicles of spindled cells with 'cigar-shaped' nuclei. In addition, leiomyosarcomas are more cellular with architectural disarray, brisk mitotic activity and necrosis. Correct diagnosis rests on an appropriate immunoprofile, such as smooth muscle actin expression or filaments with dense bodies on electron microscopy. A significant portion of intracranial leiomyosarcomas may be radiation induced, although even more frequently, smooth muscle tumours arise in the context of an immunocompromised status (often those patients infected with human immunodeficiency virus).[65] It is in this latter group where intratumoural EBV has been demonstrated.[35,57,64]

Rhabdomyosarcoma

Circumscribed dural-based lesions and rhabdomyosarcomas with more widespread leptomeningeal involvement have been described, although secondary meningeal involvement is far more common than primary disease. The variant most commonly encountered in the CNS is the embryonal type.[38,50,63] These tumours are composed of small cells with variable amounts of eosinophilic, fibril-rich cytoplasm. Cross-striations may be difficult to demonstrate. Verification of skeletal muscle differentiation is made by demonstration of desmin, myoglobin, MYOD1 or myogenenin by immunohistochemistry. Once skeletal muscle differentiation is documented, a primitive neuroectodermal tumour showing focal rhabdomyoblastic differentiation (e.g. medullomyoblastoma) should be excluded.

Miscellaneous Mesenchymal Neoplasms

Alveolar soft part sarcoma not infrequently metastasizes to the CNS, including the dura; however, primary intracranial examples are rare. Bodi and colleagues described such a lesion mimicking a meningioma in a young adult; definitive diagnosis included demonstration of the typical period acid–Schiff-positive, diastase resistant rod-like cytoplasmic inclusions and molecular confirmation of ASPCR1-TFE3 fusion.[7] Occasional cases of dural-based liposarcoma and synovial sarcoma have also been described, showing histomorphologic and immunohistochemical signatures identical to their soft tissue counterparts.[28,14,35,48] Demonstration of the t(X;18) translocation is helpful in differentiating synovial sarcoma from other morphologically similar spindle cells lesions.[28]

REFERENCES

1. Antunes NL, Lellouch-Tubiana A, Kalifa C, *et al.* Intracranial Ewing sarcoma/"peripheral" primitive neuroectodermal tumor of dural origin with molecular genetic confirmation. *J Neurooncol* 2001;**51**:51–6.
2. Ariza A, Kim JH. Kaposi's sarcoma of the dura mater. *Hum Pathol* 1988;**19**:1461–3.
3. Bar-Sela G, Tzuk-Shina T, Zaaroor M, *et al.* Primary osteogenic sarcoma arising from the dura mater: case report. *Am J Clin Oncol* 2001;**24**:418–20.
4. Bergmann M, Pinz W, Blasius S, *et al.* Chondroid tumors arising from the meninges. report of 2 cases and review of the literature. *Clin Neuropathol* 2004;**23**:149–53.
5. Bisceglia M, Galliani C, Giannatempo G, *et al.* Solitary fibrous tumor of the central nervous system: A 15-year literature survey of 220 cases (August 1996-July 2011). *Adv Anat Pathol* 2011;**18**:356–92.
6. Boccardo M, Bavaresco E, Sola S, Vitali A. Parafalcine chondrosarcoma: report of a case and review of the literature. *J Neurosurg Sci* 2009;**53**:137–40.
7. Bodi I, Gonzalez D, Epaliyange P, *et al.* Meningeal alveolar soft part sarcoma confirmed by characteristic ASPCR1-TFE3 fusion. *Neuropathology* 2009;**29**:460–5.
8. Bouvier D, Metellus P, de Paula AM, *et al.* Solitary fibrous tumors and hemangiopericytomas of the meninges: overlapping pathological features and common prognostic factors suggest the same spectrum of tumors. *Brain Pathol* 2012;**22**:511–21.
9. Cai N, Kahn LB. A report of primary brain fibrosarcoma with literature review. *J Neurooncol* 2004;**68**:161–7.
10. Carneiro SS, Scheithauer BW, Nascimento AG, *et al.* Solitary fibrous tumor of the meninges: a lesion distinct from fibrous meningioma. A clinicopathologic and immunohistochemical study. *Am J Clin Pathol* 1996;**106**:217–24.
11. Castilla EA, Prayson RA, Stevens GH, Barnett GH. Brain-invasive solitary fibrous tumors of the meninges: report of a case. *Int J Surg Pathol* 2002;**10**:217–21.
12. Chandler JP, Yashar P, Laskin WB, Russell EJ. Intradural chondrosarcoma: a case report and review of the literature. *J Neurooncol* 2004;**68**:33–9.
13. Christensen E, Lara DE. Intracranial sarcomas. *J Neuropathol Exp Neurol* 1953;**12**:41–56.
14. Cinalli G, Zerah M, Carteret M, *et al.* Subdural sarcoma associated with chronic subdural hematoma. Report of two cases and review of the literature. *J Neurosurg* 1997;**86**:553–7.
15. Dedeurwaerdere F, Giannini C, Sciot R, *et al.* Primary peripheral PNET/Ewing's sarcoma of the dura: a clinicopathologic entity distinct from central PNET. *Mod Pathol* 2002;**15**:673–8.
16. Ecker RD, Marsh WR, Pollock BE, *et al.* Hemangiopericytoma in the central nervous system: treatment, pathological features, and long-term follow up in 38 patients. *J Neurosurg* 2003;**98**:1182–7.

17. Enzinger FM, Smith BH. Hemangiopericytoma: an analysis of 106 cases. *Hum Pathol* 1976;7:61–82.

18. Fletcher CDM, Unni KK, Mertens F. *World Health Organization classification of tumours. Pathology and genetics of tumours of soft tissue and bone.* Lyon: IARC Press; 2002.

19. Fountas KN, Stamatiou S, Varvanis S, Kourtopoulos H. Intracranial falx chondroma: literature review and a case report. *Clin Neurol Neurosurg* 2008;11:8–13.

20. Furuno Y, Nishimura S, Kamiyama H, *et al.* Intracranial peripheral-type primitive neuroectodermal tumor. Case report. *Neurol Med Chir (Tokyo)* 2008;48:72–6.

21. Gaspar LE, Mackenzie IR, Gilbert JJ, *et al.* Primary cerebral fibrosarcomas. Clinicopathological study and review of the literature. *Cancer* 1993;72:3277–81.

22. Gunes M, Gunaldi O, Tugcu O, *et al.* Intracranial chondrosarcoma: a case report and review of the literature. *Minim Invasive Neurosurg* 2009;52:238–41.

23. Guthrie BL, Ebersold MJ, Scheithauer BW, Shaw EG. Meningeal haemangiopericytoma: histopathological features, treatment, and long-term followup of 44 cases. *Neurosurgery* 1989;25:514–22.

24. Hahn HP, Bundock EA, Hornick JL. Immunohistochemical staining for claudin-1 can help distinguish meningiomas from histological mimics. *Am J Clin Pathol* 2006;125:203–8.

25. Hajdu M, Singer S, Maik RG, *et al.* IGF2 over-expression in solitary fibrous tumours is independent of anatomical location and is related to loss of imprinting. *J Pathol* 2010;221:300–7.

26. Haresh KP, Chinikkatti SK, Rishi A, *et al.* A rare case of intradural extramedullary Ewing's sarcoma with skip metastasis in the spine. *Spinal Cord* 2008;46:582–4.

27. Hirato J, Nakazato Y, Sasaki A, *et al.* Intracranial malignant fibrous histiocytoma: characterization of GFAP-positive cells in the tumour. *Clin Neuropathol* 1994;13:315–22.

28. Horbinski C, Cieply K, Bejjani GK, McFadden K. Primary intracranial dural-based synovial sarcoma with an unusual SYT fluorescence in situ hybridization pattern. *J Neurosurg* 2008;109:897–903.

29. Hua W, Xu F, Mao Y, *et al.* Primary intracranial leiomyomas: report of two cases and review of the literature. *Clin Neurol Neurosurg* 2009;111:907–12.

30. Jeon YK, Chang K-H, Suh Y-L, *et al.* Inflammatory myofibroblastic tumor of the central nervous system: clinicopathologic analysis of 10 cases. *J Neuropathol Exp Neurol* 2005;64:254–9.

31. Joseph JT, Lisle DK, Jacoby LB, *et al.* NF2 gene analysis distinguishes haemangiopericytoma from meningioma. *Am J Pathol* 1995;147:1450–55.

32. Katayama Y, Kimura S, Watanabe T, *et al.* Peripheral-type primitive neuroectodermal tumor arising in the tentorium. Case report. *J Neurosurg* 1999;90:141–4.

33. Kim JH, Chang KH, Na DG, *et al.* Imaging features of meningeal inflammatory myofibroblastic tumor. *AJNR Am J Neuroradiol* 2009;30:1261–7.

34. Kim JH, Jung HW, Kim YS, *et al.* Meningeal hemangiopericytomas: long-term outcome and biological behavior. *Surg Neurol* 2003;59:47–53.

35. Kleinschmidt-Demasters BK, Mierua GW, Sze C-I, *et al.* Unusual dural and skull-based mesenchymal neoplasms: a report of four cases. *Hum Pathol* 1998;29:240–5.

36. Kocak A, Cayli SR, Onal SC, *et al.* Dural cavernous hemangioma originating from superior petrosal sinus. *J Neurosurg Sci* 2002;46:143–6.

37. Kotil K, Bilge T, Olagac V. Primary intradural myxoid chondrosarcoma: a case report and review in the literature. *J Neurooncol* 2005;75:169–72.

38. Lee JY, Kim BS, Phi JH, *et al.* Primary meningeal rhabdomyosarcoma associated with chronic subdural effusion. Case report. *J Neurosurg Pediatr* 2010;5:167–71.

39. Louis DN, Ohgaki H, Wiestler OD, Cavenee WK. *WHO classification of tumours of the central nervous system.* 4th ed. Lyon: IARC; 2007.

40. Louis DN, Richardson EP, Dickersin GR, *et al.* Primary intracranial leiomyosarcoma. Case report. *J Neurosurg* 1989;71:279–82.

41. Maran-Gonzalez A, Laquerriere A, Bigi N, *et al.* Posterior fossa solitary fibrous tumour: report of a fetal case and review of the literature. *J Neurooncol* 2011;101:297–300.

42. Maruno M, Muhammad AKMG, Taguchi J, *et al.* Giant cell type of primary intracranial malignant fibrous histiocytoma: a case report. *Brain Tumor Pathol* 2006;23:65–70.

43. Mena H, Ribas JL, Enzinger FM, Parisi JE. Primary angiosarcoma of the central nervous system. Study of eight cases and review of the literature. *J Neurosurg* 1991;75:73–6.

44. Mena H, Ribas JL, Pezeshkpour GH, *et al.* Hemangiopericytoma of the central nervous system: a review of 94 cases. *Hum Pathol* 1991;22:84–91.

45. Mobley BC, Roulston D, Shah GV, *et al.* Peripheral primitive neuroectodermal tumor/Ewing's sarcoma of the craniospinal vault: case report and review. *Hum Pathol* 2006;37:845–53.

46. Moliterno JA, Sood S, Zambrano E, *et al.* Intracranial benign fibrous histiocytomas: a case report and review. *J Neurooncol* 2009;92:203–9.

47. Moscovici S, Ramirez-DeNoriega F, Feliq Y, *et al.* Intradural extramedullary haemangiopericytoma of the thoracic spine infiltrating a nerve root: a case report and literature review. *Spine (Phila Pa 1976)* 2011;36:E1534–39.

48. Mumert MJ, Walsh MJ, Jensen EM, Jensen RL. Pleomorphic liposarcoma originating from intracranial dura mater. *J Neurooncol* 2010;97:149–53.

49. Papotti M, Abbona G, Pagani A, *et al.* Primitive neuroectodermal tumor of the meninges: an histological, immunohistochemical, ultrastructural, and cytogenetic study. *Endocr Pathol* 1998;9:275–80.

50. Paulus W, Slowik F, Jellinger K. Primary intracranial sarcomas: histopathological features of 19 cases. *Histopathology* 1991;18:395–402.

51. Perry A, Scheithauer BW, Nascimento AG. The immunophenotypic spectrum of meningeal haemangiopericytoma: a comparison with fibrous meningioma and solitary fibrous tumor of the meninges. *Am J Surg Pathol* 1997;21:1354–60.

52. Rajaram V, Brat D, Perry A. Anaplastic meningioma vs. meningeal haemangiopericytoma: Immunohistochemical and genetic markers. *Hum Pathol* 2004;35:1413–8.

53. Rosso D, Lee DH, Ferguson GG, *et al.* Dural cavernous angioma: a preoperative diagnostic challenge. *Can J Neurol Sci* 2003;30:272–7.

54. Russell DS, Rubenstein LJ. *Pathology of tumours of the nervous system.* London: Edward Arnold; 1989.

55. Schweizer L, Koelsche C, Sahm F, Pisa R, Capper D, Reuss D *et al.* Meningeal hemangiopericytoma and solitary fibrous tumors carry the NAB2-STAT6 fusion and can be diagnosed by nuclear expression of STAT6 protein. *Acta Neuropathol* 2013; 125:651–8.

56. Sibtain NA, Butt C, Connor WE. Imaging features of central nervous system haemangiopericytomas. *Eur Radiol* 2007;17:1685–13.

57. Sivendran S, Vidal CI, Barginear MF. Primary intracranial leiomyosarcoma in an HIV-infected patient. *Int J Clin Oncol* 2011;1:663–66.

58. Suzuki SO, Fukui M, Nishio S, Iwaki T. Clinicopathological features of solitary fibrous tumor of the meninges: an immunohistochemical reappraisal of cases previously diagnosed to be fibrous meningioma or haemangiopericytoma. *Pathol Int* 2000;50:808–17.

59. Tihan T, Viglione M, Rosenblum MK, *et al.* Solitary fibrous tumors in the central nervous system. A clinicopathologic review of 18 cases and comparison to meningeal haemangiopericytoma. *Arch Pathol Lab Med* 2003;127:432–9.

60. Uesaka T, Amano T, Inamura T, *et al.* Intradural, extramedullary spinal Ewing's sarcoma in childhood. *J Clin Neurosci* 2002;10:122–5.

61. Vuorinen V, Sallinen P, Haapasalo H, *et al.* Outcome of 31 intracranial hemangiopericytomas: poor predictive value of cell proliferation indices. *Acta Neurochir (Wien)* 1996;138:1399–408.

62. Weon YC, Kim EY, Kim HJ, *et al.* Intracranial solitary fibrous tumors: imaging findings in 6 consecutive patients. *AJNR Am J Neuroradiol* 2007;28:1466–9.

63. Xu F, De Las Casas LE, Dobbs LJJr. Primary meningeal rhabdomyosarcoma in a child with hypomelanosis of Ito. *Arch Pathol Lab Med* 2000;124:762–5.

64. Zevgaridis D, Tsonidis C, Kapranos N, *et al.* Epstein-Barr virus associated primary intracranial leiomyoma in organ transplant recipient: case report and review of the literature. *Acta Neurochir (Wien)* 2009;151:1705–9.

65. Zhang H, Dong L, Huang Y, *et al.* Primary intracranial leiomyosarcoma: review of the literature and presentation of a case. *Onkologie* 2012;35:609–16.

66. Zheng J, Liu L, Wang J, Wang S, Cao Y, Zhao J. Primary intracranial epithelioid hemangioendothelioma: a low-proliferation tumor exhibiting clinically malignant behavior. *J Neurooncol* 2012; 110:119–27.

Germ Cell Tumours

Marc K Rosenblum

EPIDEMIOLOGY

Germ cell tumours of the nervous system (Table 38.1) are the morphological homologues of germinal neoplasms arising in the gonads and other extragonadal sites.[65] There is considerable geographical variation in the incidence of these uncommon lesions, which occur at highest frequency among Far East Asians.[35,50,82] In Western series, they collectively account for no more than 0.5 per cent of all primary intracranial neoplasms and approximately 3.0 per cent of those that are discovered in childhood and adolescence (the periods of greatest risk).[6,10,22,26] By contrast, germ cell tumours constitute at least 2 per cent of all primary intracranial neoplasms and up to 15 per cent of paediatric examples in Taiwan and Japan, where they are most prevalent.[21,35,40] One outlying analysis of tumor registries in Japan and the United States, however, documented similar incidence rates.[43] A significantly increased incidence has also been noted in Koreans, children being preferentially affected.[36,82] In fact, 90 per cent of these tumours involve subjects below the age of 20 years (most occurring in the second decade) and case rates peak in 10–12 year olds.[6,10,21,22,40,42,74] Congenital examples (typically teratomas) account for more than half of all fetal brain tumours,[60,65] and exceptional cases come to attention in late adulthood.[26] All sites considered, the male/female ratio is at least 2–2.5:1, but the sex distribution of central nervous system (CNS) germ cell tumours varies by region: a great excess of pineal examples affects boys, whereas girls predominate among patients with suprasellar lesions. Sex differences are also apparent in the distribution of histological subtypes: a male/female ratio of 1.5–2:1 for germinomas increases to over 3:1 for non-germinomatous tumour subtypes in some series.[6,21,22,42,73]

Pure germinomas are most frequently encountered, followed by mixed germ cell tumours and teratomas.[6,10,21,22,34,42,67,73,74] One large series yielded the following percentages by histological subtype: germinomas, 41.1 per cent (including those with syncytiotrophoblastic giant cells, which accounted for 5.2 per cent of all cases); mixed germ cell tumours, 32 per cent; teratomas, 19.6 per cent (63.3 per cent of these being mature, 23.3 per cent immature and 13.3 per cent showing malignant transformation); embryonal carcinomas, 3.3 per cent; choriocarcinomas, 2 per cent; and yolk sac tumours, 2 per cent.[42]

Eighty per cent of CNS germ cell tumours arise in midline structures abutting the third ventricle.[6,10,21,22,73,74] They are the most common neoplasms originating in the region of the pineal gland, their favoured location, followed by the suprasellar compartment (including the infundibulum and hypothalamus). Germ cell tumours may also arise in the basal ganglia or thalami, ventricular system (some germinomas presenting as diffuse growths coating the ventricular surfaces), cerebral hemispheres, cerebellum, brain stem, spinal cord and sellar compartment. Congenital

TABLE 38.1 Central nervous system germ cell tumours	
Germinoma	With syncytiotrophoblastic giant cells
Teratoma	Mature
	Immature
	With malignant transformation
Yolk sac tumour	
Embryonal carcinoma	
Choriocarcinoma	
Mixed germ cell tumour	

examples (usually teratomas) may assume holocranial proportions and involve the orbit and extracranial soft tissues in complex with brain.[2,66] A bifocal presentation in the pineal region and suprasellar compartment constitutes the most common pattern of CNS germ cell tumor multicentricity,[26,42,73] followed by bilateral thalamic and basal ganglionic primaries.[31,68] Synchronous pineal and sellar involvement has been described.[7] Metachronous involvement of these and other intracranial sites is exceptional.[28,81,86] Germinomas are most prevalent in the suprasellar compartment and thalamostriatal regions, whereas non-germinomatous neoplasms predominate in other locations.

The great majority of CNS germ cell tumours arise sporadically. Klinefelter's syndrome (47 XXY), however, is associated with an increased risk of both intracranial and mediastinal germ cell tumourigenesis.[27] This susceptibility could reflect increased dosage of a chromosome X-associated gene, CNS germ cell tumours frequently exhibiting extra copies of this chromosome.[50] That the chronic elevation of serum gonadotrophins characteristic of this disorder could also contribute is suggested by the predilection of these lesions for peripubertal subjects. Intracranial germ cell tumours have also been described in association with Down's syndrome,[9,17] which carries an increased risk of testicular germ cell tumourigenesis.[98] On record are isolated accounts of CNS germ cell tumours arising in the setting of neurofibromatosis type 1[97] and involving siblings.[4,91] Multicentric germ cell neoplasia with independent intracranial and gonadal or mediastinal primaries has been communicated.[17,25,53,93] The remarkable discovery of a primary intracranial teratoma in the fetus of a mother who was diagnosed as having an independent ovarian teratoma has been reported.[58]

CLINICAL FEATURES

Clinical manifestations reflect lesion location. Pineal region examples are prone to compress the cerebral aqueduct, producing obstructive hydrocephalus with signs and symptoms of increased intracranial pressure, and to produce a paresis of upwards gaze and convergence (Parinaud syndrome) by impinging on the tectal plate. Suprasellar examples distort the optic chiasm, causing visual disturbances, and frequently result in diabetes insipidus and manifestations of pituitary failure (e.g. growth retardation and arrested sexual maturation) as a result of disruption of the hypothalamo-hypophyseal axis. Pineal or hypothalamic injury may release the immature testes from tonic inhibitory controls and produce 'precocious puberty' (isosexual pseudoprecocity) in boys, as may the secretion, by neoplastic syncytiotrophoblastic elements, of human chorionic gonadotropin (HCG), a stimulant of testosterone production.[1,63] Tumour expression of aromatase, a catalyst of oestrogen formation, may explain the rare instances of precocious puberty documented in girls with HCG-producing germinal neoplasms of the CNS.[51]

The pre-surgical assessment of suspected CNS germ cell tumours routinely includes serum and CSF alpha-fetoprotein (AFP) and beta-HCG measurements. Elevated levels of either oncoprotein constitute compelling evidence of a germ cell neoplasm and the pattern of elevation correlates, albeit imperfectly, with tumour histology and immunophenotype.[21,22,34,42] Marked elevations of AFP reliably predict the presence of yolk sac tumour elements, although modest increases in this marker may result from its expression by the enteric components of some teratomas. High beta-HCG levels, by contrast, are most suggestive of choriocarcinomatous elements, but modest increases may also be associated with tumours, including a subset of germinomas, that harbour syncytiotrophoblastic giant cells in the absence of cytotrophoblastic cells. Sampling artefact must be assumed if the assessment, including immunohistochemical evaluation, of neurosurgical specimens proves at odds with preoperative serum or CSF profiles.

RADIOLOGY

Neuroradiological features are generally non-specific.[38] Of some utility, however, is the observation that germ cell tumours arising in the region of the pineal gland may occasionally surround or displace this organ rather than obliterating it in the manner of pineal parenchymal neoplasms. The demonstration of a complex mass containing cysts, regions of calcification and foci having the signal characteristics of fat suggests a teratoma or mixed germ cell tumour with teratomatous elements. On computed tomography (CT) and magnetic resonance (MR) imaging, non-teratomatous germ cell neoplasms of the nervous system are usually solid and conspicuously contrast-enhancing, though germinomas arising in the basal ganglia and thalamus may be more prone to cystic change (as well as calcification) than their pineal and suprasellar counterparts.[20,38] On rare occasion, germinomas permeate neuroparenchyma in glioma-like fashion rather than presenting as discrete neuroradiologic lesions.[68] Germinomas tend to enhance homogeneously, whereas non-germinomatous tumours often enhance in a heterogeneous fashion. Tumour tissue is generally hypo- to iso-intense on T1-weighted sequences and iso- to hyper-intense on T2-weighted study. There may be associated oedema. Intratumoural haemorrhage is especially characteristic of choriocarcinomatous components. Ultrasonographic or fast magnetic resonance imaging may detect congenital germ cell tumours (typically teratomas) *in utero*.[39,75]

GERMINOMA

Germinomas are soft or friable, tan-white and typically solid, although some show cystic change, the rare thalamostriatal examples being prone to cyst formation and calcification. Necrosis and haemorrhage may be apparent, but if extensive raise the possibility of more aggressive components, such as embryonal carcinoma and choriocarcinoma.

Pure germinomas are populated by large cells of undifferentiated appearance that resemble primordial germinal elements. These are usually disposed in sheets or lobules, but may be forced into cords or trabeculae by a desmoplastic stromal response that can progress to regions of paucicellular fibrosis. Cytological features evident in promptly fixed tissue sections, intraoperative smear or CSF preparations include centrally placed, round and vesicular nuclei, prominent nucleoli, discrete cell membranes and relatively abundant clear cytoplasm that is glycogen-rich (Figure 38.1a) and period acid–Schiff (PAS) positive. Mitotic activity may be conspicuous. A characteristic feature is infiltration by both B- and T-lymphocytes, helper/inducer and cytoxic/suppressor cells predominating, with recent evidence suggesting a significant humoral immune response.[72,94,96] Lymphocytes may be restricted to traversing fibrovascular septa, but often mingle with tumour cells and may be so numerous as to obscure the underlying neoplastic process. The presence of these cells admixed with a second population of atypical, large and polygonal cells of undifferentiated

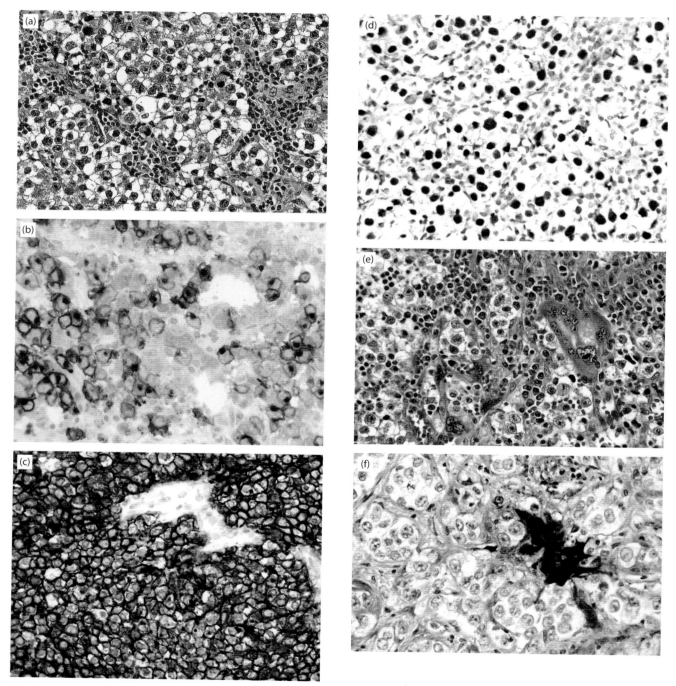

38.1 Germinoma. (a) Large tumour cells with abundant clear cytoplasm are admixed with small lymphocytes along fibrovascular septa. **(b)** Intense cell membrane and Golgi region immunoreactivty for CD117 is unique to the germinoma among germ cell tumours. **(c)** Diffuse membranous and focal dot-like immunoreactivity for D2-40 is typical. **(d)** Nuclear immunoreactivity for OCT4, a feature shared by embryonal carcinomas, is regularly seen. **(e)** Occasional germinomas feature scattered syncytiotrophoblasts. **(f)** A syncytiotrophoblast in this germinoma expresses beta HCG, but in the absence of cytotrophoblasts, this should not be interpreted as evidence of choriocarcinoma.

aspect should suggest the diagnosis in smear or crush preparations. Germinomas can also elicit a florid granulomatous reaction that may prompt considerations of sarcoidosis or tuberculosis, a particular problem in small biopsies.[35,36] It is tempting to speculate that a restraining immunological response accounts for the sometimes protracted pre-operative duration of clinical symptoms and for the rare observation of spontaneous germinoma regression on neuroradiological surveillance.[47] An exceptional sellar/suprasellar mass composed of germinoma and Burkitt-like B-cell lymphoma is on record.[88] Whether this represents a chance collison, neoplastic transformation of germinoma-associated lymphoid elements or underlying teratoma with somatic malignant transformation is unclear.

On immunohistochemical assessment, germinomas are characterized by highly variable cytoplasmic reactivity for placental alkaline phosphatase (PLAP), an oncoprotein normally expressed by primordial germ cells and syncytiotrophoblasts.[6,21,42,67] Labelling of cell membranes is typical, some cases also exhibiting a dot-like, 'Golgi' pattern of paranuclear cytoplasmic reactivity or more diffuse decoration of the cytoplasm. At least 5–10 per cent of germinomas, however, are PLAP-negative and immunoreactivity may be especially difficult to demonstrate in previously frozen material or specimens with florid inflammation. In addition, PLAP expression may be manifested by embryonal carcnomas, yolk sac tumours and choriocarcinomas. Germinomas differ from these tumour types, and are homologous to testicular seminomas, in regularly exhibiting intense cell membrane labelling (often accompanied by paranuclear Golgi region reactivity) for CD117 (Figure 38.1b), a product of the c-kit proto-oncogene, as well as membranous immunoexpression of D2-40/podoplanin (Figure 38.1c).[23] Similarly, a more constant feature of the germinoma immunoprofile than PLAP reactivty, but one shared by embryonal carcinomas, is nuclear labelling for OCT4 (Figure 38.1d), a transcription factor that is also expressed by seminomas and, normally, by embryonic stem cell populations and primordial germ cells.[23] Also shared by germinomas and embryonal carcinomas is nuclear reactivity for UTF1, another stem cell transcription factor and downstream target of OCT4.[55] Germinoma cells are further characterized by nuclear immunoexpression of HESRG,[92] NANOG[70] and SALL4[44] transcription factors, as well as the RNA-binding LIN 28 protein,[8] the latter two being widely expressed by non-germinomatous germ cell tumours as well.

A minority of germinomas show cytoplasmic labelling for cytokeratins CAM 5.2 and AE1/3.[12,21] Coupled with the ultrastructural demonstration that germinoma cells may engage in intercellular junction and true lumen formation,[46] these observations have been taken as evidence that such tumours can differentiate along epithelial or embryonal carcinomatous lines and that they may be more prone to do so than their testicular counterparts. Clinical consequences have not been attached to these phenomena. Cytokeratin immunoreactivity in germinomas is typically focal, often weak, and restricted to minor tumour populations. Embryonal carcinomas and solid variants of yolk sac tumour, differential diagnostic considerations, characteristically manifest diffuse and strong

cytokeratin labelling.[6,12,21,67] AFP-positive elements within 'germinomas' usually prove to represent minimal elements of yolk sac tumour not recognized in conventionally stained sections and beta-HCG immunolabelling is almost invariably restricted to syncytiotrophoblastic giant cells that populate a distinct subset of these lesions (Figure 38.1e,f). The presence of these syncytiotrophoblastic elements, which also show cytoplasmic reactivity for human placental lactogen (HPL) and for cytokeratins, must be noted, because germinomas harbouring such cells may be more prone to recurrence after radiation therapy (see under Biological Behaviour, p. 1841).

TERATOMAS

Teratomas recapitulate, albeit in disorganized fashion, somatic differentiation by the embryonic ectoderm, endoderm and mesoderm. On macroscopic inspection, the diagnosis is often suggested by the finding of mucus-filled cysts, cartilaginous nodules, bony spicules or fat. CNS teratomas may rarely contain hair or recognizable teeth, advanced organogenesis resulting in a curiosity that has been termed intracranial 'fetus-in-fetu'.[48] The maldevelopmental incorporation of dizygotic twins could account, however, for a subset of cases reported under the latter designation, which has been exactingly restricted by some observers to examples of demonstrably abortive twinning.[31]

Mature teratomas are defined by their content of only fully differentiated, 'adult'-type tissue elements (Figure 38.2a) that exhibit little, if any, mitotic activity. Ectodermal differentiation is commonly signalled by the presence of squamous epithelium-lined cysts with associated cutaneous adnexa, islands of glioneuronal tissue and choroid plexus. Nodules of hyalin cartilage, bony trabecula, adipose tissue and bundles of smooth or striated muscle are frequent mesodermal representatives. Endodermal participants usually include cysts lined by epithelia of respiratory or enteric type, at times organized into miniature gut- or bronchus-like structures. Hepatic and pancreatic tissue may also be found.

Only a minority of teratomatous neoplasms arising in the CNS qualify as fully mature. Most contain incompletely differentiated elements resembling fetal tissues (Figure 38.2b). The presence of such components, regardless of their relative representation, mandates classification of a teratoma as immature. At present, there is no clinically validated grading system for these lesions. Especially common are hypercellular and mitotically active stromal constituents reminiscent of embryonic mesenchyme and primitive neuroepithelial elements that often include neuroblastomatous components, rosettes of ependymoblastic or Flexner–Wintersteiner type and canalicular structures mimicking the developing neural tube in medulloepithelioma-like fashion. Clefts lined by a melanin-laden epithelium may reflect partial retinal differentiation. The spontaneous maturation of such tumours has been recorded,[78] but re-resection specimens harbouring only fully differentiated somatic tissue elements usually derive from initially immature teratomas or mixed germ cell neoplasms subjected to adjuvant therapy.[5,14,49] The apparent tumoural maturation

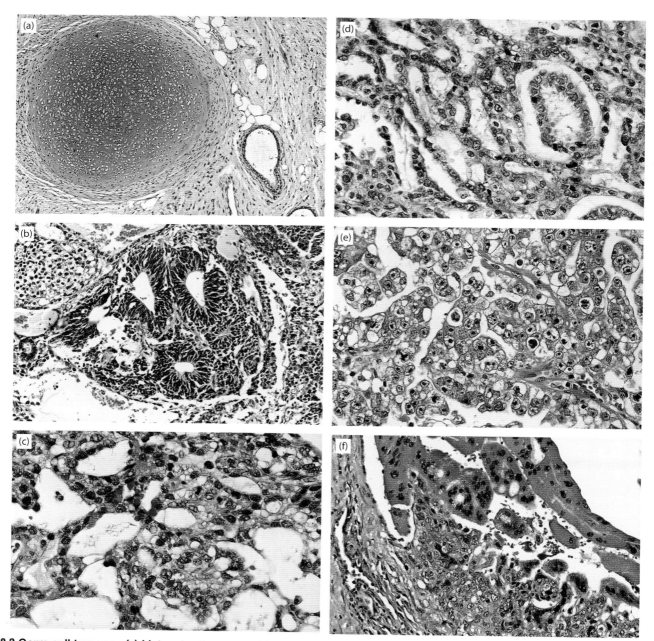

38.2 Germ cell tumours. **(a)** Mature teratoma containing well-differentiated cartilage, fibroadipose tissue and glandular structures. **(b)** Immature teratoma with primitive neuroepithelial component. **(c)** Yolk sac tumour. Primitive epithelial cells delimit irregular spaces in the reticular variant. Note eosinophilic hyaline globules. **(d)** Endodermal variant of yolk sac tumour exhibiting cytoplasmic immunolabelling for alpha-fetoprotein. **(e)** Embryonal carcinoma with large epithelial cells containing prominent nucleoli and showing abortive glandular or papillary formations. **(f)** Choriocarcinoma. Syncytiotrophoblastic giant cells drape mononucleated cytotrophoblastic elements.

in such circumstances may simply reflect the selective ablation of proliferative, incompletely differentiated cellular components. The progressive, seemingly paradoxical enlargement of these recurrent, yet ostensibly mature remnants has been referred to as the 'growing teratoma syndrome'. The expansion of tumoural cysts may account, at least in part, for this apparent growth,[54] though the cited study also demonstrated surprisingly elevated MIB-1/Ki-67 labeling fractions in fully differentiated - looking teratomatous tissues.

Cancers of conventional somatic type occasionally arise within germ cell tumours. The neoplasms in such cases almost invariably contain teratomatous components and secondary genetic events are held to account for this phenomenon—hence its designation as 'teratoma with malignant transformation'. Most often observed are sarcomatous elements of undifferentiated or rhabdomyosarcomatous appearance.[6,42,67] Teratoma-containing intracranial germ cell tumours have also spawned adenocarcinomas of enteric type,[13,30] squamous carcinomas,[42] leiomyosarcoma[80] and erythroleukaemia.[17] A carcinoid tumour has been encountered within a teratoma of the spinal neuraxis,[24] as has a malignant neoplasm interpreted as an adenocarcinoma.[57] Endodermal yolk sac tumour elements have been proposed as an alternative source for enteric adenocarcinomas arising in germinal neoplasms of the CNS.[13] As already mentioned, an account of a sellar/suprasellar mass composed of admixed germinoma and Burkitt-like B-cell lymphoma[88] is open to interpretation. Pathologists are advised to state the specific type of somatic cancer encountered in these rare neoplasms and should avoid the generic 'malignant teratoma', an imprecise term that has also been applied to tumours harbouring teratomatous and aggressive non-teratomatous germinal elements (e.g. embryonal carcinoma, choriocarcinoma or yolk sac tumour). The latter are designated as mixed germ cell tumours in the current WHO classification.[65]

The tissue components comprising teratomas will exhibit the immunotypes expected of their native somatic counterparts. AFP expression by teratomatous glands of enteric type may cause elevated serum and CSF levels of this marker oncoprotein.[21,42]

YOLK SAC TUMOURS

Yolk sac tumours are composed of primitive epithelial elements that apparently differentiate towards yolk sac endoderm and that are variably arrayed in a loose, often hypocellular and myxomatous matrix likened to extra-embryonic mesoblast. The former may be disposed in solid sheets, enclose irregular tissue spaces ('reticular' pattern) (Figure 38.2c) or line anastomosing channels ('endodermal sinus' pattern) as a cuboidal epithelium that in a subset of cases also drapes fibrovascular papillae to form pathognomonic structures known as Schiller–Duval bodies. Apparent in some examples are eccentrically constricted cysts lined by attenuated epithelial elements ('polyvesicular vitelline' pattern), glands of enteric type replete with goblet cells and foci of hepatocellular differentiation (hepatoid variant). No special clinical significance attaches to any of these morphological patterns. Eosinophilic, PAS-positive and diastase-resistant hyaline globules that may lie within the cytoplasm of its epithelial elements or appear free in its stroma are a particularly distinctive, but inconstant feature of the yolk sac tumour (Figure 38.2c). Mitotic activity may be conspicuous, but necrosis is exceptional.

Of diagnostic relevance in the identification of yolk sac tumours (though often present in only patchy distribution) is the cytoplasmic immunolabelling of their epithelial elements for AFP (Figure 38.2d), which is normally synthesized by yolk sac endoderm as well as fetal hepatocytes and intestinal epithelial cells.[6,12,21,67] Hyaline globules are also AFP-positive. AFP immunoreactivity is of particular value in distinguishing solid variants of this neoplasm from embryonal carcinomas and germinomas. Yolk sac tumours are further characterized by frequent cytoplasmic labelling for glypican-3[44] and nuclear reactivity for SALL4[44] and LIN28.[8] Epithelial components of the yolk sac tumour may label for PLAP, but unlike germinomas, are diffusely cytokeratin-positive. In only exceptional cases is any OCT4 expression apparent and CD117/c-kit

reactivity, also unusual, tends to be of diffuse cytoplasmic rather than membranous quality.[23] Beta-HCG and HPL are not expressed.

EMBRYONAL CARCINOMAS

Embryonal carcinomas are populated by large, polygonal cells with vesicular nuclei, macronucleoli and abundant clear to violet-coloured cytoplasm. These usually proliferate in cohesive nests or sheets and may fashion abortive papillae or line gland-like spaces (Figure 38.2e). The structure of the early embryo is exceptionally replicated in the form of 'embryoid bodies' possessing germ discs and diminutive amniotic cavities. A high mitotic rate and zones of coagulative necrosis are the rule.

Cytoplasmic immunoreactivty for CD30, though shared by the epithelial and mesenchymal components of some teratomas, distinguishes embryonal carcinomas from other germ cell tumours.[23] Cytoplasmic PLAP immunolabelling may be found and nuclear OCT4, SALL4, HESRG,[92] UTF1[55] and LIN28 expression are the rule, but nuclear expression of SOX2[71] and uniformly dense immunoreactivity for cytokeratins (c-kit) further distance embryonal carcinomas from germinomas, whereas the former are typically AFP-negative.[6,12,21,67] Also foreign to the embryonal carcinoma is expression of HPL and beta-HCG, though cytoplasmic CD117/c-kit labelling (usually non-membranous) may be encountered.[23]

CHORIOCARCINOMAS

The choriocarcinoma is characterized by differentiation along extra-embryonic, trophoblastic lines. Although syncytiotrophoblastic giant cells in isolation may be encountered in a variety of germ cell tumour types, the diagnosis requires the added presence of cytotrophoblastic elements (Figure 38.2f). The latter are represented by cohesive masses of large mononuclear cells with vesicular nuclei and clear or acidophilic cytoplasm that are, in turn, draped by the syncytiotrophoblasts. Giant syncytiotrophoblastic cells are recognized by their multiple and deeply hyperchromatic nuclei (which are frequently clustered) and voluminous expanses of basophilic or violaceous cytoplasm. Extensive haemorrhagic necrosis and blood lake formation are nearly constant features, preserved neoplastic elements being difficult to identify in some cases.

Syncytiotrophoblastic cells are diffusely immunoreactive for beta-HCG and HPL.[6,12,21,67] Cytokeratin labelling is also a regular feature, with a subset of choriocarcinomas being decorated by antibodies to PLAP as well. Choriocarcinomas are not immunoreactive for CD117 (c-kit) or OCT4.

MIXED GERM CELL TUMOURS

Save for the germinoma with syncytiotrophoblastic giant cells (accorded a distinct designation), germinal neoplasms composed of the foregoing histological entities in any combination are collectively termed 'mixed germ cell tumours'.[65] Pathologists are obliged in reporting such cases to specify the components identified and their relative proportion.

DIFFERENTIAL DIAGNOSIS

The histological and immunohistochemical features described previously distinguish the various CNS germ cell tumour types from one another and from a variety of neoplasms (e.g. metastatic carcinomas, lymphomas and meningiomas) that are largely theoretical considerations given the usual localization of primary germinal tumours in the neuraxis and the young age of most affected subjects. Immunoprofiling should further facilitate the exclusion of atypical teratoid/rhabdoid tumour or central neuroepithelial neoplasia in any of its forms. Emphasized again is the potential role of screening for CD117-, D2-40- or OCT4-expressing elements in the unmasking of germinomas obscured by inflammatory infiltration. Limited neurosurgical samples deriving from teratoma-bearing germ cell tumours can raise the question of epidermoid, dermoid or endodermal-type cyst, primitive neuroectodermal tumour (e.g. medulloepithelioma, ependymoblastoma and pineoblastoma) or mesenchymal neoplasia. In the absence of demonstrable differentiation along multidermal somatic lines, the diagnosis of germ cell tumour may yet be suggested on neuroradiologic grounds or established for practical purposes by detection of elevated serum/CSF AFP or β-HCG levels. Primary and secondary germ cell tumours of the CNS cannot be differentiated on morphological, immunophenotypic or genetic grounds. In fact, metastasis of a gonadal or other extraneural germ cell tumour to the midline pineal–suprasellar axis is a most exceptional event.[11]

GENETICS

Although data are limited, pure intracranial teratomas encountered as congenital or infantile lesions appear genetically different from CNS germ cell tumours presenting later in life. Normal diploid karyotypes have characterized the former in most cases,[48,66,69,95] assessment of one such tumour by comparative genomic hybridization (CGH) failing to disclose chromosomal imbalances.[61] Isolated examples have been described as exhibiting nongermline genetic anomalies, including partial duplication of chromosome 1q[18] and trisomy 1q/19p.[77] Whereas intracranial teratomas of early life resemble teratomas of the infant testis in their diploid status and chromosomal stability,[98] the more common CNS germ cell tumours arising in older children (and adults) share with their testicular homologues in young men, generally aneuploid profiles, complex chromosomal abnormalities and overlapping, non-random patterns of chromosomal imbalance. Chief among the last, irrespective of histologic subtype, are gains of 12p, 8q, 1q, 2p, 7q and X, as well as losses of 11q, 13, 5q, 10q and 18q.[50,62,76,83,85] Whether 12p gains and isochromosome 12p (i12p) formation, a signature event characterizing 80 per cent or more of testicular (and mediastinal) primaries, occur as regularly in the intracranial setting has been debated, but the weight of evidence

to date would indicate that fewer germ cell tumours of CNS origin specifically manifest the i12p.[50,62,76,83,85] In one analysis, regions of most significant gain encompassed CCND2 and PRDM14, the latter a transcriptional regulator of primordial germ cell specification, whereas the RBI locus was a prime target of copy loss, the data suggesting a role for the cyclin/CDK-RB-E2F pathway in CNS germ cell tumour pathogenesis.[85] The linkage of familial germ cell tumours to Xq27[59] and the association of the XXY (Klinefelter) genotype with elevated risk of testicular and extragonadal (including neuraxial) germ cell neoplasia underscore the relevance of increased chromosome X dosage to germinal tumourigenesis.

Studies at the single gene level implicate aberrantly activated KIT/RAS signaling, a feature of testicular and mediastinal germinomas as well as ovarian dysgerminomas, in the pathogenesis of intracranial germinomas.[16,90] A majority of the latter exhibit mutations of KIT or RAS family members, these being mutually exclusive, associated with severe chromosomal instability and only infrequently encountered in other germ cell tumour subtypes. Mutation of the negative KIT regulator CBL has also been documented in this setting.[90] Less frequent events observed in a variety of CNS germ cell tumours include mutational inactivation of the transcriptional co-repressor and tumour-suppressing BCORL1 gene and activating AKT/mTOR abnormalities.[90] Germline variants of JMJD1C, a chromatin modifier, may be associated with an increased risk of intracranial germ cell tumourigenesis among Japanese.[90] Epigenetic profiles common to gonadal and at least some neuraxial germ cell tumours include hypomethylation of the IGF2/H19 imprinting control region[79] and of the imprinted SNRPN gene.[37]

HISTOGENESIS

The histogenesis of germ cell tumours arising within the central neuraxis is a subject of debate. A time-honoured view has these deriving from primordial germ cells that either migrate aberrantly or are somehow attracted to the developing CNS rather than to the genital ridges. A germinal origin would be consonant with the observation that intracranial germ cell tumours display genetic and epigenetic alterations comparable to those that typify their gonadal homologues. The human CNS, however, has never been shown to contain primitive germ cell elements, even immunohistochemical screen of fetal pineal glands for PLAP expression proving fruitless in this search.[12] In answer, it has been proposed that an enigmatic population of skeletal muscle-type elements ('myoid' cells) known to inhabit the developing pineal gland represent the offspring of primordial germ cells in differentiated, somatic disguise.[64] Adduced in support of this seemingly far-fetched hypothesis is the fact that the thymus – like the CNS, ostensibly devoid of germ cell elements and yet a favoured site of extragonadal germ cell tumourigenesis – hosts similarly mysterious myoid cell constituents.[64]

An alternative proposal that does not require aberrant cell migration postulates the origin of CNS germ cell tumours from multipotent stem cells.[52,89] This hypothesis must invoke the selective programming of such precursors to the germ cell differentiation pathway, along with their neoplastic transformation, to explain the resemblances of intracranial and gonadal germ cell tumours at the genetic level, but *in vitro* data have been cited in theoretical support of this scenario.[52] A syncretic variation of this concept admits divergent origins for what are recognized as two fundamentally distinct neoplastic classes.[89] In this scheme, an embryonic stem cell origin is posited for the pure CNS teratomas encountered as congenital or infantile growths, these sharing the normal diploid status characteristic of infantile testicular teratomas, whereas a primordial germ cell derivation is reserved for the CNS germ cell neoplasms arising in peri- or post-pubertal subjects, which mirror the aneuploidy and, in many cases, 12p overrepresentation of their gonadal and mediastinal counterparts. The apparent divergence of these tumour types, however, could reflect distinct initiating events rather than differing cellular origins. Most recently, neural stem cells have become candidates as putative CNS germ cell tumour progenitors based in part on evidence that they share hypomethylation of the imprinted *SNRPN* gene with primordial germ cells and both testicular and extragonadal (including intracranial) germ cell neoplasms.[37] Noteworthy as well in this regard is experimental evidence that overexpression of OCT4 in neural stem cells suffices to trigger teratoma formation.[84] Whether teratomatous lesions of the spinal neuraxis, which are typically devoid of other germ cell tumour components, represent complex malformations[32] or *bona fide* neoplasms[3] is also contested.

BIOLOGICAL BEHAVIOUR

Histologic subtype has emerged from a number of multivariate analyses as the most significant predictor of CNS germ cell tumour outcome.[22,41,42,74] Non-metastasizing and typically non-invasive in their expansion, fully mature teratomas are curable by surgical means alone when amenable to gross total excision. Recurrence of initially mature and completely resected intracranial teratomas as non-teratomatous, malignant germ cell tumours is exceptional but documented.[87] Pure germinomas in localized form can be cured in most cases owing to their remarkable radiosensitivity, the addition of chemotherapy to treatment regimens facilitating tumour ablation at reduced radiation exposure to the neuraxis.[29,36,41,45,73] Given the favourable outlook of these tumour types individually, the good prognosis reported after surgery and irradiation for mixed neoplasms composed only of mature teratoma and conventional germinoma is not surprising. Germinomas harbouring syncytiotrophoblastic giant cells or associated with elevated CSF/serum β-HCG levels do not behave as aggressively as choriocarcinomas, but have been associated in some series with increased likelihood of recurrence and reduced survival following irradiation alone,[42,73] such lesions being placed in a broad 'intermediate'-risk group that appears to include immature teratomas and mixed tumours composed mainly of germinoma, teratoma or combinations thereof.[42,73] Whether syncytiotrophoblastic components or elevated HCG levels are significantly associated with poorer outcomes in the setting of otherwise pure germinoma, however, has been questioned.[29,36,45] Most aggressive are yolk sac tumours, embryonal carcinomas, choriocarcinomas, and mixed germ cell neoplasms in which these subtypes are conspicuously represented.[29,36,42,73] Aggressive treatment regimens combining radiation and intensified chemotherapy appear to substantially improve the control of intermediate risk lesions and have achieved, in some studies, modest successes in the setting of high-risk disease.[29,36,45] Although local recurrence and progression at the primary site are the most common patterns of treatment failure, CNS germ cell tumours (mature teratomas excepted) not infrequently seed the CSF, are capable of distant hematogenous metastasis (mainly to lung and bone), and can involve the abdominal cavity via ventriculoperitoneal shunts. Examples harbouring prominent choriocarcinomatous components may be especially prone to blood-borne spread. Dissemination in any form augurs poorly for affected patients, though dramatic responses to adjuvant chemotherapy are occasionally observed in this setting.

REFERENCES

1. Aguzzi A, Hedinger CE, Kleihues P, Yasargil MG. Intracranial mixed germ cell tumor with syncytiotrophoblastic giant cells and precocious puberty. *Acta Neuropathol (Berl)* 1988;**75**:427–31.
2. Alagappan A, Shattuck K, Rowe T, Hawkins H. Massive intracranial teratoma with extracranial extension into oral cavity, nose and neck. *Fetal Diagn Ther* 1998;**13**:321–4.
3. al-Sarraj ST, Parmar D, Dean AF, et al. Clinicopathological study of seven cases of spinal cord teratoma. A possible germ cell origin. *Histopathology* 1998;**32**:51–6.
4. Aoyama I, Kondo A, Ogawa H, Ikai Y. Germinoma in siblings: case reports. *Surg Neurol* 1994;**41**:313–17.
5. Bi WL, Bannykh S, Baehring J. The growing teratoma syndrome after subtotal resection of an intracranial nongerminomatous germ cell tumor in an adult: case report. *Neurosurgery* 2005;**56**:191–4.
6. Bjornsson J, Scheithauer BW, Okazaki H, Leech RW. Intracranial germ cell tumors. Pathobiological and immunohistochemical aspects of 70 cases. *J Neuropathol Exp Neurol* 1985;**44**:32–46.
7. Bohara M, Hirano H, Tokimura H, et al. Pineal mixed germ cell tumor with a synchronous sellar lesion in the sixth decade. *Brain Tumor Pathol* 2011;**28**:163–6.
8. Cao D, Liu A, Wang F, et al. RNA-binding protein LIN28 is a marker for primary extragonadal germ cell tumors: an immunohistochemical study of 131 cases. *Mod Pathol* 2011;**24**:288–96.
9. Chik K, Li C, Shing MM, et al. Intracranial germ cell tumors in children with and without Down syndrome. *J Pediatr Hematol Oncol* 1999;**21**:149–51.
10. Dearnaley DP, A'Hern RP, Whittaker S, Bloom HJ. Pineal and CNS germ cell tumors. Royal Marsden Hospital experience 1962-1987. *Int J Radiat Oncol Biol Phys* 1990;**18**:773–81.
11. Delahunt B, Teoh HH, Balakrishnan V, et al. Testicular germ cell tumor with pineal metastases. *Neurosurgery* 1990;**26**:688–91.
12. Felix I, Becker LE. Intracranial germ cell tumors in children: an immunohistochemical and electron microscopic study. *Pediatr Neurosurg* 1990;**6**:156–62.
13. Freilich RJ, Thompson SJ, Walker RW, Rosenblum MK. Adenocarcinomatous transformation of intracranial germ cell tumors. *Am J Surg Pathol* 1995;**19**:537–44.
14. Friedman JA, Lynch JJ, Buckner JC, et al. Management of malignant pineal germ cell tumors with residual mature teratoma. *Neurosurgery* 2001;**48**:518–22; discussion 522–3.
15. Fujimaki T, Matsutani M, Funada N, et al. CT and MRI features of intracranial germ cell tumors. *J Neurooncol* 1994;**19**:217–26.
16. Hashimoto T, Sasagawa I, Ishigooka M, et al. Down's syndrome associated with intracranial germinoma and

testicular embryonal carcinoma. *Urol Int* 1995;55:120–2.

17. Fukushima S, Otsuka A, Suzuki T, *et al.* Mutually exclusive mutations of KIT and RAS are associated with KIT mRNA expression and chromosomal instability in primary intracranial pure germinomas. *Acta Neuropathol* 2014;127:911–25.

18. Hecht F, Grix A, Jr., Hecht BK, *et al.* Direct prenatal chromosome diagnosis of a malignancy. *Cancer Genet Cytogenet* 1984;11:107–11.

19. Heimdal K, Evensen SA, Fossa SD, *et al.* Karyotyping of a hematologic neoplasia developing shortly after treatment for cerebral extragonadal germ cell tumor. *Cancer Genet Cytogenet* 1991;57:41–6.

20. Higano S, Takahashi S, Ishii K, *et al.* Germinoma originating in the basal ganglia and thalamus: MR and CT evaluation. *AJNR Am J Neuroradiol* 1994;15:1435–41.

21. Ho DM, Liu HC. Primary intracranial germ cell tumor. Pathologic study of 51 patients. *Cancer* 1992;70:1577–84.

22. Hoffman HJ, Otsubo H, Hendrick EB, *et al.* Intracranial germ–cell tumors in children. *J Neurosurg* 1991;74:545–51.

23. Iczkowski KA, Bulter SL, Shanks JH, *et al.* Trials of new germ cell immunohistochemical stains in 93 extragonadal and metastatic germ cell tumors. *Hum Pathol* 2008;39:275–81.

24. Ironside JW, Jefferson AA, Royds JA, *et al.* Carcinoid tumour arising in a recurrent intradural spinal teratoma. *Neuropathol Appl Neurobiol* 1984;10:479–89.

25. Iwata H, Mori Y, Takagi H, *et al.* Mediastinal growing teratoma syndrome after cisplatin-based chemotherapy and radiotherapy for intracranial germinoma. *J Thorac Cardiovasc Surg* 2004;127:291–3.

26. Jennings MT, Gelman R, Hochberg F. Intracranial germ-cell tumors: natural history and pathogenesis. *J Neurosurg* 1985;63:155–67.

27. Kaido T, Sasaoka Y, Hashimoto H, Taira K. De novo germinoma in the brain in association with Klinefelter's syndrome: case report and review of the literature. *Surg Neurol* 2003;60:553–8; discussion 559.

28. Kamoshima Y, Sawamura Y, Iwasaki M, *et al.* Metachronous mature teratoma in the corpus callosum occurring 12 years after a pineal germinoma. *J Neurosurg* 2008;109:126–9.

29. Kanamori M, Kumabe T, Saito R, *et al.* Optimal treatment strategy for intracranial germ cell tumors: a single institution analysis. *J Neurosurg Pediatr* 2009;4:506–14.

30. Kim ES, Kwon MJ, Song JH, *et al.* Adenocarcinoma arising from intracranial recurrent mature teratoma and featuring mutated KRAS and wild-type BRAF genes. *Neuropathology* 2014 Jul 11. doi: 10.1111/neup.12140 [Epub ahead of print].

31. Kim J, Park SH, Park SS, *et al.* Fetus-in-fetu in the cranium of a 4-month-old boy: histopathology and short tandem repeat polymorphism-based genotyping. *J Neurosurg Pediatr* 2008;1:410–14.

32. Kobayashi T, Yoshida J, Kida Y. Bilateral germ cell tumors involving the basal ganglia and thalamus. *Neurosurgery* 1989;24:579–83.

33. Koen JL, McLendon RE, George TM. Intradural spinal teratoma. Evidence for a dysembryogenic origin. Report of four cases. *J Neurosurg* 1998;89:844–51.

34. Kraichoke S, Cosgrove M, Chandrasoma PT. Granulomatous inflammation in pineal germinoma. A cause of diagnostic failure at stereotaxic brain biopsy. *Am J Surg Pathol* 1988;12:655–60.

35. Kuratsu J, Ushio Y. Epidemiological study of primary intracranial tumors in childhood. A population-based survey in Kumamoto Prefecture, Japan. *Pediatr Neurosurg* 1996;25:240–6.

36. Lee D, Suh YL. Histologically confirmed intracranial germ cell tumors; an analysis of 62 patients in a single institute. *Virchows Arch* 2010;457:347–57.

37. Lee SH, Appleby V, Jeyapalan JN, *et al.* Variable methylation of the imprinted gene, SNRPN, supports a relationship between intracranial germ cell tumours and neural stem cells. *J Neurooncol* 2011;101:419–28.

38. Liang L, Korogi Y, Sugahara T, *et al.* MRI of intracranial germ-cell tumours. *Neuroradiology* 2002;44:382–8.

39. Marden FA, Wippold FJ, 2nd, Perry A. Fast magnetic resonance imaging in steady-state precession (true FISP) in the prenatal diagnosis of a congenital brain teratoma. *J Comput Assist Tomogr* 2003;27:427–30.

40. Makino K, Nakamura H, Yano S, *et al.* Incidence of primary central nervous system germ cell tumors in childhood: a regional survey in Kumamoto prefecture in southern Japan. *Pediatr Neurosurg* 2013;49:155–8.

41. Matsutani M, The Japanese Pediatric Brain Tumor Study Group. Combined chemotherapy and radiation therapy for CNS germ cell tumors. The Japanese experience. *J Neurooncol* 2001;54:311–16.

42. Matsutani M, Sano K, Takakura K, *et al.* Primary intracranial germ cell tumors: a clinical analysis of 153 histologically verified cases. *J Neurosurg* 1997;86:446–55.

43. McCarthy BJ, Shibui S, Kayama T, *et al.* Primary CNS germ cell tumors in Japan and the United States: an analysis of 4 tumor registries. *Neuro-Oncology* 2012;14:1194–1200.

44. Mei K, Liu A, Allan RW, *et al.* Diagnostic utility of SALL4 in primary germ cell tumors of the central nervous system: a study of 77 cases. *Mod Pathol* 2009;22:1628–36.

45. Millard NE, Dunkel IJ. Advances in the management of central nervous system germ cell tumors. *Curr Oncol Rep* 2014;16:393. DOI 10.2007/s11912-014-0393-1 [online publication].

46. Min KW, Scheithauer BW. Pineal germinomas and testicular seminoma. A comparative ultrastructural study with special references to early carcinomatous transformation. *Ultrastruct Pathol* 1990;14:483–96.

47. Murai Y, Kobayashi S, Mizunari T, *et al.* Spontaneous regression of a germinoma in the pineal body after placement of a ventriculoperitoneal shunt. *J Neurosurg* 2000;93:884–6.

48. Naudin ten Cate L, Vermeij-Keers C, Smit DA, *et al.* Intracranial teratoma with multiple fetuses: pre- and post-natal appearance. *Hum Pathol* 1995;26:804–7.

49. O'Callaghan AM, Katapodis O, Ellison DW, *et al.* The growing teratoma syndrome in a nongerminomatous germ cell tumor of the pineal gland. A case report and review. *Cancer* 1997;80:942–7.

50. Okada Y, Nishikawa R, Matsutani M, Louis DN. Hypomethylated X chromosome gain and rare isochromosome 12p in diverse intracranial germ cell tumors. *J Neuropathol Exp Neurol* 2002;61:531–8.

51. O'Marcaigh AS, Ledger GA, Roche PC, *et al.* Aromatase expression in human germinomas with possible biological effects. *J Clin Endocrinol Metab* 1995;80:3763–6.

52. Oosterhuis JW, Stoop H, Honecker F, Looijenga LHJ. Why human extragonadal germ cell tumours occur in the midline of the body: old concepts, new perspectives. *Int J Androl* 2007;30:256–64.

53. Osumi AM, Tien RD. MR findings of pineal yolk sac tumor in a patient with testicular embryonal carcinoma. *Clin Imaging* 1994;18:203–8.

54. Oya S, Saito A, Okano A, *et al.* The pathogenesis of intracranial growing teratoma syndrome: proliferation of tumor cells or formation of multiple expanding cysts? Two case reports and review of the literature. *Childs Nerv Syst* 2014;30:1455–61.

55. Pantazis G, Harter PN, Capper D, *et al.* The embryonic stem cell factor UTF1 serves as a reliable diagnostic marker for germinomas. *Pathology* 2014;46:225–9.

56. Peoples DM, Stern BJ, Jiji V, Sahni S. Germ cell tumors masquerading as central nervous system sarcoidosis. *Arch Neurol* 1991;48:554–6.

57. Poeze M, Herpers MJ, Tjandra B, *et al.* Intramedullary spinal teratoma presenting with urinary retention. Case report and review of the literature. *Neurosurgery* 1999;45:379–85.

58. Poremba C, Dockhorn-Dworniczak B, Merritt V, *et al.* Immature teratomas of different origin carried by a pregnant mother and her fetus. *Diagn Mol Pathol* 1993;2:131–6.

59. Rapley EA, Crockford GP, Teare D, *et al.* Localization to Xq27 of a susceptibility gene for testicular germ-cell tumours. *Nat Genet* 2000;24:197–200.

60. Rickert CH. Neuropathology and prognosis of foetal brain tumours. *Acta Neuropathol (Berl)* 1999;98:567–76.

61. Rickert CH, Paulus W. No chromosomal imbalances detected by comparative genomic hybridisation in a case of fetal immature teratoma. *Childs Nerv Syst* 2002;18:639–43.

62. Rickert CH, Simon R, Bergmann M, *et al.* Comparative genomic hybridization in pineal germ cell tumors. *J Neuropathol Exp Neurol* 2000;59:815–21.

63. Rivarola M, Belgorosky A, Mendilaharzu H, Vidal G. Precocious puberty in children with tumours of the suprasellar and pineal areas: organic central precocious puberty. *Acta Paediatr* 2001;90:751–6.

64. Rosai J, Parkash V, Reuter VE. The origin of mediastinal germ cell tumors in men. *Int J Surg Pathol* 1994;2:73–8.

65. Rosenblum MK, Nakazato Y, Matsutani M. CNS germ cell tumours. In: Louis DN, Ohgaki H, Wiestler OD, Cavenee WK eds. *WHO classification of tumours of the central nervous system.* Lyon: IARC, 2007:198–204.

66. Rostad S, Kleinschmidt-DeMasters BK, Manchester DK. Two massive congenital intracranial immature teratomas with neck extension. *Teratology* 1985;32:163–9.

67. Rueda-Pedraza ME, Heifetz SA, Sesterhenn IA, Clark GB. Primary intracranial germ cell tumors in the first two decades of life. A clinical, light-microscopic, and

immunohistochemical analysis of 54 cases. *Perspect Pediatr Pathol* 1987;**10**:160–207.

68. Rushing EJ, Sandberg GD, Judkins AR, *et al.* Germinoma: unusual imaging and pathological characteristics. *J Neurosurg* 2006(2 Suppl);**104**:143–8.

69. Saiga T, Osasa H, Hatayama H, *et al.* The origin of extragonadal teratoma: case report of an immature teratoma occurring in a prenatal brain. *Pediatr Pathol* 1991;**11**:759–70.

70. Santagata S, Hornick JL, Ligon KL. Comparative analysis of germ cell transcription factors in CNS germinoma reveals diagnostic utility of NANOG. *Am J Surg Pathol* 2006;**30**:1613–18.

71. Santagata S, Ligon KL, Hornick JL. Embryonic stem cell transcription factor signatures in the diagnosis of primary and metastatic germ cell tumors. *Am J Surg Pathol* 2007;**31**:836–45.

72. Sawamura Y, Hamou MF, Kuppner MC, de Tribolet N. Immunohistochemical and in vitro functional analysis of pineal-germinoma infiltrating lymphocytes: report of a case. *Neurosurgery* 1989;**25**:454–7.

73. Sawamura Y, Ikeda J, Shirato H, *et al.* Germ cell tumours of the central nervous system: treatment consideration based on 111 cases and their long-term clinical outcomes. *Eur J Cancer* 1998;**34**:104–10.

74. Schild SE, Scheithauer BW, Haddock MG, *et al.* Histologically confirmed pineal tumors and other germ cell tumors of the brain. *Cancer* 1996;**78**:2564–71.

75. Schlembach D, Bornemann A, Rupprecht T, Beinder E. Fetal intracranial tumors detected by ultrasound: a report of two cases and review of the literature. *Ultrasound Obstet Gynecol* 1999;**14**:407–18.

76. Schneider DT, Zahn S, Sievers S, *et al.* Molecular genetic analysis of central nervous system germ cell tumors with comparative genomic hybridization. *Mod Pathol* 2006;**19**:864–73.

77. Schwartz S, Raffel LJ, Sun CC, Waters E. An unusual mosaic karyotype detected through prenatal diagnosis with duplication of 1q and 19p and associated teratoma development. *Teratology* 1992;**46**:399–404.

78. Shaffrey ME, Lanzino G, Lopes MB, *et al.* Maturation of intracranial immature teratomas. Report of two cases. *J Neurosurg* 1996;**85**:672–6.

79. Sievers S, Alemazkour K, Zahn S, *et al.* IGF2/H19 imprinting analysis of human germ cell tumors (GCTs) using the methylation-sensitive single-nucleotide primer extension method reflects the origin of GCTs in different stages of primordial germ cell development. *Gene Chromosomes Cancer* 2005;**44**:256–64.

80. Skullerud K, Stenwig AE, Brandtzaeg P, *et al.* Intracranial primary leiomyosarcoma arising in a teratoma of the pineal area. *Clin Neuropathol* 1995;**14**:245–8.

81. Sugimoto K, Nakahara I, Nishikawa M. Bilateral metachronous germinoma of the basal ganglia occurring long after total removal of a mature pineal teratoma: case report. *Neurosurgery* 2002;**50**:613–16; discussion 616–17.

82. Suh YL, Koo H, Kim TS, *et al.* Tumors of the central nervous system in Korea: a multicenter study of 3221 cases. *J Neurooncol* 2002;**56**:251–9.

83. Sukov WR, Cheville JC, Giannini C, *et al.* Isochromosome 12p and polysomy 12 in primary central nervous system germ cell tumors: frequency and association with clinicopathologic features. *Hum Pathol* 2010;**41**:232–8.

84. Tan C, Scotting PJ. Stem cell research points the way to the cell of origin for intracranial germ cell tumours. *J Pathol* 2013;**229**:4–11.

85. Terashima K, Yu A, Chow W-Y T, *et al.* Genome-wide analysis of DNA copy number alterations and loss of heterozygosity in intracranial germ cell tumors. *Pediatr Blood Cancer* 2014;**61**:593–600.

86. Tsunoda S, Sasaoka Y, Sakaki T, *et al.* Suprasellar embryonal carcinoma which developed ten years after local radiation therapy for pineal germinoma. *Surg Neurol* 1993;**40**:146–50.

87. Utsuki S, Oka H, Sagiuchi T, *et al.* Malignant transformation of intracranial mature teratoma to yolk sac tumor after late relapse. *J Neurosurg* 2007;**106**:1067–9.

88. Valdez R, McKeever P, Finn WG, *et al.* Composite germ cell tumor and B-cell non-Hodgkin's lymphoma arising in the sella turcica. *Hum Pathol* 2002;**33**:1044–7.

89. Van Meir EG, Oosterhuis JW, Looijenga LHJ. Genesis and genetics of intracranial germ cell tumors. In: Sawamura Y, Shirato H, de Tribolet N eds. *Intracranial germ cell tumours.* New York: Springer Verlag, 1998:45–76.

90. Wang L, Yamaguchi S, Burstein MD, *et al.* Novel somatic and germline mutations in intracranial germ cell tumours. *Nature* 2014;**511**:241–5.

91. Wakai S, Segawa H, Kitahara S, *et al.* Teratoma in the pineal region in two brothers. Case reports. *J Neurosurg* 1980;**53**:239–43.

92. Wanggou S, Jiang X, Li Q, *et al.* HESRG: a novel biomarker for intracranial germinoma and embryonal carcinoma. *J Neurooncol* 2012;**106**:251–9.

93. Watanabe T, Makiyama Y, Nishimoto H, *et al.* Metachronous ovarian dysgerminoma after a suprasellar germ-cell tumor treated by radiation therapy. Case report. *J Neurosurg* 1995;**83**:149–53.

94. Wei YQ, Hang ZB, Liu KF. In situ observation of inflammatory cell–tumor cell interaction in human seminomas (germinomas): light, electron microscopic, and immunohistochemical study. *Hum Pathol* 1992;**23**:421–8.

95. Weyerts LK, Catanzarite V, Jones MC, Mendoza A. Prenatal diagnosis of a giant intracranial teratoma associated with pulmonary hypoplasia. *J Med Genet* 1993;**30**:880–2.

96. Willis SN, Mallozzi SS, Rodig SJ, *et al.* The microenvironment of germ cell tumors harbors a prominent antigen-driven humoral response. *J Immunol* 2009;**182**:3310–17.

97. Wong TT, Ho DM, Chang TK, *et al.* Familial neurofibromatosis 1 with germinoma involving the basal ganglion and thalamus. *Childs Nerv Syst* 1995;**11**:456–8.

98. Woodward PJ, Heidenreich A, Looijenga LHJ, *et al.* Germ cell tumours. In: Eble JN, Sauter G, Epstein JE, Sesterhenn IA eds. *World Health Organization classification of tumours. Pathology and genetics of tumours of the urinary system and male genital organs.* IARC Press, Lyon, 2004:221–49.

Melanocytic Tumours and Haemangioblastoma

Arie Perry

PRIMARY MELANOCYTIC LESIONS

Primary benign and malignant melanocytic lesions of the nervous system include diffuse melanosis, melanocytoma and malignant melanoma. Primary melanocytic lesions originate from melanin-containing cells found in the leptomeninges. Though widespread throughout the neuraxis, these cells are normally most prominent over the lower ventral medulla oblongata, and may be grossly visible in some individuals. Meningeal melanocytic lesions may arise in association with cutaneous melanocytic lesions, for instance large congenital naevus (see later), cellular blue naevus, and naevus of Ota (oculodermal melanocytosis).[31] The rare primary leptomeningeal melanocytic tumours should be distinguished from the more common scenario of malignant melanoma spreading to the nervous system. Immunohistochemically, melanocytic lesions are positive with 'melanosome-specific' antibodies (such as HMB-45, MART-1 or Melan-A, microphthalmia transcription factor), vimentin and S-100 protein, but it is important to recall that all tumours bearing melanosomes (e.g. melanotic schwannomas) may stain with these antibodies.

DIFFUSE MELANOSIS AND NEUROCUTANEOUS MELANOSIS

Diffuse melanosis represents a benign melanocytic proliferation, diffusely involving the leptomeninges and spreading into Virchow–Robin spaces without gross tumour formation or frank brain invasion (Figure 39.1a). It is often associated with large congenital naevi of the skin, a condition termed neurocutaneous melanosis (NCM; Touraine syndrome).

In a series of 289 patients with large congenital naevi, 33 had symptomatic central nervous system (CNS) involvement, all presenting with posterior axial skin involvement, 31 of which also showed satellite naevi.[8] Such patients are at significant risk for the development of both cutaneous and leptomeningeal melanomas. Incidental forms may also be more common than previously suspected, because magnetic resonance (MR) imaging identified intracranial melanosis in 10 (23 per cent) of 43 asymptomatic children with giant congenital naevi.[10] Nonetheless, most patients with neurocutaneous melanosis present with symptoms of increased intracranial pressure and hydrocephalus in the first two years of life; roughly half develop leptomeningeal melanoma and the prognosis is poor. NCM is thought to represent an embryologic neuroectodermal defect, potentially due to aberrant hepatocyte growth factor/scatter factor expression. Other concomitant developmental abnormalities may be encountered, especially Dandy–Walker malformation.[19,44]

PRIMARY MELANOCYTIC TUMOURS

Primary meningeal melanocytic tumours comprise a spectrum, ranging from benign melanocytomas to malignant melanomas, with rare cases having histological and clinical features of an intermediate category.[4] Most of the latter are cytologically similar to melanocytoma but demonstrate CNS parenchymal invasion and/or a moderate proliferative index.

Melanocytomas are nodular, usually leptomeningeal growths composed of bland relatively uniform appearing spindled to small epithelioid melanocytes (Figure 39.1b,c). Cells have round vesicular nuclei with small nucleoli and

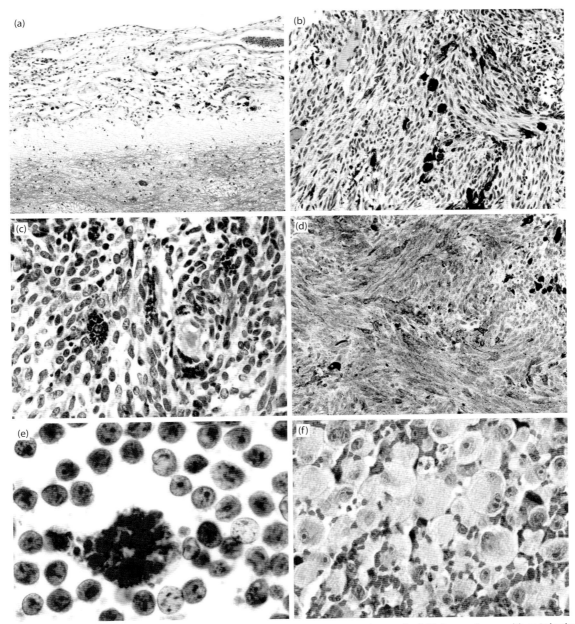

39.1 Primary melanocytic tumours. (a) Diffuse melanosis involving the leptomeninges. **(b,c)** Melanocytoma with cytologically bland spindled and scattered heavily pigmented cells. **(d)** Strong HMB-45 immunoreactivity in a melanocytoma. **(e)** Intraoperative smear from a meningeal melanoma showing malignant-appearing cells with prominent nucleoli and rare pigmented cells. **(f)** Malignant melanoma with large eosinophilic cells, vesicular nuclei, prominent nucleoli and scattered pigment.

variable cytoplasmic accumulations of melanin. However, in many, the pigment production is sufficient to impart a jet black gross appearance. Structurally, they are arranged in vague whorls, sheets, fascicles or nests, with nests being particularly characteristic. Ultrastructurally, they contain melanosomes and premelanosomes. Mitoses are rare and MIB-1 labelling indices are low (less than 1–2 per cent).[4] Although these tumours were initially mistaken in the literature for 'pigmented meningiomas', melanin is actually exceedingly rare in the latter, likely representing melanocytic colonization in such examples.[32] In the rare amelanotic forms of melanocytoma, immunoreactivity for specific melanocytic

markers (Figure 39.1d) and lack of EMA can be used to rule out meningioma. The differential diagnosis with melanotic schwannoma, however, is considerably more challenging and often relies on the presence of psammoma bodies, incorporation of neural elements, or genetic findings.[23]

Over 100 melanocytomas have been reported to date; they are typically tumours of middle-aged adults, although they can be seen at both extremes of life.[38] Roughly two-thirds occur in spinal regions, where an associated radiculopathy is common.[4] Less often, they are intracranial, particularly in the posterior fossa or Meckel's cave. The latter examples are often seen in combination with an ipsilateral naevus of Ota. Most are associated with slow growth and a protracted clinical history over several years. Prognosis is associated with extent of surgery, with most completely resected examples being cured. However, radiation therapy may reduce the risk of recurrence in subtotally resected cases and intermediate grade melanocytic tumours. Rare examples of malignant transformation to melanoma have also been reported.[46]

In contrast, malignant melanomas are usually overtly anaplastic. They grow either diffusely (meningeal melanomatosis) or in a nodular fashion. The cells tend to be large, polygonal, epithelioid or spindled, often with bizarre multinucleated giant cells and large, red nucleoli (Figure 39.1e,f). The cytoplasm may be replete with or completely devoid of pigment; as in other sites of the body, amelanotic variants are more diagnostically challenging. Useful immunohistochemical markers include S-100 protein, HMB-45 and Melan-A. Malignant melanomas have high mitotic counts and MIB-1 proliferation indices, one study showing mean mitotic and MIB-1 indices of 5.7 per 10 HPF and 8.1 per cent, respectively.[4] Necrosis and CNS invasion are common. Malignant melanomas occur at all ages, although most childhood cases are associated with neurocutaneous melanosis. These tumours usually follow an aggressive course, with most resected lesions recurring and leading to death. Nevertheless, the prognosis of primary meningeal melanoma appears to be better than metastatic melanoma, particularly if it is localized and complete resection is possible.[11]

Meningeal melanocytic neoplasms, especially melanocytomas, show considerable morphologic and genetic overlap with blue naevi, the latter including common mutations of the GNAQ and GNA11 genes.[23,30] As already stated, such mutations are useful for distinguishing these tumours from melanotic schwannomas.

HAEMANGIOBLASTOMAS

Haemangioblastomas ('capillary haemangioblastomas' or Lindau tumour) are benign, highly vascular, often cystic tumours. Although they are primarily parenchymal tumours, they may also be closely associated with the meninges. Although their histogenesis has long been controversial, recent data suggest derivation from a pluripotent mesodermal stem cell that can differentiate towards endothelial and haematopoietic cells. Haemangioblastomas may be single or multiple. The combination with angiomatosis of the retina (von Hippel's disease) forms the classic association of von Hippel–Lindau disease, a condition that may also encompass tumours and cysts of the kidneys, liver, pancreas and adrenals (see Chapter 44, Hereditary Tumour Syndromes).

Epidemiology

Haemangioblastomas account for roughly 1 to 2 per cent of intracranial and 7 per cent of posterior fossa neoplasms. Incidence is similar in men and women. Although occurring in children and the elderly, the peak incidence is between 35 and 45 years of age. Rare congenital examples have been

reported.[18] Approximately 25 per cent occur in the setting of von Hippel–Lindau disease, typically at a younger age of onset than sporadic counterparts; indeed, a haemangioblastoma in a young patient should prompt a careful workup for familial disease. In fact, all haemangioblastoma patients should undergo genetic testing, because germline VHL mutations are not uncommon, even in those failing to meet strict clinical criteria.[12,43]

The vast majority of sporadic haemangioblastomas develop in the cerebellum, although fourth ventricular (most often in the area postrema), brain stem and supratentorial cases are also reported.[28,50] Two series combining 254 von Hippel–Lindau patients reported frequencies of 43–65 per cent in the cerebellum, 24–40 per cent in the spinal cord, 10–12 per cent in the brain stem, and up to 1 per cent in the pituitary.[1,20] Other unusual locations include suprasellar region, spinal nerve roots, peripheral nerve, and even kidney, adrenal gland, soft tissue and bone;[7,9,29,34–37,47] such cases are often, but not invariably familial haemangioblastomas.

Radiology and Macroscopic Appearances

Haemangioblastomas are well-circumscribed, but unencapsulated masses. Their size varies from <1 cm to large tumours occupying most of the cerebellar hemisphere (Figure 39.2a). They are usually cystic and the cysts may be multiple and of various sizes. Most frequently, a single large cyst is associated with a solid mural nodule that enhances avidly on post-contrast neuroimaging studies. This solid component may undergo alternating periods of growth and stability, with symptoms commonly related to cyst enlargement and surrounding oedema.[42,45] The cyst content may be clear, but is often rust coloured from previous haemorrhages. The cut surface is often red to yellow because of foci of hypervascularity and high lipid contents respectively (Figure 39.2b). Angiography often highlights the highly vascular nature and demonstrates feeder vessels, mostly from the internal carotid or vertebral arterial circulations. This hypervascularity often becomes all too apparent to neurosurgeons attempting to maintain haemostasis, a challenge that then translates to the pathologist struggling to make a frozen section diagnosis on a highly cauterized specimen.

Light and Electron Microscopic Appearances

Histologically, the solid part of the tumour is formed by blood vessels of various calibre lined by a single layer of endothelium (Figure 39.2c,d). The space between the vascular channels is filled with stromal cells, which represent the principal neoplastic component. These may be relatively sparse and evenly distributed around the rich capillary meshwork (the reticular variant) or form large contiguous sheets of clear epithelioid cells (the cellular variant). Small foci of extramedullary haematopoiesis are seen in roughly 10 per cent of cases (Figure 39.2e). Stromal cells generally have bland, oval to bizarre, degenerate appearing, hyperchromatic nuclei with ample, vacuolated, clear cytoplasm containing lipid and glycogen accumulations (Figure 39.2d). The lipid is readily demonstrated in non-processed specimens by oil red O and toluidine blue

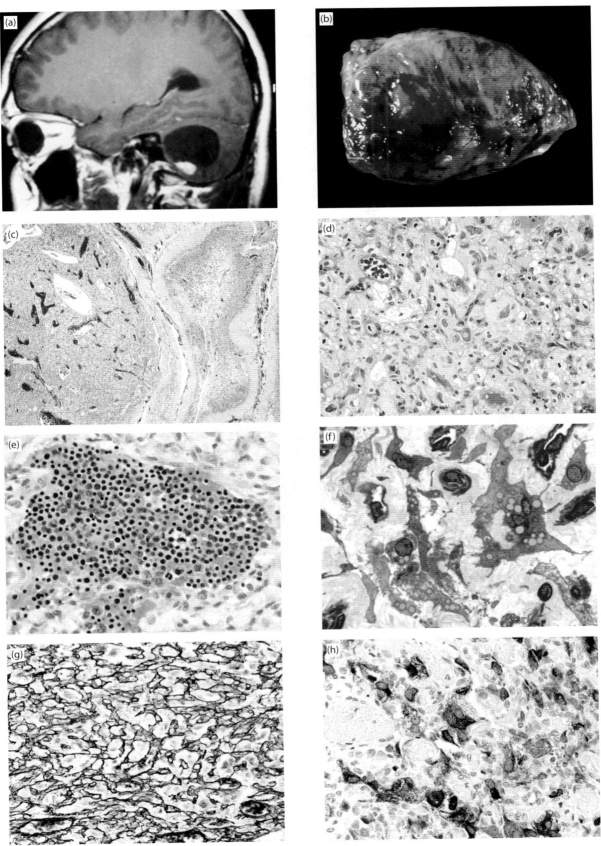

39.2 Haemangioblastoma. (a) Sagittal T1-weighted magnetic resonance image with gadolinium showing a cystic cerebellar mass with an enhancing mural nodule. **(b)** Surgical specimen showing red hypervascular and yellow lipid-rich regions on cut surface. **(c)** There is a sharp demarcation between the tumour (left) and the adjacent cerebellum (right). **(d)** Foamy stromal cells with scattered atypical nuclei are seen in association with a rich vascular network. **(e)** Extramedullary haematopoiesis. **(f)** Lipid vacuoles are evident in this toluidine blue-stained plastic section. **(g)** Rich reticulin network. **(h)** Inhibin alpha immunoreactive stromal cells.

stains (Figure 39.2f), which can be helpful for intraoperative diagnosis. However, with frozen section artefacts, stromal cells often appear fibrillar, often prompting the consideration of astrocytic neoplasms. The common finding of piloid gliosis with Rosenthal fibres at the edge exacerbates this mimicry further. Therefore, a high index of suspicion, attention to the prominent vascularity, and correlation with clinicoradiologic findings are key to proper diagnosis. In addition, there are often reactive astrocytes, mast cells and macrophages, often with haemosiderin ingested from previous microhaemorrhages. Mitotic activity is scant. The tumour is rich in reticulin, not only around blood vessels, but also outlining groups of tumour cells (Figure 39.2g).

Electron microscopy reveals three cell types: endothelial cells lining vascular channels, pericytes immediately outside the basal lamina, and stromal cells.[41] The latter contain lipid droplets and bundles of delicate filaments.

Immunohistochemistry

Immunohistochemistry has been used to address the issues of histogenesis and diagnosis of haemangioblastomas, but the findings have been controversial. For instance, variable GFAP positivity has been reported in stromal cells of some haemangioblastomas. Such cells appear to be significantly more common in the cellular variant.[15] Moreover, stromal cells occasionally show weak cytoplasmic synaptophysin positivity, a finding of unclear significance. Stromal cells are more consistently immunoreactive for neuron specific enolase (NSE) and S-100 protein, although these markers lack specificity.[27] Instead, inhibin alpha (Figure 39.2h), D2-40 (podoplanin) and brachyury have been touted as more reliable markers, particularly in the differential with the characteristically immunonegative metastatic renal cell carcinoma; in contrast, the latter are usually positive for EMA, cytokeratin, CD10, RCC, PAX8 and PAX2.[2,5,14,16,40]

Molecular Biology and Histogenesis

Molecular biological investigations, relating to the association of haemangioblastomas with von Hippel–Lindau disease, have provided the most convincing evidence for the stromal cell being the primary neoplastic cell. The responsible VHL gene is located on chromosome 3p26-p25.[24] The gene acts as a tumour suppressor in both inherited and sporadic haemangioblastomas, with either germline or somatic VHL mutations occurring in combination with allelic loss of 3p; however, whereas this gene is implicated in virtually all familial cases, its inactivation is demonstrable in only 20–50 per cent of sporadic examples.[25] Additional genes may be involved, with further regions of loss on chromosomes 6q and 22q.[3,25]

The VHL gene (see Chapter 44, Hereditary Tumour Syndromes) encodes a protein, designated pVHL, which is widely expressed and functions to regulate transcriptional elongation, mRNA stability and protein degradation. During development, it is involved in neuronal but not glial differentiation.[21] The hypoxia inducible factors (HIF), especially the alpha subunits, are regulated by pVHL and in the absence of the latter, angiogenic and erythropoietic factors, such as VEGF, PDGF-β, GLUT-1, and erythropoietin are upregulated even in normoxic conditions. These molecular changes potentially account for common findings, such as hypervascularity and extramedullary haematopoiesis in haemangioblastomas (Figure 39.2e), as well as polycythemia in haemangioblastoma patients.[13,22]

Whereas histogenesis has long been controversial and often favoured either a glial or endothelial origin, data now suggest that the neoplastic stromal cells represent pluripotent but committed mesodermal stem cells with features of true 'haemangioblasts'.[26,49] This notion is supported by the expression of early developmental markers (e.g. CD133 and OCT4 positive, but SOX2 and Nanog negative) not only on neoplastic stromal cells, but also within intratumoural endothelial cells, erythrocytes, granulocytes and mast cells; additionally, VHL deficiency has also been found within these same cell types.

Prognosis

Haemangioblastomas are benign (WHO grade I) tumours. Most present as asymptomatic masses, grow in a stuttering fashion, and never require therapy.[1] However, postresection recurrence in up to 25 per cent of cases and spontaneous intratumoural haemorrhage cause significant morbidity and mortality, particularly in patients with von Hippel–Lindau disease.[12] Recurrences have been correlated with younger age (under 30 years at the time of diagnosis), von Hippel–Lindau syndrome, and the presence of multicentricity at initial diagnosis. Histologically, the cellular variant has also been associated with higher recurrence rates.[15] Polycythemia can result from erythropoietin production by the tumour cells. This erythrocytosis may abate after resection, although its reappearance often signals tumour recurrence.[4] Moreover, despite its generally benign histology and behaviour, disseminated subarachnoid spread occurs in rare examples, a condition known as haemangioblastomatosis; the prognosis in such cases is poor.[39,48] In von Hippel–Lindau disease, haemangioblastomas and renal cell carcinomas are the two main causes of premature death.[33]

Differential Diagnosis

The most frequent differential diagnostic consideration is metastatic clear cell renal carcinoma, particularly in patients with von Hippel–Lindau disease, who are predisposed to both tumour types. In most cases, the structural patterns, as well as the differential staining of EMA, cytokeratin, CD10, RCC, PAX2 and PAX8 in renal cell carcinomas *versus* inhibin, brachyury, D2-40, S-100 protein and NSE in haemangioblastoma clearly distinguish these two tumours. Nevertheless, renal cell carcinoma metastatic to haemangioblastoma also occurs rarely and may represent a particular diagnostic challenge.[17] In cases that involve the overlying meninges, the differential may also include angiomatous meningioma, although the latter is typically EMA positive and inhibin negative.

REFERENCES

1. Ammerman JM, Lonser RR, Dambrosia J, et al. Long-term natural history of hemangioblastomas in patients with von Hippel–Lindau disease: implications for treatment. *J Neurosurg* 2006;**105**:248–55.

2. Barresi V, Vitarelli E, Branca G, et al. Expression of brachyury in hemangioblastoma: potential use in differential diagnosis. *Am J Surg Pathol* 2012;**36**:1052–7.

3. Beckner ME, Sasatomi E, Swalsky PA, et al. Loss of heterozygosity reveals non-VHL allelic loss in hemangioblastomas at 22q13. *Hum Pathol* 2004;**35**:1105–11.

4. Brat DJ, Giannini C, Scheithauer BW, Burger PC. Primary melanocytic neoplasms of the central nervous systems. *Am J Surg Pathol* 1999;**23**:745–54.

5. Carney EM, Banerjee P, Ellis CL, et al. PAX2(-)/PAX8(-)/inhibin A(+) immunoprofile in hemangioblastoma: a helpful combination in the differential diagnosis with metastatic clear cell renal cell carcinoma to the central nervous system. *Am J Surg Pathol* 2011;**35**:262–7.

6. Chishti MK, Bannister CM. Foci of extramedullary haemopoiesis in a cerebellar haemangioblastoma. *Br J Neurosurg* 1992;**6**:157–62.

7. Deb P, Pal S, Dutta V, et al. Adrenal haemangioblastoma presenting as phaeochromocytoma: a rare manifestation of extraneural hemangioblastoma. *Endocrine Pathology* 2012;**23**:187–90.

8. DeDavid M, Orlow SJ, Provost N, et al. Neurocutaneous melanosis: clinical features of large congenital melanocytic nevi in patients with manifest central nervous system melanosis. *J Am Acad Dermatol* 1996;**35**:529–38.

9. Escott EJ, Kleinschmidt-DeMasters BK, Brega K, Lillehei KO. Proximal nerve root spinal hemangioblastomas: presentation of three cases, MR appearance, and literature review. *Surg Neurol* 2004;**61**:262–73, discussion 73.

10. Foster RD, Williams ML, Barkovich AJ, et al. Giant congenital melanocytic nevi: the significance of neurocutaneous melanosis in neurologically asymptomatic children. *Plast Reconstr Surg* 2001;**107**:933–41.

11. Freudenstein D, Wagner A, Bornemann A, et al. Primary melanocytic lesions of the CNS: report of five cases. *Zentralbl Neurochir* 2004;**65**:146–53.

12. Glasker S. Central nervous system manifestations in VHL: genetics, pathology and clinical phenotypic features. *Fam Cancer* 2005;**4**:37–42.

13. Glasker S, Kruger MT, Klingler JH, et al. Hemangioblastomas and neurogenic polyglobulia. *Neurosurgery* 2013;**72**:930–5.

14. Gurses I, Scheithauer BW. Inhibin-A immunoreactivity in nervous system lesions. *Appl Immunohistochem Molec Morphol* 2012;**20**:277–84.

15. Hasselblatt M, Jeibmann A, Gerss J, et al. Cellular and reticular variants of haemangioblastoma revisited: a clinicopathologic study of 88 cases. *Neuropathol Appl Neurobiol* 2005;**31**:618–22.

16. Ingold B, Wild PJ, Nocito A, et al. Renal cell carcinoma marker reliably discriminates central nervous system haemangioblastoma from brain metastases of renal cell carcinoma. *Histopathology* 2008;**52**:674–81.

17. Jarrell ST, Vortmeyer AO, Linehan WM, et al. Metastases to hemangioblastomas in von Hippel–Lindau disease. *J Neurosurg* 2006;**105**:256–63.

18. Johnson MD, Mitchell AR, Troup EC, et al. Congenital cystic hemangioblastomas of the cerebral hemisphere in a neonate without alteration in the VHL gene. *Pediatr Neurosurg* 2004;**40**:124–7.

19. Kang SG, Yoo DS, Cho KS, et al. Coexisting intracranial meningeal melanocytoma, dermoid tumor, and Dandy–Walker cyst in a patient with neurocutaneous melanosis. Case report. *J Neurosurg* 2006;**104**:444–7.

20. Kanno H, Kuratsu J, Nishikawa R, et al. Clinical features of patients bearing central nervous system hemangioblastoma in von Hippel–Lindau disease. *Acta Neurochir* 2013;**155**:1–7.

21. Kanno H, Saljooque F, Yamamoto I, et al. Role of the von Hippel–Lindau tumor suppressor protein during neuronal differentiation. *Cancer Res* 2000;**60**:2820–4.

22. Kim WY, Kaelin WG. Role of VHL gene mutation in human cancer. *J Clin Oncol* 2004;**22**:4991–5004.

23. Kusters-Vandevelde HV, van Engen-van Grunsven IA, Kusters B, et al. Improved discrimination of melanotic schwannoma from melanocytic lesions by combined morphological and GNAQ mutational analysis. *Acta Neuropathol* 2010;**120**:755–64.

24. Latif F, Tory K, Gnarra J, et al. Identification of the von Hippel–Lindau disease tumor suppressor gene. *Science* 1993;**260**:1317–20.

25. Lemeta S, Pylkkanen L, Sainio M, et al. Loss of heterozygosity at 6q is frequent and concurrent with 3p loss in sporadic and familial capillary hemangioblastomas. *J Neuropathol Exp Neurol* 2004;**63**:1072–9.

26. Merrill MJ, Edwards NA, Lonser RR. Hemangioblastoma-associated mast cells in von Hippel–Lindau disease are tumor derived. *Blood* 2013;**121**:859–60.

27. Miller CR, Perry A. News in brief. Immunohistochemical differentiation of hemangioblastoma from metastatic clear cell renal carcinoma: an update. *Adv Anat Pathol* 2004;**11**:325–6.

28. Mills SA, Oh MC, Rutkowski MJ, et al. Supratentorial hemangioblastoma: clinical features, prognosis, and predictive value of location for von Hippel–Lindau disease. *Neuro-oncology* 2012;**14**:1097–104.

29. Mitchell A, Scheithauer BW, Wharen RE, et al. Hemangioblastoma of spinal nerve: a report of six cases. *Clin Neuropathol* 2013;**32**:91–9.

30. Murali R, Wiesner T, Rosenblum MK, Bastian BC. GNAQ and GNA11 mutations in melanocytomas of the central nervous system. *Acta Neuropathol* 2012;**123**:457–9.

31. Navas M, Pascual JM, Fraga J, et al. Intracranial intermediate-grade meningeal melanocytoma with increased cellular proliferative index: an illustrative case associated with a nevus of Ota. *J Neurooncol* 2009;**95**:105–15.

32. Nestor SL, Perry A, Kurtkaya O, et al. Melanocytic colonization of a meningothelial meningioma: histopathological and ultrastructural findings with immunohistochemical and genetic correlation: case report. *Neurosurgery* 2003;**53**:211–14, discussion 4–5.

33. Niemela M, Lemeta S, Summanen P, et al. Long-term prognosis of haemangioblastoma of the CNS: impact of von Hippel–Lindau disease. *Acta Neurochir (Wien)* 1999;**141**:1147–56.

34. Nonaka D, Rodriguez J, Rosai J. Extraneural hemangioblastoma: a report of 5 cases. *Am J Surg Pathol* 2007;**31**:1545–51.

35. Panelos J, Beltrami G, Capanna R, Franchi A. Primary capillary hemangioblastoma of bone: report of a case arising in the sacrum. *Int J Surg Pathol* 2010;**18**:580–3.

36. Patton KT, Satcher RL, Jr., Laskin WB. Capillary hemangioblastoma of soft tissue: report of a case and review of the literature. *Hum Pathol* 2005;**36**:1135–9.

37. Peker S, Kurtkaya-Yapicier O, Sun I, et al. Suprasellar haemangioblastoma. Report of two cases and review of the literature. *J Clin Neurosci* 2005;**12**:85–9.

38. Rades D, Schild SE, Tatagiba M, et al. Therapy of meningeal melanocytomas. *Cancer* 2004;**100**:2442–7.

39. Reyes-Botero G, Gallego Perez-Larraya J, Sanson M. Sporadic CNS hemangioblastomatosis, response to sunitinib and secondary polycythemia. *J Neuro-oncol* 2012;**107**:439–40.

40. Rivera AL, Takei H, Zhai J, et al. Useful immunohistochemical markers in differentiating hemangioblastoma versus metastatic renal cell carcinoma. *Neuropathology* 2010;**30**:580–5.

41. Russell DS, Rubinstein JL. *Pathology of tumours of the nervous system*, 5th edn. London: Edward Arnold, 1989.

42. Slater A, Moore NR, Huson SM. The natural history of cerebellar hemangioblastomas in von Hippel–Lindau disease. *AJNR Am J Neuroradiol* 2003;**24**:1570–4.

43. Sora S, Ueki K, Saito N, et al. Incidence of von Hippel–Lindau disease in hemangioblastoma patients: the University of Tokyo Hospital experience from 1954–1998. *Acta Neurochir (Wien)* 2001;**143**:893–6.

44. Walbert T, Sloan AE, Cohen ML, Koubeissi MZ. Symptomatic neurocutaneous melanosis and Dandy–Walker malformation in an adult. *J Clin Oncol* 2009;**27**:2886–7.

45. Wanebo JE, Lonser RR, Glenn GM, Oldfield EH. The natural history of hemangioblastomas of the central nervous system in patients with von Hippel–Lindau disease. *J Neurosurg* 2003;**98**:82–94.

46. Wang F, Qiao G, Lou X, Song X, Chen W. Malignant transformation of intracranial meningeal melanocytoma. Case report and review of the literature. *Neuropathology* 2011;**31**:414–20.

47. Wang Y, Wei C, Mou L, et al. Sporadic renal haemangioblastoma: case report and review of the literature. *Oncol Lett* 2013;**5**:360–2.

48. Weil RJ, Vortmeyer AO, Zhuang Z, et al. Clinical and molecular analysis of disseminated hemangioblastomatosis of the central nervous system in patients without von Hippel–Lindau disease. Report of four cases. *J Neurosurg* 2002;**96**:775–87.

49. Welten CM, Keats EC, Ang LC, Khan ZA. Hemangioblastoma stromal cells show committed stem cell phenotype. *Can J Neurol Sci* 2012;**39**:821–7.

50. Zhou LF, Du G, Mao Y, Zhang R. Diagnosis and surgical treatment of brainstem hemangioblastomas. *Surg Neurol* 2005;**63**:307–15, discussion 15–16.

Lymphomas and Haemopoietic Neoplasms

Martina Deckert

INTRODUCTION

The central nervous system (CNS) is affected by a wide variety of haematopoietic tumours. The term 'lymphoma' in the CNS comprises several entities that differ fundamentally in their clinical manifestation, course of disease, prognosis, morphology and underlying pathogenesis. They are strongly associated with specific clinical features, among which the immune status is of particular relevance. Careful examination to precisely classify lymphoma is a prerequisite for subsequent patient management requiring an interdisciplinary approach of neurologists, stereotactic neurosurgeons, haematologists, neuropathologists and molecular geneticists. Importantly, primary CNS lymphoma (PCNSL) has to be distinguished from systemic lymphoma secondarily spreading to the CNS, which may affect the CNS either exclusively or as part of multiorgan involvement.

PRIMARY CNS LYMPHOMA

Introduction

Primary CNS lymphoma (PCNSL) is defined as lymphoma confined to the CNS, i.e. brain parenchyma, spinal cord, eyes, the most proximal parts of the cranial nerves, and/or meninges. Establishment of diagnosis requires a comprehensive search for exclusion of extracerebral lymphoma manifestation.

Historically, the concept of a haematopoietic tumour that not only involves the CNS but also develops within the CNS has been a matter of debate for decades. Meanwhile, the haematogenous derivation of PCNSL is unequivocally accepted. PCNSL is considered a specific entity in both the current WHO Classification of Tumours of Haematopoietic and Lymphoid Tissues[72] and the WHO Classification of Tumours of the Nervous System,[37] highlighting its unique position bridging the nervous and immune systems.

Classification

PCNSLs are characterized not only by distinctive clinical, morphological, immunophenotypic, genetic and molecular features, but also by their location in the CNS, which differs from other organs, particularly lymphoid organs, in several aspects relevant for lymphomagenesis. The majority (approximately 98 per cent) are diffuse large B cell lymphoma (DLBCL), and the term PCNSL specifically refers to this subtype.[72]

The remaining minor fraction of primaries developing in the CNS corresponds to T-cell lymphomas (2 per cent), which are dealt with under Primary T-cell Lymphoma of the CNS, p. 1864.

Epidemiology

The incidence of PCNSL increased significantly over the latter part of the twentieth century but has levelled off or decreased slightly more recently. In 1989, PCNSL peaked at 6.6 per cent of all primary brain neoplasms both in immunocompetent and in immunocompromised patients.[94] Currently, it is estimated to account for 1 per cent of all lymphomas, 4–6 per cent of all extranodal lymphomas and 2.4–3 per cent of all CNS tumours (range, 1–5 per cent).[27,38,45,141] It has been debated whether this initial increase, at least in part, reflected improved diagnostic sensitivity using histological and molecular biological techniques, in particular when comparing the immunohistochemistry to the pre-immunohistochemistry era. Different classification systems used over time may also have accounted for divergent data. Finally, comparison of incidence rates reported in 2011 with those before 1978[94] raises the intriguing question of whether there is a decline towards incidence rates noticed before the acquired immunodeficiency syndrome (AIDS) era. This view is supported by a recent analysis of cases identified from the Surveillance, Epidemiology, and End Results research data set over the period of 1980 to 2008, which revealed an annual incidence rate of 0.47 per 100 000 person-years.[158] The incidence was significantly higher in males than in females, in blacks up to the age of 48 years at diagnosis as compared to whites, as well as for whites aged 50 years or greater at diagnosis. Overall, race did not affect incidence rates. The increase in incidence of PCNSL in patients of advanced age (≥75 years) is similar to the general increase of extracerebral DLBCL in this age group,[110] perhaps reflecting diminished immuno-surveillance and/or increasing genetic alterations in B lymphocytes in aged persons.

PCNSL manifests at all ages, peaking during the fifth to seventh decade with a median age of 60 years in immunocompetent patients and a male to female ratio of 3:2.[37,45] Nonetheless, PCNSL is very rare in paediatric patients. Children with congenital or acquired immune defects are at increased risk, although it also occurs in immunocompetent children. Between 1978 and 2008, a large retrospective study from 10 centres in three countries identified 29 paediatric cases with the diagnosis of PCNSL; median age was 14 years (range 2–21 years) with a male to female ratio of 2.6:1.[1] Neuropathologically, however, not all of these tumours were PCNSL but rather a mixture of DLBCL (20 patients, 69 per cent), anaplastic large T cell lymphoma (5 patients, 17 per cent), lymphoblastic lymphoma (2 patients, 7 per cent) and Burkitt-like lymphoma (2 patients, 7 per cent). Thus, these data cannot be compared directly with those obtained in adults. Interestingly, outcome was better in this paediatric age group,[1] which may, at least in part, be a result of a lack of further coexisting or underlying diseases of the brain and other organs, as occur more frequently in older patients. In this regard, it is of note that age (<60 years) unequivocally has been identified as an important prognostic factor in adult PCNSL patients.[124]

PCNSL, like other lymphomas, occurs with increased frequency in the setting of immunodeficiency, both primary and secondary, irrespective of patient age (Table 40.1).[51]

TABLE 40.1 Patient features predisposing to lymphoma

Immune deficiency
- HIV infection
- Ataxia-telangiectasia
- Wiskott–Aldrich syndrome
- IgA deficiency

Autoimmune disorders
- Systemic lupus erythematosus
- Sjögren's disease

Patients with iatrogenic immunosuppression
- Organ transplantation
- Autoimmune disorders of the peripheral nervous system
  - Autoimmune polyneuropathy
  - Polymyositis
  - Myasthenia gravis
- Rheumatoid arthritis
- Multiple sclerosis with natalizumab treatment?

Among immunosuppressed patients, human immunodeficiency virus (HIV)-infected patients are particularly prone to developing PCNSL. AIDS is associated with a 3600-fold increased incidence of PCNSL as compared with the general population.[52] In AIDS patients, PCNSL is the most frequent brain tumour[123] accounting for 15 per cent of HIV-associated lymphomas.[49] Nevertheless, its incidence has declined from 1989 to 2003,[54] which is mainly to be attributed to the introduction of highly active antiretroviral therapy (HAART) in 1996.[52] Among AIDS patients, the male to female ratio is 10:1; the mean age ranges between 30 and 40 years with a median age of 41 years, which is significantly below the median age of immunocompetent patients.[52] Ninety-six per cent of the patients are younger than 65 years. PCNSL has to be distinguished from opportunistic infections such as toxoplasma encephalitis and progressive multifocal leukoencephalopathy (PML). Of note, though, PCNSL and toxoplasma encephalitis occasionally coexist in AIDS patients.[153] Characteristically, PCNSL manifests late in AIDS when CD4 T-cell counts are extremely low.[152] This clinical observation indicates that the degree of immunosuppression plays a pathogenetic role, with T cell–mediated immunosurveillance of the CNS being critical,[81] and highlights fundamental differences not only in the clinical characteristics but also in the underlying pathogenesis in PCNSL of immunocompetent and immunodeficient patients.

In addition to HIV infection, other primary immunodeficiency states have to be considered. Autoimmune diseases including Sjögren's disease and systemic lupus erythematosus predispose to lymphoma, as do rare disorders including ataxia-telangiectasia, the Wiskott–Aldrich syndrome, and IgA deficiency. Because of the growing numbers of therapeutically immunosuppressed patients, including organ transplant patients, increased vigilance in surveillance has been recommended to prevent this complication or to treat it early when it occurs. Elderly patients who have been treated with a variety of immunosuppressive drugs for different autoimmune disorders, including autoimmune polyneuropathy, polymyositis, myasthenia gravis, and rheumatoid arthritis, similarly have an increased risk of developing Epstein-Barr virus (EBV)-associated PCNSL.[71] In addition, EBV-associated DLBCL of the elderly may manifest in the CNS in the absence of obvious immunodeficiency (discussed further in later sections). Recently, two multiple sclerosis patients developed (EBV-negative) PCNSL after natalizumab treatment. However, the issue is still unresolved whether natalizumab, which reduces lymphocyte trafficking to the CNS, is responsible for PCNSL or whether in these patients PCNSL is unrelated, occurring incidentally.[36,128,147]

Clinical Characteristics

In general, PCNSL may affect the entire neuraxis; thus, symptoms vary considerably among patients. Common presentations include cognitive dysfunction, psychomotor slowing, personality changes and disorientation; focal symptoms and increased intracranial pressure affect approximately half, whereas brain stem and cerebellar signs, cranial nerve dysfunction, and seizures are present only in a minority.[123,141] Ocular involvement, i.e. vitreous, retina, and optic nerves, occurs in 10–20 per cent of patients; however, visual complaints, mostly presenting as floaters or blurred vision, are reported in only half the patients.[11,65] Patients with meningeal involvement present with cranial nerve palsy.

Diagnosis

Neuroimaging

Neuroimaging is important in diagnostic work-up and reveals intracranial space-occupying diffuse, single or multifocal mass lesions. Magnetic resonance imaging (MRI) is the most sensitive procedure, demonstrating hypointense lesions on T1- and iso- to hypointense T2-weighted images with variable oedema and dense contrast enhancement.[78,141] Although typically deep and periventricular, meningeal enhancement is seen in 10–20 per cent.[78] In patients with meningeal lymphoma involvement, MRI shows diffuse meningeal and cranial nerve enhancement, and, later in the course of disease, enhancement of the cervical roots and the cauda equina. Unifocal parenchymal lesions on MRI in older patients (>60 years) should raise the rare differential diagnosis of sentinel lesions, i.e. demyelinating lesions preceding or associated with PCNSL (see later). A diagnostic role for ^{18}F-fluorodeoxyglucose (FDG) positron emission tomography (PET) has not been established.

Cerebrospinal Fluid Analysis

Cerebrospinal fluid (CSF) analysis can be useful in diagnostic work-up. In the minority of patients with leptomeningeal involvement, the CSF may harbour blasts, frequently mixed with reactive lymphocytes and monocytes. However, CSF often shows only a non-specific lymphomonocytic pleocytosis without lymphoma cells. In patients with meningeal seeding, detection of blasts may require repeat lumbar puncture. Based on CSF analysis, leptomeningeal involvement is diagnosed in approximately 18 per cent of patients;[48] interestingly, these patients only rarely have any symptoms suggestive of subarachnoid infiltration. However, depending on the quality of CSF preservation up to the date of analysis and the comprehensiveness of the morphological techniques employed (application of immunohistochemistry or not), wide ranges in the frequency of meningeal lymphoma cell dissemination have been reported in patients with PCNSL (7–42 per cent).[70] Fluorescence-activated cell sorting (FACS) analysis of CSF samples from 30 patients with PCNSL and 7 patients with secondary CNS lymphoma detected lymphoma cells in 29.7 per cent, with FACS being superior to conventional cytopathology alone.[144] However, CSF immunohistochemistry improves sensitivity considerably.

Polymerase chain reaction (PCR) analysis of the CDR3 region of the IGH gene without sequencing identified a monoclonal B cell population in the CSF of 6 of 37 (16 per cent) patients.[70] However, sequencing of PCR products is required to definitely establish monoclonality.

Recently, elevated CSF levels of miR-21, miR-19 and miR-92a were observed in PCNSL, which were reported to differentiate PCNSL from inflammatory and other CNS disorders.[11] However, their definite role and usefulness in the diagnostic work-up of PCNSL still needs to be investigated further.

In AIDS-associated PCNSL, detection of EBV in the CSF has been inferred as evidence of lymphoma.[16,29,30,62] EBV DNA was detected in 35 of 36 (97 per cent) of HIV-infected patients with PCNSL.[30] Sensitivity and specificity of EBV PCR in lumbar CSF were 80 and 100 per cent, respectively, in HIV-infected patients with PCNSL; thus, PCR for EBV would have allowed a correct diagnosis in 63.2 per cent of AIDS patients with PCNSL and would have excluded the diagnosis in 76.3 per cent of patients without lymphoma.[29] In contrast, in a study of 26 HIV-infected patients with brain disease, PCR detected EBV DNA in the CSF of seven patients, although only two of them actually had PCNSL, thereby revealing the positive predictive value for establishing the diagnosis of PCNSL in HIV-infected patients to be only 29 per cent with a specificity of 79 per cent.[62] Thus, these studies allow the conclusion that CSF analysis including cytomorphology, immunohistochemistry and even PCR with detection of a monoclonal B-cell population does not substitute for biopsy with morphological analysis of the tumour. Because AIDS patients may concomitantly harbour PCNSL and opportunistic CNS infections,[153] the mere demonstration of EBV in the cerebrospinal fluid (CSF) is not sufficient, and definite diagnosis should be established by neuropathological analysis of a tumour biopsy.

Neurosurgery

The diagnostic procedure of choice is stereotactic biopsy. Surgical resection does not contribute to disease control[14] and may lead to further, possibly devastating, neurological symptoms. Thus, surgical resection is not recommended. Importantly, steroid application should be strictly avoided and withheld prior to biopsy, because the lymphoma may wane, thus impairing or even preventing diagnosis. Establishment of diagnosis on tissue samples is a *sine qua non* for subsequent therapy and should be obtained if possible. Only in patients with very poor performance status and typical neuroimaging should therapy be introduced without a tissue diagnosis.

Neuropathology
Morphology
Macroscopy

PCNSL may involve the brain parenchyma, spinal cord, eye, proximal parts of the cranial nerves and meninges. The majority of cases present supratentorially (60 per cent), affecting the frontal, temporal, parietal and occipital lobes in 15, 8, 7 and 3 per cent, respectively.[37] Manifestation in the basal ganglia and periventricular brain parenchyma account for 10 per cent, with the corpus callosum involved in 3 per cent. Posterior fossa presentation is seen in 13 per cent, whereas the spinal cord is affected in only 1 per cent.[37] A single tumour is encountered in 60–70 per cent of patients, with multicentric disease in the remainder. Virtually all immunosuppressed patients have multiple lesions at initial presentation.[38] The meninges may be involved; however, exclusive meningeal manifestation is unusual.

Space-occupying mass lesions are poorly demarcated, frequently localizing to the cerebral hemispheres (often bihemispheric), the periventricular brain tissue, the basal ganglia and deep white matter. Lesions are typically grey to yellow and fleshy and may harbour focal haemorrhages and necrosis, especially in immunosuppression-associated cases. Tumour masses may bulge into the ventricles, narrowing the ventricular system, and infiltrate the ependyma and subependymal brain tissue. Based on macroscopy, the most important differential diagnosis is glioblastoma, which may look similar but is typically more heterogeneous and necrotic.

The leptomeninges may be involved throughout the entire neuraxis, including the spinal cord and cauda equina. Detection of meningeal infiltration by lymphoma cells may not be simple because, macroscopically, involved leptomeninges may appear normal. Therefore, in autopsy cases, careful and comprehensive investigation of multiple meningeal specimens is required to detect meningeal lymphomatosis. More prominent infiltration by blasts may yield cloudy, greyish or white meninges, thus raising the differential diagnosis of infectious meningitis.

Microscopy

PCNSLs are characterized by a combination of solid sheets, diffuse patternless infiltration and angiocentric growth patterns, the latter including not only perivascular cuffs of tumour cells but also invasion of blood vessel walls in a highly typical manner with argyrophilic fibres alternating with rows of tumour cells, leading to concentric layers of haematopoietic blasts in the vessel walls (Figure 40.1). In addition, lymphoma cells form perivascular cuffs. This growth pattern usually dominates in the infiltration zone at the border with surrounding brain tissue, where only relatively low numbers of tumour cells are present. The exclusive presentation of one of these growth patterns in a given biopsy reflects regional features within a tumour, i.e. infiltrative zone versus centre, and does not allow the conclusion of the existence of different PCNSL entities.

Cytologically, the tumour cells correspond to large blasts with prominent chromatin-rich nuclei, distinct nucleoli, and slightly basophilic cytoplasmic rims, thus resembling centroblasts or immunoblasts. Phenotypically, PCNSLs are mature B-cell lymphomas expressing pan–B-cell markers (PAX5, CD19, CD20, CD22, CD79a). The surface expression of IgM, but not IgG, is characteristic, because PCNSLs usually are impaired in immunoglobulin (IG) class switch recombination. κ or λ light chain restriction can be demonstrated immunohistochemically. However, the confirmation of light chain restriction is dispensable and can be misleading, not always yielding convincing results. *In situ* hybridization is superior to immunohistochemistry and preferable for this purpose. The majority of PCNSLs express BCL6 (60–80 per cent), a protein expressed by germinal centre B-cells, as well as IRF4/MUM1 (90 per cent), a marker for late germinal centre B-cells and plasma cells, whereas plasma cell markers such as CD38 and CD138 are negative. Less than 5 per cent of PCNSLs express CD10. HLA-ABC and HLA-DR expression is variable. PCNSLs frequently show a MYC[high]BCL2[high] phenotype, which is often not associated with *BCL2* or *MYC* breakpoints.[22,98] Generally, mitotic activity is very high. This is paralleled by extremely high proliferative activity, often with more than 90 per cent of the tumour cells expressing the Ki-67 antigen.[22] Although virtually all PCNSLs exhibit a Ki-67 index above 50 per cent, lower values should raise the suspicion of other lymphoma entities. Many apoptotic cells and geographic necrosis are striking features.

Blasts are intermingled with a reactive infiltrate consisting of small T and B lymphocytes and macrophages. Reactive astrogliosis and microglial activation are usually prominent.

For nodal DLBCL, distinct subgroups have been defined, originally on the basis of gene expression profiling, and later by the use of an immunohistochemical classifier as surrogate.[55,137,140] Accordingly, attempts have been undertaken to further subtype PCNSL in analogy to nodal DLBCL.[24] However, these approaches failed, which can be explained by the fact that immunohistochemical classifiers still are problematic even in nodal DLBCL, and, more importantly, that in contrast to nodal DLBCL, so far there is no evidence for distinct subgroups of PCNSL, neither with respect to clinical observations (different clinical course with differences in response to therapy and ultimate prognosis) nor with respect to pathogenesis, including gene expression profiling data (see p. 1856).[103]

Molecular Biology

PCR analysis using primers against the six VH families of the *IG* gene identifies a monoclonal B cell population that has rearranged a *VH* gene segment and also introduced somatic mutations into the rearranged *VH* gene segments.[96,154] Light chain rearrangement is also detectable. Characteristically, in PCNSL the mutation frequency is very high, exceeding that of other lymphoma entities[96]; heavily mutated IG genes may preclude primer binding, yielding false-negative results. In such cases, PCR should be performed with several primer sets directed against different DNA regions of the *IGH* gene.

In typical cases, PCR analysis is not required to establish the diagnosis. However, it may provide valuable information in difficult cases, e.g. when inflammatory disorders such as multiple sclerosis or corticosteroid-mitigated PCNSL are considered. Although PCR is highly sensitive in the detection of B-cell-derived DNA sequences, one should keep in mind that very low numbers of B cells in small biopsy samples may display pseudoclonality. Thus, a comparative analysis of molecular biological and morphological results is always mandatory.

Differential Diagnosis of PCNSL

The differential diagnosis of PCNSL is wide. All neuroepithelial tumours, in particular glioblastoma, and metastatic lesions, particularly carcinoma metastasis, as well as many other lymphoma entities need to be considered (Table 40.2). Because PCNSL cannot be distinguished from extracerebral DLBCL by morphology, immunohistochemistry, and PCR analysis of IG gene rearrangement, careful clinical work-up including physical examination, bone marrow biopsy, CT of chest and abdomen, and ultrasound of the testis is required to rule out a systemic DLBCL. In particular, testicular DLBCL, a lymphoma also manifesting in an immuno-privileged organ, has a remarkably high affinity for spread to the CNS.[17] Occult systemic lymphoma may be detected in up to 8 per cent of patients presenting with lymphoma of the CNS.[141]

In cases with large cells, which may also suggest Hodgkin's lymphoma, EBV-positive DLBCL of the elderly

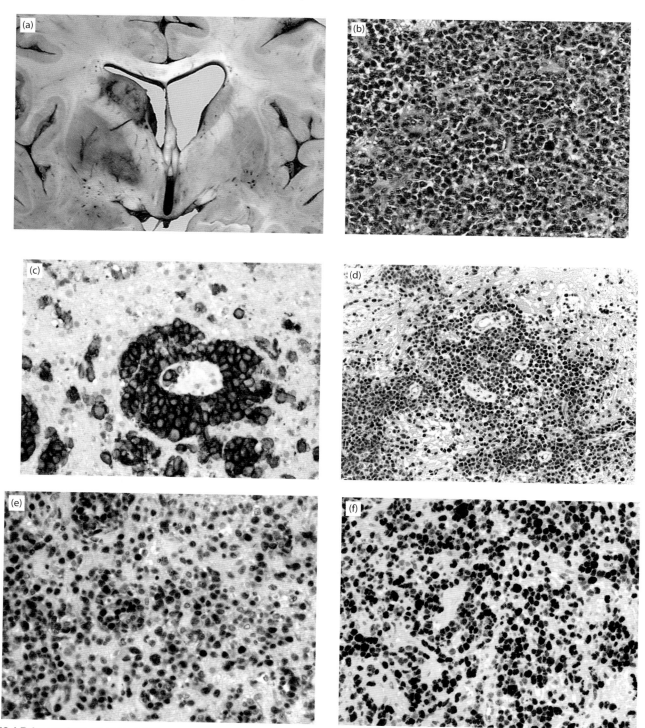

40.1 Primary CNS DLBCL. (a) Characteristic manifestation of primary central nervous system lymphoma (PCNSL) in the caudate and lentiform nuclei. **(b)** Diffuse growth pattern of blasts with chromatin-rich dark nuclei, distinct nucleoli, and small basophilic cytoplasmic rims. Mitoses are frequent. Blasts are intermingled with a reactive lymphocytic infiltrate. HE staining, original magnification ×200. **(c)** CD20+ tumour cells with an angiocentric growth pattern. In addition, single or small clusters of tumour cells diffusely infiltrate the brain tissue. Anti-CD20 immunostaining, slight counterstaining with hemalum, original magnification ×400. **(d,e)** Expression of the BCL6 protein **(d)** and of MUM1/IRF4 **(e)** identifies the germinal centre phenotype of the malignant B-cells. BCL6 **(d)** and MUM1 **(e)** immunostaining, slight counterstaining with hemalum, original magnification ×200. **(f)** High proliferative activity with more than 90 per cent of the tumour cells expressing the Ki-67 antigen. Anti-MIB-1 immunostaining, slight counterstaining with hemalum, original magnification ×400.

TABLE 40.2 Differential diagnosis of PCNSL

Non-haematopoietic tumors
- All neuroepithelial tumors, particularly glioblastoma multiforme
- Carcinoma metastasis

CNS metastasis of haematopoietic tumors
- Lymphomas
  - Extracerebral DLBCL, particularly testicular DLBCL
  - Intravascular DLBCL
  - EBV-positive DLBCL of the elderly
  - Lymphomatoid granulomatosis[a]
  - T cell/histiocyte-rich B cell lymphoma
  - CLL
  - Richter's syndrome in CLL
  - B-lymphoblastic lymphoma
  - Lymphoplasmacytic lymphoma
  - Burkitt lymphoma
  - Extranodal marginal zone lymphoma[b]
  - Follicular lymphoma[b]
  - Mantle cell lymphoma[b]
  - Plasmablastic lymphoma[a]
  - Hodgkin's lymphoma[b]
  - Anaplastic large-cell lymphoma, ALK-positive[b]
  - Anaplastic large-cell lymphoma, ALK-negative[b]
- Histiocytic tumors
  - Erdheim–Chester disease
  - Histiocytic sarcoma
  - Dendritic cell sarcoma
  - Xanthoma
- Inflammatory disorders
  - Multiple sclerosis
  - Vasculitis
  - Sentinel lesions
  - Brain abscess
  - Toxoplasma encephalitis[c]

[a]Manifestation in immunocompromised patients, particularly AIDS patients.
[b]May coexist with PCNSL in AIDS patients.
[c]Manifestation in the CNS is rare.

ALK, anaplastic lymphoma kinase; CLL, chronic lymphatic leukaemia; CNS, central nervous system; DLBCL, diffuse large B-cell lymphoma; PCNSL, primary CNS lymphoma.

needs to be considered. This aggressive subtype of DLBCL has been included as a provisional entity in the current WHO Classification of Tumours of Haematopoietic and Lymphoid Tissues;[113] it manifests in patients >50 years of age (median age, 71 years) without obvious immunodeficiency or previous lymphoma and is suggested to result from senescence of the immune system resulting in defective immunosurveillance. It accounts for 7 per cent and 8–10 per cent of DLBCL cases among Mexican and Asian patients, respectively, and is less frequent in Europe (1–3 per cent).[58,116] Involvement of extranodal sites is frequent. It may also manifest in the CNS, although the exact frequency is yet unknown. In EBV+ DLBCL of the elderly, polymorphic and monomorphic subtypes can be distinguished. Large cells reminiscent of Reed–Sternberg cells are intermingled with lymphocytes, plasma cells, and plasmablasts in the polymorphic subtype, thus raising the differential diagnosis of Hodgkin disease, whereas the monomorphic subtype is composed of sheets of large cells. Tumour cells express pan–B-cell markers with a consistent CD20 expression and frequent but not unequivocal CD30 expression. Proliferative activity is extremely high, virtually reaching 100 per cent of the tumour cells. Geographic necrosis is a characteristic feature. EBV infection is evidenced by LMP-1 and EBNA-2 expression.[4]

Furthermore, PCNSL needs to be distinguished from histiocytic lesions of the CNS. Each type of histiocytic tumour or pseudotumour may occur in the CNS. In the differential diagnosis between lymphoma and histiocytic tumours, location of the lesion may be informative because histiocytic tumours mostly are in contact with the meninges, whereas PCNSLs primarily involve the deep brain parenchyma and only rarely the meninges predominantly. In addition to tumours, inflammatory disorders need to be excluded. In this regard, multiple sclerosis (MS) is particularly important. Age is not a reliable parameter to distinguish PCNSL, because MS, although traditionally regarded as a disease of younger patients, may manifest in all age groups and not just before the sixth decade. Although demyelination is usually absent from PCNSL, it may escape detection from tiny MS biopsies, especially when the patient has received corticosteroids prior to stereotaxy. In such cases, PCR may provide a helpful tool in demonstrating polyclonality in inflammatory disorders.

So-called 'sentinel lesions', i.e. transient symptomatic contrast-enhancing brain parenchymal lesions preceding PCNSL for a period of up to 2 years,[6,19,60] pose a special problem. In rare cases, malignant lymphoma may be preceded by demyelination or may be associated with demyelination and inflammatory infiltrates consisting of CD3 and CD8 T-cells, B-cells and plasma cells with relative preservation of axons.[6,77] These lesions are indistinguishable from MS lesions by histology, in particular when biopsy was performed after initiation of high-dose corticosteroid treatment. The underlying mechanism is still unknown; a viral pathogenesis, malignant transformation of inflammatory cells, a host immune response against the tumour or demyelination due to anti-myelin antibodies secreted by the lymphoma cells are discussed.[6,77] Sentinel lesions should be considered in the differential diagnosis in patients with monofocal demyelinating lesions and/or presentation beyond 60 years of age. Currently, the issue is still unresolved whether such demyelination is a genuine feature of lymphoma or rather reflects an association of lymphoma with multiple sclerosis, which can be induced as a consequence of immunosuppressive treatment. Because most patients with sentinel lesions have received corticosteroids prior to biopsy, it is also still unclear whether they correspond to corticosteroid-mitigated PCNSL, with the morphological alterations in these cases representing reactive changes rather than autoimmune inflammation. Thus, the frequency of sentinel lesions due to primary demyelination may be overestimated.

CNS vasculitis, a heterogeneous disorder with a broad spectrum,[77] should also be considered in the differential diagnosis of CNS lymphoma. In cases that lack the full spectrum of morphological features of vasculitis, the identification of lymphocytes within blood vessel walls as B-cell blasts, which have a striking tendency to infiltrate and to split blood vessel walls, needs careful investigation. In contrast to vasculitis, PCNSL is not associated with blood vessel thrombosis and ischaemia of the respective brain tissue supplied. If morphology fails to clearly distinguish inflammatory from lymphoma lesions, PCR analysis of B- and T-cell receptors may be required and may be helpful in excluding monoclonality.

Steroid Effects on PCNSL: 'Corticosteroid-Mitigated PCNSL'

Steroids are widely used to lower increased intracranial pressure, a frequent presenting symptom of patients with PCNSL. The widely held belief that corticosteroid-mediated regression of an intracerebral lesion suspected to represent PCNSL indicates PCNSL is obsolete. On steroid application, PCNSL may vanish rapidly both on MRI and within biopsy samples. This is due to the high susceptibility of malignant as well as non-malignant lymphocytes to steroid-induced apoptosis. Thus, steroids should be strictly withheld in patients in whom PCNSL is suspected prior to stereotactic biopsy. Because the steroid effect is only temporary, corticosteroids usually delay diagnosis, and specific therapy and may even make definite diagnosis impossible. In cases of mass regression following steroid application and a non-diagnostic biopsy, close follow-up in the absence of steroids and repeat biopsy on disease progression on MRI are recommended. The 'optimal' period of corticosteroid abstinence prior to second biopsy cannot be predicted, generally because of high individual variation. In this regard, it is of note that even a repeat biopsy does not guarantee definite diagnosis. Unfortunately, in a significant proportion of patients, definite diagnosis cannot be established because non-specific histological findings may persist.

Microscopically, cellularity of the tissue may be only slightly increased, and B-cell blasts may be either totally absent or very scant. Occasionally, B cells are only slightly enlarged. Nonspecific reactive changes with sparse perivascular and parenchymal leukocytes may prevail. Reactive gliosis and microglial activation are prominent (Figure 40.2). Necrosis is variable and may or may not occur. A predominance of foamy macrophages should alert the neuropathologist to the possibility of steroid-mitigated PCNSL. In addition, some small mature lymphocytes are intermingled, forming perivascular clusters and/or scattered throughout the brain parenchyma either as single cells or within small clusters. In individual cases, the differentiation of strongly activated lymphocytes from malignant lymphocytes can be difficult, because enlargement is also characteristic of lymphocyte activation, which may acquire a 'blastic' phenotype and even express the Ki-67 antigen.

Biopsy may also show very few B-cell blasts or even single B-cells of normal or slightly increased size without mitoses within a reactive infiltrate and histiocytes of variable number. Necrosis may be extensive. PCR analysis of B- and T-cell receptors may be helpful in identifying a monoclonal cell population. However, if the number of blasts is very low in a lesion, pseudoclonality is a pitfall. If the background of the inflammatory infiltrates consists nearly entirely of T cells, the diagnosis of T-cell/histiocyte-rich, large B-cell lymphoma is frequently considered. However, manifestation of T-cell/histiocyte-rich large B-cell lymphoma in the CNS is a rarity; the diagnosis of T-cell/histiocyte-rich large B-cell lymphoma should be reserved for cases with the characteristic histology of large blasts resembling immunoblasts or plasmablasts with the genotypic and phenotypic features of DLBCL, including expression of B-cell antigens and BCL6. The latter are always scattered as single cells within a reactive inflammatory infiltrate that dominates the lesion and consists predominantly of small CD3+CD5+ T lymphocytes and, in variable number, of CD68+ histiocytes in the absence of prior corticosteroid application.

It may be virtually impossible to differentiate steroid-induced inflammatory alterations, both reactive and resorptive, from other inflammatory disorders, most importantly MS in particular, if tiny biopsies do not provide evidence for demyelination.

Biology of PCNSL

Biology of disease has been the focus of intense studies in recent years in immunocompetent patients, although it is still less well-studied in immunocompromised patients, particularly HIV-infected patients. So far, important differences have been delineated regarding pathogenesis of PCNSL in these two groups of patients, although there is evidence for a similar histogenesis.

Biology of PCNSL in Immunocompetent Patients

Histogenesis

PCNSL is a mature B-cell lymphoma, as evidenced by both genotype and immunophenotype. The expression of CD19 (100 per cent of cases), CD20 (100 per cent), CD10 (<5 per cent), BCL6 (60–100 per cent) and IRF4/MUM1 (90–100 per cent), as well as the presence of rearranged, somatically mutated IG genes with evidence for ongoing somatic mutation, suggest that the tumour cells are derived from a germinal centre B cell.[11,96,154] The remarkably high load of somatic mutations, exceeding values described for systemic DLBCL – with a mean mutation frequency two- to five-fold higher than normal peripheral B-cells – may indicate a prolonged germinal centre reaction of the tumour cells. The histogenetic origin of PCNSL is a late germinal centre exit B-cell as evidenced by the transcriptional profile.[103] Further B-cell maturation steps of the tumour cells are blocked, such as IG class switch recombination as a result of deletions of the Sμ region and low levels of activation-induced cytodeaminase.[102] In addition, mutations of the PRDM1 gene, which is required for terminal differentiation into plasma cells, are present in a substantial fraction of PCNSLs and contribute to impairment of terminal B cell maturation.[35]

Molecular Alterations

Several mechanisms may contribute to malignant transformation of B cells, including chromosomal translocations, gains and losses of genetic material, ongoing aberrant somatic hypermutation of oncogenes, mutations of tumour suppressor genes, gene inactivation by DNA methylation, and activation of the NF-κB complex.[38,104]

Chromosomal alterations with mutations and translocations in candidate oncogenes and tumour suppressor gene loci are frequent. These include translocations of the IG loci (38 per cent) and the BCL6 gene (23 per cent).[98] Although in PCNSL, IG translocations occur with similar frequency as in systemic DLBCL, the translocation partners identified for nodal DLBCL have generally not been involved in PCNSL; with the exception of BCL6, the translocation partners of the IG genes are still unknown.[99] With respect to the promiscuous BCL6 gene, HSPCA (HSP90A), GAPD, H4I and

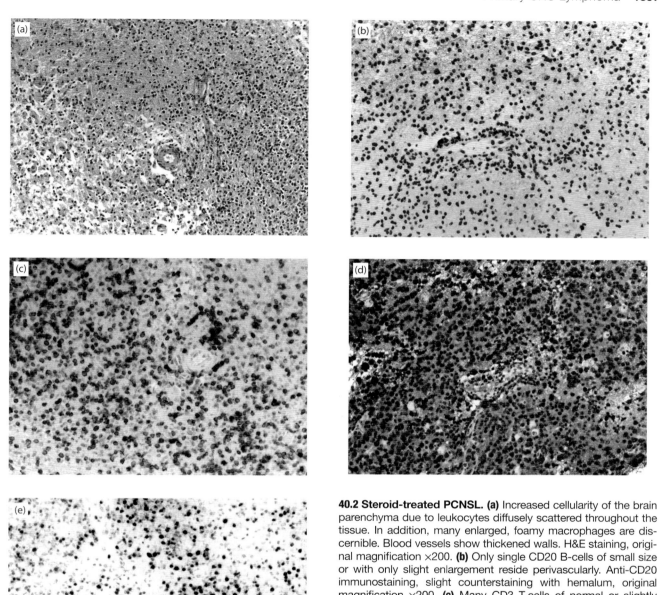

40.2 Steroid-treated PCNSL. (a) Increased cellularity of the brain parenchyma due to leukocytes diffusely scattered throughout the tissue. In addition, many enlarged, foamy macrophages are discernible. Blood vessels show thickened walls. H&E staining, original magnification ×200. **(b)** Only single CD20 B-cells of small size or with only slight enlargement reside perivascularly. Anti-CD20 immunostaining, slight counterstaining with hemalum, original magnification ×200. **(c)** Many CD3 T-cells of normal or slightly increased size are scattered throughout the brain tissue. Anti-CD3 immunostaining, slight counterstaining with hemalum, original magnification ×200. **(d)** Numerous CD68 macrophages in the brain tissue, many of which are enlarged and show a foamy cytoplasm. Anti-CD68 immunostaining, slight counterstaining with hemalum, original magnification ×200. **(e)** Proliferative activity is elevated, however, below the proliferative activity characteristic for PCNSL. Anti-Ki-67 immunostaining, slight counterstaining with hemalum, original magnification ×200.

the *LPP* genes have been identified as translocation partners in PCNSL.[99,148] In all cases, *BCL6* translocation resulted in promoter substitution with deregulated expression of the intact BCL6 protein by interruption of a negative autoregulatory feedback loop.[99]

PCNSLs carry mutations in the oncogenes *PAX5* (60 per cent), *TTF-1* (70 per cent), *PIM1* (50 per cent), and *CMYC* (60 per cent) as well as in the *CD95* (20 per cent) and *PRDM1* (19 per cent) genes.[101] Gains and losses of genetic material are recurrent. In one study, gains affected 18q21.33-q23, including both the *BCL2* and *MALT1* gene

(43 per cent) and chromosome 12 (26 per cent), whereas losses involved 6q21 (52 per cent), 8q12.1-q12.2 (32 per cent), and 10q23.21 (21 per cent).[149] Loss of 10q23 was associated with the absence of Fas mRNA, whereas gains of chromosome 12 were associated with an upregulation of STAT6 and CD27 mRNA, which may contribute to the enhanced proliferation and impaired apoptosis in tumour cells of PCNSL (Figure 40.3).[40,149]

Regarding epigenetics, silencing of genes including *RFC* (30 per cent), *DAPK* (84 per cent), *CDKN2A* (75 per cent) and *MGMT* (52 per cent) occurred as a result of

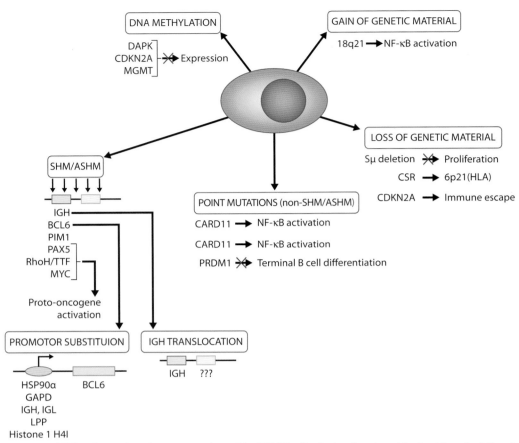

40.3 Pathogenesis of PCNSL. Several pathways are altered in PCNSL, finally leading to a block of terminal B-cell differentiation, impaired apoptosis, and uncontrolled proliferation. ASHM, aberrant somatic hypermutation; CSR, class switch recombination; SHM, somatic hypermutation.

hypermethylation of CpG islands.[28,31,47,149] Genes switched off by promoter methylation in PCNSL belong to a group of polycomb-repressing complex-regulated genes that inactivate many genes in stem cells. This methylation process may contribute to generation of the premalignant precursor cell. In addition, genes regulating tumourigenesis, lymphocyte motility, and apoptosis were inactivated by promoter methylation.[134] MiR-17-5p, which targets the pro-apoptotic *E2F1* gene, showed a significantly higher expression level in CNS lymphomas as compared with systemic DLBCL.[136]

In addition to single gene alterations, deregulation of specific pathways appears to be particularly relevant to PCNSL. Constitutive activation of the NF-κB pathway is a hallmark, as evidenced by increased expression of NF-κB regulating genes, genes of the NF-κB complex, NF-κB target genes and the nuclear Rel location in the tumour cells.[34] This can be attributed to mutations targeting components of regulatory pathways upstream of the NF-κB complex. In this regard, it is of note that the Toll-like receptor pathway is deregulated because of *MYD88* mutations in 50 per cent of PCNSLs.[106] Furthermore, crucial components of genes of the B cell receptor (BCR) signalling pathway harbour somatic mutations in a high frequency (44 per cent) of PCNSLs targeting the *SHIP*, *CD79B*, *CBL* and *BLNK* genes, finally deregulating but not abolishing BCR function.[107] BCR stimulation leads to signalling to the BCM complex, which consists of BCL10, MALT1 and CARD11. In PCNSL, which also expresses BCL10,[34]

the *MALT1* gene is amplified (37 per cent),[149] and activating mutations affect the *CARD11* gene (16 per cent).[105] Altogether, these recurrent genetic alterations may cause sustained NF-κB activity in PCNSL. With regard to the pattern of NF-κB activating mutations, PCNSLs apparently differ from nodal DLBCL, suggesting that different transforming stimuli act in these entities.

Gene expression profiling studies in nodal DLBCL identified two subtypes: the activated B-cell (ABC) and germinal centre B (GCB) subtype differ in their response to therapy and prognosis.[13,137] Different pathogenetic mechanisms underlie these subtypes, indicating that they represent distinct lymphoma entities rather than subtypes of one entity.[86] The observation that PCNSLs share characteristics with both ABC (IgM expression, lack of IG class switch recombination, activation of the NF-κB pathway) and GCB (high *IG* gene mutation frequency with ongoing somatic hypermutation, BCL6 expression) DLBCLs raised the question whether PCNSL corresponds to either one of these subtypes or whether it constitutes a distinct entity. This question encouraged gene expression profiling studies, which so far have been confined to a few because of the restricted availability of PCNSL tissue from mostly stereotactic biopsies.[18,103,138,155] However, differences in platforms and applied algorithms accounted, at least in part, for the divergent results and conclusions. One study claimed to have identified a characteristic CNS signature;[155] however, this could not be confirmed by others. Instead, the distribution of PCNSL along the spectrum of systemic DLBCL, including the ABC and GCB DLBCL, indicates its molecular heterogeneity.[103] High expression of STAT6 was associated with a shorter survival in patients treated with high-dose methotrexate (MTX) chemotherapy.[138] Combined gene-expression profiling with array CGH delineated the concept of DLBCL in immunoprivileged sites, i.e. brain and testis, as differing from DLBCL at other sites.[18] Loss of 6p21 (37 per cent) was a frequent event in PCNSL, identified in genome-wide single-nucleotide polymorphism chip analysis.[18,149] This included the HLA region (37 per cent). Interestingly, a deletion in 6p21 was associated with reduced major histocompatibility complex mRNA levels.[18] Collectively, these observations may indicate an escape mechanism of the tumour cells from the host immune response.

The impact of the microenvironment of the CNS and the interaction of the tumour cells of PCNSL with the brain are major unresolved issues. Confinement to the CNS is a curious observation. It is still unclear at what stage of (de) differentiation the cells enter the CNS, either as malignant or as premalignant cells. Tumour cells express cell adhesion molecules[121] and chemokines; however, a specific pattern that would allow their distinction from other B cells was not identified. The expression pattern of chemokines (CXCR4, CXCL12, CXCR5, CXCL13, CCR7) allows their specific interaction with cerebral endothelial cells, reactive astrocytes, and activated microglia.[21] B-cell activating factor released by astrocytes may support survival of the tumour cells in the CNS.[76] One may speculate that the interaction between the tumour cells of PCNSL and the resident cell populations of the CNS, which occurs in a cell-type-specific manner, fosters survival of the tumour cells in the CNS and supports their dissemination within the CNS. In this regard, the repeated observation of HLA-DQ, HLA-DR and HLA-A antigen losses in PCNSL[67,68,69,135] may also be important, because this may facilitate tumour cell survival in an immunologically privileged organ even in the presence of CD4 and CD8 T-cells as part of the characteristic inflammatory infiltrate. In one study, the presence of reactive perivascular T cells in PCNSL biopsy samples was associated with a better overall survival.[131] However, there is a striking regional heterogeneity in the number and density of intratumoural CD4 and CD8 T cells even within one biopsy. Thus, the question regarding the role of CD4 and CD8 T cells in PCNSL is not yet resolved. Furthermore, in this regard, corticosteroid-induced alterations in the number of intracerebral T-cells also need to be considered.

A further striking issue relates to the preferential use of the *IGHV4-34* gene segment in 50–80 per cent of PCNSLs.[96,154] The high recombination frequency of *IGHV4-34* suggests a functional role of IG encoded by this gene in the pathogenesis of PCNSL and raises the question of whether the malignant B-cells or their precursors are triggered by a specific antigen, e.g. a viral antigen. Interestingly, the *IGHV4-34* gene segment has been implicated in EBV infection. However, in immunocompetent patients, PCNSL is usually EBV-negative.[96] In addition to EBV, a potentially pathogenetic relevant role for other viruses has been discussed and was ruled out for HHV-6, HHV-8 and SV40.[97,100,122] So far, a specific (viral) antigen that might trigger the tumour cells of PCNSL has not been identified.

One may also hypothesize that the microenvironment of the CNS fosters the expansion of lymphomas using particular *IG* gene segments.

Another intriguing issue is the observation of ongoing somatic hypermutation,[96,154] a process requiring the microenvironment of a germinal centre, characteristic for secondary lymphatic organs, in the CNS, an extranodal organ. Although it cannot be excluded with certainty that B-cell transformation may have occurred outside the CNS while the clone continued to introduce somatic mutations before leaving the germinal centre of a secondary lymphoid organ, it is unlikely that several different tumour clones may leave the germinal centre simultaneously and selectively home to the CNS. This is further illustrated by patients with relapse in whom IG gene analysis demonstrated that both tumours were derived from a common ancestor that escaped elimination during therapy and achieved persistence in the brain during remission until giving rise to relapse, indicating that clonal evolution rather than subclonal selection may underlie relapse.[125]

Biology of PCNSL in Immunocompromised Patients

Because PCNSLs became a prevalent clinical problem during the AIDS era, efforts were undertaken to study the biology of PCNSL in tissue samples from HIV-infected patients. These efforts, however, were mostly disappointing because in biopsies, frozen tissue was either not available or not suitable for analysis because of infectivity, whereas autopsy-derived tissue was often too degraded for molecular studies. Thus, compared to immunocompetent patients, knowledge of the biology is rather limited. Nevertheless, there is solid evidence for fundamental differences in the pathogenesis of PCNSL in immunocompromised as opposed to immunocompetent patients.

PCNSLs in immunocompromised patients, including AIDS patients, are DLBCLs with an expression of mature B-cell markers. Somatic mutations of the *BCL6* gene in 11 of 26 (42 per cent) PCNSLs from patients with AIDS-related PCNSL and expression of the BCL6 protein by the tumour cells demonstrate that they have experienced a germinal centre reaction.[83] Thus, in this regard, PCNSLs in both groups of patients appear similar though differences are elucidated later. The effect of HIV infection in PCNSL development is indirect rather than direct and associated with various factors.

In contrast to immunocompetent patients, in which PCNSLs usually are EBV negative, EBV is expressed in virtually all AIDS-related PCNSL[83,108] and represents a major driving force for lymphomagenesis in HIV-infected patients. The powerful impact of EBV in lymphomagenesis in HIV-infected patients is not restricted to PCSNL but is a rather common feature of all HIV-associated lymphomas. In PCNSL, the LMP1 protein of EBV is expressed, which has the capacity to transform B lymphocytes,[160] activates the NF-κB pathway,[59] and increases the expression of the anti-apoptotic proteins A20 and BCL2 in infected B cells.[20] However, which of these potential effects of LMP1 on B cells are definitely involved in the pathogenesis of AIDS-associated PCNSL has not been elucidated thus far.

A virus implicated in other AIDS-associated tumours is HHV-8, although a pathogenic role was excluded in AIDS-related PCNSL.[8,97]

Biological Behaviour of PCNSL

The clinical course of patients with PCNSL differs strikingly and the prognosis is much less favourable than for patients with DLBCL outside the CNS. This observation also lends support to the concept of PCNSL's being a lymphoma entity distinct from extracerebral nodal and extranodal DLBCL. Prior to the introduction of chemoradiotherapy, survival of patients with PCNSL was approximately 2 months.[143]

Whole brain radiotherapy was the standard of care as primary therapy for PCNSL into the early 1990s, leading to complete remission rates of 80–90 per cent.[38,45,141] However, disease control was poor as a result of relapse in almost all patients. A substantial prognostic improvement was achieved within the past two decades thanks to the implementation of high-dose MTX-based chemotherapy. Nevertheless, PCNSL still runs an aggressive course and outcome is unsatisfactory. Combined chemoradiotherapy achieved complete response rates of up to 87 per cent with a median progression-free survival of up to 40 months. However, unfortunately, chemotherapy followed by radiotherapy caused delayed severe neurotoxicity, which clinically manifested as severe neurological impairment, severe cognitive dysfunction, dementia, and death, particularly in older patients (>60 years).

Macroscopy demonstrated white matter damage with diffuse pallor sparing the arcuate fibres and white matter necrosis.[157] Microscopically, cerebral hemispheric white matter damage corresponded to extensive myelin swelling and loss, axonal loss, reactive astrocytosis, spongiosis, gliosis, necrosis with oedema and abundant mononuclear cell reaction in the periventricular white matter, and necrotizing angiopathy.[9,82,142] Patients at high risk for development of white matter changes are those with a functional polymorphism that may influence methionine synthase activity.[88] Recently, a few patients, mainly those in whom aggressive therapy was precluded, received temozolomide therapy yielding encouraging results in PCNSL with MGMT promoter methylation.[3,80]

Before the introduction of HAART, the prognosis for PCNSL in AIDS patients was very poor. With HAART-induced immunologic recovery and the subsequent possibility to apply more aggressive therapy, prognosis of AIDS-associated PCNSL has remarkably improved. The treatment strategy tends to be similar to that of the immunocompetent population – high-dose MTX-based chemotherapy with or without whole brain irradiation.[52]

Regarding the search for prognostic parameters, age and performance status have been identified as the two most important independent prognostic factors for PCNSL in immunocompetent patients.[1,2,32,91] Recently, early complete tumour response assessed by MRI was shown to be highly predictive for overall survival and time to treatment failure.[126]

PCNSL relapses usually are confined to the CNS and involve anatomic sites different from initial tumour manifestation.[145] Extracerebral metastasis occurs only in very rare cases and is prone to involve the testis, illustrating the high affinity of the lymphoma cells for the microenvironment of immunoprivileged organs.[17] In a retrospective study of 209 patients treated with MTX-based chemotherapy with or without radiotherapy, 10 patients (4.8 per cent) were detected who developed isolated systemic relapse 3–94 months after initial diagnosis.[132] Early relapse, i.e. 3–8 months after diagnosis, suggests asymptomatic systemic disease that has escaped detection at the time of diagnosis. Whether manifestation of extracerebral DLBCL in a patient 10 years after PCNSL[132] represents PCNSL relapse or development of a second, independent lymphoma needs to be clarified by comparative molecular analysis of both tumours.

Analysis of the biology of PCNSL relapse is restricted to patients in whom other disorders, e.g. carcinoma metastasis or glioblastoma, are a likely differential diagnosis and need to be ruled out by biopsy. The recurrent lymphoma is usually indistinguishable from the primary tumour and keeps the morphological characteristics of PCNSL. In contrast to glial tumours, loss of differentiation is not a feature of PCNSL.

PCR analysis of *IG* gene rearrangement in a single PCNSL patient with relapse revealed that both the primary and the secondary tumour had rearranged the same *IGH* gene segment and harboured both common somatic mutations and individual somatic mutations confined to either one of the tumours. These observations demonstrate that both tumours are derived from the same ancestor[114,125] and raise the hypothesis that clonal evolution rather than subclone selection underlies the development of PCNSL recurrence.[125]

In the absence of extracerebral lymphoma manifestation, tumour-related DNA sequences have been identified in blood and/or bone marrow of some patients with PCNSL who had no evidence for systemic lymphoma.[64,92] Because the peripheral blood normally contains hundreds to thousands of related clone members of IgM/IgD memory B cells, the presence of several tumour-related clones, one of which may have entered the CNS as either a premalignant or a malignant cell, may not be specific for lymphomagenesis, but rather reflect physiological memory B-cell development.

SECONDARY INVOLVEMENT OF THE CNS BY HAEMATOPOIETIC TUMOURS

Introduction

Overall, regarding all groups and ages of patients, the CNS is more frequently involved by secondary spread of systemic lymphomas than by PCNSL (Table 4.2). Long-term retrospective studies have shown CNS involvement in 5–10 per cent of all lymphomas.[111] Virtually all lymphomas may affect the CNS. As a general rule, high-grade lymphomas more commonly spread to the CNS than do low-grade lymphomas. A small percent (2.2) of aggressive lymphomas have been reported to relapse in the CNS, which is a serious, often fatal complication, because prognosis is poor.[74,75,119] One study[53] suggested that spread of indolent lymphomas to the CNS may be underestimated in frequency and significance. A post-mortem study documented CNS affection in 13 per cent of indolent cases.[66] The authors concluded that it is not rare for indolent lymphomas to involve the CNS, although this occurs toward later phases of disease in patients with uncontrolled lymphomas and considerable systemic involvement.

Systemic Diffuse Large B-Cell Lymphoma

Between 2 and 5 per cent of extracerebral DLBCLs spread to the CNS, which is a serious and usually fatal complication. Patients with CNS relapse have a median survival of 2–6 months only.[119] At the time of diagnosis of extracerebral DLBCL, the CNS is usually not affected. Manifestation of CNS disease shortly after diagnosis raises the question whether initial involvement of the CNS may have escaped detection. CNS involvement usually manifests within 2 years of initial diagnosis with a median time of less than 1 year.[151] CNS spread is closely linked to progressive systemic disease, and improved control of systemic disease seems to be associated with fewer CNS recurrences.[75] Although 61 per cent of patients develop CNS relapse while being in complete remission, many of them also develop systemic disease within months.[151] Overall, 50 per cent of these patients also relapse systemically.[119] Molecular alterations in extracerebral DLBCL that facilitate their spread to the CNS have not yet been identified. In this regard, it is of note that patients with lymphomas of the double-hit category, who have a particularly inferior outcome with a median survival of 0.2–1.5 years, frequently have extranodal involvement, most commonly of the bone marrow and CNS, with CNS metastasis occurring in 9–50 per cent of patients.[10,139] Double-hit lymphomas show a heterogeneous morphology suggestive of DLBCL, Burkitt lymphoma or mature B-cell lymphoma not otherwise specified (NOS), and are characterized by multiple recurrent breakpoints, mostly of the *MYC* gene together with the *BCL2* or *BCL6* gene.[10]

In DLBCL metastasis to the CNS, the meninges (33–100 per cent) are affected more frequently than the brain parenchyma (10–56 per cent).[119] Meningeal blasts may be detected in the CSF by morphology. In patients with a previous diagnosis of extracerebral DLBCL, FACS analysis, which requires fewer tumour cells, was superior to conventional cytology without immunocytochemistry with regard to sensitivity in detecting occult leptomeningeal disease.[7] However, only one of 12 patients in whom FACS analysis was positive finally relapsed, thus raising a question regarding the predictive value of FACS CSF evaluation with respect to CNS relapse.[7]

Morphologically, metastasis of extracerebral DLBCL is indistinguishable from PCNSL. If in a patient with a history of extracerebral DLBCL the differential diagnosis of PCNSL versus CNS metastasis is raised, this question can only be answered by comparative *IG* gene analysis of both tumours.

Angiotropic Lymphoma (Intravascular Lymphoma)

Typically, this tumour manifests in adult patients (median, 67 years; range, 13–85 years), affecting both sexes equally. It is a B-cell lymphoma of the DLBCL type with selective intravascular growth that may affect any organ, including the CNS. The CNS is involved in more than 30 per cent of cases.[112] The brain, as well as the spinal cord, may be affected. Angiotropic lymphoma can also be confined to the spinal cord.[15]

Clinically, patients present with a broad range of neurological and psychiatric symptoms, which may fluctuate widely. Diffuse and focal neurological signs occurred in 82 and 72 per cent of patients, respectively.[15] In addition to stroke-like episodes, symptoms include seizures, dementia and impairment of consciousness. Clinically, neurological symptoms may raise the differential diagnosis of cerebral vasculitis, dementing disorders and even Creutzfeldt–Jakob disease.[15]

Neuropathology is dominated by the consequences of vascular occlusion by the tumour cells. Macroscopically, acute or old ischaemic infarcts, frequently scattered as multiple infarcts, necrosis or bleeding, including purpura cerebri with multiple haemorrhages, may be visible.[15] However, obvious neuropathology is not necessarily present in all patients; macroscopically, the CNS may even be unremarkable, and careful investigation may reveal only a few small infarcts.[15] Microscopically, small vessels (venules, capillaries and arterioles) are partially or completely occluded by neoplastic cells mixed with fibrin. Occluded vessels may be recanalized and associated with multiple recent and older anaemic infarcts.[15] Despite restriction of the tumour cells to the vascular lumen, minimal extravasation of the tumour cells may occur. The tumour cells express B-cell markers (CD19, CD20, CD22), BCL6, and CD5 and/or CD10. Virtually all CD10-negative tumours express IRF4/MUM1. The tumour cells are incapable of invading organs including the brain. The absence of β1-integrin (CD2) and ICAM-1 (CD54) on the surface of the tumour cells[130] may, at least in part, underlie their inability to cross the blood–brain barrier, thus resulting in their entrapment within the intravascular space.

Lymphomatoid Granulomatosis

Lymphomatoid granulomatosis, a rather rare lymphoma entity, frequently involves the brain (26 per cent), as well as other organs. Initially, patients may present with CNS disease, although pulmonary involvement at diagnosis is characteristic. Depending on the topography of the lesion, neurological symptoms are highly variable and include hemiparesis, ataxia, cranial nerve palsies and confusional states.[120]

Lymphomatoid granulomatosis is an EBV-driven lymphoma occurring in immunosuppressed patients with the hallmark of angiocentric and angiodestructive lesions. Blood vessel walls are infiltrated and surrounded by mature leukocytic infiltrates composed of lymphocytes, plasma cells, histiocytes and immunoblasts. EBV infection of small CD20+ B cells that may show some atypia is evidenced by Epstein–Barr virus-encoded small RNA (EBER) *in situ* hybridization. However, EBER *in situ* hybridization may yield negative results if large areas of necrosis dominate, in which tumour cell RNA is degraded. The tumour cells may express LMP1. CD30 expression is variable, although the tumour cells are CD15 negative. This immunoprofile may be helpful in the differential diagnosis of Hodgkin's lymphoma, in particular in those cases that harbour multinucleated cells. Because of the angiotropism of the lymphoma cells, vasculitis, fibrinoid blood vessel necrosis and infarct-like necrosis are prominent.

Lymphoblastic Lymphoma

B-lymphoblastic lymphoma, a precursor lymphoid neoplasm, is primarily a disease of the paediatric age group and has a particular predilection for the CNS. Although initial CNS involvement is infrequent (3–9 per cent), relapse in the CNS is common, ranging from 42–100 per cent in studies without CNS prophylaxis.[33] Interestingly, a patient with B-lymphoblastic lymphoma has been reported to develop primary T-cell lymphoma of the CNS 5 years after complete remission.[156]

Morphologically, blasts are of various size, mostly small- or medium-sized, with a narrow or moderate cytoplasm and variable, condensed or dispersed chromatin and indistinct or distinct nucleoli. A fraction of the blasts may harbour intracytoplasmic azurophilic granules. Mitotic activity is brisk. Immunohistochemically, the blasts express CD10, CD19, surface and cytoplasmic CD22, CD24, cytoplasmic CD79a, PAX5 and TdT. CD20 and CD34 expression is variable. CD45 may be absent. CD13 and CD33 may be expressed. In the differential diagnosis of PCNSL, patient age and the absence of TdT in association with the constant expression of CD20 favours PCNSL.

Chronic Lymphocytic Leukaemia

CNS involvement in chronic lymphocytic leukaemia (CLL) is rare. The incidence of CNS involvement has been estimated as 0.8–2 per cent in ante-mortem studies.[95] However, post-mortem studies detected CNS involvement at a high frequency, with a wide range of 8–71 per cent of lethal CLL cases,[95] suggesting that this complication may be significantly underestimated. CNS involvement is not confined to late stages of disease, because 48.8 per cent of patients with Rai stage 0 to II had neurological symptoms already at initial presentation.[95] Average survival of patients with CNS involvement is shorter than without CNS involvement.[95] Between 2 and 8 per cent of patients with CLL will develop DLBCL, a condition termed Richter's syndrome. Richter's syndrome may manifest in the brain as the primary location of DLBCL even in the absence of systemic DLBCL.

Patients develop diverse, nonspecific symptoms including headache, mental changes suggestive of dementia, seizures, sensory deficits, cerebellar symptoms and cranial nerve dysfunction. Overall, neurological symptoms raise the differential diagnosis of viral encephalitis or toxic-metabolic encephalopathies.[95]

Cranial imaging is insensitive to the presence of intracerebral CLL, with demonstrable pathological findings in less than 30 per cent of patients.[95] Neuroradiological findings may include diffuse coating of the leptomeninges, nodular or plaque-like meningeal lesions and intraparenchymal lesions.

CSF analysis may be uneventful because distinction of CLL tumour cells from enlarged reactive lymphocytes may be particularly difficult. Flow cytometry of CSF increases the detection rate of CLL cells considerably.[25,56] PCR analysis of *IGH* gene rearrangement may detect a monoclonal B cell population and identify this population as CLL clone by comparing *IGH* gene sequences (CDR3 region) with those derived from CLL cells in the peripheral blood.[50]

Microscopically, brain biopsy may reveal monomorphic small or slightly enlarged lymphocytes of low mitotic activity, often within blood vessels or even confined to the intravascular space. Immunohistochemistry demonstrates expression of CD5, CD19, CD20, CD22, CD23, CD79a and CD43 with a weak expression of CD11c. The tumour cells are CD10 negative. Tumour cells show a dim surface expression of IgM/IgD.

Lymphoplasmacytic Lymphoma

Lymphoplasmacytic lymphoma is a disease of older patients only rarely affecting extranodal sites. Infiltration of the CNS is uncommon but has been observed. Clinically, multifocal leukoencephalopathy with motor dysfunction, memory loss, confusion and coma has been reported.[159] In contrast to the CNS, the peripheral nervous system is frequently involved, and approximately 20 per cent of patients suffer from peripheral neuropathy with lymphoplasmacytic lymphoma-associated monoclonal IgM.

Morphologically, the tumour cells correspond to small lymphocytes, plasmacytoid lymphocytes and plasma cells. Tumour cells express B-cell antigens, i.e. CD19, CD20, CD22 and CD79a, with the plasma cells expressing CD138. Most cells show surface expression of Ig; plasmacytic cells mostly express IgM, occasionally IgG, and only seldom IgA. Tumour cells do not express CD5 or CD10, whereas CD38 expression is variable.

Plasmacytoma

Plasmacytoma frequently involves the bone of the skull and the vertebral column, where it causes lytic lesions, often multiple in number. Thoracic vertebrae are more frequently affected than cervical or lumbar levels. Neurological symptoms (paraplegia) occur when vertebral lesions progress to spinal cord compression. In the skull, tumour may invade the adjacent dura by direct extension. Infiltration of the brain parenchyma has only rarely been reported.[42,61,146]

Morphologically, cells are mature with typical plasma cell morphology harbouring eccentric nuclei with clumped chromatin and eosinophilic cytoplasm. They express plasma cell markers CD38, CD138 and IRF4/MUM1 with κ or λ light chain restriction, which can be determined either by immunohistochemistry or by *in situ* hybridization. CD20 is usually absent; however, it may be aberrantly expressed in some tumours.

Extranodal Marginal Zone Lymphoma

Twelve per cent of extranodal marginal zone lymphomas arise in the ocular adnexa. Here, the orbit is the most frequent site of origin accounting for approximately 40 per cent of cases.[12] CNS involvement occurs mostly in middle-aged women who present with a meningioma-like dural mass, mostly solitary, but multiple dural lesions have also been reported.[12] Parenchymal involvement is uncommon. Exceptionally, marginal zone lymphoma has been reported to infiltrate the basal ganglia and temporal lobe without dural involvement.[118] In a single patient, a lesion within the lateral ventricle was observed, which extended to the cavernous sinus.[12] Clinically, headache, seizures, focal sensory and/or motor deficits, and visual disturbances are common. Acute onset of symptoms raising the differential diagnosis of subdural hematoma has also been noticed.[12] The course of disease is indolent.

Morphologically, tumour cells contain small- to medium-sized nuclei with pale cytoplasm, resembling centrocytes.

Cells may also resemble small lymphocytes or monocytoid cells or may show plasmacytic differentiation. A few larger cells resembling immunoblasts or centroblasts may also be intermingled. The tumour cells exhibit a B-cell phenotype with expression of CD20, CD79a, CD21 and CD35 while being negative for CD10 and CD5; however, in rare cases, the tumour cells may express CD5. The tumour cells express surface Ig, mostly IgM and less frequently IgG and IgA. Expression of IG light chains is restricted.

Follicular Lymphoma

CNS involvement has been reported only incidentally. During late stages of follicular lymphoma, spread to the CNS was reported in a patient having already suffered from several recurrences, which manifested as a single large lesion in the parieto-occipital lobe.[53]

Morphologically, the tumour characteristically exhibits a follicular pattern, at least in a part of the tumour. The presence of diffuse areas, predominantly or totally composed of blasts, leads to classification as DLBCL, irrespective of their size. Similarly, if the tumour does not show a follicular pattern at all and consists of diffuse, patternless areas only, it is categorized as DLBCL. In the differential diagnosis, detection of follicular dendritic cells by immunohistochemical staining for CD21 and CD23 may be helpful to identify follicles. Cytologically, two types of tumour cells are discernible, i.e. centrocytes and centroblasts. Centrocytes corresponding to small- to medium-sized cells with cleaved nuclei and narrow cytoplasm usually dominate the tumour. Centroblasts are characterized by an increased size and harbour round to oval, large nuclei with prominent nucleoli and scant, basophilic cytoplasm. Immunohistochemistry reveals expression of CD10, CD19, CD20, CD22, and CD79a as well as BCL2 and BCL6, whereas CD5 and IRF4/MUM1 are absent. The tumour cells show surface Ig expression.

Mantle Cell Lymphoma

A wide variation in the frequency (4–26 per cent) of CNS involvement has been reported for patients with mantle cell lymphoma. An aggressive course of disease and relapses of systemic disease may be associated with CNS involvement, whereas usually the CNS is not affected at initial manifestation.[44]

Morphologically, the tumour is composed of small- to medium-sized monomorphic lymphocytes, which express CD5, CD43, BCL2 and cyclin D1. However, aberrant cases may show expression of CD10 and BCL6, which are usually not expressed in mantle cell lymphoma, although CD5 may be absent from such tumours. Tumour cells express surface IgM/IgD with evidence for light chain restriction with a more frequent expression of the κ than the λ light chain.

Plasmablastic Lymphoma

Plasmablastic lymphoma is an uncommon, typically extranodal lymphoma seen in immunocompromised patients, predominantly in AIDS patients. Incidental CNS involvement has been reported affecting the basal ganglia or the meninges.[90,117]

Morphology reveals cells resembling immunoblasts with large nuclei, prominent nucleoli and abundant cytoplasm. In addition, cells with plasmacytic differentiation are characteristic. Mitotic and proliferative activity is high with a Ki67 staining index usually exceeding 90 per cent of the tumour cells. Because the tumour cells are EBV infected in most cases, EBER *in situ* hybridization will confirm the presence of EBV. Although EBER *in situ* hybridization yields positive results in the majority of cases, LMP1 expression is infrequent. The tumour cells express plasma cell markers, i.e. CD38, CD138 and IRF4/MUM1 with CD79a expression in the majority (50–85 per cent) of cases, but not all. CD45, CD20 and PAX5 are negative or only weakly expressed. The tumour cells often express CD30 and epithelial membrane antigen (EMA). The majority of tumours show a cytoplasmic expression of Ig, mostly IgG.

Burkitt Lymphoma

Patients with all three clinical variants, i.e. endemic, sporadic and immunodeficiency-associated Burkitt lymphoma, are at risk for CNS involvement. The risk for CNS relapse is 30–50 per cent.[119] Because of the high risk for CNS seeding, CNS prophylaxis is routine in patients with Burkitt lymphoma.

Morphologically, the tumour cells are monomorphic and of medium size with round nuclei harbouring multiple nucleoli located paracentrally and a basophilic cytoplasm incorporating lipid vacuoles. Mitoses are frequent, and, correspondingly, proliferative activity is very high with virtually all tumour cells expressing the Ki-67 antigen. A 'starry sky' pattern is characteristic and relates to large macrophages that have phagocytosed apoptotic tumour cells. The tumour cells express CD10, CD19, CD20, CD22, BCL6 and CD38. TdT is negative as is BCL2, which, however, may be expressed weakly in a small fraction of tumours. Translocation with juxtaposition of the *MYC* oncogene and one of the *IG* loci resulting in deregulated expression of the intact *MYC* oncogene is a hallmark.[139]

Hodgkin's Lymphoma

CNS involvement by Hodgkin's lymphoma is rare; in a large cohort of 14 868 patients with both untreated and relapsed Hodgkin's disease, the incidence for CNS involvement was calculated to be below 0.02 per cent.[133] Primary CNS manifestation, which may occur incidentally,[39] should foster an intense search for primary, still silent disease outside the CNS, because exclusive CNS manifestation is unlikely.

Tumours are in contact with the dura in most cases, but location within the brain parenchyma has also been reported. Histologically, classic multinucleated Reed–Sternberg cells, characterized by large nuclei with conspicuous nucleoli and a prominent nuclear membrane, as well as a slightly basophilic cytoplasm, are embedded in a background of an inflammatory infiltrate consisting of lymphocytes, histiocytes and eosinophils. The tumour cells express CD30 and CD15, PAX5, IRF4/MUM1 and, variably, CD20 in the absence of CD45. Hodgkin and Reed–Sternberg cells are latently infected by Epstein–Barr virus in about 40 per cent of patients.[79]

In clinical practice, EBV-positive DLBCL of the elderly may be considered in the differential diagnosis of Hodgkin's lymphoma, because the latter, particularly its polymorphic subtype, may present with large cells resembling Hodgkin and Reed–Sternberg cells. The presence of geographic necrosis, a less frequent expression of CD30, together with a consistent expression of the CD20 antigen, which may be lost from Reed–Sternberg cells while they retain CD30 expression, and an extremely high proliferative index virtually reaching 100 per cent of the tumour cells in association with evidence for EBV infection (expression of LMP1 and EBNA-2) help to distinguish between these entities.

Post-transplant Lymphoproliferative Disorder

Post-transplant lymphoproliferative disorder (PTLD) is a heterogeneous group of diseases clinicopathologically, occurring in patients who have received solid organ or haematopoietic stem cell transplants.[63] DLBCL is one of several B-cell neoplasms that occurs as PTLD. The CNS is involved in about 10–20 per cent of cases.[23,26,127] The majority of these patients manifest with primary involvement as PCNSL. Age and multiorgan involvement are associated with inferior survival.[63] CNS and/or bone marrow involvement have been reported to be strongly associated with poor overall survival.[43]

Morphologically, PTLD-related PCNSL exhibits the characteristic features of DLBCL, thus in this regard being similar to other PCNSLs. Therefore, consideration of the patient's prior medical history including the immune status as well as the EBV status is important, because 50–70 per cent of all PTLD cases are associated with an EBV infection,[115] which is in contrast to EBV-negative PCNSL in immunocompetent patients.

T-Cell Lymphoma

T-cell lymphoma may involve the CNS as either a primary or a secondary tumour.

Primary T-Cell Lymphoma of the CNS

Primary T-cell lymphoma confined to the CNS is extremely rare. Approximately 2 per cent of primary CNS lymphomas with lack of systemic lymphoma at presentation are of T-cell origin.[46,150] Because of its rarity, our current knowledge mainly relies on incidental case reports.[37,161] Only a few larger retrospective studies are available, some of which date back to the 1970s.

The clinical characteristics are similar to PCNSL, i.e. primary DLBCL of the CNS. A median of age 60 years with a range of 3–84 years and a male to female ratio of 2–3:1 have been reported.[109,150] However, it has to be considered that these studies had been performed prior to the introduction of the current WHO Classification of Tumours of Haematopoietic and Lymphoid Tissues; patients with anaplastic large cell lymphoma and T-cell lymphoma in the setting of HTLV-1 infection and mycosis fungoides were also included.[150]

Brain, spinal cord and/or meninges may be involved. In the brain, the majority of cases reported manifested in the supratentorial space affecting the cerebral hemispheres (64 per cent), basal ganglia (11 per cent) and corpus callosum (13 per cent).[150] Brain stem (9 per cent), cerebellum

(7 per cent), meninges (2 per cent) and spinal cord (4 per cent) localization was rarely encountered.[150] Isolated meningeal involvement has also been reported.[87]

Macroscopically, primary T-cell lymphoma is similar to PCNSL, i.e. primary DLBCL of the CNS. Space-occupying mass lesions with greyish to yellow colour show ill-defined margins and may contain haemorrhage and necrosis.

Definite diagnosis relies on the histopathological identification of malignant T cells. CSF analysis cannot substitute for biopsy, because, similar to PCNSL (i.e. primary DLBCL of the CNS), CSF analysis may be either diagnostic, suspicious but not diagnostic of malignancy, or negative.[109]

Histologically, diffuse growth with confluent sheets of lymphoid cells and an angiocentric pattern with intra- and perivascular cuffs of tumour cells occur. Tumour cells correspond to atypical lymphoid cells of small or medium size with nuclear pleomorphism.[84] Mixed large- and small-cell lymphoma may also occur.[109] Tumour cells are admixed with a dense infiltrate of reactive small lymphocytes and plasma cells; incidentally, a granulomatous reaction with multinucleated giant cells has been reported.[109] Reactive astrocytes and activated microglial cells are particularly prominent at the edges of lymphoma.

Immunophenotypically, tumour cells may express T-cell antigens (CD2, CD3, CD4, CD8, CD5, CD7, CD45), TCRγ chain, and cytotoxic granules (granzyme B, perforin), however, at variable frequencies. Proliferative activity generally is high ($\geq$60 per cent).

With respect to differential diagnosis, secondary CNS involvement of extracerebral T-cell lymphoma needs to be excluded. As a general rule, CNS manifestation at initial presentation occurs usually in the presence of already widely disseminated systemic disease. In addition, corticosteroid-induced regression of malignant B cells may mimic T-cell lymphoma. Such cases may also show remarkably elevated proliferative activity (>30 per cent). The presence or accumulation of prominently enlarged macrophages, particularly lipid-laden macrophages, should alert one to the possibility of corticosteroid-mitigated classical PCNSL, i.e. primary DLBCL of the CNS. Monoclonal TCRγ chain amplification in the absence of monoclonal *IGH* gene rearrangements can verify the diagnosis of a monoclonal T cell population and has been proven reliable.[57]

Secondary T-Cell Lymphoma in the CNS

Peripheral T-cell lymphoma, not otherwise specified, refers to a heterogeneous group of mature T-cell lymphomas. Their definition mainly results from exclusion because they include lymphomas that do not fit into specifically defined T-cell lymphoma entities in the current WHO Classification of Tumours of Haematopoietic and Lymphoid Tissues.[129]

Peripheral T-cell lymphoma NOS may involve the CNS, which, however, is a rare event. Systemic T-cell lymphoma usually spreads to the CNS as leptomeningeal infiltrates and may cause corresponding neurological symptoms (cranial nerve palsies, paresis) or may even be clinically asymptomatic.[109]

Morphologically, patternless growing tumours show a broad cytological pattern, mostly containing pleomorphic cells of moderate to large size, whereas small cell tumours are rare. Tumour cells may grow angiocentrically. Immunohistochemically, they usually exhibit an aberrant

T-cell phenotype with expression of the T cell receptor γ chain, whereas CD4 and/or CD8 may be expressed or not. Loss of T cell antigens is a frequent event. Proliferative activity is generally high, and more than 70 per cent of the tumour cells may express the Ki-67 antigen.

Anaplastic Large Cell Lymphoma

Only a few reports have dealt with CNS manifestation of anaplastic large cell lymphoma. They stem from the time before the introduction of the current WHO Classification of Tumours of Haematopoietic and Lymphoid Tissues, which distinguishes clearly between anaplastic large cell lymphoma (ALCL), ALK (anaplastic lymphoma kinase)-positive and ALCL, ALK-negative tumours, which are regarded as separate entities of T-cell lymphomas.[41,89] Studies on the incidence, clinical manifestation and characteristics of CNS disease have, thus, to be interpreted within the confines of these limitations.

Clinically, ALCL, ALK-positive and ALCL, ALK-negative tumours differ in their age distribution, with the former manifesting predominantly in the first three decades of life, being frequent in childhood, whereas the latter usually occurs in adult patients, mainly in the fourth to sixth decade.[41,89]

In the CNS, primary manifestation of ALCL, ALK-positive tumours is rare, and only single cases have been reported; these included both ALCL, ALK-positive as well as ALCL, ALK-negative tumours.[73,93]

Neurological symptoms depend on the location of the lesion and, thus, lead to consideration of a wide spectrum of diseases including dementia and meningitis.[73] Location in the supratentorial space is encountered in most cases; one cerebellar tumour has been reported.[73] The tumour may involve the leptomeninges.[93] Secondary spread of primary extracerebral nodal or systemic ALCL to the CNS is also rare.[73]

Microscopically, ALCL, ALK-positive and ALK-negative tumours share similarities and are indistinguishable by morphology. Large cells with eccentric, horseshoe- or kidney-shaped nuclei with an eosinophilic perinuclear region are characteristic. In addition, smaller cells may be present. Overall, regarding morphology, the spectrum is broad. Several morphologic variants can be distinguished in ALCL, ALK-positive tumours;[41] all tumour cells express ALK and CD30, the most intense staining noticed in large cells. The majority of tumour cells also expresses EMA. T-cell lineage of the tumour cells is evidenced by the expression of one or more T-cell antigens (CD2, CD5, CD4); however, T-cell antigens may be lost. CD45 and CD45RO expression varies. Noticeably, CD3 is absent from the tumour cells in more than 75 per cent of cases, as is CD8, which is expressed in a few cases only. Most tumours express antigens associated with cytotoxicity, i.e. granzyme B and perforin. In rare cases, a few tumour cells may express CD15. With respect to the immunophenotype, ALCL, ALK-negative variant differs from ALCL, ALK-positive type by the absence of ALK, as well as by only a minority of cases being EMA positive.

With respect to differential diagnosis, ALCL, ALK-positive as well as ALCL, ALK-negative types have to be distinguished from primary cutaneous ALCL and other subtypes of T- or B-cell lymphomas with anaplastic features and/or expression of the CD30 antigen.

Myeloid Sarcoma

Myeloid sarcoma, also termed chloroma or granulocytic sarcoma, is defined as a tumour composed of myeloid blasts outside the bone marrow. Multiple sites may be affected. CNS involvement, mostly of the dura/leptomeninges and less frequently of the brain parenchyma, is rare and may present before, during or after diagnosis of the underlying disorder.[5,85] Clinically, disease may mimic meningioma or intracranial haemorrhage. Because patients with leukaemia may have coagulation disturbances, bleeding in an atypical location should raise the suspicion of tumourous bleeding and foster a careful search for blasts within the hematoma.

Morphologically, myeloblasts have scant cytoplasmic rims, large nuclei and prominent nucleoli and show vigorous mitotic activity. Immunohistochemically, the expression pattern of myeloperoxidase, CD68/KP1, CD68/PG-M1, CD99, CD56 and CD30, distinguishes myeloid sarcoma from DLBCL and other lymphomas that may also affect the CNS, including Burkitt lymphoma.

REFERENCES

1. Abla O, Weitzman S, Blay JY, et al. Primary CNS lymphoma in children and adolescents: a descriptive analysis from the International Primary CNS Lymphoma Collaborative Group (IPCG). Clin Cancer Res 2011;17: 346–52.

2. Abrey LE, Yahalom J, DeAngelis LM. Treatment for primary CNS lymphoma: the next step. J Clin Oncol 2000;18:3144–50.

3. Adachi J, Mishima K, Wakiya K, et al. O-methylguanine-DNA methyltransferase promoter methylation in 45 primary central nervous system lymphomas: quantitative assessment of methylation and response to temozolomide treatment. J Neurooncol 2012;107:147–53.

4. Adam P, Bonzheim I, Fend F, Quintanilla-Martinez L. Epstein–Barr virus-positive diffuse large B-cell lymphomas of the elderly. Adv Anat Pathol 2011;18:349–55.

5. Ahn JY, Kwon SO, Shin MS, Kang SH, Kim YR. Meningeal chloroma (granulocytic sarcoma) in acute lymphoblastic leukemia mimicking a falx meningioma. J Neurooncol 2002;60:31–5.

6. Alderson L, Fetell MR, Sisti M, et al. Sentinel lesions of primary CNS lymphoma. J Neurol Neurosurg Psychiatry 1996;60:102–5.

7. Alvarez R, Dupuis J, Plonquet A, et al. Clinical relevance of flow cytometric immunophenotyping of the cerebrospinal fluid in patients with diffuse large B-cell lymphoma. Ann Oncol 2012;23:1274–9.

8. Antinori A, Larocca LM, Fassone L, et al. HHV-8/KSHV is not associated with AIDS-related primary central nervous system lymphoma. Brain Pathol 1999;9:199–208.

9. Asai A, Matsutani M, Kohno T, et al. Subacute brain atrophy after radiation therapy for malignant brain tumor. Cancer 1989;63:1962–74.

10. Aukema SM, Siebert R, Schuuring E, et al. Double-hit B-cell lymphomas. Blood 2011;117:2319–31.

11. Baraniskin A, Kuhnhenn J, Schlegel U, et al. Identification of microRNAs in the cerebrospinal fluid as marker for

primary diffuse large B-cell lymphoma of the central nervous system. *Blood* 2011;**117**:3140–46.

12. Bayraktar S, Stefanovic A, Montague N, *et al.* Central nervous system manifestations of marginal zone B-cell lymphoma. *Ann Hematol* 2010;**89**:1003–9.

13. Bea S, Zettl A, Wright G, *et al.* Diffuse large B-cell lymphoma subgroups have distinct genetic profiles that influence tumor biology and improve gene-expression-based survival prediction. *Blood* 2005;**106**:3183–90.

14. Bellinzona M, Roser F, Ostertag H, Gaab RM, Saini M. Surgical removal of primary central nervous system lymphomas (PCNSL) presenting as space occupying lesions: a series of 33 cases. *Eur J Surg Oncol* 2005;**31**:100–105.

15. Bergmann M, Terzija-Wessel U, Blasius S, *et al.* Intravascular lymphomatosis of the CNS: clinicopathologic study and search for expression of oncoproteins and Epstein–Barr virus. *Clin Neurol Neurosurg* 1994;**96**:236–43.

16. Bibas M, Antinori A. EBV and HIV-related lymphoma. *Mediterr J Hematol Infect Dis* 2009;**1**:e2009032.

17. Booman M, Douwes J, Legdeur MC, *et al.* From brain to testis: immune escape and clonal selection in a B cell lymphoma with selective outgrowth in two immune sanctuaries. *Haematologica* 2007;**92**:e69–71.

18. Booman M, Szuhai K, Rosenwald A, *et al.* Genomic alterations and gene expression in primary diffuse large B-cell lymphomas of immune-privileged sites: the importance of apoptosis and immunomodulatory pathways. *J Pathol* 2008;**216**:209–17.

19. Brecher K, Hochberg FH, Louis DN, de la Monte S, Riskind P. Case report of unusual leukoencephalopathy preceding primary CNS lymphoma. *J Neurol Neurosurg Psychiatry* 1998;**65**:917–20.

20. Brinkmann MM, Schulz TF. Regulation of intracellular signalling by the terminal membrane proteins of members of the Gammaherpesvirinae. *J Gen Virol* 2006;**87**(Part 5):1047–74.

21. Brunn A, Montesinos-Rongen M, Strack A, *et al.* Expression pattern and cellular sources of chemokines in primary central nervous system lymphoma. *Acta Neuropathol* 2007;**114**:271–6.

22. Brunn A, Nagel I, Montesinos-Rongen M, *et al.* Frequent triple-hit expression of MYC, BCL2, and BCL6 in primary lymphoma of the central nervous system and absence of a favorable MYC(low) BCL2 (low) subgroup may underlie the inferior prognosis as compared to systemic diffuse large B cell lymphomas. *Acta Neuropathol* 2013;**126**:603–5.

23. Buell JF, Gross TG, Hanaway MJ, *et al.* Posttransplant lymphoproliferative disorder: significance of central nervous system involvement. *Transplant Proc* 2005;**37**:954–5.

24. Camilleri-Broet S, Criniere E, Broet P, *et al.* A uniform activated B-cell-like immunophenotype might explain the poor prognosis of primary central nervous system lymphomas: analysis of 83 cases. *Blood* 2006;**107**:190–96.

25. Cash J, Fehir KM, Pollack MS. Meningeal involvement in early stage chronic lymphocytic leukemia. *Cancer* 1987;**59**:798–800.

26. Cavaliere R, Petroni G, Lopes MB, Schiff D. Primary central nervous system post-transplantation lymphoproliferative disorder: an International Primary Central Nervous System Lymphoma Collaborative Group Report. *Cancer* 2010;**116**:863–70.

27. CBTRUS Statistical Report. *Primary brain and central nervous system tumors diagnosed in the United States in 2004–2008.* Chicago, IL: Central Brain Tumor Registry of the United States, 2012.

28. Chu LC, Eberhart CG, Grossman SA, Herman JG. Epigenetic silencing of multiple genes in primary CNS lymphoma. *Int J Cancer* 2006;**119**:2487–91.

29. Cingolani A, Fratino L, Scoppettuolo G, Antinori A. Changing pattern of primary cerebral lymphoma in the highly active antiretroviral therapy era. *J Neurovirol* 2005;**11**(Suppl 3):38–44.

30. Cinque P, Vago L, Dahl H, *et al.* Polymerase chain reaction on cerebrospinal fluid for diagnosis of virus-associated opportunistic diseases of the central nervous system in HIV-infected patients. *AIDS* 1996;**10**:951–8.

31. Cobbers JM, Wolter M, Reifenberger J, *et al.* Frequent inactivation of CDKN2A and rare mutation of TP53 in PCNSL. *Brain Pathol* 1998;**8**:263–76.

32. Corry J, Smith JG, Wirth A, Quong G, Liew KH. Primary central nervous system lymphoma: age and performance status are more important than treatment modality. *Int J Radiat Oncol Biol Phys* 1998;**41**:615–20.

33. Cortelazzo S, Ponzoni M, Ferreri AJ, Hoelzer D. Lymphoblastic lymphoma. *Crit Rev Oncol Hematol* 2011;**79**:330–43.

34. Courts C, Montesinos-Rongen M, Martin-Subero JI, *et al.* Transcriptional profiling of the nuclear factor-kappaB pathway identifies a subgroup of primary lymphoma of the central nervous system with low BCL10 expression. *J Neuropathol Exp Neurol* 2007;**66**:230–37.

35. Courts C, Montesinos-Rongen M, Brunn A, *et al.* Recurrent inactivation of the PRDM1 gene in primary central nervous system lymphoma. *J Neuropathol Exp Neurol* 2008;**67**:720–27.

36. DeAngelis LM. Natalizumab: a double-edged sword? *Ann Neurol* 2009;**66**: 262–3.

37. Deckert M, Paulus W. Malignant lymphomas. In: Louis DN, Ohgaki H, Wiestler OD, Cavenee WK eds. *WHO classification of tumours of the central nervous system*, 4th ed. Lyon: International Agency for Cancer Research, 2007:188–92.

38. Deckert M, Engert A, Bruck W, *et al.* Modern concepts in the biology, diagnosis, differential diagnosis and treatment of primary central nervous system lymphoma. *Leukemia* 2011;**25**:1797–807.

39. Deckert-Schluter M, Marek J, Setlik M, *et al.* Primary manifestation of Hodgkin's disease in the central nervous system. *Virchows Arch* 1998;**432**:477–81.

40. Deckert-Schluter M, Rang A, Wiestler OD. Apoptosis and apoptosis-related gene products in primary non-Hodgkin's lymphoma of the central nervous system. *Acta Neuropathol* 1998;**96**:157–62.

41. Delsol G, Jaffe ES, Falini B, *et al.* Anaplastic large cell lymphoma (ALCL), ALK-positive. In: Swerdlow ST, Campo E, Harris N, *et al.* eds. *WHO classification of tumours of haematopoietic and lymphoid tissues*, 4th ed. Lyon: International Agency for Research on Cancer, 2008:312–16.

42. Ellison DW, Wilkins BS. Lymphoma and the nervous system. *Curr Top Pathol* 2001;**95**:239–65.

43. Evens AM, David KA, Helenowski I, *et al.* Multicenter analysis of 80 solid organ transplantation recipients with post-transplantation lymphoproliferative disease: outcomes and prognostic factors in the modern era. *J Clin Oncol* 2010;**28**:1038–46.

44. Ferrer A, Bosch F, Villamor N, *et al.* Central nervous system involvement in mantle cell lymphoma. *Ann Oncol* 2008;**19**:135–41.

45. Ferreri AJ. How I treat primary CNS lymphoma. *Blood* 2011;**118**:510–22.

46. Ferreri AJ, Reni M, Pasini F, *et al.* A multicenter study of treatment of primary CNS lymphoma. *Neurology* 2002;**58**:1513–20.

47. Ferreri AJ, Dell'Oro S, Capello D, *et al.* Aberrant methylation in the promoter region of the reduced folate carrier gene is a potential mechanism of resistance to methotrexate in primary central nervous system lymphomas. *Br J Haematol* 2004;**126**:657–64.

48. Fischer L, Martus P, Weller M, *et al.* Meningeal dissemination in primary CNS lymphoma: prospective evaluation of 282 patients. *Neurology* 2008;**71**:1102–8.

49. Flinn IW, Ambinder RF. AIDS primary central nervous system lymphoma. *Curr Opin Oncol* 1996;**8**:373–6.

50. Garicochea B, Cliquet MG, Melo N, *et al.* Leptomeningeal involvement in chronic lymphocytic leukemia identified by polymerase chain reaction in stored slides: a case report. *Mod Pathol* 1997;**10**:500–503.

51. Goldstein J, Dickson DW, Rubenstein A, *et al.* Primary central nervous system lymphoma in a pediatric patient with acquired immune deficiency syndrome. Treatment with radiation therapy. *Cancer* 1990;**66**:2503–8.

52. Gonzalez-Aguilar A, Soto-Hernandez JL. The management of primary central nervous system lymphoma related to AIDS in the HAART era. *Curr Opin Oncol* 2011;**23**:648–53.

53. Grupka NL, Seinfeld J, Ryder J, Lillehei KO, Kleinschmidt-Demasters BK. Secondary central nervous system involvement by follicular lymphoma: case report and review of the literature. *Surg Neurol* 2006;**65**:590–94.

54. Haldorsen IS, Krakenes J, Goplen AK, *et al.* AIDS-related primary central nervous system lymphoma: a Norwegian national survey 1989–2003. *BMC Cancer* 2008;**8**:225.

55. Hans CP, Weisenburger DD, Greiner TC, *et al.* Confirmation of the molecular classification of diffuse large B-cell lymphoma by immunohistochemistry using a tissue microarray. *Blood* 2004;**103**:275–82.

56. Hanse MC, Van't Veer MB, van Lom K, van den Bent MJ. Incidence of central nervous system involvement in chronic

lymphocytic leukemia and outcome to treatment. *J Neurol* 2008;**255**:828–30.

57. Harder A, Dudel C, Anagnostopoulos I, Hummel M, Bruck W. Molecular genetic diagnosis of a primary central nervous system T cell lymphoma. *Acta Neuropathol* 2003;**105**:65–8.

58. Hofscheier A, Ponciano A, Bonzheim I, *et al.* Geographic variation in the prevalence of Epstein–Barr virus-positive diffuse large B-cell lymphoma of the elderly: a comparative analysis of a Mexican and a German population. *Mod Pathol* 2011;**24**:1046–54.

59. Huen DS, Henderson SA, Croom-Carter D, Rowe M. The Epstein–Barr virus latent membrane protein-1 (LMP1) mediates activation of NF-kappa B and cell surface phenotype via two effector regions in its carboxy-terminal cytoplasmic domain. *Oncogene* 1995;**10**:549–60.

60. Husseini L, Saleh A, Reifenberger G, Hartung HP, Kieseier BC. Inflammatory demyelinating brain lesions heralding primary CNS lymphoma. *Can J Neurol Sci* 2012;**39**:6–10.

61. Inbasekaran V, Vijayarathinam P, Arumugam S. Solitary intracerebral plasmacytoma. *J Indian Med Assoc* 1991;**89**:16–17.

62. Ivers LC, Kim AY, Sax PE. Predictive value of polymerase chain reaction of cerebrospinal fluid for detection of Epstein–Barr virus to establish the diagnosis of HIV-related primary central nervous system lymphoma. *Clin Infect Dis* 2004;**38**:1629–32.

63. Jagadeesh D, Woda BA, Draper J, Evens AM. Post transplant lymphoproliferative disorders: risk, classification, and therapeutic recommendations. *Curr Treat Options Oncol* 2012;**13**:122–36.

64. Jahnke K, Hummel M, Korfel A, *et al.* Detection of subclinical systemic disease in primary CNS lymphoma by polymerase chain reaction of the rearranged immunoglobulin heavy-chain genes. *J Clin Oncol* 2006;**24**:4754–7.

65. Jahnke K, Korfel A, Komm J, *et al.* Intraocular lymphoma 2000–2005: results of a retrospective multicentre trial. *Graefes Arch Clin Exp Ophthalmol* 2006;**244**:663–9.

66. Jellinger K, Radiaszkiewicz T. Involvement of the central nervous system in malignant lymphomas. *Virchows Arch A Pathol Anat Histol* 1976;**370**:345–62.

67. Jordanova ES, Riemersma SA, Philippo K, *et al.* Hemizygous deletions in the HLA region account for loss of heterozygosity in the majority of diffuse large B-cell lymphomas of the testis and the central nervous system. *Genes Chromosomes Cancer* 2002;**35**:38–48.

68. Jordanova ES, Philippo K, Giphart MJ, Schuuring E, Kluin PM. Mutations in the HLA class II genes leading to loss of expression of HLA-DR and HLA-DQ in diffuse large B-cell lymphoma. *Immunogenetics* 2003;**55**:203–9.

69. Jordanova ES, Riemersma SA, Philippo K, Schuuring E, Kluin PM. Beta2-microglobulin aberrations in diffuse large B-cell lymphoma of the testis and the central nervous system. *Int J Cancer* 2003;**103**:393–8.

70. Kiewe P, Fischer L, Martus P, Thiel E, Korfel A. Meningeal dissemination in primary CNS lymphoma: diagnosis, treatment, and survival in a large monocenter cohort. *Neuro Oncol* 2010;**12**:409–17.

71. Kleinschmidt-DeMasters BK, Damek DM, Lillehei KO, Dogan A, Giannini C. Epstein Barr virus-associated primary CNS lymphomas in elderly patients on immunosuppressive medications. *J Neuropathol Exp Neurol* 2008;**67**:1103–11.

72. Kluin PM, Deckert M, Ferry A. Primary diffuse large B-cell lymphoma of the CNS. In: Swerdlow SH, Campo E, Harris NL, *et al.* eds. *WHO classification of tumours of haematopoietic and lymphoid tissues,* 4th ed. Lyon: International Agency for Research in Cancer, 2008:240–41.

73. Kodama K, Hokama M, Kawaguchi K, Tanaka Y, Hongo K. Primary ALK-1-negative anaplastic large cell lymphoma of the brain: case report and review of the literature. *Neuropathology* 2009;**29**:166–71.

74. Korfel A. Prevention of central nervous system relapses in diffuse large B-cell lymphoma: which patients and how? *Curr Opin Oncol* 2011;**23**:436–40.

75. Kridel R, Dietrich PY. Prevention of CNS relapse in diffuse large B-cell lymphoma. *Lancet Oncol* 2011;**12**:1258–66.

76. Krumbholz M, Theil D, Derfuss T, *et al.* BAFF is produced by astrocytes and up-regulated in multiple sclerosis lesions and primary central nervous system lymphoma. *J Exp Med* 2005;**201**:195–200.

77. Kuhlmann T, Lassmann H, Bruck W. Diagnosis of inflammatory demyelination in biopsy specimens: a practical approach. *Acta Neuropathol* 2008;**115**:275–87.

78. Kuker W, Nagele T, Korfel A, *et al.* Primary central nervous system lymphomas (PCNSL): MRI features at presentation in 100 patients. *J Neurooncol* 2005;**72**:169–77.

79. Kuppers R. Molecular biology of Hodgkin lymphoma. *Hematology Am Soc Hematol Educ Program* 2009:491–6.

80. Kurzwelly D, Glas M, Roth P, *et al.* Primary CNS lymphoma in the elderly: temozolomide therapy and MGMT status. *J Neurooncol* 2010;**97**:389–92.

81. Kwok LY, Miletic H, Lutjen S, *et al.* Protective immunosurveillance of the central nervous system by Listeria-specific CD4 and CD8 T cells in systemic listeriosis in the absence of intracerebral Listeria. *J Immunol* 2002;**169**:2010–19.

82. Lai R, Abrey LE, Rosenblum MK, DeAngelis LM. Treatment-induced leukoencephalopathy in primary CNS lymphoma: a clinical and autopsy study. *Neurology* 2004;**62**:451–6.

83. Larocca LM, Capello D, Rinelli A, *et al.* The molecular and phenotypic profile of primary central nervous system lymphoma identifies distinct categories of the disease and is consistent with histogenetic derivation from germinal center-related B cells. *Blood* 1998;**92**:1011–19.

84. Lee DK, Chung CK, Kim HJ, *et al.* Multifocal primary CNS T cell lymphoma of the spinal cord. *Clin Neuropathol* 2002;**21**:149–55.

85. Lee SH, Park J, Hwang SK. Isolated recurrence of intracerebral granulocytic sarcoma in acute lymphoblastic leukemia: a case report. *J Neurooncol* 2006;**80**:101–4.

86. Lenz G, Wright GW, Emre NC, *et al.* Molecular subtypes of diffuse large B-cell lymphoma arise by distinct genetic pathways. *Proc Natl Acad Sci U S A* 2008;**105**:13520–25.

87. Levin N, Soffer D, Grissaru S, *et al.* Primary T-cell CNS lymphoma presenting with leptomeningeal spread and neurolymphomatosis. *J Neurooncol* 2008;**90**:77–83.

88. Linnebank M, Pels H, Kleczar N, *et al.* MTX-induced white matter changes are associated with polymorphisms of methionine metabolism. *Neurology* 2005;**64**:912–13.

89. Mason DY, Campo E, Harris N, *et al.* Anaplastic large cell lymphoma, ALK-negative. In: Swerdlow ST, Campo E, Harris N, *et al.* eds. *WHO classification of tumours of haematopoietic and lymphoid tissues,* 4th ed. Lyon: International Agency for Cancer Research, 2008:317–19.

90. Mathews MS, Bota DA, Kim RC, Hasso AN, Linskey ME. Primary leptomeningeal plasmablastic lymphoma. *J Neurooncol* 2011;**104**:835–8.

91. McAllister LD. Primary central nervous system lymphoma: a review. *Curr Neurol Neurosci Rep* 2002;**2**:210–15.

92. McCann KJ, Ashton-Key M, Smith K, Stevenson FK, Ottensmeier CH. Primary central nervous system lymphoma: tumor-related clones exist in the blood and bone marrow with evidence for separate development. *Blood* 2009;**113**:4677–80.

93. Merlin E, Chabrier S, Verkarre V, *et al.* Primary leptomeningeal ALK+ lymphoma in a 13-year-old child. *J Pediatr Hematol Oncol* 2008;**30**:963–7.

94. Miller DC, Hochberg FH, Harris NL, *et al.* Pathology with clinical correlations of primary central nervous system non-Hodgkin's lymphoma. The Massachusetts General Hospital experience 1958–1989. *Cancer* 1994;**74**:1383–97.

95. Moazzam AA, Drappatz J, Kim RY, Kesari S. Chronic lymphocytic leukemia with central nervous system involvement: report of two cases with a comprehensive literature review. *J Neurooncol* 2012;**106**:185–200.

96. Montesinos-Rongen M, Kuppers R, Schluter D, *et al.* Primary central nervous system lymphomas are derived from germinal-center B cells and show a preferential usage of the V4–34 gene segment. *Am J Pathol* 1999;**155**:2077–86.

97. Montesinos-Rongen M, Hans VH, Eis-Hubinger AM, *et al.* Human herpes virus-8 is not associated with primary central nervous system lymphoma in HIV-negative patients. *Acta Neuropathol* 2001;**102**:489–95.

98. Montesinos-Rongen M, Zuhlke-Jenisch R, Gesk S, *et al.* Interphase cytogenetic analysis of lymphoma-associated chromosomal breakpoints in primary diffuse large B-cell lymphomas of the central nervous system. *J Neuropathol Exp Neurol* 2002;**61**:926–33.

99. Montesinos-Rongen M, Akasaka T, Zuhlke-Jenisch R, *et al.* Molecular characterization of BCL6 breakpoints in primary diffuse large B-cell lymphomas of the central nervous system identifies GAPD as novel translocation partner. *Brain Pathol* 2003;**13**:534–8.

100. Montesinos-Rongen M, Besleaga R, Heinsohn S, *et al.* Absence of simian virus 40 DNA sequences in primary central nervous system lymphoma in HIV-negative patients. *Virchows Arch* 2004;**444**:436–8.

101. Montesinos-Rongen M, Van Roost D, Schaller C, Wiestler OD, Deckert M. Primary diffuse large B-cell lymphomas of the central nervous system are targeted by aberrant somatic hypermutation. *Blood* 2004;**103**:1869–75.

102. Montesinos-Rongen M, Schmitz R, Courts C, et al. Absence of immunoglobulin class switch in primary lymphomas of the central nervous system. *Am J Pathol* 2005;**166**:1773–9.

103. Montesinos-Rongen M, Brunn A, Bentink S, et al. Gene expression profiling suggests primary central nervous system lymphomas to be derived from a late germinal center B cell. *Leukemia* 2008;**22**:400–405.

104. Montesinos-Rongen M, Siebert R, Deckert M. Primary lymphoma of the central nervous system: just DLBCL or not? *Blood* 2009;**113**:7–10.

105. Montesinos-Rongen M, Schmitz R, Brunn A, et al. Mutations of CARD11 but not TNFAIP3 may activate the NF-kappaB pathway in primary CNS lymphoma. *Acta Neuropathol* 2010;**120**:529–35.

106. Montesinos-Rongen M, Godlewska E, Brunn A, et al. Activating L265P mutations of the MYD88 gene are common in primary central nervous system lymphoma. *Acta Neuropathol* 2011;**122**:791–2.

107. Montesinos-Rongen M, Schafer E, Siebert R, Deckert M. Genes regulating the B cell receptor pathway are recurrently mutated in primary central nervous system lymphoma. *Acta Neuropathol* 2012;**124**:905–6.

108. Morgello S. Pathogenesis and classification of primary central nervous system lymphoma: an update. *Brain Pathol* 1995;**5**:383–93.

109. Morgello S, Maiese K, Petito CK. T-cell lymphoma in the CNS: clinical and pathologic features. *Neurology* 1989;**39**:1190–96.

110. Morton LM, Wang SS, Devesa SS, et al. Lymphoma incidence patterns by WHO subtype in the United States, 1992–2001. *Blood* 2006;**107**:265–76.

111. Nagpal S, Glantz MJ, Recht L. Treatment and prevention of secondary CNS lymphoma. *Semin Neurol.* 2010;**30**:263–72.

112. Nakamura N, Ponzoni M, Campo E. Intravascular large B cell-lymphoma. In: Swerdlow ST, Campo E, Harris N, et al. eds. *WHO classification of tumours of haematopoietic and lymphoid tissues*, 4th ed. Lyon: International Agency for Cancer Research, 2008:252–3.

113. Nakamura S, Jaffe ES, Swerdlow ST. EBV positive diffuse large B-cell lymphoma of the elderly. In: Swerdlow ST, Campo E, Harris N, et al. eds. *WHO classification of tumours of haematopoietic and lymphoid tissues*, 4th ed. Lyon: International Agency for Research on Cancer, 2008:243–4.

114. Nayak L, Hedvat C, Rosenblum MK, Abrey LE, DeAngelis LM. Late relapse in primary central nervous system lymphoma: clonal persistence. *Neuro Oncol* 2011;**13**:525–9.

115. Nourse JP, Jones K, Gandhi MK. Epstein–Barr Virus-related post-transplant lymphoproliferative disorders: pathogenetic insights for targeted therapy. *Am J Transplant* 2011;**11**:888–95.

116. Oyama T, Yamamoto K, Asano N, et al. Age-related EBV-associated B-cell lymphoproliferative disorders constitute a distinct clinicopathologic group: a

study of 96 patients. *Clin Cancer Res* 2007;**13**:5124–32.

117. Pantanowitz L, Dezube BJ. Editorial comment: plasmablastic lymphoma: a diagnostic and therapeutic puzzle. *AIDS Read* 2007;**17**:448–9.

118. Papanicolau-Sengos A, Wang-Rodriguez J, Wang HY, et al. Rare case of a primary non-dural central nervous system low grade B-cell lymphoma and literature review. *Int J Clin Exp Pathol* 2012;**5**:89–95.

119. Patrij K, Reiser M, Watzel L, et al. Isolated central nervous system relapse of systemic lymphoma (SCNSL): clinical features and outcome of a retrospective analysis. *Ger Med Sci* 2011;**9**:Doc11.

120. Patsalides AD, Atac G, Hedge U, et al. Lymphomatoid granulomatosis: abnormalities of the brain at MR imaging. *Radiology* 2005;**237**:265–73.

121. Paulus W, Jellinger K. Comparison of integrin adhesion molecules expressed by primary brain lymphomas and nodal lymphomas. *Acta Neuropathol* 1993;**86**:360–64.

122. Paulus W, Jellinger K, Hallas C, Ott G, Muller-Hermelink HK. Human herpesvirus-6 and Epstein–Barr virus genome in primary cerebral lymphomas. *Neurology* 1993;**43**:1591–3.

123. Pels H, Schlegel U. Primary central nervous system lymphoma. *Curr Treat Options Neurol* 2006;**8**:346–57.

124. Pels H, Schmidt-Wolf IG, Glasmacher A, et al. Primary central nervous system lymphoma: results of a pilot and phase II study of systemic and intraventricular chemotherapy with deferred radiotherapy. *J Clin Oncol* 2003;**21**:4489–95.

125. Pels H, Montesinos-Rongen M, Schaller C, et al. Clonal evolution as pathogenetic mechanism in relapse of primary CNS lymphoma. *Neurology* 2004;**63**:167–9.

126. Pels H, Juergens A, Schirgens I, et al. Early complete response during chemotherapy predicts favorable outcome in patients with primary CNS lymphoma. *Neuro Oncol* 2010;**12**:720–24.

127. Penn I, Porat G. Central nervous system lymphomas in organ allograft recipients. *Transplantation* 1995;**59**:240–44.

128. Phan-Ba R, Bisig B, Deprez M, et al. Primary central nervous system lymphoma in a patient treated with natalizumab. *Ann Neurol* 2011;**69**:1060–61; author reply 1–2.

129. Pileri SA, Ralfkaier E, Wieisenburger DD, et al. Peripheral T-cell lymphoma, not otherwise specified. In: Swerdlow ST, Campo E, Harris N, et al. eds. *WHO classification of tumours of haematopoietic and lymphoid tissues*. Lyon: International Agency for Cancer Research, 2008:306.

130. Ponzoni M, Arrigoni G, Gould VE, et al. Lack of CD 29 (beta1 integrin) and CD 54 (ICAM-1) adhesion molecules in intravascular lymphomatosis. *Hum Pathol* 2000;**31**:220–26.

131. Ponzoni M, Berger F, Chassagne-Clement C, et al. Reactive perivascular T-cell infiltrate predicts survival in primary central nervous system B-cell lymphomas. *Br J Haematol* 2007;**138**:316–23.

132. Provencher S, Ferlay C, Alaoui-Slimani K, et al. Clinical characteristics and outcome of isolated extracerebral relapses of primary central nervous system lymphoma: a case series. *Hematol Oncol* 2011;**29**:10–16.

133. Re D, Fuchs M, Schober T, Engert A, Diehl V. CNS involvement in Hodgkin's lymphoma. *J Clin Oncol* 2007;**25**:3182.

134. Richter J, Ammerpohl O, Martin-Subero JI, et al. Array-based DNA methylation profiling of primary lymphomas of the central nervous system. *BMC Cancer* 2009;**9**:455.

135. Riemersma SA, Oudejans JJ, Vonk MJ, et al. High numbers of tumour-infiltrating activated cytotoxic T lymphocytes, and frequent loss of HLA class I and II expression, are features of aggressive B cell lymphomas of the brain and testis. *J Pathol* 2005;**206**:328–36.

136. Robertus JL, Harms G, Blokzijl T, et al. Specific expression of miR-17-5p and miR-127 in testicular and central nervous system diffuse large B-cell lymphoma. *Mod Pathol* 2009;**22**:547–55.

137. Rosenwald A, Wright G, Chan WC, et al. The use of molecular profiling to predict survival after chemotherapy for diffuse large-B-cell lymphoma. *N Engl J Med* 2002;**346**:1937–47.

138. Rubenstein JL, Fridlyand J, Shen A, et al. Gene expression and angiotropism in primary CNS lymphoma. *Blood* 2006;**107**:3716–23.

139. Salaverria I, Siebert R. The gray zone between Burkitt's lymphoma and diffuse large B-cell lymphoma from a genetics perspective. *J Clin Oncol* 2011;**29**:1835–43.

140. Salles G, de Jong D, Xie W, et al. Prognostic significance of immunohistochemical biomarkers in diffuse large B-cell lymphoma: a study from the Lunenburg Lymphoma Biomarker Consortium. *Blood* 2011;**117**:7070–78.

141. Schlegel U. Primary CNS lymphoma. *Ther Adv Neurol Disord* 2009;**2**:93–104.

142. Schlegel U, Pels H, Oehring R, Blumcke I. Neurologic sequelae of treatment of primary CNS lymphomas. *J Neurooncol* 1999;**43**:277–86.

143. Schlegel U, Schmidt-Wolf IG, Deckert M. Primary CNS lymphoma: clinical presentation, pathological classification, molecular pathogenesis and treatment. *J Neurol Sci* 2000;**181**:1–12.

144. Schroers R, Baraniskin A, Heute C, et al. Diagnosis of leptomeningeal disease in diffuse large B-cell lymphomas of the central nervous system by flow cytometry and cytopathology. *Eur J Haematol* 2010;**85**:520–28.

145. Schulte-Altedorneburg G, Heuser L, Pels H. MRI patterns in recurrence of primary CNS lymphoma in immunocompetent patients. *Eur J Radiol* 2012;**81**:2380–85.

146. Schwartz TH, Rhiew R, Isaacson SR, Orazi A, Bruce JN. Association between intracranial plasmacytoma and multiple myeloma: clinicopathological outcome study. *Neurosurgery* 2001;**49**:1039–44; discussion 44–5.

147. Schweikert A, Kremer M, Ringel F, et al. Primary central nervous system lymphoma in a patient treated with natalizumab. *Ann Neurol* 2009;**66**:403–406.

148. Schwindt H, Akasaka T, Zuhlke-Jenisch R, et al. Chromosomal translocations fusing the BCL6 gene to different partner loci are recurrent in primary central nervous system lymphoma and may be associated with aberrant somatic

hypermutation or defective class switch recombination. *J Neuropathol Exp Neurol* 2006;65:776–82.

149. Schwindt H, Vater I, Kreuz M, *et al.* Chromosomal imbalances and partial uniparental disomies in primary central nervous system lymphoma. *Leukemia* 2009;23:1875–84.

150. Shenkier TN, Blay JY, O'Neill BP, *et al.* Primary CNS lymphoma of T-cell origin: a descriptive analysis from the international primary CNS lymphoma collaborative group. *J Clin Oncol* 2005;23:2233–9.

151. Siegal T, Goldschmidt N. CNS prophylaxis in diffuse large B-cell lymphoma: if, when, how and for whom? *Blood Rev* 2012;26:97–106.

152. Singer EJ, Valdes-Sueiras M, Commins D, Levine A. Neurologic presentations of AIDS. *Neurol Clin* 2010;28:253–75.

153. Stenzel W, Pels H, Staib P, *et al.* Concomitant manifestation of primary CNS lymphoma and Toxoplasma encephalitis in a patient with AIDS. *J Neurol.* 2004;251:764–6.

154. Thompsett AR, Ellison DW, Stevenson FK, Zhu D. V(H) gene sequences from primary central nervous system lymphomas indicate derivation from highly mutated germinal center B cells with ongoing mutational activity. *Blood* 1999;94:1738–46.

155. Tun HW, Personett D, Baskerville KA, *et al.* Pathway analysis of primary central nervous system lymphoma. *Blood* 2008;111:3200–10.

156. Uetsuka S, Kajiwara K, Suehiro E, *et al.* T cell malignant lymphoma in the central nervous system after acute lymphoblastic leukemia in a child. *Childs Nerv Syst* 1999;15:486–9.

157. Vigliani MC, Duyckaerts C, Hauw JJ, *et al.* Dementia following treatment of brain tumors with radiotherapy administered alone or in combination with nitrosourea-based chemotherapy: a clinical and pathological study. *J Neurooncol* 1999;41:137–49.

158. Villano JL, Koshy M, Shaikh H, Dolecek TA, McCarthy BJ. Age, gender, and racial differences in incidence and survival in primary CNS lymphoma. *Br J Cancer* 2011;105:1414–18.

159. Vitolo U, Ferreri AJ, Montoto S. Lymphoplasmacytic lymphoma-Waldenstrom's macroglobulinemia. *Crit Rev Oncol Hematol* 2008;67:172–85.

160. Wang D, Liebowitz D, Kieff E. An EBV membrane protein expressed in immortalized lymphocytes transforms established rodent cells. *Cell* 1985;43(3 Part 2):831–40.

161. Wanschitz J, Hainfellner JA, Simonitsch I, *et al.* Non-HTLV-I associated pleomorphic T-cell lymphoma of the brain mimicking post-vaccinal acute inflammatory demyelination. *Neuropathol Appl Neurobiol* 1997;23:43–9.

Pituitary and Suprasellar Tumours

Sylvia L Asa

INTRODUCTION

The pituitary gland is the 'master gland' that regulates many of the functions of other endocrine glands and their target tissues throughout the body. There is virtually no organ or tissue that is not affected, directly or indirectly, by the hormones that are secreted by the anterior and posterior pituitary.

Pituitary dysfunction is a common clinical scenario. However, the manifestations of pituitary disease vary from florid clinical features that can readily be identified and recognized as pituitary in aetiology, to more subtle and nonspecific problems that are often overlooked or misdiagnosed, leaving the relationship to pituitary malfunction unnoticed. The former – conditions such as acromegaly and Cushing's disease – are rare, hence the misconception that pituitary disease is rare.

There are three types of clinical problems that can be attributed to pituitary pathology. The most common of these is insufficiency of pituitary hormones. This can be due to any number of disorders, ranging from congenital problems (see Chapter 4) to infiltrative and neoplastic diseases. Some lesions – usually pituitary adenomas, but also occasionally hyperplasias – can cause pituitary hormone excess. Mass lesions of the sella turcica can give rise to headaches, visual field defects, loss of vision, symptoms and signs due to damage of adjacent nerves, and occasionally elevations of one pituitary hormone, prolactin ('stalk effect'), that is normally maintained under tonic inhibition.

There has been significant progress in our understanding of pituitary development, physiology and pathology. The classification of pituitary disease is becoming easier and, as targeted therapies are being developed, the role of the pathologist in determining accurate diagnoses is increasingly important.

Methodology in Pituitary Pathology

The handling of the autopsy pituitary is important to ensure proper identification and characterization of lesions. When removing the brain, the hypophyseal stalk should be cut as high as possible to ensure that the gland remains intact. When there is a large lesion, the sella may be eroded and must be resected en bloc. In most patients, the sellar diaphragm can be opened and the dorsum sellae fractured to push it posteriorly, allowing the gland to be removed intact. The pituitary can be sectioned in the sagittal plane or transversely. The former allows examination of the stalk but the latter provides a more thorough examination of the gland with accurate determination of the geographic distribution of the various cell types.

The handling of the surgical specimen is usually less complex because the specimens obtained at the time of transsphenoidal surgery, with or without endoscopic approaches and image-guided intraoperative navigation, are small and often fragmented. The tissues require optimal fixation for histology and immunohistochemistry. In rare cases, there may be a need for ultrastructural analysis; because this situation is not often predicted clinically, it is recommended that a small piece of tissue be routinely fixed for electron microscopy and retained in the event that it is needed. Currently there is no indication for other techniques on a routine basis.

The distinction of pituitary adenoma from other neoplasms in the sellar region is no longer the main objective of the pathologist. The advent of targeted therapies for specific tumour subtypes mandates a more sophisticated approach.[5,10] In addition to routine haematoxylin and eosin, the reticulin stain is important in the evaluation of tissue architecture to distinguish hyperplasia from adenoma;[11] the use of type IV collagen immunohistochemistry may replace the reticulin stain.[104] The periodic acid-Schiff (PAS) stain and a panel of immunohistochemical stains are pivotal to pituitary analysis. The importance of antibody specificity for identification of hormone secretion and transcription factors cannot be overemphasized.

It is important to recognize the limitations of using nonspecific polyclonal antisera that may show extensive cross-reactivity.

The role of intraoperative consultation in the management of patients with pituitary disorders is also a controversial subject. The accuracy of pituitary frozen section is lower than that at other sites. Although most surgical pathologists achieve accuracy rates of greater than 90 per cent at frozen section, the figures for pituitary are closer to 80 per cent.[129] The reason for this low accuracy is largely technical, because of the small size of samples, freezing artefact, fibrosis and other architectural distortion. In general, intraoperative consultation should only be performed when the information it yields will alter intraoperative management. In most patients with pituitary tumours, this does not apply. Unfortunately, in many instances curiosity can result in significant freezing artefact that can compromise the ability to render an accurate histologic diagnosis. Nevertheless, if there is a suspicion of inflammation, metastatic malignancy or hyperplasia rather than a pituitary adenoma, this would indeed reduce the extent of surgery, and intraoperative pathology is critical. The use of smears rather than frozen section reduces the amount of tissue required for the intraoperative analysis, retaining suitable diagnostic tissue for histology and, in the hands of an experienced interpreter, provides adequate information for intraoperative decisions and patient management.

Synoptic reporting has been implemented in surgical pathology to ensure completeness of information and the most appropriate presentation of clinically relevant information, as well as providing a valuable mechanism to collect data. Although this has been emphasized for malignancies, its role in pituitary pathology is also being recognized. A synoptic report for primary pituitary tumours, including pituitary adenomas, hyperplasias and carcinomas, and craniopharyngiomas but excluding neural, germ cell, hematologic, mesenchymal and metastatic tumours has been proposed[144] and is included in Table 41.1.

TABLE 41.1 Synoptic report: tumours of the pituitary gland

Procedure (select all that apply)
___ Transsphenoidal resection
___ Transcranial resection
___ Other (specify): _____
___ Not specified

Clinical features
___ Functional
     Hormone excess (specify): _____
___ Clinically nonfunctioning

Tumour size (from imaging)
Greatest dimension: ___ cm
*Additional dimensions: ___ × ___ cm
___ Cannot be determined

*****Received**
*___ Fresh
*___ In formalin
*___ Other

*****Specimen integrity**
*___ Intact
*___ Fragmented

Specimen size
___ × ____ × ____cm

*****Specimen weight**
*___ grams

Histologic features
Reticulin
___ Intact
___ Expanded
___ Disrupted
PAS
___ Positive
___ Negative
Infiltrating tumour
___ Positive
     (specify tissue): _____
___ Negative
___ Cannot be determined

Immunohistochemistry (select all positive)
___ Pit-1
___ ER

___ Tpit
___ SF1
___ Alpha-subunit
___ ACTH
___ GH
___ PRL
___ β-TSH
___ β-FSH
___ β-LH
___ Keratin (CAM 5.2) Diffuse: ___
     Fibrous bodies___
     Perinuclear___
     Membranous___
___ per cent MIB-1 LI
___ p53
___ Others (specify):_____

Tumour type
Pituitary adenoma
Subtype
     ___ Densely granulated corticotroph adenoma
     ___ Sparsely granulated corticotroph adenoma
     ___ Crooke cell adenoma
     ___ Densely granulated somatotroph adenoma
     ___ Sparsely granulated somatotroph adenoma
     ___ Mammosomatotroph adenoma
     ___ Mixed somatotroph-lactotroph adenoma
     ___ Sparsely granulated lactotroph adenoma
     ___ Densely granulated lactotroph adenoma
     ___ Acidophil stem cell adenoma
     ___ Thyrotroph adenoma
     ___ Gonadotroph adenoma
     ___ Unusual plurihormonal adenoma
     ___ Null cell adenoma
     ___ Oncocytoma
     ___ Other (specify): _____
___ Typical
___ Atypical
Hyperplasia
___ Type (specify): _____
Pituitary carcinoma
___ Type (specify): _____
___Location of metastases _____
Craniopharyngioma
___ Papillary
___ Adamantinomatous

Continued

*Additional pathologic findings Nontumourous adenohypophysis: ___ Present *___ Crooke's hyaline change ___ Not identified	Neurohypophysis ___ Present ___ Not identified

*Comment(s).

NORMAL PITUITARY ANATOMY AND CYTOLOGY

The pituitary is a bean-shaped gland located in the midline at the base of the brain in the bony sella turcica that surrounds it inferiorly and laterally. Superiorly, it is covered by the diaphragma sella, a reflection of the dura mater.[11] Lateral to the sella are the cavernous sinuses; anteroinferior is the sphenoid sinus; anterosuperior is the optic chiasm; superior to it is the hypothalamus.

The average adult gland measures 0.6 cm SI × 0.9 cm AP × 1.3 cm ML and weighs 0.6 g. Females tend to have larger glands, especially during or after pregnancy, with weights up to 1 g.[11] It is surrounded by fibrous tissue that forms a capsule.

The pituitary is composed of two anatomically and functionally distinct parts: the neurohypophysis and the adenohypophysis (Figure 41.1). The neurohypophysis is composed of the infundibulum (the pituitary stalk) and the pars nervosa. These structures are made of pituicytes, modified glial cells and of the axonal processes of neurons whose cell bodies are located in the hypothalamus (Figure 41.2). The neurohypophysis stores and releases hypothalamic hormones, including oxytocin and vasopressin that have distant targets, and hypophysiotropic hormones that regulate hormone production by the epithelial cells of the adenohypophysis.

The adenohypophysis is an epithelial gland of endodermal origin. Embryologically it derives from Rathke's pouch.[14] It has three regions, the pars distalis or anterior lobe, the pars intermedia or intermediate lobe (Figure 41.1) and the pars tuberalis, an extension of epithelium that wraps around the infundibulum of the pituitary stalk. The adenohypophysis is composed of acini that contain the six specialized hormone-secreting cells within a reticulin-rich stroma (Figure 41.2). Folliculostellate cells are stromal sustentacular cells that surround the acini; they are immunoreactive for S-100 protein and glial fibrillary acidic protein (GFAP). Occasional follicular cells form around small follicles; they are thought to derive from hormone-secreting cells in response to trauma, compression or degeneration.

Adenohypophyseal development and cytodifferentiation are regulated by highly specific transcription factors.[12,188] The Rathke's pouch homeobox (Rpx) protein, Pax-6, the bicoid-related pituitary homeobox factor Ptx1 and structurally related pituitary homeobox factor 2 (Ptx2) are all required for early pituitary organogenesis. Two members of the Lhx gene family (a group of LIM homeobox genes), Lhx3 and Lhx4, as well as P-LIM, another LIM homeobox protein transcription factor, are expressed in the pituitary with highest levels at the early stages of Rathke's pouch development. Another early determinant of pituitary differentiation is the Prophet of Pit-1 (PROP-1); this paired-like

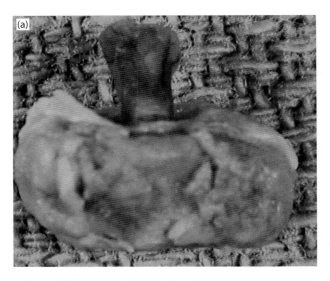

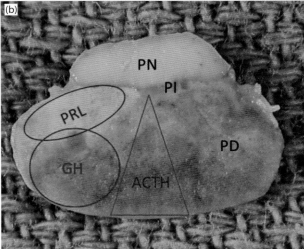

41.1 The normal pituitary. (a) A coronal section of the gland identifies the pituitary stalk or infundibulum and the tan parenchyma of the adenohypophysis inferiorly. The fibrous capsule is a reflection of dura mater. **(b)** On horizontal cross section, the gland is readily seen to have two distinct components, the posterior lobe, or neurohypophysis, known as pars nervosa (PN) that has the consistency of white matter of brain, and the anterior lobe or pars distalis (PD) representing the larger part that is a glandular, tan parenchyma. Between them is the intermediate lobe or pars intermedia (PI) that consists only of vestigial structures that are recognized grossly as tiny cysts with gelatinous contents. The anterior lobe is composed of the different hormone-secreting cell types, some of which show preferential distributions including growth hormone (GH) in the lateral lobes, prolactin (PRL) in the posterolateral wings and adrenocorticotropin (ACTH) in the median wedge.

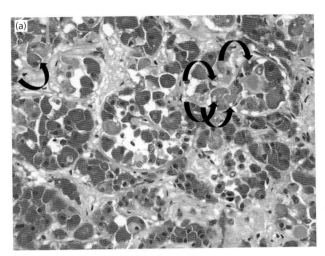

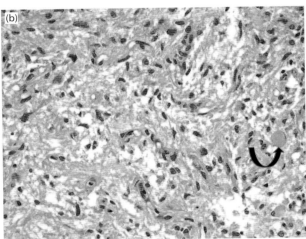

41.2 Normal pituitary histology. (a) The adenohypophysis is composed of acini of epithelial cells. In the lateral gland, acidophils predominate and there are only a few chromophobes and basophils. The latter are characterized by prominent vacuoles known as 'enigmatic bodies' (arrows). **(b)** The posterior lobe or neurohypophysis is composed mainly of axons of neurons whose cell bodies reside in the hypothalamus. They are supported by modified glia, stromal cells called 'pituicytes' whose nuclei are identified, along with those of endothelial cells. Occasional dilated axonal processes, known as 'Herring bodies' are identified (arrow).

homeodomain protein is expressed early in pituitary development. It induces expression of the next phase of development directed by the pituitary transcription factor Pit-1, and plays a role in down-regulation of Rpx that is required for cell differentiation. Id, a member of the helix-loop-helix (HLH) family of transcription factors, Isl-1, a LIM factor and several other transcription factors are also expressed early in pituitary development.

Expansion of differentiated cell populations requires the presence of hypothalamic trophic hormones, target organ hormonal feedback and growth factors. In anencephalic fetuses, adenohypophyseal cells differentiate because the transcription factors required for cytodifferentiation are expressed, but the pituitaries are small and the numbers of gonadotrophs and corticotrophs are reduced, proving the importance of hypothalamic factors in promoting expansion of those

populations.[157] Disruption of the Notch signalling pathway by deletion of the transcription factor hairy and enhancer of split 1 (Hes1) is associated with adenohypophyseal hypoplasia affecting corticotrophs and somatotrophs.[162,233] The identical pattern of maldevelopment results from deletion of the Ikaros gene,[72,73] an epigenetic regulator that plays a key role in cell proliferation and apoptosis[74] and is implicated in pituitary tumour genesis[69] as well as other aspects of neuroendocrine and immune development and disease.[62]

The molecular factors that determine cell differentiation and hormone production in adenohypophyseal cells are transcription factors that target specific hormone genes. These factors have clarified three main pathways of cell differentiation.[12]

The expression of proopiomelanocortin (POMC) that defines corticotrophs is dependent on the T-box transcription factor Tpit. Tpit interacts with Ptx1 and corticotropin upstream transcription-binding element (CUTE) proteins, including neuroD1/β2. POMC is cleaved into various derivatives that include adrenocorticotropin (ACTH), melanotropin (MSH), endorphins and lipotropin (LPH).

Corticotrophs represent approximately 15 to 20 per cent of adenohypophyseal cells. These basophilic cells are unique among adenohypophyseal cells because of their strong positivity with the periodic acid-Schiff (PAS) stain. They are concentrated mainly in the central region of the gland that is known as the 'mucoid wedge' because of its intense PAS-reactivity (Figure 41.1b). A population of these cells is the main component of the vestigial intermediate lobe that in animals is the source of MSH. In older patients the intermediate lobe corticotrophs spill into the posterior lobe, a phenomenon known as 'basophil invasion'. Corticotrophs have characteristic 'enigmatic bodies', large cytoplasmic vacuoles that represent complex lysosomes, that are identified on routine haematoxylin and eosin (H&E) staining (Figure 41.2) but can be readily seen as negative globules with the ACTH immunostain. By electron microscopy, their secretory granules are characterized by pleomorphism of size, shape and electron density, and it is not unusual to identify indentations and evaginations of granule membranes, resulting in 'heart' and 'teardrop' shapes. Small bundles of intermediate filaments identified throughout the cytoplasm by electron microscopy represent keratin filaments.

When anterior lobe corticotrophs are exposed to excess glucocorticoids, they undergo a reversible morphologic modification known as Crooke's hyaline change attributable to concentric accumulations of keratin filaments that displace the PAS-positive, ACTH-immunoreactive secretory granules to the juxtanuclear and peripheral cytoplasm (Figure 41.3). By light microscopy, the accumulated filaments have a pale, homogeneous, glassy appearance and they stain for low molecular weight cytokeratins that correspond to Moll's peptides 7 and 8 (i.e. identification using CAM 5.2 or equivalent antibodies).[61,139] Their ultrastructural appearance is characterized by massive ring-like accumulations of intermediate filaments in the cytoplasm. Corticotrophs of the pars intermedia are thought to cleave POMC differently from the ACTH-producing cells of the pars distalis and, in situations of glucocorticoid excess, do not undergo Crooke's hyaline change.

Somatotrophs, lactotrophs, mammosomatotrophs and thyrotrophs all derive from growth hormone (GH)-producing precursors that express the transcription factor Pit-1. The expression of oestrogen receptor (ER)α enhances

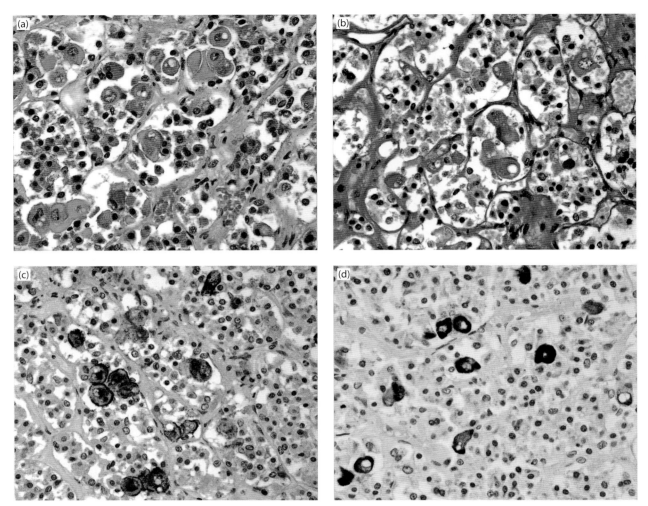

41.3 Crooke's hyaline change. (a) The nontumourous corticotrophs of patients with any form of glucocorticoid excess undergo accumulation of keratin filaments that fill the cytoplasm, creating a pale glassy appearance known as Crooke's hyaline. **(b)** With a periodic acid-Schiff (PAS) stain the positive secretory material is seen to be displaced to a juxtanuclear or peripheral location by this hyaline material. **(c)** A stain for adrenocorticotropin (ACTH) localizes the hormone in the centre of the cytoplasm and at the periphery of the cell but the hyaline material is negative for ACTH. **(d)** The hyaline material stains strongly for keratins using the CAM 5.2 antibody.

prolactin (PRL) secretion, allowing mammosomatotroph differentiation, and a silencing mechanism is thought to repress GH production to allow mature lactotrophs to develop. Thyrotroph embryonic factor (TEF) is the putative factor required for thyrotrophin (TSH)-β production, and GATA-2 appears to be an important contributor to thyrotroph development. Mature thyrotrophs also suppress GH production through an unknown mechanism. This family of cells is thought to maintain fluidity so that, in various situations, there is transdifferentiation: somatotrophs convert to mammosomatotrophs and lactotrophs during pregnancy and to thyrotrophs in hypothyroidism, and these are thought to be reversible transdifferentiation processes.

Somatotrophs that produce GH are located predominantly in the lateral wings of the anterior pituitary (Figure 41.1b) and account for approximately 50 per cent of the cell population. By light microscopy they are strongly acidophilic round cells with centrally located nuclei and diffuse cytoplasmic positivity for GH. Electron microscopy reveals abundant rough endoplasmic reticulum, well-formed Golgi complexes and numerous large dense secretory granules that store hormone. Lactotrophs that produce PRL are scattered randomly throughout the adenohypophysis; however, they can most often be found in the posterolateral aspects of the gland (Figure 41.1b). In males and nulliparous females, they constitute approximately 9 per cent of adenohypophyseal cells; in multiparous females, they can represent up to 31 per cent of that population. They are usually chromophobic polygonal cells that wrap cell processes around adjacent cells, usually gonadotrophs; some are acidophilic as a result of storage of numerous secretory granules with hormone content. The ultrastructural hallmarks of lactotrophs are the elaborate rough endoplasmic reticulum arranged in parallel arrays and occasionally forming concentric structures known as 'Nebenkern' formations, the prominent Golgi complexes, and the extrusion of secretory granules at the lateral cell border, a phenomenon known as 'misplaced exocytosis'. Mammosomatotrophs, which produce both GH and PRL, resemble somatotrophs but contain both GH and PRL by immunohistochemistry. They often have irregular, elongated and pleomorphic large granules and they exhibit the hallmark of PRL secretion, misplaced exocytosis. Thyrotrophs, which produce TSH, represent only approximately 5 per cent of adenohypophyseal cells. These angular chromophobic cells with multiple elongated cytoplasmic processes are most numerous in the anteromedial aspect of the gland. They exhibit cytoplasmic immunoreactivity for α-subunit of glycoprotein hormones and β-TSH. By electron microscopy they are characterized by short profiles of dilated rough endoplasmic reticulum and small secretory granules that are aligned along the plasma membrane.

Expression of steroidogenic factor-1 (SF-1) and GATA-2 are required for gonadotroph differentiation. Gonadotrophs, which produce the two gonadotropins, follicle-stimulating hormone (FSH) and luteinizing hormone (LH), account for 10 per cent of adenohypophyseal cells. They are scattered throughout the pars distalis and pars tuberalis. With increasing age, these cells tend to undergo oncocytic change (mitochondrial accumulation) and squamous metaplasia. These cells are reliably identified by immunoreactivity for beta-subunits of FSH and/or LH, but their ultrastructural appearance is not as characteristic as that of other adenohypophyseal cells. They are oval with eccentric spherical nuclei, and their cytoplasm contains short profiles of dilated rough endoplasmic reticulum containing flocculent electron dense material. Secretory granules are generally sparse, small and scattered throughout the cytoplasm.

Scattered cells in the gland that have features of adenohypophyseal hormone-secreting cells but cannot be classified are called null cells, and the normal gland also contains occasional oncocytes, characterized by accumulations of dilated, spherulated mitochondria; oncocytic change is most common in gonadotrophs and occurs rarely in other adenohypophyseal cells.

The pars intermedia is poorly developed in the human and is composed of small cystic spaces lined by hormone-containing cells types, predominantly corticotrophs. The pars tuberalis is the superior portion of the adenohypophysis that wraps itself around the neural stalk. It is composed primarily of gonadotrophs that with age undergo squamous metaplasia.[15]

The pituitary receives its vascular supply from the superior, middle and inferior hypophyseal arteries, all of which originate from the internal carotid arteries. The superior hypophysial arteries flow through the infundibulum of the neurohypophysis and form the portal vessels that transport regulatory hormones from the hypothalamus to the pituitary gland. The middle hypophyseal arteries supply blood directly to the adenohypophysis, whereas the inferior hypophyseal arteries supply the pars nervosa. Venous blood from the pituitary gland drains mainly into the internal jugular veins; however, there is evidence that reverse flow in the short portal vessels allows adenohypophyseal secretion to affect neurohypophyseal and hypothalamic function.

PITUITARY ADENOMAS

The most common tumours of the adenohypophysis are pituitary adenomas, benign neoplasms that arise from adenohypophyseal cells. Although classified as benign because of their inability to metastasize, these lesions can be highly invasive and may be lethal as a result of either infiltration of local structures or the complications of the metabolic effects of the hormone excess syndromes they can cause.

Epidemiology

Pituitary adenomas are present in approximately 16.9 per cent of the general population.[70] The diagnosis has become more frequent because of increased awareness and improved diagnostic techniques.[49,78] Their prevalence increases with advancing age; both sexes are affected equally. They show a wide range of biological behaviour, ranging from microscopic incidental findings to small lesions with severe hormonal manifestations, to large invasive neoplasms (Box 41.1).

Classification of Pituitary Adenomas

There are several classification schemes for pituitary adenomas: functional, anatomic/radiologic, histologic, immunohistochemical, ultrastructural and clinicopathologic.[11] The functional classification used clinically groups adenomas according to the hormonal syndromes with which they are associated. This includes the various functioning adenomas and the clinically 'silent' or nonfunctioning adenomas. The anatomic/radiologic classification categorizes pituitary adenomas based on size and degree of invasion.[90] A histologic classification, based on histochemical stains, divides adenomas into those that are acidophilic, basophilic and chromophobic; this classification is of limited value and has largely been abandoned. The immunohistochemical classification shown in Table 41.2 categorizes pituitary adenomas based primarily on hormone content with additional information provided by immunoreactivity for transcription factors and keratins.[11] Although electron microscopy can be extremely valuable in the diagnosis of certain tumours, the ultrastructural classification of adenomas is less commonly utilized.[115] Clinicopathologic classification that categorizes adenomas using both morphologic and clinical features as shown in Table 41.3 represents the most effective classification scheme.[11]

Clinical Features

The clinical manifestations of pituitary adenomas vary depending on the cell type, hormonal activity and the degree of invasiveness of the individual lesion. Clinically

---

BOX 41.1. Ectopic pituitary adenomas

Although the vast majority of these lesions arise within the sella turcica, ectopic pituitary adenomas can arise in embryonic remnants of Rathke's cleft that are found in extrasellar locations including the sphenoid sinus, parapharyngeal area, suprasellar regions, middle nasal meatus, petrous temporal bone, clivus, hypothalamus and third ventricle.[45]

Epidemiologically, these tumours resemble their intrasellar counterparts. Compared to intrasellar pituitary adenomas, higher proportions of ectopic adenomas are functional, with the most common clinical presentation being Cushing's disease. Silent ectopic adenomas usually present with mass effects and their diagnosis depends on careful examination of resected tissue specimens.

TABLE 41.2 Immunohistochemical classification of pituitary adenomas

GH–PRL–TSH family	**Pit-1**
GH-containing somatotroph adenomas	Pit-1, GH
Densely granulated somatotroph adenomas	Pit-1, GH, ± α-subunit
Sparsely granulated somatotroph adenomas	Pit-1, GH, keratin whorls
GH- and PRL-containing mammosomatotroph adenomas	Pit-1, GH, PRL, ER ± α-subunit
PRL-containing lactotroph adenomas	Pit-1, PRL, ER
Sparsely granulated lactotroph adenomas	Pit-1, PRL, ER
Densely granulated lactotroph adenomas	Pit-1, PRL, ER
PRL-cell adenomas with GH content (acidophil stem cell)	Pit-1, PRL, ER, GH, keratin whorls
TSH-containing thyrotroph adenomas	Pit-1, β-TSH, α-subunit
GH-, PRL- and TSH-containing adenomas	Pit-1, GH, PRL, ER, α-subunit, β-TSH
ACTH family	**Tpit**
ACTH-containing corticotroph adenomas	Tpit, ACTH, keratins
Densely granulated corticotroph adenomas	Tpit, ACTH, keratins
Sparsely granulated corticotroph adenomas	Tpit, ACTH, keratins
Gonadotropin family	**SF-1, ER**
FSH/LH-containing gonadotroph adenomas	SF-1, ER, β-FSH, β-LH, α-subunit
Unclassified adenomas	
Unusual plurihormonal adenomas	Multiple markers
Immunonegative adenomas	No immunohistochemical markers

TABLE 41.3 Clinicopathological classification of pituitary adenomas

Functioning Adenomas	**Nonfunctioning Adenomas**

GH-PRL-TSH family
Adenomas causing GH-excess
   Densely granulated somatotroph adenomas
   Sparsely granulated somatotroph adenomas
   Mammosomatotroph adenomas
	Silent somatotroph adenomas

Adenomas causing hyperprolactinemia
   Lactotroph adenomas
   Acidophil stem cell adenomas
	Silent lactotroph adenomas

Adenomas causing TSH excess Thyrotroph adenomas	Silent thyrotroph adenomas

ACTH family
Adenomas causing ACTH excess
   Densely granulated corticotroph adenomas
   Sparsely granulated corticotroph adenomas
	Silent corticotroph adenomas (type I)
	Silent corticotroph adenomas (type II)

Gonadotroph family Adenomas causing gonadotropin excess Gonadotroph adenomas	Silent gonadotroph adenomas (null cell adenomas, oncocytomas)
Unclassified adenomas Unusual plurihormonal adenomas	Immunonegative adenomas

functioning adenomas secrete hormones in excess, and these give rise to specific clinical manifestations. Excess secretion of GH results in gigantism in children due to the rapid growth of extremities induced by GH and its target hormone, insulin-like growth factor-1. In adults, after fusion of the epiphyseal plates, the hormone excess causes acral enlargement and prominence of facial bones, resulting in prognathism and facial deformities. In addition, these conditions result in cardiomegaly and hypertension, diabetes mellitus and an increased incidence of malignancies of various organs, all as a result of the metabolic effects of GH and IGF-1.

Prolactin hypersecretion causes gonadotropin insufficiency and sexual dysfunction; in women this is manifested as amenorrhea. Infertility is a common problem in younger patients. In women, PRL excess can ultimately cause galactorrhea, but this condition is unusual in men who lack the oestrogen priming required by breast tissue for this phenomenon. Prolonged oestrogen or androgen deficiency results in osteopenia and osteoporosis.

Thyrotropin excess is rare and manifests as clinical or subclinical hyperthyroidism. It is imperative to distinguish primary from secondary forms of thyroid hormone excess.

ACTH excess results in Cushing's disease, characterized by centripetal obesity, peripheral muscle wasting, moon facies, thinning of the skin, bruising and hirsutism. Patients with this disorder also develop osteoporosis, diabetes and immunosuppression.

Gonadotropin excess rarely manifests as a distinct entity, and most patients with tumours of a gonadotroph origin secrete an excess of subunits of FSH or LH. Hence, gonadal stimulation is rare and hypogonadism more common. Rare patients have been reported with ovarian cystic disorders.

Tumours of any type that destroy a significant proportion of pituitary parenchyma result in hypopituitarism. This is initially manifested as GH deficiency, which can be subtle in adults. In children, it may be the cause of the presenting symptom of growth failure. Loss of PRL is asymptomatic in all but lactating women. Deficiency of gonadotropins, TSH and ACTH result in target organ failure with infertility, hypothyroidism and addisonian features; the last is usually the end phase of pituitary failure and therefore is rare without almost complete pituitary destruction.

Destruction of the posterior pituitary can result in diabetes insipidus but this is rarely evident in patients with primary pituitary adenomas; instead, it usually indicates the presence of a more aggressive infiltrative tumour or an alternative diffuse tumour-like or inflammatory process.

Any pituitary mass can result in headache. With suprasellar extension, the optic chiasm can become involved, resulting in visual field deficits, usually initially a bitemporal hemianopsia. Extension well outside the sella can result in cranial nerve defects or, rarely, cavernous sinus syndrome; these are unusual features of primary pituitary adenomas (Box 41.2).

Radiology

Pituitary and sellar enlargement is found in most patients with pituitary adenomas, but microadenomas are not always identified by radiologic techniques. Macroadenomas are nearly always demonstrable on CT scanning and most

BOX 41.2. Pituitary apoplexy

Pituitary apoplexy constitutes a true endocrine emergency in which acute haemorrhagic infarction of a sellar tumour (usually an adenoma), results in rapid expansion with symptoms and signs of elevated intracranial pressure.[150] Factors predisposing to pituitary apoplexy include carotid angiography, radiation therapy, trauma, coagulopathy, temporal arteritis, diabetes mellitus and atherosclerosis. Histologic examination reveals extensive infarction and haemorrhage. These features are common as focal changes in many pituitary tumours; however, true pituitary apoplexy refers to those extreme cases where haemorrhagic infarction of the pituitary is accompanied by the appropriate clinical features.

lesions greater than 3 mm are visible with magnetic resonance imaging (MRI). Pituitary adenomas typically appear as void signals of variable intensity on MRI. T2-weighted imaging identifies heterogeneous areas within large lesions; these usually correspond to regions of haemorrhage or necrosis. Following gadolinium administration, the normal gland shows increased contrast uptake that delineates it from the adenoma that shows no or minimal contrast enhancement. The uses of lateral polytomography, air encephalography and/or carotid angiography are largely of historical interest only.

The demonstration of somatostatin receptors in pituitary tumours has led to the use of scintigraphic visualization of radiolabelled somatostatin analogues to localize some adenomas. However, in addition to identifying primary pituitary adenomas, this imaging technique has localized other lesions, such as metastatic deposits, and is therefore not as specific as originally postulated.

The localization of pituitary tumours in Cushing's disease can be exceedingly difficult, yet is necessary for appropriate transsphenoidal microsurgical resection. The use of selective venous sampling from the inferior petrosal sinus has been reported to be a reliable and useful method to establish the presence and laterality of ACTH-secreting microadenomas.[32] Because of the possibility of episodic release of ACTH, inferior petrosal sinus sampling may lead to erroneous results and the addition of CRH stimulation in combination with inferior petrosal sinus sampling has been proposed as a useful adjunctive diagnostic tool.[122]

Gross and Microscopic Pathology

The pathological features of these lesions differ according to tumour type.

Functioning Corticotroph Adenomas

Tumours composed of ACTH-secreting corticotrophs represent 10 to 15 per cent of all pituitary adenomas. There are three recognized variants: densely granulated corticotroph adenomas, sparsely granulated corticotroph adenomas and Crooke's cell adenomas. ACTH excess due to a pituitary corticotroph adenoma is known as Cushing's disease and represents one variant of Cushing's syndrome, which results from any cause of glucocorticoid excess.

The most common cause of Cushing's disease is a basophilic microadenoma.[11] These small tumours may be centrally located, because corticotrophs are most abundant in the median wedge of the anterior pituitary, but they usually exhibit lateralization of blood supply. Because they are often hard to visualize with MRI, this lateralization of vascularization allows diagnosis using inferior petrosal sinus sampling for biochemical localization. Macroadenomas are occasionally associated with Nelson's syndrome in patients who have undergone bilateral adrenalectomy as treatment for pituitary Cushing's disease without initial identification of a discrete lesion. Macroadenomas associated with Cushing's disease are seen in patients with less florid hormone excess; they are usually chromophobic or sparsely granulated adenomas.

Densely granulated corticotroph adenomas are the commonest corticotroph adenomas. These tumours are usually microadenomas composed of basophilic cells arranged in a sinusoidal architecture (Figure 41.4). The tumour cells exhibit cytoplasmic PAS positivity. They exhibit nuclear positivity for Tpit and cytoplasmic immunoreactivity for ACTH, β-endorphin and other POMC-derived peptides. Positivity for low molecular weight cytokeratins is seen in tumours associated with Cushing's disease.[61,139] In contrast, the lesions associated with Nelson's syndrome are usually

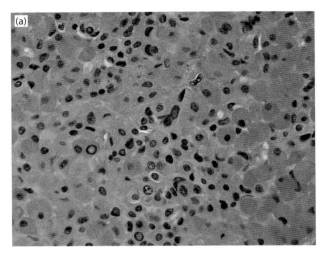

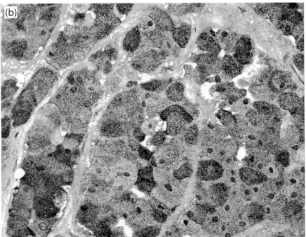

41.4 Densely granulated corticotroph adenoma. (a) These tumours are composed of large cells with basophilic granules in the cytoplasm. **(b)** The tumour cells are strongly positive for adrenocorticotropin (ACTH).

macroadenomas and the tumour cells do not accumulate keratin filaments. Ultrastructurally,[115] corticotroph cells are large and polygonal with ovoid or irregular nuclei that harbour nucleoli in contact with the inner nuclear membrane. The cytoplasm contains prominent rough endoplasmic reticulum with abundant free ribosomes, spherical Golgi complexes and perinuclear intermediate filaments composed of cytokeratins that are prominent in patients with Cushing's syndrome but are not conspicuous in Nelson's syndrome. The secretory granules range in size from 150 to 450 nm in diameter and are distinctive because of their marked variability in shape and electron density.

Sparsely granulated corticotroph adenomas are less common than the densely granulated variant. By light microscopy, the tumour cells are chromophobic and are negative or only focally positive with the PAS stain (Figure 41.5). They exhibit strong nuclear staining for Tpit, strong cytoplasmic immunoreactivity for cytokeratins and weak immunoreactivity for ACTH and other POMC-derived peptides.[11] Ultrastructurally,[115] the cells contain fewer well-developed organelles and scant secretory granules but the characteristic variability of size, shape and density of the granules characterizes them as corticotrophs.

Crooke's cell adenomas are rare tumours that exhibit Crooke's hyaline change.[77,80] Usually, Crooke's hyalinization is restricted to nontumourous corticotrophs but rarely this marker of feedback suppression by glucocorticoids is seen in adenomas. These tumours can be associated with Cushing's disease but it is generally an unusual form of the disease, such as cyclical Cushing's, in which the symptoms and biochemical abnormalities wax and wane. The tumour cells can exhibit marked cytologic and nuclear atypia (Figure 41.6). The perinuclear ring of pale hyaline material represents the accumulation of cytokeratins 7 and 8 that are intermediate filaments on electron microscopy.[61,139] The cells exhibit PAS positivity adjacent to the nucleus and at the cell periphery, corresponding to immunohistochemically detectable ACTH in secretory granules in those areas.

Differential Diagnosis

The possibility of corticotroph hyperplasia (see later) must be considered in the differential diagnosis of Cushing's disease and, again, reticulin stains should be carried out in all cases of this disorder. In patients with corticotroph hyperplasia, it is unusual to find Crooke's hyalinization of the hyperplastic cells, whereas in patients with adenomas, the nontumourous corticotrophs are usually suppressed and exhibit this alteration. In patients with tiny microadenomas, occasionally no diagnostic adenoma tissue is included in the pathology specimen. This may be attributed to loss of the adenoma during suction of a bloody operative field. The identification of Crooke's hyaline change in the nontumourous corticotrophs is critical to verify the clinical diagnosis, and the post-operative outcome will prove whether the lesion has been excised.

In patients with misdiagnosed ectopic or adrenal disease causing Cushing's syndrome, there will be Crooke's hyaline change in the pituitary specimen. In contrast, occasional patients with pseudo-Cushing's syndrome (features that mimic Cushing's syndrome together with some evidence of hypercortisolism, but attributable to depression,

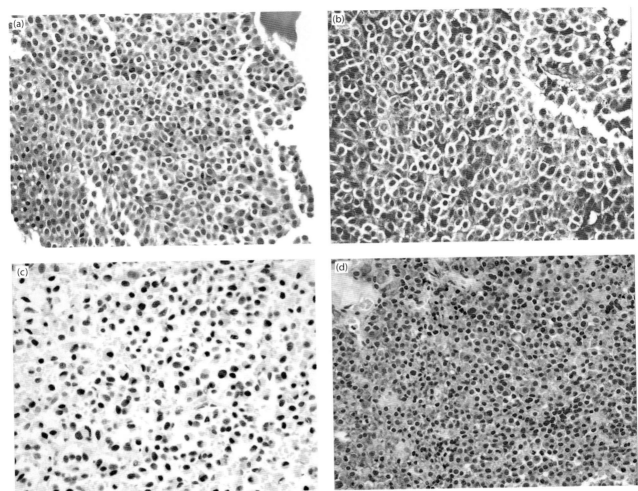

41.5 Sparsely granulated corticotroph adenoma. (a) These tumours are composed of round to cuboidal cells with chromophobic cytoplasm. **(b)** The tumour cells are weakly positive with the periodic acid-Schiff (PAS) stain. **(c)** They have strong nuclear reactivity for Tpit and **(d)** weak cytoplasmic reactivity for adrenocorticotropin (ACTH).

obesity, alcohol abuse or rarely heritable generalized glucocorticoid resistance due to mutations in the glucocorticoid receptor) will have no evidence of Crooke's hyaline change in nontumourous corticotrophs and no evidence of corticotroph hyperplasia. Tumours that exhibit significant Crooke's hyaline change can also be very atypical and can mimic ganglion cell lesions and metastases.

Functioning Somatotroph Adenomas

Somatotroph adenomas arise from GH-producing cells and represent 10 to 15 per cent of pituitary adenomas. GH excess in adults manifests as acromegaly and gigantism results from excessive GH prior to epiphyseal plate closure.[65] Hyperprolactinaemia can be prominent in some patients; it may result from stalk compression in macroadenomas, but is often due to elaboration of PRL in addition to GH by the tumour.

Grossly, these tumours are usually well demarcated and are located in the lateral wing of the adenohypophysis. They tend to be soft lesions that rarely cause compression of the surrounding gland. Microscopically, there are several subtypes of somatotroph adenomas.

Densely granulated somatotroph adenomas are composed of large round acidophilic cells arranged in a trabecular, sinusoidal, or diffuse architecture (Figure 41.7). The tumour cells show strong, diffuse cytoplasmic immunoreactivity for GH and strong nuclear immunoreactivity for Pit-1.[11] Tumour cells exhibit moderate perinuclear positivity with antibodies to low molecular weight cytokeratins. There is variable cytoplasmic immunoreactivity for α-subunit of glycoprotein hormones. By electron microscopy,[115] the tumour cells resemble nontumourous somatotrophs; they have spherical nuclei with prominent nucleoli, parallel arrays of rough endoplasmic reticulum and well-formed Golgi complexes. Secretory granules are numerous, homogeneous, dense and spherical with diameters ranging from 150 to 600 nm.

Sparsely granulated somatotroph adenomas are composed of solid sheets of poorly cohesive chromophobic cells. Unlike other pituitary adenomas, they can exhibit striking nuclear pleomorphism and have been misdiagnosed as metastatic carcinomas. The nuclei can be lobulated and harbour prominent nucleoli (Figure 41.8). Immunoreactivity for GH can be focal and weak, being easily missed; these tumours rarely stain for α-subunit. In contrast to densely granulated somatotroph adenomas, they have marked reduction of

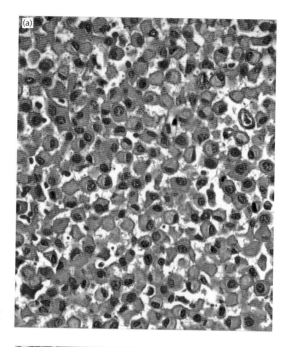

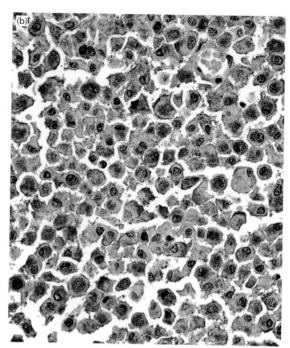

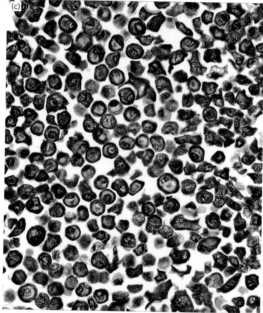

41.6 Crooke's cell adenoma. (a) The tumour cells are corticotrophs that show Crooke's hyaline change. There is marked nuclear atypia and these lesions can be mistaken for metastatic carcinoma. **(b)** They exhibit peripheral and central adrenocorticotropin (ACTH) reactivity but the hyaline material is negative. **(c)** Instead, it stains strongly for keratins with the CAM 5.2 antibody.

staining for E-cadherin and beta-catenin.[181] Nuclear immunoreactivity for Pit-1 is usually present and strong in the irregular nuclei. Immunohistochemical stains for low molecular weight cytokeratins reveal the characteristic feature of this tumour type, the fibrous body, which manifests as juxtanuclear globular reactivity.[11,140] Although some densely granulated somatotroph adenomas may show occasional globular aggregation of keratin filaments, this so-called 'mixed pattern' is of no significance and tumours with this appearance are not clinically or biochemically distinct from densely granulated somatotroph adenomas;[146] therefore the designation of sparsely granulated somatotroph adenoma should be restricted to lesions with keratin staining only in fibrous bodies. Ultrastructurally,[115] the tumour cells are irregularly shaped with eccentric, pleomorphic and multilobulated nuclei. The rough endoplasmic reticulum can be either poorly or well developed. The characteristic fibrous body is a juxtanuclear, spherical mass composed of intermediate filaments. Secretory granules are sparse and range in size from 100 to 250 nm.

Mammosomatotroph adenomas produce both GH and PRL. They are the most frequent findings in patients with gigantism and in young patients with acromegaly. Microscopically, these tumours are composed of acidophilic cells arranged in a diffuse or solid pattern, resembling densely granulated somatotroph adenomas. Immunohistochemically, the tumour cells are strongly immunoreactive for GH and variably immunoreactive for α-subunit and PRL.[11] Staining for low molecular weight cytokeratins yields a perinuclear pattern of staining similar

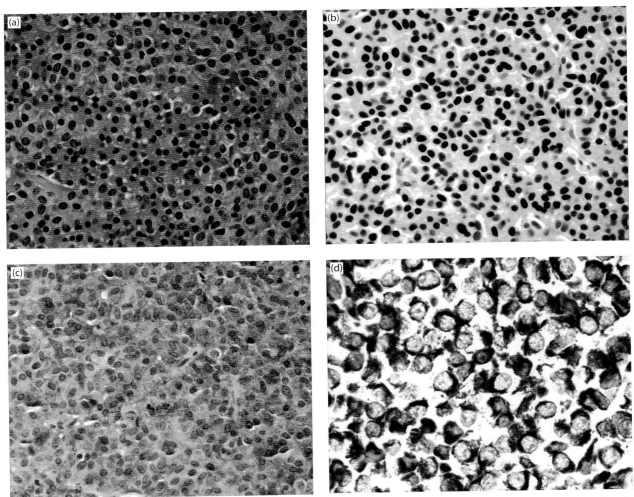

41.7 Densely granulated somatotroph adenoma. (a) These are strongly acidophilic adenomas that are usually associated with acromegaly or gigantism. **(b)** The tumour cells display intense nuclear Pit-1 reactivity. **(c)** They have abundant growth hormone (GH) reactivity in the cytoplasm of tumour cells and may also contain α-subunit of glycoprotein hormones (not shown). When they express prolactin (PRL), they are classified as mammosomatotroph adenomas. **(d)** The keratin stain with CAM 5.2 reveals a perinuclear staining pattern.

to that of normal somatotrophs and the cells of densely granulated somatotroph adenomas. There is strong nuclear immunoreactivity for Pit-1 and occasionally for ER. Very rarely, β-TSH can be demonstrated in the cytoplasm. Ultrastructurally, the tumour cells resemble densely granulated somatotrophs;[115] however, secretory granules have mottled cores, are variably pleomorphic and can measure up to 1000 nm. In addition, the cells exhibit misplaced exocytosis, which is the classic feature of PRL secretion.

Differential Diagnosis

The important differential diagnosis is between the various types of adenomas described earlier, because it is important for the subsequent management of patients who fail to achieve total surgical excision and require subsequent medical therapy to normalize GH and IGF-1 levels. The identification of PRL immunoreactivity tends to predict a possible medical response to dopaminergic agents. Treatment with somatostatin analogues is now the primary mode of treatment and often results in inhibition of GH excess,[63,65] but this is most successful in patients with densely granulated as compared

with sparsely granulated tumours.[67] Patients who fail this treatment usually have sparsely granulated adenomas[29] and are candidates for therapy with a peripheral GH antagonist, known as pegvisomant, that may block the autoregulation of GH feedback; this could be hazardous in patients with intact GH feedback in their tumours, but those with sparsely granulated somatotroph adenomas are likely to harbour mutations in the GH receptor[21] or other alterations in GH-receptor signalling that would make this a safe therapy.

Sparsely granulated somatotroph adenomas are unusual in that they exhibit significant nuclear pleomorphism and atypia that is not found in most pituitary adenomas or carcinomas. For this reason, an important differential diagnosis is metastatic malignancy. This is readily addressed by immunohistochemistry but it is important to note that GH immunoreactivity can be weak and focal in this lesion; as a result, the use of Pit-1 as a marker can be more helpful.

There is no consistent morphologic alteration attributable to medical administration of somatostatin analogues[66] that are being increasingly offered as preoperative medical therapy to reduce the surgical complications of acromegalic patients.

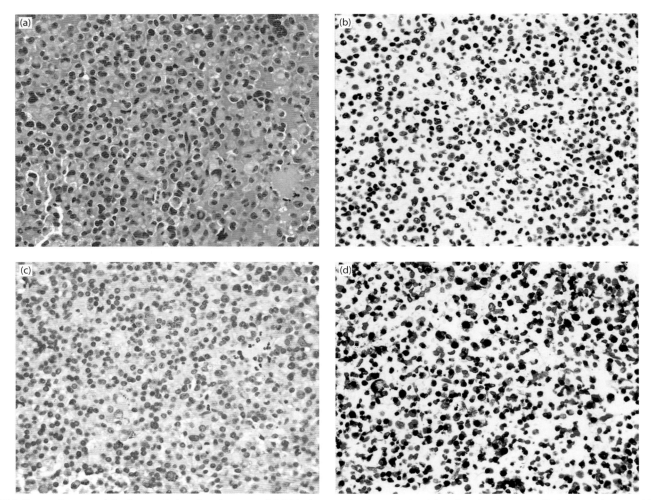

41.8 Sparsely granulated somatotroph adenoma. **(a)** This tumour is characterized by discohesive cells that have pleomorphic nuclei and chromophobic cytoplasm that may harbour juxtanuclear acidophilic round bodies. **(b)** The stain for Pit-1 highlights the marked pleomorphism of the tumour cell nuclei. **(c)** These adenomas may have only weak or focal staining for growth hormone (GH) and are usually negative for other hormones. **(d)** The hallmark of this tumour is the fibrous body, a juxtanuclear round accumulation of keratin filaments readily decorated by staining with the CAM 5.2 antibody.

Functioning Lactotroph Adenomas

Tumours arising from PRL-secreting adenohypophyseal cells ('prolactinomas') are the most common type of pituitary adenoma. Although almost half of adenomas found incidentally at autopsy are of this type,[70] the incidence is much lower in surgical series, probably because these tumours are often treated medically. Prolactinomas are more common in females, who tend to present at a younger age with hormonal disturbances. In contrast, men tend to present later, with larger tumours that more often result in mass effects and hypopituitarism secondary to adenohypophyseal destruction. Whereas this has been attributed to sexual dimorphism of the perception of the relevant symptoms, recent evidence suggests that the tumours grow faster in men.[55] There are three variants of PRL-secreting pituitary adenomas: sparsely granulated and densely granulated lactotroph adenomas and the rare but aggressive acidophil stem cell tumour.

A number of physiologic, pharmacologic and pathologic conditions may cause elevated serum PRL levels. Lactotroph adenomas tend to have a good correlation between tumour size and PRL level, so that a large tumour associated with minimal elevation of PRL levels is likely not a prolactinoma. However, patients with acidophil stem cell adenomas do not show good correlation of tumour size and circulating PRL level.

Microadenomas are most commonly located in the posterolateral portions of the gland. Macroadenomas may invade into dura mater, nasal sinuses and bone. They can be soft and red or grey and firm. Psammoma bodies may occur in pituitary adenomas and are most common in prolactinomas; they result in a gritty consistency.

Sparsely granulated lactotroph adenomas are the most common variant of adenoma arising from lactotrophs. Chromophobic tumour cells are arranged in papillae, trabeculae or solid sheets; tumour cells may form pseudorosettes around vascular spaces.[11] Calcification is occasionally present and may take the form of frank psammoma bodies. Amyloid deposition is a rare feature. The tumour cells show strong immunoreactivity for PRL in a juxtanuclear globular pattern that corresponds to the Golgi region (Figure 41.9). Nuclear staining for Pit-1 is usually

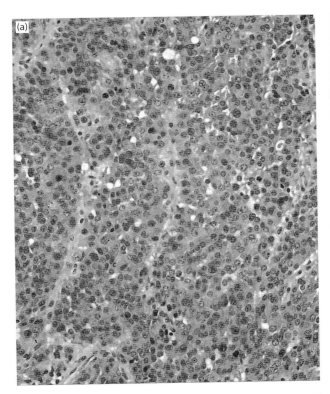

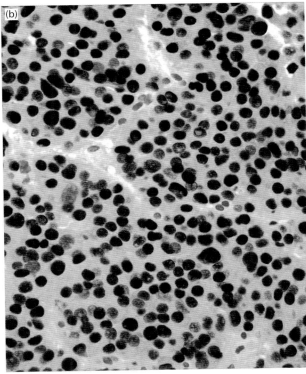

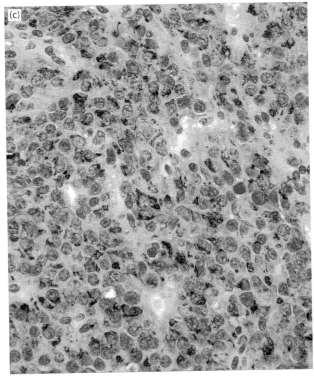

41.9 Sparsely granulated lactotroph adenoma. (a) This tumour is composed of sheets of epithelial cells that have abundant chromophobic cytoplasm. **(b)** They have intense nuclear positivity for Pit-1. **(c)** Immunostains for prolactin characteristically reveal a juxtanuclear pattern of reactivity, corresponding to the large well-developed Golgi complexes in these cells that have very few secretory granules.

present and oestrogen receptor positivity may be found by immunohistochemistry. Ultrastructurally,[115] the cells have large nuclei with prominent nucleoli. The rough endoplasmic reticulum is prominent and arranged in distinctive parallel arrays; when arranged in concentric whorls, they are known as 'Nebenkern formations'. Large, well-developed Golgi complexes harbour immature pleomorphic granules.

Secretory granules are spherical, sparse, and range in size from 150 to 300 nm. Misplaced exocytosis, or the expulsion of secretory granules from the lateral cell membrane into the extracellular space, is a diagnostic feature of PRL-producing tumours.

Densely granulated lactotroph adenomas are much less common than the sparsely granulated variant. These tumours are composed of acidophilic cells that exhibit diffuse cytoplasmic positivity for PRL, unlike the juxtanuclear Golgi pattern seen in the sparsely granulated adenoma (Figure 41.10). Ultrastructurally, densely granulated cells have abundant rough endoplasmic reticulum; secretory granules are numerous and can measure up to 700 nm. Misplaced exocytosis is a diagnostic feature.

Acidophil stem cell adenoma is composed of solid sheets of large oncocytic cells that are acidophilic because of the accumulation of mitochondria (Figure 41.11). Large cytoplasmic vacuoles corresponding to giant mitochondria can occasionally be appreciated by light microscopy.[11] The classic immunohistochemical profile shows strong diffuse immunoreactivity for PRL and scant immunoreactivity for

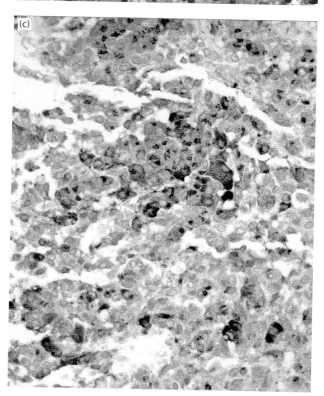

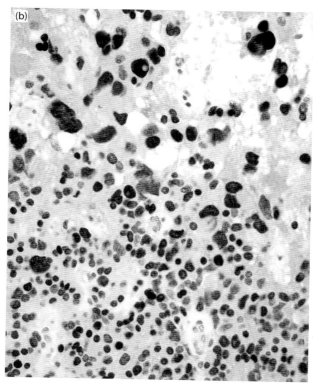

41.10 Densely granulated lactotroph adenoma. (a) This tumour is composed of epithelial cells that have variable acidophilic to chromophobic cytoplasm. The presence of large atypical nuclei is not unusual. **(b)** They exhibit nuclear positivity for Pit-1. **(c)** Immunostains for prolactin reveal cells with diffuse cytoplasmic positivity as well as some cells that have a Golgi staining pattern.

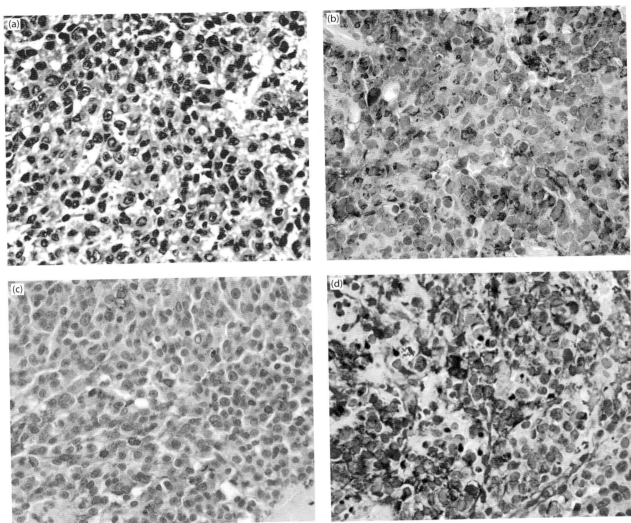

41.11 Acidophil stem cell adenoma. (a) This tumour is characterized by discohesive oncocytic cells that have pleomorphic nuclei and variable amounts of granular acidophilic cytoplasm. **(b)** They usually contain immunoreactivity for prolactin (PRL). **(c)** These adenomas may have only weak of focal staining for growth hormone (GH). **(d)** Like sparsely granulated somatotroph adenomas, these tumours contain fibrous bodies identified by the CAM 5.2 antibody, but they are few and scattered.

GH. Some tumours may lack detectable immunoreactivity for GH. Staining with low molecular weight cytokeratins allows the detection of rare fibrous bodies that may be found in this tumour, similar to but far fewer than those that characterize the sparsely granulated somatotroph adenoma.[11] Ultrastructurally, the cell cytoplasm is occupied by numerous enlarged mitochondria with scattered distinctive giant mitochondria containing electron dense tubules.[115] Juxtanuclear bundles of cytokeratin intermediate filaments, known as fibrous bodies, are scattered throughout the tumour. Secretory granules are scant and range in size from 150 to 200 nm. Misplaced exocytosis can be seen.

Differential Diagnosis

Administration of dopamine agonists such as bromocriptine, cabergoline or quinagolide results in a dramatic clinical response in patients with prolactinomas. The rapid fall in serum PRL is accompanied by an almost equally rapid reduction in tumour size that is due to tumour cell shrinkage.[204] In the absence of relevant history, the changes may

be a source of diagnostic confusion. The cytoplasm of the tumour cells shrinks, resulting in a marked increase in cellularity (Figure 41.12). The resulting picture can histologically resemble a lymphoma or metastatic small cell carcinoma and immunohistochemical studies may be required to determine the correct diagnosis. The changes are reversible upon discontinuation of therapy but a small population of tumour cells may show permanent alterations. After chronic therapy, there can be interstitial and perivascular fibrosis along with haemorrhage and hemosiderin deposition.

The importance of correct distinction of the various PRL-producing adenomas can impact therapy and outcome. Acidophil stem cell adenomas tend to be resistant to treatment with bromocriptine.[18] Surgical resection is usually necessary for these aggressive tumours; recurrence is common and radiation therapy may be required. Similarly, densely granulated lactotroph adenomas tend to behave aggressively. In contrast, the vast majority of sparsely granulated lactotroph adenomas respond well to dopamine agonist therapy.

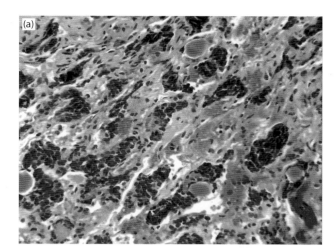

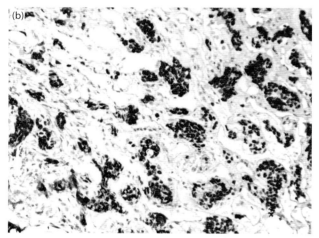

41.12 Lactotroph adenoma after long-term dopamine agonist therapy. (a) The appearance mimics inflammation, lymphoma or metastatic small cell carcinoma. **(b)** The tumour cells exhibit strong reactivity for Pit-1, confirming their differentiation.

Hyperprolactinaemia due to stalk compression of any neoplastic or non-neoplastic cause can clinically mimic prolactinoma. Lymphocytic hypophysitis is an important but readily identified mimic (see Tumour-like Lesions). In general, the levels of PRL correlate directly with tumour size in sparsely granulated lactotroph adenomas, so that a PRL level of less than 200 µg/L in a patient with a lesion larger than 1 cm usually indicates the presence of a different tumour type (Box 41.3).

Functioning Thyrotroph Adenomas

Thyrotroph adenomas are rare, accounting for less than one per cent of all pituitary neoplasms. Patients with pituitary-dependent TSH excess may exhibit features of hyperthyroidism or hypothyroidism, or may be euthyroid.[24] Because most thyrotroph tumours are invasive macroadenomas, mass effects with visual field disturbances are common.

Grossly, thyrotroph adenomas tumours tend to be invasive and fibrotic macroadenomas at the time of diagnosis. By light microscopy, these tumours are composed of chromophobic cells with indistinct cell borders and varying degrees of nuclear pleomorphism (Figure 41.13). Architecturally,

the tumours most commonly exhibit a solid or sinusoidal pattern. Stromal fibrosis is common and occasional thyrotroph adenomas form psammoma bodies. The tumour cells show immunoreactivity for α-subunit and β-TSH. Immunohistochemistry highlights the polygonal to spindled tumour cells that usually have elongated processes.[11] Ultrastructurally, thyrotroph adenoma cells resemble normal thyrotrophs.[115] The cells have euchromatic nuclei and long interdigitating cytoplasmic processes that contain abundant rough endoplasmic reticulum with prominent and spherical Golgi bodies. Secretory granules, which are spherical and range in size from 150 to 250 nm, tend to accumulate along the cell membrane. Some densely granulated tumours occasionally have larger granules measuring up to 350 nm.

Differential Diagnosis

Diffuse thyrotroph hyperplasia can mimic this disorder and it is critical to establish loss of acinar architecture using a reticulin stain (see Hyperplasia) when confronted with this clinical diagnosis. In tumours with significant nuclear atypia, the diagnosis of a metastatic lesion might be considered, but the use of immunohistochemical markers will establish the correct diagnosis.

Functioning Gonadotroph Adenomas

These tumours are mainly diagnosed in middle-aged men with no prior history of gonadal dysfunction.[194] Although they occur in women, the clinical diagnosis is often missed because elevated gonadotropins are physiological in postmenopausal women and the tumours are considered to be non-functional.[50]

Grossly, the tumours are large, soft, well vascularized, and occasionally have foci of haemorrhage or necrosis. Microscopically, they can have a trabecular, papillary, or sinusoidal pattern.[17] There is usually prominent pseudorosette formation around vascular spaces where the tumour cells show distinct polarity with nuclei aligned at the basal pole of the cell (Figure 41.14). In other areas the cells vary from columnar to cuboidal to polygonal and they tend to have scant chromophobic cytoplasm. Focal oncocytic change is common. Small PAS positive globules may be found in some tumour cells. These tumours exhibit variable and often only focal immunoreactivity for α-subunit, β-FSH and β-LH. As well, there is strong nuclear staining with steroidogenic factor-1 (SF-1).[11] It is common for gonadotroph adenomas to exhibit ultrastructural diversity.[115] Well-differentiated tumour cells are elongated with the nucleus occupying one pole and secretory granules accumulating at the opposite pole. Poorly differentiated cells are generally

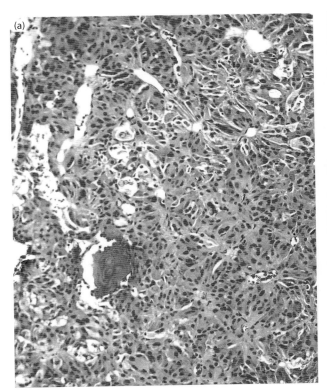

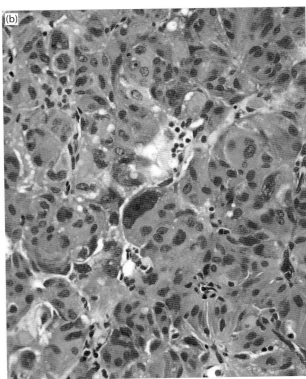

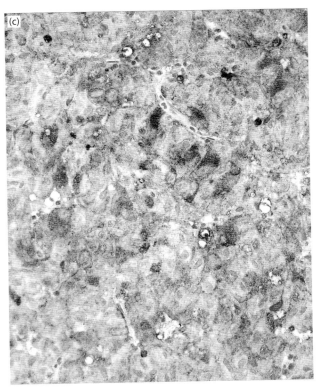

41.13 Thyrotroph adenoma. (a) The tumour cells have a spindle morphology and exhibit marked nuclear pleomorphism. There is a psammoma body, a rare finding usually associated with lactotroph or thyrotroph adenomas. **(b)** These adenomas can exhibit marked nuclear pleomorphism and multinucleate forms may be seen. **(c)** Staining for β-TSH localizes hormone in tumour cells and defines the polygonal shape of these cells.

ovoid or polygonal and lack polarity. Rough endoplasmic reticulum is usually composed of short dilated profiles that contain flocculent material. Golgi bodies are perinuclear, large and globular. Secretory granules are generally small (250 nm), variable in number and often located close to the cell membrane. Cells exhibiting oncocytic change have abundant mitochondria.

Differential Diagnosis

The histopathology of these lesions is highly characteristic and because of the formation of pseudorosettes, the lesion can be mistaken for an esthesioneuroblastoma or ependymoma. The location and immunohistochemical profile will allow a distinction between these entities in most instances, but in some adenomas, gonadotropin immunoreactivity is

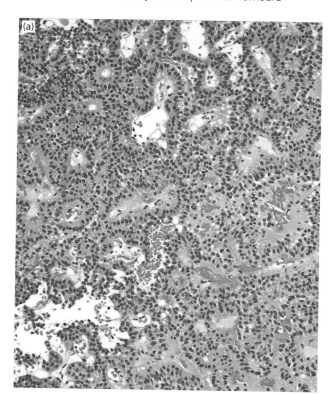

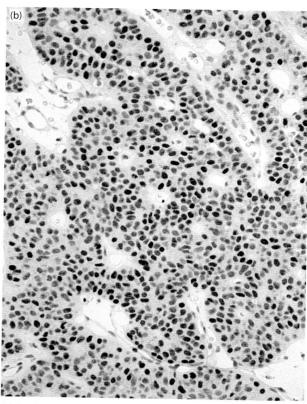

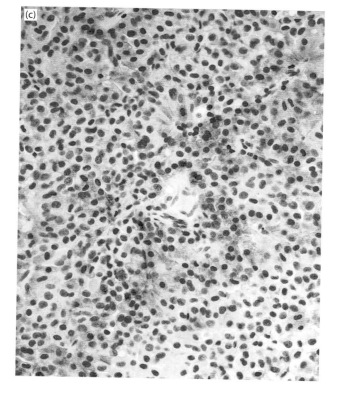

41.14 Gonadotroph adenoma. (a) The tumour cells form pseudorosettes around vascular spaces and many cells are elongated with distinct polarity. **(b)** They have strong nuclear reactivity for SF-1. **(c)** There is usually focal cytoplasmic reactivity for gonadotropin subunits, most often β-FSH.

(b) Courtesy of Dr Arie Perry, UCSF, San Francisco, CA, USA.

weak and/or focal, and the identification of SF-1 positivity may be required for diagnosis.

Clinically Non-functioning Pituitary Adenomas

These tumours account for approximately one third of all pituitary adenomas. Because of their lack of clinically detectable hormonal activity, they tend to present with mass effects.[11] If there is extensive tissue destruction, hypopituitarism results in clinical symptoms. Less commonly, pituitary apoplexy with haemorrhage into the tumour causes a medical emergency. Patients may have varying degrees of hypopituitarism depending on the amount of adenohypophyseal tissue destruction. There is no evidence of hormone excess, but stalk compression without significant adenohypophyseal destruction can result in mild hyperprolactinaemia. Diabetes insipidus is rare in patients with pituitary adenoma and usually indicates the presence of a different diagnosis.

The diagnosis of silent pituitary adenomas is based solely on morphologic and immunohistochemical features of the tumour.[11] Silent somatotroph adenomas have morphologic features similar to those of sparsely granulated somatotroph adenomas. Silent lactotroph adenomas and silent thyrotroph adenomas exhibit morphologic features corresponding to those of their functioning counterparts. Silent corticotroph adenomas are usually associated with hyperprolactinaemia even in cases without obvious stalk involvement. There are two morphologic variants. Type I silent corticotroph adenomas correspond morphologically to the functioning densely granulated corticotroph adenoma. Type II silent corticotroph adenomas are similar to the sparsely granulated functioning corticotroph adenomas. The clinical inactivity of some corticotroph adenomas may be due to aberrant cleavage of the POMC molecule. Silent gonadotroph adenomas are morphologically identical to the functioning gonadotroph adenomas and represent the largest group of clinically nonfunctioning adenomas. Most tumours classified as null cell adenomas are silent gonadotroph adenomas composed of poorly differentiated cells with scattered foci exhibiting histologic features consistent with gonadotroph differentiation; these tumours generally exhibit SF-1 staining despite lack of detectable gonadotropin content. Oncocytomas represent silent gonadotroph adenomas with extensive oncocytic change (Figure 41.15). The tumour cells are usually arranged in sheets or nests, and contain abundant granular eosinophilic cytoplasm, corresponding ultrastructurally to mitochondrial accumulation. These tumours also generally exhibit SF-1 nuclear reactivity.[11,19]

Despite advances in morphologic classification of adenohypophyseal cells that have resulted from improved tissue fixation, more specific and sensitive antibodies and transcription factors that identify cell differentiation, there remains a minority of pituitary adenomas that defy definitive classification based on histological, immunohistochemical and ultrastructural examination. Poorly differentiated adenomas (Figure 41.16) are negative for all hormones and transcription factors and exhibit no ultrastructural markers of the known adenohypophyseal cell types.[11]

The tumour identified in the literature as 'female type gonadotroph adenoma'[99] is a tumour that is usually clinically silent, immunohistochemically plurihormonal and characterized by a distinctive ultrastructural feature of dilated, saccular Golgi bodies known as 'honeycomb Golgi'. The cytogenesis of this lesion is not known, but recent information suggests that this Golgi abnormality is not specific to gonadotrophs and may be also identified in corticotroph adenomas.[179,180]

Differential Diagnosis

The most important distinction is between the various types of clinically non-functioning adenomas, because they best predict behaviour and recurrence. The vast majority of these lesions are of gonadotroph differentiation or null cell

adenomas; they tend to exhibit slow growth and delayed recurrence if any. In contrast, silent corticotroph adenomas are characteristically aggressive lesion with a high rate of early recurrence.

Other tumours, discussed below, can clinically mimic silent adenomas but are not usually difficult to classify. The one exception is metastatic endocrine carcinoma that can be easily mistaken for a pituitary adenoma. The most useful markers are the transcription factors TTF-1 and CDX-2, and hormones mostly expressed in tissues other than pituitary, such as chromogranin and gastroenteropancreatic hormones, but these are usually only considered if there is a known clinical history of previous endocrine carcinoma of the lung, gastrointestinal tract, pancreas or another site.

Plurihormonal Pituitary Adenomas

Occasionally, pituitary adenomas elaborate multiple hormones. Most often, this is due to known regulatory factors; rarely, products of different hormone families are produced. These adenomas may be fully functioning, partially functioning (in which only one component is clinically apparent), or silent. The most common combination is excessive production of GH and PRL, or GH, PRL and TSH, resulting in acromegaly/gigantism accompanied by hyperprolactinaemia and even hyperthyroidism. This pattern of plurihormonality is accounted for by the expression of Pit-1 that regulates the expression of these various hormones by related cells. Other combinations of unrelated hormones have been reported.[11] The interpretation of the individual combinations must be evaluated with caution, and may in some cases be artefacts of antibody cross-reactivity.

Monomorphous plurihormonal adenomas are composed of a single cell type that produces multiple hormones; the tumour cells contain cytoplasmic immunoreactivity for two or more hormones within the same cell. Plurimorphous plurihormonal adenomas are composed of at least two cell types, each of which exhibits a characteristic immunohistochemical and ultrastructural profile. These may represent 'collision' tumours.[105] Silent subtype III adenomas are rare and aggressive plurihormonal tumours that are identified by unique ultrastructural features.[100] They have been associated with hyperprolactinaemia that was attributed to mass effects or subtle acromegaly or may be clinically non-functioning.[60] They are histologically diffuse and exhibit focal immunoreactivity for one or more adenohypophyseal hormones, usually PRL, GH, TSH and α-subunit. The large tumour cells have nuclei that are located at one pole and may contain complex granular and lamellar inclusions known as spheridia. There is abundant well-developed rough endoplasmic reticulum with prominent, tortuous Golgi complexes and abundant groups of mitochondria. Small secretory granules are localized to attenuated, interdigitating cell processes, resembling thyrotrophs.[101] This lesion is considered to be a plurihormonal tumour of the Pit-1 lineage.[11] It is considered more aggressive and often infiltrates downwards through bone of the sphenoid area. Local recurrence is not uncommon; there may be a role for radiotherapy for this relatively radiosensitive lesion.

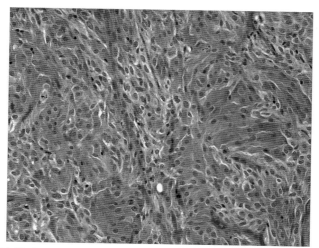

41.15 Oncocytoma. The large tumour cells have abundant granular eosinophilic cytoplasm.

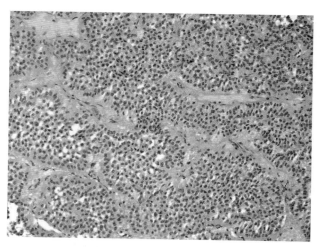

41.16 Null cell adenoma. The chromophobic cells are largely undifferentiated but at the periphery of the solid sheets, some cells show polarity, resembling cells of a gonadotroph adenoma. Occasional oncocytic cells are seen.

Pathogenesis and Molecular Genetics

The cause of sporadic pituitary adenomas is not known. A minority of these lesions is associated with familial disorders and some of the genes implicated have been identified.

Multiple endocrine neoplasia (MEN) syndromes are familial disorders in which several endocrine glands develop neoplasms or hyperplasias. Pituitary adenomas are most commonly associated with MEN-1 (Wermer's syndrome), an autosomal dominant disorder with incomplete penetrance. This syndrome is characterized by the development of para-thyroid hyperplasia or adenoma, pancreatic endocrine cell hyperplasia, dysplasia and tumour and pituitary adenoma. The various tumours develop metachronously rather than synchronously in individual patients and in no specific order. Approximately two-thirds of affected patients develop a pituitary adenoma, most often producing prolactin and/ or GH.[184] This disease results from a germline mutation of the *MEN1* gene on chromosome 11q13 that encodes the tumour suppressor protein menin.[43] Loss of heterozygos-ity of the intact allele is associated with subsequent tumour formation. However, alterations of menin are not found in the more common sporadic adenomas.[20,237]

Defects in cyclin-dependent kinase inhibitors (CDKIs) have been identified in a small number of families with multiple endocrine tumours including pituitary adenomas; this syndrome has been classified as MEN-X or MEN-4. Reports include mutations of CDKNIB/p27Kip1[83,133,154] and CDKN2C/p18INK4c.[3]

Carney's complex (CNC) is an autosomal dominant dis-order characterized by development of myxomas (mainly cardiac), spotty pigmentation due to lentigo or several types of nevi that affect mucosal surfaces and the lips, and endocrine tumours including pigmented nodular adreno-cortical disease, testicular tumours and pituitary adenoma with gigantism or acromegaly (see Chapter 44, Hereditary Tumour Syndromes).[39] These lesions share cAMP signalling pathways and the disease has been associated with germline mutations in the *PRKAR1Aα* gene that encodes the PKA regulatory subunit 1Aα.[111] Consistent with this theory, ani-mal models of PRKAR1A loss prove that this regulatory transducer is critical for pituitary tumour development.[226]

However, this gene is not implicated in the pathogenesis of sporadic pituitary tumours.[109,176]

The isolated familial somatotropinoma (IFS) and famil-ial isolated pituitary adenoma (FIPA) syndromes involve families with pituitary GH-producing adenomas (IFS)[195] or non-somatotroph lesions (FIPA); virtually all FIPA kindreds contain at least one prolactinoma or somatotropinoma.[23] Patients with FIPA are significantly younger at diagnosis and have larger tumours than sporadic counterparts. Germline mutations in the *aryl hydrocarbon receptor-inter-acting protein (AIP)* gene with loss of heterozygosity (LOH) of AIP is implicated[217] in about half of IFS kindreds and in about 15 per cent of FIPA families. In families with AIP mutations, pituitary adenomas have a penetrance of over 50 per cent.[23] In the paediatric population, where pituitary adenomas are rare, germline AIP mutations can be found in children and adolescents with GH-secreting tumours, even in the absence of a family history.[84] However, there is no evidence of AIP mutations in patients with sporadic pitu-itary tumours.[56]

The cause of sporadic pituitary tumours is unknown. A number of etiologic factors have been implicated, including genetic events, hormonal stimulation and growth factors[11,13] and it is likely that all of these interact to initiate transformation and promote tumour cell proliferation.

Somatic mutations are rare in pituitary tumours with the exception of somatotroph adenomas. Activating point mutation of the G proteins that mediate receptor signalling was one of the first genetic events identified in endocrine tumours.[209] Point mutations in two domains of Gsα, codon 201 (Arg to Cys) and codon 227 (Gln to Arg), activate ade-nylyl cyclase by interfering with GTP hydrolysis, maintain-ing Gsα in a constitutively active state.[209] These G-protein oncogenes (*gsps*), were first described in a subset of pituitary somatotroph adenomas and hormone-secreting tumours of other endocrine glands[209] and are now known to be the cause of the McCune–Albright syndrome in which there is germline mosaicism;[219] patients with this disorder develop somatotroph hyperplasia or adenoma.[116] The mutations are more frequently detected in the maternal allele, consistent with monoallelic imprinting.[93] These *gsp* mutations are identified in a subset of somatotroph adenomas, usually correlating with the phenotype of the densely granulated somatotroph adenoma;[21,196] the increased cAMP levels that are characteristic of this mutation would account for the expression of α-subunit that is regulated by CREB, and explain the clinical response of these tumours to somatostatin analogue therapy.[29,67] In contrast, sparsely granulated somatotroph adenomas have recently been reported to harbour mutations of the *GH receptor* (*GHR*) gene that reduce GH autoregulation;[21] interruption of GH autoregulation by this mutation or other mechanisms altering STAT activation may be implicated in the development of these lesions.

FGF signalling is critical in pituitary development.[103] Multiple lines of evidence implicate two FGFRs in pituitary tumourigenesis.[1] FGFR2 is expressed in the normal pituitary where it functions as a tumour suppressor that silences members of the cancer/testis-melanoma associated antigen (MAGE-A) family;[235] it is significantly down-regulated in pituitary tumours by promoter methylation.[1,234] In contrast, FGFR4 is only expressed in the developing normal gland, but is upregulated in tumours.[1] An N-terminally truncated variant, pituitary tumour-derived FGFR4 (ptd-FGFR4)[1,68] results from alternative transcription initiation from a cryptic promoter.[69,230] This oncogene displaces N-cadherin from the cell membrane to interfere with normal cell adhesion.[71] A similar mechanism may explain the relationship between expression of PSA-NCAM and tumour growth and invasiveness,[51] because PSA-NCAM would also disrupt the tri-protein complex.

Epigenetic regulators, such as the DNA methyltransferase (DNMT) enzyme family, are implicated in the silencing of the tumour suppressors pRb, p21 and p27.[236] Another epigenetic factor, Ikaros, is altered in pituitary tumours with a dominant negative isoform, Ik6, identified in nearly 50 per cent of human pituitary adenomas.[69] Forced expression of this dn form of Ikaros results in histone 3 acetylation with activation of the Bcl-XL promoter,[74] resulting in enhanced pituitary cell survival and evasion from apoptosis. Ikaros also has metabolic effects as a mediator of cholesterol uptake,[130] a factor that is required for hormone packaging and secretion. The high mobility group (HMG) proteins containing AT-hook domains (HMGA) are also involved in DNA binding and chromatin remodeling and recent studies have shown that mice overexpressing HMGA1 or HMGA2 develop pituitary tumours that secrete GH and PRL;[76] this factor upregulates cyclin B2.[53] Some human pituitary adenomas have amplification and overexpression of HMGA1 or 2.[53] Altered expression of HMGA2 may also be due to altered microRNA expression, particularly of let-7.[161]

Biological Behaviour

Previously, the only predictors of recurrence were tumour size and invasiveness that determined the success of surgical resection. However, even apparent surgical success can be followed by delayed recurrence. New technologies allow novel approaches to determine the prognosis of pituitary adenomas. The proliferative activity of pituitary tumours has been extensively investigated.[200] Studies of proliferating cell nuclear antigen (PCNA), Ki-67/MIB-1, and anti-apoptotic Bcl-2 have unfortunately demonstrated no consistent correlation with tumour invasiveness or recurrence.[7] DNA

topoisomerase II alpha (Topo II alpha), another marker of cell proliferation, was investigated in pituitary adenomas and carcinomas in relation to their biological behaviour; although invasive pituitary adenomas and carcinomas exhibit a high Topo II alpha index, this indicator has no significant advantage over MIB-1 as a prognostic marker.[215] Cyclooxygenase-2 (COX-2) expression correlates with patient age, but not with tumour size or invasiveness.[214] Detection of telomerase expression may predict recurrence in pituitary adenomas.[228] Galectin-3, a beta-galactoside-binding protein implicated in cellular differentiation and proliferation as well as angiogenesis, tumour progression and metastasis, may play a role in pituitary tumour progression.[168] The *TP53* gene does not seem to be of pathogenetic significance in pituitary tumours. Although p53 expression has been detected in adenomas of all types, and may be more common in recurrent neoplasms,[201] there is no evidence of mutation or allelic loss and the significance of the immunoreactivity remains to be established.

Unfortunately, none of these is truly a marker of biological behaviour. The WHO has recommended that invasive pituitary adenomas exhibiting increased mitotic activity, MIB-1 labelling index > 3 per cent or extensive p53 expression be classified as 'atypical adenomas'.[54] However, this terminology does not seem to reflect any biological superiority to the aggressive histological subtypes determined by the accurate classification of pituitary adenomas.[6] The diagnosis of pituitary carcinoma is restricted to adenohypophyseal proliferations that exhibit cerebrospinal and/or systemic metastasis;[54] there are no morphological criteria to distinguish locally aggressive or atypical adenomas from carcinomas when the tumour is confined to the sella.

The best predictive markers for behaviour of pituitary adenomas remain those that subclassify adenomas accurately based on hormone content and cell structure. For example, among acromegalics who fail surgical resection, response to long acting somatostatin analogues is best predicted by the subtype of somatotroph adenoma as densely or sparsely granulated.[29,67] This finding renders the value of a CAM 5.2 keratin stain more important than almost any other immunostain in this setting. A silent corticotroph adenoma will recur more often and more aggressively than a silent gonadotroph adenoma. A silent subtype 3 adenoma will almost certainly behave invasively, infiltrating the base of the skull, whereas a silent adenoma of the gonadotroph lineage will usually grow by expansion upwards.

PITUITARY CARCINOMA

Malignant tumours of adenohypophyseal origin are defined solely by their ability to metastasize.[11,54] Although many pituitary adenomas are widely invasive, destructive of adjacent tissues and lethal, they are not classified as malignancies.

Epidemiology

These lesions are extremely rare, because of the highly restrictive definition requiring distant metastases. Over 100 cases have been reported. They occur at any age and there is no gender bias. The majority are functioning lesions with a disproportionate representation of ACTH- and PRL-producing carcinomas compared to adenomas.

Clinical Features

Pituitary carcinomas generally present initially as pituitary adenoma. They can be associated with any form of hormone excess including hyperprolactinaemia, Cushing's disease, rarely acromegaly and even hyperthyroidism due to TSH excess. In some cases, they are unassociated with clinical or biochemical evidence of hormone excess and a silent subtype 3 carcinoma has been reported.[173] A single paediatric case has been described.[89] Only the subsequent development of metastases identified the lesion as malignant. The most common sites of metastasis include the subarachnoid space, brain parenchyma (not including areas of direct invasion), cervical lymph nodes, bone, liver and lungs.

Radiology

The radiology of the primary pituitary lesion is indistinguishable from pituitary adenoma. The lesions may be locally infiltrative, but that feature does not result in a diagnosis of malignancy. Radiology, however, is important to identify the metastatic foci throughout the body.

Pathology

Examination of the primary tumour usually reveals nonspecific morphologic features such as hypercellularity, haemorrhage, necrosis, mitoses, nuclear pleomorphism and invasion; none of these features, either individually or in combination, are reliable indicators of malignancy. Markers that have been suggested as helpful in predicting malignancy include a higher microvascular density,[216] high Ki67 labelling index with the MIB-1 antibody,[200] high p53 labelling,[201] loss of p27 immunoreactivity[107,114] and increased topo II alpha.[215] Overexpression of Her2/neu has been reported.[145] Despite these reported differences in number of positive cells or staining intensity of the various markers, none is able to accurately discriminate between pituitary adenoma and carcinoma and the diagnosis is only confirmed when metastatic tumour is identified.

Molecular Genetics

The pathogenesis of the rare pituitary carcinoma is not known. *H-ras* point mutations have been reported in some metastatic foci, but not in the corresponding primary tumour.[37,152] Based on immunohistochemistry alone, loss-of-function of Rb may be implicated.[94] Immunoreactivity for p53 has been reported[155,201] and mutation of this tumour suppressor gene has been documented in several tumours with more than 60 per cent of cells showing immunoreactivity for p53.[198] The clinical time course of these lesions, their histopathology and studies of several molecular markers suggest progression of an adenoma-carcinoma sequence;[82] however, some studies suggest that malignancy may arise *de novo*. The complexity of this process was highlighted by the identification of distinct clonal compositions of a primary and metastatic ACTH-producing pituitary carcinoma.[231]

Biological Behaviour

These rare tumours are uniformly lethal, usually because of tumour dissemination but also complicated by the metabolic and hormonal alterations that cannot be controlled. Precise mortality figures are not available but it is estimated that 80 per cent of patients succumb to tumour-related mortality within 8 years.[54]

CRANIOPHARYNGIOMA

This benign but locally invasive epithelial tumour has a complex, partially squamoid morphology, explained by its origin from the remnants of Rathke's pouch.

Epidemiology

Craniopharyngioma has been reported to represent from 1 to 13 per cent of intracranial neoplasms, with more recent estimates at 1.2–4.6 per cent.[132] It is the most common sellar tumour in children and accounts for 10 per cent of all childhood CNS tumours. Craniopharyngiomas can occur at all ages but the peak incidence is between 5 and 20 years old, with a second smaller peak in the sixth decade. Some series show a male predominance.

Clinical Features

These tumours do not produce adenohypophyseal hormones, but rather are hormonally inactive mass lesions. They result in headaches and can cause visual field disturbances;[191] in extreme cases with significant hypothalamic involvement they result in psychiatric disturbances, nausea, vomiting and somnolence. Because these masses interfere with hypothalamic regulation of pituitary function, hypopituitarism is identified in the majority of patients. In children, this results in a common presenting complaint, growth retardation or dwarfism. The lesion may also cause pituitary tissue destruction. In contrast to patients with large pituitary adenomas that usually compress but do not destroy the gland, patients with craniopharyngioma develop hyperprolactinaemia in less than half of patients[48,220] and about 25 per cent of patients have diabetes insipidus.

Craniopharyngioma can rarely be associated with a pituitary adenoma giving rise to marked hyperprolactinaemia with prolactinoma[48,220] or thyrotoxicosis with a thyrotroph adenoma.[227] When associated with a clinically non-functioning adenoma there is no clinical suspicion of adenoma.[87,138] Inflammation associated with craniopharyngioma may represent true lymphocytic hypophysitis as the cause of hypopituitarism[159] but more often represents a response to the tumour.

Radiology

Radiologic evaluation reveals a variably cystic lesion; only 10 per cent are entirely solid with no cystic component. An enlarged or eroded sella turcica is encountered in 50 per cent of cases; suprasellar calcification is present in more than 50 per cent of cases. MRI is the preferred technique to determine the extent of the lesion; there is often a strong

T1 signal in the absence of contrast because of high lipid content.

Craniopharyngiomas are entirely suprasellar in 85 per cent of cases; an intrasellar component is present in only 15 per cent. They can also rarely arise in ectopic pharyngeal pituitary.[113,125] The distinct localization of these lesions that differs from pituitary adenoma is explained by their proposed derivation from embryologic rests that are found in the pars tuberalis. Most of these tumours are larger than 1 cm at the time of diagnosis.

Pathology

The appearance of craniopharyngioma is usually highly distinctive. They are well circumscribed but not necessarily encapsulated and usually contain a thick oil-like fluid resembling 'black sludge'. Other features recognized grossly include the presence of cholesterol and calcification.

By light microscopy, the tumour is characterized by islands of epithelial cells punctuated by cysts and loose intercellular spaces referred to as stellate reticulum (Figure 41.17). Cholesterol clefts are common. There is often a distinctive 'wet keratin' component composed of ghost-like squamous cells lacking nuclei, which forms the nidus for calcification. A diagnosis of craniopharyngioma may be confidently rendered even in the absence of viable epithelium if wet keratin is present. Occasionally, there is a mixed chronic inflammatory infiltrate composed of lymphocytes, plasma cells and macrophages. Although grossly well delineated, microscopically these tumours frequently have infiltrative borders with associated piloid gliosis of the adjacent brain; this Rosenthal fibre-rich reaction is a known pitfall for the misdiagnosis of pilocytic astrocytoma on frozen section of a small sample obtained at the edge of the lesion. Two histologic types are identified. The adamantinomatous variant has prominent stellate reticulum, wet keratin, basal palisading and resembles the dental ameloblastic organ and adamantinomas of the bone (Figure 41.17a,b). The less common papillary variant is mostly found within the third ventricle of adults. This tumour is characterized by pseudopapillary squamous epithelium in a solid or cystic pattern (Figure 41.17c); palisading, fibrosis and cholesterol accumulation are usually absent but scattered cilia and/or goblet cells may be seen, providing some overlap with Rathke's cleft cysts that develop squamous metaplasia.

Immunohistochemistry is not usually required for the diagnosis of craniopharyngioma because the histopathology is distinctive. The epithelial component is strongly positive for cytokeratins, confirming the epithelial nature of these tumours. Craniopharyngiomas express oestrogen[202] and progesterone receptors[96] and this finding has raised the possibility that steroids may be implicated in tumour development and/or growth. Ultrastructural examination reveals tonofilaments, intercellular junctions and the absence of secretory granules.

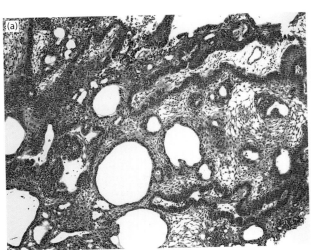

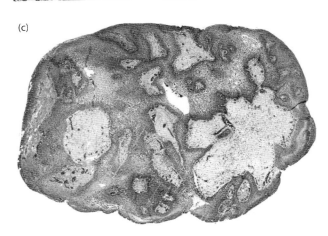

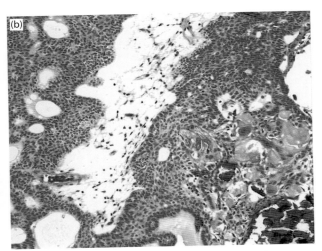

41.17 Craniopharyngioma. (a) The tumour is composed of squamous epithelium within a loose fibrous stroma forming papillae. **(b)** An adamantinomatous pattern may be present and this lesion shows focal keratin accumulation with calcification. **(c)** A papillary craniopharyngioma with non-keratinizing squamous epithelium covering fibrovascular cores.

Courtesy of Dr Arie Perry, UCSF, San Francisco, CA, USA.

Differential Diagnosis

The most difficult problem in the diagnosis of craniopharyngioma is the distinction of a cystic and hypocellular lesion from a Rathke's cleft cyst. Remnants of Rathke's pouch commonly form small cysts (<5 mm) in the vestigial pars intermedia. These small cysts occasionally enlarge into true Rathke's cleft cysts, lined by ciliated cuboidal or columnar epithelium with occasional goblet cells and areas of squamous metaplasia; as they enlarge they become symptomatic. Although this condition may occasionally be seen in children, it is most common in adults. Rathke's cleft cysts with extensive squamous metaplasia can mimic craniopharyngioma grossly, radiologically and histologically. In fact, some authors advocate a transition between these two entities, because they derive from the same precursor.[191] The development of adamantinomatous craniopharyngioma has been reported after removal of a Rathke's cleft cyst;[151] this may represent progression of the neoplasm from a cyst, but might also reflect misdiagnosis of the original lesion. The use of keratin antibodies may assist in the distinction of these lesions; it has been suggested that craniopharyngiomas do not express cytokeratins 8 and 20, whereas Rathke's cleft cysts and normal pars intermedia of pituitary glands express both of these markers.[223]

Molecular Genetics

Craniopharyngiomas are usually monoclonal.[167] Chromosomal imbalances appear rare with minimal change in the DNA copy number, regardless of their histologic subtype.[166] Only a few cases have been shown to have an increase in DNA copy number.[166]

Beta-catenin (CTNNB1) gene mutations have been documented in adamantinomatous but not papillary craniopharyngiomas,[36,148,189] suggesting a role for β-catenin in tumourigenesis. Cytoplasmic and nuclear localization of immunohistochemical reactivity for β-catenin correlates with mutation; in contrast papillary craniopharyngiomas with no mutations show exclusively membranous expression of this protein.[189] There is evidence that stromal cells may also harbour β-catenin mutations, suggesting that the stroma may be a true neoplastic component rather than a reaction to the proliferating epithelium.[189] There is no evidence of mutations of Gsα, Gi2α or patched (PTCH) genes in these lesions.[182] Craniopharyngiomas were reported in two consanguineous siblings, suggesting the possibility of genetic predisposition with autosomal recessive inheritance.[31] A craniopharyngioma has also been reported in a patient with Gardner syndrome,[128] but there is no known genetic link between familial adenomatous polyposis (FAP) and craniopharyngioma.

Biological Behaviour

The natural tendency of these lesions is towards extensive infiltration. Infiltration may involve the hypothalamus or extend as high as the third ventricle. Complete surgical resection is curative.[123] However, the highly infiltrative nature of this lesion often results in incomplete resection with subsequent high recurrence rates of 10 to 62 per cent;

this is especially true in younger patients. Post-operative radiation has been advocated to reduce recurrence.[123] Hormone replacement may be necessary for persistent hypopituitarism. Complications of untreated disease include hydrocephalus if there is extension and obstruction of the third ventricle and rupture with abscess formation or chemical meningitis resulting from the spillage of irritating cholesterol-rich fluid, the latter also occurring as a post-operative complication at times. There are reports of malignant transformation of craniopharyngioma with metastatic spread, usually via leptomeningeal seeding.[79] In some cases, malignant transformation occurred after radiotherapy,[169] but not all patients with malignancy have undergone radiotherapy.

GANGLIOCYTOMAS AND GANGLIOGLIOMAS

Neuronal tumours of the hypothalamus and pituitary are known as gangliocytomas or gangliogliomas.[11] They are composed of mature neurons, most likely derived from the ganglion cells of the hypothalamus.

Epidemiology, Clinical Features and Radiology

These are rare lesions and have no specific age or sex distribution. Clinically, the tumours can present with mass effects, hypothalamic dysregulation, hypopituitarism and hyperprolactinaemia.[160] Because these lesions have the ability to synthesize hypothalamic peptides, they may sometimes be associated with other hormonal syndromes, including acromegaly, precocious puberty or Cushing's disease.[160]

These lesions have most often been localized to the hypothalamus or tuber cinereum, with occasional involvement of the third ventricle. They may be located completely outside the hypothalamus, sometimes with a thin stalk-like connection. Some have been identified only within the sella turcica, usually within the parenchyma of the adenohypophysis or pituitary tumour; this is the most frequent localization of gangliocytomas associated with acromegaly that usually have an associated somatotroph adenoma.

Pathology

These neuronal tumours have been described to have highly heterogeneous gross appearances, because they can be nodular, pedunculated, sessile, solid or cystic and within, attached to or separate from the hypothalamus. They have been described as grey, pink, red or brown and some have exhibited necrosis.

Histologically, they are composed of mature ganglion cells with abundant cytoplasm that contains Nissl substance, and large nuclei that harbour prominent nucleoli (Figure 41.18). Binucleate or even multinucleated cells are not uncommon. The tumour cells are distributed within an abundant, highly vascular stroma composed of neuroglia or fibrous tissue. These tumours are immunoreactive for synaptophysin and neurofilaments and may contain hypothalamic peptides, including

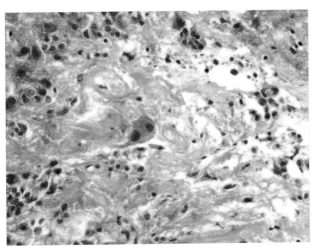

41.18 Gangliocytoma. These neuronal tumours are composed of large, often binuleate ganglion cells, resembling those of the hypothalamus. They may contain hypothalamic hormone immunoreactivity. There is abundant neuropil.

growth hormone-releasing hormone (GRH), somatostatin, gonadotropin-releasing hormone and corticotropin-releasing hormone. Ultrastructurally, the tumour cells resemble mature neurons with abundant endoplasmic reticulum, mitochondria and neurofilaments. Secretory granules are concentrated in neuronal processes.

Occasionally these lesions are associated with pituitary adenoma. The neuronal lesions associated with acromegaly have often been composite tumours with GRH reactivity and a pituitary adenoma component, usually a sparsely granulated somatotroph adenoma. Rarely other forms of composite lesions have been reported.

Histogenesis

Sellar and parasellar gangliocytomas are composed of neurons that resemble the ganglion cells of the endocrine hypothalamus. When they are found as isolated lesions, there has been little question of their histogenesis. However, their association with pituitary adenomas has raised alternative theories. There has been speculation that they may derive from pituitary adenomas by transdifferentiation, possibly induced by nerve growth factor. Alternatively, they may be the result of a pathogenetic process that exhibits a 'field effect', resulting in collision tumours. Some theories suggest that the chronic stimulation by the hypothalamic hormones results in the pituitary adenoma as a secondary phenomenon. The molecular alterations underlying these tumours are unknown.

Biological Behaviour

The behaviour of hypothalamic gangliocytomas is variable. The lesions that cause precocious puberty tend to be benign and if they are surgically resectable, cure is possible. This is often the case in lesions that are found outside the brain, hanging from the hypothalamus. In contrast, tumours that invade the brain can be infiltrative and lethal.[16]

OTHER PRIMARY NEOPLASMS OF THE SELLAR REGION

Three primary lesions of the sella — spindle cell oncocytoma, pituicytoma and granular cell tumour — are now thought to derive from 'pituicytes', glial cells of the neurohypophysis that express TTF-1,[135a] a marker of the developing and mature infundibulum.[124] Pituicytes have 5 normal variants — dark, light, oncocytic, granular and ependymal — that are reflected in the differences between these tumours, which exhibit variable degrees of oncocytic change and prominence of phagolysosomes. An unusual ependymal variant has also recently been described.[109a]

Spindle cell oncocytoma is a spindle or epithelioid, oncocytic, non-endocrine benign neoplasm of the pituitary that was initially proposed to derive from folliculostellate cells.[172] These firm lesions are composed of interlacing fascicles of bland spindled to epithelioid cells with eosinophilic, oncocytic cytoplasm (Figure 41.19 a,b);[172] occasional tumours exhibit cytologic atypia.[33] The tumour cells are negative for pituitary hormones, cytokeratins, synaptophysin and chromogranin A, but express vimentin, S-100 protein and epithelial membrane antigen (EMA). They are negative for GFAP, CD34, bcl-2, smooth muscle actin and desmin. They express TTF-1, a marker of pituicytes.[124,135a] Staining for galectin-3 is of uncertain importance.[172] The MIB-1 labelling index is usually low but cases with a higher proliferation rate have been reported.[46] By electron microscopy the tumour cells are spindled or polygonal and filled with mitochondria. They have well-formed desmosomes and intercellular junctions, but no secretory granules.

Pituicytoma is a rare low-grade spindle cell tumour composed of glial cells that originate in the neurohypophysis or infundibulum. The term has been inappropriately used for other lesions in this region, such as pilocytic astrocytomas; it should be reserved only for low grade astrocytomas of this site.[132] Other names include 'posterior pituitary astrocytoma' and 'infundibuloma'. These tumours are composed of elongated spindle-shaped cells arranged in interlacing fascicles or a storiform pattern. The tumour cells have abundant eosinophilic cytoplasm and distinct cell borders with minimal nuclear atypia (Figure 41.19c). The PAS stain is usually negative and the reticulin stain highlights perivascular fibres. They stain for vimentin, S-100 protein and GFAP, the latter only weakly, and are negative for neuronal markers (including synaptophysin, chromogranin and neurofilaments) and keratins; they may have weak patchy cytoplasmic EMA reactivity. They also stain for TTF-1.[124,135a]

Granular cell tumours of the infundibulum and posterior lobe of the pituitary[47] have also been called choristoma, granular cell myoblastoma, granular cell pituicytoma and granular cell schwannoma. They do not exhibit features of myocyte differentiation, therefore should not be considered myoblastoma. They stain for lysosomal markers, such as CD68 but are not derived from histiocytes. Whereas granular cell tumours elsewhere are thought to be of Schwann cell origin, in the pituitary, they are thought to derive from pituicytes.[47] Most of these tumours are small and are incidental autopsy findings. Occasionally, they present with visual field deficits. Diabetes insipidus is rare. These tumours are unencapsulated and composed of cells with abundant, granular,

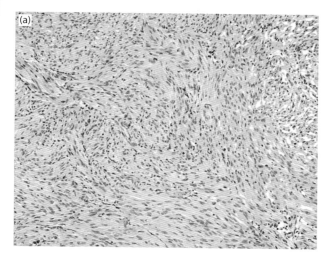

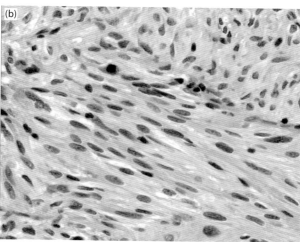

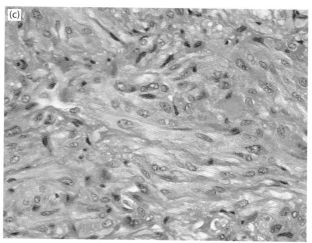

41.19 Spindle cell oncocytoma. (a) The tumour is composed of interlacing fascicles of spindle and epithelioid cells **(b)** that are thought to be derived from folliculostellate cells of the adenohypophysis but may also be tumours originating in the stromal cells of the posterior pituitary, as the lesion known as 'pituicytoma' **(c)** may not differ significantly from this lesion.

eosinophilic cytoplasm. The granules are PAS positive and diastase resistant. The tumour cells exhibit variable immunoreactivity for non-specific histiocytic markers, such as CD68, alpha-1-antitrypsin, alpha-1-antichymotrypsin and cathepsin B.[143] They may stain for S-100 protein and glial fibrillary acidic protein (GFAP), however, some are negative for these markers, casting doubt on both Schwannian and pituicyte differentiation.[208] Positivity for galectin-3 is non-specific.[170] They are positive for TTF-1, consistent with derivation from infundibular glial cells or 'pituicytes'.[124,135a] They are negative for neurofilaments, cytokeratins, synaptophysin, chromogranin A, desmin, smooth muscle actin and pituitary hormones. Electron microscopy reveals cells containing phagolysosomes with electron dense membranous debris.[121]

Pituitary blastoma is a recently described tumor of the neonatal pituitary[186] that exhibits differentiation to Rathke epithelium and adenohypophysial cells of folliculostellate and secretory type. The few tumours described have consisted of rosettes and glandular structures resembling Rathke epithelium, small undifferentiated-appearing cells (blastema) and large secretory cells. Mucin-producing goblet cells have been reported. There is immunoreactivity for synaptophysin, chromogranin, various keratins and, to a lesser extent, hormones, in secretory cells. Germ cell markers are not identified. Marked variations in cellular

proliferative activity suggest blastomas occur in low- and higher-grade form. These tumors have been interpreted to reflect arrested pituitary development and unchecked proliferation.

A number of other tumours arise in and around the region of the sella turcica and can alter pituitary function and structure. Because these lesions are not unique to the pituitary and are discussed in other chapters, only the features relevant to pituitary structure and function will be discussed here.

Paragangliomas are tumours of adrenal and extra-adrenal ganglia of the sympathetic and parasympathetic nervous system; they occur rarely in the sellar region[30] where they are thought to arise from paraganglion cells that may have been entrapped in or around the adenohypophysis or along the branches of tympanic or ciliary nerves within or close to the cavernous sinus. As in other locations, they are highly vascularized tumours with a sinusoidal growth pattern forming solid nests or 'zellballen' (Figure 41.20). The large, irregular polyhedral or elongated cells have pale eosinophilic cytoplasm that is strongly positive for synaptophysin and chromogranin but negative for cytokeratins. These lesions can be difficult to distinguish from pituitary adenoma; positivity for tyrosine hydroxylase is helpful but often negative in paragangliomas of the head and neck. Identification of neuronal markers such as neurofilaments

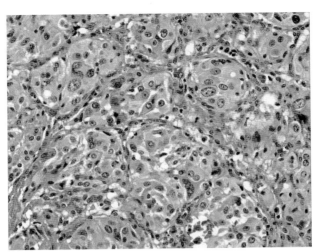

41.20 Paraganglioma. These lesions are composed of solid nests or 'zellballen' of large cells within a delicate fibrovascular stroma. The tumour cells are large, polyhedral or elongated with pale eosinophilic cytoplasm and irregular, round to oval nuclei with slight pleomorphism.

is also helpful. Malignant paragangliomas are rare but have been reported in the sella[91] and an association with von Hippel–Lindau syndrome has been reported.[185]

Esthesioneuroblastoma (olfactory neuroblastoma) is a rare, malignant neoplasm that typically arises in the nasal vault, invades adjacent tissues and causes locoregional (cervical lymph nodes) and distant metastases. Tumours of this type arising in the sellar region are rare.[127] They may arise from remnants of the nervus terminalis, which develops caudally and may have aberrant cells remaining in the sellar region. Better differentiated examples resemble pituitary adenomas but may be negative or only focally and weakly positive for cytokeratins; they usually have high Ki-67 labelling indices of 10–20 per cent and are negative for pituitary hormones.

Gliomas, including astrocytomas (Chapter 27, Astrocytic Tumours), oligodendrogliomas (Chapter 28, Oligodendroglial and Mixed Tumours), and ependymomas (Chapter 29, Ependymal Tumours), occur rarely in, but more often around, the sella.[11] The pilocytic astrocytoma, which is most common in young patients, is the most common glial tumour of the sellar or, more commonly, suprasellar region,[132] where it may be associated with predisposing syndromes, such as neurofibromatosis type 1 (NF1; see Chapter 44, Hereditary Tumour Syndromes).[164] More aggressive diffuse gliomas occur after cranial irradiation.[112,232] They are usually associated with the clinical features of a mass lesion and there is variable hypopituitarism; because they are usually suprasellar, the hypopituitarism is due to interference with hypothalamic regulation, and therefore they are associated with hyperprolactinaemia, because PRL is maintained under tonic inhibition from the hypothalamus.

Meningiomas of the sellar region account for up to 20 per cent of all meningiomas (see Chapter 36, Tumours of the Meninges). They can present with neurological deficits, visual field defects, hypopituitarism and hyperprolactinaemia due to stalk compression.[193] Completely intrasellar meningiomas are rare[193] but when they occur they generally

are not associated with hyperprolactinaemia, because there is compression of adenohypophyseal parenchyma. These lesions have also been reported following radiotherapy for pituitary adenoma.[197]

Chordomas occur in the sellar region because of their propensity to arise in the midline[134] or by direct extension from the clivus. They usually occur in patients over 30 years old. These tumours are slow growing but locally aggressive. Clinically, patients with parasellar chordomas can present with hypopituitarism. The treatment of choice is surgical excision. Tumours that are incompletely resected can be irradiated. Mean survival from time of diagnosis is approximately 5 years.

Schwannomas (see Chapter 35, Tumours of Cranial and Spinal Nerves) can present as a sellar mass with or without hypopituitarism or hyperprolactinaemia.[97] These tumours are benign and surgical resection is the treatment of choice.

Germ cell tumours (see Chapter 38, Germ Cell Tumours) also arise in the midline, including in the sellar region. These can be germinomas, embryonal carcinomas, teratomas, endodermal sinus tumours choriocarcinomas or mixed germ cell tumours. The suprasellar region is much more common than sellar, representing the second most common site of intracranial involvement after the pineal gland.[132] Mixed germ cell tumours usually contain a germinoma in combination with some other component.[165] Tumours that produce beta-hCG can mimic pituitary adenoma, because hCG can cross-react with LH and there may be elevated circulating α-subunit levels. In children, this hormonal activity may result in precocious puberty.

Vascular and other mesenchymal tumours can be benign or malignant. Involvement of the sella turcica by such neoplasms is uncommon; they usually manifest with mass effects and variable hypofunction of anterior or posterior pituitary function. Those reported in the sellar region include haemangioma,[41] glomangioma,[59] haemangioblastoma,[88] solitary fibrous tumour,[81] lipoma,[11] giant cell tumours,[222] chondromyxoid fibroma,[218] enchondroma,[136] chondroma,[9] osteochondroma,[102] osteosarcoma,[8] fibrosarcoma,[4] chondrosarcoma,[192] and alveolar soft part sarcoma.[34] They can be sporadic, or can occur as part of a clinical syndrome; haemangioblastomas may be found in patients with von Hippel–Lindau disease.[88] However, most commonly, sarcomas of the sellar region develop as a result of previous irradiation for lesions such as pituitary adenoma or craniopharyngioma.[156]

Haematopoietic neoplasms (see Chapter 40, Lymphomas and Haemopoietic Neoplasms) within the hypophysis and hypothalamus usually occur as part of a systemic disorder, but may rarely be the primary site of involvement.[175] Rarely, lymphomas, leukaemias or plasmacytomas present with sellar masses as the first lesion.[225] There is a report of a pituitary adenoma associated with a primary CNS lymphoma with hypothalamic involvement.[171] Histologically, these neoplasms are most commonly non-Hodgkin's lymphomas composed of B-cells. The differential diagnosis of these lesions includes lymphocytic hypophysitis and prolactinoma, which when treated with dopaminergic drugs can involute and resemble lymphoma.

The disorder formerly known as histiocytosis X, encompassing eosinophilic granuloma, Hand–Schüller–Christian disease, Letterer–Siwe disease, Langerhans' cell granuloma, and several other eponymic variants, is now classified as Langerhans' cell histiocytosis.[75] The classic presentation of Hand–Schüller–Christian disease involved the hypothalamus, and was known as hypothalamic granuloma, Gagel's granuloma or Ayala disease.[110] The disorder may also involve the pituitary gland itself.[142]

Non-Langerhans' cell histiocytoses include Rosai–Dorfman disease, Erdheim–Chester disease, haemophagocytic lymphohistiocytosis and juvenile xanthogranuloma, as well as rare malignant histiocytic tumours. These lesions have been rarely reported to involve the pituitary.[117]

Lesions involving the hypothalamus and pituitary cause hypopituitarism and diabetes insipidus.[117] Diabetes insipidus is the most common and usually initial manifestation. Rarely, the hypopituitarism is due to adenohypophyseal tissue destruction.[142] More commonly the disease is predominantly hypothalamic and the hypopituitarism is secondary to hypothalamic destruction; in this situation, pituitary hypofunction is associated with hyperprolactinaemia due to destruction of the dopaminergic neurons that maintain tonic inhibition of that hormone.[110,117]

Primary pituitary melanoma is a rare tumour of uncertain histogenesis in this site.[207] These lesions have the histologic and immunohistochemical profile of melanoma, but because of the well recognized variability of the histologic features of this entity, it can mimic other entities. The diagnosis is not difficult if melanoma is considered, because immunohistochemistry provides unequivocal evidence with positivity for S-100 protein, HMB-45, Melan A and tyrosinase.

Rare salivary gland neoplasms have been reported in the sella.[210] These are attributed to the origin of the adenohypophysis from the oral ectoderm and the occasional detection of salivary gland hamartomas in this region.[187]

SECONDARY NEOPLASMS

The pituitary gland, being a highly vascular organ, can be the target of blood-borne metastases from many malignancies.

Epidemiology and Clinical Features

Metastatic tumours to the pituitary gland are not an uncommon event in patients with disseminated malignancy; the frequency has been reported to be as high as 26.7 per cent at autopsy. Involvement of the neurohypophysis is more common than the adenohypophysis. The most common sites of origin are lung, breast, and gastrointestinal tract.[211]

Metastatic tumours to the pituitary gland are usually not among the most prominent clinical complaints of patients with disseminated malignancy and are usually discovered at autopsy. They may occasionally present as a sellar tumour in a patient with an occult primary. Clinically they are distinguished from primary pituitary adenomas by the prominence of diabetes insipidus, and mass effects that can include ptosis and ophthalmoplegia; these are rare in patients with pituitary adenomas. Hypopituitarism occurs only when adenohypophyseal involvement is extensive. In rare cases, metastatic involvement of a pituitary adenoma may result in rapid increase in tumour size and/or sudden worsening symptoms.[158,163]

The outcome of pituitary metastasis is usually extremely unfavourable. Rarely, the primary may be one with a targeted therapy that predicts a better prognosis, as in the case of an unusual metastatic papillary thyroid carcinoma.[25]

Pathology and Differential Diagnosis

The morphologic features of the metastatic tumour usually conform to those of the primary malignancy. The differential diagnosis of these lesions is not usually difficult on histology alone. Occasionally, however, there can be confusion. The major differential diagnosis for metastatic tumours to the hypophysis is a pituitary adenoma. Problems may arise because nuclear pleomorphism and mitotic activity can be prominent features in some adenomas; this is especially true for the sparsely granulated somatotroph adenoma.[11] Other lesions that can mimic metastatic carcinoma include thyrotroph and Crooke's cell corticotroph adenomas as well as chordomas and the rare primary melanomas that require exclusion of a primary lesion elsewhere.

Metastatic endocrine carcinomas can be difficult to distinguish from a primary pituitary neoplasm. The use of immunohistochemical markers, including transcription factors that are specific to the pituitary (Pit-1, Tpit) and those of lung or thyroid tumours (TTF-1) or pancreatic and gastrointestinal tract primaries (CDX-2) can be very helpful. Primary pituitary tumours do not usually express peptides of the gastrointestinal tract and pancreas, and the converse is also usually true; however, ACTH production is common as an ectopic phenomenon and a metastatic lesion producing ACTH could be mistaken for a primary pituitary adenoma. These extrapituitary lesions do not express Tpit.[120]

TUMOUR-LIKE LESIONS

A number of tumour-like lesions can occur in the pituitary and sellar regions. The most important are hyperplasias, inflammatory conditions and cysts. Other rare and unusual mass lesions of the pituitary region include inflammatory pseudotumours,[221] aneurysms,[58] meningoencephalocoeles,[57] hamartomas and choristomas,[149] and brown tumour of bone.[190]

Hyperplasia

Hyperplasia is an increase in the number of cells of an organ or tissue in response to a stimulus. Any endocrine cell population within the pituitary gland can undergo hyperplasia. This process can be physiological or pathological[98] and when prolonged may progress to adenoma formation.[238] Pituitary hyperplasia is a rare but important disorder. It should be considered in patients who have unusual radiological features and clinical manifestations of a primary sellar disorder.

Clinical Features

The clinical features of hyperplasia depend on the cell population involved in the hyperplastic process. Somatotroph hyperplasia results in acromegaly or gigantism that is indistinguishable from that due to a primary pituitary adenoma. It is seen in patients with ectopic production of GH-releasing hormone (GRH) by pheo-chromocytomas, endocrine tumours of lung, pancreas or other elements of the dispersed endocrine system.[64,177] Rarely, it may be associated with a gangliocytoma of the hypothalamus.[16] Mammosomatotroph hyperplasia is also associated with acromegaly or gigantism and hyper-prolactinaemia; it is the characteristic pituitary lesion in McCune–Albright syndrome[219] but it may also be due to GRH excess or it may be idiopathic.[137] Lactotroph hyperplasia is associated with hyperprolactinaemia. It is physiologic during pregnancy or other conditions of oestrogen excess, but pathological idiopathic lactotroph hyperplasia is a rare cause of hyperprolactinaemia.[153] Corticotroph hyperplasia is a cause of Cushing's disease that may be associated with a corticotroph adenoma[118] or may be idiopathic and the sole cause of pituitary-dependent Cushing's disease.[135] In rare patients, it is attributed to ectopic or eutopic excess of corticotropin-releasing hormone (CRH). It is also physiological in patients with untreated Addison's disease. Thyrotroph hyperplasia develops in patients with prolonged primary hypothyroidism.[42] Gonadotroph hyperplasia is seen in patients with prolonged primary hypogonadism.[141]

Radiology

Radiologic evaluation of patents with hyperplasia usually reveals diffuse sellar enlargement without enhancing normal tissue on contrast administration. The careful evaluation of this aspect of the MRI scan may be the only clinical feature indicating this diagnosis that can prevent unnecessary pituitary surgery. If detected, the patient should undergo evaluation for an underlying cause that can be treated, such as the identification of a tumour responsible for ectopic production of GHRH or CRH or the evaluation of primary hypothyroidism.

Pathology

The key to distinguishing adenohypophyseal hyperplasia from adenoma lies in the reticulin stain (Figure 41.21). Hyperplasia is characterized by expanded acini with an intact reticulin framework whereas adenomas have breakdown of the reticulin fibre network. Immunohistochemistry shows predominance of the hyperplastic cell type with other hormone-containing cells interspersed. Ultrastructural examination is not a reliable method to distinguish hyperplasia from adenoma; however, it was the method used to describe the cell enlargement that defines 'thyroidectomy' cells (Figure 41.22) in patients with primary hypothyroidism, and 'gonadectomy' cells in patients with primary hypogonadism. In both situations, the target cells develop abundant vacuolated cytoplasm that is occupied almost entirely by dilated rough endoplasmic reticulum with secretory material. Hyperplastic changes may be diffuse or focal. In some cases, an adenoma can co-exist with hyperplasia.[141,238]

Biological Behaviour

Hyperplasia is usually reversible if the underlying condition is appropriately treated. However, in patients with idiopathic hyperplasia, the underlying stimulus is not known. Patients with lactotroph hyperplasia can be treated with dopaminergic agonists. Those with Cushing's syndrome may require total hypophysectomy to achieve clinical control.

Inflammation

Inflammatory conditions can cause mass effects and/or hypothalamic-hypophyseal dysfunction. Primary or idiopathic inflammatory conditions include lymphocytic hypophysitis, granulomatous hypophysitis, and xanthomatous hypophysitis.[44] Secondary hypophysitis is inflammation of the pituitary gland due to a definite aetiology[86] or part of a systemic process. A number of infectious agents can involve the pituitary, including fungi, mycobacteria, brucellosis and syphilis.[27] They can result in acute or chronic hypophysitis with occasional abscess formation. Other causes of secondary hypophysitis include sarcoidosis,[213] vasculitides such as Takayasu's disease[205] and Wegener's granulomatosis,[131] Crohn's disease,[52] Whipple's disease, ruptured Rathke's cleft cyst,[38] necrotizing adenoma,[86] and meningitis.[229] The acquired immunodeficiency syndrome (AIDS) may also lead to pituitary pathology;[178] involvement is usually infectious in nature (including *Pneumocystis carinii*, toxoplasmosis and CMV) and results in acute or chronic inflammation with necrosis. Hypophysitis is one of the side effects of ipilimumab, a promising new immunotherapeutic antineoplastic agent used for the treatment of metastatic melanoma and renal cell carcinoma;[22,40] the morphology of this type of inflammation has not yet been described.

Lymphocytic Hypophysitis

Lymphocytic hypophysitis is most common in young postpartum or pregnant females.[203] The female to male ratio is 8.5:1. The mean ages of presentation are 34.5 years in females and 44.7 years in males. An autoimmune aetiology has been proposed as the basis for lymphocytic hypophysitis because of its association with a number of other autoimmune endocrine disorders such as thyroiditis, adrenalitis, atrophic gastritis and lymphocytic parathyroiditis and there is evidence for pituitary antibodies in patients with this disease.[26] Recent data suggest that the precipitating antigen is alpha-enolase, a protein that is expressed by the placenta as well as pituitary, possibly explaining pregnancy as an initiating event.

The symptoms and signs of lymphocytic hypophysitis tend to be nonspecific, mimicking adenoma. The most common manifestation is mild to moderate hyperprolactinaemia; occasional cases of isolated ACTH or GH deficiency have been reported, but isolated hormone deficiencies are rare. In addition, lymphocytic hypophysitis can present with mass effects such as headache and visual field deficits. Rarely, patients present with isolated diabetes insipidus and the inflammatory process is restricted to the posterior lobe and stalk, which can exhibit localized enlargement; this disorder has been named infundibular neurohypophysitis.[206] Radiologic findings can mimic features of an adenoma; the gland is enlarged and may even exhibit suprasellar extension. However, careful MRI examination with contrast enhancement documents diffuse involvement of the gland without discrete delineation and lacking enhancement in normal gland.

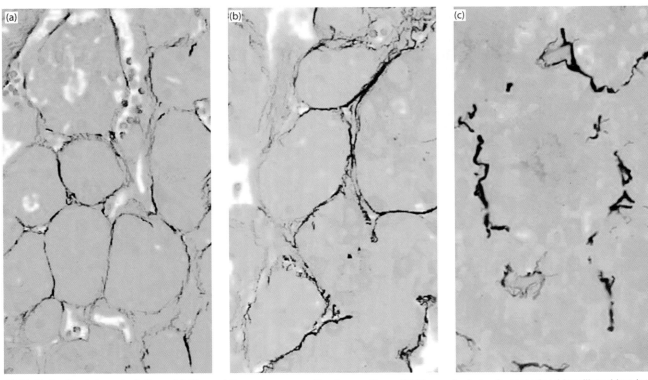

41.21 Reticulin stains of pituitary. **(a)** Normal tissue has a small acinar pattern. **(b)** Hyperplasia is characterized by dilated but intact acini that retain delineation by reticulin fibres. **(c)** Adenoma is defined by loss of the reticulin fibre network.

At surgery the gland is inflamed, enlarged and soft or may appear atrophic and fibrotic if the disease has been prolonged. Microscopic examination reveals a diffuse inflammatory infiltrate composed mainly of lymphocytes and plasma cells forming occasional lymphoid follicles (Figure 41.23), accompanied by variable numbers of neutrophils, eosinophils and macrophages. There is destruction of the adenohypophyseal tissue; the remaining parenchymal cells exhibit variable oncocytic change. Rarely, there seems to be preferential destruction of one hormone-containing cell type. The extent of fibrosis varies with the duration of the disease. The lymphocytic infiltrate is immunoreactive for both B-cell and T-cell markers. By electron microscopy, the adenohypophyseal cells exhibit degenerative changes including crinophagy and oncocytosis. Numerous lymphocytes and plasma cells can be easily identified.

Clinically, this lesion mimics prolactinoma and, if the patient is treated with dopamine agonist therapy, the morphologic features may also be difficult to distinguish from those of an involuted adenoma that also has a lymphocytic morphology. However, the immune process tends to be polymorphic with plasma cells and scattered residual adenohypophyseal cells of all types showing variable degrees of oncocytic change. Fibrosis may be a confounding feature but is unusual in hypophysitis. In contrast, adenomas exposed to dopamine agonist therapy tend to be monotonous and fibrotic. The inflammatory process can be difficult to distinguish from a primary hematologic neoplasm and immunohistochemistry may be required to establish the polyclonal nature of the infiltrate.

The natural history of untreated lymphocytic hypophysitis is variable; it may result in permanent hypopituitarism because of extensive destruction of adenohypophyseal cells, or it may run a self-limited course followed by a full recovery. Treatment for this condition is supportive with appropriate hormone replacement. Corticosteroids have been proposed to decrease inflammation, but the efficacy of this treatment has yet to be determined. Transsphenoidal surgery should be considered if the patient suffers progressive mass effects, or deterioration as evidenced by radiologic or neurologic changes. It should be noted however, that surgery has resulted in deleterious effects in occasional cases.

Idiopathic Granulomatous Hypophysitis

This rare chronic inflammatory disorder of unknown pathogenesis was first described in 1917.[165,183] The disorder represents less than one per cent of all pituitary lesions with an annual incidence of 1 in 10 million. As of 1991, only 31 cases were described in publications, 21 from autopsy material. Unlike lymphocytic hypophysitis, there is no gender predilection. The mean age of presentation in females is 21.5 years; in males it is 50 years.

Patients may present with visual field deficits, cranial nerve palsies or headaches, which may be accompanied by nausea and vomiting; this is in contrast to headaches caused by adenomas that are not associated with nausea and vomiting. Other clinical manifestations include variable degrees of adenohypophyseal failure,[92] hyperprolactinaemia,[95] diabetes insipidus and meningitis with CSF leucocytosis.[229] Radiologic evaluation usually reveals an intrasellar mass with or without suprasellar extension.[212] Sometimes, a tongue-like extension along the basal hypothalamus can be seen.

Microscopically, this condition is characterized by collections of histiocytes with scattered lymphocytes and plasma cells (Figure 41.24); multinucleated giant cells may

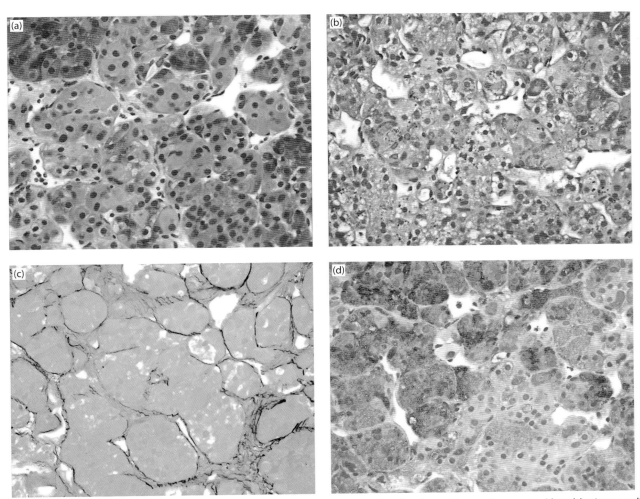

41.22 Thyrotroph hyperplasia. (a) The numerous thyrotrophs are enlarged and pale, a change known as 'thyroidectomy cells'. Scattered acidophils and basophils provide a framework defining residual acini and emphasizing the marked cellular enlargement of the dominant cell population. **(b)** The large cells contain conspicuous periodic acid-Schiff (PAS)-positive cytoplasmic droplets. **(c)** The reticulin stain reveals enlarged but intact acini. **(d)** The stain for β-TSH reveals numerous large dilated thyrotrophs that have lost their normal polygonal morphology.

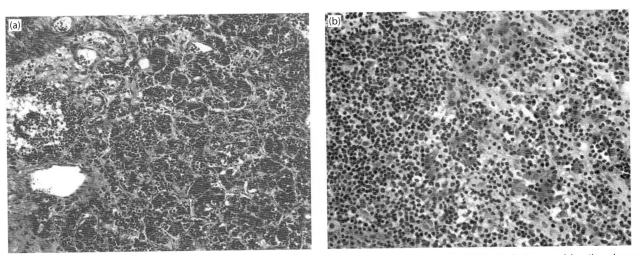

41.23 Lymphocytic hypophysitis. (a) The pituitary is distorted by a heavy lymphoplasmacytic infiltrate that resembles the changes seen in Hashimoto's thyroiditis. **(b)** The residual parenchymal cells show oncocytic change.

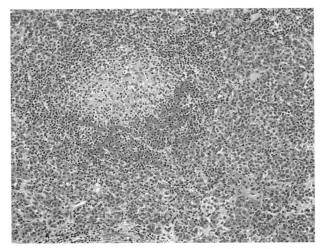

41.24 Granulomatous hypophysitis. An early granuloma composed of histiocytic cells is surrounded by a lymphocytic infiltrate.

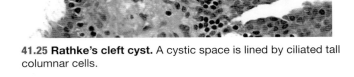

41.25 Rathke's cleft cyst. A cystic space is lined by ciliated tall columnar cells.

be present. There may be focal calcification that can take the form of psammoma bodies.[106] By definition, a diagnosis of idiopathic granulomatous hypophysitis cannot be made until systemic granulomatous disease has been excluded.

Treatment is somewhat controversial; transsphenoidal biopsy/resection with subsequent administration of corticosteroids may result in amelioration of symptoms.[44,174]

Xanthomatous Hypophysitis

Xanthomatous hypophysitis is a relatively new clinicopathologic entity characterized by a chronic inflammatory infiltrate composed mainly of foamy histiocytes with scattered lymphocytes and plasma cells. This disorder may represent a reactive process;[44] however, it remains idiopathic.

Only a handful of cases have been reported and therefore the epidemiology is not known. The first patients reported were young females[44] but subsequent reports included males.[35] Clinical presentation includes headache, nausea, menstrual irregularity and diabetes insipidus; elevated prolactin levels have been identified.[35,44,199] In most patients, a preoperative diagnosis of pituitary adenoma was suspected based on the presence of a localized lesion in the pituitary.[44] Some of the cases have had a cystic lesion identified radiologically.

Histologically, the condition is characterized by infiltration of the adenohypophysis by foamy lipid-containing histiocytes with areas of granulation tissue. The histiocytes are immunoreactive with antibodies to CD68; they are not immunoreactive for S-100 and CD1a. The presence of lipid within the infiltrating histiocytes has been confirmed by electron microscopy. A diagnosis of xanthomatous hypophysitis can only be made after causes of secondary hypophysitis are ruled out.

Cysts

A number of cysts in the parasellar region can present as mass lesions mimicking a primary pituitary tumour. Small cysts that are residua of the developing gland are present in most pituitaries at autopsy; however, they are only considered to be of clinical significance when detected as a

result of symptomatology or on imaging. The incidence of parasellar cysts seems to be increasing because of improved detection by MRI;[191] however, the exact epidemiology of these lesions is not known.

These cysts are non-functional, but may cause hypopituitarism or diabetes insipidus by compression of surrounding structures.[191] Suprasellar extension may give rise to mass effects such as visual field defects and headaches. Severe cases can lead to hydrocephalus, aseptic meningitis, and rarely, abscess formation.[147] CT scans usually reveal low-density cystic areas with peripheral enhancement; MRI findings tend to be more variable.[119]

Treatment by drainage with or without surgical excision usually results in resolution of mass effects; however, hypopituitarism and diabetes insipidus may persist, requiring permanent hormone replacement. Recurrence rates are low. Complications of dermoid and epidermoid cysts include rupture of the cyst with subsequent meningitis, or the development of squamous cell carcinoma.[2,126]

Rathke's cleft cysts are remnants of Rathke's pouch that commonly form small cysts (<5 mm) in the vestigial pars intermedia. These small cysts occasionally enlarge into true Rathke's cleft cysts, lined by ciliated cuboidal or columnar epithelium (Figure 41.25) with occasional goblet cells and areas of squamous metaplasia; as they enlarge they become symptomatic.

Arachnoid cysts originate in the arachnoid of the sellar and parasellar areas; they may be congenital or acquired. They contain clear fluid and the cyst wall is arachnoid laminar connective tissue with incomplete simple flattened epithelium.

Dermoid and epidermoid cysts (sometimes referred to as 'cholesteatomas') originate from ectopic or traumatically implanted epithelial cells. Epidermoid cysts have a lining composed of keratinizing squamous epithelium; the lining of dermoid cysts contains skin appendages such as hair follicles and sweat glands. In addition to the sellar and suprasellar regions, these cysts are also found intracranially, most often at the cerebellopontine angle.[224]

REFERENCES

1. Abbass SAA, Asa SL, Ezzat S. Altered expression of fibroblast growth factor receptors in human pituitary adenomas. *J Clin Endocrinol Metab* 1997;**82**:1160–1166.
2. Abramson RC, Morawetz RB, Schlitt M. Multiple complications from an intracranial epidermoid cyst: case report and literature review. *Neurosurgery* 1989;**24**:574–578.
3. Agarwal SK, Mateo CM, Marx SJ. Rare germline mutations in cyclin-dependent kinase inhibitor genes in multiple endocrine neoplasia type 1 and related states. *J Clin Endocrinol Metab* 2009;**94**(5):1826–1834.
4. Ahmad K, Fayos JV. Pituitary fibrosarcoma secondary to radiation therapy. *Cancer* 1978;**42**:107–110.
5. Al Brahim NY, Asa SL. My approach to pathology of the pituitary gland. *J Clin Pathol* 2006;**59**(12):1245–1253.
6. Al Shraim M, Asa SL. The 2004 World Health Organization classification of pituitary tumors: what is new? *Acta Neuropathol* 2006;**111**(1):1–7.
7. Amar AP, Hinton DR, Krieger MD, Weiss MH. Invasive pituitary adenomas: significance of proliferation parameters. *Pituitary* 1999;**2**(2):117–122.
8. Amine ARC, Sugar O. Suprasellar osteogenic sarcoma following radiation for pituitary adenoma. Case report. *J Neurosurg* 1976;**44**:88–91.
9. Angiari P, Torcia E, Botticelli RA, et al. Ossifying parasellar chondroma. Case report. *J Neursurg Sci* 1987;**31**:59–63.
10. Asa SL. Practical pituitary pathology: what does the pathologist need to know? *Arch Pathol Lab Med* 2008;**132**(8):1231–1240.
11. Asa SL. Tumors of the pituitary gland. In: Silverberg SG ed. *AFIP Atlas of Tumor Pathology*. 4[15]. Silver Spring, MD: ARP Press, 2011.
12. Asa SL, Ezzat S. Molecular determinants of pituitary cytodifferentiation. *Pituitary* 1999;**1**(3–4):159–168.
13. Asa SL, Ezzat S. The pathogenesis of pituitary tumors. *Annu Rev Pathol* 2009;**4**:97–126.
14. Asa SL, Kovacs K. Functional morphology of the human fetal pituitary. *Pathol Annu* 1984;**19**(Part 1):275–315.
15. Asa SL, Kovacs K, Bilbao JM. The pars tuberalis of the human pituitary. A histologic, immunohistochemical, ultrastructural and immunoelectron microscopic analysis. *Virchows Arch* 1983;**399**:49–59.
16. Asa SL, Scheithauer BW, Bilbao JM, et al. A case for hypothalamic acromegaly: a clinicopathological study of six patients with hypothalamic gangliocytomas producing growth hormone-releasing factor. *J Clin Endocrinol Metab* 1984;**58**:796–803.
17. Asa SL, Gerrie BM, Kovacs K, et al. Structure-function correlations of human pituitary gonadotroph adenomas *in vitro*. *Lab Invest* 1988;**58**:403–410.
18. Asa SL, Kovacs K, Horvath E, Singer W, Smyth HS. Hormone secretion *in vitro* by plurihormonal pituitary adenomas of the acidophil cell line. *J Clin Endocrinol Metab* 1992;**75**:68–75.
19. Asa SL, Bamberger A-M, Cao B, Wong M, Parker KL, Ezzat S. The transcription activator steroidogenic factor-1 is preferentially expressed in the human pituitary gonadotroph. *J Clin Endocrinol Metab* 1996;**81**:2165–2170.
20. Asa SL, Somers K, Ezzat S. The MEN-1 gene is rarely down-regulated in pituitary adenomas. *J Clin Endocrinol Metab* 1998;**83**:3210–3212.
21. Asa SL, DiGiovanni R, Jiang J, et al. A growth hormone receptor mutation impairs growth hormone autofeedback signalling in pituitary tumors. *Cancer Res* 2007;**67**(15):7505–7511.
22. Barnard ZR, Walcott BP, Kahle KT, Nahed BV, Coumans JV. Hyponatremia associated with ipilimumab-induced hypophysitis. *Med Oncol* 2012;**29**(1):374–377.
23. Beckers A, Daly AF. The clinical, pathological and genetic features of familial isolated pituitary adenomas. *Eur J Endocrinol* 2007;**157**(4):371–382.
24. Beck–Peccoz P, Brucker–Davis F, Persani L, Smallridge RC, Weintraub BD. Thyrotropin-secreting pituitary tumors. *Endocr Rev* 1996;**17**:610–638.
25. Bell CD, Kovacs K, Horvath E, Smythe H, Asa S. Papillary carcinoma of thyroid metastatic to the pituitary gland. *Arch Pathol Lab Med* 2001;**125**(7):935–938.
26. Bensing S, Fetissov SO, Mulder J, et al. Pituitary autoantibodies in autoimmune polyendocrine syndrome type 1. *Proc Natl Acad Sci U S A* 2007;**104**(3):949–954.
27. Berger SA, Edberg SC, David G. Infectious disease in the sella turcica. *Rev Infect Dis* 1986;**5**:747–755.
28. Bergeron C, Kovacs K, Bilbao JM. Primary empty sella. A histologic and immunocytologic study. *Arch Intern Med* 1979;**139**:248–249.
29. Bhayana S, Booth GL, Asa SL, Kovacs K, Ezzat S. The implication of somatotroph adenoma phenotype to somatostatin analog responsiveness in acromegaly. *J Clin Endocrinol Metab* 2005;**90**(11):6290–6295.
30. Boari N, Losa M, Mortini P, Snider S, Terreni MR, Giovanelli M. Intrasellar paraganglioma: a case report and review of the literature. *Acta Neurochir (Wien)* 2006;**148**(12):1311–1314.
31. Boch AL, van Effenterre R, Kujas M. Craniopharyngiomas in two consanguineous siblings: case report. *Neurosurgery* 1997;**41**(5):1185–1187.
32. Booth GL, Redelmeier DA, Grosman H, et al. Improved diagnostic accuracy of inferior petrosal sinus sampling over imaging for localizing pituitary pathology in patients with Cushing's disease. *J Clin Endocrinol Metab* 1998;**83**:2291–2295.
33. Borota OC, Scheithauer BW, Fougner SL, et al. Spindle cell oncocytoma of the adenohypophysis: report of a case with marked cellular atypia and recurrence despite adjuvant treatment. *Clin Neuropathol* 2009;**28**(2):91–95.
34. Bots GTAM, Tijssen CC, Wijnalda D, Teepen JLJM. Alveolar soft part sarcoma of the pituitary gland with secondary involvement of the right cerebral ventricle. *Br J Neurosurg* 1988;**2**:101–107.
35. Burt MG, Morey AL, Turner JJ, et al. Xanthomatous pituitary lesions: a report of two cases and review of the literature. *Pituitary* 2003;**6**(3):161–168.
36. Buslei R, Nolde M, Hofmann B, et al. Common mutations of beta-catenin in adamantinomatous craniopharyngiomas but not in other tumours originating from the sellar region. *Acta Neuropathol* 2005;**109**(6):589–597.
37. Cai WY, Alexander JM, Hedley–Whyte ET, et al. Ras mutations in human prolactinomas and pituitary carcinomas. *J Clin Endocrinol Metab* 1994;**78**:89–93.
38. Cannavo S, Romaon C, Calbucci F, Faglia G. Granulomatous sarcoidotic lesion of hypothalamic–pituitary region associated with Rathke's cleft cyst. *J Enocrinol Invest* 1997;**20**:77–81.
39. Carney JA, Gordon H, Carpenter PC, Shenoy BV, Go VL. The complex of myxomas, spotty pigmentation and endocrine overactivity. *Medicine (Baltimore)* 1985;**64**(4):270–283.
40. Carpenter KJ, Murtagh RD, Lilienfeld H, Weber J, Murtagh FR. Ipilimumab-induced hypophysitis: MR imaging findings. *AJNR Am J Neuroradiol* 2009;**30**(9):1751–1753.
41. Castel JP, Delorge–Kerdiles C, Rivel J. Angiome caverneux du chiasma optique. *Neurochirurgie* 1989;**35**:252–256.
42. Chan AW, MacFarlane IA, Foy PM, Miles JB. Pituitary enlargement and hyperprolactinaemia due to primary hypothyroidism: errors and delays in diagnosis. *Br J Neurosurg* 1990;**4**:107–112.
43. Chandrasekharappa SC, Guru SC, Manickam P, et al. Positional cloning of the gene for multiple endocrine neoplasia-type 1. *Science* 1997;**276**:404–407.
44. Cheung CC, Ezzat S, Smyth HS, Asa SL. The spectrum and significance of primary hypophysitis. *J Clin Endocrinol Metab* 2001;**86**(3):1048–1053.
45. Coire CI, Horvath E, Kovacs K, Smyth HS, Ezzat S. Cushing's syndrome from an ectopic pituitary adenoma with peliosis: A histological, immunohistochemical and ultrastructural study and review of the literature. *Endocr Pathol* 1997;**8**:65–74.
46. Coire CI, Horvath E, Smyth HS, Kovacs K. Rapidly recurring folliculostellate cell tumor of the adenohypophysis with the morphology of a spindle cell oncocytoma: case report with electron microscopic studies. *Clin Neuropathol* 2009;**28**(4):303–308.
47. Cone L, Srinivasan M, Romanul FCA. Granular cell tumor (choristoma) of the neurohypophysis: Two cases and a review of the literature. *Am J Neuroradiol* 1990;**11**:403–406.
48. Cusimano MD, Kovacs K, Bilbao JM, Tucker WS, Singer W. Suprasellar craniopharyngioma associated with hyperprolactinemia, pituitary lactotroph hyperplasia, and microprolactinoma. Case report. *J Neurosurg* 1988;**69**:620–623.
49. Daly AF, Rixhon M, Adam C, et al. High prevalence of pituitary adenomas: a cross-sectional study in the province of Liege, Belgium. *J Clin Endocrinol Metab* 2006;**91**(12):4769–4775.
50. Daneshdoost L, Gennarelli TA, Bashey HM, et al. Recognition of gonadotroph adenomas in women. *N Engl J Med* 1991;**324**:589–594.
51. Daniel L, Trouillas J, Renaud W, et al. Polysialylated-neural cell adhesion molecule expression in rat pituitary transplantable tumors (spontaneous mammotropic transplantable tumor in

Wistar–Furth rats) is related to growth rate and malignancy. *Cancer Res* 2000;**60**(1):80–85.

52. De Bruin WI, van't Verlaat JW, Graamans K, De Bruin TWA. Sellar granulomatous mass in a pregnant woman with active Crohn's disease. *Neth J Med* 1991;**39**:136–141.

53. De Martino I, Visone R, Wierinckx A, et al. HMGA proteins upregulate CCNB2 gene in mouse and human pituitary adenomas. *Cancer Res* 2009;**69**(5):1844–1850.

54. DeLellis RA, Lloyd RV, Heitz PU, Eng C. *Pathology and Genetics of Tumours of Endocrine Organs.* Lyons, France: IARC Press, 2004.

55. Delgrange E, Trouillas J, Maiter D, Donckier J, Tourniaire J. Sex-related difference in the growth of prolactinomas: a clinical and proliferation marker study. *J Clin Endocrinol Metab* 1997;**82**(7):2102–2107.

56. DiGiovanni R, Serra S, Ezzat S, Asa SL. AIP mutations are not identified in patients with sporadic pituitary adenomas. *Endocr Pathol* 2007;**18**(2):76–78.

57. Durham LH, Mackenzie IJ, Miles JB. Transphenoidal meningohydroencephalocoele. *Br J Neurosurg* 1988;**2**:407–410.

58. Dussault J, Plamondon C, Volpe R. Aneurysms of the internal carotid artery simulating pituitary tumours. *Can Med Assoc J* 1969;**101**:51–56.

59. Ebinu JO, Shahideh M, Ibrahim GM, et al. Sellar glomangioma. *Endocr Pathol* 2011;**22**(4):218–221.

60. Erickson D, Scheithauer B, Atkinson J, et al. Silent subtype 3 pituitary adenoma: a clinicopathologic analysis of the Mayo Clinic experience. *Clin Endocrinol (Oxf)* 2009;**71**(1):92–99.

61. Eschbacher JM, Coons SW. Cytokeratin CK20 is a sensitive marker for Crooke's cells and the early cytoskeletal changes associated with hypercortisolism within pituitary corticotrophs. *Endocr Pathol* 2006;**17**(4):365–376.

62. Ezzat S, Asa SL. The emerging role of the Ikaros stem cell factor in the neuroendocrine system. *J Mol Endocrinol* 2008;**41**(2):45–51.

63. Ezzat S, Snyder PJ, Young WF, et al. Octreotide treatment of acromegaly. A randomized, multicenter study. *Ann Intern Med* 1992;**117**:711–718.

64. Ezzat S, Asa SL, Stefaneanu L, et al. Somatotroph hyperplasia without pituitary adenoma associated with a long standing growth hormone-releasing hormone-producing bronchial carcinoid. *J Clin Endocrinol Metab* 1994;**78**:555–560.

65. Ezzat S, Forster MJ, Berchtold P, et al. Acromegaly. Clinical and biochemical features in 500 patients. *Medicine* 1994;**73**:233–240.

66. Ezzat S, Horvath E, Harris AG, Kovacs K. Morphological effects of octreotide on growth hormone-producing adenomas. *J Clin Endocrinol Metab* 1994;**79**:113–118.

67. Ezzat S, Kontogeorgos G, Redelmeier DA, et al. In vivo responsiveness of morphological variants of growth hormone-producing pituitary adenomas to octreotide. *Eur J Endocrinol* 1995;**133**:686–690.

68. Ezzat S, Zheng L, Zhu XF, Wu GE, Asa SL. Targeted expression of a human pituitary tumor-derived isoform of FGF receptor-4 recapitulates pituitary tumorigenesis. *J Clin Invest* 2002;**109**(1):69–78.

69. Ezzat S, Yu S, Asa SL. Ikaros isoforms in human pituitary tumors: distinct localization, histone acetylation, and activation of the 5′ fibroblast growth factor receptor-4 promoter. *Am J Pathol* 2003;**163**(3):1177–1184.

70. Ezzat S, Asa SL, Couldwell WT, et al. The prevalence of pituitary adenomas: a systematic review. *Cancer* 2004;**101**(3):613–619.

71. Ezzat S, Zheng L, Asa SL. Pituitary tumor-derived fibroblast growth factor receptor 4 isoform disrupts neural cell-adhesion molecule/N-cadherin signalling to diminish cell adhesiveness: a mechanism underlying pituitary neoplasia. *Mol Endocrinol* 2004;**18**(10):2543–2552.

72. Ezzat S, Mader R, Yu S, et al. Ikaros integrates endocrine and immune system development. *J Clin Invest* 2005;**115**(4):1021–1029.

73. Ezzat S, Mader R, Fischer S, et al. An essential role for the hematopoietic transcription factor Ikaros in hypothalamic-pituitary-mediated somatic growth. *Proc Natl Acad Sci U S A* 2006;**103**(7):2214–2219.

74. Ezzat S, Zhu X, Loeper S, Fischer S, Asa SL. Tumor-derived Ikaros 6 acetylates the Bcl-XL promoter to up-regulate a survival signal in pituitary cells. *Mol Endocrinol* 2006;**20**(11):2976–2986.

75. Favara BE, Feller AC, Pauli M, et al. Contemporary classification of histiocytic disorders. The WHO Committee On Histiocytic/Reticulum Cell Proliferations. Reclassification Working Group of the Histiocyte Society. *Med Pediatr Oncol* 1997;**29**(3):157–166.

76. Fedele M, Pentimalli F, Baldassarre G, et al. Transgenic mice overexpressing the wild-type form of the HMGA1 gene develop mixed growth hormone/prolactin cell pituitary adenomas and natural killer cell lymphomas. *Oncogene* 2005;**24**(21):3427–3435.

77. Felix IA, Horvath E, Kovacs K. Massive Crooke's hyalinization in corticotroph cell adenomas of the human pituitary. A histological, immunocytological and electron microscopic study of three cases. *Acta Neurochir* 1981;**58**:235–243.

78. Fernandez A, Karavitaki N, Wass JA. Prevalence of pituitary adenomas: a community-based, cross-sectional study in Banbury (Oxfordshire, UK). *Clin Endocrinol (Oxf)* 2010;**72**(3):377–382.

79. Frangou EM, Tynan JR, Robinson CA, Ogieglo LM, Vitali AM. Metastatic craniopharyngioma: case report and literature review. *Childs Nerv Syst* 2009;**25**(9):1143–1147.

80. Franscella S, Favod–Coune C-A, Pizzolato G, et al. Pituitary corticotroph adenoma with Crooke's hyalinization. *Endocr Pathol* 1991;**2**:111–116.

81. Furlanetto TW, Pinheiro CF, Oppitz PP, de Alencastro LC, Asa SL. Solitary fibrous tumor of the sella mimicking pituitary adenoma: an uncommon tumor in a rare location–a case report. *Endocr Pathol* 2009;**20**(1):56–61.

82. Gaffey TA, Scheithauer BW, Lloyd RV, et al. Corticotroph carcinoma of the pituitary: a clinicopathological study. Report of four cases. *J Neurosurg* 2002;**96**(2):352–360.

83. Georgitsi M, Raitila A, Karhu A, et al. Germline CDKN1B/p27Kip1 mutation in multiple endocrine neoplasia. *J Clin Endocrinol Metab* 2007;**92**(8):3321–3325.

84. Georgitsi M, De Menis E, Cannavo S, et al. Aryl hydrocarbon receptor interacting protein (AIP) gene mutation analysis in children and adolescents with sporadic pituitary adenomas. *Clin Endocrinol (Oxf)* 2008;**69**(4):621–627.

85. Gharib H, Frey HM, Laws ER Jr, Randall RV, Scheithauer BW. Coexistent primary empty sella syndrome and hyperprolactinemia. Report of 11 cases. *Arch Intern Med* 1983;**143**:1383–1386.

86. Glauber HS, Brown BM. Pituitary macroadenoma associated with intrasellar abscess: a case report and review. *The Endocrinologist* 1992;**2**:169–172.

87. Gokden M, Mrak RE. Pituitary adenoma with craniopharyngioma component. *Hum Pathol* 2009;**40**(8):1189–1193.

88. Goto T, Nishi T, Kunitoku N, et al. Suprasellar hemangioblastoma in a patient with von Hippel–Lindau disease confirmed by germline mutation study: case report and review of the literature. *Surg Neurol* 2001;**56**(1):22–26.

89. Guzel A, Tatli M, Senturk S, et al. Pituitary carcinoma presenting with multiple metastases: case report. *J Child Neurol* 2008;**23**(12):1467–1471.

90. Hardy J. Transsphenoidal microsurgery of the normal and pathological pituitary. In: *Clinical Neurosurgery. Proceedings of the Congress of Neurological Surgeons, 1968.* Baltimore: Williams and Wilkins, 1969:185–217.

91. Haresh KP, Prabhakar R, Anand Rajan KD, et al. A rare case of paraganglioma of the sella with bone metastases. *Pituitary* 2009;**12**(3):276–279.

92. Hassoun P, Anayssi E, Salti I. A case of granulomatous hypophysitis with hypopituitarism and minimal pituitary enlargement. *J Neurol Neurosurg Psychiatry* 1985;**48**:949–951.

93. Hayward BE, Barlier A, Korbonits M, et al. Imprinting of the G(s)alpha gene GNAS1 in the pathogenesis of acromegaly. *J Clin Invest* 2001;**107**(6):R31–R36.

94. Hinton DR, Hahn JA, Weiss MH, Couldwell WT. Loss of Rb expression in an ACTH-secreting pituitary carcinoma. *Cancer Lett* 1998;**126**(2):209–214.

95. Holck S, Laursen H. Prolactinoma coexistent with granulomatous hypophysitis. *Acta Neuropathol (Berl)* 1983;**61**:253–257.

96. Honegger J, Renner C, Fahlbusch R, Adams EF. Progesterone receptor gene expression in craniopharyngiomas and evidence for biological activity. *Neurosurgery* 1997;**41**(6):1359–1363.

97. Honegger J, Koerbel A, Psaras T, Petrick M, Mueller K. Primary intrasellar schwannoma: clinical, aetiopathological and surgical considerations. *Br J Neurosurg* 2005;**19**(5):432–438.

98. Horvath E. Pituitary hyperplasia. *Pathol Res Pract* 1988;**183**:623–625.

99. Horvath E, Kovacs K. Gonadotroph adenomas of the human pituitary: sex-related fine-structural dichotomy. A histologic, immunocytochemical, and electron-microscopic study of 30 tumors. *Am J Pathol* 1984;**117**:429–440.

100. Horvath E, Kovacs K, Smyth HS, et al. A novel type of pituitary adenoma: Morphological feature and clinical correlations. *J Clin Endocrinol Metab* 1988;**66**:1111–1118.

101. Horvath E, Kovacs K, Smyth HS, Cusimano M, Singer W. Silent adenoma subtype 3 of the pituitary–immunohistochemical and ultrastructural classification: a review of 29 cases. *Ultrastruct Pathol* 2005;29(6):511–524.

102. Inoue T, Takahashi N, Murakami K, *et al.* Osteochondroma of the sella turcica presenting with intratumoral hemorrhage. *Neurol Med Chir (Tokyo)* 2009;49(1):37–41.

103. Itoh N, Ornitz DM. Evolution of the Fgf and Fgfr gene families. *Trends Genet* 2004;20(11):563–569.

104. Jarzembowski J, Lloyd R, McKeever P. Type IV collagen immunostaining is a simple, reliable diagnostic tool for distinguishing between adenomatous and normal pituitary glands. *Arch Pathol Lab Med* 2007;131(6):931–935.

105. Jastania RA, Alsaad KO, Al Shraim M, Kovacs K, Asa SL. Double adenomas of the pituitary: transcription factors Pit-1, T-pit, and SF-1 identify cytogenesis and differentiation. *Endocr Pathol* 2005;16(3):187–194.

106. Jastania R, Nageeti T, Kovacs K, Ezzat S, Asa SL. Granulomatous hypophysitis with psammoma bodies: a diagnostic dilemma. *Endocr Pathol* 2004;15(4):359–363.

107. Jin L, Qian X, Kulig E, *et al.* Transforming growth factor-beta, transforming growth factor-beta receptor II and p27Kip1 expression in nontumorous and neoplastic human pituitaries. *Am J Pathol* 1997;151(2):509–519.

108. Kageyama N, Kobayashi T, Kida Y, Yoshida J, Kato K. Intracranial germinal tumors. *Prog Exp Tumor Res* 1987;30:255–267.

109. Kaltsas GA, Kola B, Borboli N, *et al.* Sequence analysis of the PRKAR1A gene in sporadic somatotroph and other pituitary tumours. *Clin Endocrinol (Oxf)* 2002;57(4):443–448.

109a. Kamil Z, Sinson G, Gucer H, *et al.* TTF-1 expressing sellar neoplasm with ependymal rosettes and oncocytic change: mixed ependymal and oncocytic variant pituicytoma. 2014; in press.

110. Kepes JJ, Kepes M. Predominantly cerebral forms of histiocytosis-X. A reappraisal of 'Gagel's hypothalamic granuloma', 'granuloma infiltrans of the hypothalamus' and 'Ayala's disease' with a report of four cases. *Acta Neuropathol (Berl)* 1969;14:77–98.

111. Kirschner LS, Carney JA, Pack SD, *et al.* Mutations of the gene encoding the protein kinase A type I-alpha regulatory subunit in patients with the Carney complex. *Nat Genet* 2000;26(1):89–92.

112. Kitanaka C, Shitara N, Nakagomi T, *et al.* Postradiation astrocytoma. Report of two cases. *J Neurosurg* 1989;70:469–474.

113. Koral K, Weprin B, Rollins NK. Sphenoid sinus craniopharyngioma simulating mucocele. *Acta Radiol* 2006;47(5):494–496.

114. Korbonits M, Chahal HS, Kaltsas G, *et al.* Expression of phosphorylated p27(Kip1) protein and Jun activation domain-binding protein 1 in human pituitary tumors. *J Clin Endocrinol Metab* 2002;87(6):2635–2643.

115. Kovacs K, Horvath E. Tumors of the pituitary gland. In: *Atlas of Tumor Pathology*, 2[21]. Washington, D.C.: Armed Forces Institute of Pathology, 1986.

116. Kovacs K, Horvath E, Thorner MO, Rogol AD. Mammosomatotroph hyperplasia associated with acromegaly and hyperprolactinemia in a patient with the McCune–Albright syndrome. *Virchows Arch* 1984;403:77–86.

117. Kovacs K, Bilbao JM, Fornasier VL, Horvath E. Pituitary pathology in Erdheim–Chester disease. *Endocr Pathol* 2004;15(2):159–166.

118. Kubota T, Hayashi M, Kabuto M, *et al.* Corticotroph cell hyperplasia in a patient with Addison disease: case report. *Surg Neurol* 1992;37:441–447.

119. Kucharczyk W, Peck WW, Kelly WM, Norman D, Newton TH. Rathke's cleft cysts: CT, MR imaging and pathologic features. *Radiology* 1987;165:491–495.

120. Lamolet B, Pulichino AM, Lamonerie T, *et al.* A pituitary cell-restricted T-box factor, Tpit, activates POMC transcription in cooperation with Pitx homeoproteins. *Cell* 2001;104(6):849–859.

121. Landolt AM. Granular cell tumors of the neurohypophysis. *Acta Neurochir* 1975;(Suppl 22):120–128.

122. Landolt AM, Valvanis A, Girard J, Eberle AN. Corticotrophin-releasing factor-test used with bilateral, simultaneous inferior petrosal sinus blood-sampling for the diagnosis of pituitary-dependent Cushing's disease. *Clin Endocrinol (Oxf)* 1986;25:687–696.

123. Laws ER Jr. Craniopharyngioma: Diagnosis and treatment. *The Endocrinologist* 1992;2:184–188.

124. Lee EB, Tihan T, Scheithauer BW, Zhang PJ, Gonatas NK. Thyroid transcription factor 1 expression in sellar tumors: a histogenetic marker? *J Neuropathol Exp Neurol* 2009;68(5):482–488.

125. Lewin R, Ruffolo E, Saraceno C. Craniopharyngioma arising in the pharyngeal hypophysis. *Southern Med J* 1984;77:1519–1523.

126. Lewis AJ, Cooper PW, Kassel EE, Schwartz ML. Squamous cell carcinoma arising in a suprasellar epidermoid cyst. Case report. *J Neurosurg* 1983;59:538–541.

127. Lin JH, Tsai DH, Chiang YH. A primary sellar esthesioneuroblastomas with unusual presentations: a case report and reviews of literatures. *Pituitary* 2009;12(1):70–75.

128. Link MJ, Driscoll CL, Giannini C. Isolated, giant cerebellopontine angle craniopharyngioma in a patient with Gardner syndrome: case report. *Neurosurgery* 2002;51(1):221–225.

129. Lloyd RV. Frozen sections in the diagnosis of pituitary lesions. In: Lloyd RV ed. *Surgical Pathology of the Pituitary Gland.* Philadelphia, PA: W.B. Saunders Company, 1993: 22–24.

130. Loeper S, Asa SL, Ezzat S. Ikaros modulates cholesterol uptake: A link between tumor suppression and differentiation. *Cancer Res* 2008;68(10):3715–3723.

131. Lohr KM, Ryan LM, Toohill RJ, Anderson T. Anterior pituitary involvement in Wegener's granulomatosis. *J Rheumatol* 1988;15:855–861.

132. Louis DN, Ohgaki H, Wiestler OD, Cavenee WK. *WHO Classification of Tumours of the Central Nervous System.* Lyon, France: IARC, 2007.

133. Malanga D, De Gisi S, Riccardi M, *et al.* Functional characterization of a rare germline mutation in the gene encoding the cyclin-dependent kinase

inhibitor p27Kip1 (CDKN1B) in a Spanish patient with multiple endocrine neoplasia-like phenotype. *Eur J Endocrinol* 2012;166(3):551–560.

134. Mathews W, Wilson CB. Ectopic intrasellar chordoma. *J Neurosurg* 1974;39:260–263.

135. McKeever PE, Koppelman MCS, Metcalf D, *et al.* Refractory Cushing's disease caused by multinodular ACTH-cell hyperplasia. *J Neuropathol Exp Neurol* 1982;41:490–499.

135a. Mete O, Lopes MB, Asa SL: Spindle cell oncocytomas and granular cell tumors of the pituitary are variants of pituicytoma. *Am J Surg Pathol* 2013;37(11):1694–9.

136. Miki K, Kawamoto K, Kawamura Y, *et al.* A rare case of Maffucci's syndrome combined with tuberculum sellae enchondroma, pituitary adenoma and thyroid adenoma. *Acta Neurochir* 1987;87:79–85.

137. Moran A, Asa SL, Kovacs K, *et al.* Gigantism due to pituitary mammosomatotroph hyperplasia. *N Engl J Med* 1990;323:322–327.

138. Moshkin O, Scheithauer BW, Syro LV, *et al.* Collision tumors of the sella: craniopharyngioma and silent pituitary adenoma subtype 3: case report. *Endocr Pathol* 2009;20(1):50–55.

139. Neumann PE, Horoupian DS, Goldman JE, Hess MA. Cytoplasmic filaments of Crooke's hyaline change belong to the cytokeratin class. An immunocytochemical and ultrastructural study. *Am J Pathol* 1984;116:214–222.

140. Neumann PE, Goldman JE, Horoupian DS, Hess MA. Fibrous bodies in growth hormone-secreting adenomas contain cytokeratin filaments. *Arch Pathol Lab Med* 1985;109:505–508.

141. Nicolis G, Shimshi M, Allen C, Halmi NS, Kourides IA. Gonadotropin-producing pituitary adenoma in a man with long-standing primary hypogonadism. *J Clin Endocrinol Metab* 1988;66:237–241.

142. Nishio S, Mizuno J, Barrow DL, Takei Y, Tindall GT. Isolated Histiocytosis X of the pituitary gland: case report. *Neurosurgery* 1987;21:718–721.

143. Nishioka H, Ii K, Llena JF, Hirano A. Immunohistochemical study of granular cell tumors of the neurohypophysis. *Virchows Arch* 1991;60:413–417.

144. Nose V, Ezzat S, Horvath E, *et al.* Protocol for the examination of specimens from patients with primary pituitary tumors. *Arch Pathol Lab Med* 2011;135(5):640–646.

145. Nose–Alberti V, Mesquita MI, Martin LC, Kayath MJ. Adrenocorticotropin-producing pituitary carcinoma with expression of c-erbB-2 and high PCNA index: A comparative study with pituitary adenomas and normal pituitary tissues. *Endocr Pathol* 1998;9(1):53–62.

146. Obari A, Sano T, Ohyama K, *et al.* Clinicopathological features of growth hormone-producing pituitary adenomas: difference among various types defined by cytokeratin distribution pattern including a transitional form. *Endocr Pathol* 2008;19(2):82–91.

147. Obenchain TG, Becker DP. Abscess formation in a Rathke's cleft cyst. Case report. *J Neurosurg* 1972;36:359–362.

148. Oikonomou E, Barreto DC, Soares B, *et al.* Beta-catenin mutations in craniopharyngiomas and

pituitary adenomas. *J Neurooncol* 2005;**73**(3):205–209.

149. Oka H, Kameya T, Sasano H, *et al.* Pituitary choristoma composed of corticotrophs and adrenocortical cells in the sella turcica. *Virchows Arch* 1996;**427**:613–617.

150. Pal A, Capatina C, Tenreiro AP, *et al.* Pituitary apoplexy in non-functioning pituitary adenomas: long term follow up is important because of significant numbers of tumour recurrences. *Clin Endocrinol (Oxf)* 2011;**75**(4):501–504.

151. Park YS, Ahn JY, Kim DS, Kim TS, Kim SH. Late development of craniopharyngioma following surgery for Rathke's cleft cyst. *Clin Neuropathol* 2009;**28**(3):177–181.

152. Pei L, Melmed S, Scheithauer B, Kovacs K, Prager D. H-ras mutations in human pituitary carcinoma metastases. *J Clin Endocrinol Metab* 1994;**78**:842–846.

153. Peillon F, Dupuy M, Li JY, *et al.* Pituitary enlargement with suprasellar extension in functional hyperprolactinemia due to lactotroph hyperplasia: A pseudotumoral disease. *J Clin Endocrinol Metab* 1991;**73**:1008–1015.

154. Pellegata NS, Quintanilla–Martinez L, Siggelkow H, *et al.* Germ-line mutations in p27Kip1 cause a multiple endocrine neoplasia syndrome in rats and humans. *Proc Natl Acad Sci U S A* 2006;**103**(42):15558–15563.

155. Pernicone PJ, Scheithauer B, Sebo TJ, *et al.* Pituitary carcinoma: a clinicopathologic study of 15 cases. *Cancer* 1997;**79**:804–812.

156. Piatt JH, Blue JM, Schold SC, Burger PC. Glioblastoma multiforme after radiotherapy for acromegaly. *Neurosurgery* 1983;**13**:85–89.

157. Pilavdzic D, Kovacs K, Asa SL. Pituitary morphology in anencephalic human fetuses. *Neuroendocrinology* 1997;**65**(3):164–172.

158. Post KD, McCormick PC, Hays AP, Kankji AD. Metastatic carcinoma to pituitary adenoma. Report of two cases. *Surg Neurol* 1988;**30**:286–292.

159. Puchner MJA, Lüdecke DK, Saeger W. The anterior pituitary lobe in patients with cystic craniopharyngiomas: Three cases of associated lymphocytic hypophysitis. *Acta Neurochir* 1994;**126**:38–43.

160. Puchner MJA, Lüdecke DK, Saeger W, Riedel M, Asa SL. Gangliocytomas of the sellar region–a review. *Exper Clin Endocrinol* 1995;**103**:129–149.

161. Qian ZR, Asa SL, Siomi H, *et al.* Overexpression of HMGA2 relates to reduction of the let-7 and its relationship to clinicopathological features in pituitary adenomas. *Mod Pathol* 2009;**22**(3):431–441.

162. Raetzman LT, Cai JX, Camper SA. Hes1 is required for pituitary growth and melanotrope specification. *Dev Biol* 2007;**304**(2):455–466.

163. Ramsay JA, Kovacs K, Scheithauer BW, Ezrin C, Weiss MH. Metastatic carcinoma to pituitary adenomas: a report of two cases. *Exper Clin Endocrinol* 1988;**92**:69–76.

164. Riccardi VM. Neurofibromatosis. In: Gomez MR ed. *Neurocutaneous Syndromes–A Practical Approach.* Boston: Butterworths, 1987:11–29.

165. Rickards AD, Harvey PW. Giant-cell granuloma and the other pituitary granulomata. *Quarterly J Med* 1989;**23**:425–439.

166. Rickert CH, Paulus W. Lack of chromosomal imbalances in adamantinomatous and papillary craniopharyngiomas. *J Neurol Neurosurg Psychiatry* 2003;**74**(2):260–261.

167. Rienstein S, Adams EF, Pilzer D, *et al.* Comparative genomic hybridization analysis of craniopharyngiomas. *J Neurosurg* 2003;**98**(1):162–164.

168. Riss D, Jin L, Qian X, *et al.* Differential expression of galectin-3 in pituitary tumors. *Cancer Res* 2003;**63**(9):2251–2255.

169. Rodriguez FJ, Scheithauer BW, Tsunoda S, *et al.* The spectrum of malignancy in craniopharyngioma. *Am J Surg Pathol* 2007;**31**(7):1020–1028.

170. Rodriguez FJ, Scheithauer BW, Roncaroli F, *et al.* Galectin-3 expression is ubiquitous in tumors of the sellar region, nervous system and mimics: an immunohistochemical and RT-PCR study. *Am J Surg Pathol* 2008;**32**(9):1344–1352.

171. Roggli VL, Suzuki M, Armstrong D, McGavran MH. Pituitary microadenoma and primarylymphoma of brain associated with hypopthalamic invasion. *Am J Clin Pathol* 1979;**71**:724–7.

172. Roncaroli F, Scheithauer BW, Cenacchi G, *et al.* 'Spindle cell oncocytoma' of the adenohypophysis: a tumor of folliculostellate cells? *Am J Surg Pathol* 2002;**26**(8):1048–1055.

173. Roncaroli F, Scheithauer BW, Horvath E, *et al.* Silent subtype 3 carcinoma of the pituitary: A case report. *Neuropathol Appl Neurobiol* 2010;**36**(1):90–94.

174. Rossi GP, Pavan E, Chiesura–Corona M, *et al.* Bronchocentric granulomatosis and central diabetes insipidus successfully treated with corticosteroids. *Eur Respir J* 1994;**7**:1893–1898.

175. Samaratunga H, Perry–Keene D, Apel RL. Primary lymphoma of the pituitary gland: a neoplasm of acquired MALT? *Endocr Pathol* 1997;**8**:335–341.

176. Sandrini F, Kirschner LS, Bei T, *et al.* PRKAR1A, one of the Carney complex genes, and its locus (17q22–24) are rarely altered in pituitary tumours outside the Carney complex. *J Med Genet* 2002;**39**(12):e78.

177. Sano T, Asa SL, Kovacs K. Growth hormone-releasing hormone-producing tumors: clinical, biochemical, and morphological manifestations. *Endocr Rev* 1988;**9**:357–373.

178. Sano T, Kovacs K, Scheithauer BW, *et al.* Pituitary pathology in acquired immunodeficiency syndrome. *Arch Pathol Lab Med* 1989;**113**:1066–1070.

179. Sano T, Kovacs K, Asa SL, *et al.* Pituitary adenoma with 'honeycomb Golgi' appearance showing a phenotypic change at recurrence from clinically nonfunctioning to typical Cushing disease. *Endocr Pathol* 2002;**13**(2):125–130.

180. Sano T, Mader R, Asa SL, *et al.* 'Honeycomb Golgi' in pituitary adenomas: not a marker of gonadotroph adenomas. *Endocr Pathol* 2003;**14**(4):363–368.

181. Sano T, Rong QZ, Kagawa N, Yamada S. Down-regulation of E-cadherin and catenins in human pituitary growth hormone-producing adenomas. *Front Horm Res* 2004;**32**:127–132.

182. Sarubi JC, Bei H, Adams EF, *et al.* Clonal composition of human adamantinomatous craniopharyngiomas and somatic mutation analyses of the patched (PTCH), Gsalpha and Gi2alpha genes. *Neurosci Lett* 2001;**310**(1):5–8.

183. Scanarini M, d'Ercole AJ, Rotilio A, Kitromilis N, Mingrino S. Giant-cell granulomatous hypophysitis: a distinct clinicopathological entity. *J Neurosurg* 1989;**71**:681–686.

184. Scheithauer BW, Laws ER Jr, Kovacs K, *et al.* Pituitary adenomas of the multiple endocrine neoplasia type I syndrome. *Semin Diagn Pathol* 1987;**4**(3):205–211.

185. Scheithauer BW, Parameswaran A, Burdick B. Intrasellar paraganglioma: report of a case in a sibship of von Hippel–Lindau disease. *Neurosurgery* 1996;**38**(2):395–399.

186. Scheithauer BW, Horvath E, Abel TW, *et al.* Pituitary blastoma: a unique embryonal tumor. *Pituitary* 2012;**15**(3):365–373.

187. Schochet SS Jr, McCormick WF, Halmi NS. Salivary gland rests in the human pituitary. Light and electron microscopical study. *Arch Pathol* 1974;**98**:193–200.

188. Scully KM, Rosenfeld MG. Pituitary development: regulatory codes in mammalian organogenesis. *Science* 2002;**295**(5563):2231–2235.

189. Sekine S, Shibata T, Kokubu A, *et al.* Craniopharyngiomas of adamantinomatous type harbor beta-catenin gene mutations. *Am J Pathol* 2002;**161**(6):1997–2001.

190. Shenker Y, Lloyd RV, Weatherbee L, *et al.* Ectopic prolactinoma in a patient with hyperparathyroidism and abnormal sellar radiography. *J Clin Endocrinol Metab* 1986;**62**:1065–1069.

191. Shin JL, Asa SL, Woodhouse LJ, Smyth HS, Ezzat S. Cystic lesions of the pituitary: clinicopathological features distinguishing craniopharyngioma, Rathke's cleft cyst, and arachnoid cyst. *J Clin Endocrinol Metab* 1999;**84**(11):3972–3982.

192. Sindou M, Daher A, Vighetto A, Goutelle A. Chondrosarcome parasellaire: rapport d'un cas opéré par voie ptériono-temporale et revue de la littérature. *Neurochirurgie* 1989;**35**:186–190.

193. Slavin MJ, Weintraub J. Suprasellar meningioma with intrasellar extension simulating pituitary adenoma. *Arch Ophthalmol* 1987;**105**:1488–1489.

194. Snyder PJ. Gonadotroph cell adenomas of the pituitary. *Endocr Rev* 1985;**6**:552–563.

195. Soares BS, Frohman LA. Isolated familial somatotropinoma. *Pituitary* 2004;**7**(2):95–101.

196. Spada A, Arosio M, Bochicchio D, *et al.* Clinical, biochemical and morphological correlates in patients bearing growth hormone-secreting pituitary tumors with or without constitutively active adenylyl cyclase. *J Clin Endocrinol Metab* 1990;**71**:1421–1426.

197. Sridhar K, Ramamurthi B. Intracranial meningioma subsequent to radiation for a pituitary tumor: case report. *Neurosurgery* 1989;**25**:643–645.

198. Tanizaki Y, Jin L, Scheithauer BW, *et al.* P53 gene mutations in pituitary carcinomas. *Endocr Pathol* 2007;**18**(4):217–222.

199. Tashiro T, Sano T, Xu B, *et al.* Spectrum of different types of hypophysitis: a clinicopathologic study of hypophysitis in 31 cases. *Endocr Pathol* 2002;**13**(3):183–195.

200. Thapar K, Kovacs K, Scheithauer BW, *et al.* Proliferative activity and invasiveness among pituitary adenomas and carcinomas: an analysis using the MIB-1 antibody. *Neurosurgery* 1996;38:99–107.

201. Thapar K, Scheithauer BW, Kovacs K, Pernicone PJ, Laws ER Jr. p53 expression in pituitary adenomas and carcinomas: Correlation with invasiveness and tumor growth fractions. *Neurosurgery* 1996;38:765–771.

202. Thapar K, Stefaneanu L, Kovacs K, *et al.* Estrogen receptor gene expression in craniopharyngiomas: an *in situ* hybridization study. *Neurosurgery* 1994;35(6):1012–1017.

203. Thodou E, Asa SL, Kontogeorgos G, *et al.* Lymphocytic hypophysitis: Clinicopathological findings. *J Clin Endocrinol Metab* 1995;80:2302–2311.

204. Tindall GT, Kovacs K, Horvath E, Thorner MO. Human prolactin-producing adenomas and bromocriptine: a histological, immunocytochemica, ultrastructural and morphometric study. *J Clin Endocrinol Metab* 1982;55:1178–1183.

205. Toth M, Szabo P, Racz K, *et al.* Granulomatous hypophysitis associated with Takayasu's disease. *Clin Endocrinol (Oxf)* 1996;45:499–503.

206. Tubridy N, Saunders D, Thom M, *et al.* Infundibulohypophysitis in a man presenting with diabetes insipidus and cavernous sinus involvement. *J Neurol Neurosurg Psychiatry* 2001;71(6):798–801.

207. Tuttenberg J, Fink W, Back W, *et al.* A rare primary sellar melanoma. Case report. *J Neurosurg* 2004;100(5):931–934.

208. Ulrich J, Heitz PhU, Fischer T, Obrist E, Gullotta F. Granular cell tumors: evidence for heterogeneous tumor cell differentiation. An immunocytochemical study. *Virchows Arch* 1987;53:52–57.

209. Vallar L, Spada A, Giannattasio G. Altered Gs and adenylate cyclase activity in human GH-secreting pituitary adenomas. *Nature* 1987;330:566–568.

210. van Furth W, Smyth HS, Horvath E, *et al.* Salivary gland-like tumor of the sella. *Can J Neurol Sci* 2007;34(4):478–482.

211. van Seters AP, Bots GTAM, Van Dulken H, Luyendijk W, Vielvoye GJ. Metastasis of an occult gastric carcinoma suggesting growth of a prolactinoma during bromocriptine therapy: a case report with a review of the literature. *Neurosurgery* 1985;16:813–817.

212. Vasile M, Marsot-Dupuch K, Kujas M, C *et al.* Idiopathic granulomatous hypophysitis: Clinical and imaging features. *Neuroradiol* 1997;39:7–11.

213. Veseley DL, Maldonodo A, Levey GS. Partial hypopituitarism and possible hypothalamic involvement in sarcoidosis. Report of a case and review of the literature. *Am J Med* 1977;62:425–431.

214. Vidal S, Kovacs K, Bell D, *et al.* Cyclooxygenase-2 expression in human pituitary tumors. *Cancer* 2003;97(11):2814–2821.

215. Vidal S, Kovacs K, Horvath E, *et al.* Topoisomerase II-alpha expression in pituitary adenomas and carcinomas: relationship to tumor behavior. *Mod Pathol* 2002;15(11):1205–1212.

216. Vidal S, Kovacs K, Horvath E, *et al.* Microvessel density in pituitary adenomas and carcinomas. *Virchows Arch* 2001;438(6):595–602.

217. Vierimaa O, Georgitsi M, Lehtonen R, *et al.* Pituitary adenoma predisposition caused by germline mutations in the AIP gene. *Science* 2006;312(5777):1228–1230.

218. Viswanathan R, Jegathraman AR, Ganapathy K, Bharati AS, Govindan R. Parasellar chondromyxofibroma with ipsilateral total internal carotid artery occlusion. *Surg Neurol* 1987;28:141–144.

219. Weinstein LS, Shenker A, Gejman PV, *et al.* Activating mutations of the stimulatory G protein in the McCune–Albright syndrome. *N Engl J Med* 1991;325:1688–1695.

220. Wheatley T, Clark JDA, Stewart S. Craniopharyngioma with hyperprolactinaemia due to a prolactinoma. *J Neurol Neurosurg Psychiatry* 1986;49:1305–1307.

221. Wong S, Lam WY, Wong WK, Lee KC. Hypophysitis presented as inflammatory pseudotumor in immunoglobulin G4-related systemic disease. *Hum Pathol* 2007;38(11):1720–1723.

222. Wu KK, Ross PM, Mitchell DC, Sprague HH. Evolution of a case of multicentric giant cell tumor over a 23-year period. *Clin Orthop Rel Res* 1986;213:279–288.

223. Xin W, Rubin MA, McKeever PE. Differential expression of cytokeratins 8 and 20 distinguishes craniopharyngioma from rathke cleft cyst. *Arch Pathol Lab Med* 2002;126(10):1174–1178.

224. Yamakawa K, Shitara N, Genka S, Manaka S, Takakura K. Clinical course and surgical prognosis of 33 cases of intracranial epidermoid tumors. *Neurosurgery* 1989;24:568–573.

225. Yaman E, Benekli M, Coskun U, *et al.* Intrasellar plasmacytoma: an unusual presentation of multiple myeloma. *Acta Neurochir (Wien)* 2008;150(9):921–924.

226. Yin Z, Williams–Simons L, Parlow AF, Asa S, Kirschner LS. Pituitary-specific knockout of the Carney complex gene prkar1a leads to pituitary tumorigenesis. *Mol Endocrinol* 2008;22(2):380–387.

227. Yoshida A, Sen C, Asa SL, Rosenblum MK. Composite pituitary adenoma and craniopharyngioma?: an unusual sellar neoplasm with divergent differentiation. *Am J Surg Pathol* 2008;32(11):1736–1741.

228. Yoshino A, Katayama Y, Fukushima T, *et al.* Telomerase activity in pituitary adenomas: significance of telomerase expression in predicting pituitary adenoma recurrence. *J Neurooncol* 2003;63(2):155–162.

229. Yoshioka M, Yamakawa N, Sarro H, *et al.* Granulomatous hypophysitis with meningitis and hypopituitarism. *Intern Med* 1992;31:1147–1150.

230. Yu S, Asa SL, Weigel RJ, Ezzat S. Pituitary tumor AP-2alpha recognizes a cryptic promoter in intron 4 of fibroblast growth factor receptor 4. *J Biol Chem* 2003;278(22):19597–19602.

231. Zahedi A, Booth GL, Smyth HS, *et al.* Distinct clonal composition of primary and metastatic adrencorticotrophic hormone-producing pituitary carcinoma. *Clin Endocrinol (Oxf)* 2001;55(4):549–556.

232. Zampieri P, Zorat PL, Mingrino S, Soattin GB. Radiation-associated cerebral gliomas. A report of two cases and review of the literature. *J Neursurg Sci* 1989;33:271–279.

233. Zhu X, Zhang J, Tollkuhn J, *et al.* Sustained Notch signalling in progenitors is required for sequential emergence of distinct cell lineages during organogenesis. *Genes Dev* 2006;20(19):2739–2753.

234. Zhu X, Lee K, Asa SL, Ezzat S. Epigenetic silencing through DNA and histone methylation of fibroblast growth factor receptor 2 in neoplastic pituitary cells. *Am J Pathol* 2007;170(5):1618–1628.

235. Zhu X, Asa SL, Ezzat S. Fibroblast growth factor 2 and estrogen control the balance of histone 3 modifications targeting MAGE-A3 in pituitary neoplasia. *Clin Cancer Res* 2008;14(7):1984–1996.

236. Zhu X, Mao X, Hurren R, *et al.* Deoxyribonucleic acid methyltransferase 3B promotes epigenetic silencing through histone 3 chromatin modifications in pituitary cells. *J Clin Endocrinol Metab* 2008;93(9):3610–3617.

237. Zhuang Z, Ezzat S, Vortmeyer AO, *et al.* Mutations of the MEN1 tumor suppressor gene in pituitary tumors. *Cancer Res* 1997;57:5446–5451.

238. Zimmerman D, Young WF Jr, Ebersold MJ, *et al.* Congenital gigantism due to growth hormone-releasing hormone excess and pituitary hyperplasia with adenomatous transformation. *J Clin Endocrinol Metab* 1993;76:216–222.

CHAPTER

42

Cysts and Tumour-like Conditions

Arie Perry

INTRODUCTION

Developmental cysts and other tumour-like conditions of the central nervous system (CNS) include epidermoid, dermoid, colloid, neurenteric and other benign cysts, as well as nasal glial heterotopia, inflammatory tumours and histiocytic disorders, the malignant lymphomas and other haemopoietic neoplasms covered separately in Chapter 40. Rathke cleft cysts, which are topographically and pathogenically closely associated with craniopharyngiomas, are covered separately in Pituitary and Suprasellar Tumours (Chapter 41). The epithelial cysts can be roughly divided into those of ectodermal (epidermoid, dermoid), neuroectodermal (ependymal, choroid plexus) and endodermal (Rathke cleft, colloid, neurenteric) origin. Secondary changes, such as epithelial atrophy, ulceration, squamous metaplasia and cyst rupture with haemorrhage, inflammation and granuloma formation are common and may hinder precise classification. Immunohistochemistry is helpful for further characterization, although some limited samples can only be descriptively diagnosed as 'benign epithelial cyst'. In others, both the diagnosis and patient management rely heavily on a careful radiologic workup to rule out connections between intracranial and extracranial contents.

EPIDERMOID CYSTS

Epidemiology

Developmental cysts are variably estimated to form between 0.2 and 2.0 per cent of all intracranial tumours, although these are likely gross underestimates, because many are asymptomatic, some are diagnosed purely on radiology and such lesions are not typically reported to tumour registries. Despite their congenital nature, they present at all ages with equal representation of both sexes, specific exceptions being covered later.

Sites

Common locations include the cerebellopontine angle, suprasellar region, diploic skull, floor of the fourth ventricle and spinal cord.[37] They may also rarely occur in the brain stem, corpus callosum and the pineal gland/quadrigeminal cistern. In the cranial vault, the frontal and parietal bones are most often involved and in the petrous region, they may cause facial paralysis and bone destruction. Large intradiploic variants usually break through the inner table and may also destroy the outer table to cause soft-tissue swelling under the scalp.[9] Rare examples may be found within cerebral parenchyma.[37]

Clinical Features and Neuroimaging

The clinical features of epidermoid cysts vary greatly depending on tumour localization. In addition to the usual generalized signs and symptoms of increased intracranial pressure, the common cerebellopontine variety most often presents with involvement of the facial nerve followed by unilateral hearing loss and other cranial nerve palsies.[40] Cerebellar signs, wasting of muscles of mastication and trigeminal neuralgia are also observed.

On computed tomography (CT), epidermoid cysts appear as well-demarcated, low-density, non-enhancing lesions; magnetic resonance imaging demonstrates hypointensity on T1- and hyperintensity on T2-weighted images. Usually the cyst content has a different signal from that of cerebrospinal fluid (CSF). Heterogeneous hyperintensity on fluid attenuated inversion recovery (FLAIR) and homogeneous hyperintensity on diffusion weighted imaging are characteristic.[79]

Macroscopic Appearances

Epidermoid cysts are well-demarcated, encapsulated lesions of varying size, often with a striking white capsule having a mother-of-pearl sheen, hence the synonym of pearly tumour (Figure 42.1a). The outer surface may be smooth, nodular or lobulated. They may be easily shelled out from adjacent structures or firmly anchored as a result of local inflammation. Cysts in the ventricles or in the subarachnoid space are liable to rupture and cause meningitis. The cut surface reveals an interior filled with soft, pasty to dry, flaky material. The content may be occasionally brownish-grey and viscous. Calcification is rare.

Microscopy and Immunohistochemistry

The lining is composed of stratified squamous epithelium mounted on collagenous connective tissue. This epithelial lining reproduces the normal layers of the epidermis, complete with keratohyalin granules. The progressive production and desquamation of keratin result in the formation of concentric lamellae that fill the interior of the cyst, causing gradual expansion. The lining occasionally may be papillary, but the typical squamous epithelium is maintained. Cholesterol crystals are usually present. The lining expresses EMA and cytokeratin, as well squamous markers such as CK5/6 and p63.[70]

Biological Behaviour

Epidermoid cysts originate from the ectoderm, in common with dermoids. Cerebellopontine epidermoids derive from the first branchial groove, presumably from entrapped or misplaced migratory cells; this is similar to the derivation of acquired cholesteatomas in the ear.[43] Epidermoid cysts are benign, slow-growing lesions. The treatment of choice is surgery; complete resection is more common today because of improvements in microsurgery.[40] When incompletely removed, they tend to recur. Cyst rupture is occasionally complicated by chemical meningitis.[1] An uncommon, but deadly complication is malignant transformation.[29,70]

DERMOID CYSTS

Epidemiology

Dermoid cysts are rarer than epidermoids, although their true incidence is unclear. They may be slightly more common in males and slightly younger patients than epidermoids.

Sites

These lesions usually occur in the posterior fossa, in the midline attached to the dura or embedded in the vermis. They may also

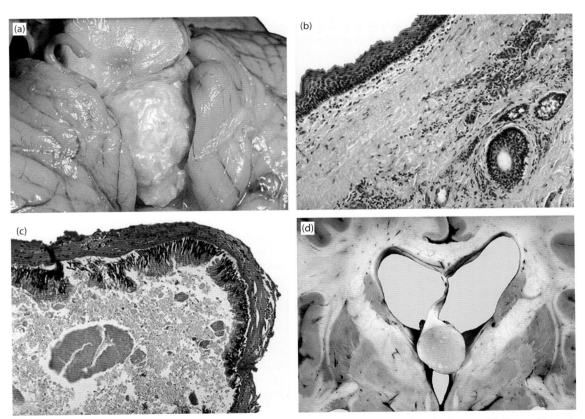

42.1 Cysts. (a) Epidermoid cyst: a 'pearly' tumour between the cerebellar hemispheres. **(b)** Dermoid cyst. Keratinizing squamous epithelium covers collagenous connective tissue containing skin adnexal structures. **(c)** Colloid cyst showing a lining of stratified columnar epithelium mounted on fibrous tissue and containing acellular debris. **(d)** Colloid cyst of the third ventricle.

(a) Courtesy of Dr HC Grant, formerly of the Middlesex Hospital, London, UK.

develop in the fourth ventricle, brain stem or the skull base, including the cavernous sinus.[2,86] Supratentorial dermoids are uncommon and are often associated with an extracranial component or dermal sinus tract.[76] Congenital variants may occur over the anterior fontanelle and these are more common than epidermoid cysts affecting the same site.[53] Dermoid cysts have been found in association with encephaloceles,[52] dermal sinuses,[54] and with Arnold–Chiari malformation.[6] In the spinal canal they most often develop in the lumbosacral regions and they may be extramedullary or intramedullary.

Clinical Features and Neuroimaging

Intracranial dermoids are often associated with fluctuating symptoms. CT scan shows well-defined, non-enhancing areas of low density. The combined use of CT and MR imaging may provide detailed information, including the presence of hair within the cyst.[51] The presence of disseminated CSF fat suggests a ruptured dermoid cyst.[47]

Macroscopic Appearances

Dermoid cysts vary in size. They are well-demarcated, smooth-contoured, round or oval masses. Their wall thickness varies, including occasional papillary projections and rarely calcified plaques. The cyst contains thick, cheesy, yellowish material that results from the secretory activity of sebaceous glands and from desquamated epithelium. Hair is often found, but teeth are rare. The connection of dermoid cysts with dermal sinuses is known to occur in both intracranial and spinal examples.[76]

Microscopy

Dermoid cyst lining is similar in places to that of epidermoid cysts (see earlier), comprising simple stratified squamous epithelium supported by collagen. However, in thicker parts of the wall, this simple structure is augmented by more complex dermis; hair follicles, sebaceous and sweat glands may all be present (Figure 42.1b). Bone and cartilage are rare, their presence being more typical of classic teratomas.

Biological Behaviour

These lesions are slow growing and benign, but are likely to recur when incompletely removed. Dermal sinuses penetrating the dura may be the route of pyogenic infection, a potentially serious complication, which can be prevented by early surgery.[76] Rupture of a dermoid cyst into the CSF is a potentially serious complication, potentially leading to granulomatous meningitis with foreign body-type giant cells. Rarely, chronic inflammation destroys the cyst wall, causing gliosis in the adjacent cerebral tissue. Cyst rupture may also lead to a surprisingly indolent dissemination of fat into the CSF.[47] Malignant transformation is extremely rare.[29]

COLLOID CYSTS

Epidemiology

In surgical series, colloid cysts constitute 0.5–2.0 per cent of all intracranial tumours.[33,80] They occur most commonly between the third and fifth decades of life; although all ages are affected, they are uncommon in children. The male to female ratio has been estimated at 1.5:1.[19,69] The mean age of individuals with asymptomatic lesions is considerably higher than those with symptomatic tumours: 57 years and 44 years, respectively. Colloid cysts have been reported in association with astrocytoma,[26] the naevoid basal cell carcinoma syndrome,[58] nasal dermoid sinus,[16] and agenesis of the corpus callosum.[18] Also, a colloid cyst of the third ventricle was diagnosed *in vitro* by sonography in a male foetus of 21 weeks' gestation with the XYY syndrome.[24] Whether these rare cases represent true biological associations or mere coincidence remains to be determined. Familial colloid cysts are rare, although families with two or more affected members should be screened, because an autosomal dominant inheritance has been suggested.[61]

Sites

By definition, colloid cysts are in the third ventricle, typically arising from the anterosuperior portion (Figure 42.1d). Rare examples in the lateral ventricles, fourth ventricle, and outside the ventricular system have been reported, although they are perhaps better regarded as neurenteric cysts because the histology of these two lesions is identical (discussed later).

Clinical Features and Neuroimaging

Symptoms depend on the lesion's size and site. Small examples may remain silent, detected incidentally on imaging or autopsy. At the other extreme, large cysts splay the fornices causing memory deficits and occlude the foramina of Monro, causing obstructive hydrocephalus. The most common symptom is headache, which is often episodic and positional, such that it is exacerbated when the patient lies down to sleep and improves upon standing. A comparative study of symptomatic and asymptomatic patients revealed four factors associated with symptoms: younger age, larger cyst size, ventriculomegaly and increased signal on T2-weighted MR imaging.[69] Colloid cysts are occasionally associated with marked psychiatric disturbances pre- or post-operatively, even in the absence of hydrocephalus; these include depression, personality changes, psychosis, and olfactory/gustatory hallucinations.[12] These symptoms and signs may be attributed to aqueductal compression or vascular compromise of the diencephalon with dysfunction of major limbic system structures. Moreover, forniceal damage is associated with anterograde amnesia.[1] Colloid cysts may also cause acute neurological deterioration and sudden death, not only in adults, but also in children.[13] Autopsy in most cases reveals hydrocephalus and severe cerebral swelling with tonsillar herniation. However, acute cerebral hydrocephalus leading to neurogenically 'stunned' myocardium and cardiac arrest has been proposed as an alternate mechanism.[32]

Unenhanced CT scan usually shows the cyst to be hypodense in relation to the periphery.[5] On MR imaging, roughly half are hyperintense on T1-weighted images with the other half being either hypointense or isointense to brain. T2-weighted images may show a reversal of the T1 pattern, although often, there is a hyperintense periphery and a hypointense core. A thin rim of contrast enhancement represents the capsule and intracystic fluid levels are occasionally seen. MR imaging is useful for surgical planning, because the relative signal intensities correlate with the viscosity of the cyst content. For example, a hypodense CT appearance suggests a liquid consistency amenable to aspiration, whereas a hyperdense core on CT or hypointense T2 MR signal suggests a viscous content that may require surgical excision.[5]

Macroscopic Appearances

Colloid cysts are smooth and spherical (Figure 42.1d). The wall is usually thin, surrounding a homogeneous, soft, opaque or occasionally denser, hyaline-like material. Size varies from millimetres to centimetres. The cyst may be firmly anchored to surrounding brain structures, including the foramina of Monro, the wall of the lateral ventricle or the columns of the fornix. The fibrous capsule of the lesion may be intricately associated with the connective tissue stroma of the choroid plexus of the third ventricle.

Light and Electron Microscopy

The lining of the cyst is variable, even within the same specimen. Stretches of cuboidal or flattened columnar epithelium may alternate with ciliated, simple or pseudostratified columnar epithelium. Completely denuded areas are common. Occasional goblet cells with intracytoplasmic mucin may be found. The cyst content is PAS positive and composed of amorphous debris with necrotic leukocytes and occasional lipid droplets (Figure 42.1c). A xanthogranulomatous reaction occasionally develops because of desquamation of lining cells, exposure of colloid material, and microhaemorrhages: epithelioid cells and macrophages contain refractile material and haemosiderin. Small microcysts in the surrounding fibrovascular stroma may occasionally be seen.[50]

Electron microscopy of colloid cysts reveals ciliated and non-ciliated epithelial cells, goblet cells, basal cells and intermediate forms, some with evidence of early squamous differentiation. Occasional colloid cysts may display mainly squamous differentiation and basally located cells may resemble myoepithelial cells. There are six cell types in the lining epithelium: ciliated cells with occasional abnormal cilia, non-ciliated cells with microvilli coated with granulofibrillary material, goblet cells with secretory activity, basal cells with tonofilaments and desmosomes, basally located, elongated cells with scattered, membrane-bound secretory granules in the electron-lucent cytoplasm and small, undifferentiated cells poor in organelles. These cell types and their distribution within the lining are similar to normal upper respiratory epithelium and the lining of spinal neuroenteric cysts, suggesting that colloid cysts originate from the endoderm.[30,44]

Immunohistochemistry and Histogenesis

The immunohistochemical profile of colloid cysts resembles that of respiratory epithelium: positive for cytokeratins (including CK7), EMA and vimentin. Occasional cells are positive for Clara cell-specific antigens. Carcinoembryonic antigen is expressed on the apical surface of scattered cells. Unlike choroid plexus tumours, they are negative for prealbumin (transthyretin), S-100 protein, glial fibrillary acidic protein (GFAP) and neuron specific enolase (NSE). Thus, the immunoprofile of colloid cysts is virtually identical to that of both respiratory tract mucosa and histologically similar developmental cysts, such as Rathke's cleft and neurenteric cysts; these data further support an endodermal rather than neuroepithelial derivation.[28,45]

Biological Behaviour and Prognosis

Colloid cysts are benign. Asymptomatic patients can be managed with observation and serial neuroimaging.[68,69] If symptoms appear, the cyst enlarges or hydrocephalus develops, the treatment of choice is surgical removal: stereotactic surgery can be offered to selected patients as the initial procedure of choice, whereas craniotomy is reserved for those whose imaging predicts failure or complications, and for those whose cyst cannot be aspirated. Endoscopic removal has also gained popularity because of its reduced morbidity, intra-operative time and length of hospitalization.[15] Preoperative neuroimaging accurately predicts viscosity, helping to identify those patients for whom stereotactic aspiration is likely to be successful. Unsuccessful stereotactic aspiration is usually related to high viscosity or deflection of the cyst away from the aspiration needle as a result of small size.[42] An exceptional example of malignant transformation to mucinous papillary cystadenoma has been reported.[20]

NEURENTERIC (ENTEROGENOUS) CYSTS

Epidemiology

Neurenteric cysts are rare, comprising anywhere from 0.3 per cent to 5 per cent of spinal tumours.[77] A comparative analysis of 80 histologically verified cases without vertebral, skin or visceral malformation, and 56 cases with associated spinal dysraphism revealed a male preponderance (>60 per cent) for both groups.[59] The age at presentation ranges from 8 days to 72 years, but cysts associated with additional malformations present at a significantly younger age than isolated cysts: 16.5 years versus 25.2 years.[59]

Clinical Features and Neuroimaging

Patients with associated malformations usually present with symptoms caused by the particular defect (e.g. vertebral deformity, visceral or cardiac anomalies). In rare cases, it may be associated with Currarino syndrome.[84] The clinical symptoms of patients with solitary neurenteric cysts results chiefly from compression of the spinal cord and adjacent nerve roots. In infancy the lesion may present with chronic fever and myelopathy, the fever thought to result from inflammation and secretion of TNF-α elicited by degenerative changes in the cyst.[36] CT scan shows a hypodense or rarely a mixed density mass. In 90 per cent of the cases, T1-weighted MR imaging demonstrates a lesion that is hypointense to spinal cord and isointense or hypointense to the CSF; this corresponds to clear cyst fluid whereas cases with cloudy or haemorrhagic fluid are usually hyperintense to CSF.[59]

Sites, Macroscopical Appearances and Microscopy

Most cases are encountered in the intradural extramedullary spinal compartment. Solitary cysts occur most frequently in the cervical region, whereas the lumbosacral cases are often associated with dysraphic defects. For both groups, ventral location is more common, followed by dorsal lesions and the relatively rare intramedullary examples.[59] Neurenteric cysts outside the spinal canal have also been reported, including the lateral and fourth ventricles, the cerebellopontine angle, the brain stem and supratentorially in the cerebral hemispheres.[35,64] Some are incidental findings unassociated with symptoms.

Histologically, neurenteric cysts may be lined by a single-layered or pseudostratified cuboidal or columnar, ciliated or non-ciliated epithelium, resembling gastrointestinal or respiratory epithelium, mounted on a basement membrane. In addition, some contain mucous or serous glands, smooth muscle, various connective tissue components, lymphoid tissue and even ganglia, while rare examples additionally show glioependymal elements.[89]

Electron Microscopy, Immunohistochemistry and Histogenesis

Ultrastructural examination of neurenteric cysts shows striking similarities with colloid cysts, Rathke's cleft cysts and follicular cysts of the normal pituitary gland.[44] Their immunophenotype is also analogous to that of other endodermal cysts. The epithelial cells of neurenteric cysts are positive for cytokeratins, EMA, secretory component and vimentin, but fail to stain with antibodies to prealbumin (transthyretin), S-100 protein, GFAP and NSE.[45] They also express the common CK7-positive, CK20-negative pattern of respiratory epithelium.[35,66]

During the first 3 weeks of embryonic life, the cells of the notochord are in close contact with the endoderm (primitive foregut). Although the origin of neurenteric cysts is not known, a favoured theory states that incomplete separation of these two embryonic layers hinders the development of the mesoderm, trapping a portion of the primitive foregut in the developing spinal canal. However, this hypothesis does not account for intracranial examples.

Given the rarity of these lesions, it is difficult to establish accurate recurrence rates, which have ranged from 0 to 37 per cent in relatively small series.[59,77] The risk of recurrence clearly increases with subtotal resection. Overall prognosis is best in patients presenting with a long or intermittent clinical course, no pre-operative neurologic deficits, no evidence of spinal atrophy on MR imaging, and complete cyst removal.[59] Rare multifocal disease has also been reported. In one case, multiple, relentlessly progressive, but benign-appearing supratentorial, infratentorial and spinal enterogenous cysts appeared 14 years after incomplete removal of a posterior fossa cyst, suggesting the possibility of subarachnoid dissemination.[66] Malignant transformation to adenocarcinoma is extremely uncommon.[27]

NEUROEPITHELIAL CYSTS

The term neuroepithelial cyst has been used rather loosely in the past for a wide range of entities; this category is currently reserved for cysts lined by epithelial cells with features of ependyma, choroid plexus, or both. Most hemispheric examples are asymptomatic and the cyst fluid is typically CSF-like. Of 57 posterior fossa neuroepithelial cysts, 32 were symptomatic and 25 were incidental. Both sexes were equally affected and the mean age of 35 patients was 30 years, ranging from 5.5 months to 65 years.[78] Roughly half of reported thalamic neuroepithelial cysts have been symptomatic.[75]

Ependymal (Glioependymal) Cysts

Ependymal cysts are intraventricular and extraventricular, parenchymal cysts that are simple or multiloculated and are lined by a thin layer of cuboidal to columnar ependymal cells, resting on a gliotic stroma with no intervening fibrous capsule; there are no intraepithelial mucin-producing goblet cells. They may also be found in the lateral convexities, posterior fossa, brain stem, spinal cord, and within the subarachnoid space.[73,85] In rare cases, they are associated with other developmental abnormalities such as tethered cord or agenesis of the corpus callosum.[7] The lining of these cysts is negative for cytokeratin and is positive for both GFAP and S-100 protein, distinguishing these lesions from other developmental cysts of the CNS. A collagen type IV-immunoreactive subependymal basement membrane is either entirely lacking or thin and less well developed than that of endodermal cysts.

These cysts are thought to originate from ectopic or pinched off remnants of neural tube. In subarachnoid examples, a derivation from leptomeningeal neuroglial heterotopias is favoured. Consistent with its congenital nature, a large example has been reported in a 22-week estimated gestational age fetus and mimicked holoprosencephaly on ultrasound.[63]

Choroid Plexus Cysts

Cysts of the choroid plexus are extremely common, encountered as incidental findings in up to half of all autopsies.[34] They are most often multiple and found in the lateral ventricles. The vast majority are asymptomatic and smaller than 1 cm. Symptomatic cysts are most common in the trigone of the lateral ventricles in young boys, the symptoms are intermittent, possibly as a result of a ball valve obstruction of the foramen of Monro, and they are typically large (2–8 cm). Fetal cysts may be associated with trisomies of chromosomes 18 and 21,[60] but are typically asymptomatic and resolve spontaneously. As with normal choroid plexus, the lining epithelium is immunoreactive for cytokeratin, prealbumin (transthyretin) and S-100 protein.

ARACHNOIDAL CYSTS

Arachnoidal cysts may be either congenital or acquired, the latter following bouts of inflammation, subarachnoid chemical irritation, trauma, or haemorrhage. Those involving the Sylvian fissure are thought to be associated with cerebral hypoplasia secondary to abnormal development of the overlying arachnoid membrane. Other proposed mechanisms of cyst formation include the creation of diverticuli, duplication, splitting or lack of fusion of arachnoid membranes, resulting in chambers that have lost their communication with the subarachnoid space.

Arachnoid cysts are estimated to represent roughly 1 per cent of intracranial masses and may occur at any age, although symptomatic cases predominantly involve children. In 234 cases from two large series, the mean age at presentation was approximately 5 years, with half to two-thirds of cases involving the middle fossa/Sylvian fissure.[23,88] At this site, there is a marked male predilection with the M:F ratio approaching 5 to 1; in contrast, other regions show even sex distributions. Other sites include the cisterna magna, cerebellopontine angle, quadrigeminal region, optic chiasm, sylvian fissure, pineal gland and interhemispheric fissure. Rare suprasellar examples present with precocious puberty and other endocrine abnormalities.[81] In the spinal canal, extradural and intradural forms are distinguished.[11,14,21] They most commonly arise in the posterior thoracic or anterior cervical regions. Ventral extradural examples represent dural defects, suggesting a mild form of spinal dysraphism or 'ventral spinal intradural dissecting meningoceles' as suggested by one group.[8]

Other concomitant developmental defects include agenesis of the corpus callosum and anterior commissure, fornix dysgenesis, neuroglial heterotopias, cerebral and cerebellar dysplasias, Chiari type II malformation and cavernous angioma.[67,83,87] They have also been reported in association with genetic syndromes, including Chudley–McCullough syndrome, an autosomal recessive disorder with sensorineural deafness and obstructive hydrocephalus, as well as glutaric aciduria type 1 (GAT1), an autosomal recessive metabolic disease associated with glutaryl-CoA-dehydrogenase deficiency, macrocephaly, bitemporal arachnoid cysts, and a progressive encephalopathy associated with neuronal loss and gliosis in the basal ganglia.[49,83,87] The latter disorder is particularly important to recognize, not only so the appropriate low-protein diet can be initiated, but also because surgery should be avoided because of its potential to induce a catabolic state that can exacerbate the neurologic problems. In a study of 147 patients with arachnoid cysts, 8 (5 per cent) had bitemporal disease and GAT1 was diagnosed in 2 of 7 patients tested with urine screening.[49] Lastly, it should be noted that sometimes even minor trauma can cause intracystic haemorrhage or cyst rupture with subdural hygroma or haematoma; these complications lead to acute hydrocephalus and may require emergent surgery.[3]

Macroscopically, arachnoid cysts have a thin, collapsible, translucent membrane, containing clear fluid, the content occasionally being xanthochromic. Their size varies considerably, and larger examples may cause compression and gliosis of underlying brain tissue. Uncomplicated arachnoid cysts are easily separated from the dura and from the surrounding leptomeninges. Histologically, the wall is composed of an inner layer of arachnoid cells and an outer collagenous membrane. Electron microscopy shows an absence of the normal trabeculation of the subarachnoid space and a discontinuous inner layer.[74] The presence of chronic inflammatory cells, excess collagen or haemosiderin-containing macrophages suggests an inflammatory or a traumatic aetiology. Arachnoidal cysts give a positive reaction with antibody to EMA, but are negative for cytokeratin, GFAP, S-100 protein, prealbumin (transthyretin) and CEA.

The radiologic differential diagnosis includes other cystic lesions, including craniopharyngiomas, dermoid/epidermoid cysts, astrocytomas and chronic subdural haematomas. However, on MR imaging, the combination of site, morphological features and a signal intensity matching that of the CSF allows the diagnosis of uncomplicated arachnoid cyst to be made.[41] Surgical excision or cyst fenestration/shunting are common in symptomatic cases, although rare examples of idiopathic intracranial hypertension have been reported as a post-operative complication.[38]

GLIAL CYSTS OF THE PINEAL GLAND

Glial cysts of the pineal gland, often referred to simply as pineal cysts, are seen in 21 to 41 per cent of autopsies, most examples being <1 cm.[62] Larger cysts are detected by MR imaging in 1.0 to 4.3 per cent, although even most of these are incidental;[4] symptomatic cases average 1 to 2 cm. They are typically dark on T1- and bright on T2-weighted images, with a thin contrast-enhancing capsule. Symptoms result from either obstructive hydrocephalus or compression of adjacent structures. In 478 adult cases from one series, the female to male ratio was 2:1.[4] Symptoms include headache, diplopia, nausea and vomiting, papilloedema, seizures, Parinaud's syndrome, ataxia and hemiparesis. Analogous to colloid cyst of the third ventricle, sudden death is a potential complication, but is rare. Additionally, pineal apoplexy has been reported in 19 cases and is characterized by sudden worsening of symptoms with signs of acute hydrocephalus and often a fluid-fluid level on MR imaging, consistent with intracystic haemorrhage.[62] As in the pituitary, apoplexy can be a medical emergency with rare fatalities reported.

Pathologically, pineal cysts are perhaps more accurately considered pseudocysts, because there is no true epithelial, ependymal or meningothelial lining. Instead, the cyst wall is 0.5 to 2 mm thick, composed of an inner gliotic rim, adjacent pineal parenchyma, and an external fibrous layer.[22,56] The hypocellular astrocytic lining is characteristically rich in Rosenthal fibres, with occasional eosinophilic granular bodies and scattered hemosiderin. Because of this piloid appearance and the normal hypercellularity of pineal parenchymal cells, pineal cysts are often misdiagnosed as either pilocytic astrocytoma or pineocytoma.[22] However, they lack the classic biphasic appearance of the former and the pineocytic rosettes with loss of native nodular pineal architecture of the latter. In cases of apoplexy, there is often greater evidence of haemorrhage.[62] A number of hypotheses have been rendered for the pathogenesis of pineal cysts, although the spontaneous involution of some and the frequent hemosiderin deposition perhaps favour a degenerative over a developmental origin.

NASAL GLIAL HETEROTOPIA AND NASAL ENCEPHALOCELES

Although heterotopic glial tissues may rarely occur in other regions of the head and neck, nasal glial heterotopia is best recognized. Despite the common misnomer 'nasal glioma', there is no evidence of a neoplasm. The main distinction is with nasal encephalocele (see Malformations, Chapter 4),

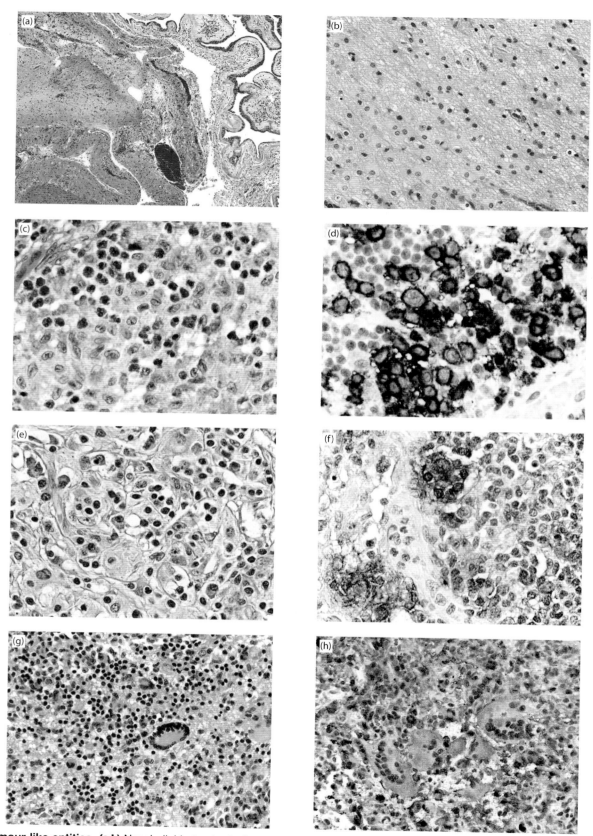

42.2 Tumour-like entities. (a,b) Nasal glial heterotopia ('nasal glioma') with islands of neuroglial tissue (a: left) beneath respiratory mucosa (a: right); rare ganglion cells were also present **(b)**. **(c,d)** Langerhans cell histiocytosis with numerous eosinophils and histiocytic cells with grooved reniform nuclei **(c)**, the latter highlighted with a CD1a immunostain **(d)**. **(e,f)** Rosai–Dorfman disease with a prominent lymphoplasmacytic infiltrate and large, pale histiocytic cells displaying emperipolesis **(e)** and S-100 immunoreactivity **(f)**. **(g,h)** Juvenile xanthogranuloma with wreath-like Touton giant cells **(g)** and factor XIIIa expression **(h)**.

a developmentally related entity that has an intracranial connection and is similarly rare, but affects as many as 1 in 5000 births in Southeast Asia.[31,71] Because the histopathology is virtually identical, an encephalocele must be excluded based on clinical and radiologic grounds; the distinction is critical to therapeutic planning and to avoid the risk of CSF leak and meningitis. For similar reasons, aspiration and biopsy are contraindicated. Unlike the heterotopias, encephaloceles are often pulsatile with crying, straining or compression of the jugular vein (Furstenberg test). Embryologically, both are thought to originate from faulty closure of the anterior neuropore during the fourth gestational week. However, in the case of glial heterotopia, a stalk-like connection with the brain degenerates. This hypothesis is supported by the presence of a fibrous stalk extending towards the skull in 10 to 25 per cent of patients with glial heterotopia.

These lesions are both present at birth, but may not become manifest until years to decades later. Nasal glial heterotopias are rare with roughly 250 cases reported and a slight male preponderance (male/female ratio 3:2).[71] There is no known familial predisposition and they are divided into extranasal (60 per cent), intranasal (30 per cent) and combined (10 per cent) variants. Extranasal cases are usually detected early because of disfigurement, whereas intranasal examples present with nasal congestion or difficulty feeding. The clinical differential often includes other midline congenital lesions, such as dermoid cysts and haemangiomas.

Histologically, they are composed of a mixture of neuroglial tissue and fibrovascular septae (Figure 42.2a,b).

BOX 42.1. Diagnostic approach to inflammatory and histiocytic tumours

Inflammatory pseudotumours (plasma cell granulomas) represent a spectrum of lymphoplasmacyte-rich myofibroblastic proliferations of unknown etiology, although more recently reported examples of CNS or peripheral nerve have features suggestive of **IgG4-related disease**, a sclerosing, potentially systemic, autoimmune disorder rich in IgG4 producing plasma cells.[39,48,55] Although initially described in the lung, extra-pulmonary sites have been encountered, including intracranial and orbital examples. Over half present as dural, meningeal-based or cranial nerve–associated masses, often in children or young adults. They present as either isolated primary CNS lesions or secondary involvement in patients with systemic disease. Histologically, they are characterized by loose spindle cell and polyclonal plasma cell proliferations with dense collagen deposition. IgG and IgG4 immunostains should be performed to rule out IgG4-related disease. Additionally, given overlapping features with other lesions, it is important to rule out the lymphoplasmacyte-rich variant of meningioma (see Chapter 36), Rosai–Dorfman disease (extranodal sinus histiocytosis with massive lymphadenopathy), low-grade lymphoma (especially the marginal zone/MALT-type variant), infection and collagen vascular diseases. Helpful features include the presence of numerous actin-positive myofibroblasts, a lack of large EMA-positive meningothelial clusters, S-100/CD1a-negative histiocytic cells lacking emperipolesis, a polyclonal κ/λ pattern, negative microorganism stains, and lack of necrobiotic debris. A subset express the ALK-1 (anaplastic lymphoma kinase) protein in the myofibroblastic component, presumably reflecting gene fusions of the *ALK* gene on 2p23;[82] based on clonal genetic alterations and the potential for recurrence, metastasis and sarcomatous transformation, this subset is now considered neoplastic and the term **inflammatory myofibroblastic tumour** (IMT) is utilized for such cases. In the CNS, recurrence rates have been high in subtotally resected tumours.[82]

Langerhans cell histiocytosis (LCH), also known as histiocytosis X and eosinophilic granuloma has a predilection for children less than 10 years of age. Involvement of the CNS or meninges usually represents contiguous spread from bony lesions of the skull.[65] However, pure suprasellar localization has also been described and may be associated with diabetes insipidus. The cellular infiltrate is often rich in eosinophils and the histiocytes or Langerhans cells are characterized by prominent nuclear grooves (Figure 42.2c). Ultrastructurally, these cells contain pentalaminar Birbeck granules and they are strongly immunoreactive for S-100 protein and CD1a (Figure 42.2d). Most cases with CNS involvement are self-limited, although long-term neurodegeneration has been reported in as many as 24 per cent of patients.[46,57]

Rosai–Dorfman disease (RDD) with CNS involvement nearly always mimics meningioma on neuroimaging and grossly.[65] Although the CNS may be affected in systemic cases, isolated cerebral disease occurs, usually in adults. The typical microscopic appearance is that of a lobulated dural mass with a plasma cell-rich inflammatory infiltrate and large, pale S-100-positive, CD1a-negative histiocytic cells displaying emperipolesis (i.e. phagocytosis of lymphoplasmacytic cells) (Figure 42.2e). In the dura, the latter may be subtle and are often best appreciated with S-100 protein stains (Figure 42.2f); this immunoreactivity is generally stronger and more diffuse than in juvenile xanthogranuloma and Erdheim–Chester disease. Most cases have behaved in a benign fashion following surgery with or without adjuvant radiotherapy.

Juvenile xanthogranuloma (JXG) is a non-Langerhans cell proliferation, which most often occurs in the first four years of life as a solitary cutaneous lesion. The CNS may be involved in those with systemic disease or rarely as an isolated intraparenchymal, ventricular or dural-based mass.[65] They may consist exclusively of mononuclear cells with or without xanthomatous features or associated with spindle cells and multinucleated cells, with or without classic Touton features (wreath-like nuclear arrangement) (Figure 42.2g). The cells are immunoreactive for CD68 and factor XIIIa (Figure 42.2h); the latter helps to further distinguish JXG from simple xanthomas formed by foamy macrophages containing cholesterol debris. Occasional cases also show focal or patchy S-100 immunoreactivity, overlapping with RDD and LCH. Unlike the latter however, the histiocytes of JXG are negative for CD1a and do not contain Birbeck granules ultrastructurally. Although cutaneous JXG is typically benign or self limited, intracranial involvement may be associated with recurrence or other manifestations of aggressive clinical behaviour.

Erdheim–Chester disease represents another rare form of systemic non-Langerhans cell histiocytosis, predominantly affecting middle-aged adults and diagnosed by symmetric, radiologically characteristic metaphyseal osteosclerotic lesions of long bones, pulmonary disease, cutaneous lesions and fever.[10,72] CNS lesions are common and involve the hypothalamic-pituitary axis (as diabetes insipidus), retrobulbar space (as exophthalmos), and the meninges/parenchyma of the cerebellum, cerebrum, brain stem and spinal cord. Most patients with extraosseous disease die within 2–3 years of diagnosis from pulmonary fibrosis, CNS disease, congestive heart failure or renal failure. Solitary CNS involvement has been postulated in very rare cases.[17] In CNS parenchymal lesions, the infiltrating histiocytic cells may be difficult to distinguish from atypical astrocytes or microglia, raising the differential with diffuse glioma. However, they may also appear foamy or contain Touton giant cells, similar to those of JXG. The histiocytes are typically CD68-positive, CD1a-negative and variable for S-100 protein. Histiocytic monoclonality has been demonstrated in some cases, but not others.

The neuroglia contain mature, GFAP-positive astrocytes, including gemistocytes and occasional multinucleated giant cells. Ganglion cells and ependymal elements may also be seen, but are less common in heterotopias. Depending on the extent of neuropil formation, there is variable NSE and synaptophysin immunoreactivity. Occasionally, all three types of neuroepithelial tissue, leptomeninges, glia and neurons are intermingled with hyperplastic sweat glands.[25] Ki-67 and p53 stains are typically negative and recurrence suggests incomplete removal rather than neoplastic transformation.

INFLAMMATORY AND HISTIOCYTIC TUMOURS

The common denominator for this group of enigmatic disorders is an inflammation-rich CNS mass. They do not fit neatly into any single etiologic category and the biological behaviour may be difficult to predict purely on histological grounds (Box 42.1). For example, whereas the entity of plasma cell granuloma has long been considered reactive ('inflammatory pseudotumour'), clonal examples with the potential to recur and metastasize ('inflammatory myofibroblastic tumour') are now well recognized, highly suggestive that some are neoplastic. Similarly, a spectrum of histiocytic disorders may be encountered in conditions ranging from isolated, self limited masses to disseminated multisystem proliferations with considerable morbidity and mortality (see Box 42.1). These entities commonly afflict children and young adults and have a predilection for the meninges, although parenchymal examples are also encountered.[65] The inflammatory constituents vary with each entity, but often include lymphocytes, plasma cells, and macrophages; eosinophils are most common in Langerhans cell histiocytosis and variable numbers of neutrophils may also be encountered. Fibrosis is similarly common and epithelioid histiocytes may be seen, although they usually do not aggregate into well formed granulomas, the latter expanding the differential to include sarcoidosis and mycobacterial or fungal infections.

REFERENCES

1. Aggleton JP, McMackin D, Carpenter K, et al. Differential cognitive effects of colloid cysts in the third ventricle that spare or compromise the fornix. *Brain* 2000;**123** (Part 4):800–15.
2. Akdemir G, Daglioglu E, Ergungor MF. Dermoid lesion of the cavernous sinus: case report and review of the literature. *Neurosurg Rev* 2004;**27**(4):294–8.
3. Albuquerque FC, Giannotta SL. Arachnoid cyst rupture producing subdural hygroma and intracranial hypertension: case reports. *Neurosurgery* 1997;**41**(4):951–5; discussion 5–6.
4. Al-Holou WN, Terman SW, Kilburg C, et al. Prevalence and natural history of pineal cysts in adults. *J Neurosurg* 2011;**115**(6):1106–14.
5. Armao D, Castillo M, Chen H, Kwock L. Colloid cyst of the third ventricle: imaging–pathologic correlation. *AJNR Am J Neuroradiol* 2000;**21**(8):1470–7.
6. Baecque CD, Snyder DH, Suzuki K. Congenital intramedullary spinal dermoid cyst associated with an Arnold–Chiari malformation. *Acta Neuropathol (Berl)* 1977;**38**:239–42.
7. Balasubramaniam C, Balasubramaniam V, Santosh V. Intramedullary glioependymal cyst and tethered cord in an infant. *Childs Nerv Syst* 2004;**20**(7):496–8.
8. Ball BG, Luetmer PH, Giannini C, et al. Ventral 'spinal epidural meningeal cysts' – not epidural and not cysts? Case series and review of the literature. *Neurosurgery* [Case Reports Review] 2012;**70**(2):320–8; discussion 328.
9. Bikmaz K, Cosar M, Bek S, et al. Intradiploic epidermoid cysts of the skull: a report of four cases. *Clin Neurol Neurosurg* 2005;**107**(3):262–7.
10. Bisceglia M, Cammisa M, Suster S, Colby TV. Erdheim–Chester disease: clinical and pathologic spectrum of four cases from the Arkadi M. Rywlin slide seminars. *Adv Anat Pathol* 2003;**10**(3):160–71.
11. Bond AE, Zada G, Bowen I, McComb JG, Krieger MD. Spinal arachnoid cysts in the pediatric population: report of 31 cases and a review of the literature. *J Neurosurg Pediatr* [Comparative Study Review] 2012;**9**(4):432–41.
12. Brand M, Kalbe E, Kracht LW, et al. Organic and psychogenic factors leading to executive dysfunctions in a patient suffering from surgery of a colloid cyst of the foramen of Monro. *Neurocase* 2004;**10**(6):420–5.
13. Buttner A, Winkler PA, Eisenmenger W, Weis S. Colloid cysts of the third ventricle with fatal outcome: a report of two cases and review of the literature. *Int J Legal Med* 1997;**110**(5):260–6.
14. Chang IC, Chou MC, Bell WR, Lin ZI. Spinal cord compression caused by extradural arachnoid cysts. Clinical examples and review. *Pediatr Neurosurg* 2004;**40**(2):70–4.
15. Charalampaki P, Filippi R, Welschehold S, Perneczky A. Endoscope–assisted removal of colloid cysts of the third ventricle. *Neurosurg Rev* 2006;**29**(1):72–9.
16. Cheng ML, Chang SD, Pang D, Adler JR. Intracranial nasal dermoid sinus cyst associated with colloid cyst of the third ventricle. Case report and new concepts. *Pediatr Neurosurg* 1999;**31**(4):201–6.
17. Conley A, Manjila S, Guan H, et al. Non-Langerhans cell histiocytosis with isolated CNS involvement: an unusual variant of Erdheim–Chester disease. *Neuropathology* [Case Reports]. 2010;**30**(6):634–47.
18. del Carpio–O'Donovan R, Cardinal E. Agenesis of the corpus callosum and colloid cyst of the third ventricle: magnetic resonance imaging of an unusual association. *Can Assoc Radiol J* 1990;**41**(6):375–9.
19. Desai KI, Nadkarni TD, Muzumdar DP, Goel AH. Surgical management of colloid cyst of the third ventricle – a study of 105 cases. *Surg Neurol* 2002;**57**(5):295–302; discussion –4.
20. Dunham CP, Curry B, Hamilton M. Malignant transformation of an intraaxial–supratentorial neurenteric cyst – case report and review of the literature. *Clin Neuropathol* [Case Reports Review] 2009;**28**(6):460–6.
21. Evangelou P, Meixensberger J, Bernhard M, et al. Operative management of idiopathic spinal intradural arachnoid cysts in children: a systematic review. *Childs Nerv Syst* 2012;**29**(4):657–64.
22. Fain JS, Tomlinson FH, Scheithauer BW, et al. Symptomatic glial cysts of the pineal gland. *J Neurosurg* 1994;**80**(3):454–60.
23. Fewel ME, Levy ML, McComb JG. Surgical treatment of 95 children with 102 intracranial arachnoid cysts. *Pediatr Neurosurg* 1996;**25**(4):165–73.
24. Gaertner HJ, Prager B, Hinkel GK. Colloid cyst of the third ventricle with XYY-syndrome. *J Hirnforsch* 1993;**34**:555–60.
25. Gambini C, Rongioletti F, Rebora A. Proliferation of eccrine sweat ducts associated with heterotopic neural tissue (nasal glioma). *Am J Dermatopathol* 2000;**22**(2):179–82.
26. Gelabert M, Bollar A, Martinez R, Allut AG. Coincidence of a frontal lobe astrocytoma and colloid cyst of the third ventricle. *Neurochirurgia (Stuttg)* 1991;**34**(2):69–70.
27. Gessi M, Legnani FG, Maderna E, et al. Mucinous low-grade adenocarcinoma arising in an intracranial enterogenous cyst: case report. *Neurosurgery* [Case Reports] 2008;**62**(4):E972–3; discussion E3.
28. Graziani N, Dufour H, Figarella–Branger D, et al. Do the suprasellar neurenteric cyst, the Rathke cleft cyst and the colloid cyst constitute a same entity? *Acta Neurochir (Wien)* 1995;**133**(3–4):174–80.
29. Hamlat A, Hua ZF, Saikali S, et al. Malignant transformation of intra-cranial epithelial cysts: systematic article review. *J Neurooncol* 2005;**74**(2):187–94.
30. Ho KL, Garcia JH. Colloid cysts of the third ventricle: ultrastructural features are compatible with endodermal derivation.

Acta Neuropathol (Berl) 1992;83(6):605–12.

31. Hoving EW. Nasal encephaloceles. *Childs Nerv Syst* 2000;16(10–11):702–6.

32. Jarquin–Valdivia AA, Rich AT, Yarbrough JL, Thompson RC. Intraventricular colloid cyst, hydrocephalus and neurogenic stunned myocardium. *Clin Neurol Neurosurg* 2005;107(5):361–5.

33. Jeffree RL, Besser M. Colloid cyst of the third ventricle: a clinical review of 39 cases. *J Clin Neurosci* 2001;8(4):328–31.

34. Jeon JH, Lee SW, Ko JK, et al. Neuroendoscopic removal of large choroid plexus cyst: a case report. *J Korean Med Sci* 2005;20(2):335–9.

35. Kachur E, Ang LC, Megyesi JF. Intraparenchymal supratentorial neurenteric cyst. *Can J Neurol Sci* 2004;31(3):412–6.

36. Kadhim H, Proano PG, Saint Martin C, et al. Spinal neurenteric cyst presenting in infancy with chronic fever and acute myelopathy. *Neurology* 2000;54(10):2011–5.

37. Kaido T, Okazaki A, Kurokawa S, Tsukamoto M. Pathogenesis of intraparenchymal epidermoid cyst in the brain: a case report and review of the literature. *Surg Neurol* 2003;59(3):211–6.

38. Kaliaperumal C, O'Connor B, Marks C. Development of intracranial hypertension after surgical management of intracranial arachnoid cyst: report of three cases and review of the literature. *World Neurosurg* 2012;80(1–2):222.

39. Katsura M, Morita A, Horiuchi H, Ohtomo K, Machida T. IgG4-related inflammatory pseudotumor of the trigeminal nerve: another component of IgG4-related sclerosing disease? AJNR Am J Neuroradiol [Case Reports]. 2011;32(8):E150–2.

40. Kaylie DM, Warren FM 3rd, Haynes DS, Jackson CG. Neurotologic management of intracranial epidermoid tumours. *Laryngoscope* 2005;115(6):1082–6.

41. Kirollos RW, Javadpour M, May P, Mallucci C. Endoscopic treatment of suprasellar and third ventricle-related arachnoid cysts. *Childs Nerv Syst* 2001;17(12):713–8.

42. Kondziolka D, Lunsford LD. Stereotactic techniques for colloid cysts: roles of aspiration, endoscopy and microsurgery. *Acta Neurochir Suppl* 1994;61:76–8.

43. Kountakis SE, Chang CY, Gormley WB, Cabral FR. Migration of intradural epidermoid matrix: embryologic implications. *Otolaryngol Head Neck Surg* 2000;123(3):170–3.

44. Lach B, Scheithauer BW. Colloid cyst of the third ventricle: a comparative ultrastructural study of neuraxis cysts and choroid plexus epithelium. *Ultrastruct Pathol* 1992;16(3):331–49.

45. Lach B, Scheithauer BW, Gregor A, Wick MR. Colloid cyst of the third ventricle. A comparative immunohistochemical study of neuraxis cysts and choroid plexus epithelium. *J Neurosurg* 1993;78(1):101–11.

46. Laurencikas E, Gavhed D, Stålemark H, et al. Incidence and pattern of radiological central nervous system Langerhans cell histiocytosis in children: a population based study. *Pediatr Blood Cancer* 2011;56(2):250–7.

47. Liu JK, Gottfried ON, Salzman KL, Schmidt RH, Couldwell WT. Ruptured intracranial dermoid cysts: clinical, radiographic, and surgical features. *Neurosurgery* [Case Reports] 2008;62(2):377–84; discussion 84.

48. Lui PC, Fan YS, Wong SS, et al. Inflammatory pseudotumors of the central nervous system. *Hum Pathol* 2009;40(11):1611–7.

49. Lutcherath V, Waaler PE, Jellum E, Wester K. Children with bilateral temporal arachnoid cysts may have glutaric aciduria type 1 (GAT1); operation without knowing that may be harmful. *Acta Neurochir (Wien)* 2000;142(9):1025–30.

50. Macaulay RJ, Felix I, Jay V, Becker LE. Histological and ultrastructural analysis of six colloid cysts in children. *Acta Neuropathol (Berl)* 1997;93(3):271–6.

51. Markus H, Kendall BE. MRI of a dermoid cyst containing hair. *Neuroradiology* 1993;35(4):256–7.

52. Martinez–Lage JF, Poza M, Ramos J, et al. Occipital encephalocele associated with a dermoid cyst. *J Child Neurol* 1992;7:427–30.

53. Martinez–Lage JF, Quiñonez MA, Poza M, et al. Congenital epidermoid cysts over the anterior fontanelle. *Childs Nerv Syst* 1985;1:319–23.

54. Martinez–Lage JF, Ramos J, Puche A, Poza M. Extradural dermoid tumours of the posterior fossa. *Arch Dis Child* 1997;77(5):427–30.

55. Mauermann ML, Scheithauer BW, Spinner RJ, et al. Inflammatory pseudotumor of nerve: clinicopathological characteristics and a potential therapy. *J Peripher Nerv Syst* 2010;15(3):216–26.

56. Mena H, Armonda RA, Ribas JL, Ondra SL, Rushing EJ. Nonneoplastic pineal cysts: a clinicopathologic study of twenty-one cases. *Ann Diagn Pathol* 1997;1(1):11–8.

57. Nanduri VR, Pritchard J, Levitt G, Glaser AW. Long term morbidity and health related quality of life after multi-system Langerhans cell histiocytosis. *Eur J Cancer* 2006;42(15):2563–9.

58. Nishino H, Gomez MR, Kelly PJ. Is colloid cyst of the third ventricle a manifestation of nevoid basal cell carcinoma syndrome? *Brain Dev* 1991;13:368–70.

59. Paleologos TS, Thom M, Thomas DG. Spinal neurenteric cysts without associated malformations. Are they the same as those presenting in spinal dysraphism? *Br J Neurosurg* 2000;14(3):185–94.

60. Papp C, Ban Z, Szigeti Z, et al. Role of second trimester sonography in detecting trisomy 18: a review of 70 cases. *J Clin Ultrasound* 2007;35(2):68–72.

61. Partington MW, Bookalil AJ. Familial colloid cysts of the third ventricle. *Clin Genet* 2004;66(5):473–5.

62. Patel AJ, Fuller GN, Wildrick DM, Sawaya R. Pineal cyst apoplexy: case report and review of the literature. *Neurosurgery* 2005;57(5):E1066; discussion E.

63. Pelkey TJ, Ferguson JE 2nd, Veille JC, Alston SR. Giant glioependymal cyst resembling holoprosencephaly on prenatal ultrasound: case report and review of the literature. *Ultrasound Obstet Gynecol* 1997;9(3):200–3.

64. Perrini P, Rutherford SA, King AT, du Plessis D, Di Lorenzo N. Enterogenous cysts of the cerebellopontine angle: short review illustrated by two new patients. *Acta Neurochirurgica* [Case Reports Review] 2008;150(2):177–84; discussion 84.

65. Perry A, Dehner LP. Meningeal tumours of childhood and infancy. An update and literature review. *Brain Pathol* 2003;13(3):386–408.

66. Perry A, Scheithauer BW, Zaias BW, Minassian HV. Aggressive enterogenous cyst with extensive craniospinal spread: case report. *Neurosurgery* 1999;44(2):401–4; discussion 4–5.

67. Piatt JH Jr, D'Agostino A. The Chiari II malformation: lesions discovered within the fourth ventricle. *Pediatr Neurosurg* 1999;30(2):79–85.

68. Pollock BE, Huston J 3rd. Natural history of asymptomatic colloid cysts of the third ventricle. *J Neurosurg* 1999;91(3):364–9.

69. Pollock BE, Schreiner SA, Huston J 3rd. A theory on the natural history of colloid cysts of the third ventricle. *Neurosurgery* 2000;46(5):1077–81; discussion 81–3.

70. Raghunathan A, Barber SM, Takei H, et al. Primary intracranial sarcomatoid carcinoma arising from a recurrent/residual epidermoid cyst of the cerebellopontine angle: a case report. *Am J Surg Pathol* [Case Reports] 2011;35(8):1238–43.

71. Rahbar R, Resto VA, Robson CD, et al. Nasal glioma and encephalocele: diagnosis and management. *Laryngoscope* 2003;113(12):2069–77.

72. Rushing EJ, Kaplan KJ, Mena H, et al. Erdheim–Chester disease of the brain: cytological features and differential diagnosis of a challenging case. *Diagn Cytopathol* 2004;31(6):420–2.

73. Saito K, Morita A, Shibahara J, Kirino T. Spinal intramedullary ependymal cyst: a case report and review of the literature. *Acta Neurochir (Wien)* 2005;147(4):443–6; discussion 6.

74. Schachenmayr W, Friede RL. Fine structure of arachnoid cysts. *J Neuropathol Exp Neurol* 1979;38:434–46.

75. Schmidt K, Coimbra C. Endoscopic treatment of thalamic neuroepithelial cysts. Report of three cases. *J Neurosurg* 2005;103(2):342–6.

76. Scolozzi P, Lombardi T, Jaques B. Congenital intracranial frontotemporal dermoid cyst presenting as a cutaneous fistula. *Head Neck* 2005;27(5):429–32.

77. Shenoy SN, Raja A. Spinal neurenteric cyst. Report of 4 cases and review of the literature. *Pediatr Neurosurg* 2004;40(6):284–92.

78. Shuangshoti S. Neuroepithelial cyst of the cerebellopontine angle: case report with a review of the literature. *Neuropathology* 1998;18:328–35.

79. Sirin S, Gonul E, Kahraman S, Timurkaynak E. Imaging of posterior fossa epidermoid tumors. *Clin Neurol Neurosurg* 2005;107(6):461–7.

80. Solaroglu I, Beskonakli E, Kaptanoglu E, et al. Transcortical-transventricular approach in colloid cysts of the third ventricle: surgical experience with 26 cases. *Neurosurg Rev* 2004;27(2):89–92.

81. Starzyk J, Kwiatkowski S, Urbanowicz W, et al. Suprasellar arachnoidal cyst as a cause of precocious puberty – report of three patients and literature

overview. *J Pediatr Endocrinol Metab* 2003;**16**(3):447–55.

82. Swain RS, Tihan T, Horvai AE, *et al*. Inflammatory myofibroblastic tumor of the central nervous system and its relationship to inflammatory pseudotumor. *Hum Pathol* 2008;**39**(3):410–9.

83. Tatli M, Guzel A, Keklikci U, Guzel E. Pediatric orbital multifocal cavernous hemangiomas associated with bilateral arachnoid cysts of the middle cranial fossa. Case report and review of the literature. *J Neurosurg* 2005;**103** (5 Suppl):454–7.

84. Thambidorai CR, Muin I, Razman J, Zulfiqar A. Currarino triad with dual pathology in the presacral mass: report of a case. *Dis Colon Rectum* 2003;**46**(7):974–7.

85. Tsuchida T, Kawamoto K, Sakai N, Tsutsumi A. Glioependymal cyst in the posterior fossa. *Clin Neuropathol* 1997;**16**(1):13–6.

86. van Calenbergh F, Demaerel P, Sciot R, van Gool S. Long-term survival in a child with a brain stem dermoid cyst. *Surg Neurol* 2005;**63**(3):261–3; discussion 3–4.

87. Welch KO, Tekin M, Nance WE, *et al*. Chudley–McCullough syndrome: expanded phenotype and review of the literature. *Am J Med Genet A* 2003;**119**(1):71–6.

88. Wester K. Peculiarities of intracranial arachnoid cysts: location, sidedness and sex distribution in 126 consecutive patients. *Neurosurgery* 1999;**45**(4):775–9.

89. Wilkins R, Odom G. Spinal intradural cysts. In: Vinken P, Bruyn G eds. *Handbook of Clinical Neurology*. Amsterdam: North-Holland, 1976; 55–102.

Metastatic Disease

Matthew D Cykowski and Gregory N Fuller

INTRODUCTION

The most common malignancy of the central nervous system (CNS) is metastatic disease,[10,36] which accounts for approximately 20 per cent of clinically significant brain neoplasms.[25] CNS metastases affect more than 100 000 patients in the United States alone each year,[23] with an annual incidence of at least 11 individuals per 100 000 in the population.[36] Consequently, metastases are among the most common neuropathology specimens submitted to the anatomic pathology laboratory for the adult patient population.[3]

This chapter provides a broad overview of the clinical, imaging and general pathologic features of CNS metastasis, including cancer of unknown primary (CUP) site and the increasing use of molecular profiling approaches in CUP evaluation.

CLINICAL PRESENTATION

Although a majority of patients with brain metastasis have a well-documented history of a primary neoplasm, CNS metastasis may occur in patients with no previous cancer history, and less than half of patients with metastatic disease have systemic metastasis at presentation.[27] Moreover, a primary site is not revealed by clinical work-up in approximately 10 per cent of CNS metastasis cases.[36] Non-pulmonary primary tumours often metastasize to the lungs antecedent to CNS metastasis;[10] thus, the synchronous presentation of pulmonary and CNS lesions cannot be automatically assumed to indicate a lung primary *a priori*, and biomarker evaluation may be indicated for confirmation.

Presenting clinical signs and symptoms vary by anatomic site of involvement, and may include localizing symptoms and/or non-specific sequelae of increased intracranial pressure (headache, nausea, vomiting, mental status changes); all symptoms are typically progressive.[1]

Seizures constitute a presenting feature seen in about 16 per cent of patients.[23] Approximately 6 per cent of patients present with symptoms related to acute intratumoral haemorrhage,[23] which can lead to acute mass effect, rapid increase in intracranial pressure, herniation and death.[15] Other relatively common presenting symptoms include paresis and gait disturbance, vision alterations, dysphasia[23] and cognitive decline.

Based on sheer numbers of CNS metastases, lung carcinoma predominates (35–50 per cent of all CNS metastases).[18,36] Other common primary sites for metastatic carcinoma include breast (15–20 per cent of CNS metastases), melanoma (10–11 per cent), gastrointestinal tract (5–6 per cent), kidney (6–10 per cent) and uterus/vulva (5 per cent).[18,23,36] Less common primaries include prostatic (2 per cent), urothelial (2 per cent) and ovarian (2 per cent) carcinomas. Thyroid carcinoma, hepatocellular carcinoma and choriocarcinoma metastases are relatively uncommon, but are recognized.[4,23] Primary tumours with a high *proclivity* for CNS metastasis include melanoma, testicular germ cell tumours and choriocarcinoma.[1,15] Metastatic cancers (primarily carcinomas) of unknown primary site constitute a unique group and are discussed later under Cancer of Unknown Primary, p. 1924.

ANATOMIC COMPARTMENTS AND NEUROIMAGING

The specific anatomic site(s) involved by metastatic disease is very important, both clinically and biologically. Metastases may localize to one or more of the following anatomic compartments: bone (cranium or vertebrae), dura, subarachnoid space, subpial/perivascular space, and/or the CNS parenchyma, including specialized sites such as the choroid plexus, pineal gland and pituitary gland.

Subsets of tumours from some primary sites exhibit a proclivity for specific CNS regions or anatomic compartments; for example, a subset of breast carcinomas show solitary metastasis involving the dura and subarachnoid space with invasion into the underlying brain along the perivascular Virchow–Robin spaces. Preoperative MR imaging provides the pathologist with a highly informative first view of the 'gross pathology' of the patient's metastatic disease (Figure 43.1).

The ratio of supratentorial to infratentorial metastases in adults is approximately 3–4:1,[16,27] with specific primary sites, such as the pelvic organs (colorectal, ovarian and uterine carcinomas) and breast being overrepresented in the infratentorial (posterior fossa) compartment.[36] Some primary sites most frequently give rise to *solitary* metastases (53 per cent overall; the most common pattern for prostatic and colorectal metastases), whereas others are more frequently associated with *multiple* metastases (47 per cent overall; the most common pattern for small cell lung carcinoma and melanoma).[10,16,23] Innumerable (often dozens to hundreds) of discrete minute CNS metastases comprise the *miliary* brain metastasis pattern, discussed in more detail later under Miliary Metastasis, p. 1922.[10]

Intraparenchymal metastases are well demarcated and show solid (for small diameter metastases) or irregular ('ragged') ring enhancement (for large metastases) following gadolinium administration on T1-weighted sequences (see Figure 43.1).[36] The central area of larger metastases typically exhibits the imaging correlates of necrosis, being hypointense, non-enhancing and without restricted diffusion. An additional imaging feature associated with metastases is the presence of vasogenic oedema that is often dramatically extensive and out of proportion to tumour size.[3,25] Vasogenic oedema is seen on MR imaging as T2/T2-FLAIR hyperintensity that preferentially affects the white matter, extending 'fingers' into the cortical gyri and deep grey matter myelinated fibre capsules and medullary laminae. T2-weighted gradient echo (T2-GRE, T2*) sequences are very sensitive to intratumoral haemorrhage and to the presence of hemosiderin,[16] which can be diagnostically helpful; some CNS metastases particularly prone to intratumoral haemorrhage include melanoma, choriocarcinoma, testicular germ cell tumours, renal cell carcinoma (RCC), lung carcinoma, ovarian carcinoma[1,23] and thyroid carcinoma.[16,19] Melanoma metastases may show T1-weighted sequence intrinsic hyperintensity secondary to either haemorrhage or high melanin content.[16]

GENERAL PATHOLOGIC CONSIDERATIONS

Anatomic Sites of Involvement by Metastatic Carcinoma

The cerebral parenchyma is the most common site of metastasis, with the arterial border zones and cortical grey–white junction of the frontal lobe (19 per cent) and parietal lobe (13 per cent) being most frequently affected by virtue of their large spatial volume and blood supply,[23,36] followed by the temporal and occipital lobe (11 per cent combined) and the cerebellum (10–15 per cent).[23,36] Multiple metastases

are identified in approximately 50 per cent of patients as either multiple cerebral foci (33 per cent) or combined cerebral and cerebellar foci (12 per cent).[23] The brain stem is involved in only 1 per cent of cases.[4,23] Metastases to spinal cord parenchyma are also rare, with the majority arising from primary sites in the lung, and less commonly from breast, kidney or skin (melanoma).[26]

Metastases may also involve the choroid plexus, the ependymal/ventricular lining,[4] and the pineal and pituitary glands. RCC has a predilection to metastasize to choroid plexus,[10] whereas in the pituitary/sellar region, lung and breast metastases are most common. Sellar metastases may cause either diabetes insipidus or anterior pituitary insufficiency, as reflected by low thyroxine and cortisol levels.[21] Rapid progression of diabetes insipidus and painful ophthalmoplegia are suggestive of a pituitary metastasis.[21] Metastases to the pituitary stalk and hypothalamus are most often associated with endocrine disturbances.[25]

Metastatic tumour may also be limited to the cranial and spinal leptomeninges. This pattern was historically termed *neoplastic meningitis* (subsuming the terms leptomeningeal carcinomatosis and melanomatosis, carcinomatous meningitis, lymphomatous meningitis, and leukemic meningitis[6]) and occurs in 4–8 per cent of CNS metastases.[1,7] Leptomeningeal spread is typically most prominent over the base of the brain and posterior spinal cord.[25] Magnetic resonance imaging (MRI) studies demonstrate diffuse and/or nodular contrast-enhancing leptomeningeal thickening,[36] which may be associated with secondary parenchymal invasion.[16] Primary tumours likely to spread in this fashion include melanoma, acute leukaemias and non-Hodgkin lymphomas, and breast, lung (small cell lung cancer [SCLC]), and gastric carcinomas.[1,7,16] For non-haematologic cancers, approximately one-third of cases involving the leptomeninges will also have imaging evidence of parenchymal involvement.[6] Because of spread of tumour cells into the subarachnoid space, a diagnosis may be made by cytologic examination of cerebrospinal fluid (CSF), accounting for >90 per cent of positive CSF samples.[7] However, CSF cytology, and flow cytometry in the case of haematologic malignancies, may be negative, necessitating a presumptive diagnosis based on clinicoradiologic features.[6]

Metastases to the skull and dura occur in 8–9 per cent of patients.[36] Among all metastatic carcinomas, those arising in the breast are distinctive in their affinity for the dura, accounting for approximately half of all dural-based metastases.[26] These skull/dura tumours may access the CNS via communications between the external and internal vertebral venous plexuses[1] where bidirectional flow through a valveless system is possible.[6] Additional common histologic types to involve dura and skull are prostate carcinoma and multiple myeloma.[1] Vertebral osseous metastases are also common, in which the ventral elements (vertebral bodies) are more frequently involved compared to the dorsal elements (pedicles and laminae).[6]

Epidural soft tissues of the spine may be invaded by local spread of tumour out of involved vertebrae, paravertebral soft tissues, or lymph nodes. In contrast, primary CNS tumours of cord parenchyma only exceptionally

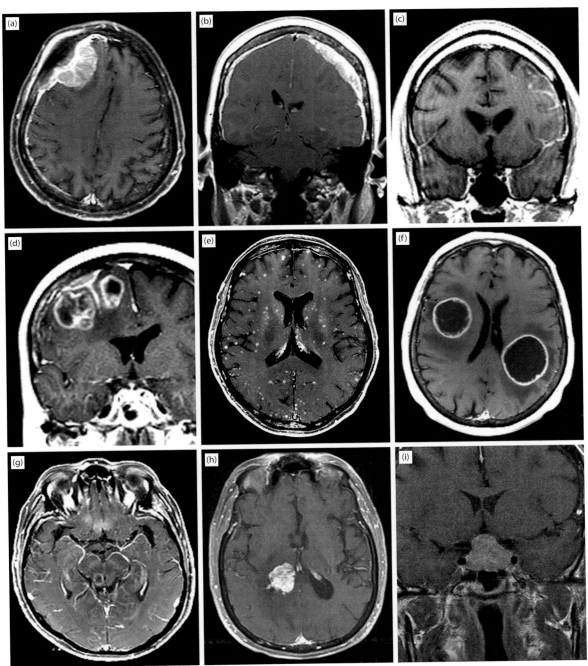

43.1 Magnetic resonance imaging of CNS metastatic disease: the pathologist's 'gross anatomy'. MR imaging permits exquisite delineation of the specific pattern of central nervous system (CNS) metastatic disease ('gross anatomy') in living patients, particularly with respect to the anatomic compartment(s) involved, which has important treatment ramifications. Illustrated here are nine patterns of metastasis, ordered from superficial to deep: **(a)** Cranial bone metastasis to the calvarium with intra- and extra-cranial extension; **(b)** dural metastasis; **(c)** subarachnoid space (leptomeningeal) metastasis ('leptomeningeal carcinomatosis', 'carcinomatous meningitis'). Note the extension of contrast-enhancing tumour as finger-like projections into the sulci, in contrast to the purely dural metastatic pattern seen in (b), in which subarachnoid space involvement, and hence sulcal extension, is absent; **(d)** dural metastasis with subsequent leptomeningeal extension (note the sulcal involvement) and invasion of the underlying cerebral initially via the perivascular (Virchow–Robin) spaces and ultimately leading to 'blooming' of large parenchymal metastatic nodules with centrally necrotic (hypodense) core; **(e)** miliary metastasis, with innumerable (literally hundreds) of punctate, contrast-enhancing foci, primarily superficially located in the cerebral cortex but also involving the deep grey matter (basal ganglia and thalamus); **(f)** classic CNS metastases to the grey–white junction, which exhibit ring enhancement with central necrosis (hypointense) and are surrounded by vasogenic oedema (visualized as mild hypointensity on this T1-weighted sequence); **(g)** isolated metastasis to the midbrain tectum. Although the vast majority of solitary metastases are found in the cerebral hemisphere, any part of the CNS may be affected, often with specific localizing presenting symptoms; **(h)** isolated metastasis to the choroid plexus (glomus choroideum) of the lateral ventricle. Among primary site carcinomas, renal cell carcinoma in particular exhibits a tendency for choroid plexus metastasis; **(i)** isolated metastasis to the pituitary gland (sella turcica), with suprasellar extension mimicking pituitary macroadenoma.

extend through leptomeninges and dura to involve the epidural space.[4,25] Spinal epidural metastases are most common with carcinomas of the prostate, breast, kidney and lung, as well as non-Hodgkin lymphoma,[36] with the thoracic spine most frequently involved.[26] There are a few noteworthy clinicopathologic points that distinguish epidural metastasis from intramedullary metastasis. First, the clinical presentation of epidural metastasis often reflects cord and nerve root compression, leading to findings of extremity weakness and sensory loss.[26,36] Second, epidural metastases rarely penetrate through the spinal dura to invade cord parenchyma. This is unlike leptomeningeal metastatic disease, in which invasion into parenchyma is common.[16] Third, *compressive myelopathy* is a significant complication of epidural metastases that is often progressive and irreversible.[25] These patients may present acutely with features of paraparesis and paraplegia, with incontinence occurring later in the course.[6] Histologic examination shows myelopathy, with white matter spongiosis and vacuolation in ascending/descending tracts that may progress to cavitation and parenchymal necrosis.[25] This may result from compression of radicular arteries or veins by tumour at affected cord levels.[25]

Macroscopic Features of Metastasis

The macroscopic features of metastatic tumours reflect their preoperative imaging attributes. Prototypical parenchymal metastases are well demarcated, with the epicentre commonly located at the cortical grey–white junction in the vascular distribution territory of the middle cerebral artery, particularly in the arterial border zone area ('watershed zone').[4,10,26] The tendency of metastases to localize to the grey–white junction has been attributed to narrowing of the calibre and acute branching of cortical vessels at this site.[10] Larger tumours usually exhibit a necrotic centre, which correlates with preoperative MR imaging findings. Cystic tumours with prominent myxoid material may be seen in various types of metastatic adenocarcinoma.[25] Metastatic melanoma exhibits a more variable appearance grossly, ranging from fleshy pink-tan in amelanotic, non-haemorrhagic examples, to dark red-black in tumours with haemorrhage and/or high melanin content.[36] Leptomeningeal involvement by melanoma may be reflected by thickening and/or red-purple to black-brown discoloration of the meninges.

Secondary changes in tumour metastases may be associated with high morbidity and mortality; chief among these is acute intratumoral haemorrhage, which, through acute mass effect, may lead to herniation, secondary brain stem (Duret) haemorrhage and death.[15] Intratumoral haemorrhage is also common in secondary leukaemia, with multiple parenchymal haemorrhages seen in patients with blast crisis.[26] Even in the absence of a dominant tumour mass, emboli of tightly cohesive tumour cells (e.g. squamous cell carcinoma) may cause multifocal parenchymal infarcts distal to points of vessel occlusion.[25] Metastases to the brain stem, fourth ventricle choroid plexus and cerebellum may result in significant compression of vasomotor and respiratory centres in the pons and medulla.[15]

Microscopic Features of Metastasis

Cytologic specimens from metastases often reveal cohesive tissue fragments of pleomorphic epithelial-appearing cells with prominent nucleoli in a background of blood and necrotic debris.[3] Cell cohesion on cytologic preparations reflects the presence of junctional complexes and desmosomes.[8] Not all metastases appear high-grade; mildly pleomorphic or even bland nuclear features may be seen with metastatic melanoma, and prostatic, renal cell and breast carcinomas.[3]

Frozen and formalin-fixed paraffin-embedded (FFPE) histologic sections of metastases typically show a relatively sharply circumscribed 'pushing' border[4] with gliotic adjacent parenchyma. A less common microscopic pattern is parenchymal infiltration by small cohesive groups of tumour cells or, rarely, even single cells;[3] this feature may be exhibited by some cases of SCLC or melanoma.[4] Prominent vascular proliferation is often seen in the neuropil adjacent to metastases, especially with renal cell carcinoma.[3,36]

Differential Diagnosis

Patient history and imaging are critical in the setting of metastatic tumour. In some cases, clinical features do not resolve the differential diagnosis and additional ancillary studies (immunohistochemical, molecular) are required. Moreover, even in patients with a known cancer history and disseminated systemic disease, a primary CNS tumour, such as glioblastoma, or a non-neoplastic mimic of metastatic disease (e.g. abscess, tumefactive demyelinating disease, subacute infarct, lobar haemorrhage) may arise independently, and this possibility must always be entertained.[16,27] Reviews of the microscopic and immunohistochemical features of primary CNS tumours and of metastases from different primary sites with diagnostic algorithms are available,[10,29] but these rapidly become outdated secondary to the continual advance in biomarker discovery and clinical implementation; there is no substitute for vigilant monitoring of the current literature.

MILIARY METASTASIS

Miliary metastasis, termed 'carcinomatous encephalitis' by Madow and Alpers in 1951,[4,17,25,30] constitutes a unique form of CNS metastatic involvement that has been described in the setting of several different primary tumours, including lung carcinoma,[13] melanoma, and cancer of unknown primary (see later under CUP, p. 1924).[13] Miliary metastasis is characterized by dozens to hundreds of minute micrometastases distributed throughout the brain, with a distinct proclivity for the middle and upper layers of the cerebral cortex, rather than for the grey–white junction as seen in classical cerebral metastasis.[14,30] Non-contrast CT imaging may fail to identify the minute foci of tumour and MR imaging (T2-weighted and/or T1-weighted with gadolinium) is far more sensitive. The characteristic pattern of miliary metastasis is innumerable, superficially located, punctate enhancing nodules (Figures 43.1 and 43.2). This pattern can mimic neurocysticercosis,[2] toxoplasmosis or

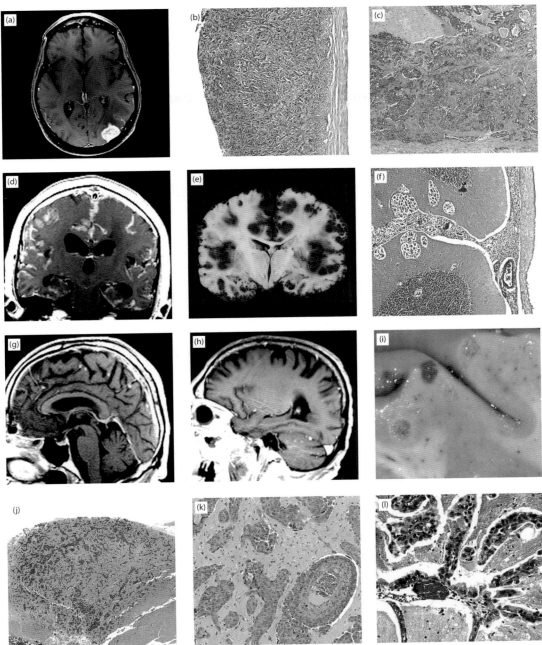

43.2 Histologic patterns of central nervous system (CNS) metastatic disease: Anatomic compartments. (a–c) Dural metastasis from breast adenocarcinoma with secondary invasion of underlying subarachnoid space, perivascular Virchow–Robin spaces and cerebral parenchyma. **(a)** Solitary dural metastasis often mimics meningioma, including the presence of tapering lateral extensions ('dural tail'), as seen in this example. Also note the focal 'fuzzy' extension into the deep cerebral parenchyma, which corresponded to perivascular invasion microscopically. **(b)** Dural metastasis (same case as panel [a]) showing the thicker part of the dural tail. Note the reactive sclerosis with abundant collagen deposition. There was no invasion of the underlying subarachnoid space in this area. **(c)** Dural metastasis (same case as panel [a]) showing focal invasion into the subarachnoid space with sulcal spread. (d–f) Leptomeningeal melanomatosis. **(d)** Coronal T1-weighted image with contrast shows diffuse involvement of the subarachnoid space of the convexity and sulci by melanoma. **(e)** Gross photo (same case as panel [d]) showing diffuse leptomeningeal melanomatosis, identical to the antemortem MRI findings. **(f)** Leptomeningeal melanomatosis (same case as panel [d]) is seen filling the subarachnoid space overlying the cerebellum with spread into the sulci between the folia and early invasion along the perivascular Virchow Robin spaces. **(g–l)** Miliary metastasis. (g–i) Multiple punctate metastases primarily localized to the superficial cerebral and cerebellar cortex ([g,h] sagittal T1-weighted images with contrast; [i] gross specimen photograph). (j–l) At increasing magnification, miliary metastasis displaying the characteristic anatomic localization with an epicentre in cortical lamina III (j), and anatomic involvement confined to the perivascular (k, l) and subpial (l) compartment. In panel (l), the pia has artefactually separated from the underlying glia limitans, expanding the subpial space. Note that a layer of tumour cells remains adherent to the inner surface (subpial space side) of the pia; the subarachnoid space, seen here as the small triangular spaces on either side of a venule, is not involved by tumour, which explains the absence of subarachnoid space spread pattern on the antemortem magnetic resonance imaging studies (g, h).

Cryptococcus meningitis.[30] Presenting symptoms in miliary metastasis may be very atypical compared to the usual focal motor and/or sensory complaints seen with ordinary metastasis, and include such dramatic presentations as rapid onset dementia, mutism or visual hallucinations.[31]

Microscopically, miliary metastasis foci are seen as minute intracortical tumour deposits characteristically confined to the perivascular–subpial space compartment, with the smallest foci epicentred in cortical lamina III. Subsequent enlargement of individual metastatic foci occurs by centrifugal perivascular spread, including into the contiguous subpial space,[24] but typically not into the subarachnoid space. The perivascular/subpial space, which has received relatively little attention in the neuropathology literature, is a well-documented anatomic compartment[5,12,35,37] for which miliary metastasis is a striking example of clinical relevance. Although involvement of the grey–white junction, white matter, deep grey nuclei, pineal gland, mammillary bodies and meninges can be seen[30] in miliary metastasis, it is the involvement of the perivascular/subpial space compartment that is distinctive. One hypothesis[24] postulates an affinity between tumour cells and the pia, including the arteriolar pial sheath and the pial membrane, as the critical pathophysiologic feature common to all tumours that present with miliary metastasis; however, the pathobiology underlying this distinctive tropism has yet to be elucidated, and this represents but one of the many intriguing and clinically important areas of CNS metastatic disease begging for additional investigative scrutiny.

CANCER OF UNKNOWN PRIMARY

In approximately 10 per cent of brain metastases, a primary site is not identified even after comprehensive clinical evaluation, yielding a working clinical diagnosis of CUP. CUP is defined as a malignant tumour, most commonly a carcinoma, for which no primary site has been identified after an exhaustive clinical (e.g. medical history, physical examination), laboratory (e.g. urinalysis, occult blood in stool), serologic, endoscopic[34] and imaging search.[28,32] The imaging search typically entails computed tomography (CT) scan of the chest, abdomen and pelvis, and/or 18-fluorodeoxyglucose positron emission tomography (FDG-PET). Serologic work-up typically includes, among others, prostate-specific antigen and other cancer antigen markers (e.g. CA 19-9, CA-125) and alpha-fetoprotein.[22] The clinical CUP work-up does not ensure localization of a very small (or, in the case of melanoma, regressed) primary site tumour, with even FDG-PET scanning having a tumour detection rate of only approximately 50 per cent in this setting.[22] The majority of CUPs are adenocarcinomas or poorly differentiated carcinomas (approximately 80 per cent),[28] with the remainder largely consisting of squamous cell carcinoma (10 per cent) and neuroendocrine carcinoma (5 per cent).[32] For brain metastases specifically, CUP most commonly occurs in patients with a median age of 51–55 years, with a slight male predilection.[28]

More recently, molecular profiling approaches to the characterization of CUP for diagnostic and treatment purposes have been explored. One operating assumption of this approach is that the gene expression pattern of a metastasis reflects that of the primary tumour.[22] The earliest studies used gene expression microarrays to predict primary site ('tissue of origin'). Subsequently, more limited gene panels amenable to FFPE tissue testing, such as quantitative reverse transcriptase PCR (qRT-PCR),[20] were explored. Most recently, microRNA expression assays have been used to identify primary site-specific alterations.[9] Determinants of normal development, microRNAs are short, 21–23 nucleotide in length, non-translated RNA molecules that regulate gene expression at the mRNA level.[22] The resulting mRNA degradation or inhibition in tumour cells may be oncogenic.[22] As with other gene expression studies, a variety of clustering algorithms have been used to determine the similarities of microRNA expression across tumours from a primary site, develop classifiers, and 'assign' a tumour one of a finite number of tumour diagnoses,[34] typically after 'training' the algorithm on test data sets of known primary site malignancies.[11] These studies have shown that microRNA expression profiling can assign a primary site in approximately 80 per cent of CUP, including CUP for which immunohistochemical evaluation is non-informative or equivocal.

Determination of primary site in CUP through immunophenotyping and/or molecular profiling will likely become increasingly prevalent as more precisely targeted agents tailored to specific primary site malignancies yields efficacious results. This CUP treatment approach is based on the tenet that even poorly differentiated metastases respond better to a primary-specific therapeutic regimen, as opposed to the empiric platinum or taxane-based chemotherapy that has historically been the mainstay for CUP.[28] The traditional binary algorithm approach using immunophenotypic profiling may be supplemented by molecular profiling in diagnostically refractory cases to provide a more confident estimate of tumour origin and allow the oncologist to pursue optimal therapy. For example, in the setting of a brain metastasis, this might include molecular profiling of a poorly differentiated carcinoma with an otherwise non-informative immunophenotyping work-up. Conversely, molecular profiling of CUP may also be of use when immunohistochemical findings do strongly suggestive of a specific anatomic origin, e.g. a CK7–, CK20+, CDX2+ metastatic adenocarcinoma, when there is an absence of confirmatory clinical, endoscopic and radiologic evidence for a colorectal primary.[34] This therapeutic approach has been used for poorly differentiated CUP presenting in a variety of body sites in which molecular characterization identifies a 'colorectal profile'. Even in the absence of a confirmed colorectal primary, patients with a CUP so identified respond better to site-specific chemotherapy compared to empiric chemotherapy.[33] This may not be a universally applicable assumption, however. By definition, all CUPs, regardless of site of origin, exhibit in common the property of early metastasis, and thus share this important aspect of tumour biology, the pathophysiological basis for which is an area requiring additional investigation.

REFERENCES

1. Adams RD, Victor M. Intracranial neoplasms. In: *Principles of neurology*, 4th edn. New York: McGraw-Hill, 1989: 516–53

2. Bhushan C. 'Miliary' metastatic tumors in the brain. Case report. *J Neurosurg* 1997; **86**: 564–6.

3. Burger PC. *Smears and frozen sections in surgical neuropathology: a manual.* Baltimore, MD: PB Medical, 2009

4. Burger PC, Scheithauer BW, Vogel FS. *Surgical pathology of the nervous system and its coverings*, 4th edn. New York: Churchill Livingstone, 2002

5. Cerase A, Vallone IM, Muccio CF, *et al.* Regression of dilated perivascular spaces of the brain. *Surg Radiol Anat* 2010; **32**: 555–61

6. Chamberlain MC. Neoplastic meningitis and metastatic epidural spinal cord compression. In: Lacy J, Baehring JM eds. *Central nervous system malignancies*, vol. 26. Philadelphia: WB Saunders, 2012: 917–32

7. Cibas ES. Cerebrospinal fluid. In: *Cytology: diagnostic principles and clinical correlates*, 3rd edn. Philadelphia: Elsevier, 2009: 171–96

8. Dickersin GR. Large cell undifferentiated neoplasms. In: *Diagnostic electron microscopy: a text/atlas.* New York: Igaku-Shoin, 1988: 26–79

9. Ferracin M, Pedriali M, Veronese A, *et al.* MicroRNA profiling for the identification of cancers with unknown primary tissue-of-origin. *J Pathol* 2011; **225**: 43–53

10. Fuller GN. Epithelial, neuroendocrine, and metastatic lesions. In: Perry A, Brat DJ eds. *Practical surgical neuropathology: a diagnostic approach*, 1st edn. Philadelphia: Churchill Livingstone, 2010: 287–314

11. Greco FA, Oien K, Erlander M, *et al.* Cancer of unknown primary: progress in the search for improved and rapid diagnosis leading toward superior patient outcomes. *Ann Oncol* 2012; **23**: 298–304

12. Hutchings M, Weller RO. Anatomical relationships of the pia mater to cerebral blood vessels in man. *J Neurosurg* 1986; **65**: 316–25

13. Iguchi Y, Mano K, Goto Y, *et al.* Miliary brain metastases from adenocarcinoma of the lung: MR imaging findings with clinical and post-mortem histopathologic correlation. *Neuroradiology* 2007; **49**: 35–9

14. Inomata M, Hayashi R, Kambara K, *et al.* Miliary brain metastasis presenting with calcification in a patient with lung cancer: a case report. *J Med Case Rep* 2012; **6**: 279

15. Itabashi HH. *Forensic neuropathology: a practical review of the fundamentals.* Boston: Elsevier Academic Press, 2007

16. Keogh BP, Henson JW. Clinical manifestations and diagnostic imaging of brain tumors. In: Lacy J, Baehring JM eds. *Central nervous system malignancies*, vol. 26. Philadelphia: WB Saunders, 2012: 733–56

17. Madow L, Alpers BJ. Encephalitic form of metastatic carcinoma. *AMA Arch Neurol Psychiatry* 1951; **65**: 161–73

18. McKeever PE. The brain, spinal cord, and meninges. In: Mills SE ed. *Sternberg's diagnostic surgical pathology*, vol. 1, 5th edn. Philadelphia: Lippincott Williams & Wilkins, 2010: 351–448

19. McWilliams RR, Giannini C, Hay ID, *et al.* Management of brain metastases from thyroid carcinoma: a study of 16 pathologically confirmed cases over 25 years. *Cancer* 2003; **98**: 356–62

20. Monzon FA, Koen TJ. Diagnosis of metastatic neoplasms: molecular approaches for identification of tissue of origin. *Arch Pathol Lab Med* 2010; **134**: 216–24

21. Morita A, Meyer FB, Laws ER, Jr. Symptomatic pituitary metastases. *J Neurosurg* 1998; **89**: 69–73

22. Natoli C, Ramazzotti V, Nappi O, *et al.* Unknown primary tumors. *Biochim Biophys Acta* 2011; **1816**: 13–24

23. Nussbaum ES, Djalilian HR, Cho KH, Hall WA. Brain metastases. Histology, multiplicity, surgery, and survival. *Cancer* 1996; **78**: 1781–8

24. Ogawa M, Kurahashi K, Ebina A, *et al.* Miliary brain metastasis presenting with dementia: progression pattern of cancer metastases in the cerebral cortex. *Neuropathology* 2007; **27**: 390–5

25. Okazaki H. *Fundamentals of neuropathology: morphologic basis of neurologic disorders*, 2nd edn. New York: Igaku-Shoin, 1989

26. Parisi JE, Mena H, Scheithauer BW. CNS tumors (excluding pituitary, PNET, and embryonal tumors). In: Nelson JS, Mena H, Parisi JE, Schochet SS eds. *Principles and practice of neuropathology*, 2nd edn. New York: Oxford University Press, 2003: 298–382

27. Patchell RA, Tibbs PA, Walsh JW, *et al.* A randomized trial of surgery in the treatment of single metastases to the brain. *New Engl J Med* 1990; **322**: 494–500

28. Pavlidis N, Pentheroudakis G. Cancer of unknown primary site. *Lancet* 2012; **379**: 1428–35

29. Pekmezci M, Perry A. Neuropathology of brain metastases. *Surg Neurol Int* 2013; **4**(Suppl 4): S245–55

30. Ribeiro HB, Paiva TF, Jr, Mamprin GP *et al.* Carcinomatous encephalitis as clinical presentation of occult lung adenocarcinoma: case report. *Arq Neuropsiquiatr* 2007; **65**: 841–4

31. Rivas E, Sanchez-Herrero J, Alonso M, *et al.* Miliary brain metastases presenting as rapidly progressive dementia. *Neuropathology* 2005; **25**: 153–8.

32. Taylor MB, Bromham NR, Arnold SE. Carcinoma of unknown primary: key radiological issues from the recent National Institute for Health and Clinical Excellence guidelines. *Br J Radiol* 2012; **85**: 661–71

33. Varadhachary GR, Talantov D, Raber MN, *et al.* Molecular profiling of carcinoma of unknown primary and correlation with clinical evaluation. *J Clin Oncol* 2008; **26**: 4442–8

34. Varadhachary GR, Spector Y, Abbruzzese JL, *et al.* Prospective gene signature study using microRNA to identify the tissue of origin in patients with carcinoma of unknown primary. *Clin Cancer Res* 2011; **17**: 4063–70

35. Weller RO. Microscopic morphology and histology of the human meninges. *Morphologie* 2005; **89**: 22–34

36. Wesseling P, von Deimling A, Aldape KD. Metastatic tumours of the CNS. In: Louis D, Ohgaki H, Wiestler O, Cavenee W eds. *WHO Classification of Tumours of the Central Nervous System*, 4th ed. Geneva: Distributed by WHO Press, World Health Organization; 2007: 309

37. Zhang ET, Inman CB, Weller RO. Interrelationships of the pia mater and the perivascular (Virchow–Robin) spaces in the human cerebrum. *J Anat* 1990; **170**: 111–23

Hereditary Tumour Syndromes

Arie Perry

INTRODUCTION

The nervous system is affected in many hereditary tumour syndromes, with the most important manifestations listed in Table 44.1. Most are autosomal dominant and are typically caused by the inactivation of a tumour suppressor gene, so that a growth suppressing gene is either inherited in a mutant form from a parent or mutated in the germline. Therefore, with the exception of somatic mosaics that carry a mutation in only a portion of their body, the patient carries a germline mutation in all cells; once the second allele is inactivated (somatic mutation), tumourigenesis ensues. Approximately half of cases in common syndromes, such as neurofibromatosis 1 (NF1) and tuberous sclerosis, arise sporadically, without a family history, as new germline mutations. Very rarely, two syndromes may occur in the same individual or family, e.g. combined NF1 and tuberous sclerosis[5,131] or von Hippel–Lindau with neurofibromatosis[118a] or multiple endocrine neoplasia.[92]

The study of these syndromes has proved essential in the identification of tumour suppressor genes involved in nervous system neoplasia. Indeed, more tumour suppressors have been identified through investigations of these rare syndromes than through studies of the more common, sporadic tumours. Nonetheless, these same syndromic tumour genes are also involved in the sporadic counterparts. For instance, although neurofibromatosis 2 (NF2) is an uncommon condition, the *NF2* gene is inactivated in the majority of sporadic schwannomas and meningiomas, both common human tumours. The correlation between genetic defects in hereditary syndromes and sporadic tumours, however, is not exact; for instance, although germline defects in DNA mismatch repair genes underlie some of the glioblastomas arising in Turcot's syndrome, evidence of DNA mismatch repair is only rarely noted in sporadic glioblastomas.

NEUROFIBROMATOSIS

The term neurofibromatosis (NF) historically encompassed a spectrum of syndromes: NF1 (von Recklinghausen's disease, peripheral NF), NF2 (central, bilateral acoustic NF), NF3 (overlapping NF1 and NF2), NF5 (segmental NF), NF6 (café-au-lait lesions only), NF7 (late-onset NF), NF8 (gastrointestinal NF) and NF9 (NF with Noonan syndrome).[39,95] Of these, however, only NF1 and NF2 are distinct. Most cases previously considered NF3 to NF9 are nosologically related to either NF1 or NF2 on the basis of molecular genetics;[22,104] for instance, many regionally localized examples are now recognized as either a third genetic disorder, schwannomatosis or mosaic/segmental forms of NF1 or NF2.

NEUROFIBROMATOSIS 1

The most common genetic disorder, NF1, predisposes to hyperplasias, hamartomas, malformations and neoplasms of multiple organs that vary by patient age and disease severity.[99] Malignancies are nearly three-fold as common in NF1 patients than in the general population, represent the leading cause of death, and reduce life expectancy by an average of 10–15 years.[85]

Diagnostic Criteria

A definitive diagnosis of NF1 is made when ≥2 of the following are present: (1) ≥6 café-au-lait macules (≥1.5 cm in

TABLE 44.1 Synopsis of hereditary tumour syndromes involving the nervous system

Syndrome	Gene	Chromosome	Protein and major functions	Major manifestations		
				Nervous system	Skin	Other organs
Neurofibromatosis 1	NF1	17q11.2	Neurofibromin: KRAS suppressor	Neurofibromas (especially plexiform), MPNST, learning disabilities, cerebral arteriopathies, 'optic glioma', and pilocytic, pilomyxoid, and diffuse astrocytomas; less commonly, ganglioglioma, dysembryoplastic neuroepithelial tumour, rosette-forming glioneuronal tumour	Café-au-lait spots, axillary freckling (virtually pathognomonic)	Lisch nodules of the iris (virtually pathognomonic), pulmonary stenosis, phaeochromocytoma, osseous lesions, rhabdomyosarcoma, CML, ALL, lymphomas, JXG, GIST, duodenal carcinoid, breast carcinomas, melanoma, medullary thyroid carcinoma, glomus tumour
Neurofibromatosis 2	NF2	22q12.2	Merlin: member of protein 4.1 family thought to mediate signals between cell membrane and actin cytoskeleton	Bilateral schwannoma (VIIIth nerve), meningioma, ependymoma, glial microhamartomas, non-vestibular schwannomas, meningioangiomatosis, peripheral neuropathies, cerebral calcifications	Café-au-lait spots (rare), hairy plaque-like lesions, cutaneous schwannoma. Less often neurofibroma	Cataract, retinal hamartoma, epiretinal membranes
Schwannomatosis (± rare forms of familial meningiomas)	INI1/ hSNF5/ BAF47/ SMARCB1	22q11.2	INI1/hSNF5/BAF47 SMARCB1: SWI/SNF chromatin-remodelling complex subunit	Non-vestibular, non-dermal schwannomas. Rarely, meningiomas and/or unilateral vestibular schwannoma	Rare examples of dermal neurofibroma reported	None
von Hippel–Lindau	VHL	3q25	pVHL: regulates hypoxia-inducible factors, such as HIF, VEGF, and erythropoietin	Haemangioblastomas of brain, spinal cord, or nerve roots; paraganglioma; brain involvement from regional spread or metastatic disease of other primaries (see other organs)	None	Retinal angiomatosis, renal cysts and carcinoma, epididymal cystadenoma, pancreatic microcystic adenoma, pancreatic neuroendocrine tumours, phaeochromocytoma, endolymphatic sac tumour, rare extraneural haemangioblastomas
Tuberous sclerosis	TSC1	9q34	Hamartin: complexes with tuberin to regulate PI3K-mTOR pathway	Subependymal giant-cell tumour, subependymal nodules, cortical tubers, radial white matter migration lines, transmantle cortical dysplasia, other malformations and dysplasias, including vascular aneurysms	Cutaneous angiofibromas ('adenoma sebaceum'), hypomelanotic macules, subungual fibromas, shagreen patches	Cardiac rhabdomyomas, hamartomatous gastrointestinal polyps, cysts of the kidney, angiomyolipoma of the kidney, lymphangioleiomyomatosis of the lung, retinal hamartomas, bone cysts, dental enamel pits, gingival fibromas
	TSC2	16p13	Tuberin: complexes with hamartin to regulate PI3K-mTOR pathway			
Li-Fraumeni	TP53	17p13	p53: transcriptional regulator regulating cell cycle arrest and apoptosis during DNA damage	Astrocytomas including glioblastoma, medulloblastoma/PNET, choroid plexus papilloma, choroid plexus carcinoma	Malignant melanoma; cutaneous carcinomas or sarcomas (rare)	Breast cancer, bone and soft-tissue sarcoma, adrenocortical carcinoma, leukaemia, other carcinomas, Wilms tumour

TABLE 44.1 Synopsis of hereditary tumour syndromes involving the nervous system (*Continued*)

Syndrome	Gene	Chromosome	Protein and major functions	Major manifestations		
				Nervous system	Skin	Other organs
Cowden	*PTEN*	10q23.2	PTEN: regulates PI3K-mTOR pathway	Dysplastic gangliocytoma of the cerebellum (Lhermitte–Duclos), macrocephaly. Possibly meningioma, pseudotumour cerebri, dural AVM, subcutaneous neuromas, ganglioneuromas, neurofibromas, oral neuromas, granular cell tumour, myasthenia gravis	Multiple tricholemmomas, fibromas	Breast, thyroid, endometrial, renal and colorectal carcinoma, multiple hamartomas, gastrointestinal polyps/ganglioneuromatosis, fibrocystic breast disease, lipomas, uterine leiomyomas, oral papillomas
Turcot type 2	*APC*	5q21	APC: regulates β-catenin pathway	Medulloblastoma, pineoblastoma	None	Familial adenomatous polyposis
Turcot type 1	Mismatch repair genes	Multiple loci	DNA mismatch repair enzymes	Glioblastoma	NF1-like manifestations	Hereditary non-polyposis colorectal cancer, NF1-like manifestations, leukaemias/lymphomas
Gorlin-Goltz (naevoid basal cell carcinoma) syndrome	*PTCH*	9q22.3	Patched: regulates sonic hedgehog pathway	Medulloblastoma, dural calcifications, other CNS and skull malformations, meningioma,* glioblastoma*	Basal cell carcinomas, palmar/plantar pits	Jaw cysts, ovarian tumours, dysmorphic features, skeletal anomalies
Rhabdoid tumour predisposition syndrome	*INI1/hSNF5/BAF47/SMARCB1*	22q11.2	INI1/hSNF5/BAF47: SMARCB1: SWI/SNF chromatin-remodelling complex subunit	Atypical teratoid/rhabdoid tumour, schwannoma,* meningioma*	None	Malignant rhabdoid tumours of kidney and soft tissue, chondrosarcoma*
Carney complex	*PRKAR1A*	17q24	PRKAR1A: regulates cyclic AMP signalling	Psammomatous melanotic schwannoma, somatotrophic pituitary adenoma	Spotty pigmentation, myxomas, epithelioid blue naevi	Cardiac myxoma, pigmented nodular adrenocortical dysplasia, fibromyxoma of breast, ductal breast adenoma, large cell calcifying Sertoli cell tumor, thyroid carcinoma, osteochondromyxoma
DICER1 syndrome	*DICER1*	14q32.13	Member of RNaseIII family, involved in generating miRNAs that regulate gene expression	CNS primitive neuroectodermal tumours including pineoblastoma, pituitary blastoma	None	Pleuropulmonary blastoma, cystic nephroma, embryonal rhabdomyosarcoma, ovarian. Sertoli-Leydig cell tumour, intraocular medulloepithelioma, Wilms tumour, and multinodular goiter
Familial spinal/clear cell meningioma*	*SMARCE1*	17q21.2	SMARCE1: SWI/SNF chromatin-remodelling complex subunit	Spinal meningiomas of clear cell type	Not known	Not known
Familial meningioma*	*SUFU*	10q24.32	SMARCE1: SWI/SNF chromatin-remodelling complex subunit	Multiple intracranial meningiomas	Not known	Not known

*Based on limited data.

ALL, acute lymphocytic leukaemia; AVM, arteriovenous malformation; CML, chronic myelogenous leukaemia; GIST, gastrointestinal stromal tumour; JXG, juvenile xanthogranuloma; MPNST, malignant peripheral nerve sheath tumour; PNET, primitive neuroectodermal tumour; VEGF, vascular endothelial growth factor.

post-pubertal or ≥0.5 cm in pre-pubertal individuals); (2) ≥2 neurofibromas of any type or ≥1 plexiform neurofibromas; (3) freckling of armpits or groin; (4) pilocytic astrocytoma of optic pathway ('optic glioma'); (5) ≥2 Lisch nodules (iris hamartomas); (6) dysplasia/absence of the sphenoid bone or dysplasia/thinning of long bone cortex; (7) first-degree relative with NF1.[43] By adulthood, about 95 per cent of patients manifest café-au-lait spots as lightly pigmented, flat, approximately symmetrical cutaneous patches. These may be present at birth, as the first manifestation, and increase in size and number until puberty. A related cutaneous lesion that usually develops later in about half of cases is the formation of freckles within intertriginous zones of the axilla or groin. About 90 per cent will develop Lisch nodules by adulthood. Skeletal lesions primarily involve dysplasias of the skull, spine and long bones, including macrocephaly, absence of the sphenoid, vertebral scalloping, scoliosis, pseudoarthrosis (mostly tibia or other long bones after non-union fractures) and long bone thinning.[120] Optic gliomas affect 1.5 to 7.5 per cent of the NF1 paediatric group and are mostly indolent.[63]

On T2-weighted magnetic resonance (MR) sequences, up to 93 per cent of affected children between 4 and 10 years of age have focal increases in signal intensity referred to as 'unidentified bright objects' (UBOs), corresponding to vacuolated myelin in the basal ganglia, brainstem and cerebellum. These are typically transient, but relatively characteristic and may be particularly helpful in diagnosing NF1 in young children who have not yet developed other pathognomonic features.[21] Apparent diffusion coefficients are also elevated in children with NF1, both in the UBOs and even in normal appearing white matter, suggesting higher water content.[119] Lastly, white matter volumes are often increased, contributing to the megalencephaly commonly noted and further supporting the presence of a myelinopathy in NF1.[19] Whether or not these alterations correlate with the learning deficits often encountered in NF1 patients remains uncertain.

Systemic tumours also occur in association with NF1 (Table 44.1), accounting for considerable morbidity and mortality.[138]

Nervous System Tumours

Tumours of the nervous system associated with NF1 include: (1) multiple neurofibromas at any site, particularly cutaneous and paraspinal examples; (2) the hallmark plexiform neurofibroma, most often affecting larger, deep nerves; (3) malignant peripheral nerve sheath tumours (MPNSTs); (4) optic pathway pilocytic and pilomyxoid astrocytomas; (5) other astrocytoma subtypes, WHO grades II–IV; (6) glioneuronal neoplasms, such as ganglioglioma, dysembryoplastic neuroepithelial tumour, and rosette-forming glioneuronal tumour.[85]

The neurofibromas that affect NF1 patients are pathologically similar to sporadic neurofibromas, with some notable exceptions. The presence of paraspinal neurofibromas, particularly multiple tumours, is essentially diagnostic and often associated with significant peripheral neuropathy.[24] Furthermore, both 'rope-like' expansions of multiple deep peripheral nerve fascicles by plexiform neurofibroma and massive diffuse appearing soft tissue neurofibromas are virtually restricted to NF1 (Figure 44.1a–d).[99]

Malignant transformation of nerve sheath tumours in NF1 patients is a major cause of morbidity and mortality, with plexiform neurofibromas being most prone. Lifetime risks of developing MPNST have been estimated at 8–13 per cent,[85] with patients harbouring large germline deletions at even greater risk.[23] Additionally, there are 3- and 20-fold increased risks of malignant transformation to MPNST in NF1 patients with subcutaneous and plexiform neurofibromas, respectively.[85] Such NF1 associated MPNSTs represent 10–50 per cent of cases, with the remainder considered *de novo*. These tumours may be histologically identical to sporadic MPNSTs (Figure 44.1e), but there is a greater tendency for malignant Triton tumour (MPNST with rhabdomyosarcomatous differentiation), glandular MPNST and nerve sheath tumour with angiosarcoma in NF1.[134] Five-year survival is also worse in NF1-associated (16–38 per cent) than sporadic MPNST (42–57 per cent), possibly because of later presentations and difficulties in clinically distinguishing malignant from benign tumours in NF1.[85]

Optic gliomas have an incidence of 1.5–20 per cent in NF1 patients, most commonly presenting in the first 6 years of life;[64,85] they show classic features of pilocytic astrocytoma, although with greater propensity towards leptomeningeal invasion and meningothelial hyperplasia than sporadic counterparts (Figure 44.1f,g).[103] These are often remarkably indolent tumours; many resolve

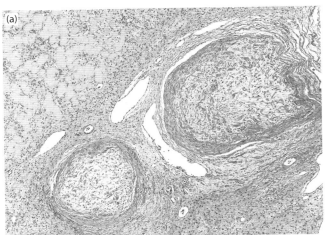
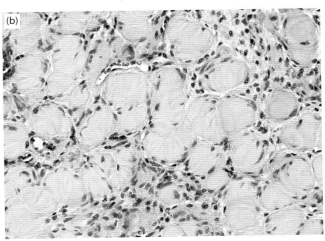

44.1 Representative tumours encountered in NF1 patients. *See next page for legend.*

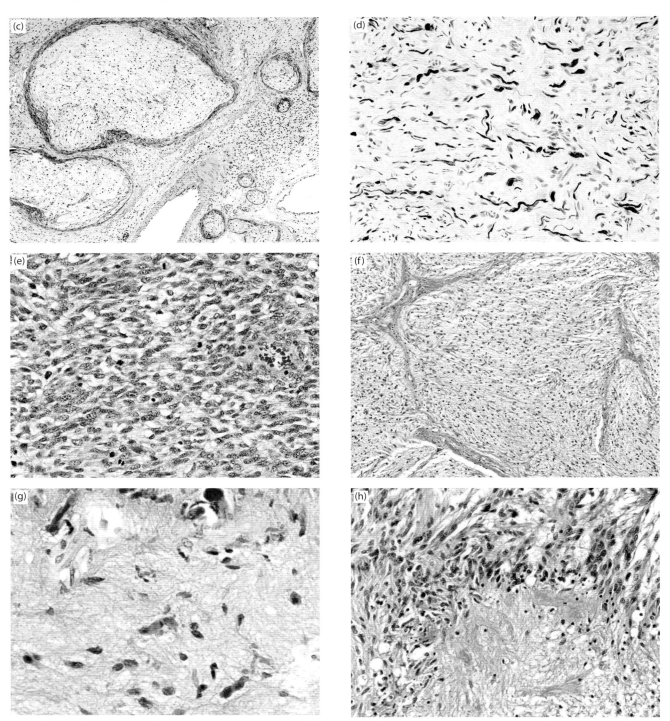

44.1 (*Continued*) Representative tumours encountered in NF1 patients. Plexiform neurofibroma **(a–d)**, showing expansion of multiple nerve fascicles (a, c: EMA highlighting perineurium), formation of tactile-like bodies (a: upper left, b), and a subset of S-100 protein positive Schwann cells **(d)**. Intraneural malignant peripheral nerve sheath tumour (MPNST) with non-specific fibrosarcoma-like spindle cell proliferation **(e)**. Optic glioma with infiltration between the normal collagenous septae of the optic nerve simulating diffuse astrocytoma **(f)**, but with presence of Rosenthal fibres elsewhere **(g)**, consistent with pilocytic astrocytoma. Glioblastoma with focus of necrosis **(h)**.

without therapy. NF1-associated pilocytic astrocytomas are frequently in the cerebellum and brain stem, especially the medulla. Patients also have increased risks of developing malignant astrocytomas,[44] particularly in those over 10 years of age or those whose optic gliomas have been treated with irradiation; such tumours are often highly aggressive (Figure 44.1h). In contrast, some seemingly diffuse parenchymal lesions appear to resolve spontaneously. The expansive pontine lesions in NF1 patients that resemble pontine gliomas on neuroimaging often follow a surprisingly indolent course.[123] However, symptomatic presentation, adult onset, and extra-optic location appear independently associated with decreased survival in NF1 patients with central nervous system (CNS) tumours.[42]

Molecular Genetics and Biology of Disease

NF1 is an autosomal dominant disorder with an estimated incidence of 1 in 3000. Half, however, have no family history, representing new mutations.[102] Penetrance is nearly 100 per cent by 5 years of age,[85] but a definitive determination is difficult, owing to intrafamilial variability of manifestations and the number of new mutations. Linkage studies demonstrate that the majority of mutations occur in the parental germline. The high mutation rate, estimated at 1 per 10 000 alleles per generation, may relate to the large size of the *NF1* gene, which is located on chromosome 17q11.2, spans about 350 kb of genomic DNA and contains 59 exons. This large size has frustrated extensive mutation screening, although over 500 pathogenic mutations have now been identified, most being kindred specific.[85] No hotspots have been identified; however, a common 1.5 Mb microdeletion involving the entire *NF1* gene is seen in 5–10 per cent of patients and is generally associated with more severe phenotype, including facial dysmorphism, mental retardation, developmental delay, increased neurofibroma burden and enhanced risk of MPNST.[23]

The *NF1* transcript is approximately 13 kb long and includes three alternatively spliced isoforms (exons 9a, 23a and 48a), thought to reflect tissue-specific and differentiation-associated regulation.[102] The gene encodes a widely expressed 220–250 kDa protein, designated neurofibromin. One major functional role for neurofibromin appears to be related to its activity as a RAS GTPase activator protein (GAP), as suggested by sequence homology to the catalytic subunits of a variety of GAP and by functional assays with the GAP-related domain (GRD). Neurofibromin loss may specifically activate the KRAS, but not the HRAS isoform, thereby activating various downstream signaling cascades and mitogenic mediators, such as AKT, ERK1/2, RAF, PI3K, mTOR and S6K.[102] There is also evidence for growth-regulatory functions outside the neurofibromin GRD.

Inactivation of the wild-type *NF1* allele with loss of neurofibromin expression is considered a critical early event in tumourigenesis. It was therefore surprising that genetically engineered mouse models with conditionally knocked out *NF1* in either Schwann cells or astrocytes do not form neurofibromas or optic gliomas respectively. In both cases, a heterozygous Nf1± state of non-neoplastic elements (similar to the human condition) was required for tumour formation.[9,137] These data suggest that growth factors secreted by mast cells, microglia or other NF1 haploinsufficient stromal elements are needed for a permissive tumourigenic environment, possibly progressing through a hyperplastic proliferation initially.[102,114] By the time neurofibromas transform to MPNSTs, numerous additional alterations have taken place, including the loss of other tumour suppressor genes, such as *TP53* and *CDKN2A/p16* and overexpression of various oncogenes, growth factors, growth factor receptors, and chemokines, such as EGFR, HER-2/neu, neuregulin-1 (NRG1), topoisomerase IIα, hepatocyte growth factor (HGF), c-Met, PDGF and CXCR4.[15,76,136]

NEUROFIBROMATOSIS 2

NF2 (synonyms: bilateral acoustic neurofibromatosis or central neurofibromatosis) is an autosomal dominant syndrome with high penetrance (0.95), an estimated incidence of 1 in 25 000 and prevalence of 1 in 60 000.[26] Over half are due to *de novo* gene mutations and therefore, have no family history; of those, 20–30 per cent represent somatic mosaics, often with too few mutation-bearing cells in the blood to be detected by standard techniques. Life expectancy is reduced considerably.

Diagnostic Criteria

Patients with NF2 develop hyperplastic/hamartomatous lesions and benign Schwann cell (schwannomas and schwannosis; less commonly, neurofibromas), meningothelial (meningiomas and meningioangiomatosis), and glial (ependymomas and glial hamartomas) proliferations. In addition, NF2 patients are susceptible to posterior lens opacities/cataracts, cerebral calcifications and peripheral neuropathies, the latter resulting not only from schwannomas, but from also tumourlets, neurofibroma-like reactive proliferations, onion bulb formation, and functional deficits related to NF2 haploinsufficiency.[8,109] Bilateral VIIIth nerve schwannomas are pathognomonic. However, given that many patients have no family history and present with other manifestations initially, the Manchester criteria have been devised to increase diagnostic sensitivity without significant loss in specificity. Other diagnostic criteria include: (1) a first-degree relative with NF2 and either a unilateral vestibular schwannoma or two of the following: meningioma, schwannoma, glioma (ependymoma), neurofibroma, posterior subcapsular lens opacity; (2) unilateral vestibular schwannoma and any two additional lesions listed in point (1); (3) multiple meningiomas and unilateral vestibular schwannoma or any two of the following: schwannoma, glioma, neurofibroma, cataract.[10] The mean age of onset, related to symptoms from VIIIth nerve schwannomas is about 22 years. Although NF2 may have manifestations in the paediatric population, its onset typically does not extend beyond the sixth decade. Café-au-lait spots can occur but are usually fewer than six; superficial plaque-like cutaneous or nodular subcutaneous lesions (typically schwannomas and only rarely neurofibromas) occur in 68 per cent and cataracts in about 38 per cent of cases.[100] The latter may be among the first detectable lesion in the paediatric group.[105] Death is often due to the disease and may be as early as the fourth decade, with worse prognosis associated with younger age at diagnosis, numerous meningiomas, and truncating *NF2* mutations.[26] There is, however, marked variability with two ends of the severity spectrum: the Gardner (mild) and Wishart (severe) variants, based on the number and types of tumours. The mild form commonly presents with bilateral vestibular schwannomas in adults, whereas the severe form often presents during childhood with other tumour types, including meningiomas.[87] There is a tendency for these variants to cluster within families and to segregate with distinct types of *NF2* gene mutations, such that nonsense and frameshift mutations are more often seen in patients with the severe phenotype. Because of the complex multiorgan manifestations, NF2 patients and their families do better with both quality and quantity of life issues when receiving care at specialized multidisciplinary centres.[27]

Vestibular Schwannomas

The most common and diagnostic neuroimaging features in NF2 are bilateral vestibular schwannomas. When small, they may require thin MR cuts through the internal auditory meatus for detection; without such detailed neuroimaging, NF2 cannot be excluded. Vestibular schwannomas in NF2 are histologically similar to sporadic schwannomas, except NF2 vestibular schwannomas tend to be multicentric, have a multinodular ('cluster of grapes') appearance, demonstrate more entrapped nerve fibres, and more often display a mosaic pattern (mixed positive and negative nuclei) of INI1 expression.[45,86] In rare cases, irradiation may be necessary to control tumour growth, although this option should be considered with caution because secondary radiation-induced malignancies are more common in NF2 than in the general population.[26]

Peripheral Schwannomas

In addition to the vestibular nerves, schwannomas may arise at any site of the body in patients with NF2. Other cranial nerves may be affected, such as the Vth, VIIth and XIIth, as well as paraspinal and cutaneous nerves. Unlike the deep-seated neurofibromas of NF1, however, peripheral schwannomas rarely involve deep nerves in a plexiform manner or undergo malignant change. Paraspinal schwannomas appear to arise from minute precursor neoplasms, dubbed 'tumourlets', that may stud the rootlets and proximal nerves.[26,113] Peripheral NF2-associated schwannomas are histologically identical to sporadic schwannomas, although the former similarly appear more infiltrative, with entrapped axons evident using neurofilament immunohistochemistry.[130] Also, the presence of a mosaic pattern of INI1 expression favours a syndromic (NF2 or schwannomatosis) schwannoma.[86] Lastly, there is a link between plexiform cutaneous schwannomas and NF2;[62] indeed, most tumours diagnosed as 'plexiform neurofibromas' in NF2 patients turn out to be plexiform schwannomas on review (Figure 44.2a,b). In contrast the majority of deep-seated plexiform schwannomas have no association with either NF1 or NF2, although their increased cellularity, proliferative activity and large size may be misinterpreted as MPNST.[3,135]

Schwannosis

Schwannosis is a non-neoplastic proliferation of Schwann cells that occurs in both NF2 and non-NF2 patients. It is typically found in the spinal cord, either at the dorsal root entry zones or in the parenchyma of the cord, but is most commonly noted in NF2 patients. In non-NF2 patients, schwannosis occurs in response to infarction or trauma, although such inciting events are not usually identifiable in NF2 patients. Clonality studies have to be performed, although a reactive process is favoured.

Meningiomas

Multiple meningiomas are also a common feature of NF2 and represent a major source of morbidity and mortality. They occasionally precede the detection of vestibular schwannomas, being the presenting feature in 20–30 per cent of patients.[26] Evidence suggests that fibroblastic or transitional meningiomas are more common in NF2 patients. However, the full range of both benign and aggressive subtypes is seen. Additionally, larger series suggest an increased incidence of atypical and malignant subtypes (Figure 44.2c,d),[87] although it is unclear whether this might represent a selection bias given that slow-growing meningiomas are less likely to be resected. Furthermore, whereas NF2 accounts for only a small fraction of adult meningiomas, up to 40 per cent of paediatric meningioma patients ultimately fulfil criteria for NF2. Therefore, it is important to screen children with meningioma for this possibility, particularly if multiple tumours are present.

Meningioangiomatosis

Meningioangiomatosis is an uncommon plaque-like cerebral mass characterized by meningothelial and fibroblastic proliferations in association with angiomatous microvascular formation (Figure 44.2e).[88] These masses may develop in the meninges, cortex or both. The relative composition of meningothelial and vascular components varies among lesions such that they may appear principally as a vascular malformation or as a primary meningothelial/fibroblastic lesion. Low or absent MIB-1 labelling and lack of meningioma-associated genetic alterations suggest a hamartomatous aetiology. The adjacent brain may manifest a spectrum of reactive and degenerative changes. Importantly, in NF2 patients, these lesions are often multiple, associated with adjacent glial microhamartomas, and are incidental findings; in contrast, sporadic meningioangiomatosis is typically single and symptomatic, presenting with seizures. Some may be associated with an overlying meningioma, although genetic data suggest that most such cases actually represent meningiomas with extensive perivascular spread, mimicking meningioangiomatosis.[88]

Gliomas

The association of NF2 with gliomas is infrequent, with the exception of spinal ependymomas. These are typically indolent, well-demarcated, intramedullary masses that are amenable to surgical excision. They nearly always affect the cervical cord, but may be multicentric. The occurrence of other gliomas, usually low-grade pilocytic astrocytomas, has been reported in NF2 patients, but some of these may represent misdiagnoses of tanycytic ependymomas.[59,121]

Glial Microhamartomas

These circumscribed clusters of cytologically atypical cells with S-100 immunoreactivity are common in the molecular and deeper layers of the cerebral cortex, basal ganglia, thalamus and cerebellum (Figure 44.2f). They are pathognomonic of NF2 and do not resemble the hamartomas seen in other neurological diseases, such as tuberous sclerosis.[88,132]

Molecular Genetics and Biology of Disease

The *NF2* gene is located on chromosome 22q12.2 and appears to act as a classic tumour suppressor.[8,26] It

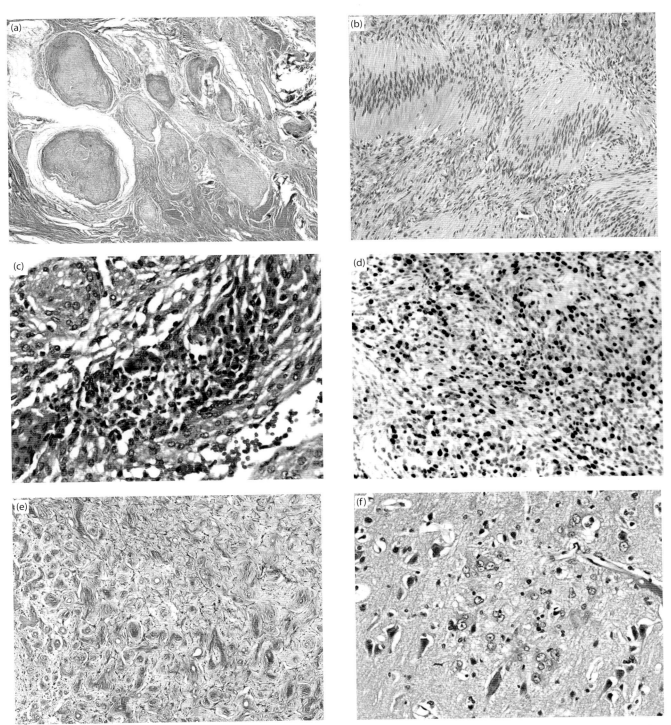

44.2 Representative lesions in NF2 patients. Cutaneous plexiform schwannoma **(a,b)**, with involvement of multiple fascicles **(a)** and foci showing Verocay bodies **(b)**. Meningioma with aggressive features includeing spontaneous necrosis **(c)** and high Ki-67 labelling index **(d)**. Meningioangiomatosis with markedly hyalinized vascular proliferations and thin ribbons of epithelioid meningothelial cells **(e)**. Glial microhamartomas consisting of clusters of bizarre-appearing astrocytes in the cortex **(f)**.

encompasses about 110 kb, including 16 constitutive and one alternatively spliced exons. The *NF2* gene is expressed in most tissues, including the nervous system, where it is present at high levels during development. The gene product, designated merlin or schwannomin, is a member of the protein 4.1 family of cytoskeletal-associated proteins, impacting PI3 kinase/Akt, Raf/MEK/ERK and mTOR signaling pathways.[26] Two merlin isoforms exist, with only isoform 1 thought to have tumour suppressor qualities.[8] Point mutations are most common, with the majority of mutations leading to truncated protein products; large deletions, duplications, and insertions may be more difficult to detect. Mutations resulting in abnormal protein expression lead to a more severe phenotype than the mutations/large deletions resulting in complete merlin loss or retention.[100] Using current multimodality approaches, mutations are detectable in nearly all familial and 59 per cent of sporadic NF2 cases.[58,128] The similarity of merlin to the 4.1 protein family of cytoskeletal-associated proteins suggests that it may play a role in mediating communication between surface membrane signalling and the cytoskeleton matrix, with its normal role in contact-dependent inhibition being a key tumourigenic function.[100] Indeed, merlin interacts with transmembrane molecules, such as CD44, in addition to having actin-binding sites. Through its interaction with a variety of other submembrane proteins, such as Na+-H+ exchanger-regulatory factor (NHE-RF), merlin probably acts to transmit growth and motility signals to the underlying cytoskeleton. In this manner, the absence of merlin in NF2-associated tumours leads to their growth potential. Conditional knockout mouse models of the *NF2* gene in Schwann cells have similarly yielded examples of schwannosis and schwannomas.[35]

SCHWANNOMATOSIS

Schwannomatosis, sometimes referred to as the third form of neurofibromatosis, is characterized by the development of multiple, mostly non-vestibular, non-dermal schwannomas in the absence of other NF2 features. The true incidence is difficult to determine, although it may be as common as NF2, accounting for up to 2.4–5 per cent of all schwannoma resections.[70] Familial (inherited) cases only account for 15–20 per cent, with the majority representing sporadic (non-inherited) examples.[90] Segmental forms involving a single limb or region of the spine represent up to a third of cases. Patients often present with localized and sometimes debilitating chronic pain, a feature not frequent in typical NF2.[100]

Notably, patients with schwannomatosis do not have germline NF2 mutations, although somatic mutations are involved in tumourigenesis. Although when originally described, neither vestibular schwannomas nor meningiomas were allowed, rare occurrences of both have now been described,[75,90,111,124] complicating the distinction from NF2. Nonetheless, bilateral vestibular schwannomas are still definitional of NF2 and are therefore, not allowed in schwannomatosis. Additionally, rare examples including cutaneous neurofibromas have also been reported.[98]

Diagnostic criteria for schwannomatosis are still developing, but the diagnosis can currently be made either molecularly or clinically. The latter require (1) ≥2 non-intradermal schwannomas, one with pathological confirmation, but no evidence of bilateral vestibular schwannomas on high-quality magnetic resonance imaging (MRI); (2) one pathologically confirmed schwannoma or intracranial meningioma and an affected first-degree relative or (3) a possible diagnosis if there are two or more nonintradermal tumours, but none are pathologically proven schwannomas, especially in association with chronic pain.[90] A cut-off age of 30 years has also been proposed to exclude bilateral vestibular schwannomas (and therefore NF2).[100] The schwannomas generally resemble their non-syndromic counterparts, but more frequently feature prominent myxoid changes, intraneural growth, peritumoural oedema and mosaic INI1 immunoreactivity.

Molecular Genetics and Biology of Disease

The gene considered responsible for schwannomatosis is the *SMARCB1* (*INI1/hSNF5/BAF47*) gene on chromosome 22q11.2, centromeric to the *NF2* gene.[49] This gene is involed in the ATP-dependent SWI/SNF chromatin remodelling complex and functional alterations are thought to lead to secondary transcriptional and epigenetic changes.[90] The protein product interacts with the E1 protein of human papilloma virus 18 and the EBNA-2 protein of Epstein–Barr virus, as well as with cellular proteins MYC, MLL (HXR), GADD34 and AKT. It is also involved in HIV-1 viral replication. Studies suggest that tumour suppressor activities include: (1) the induction of G1 arrest; (2) mitotic arrest; (3) inhibition of aneuploidy and (4) the induction of senescence.

Germline *SMARCB1* mutations are detectable in 40–50 per cent of familial and 8–10 per cent of sporadic schwannomatosis cases, where a four-hit, three-step model has now been touted.[90] The latter starts with a germline mutation (step 1, hit 1), followed by a variably sized chromosome 22q deletion that includes both *SMARCB1* and *NF2* (step 2, hits 2 and 3), culminating in a somatic mutation of the remaining *NF2* allele (step 3, hit 4). This same model has also been implicated in rare familial meningiomas.[17] Given that there is considerable overlap between sporadic schwannomatosis and mosaic NF2, genetic analysis of both *SMARCB1* and *NF2* genes in multiple tumours from the same individual is sometimes required to definitively distinguish these two possibilities.[90] A molecular diagnosis can be made by (1) ≥2 pathologically proven schwannomas or meningiomas with genetic studies showing loss of heterozygosity (LOH) for chromosome 22 and two different *NF2* mutations but a common *SMARCB1* mutation or (2) one pathologically proven schwannoma or meningioma and a germline *SMARCB1* pathogenic mutation.[90]

Given that germline *SMARCB1* mutations are also responsible for rhabdoid predisposition syndrome (RPS), it remains unclear which additional factors predispose to these very different syndromes. Because, in contrast to RPS, the germline mutations in schwannomatosis tend be non-truncating, it has been postulated that the resulting milder phenotype underlies the differences. Nonetheless, it is interesting to note that combined manifestations of both syndromes are encountered rarely.[90,116]

VON HIPPEL–LINDAU DISEASE

This autosomal dominant tumour syndrome manifests in many tissues, including the CNS, eye, kidney, adrenal medulla, pancreas, middle ear and epididymis. The incidence is estimated at 1 in 36 000 live births, up to 20 per cent representing new mutations, with penetrance over 90 per cent by 65 years of age.[53,127] As with the neurofibromatoses, it is a complex disorder with significant morbidity and mortality, which is most effectively treated at multidisciplinary specialty centres.

Diagnostic Criteria

Von Hippel–Lindau (VHL) disease is defined by the presence of retinal angiomatosis (25–60 per cent), CNS haemangioblastomas (44–72 per cent), phaeochromocytoma (10–20 per cent), pancreatic cysts (35–70 per cent), renal cysts and renal cell carcinomas (RCC; 25–60 per cent), endolymphatic sac tumours (10 per cent), and in males, bilateral papillary cystadenoma of the epididymis (25–60 per cent). Families with and without pheochromocytomas are broadly divided into type 2 and type 1 variants of VHL, respectively. The type 2 category is further stratified into 2A (haemangioblastomas, low risk of RCC), 2B (haemangioblastomas, high risk of RCC) and 2C (phaeochromocytomas only). The minimal diagnostic criteria are (1) a family history plus CNS haemangioblastoma, phaeochromocytoma or clear cell RCC, (2) ≥2 CNS haemangioblastomas or (3) one CNS haemangioblastoma plus one of the visceral tumours mentioned earlier.[66] Most lesions can be identified by computed tomography (CT) or MR imaging in patients known to be at risk, but ophthalmological screening for retinal angiomatosis is considered the least invasive early detection approach. The mean ages at clinical manifestation are 22 for endolymphatic sac tumour, 25 for retinal angiomatosis, 33 for CNS haemangioblastoma, 30 for phaeochromocytoma and 39 years for RCC.[66] Until recently, life expectancy was estimated at 50 years, with death commonly resulting from complications of RCC and CNS haemangioblastoma; however, modern screening and surveillance programmes have led to earlier detection, improving morbidity and mortality figures considerably.[127]

Central Nervous System Manifestations

Solitary or multiple haemangioblastomas are hallmarks of VHL and are seen in 80 per cent of patients.[127] As in sporadic haemangioblastomas, in VHL most are located infratentorially. In a study of 1921 CNS hemangioblastomas from 225 patients, tumours were localized to cerebellum (45 per cent), spinal cord (36 per cent), cauda equina (11 per cent), brain stem (7 per cent), supratentorial region (1 per cent) and nerve roots (0.3 per cent).[67] Roughly half remained stable over time, although the other half grew in a saltatory (most common), exponential or linear pattern; however, it was difficult to predict future behaviour. Rare extraneural examples have also been reported.[20,83] During the course of disease, additional haemangioblastomas may develop, either at the same site or remotely. Symptoms most often correlate with cyst enlargement. CNS haemangioblastomas may produce sufficient erythropoietin to induce polycythaemia. In rare cases, VHL patients develop other brain neoplasms, including cerebellar astrocytoma,[78] medulloblastoma/PNET[11] and meningioma.[51] In addition, papillary middle ear tumours, known as endolymphatic sac tumours, are relatively common and may involve the cerebellopontine angle with resultant hearing loss, tinnitus and vertigo.[52] Lastly, CNS metastases are encountered, most commonly from RCC, but occasionally from phaeochromocytoma, paraganglioma or pancreatic neuroendocrine tumour.[127]

Molecular Genetics and Biology of Disease

The *VHL* tumour suppressor gene maps to chromosome 3p25. The 852 nucleotide coding sequence is divided into three highly conserved exons and encodes a 213 amino-acid, 30-kDa protein (pVHL) that is widely expressed in both fetal and adult tissues.[53] A second 19-kDa isoform results from internal translational initiation at codon 54. Both isoforms have tumour suppressor activity, with dysfunction leading to developmental arrest.[127] The pVHL protein forms oligomeric complexes with several cellular proteins, including the elongin B and C subunits, Cul2 and Rbx1. Elongin is a transcription factor that regulates mRNA elongation, particularly during pauses in transcription. Even in the earliest tumour precursors, VHL protein dysfunction leads to hypoxia inducible factor (HIF) accumulation and activation, which then increases expression of VEGF, erythropoietin (Epo), nitric oxide synthase and glucose transporter 1.[127] In normoxic conditions, the pVHL complex targets HIF for degradation by ubiquitination, whereas in the setting of hypoxia or loss of pVHL function, HIF levels increase. The subsequent overexpression of angiogenic downstream targets, such as VEGF and PDGF-B, likely account for the hypervascularity of VHL-associated tumours and represent attractive candidates for targeted therapies, along with TGFα and EGFR, which are also overexpressed in haemangioblastomas and RCCs. In addition to its interactions with HIF, alternative functions of pVHL relate to regulation of extracellular matrix, cytoskeletal stability, cell cycle control and cellular differentiation.[53]

Mutations of the *VHL* gene occur in affected family members, as well as in roughly 30 per cent of sporadic CNS haemangioblastomas and 50 per cent of clear cell RCCs.[53,66] Promoter region hypermethylation is found in 10–20 per cent of sporadic RCC, but not in haemangioblastomas. In VHL patients, the gene is typically affected by insertions, deletions or missense mutations with subsequent loss of the wild-type allele in tumours. Genotype–phenotype associations exist, such that the vast majority of families with phaeochromocytomas (VHL type 2) harbour missense mutations, whereas most type 1 families demonstrate deletions or nonsense mutations. Molecular testing now enables detection of a germline mutation in blood from virtually all affected families, with the exception of rare mosaic patients.[33,66] The mechanism of somatic loss of the wild-type allele in tumours and benign cysts is highly variable, ranging from small deletions to monosomy 3.[36] Because even preneoplastic lesions, known as tumourlets or developmentally arrested structural elements (DASE), demonstrate biallelic inactivation, it is likely that additional genetic or epigenetic events are necessary for neoplastic transformation.[127] Another common denominator in these early lesions is the presence of haemangioblast progenitor cells, which may also represent the origin of the neoplastic 'stromal cells' in haemangioblastoma.

TUBEROUS SCLEROSIS

Tuberous sclerosis complex (TSC) is an autosomal dominant disease with high penetrance, in which hamartomatous lesions involving multiple organ systems develop at different stages of the disease.[25,40,82] TSC is the second most common hereditary tumour syndrome of the nervous system, with an incidence of 1 in 6000. Roughly 70 per cent occur sporadically as new cases and about 2 per cent are thought to be mosaic.

Diagnostic Criteria

TSC affects tissues derived from all three embryonal germ layers and invariably involves the CNS with various dysplastic and benign neoplastic lesions. The presence of multiple facial angiofibromas (previously known as 'adenoma sebaceum') and subungual fibromas ('Koenen tumours') are characteristic cutaneous lesions; however, hypomelanotic macules ('ashleaf spots') are most common and appear earliest. Shagreen patches and fibrous plaques on the forehead are also typical, but not specific. TSC was once defined by a classic triad of adenoma sebaceum, seizures and mental retardation. However, revised diagnostic criteria are more accurate and cite major features as facial angiofibromas or forehead plaques, subungual/periungual fibroma, hypomelanotic macules (at least three), shagreen patch (connective tissue naevus), retinal nodular hamartomas, tubers, subependymal nodules, subependymal giant cell astrocytoma (SEGA), cardiac rhabdomyoma, and lymphangiomyomatosis and/or renal angiomyolipoma.[40,97] Minor diagnostic features include dental enamel pits, hamartomatous rectal polyps, bone cysts, cerebral white-matter migration lines, gingival fibromas, non-renal hamartomas, retinal achromic patch, multiple renal cysts and 'confetti' skin lesions. Definite TSC can be diagnosed with two major or one major plus two minor features. Probable TSC requires one major and one minor feature, although the designation of possible TSC requires a major feature or two or more minor features. Dental examination may be particularly helpful, because enamel pits/craters and gingival fibromas are seen in nearly all TSC patients.[72] RCC, angiomyolipomas, oncocytomas, high-grade astrocytomas and chordomas have also been associated.[6,61] Angiomyolipomas occur in approximately 80 per cent of patients, representing the leading cause of death due to hemorrhage.[82]

Neurological manifestations vary considerably, but are clinically apparent in about 90 per cent. Seizure disorders (including infantile spasms) often manifesting within the first year of life (60–90 per cent), mental retardation (45 per cent) and autism (25 per cent) are most common and are roughly correlated with the location, number and size of tubers, although data also suggest functional deficits in tuber-free cortex.[25,82] Progressive signs of elevated intracranial pressure (ICP) often herald the presence of a SEGA near the foramen of Monro.

CNS Manifestations

The hallmark lesions are focal cortical dysplasias or tubers, typically centred around the corticomedullary junction, along with subependymal nodules, SEGA, radial white matter migration lines, transmantle cortical dysplasia, and less often, other malformations, such as agenesis of the corpus callosum, schizencephaly, cerebellar dysplasias and vascular aneurysms.[40] Cortical tubers are usually detectable by MRI, most being supratentorial, with cerebellar examples

seen in 8–15 per cent.[40,50] In infants, they are T1-bright and T2-dark compared to unmyelinated white matter, although in older patients, they are mostly T1-hypodense to isodense and hyperintense on T2-weighted and FLAIR sequences, with variable calcification, the latter best detected on CT scan. Positron emission tomography (PET) scans reveal increased N-acetylaspartate (NAA) and myo-inositol, consistent with neuronal reduction, gliosis and the presence of immature neurons. Grossly, they are mushroom-shaped, firm cortical expansions ('tuber' reflecting potato-like consistency) limited to one or two gyri (Figure 44.3a), although more diffuse examples manifest as hemimegalencephaly. Cortical tubers and radially oriented heterotopias are composed of enlarged, atypical and disorganized glial, neuronal and mixed glioneuronal elements (e.g. neuronomegaly, balloon cells), with astrocytosis and variable calcification (Figure 44.3b). Demonstrably epileptogenic tubers are often excised for seizure control.[84] Dysplastic cells abnormally regulate gamma-aminobutyric acid (GABA) and may overexpress glutamate transporters, such as EAAC1, potentially contributing to epilepsy.[25,40] A potential diagnostic pitfall in a subset includes increased proliferative indices and astrocytoma-like histology.[29] In the developing fetus, such dysplastic cells are often found in deep white matter, suggesting a migrational defect as part of the lesion. Distinctive CD34-immunoreactive cells are also seen in a subset of tubers, possibly representing a progenitor cell (Figure 44.3c).

The subependymal nodules and SEGAs are also characterized histologically by atypical, enlarged glioneuronal cells, and often by dystrophic calcification (Figure 44.3d). The smaller 'candle guttering' lesions are seen in about 80 per cent of patients, grossly resemble wax drippings, line the lateral ventricular walls, but only become symptomatic if they enlarge to form SEGA (5–10 per cent of patients), with hydrocephalus resulting from obstruction of the foramen of Monro. In contrast to the subependymal nodules, SEGAs are >1 cm in size and are usually contrast enhancing on MR imaging. They are composed of polygonal, epithelioid, gemistocytic or spindle-shaped cells with marked pleomorphism, abundant pink cytoplasm, eccentric nuclei, prominent nucleoli and nuclear pseudo-inclusions, often forming sweeping fascicles or ependymoma-like perivascular pseudo-rosettes (Figure 44.3d). Whereas resection is the treatment of choice, medical therapy with everolimus or other mTOR inhibitors represents a successful alternative for nonresectable cases and those with residual/recurrent masses following surgery.[18,32] Retinal astroglial hamartomas are present in about 50 per cent and may undergo calcification and cystic degeneration. However, visual impairment only accompanies macular involvement or secondary haemorrhage.

Molecular Genetics

Two genes have been identified.[73] The first, designated *TSC1*, resides on 9q34 and encodes a 8.6-kb transcript for a 1164 amino-acid hydrophilic protein, hamartin, with no clear homology to known vertebrate proteins. The second, designated *TSC2*, maps to 16p13.3 and encodes a 5.5-kb transcript for a 1807 amino-acid protein, tuberin, with partial homology to the Rap1 activator Rap1-GAP. Over 1000 mutations have been identified, with *TSC2* mutations

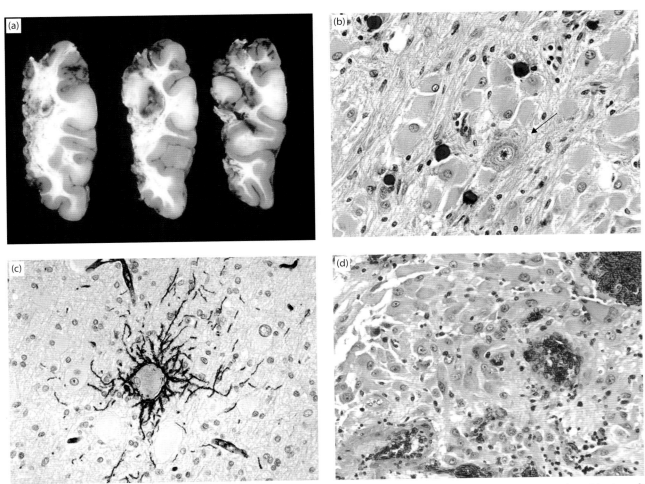

44.3 Central nervous system (CNS) lesions in patients with tuberous sclerosis. Multiple tubers are grossly evident as foci of cortical pallor and blurring of the corticomedullary junctions in this seizure resection specimen **(a)**. Microscopically, there are numerous balloon cells with glassy eosinophilic cytoplasm, neuronomegaly (arrow), and microcalcifications **(b)**. Distinctive CD34-positive cells with highly ramified cellular processes were evident, potentially representing progenitor cells **(c)**. Similar dysmorphic glioneuronal cells are seen in subependymal giant cell astrocytoma; ependymoma-like perivascular pseudorosettes (right) are also common **(d)**.

roughly five times as common as *TSC1* mutations in sporadic cases, but with equal representation in familial examples.[77] Mutations are detectable in 80–90 per cent of TSC patients, nearly all *TSC1* mutations being truncating, although 20 per cent of *TSC2* mutations are missense. *TSC2* mutations may be associated with a more severe phenotype, particularly in terms of CNS disease.[77] In tubers and SEGAs, classic second hits are often absent, although targeting of other genes in the pathway, epigenetic mechanisms and haploinsufficiency alone may play roles.[25,40,47]

Both proteins are widely expressed in human tissues. Hamartin and tuberin form heterodimers via coiled-coil regions and function together at a critical point in the PI3K signalling pathway. The tuberin–hamartin complex normally inhibits Rheb (a Ras-like GTPase) and mTOR, with these downstream regulators overexpressed in TSC. TSC1 and TSC2 proteins function in cell body size, proliferation, dendritic arborization, axonal outgrowth and targeting, neuronal migration, cortical lamination and spine formation.[77,82] This correlates well with the observed pathology including giant cells, an immature glioneuronal phenotype,

proliferative potential and migrational defects. Most studies have found remarkably similar genotypic and phenotypic features among the giant cells of SEGA, tubers and focal cortical dysplasia type IIb, suggesting that these morphologically similar cell types arise from a single CNS progenitor, most likely originating from the periventricular region. Progress has also been made using animal models, including Eker rats that harbour a natural *TSC2* mutation and genetically engineered mice.[25] For example, conditional knockout of Tsc1 in astrocytes produces not only astrocytic proliferation, but also abnormal neuronal migration and differentiation, as well as a distinct clinical phenotype that includes seizures.[122] A knockout model involving Tsc2 in Purkinje cells potentially models autism.[94]

LI–FRAUMENI SYNDROME

Li–Fraumeni syndrome (LFS) is an autosomal dominant condition in which affected family members are prone to develop a wide variety of neoplasms. Although bone and soft tissue sarcomas, breast cancer, adrenocortical carcinoma (ACC), brain tumours and leukaemia remain the classical hallmarks, further studies reveal a wider spectrum, including cancers of the lung, colorectum, stomach, prostate, ovary, pancreas, as well as lymphoma, melanoma and choroid plexus carcinoma (Table 44.1).[71,81] Penetrance is less than 20 per cent in children, but 100 per cent by age 70, with earlier onset in women, mostly due to breast cancer. The responsible gene in most families is the *TP53* gene, a tumour suppressor that is mutated somatically in many sporadic human cancers. Conversely, the majority of families with *TP53* germline mutations meet diagnostic criteria for Li–Fraumeni syndrome.[56]

Diagnostic Criteria

The diagnostic criteria used to identify LFS are (1) a proband with a sarcoma before 45 years of age; (2) at least one first-degree relative with any tumour before age 45 and (3) a second- (or first-) degree relative with cancer before age 45 or a sarcoma at any age. A modification of this definition designated Li–Fraumeni-like syndrome (LFL) is defined by (1) a proband with any childhood tumour or a sarcoma, brain tumour or adrenocortical tumour under age 45; (2) a first- (or second-) degree relative with a typical LFS tumour at any age and (3) an additional first- (or second-) degree relative with any cancer under 60 years of age. Lastly, in order to guide which individuals should be referred for genetic testing, the Chompret criteria include (1) a proband with a tumour in the LFS spectrum before age 46 and at least one first- or second-degree relative with an LFS tumour (except breast cancer if the proband has breast cancer) before age 56 or with multiple tumours; (2) a proband with multiple tumours (except multiple breast tumours), two of which are in the LFS spectrum, the first of which occurred before age 46 or (3) a proband who is diagnosed with childhood ACC or choroid plexus tumour, irrespective of family history.[71,118]

In a review of 475 tumours in 91 reported families with *TP53* germline mutations, breast carcinomas were most frequent, accounting for 24 per cent of all tumours, followed by bone sarcomas (12.6 per cent), brain tumours (12.0 per cent) and soft-tissue sarcomas (11.6 per cent).[56] ACCs are uncommon (3.6 per cent) but, if occurring in children, are nearly pathognomonic of LFS. Given the increased risk of secondary malignancies, irradiation should be avoided if at all possible.[71]

Central Nervous System Manifestations

Of a total of 475 tumours reported in families with *TP53* germline mutations, 57 were located in the nervous system. Of those classified histopathologically, 69 per cent were astrocytic (diffuse astrocytoma, anaplastic astrocytoma and glioblastoma), followed by medulloblastomas and other CNS PNETs (17 per cent). This corresponds to the observation that in sporadic brain tumours, *TP53* mutations occur preferentially in astrocytic tumours and less frequently in medulloblastomas. As in sporadic brain tumours, the age of patients with CNS tumours due to *TP53* germline mutations shows a bimodal distribution, with a first peak in childhood and a second peak in the third to fourth decades.

Molecular Genetics and Biology of Disease

The highly conserved *TP53* tumour suppressor gene, which maps to 17p13, encodes the p53 protein with five conserved domains, an N-terminal acidic domain and a C-terminal oligomerization domain. It binds in a sequence-specific manner to DNA acting as a transcriptional regulatory element. The biological functions of p53 are manifold and include growth arrest through suspension of cell-cycle progression from G1- to S-phase and induction of apoptosis as a response to DNA damage. An international IARC website has been created for cataloguing the large number of familial and sporadic *TP53* mutations, which is updated annually (http://p53.iarc.fr). Germline *TP53* mutations are detected in roughly 70 per cent of LFS, 40 per cent of LFL and 30 per cent of Chompret criteria positive individuals, the most common types being missense mutations (75 per cent), followed by small 1–4 bp deletions resulting in a frameshift (10 per cent).[71,81] A similar spectrum of somatic mutations is encountered in sporadic neoplasms. Additionally, about 80 per cent of all paediatric ACC patients carry a germline *TP53* mutation, most often involving mutations at codons 152 or 158.[71]

A number of genotype–phenotype associations exist. For instance, most LFS/LFL families with brain tumours have missense mutations in the DNA-binding loop that contacts the minor groove of DNA, whereas those with null phenotype mutations present with significantly earlier onset brain tumours.[81] In contrast, LFS/LFL families lacking *TP53* mutations rarely develop brain tumours. Lastly, families with mutations in the central core domain typically suffer more cancers and earlier onsets. Similar to somatic mutations, *TP53* germline mutations are most commonly in exons 5–8, with clusters at codons 248, 273, 245, 175 and 182. However, as many as 27 per cent of germline and 14 per cent of somatic mutations fall outside these regions. Tumours often show a loss of the wild-type allele, consistent with the classic two-hit model. Of interest, LFS associated astrocytomas often develop a rare form of *IDH1* gene mutation (R132C), in contrast to the common R132H mutation seen in sporadic counterparts.[129] In LFS-associated medulloblastomas, *CTNNB* mutations and *MYCN* gene amplifications may be more common, although not many tumours have been studied to date.[89]

COWDEN DISEASE

Cowden disease (CD; or multiple hamartoma syndrome) is an autosomal dominant disorder featuring a wide range of benign and malignant tumours. Adult onset Lhermitte–Duclos disease (LDD; dysplastic gangliocytoma of the cerebellum) is now considered pathognomonic. Other features include mucocutaneous lesions (facial trichilemmomas, acral keratoses, papillomatous papules, mucosal lesions), as well as major (macrocephaly (≥97th percentile); breast, thyroid and endometrial cancers), and minor (benign thyroid lesions, IQ ≤75, gastrointestinal (GI) hamartomas, fibrocystic breast disease, lipomas, fibromas, renal cell carcinoma or other genitourinary (GU) tumours, uterine leiomyomas, and GU malformations) diagnostic criteria.[28,96] Colorectal carcinomas have been more recently reported in roughly 16 per cent of patients.[96] Additionally, meningioma, pseudotumour cerebri, dural arteriovenous malformation, subcutaneous neuromas, ganglioneuromas, neurofibromas, oral neuromas, granular cell tumour, and myasthenia gravis have all been reported, although it is not entirely clear whether these associations are beyond chance.[28]

Roughly half are familial and half are sporadic. In the absence of a family history, classic mucocutaneous lesions, two major criteria, one major and three minor criteria, or four minor criteria are necessary for diagnosis. In patients with at least one family member involved, the diagnosis requires mucocutaneous lesions, one major criterion, two minor criteria, or a history of Bannayan–Riley–Ruvalcaba syndrome (BRRS). The cumulative risk of developing any cancer and/or LDD by age 60 is 56 per cent for men and 87 per cent for women;[79] there is an 81 per cent lifetime risk for breast cancer in women and 32 per cent risk of LDD overall.[96] In the CNS, LDD is the major manifestation. Most patients with LDD either eventually fulfill diagnostic features of CD or harbour at least one other characteristic feature. Interestingly, a subset with childhood onset LDD neither acquire other features nor have the typical germline mutations of CD.

CD is caused by germline mutations in the *PTEN* (*MMAC1/TEP1*) gene on chromosome 10q23.2, evident in roughly 80 per cent of patients, with an additional 10 per cent showing mutations in the promoter region. Nearly 100 different point, nonsense, frame shift, splice site, missense and deletion/insertion germline mutations have been reported.[28] Related disorders with similar germline mutations include BRRS (macrocephaly, lipomatosis and pigmented macules of the glans penis), proteus syndrome, proteus-like syndrome and CD-like syndrome (not fully meeting the diagnostic criteria of CD). *PTEN* encodes a molecule with phosphatase activity and homology to tensin and auxilin that functions in several cell signalling pathways, including the AKT-mTOR-S6K pathway involved in cell size regulation as also implicated in TSC. There are also at least two microRNA modifiers, miR-19a and miR-21 that may play a biologic role in determining phenotype.[28] As a tumour suppressor, *PTEN* is widely involved in sporadic malignant tumours, including malignant gliomas. Notably, however, patients with CD are not predisposed to malignant gliomas, perhaps because *PTEN* inactivation is a progression-associated, rather than an early event in sporadic glioma tumourigenesis. Biallelic inactivation is suspected in LDD: the large dysplastic neurons in most examples lose PTEN immunoreactivity and strongly express downstream regulators, such as phospho-AKT and phospho-S6K.[2] Interestingly, conditional *Pten* knockout mice develop cerebellar lesions virtually identical to human LDD and this phenotype is rescued using an mTOR inhibitor.[60]

TURCOT SYNDROME

Also known as brain tumour-polyposis syndrome, Turcot syndrome (TS) is a rare autosomal dominant or recessive disease characterized by combined tumours of the colon and brain.[46] The majority of patients have TS type 2, with colonic disease identical to familial polyposis (FAP). Accordingly, these patients have germline defects in the *APC* gene on chromosome 5q21, which is implicated in FAP. In these kindreds, the predominant CNS lesions are medulloblastomas, which develop at an incidence nearly 100-fold higher than the general population.[46] However, *APC* mutations and chromosomal 5q loss are rare in sporadic medulloblastomas.[93] Rare pineoblastomas have also been reported.[34] In contrast, a smaller number of TS type 1 families feature colonic disease similar to hereditary non-polyposis colorectal carcinoma (HNPCC), and have germline defects in DNA mismatch repair (MMR) genes (e.g. *MLH1*, *PMS2*), often yielding microsatellite instability (MSI) in associated neoplasms. In these families, glioblastoma is the primary CNS manifestation. The risk of gliomas appears greater in patients with *MSH2* than with *MLH1* mutations.[68] In addition, *PMS2* mutations are rare, but associated with a particularly severe phenotype, including gliomas. Studies suggest that the giant cell variant of glioblastoma and gliosarcomas may be overrepresented, but that associated survival times can be surprisingly long.[69] Furthermore, patients with homozygous MMR gene mutations often display NF1-like manifestations (café-au-lait spots, axillary freckling, neurofibromas, tibial pseudoarthrosis), one potential explanation being coexistent *NF1* mutations resulting from the global mismatch repair and genomic instability.[4,68] These rare patients often die of childhood leukaemias or lymphomas, rather than brain tumours. Data also suggest a possible link between TS type 1 and Muir-Torre syndrome, the latter similarly associated with germline MMR gene mutations.[41,57] Finally, it is important to note that cases do not always fall neatly into the FAP or HNPCC phenotype, with rare families having both medulloblastomas and glioblastomas.

GORLIN-GOLTZ SYNDROME

This autosomal dominant condition, also referred to as naevoid basal cell carcinoma syndrome (NBCCS), has an estimated prevalence of up to 1 in 60 000.[55] It is diagnosed by the presence of two major or one major and two minor criteria.[38,54] Major criteria are ≥2 basal cell carcinomas or a basal cell carcinoma under 20 years of age, medulloblastoma, odontogenic keratocysts of the jaw, ≥3 palmar or plantar pits, lamellar calcification of the falx cerebri, characteristic rib anomalies, ovarian fibroma, phalangeal flame-shaped radiolucencies, brachymetacarpaly in all four limbs, and a first-degree relative with NBCCS. Minor features include spina bifida, brachymetacarpaly in at least one limb, hypertelorism or telcanthus, and frontal bossing. Additionally, neuroimaging studies have demonstrated increased frequencies of falx calcification (79 per cent), bridging of the sella (68 per cent), tentorial calcification (20 per cent), abnormal frontal sinus aeration (18 per cent), asymmetric or dilated ventricles (24 per cent), cavum septum pellucidum (19 per cent), cerebral atrophy (10 per cent), agenesis/dysgenesis of the corpus callosum (10 per cent) and meningiomas (5 per cent).[54] Cystic mesenchymal hamartomas involving the skull are occasionally misinterpreted as metastatic medulloblastoma.[38] Patients are particularly hypersensitive to therapeutic irradiation and may develop secondary carcinomas. Less commonly, other CNS tumours may be radiation-associated, possibly including meningioma, astrocytoma, oligodendroglioma, and craniopharyngioma. As a result, cranial CT scans are discouraged. Roughly 2–5 per cent of NBCCS patients develop medulloblastoma and the male to female ratio is 3:1, with mean age of onset being 2 years, as opposed to 7 years in sporadic counterparts.[54,55] The possibility of NBCCS should therefore be explored in any medulloblastoma patient under 5 years of age. The vast majority belong to the desmoplastic/nodular subtype and follow a more indolent course than conventional counterparts. For this reason and the hypersensitivities already discussed, irradiation should be avoided. As with other complex syndromes, multidisciplinary care is critical for optimal management.[55]

The gene responsible for NBCCS is the *PTCH1* gene on chromosome 9q22.3, although 20–40 per cent represent *de novo* (sporadic) mutations.[55] Germline mutations are detectable in the rest, most of which result in a truncated protein.[38] The *PTCH* gene product functions in a growth signalling pathway that involves the sonic hedgehog (SHH) protein and the smoothened (SMO) protein. Accordingly, *PTCH* and *SMO* mutations have been detected in sporadic medulloblastomas; however, germline alterations leading to NBCCS have only been detected in the *PTCH* gene.

RHABDOID TUMOUR PREDISPOSITION SYNDROME

This complex familial disorder is usually characterized by germline mutations of the *INI1/hSNF5/BAF47/SMARCB1* gene on 22q11.2, predisposing patients to the formation of malignant rhabdoid tumours (MRT) of the kidney and soft tissue, as well as to atypical teratoid/rhabdoid tumours (AT/RT) and, to a lesser extent, schwannomas, meningiomas and chondrosarcomas later in life.[7,13,14,30,107] In very rare examples, germline mutations for other SWI/SNF chromatin remodelling members are implicated, notably the *SMARCA4/BRG1* gene on 19p13.2.[108,133] Most AT/RTs occur in children under 4 years of age, roughly a third being associated with germline mutations and up to 60 per cent in those presenting during the first 6 months of life.[13,14] Given these high rates of germline mutations, genetic screening is probably warranted in all newly diagnosed patients. Nevertheless, only a minority have a positive family history, with occasional parents being silent carriers. New mutations and gonadal mosaicism are thought to be the most likely explanations for this finding. Sporadic AT/RTs similarly demonstrate biallelic *INI1* inactivation and loss of protein expression in the vast majority. In comparison, however, the familial forms present at earlier ages with more extensive disease and shorter survival times.[13,14] *Smarcb1* heterozygote mouse models develop rhabdoid tumours in 5–35 per cent, as well as other often highly aggressive tumour types.[90] Lastly, rare families with both rhabdoid tumour predisposition syndrome (RPS) and schwannomatosis have been reported, providing some link between these two disorders.[116]

CARNEY COMPLEX

This autosomal dominant disorder is considered a form of multiple endocrine neoplasia (MEN) in that two or more endocrine tumours are often present. However, it is considerably more complex with additional manifestations. Approximately 70 per cent of cases are familial.[100] The diagnosis requires at least two of the following: spotty pigmentation (70–75 per cent), cutaneous or mucosal myxomas, cardiac myxoma (potentially fatal), fibromyxoma of the breast, Cushing syndrome associated with primary pigmented nodular adrenocortical dysplasia (25–30 per cent), acromegaly or gigantism from a growth hormone adenoma (10 per cent), large cell calcifying Sertoli cell tumour (often bilateral; 50 per cent of men), thyroid carcinoma, psammomatous melanotic schwannoma (PMS in 8 per cent; potentially malignant), blue naevi (especially epthelioid), ductal breast adenoma, osteochondromyxoma, an affected first-degree relative or a mutation of the *PRKAR1A* gene. Neuropathological features include psammomatous melanotic schwannoma (10 per cent) (Figure 44.4) and cerebral infarcts associated with emboli from cardiac myxomas. Additionally, pituitary abnormalities are relatively frequent and recent data suggest that somatomammotroph hyperplasia precedes growth hormone adenomas.[115] The *PRKAR1A* tumour suppressor gene (representing the CNC1 locus) maps to chromosome 17q24.2 and encodes the R1α regulatory subunit (RI-A) of protein kinase A, the main mediator of cyclic AMP signalling. Over 100 mutations in the RI-A subunit have been detected, mostly leading to R1A haploinsufficiency and involving about 60 per cent of CNC patients.[101] Most mutations are base substitutions, small deletions/insertions, or rearrangements and are either patient or family specific.[100] *PRKAR1A* mutations are found in 80 per cent of familial and 37 per cent of sporadic CNC patients. Those with mutations present earlier and more often have myxomas, skin lesions, thyroid and gonadal tumours. Exonic mutations are more often associated with acromegaly, cardiac myxoma, lentigines and PMS. Important downstream tumourigenic mediators involve Wnt signalling and cell cycle dysregulation.[101] Other disease-causing genes have yet to be identified, including a CNC2 locus on chromosome 2p16.

DICER1 SYNDROME

Also known as familial pleuropulmonaryblastoma (PPB) tumour predisposition, this syndrome is associated with the development of multiple developmental and neoplastic lesions, especially PPB, cystic nephroma (CN), ovarian Sertoli-Leydig cell tumour and multinodular goiters.[31] Congenital malformations such as pulmonary sequestration and transposition of the great arteries (TGA) are also described rarely. Nonetheless, the spectrum of associated alterations continues to expand, including occasional intracranial manifestations, such as CNS primitive neuroectodermal tumour (PNET), pineoblastoma and pituitary blastoma, the latter typically presenting as Cushing disease in infants under 2 years of age with a histologically distinctive pituitary mass characterized by proliferation of developmentally arrested corticotroph cells.[16,31,106,110] Over 40 different germline mutations have been identified in the *DICER1* gene on 14q32.13. Despite the germline alteration, family history is often negative or inconclusive.[107] The *DICER1* gene transcribes a member of the RNaseIII family, cleaving precursor molecules into small mature double-stranded noncoding RNAs (miRNAs)

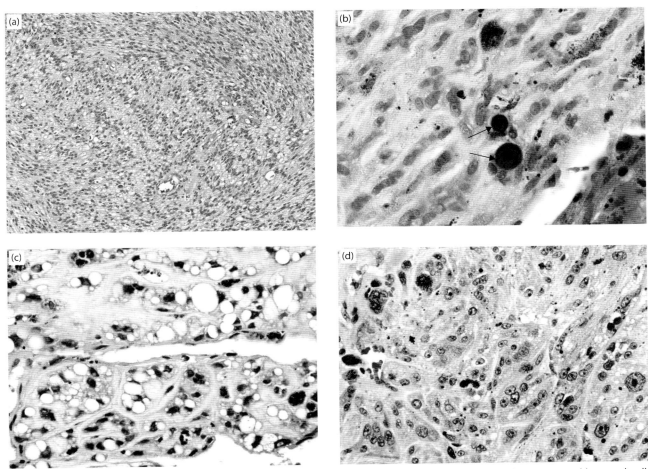

44.4 Psammomatous melanotic schwannoma in a patient with Carney complex. Like ordinary schwannomas, Verocay bodies were seen focally **(a)**. Unlike conventional schwannomas, there was melanin pigment **(b–d)**, psammoma bodies (b, arrows), lipidization **(c)** and foci showing malignant cytologic features **(d)**.

that regulate gene expression in a wide variety of pathways, particularly during early development. Although homozygous knockout is embryologically lethal, hemizygous knock-out animal models yield phenotypes resembling the human counterpart.

OTHER HEREDITARY BRAIN TUMOUR SYNDROMES

Pituitary adenomas are common endocrine neoplasms that may be seen in a number of hereditary syndromes,[12,48,80] including some that have already been discussed (see Chapter 41). In rare examples, patients with familial retinoblastoma develop pineoblastomas or other central PNETs

('trilateral retinoblastoma') associated with inactivation of the *RB* gene.[91] Patients with one form of progeria, Werner's syndrome, have been reported to have a slightly higher likelihood of developing meningiomas. Also, a prostate and brain cancer susceptibility gene (*CAPB*) has been localized to chromosome 1p36.[125] A number of families have been described with isolated predisposition to brain tumours, particularly malignant gliomas, or with predispositions to brain and systemic neoplasms that do not fall clearly into a known syndrome.[126] Some of these are associated with specific high-risk single nucleotide polymorphisms.[37,65] Rare *CDKN2A* germline mutations have also been described.[117] Lastly, familial meningiomas have been described outside the setting of NF2 or schwannomatosis; rare associations have included germline mutations of *SUFU* and *SMARCE4*.[1,112]

REFERENCES

1. Aavikko M, Li SP, Saarinen S, *et al.* Loss of SUFU Function in familial multiple meningioma. *Am J Hum Genet* 2012;**91**:520–6.
2. Abel TW, Baker SJ, Fraser MM, *et al.* Lhermitte–Duclos disease: a report of 31 cases with immunohistochemical analysis of the PTEN/AKT/mTOR pathway. *J Neuropathol Exp Neurol* 2005;**64**:341–9.
3. Agaram NP, Prakash S, Antonescu CR. Deep-seated plexiform schwannoma: a pathologic study of 16 cases and comparative analysis with the superficial variety. *Am J Surg Pathol* 2005;**29**:1042–8.
4. Agostini M, Tibiletti MG, Lucci-Cordisco E *et al.* Two PMS2 mutations in a Turcot syndrome family with small bowel cancers. *Am J Gastroenterol* 2005;**100**:1886–91.
5. Alaraj AM, Valyi-Nagy T, Roitberg B. Double phakomatosis; neurofibromatosis type-1 and tuberous

sclerosis. *Acta Neurochir (Wien)* 2007;**149**:505–9; discussion 9.

6. Al-Saleem T, Wessner LL, Scheithauer BW, *et al.* Malignant tumors of the kidney, brain, and soft tissues in children and young adults with the tuberous sclerosis complex. *Cancer* 1998;**83**:2208–16.

7. Ammerlaan AC, Houben MP, Tijssen CC, Wesseling P, Hulsebos TJ. Secondary meningioma in a long-term survivor of atypical teratoid/rhabdoid tumour with a germline INI1 mutation. *Childs Nerv Syst* 2008;**24**:855–7.

8. Asthagiri AR, Parry DM, Butman JA, *et al.* Neurofibromatosis type 2. *Lancet* 2009;**373**:1974–86.

9. Bajenaru ML, Hernandez MR, Perry A, *et al.* Optic nerve glioma in mice requires astrocyte Nf1 gene inactivation and Nf1 brain heterozygosity. *Cancer Res* 2003;**63**:8573–7.

10. Baser ME, Friedman JM, Wallace AJ, *et al.* Evaluation of clinical diagnostic criteria for neurofibromatosis 2. *Neurology* 2002;**59**:1759–65.

11. Becker R, Bauer BL, Mennel HD, Plate KH. Cerebellar primitive neuroectodermal tumor with multipotent differentiation in a family with von Hippel–Lindau disease. Case report. *Clin Neuropathol* 1993;**12**:107–11.

12. Beckers A, Aaltonen LA, Daly AF, Karhu A. Familial isolated pituitary adenomas (FIPA) and the pituitary adenoma predisposition due to mutations in the aryl hydrocarbon receptor interacting protein (AIP) Gene. *Endocr Rev* 2013;**34**:239–77.

13. Bourdeaut F, Lequin D, Brugieres L, *et al.* Frequent hSNF5/INI1 germline mutations in patients with rhabdoid tumor. *Clin Cancer Res* 2011;**17**:31–8.

14. Bruggers CS, Bleyl SB, Pysher T, *et al.* Clinicopathologic comparison of familial versus sporadic atypical teratoid/rhabdoid tumors (AT/RT) of the central nervous system. *Pediatr Blood Cancer* 2011;**56**:1026–31.

15. Carroll SL. Molecular mechanisms promoting the pathogenesis of Schwann cell neoplasms. *Acta Neuropathol* 2012;**123**:321–48.

16. Choong CS, Priest JR, Foulkes WD. Exploring the endocrine manifestations of DICER1 mutations. *Trends Mol Med* 2012;**18**:503–5.

17. Christiaans I, Kenter SB, Brink HC, *et al.* Germline SMARCB1 mutation and somatic NF2 mutations in familial multiple meningiomas. *J Med Genet* 2011;**48**:93–7.

18. Curran MP. Everolimus in patients with subependymal giant cell astrocytoma associated with tuberous sclerosis complex. *Paediatr Drugs* 2011;**14**:51–60.

19. Cutting LE, Cooper KL, Koth CW, *et al.* Megalencephaly in NF1: predominantly white matter contribution and mitigation by ADHD. *Neurology* 2002;**59**:1388–94.

20. Deb P, Pal S, Dutta V, *et al.* Adrenal haemangioblastoma presenting as phaeochromocytoma: a rare manifestation of extraneural hemangioblastoma. *Endocr Pathol* 2012;**23**:187–90.

21. DeBella K, Poskitt K, Szudek J, Friedman JM. Use of 'unidentified bright objects' on MRI for diagnosis of neurofibromatosis 1 in children. *Neurology* 2000;**54**:1646–51.

22. De Luca A, Bottillo I, Sarkozy A, *et al.* NF1 gene mutations represent the major molecular event underlying neurofibromatosis-Noonan syndrome. *Am J Hum Genet* 2005;**77**:1092–101.

23. De Raedt T, Brems H, Wolkenstein P, *et al.* Elevated risk for MPNST in NF1 microdeletion patients. *Am J Hum Genet* 2003;**72**:1288–92.

24. Drouet A, Wolkenstein P, Lefaucheur JP, *et al.* Neurofibromatosis 1-associated neuropathies: a reappraisal. *Brain* 2004;**127**:1993–2009.

25. Ess KC. Tuberous sclerosis complex: a brave new world? *Curr Opin Neurol* 2010;**23**:189–93.

26. Evans DG. Neurofibromatosis type 2 (NF2): a clinical and molecular review. *Orphanet J Rare Dis* 2009;**4**:16.

27. Evans DG, Baser ME, O'Reilly B, *et al.* Management of the patient and family with neurofibromatosis 2: a consensus conference statement. *Br J Neurosurg* 2005;**19**:5–12.

28. Farooq A, Walker LJ, Bowling J, Audisio RA. Cowden syndrome. *Cancer Treat Rev* 2010;**36**:577–83.

29. Fischer I, Cunliffe C, Bollo RJ, *et al.* Glioma-like proliferation within tissues excised as tubers in patients with tuberous sclerosis complex. *Acta Neuropathol* 2008;**116**:67–77.

30. Forest F, David A, Arrufat S, *et al.* Conventional chondrosarcoma in a survivor of rhabdoid tumor: enlarging the spectrum of tumors associated with SMARCB1 germline mutations. *Am J Surg Pathol* [Research Support, Non-U.S. Gov't]. 2012;**36**:1892–6.

31. Foulkes WD, Bahubeshi A, Hamel N, *et al.* Extending the phenotypes associated with DICER1 mutations. *Hum Mutat* 2011;**32**:1381–4.

32. Franz DN, Agricola KD, Tudor CA, Krueger DA. Everolimus for tumor recurrence after surgical resection for subependymal giant cell astrocytoma associated with tuberous sclerosis complex. *J Child Neurol* 2013;**28**:602–7.

33. Friedrich CA. Genotype-phenotype correlation in von Hippel-Lindau syndrome. *Hum Mol Genet* 2001;**10**:763–7.

34. Gadish T, Tulchinsky H, Deutsch AA, Rabau M. Pinealoblastoma in a patient with familial adenomatous polyposis: variant of Turcot syndrome type 2? Report of a case and review of the literature. *Dis Colon Rectum* 2005;**48**:2343–6.

35. Giovannini M, Robanus-Maandag E, van der Valk M, *et al.* Conditional biallelic Nf2 mutation in the mouse promotes manifestations of human neurofibromatosis type 2. *Genes Dev* 2000;**14**:1617–30.

36. Glasker S, Sohn TS, Okamoto H, *et al.* Second hit deletion size in von Hippel–Lindau disease. *Ann Neurol* 2006;**59**:105–10.

37. Goodenberger ML, Jenkins RB. Genetics of adult glioma. *Cancer Genet* 2012;**205**:613–21.

38. Gorlin RJ. Nevoid basal cell carcinoma (Gorlin) syndrome. *Genet Med* 2004;**6**:530–9.

39. Gorlin R, Cohen MJ, Levine M. The neurofibromatoses (NfI Recklinghausen type, NfII acoustic type, other types). In: Gorlin R, Cohen MJ, Levine M, editors. *Syndromes of the head and neck.* Oxford: Oxford University Press; 1992: 392–9.

40. Grajkowska W, Kotulska K, Jurkiewicz E, Matyja E. Brain lesions in tuberous sclerosis complex. Review. *Folia Neuropathol* 2010;**48**:139–49.

41. Grandhi R, Deibert CP, Pirris SM, Lembersky B, Mintz AH. Simultaneous Muir–Torre and Turcot's syndrome: A case report and review of the literature. *Surg Neurol Int* 2013;**4**:52.

42. Guillamo JS, Creange A, Kalifa C, *et al.* Prognostic factors of CNS tumours in neurofibromatosis 1 (NF1): a retrospective study of 104 patients. *Brain* 2003;**126**:152–60.

43. Gutmann DH, Aylsworth A, Carey JC, *et al.* The diagnostic evaluation and multidisciplinary management of neurofibromatosis 1 and neurofibromatosis 2. *JAMA* 1997;**278**:51–7.

44. Gutmann DH, James CD, Poyhonen M, *et al.* Molecular analysis of astrocytomas presenting after age 10 in individuals with NF1. *Neurology* 2003;**61**:1397–400.

45. Hamada Y, Iwaki T, Fukui M, Tateishi J. A comparative study of embedded nerve tissue in six NF2-associated schwannomas and 17 nonassociated NF2 schwannomas. *Surg Neurol* 1997;**48**:395–400.

46. Hamilton SR, Liu B, Parsons RE, *et al.* The molecular basis of Turcot's syndrome. *N Engl J Med* 1995;**332**:839–47.

47. Han S, Santos TM, Puga A, *et al.* Phosphorylation of tuberin as a novel mechanism for somatic inactivation of the tuberous sclerosis complex proteins in brain lesions. *Cancer Res* 2004;**64**:812–6.

48. Horvath A, Stratakis CA. Clinical and molecular genetics of acromegaly: MEN1, Carney complex, McCune–Albright syndrome, familial acromegaly and genetic defects in sporadic tumors. *Rev Endocr Metab Disord* 2008;**9**:1–11.

49. Hulsebos TJ, Plomp AS, Wolterman RA, *et al.* Germline mutation of INI1/SMARCB1 in familial schwannomatosis. *Am J Hum Genet* 2007;**80**:805–10.

50. Kalantari BN, Salamon N. Neuroimaging of tuberous sclerosis: spectrum of pathologic findings and frontiers in imaging. *AJR Am J Roentgenol* 2008;**190**:W304–9.

51. Kanno H, Yamamoto I, Yoshida M, Kitamura H. Meningioma showing VHL gene inactivation in a patient with von Hippel–Lindau disease. *Neurology* 2003;**60**:1197–9.

52. Kim HJ, Butman JA, Brewer C, *et al.* Tumors of the endolymphatic sac in patients with von Hippel-Lindau disease: implications for their natural history, diagnosis, and treatment. *J Neurosurg* 2005;**102**:503–12.

53. Kim WY, Kaelin WG. Role of VHL gene mutation in human cancer. *J Clin Oncol* 2004;**22**:4991–5004.

54. Kimonis VE, Mehta SG, Digiovanna JJ, Bale SJ, Pastakia B. Radiological features in 82 patients with nevoid basal cell carcinoma (NBCC or Gorlin) syndrome. *Genet Med* 2004;**6**:495–502.

55. Kiwilsza M, Sporniak-Tutak K. Gorlin–Goltz syndrome – a medical condition requiring a multidisciplinary approach. *Med Sci Monit* 2012;**18**:RA145–53.

56. Kleihues P, Schauble B, zur Hausen A, Esteve J, Ohgaki H. Tumors associated with p53 germline mutations: a synopsis of 91 families. *Am J Pathol* 1997;**150**:1–13.

57. Kleinerman R, Marino J, Loucas E. Muir–Torre syndrome/Turcot

syndrome overlap? A patient with sebaceous carcinoma, colon cancer, and a malignant astrocytoma. *Dermatol Online J* 2012;**18**:3.

58. Kluwe L, Nygren AO, Errami A, *et al.* Screening for large mutations of the NF2 gene. *Genes Chromosomes Cancer* 2005;**42**:384–91.

59. Kobata H, Kuroiwa T, Isono N, *et al.* Tanycytic ependymoma in association with neurofibromatosis type 2. *Clin Neuropathol* 2001;**20**:93–100.

60. Kwon CH, Zhu X, Zhang J, Baker SJ. mTor is required for hypertrophy of Pten-deficient neuronal soma *in vivo. Proc Natl Acad Sci U S A* 2003;**100**:12923–8.

61. Lee-Jones L, Aligianis I, Davies PA, *et al.* Sacrococcygeal chordomas in patients with tuberous sclerosis complex show somatic loss of TSC1 or TSC2. *Genes Chromosomes Cancer* 2004;**41**:80–5.

62. Lim HS, Jung J, Chung KY. Neurofibromatosis type 2 with multiple plexiform schwannomas. *Int J Dermatol* 2004;**43**:336–40.

63. Listernick R, Louis DN, Packer RJ, Gutmann DH. Optic pathway gliomas in children with neurofibromatosis 1: consensus statement from the NF1 Optic Pathway Glioma Task Force. *Ann Neurol* 1997;**41**:143–9.

64. Listernick R, Ferner RE, Liu GT, Gutmann DH. Optic pathway gliomas in neurofibromatosis-1: controversies and recommendations. *Ann Neurol* 2007;**61**:189–98.

65. Liu Y, Melin BS, Rajaraman P, *et al.* Insight in glioma susceptibility through an analysis of 6p22.3, 12p13.33-12.1, 17q22–23.2 and 18q23 SNP genotypes in familial and non-familial glioma. *Hum Genet* 2012;**131**:1507.

66. Lonser RR, Glenn GM, Walther M, *et al.* von Hippel–Lindau disease. *Lancet* 2003;**361**:2059–67.

67. Lonser RR, Huntoon K, Butman JA, *et al.* 145 Natural history of central nervous system hemangioblastomas in von hippel-lindau disease. *Neurosurgery* 2013;**60**:168.

68. Lucci-Cordisco E, Zito I, Gensini F, Genuardi M. Hereditary nonpolyposis colorectal cancer and related conditions. *Am J Med Genet A* 2003;**122**:325–34.

69. Lusis EA, Travers S, Jost SC, Perry A. Glioblastomas with giant cell and sarcomatous features in patients with Turcot syndrome type 1: a clinicopathological study of 3 cases. *Neurosurgery* 2010;**67**:811–7.

70. MacCollin M, Chiocca EA, Evans DG, *et al.* Diagnostic criteria for schwannomatosis. *Neurology* 2005;**64**:1838–45.

71. Mai PL, Malkin D, Garber JE, *et al.* Li-Fraumeni syndrome: report of a clinical research workshop and creation of a research consortium. *Cancer Genet* 2012;**205**:479–87.

72. Maria BL, Deidrick KM, Roach ES, Gutmann DH. Tuberous sclerosis complex: pathogenesis, diagnosis, strategies, therapies, and future research directions. *J Child Neurol.* 2004;**19**:632–42.

73. McCall T, Chin SS, Salzman KL, Fults DW. Tuberous sclerosis: a syndrome of incomplete tumor suppression. *Neurosurg Focus* 2006;**20**:E3.

74. Menon AG, Anderson KM, Riccardi VM, *et al.* Chromosome 17p deletions and p53 gene mutations associated with the formation of malignant neurofibrosarcomas in von Recklinghausen neurofibromatosis. *Proc Natl Acad Sci U S A* 1990;**87**:5435–9.

75. Merker VL, Esparza S, Smith MJ, Stemmer-Rachamimov A, Plotkin SR. Clinical features of schwannomatosis: a retrospective analysis of 87 patients. *Oncologist* 2012;**17**:1317–22.

76. Mo W, Chen J, Patel A, *et al.* CXCR4/CXCL12 mediate autocrine cell-cycle progression in NF1-associated malignant peripheral nerve sheath tumors. *Cell* 2013;**152**:1077–90.

77. Napolioni V, Moavero R, Curatolo P. Recent advances in neurobiology of tuberous sclerosis complex. *Brain Dev* 2009;**31**:104–13.

78. Ng HK, Tse JY, Poon WS. Cerebellar astrocytoma associated with von Hippel-Lindau disease: case report with molecular findings. *Br J Neurosurg* 1999;**13**:504–7.

79. Nieuwenhuis MH, Kets CM, Murphy-Ryan M, *et al.* Cancer risk and genotype-phenotype correlations in PTEN hamartoma tumor syndrome. *Fam Cancer* 2014;**13**:57–63.

80. Nunes VS, Souza GL, Perone D, Conde SJ, Nogueira CR. Frequency of multiple endocrine neoplasia type 1 in a group of patients with pituitary adenoma: genetic study and familial screening. *Pituitary* 2014;**17**:30–7.

81. Olivier M, Goldgar DE, Sodha N, *et al.* Li-Fraumeni and related syndromes: correlation between tumor type, family structure, and TP53 genotype. *Cancer Res* 2003;**63**:6643–50.

82. Orlova KA, Crino PB. The tuberous sclerosis complex. *Ann N Y Acad Sci* 2010;**1184**:87–105.

83. Panelos J, Beltrami G, Capanna R, Franchi A. Primary capillary hemangioblastoma of bone: report of a case arising in the sacrum. *Int J Surg Pathol* 2010;**18**:580–3.

84. Pascual-Castroviejo I. Neurosurgical treatment of tuberous sclerosis complex lesions. *Childs Nerv Syst* 2011;**27**:1211–9.

85. Patil S, Chamberlain RS. Neoplasms associated with germline and somatic NF1 gene mutations. *Oncologist* Review 2012;**17**:101–16.

86. Patil S, Perry A, Maccollin M, *et al.* Immunohistochemical analysis supports a role for INI1/SMARCB1 in hereditary forms of schwannomas, but not in solitary, sporadic schwannomas. *Brain Pathol* 2008;**18**:517–9.

87. Perry A, Giannini C, Raghavan R, *et al.* Aggressive phenotypic and genotypic features in pediatric and NF2-associated meningiomas: a clinicopathologic study of 53 cases. *J Neuropathol Exp Neurol* 2001;**60**:994–1003.

88. Perry A, Kurtkaya-Yapicier O, Scheithauer BW, *et al.* Insights into meningioangiomatosis with and without meningioma: a clinicopathologic and genetic series of 24 cases with review of the literature. *Brain Pathol* 2005;**15**:55–65.

89. Pfaff E, Remke M, Sturm D, *et al.* TP53 mutation is frequently associated with CTNNB1 mutation or MYCN amplification and is compatible with long-term survival in medulloblastoma. *J Clin Oncol* 2010;**28**:5188–96.

90. Plotkin SR, Blakeley JO, Evans DG, *et al.* Update from the 2011 International Schwannomatosis Workshop: From genetics to diagnostic criteria. *Am J Med Genet A* 2013;**161**:405–16.

91. Plowman PN, Pizer B, Kingston JE. Pineal parenchymal tumours: II. On the aggressive behaviour of pineoblastoma in patients with an inherited mutation of the RB1 gene. *Clin Oncol (R Coll Radiol)* 2004;**16**:244–7.

92. Probst A, Lotz M, Heitz P. Von Hippel-Lindau's disease, syringomyelia and multiple endocrine tumors: a complex neuroendocrinopathy. *Virchows Arch A Pathol Anat Histol* 1978;**378**:265–72.

93. Raffel C. Medulloblastoma: molecular genetics and animal models. *Neoplasia* 2004;**6**:310–22.

94. Reith RM, McKenna J, Wu H, *et al.* Loss of Tsc2 in Purkinje cells is associated with autistic-like behavior in a mouse model of tuberous sclerosis complex. *Neurobiol Dis* 2012;**51**:93–103.

95. Riccardi V. *Neurofibromatosis: phenotype, natural history and pathogenesis,* 2nd edn. Baltimore, MD: Johns Hopkins University Press, 1992.

96. Riegert-Johnson DL, Gleeson FC, Roberts M, *et al.* Cancer and Lhermitte–Duclos disease are common in Cowden syndrome patients. *Hered Cancer Clin Pract* 2010;**8**:6.

97. Roach ES, DiMario FJ, Kandt RS, Northrup H. Tuberous Sclerosis Consensus Conference: recommendations for diagnostic evaluation. National Tuberous Sclerosis Association. *J Child Neurol* 1999;**14**:401–7.

98. Rodriguez FJ, Scheithauer BW, George D, *et al.* Superficial neurofibromas in the setting of schwannomatosis: nosologic implications. *Acta Neuropathol* 2011;**121**:663–8.

99. Rodriguez FJ, Folpe AL, Giannini C, Perry A. Pathology of peripheral nerve sheath tumors: diagnostic overview and update on selected diagnostic problems. *Acta Neuropathol* 2012;**123**:295–319.

100. Rodriguez FJ, Stratakis CA, Evans DG. Genetic predisposition to peripheral nerve neoplasia: diagnostic criteria and pathogenesis of neurofibromatoses, Carney complex, and related syndromes. *Acta Neuropathol* 2012;**123**:349–67.

101. Rothenbuhler A, Stratakis CA. Clinical and molecular genetics of Carney complex. *Best Pract Res Clin Endocrinol Metab* 2010;**24**:389–99.

102. Rubin JB, Gutmann DH. Neurofibromatosis type 1 – a model for nervous system tumour formation? *Nat Rev Cancer* 2005;**5**:557–64.

103. Rubinstein LJ. Pathological features of optic nerve and chiasmatic gliomas. *Neurofibromatosis* 1988;**1**:152–8.

104. Ruggieri M. The different forms of neurofibromatosis. *Childs Nerv Syst* 1999;**15**:295–308.

105. Ruggieri M, Iannetti P, Polizzi A, *et al.* Earliest clinical manifestations and natural history of neurofibromatosis type 2 (NF2) in childhood: a study of 24 patients. *Neuropediatrics* 2005;**36**:21–34.

106. Sabbaghian N, Hamel N, Srivastava A, *et al.* Germline DICER1 mutation and associated loss of heterozygosity in a pineoblastoma. *J Med Genet* 2012;**49**:417–9.

107. Schiffman JD, Geller JI, Mundt E, *et al.* Update on pediatric cancer predisposition syndromes. *Pediatr Blood Cancer* 2013;**60**:1247–52.

108. Schneppenheim R, Fruhwald MC, Gesk S, et al. Germline nonsense mutation and somatic inactivation of SMARCA4/BRG1 in a family with rhabdoid tumor predisposition syndrome. *Am J Hum Genet* 2010;**86**:279–84.

109. Schulz A, Baader SL, Niwa-Kawakita M, et al. Merlin isoform 2 in neurofibromatosis type 2-associated polyneuropathy. *Nat Neurosci* 2013;**16**:426–33.

110. Slade I, Bacchelli C, Davies H, et al. DICER1 syndrome: clarifying the diagnosis, clinical features and management implications of a pleiotropic tumour predisposition syndrome. *J Med Genet* 2011;**48**:273–8.

111. Smith MJ, Kulkarni A, Rustad C, et al. Vestibular schwannomas occur in schwannomatosis and should not be considered an exclusion criterion for clinical diagnosis. *Am J Med Genet A.* 2012;**158A**:215–9.

112. Smith MJ, O'Sullivan J, Bhaskar SS, et al. Loss-of-function mutations in SMARCE1 cause an inherited disorder of multiple spinal meningiomas. *Nat Genet* 2013;**45**:295–8.

113. Stemmer-Rachamimov AO, Ino Y, Lim ZY, et al. Loss of the NF2 gene and merlin occur by the tumorlet stage of schwannoma development in neurofibromatosis 2. *J Neuropathol Exp Neurol* 1998;**57**:1164–7.

114. Stemmer-Rachamimov AO, Louis DN, Nielsen GP, et al. Comparative pathology of nerve sheath tumors in mouse models and humans. *Cancer Res* 2004;**64**: 3718–24.

115. Stergiopoulos SG, Abu-Asab MS, Tsokos M, Stratakis CA. Pituitary pathology in Carney complex patients. *Pituitary* 2004;**7**:73–82.

116. Swensen JJ, Keyser J, Coffin CM et al. Familial occurrence of schwannomas and malignant rhabdoid tumour associated with a duplication in SMARCB1. *J Med Genet* 2009;**46**:68–72.

117. Tachibana I, Smith JS, Sato K, et al. Investigation of germline PTEN, p53, p16(INK4A)/p14(ARF) and CDK4 alterations in familial glioma. *Am J Med Genet* 2000;**92**:136–41.

118. Tinat J, Bougeard G, Baert-Desurmont S, et al. 2009 version of the Chompret criteria for Li Fraumeni syndrome.

J Clin Oncol 2009;**27**:e108–9; author reply e10.

118a. Tishler PV. A family with coexistent von Recklinghausen's neurofibromatosis and von Hippel-Lindau's disease. Diseases possibly derived from a common gene. *Neurology* 1975 Sep;25(9):840–4.

119. Tognini G, Ferrozzi F, Garlaschi G, et al. Brain apparent diffusion coefficient evaluation in pediatric patients with neurofibromatosis type 1. *J Comput Assist Tomogr* 2005;**29**:298–304.

120. Tsirikos AI, Saifuddin A, Noordeen MH. Spinal deformity in neurofibromatosis type-1: diagnosis and treatment. *Eur Spine J* 2005;**14**:427–39.

121. Ueki K, Sasaki T, Ishida T, Kirino T. Spinal tanycytic ependymoma associated with neurofibromatosis type 2 – case report. *Neurol Med Chir (Tokyo)* 2001;**41**:513–6.

122. Uhlmann EJ, Wong M, Baldwin RL, et al. Astrocyte-specific TSC1 conditional knockout mice exhibit abnormal neuronal organization and seizures. *Ann Neurol* 2002;**52**:285–96.

123. Ullrich NJ, Raja AI, Irons MB, Kieran MW, Goumnerova L. Brainstem lesions in neurofibromatosis type 1. *Neurosurgery* 2007;**61**:762–6; discussion 6–7.

124. van den Munckhof P, Christiaans I, Kenter SB, Baas F, Hulsebos TJ. Germline SMARCB1 mutation predisposes to multiple meningiomas and schwannomas with preferential location of cranial meningiomas at the falx cerebri. *Neurogenetics* 2012;**13**:1–7.

125. Verhage BA, Aben KK, Witjes JA, et al. Site-specific familial aggregation of prostate cancer. *Int J Cancer* 2004;**109**:611–7.

126. von Koch CS, Gulati M, Aldape K, Berger MS. Familial medulloblastoma: case report of one family and review of the literature. *Neurosurgery* 2002;**51**:227–33; discussion 33.

127. Vortmeyer AO, Falke EA, Glasker S, Li J, Oldfield EH. Nervous system involvement in von Hippel-Lindau disease: pathology and mechanisms. *Acta Neuropathol* 2013;**125**:333–50.

128. Wallace AJ, Watson CJ, Oward E, Evans DG, Elles RG. Mutation scanning of the NF2 gene: an improved service based on meta-PCR/sequencing, dosage analysis,

and loss of heterozygosity analysis. *Genet Test* 2004;**8**:368–80.

129. Watanabe T, Vital A, Nobusawa S, Kleihues P, Ohgaki H. Selective acquisition of IDH1 R132C mutations in astrocytomas associated with Li-Fraumeni syndrome. *Acta Neuropathol* 2009;**117**:653–6.

130. Wechsler J, Lantieri L, Zeller J, et al. Aberrant axon neurofilaments in schwannomas associated with phacomatoses. *Virchows Arch* 2003;**443**:768–73.

131. Wheeler PG, Sadeghi-Nejad A. Simultaneous occurrence of neurofibromatosis type 1 and tuberous sclerosis in a young girl. *Am J Med Genet A* 2005;**133**:78–81.

132. Wiestler OD, von Siebenthal K, Schmitt HP, Feiden W, Kleihues P. Distribution and immunoreactivity of cerebral micro-hamartomas in bilateral acoustic neurofibromatosis (neurofibromatosis 2). *Acta Neuropathol (Berl)* 1989;**79**:137–43.

133. Witkowski L, Lalonde E, Zhang J, et al. Familial rhabdoid tumour 'avant la lettre' – from pathology review to exome sequencing and back again. *J Pathol* 2013;**231**:35–43.

134. Woodruff JM. Pathology of tumors of the peripheral nerve sheath in type 1 neurofibromatosis. *Am J Med Genet* 1999;**89**:23–30.

135. Woodruff JM, Scheithauer BW, Kurtkaya-Yapicier O, et al. Congenital and childhood plexiform (multinodular) cellular schwannoma: a troublesome mimic of malignant peripheral nerve sheath tumor. *Am J Surg Pathol* 2003;**27**:1321–9.

136. Wu J, Patmore DM, Jousma E, et al. EGFR-STAT3 signaling promotes formation of malignant peripheral nerve sheath tumors. *Oncogene* 2014;**33**:173–80.

137. Zhu Y, Ghosh P, Charnay P, Burns DK, Parada LF. Neurofibromas in NF1: Schwann cell origin and role of tumor environment. *Science* 2002;**296**:920–2.

138. Zoller ME, Rembeck B, Oden A, Samuelsson M, Angervall L. Malignant and benign tumors in patients with neurofibromatosis type 1 in a defined Swedish population. *Cancer* 1997;**79**:2125–31.

Paraneoplastic Syndromes

Marc K Rosenblum

INTRODUCTION

'Paraneoplastic' is a designation reserved for tumour-associated neurologic disorders that cannot be ascribed to compression or infiltration of the nervous system by tumour cells or attributed to the metabolic derangements, unwanted effects of therapy, disturbances of coagulation or opportunistic infections that potentially complicate the course and management of systemic neoplasia. Though rare, paraneoplastic phenomena compel attention because these frequently constitute the first manifestations of otherwise occult tumours. Paraneoplasia, furthermore, looms large in the differential diagnosis of certain symptom complexes that, in turn, have come to be associated with offending cancers of relatively restricted types. Thus, 60–70 per cent of patients developing the Lambert–Eaton myasthenic syndrome harbour small-cell carcinomas of the lung,[13] whereas over 50 per cent of women presenting with subacute pancerebellar dysfunction will be found to have adenocarcinomas of mullerian or mammary duct origin.[66] Paraneoplastic injury may affect any division of the central or peripheral (including autonomic) neuraxis and often proves a greater threat to the patient than its inciting tumour, which is often relatively confined on discovery and which may remain in abeyance even as neurological symptoms progress to devastating disability.

Investigations conducted over the last several decades have demonstrated that many paraneoplastic neurological disorders are attributable to an immune attack, provoked by the tumoural expression of native neuronal antigens, that comes to be misdirected against the nervous system.[58] Surveyed here are the more prevalent and best characterized of this autoimmune group, the members of which have come to be defined by their association with antibodies to specific 'onconeural' antigens. These antibodies can be divided into two broad classes depending on whether the target is an intracellular or cell membrane-associated/extracellular epitope. Antibodies of the first type are more tightly correlated with underlying neoplastic disease, but the evidence amassed to date indicates that these do not suffice to cause nervous system injury. Antibody-depleting strategies are typically of no benefit to affected patients, as both experimental and neuropathological studies (reviewed later) implicate cell-mediated cytotoxic mechanisms. On the other hand, both favourable responses to antibody depletion and experimental models implicate autoantibodies to cell membrane-associated and extracellular neuronal antigens as directly pathogenic agents in nervous system injury.

SYNDROMES ASSOCIATED WITH ANTIBODIES TO INTRACELLULAR NEURONAL ANTIGENS

Hu Antigen

The most prevalent of paraneoplastic neurological disorders in the intracellular neuronal antigen group is a syndrome of potentially widespread injury to the central and peripheral neuraxes associated with high-titre anti-Hu[20,39] (a.k.a. anti-neuronal nuclear autoantibody type 1)[54] antibodies. The offending tumour in over 75 per cent of cases is a small-cell carcinoma of the lung, the most common presenting manifestation (and dominant clinical feature in many cases) being peripheral sensory loss that involves all modalities and progresses inexorably to crippling deafferentation over a few weeks or months. Some 70–80 per cent of patients develop evidence of central nervous system (CNS) injury as well, this often being multifocal and including (singly or in any combination) bulbar and cerebellar dysfunction, limbic encephalopathy (seizures, disturbances of cognition, affect and short-term memory) and myelopathy (particularly a paralyzing lower motor neuron syndrome). Autonomic damage may produce gastrointestinal pseudo-obstruction, urinary retention, impotence, severe orthostatic hypotension and life-threatening cardiac arrhythmias. Treatment of the underlying neoplasm, plasmapheresis and immunosuppressive regimens usually fail to effect neurologic improvement.

Predominantly of IgG1 subtype and found in both the serum and cerebrospinal fluid (CSF) of symptomatic patients, anti-Hu antibodies identify a family of highly conserved RNA-binding proteins that are involved in the post-transcriptional regulation of gene expression and that are integral to neuronal differentiation and maintenance.[41] In addition to labelling the nuclei and, to a lesser extent,

perikarya of neurons throughout the central and peripheral nervous systems,[4,19] anti-Hu antibodies consistently label small-cell carcinomas of the lung (including those unassociated with paraneoplastic disease) – a phenomenon reflecting their ubiquitous expression of the major immunogen, HuD, in non-mutated form (Figure 45.1a–c).[15,56] The triggering mechanism of injurious immune reactions

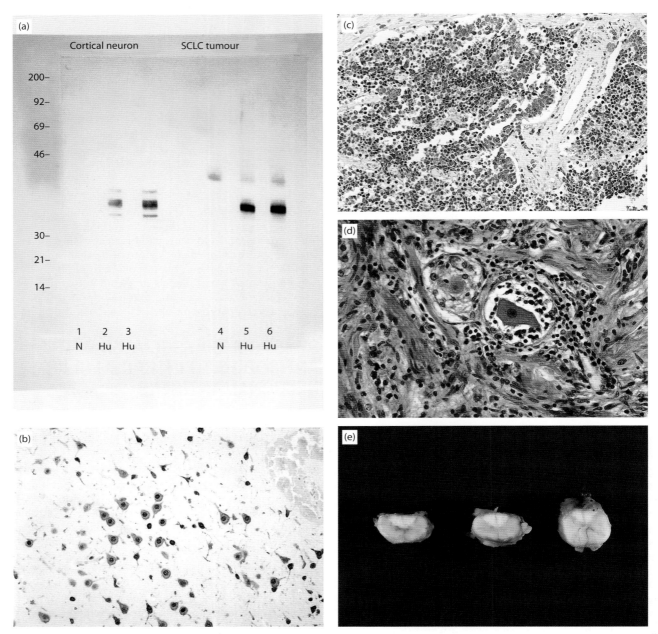

45.1 Paraneoplastic sensory neuropathy/encephalomyelitis. (a) Expression of Hu antigen in central nervous system and small-cell lung carcinomas. Western blot study demonstrating bands in the 35–40 kDa region on assay of purified cortical neuronal protein preparations (lanes 2 and 3) or small-cell lung cancer extracts (lanes 5 and 6) against anti-Hu IgG from patients with paraneoplastic sensory neuropathy/encephalomyelitis. Normal human IgG (lanes 1 and 4) does not yield such bands. **(b)** Hu expression is concentrated in neuronal nuclei, as shown in this immunohistochemical study of normal human cerebral cortex. Perikaryal labelling is also apparent. (Immunohistochemistry for Fab GLN 495 recombinant anti-Hu.) **(c)** Small-cell carcinoma of the lung showing anti-Hu immunoreactivity. (Immunohistochemistry for Fab GLN 495 recombinant anti-Hu.) **(d)** Paraneoplastic sensory neuropathy. Note the dorsal root ganglion cell surrounded by small lymphocytes. A residual nodule of Nageotte marks the adjacent ganglion cell bed. **(e)** The selective pallor of the dorsal columns demonstrated in these spinal cord sections reflects advanced dorsal root ganglion cell loss with secondary degeneration of ascending sensory fibres.

in affected patients is unclear, with only 15–20 per cent of subjects with small-cell lung cancers developing Hu seropositivity and only a fraction of these suffering paraneoplastic consequences.[18,36] Studies have found HuD-specific CD8+ T-lymphocytes to be normal components of the T-cell repertoire in mice, which display a high level of immune tolerance to this antigen.[29] A patient in the subacute phase of the anti-Hu syndrome, on the other hand, was found to harbour circulating HuD-specific T-cells of classic, CD8+ cytotoxic type that could not be detected in neurologically normal controls.[73] Two chronically impaired patients in this study had, instead, HuD-specific 'type 2' CD8+ lymphocytes sharing properties of CD4+ type (Th2) helper cells. Having attenuated cytolytic capacity, T-cells of this kind were speculated to downregulate cytotoxic T-cell activity following the initial nervous system assault and to possibly augment anti-Hu IgG production. Production of antibody alone does not suffice to cause neurological disease in the experimental setting.[79]

The clinical manifestations of the anti-Hu syndrome reflect an inflammatory attack on neurons.[7,20,45] Lymphocytes flood the dorsal root ganglia of patients with sensory neuropathy, surrounding ganglion cells and sometimes appearing to invade their degenerating or necrotic perikarya (Figure 45.1d). Nests of reactive satellite cells known as nodules of Nageotte come to mark, in tombstone-like fashion, the positions formerly occupied by ganglion cells, the end stage being a 'burned out' ganglion devoid of neuronal elements but deceptively free of inflammatory invaders. The consequences of advanced ganglion cell extinction may be appreciated at autopsy as atrophy of the posterior spinal roots and pallor of the dorsal columns of the spinal cord (Figure 45.1e). A comparable sequence of events is observed in affected myenteric plexi and CNS, where lymphocytes cuff regional blood vessels, migrate into the neuropil, converge on neurons and participate, along with histiocytes, in the formation of microglial or 'neuronophagic' nodules. Neuronal loss, highly variable in extent, is typically accompanied by striking astrogliosis.

Immunopathological analyses support a primary role for cytotoxic T-cells in anti-Hu-associated neuronal damage.[7,45] Although B- and T- (predominantly CD4+) lymphocytes cuff intraparenchymal blood vessels, the lymphoid elements that infiltrate the neuropil and surround neurons are principally CD8+ T-cells that have been shown to express the TIA-1 component of cytotoxic granules.[7] Upregulated regional expression of the ICAM-1 intercellular adhesion molecule may contribute to a pro-inflammatory environment and augment lymphocyte-neuron interactions in dorsal root ganglia and the CNS of affected patients.[7] This cited study could not marshal evidence for antibody-mediated complement activation.

Of note, the Hu-expressing neoplasms associated with paraneoplastic sensory neuropathy and encephalomyelitis are often occult and localized. Neurological complaints precede the diagnosis of cancer in over 70 per cent of patients, most of whom have small-cell lung carcinomas that not only are limited to the thorax upon discovery but often remain so through the course of their illnesses.[20,39,54] A majority die of neurological complications. This may not reflect early tumour detection alone, as an unexpectedly low incidence of extrathoracic metastasis, enhanced treatment

responsiveness and improved survival seem to characterize small-cell lung cancers deriving from a subset of patients having low-titre anti-Hu seropositivity unattended by paraneoplastic phenomena.[18,36] 'Spontaneous' regression of small-cell lung carcinoma in the setting of Hu-seropositive paraneoplastic disease has been documented,[26] as has growth inhibition of Hu-expressing neuroblastoma cells in mice following vaccination with HuD-encoding DNA.[14] The presence within syndrome-associated tumours of lymphocytes that include recombinant HuD-binding elements[83] further suggests that immune reflexes, while wreaking havoc on the nervous system, serve to check the growth and spread of these neoplasms.

Nova Proteins/Ri Antigen

High-titre anti-Ri[55] or antineuronal nuclear autoantibody type 2[53] antibodies are associated with an encephalomyelitic syndrome occurring mainly in patients with small-cell carcinomas of the lung and mammary adenocarcinomas.[55,68,70] As additional autoantibodies to other onconeural antigens (e.g. Hu, CRMP-5, calcium channel proteins, *etc.*) may be found, a wide variety of neurologic manifestations can be encountered in anti-Ri seropositive patients. Brain stem and cerebellar involvement are particularly common, the most distinctive features of the anti-Ri syndrome including a relatively high frequency of opsoclonus, myoclonus, jaw dystonia and laryngospasm.

Anti-Ri antibodies identify RNA-binding 55 and 80kDa proteins, termed Nova 1 and Nova 2, that regulate pre-mRNA alternative splicing in neurons[25] and that are co-expressed in tumour cells and the nuclei of neuronal subpopulations restricted to the CNS.[35] Autopsy studies have demonstrated that anti-Ri-associated neurologic dysfunction reflects a potentially widespread encephalomyelitic process in which the cerebellum, brain stem and spinal cord are targets of particularly severe injury.[10,42,70,71] Purkinje cell loss, destruction of bulbar (especially pontine) and spinal cord neurons, ventrolateral spinal tract degenerations, accompanying astrogliosis, microglial nodule formation and lymphocytic infiltrates composed principally of CD8+ cytotoxic/suppressor T-cells with cuffing of regional blood vessels by mixed T- and B-cell populations have all been documented. Ocular movement abnormalities may specifically reflect involvement of the pontine paramedian reticular formation.[42,70] Complement deposition and natural killer cell infiltration were identified in one case.[42] The absence of conspicuous inflammatory change in some affected regions of the CNS may simply reflect disease chronicity.

Collapsin Response-Mediator Protein-5

IgG antibodies to the 62kDa collapsin-response mediator-protein-5 (CRMP-5), member of a protein family that mediates axonal guidance and axon–Schwann cell interactions[12] among other functions, define a paraneoplastic neurologic disorder associated with small-cell carcinomas of the lung (over 75 per cent of cases) and occasionally with thymomas and tumours of other types.[17,46,94] The antigen is expressed widely within the central and peripheral neuraxes, localizing to synapse-rich neuropil and some neuronal perikarya, as well as the retina, where expression is found by photoreceptor and ganglion cell elements.[17] Clinical manifestations commonly include peripheral and autonomic neuropathy, cerebellar dysfunction, cognitive impairment and cranial neuropathy (particularly loss of olfaction and taste as well as visual loss due to optic neuritis and retinitis).[17] Chorea and other movement abnormalities referable to basal ganglionic injury may be encountered in this setting[94] as may progressive myelopathy.[46] Autopsy examination of an affected patient with encephalomyelopathy, optic neuritis and retinitis demonstrated lymphoid infiltrates of predominantly CD8+ T-cell type within the optic nerves in association with nerve fibre and myelin loss.[17] Microglial activation, isolated microglial nodules and perivascular lymphoid cuffing (again principally by CD8+ T-cells) were also widely distributed in the CNS, being most prominent in the mesial temporal lobes, brain stem, cerebellum and spinal cord. Spinal roots, dorsal root ganglia and peripheral nerves exhibited mild loss of myelinated axons.

Cdr2 Protein/Yo Antigen

High serum and CSF titres of an IgG antibody initially designated anti-Yo[66] and subsequently termed anti-Purkinje cell cytoplasmic antibody type 1[53] are strongly associated with a subacutely evolving and relentlessly progressive syndrome of paraneoplastic cerebellar dysfunction.[60,66] Evidence of bulbar, spinal cord and peripheral nervous system injury may also be encountered in this setting. Over 95 per cent of affected patients are women, the great majority of whom harbour adenocarcinomas of mullerian (usually ovarian) or mammary origin. Neurologic complaints typically precede the identification of these neoplasms, which tend to be relatively confined on discovery and which may be minute.[40,66] Treatment of the underlying tumour and immunosuppressive therapy benefit only a small minority of patients and many succumb to complications of nervous system damage rather than progression of neoplastic disease.[60,66,74]

Anti-Yo antibodies characteristically yield a major band at 52 or 62 kDa and minor band at 34 kDa on Western blotting against purified Purkinje cell proteins (Figure 45.2a), immunohistochemical preparations demonstrating perikaryal distribution of the antigen in Purkinje cells (Figure 45.2b). Yo expression by select neuronal subpopulations in the human cerebral cortex, brain stem, spinal cord, dorsal root ganglia and autonomic plexi has been demonstrated.[1,4,56] Shared cytoplasmic expression of the immunogen – a 52 kDa leucine zipper protein that is designated cdr2 and that displays c-Myc binding with resultant inhibition of c-Myc transcriptional activity[63] – is a constant feature of syndrome-associated cancers, but has also been detected in mammary and ovarian carcinomas unattended by neurologic dysfunction.[27] It has been suggested that Her 2 overexpression, a regular feature of associated breast cancers, acts to facilitate immune responses to cdr2.[75] Anti-Yo antibodies have not been shown to cause nervous system injury. Although these could, in theory, interfere with the down-regulatory binding of cdr2 to c-Myc, resulting in excess c-Myc activation and consequent neuronal apoptosis,[63] anti-Yo IgG does not suffice to produce neurologic disease in animals[34,77,84-86] and is occasionally demonstrable in cancer patients without neurologic manifestations.[30] The detection of Yo peptide/cdr2–specific cytotoxic

T-lymphocytes in the blood of affected subjects[3,87] and recovery of activated T-cells from their CSF[2] support a role for cell-mediated immune responses in this disorder. *In vitro* data indicate that dendritic cells bearing apoptotic tumour cell fragments to lymph nodes could initiate cdr2-specific T-cell activation.[72]

At autopsy, the hallmark of anti-Yo-associated cerebellar dysfunction is Purkinje cell loss that affects all portions of the cerebellum, which is severe and may be total. (Figure 45.2c).[1,60,66,81,91] Variable thinning of the granule cell layer may be encountered and reactive Bergmann astrogliosis is the rule. The appearance in most cases is that of a non-inflammatory degeneration but this likely reflects the end-stage, 'burned out' nature of the process. In some cases, microglial nodules have been identified in the Purkinje cell layer[1,81] and in one example cytotoxic T-lymphocytes with polarized granzyme B-labelling granules were noted to surround residual, MHC class I-expressing Purkinje cells.[1] Bulbar inflammation is not uncommonly found, even in the absence of brain stem signs, and cytotoxic T-cell infiltrates may be widely distributed in the brain, spinal cord and dorsal root ganglia.[1,60] The gracile, cuneate, spinocerebellar and corticospinal tracts may exhibit pronounced rarefaction, vacuolar change and myelin loss.[81,91] Carcinomas provoking anti-Yo-associated neurological injury are typically infiltrated by lymphocytes in large numbers, these including cytotoxic T-cells,[1] and may also harbour prominent plasmacellular infiltrates.[66,91] Thus, immune mechanisms may act to restrain their growth.

Ma Antigens

Paraneoplastic syndromes having prominent components of limbic and bulbar encephalitis, hypothalamic dysfunction and cerebellar injury are associated with antibodies to the Ma (also termed paraneoplastic Ma (PNMA)) protein family.[21,76,92] Patients seropositive against Ma2 (42 kDa) alone are usually men with underlying testicular germ cell tumours, whereas women with carcinomas of varying origin (including breast, lung, colon and ovary) predominate among a group of patients having antibodies to Ma1 (40 kDa) as well.[76] Neurological responses to anti-cancer therapy and immunosuppression may be seen in the former group. Ma1 and Ma2 are co-expressed by syndrome-associated neoplasms and neurons throughout the nervous system, Ma1 expression also being a feature of testicular germ cells.[21] Applied to tissue sections of CNS, patient sera yield neuron-specific immunolabelling in a dot-like pattern that is predominantly nuclear and that includes labelling of nucleoli.[76] Speculations regarding Ma protein function include roles in RNA transcription[76] and apoptosis.[78]

As has been the case in other paraneoplastic neurological disorders associated with immune responses to intracellular antigens, biopsy and autopsy studies of Ma-seropositive patients have consistently demonstrated infiltration of clinically affected CNS structures by lymphoid elements with variable degrees of microglial nodule formation, gliosis and neuronal loss (the last especially prominent at brain stem and cerebellar levels in post-mortem specimens).[5,21,82,92] Immunophenotyping of the lymphoid infiltrates observed has shown these to be composed overwhelmingly of T-cells and to be heavily dominated by CD8+ cytotoxic

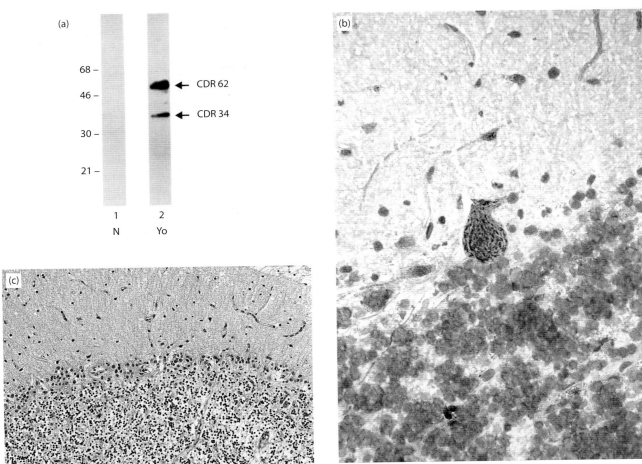

45.2 Paraneoplastic cerebellar degeneration. (a) Western blot demonstrating 62 and 34 kDa bands apparent when anti-Yo IgG from an afflicted patient is applied to purified Purkinje cell proteins (lane 2). Normal IgG does not produce corresponding bands (lane 1). **(b)** The perikaryon of this Purkinje cell is selectively labelled by anti-Yo IgG in a characteristically coarse, 'tigroid' fashion. Immunohistochemistry for anti-Yo. **(c)** Typical of anti-Yo-associated paraneoplastic cerebellar degeneration is the diffuse loss of Purkinje cells and reactive Bergmann astrogliosis shown in this autopsy specimen of affected cerebellar cortex.

T-lymphocytes.[21] The surrounding of neurons by granzyme B-expressing cytotoxic T-cells has been depicted.[6] In further support of cell-mediated immune mechanisms as affecting Ma-associated CNS injury is a rat model in which adoptive transfer of CD4+ T-helper cells specifically sensitized to autologous Ma1 induced meningoencephalitic inflammatory alterations (though unassociated with neurologic dysfunction) whereas immunization with recombinant Ma1 prompted anti-Ma1 antibody production but not neuropathologic abnormalities.[65]

Amphiphysin

Antibodies to amphiphysin, a 128 kDa presynaptic protein that acts to inhibit neurotransmission through the endocytosis of synaptic vesicles released at axon terminals, are associated with a paraneoplastic syndrome having, as its hallmark, muscle stiffness, rigidity and spasms affecting the neck, trunk and limbs.[61,62,69] The inciting neoplasm is typically a small-cell carcinoma of lung or adenocarcinoma of the breast. Whereas women with underlying mammary cancers are usually seropositive for anti-amphiphysin

alone, patients with small-cell carcinomas often evidence circulating antibodies to other onconeural antigens such as Hu, CRMP-5 and voltage-gated calcium channel proteins. The latter may contribute to accompanying clinical manifestations that can include encephalopathy, cerebellar dysfunction and neuropathies. Though the anti-amphiphysin antibody-associated disorder is often referred to as 'stiff man' or 'stiff person' syndrome, the classic stiff man syndrome occurring in patients with antibodies to the 65 kDa isoform of glutamic acid decarboxylase (GAD65) differs in its far less frequent involvement of the cervical musculature and upper extremities, common occurrence in complex with extraneural autoimmune disease (especially type 1 diabetes mellitus) and only exceptional association with neoplasia.[61,62]

Adduced in support of a directly pathogenic role for antibodies to amphiphysin in neurologic injury are the observations that some afflicted patients benefit from antibody-depleting plasmapheresis[93] and the induction of stiff man syndrome-like disorders in rats by passive transfer of human anti-amphiphysin IgG.[33,80] Intrathecally administered anti-amphiphysin IgG was found in one such model to co-localize with several presynaptic antigens and to result in reduced presynaptic GABAergic inhibition, the authors also reporting the internalization of this IgG by cultured hippocampal neurons.[33] Autopsy examinations of amphiphysin-seropositive patients without potentially confounding autoantibodies of other types, although limited to isolated cases, suggest, however, that cell-mediated immune reflexes are also activated in this setting.[69,93] Major findings, principally observed within the pons, medulla and spinal cord, have included perivascular cuffing by lymphocytes of both B- and T-cell types with neuroparenchymal infiltration primarily by CD8+ T-cells and accompanying neuronal loss, gliosis and microglial nodule formation. Deposition of the terminal component of complement C5b9 was observed in one case.[93]

SYNDROMES ASSOCIATED WITH ANTIBODIES TO SYNAPTIC AND OTHER CELL MEMBRANE–ASSOCIATED NEURONAL PROTEINS

N-Methyl-D-Aspartate Receptors

By far the most prevalent disorder in this group is an encephalitis associated with antibodies of predominantly IgG1 and IgG3 subtypes to an extracellular epitope localized to the N-terminal domain of the N-methyl-D-aspartate receptor (NMDAR) NR1 subunit.[22,24] These antibodies produce a pattern of neuropil immunolabelling that is particularly concentrated in the hippocampal region when applied to sections of rodent brain. The target is one of a group of ionotropic glutamate receptors. Often unassociated with underlying neoplastic disease, anti-NMDAR paraneoplastic encephalitis principally affects women (80 per cent of cases) and the inciting tumour is typically an ovarian teratoma. Approximately 70 per cent of patients experience a virus infection-like prodrome of fever, headache and, in some cases, vomiting, diarrhoea or upper respiratory tract symptoms. This is shortly followed by psychiatric manifestations (anxiety, insomnia, manic hyper-religiosity, bizarre behaviour, delusions or hallucinations), short-term memory loss and language deterioration ranging from reduced verbal output with echolalia to frank mutism. The affected then develop movement abnormalities (limb and orofacial dyskinesias, choreoathetosis, dystonia, rigidity and opisthotonic posturing) and decline into catatonia and coma attended by disturbances of autonomic function and breathing. Remarkably, antibody-depleting immunotherapy and tumour resection completely reverse or substantially alleviate neurologic dysfunction in 75–80 per cent of patients.

Neuropathological and immunopathological assessment of paraneoplastic anti-NMDAR encephalitis has been limited.[22,57,89] Prominent findings at autopsy have included gliosis, conspicuous microglial proliferation and IgG deposition predominantly affecting the hippocampi, basal forebrain, basal ganglia and cervical spinal cord. Reduced immunoexpression of NMDAR NR1 characterized the hippocampal regions of two autopsied patients.[43] Modest infiltration of the leptomeninges, perivascular spaces and neuroparenchyma by lymphocytes of T and B types as well

as plasma cells has been documented, but complement deposition has not been seen and lymphocytes expressing cytotoxic T-cell markers (TIA-1, perforin, granzyme B, Fas/Fas ligand) have been absent or constituted only about 1 per cent of inflammatory cells present.[57,89] Neuronal loss was conspicuous in Sommer's sector of the hippocampus in one case, but was not otherwise striking.[89] Examination of teratomas from affected patients has shown these to consistently harbour central nervous system-type tissues that include NMDAR-expressing neuronal elements and to manifest infiltration by T-lymphocytes, macrophages and, in smaller numbers, B-cells and plasma cells.[89] Complement deposition in neuron-containing regions of these tumours has also been documented.[57] Anti-NMDAR encephalitis emerges from the clinical and pathologic studies cited previously as differing fundamentally from paraneoplastic syndromes associated with antibodies to cytoplasmic and nuclear neuronal proteins (such as Yo and Hu, respectively) in its responsiveness to antibody-depleting therapeutic strategies and a pathogenesis that does not seem to depend on the cytotoxic T-cell-mediated destruction of target neuronal populations. Additional evidence for the direct pathogenicity of anti-NMDAR antibodies includes experimental observations that the exposure of rodent hippocampal neurons to the CSF or purified IgG of affected patients causes a reduction of synaptic NMDAR clusters and protein that is titre-proportional, selective (i.e. sparing of other synaptic components), reversed on antibody removal and associated with specific dampening of excitatory NMDAR-mediated post-synaptic currents.[23,43] NMDAR cluster reduction appears to reflect internalization following capping and bivalent IgG antigenic cross-linking.[43]

Other Ionotropic Glutamate Receptors

Infrequently, ionotropic glutamate receptors other than NMDARs are implicated in paraneoplastic CNS dysfunction but the GluR1 and GluR2 subunits of the α-amino-3hydroxy-5-methyl-4-isoxazolepropionic acid (AMPA) receptor and the B1 subunit of the gamma-aminobutyric acid-B (GABA-B) receptor are targets of antibody responses that have been associated with limbic encephalitis.[48,50] Anti-AMPA receptor limbic encephalitis has been seen in patients with lung carcinomas of both small and non-small-cell types, thymomas and mammary adenocarcinomas. The antibodies preferentially label those brain regions richest in GluR1/2 and GluR2/3 receptors, including the CA3-CA1 zones of the hippocampus, amygdala, cerebellum, caudate, putamen and cerebral cortex, causing a reversible decrease in AMPA receptor clusters through receptor cross-linking and internalization. Such patients may harbour antibodies to other neuronal antigens (e.g. CRMP-5, GAD65 and voltage-gated calcium channel-associated proteins), complicating treatment as well as interpretation of the scant neuropathological data available. One autopsied patient with coexisting SOX1 and N-type calcium channel antibodies had only mild perivascular lymphocytic cuffing, foci of lymphocytic infiltration of the hippocampus (mainly involving CA4) and only rare microglial nodules.[48] A second fatal case, involving a patient who also harboured CRMP-5 antibodies, was characterized by perivascular and interstitial infiltrates dominated by CD8+ cytotoxic T-lymphocytes, astrogliosis and microglial nodules principally localized to the hippocampi.[48] The neuropathologic substrate of anti-GABA-B receptor limbic encephalitis, seen mainly in the setting of small-cell lung cancer and also potentially complicated by production of other antineuronal antibodies, is yet to be elucidated. Anti-GABA-B receptor antibodies block receptor function, but do not appear to cause receptor internalization.[51]

Tr Antigen; Delta/Notch-like Epidermal Growth Factor-Related Receptor

IgG autoantibodies to an antigen designated Tr are powerful markers of paraneoplastic cerebellar dysfunction occurring in complex with Hodgkin's lymphoma,[8,9,37] but have also been detected in select patients with cerebellar degeneration and lymphomas of non-Hodgkin type.[9] Anti-Tr IgG diffusely labels the cytoplasm and proximal dendrites of Purkinje cells, producing, as well, a punctate pattern of immunoreactivity in the overlying molecular layer.[37] In rat studies, Tr expression appeared localized to Purkinje cell perikarya and dendrites, as well as the cytosol and outer surfaces of the endoplasmic reticulum in molecular layer neurons.[38] Recent investigations, however, have provided evidence that the principal, if not sole, Tr immunogen resides in the extracellular domain of the Delta/Notch-like epidermal growth factor-related receptor (DNER),[28] which may mediate neuronal-glial interactions through Notch signalling.[32]

The trigger of anti-Tr-associated cerebellar injury is unclear. Only exceptionally has a syndrome-associated Hodgkin's lymphoma been shown to label with anti-Tr IgG[8] and preliminary studies failed to detect DNER protein within tumour biopsies from Tr-seropositive patients.[28] Severe loss of Purkinje cells and Bergmann gliosis with only sparse infiltration of the cerebellum by CD3-labelling T-lymphocytes and CD68-labelling histiocytes/microglia have been documented at autopsy,[8] but the role of anti-Tr antibodies in this picture is obscure. Exposure to anti-Tr-positive sera *in vitro* reportedly yielded endogenous labelling of Purkinje cells and hippocampal neurons but failed to affect obvious morphological alterations in these cells.[28] Impaired cerebellar development and function are features of a DNER knockout mouse model.[88]

Voltage-Gated Potassium Channel–Interacting Proteins

Proteins that interact with voltage-gated potassium channels (VGKCs) have also been implicated as targets of pathogenic antibody formation, including leucine-rich glioma-inactivated 1 (LGI1) and contactin-associated protein 2 (CASPR2), though only a minority of affected patients have demonstrable neoplastic disease. Limbic encephalitis, brief tonic-myoclonic seizures and hyponatremia have been associated with anti-GLI1 antibodies in patients having small-cell carcinoma of the lung, thymoma and other epithelial neoplasms,[49] whereas neuromuscular hyperexcitability, dysautonomia and encephalopathy have been recorded in thymoma-related anti-CASPR2 cases.[44] Paraneoplastic examples of these immunotherapy-responsive syndromes have not been subject to neuropathologic study, though three tumour-unassociated autopsy cases of 'VGKC antibody-associated' limbic encephalitis probably corresponding to the anti-LGI1 syndrome have been communicated.[31,47,64] Findings included variable degrees of T-lymphocytic infiltration, astrogliosis and microglial proliferation in the amygdaloid nuclei and hippocampi, one report describing perivascular lymphoid infiltrates dominated by CD20+ B-cells[47] and two describing neuronal loss in these regions.[31,47]

Other Membrane Channel and Receptor Proteins

Antibodies to voltage-gated calcium channels cause the Lambert–Eaton myasthenic syndrome, most of the offending neoplasms in this setting being small-cell carcinomas of lung origin.[13] Antibody-mediated blockage of calcium influx prevents quantal acetylcholine release, producing weakness and electrophysiological disturbances that remit on removal of the offending immunoglobulins from patient sera and that are replicated in animals by passive antibody transfer.[52] Myasthenic syndromes may also be encountered in patients with thymoma and antibodies to muscle-associated acetylcholine receptors,[90] whereas patients with a variety of neoplasms (particularly adenocarcinomas of mammary, prostatic, pulmonary and gastrointestinal types) can manifest dysautonomia, peripheral neuropathy and encephalopathy in association with antibodies to neuronal/ganglionic acetylcholine receptors.[59] Thymic epithelial neoplasms and carcinomas of diverse (principally breast) origin have been documented in optic neuritis and transverse myelitis patients with astrocytic aquaporin-4 water channel antibodies of the type that characterize neuromyelitis optica.[67] Isolated reports describe progressive muscle rigidity, brain stem dysfunction and stimulus-sensitive myoclonus (the 'progressive encephalomyelitis with rigidity and myoclonus' or PERM syndrome) in one patient with thymoma and antibodies to glycine receptors[16] and a second harbouring an undifferentiated carcinoma that presented in the mediastinum and was associated with antibodies to gephyrin, which interacts with glycine and GABA receptors in the postsynaptic membrane component of inhibitory synapses.[11]

REFERENCES

1. Aboul–Enein F, Hoftberger R, Buxhofer–Ausch V, *et al*. Neocortical neurones may be targeted by immune attack in anti-Yo paraneoplastic syndrome. *Neuropathol Appl Neurobiol* 2008;34:248–52.

2. Albert ML, Austin LM, Darnell RB. Detection and treatment of activated T-cells in the cerebrospinal fluid of patients with paraneoplastic cerebellar degeneration. *Ann Neurol* 2000;47:9–17.

3. Albert ML, Darnell JC, Bender A, *et al*. Tumour-specific killer cells in paraneoplastic cerebellar degeneration. *Nat Med* 1998;4:1321–4.

4. Altermatt HJ, Rodriguez M, Scheithauer BW, et al. Paraneoplastic anti-Purkinje and type I anti-neuronal nuclear autoantibodies bind selectively to central, peripheral and autonomic nervous system cells. *Lab Invest* 1991;65:412–20.

5. Barnett M, Prosser J, Sutton J, et al. Paraneoplastic brainstem/limbic encephalitis in a woman with anti-Ma2 antibody. *J Neurol Neurosurg Psychiatry* 2001;70:222–5.

6. Bauer J, Bien CG. Encephalitis and epilepsy. *Semin Immunopathol* 2009;31:537–544.

7. Bernal F, Graus F, Pifarre A, et al. Immunohistochemical analysis of anti-Hu-associated paraneoplastic encephalomyelitis. *Acta Neuropathol* 2002;103:509–515.

8. Bernal F, Shams'ili S, Rojas I, et al. Anti-Tr antibodies as markers of paraneoplastic cerebellar degeneration and Hodgkin's disease. *Neurology* 2003;60:230–234.

9. Briani C, Vitaliani R, Grisold W, et al. Spectrum of paraneoplastic disease associated with lymphoma. *Neurology* 2011;76:705–710.

10. Brieva-Ruiz L, Diaz-Hurtado M, Matias-Guiu X, et al. Anti-Ri-associated paraneoplastic cerebellar degeneration and breast cancer: an autopsy case study. *Clin Neurol Neurosurg* 2008;110:1044–1046.

11. Butler MH, Hayashi A, Ohkoshi N, et al. Autoimmunity to gephyrin in stiff-man syndrome. *Neuron* 2000;26:307–312.

12. Camdessanche JP, Ferraud K, Boutahar N, et al. The collapsing response mediator protein 5 onconeural protein is expressed in Schwann cells under axonal signals and regulates axon-Schwann cell interactions. *J Neuropathol Exp Neurol* 2012;71:298–311.

13. Carpentier AF and Delattre JY. The Lambert–Eaton myasthenic syndrome. *Clin Rev Allergy Immuno* 2001;20:155–8.

14. Carpentier AF, Rosenfeld MR, Delattre JY, et al. DNA vaccination with HuD inhibits growth of neuroblastoma in mice. *Clin Cancer Res* 1998;4:2819–24.

15. Carpentier AF, Voltz R, DesChamps T, et al. Absence of HuD gene mutations in paraneoplastic small-cell lung cancer tissue. *Neurology* 1998;50:1919.

16. Clerinx K, Breban T, Schrooten M, et al. Progressive encephalomyelitis with rigidity and myoclonus: resolution after thymectomy. *Neurology* 2011;76:303–304.

17. Cross SA, Salomao DR, Parisi JE, et al. Paraneoplastic autoimmune optic neuritis with retinitis defined by CRMP-5-IgG. *Ann Neurol* 2003;54:38–50.

18. Dalmau J, Furneaux HM, Gralla RJ, et al. Detection of the anti-Hu antibody in the serum of patients with small-cell lung cancer – a quantitative western blot analysis. *Ann Neurol* 1990;27:544–52.

19. Dalmau J, Furneaux HM, Cordon Cardo C, Posner JB. The expression of the Hu (paraneoplastic encephalomyelitis / sensory neuronopathy) antigen in human normal and tumour tissues. *Am J Pathol* 1992;141:881–6.

20. Dalmau J, Graus F, Rosenblum MK, Posner JB. Anti-Hu–associated paraneoplastic encephalomyelitis/ sensory neuronopathy. A clinical study of 71 patients. *Medicine (Baltimore)* 1992;71:59–72.

21. Dalmau J, Gultekin SH, Voltz R, et al. Ma1, a novel neuron-and testis-specific protein, is recognized by the serum of patients with paraneoplastic neurological disorders. *Brain* 1999;122:27–39.

22. Dalmau J, Tuzun E, Wu HY, et al. Paraneoplastic anti-N-methyl-D-aspartate receptor encephalitis associated with ovarian teratoma. *Ann Neurol* 2007;61:25–36.

23. Dalmau J, Gleichman AJ, Hughes EG, et al. Anti-NMDA-receptor encephalitis: case series and analysis of the effects of antibodies. *Lancet Neurol* 2008;7:1091–8.

24. Dalmau J, Lancaster E, Martinez-Hernandez E, et al. Clinical experience and laboratory investigations in patients with anti-NMDAR encephalitis. *Lancet Neurol* 2011;10:63–74.

25. Darnell RB. RNA regulation in neurologic disease and cancer. *Cancer Res Treat* 2010;42:125–129.

26. Darnell RB and DeAngelis LM. Regression of small-cell lung carcinoma in patients with paraneoplastic neuronal antibodies. *Lancet* 1993;341:21–2.

27. Darnell JC, Albert ML, Darnell RB. Cdr2, a target antigen of naturally occurring human tumour immunity, is widely expressed in gynaecological tumours. *Cancer Res* 2000;60:2136–9.

28. de Graaff E, Maat P, Hulsenboom E, et al. Identification of delta/notch-like epidermal growth factor-related receptor as the Tr antigen in paraneoplastic cerebellar degeneration. *Ann Neurol* 2012;71:815–24.

29. DeLuca I, Blachere NE, Santomasso B, Darnell RB. Tolerance to the neuron-specific HuD antigen. *PloS One* 2009;4:e5739.

30. Drlicek M, Bianchi G, Boglium G, et al. Antibodies of the anti-Yo and Anti-Ri type in the absence of paraneoplastic neurological syndromes: a long-term survey of ovarian cancer patients. *J Neurol* 1997;244:85–9.

31. Dunstan EJ, Winer JB. Autoimmune limbic encephalitis causing fits, rapidly progressive confusion and hyponatremia. *Age Ageing* 2006;35:536–537.

32. Eiraku M, Tohgo A, Ono K, et al. DNER acts as a neuron-specific Notch ligand during Bergmann glial development. *Nat Neurosci* 2005;8:873–880.

33. Geis C, Weishaupt A, Hallermann S, et al. Stiff person syndrome-associated autoantibodies to amphiphysin mediate reduced GABAergic inhibition. *Brain* 2010;133:3166–80.

34. Graus F, Illa I, Agusti M, et al. Effect of intraventricular injection of an anti-Purkinje cell antibody (anti-Yo) in a guinea pig model. *J Neurol Sci* 1991;106:82–7.

35. Graus F, Rowe G, Fueyo J, et al. The neuronal nuclear antigen recognized by the human anti-Ri autoantibody is expressed in central but not peripheral nervous system neurons. *Neurosci Lett* 1993;150:212–4.

36. Graus F, Dalmau J, Rene R, et al. Anti-Hu antibodies in patients with small-cell lung cancer: association with complete response to therapy and improved survival. *J Clin Oncol* 1997;15:2866–72.

37. Graus F, Dalmau J, Valldeoriola F, et al. Immunological characterization of a neuronal antibody (anti-Tr) associated with paraneoplastic cerebellar degeneration and Hodgkin's disease. *J Neuroimmunol* 1997;74:55–61.

38. Graus F, Gultekin SH, Ferrer I, et al. Localization of the neuronal antigen recognized by anti-Tr antibodies from patients with paraneoplastic cerebellar degeneration and Hodgkin's disease in the rat nervous system. *Acta Neuropathol* 1998;96:1–7.

39. Graus F, Keime-Guibert F, Rene R, et al. Anti-Hu-associated paraneoplastic encephalomyelitis:analysis of 200 patients. *Brain* 2001;124:1138–48.

40. Hetzel DJ, Stanhope CR, O'Neill BP, Lennon VA. Gynaecologic cancer in patients with subacute cerebellar degeneration predicted by anti-Purkinje cell antibodies and limited in metastatic volume. *Mayo Clinic Proc* 1990;65:1558–63.

41. Hinman MN and Lou H. Diverse molecular functions of Hu proteins. *Cell Mol Life Sci* 2008;65:3168–3181.

42. Hormigo A, Dalmau J, Rosenblum MK, et al. Immunological and pathological study of anti-Ri-associated encephalopathy. *Ann Neurol* 1994;36:896–902.

43. Hughes EG, Peng X, Gleichman AJ, et al. Cellular and synaptic mechanisms of anti-NMDA receptor encephalitis. *J Neurosci* 2010;17:5866–5875.

44. Irani SR, Alexander S, Waters P, et al. Antibodies to Kv1 potassium channel-complex proteins leucine-rich, glioma inactivated 1 protein and contactin-associated protein-2 in limbic encephalitis, Morvan's syndrome and acquired neuromyotonia. *Brain* 2010;133:2734–2748.

45. Jean WC, Dalmau J, Ho A, Posner JB. Analysis of the IgG subclass distribution and inflammatory infiltrates in patients with anti-Hu-associated paraneoplastic encephalomyelitis. *Neurology* 1994;44:140–7.

46. Keegan BM, Pittock SJ, Lennon VA. Autoimmune myelopathy associated with collapsin response-mediator protein-5 immunoglobulin G. *Ann Neurol* 2008;63:531–534.

47. Khan NL, Jeffree MA, Good C, et al. Histopathology of VGKC antibody-associated limbic encephalitis. *Neurology* 2009;72:1703–1705.

48. Lai M, Hughes EG, Peng X, et al. AMPA receptor antibodies in limbic encephalitis alter synaptic receptor location. *Ann Neurol* 2009;65:424–34.

49. Lai M, Hujibers MGM, Lancaster E, et al. Investigation of LGI1 as the antigen in limbic encephalitis previously attributed to potassium channels: a case series. *Lancet Neurol* 2010;9:776–785.

50. Lancaster E, Lai M, Peng X, et al. Antibodies to the GABA (B) receptor in limbic encephalitis with seizures: case series and characterisation of the antigen. *Lancet Neurol* 2010;9:67–76.

51. Lancaster E, Martinez-Hernandez E, Dalmau J. Encephalitis and antibodies to synaptic and neuronal cell surface proteins. *Neurology* 2011;77:179–189.

52. Lang B, Newsom-Davis J. Immunopathology of the Lambert–Eaton myasthenic syndrome. *Springer Semin Immunopathol* 1995;17:3–15.

53. Lennon VA. Paraneoplastic autoantibodies: the case for a descriptive generic nomenclature [see comments]. *Neurology* 1994;44:2236–2240.

54. Lucchinetti CF, Kimmel DW, Lennon VA. Paraneoplastic and oncologic profiles of patients seropositive for type 1 antineuronal nuclear autoantibodies. *Neurology* 1998;50:652–7.

55. Luque FA, Furneaux HM, Ferziger R, *et al.* Anti-Ri: an antibody associated with paraneoplastic opsoclonus and breast cancer. *Ann Neurol* 1991;29:241–51.

56. Manley GT, Smitt PS, Dalmau J and Posner JB. Hu antigens: reactivity with Hu antibodies, tumour expression and major immunogenic sites. *Ann Neurol* 1995;38:102–10.

57. Martinez–Hernandez E, Horvath J, Shiloh–Malawsky Y, *et al.* Analysis of complement and plasma cells in the brain of patients with anti-NMDAR encephalitis. *Neurology* 2011;77:589–593.

58. McKeon A, Pittock SJ. Paraneoplastic encephalomyelopathies: pathology and mechanisms. *Acta Neuropathol* 2011;122:381–400.

59. McKeon A, Lennon VA, Lachance DH, *et al.* Ganglionic acetylcholine receptor autoantibody: oncological, neurological and serological accompaniments. *Arch Neurol* 2009;66:735–741.

60. McKeon A, Tracy JA, Pittock SJ, *et al.* Purkinje cell cytoplasmic autoantibody type 1 accompaniments: the cerebellum and beyond. *Arch Neurol* 2011;68:1282–1289.

61. McKeon A, Robinson MT, McEvoy KM, *et al.* Stiff-man syndrome and variants: clinical course, treatments, and outcomes. *Arch Neurol* 2012;69:230–238.

62. Murinson BB, Guarnaccia JB. Stiff-person syndrome with amphiphysin antibodies: distinctive features of a rare disease. *Neurology* 2008;71:1955–8.

63. Okano HJ, Park WY, Corradi JP, Darnell RB. The cytoplasmic Purkinje onconeural antigen cdr2 down-regulates c-Myc function: implications for neuronal and tumour cell survival. *Genes Dev* 1999;13:2087–97.

64. Park DC, Murman DL, Perry KD, *et al.* An autopsy case of limbic encephalitis with voltage-gated potassium channel antibodies. *Eur J Neurol* 2007;14:e5–e6.

65. Pellkofer H, Schubart AS, Hoftberger R, *et al.* Modelling paraneoplastic CNS disease: T-cells specific for the onconeural antigen PNMA1 mediate autoimmune encephalomyelitis in the rat. *Brain* 2004;127:1822–1830.

66. Peterson K, Rosenblum MK, Kotanides H, Posner JB. Paraneoplastic cerebellar degeneration. I. A clinical analysis of 55 anti-Yo antibody- positive patients. *Neurology* 1992;42:1931–7.

67. Pittock SJ, Lennon VA. Aquaporin-4 autoantibodies in a paraneoplastic context. *Arch Neurol* 2008;65:629–632.

68. Pittock SJ, Lucchinetti CF, Lennon VA. Anti-neuronal nuclear autoantibody type 2: paraneoplastic accompaniments. *Ann Neurol* 2003;53:580–587.

69. Pittock SJ, Lucchinetti CF, Parisi JE, *et al.* Amphipysin autoimmunity: paraneoplastic accompaniments. *Ann Neurol* 2005;58:96–107.

70. Pittock SJ, Parisi JE, McKeon A, *et al.* Paraneoplastic jaw dystonia and laryngospasm with antineuronal nuclear autoantibody type 2 (Anti-Ri). *Arch Neurol* 2010;67:1109–1115.

71. Prestigiacomo CJ, Balmaceda C, Dalmau J. Anti-Ri-associated paraneoplastic opsoclonus-ataxia syndrome in a man with transitional cell carcinoma: A case report. *Cancer* 2001;91:1423–8.

72. Roberts WK, Darnell RB. Neuroimmunology of the paraneoplastic neurological degenerations. *Curr Opin Immunol* 2004;16:616–22.

73. Roberts WK, DeLuca IJ, Thomas A, *et al.* Patients with lung cancer and paraneoplastic Hu syndrome harbour HuD-specific type 2 CD8+ T-cells. *J Clin Invest* 2009;119:2042–51.

74. Rojas I, Graus F, Keime–Guibert F, *et al.* Long-term clinical outcome of paraneoplastic cerebellar degeneration and anti-Yo antibodies. *Neurology* 2000;55:713–5.

75. Rojas–Marcos I, Picard G, Chinchon D, *et al.* Human epidermal growth factor receptor 2 overexpression in breast cancer of patients with anti-Yo-associated paraneoplastic cerebellar degeneration. *Neuro Oncol* 2012;14:506–510.

76. Rosenfeld MR, Eichen JG, Wade DF, *et al.* Molecular and clinical diversity in paraneoplastic immunity to Ma proteins. *Arch Neurol* 2001;50:339–348.

77. Sakai K, Gofuku M, Kitagawa Y, *et al.* Induction of anti-Purkinje cell antibodies *in vivo* by immunizing with a recombinant 52-kDa paraneoplastic cerebellar degeneration-associated protein. *J Neuroimmunol* 1995;60:135–41.

78. Schuller M, Jenne D, Voltz R. The human PNMA family: novel neuronal proteins implicated in paraneoplastic neurological disease. *J Neuroimmunol* 2005;169:172–176.

79. Sillevis Smitt P, Manley GT, Posner JB. Immunization with the paraneoplastic encephalomyelitis antigen HuD does not cause neurologic disease in mice. *Neurology* 1995;45:1873–8.

80. Sommer C, Weishaupt A, Brinkhoff J, *et al.* Paraneoplastic stiff-person syndrome: passive transfer to rats by means of IgG antibodies to amphiphysin. *Lancet* 2005;365:1406–1411.

81. Storstein A, Krossnes BK, Vedeler CA. Morphological and immunohistochemical characterization of paraneoplastic cerebellar degeneration associated with Yo antibodies. *Acta Neurol Scand* 2009;120:64–67.

82. Sutton I, Winer J, Rowlands D, Dalmau J. Limbic encephalitis and antibodies to Ma2: a paraneoplastic presentation of breast cancer. *J Neurol Neurosurg Psychiatry* 2000;69:266–8.

83. Szabo A, Dalmau J, Manley G *et al.* HuD, a paraneoplastic encephalomyelitis antigen, contains RNA-binding domains and is homologous to Elav and Sex-Lethal. *Cell* 1991;67:325–33.

84. Tanaka K, Tanaka M, Onodera O, *et al.* Passive transfer and active immunization with the recombinant leucine-zipper (Yo) protein as an attempt to establish an animal model of paraneoplastic cerebellar degeneration. *J Neurol Sci* 1994;127:153–8.

85. Tanaka M, Tanaka K, Onodera O, Tsuji S. Trial to establish an animal model of paraneoplastic cerebellar degeneration with anti-Yo antibody. 1. Mouse strains bearing different MHC molecules produce antibodies on immunization with recombinant Yo protein, but do not cause Purkinje cell loss. *Clin Neurol Neurosurg* 1995b;97:95–100.

86. Tanaka K, Tanaka M, Igarashi S, *et al.* Trial to establish an animal model of paraneoplastic cerebellar degeneration with anti-Yo antibody. 2. Passive transfer of murine mononuclear cells activated with recombinant Yo protein to paraneoplastic cerebellar degeneration lymphocytes in severe combined immunodeficiency mince. *Clin Neurol Neurosurg* 1995a;97:101–5.

87. Tanaka M, Tanaka K, Tsuji S, *et al.* Cytotoxic T-cell activity against the peptide, AYRARALEL, from Yo protein of patients with the HLA A24 or B27 supertype and paraneoplastic cerebellar degeneration. *J Neurol Sci* 2001;188:61–5.

88. Tohgo A, Eiraku M, Miyazaki T, *et al.* Impaired cerebellar functions in mutant mice lacking DNER. *Mol Cell Neurosci* 2006;31:326–333.

89. Tuzun E, Zhou L, Baehring JM, *et al.* Evidence for antibody-mediated pathogenesis in anti-NMDAR encephalitis associated with ovarian teratoma. *Acta Neuropathol* 2009;118:737–43.

90. Vernino S, Lennon VA. Autoantibody profiles and neurological correlations of thymoma. *Clin Cancer Res* 2004;10:7270–7275.

91. Verschuuren J, Chuang L, Rosenblum MK, *et al.* Inflammatory infiltrates and complete absence of Purkinje cells in anti-Yo-associated paraneoplastic cerebellar degeneration. *Acta Neuropathol (Berl)* 1996;91:519–25.

92. Voltz R, Gultekin SH, Rosenfeld MR, *et al.* A serologic marker of paraneoplastic limbic and brain-stem encephalitis in patients with testicular cancer. *N Engl J Med* 1999;340:1788–95.

93. Wessig C, Klein R, Schneider MF, *et al.* Neuropathology and binding studies in anti-amphiphysin-associated stiff-person syndrome. *Neurology* 2003;61:195–198.

94. Yu Z, Kryzer TJ, Griesmann GE, *et al.* CRMP-5 neuronal autoantibody: marker of lung cancer and thymoma-related autoimmunity. *Ann Neurol* 2001;49:146–154.

CNS Reactions to Anti-neoplastic Therapies

Arie Perry

INTRODUCTION

The management of brain tumour patients poses formidable challenges because the same therapies used to enhance survival can cause severe central nervous system (CNS) toxicities.[37] Unfortunately, as therapeutic options increase over time, so do the frequencies of neurotoxicity. Potential surgical complications are mostly acute in nature and consist of haemorrhage, vascular damage, infarcts, coagulopathies, malignant cerebral oedema with herniation and post-operative infection. In contrast, serious side effects of radiation and chemotherapy, such as radiation necrosis, chemotherapy-associated leukoencephalopathy and secondary neoplasms, are typically more subacute to chronic in nature. Therapy-induced peripheral neuropathies and pituitary changes are also common, but are covered in Chapter 24, Diseases of Peripheral Nerve, and Chapter 41, Pituitary and Suprasellar Tumours, respectively. Individual predisposing factors remain poorly understood. Nonetheless, it is clear that the developing nervous system is particularly vulnerable, especially to the effects of radiation.[38] Other known risk factors include the specific therapeutic modality and dosage, combined radiochemotherapy, genetic background and idiosyncratic predilections.[21,38,51,58]

RADIATION NECROSIS AND OTHER FORMS OF RADIATION INJURY

Injury to the nervous system is a common complication of radiation therapy, with acute, early delayed and late delayed forms.[52] The acute and early delayed forms are thought to primarily represent blood–brain barrier disruption and cerebral oedema, with neurologic deficits being mostly transient and reversible. In contrast, the late delayed effects occur months to years after therapy and are often irreversible, sometimes fatal injuries. In adults, the incidence of radiation necrosis after conventional doses for CNS therapy ranges from 5–24 per cent and is rarely encountered with cumulative doses of standard fractionated radiation under 50–60 Gy to the brain or 45 Gy to the spinal cord.[37] However, a non-necrotizing form of encephalopathy with neurobehavioural manifestations is even more common and is seen with lower dosages as well. Some data suggest that neuroprotective agents, such as lithium, have the potential to reduce this complication.[23] Although less severe than radiation necrosis and not life threatening, this form of encephalopathy tends to progress over many years and significantly alters quality of life. Individual risk factors for radiation damage are inadequately understood, but may include superimposed vascular disorders due to diabetes, hypertension and old age. Paediatric patients are even more vulnerable and generally, the younger the patient, the more susceptible they are to radiation-induced neurotoxicity. Long-term survivors of irradiated childhood brain tumours often suffer moderate to marked cognitive deficits, learning disabilities, hormonal deficits, growth retardation and psychomotor retardation. For instance, in an autopsy study of 22 paediatric glioma patients treated with radiation, there were foci of demyelination in 7, necrosis in 6 and cortical atrophy in 4 cases, respectively.[34]

Clinically, the need to distinguish radiation necrosis from tumour recurrence is common and critical, because the two are managed quite differently. On routine magnetic resonance (MR) imaging, a 'soap bubble' or 'Swiss cheese-like' interior favours radiation necrosis, although this sign is neither sufficiently sensitive nor specific.[26] Other examples display features that are indistinguishable from high-grade glioma. Newer radiologic modalities, such as diffusion weighted imaging (DWI), perfusion studies, proton magnetic resonance spectroscopy (H-MRS), and positron emission tomography (PET) have further enhanced the clinical distinction, although false positives and negatives remain common. Therefore, tissue diagnosis remains the gold standard. The clinical, radiographic and histological features that favour treatment effects or tumour progression are summarized in Table 46.1. Most commonly, however, there is a mixture of both; nonetheless, some data suggest that the ratio of the two may provide additional prognostic information.[13,18,56,63] Specimens composed predominantly of radiation necrosis indicate a favourable response to therapy, whereas cellular tumour specimens with little necrosis suggest minimal cytotoxic effects.

Gross Pathology

Radiation effects and radio-necrosis may involve any CNS site, although cerebral white matter commonly bears the brunt of the injury. Subcortical U-fibres are mostly spared, although lesions may extend into adjacent cortex or deep grey matter. Depending on the relative proportions of necrosis, vasculopathy/haemorrhage, oedema and gliosis, lesions may appear as firm, ill-defined, glioma-like masses or soft, friable, infarct-like regions of cystic degeneration (Figure 46.1a). Grey-white junctions may be blurred, with necrotic foci showing yellow to tan–brown discolouration. Areas of dystrophic calcification appear white and chalky. Superimposed petechial haemorrhages may produce a variegated appearance similar to that of glioblastoma, although more advanced cases show marked white matter loss and cerebral atrophy with hydrocephalus *ex vacuo*, rather than mass effect.

Histopathology and Proposed Mechanisms of Injury

Vascular changes are prominent in radiation injury and likely play an important pathogenic role. As one of the few actively proliferating sites in the brain, it is not surprising that the endothelial cell is particularly susceptible to radiation damage. Early disruptions in the blood–brain barrier are likely responsible for the vasogenic oedema seen in the transient acute and early delayed, often steroid responsive forms of radiation toxicity.[53] In contrast, more permanent forms of endothelial damage likely account for many of the classic changes of late delayed radiation injury seen in roughly 3–24 per cent of patients, including coagulative necrosis, thrombosis, haemorrhage, telangiectasia, vascular fibrosis/hyalinization with luminal stenosis and necrotising vasculopathy (Figure 46.1b), all of which facilitate hypoxic injury, white matter damage and parenchymal necrosis.[20,53] Other common findings include dystrophic calcifications and variable macrophage-rich infiltrates. Occasionally, neurodegenerative changes in the adjacent cortex or malformation-like vasculature are seen. Besides endothelial damage, other proposed mechanisms of radiation damage include coagulopathies and immune mechanisms, such as autoimmune vasculitis. The disseminated form of white matter damage from whole brain irradiation is known as radiation leukoencephalopathy.[7,41]

Although it is generally assumed that the radiation effects from newer modalities (e.g. stereotactic radiosurgery) are essentially identical to those of conventional external beam therapy, there is considerably less experience with

TABLE 46.1 Changes favouring therapy effects* vs recurrent/progressive tumour

Clinical feature	Therapy effects	Tumour recurrence/progression
Patient symptoms	No new symptoms	Worsening neurological status
Imaging feature		
Standard MRI	Swiss cheese or soap bubble patterns, limited mass effect	New enhancement outside 80%% isodose line, multifocality, corpus callosum spread, subependymal disease
DWI/ADC/DTI	High ADC values, low fractional anisotropy	Restricted DWI, low ADC, high fractional anisotropy
DSC	rCBV <0.6	rCBV >2.6
H–MRS	Low NAA, low Cr, Cho/Cr and NAA/Cr ratios	Increased Cho, high Cho/Cr and NAA/Cr ratios
PET	Metabolically inactive	Metabolically active
Histologic feature		
Necrosis	Large infarct like zones with hypocellular edges and dystrophic calcifications	Large or microscopic foci with hypercellular or pseudopalisading edges
Blood vessels	Telangiectatic Hyalinized Angionecrotic	Microvascular proliferation with enlarged and multilayered endothelial lining
Adjacent brain parenchyma	Rarefied or vacuolated, pale, and gliotic with vascular changes listed earlier	Nearly normal or infiltrated by individual tumour cells
Cytologic atypia	Bizarre bubbly nuclei and abundant cytoplasm	High N/C ratio
Mitotic figures	Rare	Frequent (if tumour is high grade)

*Given overlapping features, 'therapy effects' refers to changes seen with radiation, chemoradiation or pseudoprogression.

ADC, apparent diffusion coefficient; Cho, choline; Cr, creatine; DSC, dynamic, susceptibility-weighted, contrast-enhanced MR imaging; DTI, diffusion tensor imaging; DWI, diffusion weighted imaging; NAA, N-acetyl aspartate; rCBV, relative cerebral blood volume; H–MRS, proton magnetic resonance spectroscopy; PET, positron emission tomography (fluorine–18 fluorodeoxyglucose is most common but may be less sensitive and specific than 11C–methionine, 3,4–dihydroxy–6–18F–fluoro–L–phenylalanine, O– (2–18F–fluoroethyl)–L–tyrosine and 3'–deoxy–3'–18F–fluorothymidine forms of PET).

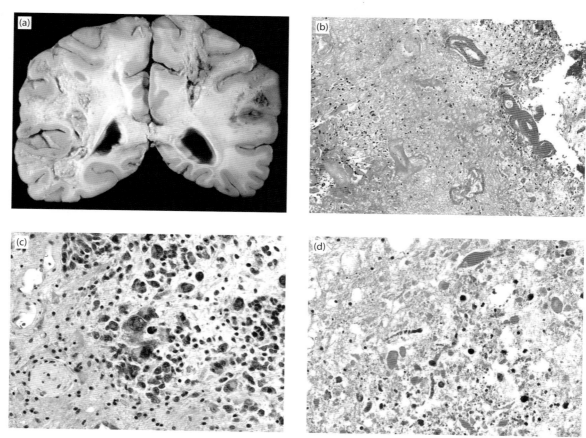

46.1 (a) Autopsy specimen from a patient with radiation leukoencephalopathy displaying predominantly white matter foci of radiation necrosis, cystic degeneration and atrophy. **(b)** Example of radiation necrosis with large zone of coagulative necrosis and extensive vasculopathy, including fibrinoid vascular necrosis and markedly hyalinized vessel walls. **(c)** Marked radiation-induced cytologic atypia in an irradiated, previously classic appearing oligodendroglioma, characterized by increased quantities of eosinophilic cytoplasm and large bizarre nuclei with bubbly chromatin. These changes resemble astrocytic differentiation, although in this case, both the original tumour and the post-radiation recurrence showed the 1p and 19q chromosomal co-deletions typical of oligodendroglioma. **(d)** Case of disseminated necrotizing leukoencephalopathy with prominent white matter vacuolation, foci of necrosis, diminished numbers of oligodendrocytes, and collections of swollen, dystrophic axons, many of which are calcified.

such post-therapy biopsies. Generally, observed pathological changes have been similar to those of conventional external beam radiotherapy, although the severity is often exaggerated and findings may be seen beyond high dose margins.[41] Foci of paucicellular, congealed fibrin-rich tissue are common. Viable tumour may be scant or totally absent and the peritumoural brain is often highly gliotic, sometimes with inflammation and considerable radiation-induced atypia.

Radiation-induced cytologic atypia and its potential for mimicking cancer is more commonly emphasised in other parts of the body. Nevertheless, it can be dramatic in the CNS as well, involving tumour cells, endothelial cells and adjacent brain parenchymal cells, such as reactive astrocytes and even neurons. Such changes can pose substantial diagnostic challenges in terms of glioma classification and grading. For example, because both increased nuclear pleomorphism and the accumulation of eosinophilic cytoplasm may be seen, oligodendroglial neoplasms may appear 'astrocytoma-like' after therapy (Figure 46.1c). In general, isolated cytomegalic cells with bizarre appearing bubbly nuclei are more likely to be radiation-induced, particularly if they are seen in hypocellular regions. Nevertheless, it is sometimes impossible to distinguish radiation from true atypia. Furthermore, when this

increased pleomorphism is coupled with radiation necrosis and telangiectatic vessels that may resemble the microvascular proliferation of glioblastoma, a previously radiated low-grade glioma can easily be overgraded if the radiation changes are not recognized as such. Therefore, one should use strict diagnostic criteria for endothelial hyperplasia (multilayering of hypertrophic cells) and spontaneous tumour necrosis (e.g. pseudopalisading pattern) before upgrading a previously irradiated low-grade glioma. In contrast, an increased mitotic or proliferative index is not a radiation effect and is therefore a reliable indicator of tumour progression in this setting.

THERAPY-INDUCED LEUKOENCEPHALOPATHIES AND VASCULOPATHIES

Radiation

The vulnerability of both endothelial cells and oligodendrocytes to radiation injury likely accounts for the radiation leukoencephalopathy seen in some patients. However, the risk of encephalopathy is enhanced about 3-fold[20,53] and the timing is shortened when chemotherapy is added, one study finding roughly a fourth of glioma patients with radiographic evidence of 'progression' after combined radiation/temozolomide therapy showing early (3–20 weeks post-therapy) radiation necrosis (also see section on Pseudoprogression and Pseudoresponse).[61] Pure radiation leukoencephalopathy is rarely seen today, as a result of the therapeutic shifts towards more localized forms of radiation over whole brain irradiation. Nonetheless, the clinical and radiologic features are essentially identical to those encountered with chemoradiation, despite a few histopathologic differences. Injury of small to medium sized vessels with superimposed oligodendroglial and stem cell/progenitor cell toxicities are thought to account for this leukoencephalopathy. The histopathology shows a spectrum of changes ranging from myelin pallor and gliosis to demyelination to coagulative necrosis, typically superimposed on the classic radiation-induced vascular changes already described. Arterial infarcts, vascular malformations and large vessel vasculopathies are less common complications, but have also been reported, including aneurysm formation, haemorrhage, arterial dissection, accelerated atherosclerosis and thrombosis.[37]

Methotrexate and Other Chemotherapeutic Agents

White matter toxicity is a potentially serious complication of chemotherapy. This is particularly true for regimens including methotrexate, although drugs of virtually all mechanistic categories have been implicated, including temozolomide, vincristine, lomustine (CCNU), carmustine (BCNU), melphalan, fludarabine, cytarabine (Ara–C), 5–fluorouracil (5–FU), levamisole, doxorubicin, cyclophosphamide, ifosfamide, thioTEPA, oxaliplatin, paclitaxel, vinblastine and cisplatin.[51] The frequency of pure chemotherapy-induced cognitive dysfunction in learning, memory, information processing speed and executive function is increasingly reported, especially in breast cancer patients where no confounding CNS factors exist; estimated frequencies range widely from 15–80 per cent.[51,58] Synergistic or additive effects are also seen with combined chemotherapies and because this is the current direction of medical oncology, it is likely that neurotoxicities will continue to increase in the future. Commonly disrupted processes include neurogenesis, gliogenesis and maintenance of myelin fibre integrity, with damage to neural progenitor cells thought to be particularly important in delayed neurotoxic disorders. Oxidative stress, inflammation, angiogenic changes, apoptotic dysregulation, altered transcriptional expression and histone acetylation likely play important roles as well. Potentially, neuroprotective agents may be useful in reducing neurotoxicity in the future, although some may potentially also reduce therapeutic efficacy and further study is therefore needed.[51] Additionally, because molecularly targeted strategies may also affect critical signalling in progenitor cells, there is growing concern over potential long term CNS effects using these newer agents.

In many cases, a mild and reversible form of injury is seen acutely, although in up to a third, deficits persist for months to years.[21] Other clinical manifestations include reversible posterior leukoencephalopathy (see later), subcortical dementia, incontinence, gait disturbances, stroke-like episodes, and a cerebellar syndrome, with white matter pathology predominating.[58] The risk of serious or permanent damage appears to be greatest when methotrexate is combined with radiation therapy and therefore, it is difficult to dissect the precise contribution of each modality to this type of pathology. Nevertheless, methotrexate and other drugs have occasionally been shown to cause the same leukoencephalopathy in the absence of radiation, particularly in cases with intrathecal or intraventricular administration.[27,30] Additional evidence for its pathogenic role comes from occasional examples where the injury is exacerbated around a leaky or misplaced ventriculostomy tube used to administer cerebrospinal fluid (CSF) methotrexate.[37] The mechanisms of chemotherapy neurotoxicity are elusive, but may include direct toxic effects on axons, oligodendrocytes and progenitor cells, as well as secondary immunologic reactions, oxidative stress and microvascular injury.[5,7,35] Risk factors for chemotherapy toxicity are also poorly understood, but likely depend on treatment modalities, nutritional deficiencies, patient age, cognitive reserve, co-morbidities and idiosyncratic predispositions, including genetic variability in multi-drug resistance pumps, DNA repair mechanisms, telomere maintenance, cytokine regulation, neurotransmitter activity, Alzheimer disease risk factors (e.g. ApoE alleles), and hormone status/endocrine therapy.[21,51,58]

A fairly wide spectrum of pathologic changes may be seen. In some, the pathology appears to be partially or entirely reversible, whereas others suffer permanent, potentially fatal deficits. For example, an acute asymptomatic form of white matter disease is commonly detected radiologically in medulloblastoma and supratentorial primitive neuroectodermal tumour (PNET) patients receiving multiagent chemotherapy regimens, with or without concomitant radiation.[14,47] In most, lesions are transient, although there is increased risk of subsequent neurocognitive deficits, suggesting that permanent damage occurs in a subset. Because such cases are rarely biopsied, however, the pathogenesis of this milder form of leukoencephalopathy is unclear. A disruption of the blood–brain barrier with oedema is suspected. In slightly more severe examples, myelin pallor, vacuolation, axonal spheroids, modest macrophage infiltrates and gliosis are common.[33,37]

The most dramatic examples of chemotherapy-induced leukoencephalopathy present with miliary, small rounded to large confluent foci of predominantly non-inflammatory demyelination or, more commonly, frank white matter necrosis. Rubinstein and colleagues coined the term disseminated necrotizing leukoencephalopathy (DNL) for this severe, progressive and often fatal form that they and others described originally in children with metastatic meningeal acute lymphoblastic leukaemia (ALL) treated with high-dose methotrexate based chemotherapy and whole brain irradiation.[45,46] Similar examples have subsequently been reported both in adults and patients with other tumour types.[37] This complication has also been encountered in cases of meningeal carcinomatosis,[16] which makes sense given that DNL is mostly encountered with whole brain irradiation. Lastly, a similar pathology has been reported in glioma patients treated with intra-arterial BCNU, either in combination with brain irradiation or less often, administered in isolation.[44] However, the latter pathology is generally limited to the vascular distribution of drug administration and shows a greater degree of vasculopathy than classic DNL.

Grossly, DNL is characterized by small, discrete, grey-brown foci of softened oedematous white matter, a chalky to friable consistency and petechial or ring-shaped haemorrhages in larger coalescent lesions. The pathology is most prominent in cerebral white matter, but can also affect the cerebellum and brain stem. Microscopically, lesions range from ill-defined zones of myelin pallor, oligodendrocyte loss and prominent spongiosis to discrete rounded foci of coagulative necrosis with numerous microcalcifications, a surprising paucity of inflammation and collections of markedly swollen axons with dystrophic calcifications (Figure 46.1d). Ultrastructurally, dystrophic axons are stuffed with mitochondria, autophagic vacuoles and microfilaments, with this prominent axonopathy considered one of the key distinguishers of DNL from pure radiation leukoencephalopathy. Only rare cases of DNL have included superimposed features of radiation damage, such as fibrinoid vascular necrosis, vascular hyalinization, telangiectasias and fibrinous exudates.

In a series of 185 primary CNS lymphoma patients treated at Memorial Sloan–Kettering Cancer Center, the estimated 5-year incidence of DNL was 24 per cent.[35] Clinically, it was characterized by a rapidly progressive subcortical dementia, similar in type to arteriosclerotic encephalopathy (Binswanger's disease), cerebral autosomal dominant arteriopathy with subcortical infarcts and leukoencephalopathy (CADASIL) and normal pressure hydrocephalus. Symptoms begin shortly after therapy to many months later, including irritability, somnolence, ataxia, memory deficits, apathy, psychomotor retardation and psychiatric disturbances. Over time, cognitive deficits progress to frank dementia, with motor and autonomic deficits increasingly apparent. Most progress further to seizures, coma and death, often within a few months of onset.

Neuroimaging studies of DNL may be unremarkable at presentation, but later reveal variably calcified, progressively confluent white matter lesions. On computed tomography (CT), the calcifications are among the earliest findings, followed by low density lesions and contrast enhancing masses that may be difficult to distinguish from tumour recurrence or progression. MR imaging is more sensitive in early lesions, with white matter pathology showing decreased T1-weighted signal intensity and increased signal on T2-weighted and fluid attenuated inversion recovery (FLAIR) studies.[28,35] Large advanced lesions commonly demonstrate contrast enhancement that may mimic tumour initially, although cerebral atrophy and hydrocephalus *ex vacuo* typically develop as the disease progresses.

Pseudoprogression and Pseudoresponse

These two terms have been introduced to reflect increasing challenges in accurately distinguishing tumour progression and therapeutic responses from radiological mimics using current chemoradiation approaches. For instance, since the 2005 publication by Stupp, *et al.* of their phase III trial showing a survival benefit for combined radiation and temozolomide chemotherapy in glioblastoma patients,[55] this has become the standard of care.[11,20,53] In early follow-up imaging (2–6 months), roughly half develop contrast enhancing lesions consistent with tumour progression using standard MacDonald criteria.[31] On follow-up imaging of patients continuing this therapeutic regimen however, 28–64 per cent show stabilization, improvement or resolution,[11] a process termed 'pseudoprogression'. As such, this is now considered an exaggerated favourable response to therapy and correlates well with the finding that patient survival is improved in pseudoprogression when compared with true progression. This phenomenon appears to be even more commonly associated with tumours displaying *MGMT* hypermethylation.[2,9,36] One study suggested that glioblastomas with high proliferative indices (Ki–67 labelling >20 per cent) are also more likely to undergo pseudoprogression.[39]

The mechanism of pseudoprogression remains poorly understood, but is sometimes explained as transient disruptions in blood-brain barrier or endothelial function, with or without associated inflammation.[10,20,53] However, this premise conflicts with the nearly invariable reports of necrosis in the rare cases undergoing biopsy.[18,56,61,63] Similarly, the proposed notion that pseudoprogression affects the tumour while radiation necrosis affects adjacent brain parenchyma seems overly simplistic, as simultaneous changes involving both are often seen histologically. Therefore, it is possible that despite perceived clinical differences, pseudoprogression and chemoradiation necrosis represent a single spectrum, with a preferable all-encompassing term being 'therapy effects'. Features favouring treatment effects or progression are summarized in Table 46.1, although none are completely reliable. The great conundrum for oncologists is that in the setting of a worrisome post-therapy imaging change, they must wait until the next MRI to determine whether the current therapy was actually working (pseudoprogression) or whether a true progression occurred, in which case an earlier switch in therapy might have been warranted. As such, repeat surgery for pseudoprogression vs progression has become more common. Unfortunately, even with tissue examination, this question may be challenging, because most samples contain a combination of both viable tumour and treatment effects. As such, additional studies are sorely needed to better predict patient outcome based on post-therapy findings.

In contrast, the term pseudoresponse refers to apparent 'normalization' of tumour associated vasculature, such that seemingly dramatic responses to enhancing foci on MR imaging occur despite a lack of reduction in tumour burden.[10,11,19,20] This phenomenon is mostly seen with anti-angiogenic therapy, such as the *VEGF* inhibitor, bevacizumab. Further complicating interpretations, the reduction in contrast enhancement is accompanied by marked expansion of the T2-weighted and FLAIR abnormalities, sometimes resulting in a gliomatosis-like pattern. Given these pitfalls and the lack of reliability of post-contrast measurements alone, the MacDonald criteria were replaced by the response assessment in neuro-oncology (RANO) criteria in 2010 in order to obtain more accurate response determinations in the setting of anti-angiogenic therapy.[20,53,59]

Posterior Reversible Encephalopathy Syndrome (PRES)

The term reversible posterior leukoencephalopathy syndrome was first coined by Hinchey, *et al.* in 1996[17] and refers to a disorder presenting with acute cortical blindness, headaches, mental status changes and sometimes seizures, typically associated with malignant hypertension and T2-weighted/FLAIR MRI signal abnormalities in the occipital and posterior parietal lobes. Given that changes may be irreversible, lesions may not be limited to the posterior circulation and that grey matter may also be involved, some have advocated alternate names, such as posterior reversible encephalopathy (PRES) or occipital–parietal encephalopathy.[50,54] PRES has been associated with a wide variety of inciting factors, including the use of high-dose corticosteroids and various single or multiagent chemotherapy regimens.[60] The latter have included cisplatin, cytarabine, cyclophosphamide and methotrexate.

Symptoms and signs may develop during therapy or be delayed for days to weeks. In most cases, the neurotoxicity is completely reversible, although the importance of controlling the hypertension in order to prevent permanent damage has been emphasized. The mechanism of toxicity is also poorly understood, although radiologic studies, particularly those utilizing diffusion weighted imaging with apparent diffusion coefficient measurements, are consistent with vasogenic oedema. This pattern differs from that of the cytotoxic oedema encountered in classic cerebral infarcts and could explain the reversible nature of most examples. Proposed mechanisms have included endothelial damage with blood–brain barrier disruption, transient episodes of hypertension overloading the autoregulatory capabilities of the posterior circulation, and electrolyte imbalances with hypomagnesaemia.[37,50,54]

Because PRES is predominantly a clinicoradiological diagnosis, few descriptions of the neuropathology exist. However, a biopsied example found evidence of vasogenic oedema without overt vascular damage or infarct.[50] A rare fatal example found dilated perivascular spaces with proteinaceous exudates, macrophages, fibrinoid necrosis and acute haemorrhage reminiscent of acute hypertensive encephalopathy.[24] Even so, the permanent deficits occasionally encountered suggest that ischemic damage is possible in severe cases or those in whom diagnostic delay leads to inadequate control of the hypertension.

THERAPY-INDUCED SECONDARY NEOPLASMS

Given that both radiation and chemotherapy induce DNA mutations, it is not surprising that a potential complication is therapy-induced secondary neoplasms. In fact, as oncology becomes more successful at prolonging the survival of cancer patients, secondary neoplasms are increasingly encountered (see[25,32] for reviews). Epidemiological data links the risk of secondary brain tumours with ionizing radiation much more than with chemotherapy, although given their mutagenic properties, it is likely that the latter increases risk as well, either alone or in combination with radiation.

Cahan's criteria for a radiation-induced neoplasm state that the tumour must differ histologically from the original lesion being treated and should arise within the irradiation field over a sufficient latency period, typically years.[4] In the CNS, the most common secondary tumours are meningiomas, nerve sheath tumours, pituitary adenomas, gliomas, sarcomas and embryonal neoplasms, with latency periods varying greatly, but typically presenting years to decades after therapy.[25,32] The greatest risks have been associated with irradiation during childhood, suggesting that there are critical windows of enhanced susceptibility, perhaps associated with active CNS development and growth in general, increased proliferation rates in various progenitor cell types or an increased number of progenitor cells overall in comparison to adult brains. The data also suggest a dosage effect, such that greater exposures are associated with shorter latency periods and higher risks of malignancy. For instance, the British Childhood Cancer Survivor Study of nearly 18 000 paediatric cancer survivors found subsequent primary neoplasms to be 4 times greater than expected, with the most frequently observed second neoplasms at a median follow-up of 24.3 years being located in the CNS.[42]

Additional epidemiologic data come from follow-up studies of paediatric patients receiving CNS irradiation for ALL or other common childhood malignancies, Israeli immigrants treated with radiation for tinea capitis between 1948 and 1960, and atomic bomb survivors from Hiroshima and Nagasaki.[43,48,62] For example, Ron and colleagues estimated relative risks among nearly 11 000 children treated with low-dose scalp irradiation (mean 1.4–1.8 Gy) for tinea capitis as 9.5 for meningiomas, 2.6 for gliomas and 18.8 for nerve sheath tumours (mostly schwannomas) when compared with non-irradiated controls from the general population.[43] The relative risk of developing a meningioma increased to nearly 20 for patients treated with doses of roughly 2.5 Gy.[48] Similarly, the latency period is inversely associated with dosage, such that those with greater exposures present earlier, potentially developing tumours as soon as 12 months after therapy.[5] In studies of atomic bomb survivors, meningiomas, schwannomas and pituitary tumours were most common and there was generally an inverse relationship between the patient's distance from the epicentre of the blast and the relative risk of tumour development.[62]

Pathology and Genetics

Although some have emphasized features such as nuclear atypia and vascular hyalinization as being common in radiation-induced brain tumours, the histology of secondary neoplasms is usually indistinguishable from sporadic counterparts. Nevertheless, there may be genetic and biologic differences, most notably in meningiomas. There has been a debate as to whether or not radiation-induced meningiomas (RIMs) are more aggressive as a group, with increased numbers of high grade examples.[8,15,57] Although it is clear that most reported examples are both histologically and biologically benign, most data now support this hypothesis, particularly in patients that received high-dose (>20 Gy) radiation at a young age. Additionally, the RIMs are more likely to present with multicentric disease, unusual histologic subtypes and calvarial involvement, often with associated alopecia, atrophy and poor vascularization of previously irradiated scalp. In contrast to sporadic counterparts, RIMs are less likely to harbour alterations of the *NF2* gene, instead being characterized genetically by frequent losses and structural alterations of chromosome 1.[8,29,40] Lastly, there is evidence to suggest that genotypic patterns may be able to predict higher or lower predispositions for RIMs in individual patients.[12]

Radiation-induced gliomas (RIGs) are also similar to their sporadic counterparts, with high-grade astrocytomas encountered most frequently.[3,49] However, these tumours characteristically present at younger ages of onset than sporadic glioblastomas, especially for patients irradiated during childhood. Genetically, Brat and colleagues examined nine examples for alterations of the *TP53*, *p16*, *MTAP*, *PTEN*, *KRAS* and *EGFR* genes, finding similar alterations to those of sporadic gliomas, particularly *de novo* glioblastomas.[3] One potential difference was the lack of *PTEN* mutations in the RIGs; however, the numbers of cases examined were insufficient for statistical significance. Additionally, an expression profiling and Western blot study comparing RIGs and paediatric glioblastomas found a less complex pattern in the former with increased expression levels of ErbB3, Sox10 and platelet-derived growth factor receptor–α proteins.[6]

Therapy-Induced Malignant Transformation

Recent data suggest that temozolomide chemotherapy can induce a characteristic 'hypermutator phenotype' associated with malignant progression of lower grade gliomas to glioblastoma.[22] It remains unclear whether or not irradiation can promote or enhance the rate of malignant transformation within benign or low-grade primary CNS tumours. Malignant progression in such tumours may be mediated by additional mutations, which could conceivably be facilitated by irradiation. This hypothesis is difficult to prove in tumours that normally undergo malignant progression even in the absence of therapy. However, there is some support for this notion in benign tumour types that almost never progress otherwise, such as pilocytic astrocytoma, ganglioglioma, dysembryoplastic neuroepithelial tumour and schwannoma.[37]

Nevertheless, such examples remain rare. Considerably fewer data are available regarding the risks of secondary neoplasms or malignant transformation induced by newer modalities of radiation therapy, although examples are increasingly being reported as experience is gained, particularly with various forms of stereotactic neurosurgery, such as gamma knife.[25,37]

GENETIC PREDISPOSITIONS TO THERAPEUTIC NEUROTOXICITY

Given that familial cancer predisposition syndromes are caused by germline mutations in tumour suppressor genes, patients with these syndromes may be even more susceptible than other patients to the mutagenic effects of radiation and chemotherapy (see Chapter 44, Hereditary Tumour Syndromes). Examples include neurofibromatosis 1 (NF1) patients developing malignant peripheral nerve sheath tumours (MPNST) or other sarcomas within radiation fields.[25,32,37] Because MPNSTs are uncommon in the head and orbital regions where optic pathway gliomas have been radiated, it seems unlikely that such cases are coincidental, although admittedly such patients are already at risk for this tumour type. NF1 patients also appear at greater risk for developing post-irradiation strokes and other vasculopathies, especially moyamoya syndrome. Similarly, increased risks of radiation-induced sarcomas have been reported in children with Li–Fraumeni syndrome and familial retinoblastoma.[25,37] Lastly, secondary glial, meningothelial and neural (e.g. MPNST) malignancies have been reported in NF2 patients receiving radiosurgery for vestibular schwannomas.[1] Although the tumour types that have developed within the radiation fields in these patients have often been the types to which the patients are already at risk, such studies nevertheless suggest an increased susceptibility to the transforming effects of radiation. This could be true for various forms of chemotherapy as well, although there are currently no clear data to prove this.

REFERENCES

1. Balasubramaniam A, Shannon P, Hodaie M, *et al.* Glioblastoma multiforme after stereotactic radiotherapy for acoustic neuroma: case report and review of the literature. *Neuro Oncol* 2007;9(4):447–53.
2. Brandes AA, Franceschi E, Tosoni A, *et al.* MGMT promoter methylation status can predict the incidence and outcome of pseudoprogression after concomitant radiochemotherapy in newly diagnosed glioblastoma patients. *J Clin Oncol* 2008;26(13):2192–7.
3. Brat DJ, James CD, Jedlicka AE, *et al.* Molecular genetic alterations in radiation-induced astrocytomas. *Am J Pathol* 1999;154(5):1431–8.
4. Cahan WG, Woodard HQ, Higinbotham NL, Stewart FW, Coley BL. Sarcoma arising in irradiated bone: report of eleven cases. 1948. *Cancer* 1998;82(1):8–34.
5. Choudhary A, Pradhan S, Huda MF, Mohanty S, Kumar M. Radiation-induced meningioma with a short latent period following high dose cranial

irradiation – Case report and literature review. *J Neurooncol* 2006;77(1):73–7.
6. Donson AM, Erwin NS, Kleinschmidt–DeMasters BK, *et al.* Unique molecular characteristics of radiation-induced glioblastoma. *J Neuropathol Exp Neurol* 2007;66(8):740–9.
7. Ebi J, Sato H, Nakajima M, Shishido F. Incidence of leukoencephalopathy after whole-brain radiation therapy for brain metastases. *Int J Radiat Oncol Biol Phys* 2013;85(5):1212–7.
8. Elbabaa SK, Gokden M, Crawford JR, Kesari S, Saad AG. Radiation-associated meningiomas in children: clinical, pathological, and cytogenetic characteristics with a critical review of the literature. *J Neurosurg Pediatr* 2012;10(4):281–90.
9. Fabi A, Russillo M, Metro G, *et al.* Pseudoprogression and MGMT status in glioblastoma patients: implications in clinical practice. *Anticancer Res* 2009;29(7):2607–10.

10. Fatterpekar GM, Galheigo D, Narayana A, Johnson G, Knopp E. Treatment-related change versus tumor recurrence in high-grade gliomas: a diagnostic conundrum—use of dynamic susceptibility contrast-enhanced (DSC) perfusion MRI. *AJR Am J Roentgenol* 2012;198(1):19–26.
11. Fink J, Born D, Chamberlain MC. Pseudoprogression: relevance with respect to treatment of high-grade gliomas. *Curr Treat Options Oncol* 2011;12(3):240–52.
12. Flint–Richter P, Sadetzki S. Genetic predisposition for the development of radiation-associated meningioma: an epidemiological study. *Lancet Oncol* 2007;8(5):403–10.
13. Forsyth PA, Kelly PJ, Cascino TL, *et al.* Radiation necrosis or glioma recurrence: is computer-assisted stereotactic biopsy useful? *J Neurosurg* 1995;82(3):436–44.
14. Fouladi M, Chintagumpala M, Laningham FH, *et al.* White matter lesions detected by magnetic resonance imaging after radiotherapy and high-dose chemotherapy

in children with medulloblastoma or primitive neuroectodermal tumor. *J Clin Oncol* 2004;**22**(22):4551–60.

15. Galloway TJ, Indelicato DJ, Amdur RJ, *et al.* Favorable outcomes of pediatric patients treated with radiotherapy to the central nervous system who develop radiation-induced meningiomas. *Int J Radiat Oncol Biol Phys* 2011;**79**(1):117–20.

16. Grossman SA, Krabak MJ. Leptomeningeal carcinomatosis. *Cancer Treat Rev* 1999;**25**(2):103–19.

17. Hinchey J, Chaves C, Appignani B, *et al.* A reversible posterior leukoencephalopathy syndrome. *N Engl J Med* 1996;**334**(8):494–500.

18. Hu LS, Eschbacher JM, Heiserman JE, *et al.* Re-evaluating the imaging definition of tumor progression: perfusion MRI quantifies recurrent glioblastoma tumor fraction, pseudoprogression, and radiation necrosis to predict survival. *Neuro Oncol* 2012;**14**(7):919–30.

19. Hygino da Cruz LC Jr, Rodriguez I, Domingues RC, Gasparetto EL, Sorensen AG. Pseudoprogression and pseudoresponse: imaging challenges in the assessment of posttreatment glioma. *AJNR American Journal of Neuroradiology* 2011;**32**(11):1978–85.

20. Jahangiri A, Aghi MK. Pseudoprogression and treatment effect. *Neurosurg Clin N Am* 2012;**23**(2):277–87, viii–ix.

21. Janelsins MC, Kohli S, Mohile SG, *et al.* An update on cancer- and chemotherapy-related cognitive dysfunction: current status. *Semin Oncol* 2011;**38**(3):431–8.

22. Johnson BE, Mazor T, Hong C, *et al.* Mutational analysis reveals the origin and therapy-driven evolution of recurrent glioma. *Science* 2014 Jan 10;343:189–93.

23. Khasraw M, Ashley D, Wheeler G, Berk M. Using lithium as a neuroprotective agent in patients with cancer. *BMC Med* 2012;**10**:131.

24. Kheir JN, Lawlor MW, Ahn ES, *et al.* Neuropathology of a fatal case of posterior reversible encephalopathy syndrome. *Pediatr Dev Pathol* 2010;**13**(5):397–403.

25. Kleinschmidt–Demasters BK, Kang JS, Lillehei KO. The burden of radiation-induced central nervous system tumors: a single institutions experience. *J Neuropathol Exp Neurol* 2006;**65**(3):204–16.

26. Kumar AJ, Leeds NE, Fuller GN, *et al.* Malignant gliomas: MR imaging spectrum of radiation therapy – and chemotherapy-induced necrosis of the brain after treatment. *Radiology* 2000;**217**(2):377–84.

27. Lai R, Abrey LE, Rosenblum MK, DeAngelis LM. Treatment-induced leukoencephalopathy in primary CNS lymphoma: a clinical and autopsy study. *Neurology* 2004;**62**(3):451–6.

28. Laxmi SN, Takahashi S, Matsumoto K, *et al.* Treatment-related disseminated necrotizing leukoencephalopathy with characteristic contrast enhancement of the white matter. *Radiat Med* 1996;**14**(6):303–7.

29. Lillehei KO, Donson AM, Kleinschmidt–Demasters BK. Radiation-induced meningiomas: clinical, cytogenetic, and microarray features. *Acta Neuropathol* 2008;**116**(3):289–301.

30. Lovblad K, Kelkar P, Ozdoba C, *et al.* Pure methotrexate encephalopathy presenting with seizures: CT and MRI features. *Pediatr Radiol* 1998;**28**(2):86–91.

31. Macdonald DR, Cascino TL, Schold SC, Jr., Cairncross JG. Response criteria for phase II studies of supratentorial malignant glioma. *J Clin Oncol* 1990;**8**(7):1277–80.

32. Marks AM, Packer RJ. A review of secondary central nervous system tumors after treatment of a primary pediatric malignancy. *Semin Pediatr Neurol* 2012;**19**(1):43–8.

33. Moore–Maxwell CA, Datto MB, Hulette CM. Chemotherapy-induced toxic leukoencephalopathy causes a wide range of symptoms: a series of four autopsies. *Mod Pathol* 2004;**17**(2):241–7.

34. Oi S, Kokunai T, Ijichi A, Matsumoto S, Raimondi AJ. Radiation-induced brain damage in children – histological analysis of sequential tissue changes in 34 autopsy cases. *Neurol Med Chir* (Tokyo) 1990;**30**(1):36–42.

35. Omuro AM, Ben–Porat LS, Panageas KS, *et al.* Delayed neurotoxicity in primary central nervous system lymphoma. *Arch Neurol* 2005;**62**(10):1595–600.

36. Park CK, Kim J, Yim SY, *et al.* Usefulness of MS–MLPA for detection of MGMT promoter methylation in the evaluation of pseudoprogression in glioblastoma patients. *Neuro Oncol* 2011;**13**(2): 195–202.

37. Perry A, Schmidt RE. Cancer therapy-associated CNS neuropathology: an update and review of the literature. *Acta Neuropathol* (Berl) 2006;**111**(3):197–212.

38. Pimperl LC. Radiation as a nervous system toxin. *Neurol Clin* 2005;**23**(2):571–97.

39. Pouleau HB, Sadeghi N, Baleriaux D, *et al.* High levels of cellular proliferation predict pseudoprogression in glioblastoma patients. *Int J Oncol* 2012;**40**(4):923–8.

40. Rajcan–Separovic E, Maguire J, Loukianova T, Nisha M, Kalousek D. Loss of 1p and 7p in radiation-induced meningiomas identified by comparative genomic hybridization. *Cancer Genet Cytogenet* 2003;**144**(1):6–11.

41. Rauch PJ, Park HS, Knisely JP, Chiang VL, Vortmeyer AO. Delayed radiation-induced vasculitic leukoencephalopathy. *Int J Radiat Oncol Biol Phys* 2012;**83**(1):75.

42. Reulen RC, Frobisher C, Winter DL, *et al.* Long-term risks of subsequent primary neoplasms among survivors of childhood cancer. *JAMA* 2011;**305**(22):2311–9.

43. Ron E, Modan B, Boice JD Jr, *et al.* Tumors of the brain and nervous system after radiotherapy in childhood. *N Engl J Med* 1988 ;**319**(16):1033–9.

44. Rosenblum MK, Delattre JY, Walker RW, Shapiro WR. Fatal necrotizing encephalopathy complicating treatment of malignant gliomas with intra-arterial BCNU and irradiation: a pathological study. *J Neurooncol* 1989;**7**(3):269–81.

45. Rubinstein JL, Herman MM, Long TF, Wilbur JR. Leukoencephalopathy following combined therapy of central nervous system leukemia and lymphoma. *Acta Neuropathol Suppl* (Berl) 1975;**Suppl** 6:251–5.

46. Rubinstein LJ, Herman MM, Long TF, Wilbur JR. Disseminated necrotizing leukoencephalopathy: a complication of treated central nervous system leukemia and lymphoma. *Cancer* 1975;**35**(2): 291–305.

47. Rutkowski S, Bode U, Deinlein F, *et al.* Treatment of early childhood medulloblastoma by postoperative chemotherapy alone. *N Engl J Med* 2005;**352**(10):978–86.

48. Sadetzki S, Flint–Richter P, Ben–Tal T, Nass D. Radiation-induced meningioma: a descriptive study of 253 cases. *J Neurosurg* 2002;**97**(5):1078–82.

49. Salvati M, D'Elia A, Melone GA, *et al.* Radio-induced gliomas: 20-year experience and critical review of the pathology. *J Neurooncol* 2008;**89**(2):169–77.

50. Schiff D, Lopes MB. Neuropathological correlates of reversible posterior leukoencephalopathy. *Neurocrit Care* 2005;**2**(3):303–5.

51. Seigers R, Schagen SB, Van Tellingen O, Dietrich J. Chemotherapy-related cognitive dysfunction: current animal studies and future directions. *Brain Imaging Behav* 2013;**7**(4):453–9.

52. Sheline GE. Radiation therapy of brain tumors. *Cancer* 1977;**39**(2 Suppl):873–81.

53. Siu A, Wind JJ, Iorgulescu JB, *et al.* Radiation necrosis following treatment of high grade glioma – a review of the literature and current understanding. *Acta Neurochir* (Wien) 2012;**154**(2):191–201; discussion.

54. Stott VL, Hurrell MA, Anderson TJ. Reversible posterior leukoencephalopathy syndrome: a misnomer reviewed. *Intern Med J* 2005;**35**(2):83–90.

55. Stupp R, Mason WP, van den Bent MJ, *et al.* Radiotherapy plus concomitant and adjuvant temozolomide for glioblastoma. *N Engl J Med* 2005;**352**(10):987–96.

56. Topkan E, Topuk S, Oymak E, Parlak C, Pehlivan B. Pseudoprogression in patients with glioblastoma multiforme after concurrent radiotherapy and temozolomide. *Am J Clin Oncol* 2012;**35**(3):284–9.

57. Umansky F, Shoshan Y, Rosenthal G, Fraifeld S, Spektor S. Radiation-induced meningioma. *Neurosurg Focus* 2008;**24**(5):E7.

58. Wefel JS, Schagen SB. Chemotherapy-related cognitive dysfunction. *Curr Neurol Neurosci Rep* [Review] 2012;**12**(3):267–75.

59. Wen PY, Macdonald DR, Reardon DA, *et al.* Updated response assessment criteria for high-grade gliomas: response assessment in neuro-oncology working group. *J Clin Oncol* 2010;**28**(11):1963–72.

60. Won SC, Kwon SY, Han JW, Choi SY, Lyu CJ. Posterior reversible encephalopathy syndrome in childhood with hematologic/oncologic diseases. *J Pediatr Hematol Oncol* 2009;**31**(7):505–8.

61. Yaman E, Buyukberber S, Benekli M, *et al.* Radiation-induced early necrosis in patients with malignant gliomas receiving temozolomide. *Clin Neurol Neurosurg* 2010;**112**(8):662–7.

62. Yonehara S, Brenner AV, Kishikawa M, *et al.* Clinical and epidemiologic characteristics of first primary tumors of the central nervous system and related organs among atomic bomb survivors in Hiroshima and Nagasaki, 1958–1995. *Cancer* 2004;**101**(7):1644–54.

63. Young RJ, Gupta A, Shah AD, *et al.* Potential utility of conventional MRI signs in diagnosing pseudoprogression in glioblastoma. *Neurology* 2011;**76**(22):1918–24.

Index

immunohistochemistry, 1682f, 1683
incidence, 1681
macroscopy, 1682, 1682f
microscopy, 1682–1683, 1682f
molecular genetics, 1683–1684
prognosis, 1684–1685
biological behavior, 1681
clinical features, 1673–1674, 1674f
defined, 1673
differential diagnosis, 1675f, 1676, 1677–1678
electron microscopy, 1677
genetic susceptibility, 1680–1681
grading, 1675–1676
histogenesis, 1678–1679
immunohistochemistry, 1675f, 1676–1677
incidence, 1673
macroscopy, 1674
microscopy, 1674–1675, 1675f
molecular genetics, 1679–1680, 1679f, 1680f
prognosis, 1681
radiological features, 1673–1674, 1674f
Oligodendrogliopathy, dying back, MS, 1327
Oligoependymomas, 1689
Olivary heterotopia, 356f, 357
Olivopontocerebellar atrophy (OPCA), 801f
with prominent cerebellar ataxia, 763
Onchocerciasis, 1262, 1262f
Oncocytic meningioma, 1814
Oncocytoma, 1889, 1890f
spindle cell, 1895, 1896f
Oncogenic viruses, animal models, 1629–1630
OPCA. See Olivopontocerebellar atrophy
OPDM. See Oculopharyngodistal myopathy
Ophthalmic zoster, 1115
Ophthalmomyiasis, 1275, 1276f
OPMD. See Oculopharyngeal muscular dystrophy
Optic gliomas, in NF1 patients, 1929–1930, 1930f
Optic nerve, MS lesion localization pattern, 1343f, 1354–1355, 1355f
Optic neuritis, MS, 1343f, 1354, 1355f
Optico-spinal multiple sclerosis (OSMS), 1357
Asian, 1375
Orbit, fungal infections, 1294, 1294f
Organelle(s)
neuronal, 2–3, 8
staining, 2, 3
Organic mercury, toxicity, 617
Organophosphates, toxicity, 620, 621f
Organophosphorus compounds, neurotoxicity, 615
Organophosphorus esters, 1492t, 1494
Ornithine transcarbamylase (OTC) deficiency, 607
Orofacial–digital syndrome, X-linked, 377
Oroya fever, 1225
Orthomyxoviruses, 1127, 1128f
OSMS. See Optico-spinal multiple sclerosis
Osteogenic tumours, 1831
Osteosclerotic myeloma, 1484–1485
OTC deficiency. See Ornithine transcarbamylase (OTC) deficiency
Oxidative phosphorylation (OXPHOS), 1602
Oxidative stress
aetiology, 859–860
diabetic neuropathy–related, 1490–1491, 1491t
FCI pathophysiology, 146
OXPHOS. See Oxidative phosphorylation

P

Pachygyria, 318–320, 319f, 321f
Pachymeningitis, hypertrophic, 1209
Paclitaxel, 1492t, 1498

PACNS. See Primary angiitis of central nervous system
Paget's disease of bone, inclusion body myopathy with, 922t, 923
Pallister–Hall syndrome, 278t
PAN. See Polyarteritis nodosa
Pan-dysautonomia, 1457
Pan-encephalitis, 1095t, 1096
progressive rubella, 1147–1149, 1150f
subacute sclerosing, 1146, 1148f
Pan-myelitis, 1095t, 1096
Pan-necrosis
axonal swelling, 78, 79f
infarction, 76f, 78, 78f
neuronal, 76–77, 76f
Pancreas, bone marrow, 526t, 527t, 528
Pancreatitis, acute, 134, 135f
Panhypopituitarism, Russell's viper envenoming bite and, 623, 623f
Panniculitis, fasciitis/myofasciitis with, 1522–1523, 1610f
Pantothenate kinase–associated neurodegeneration (PKAN), 404–406, 404t, 406f, 780t, 781, 781f
Papillary meningioma, 1807t, 1813f, 1814
Papillary tumour of pineal region (PTPR), 1760–1762, 1761f
Papp–Lantos bodies, 763
Paracoccidioidomycosis, 1289, 1290f
Paragangliomas, 1896–1897, 1897f
CNS, 1745–1748, 1746f
biological behaviour, 1747
classification, 1745
clinical features, 1745
differential diagnosis, 1747–1748
epidemiology, 1745
histogenesis, 1747
macroscopic appearances, 1746
microscopy, electron microscopy and immunohistochemistry, 1746–1747, 1746f
molecular biology and genetics, 1747
prognosis, 1747
radiology, 1745–1746
Paragonimiasis, 1267, 1268f
Parahippocampal gyrus region, HS, 706
Paramyxoviruses, 1127–1129
Paraneoplasia, defined, 1945
Paraneoplastic, defined, 1945
Paraneoplastic syndromes, 1945–1953
antibodies to intracellular neuronal antigens–related, 1945–1950
amphiphysin, 1949–1950
Cdr2 protein/Yo antigen, 1948, 1949f
cerebellar degeneration, 1948, 1949f
collapsin response-mediator protein-5, 1947–1948
Hu antigen, 1945–1947, 1946f
Ma antigens, 1948–1949
nova proteins/Ri antigens, 1947
sensory neuropathy/encephalomyelitis, 1945–1947, 1946f
introduction, 1945
neuropathy, 1500–1501, 1501f, 1502f
synaptic/other cell membrane–associated neuronal proteins–related, 1950–1951
delta/notch-like epidermal growth factor–related receptor, 1951
ionotropic glutamate receptors, 1950–1951
membrane channel and receptor proteins, 1951
N-methyl-D-aspartate receptors, 1950
Tr antigen, 1951
voltage-gated potassium channel-interacting proteins, 1951
Paranode, molecular constituents, 1323, 1323f
Paranodin, 1323, 1323f
Paraprotein-associated neuropathies, 1480t

Paraproteinaemia
CIDP–related, 1481–1482
IgM, 1481, 1482f, 1483f, 1485f
Parasagittal cerebral injury, combined grey and white matter lesions, 242
Parasitic infections, 1230–1280, 1231t, 1232t. See also specific types
arthropod infections, 1275, 1276f
cestode infections, 1267–1274
CNS, 1231t
eye, 1232t
information resources, 1231
introduction, 1230–1231
muscle, 1232t
nematode, 1259–1263
pathogenesis, 1230–1231
perinatal period, 255
protozoal, 1231–1257. See also specific types and Protozoal infections
routes, 1230–1231
Parasitized erythrocyte sequestration, 1237f, 1238
Parechovirus (HpeV), 1098–1099
Parenchymal brain haemorrhage (PBH), 174–181
aetiology, 174
anatomical aspects, 175t, 178–179, 179f, 179t
aneurysms, 177–178, 178f
angiomas, 177–178, 178f
anticoagulants/antithrombolytics–related, 176
AVMs, 177–178, 178f
CAAH, 176
clinical features/imaging, 175f, 178
drug-related intraparenchymal haemorrhage, 176, 177
epidemiology, 174, 174f, 175t
hypertensive, 174, 176, 176t
infratentorial, 175t, 179
pathology/pathogenesis, 179–180
supratentorial, 178–179
Parenchymal neurosyphilis, 1216–1217, 1218f
Parietal encephalocele, 294f, 298
Parietal meningocele, 294f, 298
Parkin gene, 743–745, 744t
Parkinsonism, 752–755, 754f, 754t
arteriosclerotic disease–related, 754
autosomal dominant, 743, 745
dementia-related, 754, 755t
drug-/toxin-induced, 753–754
Guamanian, 754–755, 759t
'lower body,' 754
postencephalitic, 752–753, 754f, 754t, 759t
predominant, SND, 763
pseudo-
arteriosclerotic, 754
vascular, 754
sporadic, with neurofibrillary tangles, 756, 757, 759t
vascular, 754
western Pacific, 754–755
Parkinson's disease (PD), 741–752, 742f, 743t, 744t, 747f–749f, 750t, 751f, 753f
age of onset, 742
BBB abnormalities, 46
diagnosis, 741
epidemiology, 742–743
genetics, 743–745, 744t
glial pathology, 752, 753f
GWA studies, 745
neuropathology, 741, 742f, 746–752, 747f–749f, 750t, 751f, 753f
Lewy pathologies, 746–752. See also Lewy body pathologies, PD
pathological definition, 741, 742f, 743t, 746–747, 748f
pathogenesis, 745–746
risk factors, 742–743
α-synuclein, 743–745, 743t

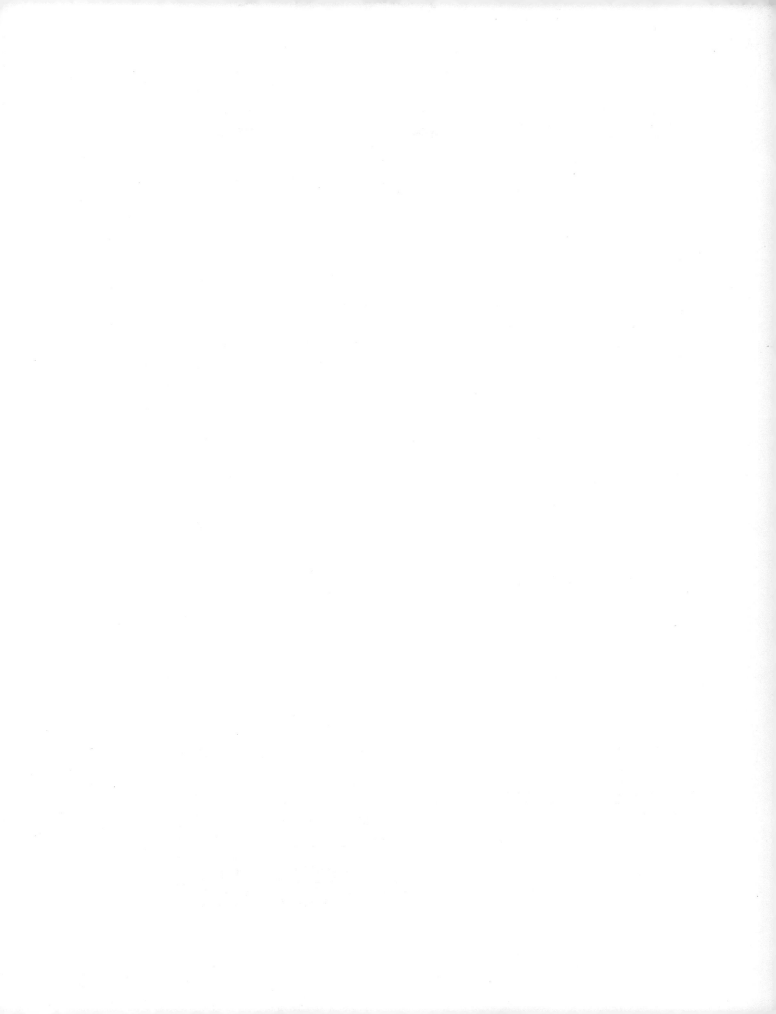

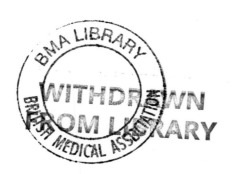